Nutrition, Altered: High risk for more than body requirements

Oral Mucous membrane, Altered

Pain [Acute]

Pain, Chronic

Parental role conflict

Parenting, Altered

Parenting, Altered: High risk

Peripheral neurovascular dysfunction: High risk[1]

Personal identity disturbance

Poisoning: High risk

Post-trauma response

Powerlessness

Protection, Altered

Rape-trauma syndrome

Rape-trauma syndrome: Compound reaction

Rape-trauma syndrome: Silent reaction

Relocation stress syndrome[1]

Role performance, Altered

Self-care deficit: Bathing/hygiene

Self-care deficit: Dressing/grooming

Self-care deficit: Feeding

Self-care deficit: Toileting

Self-esteem disturbance

Self-esteem, Low: Chronic

Self-esteem, Low: Situational

Self-mutilation: High risk[1]

Sensory/perceptual alterations: Visual, auditory, kinesthetic, gustatory, tactile, olfactory (specify)

Sexual dysfunction

Sexuality patterns, Altered

Skin Integrity, Impaired

Skin Integrity, Impaired: High risk

Sleep pattern disturbance

Social interaction, Impaired

Social isolation

Spiritual distress

Spontaneous ventilation: Inability to sustain[1]

Suffocation: High risk

Swallowing, Impaired

Therapeutic Regimen Management (Individual), Ineffective[1]

Thermoregulation, Impaired

Thought processes, Altered

Tissue integrity, Impaired

Tissue perfusion, Altered: Renal, cerebral, cardiopulmonary, gastrointestinal, peripheral (specify type)

Trauma: High risk

Unilateral neglect

Urinary elimination, Altered

Urinary incontinence, Functional

Urinary incontinence, Reflex

Urinary incontinence, Stress

Urinary incontinence, Total

Urinary incontinence, Urge

Urinary retention

Violence, High risk: Self-directed or directed at others

1. Diagnosis accepted in 1992

The Nurse, Pharmacology, and Drug Therapy:

A Prototype Approach, Second Edition

The Nurse, Pharmacology, and Drug Therapy:

A Prototype Approach, Second Edition

Marshal Shlafer, PhD

Professor, Department of Pharmacology
Associate Dean for Student Programs
The University of Michigan Medical School
Ann Arbor, Michigan

ADDISON-WESLEY NURSING

A Division of The Benjamin/Cummings Publishing Company, Inc.
Redwood City, California • Menlo Park, California • Reading, Massachusetts
New York • Don Mills, Ontario • Workingham, U.K. • Amsterdam • Bonn
Sydney • Singapore • Tokyo • Madrid • San Juan

Dedication

I dedicate this book with love, devotion, and appreciation to Jeannie—a dynamite mother, wife, friend, and nurse—and to our wonderful kids Beth, RJ, and Jon. It was written with fond memories of Ray Ahlquist. Ray "invented" adrenergic receptors, which came to be one of the curses of students who had to learn about them, and which set the stage for the development of many drugs that have helped countless patients. Ray's legacy instilled the love of teaching, and recognition of teaching's many intangible rewards and satisfactions. Importantly, the book is dedicated to the several thousand motivated and knowledge-thirsty nursing students to whom I have had the privilege of teaching the subjects that are the essence of this book. Lastly, it is dedicated to the memory of my late and beloved parents.

Executive Editor: *Patti Cleary*
Sponsoring Editor: *Mark McCormick*
Editorial Assistant: *Bob Bledsoe*
Production Supervisor: *Anne Friedman*
Manufacturing Supervisor: *Merry Free Osborn*
Interior Designer: *Jeanne Calabrese*
Copyeditors: *Melissa Moore, Sharon Cloud Hogan, Sally Peyrefitte*
Proofreaders: *Holly McLean-Aldis, Eleanor R. Brown, Anita Wagner*
Indexer: *Katherine Pitcoff*
Typesetter: *G&S Typesetters, Inc., Austin, Texas*
Artwork: *Betsy Palay, Linda Harris, Lynne Larson, Susan Strawn, Susan Gemmell, Victor Royer, and Irene Imfeld.*

Library of Congress Cataloging-in-Publication Data
Shlafer, Marshal.
The nurse, pharmacology, and drug therapy : a prototype approach / Marshal Shlafer. — 2nd ed.
p. cm.
Includes bibliographical references and index.
ISBN 0-8053-7241-5
1. Pharmacology. 2. Chemotherapy. 3. Nursing. I. Title.
[DNLM: 1. Drug Therapy—nurses' instruction. 2. Pharmacology—nurses' instruction. QV 4 S558n 1993]
RM301.S565 1993
615.5′8—dc20
DNLM/DLC
for Library of Congress 92-48493
CIP

ISBN 0-8053-7241-5
2 3 4 5 6 7 8 9 10 -RM- 97 96 95 94 93

The authors and publishers have exerted every effort to ensure that drug selection and dosage set forth in this text are in accord with current recommendations and practice at the time of publication. However, in view of ongoing research, changes in government regulations and the constant flow of information relating to drug therapy and drug reactions, the reader is urged to check the package insert for each drug for any change in indications of dosage and for added warnings and precautions. This is particularly important where the recommended agent is a new and/or infrequently used drug. Mention of a particular generic or brand name drug is not an endorsement, nor an implication that it is preferable to other named or unnamed agents.

Addison-Wesley Nursing
A Division of The Benjamin/Cummings Publishing Company, Inc.
390 Bridge Parkway
Redwood City, California 94065

Contributors

To the First Edition

Elaine N. Marieb, RN, PhD
Robyn Nelson, RN, DNSc
Norman L. Keltner, RN, EdD, CS
Betsy Todd, RN, BSN

Jeffrey N. Baldwin, PharmD
Patricia G. Beare, RN, PhD
Nancy J. Brent, RN, JD
Maureen Groër, RN, PhD
Mark Hamelink, CRNA, MSN, CCRN
Jennifer Holmes, RN, BSN
Patricia Horrigan-Creahan, RN
Linda S. Jones, RN, CS, MS, OCN
Robert Julien, MD, PhD
Amy Karch, RN, MS
Joyce Keithley, DNSc, RN
Carol A. Kilmon, RN, PhD
Michael J. Norvell, PharmD
Gaye W. Poteet, RN, EdD
Margaret A. Reilly, MS, PhD
Dorothy Russo, RN, MEd
Judith Shockley, RN, MSN
Cherie Whitmore, PharmD
Stephen E. Williams, PharmD

To the Second Edition

Rosalinda Alfaro-LeFevre, MSN, RN
President
NDNP Consultants
Malvern, Pennsylvania
Prototype Drug Cards

Jeffrey N. Baldwin, PharmD
Associate Professor
College of Pharmacy
University of Nebraska Medical Center
Chapters 57 and 58

Nancy J. Brent, RN, MS, JD
Attorney at Law
Chicago, Illinois
Chapter 3

Margaret Z. Cassey, MPH, RN
Lecturer
Wayne State University
Prototype Drug Cards

Nancy M. Flynn, MSN, RNC
Clinical Educator
Bryn Mawr Hospital
Bryn Mawr, Pennsylvania
Prototype Drug Cards

Maureen W. Groër, RN, PhD
Graduate Nursing Program Director
Massachusetts General Hospital Institute of Health Professions
Chapter 60

Robert M. Julien, MD, PhD
Staff Anesthesiologist
St. Vincent Hospital & Medical Center
Portland, Oregon
Chapter 20

Joyce K. Keithley, DNSc, FAAN
Chairperson and Professor
Department of O. R. and Surgical Nursing
Rush-Presbyterian-St. Luke's Medical Center
Chicago, IL
Chapter 61

Norman L. Keltner, EdD, RN
Associate Professor
School of Nursing
University of Alabama at Birmingham
Chapters 23, 24, 25 and 26

Carol A. Kilmon, PhD, RN
Assistant Professor
School of Nursing
The University of Texas at Galveston
Chapter 2

Elaine N. Marieb, RN, PhD
Holyoke Community College

Lori A. Martell, PhD
Research Investigator
Department of Surgery
University of Michigan Medical School
Chapters 43, 44, 47 and 48

Jonathan Maybaum, PhD
Associate Professor of Pharmacology
University of Michigan Medical Center

Robyn Nelson, RN, DNSc
Professor
California State University at Sacramento
Nursing Implications

Michael J. Norvell, PharmD
Assistant Professor
College of Pharmacy
University of Nebraska Medical Center
Chapters 57 and 58

Margaret Reilly, PhD
Adjunct Associate Professor of Pharmacology
Nathan Kline Research Institute
Orangeburg, New York
Chapters 50 and 54

Judith S. Shockey, RN, MSN
Associate Professor
University of Texas Health Science Center at San Antonio School of Nursing
Chapter 1

Debbie Storm, PhD, RN
Post-Doctoral Fellow
Hypertension Research Center
Department of Pediatrics
University of Medicine and Dentistry of New Jersey
"Trends and Controversies in Pharmacology" and "Spotlight on Nursing Research" boxes

Burgunda Sweet, PharmD
Clinical Assistant Professor of Pharmacy
College of Pharmacy
Chief, Drug Information Services, Pharmacy Services
University of Michigan Hospitals
Consultant, Drug Tables

Gail Winger, MS, PhD
Associate Research Scientist
Department of Pharmacology
University of Michigan Medical School
Chapter 28

Alvin F. Wong, PharmD
Associate Clinical Professor
Division of Clinical Pharmacology
The Medical Center at the University of California, San Francisco
Pharmacology Consultant

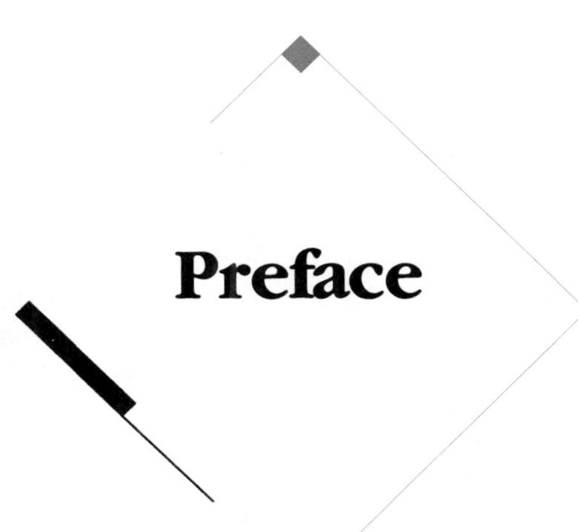

Preface

TO THE STUDENT

This part of the preface—and in fact all of THE NURSE, PHARMACOLOGY, AND DRUG THERAPY: A Prototype Approach, Second Edition—was written for *you.* Before you start using this book, I think I owe you a little insight into how the book came about. First, I should tell you that I'm not a nurse and I'm not a physician. I'm a pharmacologist. And, since 1977 I've been teaching pharmacology and therapeutics to nursing students and nurses like you. I also do much teaching to future and current physicians and clinical pharmacists. Eventually they will be your coworkers in drug therapy, and they will rely on your knowledge.

My students have done remarkably well. I've had students remark that their pharmacology course is the best (of any) course they've taken. One reason for that, I believe, is that I've tried to turn the complex world of pharmacology and therapeutics into words my students can understand, appreciate, think about, and then apply in their day-to-day practice. (The fact that my wife of nearly 20 years is an extremely competent nurse, and an invaluable source of advice concerning my teaching and writing, has helped immensely in terms of what I present and how I present it.)

I ask my students to learn many facts about many drugs, and that will certainly be an expectation of your instructors. But I've always done that with the goal of having students see how they will eventually blend the facts into concepts, principles, and practical use. Indeed, within weeks of the course starting I've had students tell me how they've put into use (for their patients, families, or for themselves) many of the things we've discussed.

I've tried to reduce what's known as "information overload" by focusing on **prototype drugs**—a relatively small number of drugs that are most representative of their potentially very large overall class. You'll find the prototypes identified clearly in your book. Prototypes are drugs that are "most representative" of their class. Learn their major characteristics—their actions, uses, unwanted effects, and the ways in which they interact with other drugs—and you'll have learned most of what you need to know about many other drugs that are similar to the prototype (in ways that you will read and learn about from the related drugs sections).

What you'll learn from this book is only a small part of what my contributors and I have learned and put into use over many years. It's not easy to sort and summarize all that information and I know that nursing curricula differ from place to place. I can't write a book just for "your course." But I've tried to condense that information into a manageable whole that you will be able to use for your initial course-based learning, and for future reference as your career develops. Your instructor will help focus your learning even more.

Good luck and best wishes in your learning and career.

TO THE INSTRUCTOR

Welcome to the second edition of THE NURSE, PHARMACOLOGY, AND DRUG THERAPY: A Prototype Approach. The goal of this award-winning book is to provide your students with a basic knowledge of pharmacology, with an emphasis on how drugs act in humans in ways that relate to nursing. It was written with the educational needs of nursing students and practicing nurses needing a review or update in mind. In fact, although I've already told your students about the importance of this subject, and how this book can help them, I place the responsibility for mentorship, encouragement, and educational guidance squarely on your shoulders. Learning, appreciating, and applying the subject matter cannot succeed fully without your interest, enthusiasm, motivation, knowledge, and help. Therefore, this book was also written for you, the instructor, and with an acknowledgment of your crucial role.

Like all other nursing pharmacology books, you'll find the factual information about drugs and their classifications and uses. But this text goes beyond other books in a way no other nursing pharmacology text has. It identifies and describes concepts, principles, therapeutic decision-making processes, and nursing-related actions that will help your students understand the importance, meaning, rationales, and applications of the facts. Indeed, it expects that your students will go beyond memorization of facts. All this, in turn, should provide a solid foundation for your student to become a knowledgeable participant in nearly all aspects of common drug therapy.

In the past, instructors have found that this text strikes a unique and necessary balance between "basic pharmacology," general therapeutic applications of that knowledge, and "nursing." They felt comfortable using it, and confident of the information it contains, regardless of whether their background is mainly in pharmacology or nursing. Indeed, we have strived to improve on the acknowledged qualities of this book, and to correct any limitations that were identified.

This Book's Background

This book evolved from the content of a one-term, 42-hour nursing pharmacology and therapeutics course I directed and taught at the University of Michigan for 16 years. These students have had no formal introduction to the fields of pharmacology and therapeutics, and little, if any, clinical experience. The course has been overwhelmingly successful in terms of students' academic performance and motivation to learn.

Frankly, the content and approach of my teaching and writing also evolved from many years of teaching pharmacology and therapeutics to medical and clinical pharmacy students. During that time it became clear that nurses play an essential (and often underestimated and underappreciated) role in a checks-and-balances system of health care delivery; that nurses, physicians, and pharmacists must have not only a collegial relationship, but also a common knowledge base on which to make therapeutic assessments and recommendations. It also became clear that subspecialization has become a trend in medical education, and that a general knowledge base such as that which we can expect of nurses (and the all-too-few primary care physicians that are being graduated from medical schools) can be an important (if not essential) asset to health care recipients. Finally, the importance of a book such as this becomes greater with a growing role of nurses as prescribers of medications.

Why I Wrote This Book

Until THE NURSE, PHARMACOLOGY, AND DRUG THERAPY, 1st edition, was introduced, students in my course were not satisfied with available textbooks. They complained about long lists of facts to memorize. Which of all the drugs, uses, side effects, or interactions were really important? Students often became overwhelmed and scared that the texts weren't preparing them well to be active and knowledgeable participants in the health care system. In addition, the students often failed to appreciate and be motivated by the marvelous ways in which drugs can alter our bodies and our lives, desirably or otherwise. I trust that the information I got was not unusual, and that it applied elsewhere.

I was equally dissatisfied with the existing nursing pharmacology texts. Some had reasonable pharmacology content, but little or none of the practical relevance that nurses need (and that is essential for motivating student learning). Some texts had a strong nursing orientation, but little solid information on pharmacology.

In order to write a book with the right balance of nursing information and pharmacology content, the publisher and I put together a very special author/contributor team. It includes educators of nursing, medical, and pharmacy students as well as nurses, physicians, pharmacists, and other health care providers. These individuals include scientists and clinicians in academia, hospitals, industry, and private practice.

This is a multiauthored book because no one person can or should write a text of this type. Importantly, however, you will still also find consistency of style and content throughout the book. That was a hallmark of the first edition. The contributors and I have been very selective in arriving at the content of the text and each of its chapters. In my dual role as author and editor, I have reviewed, critiqued, and edited each step of preparation for every part of this book. That process has been done in conjunction with our expert contributors, external reviewers, student-readers, and the publishing and educational professionals at Addison-Wesley.

The Philosophy Behind the Book

Thorough, Clear, and Current Coverage

I think too many pharmacology texts underestimate or incorrectly interpret the educational and professional needs of nursing students (and nurses) to learn and really understand this material. Moreover, I believe that through a paucity of information and a lack of accurate but clear explanations of what's behind the facts, other texts underestimate the educational abilities of students who have a tremendous capacity and desire to learn when provided with the right information in the right way.

THE NURSE, PHARMACOLOGY, AND DRUG THERAPY: A Prototype Approach, 2nd edition presents what contemporary nursing students and nurses need to know in today's clinical environment. Experience tells us that it is important to explain pharmacology to students so that they learn and understand, not just memorize facts.

It is also important that drug information be current. The rewriting efforts on this new edition have been primarily focused on updating information about new drugs and proper uses for them.

Variability of Drug Therapy

Drug therapies, like the patients who receive drugs, are not fixed or rigid. The variability may be necessitated by patient-related factors, or by physician preferences or hospital policy. There may be no single "right" therapeutic approach in every case. And, even though a particular drug or drug combination is being prescribed for a patient does not necessarily mean that it is the best or is even safe. This book cannot identify all therapeutic alternatives, but it tries to identify and explain those generally regarded as acceptable, reasons alternative therapies may be indicated, and drug treatment plans generally held to be unacceptable or dangerous.

The Nurse's Role in Drug Therapy

In most hospital and outpatient settings the nurse has the greatest contact with most patients, and is usually responsible for administering medications. This means more opportunity for detecting changes—good or bad—in a patient's condition. Some changes in a patient's condition may require no action at all; some may be dealt with easily; and still others may be life-threatening and progress with great speed, and require prompt and proper intervention. Some changes requiring nursing action can be predicted or anticipated. This book helps the reader understand what to predict and anticipate, and how to assess accordingly.

The nurse also has the greatest opportunity for educating patients and their families about medications.

FEATURES OF THIS BOOK

The Prototype Approach

It is impossible for students to learn and understand the thousand or so drugs that are commonly used today. Therefore, each drug-oriented chapter emphasizes one (or at most a few) drugs that are the most representative of their class. For example, we use propranolol as the prototype for the β-adrenergic blockers. Other books claim to use the prototype approach—after we set the standard. Still, this is the only nursing pharmacology book that identifies the prototypes in an explicit, readily identifiable way, in both the text and in the tables.

Within every discussion of a prototype there is consistent format so students and instructors will have a familiar organization to follow from chapter to chapter:

- *Absorption, distribution, metabolism, and excretion*
- *Major pharmacologic effects*
- *Clinical indications and administration*
- *Side effects, adverse reactions, and contraindications*
- *Interactions with other drugs*
- *Overdoses and toxicity*

Drugs related to the prototype are then discussed briefly in terms of the important ways in which they are similar to or different from the prototype.

Nursing Implications and a *Holistic* Approach

Nursing implications and interventions are integrated throughout the book following each major chapter section as needed. These sections relate to the material just presented, and include information about such topics as administration techniques, dosage adjustments, precautions, assessment, and treatment guidelines. They help the reader and practitioner anticipate and manage side effects and adverse reactions. And, they give practical advice important to patient monitoring and patient teaching. These sections address both drug-related considerations and important *nondrug* interventions, which often can be the critical difference between successful and unsuccessful drug therapy.

The discussions encompass a holistic approach to patients and their care in both illness and wellness—an approach that is essential for and perhaps unique to contemporary nursing.

In addition each chapter ends with a Summary of Nursing Implications that is organized by the nursing process. Headings identify assessment, nursing diagnoses, planning, implementation, patient/family teaching, and evaluation. The Summary of Nursing Implications sections were written by Dr. Robyn Nelson, Professor of Nursing at California State University, Sacramento.

A Lifespan Approach

One of the major variables affecting the response to drug therapy is age. Chapter 8, a new chapter for the second edition, is devoted entirely to this subject. It spans pregnancy through old age. Further, this text presents information about drug therapy in the settings of pediatrics, pregnancy and lactation, and geriatrics, in every chapter. For ease of use, especially in integrated curricula, this material is identified with separate headings. Many chapters have expanded coverage of general and special aspects of drug therapy for adults, children, pregnant women, the elderly, and other patient populations. Chapter 33, on Antihypertensive Drugs, is a good example.

Tables

Tables throughout the book serve as a useful reference source for students. The tables are set up with consistent headings. Each gives basic information on the prototype drug and others related to it. Three tables found in virtually all drug-related chapters are devoted to clinical uses and administration (the "C" tables, which include dosages), major side effects and contraindications (the "S" tables), and major interactions with other drugs (the "I" tables). These three main tables have been moved to the back of each chapter so they won't interfere with reading the text. The side effects tables will be particularly useful for quick reference because of logos that show at a glance which body systems are affected by a drug or drug group. In addition, the side effects and drug interactions tables include brief but valuable points about relevant nursing implications and interventions, suitability of alternative drugs, and explanations or rationales for the comments.

Most chapters include several other tables that summarize important text information, such as comparisons of drug characteristics' summaries of different drugs or drug classes that might be used to treat a particular condition, other drug classes that share a particular property, or drugs to be avoided by persons with a particular condition.

Spotlight on Nursing Research, and Trends and Controversies Boxes

These are placed throughout the book, and most of them are new replacements for boxes in the first edition, some of which are no longer contemporary. First edition boxes that we consider to be important, regardless of their publication date, remain but are updated.

Nursing Research boxes describe important findings of nurse-researchers that apply to drug development or drug therapy. Trends and Controversies boxes serve two main purposes. They highlight likely changes in drug therapy and they identify current and future issues with which not all healthcare providers or educators agree. Like the Nursing Research boxes, most of the Trends boxes are new to reflect current thinking in the field. All the boxes were written to stimulate critical thinking and judgment-making.

New to This Edition: Removable Prototype Drug Cards

Though we believe it's counterproductive for students to memorize lists and lists of drug information, we do recognize the importance of having key points about prototype conveniently available. So we designed detachable prototype drug cards that can be used as a study aid or clinical reference.

Annotated Bibliographies

Each chapter includes an Annotated Bibliography. This section identifies selected articles that are considered to be unusually meritorious for reasons cited in the annotation—for example, a timely review; lucid diagrams; controversies or therapeutic trends; special relevance to clinical nursing or a specialty, and so on.

Review of Anatomy and Physiology

Drug-related units of the book begin with a brief review of pertinent anatomy, physiology, and pathophysiology of body systems or processes. While most students will have taken an anatomy and physiology course, and many will have had a pathophysiology course, they often need to refresh their knowledge. Our introductory chapters provide this, plus the important insights into physiology and pathophysiology related to drug actions and drug therapies discussed in following chapters. Chapters that follow the unit introductions provide more focused information about pathophysiology as it relates to the actions and uses of a particular drug.

An Overview of the Book

Unit One

The book starts with three chapters devoted to *nursing roles and responsibilities in drug therapy, application of the nursing process to drug therapy,* and *legal considerations.*

Unit Two

The chapters in this unit address the *fundamental principles that govern the actions of virtually every drug:* how they enter the body; what happens to them once they do; general ways in which they alter functions of biologic systems; and time-related aspects of drug administration and responses. One chapter is devoted to the effects of age on drug actions and use.

Unit Three

This critically important unit discusses the *autonomic nervous system* and drugs that affect it. That system has unquestionable importance to body function and dysfunction, and so has considerable therapeutic implications. The student is introduced early to the fact that many drugs to be discussed in other units have crucial autonomic actions. That is a prime reason for placing this unit in the early part of the book.

Unit Four

The many important classes of drugs given or used to affect the *central nervous system* are discussed. Such agents have not only obvious therapeutic value, but also great potential for misuse and abuse. Characteristics of abuse pertaining to a particular class of drugs are discussed in each chapter. The general issue of substance abuse is summarized, and new perspectives presented, in the unit's last chapter.

Unit Five

This discusses the many classes of drugs that affect *the cardiovascular system:* the heart, the vasculature, and the blood. This unit is particularly important in view of the fact that cardiovascular diseases are the number one killer in western society. The chapter on the therapy of essential hypertension is one of the most obvious chapters in the book in which the recent changing trends in drug therapy are highlighted and explained.

Unit Six

This short but important unit covers drugs that affect the *respiratory system.* Its emphasis is on asthma and obstructive pulmonary disease, mainly because these disorders are so common and debilitating. It integrates information about the many drugs that may need to be used together for some patients, explains the rationales for such use, and identifies drug-related problems that may arise when the pulmonary patient has unique therapeutic needs.

Unit Seven

This short unit discusses the actions and uses of drugs given mainly for effects on the *gastrointestinal tract* for treating ulcers, altering gut motility (as in diarrhea or constipation), and suppressing or causing vomiting. Since many of the drugs are available over-the-counter, and are often misused, that issue is given considerable attention.

Unit Eight

This unit focuses on the *endocrine system.* Chapters cover basic endocrine control systems and factors, as well as endocrine derangements and the drugs used to treat them. Some chapters, such as those covering diabetes and hyperthyroidism, relate to many patients regardless of their sex. Others focus on hormones or drugs that mainly affect or are used for females or males.

Unit Nine

Unit nine covers the *immune system and mediators of inflammation,* and drugs that have important actions on these systems and processes. Important elements include full discussions of the over-the-counter drugs aspirin, acetaminophen, and ibuprofen, as well as prescription drugs for arthritic states, including gout; histamine, serotonin, and their antagonists; immunosuppressants, particularly as they relate to the increasing prevalence of organ transplantation; vaccines;

and immunostimulants and features of disorders such as AIDS.

Unit Ten

The three chapters of this unit cover *antimicrobial therapy;* actions and uses of the major groups of antibiotics, including the newer quinolones; and chemotherapeutic agents for other microbial infections, including those used for the resurgence of tuberculosis.

Unit Eleven

This unit begins focuses on principles of *cell growth and neoplasia,* and the principles of *cancer chemotherapy.* It continues with focused coverage of specific anticancer drugs and their use alone or in combination.

Unit Twelve

The final unit includes one chapter on *fluid and electrolyte therapy,* and another on *nutrients*—vitamins, minerals, and their relationship to health, illness, and drug therapy. These chapters contain much more information that relates to the overall issue of nutrition and nutrient status as a factor that modifies wellness, illness, and the response to many drugs discussed earlier.

The Appendixes and Glossary

We are equally proud of the material presented in the appendixes and following sections. Here you will find:

- A summary of techniques of drug administration, written at a level to refresh knowledge learned in other venues
- A concise and unique section that integrates and summarizes, through text and tables cross-referenced to the chapters, key points about the use, misuse, and dangers of major classes of over-the-counter drugs
- A section on poisoning emergencies. It reviews identification of and contemporary treatments for these life-threatening situations; summarizes related information from throughout the text; and identifies poison "syndromes" that should help the nurse and the rest of the treatment team diagnose and then properly treat poisonings
- Tables summarizing physical and chemical compatibilities of parenteral drugs and fluids
- Tables that summarize some common normal values for blood and urine analyses, with values given in the new SI units system.

To aid student understanding and communication, there is a comprehensive *glossary* that includes both terms specific to pharmacology, and those likely to arise in therapeutics. Terms in the text that are defined in the glossary are in bold face. Some terms are defined "formally," whereas others are provided as working definitions. All are written to facilitate comprehension.

Supplements

We provide several supplements for the book. We hope they will be helpful to faculty as they prepare for their teaching assignments.

Test Item File

Available to faculty only, the test bank includes nearly 1,000 multiple choice items, most in scenario format. Questions are coded by the appropriate step of the nursing process and by cognitive level.

Instructor's Manual

The *Instructor's Manual* presents outlines for each chapter; questions and suggestions to foster student discussion, thought, and interest; teaching strategies that have been used successfully to help explain difficult concepts or link facts and concepts with clinical applications; and suggestions for varying the sequence of chapter presentation to fit special course-related needs. The Instructor's Manual has been updated to reflect new content in the text. It includes 20 transparency masters chosen from art in the book.

I offer best wishes for success to all who use this book. Do not hesitate to contact me in writing (Department of Pharmacology, University of Michigan Medical School, Ann Arbor 48109-0626) or by phone (313-764-0346, 8 am to 5 pm, Eastern Time) with suggestions, criticisms, other comments, or questions. I'll answer all your inquiries.

Marshal Shlafer, Ph.D.
Ann Arbor, Michigan

LIST OF BOXES

TRENDS AND CONTROVERSIES IN PHARMACOLOGY

SPOTLIGHT ON NURSING RESEARCH

Reviewers

To the First Edition

Dan Baker
Barbara Ross RN, PhD
Diane Sadler Benson, MEd, MS, RN
Billie F. Bond, BSN, MSN
Patricia Brien, BSN, MEd
Barbara Buchen, BA, MA, RN
R. Keith Campbell, PharmD, MBA
Sandra Carden, BS, RD
Bruce Clayton, PharmD
Susan C. deWit, BA, MSN, EdD
Phyllis Drumond, BSN, MSN
Mary-Lou Ellerton, MN, BScN
Elizabeth A. Farren, BSN, MSN, PhD
Nancy Fairchild, BS, MS
Darlene Fishman, RN, MSN
Diana Foley, BS, MSN
Roxie Foster, BSN
Lynn Genter
Diana Graham, MSN, CSNP, RN
Kathy Gutierrez, BSN, MSN
Marion R. Hale, BS, MN
Janice Hassell, PhD, RN
Rhoda Lea Headley, BSN, MSN
Anita Hupy, BSN, MEd
Barbara Jester, BS, MS
Bonnie Johnson, BSN, MSN
Karen Jones, MSN
Robert Julien, MD, PhD
Norman Keltner, EdD, RN
Jean Kijek, RN, PhD
Linda Krebs
Dolores LaMothe, BSN, MS
Patricia S. Lisk, BSN, MS
Barbara MacDermott, MS, RN
Esther Matassarin-Jacobs, BSN, MSN, MEd
Andrea Matz, BSN
Jean Maurer, MSN, MA, RNC
Bernice Metcalf, BSN, MSN, MEd
Patricia O'Connell, MSN, OCN, RN
Margaret Parsons, MN, RN
Margaret A. Reilly, PhD
Suzanne Resner, DNSc, RN
Mary L. Richards, BSN, MS, PhD
Neil Rote, MD
Elaine Sampson
Jean Shlafer, BSN, RN
Judith Shockley, MSN, RN
Donald Stanski, MD
Betsy Todd, BSN, RN
Carolyn Van Couwenberghe
Janice Weems, MN, RN
Bruce Woolley, MD
Kathy Wruk, BSN

To the Second Edition

Robert Ertel, PhD
Department of Physiology/Pharmacology
School of Dental Medicine
University of Pittsburgh

Jean Kijek, PhD
Nursing Department
University of Central Florida

Peter Lamy, PhD
School of Pharmacy
The University of Maryland and Baltimore

Mildred Marion, MA, MS
Department of Nursing
Fitchburg State College

Esther Matassarin-Jacobs, PhD, RN, OCN
Department of Med/Surg
Loyola University Chicago

David Reinke, PhD
Department of Pharmacology and Toxicology
Michigan State University

Jean Shlafer, BSN, RN
Surgical Nursing
University of Michigan Hospitals

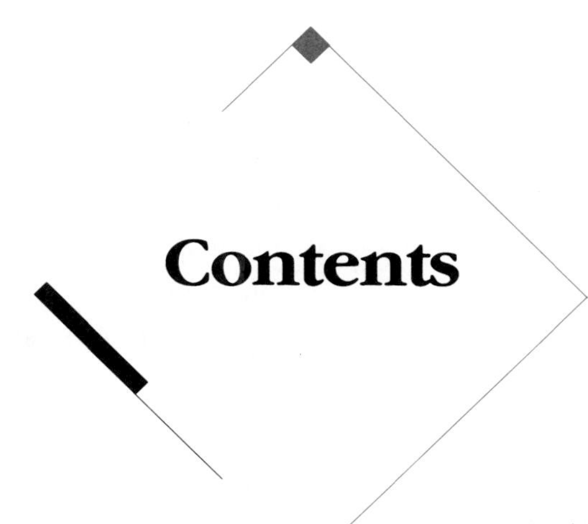

Contents

Chapter 15 Adrenergic Receptor Blocking Drugs 224

Chapter 16 Ganglionic Blockers and Stimulants 251

Chapter 17
Neuromuscular Blockers and Miscellaneous Skeletal Muscle Relaxants 264

UNIT 4 *Drugs That Affect the Central Nervous System*

Chapter 18
Structure and Function of the Central Nervous System 284

Chapter 19
Local Anesthetic Agents 290

UNIT 6 *Drugs That Affect the Respiratory System*

UNIT 7 *Drugs That Affect the Gastrointestinal Tract*

UNIT 8 *Hormones, Hormone Antagonists, and Drugs That Affect Endocrine Disorders*

UNIT 9 *Drugs That Affect the Immune System*

UNIT 10 *Antimicrobial Agents*

UNIT 11 *Chemotherapy of Neoplastic Diseases*

The Nurse, Pharmacology, and Drug Therapy:
A Prototype Approach, Second Edition

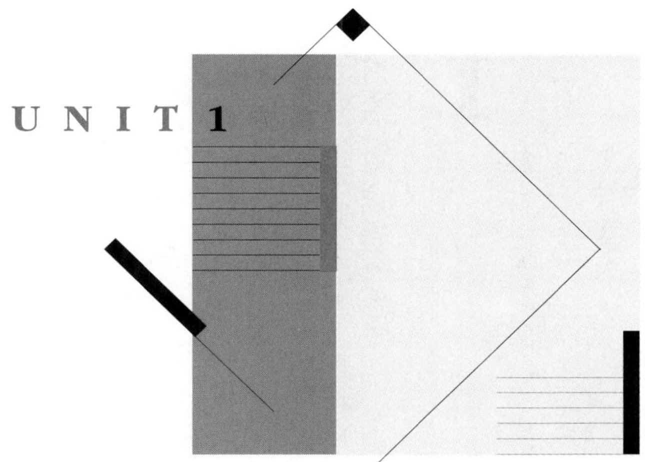

The Nurse, Pharmacology, and Therapeutics

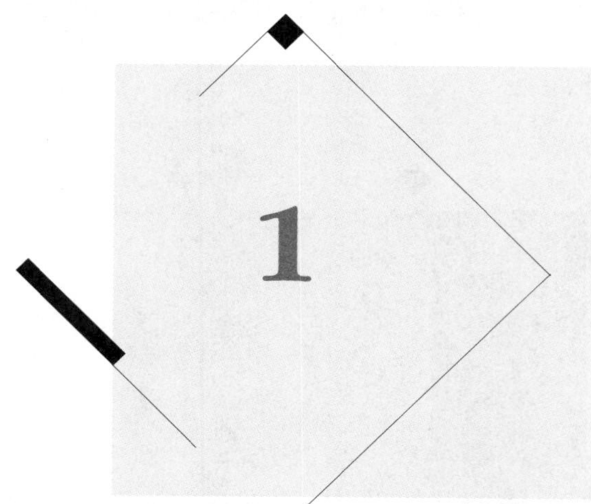

Nursing Roles and Responsibilities in Drug Therapy

The administration of drugs for the diagnosis, treatment, and prevention of disease is basic to the practice of nursing. A drug is defined as any chemical compound of synthetic, semisynthetic, or natural origin that interacts with animal or human tissue. The Food and Drug Administration (FDA) further defines a drug as any substance for use in the diagnosis, cure, mitigation, treatment, or prevention of a disease or condition.

The past two decades have seen a dramatic increase in the development of new drugs and methods of drug delivery. The new drugs reflect major biomedical breakthroughs as well as modifications of older drugs to strengthen their therapeutic effects or minimize side and adverse effects. Pharmacology, the study of the effect of chemical substances on living systems, provides the basis for the nurse's understanding of drug effects in individuals.

Current trends in health care, including increased public concern about the effects of drugs on the body, have contributed to the growing involvement and responsibility of today's nurse in every aspect of drug therapy. Nurses have the most contact with patients, both in the institutional setting and in the home-care setting, and thus they have a major role in evaluating the therapeutic effects of drugs as well as the undesired or unexpected effects (adverse reactions, allergic responses, and drug interactions). Nurses are increasingly responsible not only for administering drugs by newer and more dangerous routes, but also for educating patients about drug use and detecting potential drug interactions. The nurse's role can be carried out only with a proper knowledge of pharmacology.

Portions of this chapter were adapted with permission from Kozier B, Erb G. Techniques in Clinical Nursing. 4th ed. Menlo Park, CA, Addison-Wesley, 1993.

Historic Perspective

The use of drugs dates back to primitive times, when sickness was treated with mixtures of various plant and animal substances, although treatment was dominated by spiritual beliefs. As more became known about the effects of drugs, use of drugs moved from the supernatural to a scientific base. By the end of the eighteenth century, scientific advances enabled the isolation of active ingredients from crude drugs and the synthesis of chemical compounds that produced predictable biologic results.

The Middle East had the earliest systematic approach to the use of drugs to treat illness. Records from Egypt and Arabia reveal early attempts to codify and standardize remedies. The Ebers Papyrus (1550 BC) contains about 800 prescriptions, in which many of the active substances are the same as those used today.

In European countries "folk remedies" dominated and were formulated and recorded by the religious orders who provided nursing care during the Middle Ages. It was not until the later Middle Ages that doctors and apothecaries in Europe began to assume a major role in the preparation and selection of drugs.

In the Western Hemisphere the use of drugs had a major role in the rites of most Indians of North, South, and Central America. Combinations of herbal remedies and appeals to various gods were the mainstays of early treatment. In Europe, country women frequently developed and used herbal potions to treat illness. In the eighteenth century, William Withering isolated digitalis, and Edward Jenner developed and used cowpox vaccine to prevent smallpox.

The nineteenth century marked the beginning of rational scientific practice, as evidenced by more accurate studies of drug dosages and more precise knowledge of the expected action of drugs. Representative discoveries include the extraction of morphine from opium and the introduction of aspirin.

The twentieth century has seen explosive advances in the field of pharmacology, including the extraction of insulin to treat diabetes, the development of site-specific autonomic nervous system drugs to treat cardiovascular disease, the discovery of antineoplastic agents to treat cancer, and, most recently, the development of genetically engineered biologic substances.

Sources of Drugs and New Drug Development

Drugs are derived from three main sources: plants, animals, and synthetic chemicals. Plants were the earliest source of drugs; their use dates back to primitive times. Commonly used drugs derived from plant sources include digitalis (purple foxglove), vincristine (periwinkle), and morphine (opium poppy). Drugs derived from plants are classified according to their physical and chemical properties and include alkaloids, glycosides, oils, gums, and resins. Drugs derived from animal sources include agents such as insulin and pituitary hormone. Most drugs used today are chemical compounds, either inorganic or organic, that have been produced in the laboratory. As technology has advanced, so has our ability to develop synthetic versions of drugs that were originally derived from plants and animals and to develop genetically engineered drugs. Synthetic drugs are far more standardized and less frequently associated with allergic reactions.

The effectiveness and safety of drugs derived from any of the three main sources is based on uniformity of strength, purity of the drug, and consistency of the drug's action within the organism. Chemical and biologic tests called *assays* are used to determine effectiveness and safety. A chemical assay measures the amount and type of substances in a drug; biologic assays (bioassays) measure the amount of drug required to produce a predetermined biologic effect.

Pharmaceutical Research

The pharmaceutical industry continually screens new substances for potential usefulness. The testing required is both extraordinarily expensive and time-consuming. The process of getting a prospective drug to the marketplace begins with animal studies and ends with postmarketing surveillance studies. Screening studies in animals involve the administration of promising new drugs to several species of animals to provide as much information as possible on the pharmacologic uses and adverse and **toxic** effects. Many of these drugs are modifications of available drugs that are thought to be more effective or less toxic. The FDA requires testing with both male and female animals of at least two different mammalian species. Detailed measurements and observations of all body systems are made. Special emphasis is placed on the incidence of toxic effects, reversibility of toxic effects, carcinogenicity, and reproductive toxicity. Toxicity testing includes determination of dosage levels that produce toxicity.

Finally, extensive data on the drug's **pharmacokinetics** in animals are collected and analyzed. Although no animal can stand as a substitute for a human being, particularly for subjective symptoms such as nausea, dizziness, nervousness, drowsiness, or fatigue, or for psychopathologic conditions, the extensive studies with animals provide the basis for consideration of human studies.

Once the animal studies have been completed, the drug company applies for an Investigational New Drug (IND) Exemption from the FDA. Following approval of the IND Exemption, the drug undergoes four phases of clinical evaluation using human subjects. Most of the clinical trials associated with each of the phases employ a randomized controlled experimental design. This design involves selection of subjects who meet the clinical trial criteria, random assignment of the subjects to experimental groups, and administration of the test drug to one group and a control substance to at least one other group. The outcomes are then evaluated to determine whether the effects produced can be attributed to the test drug.

Phase I

Phase I studies are the initial pharmacologic evaluation of a drug; they are limited investigations in human beings carried out on a small number of healthy volunteers. Emphasis is placed on determining toxicity, absorption, metabolism, excretion, and preferred route of administration, and on establishing a safe dosage range. Certain drugs, such as antineoplastic agents, may not be used in normal subjects owing to the high risk of adverse effects. In general, Phase I studies consist of administration of a single dose of the new drug. If no adverse effects are observed, additional doses, possibly in increasing amounts, are administered until a predetermined dose or serum level is reached or toxicity occurs.

Phase II

If the Phase I studies provide evidence that the new drug is safe, Phase II studies are initiated. A Phase II study is a limited controlled evaluation of a new drug conducted with a small, select group of subjects to determine the potential use of the drug with respect to the actual disease. Phase II studies evaluate the same factors as Phase I studies, with emphasis on comparing the effects of the drug in a healthy subject and a subject with the disease. Patient responses are closely monitored, particularly side effects and toxic effects. Therapeutic dosage levels are also refined during this phase.

Phase III

When effective dose ranges have been established, and if no serious adverse reactions have occurred, extended clinical evaluation of the drug is undertaken in Phase III studies. Phase III studies are conducted with large numbers of patients who are treated with the new drug in facilities that include research physicians, such as health science centers. Since a much larger and more representative population is exposed to the drug, this phase verifies the therapeutic effectiveness of the drug as well as provides information concerning infrequent or rare adverse effects.

The experimental design used in Phase III studies focuses on methods that will minimize bias, including the use of double-blind studies, crossover studies, control studies, and subject matching. In the *double-blind studies,* half the patients receive a **placebo** (an inactive substance) and half receive the new drug; the actions of the two substances are then compared. Neither the physician nor the patient knows which therapy was received until after the study is complete. This type of study reduces much of the bias associated with drug evaluation.

In *crossover studies* the patient receives the new drug during half of the study and a placebo during the other half. This allows each patient to serve as his or her own control.

Control studies are similar to double-blind studies except that, instead of a placebo, some of the patients receive a known drug. In some studies, each experimental group of patients will be matched on key parameters, such as type of surgery, sex, weight, or age, to allow a comparison in which the effects of individual patient differences are minimized; this is referred to as *subject matching.*

Most risks associated with therapy with the new drug will be determined during Phase III studies, concluding with data that help determine whether the benefits of the drug outweigh the risks.

Phase IV

Before a drug is marketed, the FDA evaluates the data from the first three phases. If there is reasonable evidence that the new drug is safe and effective the drug is approved and marketed. Then, Phase IV (postmarketing) studies are initiated. During Phase IV, the drug company controls the release of the drug, monitors patients via reports provided by medical professionals on the results and effects of therapy, and maintains communication with the FDA on adverse effects and updates on therapy. The drug company has a continuing responsibility to protect the public by providing information on the product, even after years of use. Some medications have been shown during the postmarketing phase to be toxic in some patients. Of particular importance in Phase IV is information on effects of the drug in women, children, and the elderly, since these groups frequently are excluded from the clinical trials in Phases I, II, and III.

Although the studies required by the FDA are intended to provide evidence of the efficacy, safety, and risk–benefit ratio of new drugs, the time needed to conduct these studies has produced a "drug lag." In 1988, the FDA established new procedures to make promising investigational drugs available to patients with serious diseases as early in the drug development process as possible.

Classification of Drugs

Drugs can be classified in many ways, but the two types of greatest interest to the nurse are the pharmacologic and legal classifications. Pharmacologically, drugs are commonly classified by name and by function. Legally, drugs are classified as prescription and nonprescription.

Pharmacologic Classification

Classification by Name

Systematic study in any field requires the use of a standardized nomenclature. This is no less true for the study of pharmacology, in which there are three conventions for naming drugs: chemical, generic, and trade.

The *chemical name* is the most formal of a drug's names, consisting of a precise description of the drug's chemical composition and molecular structure.

The *generic,* or nonproprietary, name is selected by the United States Adopted Name (USAN) Council. This name is the official drug name and is listed in the *United States Pharmacopeia* (USP), the official United States drug compendium. The generic name is simpler than the chemical name (eg, the chemical name for diazepam is 7-chloro-1,3-dihydro-1-methyl-5-phenyl-2H-1,4-benzodiazepin-2-one). As is obvious, chemical names are complex and virtually meaningless except to a chemist.

The *trade name, brand name,* or *proprietary name* is the name designated and copyrighted by the drug company that produces or markets it (eg, the trade name for diazepam is VALIUM).

The generic name is the name that is most clinically useful. It provides a means to determine chemical equivalence of preparations manufactured by different companies. However, there may be biologic or therapeutic variability among the same generic drugs sold or marketed by different companies, even though each individual company's drug is within the standards established by the FDA. These differences are largely attributable to differences in bioequivalence. *Bioequivalence* is the therapeutic efficacy of chemically equivalent drugs, assessed in the intact organism. Although purchase of generic equivalents of trade name drugs can produce sizable savings, there are some drugs, such as insulin, whose action may be influenced by switching manufacturers. Unless the physician notes "substitution permissible," a prescription written using the trade name must be filled with the brand name drug produced by the specific manufacturer.

Some trade names are so well known that it is easy to confuse them with the generic name for the drug. This text indicates the generic name in lower case letters followed, when appropriate, by the trade name in capital letters. For example: meperidine hydrochloride (DEMEROL).

Classification by Function

The three most common methods of functional drug classification are clinical indication (eg, antineoplastic agents, antihypertensives, laxatives); body system (eg, drugs affecting the autonomic nervous system or the gastrointestinal tract); and chemical or pharmacologic (eg, barbiturates, digitalis glycosides).

Legal Classification

Legally, drugs are classified as being prescription or nonprescription. Prescription drugs require an order by a health professional (usually, but not always, a physician) who is licensed to prescribe drugs. Prescription drugs are dispensed by a licensed pharmacist. Nonprescription drugs are better known as over-the-counter (OTC) drugs and may be purchased without a prescription from a variety of commercial sources. Prescription drugs are further classified into controlled and noncontrolled substances. Controlled substances are prescription drugs that have a potential for causing drug dependence, abuse, or both, such as barbiturates, morphine, and amphetamines.

A final legal consideration relates to drugs and other chemical substances that may be illegally used. These include legal drugs used for nontherapeutic purposes, legal drugs that are illegally obtained (eg, cocaine, steroids), and substances that are illegal or have not been approved for use (eg, heroin, and phencyclidine [PCP]). Chapter 3 includes additional information on the legal aspects of drug classification.

Over-the-Counter Drugs

Over-the-counter drugs are also subject to scientific and government review. They are drugs that do not require a prescription for purchase, and are intended for the treatment of minor discomforts. Since 1968, FDA advisory panels have been in the process of reviewing the safety and effectiveness of all OTC drugs. The panels include pharmacists, pharmacologists, physicians, and persons representing consumers and the drug industry. Appendix B includes a more detailed discussion of some of the important aspects of OTC drugs.

Orphan Drugs

A special category of drugs is the orphan drugs. *Orphan drugs* are drugs that have been found to be useful in the treatment of certain rare diseases but that, because of patent laws or a limited market, are not considered a good financial investment by drug manufacturers. Since the cost of research, development, and marketing of new drugs is high, drug manufacturers normally select for development only drugs for which there is reasonable evidence that the investment will bring an adequate financial return. The Orphan Drug Act of 1983 provides drug manufacturers with tax credits so they are able to recover a substantial portion of the development costs of drugs. The goal is to help make drug companies more willing to develop drugs with a limited market.

Sources of Drug Information

New drugs are continually being developed, and new uses are being discovered for existing drugs. Awareness of available drug information resources and the specific type of information each source can provide enables nurses to be fully informed about new developments. In addition to this textbook, many sources of information are available to provide nurses with the knowledge required for safe administration of drugs.

The resource that sets the standards for drugs used in the United States is the *United States Pharmacopeia.* The USP includes standards related to efficacy, safety, strength, purity, packaging safety, labeling, and dosage forms. Drugs that meet these standards can be identified by the designation "USP" after the drug name. The USP also specifies the official drug name, which is frequently the same as the generic drug name. Many other countries have their own pharmacopeias, such as the *British Pharmacopoeia* (BP) and the *Canadian Formulary* (CF). However, these books are of little value to the practitioner on a day-to-day basis.

The *United States Pharmacopeia Dispensing Information* (USPDI) is a two-volume supplement to the USP that provides information to individuals dispensing, administering, or taking prescribed drugs. Volume 1, *Drug Information for the Health Care Provider,* includes information oriented toward persons dispensing or administering prescribed drugs; Volume 2, *Advice for the Patient,* contains drug information expressed in lay terms. It is a definitive source of information for planning nursing care related to drug therapy, and is especially useful as a resource for teaching patients about drugs prescribed for them. An update to the USPDI is published monthly.

The most commonly available sources of drug information for use in clinical settings include package inserts, the *Physician's Desk Reference* (PDR), and the clinical pharmacist. The PDR (also available in versions for nonprescription drugs and ophthalmologic drugs) is organized for quick reference, with indexes listing products by trade name, generic and chemical name, and use category. One section contains photographs of commonly used drugs, facilitating identification of unlabeled drugs that patients may bring into the healthcare setting. The information is primarily derived from package inserts, and, like them, provides extensive data on the clinically significant therapeutic, side, and adverse effects, as well as information on dosage and administration. A drawback of both the PDR and package inserts is that they list virtually all side effects ever reported, without always identifying those that are common or clinically significant. Another drawback of the PDR is that it is not organized in a way that makes it easy to compare one drug or product with similar ones. Use additional sources to obtain information that reflects the knowledge and judgment of experts.

The *Handbook of Nonprescription Drugs,* published periodically by the American Pharmaceutical Association, is a valuable resource for nurses who require information about nonprescription drugs. The book is organized into chapters for all classes of OTC drugs. Each chapter gives a background on the disorder for which the drugs are used and an overview of the ingredients in common products, including the rationale for their inclusion and possible negative responses. Its greatest value is the tables, which, in one place, list the ingredients in virtually all OTC products for a given use. This allows easy access to pertinent information. It is also a quick way for the nurse to recommend a specific product best suited to a particular patient based on its ingredients (or lack of certain chemicals). The *Handbook of Nonprescription Drugs* is not updated often enough to reflect the frequent changes in the composition of some OTC medications, or to keep pace with products that are removed from or added to the marketplace. Nevertheless, the background information it provides is always very useful.

Drug Facts and Comparisons (published by Facts & Comparisons, Inc.) provides more concise information about drugs than can be found in the PDR. It conveniently organizes drugs by category or class, begins each section with overviews and comparisons of the drugs (including OTC products), then covers the agents thoroughly in sequence. A subscription to the loose-leaf version provides monthly updates of important changes in drugs and drug therapy. Another resource from the same publisher is *Drug Interaction Facts.* Also available by subscription with updates, this reference gives easy to find information about whether a particular interaction is likely to be major, moderate, or minor; whether it is likely to occur quickly or be delayed; and whether it ranges anywhere from well established to theoretical, but unlikely. *Drug Interactions Facts* also gives reasons for the interaction, and practical advice about how to prevent or assess interactions.

The *AMA Drug Evaluations* (published yearly by the AMA), and *The Medical Letter on Drugs and Therapeutics* (published roughly twice-monthly by The Medical Letter, Inc.), give current, unbiased information about the clinical use of drugs. Each issue of *The Medical Letter* may contain only a few pages, but the content will help the practitioner keep updated on new drugs, and assess whether and how new drugs differ from older ones. Occasional issues of the *Letter* are devoted to a particular theme, such as drugs for hypertension, arrhythmias, or infections. These are especially useful.

The use of electronic databases for current drug related information is increasing. Many of these (e.g. TOXLINE and MEDLINE) are available through the National Library of Medicine's on-line services and can be accessed at little or no cost from anywhere in the country. Other databases such as CINAHL, a cumulative index to nursing and allied health literature, can be accessed through private on-line services such as CompuServe and BRS. Many libraries and schools also have access to the complete CINAHL listings using CD-ROM disks and a personal computer. Electronic databases enable the user to search through years of publications in virtually all the major health care journals using key terms to narrow the search to articles in highly specific areas. Abstracts are available for many of the articles.

There are also many journals for health professionals that include current information on drugs of interest to the particular professional group. For example, most nursing journals include a section devoted to new drugs in each of its issues, as well as occasional articles that provide information on new or older drugs and clinical considerations of particular interest to nurses. The *Journal of the American Pharmaceutical Association* identifies, in its monthly issues, newly approved or marketed drugs and new FDA-approved indications for existing drugs before they are published in the PDR.

The principal criteria used to select any source of information should be the purpose of the desired information and the currency and accuracy of the source.

Nursing Roles in Drug Administration

Nurses are expected to assume increasing responsibility in drug administration, although the specific nursing responsibilities for prescribing, ordering, and administering drugs and monitoring their effects are far less well defined than in the past. No longer is the nurse relied on only for administration and monitoring of drug effects. In some areas, nurses in primary care and independent nursing practice settings are also responsible for prescribing drugs.

Systematic nursing practice with respect to drug administration began in earnest in the nineteenth century under the influence and direction of Florence Nightingale. Nightingale was instrumental in providing guidelines for assessing the action of medications, measuring medications, and establishing a basis for ethics in drug administration.

With the establishment of formal schools of nursing in the late nineteenth and early twentieth centuries, systematic guidelines regarding drug administration were developed.

The introduction of the sulfonamide and penicillin antibiotics in the mid twentieth century and the increased use of the parenteral route of drug administration significantly altered the nurse's role.

The practice of nursing as it is known today began in the 1960s. Advanced nursing education was promoted, including more specialized knowledge in the area of drug therapy. The role of nurse practitioner gained prominence and was associated with increasingly more independent functions, including selected writing of drug prescriptions. More emphasis was placed on patient involvement in their own care. As a result, nurses assumed more responsibility in providing drug-related information. Physician shortages and public demands for good health care broadened the responsibilities of the nurse in the area of drug administration. Nurses moved from performing intramuscular, intradermal, and subcutaneous injections to intravenous and intraarterial administration of drugs.

Most alarming in the modern era has been the increased evidence of adverse drug reactions in patients, and the economic implications of these reactions. This increase in drug-related adverse effects has focused attention on the role of the nurse in systems of drug delivery, especially on the need to establish minimum levels of knowledge of pharmacology. Increased litigation has also refocused attention on the legal implications associated with the administration of medications.

General Nursing Responsibilities Associated with Drug Administration

The role of the contemporary nurse in drug therapy is diverse, and in all aspects is guided by the nursing process. Although drugs are usually prescribed by a physician, they may also be ordered by other health-care professionals, such as dentists or osteopaths, who are licensed to prescribe medications. In some states the law permits nurse practitioners to prescribe certain drugs, such as laxatives, under specific circumstances. Although pharmacists are responsible for preparing and dispensing a prescribed drug, it is almost always the nurse who either administers the drug or instructs the patient on self-administration.

To provide good care the nurse must have comprehensive knowledge of both the drug and the patient. The nurse must be aware of the general characteristics of the drug, its biochemical action within the organism, its usual dosage and route of administration, its therapeutic and adverse effects, and other drugs with which it interacts. Nurses must further understand the purpose of the drug in the specific patient, as well as how the patient's present condition affects the use of the drug.

Successful drug therapy depends on nursing care that is careful and thorough and spans each step in the nursing process. Assessment includes careful data gathering both before and during therapy. A careful history, for instance, will help to reveal other drugs that may cause interactions, as well as a health condition, such as diarrhea, that may interfere with drug absorption. Past adverse reactions, as well as current responses and reactions to therapy, all need to be noted. With such data, appropriate nursing diagnoses can be made to guide the development of an optimal care plan. Planning may include the development of schedules and follow-up for evaluation and additional intervention if needed. Implementation includes not only administering drugs, but also teaching patients about their medications. Throughout drug therapy the nurse must evaluate the patient's response and alter the care plan as necessary.

Systems of Measurement

There are three systems of measurement used in North America: the metric system, the apothecaries' system, and the household system. The metric system is the system most frequently used by health professionals. It is often necessary for the nurse to convert from one system to another (as, for example, when the medication order is written in drams or ounces [apothecary] and the drug is labeled in milligrams [metric]), and the nurse must be aware of approximate equivalents within each system of measurement and between systems (Tables 1–1 and 1–2). Conversion charts are usually available on clinical units. It is recommended that conversions be double-checked by another nurse or by a pharmacist.

Table 1–1 Approximate Volume Equivalents: Metric, Apothecary, and Household Systems

Metric		Apothecaries'		Household
1 mL	=	15 minims (min or m)	=	15 drops (gtt)
15 mL	=	4 fluid drams (f3)	=	1 tablespoon (tbsp)
30 mL	=	1 fluid ounce (f3)	=	1 (f3)
500 mL	=	1 pint (pt)	=	1 pt
1000 mL	=	1 quart (qt)	=	1 qt
4000 mL	=	1 gallon (gal)	=	1 gal

Source: From Kozier B, Erb G. *Fundamentals of Nursing: Concepts and Procedures*. 4th ed. Menlo Park, CA, Addison-Wesley, 1991. Reprinted with permission.

Table 1–2 Approximate Weight Equivalents: Metric and Apothecary Systems

Metric		Apothecary
1 mg	=	1/60 grain (gr)
60 mg	=	1 gr
1 g	=	15 gr
4 g	=	1 dram (dr)
30 g	=	1 ounce
500 g	=	1.1 pound (lb)
1000 g (1 kg)	=	2.2 lb

Source: From Kozier B, Erb G. *Fundamentals of Nursing: Concepts and Procedures*. 4th ed. Menlo Park, CA, Addison-Wesley, 1991. Reprinted with permission.

Drug Distribution Systems

Systems for delivering medications to patients vary among health-care agencies in accordance with their facilities and equipment, supply systems, and defined procedural policies. All systems are designed to ensure the safe storage and administration of medications. No

TRENDS AND CONTROVERSIES IN PHARMACOLOGY

Changing Nursing Practice Through Research

A great deal of nursing care—and nursing time—focuses on practices surrounding drug therapy. Nursing care is not limited to the safe administration of medication. Nurses assess the need for medications and monitor drug effects, side effects, and adverse reactions. Care plans include interventions to minimize side effects and to help patients cope with these problems. Nurses are concerned with helping patients and their families learn about prescribed treatment and assume responsibility for self-medication at home. Home health care nurses are becoming increasingly involved in the delivery of intravenous drug therapy that used to be confined to the hospital setting.

These aspects of nursing care provide only a brief outline of the scope and depth of nursing practice in the area of drug therapy, an area that is an important topic for nursing research. In this textbook, the studies described in Spotlight on Nursing Research boxes illustrate the variety of some of the topics that are being addressed. It should be emphasized that although a single study may be sufficient to document a problem or need in a specific setting, generalized changes in nursing practice require replicated research in different settings and populations.

A topic that has been the subject of a number of recent nursing studies is the maintenance of intermittent intravenous devices. These devices, often referred to as "heparin locks," are used when there is a need for repeated intravenous access without a need for continuous infusion. As their use has become increasingly widespread, questions have been raised about appropriate nursing management. Traditionally, patency of intermittent intravenous devices has been maintained by infusion of a small amount of dilute heparin. Concerns regarding this practice include the potential for heparin-drug incompatibilities as well as local and systemic side effects related to the anticoagulant effects of heparin. In addition, the costs associated with the drug itself and the nursing time required for its administration have received attention.

Recent studies have demonstrated that the infusion of a 0.9% normal saline provides an effective alternative for heparinized saline in the maintenance of peripheral intermittent intravenous lines. A metanalysis of existing research by Peterson and Kirchhoff (1991) supports this conclusion. The substitution of normal saline does not appear to increase the rate of selected local complications: site loss due to coagulation, phlebitis, or infiltration—although these variables were not reported in every study. Annual cost savings per hospital ranging from $10,000 to $66,000 have been reported. These findings have provided the basis for changes in nursing practice in many institutions.

Based on their review of 20 studies, Peterson and Kirchhoff (1991) note that there is a great deal of variability in the irrigation procedures that have been examined. Consensus regarding a single protocol has not yet developed, and questions remain to be answered. Is the incidence of complications affected by flush technique or patient condition? Does the solution or flush technique used affect patient comfort? Furthermore, replication is needed, particularly in pediatric populations and to address appropriate maintenance procedures for central lines and intraarterial catheters.

Research about the maintenance of intermittent intravenous devices illustrates that generalized changes in nursing interventions rarely stem from a single piece of work but that even very simple studies can make an important contribution. The scope of nursing roles in pharmacotherapy make this topic the source of many different questions and issues for nursing research aimed at the change and development of nursing practice.

Peterson FY, Kirchhoff KT: Analysis of the research about heparinized versus nonheparinized intravascular lines. *Heart Lung* 1991;20:631–640.

one drug distribution system is consistently associated with any significant decrease in medication errors.

Facilities and Equipment

All agencies have in each nursing unit at least one area designated for stocking drugs ready to dispense to patients. Many agencies have specially designed central medication rooms with locked cupboards in which the medications are kept. Other agencies have locked wall cupboards near patients' rooms or mobile carts with locked drawers. In all facilities narcotics and other controlled substances are kept in a double-locked drawer, box, or cupboard.

Supply Systems

Procedures for delivering medications are based on three types of supply systems:

1. the stock supply system;
2. the individual patient supply system; and
3. the unit-dose system.

In the *stock supply system,* individual doses are taken from medications kept on the unit in relatively large quantities. For example, individual doses of a laxative or an antibiotic may be taken from a large stock supply bottle. Sedatives and narcotics are commonly provided as stock supply medications on each nursing unit.

In the *individual patient supply system* the medications for each patient are supplied separately in specified doses and quantities for a specified period of time. For example, twenty 250-mg tetracycline capsules may be supplied in a separate container or envelope intended only for Mr John Brown. This supply is not used for other patients.

Use of the *unit-dose system* has increased since pharmacy personnel have begun to participate in administering medications to patients and in evaluating their effects. In this system, pharmacy personnel prepackage and label an individual dose, called the *unit dose,* for each patient. The unit dose is the ordered amount of medication the patient is to receive at a prescribed hour. Depending on the agency, the medications are administered either by pharmacy personnel or by nursing personnel from the pharmacy or the nursing unit. Studies have shown a lower medication error rate with the unit-dose system than with other traditional systems.

The Medication Order

The complete medication order is written in four parts:

1. the name of the drug;
2. the dosage;
3. the route of administration; and
4. the frequency or time of administration.

A drug may be ordered by its *trade name* or *generic name.* If the trade name is used and the drug is available at a reduced price in the generic form, it is appropriate for the nurse or pharmacist to inform the physician. If the ordered drug name is not clearly written, the nurse should request clarification or rewriting of the order.

Dosage is generally indicated in some unit of measurement (milligrams [mg], milliliters [mL], or units [U]) or by the number of tablets or capsules that are to be administered.

A drug ordered using both unit of measurement and number of tablets (eg, diazepam 20 mg 2 tablets) is subject to misinterpretation. An order calling for diazepam 20 mg 2 tablets could be interpreted in one of two ways if the drug were available in both 10-mg and 20-mg tablets: administer two 20-mg tablets or administer two 10-mg tablets, with the dosages differing by a factor of two.

Ambiguous orders must be clarified and rewritten to avoid potentially disastrous consequences. Another common dosage error is associated with the placement of the decimal point; every misplaced decimal point alters a dose by a factor of 10 (eg, digoxin 1.25 mg vs digoxin 0.125 mg).

The *route of administration* is generally specified with an abbreviation, such as PO for oral or IV for intravenous. Table 1–3 lists common abbreviations used in medication orders. Unless a drug can be given by only one route, medication orders that omit the route must be rewritten.

Medication orders can be one of several types with respect to the *frequency* or *time of administration:* a standing order, a single order, a stat order, or a prn order.

A standing order is the most common type of medication order. It provides a specified frequency of administration and may or may not have a termination date. For example, the order could be carried out indefinitely (eg, multiple vitamins daily). The drug could also be administered until an order is written to cancel it, or it could be ordered for a specified number of days (eg, DEMEROL 100 mg IM q4h × 5 days). In some agencies, standing orders are automatically canceled after a specified number of days.

A stat order states that the medication is to be given immediately and only once (eg, DEMEROL 100 mg IM stat). A single order is for a medication to be given once at a specified time (eg, atropine 0.6 mg SC on call to OR).

A prn order permits nurses to give a medication when in their judgment the patient requires it (eg, AMPHOJEL 15 mL PO prn). The nurse must consider the purpose of the drug and the patient's condition when deciding when a medication is needed and can be safely administered.

Frequency of administration is generally expressed using one of the common abbreviations listed in Table 1–3 (eg, DEMEROL 50 mg IM q4h prn, or erythromycin 250 mg PO q6h × 10 days). The nurse must be aware of the nature of the medication ordered to ensure that

Table 1–3 Abbreviations Used in Medication Orders

Abbreviation	Explanation	Example of Administration Time
ā	before	
ac	before meals	0700, 1100, and 1700 hours
ad lib	freely, as desired	
agit	shake, stir	
AM	morning	
Aq	water	
Aq dist	distilled water	
bid	twice a day	0900 and 2100 hours
c̄	with	
cap	capsule	
cc	cubic centimeter	
comp	compound	
D_5NS	dextrose 5% normal saline	
D_5W	dextrose 5% water	
dil	dissolve, dilute	
disp, dis	dispense	
dL	deciliter	
elix	elixir	
ext	extract	
g	gram	
gr	grain	
gtt	drop	
h	an hour	
H	hypodermic, subcutaneous	
hs	at bedtime	
IA	intraarterial	
IM	intramuscular	
IV	intravenous	
IVPB	IV piggyback	
kg	kilogram	
KVO	keep vein open	
L	liter	
m	minim	
M, m	mix	
mcg	microgram; see µg	
mEq	milliequivalent	
mg	milligram	
mL	milliliter	
no	number	
non rep	do not repeat	
OD	right eye	
OS, OL	left eye	
OTC	over-the-counter	
OU	both eyes	
p̄	after	
pc	after meals	0900, 1300, and 1900 hours
PM	after noon	
PO	by mouth	
prn	when needed	
q	every	
qam, om	every morning	1000 hours
qd	every day	
qh, q1h	every hour	
q2h	every 2 hours	0800, 1000, 1200 hours, etc
q3h	every 3 hours	0900, 1200, 1500 hours, etc
q4h	every 4 hours	1000, 1400, 1800 hours etc
q6h	every 6 hours	0600, 1200, 1800, and 2400 hours
qhs	every night at bedtime	
qid	four times a day	1000, 1400, 1800, and 2200 hours
qod	every other day	0900 hours on odd dates
qs	sufficient quantity	
rep	may be repeated	
Rx	take	
s̄	without	
SC, SQ	subcutaneous	
Sig, S	label	
sos	if needed	
ss, s̄s̄	one half	
stat	at once	
sup, supp	suppository	
susp	suspension	
tbsp, T	tablespoon	
tid	three times a day	1000, 1400, and 1800 hours
TKO	to keep (vein) open	
tr, tinct	tincture	
tsp	teaspoon	
U	unit	
µg	microgram	
ī	one	
īī	two	
ʒ	dram	
℥	ounce, fluid ounce	

the frequency of administration provides maximal effectiveness with minimal patient discomfort. For example, antibiotics require a constant blood level and therefore must be administered at even intervals, while oral iron preparations may irritate the stomach and should be administered after meals. Specific time schedules are usually a nursing prerogative, so that drugs can be scheduled to minimize patient discomfort (for example, a drug ordered three times a day [tid] is scheduled during the patient's waking hours, or a q6h schedule is set up to be 6 AM–12 noon–6 PM–12 midnight instead of 9 AM–3 PM–9 PM–3 AM, which would disturb the patient's sleep). The importance of administering most drugs at specified time intervals is discussed in greater depth in Chapter 5.

Contraindicated Orders

The patient's medical condition or other drugs he or she is taking may **contraindicate** the use of some drugs. If the patient is taking many medications (polypharmacy), as is often the case with elderly persons, or if the patient has multiple medical problems, the likelihood is even greater of administering drugs that are contraindicated. Although pharmacists monitor the drugs a patient is receiving and are alert for drug–drug interactions, they are usually not aware of the patient's medical condition or of nonprescription drugs the patient may be taking. The nurse, as the person who has the broadest knowledge of the patient's condition and total care plan, must therefore be aware of how to identify and deal with potential contraindications. The assessment process regarding drug administration includes assessment both of the patient's medical condition and of the drugs the patient is taking.

If the nurse suspects that a drug that is contraindicated has been ordered, he or she needs to validate that suspicion. This involves consulting resource materials on drug interactions, effects, and contraindications, and contact with the registered pharmacist. The pharmacist usually has access to the most current information on drug contraindications.

Once the nurse has verified that the drug is contraindicated, the physician should be informed of the situation. It is particularly important to include the factual information derived from the resource materials and the pharmacist. In the event the physician still wants the drug to be administered, the nurse must decide the appropriate course of action. Ultimately, the nurse who administers the drug in question is responsible and can be charged with negligence when a drug known to be contraindicated is administered. In most settings, the policies and procedures of the institution will guide the nurse. Such policies commonly require notification of the nursing supervisor and documentation in the patient's chart.

Drug Preparation or Formulation

The effective delivery of a drug is a three-stage process.

1. Selection of a drug form based on the patient's medical condition.
2. Administration of the drug by a route that will effect release of the active drug ingredients.
3. Transport of the active ingredient to the desired site of action.

Both the form of the drug and the route of administration alter the speed of onset and the intensity of the drug response.

Medications are manufactured as different types of preparations. The type of preparation can determine the method of administration (eg, an elixir is taken by mouth, an ointment is applied to the skin). Some medications are prepared in several forms. Penicillin, for example, is prepared as a tablet for oral administration and as an aqueous suspension for intramuscular (IM) injection. The different types of preparations are described in Table 1–4.

The effectiveness of a drug, and the speed with which it causes its effects, can be affected by the materials and methods used to manufacture the drug. Drug carriers, or additives, are used to increase palatability, stabilize the active drug ingredient, affect disintegration speed, and serve as binding agents. As mentioned, generic equivalent drugs (those that contain an equivalent quantity of the active drug) may not produce identical effects. Since many states have legislation that permits generic substitution for trade name drugs, the nurse must be aware that a patient may experience an alteration in drug response as a result of generic substitution. This is particularly important for drugs with a low **therapeutic index**, or margin of safety, in which minor dosage or absorption changes can result in toxicity or therapeutic failure. (Chapter 4 discusses drug absorption and the various factors affecting it.)

Prolonged-Release Preparations

Prolonged-release medications are drugs in which a carrier or a special formulation is used to allow sustained and consistent release of a drug, in order to maintain a stable drug concentration in the bloodstream. Methods of achieving sustained release in nonparenteral medications include the use of certain carrier substances that can bind the active drug in such

Table 1–4 Types of Drug Preparations

Type	Description
Aerosol spray or foam	A liquid, powder, or foam deposited in a thin layer on the skin by air pressure
Capsule	A gelatinous container to hold a drug in powder, liquid, or oil form. When swallowed the gelatin in the capsule is dissolved by gastric juices
Cream	A nongreasy, semisolid preparation used on the skin
Elixir	A sweetened and aromatic solution of alcohol used as a vehicle for medicinal agents
Extract	A concentrated form of a drug made from vegetables or animals
Fluid extract	An alcoholic solution of a drug from a vegetable source; the most concentrated of all fluid preparations
Gel or jelly	A clear or translucent semisolid that liquefies when applied to the skin
Liniment	An oily liquid used on the skin
Lotion	An emollient liquid that may be a clear solution, suspension, or emulsion used on the skin
Lozenge (troche)	A flat, round, or oval preparation that dissolves and releases a drug when held in the mouth
Ointment	A semisolid preparation used to apply one or more drugs to the skin or mucous membrane
Paste	A preparation like an ointment but thicker and stiffer, which penetrates the skin less than an ointment
Pill	One or more drugs mixed with a cohesive material, in oval, round, or flattened shapes
Powder	A finely ground drug or drugs; some are used internally, others externally
Solution	One or more drugs dissolved in a liquid carrier; *aqueous* solutions are those in which the liquid carrier is water.
Spirit	A concentrated alcoholic solution of a volatile substance
Suppository	One or several drugs mixed with a firm base such as gelatin and shaped for insertion into the body; the base dissolves gradually at body temperature, releasing the drug
Suspension	One or more drugs in small particles that are suspended in a liquid carrier. *Aqueous* suspensions are those in which the liquid carrier is water. Suspensions are never used for intravenous or intraarterial routes of administration
Syrup	An aqueous solution of sugar often used to disguise unpleasant-tasting drugs
Tablet	A powdered drug compressed into a hard small disk; may contain other substances that contribute to disintegration and dissolution of the drug. Tablets are the most common oral drug preparation form. *Enteric coated tablets* have a coating that delays disintegration until the tablet reaches the small intestine. They are useful if a drug is irritating to the stomach or if the acidity of gastric juices interferes with drug absorption
Tincture	An alcoholic or water-and-alcohol solution prepared from drugs derived from plants

Source: Adapted from Kozier B, Erb G., *Fundamentals of Nursing: Concepts and Procedures.* 4th ed. Menlo Park, CA, Addison-Wesley, 1991. Reproduced with permission.

a way that it is gradually released, rather than immediately released on disintegration of the tablet.

Development of prolonged-release parenteral preparations and delivery systems is an area in which rapid changes are taking place. Formulation of substances for intravenous (IV), IM, and subcutaneous (SC) administration uses materials such as serum albumin beads, liposomes (tiny drug-containing lipid droplets), and polymers to provide for sustained drug release as well as extended biodistribution. A wide variety of devices for delivery of parenteral drugs is used, including portable and implantable infusion pumps. These devices use both osmotic gradient and electrodiffusion technology and mechanical means to deliver drugs in continuous steady doses. The ability of the new devices and solutions to control the speed and volume of drug release has greatly improved the safety of administration as compared with drug delivery using motor-driven syringe pumps, which are more easily affected by malfunction. Motor-driven syringe pump systems require frequent monitoring because malfunction can result in release of much higher or lower amounts of drug than expected.

Routes of Administration

Pharmaceutic preparations are designed for a specific route of administration. Normally, the route of administration is specified when the drug is ordered. When a nurse is administering the drug, it is essential that the preparation be appropriate to the route ordered. For example, phenobarbital is taken orally; phenobarbital sodium may be taken parenterally.

Oral

Most commonly, drugs are administered orally. Oral administration is usually the least expensive and most convenient method for patients. It is also a safe method of administration in that the skin is not broken, as it is with an injection.

The major disadvantages of oral administration are that the drug may have an unpleasant taste or be difficult to swallow, irritate the gastric mucosa, be absorbed irregularly from the gastrointestinal tract, be absorbed slowly, and in some cases harm the teeth. A step-by-step procedure for administration of oral medications is given in Appendix A.

Sublingual

A drug may be given sublingually, that is, placed under the tongue, where it dissolves. The drug is absorbed into the blood vessels on the underside of the tongue in a relatively short time. The medication should not be swallowed. Drugs such as nitroglycerin are commonly given in this manner.

Buccal

Buccal means pertaining to the cheek. In buccal (transmucosal) administration, a medication is held in the mouth against the mucous membranes of the cheek until the drug dissolves. The drug may act locally on the mucous membranes of the mouth or systemically when it is absorbed through the buccal mucosa or swallowed in the saliva. Nitroglycerin may be given by buccal administration.

Topical

Topical application is a general route of administration in which a drug is applied directly to a circumscribed area of the body, or to an easily accessible body cavity. Special types of topical administration include drug instillation and inhalation.

Dermatologic preparations are frequently applied to the skin. The active drug must be in a vehicle that allows release of the drug and diffusion through the skin. Topical preparations applied to the skin include ointments, pastes, liniments, and tinctures. In many cases the intent of topical administration is to restrict drug effects to nearby structures. However, active drug may diffuse through the skin (**percutaneous absorption**) and underlying structures and be absorbed in the bloodstream. The resulting systemic effects may be unwanted. Some drugs (eg, nitroglycerin to alleviate angina pectoris, and scopolamine to prevent motion sickness) are formulated specifically to enhance their percutaneous absorption, and are administered on the skin for effects on internal body structures. Accurate measurement of doses for percutaneous administration can be problematic when the drug form is an ointment in a tube or jar. Newer preparations of drugs for percutaneous absorption come in unit-dose patches, each of which provides a precise dose of drug released over a specified time. Procedures for topical drug administration are given in Appendix A.

Instillation

Instillation involves the application of a drug into a body cavity or orifice, such as the urinary bladder, rectum, vagina, ears, nose, or conjunctival sac of the eye. Rectal and vaginal suppositories are often used for drug administration. Drug dissolution and absorption from a rectal suppository is influenced by defecation and the presence of fecal matter in the rectum. The use of an enema prior to rectal instillation can improve absorption. Solutions are generally used to administer drugs through the nonparenteral routes of the nose, ears, and eyes. Appendix A describes the step-by-step procedure for ophthalmic, nasal, vaginal, and ear irrigations and instillations.

Inhalation

Drugs can be administered directly to, or absorbed through, the respiratory passages by inhalation. This is achieved by drug delivery with devices such as nasal cannulas, face masks, positive-pressure breathing machines, and hand-held nebulizers that break up the drug (usually in some liquid carrier) into finely dispersed particles or aerosols that can penetrate deep into the respiratory passages.

Some inhaled drugs, whether because of their chemical makeup or their pharmaceutical formulation, will be largely restricted to the respiratory passages and will exert their desired effects there. Many drugs used for treating asthma are administered that way. However, although local effects may be intended, the large absorptive surface of the alveoli and mucosae in the upper parts of the respiratory tree can provide a route for appreciable drug absorption into the systemic circulation. Clinically significant systemic side effects can thus occur. Other drugs, notably general anesthetic gases and volatile liquids that are administered solely for their effects in the brain, are given by inhalation. This route capitalizes on their quick and efficient systemic absorption through the lungs.

Parenteral

Parenteral administration refers to all routes of administration that involve injection of a drug into some structure under the skin. Some of the more common routes for parenteral administration are

1. Subcutaneous (hypodermic): into the subcutaneous tissue, just below the skin
2. Intramuscular: into a muscle
3. Intradermal: under the epidermis (into the dermis)
4. Intravenous: into a vein

Some of the less commonly used routes for parenteral administration are intraarterial (into an artery), intracardiac (into the heart muscle), intraosseous (into a bone), **intraperitoneal** (into the peritoneal cavity), and intraspinal (into the spinal canal). These less common injections are normally carried out by physicians. All parenteral therapy uses sterile equipment and sterile drug solutions. Parenteral therapy has the primary advantage of fast absorption of a measured amount of drug. Its primary disadvantage is that it allows little or no margin for error because the drug is irretrievable after administration.

Drugs used for parenteral administration are usually solutions, although some agents for IM, SC, and intradermal injection, such as insulin and penicillin, may be in the form of a suspension. Two major concerns are the compatibility of the solution with the body fluid into which it is administered and the sterility of the solution.

A variety of methods are used to package solutions for parenteral administration. Drugs that are unstable in solution are generally packaged in dry form with instructions to add a liquid carrier or diluent at the time of administration. The nature of the liquid carrier is a critical factor for some substances, such as those that require a narrow pH range for activity, or those that may precipitate on contact with certain solutions. For drugs that are highly toxic to the skin or the lungs if inhaled (eg, doxorubicin and a number of other antineoplastic agents), vials with deep negative pressure (a vacuum) may be used. When mixing the drug with a diluent, the vacuum results in a "sucking in" of the diluent, thus greatly reducing the likelihood of escape of the active drug from the vial into the atmosphere. Proper mixing and handling instructions are given in the package insert, and they should always be checked and followed explicitly.

Equipment for Injections

Syringes

All syringes have three parts: the tip, which connects with the needle; the barrel, or outside part, on which the scales are printed; and the plunger, which fits inside the barrel.

Types of Syringes

There are several kinds of syringes, differing in size, shape, and material. The three most commonly used types are the standard hypodermic syringe, the insulin syringe, and the tuberculin syringe.

Hypodermic syringes come in 2, 2.5, and 3 mL sizes. They usually have two scales marked on them: the minim and the milliliter. The milliliter scale is the one normally used; the minim scale is used for very small dosages, such as "epinephrine minims iii H."

Insulin syringes are similar to hypodermic syringes except that they have a scale especially designed for insulin: a 100-unit calibrated scale intended for use with U-100 insulin.

The tuberculin syringe was designed to administer tuberculin. It is a narrow syringe, calibrated in tenths and hundredths of a milliliter (up to 1 mL) on one scale and in sixteenths of a minim (up to 1 minim) on the other scale. This type of syringe can also be useful in administering other drugs, particularly when small or precise measurement is indicated, as, for example, for pediatric dosages.

Syringes are made in other sizes as well, including 5, 10, 20, and 50 milliliters. These are not generally used to administer drugs directly to patients but can be useful for adding sterile solutions to intravenous flasks or for irrigating wounds.

Disposable Plastic Syringes

The syringe most frequently used today is the disposable plastic syringe. The syringe and needle may be packaged together or separately, either in a paper wrapper or in a rigid plastic container for sterility.

Disposable Prefilled Syringes and Cartridges

Some injectable medications are supplied in disposable prefilled unit-dose syringes with needles or cartridge-needle units. These devices come with manufacturer's directions for use.

Glass Syringes

Nondisposable glass syringes are less widely used now that disposable plastic syringes are available. However, because glass syringes can be sterilized, they are often placed in sterile treatment sets for special procedures, such as administering a local anesthetic.

Needles

Needles are made of stainless steel. The vast majority of needles used for drug administration are disposable. Reusable needles are used primarily for special procedures (eg, bone marrow aspiration). They need to be sharpened periodically before resterilization because the points become dull with use and are occasionally damaged or acquire burrs on the tips. A dull or damaged needle should never be used.

A needle has three parts: the hub, which fits onto the syringe; the cannula, or shaft, which is attached to the hub; and the bevel, which is the slanted part at the tip of the needle.

Needles used for injections have three variables: the slant or length of the bevel, the length of the shaft, and the gauge (or diameter) of the shaft. The bevel of the needle may be short or long. Longer bevels provide the sharpest needle and are commonly used for SC and IM injections. Short bevels are used for intradermal and IV injections, because a long bevel can become occluded if it rests against the side of a blood vessel.

The shaft length of commonly used needles varies from ¼ in. to 5 in., and the gauge varies from 14 to 27. The larger the gauge number, the smaller the diameter of the shaft. Smaller gauges produce less tissue trauma, but larger gauges are necessary for viscous medications, such as penicillin. Obese patients may require a needle with a longer shaft.

Ampules and Vials

Ampules and vials are frequently used to package sterile parenteral medications. An *ampule* is a container usually designed to hold a single dose of a drug. It is made of clear glass and has a particular shape with a constricted neck. Some ampule necks have colored marks around them, and some are scored for easy opening. If the neck is not scored, it is filed with a small file, then broken off at the neck.

Vials are small glass bottles with sealed rubber caps. They come in different sizes, from single to multidose vials. Vials usually have a metal cap that protects the rubber seal; it is easily removed.

Types of Injections

Subcutaneous

Subcutaneous (SC) injection involves injection of a drug solution below the dermis of the skin into the fat and connective tissue. Almost any area of the body surface can be used as a site for subcutaneous injection, although the most common sites are the upper lateral aspect of the arm, the anterior thigh, and the abdomen. Insulin is an example of drug that is commonly administered subcutaneously. A step-by-step procedure for SC injections is given in Appendix A.

Intradermal

Intradermal injection involves injection of a small amount of a drug solution between the dermal and epidermal layers of the skin. Absorption is slow and often confined to the injected area. The intradermal route is most commonly used for skin testing, and for initial injection of local anesthetics to prevent serious adverse effects if too much of the drug reaches the bloodstream. Common sites for intradermal injections are the inner lower arm, the upper chest, and the back beneath the scapulae. A step-by-step procedure for intradermal injection can be found in Appendix A.

Intravenous and Intraarterial

Intravenous (IV) or intraarterial (IA) administration causes rapid results, usually within seconds. For this reason, speed of administration and drug concentration are critical factors in both therapeutic effectiveness and adverse drug effects. Toxic effects can develop rapidly, especially if the speed of administration is too rapid. Nurses seldom administer drugs intraarterially because of the added skills required and the potential dangers. Intravenous or intraarterial administration is especially effective for drugs with short half-lives, drugs that are extremely irritating to tissues, and drugs that require controlled blood concentrations. For example, many neoplastic agents are irritating to body tissues, and sustained blood levels of antimicrobials are critical in certain conditions, such as subacute bacterial endocarditis.

The two principal methods of administering IV drugs are bolus (direct) injection and slow infusion with the drug diluted in a compatible IV fluid. Increasingly, infusion pumps are used to administer IV drugs, particularly potent drugs and drugs with a short duration of action. Step-by-step procedures for the following IV administrations can be found in Appendix A: adding medication to an IV bottle or bag, adding medication to a volume-control IV administration set, adding IV medication using additional containers, and IV push, or bolus, procedure.

Intraspinal

Intraspinal administration of drugs involves injection of drugs into the spinal canal. *Intrathecal* administration is injection of a drug into the subarachnoid space around the spinal cord. *Epidural* administration is the injection of a drug between the vertebral spines into the extradural space. These routes are used to minimize systemic side effects when high local concentrations of a drug are desired. For example, antibiotics may be administered intrathecally to treat an acute infection of the nervous system. Anesthetic and analgesic agents may be administered via the epidural route. Various delivery systems are used to administer drugs by the intrathecal or epidural route, including external catheters and implanted ports and pumps.

General Guidelines for Drug Administration

Arrange a time when you will not be interrupted to prepare medications. Quiet and concentration are necessary to prevent drug errors. Before administering a medication, make sure that you are knowledgeable about the drug. If necessary, refer to drug information resources.

The "Five Rights"

Use the "five rights" as a guide while preparing and administering medications: the right *drug,* right *dose,* right *route,* right *patient,* and right *time.* Adhering to the following guidelines should ensure that the "five rights" are achieved.

1. To prevent an error when preparing medications, read the label on the container three times: before taking it off the shelf, while pouring the medication, and after placing it back on the shelf.
2. Ensure that the drug preparation is appropriate to the route prescribed.
3. If you prepare medications, you must also administer and chart them. You are the only person who can verify the medication. The record should include the time, the name of the drug, the dosage, the route of administration, and any related data.
4. Identify the patient correctly and carefully, using the appropriate means of identification (eg, the identification bracelet).
5. Give medications within 30 minutes of the time ordered, except for preoperative medications, which must be given at the exact time ordered, or medications that are ordered to be given hourly or every 2 hours.
6. Certain drugs require special precautions. Most agencies require that two qualified nurses double-check the dosages of anticoagulants, insulin, digitalis preparations, and certain IV medications. Dosage calculations and conversions should also be double-checked.
7. Never return a medication to a container or transfer a medication from one container to another. This practice avoids mixing drugs or placing a drug in the wrong container.

8. When preparing medications, do not use the following:
    a. Medications from unmarked containers or containers with illegible labels—even if you think you can identify the drug.
    b. Medications that are cloudy or have changed color.
    c. Medications that have a sediment at the bottom, unless the medication normally requires shaking before use.

    Return such medications to the pharmacy. Write the reason for their return on the label.
9. Do not leave medications at the bedside, with the exception of antacids, nonnarcotic cough syrups, nitroglycerin, lotions or ointments, certain eye medications, and inhalants. Check agency policies about each of these. When medications are left at the bedside, determine from the patient when she or he takes or applies them.
10. With rare exceptions, patients have the right to know the name and the action of the drug they are taking, and they have the right to refuse a medication. Medications that are refused must be discarded and the reason for refusal charted. Recheck the medication if the patient claims it is not the proper drug, or the one he or she has been taking.
11. If a patient vomits after taking an oral medication, report it and state the names of all medications given. Withhold further medication(s). Often the physician will reorder the same drug by a different route.
12. When medication dosages are intentionally omitted, as before surgery or a diagnostic test, record the omission and the reason on the patient's chart. It may also be necessary to notify the prescriber.
13. Evaluate the effectiveness of a medication a suitable time after its administration. For example, the initial effectiveness of an intramuscularly injected analgesic can be evaluated 10 to 20 minutes after administration. The duration of its effectiveness must also be evaluated.

Medication Errors and Incident Reports

Unfortunately, medication errors are an all too frequent occurrence. The most common medication error is omission, but dosage errors also may result from calculation errors, ordering the wrong dosage, or dispensing the wrong dosage. Calculation errors can be especially dangerous in neonatal and pediatric patients and with drugs having a low therapeutic index, such as digoxin, for which minor changes in dosage can produce major changes in action. Studies have found that 50% of the medication errors committed by pediatric and neonatal personnel resulted in a tenfold increase or decrease in dosage, which certainly makes a case for careful attention to decimal places.

Many calculation errors can be prevented by listening to the patient when he or she says, "That isn't what I got last time" or "I only took one pill at home and it was pink"; double-checking when the dose prepared seems to be unusually large or small; reading the package label for information on drug preparation; and having all conversions and calculations double-checked by a peer. With few exceptions, most oral drugs involve administration of one or two tablets or capsules and most parenteral drugs involve administration of less than 2 mL of a solution.

Administration of the wrong drug is commonly a result of failure to follow safe administration procedures (that is, to observe the "five rights" of medication administration), although it may be the result of labeling errors in which the pharmacy has incorrectly labeled the drug form, drug, or dosage. One common cause of a very serious drug error is the result of switching medications (for example, preparing two IV solutions with additives and mixing up the labels). Other causes include failure to follow accepted patient identification procedures, inadequate labeling and placement of medications after they are poured, and failures in communication.

Errors associated with administration are frequently due to the nurse's lack of knowledge about proper handling of the drug, administration techniques, or both. Certain drugs require special handling to retain their potency and to achieve effective absorption. Special handling may include control of storage temperature, light, or humidity, or the use of specified liquid carriers when reconstituting the powder form of a drug into a solution. For example, many antineoplastic drugs are light-sensitive; other drugs require the use of water as a liquid carrier instead of normal saline, which could cause precipitation of drug into an inactive form. Many tablets, such as common aspirin, disintegrate when exposed to excess humidity. Some drugs, especially those administered parenterally, require special administration techniques (eg, iron-dextran must be given by deep IM injection using a Z-tract technique to prevent leakage into the subcutaneous tissues). Vincristine must be well diluted and given in a large vein to minimize the chance of contact of the drug with blood vessels, which would cause vascular damage and tissue sloughing. Indwelling IV lines and devices require special attention to placement and calibration, particularly when a patient is discharged with one in place.

Medication errors are usually documented on incident report forms that become part of the agency's permanent record. The form and procedures used to file an incident report vary from one agency to another. In all cases, however, incident reports are intended to provide a record of the facts of a situation. The facts include patient name, time, place, name of the person preparing the report, and the circumstances surrounding the medication error, as well as a report of the actual incident. The incident report will also include a section for a statement of the action that was taken, including not only any medical treatment rendered but also information on who was notified of the incident (eg, physician, patient, patient's family).

Procedural Policies and Practices

Procedures and policies may vary from one agency to another, and it is important to know your agency's guidelines. General guidelines, however, are reviewed here. The initial medication order is usually written, but under certain circumstances may be given by telephone or verbally. An order is not considered legal, however, until it has been written and signed. Most agencies require that verbal orders be written and signed by the physician within a specified time period. The availability of communication technologies such as facsimile and voice mail provide for rapid documentation of medication orders given from a remote location. Agency policies dictate which nursing personnel are permitted to accept telephone and verbal orders from a physician. Usually only registered nurses are allowed to accept them, and some agencies require two nurses to listen to verbal or telephone orders.

The nurse is responsible for ensuring that the medication order is complete, correct, appropriate, and contains a valid signature before administering the first dose. Incorrect or inappropriate drugs include those that are not indicated on the basis of the patient's condition or that would produce adverse effects (eg, administration of aspirin to a patient with a bleeding gastric ulcer).

A valid medication order requires that the order be written and signed by an appropriate licensed professional. In a teaching hospital, where unlicensed medical students may order drugs, the order is not legal until countersigned by a licensed physician. Nurses have the right, indeed the legal obligation, to refuse to administer a drug that is not accompanied by a complete written medication order or which, in their judgment, would harm the patient.

Dispensing medications is the responsibility of the pharmacist, although in some agencies a senior nurse may be given the responsibility of dispensing drugs in the absence of a pharmacist.

In most agencies registered nurses are permitted to administer all types of medications (oral, topical, and parenteral) unless the unit-dose system is used and pharmacy personnel have been delegated this function. Practices may vary about who is permitted to administer medications by venipuncture. Licensed vocational nurses are often permitted to administer oral medications only, while nursing students are generally allowed to administer all types of medications after competence is achieved. It is essential that the new nurse, either student or graduate, check the appropriate policies and practices in each agency before administering medications. An agency's policies and procedures on medication administration are usually an integral component of the new nurse's orientation.

Some agencies also have procedures that govern the administration of selected, potentially dangerous drugs. Examples of these are policies stating that all doses of insulin and all pediatric parenteral drugs must be checked by two licensed nurses.

All agencies have procedures for recording the administration of drugs and for reporting medication errors. Although the forms and procedures vary, all systems provide for the completion of drug records that become part of the permanent patient record.

Drug Therapy in Long-Term-Care Facilities

Mentally and physically competent patients in long-term-care facilities may self-administer their drugs. In rehabilitation facilities, where the focus is on the development of self-reliance, self-administration may be a mechanism for achieving self-care. The nurse in long-term-care facilities has a major responsibility for meeting the legal and safety factors associated with self-administration of medications, including

1. Using written physicians' orders.
2. Comprehensive patient drug teaching, preferably with the use of written guides.
3. Providing safe locations for storing drugs.
4. Providing mechanisms for accurate record-keeping by the patient and in the patient record.
5. Maintaining professional accountability through regular checking of patient records and continual reassessment of the patient.

The increased number of long-term-care facilities for geriatric patients is an area of special concern. Polypharmacy, complex medication schedules, and poor vision and other diminished sensory abilities all contribute to a high rate of noncompliance and incidence of adverse effects. It is incumbent upon the nurse to develop teaching programs and systems of monitoring drug compliance that address the special needs of this growing segment of the population.

Drug Therapy in Home and Community Settings

Intravenous therapy, which for years has been used only in institutional settings, has moved into the home and community. Patients receiving long-term antibiotic or antineoplastic therapy are being taught to administer their own medications using a variety of portable IV drug infusion devices. One of the critical factors associated with IV drug administration in the home is the need for immediate assistance should any adverse reactions occur. This is frequently accomplished through the use of on-call medical personnel, such as home health nurses; restrictions on the distance between the patient's home and the nearest medical facility; or both. Teaching the patient and family not only about the drug and its side effects, but also about the correct preparation and administration of the drug and care of the intravenous site, are essential responsibilities of the nurse.

The greatest role of the nurse with respect to administration of medications in the home and community setting is teaching. In addition to providing specific drug information to patients and their families, the nurse plays a major part in the education of the community as a whole, especially regarding the appropriate use of OTC drugs and avoidance of drug quackery. With the availability of generic substitution for prescribed drugs, the community needs to be better informed not just of the potential economic advantages of substitution, but also of the potential adverse consequences.

The goal of teaching is to help patients become informed consumers who question any change in their medications. Patients need to be taught to question and to verify their medications with all health-care professionals: nurses, pharmacists, and physicians.

Investigational Drugs

Patients participating in clinical drug trials are at added risk, not only from the drug's potential adverse effects but also from the possibility of failure of the drug to improve the condition for which it is being administered. The nurse who is serving as a research coinvestigator must be particularly sensitive to both the legal aspects associated with use of investigational drugs and the special concerns associated with administering and monitoring a new drug.

Informed consent is the primary legal concern. Informed consent is a written contract in which the patient is given information by the physician investigator on the risks, benefits, and alternatives to the experimental therapy. The consent document should also state what financial compensation (if any) will be paid for participating in the study, and any compensation or follow-up medical care that will be provided in the event of untoward reactions or responses. During this process the nurse serves as a patient advocate, a recorder of the information provided to the patient, and a witness to the signing of the informed consent form.

Several special concerns arise when providing care for the patient receiving an investigational drug. In addition to the usual measures, such as providing the patient and family with information about the drug, the nurse must also be aware of the secondary costs to the patient in time and money. (The patient may or may not be reimbursed fully.) The patient's response to an investigational drug is monitored with a battery of laboratory tests and extensive evaluation, which generally require that the patient make frequent time-consuming visits to the health-care facility. Another major role of the nurse in investigational drug studies is data collection and record-keeping. Future marketing of investigational drugs that prove to be safe and efficacious depends on accurate recording and reporting of the data obtained during the investigational phases.

Illegal Drugs

The majority of the drugs used illegally exert their primary effects on the central nervous system and result in physical dependence (addiction), psychologic dependence (habituation), or both. It is common for drug abusers to use several substances concurrently. Alcohol, barbiturates, and sedative-hypnotic drugs are frequently taken along with the illegal substance. The nurse's role with respect to illegal drug use includes:

1. Primary prevention through patient and public education.
2. Identification of drug abusers through careful assessment and knowledge of the abuse potential of certain drugs.
3. Development and implementation of policies and procedures in the health-care setting for handling drugs with high abuse potential.
4. Nursing management of patients experiencing the consequences of illegal drug use.

Annotated Bibliography

Alford DM, Moll JA. Helping elderly patients in ambulatory settings cope with drug therapy. *Nurs Clin North Am* 1982;17:275–282. *This article describes methods of helping elderly patients manage their own drugs safely and effectively. Discussed are the use of a drug profile, the role of the pharmacist, family teaching, drug labeling, drug monitoring, and management of the assertive elderly patient.*

Carr DS. New strategies for avoiding medication errors. *Nursing '89* 1989;19:39–45. *This article reviews the basics of medication administration in the context of today's rapid changes in drug delivery methods, drug packaging, and technology.*

Corbett KM, Lynch LC. Professional nursing issues in the administration of investigational antiarrhythmic medications. *Heart Lung* 1984;13:395–399. *This is an excellent discussion of the role of nurse coinvestigator in supervising drug protocols. Detailed information on the legal aspects of investigational drugs is provided, and there is an extensive discussion of nursing considerations associated with the care of the patient who is receiving an investigational drug.*

Faut-Callahan M (Guest editor). Update on nursing interventions. *Nurs Clin North Am* 1991;26(2). *An entire issue devoted to a series of articles providing both a review of basic care associated with the nurses' role in drug administration, and an update on new developments. Topics include nursing implications of new methods of drug administration, changes in client demographics (eg, increased elderly population), changes in nursing practice settings (eg, home health care), and changing areas of health concern (AIDS, organ transplantation, etc.).*

Gardner C. Risk management of medication errors (Part 1). *NITA* 1987;3:187–196.

Gardner C. Risk management of medication errors (Part 2). *NITA* 1987;4:266–278. *These two articles provide a comprehensive review of the problem of medication errors, including the extent of the problem, lawsuits filed, developing patient risk profiles, and a detailed listing of reported causes of medication errors.*

Hyssey LC. Overcoming the clinical barriers of low literacy and medication noncompliance among the elderly. *J Gerontol Nurs* 1991; 17(3):27–29. *A discussion of common barriers to medication compliance, including that of low literacy. The article offers methods to improve compliance derived from theories of behavioral modification, including tailoring and cuing.*

Lesar TS, Briceland LL, Delcoure K, Parmalee JC, Masta-Gornic V, Pohl H. Medication prescribing errors in a teaching hospital. *JAMA* 1990;263(17):2329–2334. *In one tertiary-care hospital, nearly 300,000 prescriptions were written over a 1-year period. About 900 prescribing errors were detected, of which nearly 60% were rated as having the potential for adverse consequences—a "significant risk to patients." Among other things, the authors conclude that the data confirm "the importance of checks and balances with health care systems." As we maintain throughout this book, nurses, through their roles and responsibilities, are an essential part of that system.*

Young FC, Norris JA, Levitt JA, Nightingale SL. The FDA's new procedures for the use of investigational drugs in treatment. *JAMA* 1988;259(15):2267–2270. *This article provides an excellent description of the 1988 FDA regulations that established new procedures for making investigational drugs available for treatment of patients with immediately life-threatening or serious diseases as early in the drug development process as possible.*

Ziporyn T. The Food and Drug Administration: How those regulations came to be. *JAMA* 1985;254:2037–2039, 2043–2046. *An excellent historical account and discussion of the evolution of federal regulations on food and drugs in the United States.*

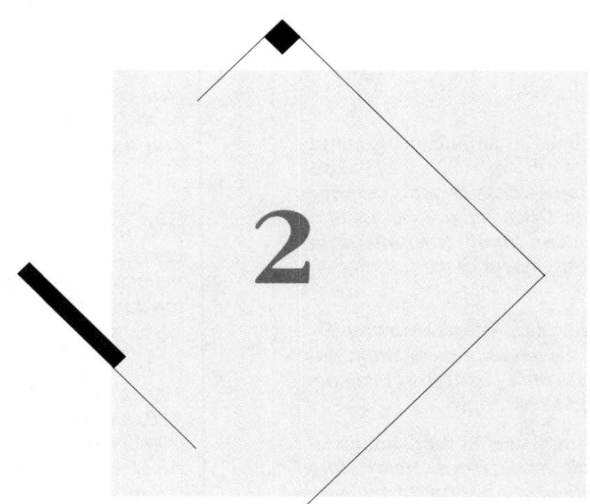

Application of the Nursing Process to Drug Therapy

Nurses have always had a significant role in the management of drug therapy, but never has it been more critically important than today. Technologic advances have led to the development of increasingly sophisticated drugs and made possible the survival of patients who are critically ill. This combination of critically ill patients and potent drugs creates a situation in which the nurse must be especially alert to subtle physiologic changes in the patient's condition that may indicate a need to alter drug therapy or provide additional interventions to support the patient who is experiencing complications of drug therapy.

In addition, many patients are treated outside the traditional hospital setting. They depend on nurses to educate them about their drug therapy and assist them in implementing it successfully. Therefore, nurses must be able to assume responsibility for seeing that drug therapy is managed effectively at home as well as assuming direct responsibility for the implementation of the medication regimen in the hospital.

The nurse's holistic approach to care is also very important in drug therapy. Patients in any setting often have more than one health problem. Thus, they may receive a number of drugs, some of which may interact with one another. In many cases, patients are treated by various specialists, each prescribing drugs for the treatment of one disease without being aware of other drugs that the patient is taking. Individual factors related to the patient's physiology or lifestyle can compound the problem of drug interactions and necessitate alterations in drug therapy. The nurse, by taking a holistic approach to patient care, is often the first to become aware of problems or potential problems. Thus, the nurse's role is frequently crucial to the success of drug therapy.

This chapter explains the nursing responsibilities in drug therapy as they apply to each step of the nursing process. Because each step of the process is important to the entire drug regimen, a nurse who is careful and thorough in the performance of every step will greatly improve the patient's chances for successful drug therapy. At the end of the chapter, two case studies are presented to illustrate the use of the nursing process in drug therapy.

Assessment

The first step in the nursing process, assessment, includes not only the patient but also the patient's environment and the drug or drugs the patient is taking.

Although this step is an especially important one in drug therapy, it is often hurriedly done. It is important for the nurse to understand at the outset that adequate attention to assessment will not only improve the effectiveness of the drug therapy but also save time later when providing care and performing other steps of the nursing process.

The Patient and the Patient's Environment

Assessment of the patient and his or her environment is outlined in Table 2–1.

Current Health History

Much of the information about the patient's health history can be found in the health record. The current health history should include information about pathophysiologic conditions that may affect the absorption, distribution, metabolism, or excretion of a drug, or, more importantly, the overall response to a new medication. For instance, diarrhea will probably reduce the absorption of an oral medication. Patients with liver or kidney dysfunction are at risk for accumulation of drugs or their waste products that are broken down or excreted by those organs. When evaluating the current health history the nurse should also obtain information about problems that could affect the patient's ability to manage the drug regimen successfully. Individuals with memory problems should be assessed for their ability to remember doses.

Because many drugs interact with each other, it is important to know about any other drugs the patient is currently taking. Thus, assessment should include information about prescription drugs, nonprescription drugs, street drugs, alcoholic beverages, and smoking. Information about smoking is included because of the effects of nicotine on the body. Many patients are not aware of the interactions between drugs, and so it is the nurse's responsibility to ask specific questions about the use of all types of drugs. Some drugs also interact with certain foods; therefore, it is important to assess the patient's diet so that information about possible food–drug interactions can be obtained.

Table 2–1 | Assessment of the Patient Receiving Drug Therapy

Current health history

- Current diseases or disabilities
- Other drugs currently used
  - Prescribed
  - Over-the-counter
  - Recreational

Past health history

- Prior episodes of illness and drug therapy
  - Medications stored at home after previous illness
- Allergies

Lifestyle and resources

- Members of household
- Daily schedule, including dietary patterns
- Physical resources
- Human resources

Patient's knowledge level and desire for information

Past Health History

The past health history may alert the nurse to a patient who may experience an adverse response to a drug. It is a good practice to ask if the patient has ever taken this drug or one like it and if it had any effect other than the desired therapeutic effect. This is easily accomplished in conjunction with the history of the present illness, and may include such questions as "Have you ever had this type of problem before?"; "Did you take any medications for it at that time?"; "Do you remember the name of the medication(s) that you took?"; "Was the medication helpful in relieving the problem?"; and "Did the medication have any effects other than relieving the problem?" The nurse may then question the patient about specific side effects of the prescribed drug. It is also important to obtain information about allergies to foods, drugs, or environmental factors.

Lifestyle and Resources

The patient's and family's lifestyle should be considered when planning a medication regimen. Assessment should include information about the members of the patient's household and their relationship to the patient. The assessment should include the patient's daily schedule, and whether part of each day is spent at work, school, a day care facility, with a babysitter, or at another location away from the patient's home. If the medication schedule is planned so that any doses of the drug must be taken while the patient is away from home, it is important that provisions be available for proper drug storage and administration. If some doses of medication are to be given at a day care facility, family members may find it helpful to have the medication dispensed in two bottles so that one may be kept at each location. This may reduce the number of missed doses caused by failure to transport the medication to or from the day care center.

Assessment of lifestyle also includes the timing and number of meals eaten by the patient. This is especially important if the medication must be given at a particular time in relation to a meal. The patient's sleep schedule can be important as well, because in many cases compliance can be improved by scheduling medications so that the patient does not have to get up during the night to take a dose. Eliminating night doses is also likely to reduce the possibility of medication error or poisoning by a sleepy patient or family member who mistakes one bottle for another or pours the wrong amount of medication.

One of the most easily overlooked factors to be considered when a drug is selected for use with a particular patient is whether the patient has the material resources to enable safe and appropriate use of the drug. For example, it is inappropriate to prescribe an antibiotic suspension that must be kept refrigerated if the patient does not have access to a refrigerator. This problem is more common than many nurses realize, especially among low-income families and families who are staying in a hotel or other temporary lodgings. Another example of this type of consideration is the patient's ability to store the drug safely out of the reach of small children. In most cases, there are facilities in the home for proper storage of medications. However, a momentary lapse of vigilance can result in a medication left within a child's reach for a few minutes; a child can swallow a significant amount of drug in that period of time. Thus, if there are small children in the household, smaller amounts of the drug may be dispensed with provision for refills so that small children cannot accidentally ingest a large amount of the drug. Dispensing of small quantities of medication may also be appropriate when there are individuals in the home who are at risk for using the medication in a suicide attempt.

In some cases, it may be relevant to consider the patient's financial state. Sometimes a less expensive drug can be used if the cost of the most desirable drug will be a financial hardship for the family. This may be done by indicating that a generic drug may be substituted for the brand name drug if the patient so desires. Generic drugs must meet FDA standards of quality and, in most cases, they can be expected to have the same therapeutic effect as their brand name equivalents. They may not look or taste the same, however, and some differ in the rate at which the active ingredient is absorbed in the body. Those that differ in absorption rate cannot be considered therapeutically equivalent and should not be substituted for each other. If there is any question, a pharmacist should have the most up-to-date information about the therapeutic equivalence of specific generic products.

The support system available to the patient may also be an important consideration in the selection of drug therapy, especially if the patient has a problem that would make self-administration of the medication difficult or impossible. In these cases, the nurse should assess the availability of assistance to the patient. Household members are an obvious source of assistance, but home-care nurses, neighbors, relatives, or domestic workers employed by the family may also be significant resources.

Knowledge Level and Desire for Information

The patient's knowledge, attitudes, and desire for information may influence compliance with the medication regimen. The patient should understand the purpose of the medication, the rationale behind the scheduling of doses, the expected treatment effects, any side effects that may be experienced, and what should be done if side effects occur. It is necessary to ensure that the patient understands when the medication should be taken. For example, persons who think medicine should be taken only when symptoms are present will probably take pain or fever medications appropriately, but may need an explanation of the necessity to take blood pressure medications when they feel well.

If the drug therapy includes any medication that must be administered by a special technique (such as eye drops, injections, or inhalants), the nurse should assess the patient's ability to self-administer the medication correctly. If this is the patient's first experience with this type of drug, a demonstration of the proper technique for administration is appropriate, followed by a return demonstration by the patient. This process can be done with practice materials until the patient demonstrates the ability to administer the drug correctly. Because experience with a technique does not guarantee that the patient will continue to perform it correctly, the patient should be observed periodically during the course of treatment so that errors in technique can be noted and corrected.

Patients vary in their desire for information and their ability to absorb detailed information about their therapy. An assessment of these factors will help the nurse plan the right amount of detail to include in each teaching session for progressive learning to take place.

TRENDS AND CONTROVERSIES IN PHARMACOLOGY

Drug Advertisements—Informational or Misleading??

Truth in advertising is often taken for granted by health professionals when it comes to prescription drugs. According to Food and Drug Administration (FDA) regulations (1981), advertisements must be accurate and include information about side effects, contraindications, and effectiveness. Advertised information should not be one-sided. Material concerning a drug's effectiveness must be balanced by information about side effects and contraindications.

A recent study by Wilkes and colleagues (1992) indicates that many pharmaceutical advertisements in peer-reviewed medical journals fall short of these standards. The findings are disturbing, because product advertisements provide an important source of information for busy clinicians and may influence prescribing practices. By affecting these practices, misleading advertisements could adversely affect patient outcomes and/or increase health care costs.

Greater use of selected drugs without support for their therapeutic advantage demonstrates the potential power of marketing strategies. An illustration of this involved a nonsteroidal antiinflammatory drug (NSAID) approved by the FDA a few years ago. The drug had been used so extensively outside the United States that the manufacturer claimed it to be the #1 prescription antiarthritic drug worldwide. Despite this claim, studies comparing this drug with other NSAIDs, including aspirin, indicated that the drug did not appear to be more efficacious for the treatment of several inflammatory conditions.

Each year, companies spend millions of dollars advertising drug products in professional journals. These advertisements are directed primarily at physicians. It is interesting to note that many research-focused nursing journals do not include drug advertisements, but they are often seen in clinical and combined clinical/research publications. Although most nurses do not directly prescribe medications, misleading advertisements could influence nursing care by affecting medication choices, knowledge about specific drugs, and the information given to patients about selected products.

The editorial policies of most journals include some guidelines about advertisements. But responsibility for evaluating the content of specific advertisements rests with the FDA, and it has been pointed out that it would be inappropriate and inefficient for professional journals to assume this role (Fletcher & Fletcher, 1992). There does appear to be general agreement that the problem of misleading claims in advertisements can be addressed effectively by a variety of actions from those involved: the pharmaceutical industry, FDA, and professional journals. However, it will always be important for health care providers to remember that drug advertisements may be informative, but they are designed to persuade. Therefore, a critical eye, knowledge, and some degree of skepticism, are warranted when reading these advertisements and when evaluating manufacturers' claims for their products.

Code of Federal Regulations. Title 21: Food and Drugs. Part 202, Prescribing drug advertising. Washington DC: U.S. Government Printing Office, 1981.

Fletcher RH, Fletcher SW: Pharmaceutical advertisements in medical journals. *Ann Intern Med* 1992; 116:951–952.

Wilkes MS, Doblin BH, Shapiro MF: Pharmaceutical advertisements in leading medical journals: experts' assessments. *Ann Intern Med* 1992; 116:912–919.

The Drug

Having obtained information about the patient, the nurse should become familiar with the drug. This includes knowledge about the mechanism of action of the drug and its expected effects, both desired and adverse. Because the nurse is often the first health-care provider to observe side effects or toxic effects, it is important to know specifically what these may be. If the patient is receiving more than one drug, the nurse must know how each drug interacts with the other drugs. It is important to check the expiration date on the label of a medication before giving a dose to a patient. This is especially necessary if a drug is one that is stocked in the clinical area but rarely used. Expiration of medications may also occur when medications are locked in an emergency cart. For this reason, hospitals require that medications be checked on a regular basis, with replacement of any that will expire before the next scheduled check.

It is also important to inspect all medications for any signs of contamination or decomposition. Medications may decompose before their stated expiration date if they are stored improperly or contaminated with bacteria or other medications. Signs of contamination or decomposition include discoloration, changes in the texture of tablets, the presence of crystals in liquid medications, or any indication that someone may have tampered with the medication. If any of these findings are present, the medication should be returned to the pharmacy at once and exchanged for fresh medication.

Nursing Diagnosis

A comprehensive assessment will lead to the identification of nursing diagnoses specific to the patient and the drug therapy. Some nursing diagnoses may relate to the drug therapy itself. For example, steroid drugs may interfere with the body's defense mechanisms so that the patient has a high risk for infection. Antihypertensive drugs may cause altered sexuality patterns related to impotence. High risk for injury may be related to the patient's lack of knowledge about the drug, the potency and possible side effects of the drug, or the presence of small children in the home. Noncompliance is another problem that may relate either to knowledge deficit or to other factors, including a lack of fit between the drug therapy and the patient's lifestyle, problematic side effects, or the patient's denial of the illness.

Other pertinent nursing diagnoses relate to characteristics of the patient or family that make compliance with drug therapy difficult. These include defensive coping by an individual or family, or impaired adjustment of an individual. An illustration of this type of problem is an individual who denies the existence of a health problem. Patients with sensory/perceptual alterations, such as mentally ill patients, may not be able to plan or implement drug therapy, or may forget to take their medications.

Impaired physical mobility (specifically joint mobility) is a problem for many elderly persons who may have difficulty opening and closing childproof containers. Impaired mobility is also a problem for the patient who receives a diuretic but has difficulty ambulating to the bathroom. Persons who have visual problems may have difficulty reading the small print on standard prescription labels. Finally, impaired swallowing affects the patient's ability to take oral medication and may indicate the need to change to another form of medication. Table 2–2 presents a selection of potential nursing diagnoses with examples.

Table 2–2 Examples of Nursing Diagnoses Related to Drug Therapy

Diagnosis	Example
Impaired adjustment	A 13-year-old male is a newly diagnosed diabetic. He frequently misses insulin doses and does not comply well with his diet. When questioned, he says he can handle this himself and does not want others always telling him what to do.
Defensive coping	A 45-year-old female was recently found to be hypertensive. She is asymptomatic. She does not take her medication because she feels fine and does not believe that she has a significant health problem.
Altered family processes	A family of four usually functions quite well. However, owing to a recent natural disaster they are living in a temporary shelter. They lost some of their medications and have been unable to contact their family physician.
Ineffective family coping: compromised	A mother was treating her child's ear infection by pouring the antibiotic into the child's ear. She did not realize that the child should take the drug by mouth.
Noncompliance	A 40-year-old hypertensive male stopped taking his medication when he became impotent. He realizes that this can have serious consequences, but states that the effects of the medication are intolerable.
Impaired skin integrity	A 30-year-old male was given penicillin for treatment of streptococcal pharyngitis. He now has a generalized rash that itches.
Potential for injury	A 32-year-old female with epilepsy is taking medications that make her drowsy. She often stumbles, has had several minor falls, and is afraid to drive her car, but says she has to drive sometimes.
Potential for poisoning	A young mother of a toddler keeps tranquilizers in a dish on her bedside table.

Planning

Having assessed factors that affect the administration, effectiveness, and safety of the planned drug therapy for a particular patient, and having identified pertinent nursing diagnoses, the nurse now begins planning the medication regimen. Planning includes the development of a medication schedule and making arrangements for follow-up and evaluation of the effectiveness of drug therapy.

A patient who is receiving several drugs may need assistance with the development of a dosage schedule. Doses must be planned so that drugs are given at the appropriate time in relationship to meals and other drugs. The rationale for timing drug doses in relation to each other should be explained so the patient will see this as a necessary part of therapy rather than a nuisance. Timing of therapeutic or side effects also may be a consideration. For example, a patient may be able to tolerate a drug that causes drowsiness if it can be given at bedtime. The schedule should be planned to produce minimal interference with the patient's lifestyle. This type of planning is often a cooperative effort between patient and nurse, with the patient supplying information about lifestyle and preferences and the nurse supplying information about the drugs.

Expected patient outcomes from this planning are that the patient will receive all required doses of each medication, side effects and adverse drug–drug or drug–food interactions will be minimized or avoided, and the patient will express satisfaction with the scheduling of drug doses.

Planning also includes arranging for follow-up for evaluation, further intervention, or both. When the object of the therapy is rapid or short-term relief of a problem, it is appropriate for the nurse to arrange prompt evaluation of the drug's effectiveness. For example, 20 or 30 minutes after giving an injection for the relief of pain, the nurse should check with the patient to see whether the pain has been relieved. With longer-term therapy, the nurse and patient should arrange for a convenient time for evaluation; the patient should be instructed to write down any concerns so that they will not be forgotten during the follow-up visit. The patient should also be given a telephone number to call in case questions or problems arise prior to the follow-up visit.

The expected outcomes from this type of planning are that the patient will show evidence of using the drug appropriately and that any problems or concerns will be brought to the nurse's attention promptly. Methods of evaluating drug use and the effectiveness of therapy are discussed in the section on evaluation.

Implementation

Two key nursing responsibilities in drug therapy are performed during the implementation stage of the nursing process: patient education and, for nurses in an inpatient setting, drug administration.

Patient Education

Patients receiving a prescription for a new medication need to obtain a certain amount of information to use the drug effectively. The amount of information needed depends both on the drug and on prior assessment of the patient. In some situations, teaching may consist of a brief explanation of the drug therapy and directions for taking the drug. This type of teaching is often seen in outpatient settings when the patient will be receiving a short-term course of therapy for a simple health problem. In other situations, there may be a sequence of sessions to provide the patient with detailed information and directions for use of the drug. This is often necessary when the patient has a complex or chronic condition requiring the use of multiple drugs, the acquisition of new skills, or alterations in habits or lifestyle.

Decisions about the amount of information to cover in each teaching session and the number of sessions needed by a particular patient usually are based on the information the nurse gained during the assessment phase and the patient's response to instruction. If the patient already has experience with this type of drug and demonstrates knowledge about it, one brief review may be all that is needed. On the other hand, if the patient is expected to learn a great deal of information, or several skills, it may be better to plan a series of sessions covering one topic or one new skill at each session.

The patient's attention span and response to instruction should be considered when planning the length of sessions and the amount of content presented in each session. Ideally, sessions should not be scheduled when the patient is tired or uncomfortable. However, if they must be, it is best to make the sessions short and not expect the patient to remember a lot of new material. Plans should be flexible to accommodate the patient's condition at the time of teaching. For example, the patient may become tired or frustrated, in which case the teaching session should halt. Additional sessions can be planned if the patient needs more information or practice with a new technique of drug administration. Assessment, evaluation, and implementation are ongoing as the nurse constantly observes the

TRENDS AND CONTROVERSIES IN PHARMACOLOGY

Teaching on the Run

How can nurses effectively teach patients about their medications when time is limited? On a typical hospital unit, patients receive well-intentioned but hurried medication instructions on the day of discharge. They are then left to make a very abrupt transition from total dependence on others for medication management to total responsibility for the drugs at home.

Patient education is an ongoing process. If we free ourselves from the idea that teaching and learning take place only within structured educational sessions, and if every contact with a patient is a thoughtful one, there are many opportunities for good patient teaching.

In the hospital or long-term– care facility, drug administration rounds provide a perfect time for teaching. You can share information, elicit feedback, and avoid medication errors, all at the same time!

Medication education begins with the very first drug dose administered. Start small, and progress to more information in future contacts with the patient. Determine the patient's present level of knowledge by asking a question: "Mrs Jones, this is your XYZ drug. What have you been told about it?"

Your initial goal may be to help the patient recognize the medicine, and to know what it's for. This sets the stage for further teaching and demonstrates to the patient that you are open to discussing medication concerns.

Basic information is important, even with a patient who is confused. "Hi, Mr Jones. I have your 9 AM heart medicine. Remember? It's the small white pill I bring you every morning." This approach helps orient and reassure the confused person, and imparts information as well.

Relate the drug to the condition being treated. "I know this potassium elixir tastes awful. But since your water pill flushes too much potassium out of your system, you need this medicine to replace it." Use terms—simple or complex—that are meaningful to the individual. The ability to modify patient teaching on the spot, within a range from basic to very detailed, is part of the art of nursing.

As appropriate, point out the relationship between various drugs in the regimen. "We hope that this prednisone, by reducing the inflammation in the tiny air spaces in your lungs, will work with your theophylline to ease your breathing."

The patient may initiate a discussion of potential adverse reactions by reporting symptoms that you recognize as drug side effects. Alternatively, you might ask the patient about common side effects. "Have you noticed any lightheadedness since you started this medicine?" Depending on the patient's answer, your response might be to provide information on avoiding or coping with the side effect; to ask more questions to better assess the problem; or to speak with the prescriber about the need to modify the dose or try a different drug.

Encourage the patient to write down questions to ask during your next medication rounds. Remember: a fundamental goal of teaching should be to help patients develop an active role in understanding their medications, and to identify sources of information (eg, local pharmacists) that are available to them once they leave the hospital. Because it is difficult to give patients complete information while they are hospitalized, teaching them how to ask good questions and how to learn about medications on their own are probably among the most important elements of effective teaching on the run.

patient's response to instruction and makes appropriate modifications in the teaching plan until the desired outcome is achieved.

If outpatients are unable to self-administer a drug or are too ill to tolerate instruction, it is necessary to teach someone else to administer and monitor the patient's drug therapy. This person will usually be the person identified in the assessment phase as being available to assist the patient. Often it is desirable to include other family members in the teaching sessions, even when the patient is not disabled. This is especially true if another family member needs to cooperate in some way, such as by altering methods of food preparation. The "significant other" may also be of assistance in providing support and encouragement and observing for side or toxic effects.

When making decisions about specific content to include in teaching sessions, it is important for nurses to tailor the information to the patient's interest and ability to understand. Some patients are eager and able to learn everything possible, while others seem disinterested or overwhelmed by a great deal of detailed information. Any patient should be able to understand a simple explanation of the nature of the problem being treated and the rationale for the drug therapy. This explanation may be followed by directions for use of the medication and the reasons for any special instructions. If the drug may interact with any foods or other drugs, this information should be given. The expected therapeutic effects should be explained and the patient should be alerted to side effects and toxic effects that may occur. The patient should be instructed what to do if side effects or toxic effects occur. The patient should be taught any special skills that may be needed to administer a medication. This includes instruction to parents about how to measure liquid medications correctly. Finally, instruction should be given about how to store the medication safely. In many cases, this may be too much information to expect an ill patient or fatigued parent to remember, especially if the patient is receiving more than one drug. Written instructions are advocated because they provide the patient with a continuous source of information for reference. Of course, such instructions must be geared to the patient and family's reading ability and level of comprehension.

Drug Administration

For most nurses in the inpatient setting, implementation includes drug administration. As discussed in Chapter 1, nurses who administer drugs must be careful to check the "five rights": ***right drug, right dose, right route, right patient,*** and ***right time.*** Most institutions have policies to ensure that the medication card or worksheet used by the nurse accurately reflects the information contained in the physician's order for the drug. Having verified that information, the nurse checks the medication three times: when taking it from the location where it is stored, when preparing it for administration, and when returning it to its storage location. This check should include the name of the drug and, when appropriate, its concentration and expiration date. When dosages must be calculated, many agencies require that a colleague check the calculations to ensure their accuracy. Verifying that the drug is being given at the appropriate time is especially important when the patient's schedule has been disrupted by treatments or laboratory tests. Sometimes a dose must be delayed and subsequent doses made on an adjusted time schedule until the original schedule can be reinstated.

The use of computers and the expanding role of the hospital pharmacist have made the job of giving medications much easier for many nurses. Using a computerized system, the nurse can generate current and accurate listings of medications to be given each hour. Using the same list, the hospital pharmacist can stock unit medication carts with the correct medications for each patient. Each dose can be calculated by the pharmacist and individually labeled. Once all medications have been given, the nurse can use the computer to document administration of the medication and the patient's reaction to the dose. This system has the potential to save many hours of the nurse's time, as well as reduce medication errors.

When administering medication, it is important to ensure that it is given by the right route. Giving some drugs by the wrong route can have severe consequences. For example, the packaging of some drugs designed to be inhaled through a nebulizer is similar to that of the same drug formulated for injection.

Having verified that the drug is correctly prepared for administration, it is important to verify that it will be administered to the right patient. In hospitalized patients this is done by checking the hospital identification bracelet. Addressing the patient by name is not an adequate substitute for the identification bracelet check. Many times a patient, stressed by illness and hospitalization, will respond when addressed by another name.

If the patient looks at the medication and remarks that it is not the same as the medication he or she had been receiving, make another check. The patient may be receiving the first dose of a newly prescribed drug, or it may be a different dose, form, or brand of the drug. But in some situations the problem may be a medication error. The nurse may have dropped a pill into the wrong cup while preparing medications, or may have picked the wrong cup off a medication tray while administering medications to several patients. The knowledgeable patient can be an ally in preventing medication errors.

After giving the medications to the patient, the nurse should stay with that patient while each medication is swallowed. Psychiatric patients may need to be checked to ensure that they have not held the medications in their cheeks rather than swallowed them. Other patients may have difficulty swallowing or may simply not have enough water at the bedside to take their medications.

In addition to verifying that the medication is given correctly, the nurse must provide supportive nursing care to enhance the therapeutic effect or prevent complications from certain types of drugs. For instance, when a series of injections is given, the nurse uses different (but proper) injection sites to minimize trauma and damage to tissues in any one area of the body. Also, certain drugs administered orally may cause damage to the teeth if administered carelessly. Many syrups and suspensions contain significant amounts of sugar, so the nurse must emphasize the importance of brushing the teeth after each dose of the medication. Other medications may stain the teeth. The nurse or caretaker should administer these through a straw to minimize contact with the teeth.

In contrast, some medications have a therapeutic local effect as well as a systemic effect. For this reason, patients taking an oral suspension of nystatin, for example, should be instructed to "swish and swallow" to maximize the drug's contact with lesions on the oral mucosa.

Other types of supportive nursing measures may include providing a quiet environment for a patient who has taken a sedative, or encouraging fluid intake for a patient who is taking a medication that may cause crystal formation in the kidneys or ureters.

Prompt and complete charting of medication administration is critically important for both legal and practical reasons. Such written documentation is the only legal proof that a medication was actually administered. When legal questions arise, there is often a long time between the incident in question and the legal proceedings. The nurse may no longer remember the incident itself or the events surrounding it. In addition, prompt documentation helps ensure accuracy and prevent a colleague from unknowingly administering another dose before the required time interval has elapsed.

Evaluation

The evaluation of drug therapy can be organized around four key questions:

1. Has the drug produced the desired therapeutic effect?
2. Is the patient using the drug appropriately?
3. Has the patient experienced any side effects or adverse effects?
4. How satisfied is the patient with the drug?

A problem in any of these areas may necessitate further nursing interventions or modification of the drug therapy.

Table 2–3 describes methods that may be used to obtain the information needed to answer the four questions. Methods should be chosen by considering the advantages and disadvantages of each for obtaining the type of information needed. Also consider that some methods may work well with some patients but not with

Table 2–3 Methods Used to Assess Compliance with Prescribed Medication Regimen

Method	Description	Comments
History	Asking whether medication doses were taken as prescribed	May be inaccurate if the patient has a memory problem or is reluctant to admit that the medication was not taken
Physical assessment	Monitoring physical effect(s) of the prescribed drug (e.g., blood pressure or hemoglobin level.)	Necessary to determine effectiveness of therapy, but not a guarantee that change(s) were produced as a result of the drug (other factors may have produced the changes, eg, decreased stress or change in diet)
Medication diary or chart	Patient records each medication dose as it is taken, either in diary form or by marking it on a chart	Can be posted in the home to serve as a reminder for the patient; can help patient remember whether a particular dose was taken or not, thus helping to eliminate missed doses and double doses; requires effort and consistency by the patient
Serum drug concentration	Measurement of blood levels of prescribed drugs	Most useful for drugs with a long half-life; for drugs with a short half-life, this method provides information only about the past few hours; involves additional cost to the patient
Pill counts	Counting the pills remaining in the bottle to determine how many doses have been taken since the last visit	Easy and relatively inexpensive; provides no information about timing of doses; misplaced bottles, dropped pills, and leftover doses from a previous prescription can make the count inaccurate
Microprocessors in medication bottle caps	The time and date is recorded every time the bottle is opened	Provides information about timing of doses; does not rely on patient memory; assumes that a dose was taken every time the bottle was opened; involves additional cost to the patient.

TRENDS AND CONTROVERSIES IN PHARMACOLOGY

PRN Drug Administration

"PRN" drugs are "just what the nurse ordered"—or almost, at any rate. Nurses control the patient's access to these drugs, and should carefully avoid making prn drug administration a reflex act.

Long before medications were widely available, Florence Nightingale recognized our tendency to rely on drugs: ". . . so deep-rooted and universal is the conviction that to give medicine is to be doing something, or rather everything; to give air, warmth, cleanliness, and so on is to do nothing." Never undervalue nursing interventions.

Always consider measures that could alleviate the patient's symptoms without drugs, or could enhance drug effects. People in pain need proper positioning and rest, and may benefit from the use of guided imagery or relaxation techniques. The person with gastrointestinal distress may need a change in diet or better-fitting dentures. Carefully assess the patient's complaints *each time* a prn drug is requested. Never assume that the condition for which a drug is prescribed is static. The complaint of stomach distress may warrant more than simple antacid treatment; for example, if the patient suddenly notices blood in the stool. For the person with chronic pain, pain in a new area or of a different quality could signal thrombophlebitis, pneumonia, or other medical complications.

PRN psychotropic drugs demand special consideration. The evaluation of agitation, anxiety, or the need for a sleeping pill depends a great deal on the individual nurse's perception of events. At times, one could say that a prn drug is given to the patient to relieve the nurse's distress. When staffing is short and an anxious preoperative patient needs information and reassurance, or an angry patient needs to be listened to, nurses sometimes employ prn medications when they know that what the patient needs most is attentive nursing care.

Assessment doesn't stop with drug administration. What happened after the drug was given? Was the problem relieved, or at least ameliorated? How long did this take? Were any adverse effects apparent? Did non-drug measures contribute to the patient's comfort?

Charting should clearly support the decision to administer prn drugs, and should describe the effects of therapy. If the drug isn't working, or if the patient is dissatisfied with the results, this fact should be documented. Some prescribers are not easily convinced that a patient isn't responding to a "good" drug. Clear documentation of the patient's need for and response to the drug may be the determining factor in revising a prn regimen.

Nightingale F. *Notes on Nursing: What It Is and What It Is Not.* East Norwalk, CT: Appleton, 1918:9 .

others. Many clinicians use a combination of methods, based on their knowledge of the individual patient and the specific drug therapy.

Has the Drug Produced the Desired Therapeutic Effect?

The answer to this question is obtained by asking the patient about the drug's effectiveness in relieving symptoms, examining the patient to obtain objective evidence of problem resolution, or obtaining laboratory studies when appropriate. The nature of the patient's problem will determine what method of evaluation is most appropriate. In some cases, such as evaluation of drug therapy to relieve pain, questioning the patient may be the only evaluation method used. However, if the patient is taking medication for an asymptomatic condition, such as hypertension, the most appropriate assessment might be measuring the blood pressure. Laboratory studies are important assessment tools for other situations. Whatever the method used, absence of therapeutic effectiveness is an indication that something must be changed. Often the change involves an increased dosage of the current drug, or the use of another drug in addition to, or in place of, the current medication(s). Before this is done, however, an assessment is usually made of how the patient is using the drug.

Is the Patient Using the Drug Appropriately?

Again, the answer comes from both subjective and objective evidence. For the patient in an inpatient setting, the nurse should review the medical record and the practices used in administering medications to ensure that each dose has been given correctly and that the

Case Study **Mrs Yin**

Mrs Yin is a 45-year-old woman who was hospitalized for removal of her gallbladder. Her surgery was performed yesterday and she has been experiencing a great deal of pain. She is receiving meperidine (DEMEROL) 50 mg q4h prn. Her last dose was 5 hours ago and she has just asked for another dose.

Assessment	Nursing Diagnosis	Planning	Implementation	Evaluation
Amount of pain: "Very uncomfortable, especially when I take a deep breath."	Pain	Plan timing of dose to allow for pain control when doing deep breathing exercises	Check the "five rights"	Check in 20 min to see if pain relief has been obtained
Location of pain: operative site			Check drug's expiration date	
Type of pain: "Dull and aching"				Check for adverse reactions or side effects (decreased blood pressure, excessive drowsiness)
Condition of operative site: sutures intact, T-tube draining, no distention, hypoactive bowel sounds		Develop rotation plan for injection sites	Document medication administration on medical record	Rotate injection sites according to plan
Vital signs: temp. = 98.4°F pulse = 80 resp. = 20 (shallow) bp = 130/84				
Effectiveness of last dose: "It helped a lot"				
Environment: bothered by noise due to street repairs	Ineffective individual coping related to noise in environment	Check availability of quieter room	Move to quieter room	Note amount of relief obtained and time between doses after room change

patient has taken it. The patient on self-medication should be questioned about use of the drug. If the patient has kept a medication diary, log, or chart, the nurse may use it to assess proper drug use. The nurse may also count pills or measure the amount of liquid medication remaining in the patient's medication bottle and compare that with the amount that should remain if the patient had taken the medication correctly. In addition, some drugs produce changes in the color of urine or stool. This may be looked for, or the patient may be questioned about these changes.

When drugs are being given improperly, the cause of the problem must be ascertained and corrected. Sometimes the cause is a misunderstanding or lack of information. At other times the problem is the patient's inability to tolerate undesirable side effects, which brings up assessment of the side effects or adverse effects of the drug.

Has the Patient Experienced Any Side Effects or Adverse Effects?

Most drugs have the potential to produce effects other than those desired for therapy. The nurse should be knowledgeable about these effects and assess the patient for them by the most appropriate means. Usually questioning the patient and observing for physical or behavioral evidence of side effects will provide the answer. Questioning should be guided by a knowledge of the potential side effects of the patient's drug therapy. If the drug produces side effects that interfere with sexual desire or performance, the patient may not volunteer that information. However, a skilled nurse will be able to inquire about this in a sensitive manner so that the patient can be helped with the problem.

Medication side effects may be sufficiently problematic that the patient perceives the therapy to be

Case Study | **Jerry Thomas**

Jerry Thomas is a 2-year-old boy who was seen 2 weeks ago in the pediatric clinic for a middle-ear infection. He received a prescription for ampicillin suspension 1 tsp PO qid for 10 days. His mother says that she gave the medication for 3 days. At that time his ears no longer hurt, so she stopped giving the antibiotic. Now his ears are hurting again. She would like "to get some more medicine."

Assessment	Nursing Diagnosis	Planning	Implementation	Evaluation
Mother's knowledge of ear infection and antibiotic therapy: mother can explain what otitis media is, but thought that the antibiotic could be stopped after symptoms had resolved	Knowledge deficit related to antibiotic therapy	Arrange for quiet location, time, and audio-visual resources for teaching session Plan content of session: how antibiotics work, measurement and timing of doses, administration of drug, side effects, what to do if problems occur, what happens if drug is stopped too soon	Conduct teaching session Give written instructions Answer mother's questions Give mother a telephone number to call if she has questions or problems	Ask mother questions to assess her understanding of content presented Evaluate knowledge at follow-up visit
	Noncompliance related to antibiotic therapy		Have mother keep a medication diary or chart	Check diary at follow-up to see if all doses were given
Ability to store and give drug appropriately: family just moved here, staying in motel while house hunting, no refrigerator in hotel room	Impaired home maintenance management	Recommend use of another drug or form of drug that does not require refrigeration		

more difficult to live with than the health problem itself. If side effects are sufficiently unacceptable to the patient that the medication is discontinued, intervention is always called for. Possible interventions might include reinforcing the importance of taking the medication, teaching the patient interventions to minimize or cope more effectively with side effects, or informing the physician of the problem so that the dosage can be changed or another medication substituted.

Some drugs produce side effects that occur in most patients who receive them. These side effects may be anticipated and the patient prepared in advance to cope with them. For example, the patient who is told that a drug will cause urine to change color will be less likely to panic and discontinue the drug when that happens than the patient who isn't prepared for that side effect. Outpatients should also be given the office or clinic telephone number so that they can call for advice before discontinuing a drug.

How Satisfied Is the Patient with the Drug?

In addition to curing or controlling health problems, it is important to promote the best possible quality of life for patients. Medications that are expensive, difficult to administer, or inconvenient to store or prepare can cause dissatisfaction with drug therapy. Dissatisfaction may lead to noncompliance and failure of otherwise adequate drug therapy. This type of problem can frequently be prevented if therapy is designed to fit the patient's lifestyle, resources, and preferences. The patient should be asked about satisfaction with the drug therapy and assisted with problems that are identified.

ANNOTATED BIBLIOGRAPHY

Bell SK. Guidelines for taking a complete drug history. *Nursing '80* 1980;10(3):10–11. *This short article outlines the compon-*

ents of a drug history and gives the significance of each piece of information.

Beyond instructions for use: How to counsel your patients about their prescriptions. *Ohio Med* 1990;86(10):711–712. *The National Council on Patient Information and Education suggests that patients be given basic oral and written information about their prescribed medications: the drug name; expected effects; possible side effects and actions to take if these occur; scheduling and duration of drug administration; avoidance of other medications and/or foods; potential benefits and risks; and where to obtain more information.*

Carpenito LJ. *Nursing diagnosis: Application to clinical practice.* 4th ed. Philadelphia: J. B. Lippincott, 1992. *This book provides basic information about nursing diagnosis. Nursing diagnoses are listed by category. Each diagnosis is defined and its defining characteristics identified. Related factors, diagnostic considerations, interventions, and outcome criteria are provided.*

Col N, Fandale JE, Kronholm P. The role of medication noncompliance and adverse drug reactions in hospitalizations of the elderly. *Arch Intern Med* 1990;150:841–845. *Interviews of elderly hospitalized patients revealed that 28% of the admissions were drug-related. Noncompliance (11% of admissions) and adverse drug reactions (17%) were the leading causes of drug-related admissions. Risk factors for medication problems are identified.*

Cramer JA, Mattson RH, Prevey ML, Scheyer RD, Ouellette VL. How often is medication taken as prescribed? *JAMA* 1989;261:3273–3277. *Pill bottles with microprocessors in the cap to record every bottle opening were used to assess epileptic patients' compliance with their medication regimens. Only 76% of the patients in this study took their medication as prescribed. Pros and cons of various methods to assess compliance are discussed.*

Fuqua RA, Stevens KR. What we know about medication errors: A literature review. *J Nurs Qual Assur* 1988;3(1):1–17. *This article summarizes the most common types of reported medication errors, and stresses that most errors are the result of multiple causes. The discussion of each type of error includes information about contributing factors and measures that can be taken to prevent it. A useful table summarizes recommendations for reducing medication errors.*

Gardner M, Hurd PD, Slack M. Effect of information organization on recall of medication instructions. *J Clin Pharm Ther* 1990;15(1):13–19. *A highly structured format for presenting prescription information seems to facilitate immediate recall of that information.*

Kay EA, Bailie GR, Bernstein A. Patient knowledge of cardiorespiratory drugs. *J Clin Pharm Ther* 1988;13(4):263–268. *Interviews of 85 patients revealed that 85% knew the reason for use of their medications and 73% knew the frequency of use. However, only 16% knew the anticipated duration of use and a mere 8% had been warned of adverse effects. Patients changed the doses of 34% of their medications without consulting their health-care provider. The majority of patients interviewed (68%) had questions about their treatment.*

McGovern KA. 10 golden rules for administering drugs safely. *Nursing '88* 1988;18(8):34–41. *A discussion of rules for safe medication administration—the "5 rights"—is provided. Patient education, taking a complete drug history, and evaluating the potential for adverse effects are also emphasized.*

Morrow D, Leirer V, Sheikh J. Adherence and medication instructions: Review and recommendations. *J Am Geriatr Soc* 1988;36(12):1147–1160. *Among the elderly, nonadherence with prescription medication regimens is caused primarily by poor communication with health-care providers. The problem stems from an inability to understand and remember medication instructions. A proposed solution is to help the elderly construct a clear and simple mental model of how to take their medications.*

Rost K, Roter D, Bertakis D, Quill T. Physician–patient familiarity and patient recall of medication changes. The collaborative study group of the SGIM task force on the doctor and patient. *Fam Med* 1990;22(6):453–457. *For "new" patients in primary care settings, the more drug information given during the concluding part of a visit, the less the patient remembered. However, this relationship was reversed for patients who were familiar with the physician. Elderly patients tended to remember less, regardless of their familiarity with the physician. Asking patients to restate instructions is recommended to enhance recall.*

Sandler DA, Mitchell JR, Fellows A, Garner ST. Is an information booklet for patients leaving hospital helpful and useful? *BMJ* 1989;298(6677):870–874. *Sixty-five patients received informational booklets upon discharge from a large teaching hospital, and 66 patients served as controls. At the time of their follow-up outpatient visit, patients who received booklets recalled important medical details concerning their illness with greater accuracy and thoroughness than did controls.*

Tinetti ME, Speechley M. Prevention of falls among the elderly. *N Engl J Med* 1989;320:1055–1059. *An extraordinarily well written discussion of the many often-overlooked physiologic and drug-induced causes of significant morbidity and mortality in the elderly. Noteworthy not only for its timeless content and ease of reading, but also because a topic that has been of concern to nurses for years has now been presented to a wide physician readership.*

Vincer MJ, Murray JM, Yuill A, Allen AC, Evans JR, Stinson DA. Drug errors and incidents in a neonatal intensive care unit. *Am J Dis Child* 1989;143:737–740. *A regular audit of all medication errors and incidents was established as a quality assurance and staff education activity. The most frequent causes of medication incidents were neglecting to give a drug at the scheduled time, and failing to regulate an intravenous infusion properly. Errors in physician's orders tended to result in more serious incidents than did other types of errors. The patient acuity level increased the risk of errors.*

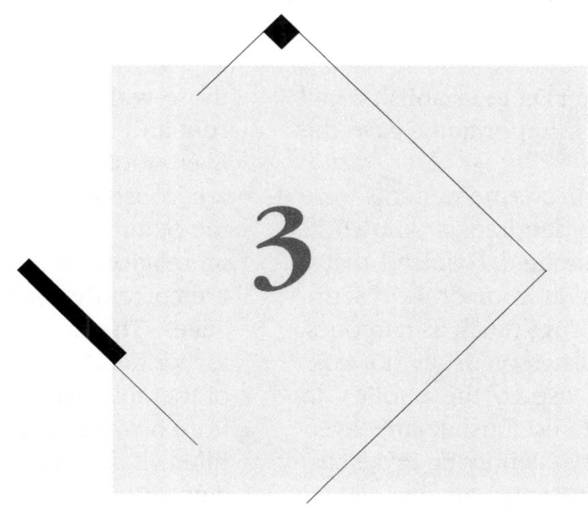

Legal Considerations in Drug Therapy

Nurses are responsible not only for being knowledgeable about the many agents used in drug therapy, but also for understanding and abiding by the professional ethics and laws that govern this part of nursing practice. This chapter presents a brief overview of the federal and state laws that govern the development, manufacture, and distribution of drugs; a discussion of the legal concept of professional negligence or malpractice and its application to medication administration; and a discussion of current trends and controversies arising from the expanded role of the nurse. This chapter provides only general information concerning the legal aspects of drug therapy. It is not intended to be a source of specific legal or professional advice. If such advice is needed, the reader is encouraged to seek specific legal or other professional services.

Legal Regulation of the Development, Manufacture, and Distribution of Drugs

Federal Laws Concerning the Quality, Labeling, Effectiveness, and Safety of Drugs

One of the first federal laws dealing with drugs was the Pure Food and Drugs Act of 1906. This act was aimed at improving the quality and labeling of drugs, which until then were being manufactured and sold in unsafe, mislabeled, and often adulterated conditions. The act covered all National Formulary (NF) and United States Pharmacopeia (USP) medicines.

Despite its attempt at reform, the 1906 act did not have a provision that allowed the government, specifically the Food and Drug Administration (FDA), to enforce it. Nor did it specify premarket safety standards that had to be met before a drug could be placed on the market. As a result, the Federal Food, Drug, and Cosmetics Act of 1938 was passed. The 1938 act, in addition to preserving the requirements of the 1906 act, required drug manufacturers to test drugs for toxicity on non-human subjects prior to seeking FDA approval to market them. It also allowed the FDA to establish recall procedures for drugs, and, most importantly, gave the FDA the power of enforcement.

In 1951 the Durham–Humphrey Amendments were added to the 1938 act. These amendments, known as the "prescription drug amendments," required that a pharmacist have a physician's written or oral prescription before dispensing certain drugs (such as narcotics, hypnotics, and investigational drugs or drugs not considered safe for indiscriminate use by the public). In addition, the 1951 amendments established the over-the-counter (OTC) drug category, identifying drugs that could be dispensed without a prescription.

In 1962, the thalidomide tragedies that occurred in the United States and Europe prompted the passage of the Kefauver–Harris Act. Prior to this time, an application for a new drug was approved by the FDA when the drug was shown to be safe for use in human beings. With the passage of the Kefauver–Harris Act, evidence not only of safety, but also of effectiveness, was needed before the drug could be marketed.

Federal Laws Concerning Abuse of Drugs and Drug Addiction

At the same time the government was realizing the need to regulate the quality, labeling, effectiveness, and safety of drugs used to treat human illness, the government and the public became increasingly concerned about drug abuse and the potential for drug addiction. As a result, the Harrison Narcotic Law was passed in 1914 to regulate the importation, manufacture, sale, and use of certain drugs (opium, cocaine, marijuana, synthetic analgesics, and any and all derivatives of these groups of drugs) that could result in addiction, habituation, or both.

In 1970 the Comprehensive Drug Abuse Prevention and Control Act (also called the Controlled Substances Act) was passed. It provided for control of drug abuse and the enforcement of its provisions by the FDA and the Drug Enforcement Agency of the Department of Justice. The classification of controlled substances into schedules, and requirements regarding documentation and storage of drugs, are important aspects of this act for nurses.

Drug Schedules

The Controlled Substances Act set up five schedules of controlled substances (Schedules I through V), based on three main criteria: potential for abuse, accepted medical uses, and potential for physical or psychologic dependence. Under this scheme, Schedule I drugs are those with a high potential for abuse and with no current and accepted therapeutic use in the United States. Even under professional supervision, Schedule I drugs are considered unsafe for use. Schedule V drugs, on the other hand, are those with a low potential for abuse in relation to the other drugs in the schedules, and are currently used for medical treatment in the United States. The drug schedules also regulate requirements for written or verbal prescriptions, the number of days of therapy that can be provided for by a given prescription, how many times a single prescription can be refilled, if any, and the time after which a prescription automatically expires. Some examples of drugs found on each of the five schedules are listed in Table 3–1.

It is important to note that the attorney general and the Drug Enforcement Agency may change the schedule in which a drug is listed (rescheduling), may place a previously unscheduled drug in the schedule, or may remove a drug from the schedule. Thus, it is essential that the nurse stay abreast of changes that may occur as a result of revisions in the Controlled Substances Act. The act requires that the pharmacist label all controlled substances with an identifying symbol indicating the schedule in which the drug is listed. This symbol, the letter "C" with the number of the schedule following it (C-III, for example), either is located in the upper right corner of the label in large type, or is overprinted on the label in an easily seen and contrasting color. Even with these precautions, it is still important that the nurse also be aware of changes in the schedules.

Record-Keeping and Storage of Scheduled Drugs

In addition to the schedules, the act also mandates extensive record-keeping and storage requirements for scheduled drugs. Although many of its provisions are specific to pharmacists and pharmacies, the nurse must be aware of certain of these requirements. For example, in addition to careful documentation of the administration of a controlled substance, the medical record must also contain the physician's order for that drug. All scheduled drugs kept on nursing units must be securely locked, and access to these drugs is limited to certain members of the nursing staff. If an institution uses medication carts, the carts must be equipped with locks.

Other Governmental Regulation of Drugs

Besides the Drug Enforcement Agency and the FDA, other government agencies may be responsible for enforcement of the many laws dealing with medications.

Table 3–1 Controlled Substances

Schedule	Examples	Comments	Prescription Details
C-I	Opiates not covered in other schedules, including heroin. Hallucinogens, including LSD, mescaline, peyote, and phencyclidine (PCP); methaqualone; marijuana (excluding some oral derivatives)	Abuse potential high; no currently accepted medical use in the US; no accepted standards for safe use, even under medical supervision; drugs may be obtained for research if proper forms are filed	
C-II	*Opium and related drugs:* alfentanyl, opium (raw extracts, fluid extracts, powdered, granulated, tincture), codeine, fentanyl, hydrocodone, hydromorphone, methadone, morphine, oxycodone, oxymorphone. *Stimulants:* amphetamine, methamphetamine, methylphenidate, phenmetrazine. *Depressants:* amobarbital, glutethimide, pentobarbital, secobarbital; any preparation containing amobarbital or secobarbital combined with one or more other controlled substances	High potential for abuse; abuse may cause severe psychologic or physical dependence; currently accepted medical uses in US, with severe restrictions	Prescription must be written (ink, typewriter, indelible pencil); signed personally by licensed prescriber (rubber stamp not allowed); entire prescribed amount usually must be dispensed within 72 h by pharmacist. Verbal orders for oral C-II prescriptions acceptable if all three conditions are met: immediate administration necessary for patient care; no suitable alternative available; prescriber cannot present written prescription; amount to be dispensed in emergency should be limited to 72 h of treatment. Refill prescriptions not allowed. Container must have suitable warning label
C-III	Anabolic steroids: stimulants not covered in other schedules, including benzphetamine, chlorphentermine, clortermine, phendimetrazine. Depressants not covered in other schedules; combinations of amobarbital, secobarbital, or pentobarbital with another medicinal ingredient that is not a controlled substance; products containing amobarbital, secobarbital, pentobarbital for administration as rectal suppository; products containing low amount of codeine per unit dose	Abuse potential less than substances in C-I or C-II; abuse may lead to moderate to low physical dependence or high psychologic dependence	Written or oral prescription is acceptable. Prescription may be refilled if so authorized by prescriber, but may not be refilled more than 5 times or more than 6 months after issue date, whichever comes first. Container must have suitable warning label
C-IV	Barbital, chloral betaine or hydrate, chlordiazepoxide, clonazepam, clorazepate, dextropropoxyphene, diazepam, ethchlorvynol, ethinamate, flurazepam, lorazepam, meprobamate, methohexital, oxazepam, paraldehyde, pentazocine, phenobarbital, prazepam, temazepam	Low potential for abuse relative to substances in C-III; abuse may cause limited physical or psychologic dependence	Restrictions noted for C-III drugs apply also to C-IV agents

(*continued*)

Table 3–1 Controlled Substances (*Continued*)

Schedule	Examples	Comments	Prescription Details
C-V	Loperamide; products containing no more than 200 mg codeine per 100 mL or per 100 g, and not more than 10 mg per dosage unit; products containing not more than 100 mg of opium per 100 mL or 100 g, and not more than 5 mg per dosage unit (eg, many antitussive and antidiarrheal agents)	Low potential for abuse; abuse may cause limited psychologic or physical dependence compared with C-IV agents	Some C-V agents may be sold OTC without prescription, others may require written prescription. State laws may vary; most restrictions focus on limiting amount and frequency of requested drug and identifying age and identity of purchaser

All prescriptions for controlled substances require the full name and address of the patient; name, address, and registration number of the prescriber; and the date of issue. Substances in C-II to C-IV cannot be transferred to a person other than the one for whom the substance was prescribed. States may place some substances in a schedule more restrictive than that assigned by federal law.

The Public Health Service, for example, through its Division of Biological Standards of the National Institutes of Health (NIH), sets control requirements for biologic products such as antitoxins, blood derivatives, immune serums, and immunologic diagnostic aids. The Federal Trade Commission (FTC) is charged with monitoring and protecting the public from false advertising and deceptive trade practices.

State and Local Laws, and Institutional Policies Governing the Use of Drugs

Although a state cannot pass a law that conflicts with federal drug laws, it may pass additional provisions concerning the regulation of drugs and medications within that state. As a result, most of the federal laws just discussed have either been adopted as the only state law, or been included in more extensive state laws.

Some states have also adopted model uniform laws. Two such laws are the Uniform State Food, Drug, and Cosmetic Act and the Uniform Controlled Substance Act. The benefit in adopting uniform state laws is the ease with which the laws can be enforced between states. Each state is further responsible for establishing its own agency to regulate and enforce the provisions of its own acts. Such agencies are also responsible for setting up procedures required by state laws.

Local governments may also pass specific ordinances, regulations, or other laws that specifically cover drug administration. Both state and local regulations vary considerably in the additional constraints that may be placed on the administration of medications by the health professional, and a thorough knowledge and understanding of them is necessary.

In addition to government regulations, institutions that provide health care have their own policies and procedures covering medications. These policies and procedures must conform to current federal, state, and local laws, but may be even more restrictive. Institutional policies often regulate the renewal or automatic expiration of prescriptions for certain medications, or may regulate the administration of medications by a particular route (usually intravenous). For example, an institution may regulate the use of certain antibiotics, since indiscriminate antibiotic use may increase the chance of drug-induced infections that are very difficult to treat. Although these constraints may not be required by state or federal law, they are the institution's attempt to avoid drug abuse, violation of existing laws, or potential harm to patients, and to encourage frequent assessment of the patient's true needs for drug therapy. Thus, it is exceedingly important that the nurse be familiar with the institution's specific policies concerning drug administration. Out-of-date policies, or ones that do not conform with federal, state, and local laws, must be changed, and it is the nurse's professional responsibility to be sure that an institution's policies are in compliance with the law. Nursing representation on policy and procedure committees is essential to ensure that the regulations concerning drug and medication administration also conform with nursing standards and the delivery of high-quality nursing care.

State Practice Acts

Three additional state laws that the nurse must be familiar with are the practice acts of nursing, pharmacy, and medicine. These are the acts that govern the prac-

TRENDS AND CONTROVERSIES IN PHARMACOLOGY

The Nurse as Prescriber

The expansion of nursing roles to include the prescription of medication began in the 1960s. Today, nurse practitioners in 40 states have been granted some level of prescriptive authority. Existing regulations vary widely, with some states granting direct authority to nurse practitioners through nurse–practice acts, whereas others mandate that prescribing roles are carried out as an extension of physician authority (Mahoney, 1992).

Authorization to prescribe medications has been important to the successful role development of nurse practitioners, allowing them to provide comprehensive health care for their patients and to compete effectively with other health care providers. Despite initial concerns regarding the appropriateness of this function for nurses, evidence indicates that nurse practitioners use the prescription of medications as an adjunct to, not a substitute for, nursing care. For example, studies have reported that practitioners rely less on medications and prescribe more nondrug therapies than their physician counterparts (Simborg et al, 1978; Munroe et al, 1982). Moreover, nurse practitioners have been accepted as safe, effective prescribers who adhere to accepted protocols.

A recent review by Mahoney (1992) points out that while there have been numerous studies of nurse practitioners, relatively few have examined prescribing roles in depth. Prescribing practices of physicians are influenced by many factors, including peer pressure, type of reimbursement, sources of drug information, and limitations placed by employers or insurers. Nurses may be influenced by similar factors, but this remains to be determined. In addition, it has not been established how nursing care or nursing philosophies affect prescriptive practices. Mahoney also notes that little attention has been given to the effects of regulatory constraints on the practice of nurse practitioners. This is an important topic, since nurses may be faced with complex but unnecessary regulation, and some states have yet to grant prescriptive authority to nurses.

The ability to prescribe medication enhances nurses' abilities to meet the needs of their patients. Although we need more research, differences noted between the prescribing practices of physicians and nurses suggest that nurses are using nursing expertise to redefine this role.

Mahoney DF: Nurse practitioners as prescribers: past research trends and future study needs. *Nurse Practitioner* 1992;17:44–51.

Simborg DW, Starfield B, Horn SD: Non physician health practitioners: the characteristics of their practices and their relationships. *Am J Public H* 1978;68:44–48.

Munroe D, Pohl J, Gardner H, et al.: Prescribing patterns of nurse practitioners. *Am J Nurs* 1982;10:1538–1542.

tices of these professions and specifically state who can administer, dispense, and prescribe medications.

State nurse practice acts define the practice of professional and licensed practical nursing within that state. Although nurse practice acts vary widely from state to state, most cover the nurse's role in the administration of medications and treatments (pursuant to a physician's order or that of another licensed health professional) in addition to other roles of the nurse.

Like the nurse practice act, the pharmacy act defines the scope of pharmacy practice. *Pharmacy* is defined in most states as the compounding, dispensing, recommending, or advising concerning medicines, drugs, or poisons, as well as the selling of these substances. In addition, the act defines certain key terms in pharmacy. Dispensing may be defined as the labeling, delivering, and distribution of drugs and medications. Administration, on the other hand, is defined as the distribution of a single dose of medication.

In most states the medical practice act defines the practice of medicine as including, among other things, the prescribing, dispensing, and administration of medications. Some medical practice acts state that no one except physicians or nurses may administer medications.

Nurses administering medications must be very clear about the scope of nursing practice in the states in which they practice. This familiarity includes knowing whether the state's attorney general or the boards of nursing, pharmacy, or medicine have declared any state attorney general opinions, joint practice statements, rules, or regulations that might allow nurses to dispense medications in certain situations. If no such opinions or rules or regulations are in effect, it is essential not to dispense medications, as it would be a violation of the pharmacy act. To avoid this possibility the nurse should not transfer medication from its original container to another container, should not label or relabel medication containers, and should not go into the pharmacy when a pharmacist is not available to take medication to the nursing unit. These are the functions of a licensed pharmacist; a nurse who carries out these functions could be charged with practicing pharmacy without a license. Similarly (unless the law specifically states otherwise; see the section below on the expanded role of the nurse), the nurse may not prescribe medications; to do so could result in charges being filed against the nurse for practicing medicine without a license.

State Criminal Laws

The laws discussed thus far have been concerned with civil liability—noncriminal violations. However, the nurse must also be aware of actions that could lead to criminal liability. State criminal laws vary, but in general they are similar or identical to federal laws dealing with controlled drugs. Therefore, in most states it is a felony to be found guilty of illegal possession of a controlled substance; forgery (eg, signing another nurse's name in a patient's record as having administered a controlled substance); or the manufacture or distribution of controlled substances.

Canadian Laws

Canadian laws dealing with the administration, manufacture, and distribution of drugs do not differ significantly from those of the United States. There have been laws regulating drugs in Canada since 1875, when the Canadian Parliament passed an act in an attempt to control the sale of adulterated food, drink, and drugs.

The current Canadian Food and Drug Act was passed in 1953. It established several schedules of drugs that require certain standards for advertising, labeling, and quality; controls the manufacture of drugs; and sets standards that must be met before a drug can be sold. The Health Protection Branch of the Department of National Health and Welfare is responsible for the administration and enforcement of this act.

The Canadian Narcotic Control Act was passed in 1961 to deal with the manufacture, sale, possession, and distribution of narcotics. Like the American counterpart, it states that only authorized individuals can possess a narcotic, mandates strict record-keeping, and requires prescriptions for all narcotics.

Nurses practicing in Canada must also be aware of local and provincial laws that may require additional safeguards concerning medication administration.

Nurses' Legal Responsibilities in Drug Therapy

The laws briefly presented here have a clear impact on the responsibilities of the nurse administering drug therapy. The nurse must be familiar with both state and federal laws dealing with criminal causes of action, and must conform to their requirements. This responsibility can be met by attending continuing education or in-service programs on drug and medication administration and through active cooperation with a hospital's pharmacy department. Knowledge and understanding of the applicable laws, and incorporation of their precepts into the nurse's everyday practice, is necessary both for the public's protection and for the nurse's protection.

The nurse who violates these laws is subject not only to criminal charges, but also to disciplinary action by the state's regulatory licensing agency. Disciplinary action frequently follows conviction on felony charges for the unlawful use, possession, or distribution of a controlled substance. In most states a felony conviction is grounds for the regulatory agency to file a complaint against a nurse. However, disciplinary actions also may be initiated against a nurse without a felony conviction, if the regulatory agency finds that there is enough evidence to support a complaint of unlawful use, possession, or distribution of drugs, or if such conduct violates other provisions of the act (eg, unprofessional conduct).

The Impaired Nurse

Recently, many state nurse practice acts have been amended to include habitual intoxication or addiction that affects the practice of nursing as grounds for initiating an action against a nurse. In addition, some states *require* that nurse executives or other nurses report to the state Board of Nursing any nursing staff who are diverting, using, or converting for their own use habit-forming drugs belonging to the facility. These acts usually provide immunity from civil or criminal prosecution to nurse executives and others who in good faith provide information or assist in the determination that a nurse is illegally using facility drugs.

The mandatory reporting provisions of nurse practice acts were initially a response to the public's concern about "impaired health professionals," that is, those working under the influence of chemicals, and was consistent with a provision in the Controlled Substances Act concerning the responsibility of employees to report to their employers any knowledge of diversion of drugs by fellow employees. However, the reasons for mandatory reporting have changed recently. Owing to the efforts of many professional nursing groups, such as the American Nurses' Association (ANA) and the National Nurses Society on Addictions, the mandatory reporting requirements have also included a rehabilitative focus. Currently, many nurse practice acts have been amended to provide continued licensure for the impaired or recovering nurse as long as active and continuing treatment for chemical use is successfully undertaken (Haack and Hughes, 1989, pp. 35–63).

Negligence and Malpractice

In addition to knowing the laws that govern the manufacture, distribution, and administration of drugs, the nurse must also know the laws about malpractice and negligence, and understand the laws and precedents that may determine potential legal liability in relation to drug administration.

Definition of Negligence

Negligence is part of the law of torts (the law of civil wrongs) that involves injury or damages to a person, a person's property, or both, for which some type of compensation is awarded by the court when the allegations are proved. When found to be negligent by a judge or jury, the persons or institutions responsible are liable for damages for which they are found responsible and for those recognized by law as compensable (Prosser and Keeton, 1984, p. 345). Although *negligence* has been defined in many ways, it can generally be held to be either the failure to do something that could reasonably be expected would be done by an individual in a given situation, or the performance of an act that a reasonable and prudent person would not do. The concept of liability does exist in each state, although the wording of definitions varies. The professional's behavior in a particular situation will be compared with that of other professionals in the same or a similar situation.

Specifically, there are four elements of negligence, and all four must be proved in a court of law for a cause of action in negligence to be successful (Prosser and Keeton, 1984, pp. 164–165).

1. A duty exists, usually established or recognized by law, to which behavior must conform to avoid unreasonable and foreseeable risk of harm to others.
2. A breach of that duty, or a failure to conform behavior to that duty, has occurred.
3. The breach of duty is the "proximate" or "legal cause" of injury.
4. Actual damages have been suffered and the damages are ones recognized by law.

Negligent behavior is always measured by comparing the behavior alleged to be negligent with what would have been done by an "ordinary, reasonable, and prudent person in the same or similar circumstances." A professional's (eg, a nurse's) behavior in a particular situation will be compared with other professional nurses in the same or similar situation.

A key concept in a negligence action is that each person is responsible for his or her own negligence. For the most part it is very difficult in a negligence action to shift all the "blame" to another individual or to an institution. Although the doctrine of *respondeat superior* ("let the master speak") states that an employer is indirectly liable for the alleged negligent action of employees if the negligent act is committed during the course and within the scope of employment, it does not shift the blame for the alleged negligent act (Prosser and Keeton, 1984, pp. 499–500). This doctrine simply allows the injured party to sue the employer alone, or both the employer and employee. Although several individuals and an institution may be included in a suit alleging negligence, this inclusion usually does not shift the responsibility for one's own negligent conduct.

Corporate or institutional liability is a relatively new doctrine in malpractice law. This doctrine establishes certain direct duties of the institution that, if breached, allow the injured party to sue the institution directly. This doctrine is in contrast to *respondeat superior,* which holds the institution indirectly liable for the negligent acts of its employees.

Professional Negligence or Malpractice

The nurse must possess a basic understanding of negligence and its impact on professional practice. Although professional negligence or malpractice is included within the general category of negligence, it involves alleged breaches of duty of professionals (nurses, physicians, attorneys, and so on) whose conduct in a particular situation cannot be measured by the behavior of an ordinary, reasonable, and prudent person in the same or similar circumstances.

Because professionals have advanced training, education, and experience, the conduct in question is measured by the degree of skill and knowledge customarily used by a professional in the same or similar circumstances in the same or similar community (Prosser and Keeton, 1984, pp. 185–193). The "community" portion of the standard is a national community, and the professional must be practicing as others in that profession do across the country.

It is also important to note that if the professional claims to be a specialist, the law will hold that individual to the standard of care of the specialist. For example, if a nurse claims to be a clinical specialist in psychiatric/mental health nursing, then the standard by which behavior will be measured will be the degree of skill and knowledge customarily used by the specialist in psychiatric or mental health nursing in the same or similar circumstances in the same or similar community.

Clearly, professional negligence imposes individual legal accountability and responsibility on the nurse. The nurse must keep abreast of established nursing standards across the country. Such standards would include, but would not necessarily be limited to, the standards developed by the ANA and other professional organizations. Attending continuing education programs and updating skills are essential if the nurse is to practice safely and effectively, ensuring the provision of high-quality care to patients.

It is also important for nurses to be familiar with institutional policies and procedures and to participate in their development. For example, if the nurse knows that a particular procedure for administering medication is not safe or not in compliance with the law, that procedure should be reviewed with the supervisor and others in the institution so it can be modified to avoid harm to any patient and possible liability on both the nurse's and the institution's part.

Medication Administration, Storage, and Documentation

Because the administration of medications has great potential for error and subsequent injury to patients, it is especially important to carry out this aspect of practice carefully and to follow safe and accurate medication administration techniques. The nurse must be knowledgeable about the medication given; be certain that the medication is given to the correct patient; and be certain that it is administered properly, in the correct dose, and in a timely fashion. Unclear or uncertain orders, written or verbal, must be challenged. If a nurse knows that an ordered drug is contraindicated for some reason, the nurse must notify the physician of the contraindication. Nurses can also be held responsible if they *should have known* that a drug was contraindicated.

Although drug administration techniques vary depending on the type, route, and dosage of the medication, certain general safeguards should be followed at all times.

The storage of medications must ensure limited access to them. When controlled substances are stored on the unit, they must be kept under a double lock-and-key system, with access to the drugs limited to certain staff members only. Two staff members should bear the responsibility for the narcotics counts at the beginning and end of each shift. When not in use, cabinets or medication cart drawers where controlled substances are kept should be locked.

The medicine room or medication cart must be carefully organized, especially if stock medicines are kept. Consultations with nursing and pharmacy staff, and any state agencies, can help to determine whether guidelines or specific requirements for the orderly arrangement of stock medications exist. For example, it is a good practice to separate medications taken internally from those used externally. If storage procedures do not properly protect patients against mistakes, how medication is stored may be just as important as how it is administered in determining negligence.

Regardless of storage procedures, the nurse must take certain steps to ensure that the medication being administered is correct, and that the "five rights" (right drug, right dose, right route, right patient, right time) are safeguarded. It is very important to prepare and administer medication in an area where distractions are minimal, to be certain that there is a valid order for the medication, and to read the medication label three times (once before removing the drug from the storage area, once before removing the specific dose, and once before returning the drug to its original storage container and area).

In addition to the procedural aspects of giving medications, the nurse should be knowledgeable about the medication to be given. Before administering any medication, the nurse should understand the action, expected results, side effects, possible complications, and proper dose and route of administration. Even with a written order, nurses should *not* administer medications with which they are unfamiliar or about which they have a question until the prescribing physician has been consulted.

The nurse must also be certain to administer the medication properly to avoid any foreseeable harm to the patient. Giving the right medication but by the wrong route may result in significant injury. Nursing judgment must be used when giving medications; an unclear or nonspecific order cannot be used to shift the blame from the nurse to another person when good judgment is not exercised.

A nurse may also be held to be negligent if injury results from a delay in administering medication that is ordered to be given "stat," or immediately. In fact, the nurse may be held responsible for any injury that results from not administering a medication pursuant to a correct order.

TRENDS AND CONTROVERSIES IN PHARMACOLOGY

What If the Patient Refuses Medication?

What do you do when a patient refuses a medication? For many nurses, the annoyance of an interruption in a crammed drug administration schedule overshadows the opportunity of the moment.

A patient's refusal is a signal for the nurse to stop and review the situation. Perhaps the person wasn't told that a new medication was prescribed, and simply needs some information or clarification. This is a good opportunity for patient teaching. Or it may be that the patient is experiencing some discomfort that he or she believes is due to the medication. In this case, the nurse needs to evaluate the symptoms, decide whether they are drug-related, and confer with the prescriber as necessary.

Sometimes a misunderstanding exists, and a brief discussion can elicit a perfectly reasonable basis for the patient's refusal. A regularly scheduled drug may not, in fact, be needed. Occasionally, for example, a physician may respond to the patient's complaint of incidental gastric distress with an order for an antacid qid. If the patient declines a dose, it's not constructive for the nurse to insist that the patient follow the doctor's order. In this case, the problem is not the patient; it's the medication order.

Some patients are adamant in refusing medication because they are convinced that the doctor or nurse has made a mistake. Rather than try to maintain the (impossible) role of infallible authority figure, objectively consider this possibility. There are so many points at which an error can be made. The physician may have written an order in the wrong chart, or may have been interrupted while writing an order, subsequently misstating a dosage. A busy clerk or nurse may have transcribed an order incorrectly. The order may have been filled incorrectly in the pharmacy. The nurse might miss the revision of a previous order, or pour the wrong medication, or simply pick up the wrong cup from the medication cart. It is not uncommon for a patient's refusal to prevent a medication error!

What about the confused patient who refuses medication? People who are not mentally clear need structure and reassurance, so the nurse's approach is vitally important. A hurried, abrupt encounter is not likely to yield good results. The nurse can explain to the patient that "I've brought your usual morning medicine" (or whatever). A choice should be offered, if possible, to give the patient some sense of control. "Would you like to take this with water or juice?" or "Do you want the chewable pill first or the big one?"

All this can be done in a pleasant and positive manner, and should never be intimidating or punishing. The use of force in medication administration is never justified. Remember, too, that a confused patient cannot provide the safeguard of a double-check on medication, as an alert person can, so be certain that the right drugs are administered!

Document a patient's refusal of medicine, including the reasons given, any attempts to clarify the situation for the patient, and any additional nursing actions taken.

The nurse is responsible for documenting drug administration according to the institution's policies. This is especially important when the medication administered is a controlled substance.

The Expanded Role of the Nurse

The expanded role of the nurse and independent practice bring with them changes in the potential legal liabilities of the nurse practicing in today's health-care environment. With more nurses working outside the hospital setting and taking on responsibilities that were formerly the prerogative of physicians only, the charge of practicing medicine without a license is a major legal liability nurses may face. The state's nursing act, if it includes an expanded definition of professional nursing, can have a key role in ensuring that this expanded role is afforded strong legal footing.

Prescribing

With regard to pharmacology and medications, one area in which the nurse will be exposed to an increase in potential liability is in the prescribing of medications. Most of the laws or rules passed by the 34 states noted in a 1990 article relating to nurse practitioners (Pearson, 1990) indicated that the states have some authority, albeit under varying requirements, to allow nurse practitioners to prescribe medications. Other advanced nurse practitioners, such as nurse midwives and nurse anesthetists, have been given prescriptive ability as well. And, with recent Medicare and Medicaid changes allowing advanced nurse practitioners to prescribe medications, where consistent with state law, the continued growth of prescriptive authority for nurses will likely continue. Concerned about uniformity in state nursing acts and prescriptive authority, the ANA has suggested a model act (ANA, 1990).

Legal concerns that accompany the responsibility of prescribing medications include obtaining informed consent prior to the prescription of a particular medication (now the legal responsibility of the physician), and, of course, liability for negligent prescription. If the nurse prescribes, these potential liabilities will rest solely with the nurse. Potential liability in this area can be minimized by being properly educated and by following standing orders and protocols developed in conjunction with a physician supervisor/collaborator. The development of protocols can also help the nurse avoid a charge of practicing medicine without a license.

Medication Administration in the Home

Another area of potential liability for the nurse is administration of medications and drugs in the home. Although this procedure has a long history, it has become noticeably more complex with recent technologic advances. The nurse administering medications in the home must be diligent about staying up-to-date by attending continuing education programs, obtaining graduate or postgraduate training, or both. To avoid allegations of negligence, all principles of medication administration used in the acute-care setting should also be used in the home setting.

The nurse must be certain that the care being undertaken is within the scope of the state's nurse practice act. If there is no legal foundation for prescribing medications or treatments, standing orders or written protocols are needed. Adequate documentation concerning decisions made by the nurse is essential, as is documentation of any referrals or follow-up. In addition, nurses administering controlled substances in the home must adhere to applicable storage, documentation, and disposal requirements to avoid allegations of diversion of the controlled substances, and to account accurately for controlled substances administered in the home (Brent, 1989).

Administration Based on Orders by Other Professionals

Another area of concern is the administration of medications ordered by a licensed individual not specifically listed in the state's nurse practice act. Historically, only licensed physicians or dentists were authorized by state law to prescribe. Many states now allow osteopaths, podiatrists, physicians' assistants, and other health-care professionals to prescribe. If the nurse is unclear about whether to carry out such orders, it is wise to seek an opinion from the state board of nursing, the state attorney general, or the regulatory agency responsible for enforcing the nurse practice act. Amendments of nursing acts to provide broader definitions of who can order medications and treatments may be one way to solve this difficulty (ANA, 1990).

Although it is easy to see that drug therapy is fraught with potential legal liability for the nurse, knowledge of the laws and regulations that affect this aspect of nursing practice will allow the nurse to practice in a safe and legal manner.

Annotated Bibliography

American Nurses' Association. *Suggested state legislation: Nursing practice act, nursing disciplinary diversion act, prescriptive authority act.* Kansas City, Missouri: ANA, 1990. *This is an excellent reference booklet.*

Brent N. Administering controlled substances in the home: Minimizing the risk of potential diversion. *Home Healthcare Nurse* 1989;7: 6–7.

DeMarco C: *Pharmacy and the law,* 2nd ed. Rockville, MD: Aspen Systems, 1984. *This is an excellent reference text.*

Goldstein A, Perdew S, Pruitt S. *The nurse's legal advisor: Your guide to legally safe practice.* Philadelphia: J.B. Lippincott, 1989. *A handy quick reference to general information on the law.*

Gruber M, Gruber JM. Nursing malpractice: The importance of documentation, or saved by the pen! *Gastroenterol Nurs* 1990;12: 255–259. *The authors identify why accurate, complete documentation is necessary, discuss the elements of documentation, and give methods about how to do it. The article describes several examples of nursing malpractice involving improper documentation.*

Haack M, Hughes T, eds. *Addiction in the nursing profession.* New York: Springer, 1989. *A comprehensive compilation of issues concerning addiction in the nursing profession.*

Pearson LJ. How each state stands on legislative issues affecting advanced nursing practice. *Nurse Pract* 1990;15:11–18.

Prosser WL, Keeton WP. *Prosser and Keeton on the law of torts.* 5th ed. Keeton WP, ed. St. Paul, MN: West Publishing, 1984 (with a 1988 supplement).

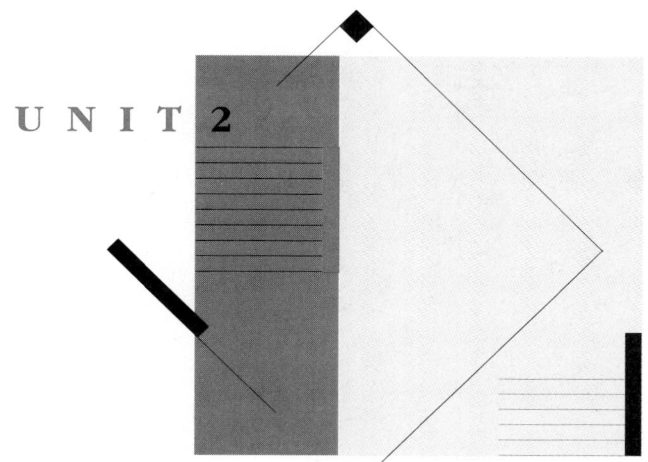

Principles That Predict or Alter Drug Action

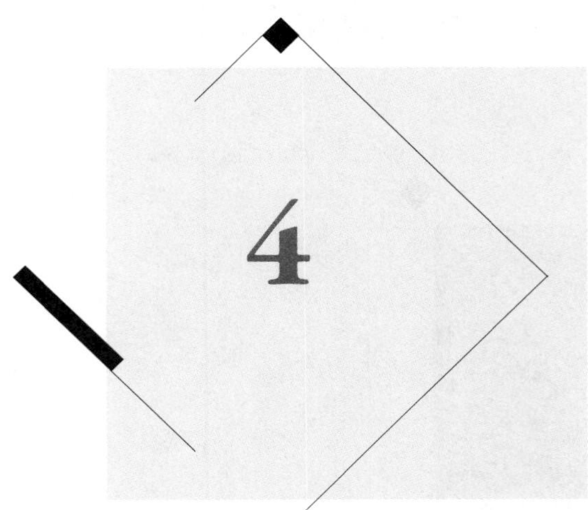

Absorption, Distribution, Metabolism, and Excretion

It should be obvious from personal experience that drugs are administered in different ways, that some drugs may need to be taken more often than others, and that people respond differently to particular doses of a given drug. To understand these differences, it is first necessary to understand the general principles that govern drugs' actions. In simple terms, drugs produce effects of various intensities. The intensity is related to the amount of drug molecules reaching their sites of action, which, in turn, is related to the **dose** of the drug. There are four basic processes that determine both the intensity and duration of a drug's actions: **absorption, distribution, metabolism,** and **excretion.**

Once a drug is administered at some place on or within the body it is usually *absorbed* into the bloodstream. This process is responsible for increasing the amount of drug in the circulatory system. Once absorbed, drug molecules are *distributed* throughout the body, which enables them to reach various sites of action that are often distant from where they were administered. Both processes contribute to the appearance of pharmacologic effects. Distribution also delivers drug molecules to sites at which they may be chemically changed, or *metabolized,* into other active or inactive compounds. Metabolism usually occurs in the liver. The metabolites, or the original unmetabolized drug, can also be *excreted* from the body, usually by the kidneys. Metabolism and excretion generally are responsible for the decrease or disappearance of a drug's actions. These four processes may occur simultaneously (Fig. 4–1).

The ever-changing balance between processes that increase blood levels of active drug and opposing processes that reduce active drug levels determines how soon the drug's actions will appear, how intense and widespread they will be, and how long they will last. The branch of pharmacology that is concerned with these four processes is called **pharmacokinetics,** and it is the topic of this chapter.

Cell Membranes

Before discussing pharmacokinetics, it is important to review the general characteristics of cell membranes, which are the primary structures that affect a drug's ability to be absorbed, distributed, excreted, and, to some extent, metabolized. Cell membranes are the structures through which drugs must pass to reach their sites of action, and in many cases they are also the targets of drug action. Most drugs must not only enter the blood-

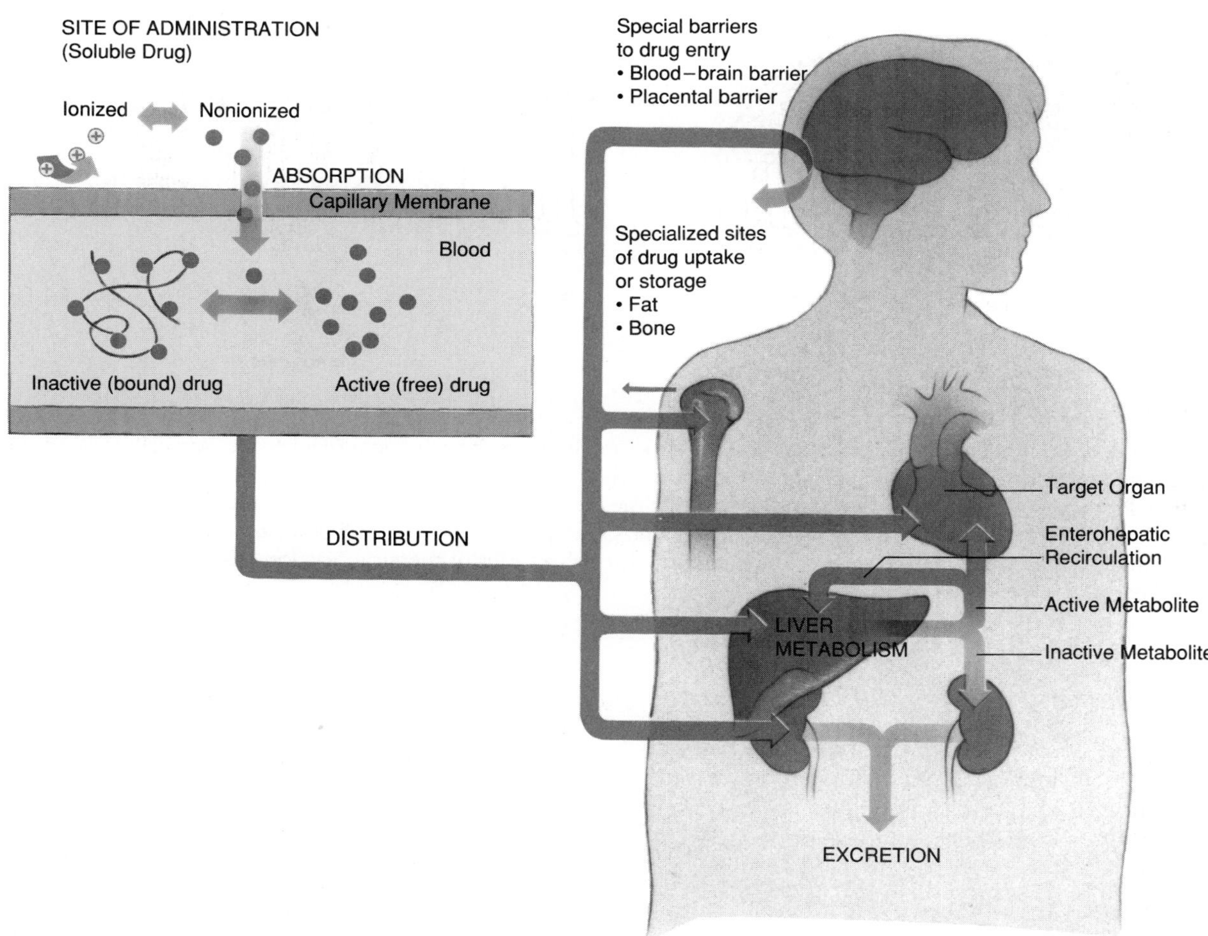

Figure 4–1

An overview of the fate of drugs in the body. All these processes can occur simultaneously.

stream, but must also leave it to reach sites of action and organs of metabolism or excretion. These processes involve drug movement through many cell membranes.

Membranes are dynamic structures composed of proteins, lipids, and carbohydrates. Besides simply surrounding every cell in the body, membranes have special properties that help regulate the composition of the intracellular environment, which must be kept separate and different from that of the extracellular fluid that bathes each cell. Membranes also have specialized structures that recognize drug molecules and initiate the cell's response to the drug.

Figure 4–2 shows a generalized concept of membrane structure. Much of the membrane is composed of a double layer (bilayer) of closely associated lipids and proteins, known as *lipoproteins*. Embedded within this lipoprotein envelope are large proteins, some of which may extend completely through the membrane from its outer surface to the intracellular surface. Other proteins appear to float on the membrane's surface. Most of these proteins are *functional proteins;* for example, enzymes specialized to transport certain kinds of molecules into the cell. Others are the **receptor** sites for drugs. There are specialized parts of the cell to which a drug molecule binds, eventually triggering chemical events that lead to the effects associated with a particular drug. Drug receptor sites and how they function in a drug's mechanism of action are discussed in Chapter 6. Some membrane proteins are organized into specialized "channels" through which certain molecules or ions can pass. Certain drugs, through interactions with membrane-bound receptors, are able to open or close the channels, thus controlling the flow of ions and molecules into the cell.

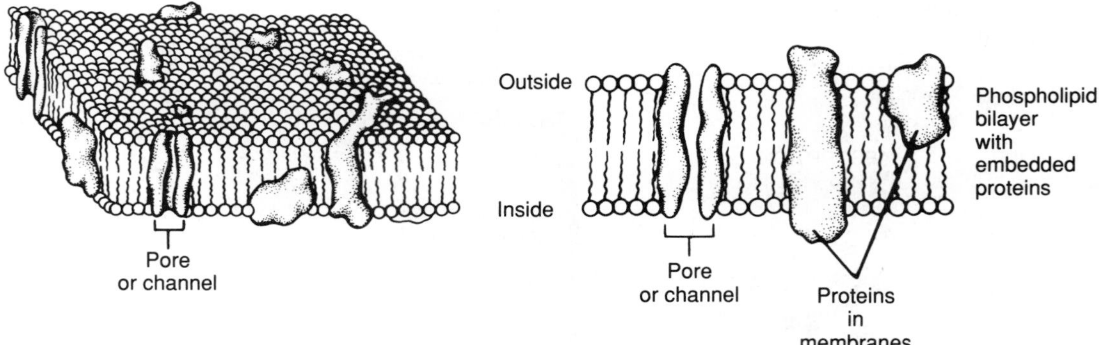

Figure 4–2

Schematic view of a cell membrane. Membranes provide structural integrity for cells; help regulate the intracellular environment by regulating movement of water and metabolites; serve as barriers to or passageways for drug diffusion; and can be sites of drug action. Proteins with open cores that span both sides of the membrane can be pores, which control movement of substances such as water, or channels that regulate ion movement. Other proteins serve as receptor sites for drugs, can communicate a chemical message from the cell surface to the interior, through a series of chemical reactions, to change cell function (cause and effect).

Drug Movement Across Cell Membranes

There are several ways by which drugs can cross cell membranes. They include passive diffusion, active transport, filtration, and pinocytosis. Figure 4–3 shows a general representation of each of these processes.

Passive Diffusion

The major process by which drugs cross membranes and are absorbed into the bloodstream is passive diffusion. Diffusion also regulates the movement of drugs out of the bloodstream into target cells, and the entry of drugs to sites of metabolism and excretion. *Passive diffusion* means that drug movement is not dependent on cellular energy. A drug must have certain chemical properties to diffuse through membranes easily: relatively small size, adequate solubility in both water and lipids, and lack of electric charge. Each of these properties is described in more detail below. Drugs that diffuse across membranes move down a concentration gradient, from the side of the membrane that has the highest drug concentration to the side with the lowest concentration. Diffusion cannot occur in the opposite direction. Once the concentration of drug on both sides of the membrane is equal, passive diffusion stops.

Drugs can also pass from one side of a cell to another by passing *between* adjacent cells, not just by crossing *through* them. This occurs mainly at the endothelial cells that line the blood vessels and make up the capillaries. Unusually "tight" cell-to-cell junctions in capillaries that make up the blood–brain barrier probably explain why this structure limits entry of drugs into the brain so well (see p. 58).

Active Transport

Some of the large proteins that are embedded in the cell membrane are specialized transport proteins that can actively "pump" a molecule from one side of the membrane to the other. *Active transport* moves molecules against concentration gradients by a process that requires a driving force, cell metabolic energy, usually in the form of adenosine triphosphate (ATP). Good examples of transport proteins are the ion pumps that are essential for the function of electrically excitable cells, such as nerve and muscle. Active transport is not very important for the absorption or distribution of most drugs, but it has a key role in drug excretion from the kidneys.

Filtration

Filtration is a process by which a drug or other molecule passes through membrane pores from one side of a membrane to the other down a concentration gradient, but driven by a pressure gradient. The pressure can be either *osmotic* or *hydrostatic*. The pores can be thought of as sieves for some substances that are small enough to pass through; molecules that are too large

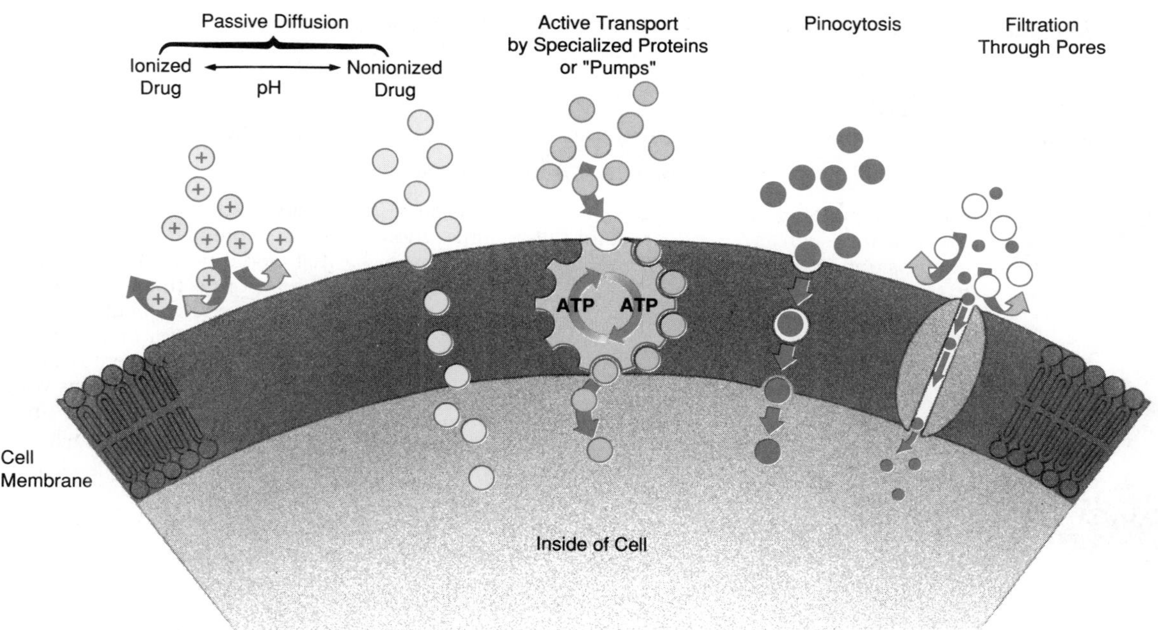

Figure 4–3

Ways for drugs to cross cell membranes. Most drugs cross cell membranes by passive diffusion. Only nonionized (uncharged), lipid-soluble drug molecules can diffuse well. Other processes are important to specific drugs, or may be important in specific organs (for example, the active transport and filtration of drugs in the kidney).

will not be filtered. Like active transport, filtration has a minor role in drug absorption, but it is an essential component in the excretion of many drugs and metabolic wastes.

Other Processes

Several minor processes regulate the ability of drugs to cross membranes. One is *facilitated diffusion,* in which a substance, for example, glucose, binds to a membrane-bound carrier protein and crosses the membrane from the side with the highest concentration to the side with the lowest concentration. Another process is *pinocytosis,* in which the cell membrane surrounds and engulfs a substance on the outer surface of the membrane and carries it inside the cell. Pinocytosis is a major process by which leukocytes and other cells in the immune system destroy bacteria, but it is not an important way of moving drugs across membranes. *Exocytosis* can be thought of as the reverse of pinocytosis. It is a mechanism by which substances synthesized in cells and stored inside membrane-bound vesicles are eventually released into the extracellular environment.

Pharmacokinetics

Absorption

Drug absorption is the process by which a drug moves across one or more cell membranes from its site of administration into the bloodstream. The basic processes that control the ability of a drug to cross biologic membranes, and the chemical properties of each drug, determine whether the drug can be absorbed after it is given orally or whether it must be given by other routes of administration. Drugs that are taken orally or are injected into tissues other than blood, and even many drugs that are applied topically or into body orifices, have to be absorbed into the bloodstream before they can reach distant sites of action. Since absorption implies entry into the bloodstream, the processes that influence it are irrelevant to drugs that are injected directly into the circulatory system, either intravenously or intraarterially. The unique characteristics of drug absorption from all these sites affect the suitability of using a particular route of administration to give a drug to a patient (Table 4–1).

Table 4–1 Comparison of Drug Administration Routes as They Relate to Absorption

Route of Administration	Absorption Characteristics	Advantages	Disadvantages
		Major or Most Common Routes	
Oral	Variable, depending on many factors such as composition of drug, gut pH and motility, simultaneous use of other drugs that interact to alter absorption (see text), timing of dose with respect to meals	Convenient; economical; best for self-administration	Self-administration requires good patient compliance or assurance that medication was taken; unsuitable for drugs that are insoluble, poorly or erratically absorbed; usually unsuitable for infants; may be unsuitable for children, adults with dysphagia, other problems with swallowing; unsuitable for unconscious patients, patients with frequent vomiting
Parenteral			
Intramuscular	Rapid if aqueous solutions are used; slow and prolonged if oily or other depot preparation or suspension is used; absorption speed depends on local blood flow	Requires administration by nursing or other medical personnel or training of patient for self-administration; suitable for small to moderate drug volumes	May be painful; may cause muscle damage that can increase bleeding risk during anticoagulant therapy, or can interfere with some diagnostic tests that measure organ or tissue damage; risk of infection, incompatibility with diluents, other drugs
Intravenous	Absorption is immediate	Ideal for emergency use since desired effects usually appear quickly; useful for large volumes of drug, or irritating drugs if suitably diluted	Adverse effects, whether due to overdose or otherwise, appear rapidly; effects may be of short duration, requiring frequent administration; insoluble substances (eg, suspensions) cannot be given; risk of infection, pain, vasculitis, extravasation; not suitable for self-administration
Subcutaneous	See Intramuscular	See Intramuscular	May cause pain, irritation, tissue necrosis, especially if irritating drugs are used; risk of infection; limited to small volumes of drug; risk of incompatibility with other drugs, solutions, as noted for intramuscular injection
		Other Routes	
Inhalation	Rapid absorption unless drug is specifically formulated for local effects in respiratory tract (eg, steroids used for asthma)	Common route for bronchodilators to affect the desired site of action directly; or for some general anesthetics to enable giving a gaseous or volatile liquid drug that cannot be given in another form	Drugs packaged for self-administration (eg, bronchodilator aerosols) must be administered properly for optimal effect, which requires manual dexterity, coordination on part of patient; careful patient teaching is essential; some inhaled drugs may cause coughing, wheezing, etc; inhalational drugs to be given by professional personnel may require advanced training, special equipment for proper administration

Table 4–1 Comparison of Drug Administration Routes as They Relate to Absorption (*Continued*)

Route of Administration	Absorption Characteristics	Advantages	Disadvantages
Percutaneous or transdermal	Incomplete, erratic unless drug specifically formulated for this route	Drugs specifically formulated for percutaneous/transdermal administration offer convenience for and acceptance by many patients, and availability of a product with standardized amount of drug	Of limited value unless drug is specifically formulated and/or packaged for percutaneous administration
Rectal	Absorption may be erratic	Useful for small children or unconscious patients who cannot take or need not receive drugs by other routes; may be used for either locally or systemically acting drugs	Conscious patients may find rectal administration uncomfortable; some drugs administered rectally require effort to retain suppository until it dissolves; drugs given for local effects may be absorbed sufficiently to cause systemic effects
Sublingual, buccal	Absorption is usually rapid, complete (depending on product's formulation)	Preferred route for some drugs that are inactivated by first-pass metabolism when given orally and are impractical to administer by other routes (eg, nitroglycerin)	Efficacy, speed, duration of effects depend on retaining tablet at administration site; eating, drinking may interfere with absorption
Topical (on skin)	Generally incomplete, erratic	Often useful for drugs used to treat dermatologic problems	Prolonged topical administration of some drugs may cause rashes or allergic reactions; chronic or excessive use on skin, or drug use on damaged skin, may cause adverse systemic effects; precise dose may be difficult to achieve consistently

Absorption from the Gastrointestinal Tract

Drug Solubility

The factors that control the rate and amount of drug that is absorbed from its site of administration depend partly on the chemical nature of the drug itself. To be absorbed, drugs must be both water soluble and, to some extent, lipid soluble.

Solubility in Water If a drug is taken orally as a tablet, capsule, or some similar preparation of solid or undissolved drug, it must dissolve in the aqueous contents of the digestive tract before it can be absorbed. There are many pharmaceutic factors that determine where in the gastrointestinal (GI) tract the drug will dissolve, and how completely and how fast it will dissolve; for example, the use of **enteric-coated** tablets, the composition of binders used to compress tablets, and the composition of materials used to formulate "**timed-release**" (**sustained-release**) medications. In general, however, the faster and more completely a drug dissolves at the site where it will be absorbed, the more rapidly it will be absorbed and the faster its effects will appear. For this reason, drugs that are already dissolved in a liquid (solutions) are usually absorbed more rapidly than the same drug swallowed in a form that must first dissolve.

The need for a drug to dissolve before being absorbed also applies to drug **suspensions,** which are preparations of solid drug particles suspended in some liquid. All other factors being equal, drugs in suspensions dissolve (go into solution) faster than larger solid forms of drugs (e.g., whole tablets), but slower than drugs administered as true solutions.

Solubility in Lipids Although solubility of a drug in water is important for dissolution of a solid form of a drug administered orally, solubility in lipid (fat) is essential for any drug to diffuse across lipid-rich biologic membranes, regardless of the route of administration. Lipid solubility affects all four of the major pharmacokinetic processes that govern the movement and fate of drugs. A drug's lipid solubility depends in part on the drug's chemical structure, and is greatly influenced by the local environment around the drug at its site of absorption.

Drug Ionization and the Effects of pH A drug in solution, regardless of the body fluid in which it is dissolved, can be present as ionized (sometimes referred to as *electrically charged* or *polar*) molecules or nonionized (*neutral* or *nonpolar*) molecules.

Ionized molecules do not diffuse easily across lipid membranes and so they are absorbed poorly, if at all. In contrast, nonionized drug molecules are quite soluble in lipids and can diffuse through lipid membranes and be easily absorbed.

It is rare that all molecules of a drug are in either the ionized or the nonionized form. Instead, some of the molecules are in the ionized form, the remainder are nonionized, and an equilibrium between the two forms exists (Fig. 4–4). Depending on the composition of the local environment, ionized drug molecules can be converted rapidly to the nonionized form, and vice versa.

The major property of the local environment that determines the amount of drug molecules that will be in the ionized or nonionized forms, and therefore whether the drug will be absorbed poorly or easily, is the *pH* (relative acidity or alkalinity) of the environment.

Aspirin, for example, has chemical properties that make it a "weak acid," meaning that if it is dissolved in a neutral liquid the solution becomes weakly acidic. When aspirin is dissolved in the acidic environment of the stomach, only a small fraction of the total number of aspirin molecules are ionized. The remaining molecules—the majority—are in the nonionized form. Since they do not carry an electric charge, they can diffuse easily across the membranes that line the gastric mucosa and enter the bloodstream readily. In contrast, the duodenum contains a variety of enzymes and other secretions that make its contents quite alkaline (high pH). In this environment, the equilibrium shifts so that most of the aspirin molecules become ionized, reducing absorption.

The effects of pH on drug absorption can be shown by administering a large dose of an alkaline drug, such as an antacid, before administering aspirin. The increased pH of the stomach contents shifts the equilibrium, converting many of the nonionized molecules to the ionized and less readily absorbed form. This reduces aspirin absorption from the stomach, and could reduce the drug's effects.

Not all drugs are weak acids like aspirin. Others, such as the amphetamines, are "weak bases." The effects of pH on the equilibrium between ionized and nonionized forms of weak bases are the opposite of those noted for weak acids. In the acidic gastric contents, most amphetamine molecules are ionized, so drug absorption from the stomach is low. Once amphetamine molecules pass into the alkaline duodenum, however, the equilibrium shifts to convert many of the ionized molecules into the nonionized form, and absorption increases. Thus, most molecules of a weak base will be nonionized in alkaline pH, and most molecules of a weak acid will be nonionized in acid pH.

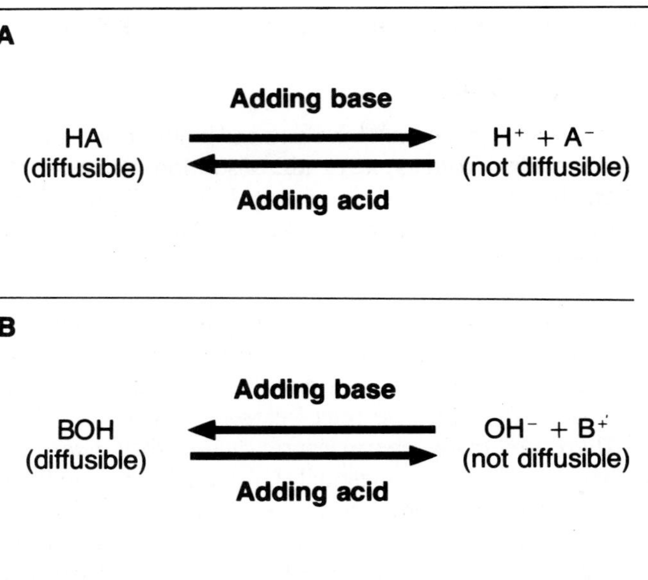

Figure 4–4

Effect of pH on the ionization of drug molecules. **A.** Drug A is a weak acid. In an acidic environment most molecules of a weak acid are nonionized (HA), and so diffuse easily across membranes. If the pH is raised by adding base, the molecule dissociates to the poorly diffusible anion (A^-), and protons (H^+). Add acid, and more nonionized (diffusible) molecules form. **B.** Drug B is a weak base. Changes of pH on ionization of a weak base are the opposite of those for weak acids: Raise the pH by adding base and more drug molecules will be in the more diffusible, nonionized form (BOH); lower pH (add acid) and more nondiffusible ionized molecules (B^+) are formed.

NURSING IMPLICATIONS

It is not important to memorize which drugs are weak acids and which are weak bases. However, it is important to understand the concept that drugs can exist in both ionized and nonionized forms, that the relative proportion of each is affected by local pH, and that this can have significant effects on the diffusion or absorption of drugs across cell membranes. The local environment can be the GI tract for drugs that are given orally, or the extracellular fluid in the tissues into which a drug might be injected. This concept is also important in understanding how one drug can markedly influence the absorption or excretion of other drugs.

Stability of Drugs in Acid

Some drugs cannot be taken orally because they are inactivated (metabolized) by acid and enzymes in the stomach. This is particularly true of drugs that are proteins, a category that includes most hormones. Other drugs are only partly inactivated in the stomach. Still others precipitate in the stomach and so cannot be absorbed. If a drug is unstable in gastric acid it must be given by another route, or some way to protect it from the damaging effects of stomach acid must be devised. One way to protect an orally administered drug is to surround a drug tablet with a special **enteric coating.** These coatings do not dissolve in acid, but dissolve well in the alkaline environment of the duodenum, exposing the drug inside so it can dissolve and be absorbed from that site. Enteric coatings are also placed around some drugs that are irritating to the stomach lining, to protect the gastric mucosa.

Local Blood Flow

The blood flow in the vicinity of the drug administration or absorption site affects the rate of drug absorption. Blood flow carries drug molecules away from the site of absorption, thereby increasing the concentration difference (and therefore the diffusion rate) across the membrane. The lining of the GI tract has a relatively high blood flow, which favors absorption. Disease states, trauma, or drugs that reduce blood flow can reduce drug absorption.

Other Factors Affecting Drug Absorption from the Gastrointestinal Tract

The *motility* of the GI tract can greatly influence absorption of orally administered drugs. For example, increases of gut motility associated with diarrhea or vomiting decrease the amount of time available for drug absorption. Therefore, methods of drug administration that avoid the GI tract may need to be used in patients with excessive vomiting or diarrhea, to achieve and maintain effective blood levels of a drug. In contrast, decreased gut motility, as with constipation, can allow extra time for a drug to be absorbed, perhaps in toxic amounts.

Some drugs that irritate the stomach when taken orally are intentionally given with *food,* which can act as a natural protectant against discomfort. However, food can also inhibit the absorption of some drugs, so that effective blood levels may not be reached. For example, virtually all dairy products contain large amounts of calcium, which binds with tetracycline antibiotics, preventing the antibiotic from reaching the bloodstream.

Absorption from Other Parts of the Gastrointestinal Tract

The small intestine is also an important site of drug absorption. Its considerable length provides a large surface area across which drugs can be absorbed. The plentiful intestinal villi and microvilli that are closely associated with blood capillaries and lymphatic channels increase the absorptive surface area even more. The surface area is so great that large amounts of aspirin molecules, for example, can be absorbed from the small bowel, even though many of the molecules are in the poorly diffusible, ionized form.

Drugs can also be absorbed through the mucosa of the large intestine and rectum. Drug administration per rectum is sometimes used for patients who are vomiting, who experience severe GI upset from oral medications, or who are unconscious and cannot swallow drugs.

As noted later, some drugs that have already been absorbed (whether from the gut or other administration sites) can be excreted into the small bowel, then reabsorbed back into the circulation. This process, called *enterohepatic recirculation,* is discussed on page 64.

Absorption After Subcutaneous or Intramuscular Injection

Many parenteral injections are given by subcutaneous (SC) or intramuscular (IM) routes, since these tissue sites contain large capillary networks across which drug molecules can diffuse and be absorbed quite readily.

The major factors that determine the rate and extent of drug absorption after SC or IM injection are basically the same as those that regulate absorption from the GI tract: local pH, physical and chemical properties of the drug, local blood flow, and so on.

SPOTLIGHT ON NURSING RESEARCH

The bioavailability of many cardiovascular medications is affected by food–drug interactions. Administering medication with food can increase or decrease bioavailability, depending on the medication and the individual. By affecting bioavailability—sometimes by as much as 50%—food–drug interactions may have a significant impact on the therapeutic responses.

These investigators examined the relationship between drug administration and mealtimes. The medications were cardiovascular drugs with published recommendations for timing in relation to meals. Using a retrospective chart review of records from 183 medical patients, adherence to timing recommendations was evaluated for five different drugs: hydralazine, phenytoin, propranolol, captopril, and quinidine sulfate. It has been recommended that hydralazine, phenytoin, and propranolol be given in the fed state; captopril in the unfed state; and that quinidine sulfate be administered in consistent relationship to meals.

Records from four health care agencies—two short-term care and two long-term care—were reviewed for medication dosages administered over a 24 hour period. Medication dosages from at least 30 patients were evaluated for each of the study drugs. During data collection, food–drug relationships were assumed to be casual, if a relationship to meals was not specified on medication sheets. Drugs given in the fed state were administered less than 30 minutes before and not more than 90 minutes after scheduled meal tray delivery times. At all other times, drug administration was considered to be in the unfed state.

For medications specifically recommended to be given in the fed state, 50% of dosages were administered correctly. Similarly, 53% of captopril dosages—which should be administered in the unfed state—were given at the recommended time. Among 30 patients receiving quinidine, only two received the drug in a consistent relationship with meals—both in the unfed state. The authors point out that most patients received their medication at inconsistent times. Only 15% received all medication dosages in the recommended relationship to meals. Indeed, 15% of patients received all dosages at times that would result in the *lowest* drug bioavailability.

The findings suggest that recommendations for medication administration in relation to meals do not affect dosage schedules in the institutions studied. Schedules were consistent within agencies. In one agency most medications were given in the fed state, whereas in the other three facilities most dosages were given in the unfed state. Interestingly, physician orders for medication frequency appeared to determine administration times, based on standard hospital policy, but *only one out of 183 physician orders* specified a relationship to meals.

Retrospective chart reviews can offer a variety of insights into clinical practices. The authors of this study conclude that published recommendations for the administration of medications in relation to food are disregarded by health care professionals in institutional settings—at least for selected cardiovascular drugs. Additional work is needed to determine why these recommendations are not followed and to evaluate their impact on patient outcomes and health care costs. In the meantime, the authors suggest that nurses obtain information about timing of administration when taking medication histories and make efforts to promote a consistent pattern of drug dosing in relation to food intake.

Strong A, Wolff H, Kinder S, Lubischer A: Drug administration in relation to meals in the institutional setting. *Heart Lung* 1991;20:39–44.

The absorption of drugs from injection sites can be modified in several ways. For example, reducing local blood flow at the injection site can slow systemic absorption. For this reason, many local anesthetic drugs that are used to reduce pain, as when suturing a wound, are mixed with a vasoconstrictor drug. The vasoconstrictor reduces blood flow to the injection site, preventing the local anesthetic from being washed away by the bloodstream, thus keeping the anesthetic at its desired site of action longer. This not only prolongs and intensifies the pain-relieving actions of the anesthetic, but also reduces its circulation throughout the body, thereby minimizing the chance of causing adverse effects elsewhere.

Drug absorption from SC or IM injection sites is generally rapid compared with absorption after oral administration, especially if the drug is in an aqueous solution. More gradual absorption after SC or IM injection can be achieved by changing the formulation of the drug. For example, some parenteral medications are manufactured as fine suspensions of solid drug particles in an aqueous or oily solution. This formulation slows absorption so that effects appear more gradually and last longer than if the same drug were given as a solution. Some drugs are formulated in special tablets that are surgically implanted in the subcutaneous tissues, where the drug dissolves slowly and provides longlasting effects.

Absorption from Other Sites

Any mucosal surface on or in the body offers a potentially effective pathway for the absorption of some drugs. Such sites include the *mucous membranes* lining the respiratory tract, the mouth, and the conjunctiva of the eye. The routes of administration at each of these sites are given unique names (for example, *inhalation* or *insufflation* into the respiratory tract; *sublingual* or *buccal* in the oral cavity; *instillation* into the conjunctival sac), but each one is a variation of **topical** drug administration. These routes can be used to produce either local or systemic effects, depending on the drug, how it is formulated, and how well it can be absorbed. For example, general anesthetics produce loss of consciousness solely through actions in the brain, but they are routinely administered via the lungs (inhalation). That these agents can anesthetize a patient completely within minutes attests to the ability of the respiratory tract to absorb some drugs readily. Nitroglycerin, the primary drug used to treat angina pectoris, is usually administered sublingually. Rapid absorption from this site, however, causes prompt effects on the heart and blood vessels. Although drugs applied to the conjunctiva of the eye are often given specifically for their local effects, these mucous membranes also serve as effective pathways for drug absorption into the bloodstream. It is important to remember the possibility of systemic absorption when using these routes of administration, because of the possibility of causing unwanted effects elsewhere.

Most drugs used therapeutically are not absorbed well, completely, or predictably when applied to intact skin because the skin's thick outer layer serves as a natural barrier to drug diffusion. This route of absorption through the skin, called *percutaneous,* can be increased if the skin is altered by a laceration, burn, or some other insult. However, if high concentrations or large amounts of drugs are applied to the skin, especially if it is done repeatedly, sufficient amounts of drug can enter the bloodstream to cause systemic effects, usually undesirable ones.

Traditionally, topical application of drugs to the skin was limited to medications intended to produce a local effect at the administration site. However, several drugs, including nitroglycerin and scopolamine, have been "packaged" in special **transdermal** delivery systems that gradually release a predictable amount of active substance into the bloodstream for as long as a week.

Percutaneous absorption of petroleum products, oils, and organic solvents, as well as drugs dissolved in them (such as insecticides), is often rapid and complete. It is an important cause of industrial and environmental poisoning.

Distribution

Once a drug is absorbed into the bloodstream it will be distributed throughout the body and can produce a variety of effects. Unless a drug is given for its effects on the blood's components, drug molecules in the bloodstream must leave that fluid, cross capillary membranes, and eventually reach their sites of action. This movement out of the blood is generally a much quicker and easier task than absorption, and usually involves only simple diffusion of drug molecules across capillary membranes.

Once the drug enters the extracellular space it can then easily diffuse to cell membranes in the various organs. Theoretically, since blood is delivered to all regions of the body, a drug can produce effects anywhere, not only at its intended sites of action.

Several important factors influence what sites a drug will actually reach, how long will be required for effects to occur, how long they will last, and how intense they will be. Many of these factors are the same ones that regulate drug absorption into the bloodstream.

Local Blood Flow

Blood flow to an organ affects how much of a drug reaches that organ and how fast drug effects will occur. If blood flow to a particular region is very low, as might result from tissue or organ **ischemia,** the ability of drug molecules to reach the affected sites will be hindered and the drug's effects will be limited.

Plasma Protein Binding

Not all drug molecules circulating in the bloodstream are free to interact with the cells of the body. Blood plasma contains a variety of proteins, the most impor-

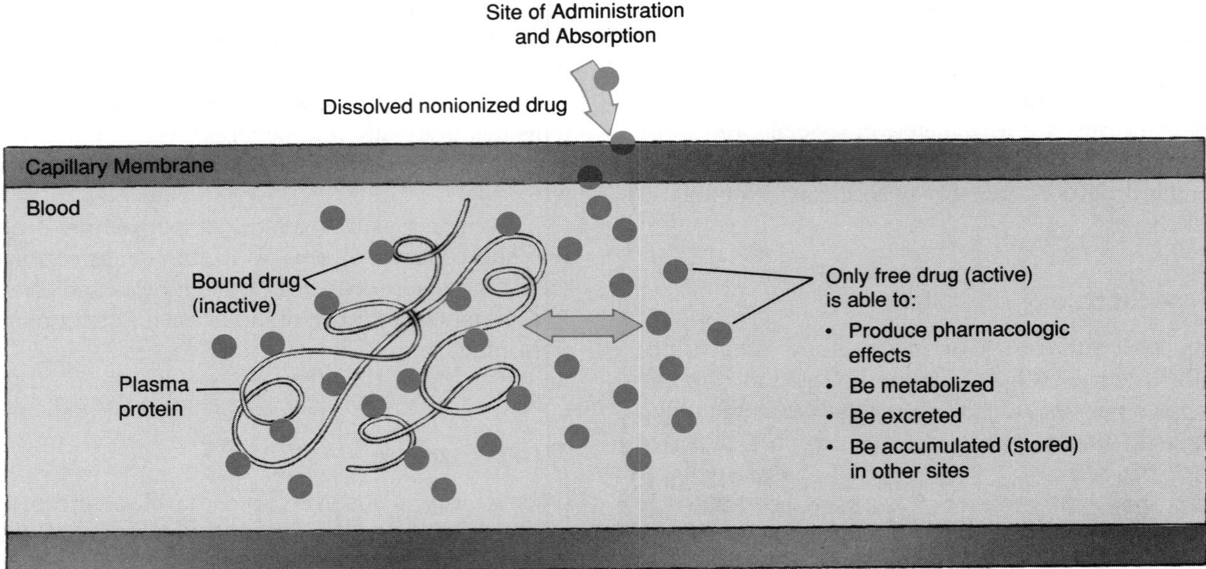

Figure 4–5

Drug distribution and the concept of bound versus free drug in the bloodstream. Once absorbed, some of the drug molecules may become reversibly bound to proteins in the blood, especially to albumin. The percentage of total drug molecules that are bound or free depends on the drug itself and on the availability of protein binding sites. Some drugs produce a response even though the percentage of free drug molecules is very low. Others are almost completely free in the bloodstream, with little or none bound.

cules can bind (Fig. 4–5). Plasma proteins therefore serve as reservoirs for drugs. To some extent they provide a means to prolong the actions of a drug in the body.

For a given total amount of drug in the blood, a certain percentage of its molecules will bind to plasma proteins, and the remainder will be free. However, *only those drug molecules that are not bound to plasma proteins are able to produce pharmacologic effects.* Likewise, *only unbound (free) drug molecules can be metabolized or excreted.* Drug molecules that are bound to plasma proteins or other storage sites are pharmacologically inactive, and remain that way until freed.

The percentage of drug molecules in the bloodstream that will be bound to plasma proteins depends largely on the chemical structure of the drug. The chemical structure affects not only how much drug will bind to storage sites, but also how strong the interaction between drug molecules and their plasma protein binding sites will be.

Depending on the drug, the fraction of total molecules that is bound (or unbound) can range from nearly zero to nearly 100%. For example, when a therapeutic dose of the nonprescription pain-reliever acetaminophen is given, virtually all the acetaminophen molecules in the bloodstream are unbound (free) and therefore pharmacologically active. In contrast, a drug such as the antidiabetic agent tolbutamide is extensively bound to plasma protein. Of the total number of tolbutamide molecules in the blood, about 98% are bound to plasma protein and are, therefore, inactive. The effects produced by tolbutamide at any given time are due solely to the remaining 2% of free molecules.

The binding of drug molecules to plasma protein is generally *nonspecific, competitive,* and *reversible.* Nonspecific binding simply means that the proteins will bind many different kinds of drugs. Competitive binding means that molecules of different drugs, each of which can bind to plasma protein, will compete with one another for the binding sites. If one drug is only slightly or weakly bound to protein it will not offer much competition to molecules of a drug that can bind more strongly. However, if the two are roughly equivalent in terms of their binding ability, the one that interacts the strongest with protein, or the one that is present in the higher concentration (somewhat related to the dose that is given), will be most extensively bound.

Reversible binding simply means that the interaction between a drug molecule and an attachment site, such as plasma protein, is not permanent. As some drug molecules in the body leave the circulatory system through metabolism or excretion, either of which reduces free drug concentration in the blood, previously bound drug molecules will be released from their binding sites. This release from binding sites helps maintain a relatively constant fraction or percentage of free drug molecules as the total number of molecules (bound plus unbound) changes.

The properties of nonspecific, competitive, and reversible binding can account for clinically important interactions between drugs. If a patient receives a drug that binds to plasma proteins, and then receives a second drug that also binds to plasma proteins, the second drug can compete with the first for the limited number of protein binding sites. In doing so the second drug *displaces* the first drug from its binding sites, causing a sudden increase in its free concentration in the blood. Since free drug molecules are pharmacologically active, the result may be a sudden and potentially dangerous increase of its actions (Fig. 4–6).

An example of this phenomenon involves the clinically important interaction between aspirin and the anticoagulant drug warfarin. When warfarin is present in the bloodstream, 99% of its molecules are bound to plasma proteins. Its therapeutic effect, inhibiting synthesis of factors needed to cause blood clotting, is therefore due to only the 1% of free warfarin molecules. If the concentration of free warfarin is too high, potentially fatal hemorrhage may occur. Aspirin molecules bind to the same plasma protein binding sites as warfa-

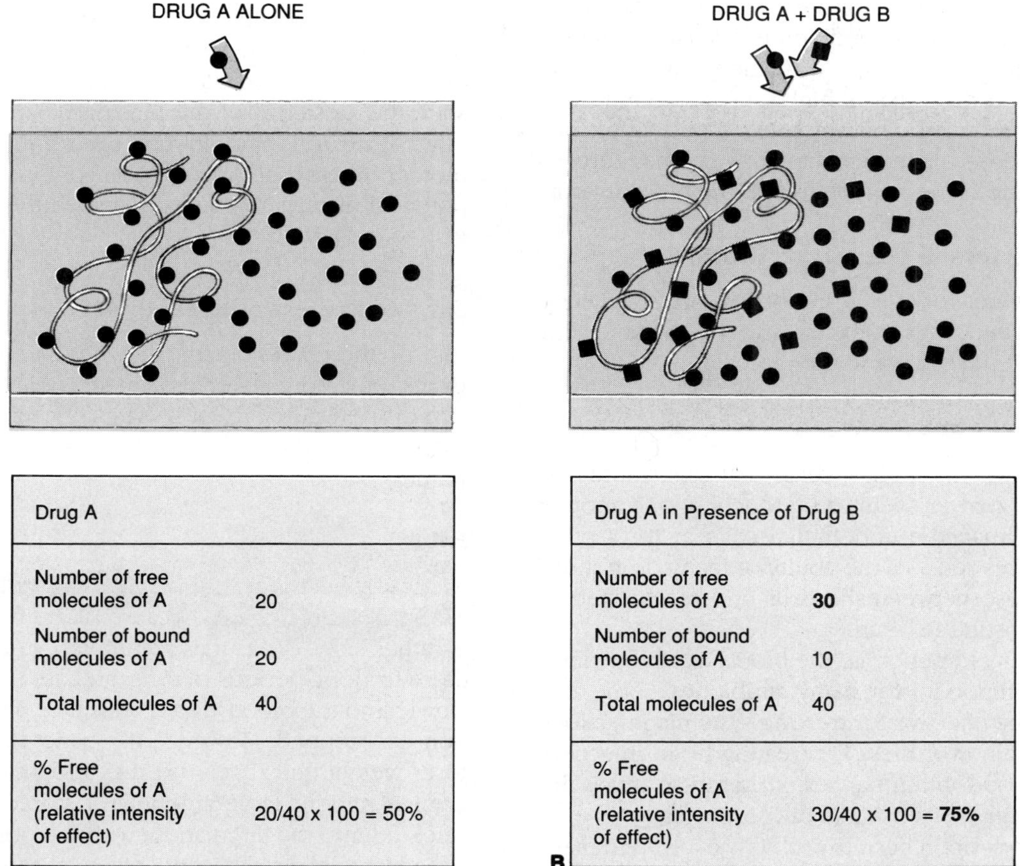

Figure 4–6

Effects of one drug displacing another from protein binding sites. **A.** Drug A alone: When drug A is administered alone, 50% of the molecules in the blood are bound to plasma protein. The remaining 50% are sufficient to produce the desired effect. **B.** Drugs A and B together: If molecules of drug B have a greater ability to bind to protein than molecules of drug A, some previously bound molecules of drug A will be displaced from their binding sites. In this example 75% of the total number of drug A molecules are now free. This causes a 50% increase in the concentration of free and therefore active drug A. Although the *dose* of drug A was not changed, its effects will be intensified. Excessive or toxic effects might occur.

rin, and in doing so displace warfarin. This elevates free warfarin concentrations and increases the anticoagulant's effects. If a person maintained on a "therapeutic" dose of warfarin were to take one or two aspirin tablets, which might displace only 1% of the bound warfarin molecules, the free warfarin concentration will have doubled. The patient could experience serious and perhaps fatal internal bleeding.

This dramatic example of a serious drug–drug interaction stresses the importance of carefully monitoring responses to drug therapy and knowing which medications are apt to produce these kinds of problems.

Other potential therapeutic problems relate to the ability of drugs to bind to plasma protein. In some diseases the liver is unable to manufacture normal amounts of plasma protein, and in others there may be kidney damage that causes excessive loss of plasma proteins into the urine. Both of these situations cause **hypoalbuminemia.** This condition is relatively common in the elderly and in pregnant women. Giving a "normal" dose of a drug that is highly protein-bound to a patient with reduced albumin levels could result in a serious overdose, since a greater than normal percentage of drug molecules will be free in the bloodstream.

Special Barriers to Drug Distribution

The capillary networks in some organs are specialized to prevent some drugs from crossing. The two most important are in the brain and the placenta.

The Blood–Brain Barrier

The capillary endothelial cells that constitute the *blood–brain barrier* seem to be touching one another more tightly than the endothelial cells in most other capillaries. This reduces the ability of many drug molecules to diffuse between the cells and reach effective concentrations in the brain.

An inability to penetrate the blood–brain barrier is particularly important for many antibiotics. Some antibiotics may be effective for treating systemic infections, but are virtually worthless for treating brain infections unless the blood–brain barrier is altered so much that it no longer serves its original purpose well.

The blood–brain barrier probably evolved to maintain homeostasis of the brain, which is the body's most critical integrative center. Its role includes keeping foreign substances, including many drugs, from reaching the brain. Only drugs that are very lipid soluble and not tightly bound to plasma protein can cross the blood–brain barrier well and produce appreciable actions in the central nervous system. Such drugs include the anesthetic gases, alcohol, some steroid hormones, and drugs that are used to calm an anxious patient or to promote sleep.

When it is essential to have high brain concentrations of a drug that does not cross the blood–brain barrier well, it can be injected directly into the cerebrospinal fluid (intrathecally). Since cerebrospinal fluid circulates very slowly, and intrathecal injection of any drug is potentially dangerous, this route of administration is seldom used for drugs other than local anesthetics and some antibiotics or anticancer agents.

The Placental Barrier

The capillary network of the placenta limits the ability of some drugs in the maternal circulation to reach the fetal circulation. This barrier serves as a means to protect the fetus against potentially harmful drug effects. Nevertheless, many drugs and substances that may enter the maternal circulation, including alcohol and nicotine, can cross the placenta and may cause fetal toxicity or birth defects (**teratogenic** effects). Therefore, despite the existence of the placental barrier, drugs and other chemicals should not be administered to the mother unless there is a medical condition in which the potential maternal benefits outweigh the potential dangers to the fetus.

Sites of Preferential Drug Accumulation

Just as there are organs that tend to exclude some drugs, other organs or tissues tend to accumulate certain drugs, leading to local drug concentrations that are higher than those in the bloodstream or in other tissues.

Fat

Fatty (adipose) tissues can serve as a "sponge" or **depot** for lipid-soluble drugs. Because blood flow through fat is rather slow, drugs that accumulate in fat tend to stay there for long periods of time, and are usually released slowly into the bloodstream only after drug administration has stopped. However, if a patient becomes ill or loses weight quickly so that the amount of body fat decreases rapidly, large amounts of stored drugs can be released into the circulation, with the potential of causing adverse effects. Poisoning from chronic exposure to highly lipid-soluble insecticides such as DDT can be explained in this way.

Bone and Teeth

Bone and teeth, structures that are made primarily of calcium, can accumulate substances that bind calcium. For example, if tetracycline antibiotics are administered

Figure 4–7

Metabolic fates of a drug. Some drugs are excreted without any prior metabolism. Others are inactivated by various metabolic reactions and then eliminated. Most drugs are partially metabolized to other compounds, while the rest of the unmetabolized drug is eliminated unchanged. Some drugs are either totally inactive or cause only weak effects in the body; metabolism may change them to more active compounds.

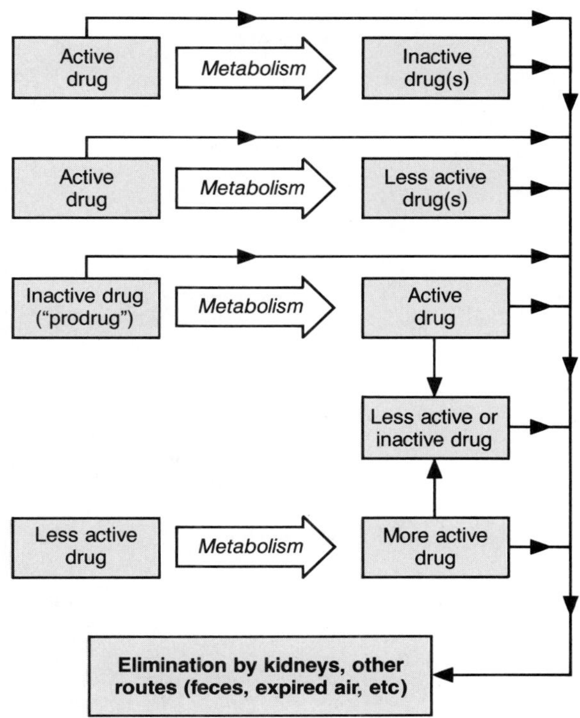

to children, in whom calcium deposition in developing teeth is high, the drug will accumulate in the teeth and permanently stain them.

Kidneys

Almost one quarter of the heart's output of blood passes through the kidneys every minute. This large blood flow exposes the kidneys to large amounts of drugs in the bloodstream. Although few therapeutic agents accumulate in the kidney, levels of metallic environmental poisons, such as lead and mercury, may reach high concentrations in renal tissues. Renal toxicity is a serious consequence of poisoning with these substances.

Metabolism

Many drugs and other foreign substances that enter the body are changed by a series of chemical reactions known as metabolism or **biotransformation.** It is one of the two basic processes responsible for reducing the amount of active drug in the body (the other is excretion). The major site of drug metabolism is the liver.

Drug metabolism serves two basic functions: (1) it transforms a drug (often called the *parent drug*) to one or more other substances (metabolites) that are less active pharmacologically and therefore potentially less toxic to the body; and (2) it converts drugs to metabolites that are more water soluble (or less lipid soluble) so they can be eliminated more readily. Only free (unbound) drugs can be metabolized.

Some drugs are totally metabolized to other compounds before they are excreted. Others undergo virtually no metabolism and are excreted unchanged, in the same chemical form in which they were administered. However, most drugs undergo both processes, with some of the drug molecules being metabolized and the rest being excreted without prior metabolism.

Some drugs are converted via a sequence of chemical reactions to a dozen or more metabolites. Others are converted to only one principal metabolite. Some drugs, called **prodrugs,** are converted from the inactive form in which they were administered to metabolites that produce the desired pharmacologic effect. The various ways that a drug can be affected by metabolism are summarized in Figure 4–7.

Hepatic Drug Metabolism

Most liver cells (hepatocytes) contain many complex and efficient enzyme systems that metabolize drugs. These enzymes are found primarily in the endoplasmic reticulum of the hepatocyte. The endoplasmic reticulum is sometimes referred to as the microsomal fraction of the liver cell, so the enzymes are sometimes called *microsomal enzymes.* The ability of these enzymes to metabolize drugs is affected by a patient's age, by genetic factors, by environmental chemicals, and even by other drugs.

The liver is supplied with blood via hepatic arteries and the hepatic portal circulation. The portal circulation delivers all drugs that have been administered orally and absorbed in the GI tract. Drugs administered orally pass through the hepatic portal circulation before they reach the systemic circulation, which provides the liver cells with an early opportunity to transform drugs that have just entered the body.

Many orally administered drugs can be significantly or even completely inactivated the first time they pass through the liver, so that their concentration in the

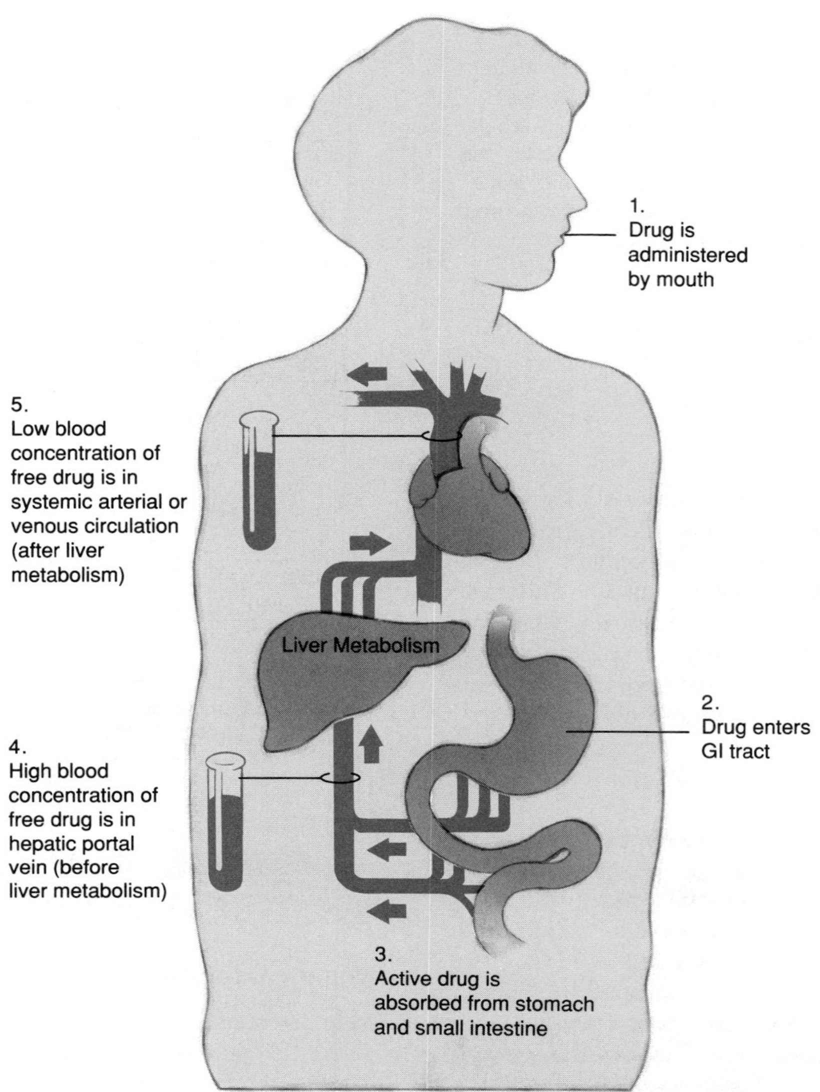

Figure 4–8

The "first-pass" effect. Some drugs that are absorbed from the GI tract and pass through the liver via the portal circulation are extensively metabolized before reaching the systemic circulation. Therefore, drug concentrations in the systemic venous and arterial systems are much lower than those in the portal vein, and drug effects are minimal. Initial administration of large doses may overcome this first-pass effect, or it can be avoided altogether by using alternate administration routes.

blood, and hence their therapeutic actions, are negligible. This phenomenon is appropriately called the **first-pass effect** (Fig. 4–8).

Some drugs undergo such extensive first-pass metabolism that they are virtually ineffective when given orally. Others can be given orally, but their initial first-pass metabolism is so great that repeated oral doses or high oral starting doses are required to overcome the effects of hepatic metabolism and to produce effective drug concentrations in the bloodstream.

If rapid effects from drugs that undergo extensive first-pass metabolism are needed, they must usually be given by injection. First-pass metabolism of almost any drug can be greatly reduced by using any route of administration other than oral. Once the liver enzymes are saturated ("loaded") with drug molecules, as occurs with repeated administration of the drug, they become less able to metabolize more drug molecules presented to them. As a result, the importance of the first-pass effect progressively decreases with repeated drug administration.

Basic Types of Metabolic Reactions

Microsomal enzymes perform two basic types of chemical reactions on drugs: *synthetic* and *nonsynthetic*. Synthetic reactions involve chemically combining the parent drug or some of its metabolites with another naturally occurring compound, such as an amino acid or sugar. These are sometimes called *conjugation* reactions.

Nonsynthetic reactions *oxidize, reduce,* or *hydrolyze* the parent drug or its metabolites. In most instances, the conjugated, oxidized, reduced, or hydrolyzed drug is more water soluble and therefore excreted more readily.

Drug-metabolizing reactions are often referred to as *detoxification* reactions, which implies that the drug is metabolized to less active and therefore less toxic compounds. Sometimes, however, drug metabolites may be more active than the parent drug. For example, codeine, which is widely used to relieve pain, is metabolized to morphine, a much better pain-relieving drug. Some drugs, called *prodrugs,* are administered in an inactive form and depend on liver metabolism for their conversion to active substances that produce the desired therapeutic effects.

In addition, some drugs can be converted to metabolites that are clearly more toxic than the parent compound. For example, the mild pain reliever and fever-reducing drug acetaminophen is pharmacologically active but also rather innocuous. However, one of its metabolites is very toxic to liver cells. If large amounts of this metabolite accumulate, as after taking a large overdose of acetaminophen, the metabolite may cause fatal liver damage.

Factors Modifying Hepatic Drug Metabolism

Several important factors can alter the ability of the liver's enzymes to metabolize drugs, and therefore can dramatically influence a patient's response to drug therapy. Such factors include the patient's age, nutritional status, and genetic makeup; the presence of liver disease; and the effects of hormones in the body. These factors will be discussed in more detail in Chapters 7 and 8. However, the general ways in which one drug can affect the hepatic metabolism of another drug, whether by inhibiting or stimulating the metabolism of the other agent, is presented here. They have considerable importance to drug therapy.

Drugs That Inhibit Hepatic Drug Metabolism Many different drugs are metabolized by the same hepatic enzyme systems. These drugs can compete with one another for the limited amount of enzymes available. The competition can result in one drug inhibiting the metabolism of another, which can lead to some important drug–drug interactions.

Other substances that suppress hepatic drug metabolism may do so by exerting toxic effects on the liver cells, thus diminishing the ability of hepatocytes to carry out necessary drug-metabolizing reactions. Hepatotoxic substances include industrial solvents such as carbon tetrachloride, therapeutic agents such as the monoamine oxidase inhibitors used to treat psychiatric depression, and large doses of alcohol ingested acutely.

Drugs That Stimulate Hepatic Drug Metabolism Some drugs can dramatically stimulate the liver's ability to metabolize other drugs, a process that also may lead to important drug–drug interactions. They do so by inducing liver cells to synthesize increased amounts of drug-metabolizing enzymes. Thus, the liver cell has more of the chemical machinery capable of altering a drug, enabling greater amounts of drug to be metabolized in a given time.

Enzyme inducers not only stimulate the metabolism of other drugs, but also may stimulate their own rate of metabolism. Examples of enzyme-inducing drugs are the barbiturate sedative phenobarbital and the anticonvulsant drug phenytoin. Chronic alcohol ingestion, in amounts that do not damage the liver cells, can also induce enzymes. Drug-related enzyme induction appears to be a reversible process that disappears days or weeks after discontinuing administration of the inducer.

It is important to remember the concept of enzyme induction when caring for patients who are being treated with two or more drugs that can interact in this way. Since responses to a particular drug are usually caused by unmetabolized drug in the bloodstream, simultaneous administration of another drug that induces drug-metabolizing enzymes can make it appear as if the patient was given too little of the first drug. Stimulation of drug metabolism is one cause for the development of drug tolerance. If tolerance develops because of the concurrent use of an enzyme-inducing drug, it may be necessary to increase carefully the dose of the other drug. Similarly, if a patient is taking two or more drugs, one of which is an enzyme inducer, and therapy with the inducer is stopped, the metabolic rates of the other drugs will eventually decrease to normal. Toxicity could

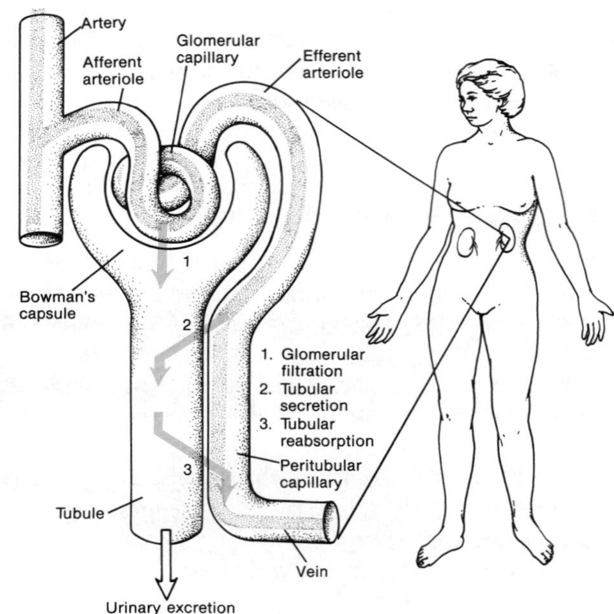

Figure 4–9

The kidney uses glomerular filtration, tubular secretion, and tubular reabsorption to regulate the excretion of drugs into the urine. A drug that is filtered may also be secreted. Also, varying amounts of some drugs that are filtered, secreted, or both may undergo tubular reabsorption, which returns drug molecules to the bloodstream via the peritubular capillaries and renal veins.

(*Source:* Adapted from Vander AJ, et al. *Human Physiology.* New York: McGraw-Hill, 1990. Reprinted with permission.)

occur if their doses are not reduced properly. Lastly, if the metabolites of a drug are more toxic than the parent drug, administration of an enzyme inducer can increase the risk of adverse effects if the metabolites cannot be eliminated quickly by other pathways.

NURSING IMPLICATIONS

It is relatively easy to predict that two drugs might interact because of enzyme induction, but it is difficult to predict how great the effect will be. Therefore, careful observation of the patient's responses to the drugs is necessary for optimal and safe drug therapy. Often it is best to measure the actual levels of the drugs in the patient's blood, and use that information to guide treatment.

Other Sites of Drug Metabolism

Drugs can be metabolized by organs and tissues other than the liver, including the lungs, the GI mucosa (and some microbes found within the GI tract), the kidneys, and even the blood. Although these sites have minor drug-metabolizing roles in general, they may be very important in metabolizing specific drugs, as will be discussed in other chapters.

Excretion

Most drugs and their metabolites are excreted by the kidneys and eliminated from the body in the urine.

Renal Excretion

The kidneys receive about 20% of the total cardiac output every minute. The basic functional unit of the kidney, the nephron, contains an extensive capillary network that is closely associated with the kidney tubules, where urine is formed.

There are two major processes by which the kidneys eliminate drugs: *glomerular filtration* and *tubular secretion* (Fig. 4–9). Often, after drug molecules have reached the urine by filtration or secretion, they may be returned to the bloodstream by the process of *tubular reabsorption.*

All three processes affect the fate of a drug in the body. Glomerular filtration and tubular secretion increase the amount of drug eliminated from the body, while tubular reabsorption reduces the amount of drug eliminated.

Glomerular Filtration

Glomerular filtration is the process by which small drug molecules (or their metabolites) pass from the bloodstream into what will become the urine. The major driving force is glomerular filtration pressure, which in turn depends on blood pressure. Blood pressure and blood flow both affect the glomerular filtration rate (GFR), which can be measured clinically as one index of renal function. Only drug molecules that are not bound to plasma protein will be filtered. Ionized drug molecules are less likely to be filtered than nonionized molecules.

Drugs or pathologic conditions that reduce renal blood flow or the GFR will diminish the elimination of drugs that depend heavily on glomerular filtration, and may have similar effects on tubular secretion and reabsorption. Factors that increase the GFR may, conversely, increase drug elimination.

Tubular Secretion

Parts of the kidney tubules, particularly those in the proximal parts of the nephron, contain specialized transport systems, or "pumps," that secrete drug molecules into the urine. The pumps require metabolic energy (adenosine triphosphate, ATP) to function. They efficiently remove drugs and their metabolites from the bloodstream.

The kidney tubular cells contain several different transport pumps, some of which are specialized to transport only drugs having certain chemical properties. However, many drugs have similar chemical properties and so share the same pumps. These drugs can compete with one another for transport into the urine, with one inhibiting the secretion (and hence the elimination) of the other.

Like the situation with two drugs that compete for a particular hepatic enzyme for metabolism, competition for renal transport processes can cause important drug–drug interactions that may lead to toxicity or other unwanted effects. For example, the drug probenecid, which is frequently used to treat patients with high blood levels of uric acid, is secreted by the same transport process as the toxic chemotherapeutic agent methotrexate, used to treat some cancers. Through competition for the same transport processes, probenecid can markedly decrease renal elimination of methotrexate, leading to side effects or outright toxicity. Probenecid also inhibits renal elimination of penicillin; this interaction can be used intentionally to cause the high and prolonged penicillin blood levels needed to treat some infections.

Tubular Reabsorption and the Effects of Urine pH

Tubular reabsorption returns to the bloodstream drug molecules that have already been filtered or secreted into the urine. The same factors that affect drug absorption into the blood from the GI tract—lipid solubility, ionization, and pH—affect the extent to which a drug will be reabsorbed. Nonionized and highly lipid-soluble drugs will be reabsorbed in considerable amounts, and therefore will not be eliminated from the body quickly. (As noted above, one of the major roles of drug metabolism is to form metabolites that are ionized and less lipid soluble so they are less able to undergo tubular reabsorption and can be better excreted.)

Whether a drug molecule in the urine is ionized and therefore unlikely to be reabsorbed, or nonionized and able to be reabsorbed well, depends on urine pH (Fig. 4–10). The relation between urine pH and drug

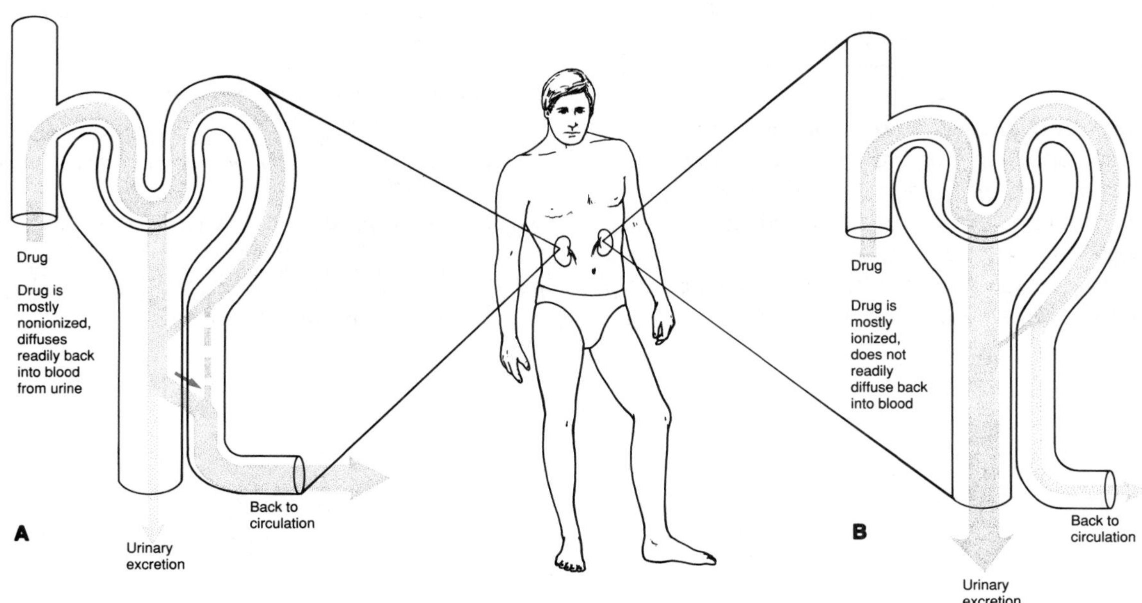

Figure 4–10

Effects of drug ionization and urine pH on renal excretion or reabsorption of drugs. **A.** Nonionized drug molecules in the urine freely diffuse (are reabsorbed) back into the peritubular capillaries. Little of this drug will be excreted. The degree of ionization, and therefore the degree of reabsorption, is influenced by the pH of the urine. **B.** Alkalinizing or acidifying the urine can have dramatic effects on the renal elimination of drugs. Done intentionally, changing urine pH can help speed the elimination of certain drugs that might be present in the body in toxic levels. Done unknowingly, it may adversely elevate or lower blood levels of a drug.

reabsorption explains how a change in urine pH can dramatically increase or reduce the renal excretion of drugs. For example, most aspirin molecules in normally acidic urine are nonionized, favoring aspirin reabsorption into the bloodstream. If a patient were to ingest an excessive dose of aspirin, and toxicity occurred, aspirin elimination in the urine could be increased by increasing urine pH, as by giving the urinary alkalinizer sodium bicarbonate. This would cause more aspirin molecules to be converted to the ionized form, which are less able to be reabsorbed.

Other Routes of Drug Excretion

Drugs may be eliminated by pathways other than through the kidneys. Although these pathways are not important for eliminating most drugs, they have important roles for a few. Their importance may also increase if a patient's renal function is reduced. The two major alternate routes of elimination are the GI tract and the lungs. Minor routes include sweat and saliva.

Elimination via the Feces

Some drugs are concentrated in bile, excreted into the intestines, and eventually eliminated from the body in the feces. However, sometimes drug molecules that are excreted in bile can be reabsorbed into the bloodstream from the lower GI tract. This process is called **enterohepatic recirculation.** It is somewhat analogous to the manner in which drugs that are filtered or secreted into urine can undergo tubular reabsorption. Drugs that undergo extensive enterohepatic recirculation may stay in the body and exert their effects for a very long time, especially if other pathways that help eliminate the drug are impaired.

Elimination via the Lungs and Expired Air

Some drugs or their metabolites will diffuse out of the bloodstream across the thin capillary membranes of the lung's alveoli. Alcohol and some of the inhaled general anesthetics are eliminated in the expired air, even though the major portion may be metabolized by the liver, excreted by the kidneys, or both. The characteristic breath odor of an individual who has been drinking alcohol is due to respiratory excretion of the drug. Alcohol concentrations in the breath are so closely related to blood alcohol levels that they are used to determine whether a person has a blood alcohol concentration above the legal limit for operating a motor vehicle.

Annotated Bibliography

American Academy of Pediatrics Committee on Drugs. Transfer of drugs and other chemicals into human milk. *Pediatrics* 1989;84(5):924–936. *Breast-feeding is a unique and important situation in which drugs are being excreted by one individual and simultaneously administered to and absorbed by another. This article provides comprehensive insight into drugs and other chemicals transferred in this way.*

Bakutis AR. The P450 enzyme system: A key to understanding the metabolism of drugs. *J Am Assoc Nurs Anes* 1983;51:272–274. *A concise summary of the major hepatic drug metabolizing system, the microsomal P450 system. This paper presents a complex topic in an understandable way, and highlights the major drugs that alter this system with potential clinically significant outcomes.*

Smith S. How drugs act. I. How drugs are absorbed and reach their destination. *Nurs Times* 1984;80:24–27. *This short article uses excellent diagrams to show how drugs are absorbed from various sites of administration, and explains why proper administration techniques are so important to help obtain predictable drug effects.*

Smith S. How drugs act. II. Elimination and cumulation. *Nurs Times* 1984;80:44–46. *A companion to the article cited above, this paper summarizes and diagrammatically depicts drug metabolism and excretion, and helps convey the importance of administering drugs at their scheduled times.*

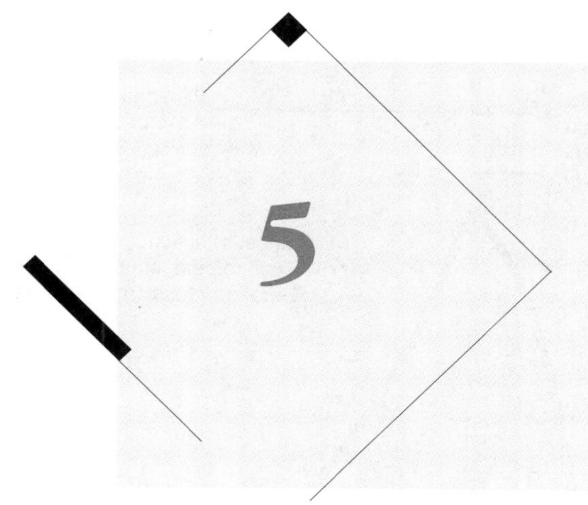

Time–Response Aspects of Drug Actions

Although there are instances in which a drug may be administered only once, it is much more common for a drug to be given repeatedly, whether for a few doses or for the remainder of the patient's life. Once the proper drug, dose, and route of administration have been selected, it is then essential to know how often the drug should be given to produce effects that are consistent, sufficient to achieve the desired therapeutic goal, and not likely to cause excessive or adverse effects. There are recommended dosage schedules for all drugs. However, it is valuable for the nurse to understand, in general, why the recommendations are important, the possible undesired consequences of deviating from the recommendations, and why changing the frequency of drug administration may actually be desirable in some cases.

The frequency with which a drug should be administered to achieve consistent, predictable effects is determined by the interaction between absorption, distribution, metabolism, and excretion. The simplest way to consider this relationship is to examine what happens when a single dose of a drug is administered to a normal individual by two of the most common routes, oral and intravenous (IV). The time–response relationships obtained with other routes of administration will not be discussed; they fall between the extremes produced by oral and IV administration.

Pharmacokinetic Aspects of Single-Dose Administration

General Time–Response Relationships

Oral Administration

The time between the administration of a drug and the first appearance of its effects is called the drug's *time to onset of action, lag time,* or *latent period.* The relationship between blood concentration and effect for an orally administered drug is illustrated in Figure 5–1. This graph shows the results of an experiment in which a patient has swallowed a drug that is absorbed from the gastrointestinal (GI) tract. At various times a small blood sample is taken from an indwelling venous catheter for measurement of the concentration of free drug. (In this example the concentration is expressed as some arbitrary unit per milliliter of blood.) During the experiment some aspect of the drug's effect in the body is

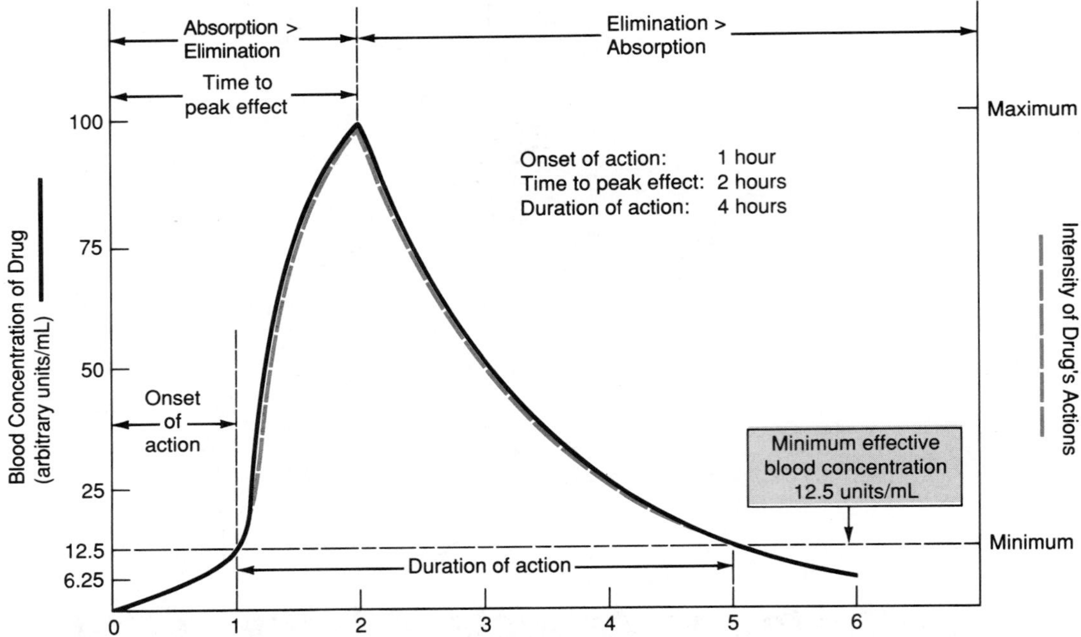

Figure 5–1

Relationship between blood concentration and effect for a single dose of an orally administered drug. Once the drug is administered and absorption begins, blood levels (solid line) start to rise. However, there will be no measurable response (dashed line) until a *minimum effective concentration* of free drug molecules in the blood is reached. The *onset of action* is the time needed for the drug concentration to reach this minimum level. While blood concentration and the intensity of the response are rising toward the peak, absorption rates are greater than elimination rates. The *time to peak effect* is the time required for the maximum effect to occur after administration. The fall of blood levels and decreased response intensity reflect metabolism, excretion, or both, at rates faster than rates of absorption. The *duration of action* is the time during which blood levels are above the minimum effective concentration.

also measured, so that time, drug concentration in the bloodstream, and biologic response to the drug can be compared.

For a short time after the drug was swallowed there is little measurable drug in the bloodstream. This delay represents the time needed for the drug to be absorbed through the various membranes in the GI tract, pass through the hepatic portal circulation, and eventually reach the systemic circulation and the target of drug action. A close look at Figure 5–1 shows that although blood levels of the drug soon become measurable, no measurable response occurs until 1 hour after administration. Thus, the onset of action is 1 hour. Figure 5–1 also shows that a certain minimum concentration of free drug in the blood—in this example, 12.5 units/mL—is necessary for a response to occur.

Once the initial response appears, its intensity increases greatly in a relatively short time, paralleling the rise of blood concentration, and eventually reaches a peak at a blood concentration of 100 units/mL. The time from drug administration to the development of the maximum effect is called the *time to peak effect.* In the example, it is about 2 hours. The rise in both drug concentration and intensity of response up to this peak indicates that active drug is being absorbed and distributed to its site of action faster than it is being eliminated.

Once the peak effect and concentration are reached, they begin to decline. The disappearance of active drug from the bloodstream can represent loss of drug through metabolism, excretion, or, as is the case for most drugs, the combined effects of both processes. Eventually, if the drug is not given again, it will completely disappear from the bloodstream. When the blood concentration falls below 12.5 units/mL, about 5 hours after administration, no measurable response remains. Since the response appeared 1 hour after the drug was given, and it disappeared 5 hours after administration, the difference—4 hours—is the drug's *duration of action.*

TRENDS AND CONTROVERSIES IN PHARMACOLOGY

How Much Do Drug Serum Levels Tell Us About Actual Patient Response?

Because it is difficult to monitor the therapeutic effects of many drugs, drug serum levels are often relied on for information about the progress of therapy. However, this technology has limitations that clinicians do not always consider.

Reynolds (1980) notes that "The major pitfall in the utilisation of blood-level monitoring is the widespread misconception that the so-called therapeutic or optimum ranges should be rigidly applied to *every* patient."

Pharmacokinetic processes are highly variable from person to person, and even in the same person over time. Some people are unusually sensitive to "therapeutic" serum levels of a particular drug, and will manifest classic signs and symptoms of drug toxicity with serum levels within the therapeutic range. In other people, serum levels will suggest drug toxicity while the person experiences an excellent therapeutic effect and no untoward reactions to the drug.

Sloan and Luderer (1981) point out several potential problems with drug serum levels. Many drugs have effects that outlast their serum levels. For example, the hypotensive effect of methyldopa and reserpine extends beyond the presence of these drugs in the serum. Cytotoxic drugs will continue to affect cells long after serum levels have subsided.

Some drugs are concentrated outside the bloodstream and are not readily measurable. Antihypertensive drugs that concentrate at adrenergic nerve terminals are a common example of this phenomenon.

It's difficult to correlate serum levels with drug effect when drugs have more than one active metabolite. Examples of drugs with active metabolites that extend their effects include diazepam, chlordiazepoxide, amitriptyline, procainamide, and phenylbutazone.

Serum levels won't always accurately reflect the effects of highly protein-bound drugs. Normally, a serum assay measures both the bound and free portions of a protein-bound drug. Because the bound-to-free ratio remains relatively constant, this presents no problem. However, when a patient is hypo-albuminemic or uremic, or when other protein-bound drugs are also present in the bloodstream, serum levels are a less accurate reflection of drug effect.

Other factors can influence toxicity at a given serum level. For example, age and disease are two variables that can affect the accuracy with which serum levels reflect pharmacologic response. In digitalis therapy, many "outside influences" make serum levels alone inadequate in assessing possible toxicity. Factors that potentiate digitalis toxicity include hypokalemia, hypercalcemia, hypomagnesemia, hypoxemia, myocardial ischemia, and acid–base disturbances. These factors must be considered when interpreting digitalis serum levels.

Koch-Weser (1981) emphasizes that, when available, "good clinical endpoints are intrinsically superior to serum concentration information." Serum levels have to be interpreted within a framework of good clinical observation. The most important information about a patient's response to drug therapy will always be the information gathered through careful assessment and questioning.

Koch-Weser J: Serum drug concentrations in clinical perspective. *Ther Drug Monitor* 1981;3:3–16.

Reynolds EH: Serum levels of anticonvulsant drugs: Interpretation and clinical value. *Pharmacol Ther* 1980;8:217–235.

Sloan RW, Luderer JR: Rational use of drug levels. *Am Fam Physician* 1981;23(4):123–126.

Intravenous Administration

Figure 5–2 illustrates the time course of action of a drug injected intravenously. Using the IV route avoids all the barriers that hinder absorption when a drug is administered by another route. Blood levels rise immediately, reach a peak, and then decline.

The peak blood concentration, 200 units/mL, is clearly higher than that achieved when the same dose was taken orally. This could indicate that not all of the oral form of the drug was absorbed, meaning that it was not completely bioavailable. This is true for many drugs, and indicates that administration of a given dose by any route other than IV may not achieve the peak blood level and intensity of response that occur when the drug is injected directly into the bloodstream.

The higher blood levels achieved with IV administration may also reflect the fact that some of the orally

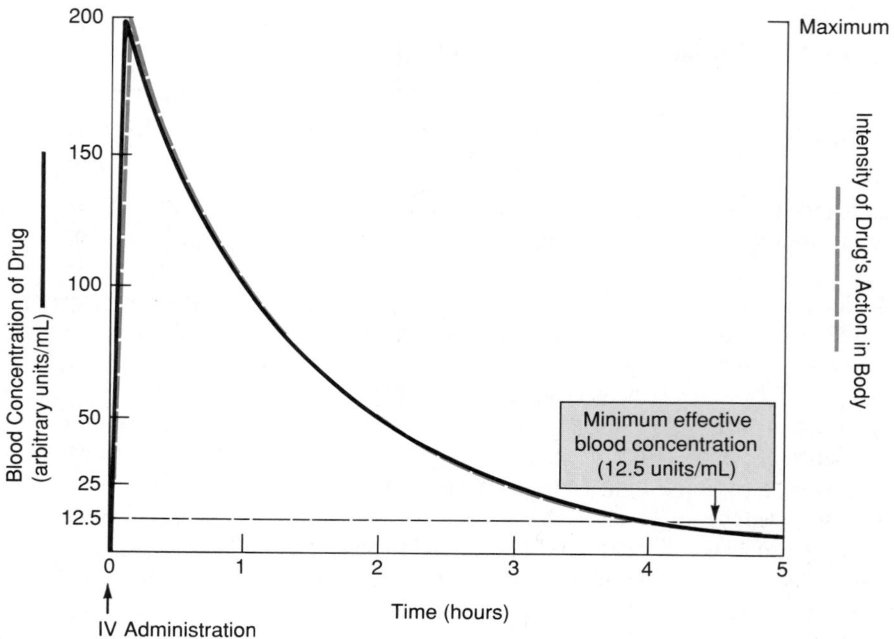

Figure 5–2

If a single dose of drug is given intravenously, thus avoiding absorption barriers, the onset of drug action and often the time to peak action are almost instantaneous. Blood levels (solid line) and the intensity of the response (dashed line) may start to fall almost immediately.

administered drug molecules were being eliminated as other molecules were still entering the bloodstream.

The fall of blood concentration after the peak was reached reflects rates of metabolism and excretion, as was the case with oral absorption.

Half-Life of a Drug

In general, the term *plasma half-life* (abbreviated $t_{1/2}$) indicates the time needed for the plasma concentration of a drug to fall to 50% (exactly one-half) of its previous concentration. Figure 5–3 compares the concentration–time effects of giving a drug orally and by the IV route. (The data are the same as shown in Figures 5–1 and 5–2. They show that the response, or blood concentration, to oral administration develops more gradually, and the peak is lower.)

It appears that blood concentrations of the drug fall more slowly when the drug is given orally. A closer look, however, shows otherwise. Note that with IV administration the peak blood concentration is 200 units/mL. One hour later it has fallen by 100 units/mL to 100 units/mL, or exactly half what it was 1 hour earlier. After another hour the blood concentration has fallen from 100 units/mL to 50 units/mL. This is a fall of only 50 units/mL in 1 hour, but it represents, exactly, another 50% decrease in the concentration from what was measured 1 hour before.

The decline is consistent, as long as no more drug is given and other factors are unchanged. The data for the same drug given orally are similar. Even though the peak blood concentration with oral administration is lower and occurs later, 1 hour after the peak concentration of 100 units/mL occurs the concentration has fallen by exactly half, and by another 50% after another hour has passed.

The comparison shows that the half-lives for the same drug given by two routes of administration are identical. This indicates that although the route of administration affects the maximum amount of drug in the bloodstream, the response intensity, and the time to onset and peak action, it has little or no effect on rates of metabolism and excretion, which account for the disappearance of drug or its effect from the body. In addition, the data show that regardless of the blood concentration at any given time, a constant *fraction* (percentage) of drug is eliminated with the passing of each $t_{1/2}$. That is, the rates of metabolism or excretion (or both) are not dependent on the blood concentration.

This generally applies to many drugs, but not to all.

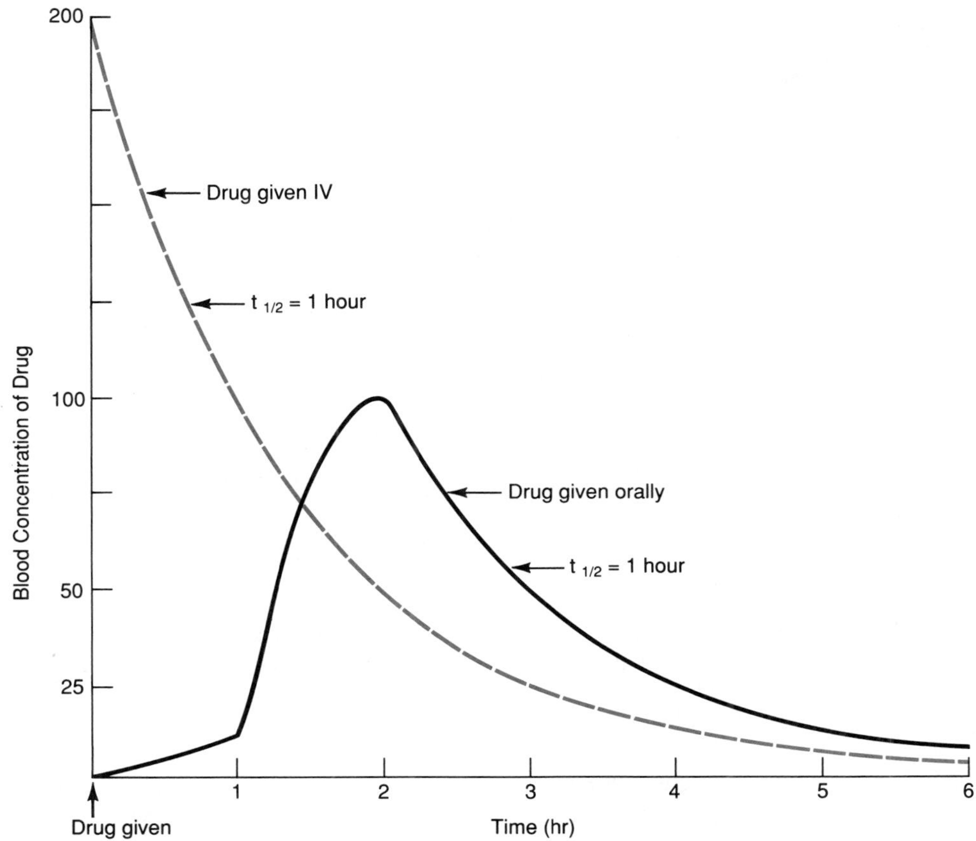

Figure 5–3

Comparison of effects on blood levels and response intensities of drugs given orally (solid line) and intravenously (dashed line). IV administration produces higher peak blood levels and a faster onset of action. The lower peak blood level for the orally administered drug could mean that some of the drug is not being absorbed, that some is being eliminated at the same time some is still being absorbed, or both. However, the rates at which blood concentrations fall after the peak, which reflect the drugs' half-lives, are identical (1 hour). This indicates that the route of administration has little or no effect on the rate at which drug molecules are eliminated.

With some drugs, and particularly when their blood concentrations are very high, processes of metabolism or excretion are operating at maximum capacity (they are said to be "saturated") and can eliminate only a constant *amount* per unit time. Only after blood levels have fallen to a certain lower level will a constant *percentage* be eliminated over time. Aspirin and alcohol (ethanol) are good examples of drugs that behave in this way.

Lastly, the $t_{1/2}$ measurement discussed above does not indicate whether elimination is occurring only by metabolism, only by renal excretion, or by a combination of these or other elimination pathways.

Figure 5–4 shows the elimination curves for three different drugs, A, B, and C, each given intravenously. The curves show that although each drug may initially produce the same plasma concentration, drugs can be metabolized or excreted at different rates. Drug A has a $t_{1/2}$ of 1 hour, drug B has a $t_{1/2}$ of 3 hours, and drug C has a $t_{1/2}$ of 8 hours. This graph provides no information about the kinds or intensities of pharmacologic effects produced by each drug, nothing about how well each drug would be absorbed if it were given orally, and nothing about the potential adverse effects each might produce. It only shows that the half-lives are different, implying that the drugs are metabolized or excreted at different rates.

Knowing only that the same blood levels of each drug produce the same desirable pharmacologic effect does not help determine which drug is "better" than another. Since drug C has the longest $t_{1/2}$ it might be preferred to drugs A and B because it does not need to

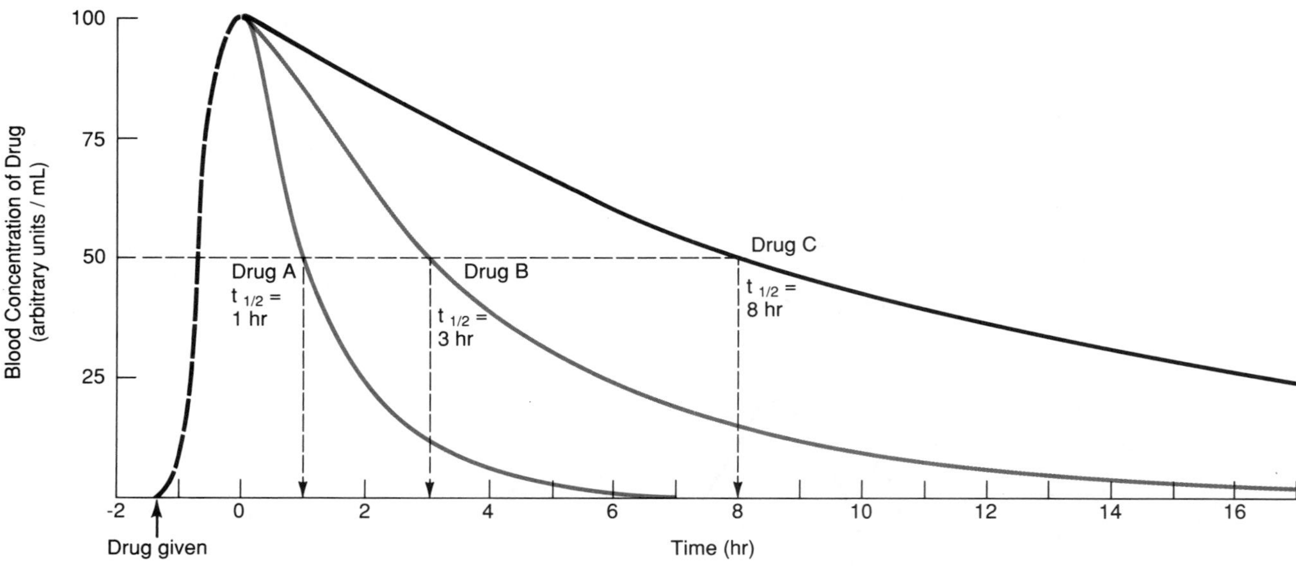

Figure 5–4

This example shows three drugs (A, B, and C) that are absorbed at the same rate and reach identical peak blood levels. However, their different elimination rates result in different half-lives. The faster the rate of metabolism, excretion, or both, the shorter the half-life.

be injected as often for the patient to obtain beneficial effects. However, if the patient accidentally received a toxic dose of one of these drugs, drug A might be preferred because its shorter $t_{1/2}$ would allow its blood levels to fall into the safe range faster. Without more information it is impossible to make an intelligent decision about which drug is better or worse. This problem will be considered in more detail in the next chapter.

Pharmacokinetic Aspects of Repeated Drug Administration

The duration of action of most drugs is relatively short compared with the length of time drug effects are often required. Many drugs have half-lives of only a few hours, yet drug therapy may need to be maintained for days, weeks, or months. Repeated drug administration is therefore necessary. During this time enough free drug must be present in the bloodstream to produce the desired effect, yet excessive or toxic drug levels, or large fluctuations in blood levels, must be avoided.

The "Plateau Principle"

When a constant dose of a drug is given at regular intervals, the concentration of drug in the blood will eventually reach a constant level (a *plateau*) and remain there until something changes:

- the dose of the drug;
- the time between doses;
- administration or discontinuation of other medications;
- or patient-related factors that affect absorption, distribution, metabolism, or excretion.

Figure 5–5 shows what happens with repeated administration of a hypothetical drug that has a $t_{1/2}$ of 4 hours. Assume for this example that the drug is given intravenously, so there is no question of incomplete absorption. The graph shows that each dose increases the drug's blood concentration by 2 μg/mL. After giving the first dose, subsequent doses are given every 4 hours, a time exactly equal to the drug's half-life.

The graph shows that after approximately four to five half-lives (or about 16 to 20 hours after the first dose), the peak blood concentration (obtained just after a dose is administered) and the minimum or "trough" concentration (obtained just before another dose is administered) are relatively constant. More importantly, the average blood concentration also becomes constant. If, as is generally true, the intensity of a drug's effects are related to the drug's concentration in the blood, then once the average blood level has stabilized the response to the drug will also be relatively stable.

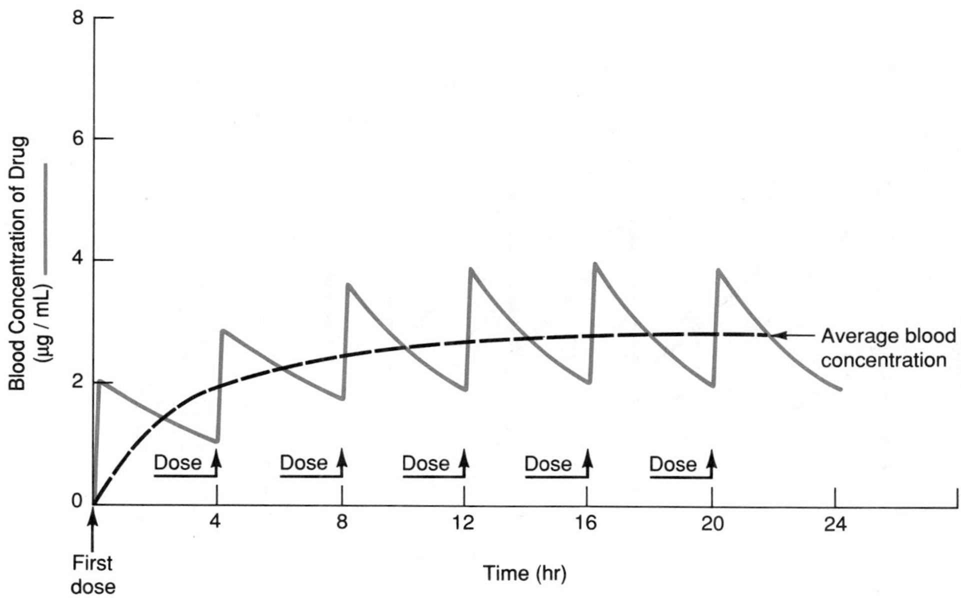

Figure 5–5

The "plateau principle" and the effects of giving a fixed dose of a drug at regular intervals. Repeated doses usually must be administered to maintain a drug's effects. In this example the drug has a half-life of 4 hours, the same dose is given every 4 hours, all the drug is "absorbed" instantaneously (that is, it is given intravenously), and each dose increases blood levels by 2 μg/mL. The **plateau principle** states that it takes about four to five half-lives (about 16 hours for this drug) for the average blood concentration (dashed line) and the related intensity of response to reach a steady (plateau) level. If the dose replaces an identical amount of drug lost through metabolism or excretion each day, the average daily blood concentration, and the resulting effect, will be constant. Such a steady response is usually desirable.

This *plateau principle* applies to virtually all drugs that are given at fixed doses at fixed time intervals. It provides the reason for giving drugs according to a specific, consistent schedule.

Implications of the "Recommended" Dosing Schedule

The situation shown in Figure 5–5 involves giving the patient a particular dose of a drug at regular intervals, intervals recommended by the drug's manufacturer. What happens when this schedule is changed? Are the same results achieved if the patient receives twice the dose half as often (that is, every 8 hours)? What would be the result if half the dose were given twice as often?

Figure 5–6 compares the results obtained with these other dosing schedules with the results obtained after giving the regular dose at the proper time. The graphs show that no matter how frequently the drug is given, the plateau (that is, the average blood concentration) is reached in about four to five half-lives (16 to 20 hours), as predicted by the plateau principle. Although the average blood levels of drug also seem to be roughly the same, regardless of how the drug is given, a closer look at the graphs indicates that the peak, trough, and average blood levels are different.

These differences are very important because a drug produces its desirable effects only when blood levels rise above a certain minimum concentration. Even more important, perhaps, is that the same drug is likely to produce unpleasant or even dangerous effects if blood levels exceed another, higher, concentration. If, in this example, beneficial or therapeutic effects do not occur if the drug's blood concentration is below 2 μg/mL, and unpleasant or toxic effects are apt to occur if the blood concentration rises above 4 μg/mL, changing the dosing schedule would produce effects in the patient very different from those associated with the recommended dosing schedule.

Doubling the Dose

In the example, doubling the dose, but giving it less often, causes the therapeutic range to be reached very quickly, immediately after giving the first dose, in fact. When the drug was given as recommended, blood con-

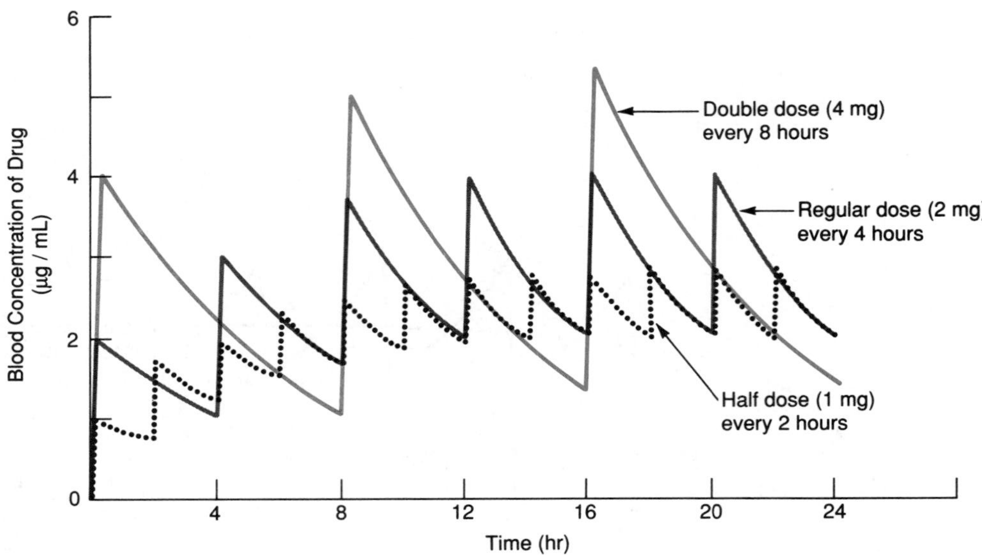

Figure 5–6

Deviations from the recommended dosing schedule produce different outcomes. Giving twice the recommended dose half as often (green line) produces large fluctuations between the peak blood concentration achieved shortly after giving each dose and the lowest ("trough") concentration achieved before the next dose is given. The average blood concentration is also increased. Giving half the usual dose twice as often (dotted line) produces more gradual effects and a lower average blood concentration. The response to the recommended schedule (gray line) is provided for comparison. Regardless of the dosage schedule, the average blood concentration will be achieved in four to five half-lives.

centrations did not reach the desired range until after the second dose, but they remained in the therapeutic range with following doses. When the dose is doubled but not repeated until 8 hours (two half-lives) later, blood levels fall below effective levels 4 hours after giving the first dose, and they stay there until the next dose is given. When the next dose is given (8 hours after the first in this example), toxic blood levels occur, at least for a while. Blood levels then fall into the desired range, and then become subeffective again. With every subsequent dose the cycle of toxic levels, desired levels, and subeffective levels is repeated. Thus, it can be seen that giving twice the usual dose half as often as recommended not only may be ineffective—at least part of the time—but also can be dangerous.

Halving the Dose

When only half the usual dose is given, but is administered twice as often as recommended, it takes much longer for blood levels to reach and then stay within the therapeutic range. With subsequent doses, the fluctuations of blood levels and the intensity of drug effects are less than those occurring with the other two administration schedules. This plan might be desirable if the toxic blood level of the drug is very close to the therapeutic blood level, if the patient experiences some discomfort at high but nontoxic blood levels, or if it is not essential to achieve a therapeutic effect quickly. In most cases, however, this approach is not suitable either.

It can be seen that improper drug administration schedules generally cause unacceptable results, either wide fluctuations between toxic and subtherapeutic blood levels or a delay in reaching and maintaining a desired blood level.

The examples shown earlier indicate the results of consistent but improper administration. As long as some consistency is maintained it might be possible to make dosage adjustments to overcome the problems. More common, however, especially for patients who self-medicate with orally administered drugs, is timing that is not only incorrect but also *inconsistent.* Other potential problems include the ingestion of food that could slow or decrease absorption from the GI tract, or the use of interacting drugs. All these factors combine to make the results of drug therapy unpredictable, and it may be impossible to achieve consistent responses. The patient's condition might not improve as well or as quickly as it should, or it might actually worsen as a result of excessive drug effects, particularly if the margin between therapeutic and toxic blood levels of the drug is narrow.

Some patients may get away with such a self-determined protocol, but others may not be so fortunate. As a result, it is important for the nurse to administer drugs properly, and to teach patients who will self-administer drugs the importance of following the treatment plan precisely. Written instructions should be provided, or another reliable person should be designated to administer the drugs. In evaluating a patient's response to a drug, assessment of compliance with schedules is very important.

An obvious question is what to do if a drug is not administered at the proper time. The most common options are to

1. give the usual dose as soon as the error is realized;
2. administer a higher dose as soon as possible;
3. give a higher dose at the next scheduled time; or
4. do nothing other than administer the regular dose at the next scheduled time.

The correct action depends on many factors, including how urgent it is to get the blood levels of drug back into an effective range and whether taking a higher dose all at once might produce toxicity. In general, if a drug has a very long half-life or there is a narrow margin between safe and toxic blood levels, a higher or double dose either need not or should not be given; the regular dose should be taken at the next scheduled time.

Alternatively, if a drug has a short duration of action (or a short half-life), its margin of safety is great, or it is essential to maintain therapeutic blood levels at all times to ensure the patient's well-being, taking either the regular dose or a higher dose may be appropriate.

When the choice makes a critical difference, consult a pharmacist or review the manufacturer's package information. It is always important to assess the patient's condition carefully to help determine whether additional drug effects provided by an increased dose are necessary, or whether continuing with the regular administration schedule is acceptable. In the hospital, all deviations from the scheduled administration plan should be documented on the patient's chart.

Alternatives to Giving Fixed Doses at Fixed Times

Many times an effective blood level of a drug must be reached quickly to manage a patient's condition, but the best drug for the condition has a very long half-life. If, for example, the preferred drug has a half-life of 24 hours, and therapy is started with the correct dose given orally at regular intervals, it will take roughly 4 to 5 days (four to five half-lives) until blood levels stabilize. If this is not satisfactory, one of several alternative dosing schedules could be used (Fig. 5–7). One way to reach

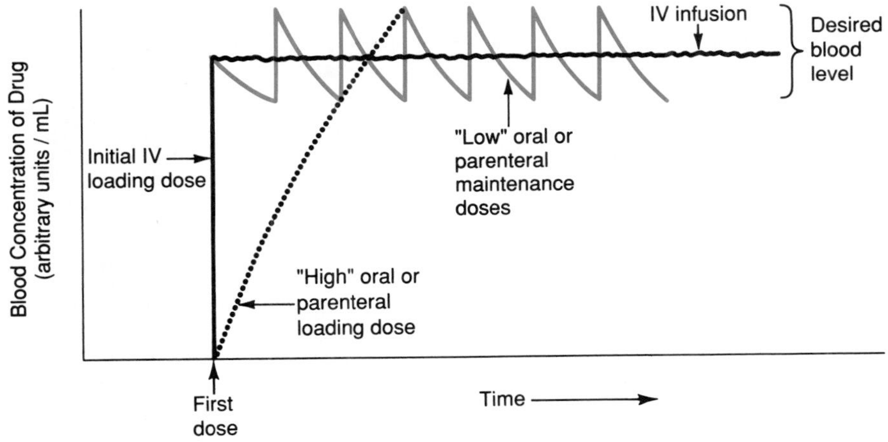

Figure 5–7

Alternatives to administering a fixed dose at fixed times. An initial IV loading dose elevates blood levels and produces the fastest response. The loading dose can also be given by other parenteral routes or by mouth (dotted line). Maintenance doses can then be used to achieve relatively constant average blood levels (green line). Intravenous infusions of a drug at rates that precisely match the amount of drug that is eliminated (wavy line) will provide constant blood levels and responses. Such a route is often essential for maintaining constant blood levels of drugs with extremely short half-lives (several minutes or less).

effective blood levels quickly is to give the drug parenterally, often by the IV route. Subsequent doses could then be given orally, with the actual doses calculated to keep blood levels stable at the plateau. Alternatively, a larger-than-usual first dose could be given orally, with subsequent doses being the usual (lower) recommended dose. In either case, the first dose that is given to elevate blood levels rapidly is called the **loading** (or **priming**) **dose,** and the subsequent doses given to maintain a relatively constant effect are referred to as **maintenance doses.**

In some critical-care situations in which IV drug administration is necessary, a loading dose (for example, a bolus injection) can be given first, followed by a slow IV infusion in which the drug is given continuously at a rate that matches its disappearance from the bloodstream. Drug infusion is also necessary when the half-life of a drug is extremely short (only a few seconds or minutes at most). For drugs with such short durations of action, the only way to maintain their effect is to infuse them continuously for as long as necessary. In other instances, when quick but prolonged effects are needed, a loading dose can be given parenterally to reach desired blood levels quickly, followed by a switch to oral maintenance doses.

The frequency with which a dose of drug must be given to maintain a relatively steady blood level (and, therefore, a relatively steady effect) can be predicted mathematically. Formulas are available to account for many other important factors, such as impaired renal excretory function or altered hepatic metabolism. Some of these equations require a computer to solve. However, a person's response to a drug does not always follow a neat mathematic formula. The body is complex and often unpredictable, and although many patients may respond to drug therapy in similar ways, *no two patients are alike.*

Regardless of whether the doses given to a patient are calculated from actual laboratory test results or other data, based on manufacturers' recommendations, or "guesstimated," if the patient does not respond appropriately to what should be the right dose given at the right time, the "proper" dose can be determined only by carefully observing the patient's responses (both beneficial and adverse) and adjusting the dose based on that response.

Annotated Bibliography

Smith S. How drugs act. II. Elimination and cumulation. *Nurs Times* 1984;80(Dec):44–46. *Summarizes and diagrammatically depicts drug metabolism and excretion, and helps convey the importance of administering drugs at their scheduled times.*

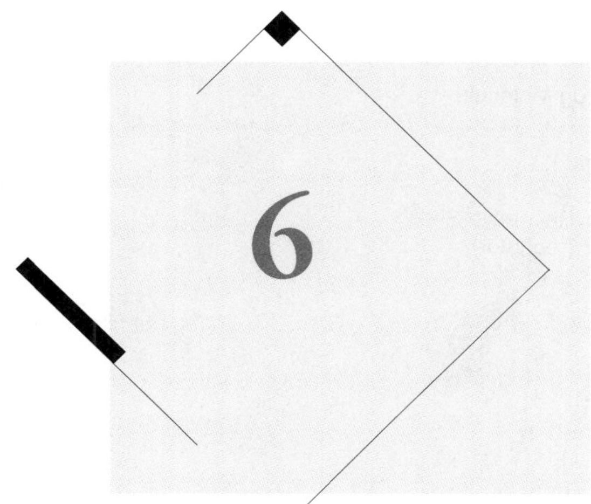

Mechanisms of Drug Action

Chapters 4 and 5 introduced two key principles governing the actions of all drugs: only drug molecules that are free in the bloodstream can produce pharmacologic effects; and the amount of free drug in the blood, and therefore the intensity of the response, is related to the dosage. This chapter discusses **pharmacodynamics,** the study of *how* the vast majority of drugs exert their effects. It focuses on how drug molecules interact with target cells, how a biologic response occurs, why the dose–response relationship applies to most drugs, and the ways in which one drug can alter the dose–response relationship of another.

Drug Receptors, Agonists, and Antagonists

Receptors

Many drugs, but certainly not all, produce their effects by interacting with specific proteins that are usually located on a cell's outer membrane. These specific interaction sites are called **receptors,** and each cell membrane may have tens of thousands of them (Fig. 6–1). The receptor is generally named according to the type of drug (or chemical class to which the drug belongs) that interacts with it. For example, receptors for histamine are called *histamine receptors.* Receptors have shapes that are specific for particular drugs. The importance of a receptor's shape, its relation to the structure of drugs, and how shape allows some drugs to interact but prevents others from doing so, are discussed later.

Second Messengers

The binding of a drug molecule to its receptor is the first step leading to a response. In many cases receptors are, or are near, enzyme systems that control some basic biochemical process of the cell. A "second messenger," a chemical synthesized as a result of the drug–receptor interaction, is often the link between drug binding and the eventual response. Cyclic adenosine monophosphate (cAMP) in muscle cells is a good example of a second messenger. When certain drugs are administered, the drug–receptor interaction on the muscle cell activates adenylate cyclase, an enzyme that increases formation of cAMP. In turn, cAMP increases the flow of calcium ions into the cell, activating the contractile proteins and causing muscle contraction. Drugs that can interrupt this sequence of events at any point can therefore affect muscle contraction.

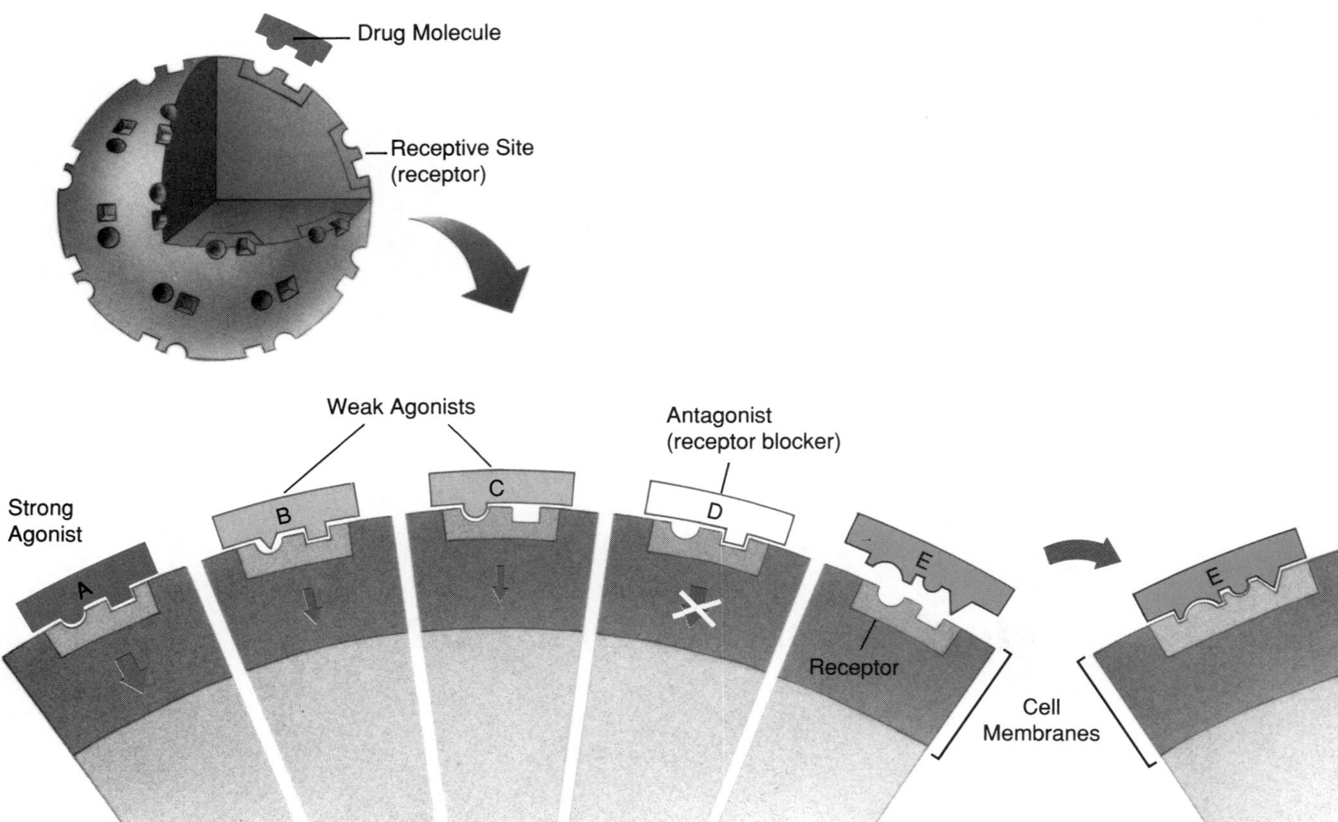

Figure 6–1

A typical cell, showing drug receptive sites (receptors). The shape, size, electric charge, and other properties of the receptor surface complement those of drug molecules that interact with it, like a lock and key. Agonists interact with the receptor to form a drug–receptor complex, and in doing so alter cell function to cause a response. Agonists with shapes that precisely match those of a particular receptor (**A**) are very efficacious. Those with somewhat different structures that do not allow precise interaction are weaker agonists (**B, C**). Drugs may have shapes that allow them to bind to a receptor, or to only part of the receptor's complex shape, but they produce no response (**D**). When they occupy the receptor they prevent formation of the agonist–receptor complex and the resulting response. These are pharmacologic antagonists, or receptor blockers. Drugs with structures that bear no resemblance to one receptor type (**E**) may be able to interact with other types of receptors on other cells, and may be agonists or antagonists for those receptors.

Agonists

Drugs that bind to a receptor and then alter some biologic function to produce an effect are called **agonists.** The type of response depends on the characteristics of the receptors, on the type of cell where the receptors are found, and, of course, on the drug. Many important agonists are found naturally (**endogenously**) within the body, including all the neurotransmitters, hormones, and local mediators ("autacoids") that normally control body functions. When a nerve or gland is activated by the proper stimulus, the endogenous agonist is released, and the activity of some other cell is changed. Many therapeutic agents act as agonists, and have chemical structures very similar to those of naturally occurring neurotransmitters or hormones. Some have exactly the same structures. Administering such drugs can be useful to intensify certain effects that might be caused by a deficiency of endogenous agonists.

To be classified as an agonist, a drug must have two major properties: **affinity** and **efficacy.**

Affinity

Affinity simply means that the agonist molecule can interact with, bind to, or occupy a specific receptor site. Although two drugs may bind to the same receptor (at different times), they may have different abilities to do so (that is, they have different affinities), similar to the way in which a strong magnet and a weak magnet differ in their ability to attract a particular metallic object.

The interaction between an agonist and its receptor is not permanent. Instead, it is a dynamic, reversible process involving weak ionic bonds between electrically charged structures on the agonist molecule and oppositely charged structures on the receptor. This allows a brief association between the drug and receptor to form a drug–receptor complex, followed promptly by separation (disassociation) of the drug molecule from its receptor.

The brief time during which the complex is formed is nevertheless sufficient to change the cell's properties and cause a response, provided that adequate numbers of drug molecules (reflecting the drug dose) interact with a comparable number of receptors. This association–disassociation process enables a particular agonist molecule in the vicinity of a receptor to stimulate that receptor, or others nearby, many times in a relatively brief time.

When a drug receptor is occupied by an agonist molecule, no other molecule can interact with it. Since the interaction is brief and reversible, it provides ample time for other nearby drug molecules to compete with the agonist and form a complex with the receptor.

Efficacy

Efficacy can be defined as the ability of an agonist to cause a response. Just as different drugs may interact with the same receptor with different affinities, they may also have different efficacies, or the ability to cause a response of a greater or lesser intensity.

Antagonists

Drugs that are called **antagonists** can interact with cell receptors, but they do not cause a response. That is, *antagonists have affinity for a receptor, but no efficacy.* They merely prevent or inhibit the binding of—and thus the response to—agonist molecules. Therefore, they can also be called *receptor blockers.*

Antagonists do not create new effects; rather, they simply increase or decrease the level of activity of ongoing biologic processes that are being regulated by some agonist. (The words *efficacy* and *effect* can be confusing when used to describe antagonists. Alone, and in the absence of any agonist molecules, the interaction between an antagonist and a receptor causes no effect. When agonist molecules are present, antagonists can be said to have an "effect," but that effect is only inhibition of the response caused by the agonist.)

There must be some similarities between two drugs, one an agonist and the other an antagonist, because they can bind to the same receptor. However, there must also be differences, if agonists produce an effect but antagonists do not. The essential difference is the chemical structure of the molecules, which determines their shape, surface electrical charges, and other properties that influence drug–receptor interactions.

The lock-and-key analogy used in biochemistry to describe the interaction between enzymes and substrates is useful for describing how drugs and receptors interact. Keys (the drug molecules) have special shapes that enable them to fit into a lock (the receptor), but only keys that have notches and peaks that exactly mirror those of the lock will open it. Keys that are slightly out of shape may require some effort to open the lock, but they too will work. Some "master keys" open many locks, whereas other keys can open only a few of the locks that are opened by the master. Keys that fit in the lock well enough to open it are like agonists.

Antagonists can be viewed as keys that fit in but do not open a lock. If an "antagonist key" is already in the lock, it prevents the "agonist key" from entering, and so prevents the lock from opening, even though the proper key may be nearby.

Structural differences between two drugs determine much more than whether one will act as an agonist or antagonist. Two drugs with slightly different chemical structures may both be agonists (or antagonists), but one may have a stronger ability to produce (or block) a particular response.

Specificity of Interactions Between Drugs and Receptors

The shapes of receptors and the drugs that act on them are responsible for the relatively specific interactions between the two. For example, histamine, an important mediator in the inflammatory response, is an agonist *only* for histamine receptors; acetylcholine, a crucial neurotransmitter that has a very different structure, is an agonist *only* for acetylcholine receptors.

Many receptors have *subtypes,* often designated with numbers, Greek letters, or other names. The subtypes have slightly different shapes, which account for even more selective or specific interactions with agonists or antagonists that have slight but important shape differences. There are at least three receptor subtypes for acetylcholine and similar drugs, and at least six for the adrenal hormone epinephrine (adrenaline). The existence of subtypes of a particular receptor has enabled development of drugs with structures specific enough to stimulate or block only one or a few of the subtypes, thereby producing only a few desired responses in the body.

Some antagonists are very specific in terms of the receptors they can block. For example, drugs that block receptors for epinephrine cannot block receptors for agonists such as acetylcholine. However, other receptor blockers, such as those classified as antihistamines (drugs that block some histamine receptors) are much less specific; they can also block some receptors for acetylcholine. Like agonists, the specificity (or lack of specificity) of antagonists has tremendous clinical importance.

The Dose–Response Relationship

A **dose-response curve** shows the relationship between the drug response and the amount (dose) of a drug given. Figure 6–2 is a type of dose–response

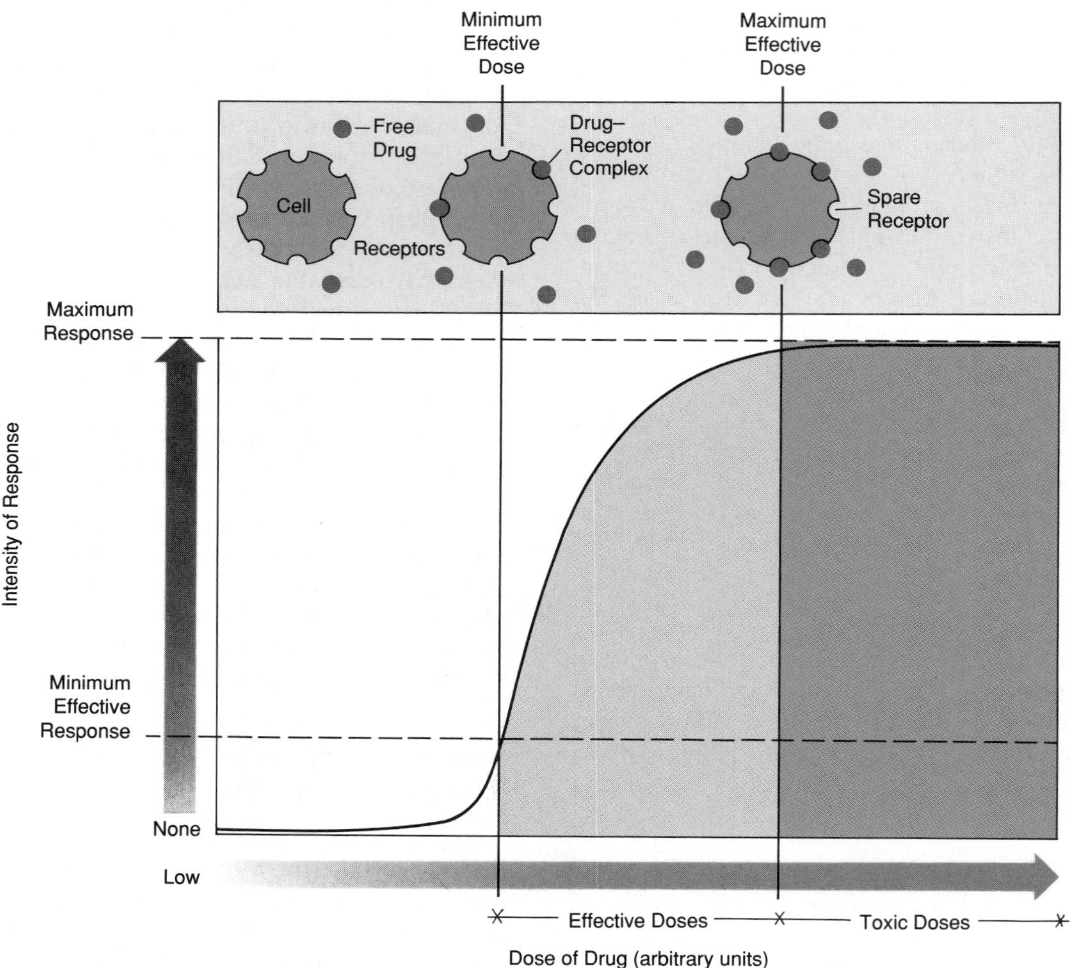

Figure 6–2

Graded dose–response curve for a hypothetical agonist. The intensity of the response depends on the dose, which, in turn, affects the concentration of drug molecules that are free (unbound) in the blood and therefore able to interact with receptors. A minimum (or threshold) dose of drug must be given to cause a measurable effect. Increasing the dose increases the number of drug–receptor complexes, and the intensity of the response increases. The maximum response coincides with the maximum effective dose. All available receptors need not be occupied by drug molecules for the maximum response to occur. Receptors that are unoccupied when the maximum response occurs are called *spare* receptors. Further dose increases may cause excessive, adverse responses (toxicity).

curve that relates drug doses to the intensity of the response caused by each dose. Because the intensity of the response is variable, or graded (ranging from no response at all to a maximum response), the curve is called a **graded dose–response curve.**

How does the agonist–receptor interaction account for this relationship? As shown in the figure, the interaction of a relatively small number of agonist molecules with their receptors produces a relatively small change of cell function (ie, the response). As more agonist molecules interact with the receptors (as occurs with further increases of drug concentration or dose), the response increases until cell function will eventually be changed maximally—the peak effect will occur. No greater effect can be produced even if the amount of drug available (the dose) is increased further. In fact, with most drugs further increases of dose or concentration will no longer produce beneficial changes of cell function, but will cause undesirable and potentially dangerous effects because the cells are stimulated excessively or other body systems are affected.

Figure 6–2 also shows that the maximum response does not necessarily occur only when all the available receptors on a cell are occupied by agonist molecules. Most cells have far more receptors than are needed for an effective agonist to cause the maximum response. These extra or "spare" receptors help explain how some agonists can still exert their maximum effect even though many of the cell's receptors for it are blocked by antagonist molecules.

In addition, a minimum concentration or dose of drug is necessary to change cell function. The amount of drug that produces this minimal observable effect is called the *threshold concentration* (*threshold dose*). If a patient's blood level of a drug is below the threshold, whether because the dose was too small or was given too infrequently, or the drug molecules were removed from the bloodstream by metabolism or excretion, there will be no therapeutic effect. It is important to remember, however, that although subtherapeutic doses or blood levels may not cause any desirable responses, they may be sufficient to cause undesirable side effects elsewhere, or interactions with other medications.

The Logarithmic Dose–Response Curve

For various reasons, graphs that plot the intensity of drug responses as a function of drug dose are difficult to analyze, especially when comparing two or more drugs. More often, to analyze the data more easily, graphs are drawn to show the intensity of the response as it relates to the logarithm of the drug dose; it is called the **log dose–response curve.**

Figure 6–3 shows a log dose–response curve for a hypothetical drug, drug A. In this example drug A is an analgesic—a drug used to prevent or relieve pain. For reasons that will be noted shortly, the dose–response relationship was measured in laboratory rats. (Assume that the doses effective in rats can be modified appropriately for human beings.)

The Concept of Effective Doses

Three points on the log dose–response curve shown in Figure 6–3 are of interest. The first, at the lower left, shows that below a certain dose no effect is produced. The lowest dose that does cause a measurable effect (relief of minor pain) is the minimum effective dose, or the threshold dose. In this example it is about 1 mg. The second point, at the upper right, is that at which further increases of dose produce no further increase of pain relief. This corresponds to the dose needed to produce the maximum effect (relief of severe pain), and the graph shows that it is approximately 100 mg. Between the minimum and maximum effective doses, the intensity of the response increases sharply as the dose is increased. The third major point is the dose that produces half (50%) of the maximal possible effect, which in this example might indicate relief of moderate pain. This dose is called the **effective dose–50%,** or **ED_{50}.** It is defined as the dose of drug needed to produce 50% of the maximum response. In this example the ED_{50} for drug A is 10 mg. The ED_{50} is often used as a guideline for determining the "average" dose that will be given to patients to produce a desired therapeutic effect, and as a reference point for comparing the effects of more than one drug.

Efficacy and Potency

Two additional concepts in the dose–response relationship are **efficacy** and **potency.** Efficacy was previously defined simply as the ability of a drug to cause a response, regardless of how intense the response is. This definition can now be expanded to indicate that efficacy also provides some information about the maximum *intensity* of the response. *Potency* indicates the dose of a drug needed to produce a response, compared with the dose of another drug needed to cause the same response at the same intensity.

In Figure 6–4 the log dose–response curve for drug A is compared with curves for two other analgesics, drug B and drug C. A threshold dose, a maximum effective dose, and an ED_{50} can be identified for each. It can be seen that drug A and drug B are capable of producing responses of identical maximum intensity (com-

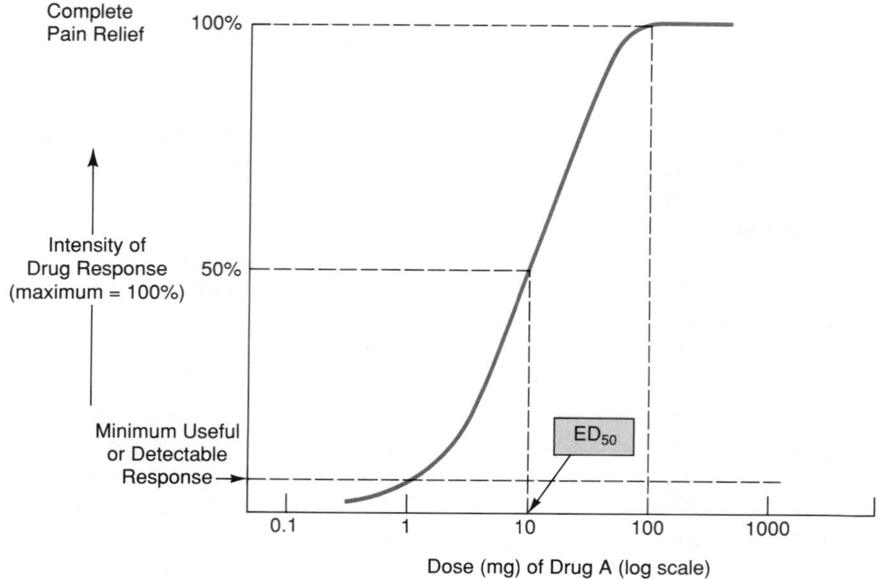

Figure 6–3

Logarithmic dose–response curve. The intensity of the response, expressed as a percentage of the maximum possible response, is plotted against the logarithm (log) of the dose. In this example, an analgesic (pain-relieving) drug, drug A, is given to a large population of animals, and its ability to alleviate or prevent pain is measured. The minimum effective dose is approximately 1 mg; lower doses do not relieve pain. Complete pain relief (the maximum response) is achieved by the maximum effective dose, 100 mg. The dose that causes half-maximal (50%) pain relief, 10 mg, is defined as the effective dose–50%, or ED_{50}. The ED_{50} is useful for comparing the doses of other agonists needed to produce a particular intensity of response.

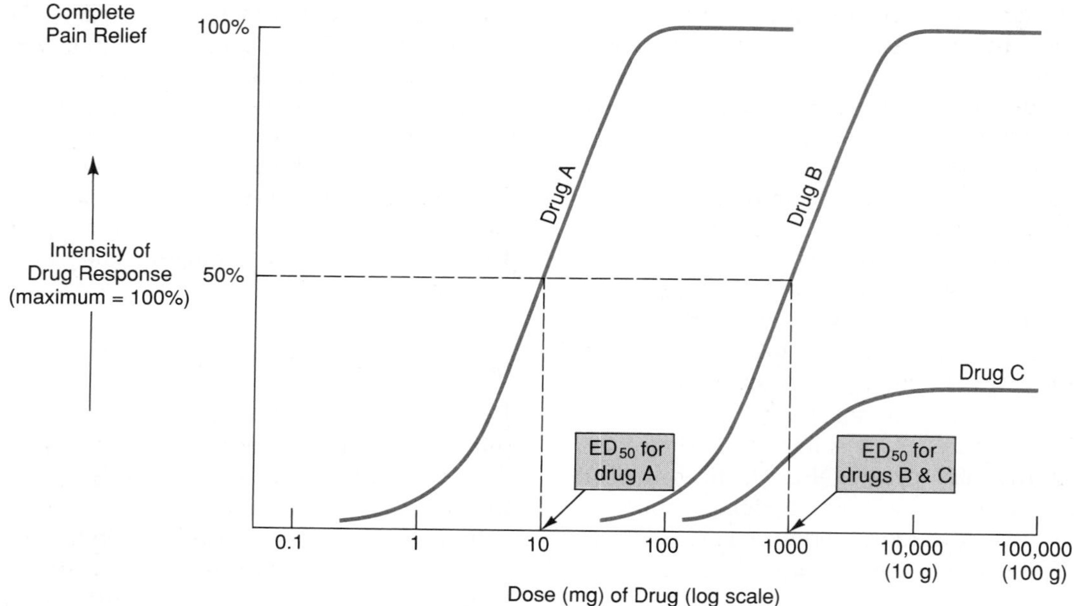

Figure 6–4

Log dose–response curves for three agonists, drugs A, B, and C. Since drug A and drug B cause identical responses by acting on the same receptor, their efficacies and potencies can be compared. Both drug A and drug B cause the same maximum response (100% relief of pain); therefore, they have equal efficacy. However, higher doses of drug B (ED_{50} = 1000 mg) than of drug A (ED_{50} = 10 mg) are needed to produce a response of given intensity. The ED_{50} values can be compared to indicate the potency ratio: drug A is 100 times as potent as drug B (1000 mg/10 mg). Drug C has lower efficacy than drugs A or B, because no matter how large a dose of drug C is given, it cannot produce the same maximum response as that caused by drug A or B (this is true even though drug C's ED_{50} is 1000 mg, the same as the ED_{50} for drug B). Therefore, its potency cannot be compared with the other two. The graph gives no indication about the relative safety of the drugs.

plete relief of severe pain), but they differ in terms of the dose needed to cause this maximum response. The ability to cause responses of equal maximum intensity indicates that drugs A and B have equal efficacy.

Since the ED_{50} is a useful reference point, we can use it to compare the ED_{50} values for drug A and drug B. The ED_{50} for drug A is 10 mg, and that of drug B is 1000 mg (1 g). This means that it takes 100 times more drug B than drug A (1000/10 = 100) to produce an effect of a given intensity, chosen here as 50% of maximum. Therefore, drug A is said to be 100 times more *potent* than drug B. (The drug with the lower ED_{50} is the one with greater potency, and the **potency factor** is simply the ratio of the two ED_{50} values, placing the higher ED_{50} in the numerator and the lower value in the denominator. It is equally correct to say that drug B has one one-hundredth the potency of drug A.)

Now the ability of a third hypothetical pain-reliever, drug C, is evaluated. Figure 6–4 shows that no matter how high a dose is given, drug C cannot completely relieve severe pain, as drugs A and B can. Drug C, therefore, has a lower efficacy (is less efficacious) than either drug A or B.

It should be understood that efficacy and potency are different concepts, and the terms cannot be used synonymously. In fact, unless two drugs have the same efficacy (that is, they can produce the same maximum effect), their potencies cannot (and should not) be compared. Potency can be a misleading term, especially as it is used in advertisements for nonprescription drugs. In therapeutics, efficacy is almost always more important than potency. For the person seeking relief from pain of a headache, for example, it makes little difference whether pain is alleviated by 10 mg of drug A or 1000 mg of drug B, as long as the drugs are equally effective and safe.

Safety

Efficacy is one of the two most important factors when a drug is considered (and approved by the government) for use in humans. The other is safety. The isolated cell or organ systems commonly used to determine how most drugs work on cells give very little insight into how a drug will act when given to a whole organism such as a human being, particularly in regard to safety. A drug studied on isolated heart cells may produce cardiac-stimulating actions that might be clinically useful, but if given to a whole animal it might produce violent illness or even death because of other effects.

When there is a choice between two similar drugs, one of which is claimed to be more potent or effective than the other, the selection is usually based on safety and on other effects that the drug may (or may not) produce. In the example presented in Figure 6–4, is drug A "better" because it is more potent than drug B or because it is more convenient to give 10 mg of drug A than 1000 mg of drug B? The information given so far about these two drugs has addressed efficacy and potency, but has provided no clue about whether they are safe or can cause unpleasant side effects when effective doses are taken. Moreover, if two drugs produce the same side effects, or even lethal effects, how do the doses needed to produce those unwanted actions compare with the doses needed to produce a desirable effect?

Relative Efficacy Versus Relative Safety

Drugs that are developed for use in humans are first tested in animals, not only to assess their ability to produce beneficial effects but also to assess their possible adverse or toxic effects. One important piece of information obtained from animal testing is the relationship between the dose needed to produce a desired effect and the dose required to cause another easily measured effect—death. (This is why our hypothetical experiment was done in rats, not human beings.)

The graph in Figure 6–5 shows the effects of drug D on two groups of animals. In the first group the relationship between the dose of drug D and the desired response was measured. In this example the desired response was arbitrarily set at a 25-mm Hg increase of blood pressure. The relationship between the dose of drug D and another, clearly undesirable effect, death, was evaluated in a second group of animals presumed to be identical to the first.

The units for the y-axis in Figure 6–5 are different from the units on the previous graphs. They represent a **quantal** (all-or-none) **dose–response curve,** or one in which the percentage of animals experiencing an effect of a specified intensity is related to the dose. The graph in Figure 6–5 shows that (1) half the rats had the desired response with a 10-mg dose of drug D; (2) a dose of 100 mg kills half the rats; and (3) a 1000-mg (1 g) dose kills all the rats.

Just as the ED_{50} was defined as the dose needed to produce 50% of the maximum desired effect, another term can be defined: the **lethal dose–50% (LD_{50})**, or the dose that kills 50% of the animals given the drug.

The LD_{50} and ED_{50} values can now be compared. The LD_{50} is 100 mg and the ED_{50} is 10 mg. The ratio of the LD_{50} and the ED_{50} (100/10), 10, defines the **therapeutic index** of drug D. The therapeutic index is a rough indicator of the drug's **margin of safety.** The term *therapeutic index* is relative, and there is no "magic value"

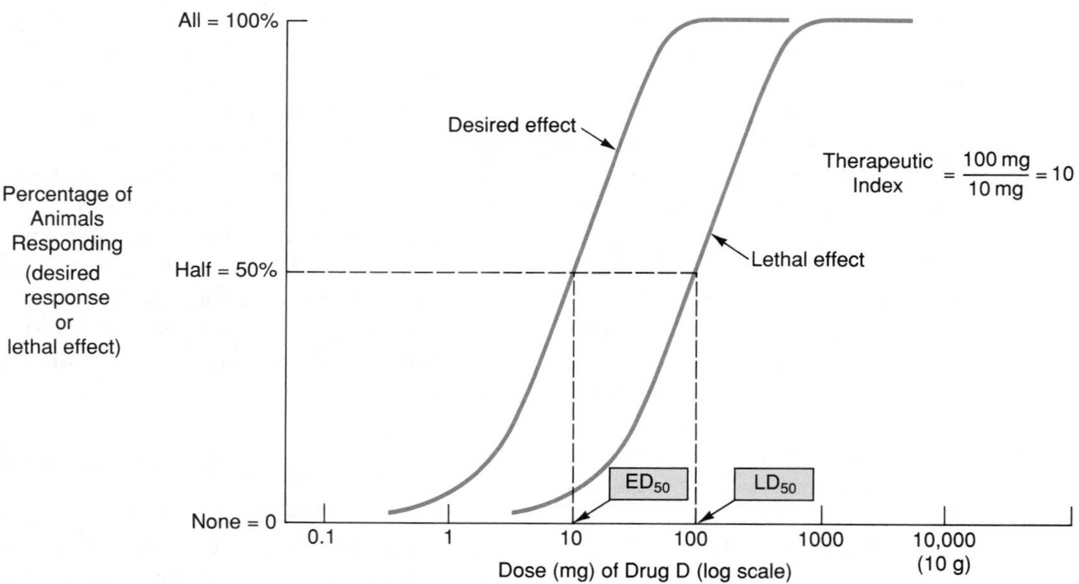

Figure 6–5

Relative efficacy versus relative safety (therapeutic index). The *y*-axis indicates the *percentage* of animals experiencing a response, desired or lethal, expressed in all-or-none terms. The curve on the left shows the desired response to drug D, a 25-mm Hg increase of blood pressure. When the dose is 10 mg, the ED_{50}, 50% of animals will experience this blood pressure rise. When the dose is 100 mg or more, 100% of the animals will respond in this way. The curve on the right relates the dose to the lethal response. The lethal dose–50% (LD_{50}), the dose that kills half the animals, is 100 mg. The ratio of the LD_{50} and ED_{50} (100 mg/10 mg = 10) is the therapeutic index, or an estimate of the drug's margin of safety. Note that the dose that raises blood pressure by 25 mm Hg in half the subjects (10 mg) is sufficient to kill a small percentage of others, and that the dose needed to ensure the desired blood pressure rise in all the animals may kill about half of them.

above which a drug can be considered safe and below which it cannot. However, when comparing two or more drugs that can cause the same kinds of effects, the drug with the greater therapeutic index or margin of safety is less likely to produce adverse or fatal effects if an overdose is taken than a drug with a lower therapeutic index. In general, although other factors must be considered, the drug with a greater therapeutic index or margin of safety should be chosen when two effective drugs can be used for the same purpose to prevent, diagnose, or treat a human disease.

Before continuing it is essential to reexamine the data for drug D, shown in Figure 6–5. Note that large parts of the dose–response curve for the desired effect overlap the lethal dose–response curve. This indicates that the drug doses needed to increase blood pressure in some of the animals (for instance, 50%, at the ED_{50} of 10 mg) are high enough to kill some others. Assume that drug D behaves in human beings as it does in rats, and the ED_{50} and the LD_{50} had the same relationship. If the ED_{50} were given, 50% of the patients would experience a certain increase of blood pressure, but a small percentage of other patients would die! If the dose of drug D were increased, either accidentally or to ensure that more than 50% of the patients experienced the desired effect, the risk of a lethal result would increase significantly.

The explanation for why some animals (or patients) experience a desired response to a given dose of a particular drug, while others may be harmed or even killed, lies in a phenomenon known as *natural biologic variability*. Just as there is variability in body weight or height, there is variability in the response to a given dose of a drug. This topic is discussed in more detail in Chapters 7 and 8.

Figure 6–6 shows the therapeutic and lethal effect curves for drug E, another imaginary blood pressure-elevating drug. Tests show that its ED_{50} is 100 mg and its LD_{50} is 10,000 mg (10 g). The therapeutic index for drug E (LD_{50}/ED_{50}) is 100. Although drug E has an ED_{50} that is higher than that for drug D (that is, drug E is less potent), the greater therapeutic index of drug E implies that it is relatively safer than drug D. Indeed, comparing the two curves shows that there is much less overlap

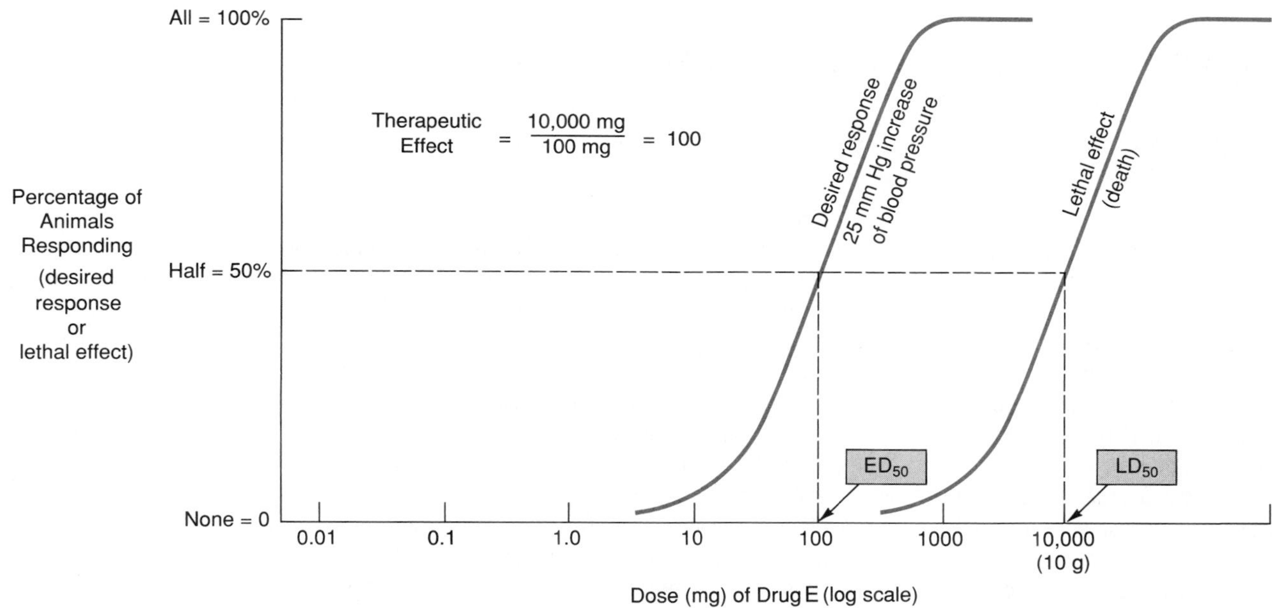

Figure 6–6

The ED_{50} of drug E is 100 mg. The LD_{50} is 10,000 mg. This drug's therapeutic index is 10,000/100, or 100. Although the ED_{50} of drug E is higher than that of drug D (see Fig. 6–5), indicating that drug E is less potent, its higher therapeutic index (or margin of safety) suggests that it is less likely to cause death if therapeutic or excessive doses are given.

between the desired and lethal effect curves. Giving an overdose of drug E would be less likely to cause a fatal outcome than if the same error were made with drug D.

The examples above compared drugs and their doses only in terms of a therapeutic effect and the most extreme adverse effect, death. Many other drug actions must be considered when comparing medications that will be given to human beings. Although one drug may be generally safer or less likely to kill someone if an overdose is given, compared with another, it is entirely possible (for example) that an effective dose causes severe nausea and vomiting in most of the patients who take it, but the other does not. In addition, one drug might also cause devastating interactions when given with another drug that the patient must also take, but the other does not.

All these variables must be taken into account when a drug is being selected for use. Careful assessment of factors such as side effects, drug–drug interactions, and even cost, help assure that drug therapy is effective and safe, and also acceptable to the patient.

Effects of Pharmacologic Antagonists

Antagonists, as described above with the lock-and-key analogy, are more precisely called **pharmacologic antagonists.** Pharmacologic antagonism accounts for many important interactions between drugs, some of which are undesirable. However, many pharmacologic antagonists are clinically useful because they can modify the activity of a body system that is reacting to the presence of excessive amounts of an agonist, regardless of whether the agonist is an endogenous substance, such as a neurotransmitter or a hormone, or another "drug." For example, if a patient has accidentally received an excessive dose of the agonist morphine, which can cause fatal respiratory depression, an antagonist for morphine receptors can be given.

There are two major types of pharmacologic antagonism: competitive and noncompetitive. They differ in terms of the manner in which antagonist molecules prevent agonists from interacting with their receptors. The most common type is competitive antagonism.

Competitive or Surmountable Antagonism

If agonist and antagonist molecules interact with the same receptors, the two drugs will be competing for a limited number of receptor sites. The presence of the antagonist prevents some of the agonist molecules from acting on their receptors, and so the intensity of the response will be decreased. If the diminished response can be overcome by increasing the dose of the agonist, the antagonism is called **competitive.**

TRENDS AND CONTROVERSIES IN PHARMACOLOGY

Product-to-Product Variability

A person's response to drug therapy sometimes changes for no apparent reason. Over time, an improved therapeutic effect, a decreased response, or a change in the pattern of adverse reactions may occur. One possible cause of altered drug response is a change in the source of the patient's drug product.

No drug consists solely of an active ingredient. Dissolving agents, fillers, binders, emulsifiers, stabilizers, preservatives, and flavors are some of the "inactive" substances added to drugs. The Food and Drug Administration (FDA) regards these additives as inert, despite longstanding evidence to the contrary. For example, the antimicrobial agent benzyl alcohol, used as a preservative in many injectable drugs, has been associated with a number of neonatal deaths and metabolic complications (Brown et al., 1982). Many aspirin-sensitive individuals are also allergic to the coloring agent tartrazine (FD&C Yellow no. 5), and serious reactions, including acute bronchospasm, led the FDA in 1980 to institute special labeling requirements for all products containing this dye. Sulfites—widely used in foods and drugs as preservatives—have been associated with several deaths from anaphylaxis (FDA Drug Bulletin, 1984). They continue to be used in some nebulizer solutions for antiasthma drugs, and in some parenteral drug products.

The United States Pharmacopoeia (USP) and National Formulary (NF) set chemical and physical standards for drugs, but they don't specify standards for manufacturing processes or inert ingredients. Consequently, when the same drug is made by two different companies, both products may be pure, consistent from dose to dose, and therapeutically active; but they are not necessarily interchangeable. Many studies have confirmed that different versions of the same drug often differ in their bioavailability. This variability has been reported with a wide range of drugs including digitalis, furosemide, insulin, oral hypoglycemics, lithium, and phenytoin.

The FDA began bioequivalence testing for certain drugs in order to eliminate interchangeability problems. But clinical studies are not conducted for every drug. And even when they are performed, there is ongoing discussion of the methods by which data should be analyzed to determine bioequivalence (Schulz and Steinijans, 1991). Furthermore, some compounds, such as pancreatic enzyme replacements used to treat cystic fibrosis patients, are not subject to regulation, because they were available before the passage of the Food, Drug, and Cosmetic Act in 1938. Yet a recent report indicates that variability in enzymatic activity among different products may lead to treatment failure in some individuals (Hendeles et al., 1990).

Cost containment efforts have led to generic substitution in hospitals and long-term care facilities. This has raised concerns that less expensive may mean less effective (Brook, 1990). This concern has not been generally supported by experience, but in view of the difficulty inherent in determining that different types of therapy are equally effective, the possibility should not be overlooked.

Problems associated with product-to-product variability are most likely during drug changes that patient and health care providers may not be aware of—changes associated with admission or discharge from the hospital, changes occurring when a patient frequents several pharmacies and refills prescriptions at different places, or when an institution or local pharmacy replaces a brand name product with a generic substitute. Clearly, not every patient who changes drug brands will experience a dramatically different effect. However, because changes can occur, health care providers should be alert to this potential problem.

Brooks I: The risks of substitution of therapeutic modalities by cheaper and sometimes less effective agents. *Arch Int Med* 1990; 150:688–689.

Brown WJ, et al.: Fatal benzyl alcohol poisoning in a neonatal intensive care unit. *Lancet* 1982;1:1250.

Hendeles L, Dorf A, Stencko A, Weinberger M: Treatment failure after substitution of generic pancrelipase capsules: Correlation with in vitro lipase activity. *JAMA* 1990;263:2459–2461.

Schulz HU, Steinijans VW: Striving for standards in bioequivalence assessment: A review. *Int J Clin Pharmacol Therap Toxicol* 1991;29:293–298.

Sulfite update. *FDA Drug Bull* 1984;14:24.

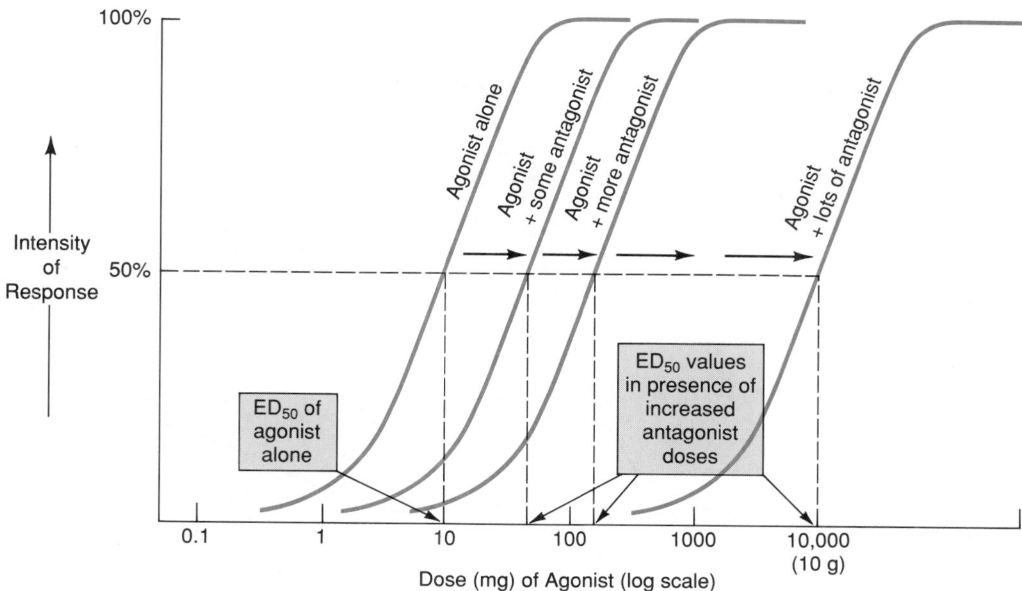

Figure 6–7

Competitive antagonism. Competitive (surmountable) antagonists temporarily occupy (block) receptors for agonists that act on the same receptor, thereby reducing the intensity of the response. The maximum response to the agonist can be produced (that is, antagonism can be overcome) if the agonist's dose is raised sufficiently. In the absence of any agonist molecules, antagonists produce no effect.

Competitive antagonism is depicted in Figure 6–7. In this example, the ED_{50} of the agonist, given in the absence of any antagonist, is about 10 mg. In the presence of a "low" dose of antagonist, the intensity of responses to most doses of the agonist is reduced, and the ED_{50} is increased to about 50 mg. That is, when the antagonist is present, a higher dose of agonist is needed to cause a response of given intensity. If still greater doses of antagonist are given, the ED_{50} for the agonist is shifted farther to the right. Increasing the dose of agonist sufficiently, however, allows it to compete successfully for receptor sites and overcome the inhibited response caused by the antagonist. With further increases in dose of the agonist, a response of maximum intensity can be produced. Since the effects of the antagonist can be overcome or surmounted, competitive antagonism is also called **surmountable antagonism.** There are two major reasons to explain the phenomenon. First, the cell has spare receptors; even though some receptors are blocked by antagonist molecules, enough are unoccupied (not blocked) to allow the agonist to produce its maximum response if sufficiently high doses are given. Second, molecules of competitive antagonists, like molecules of agonists, do not bind to the receptor permanently. Their brief interaction, followed by "unbinding" from the receptors, gives ample time for agonist molecules to have access to the receptors.

In terms of outcome, it makes no difference whether the agonist or antagonist is given first. This is clinically desirable. If a patient receives an excessive dose of an antagonist, its effects can be overcome by administering the proper agonist. Conversely, too much agonist can be managed by giving more of the antagonist.

Noncompetitive Antagonism

The blockade or inhibition produced by some antagonists cannot be overcome. This kind of pharmacologic antagonism is called **noncompetitive antagonism;** it is depicted in Figure 6–8. This illustration shows that no matter how high the dose of the agonist is raised, the same maximum intensity of response as produced in the absence of the antagonist cannot be reached. Although both competitive and noncompetitive antagonists reduce the responses to a given dose of agonist, the shape of the dose–response curves in the presence of a competitive antagonist are different (compare Figs. 6–7 and 6–8).

One explanation for noncompetitive antagonism is that noncompetitive antagonists bind to receptors more

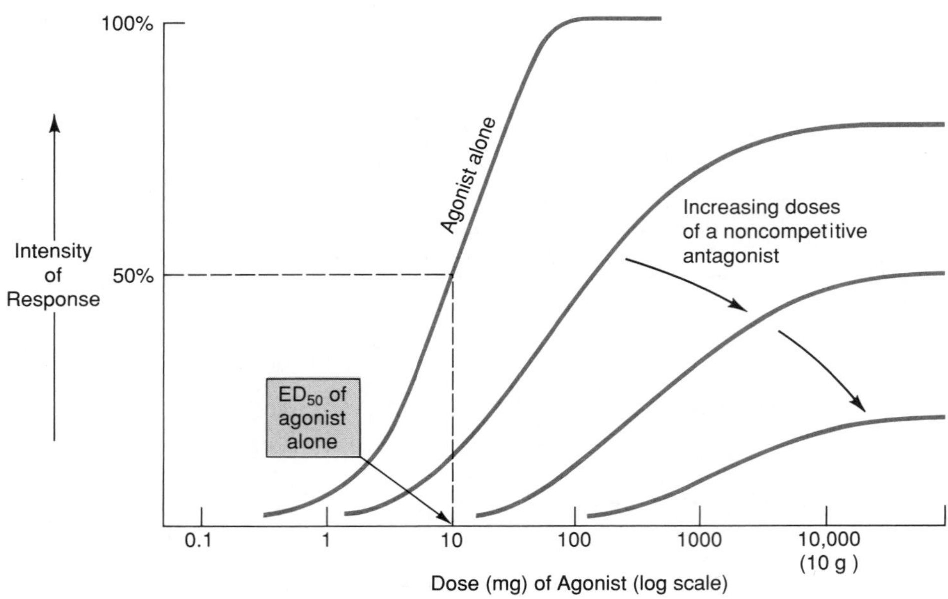

Figure 6–8

Noncompetitive antagonism. Noncompetitive antagonists bind tightly to receptors, or otherwise reduce the ability of an agonist to form a complex with the receptor. Unlike the situation with competitive antagonists, no matter how much the dose of the agonist is increased, the same maximal response cannot be achieved. The greater the dose of antagonist, the greater the agonist's maximum response can be inhibited.

tightly or for a much longer time, so the ability of agonist molecules to interact with the receptors is lost. Some noncompetitive antagonists may bind to a cell's membrane at places immediately adjacent to receptor sites for the agonist, and in doing so change the shape of the receptor so that it no longer "recognizes" the agonist. Few antagonists used clinically are noncompetitive, because it would be difficult to overcome their effects if an overdose were taken.

Other Types of Drug Antagonism

Both competitive and noncompetitive antagonism involve the ability of one drug to interfere with the drug–receptor interaction of another. Other forms of antagonism do not involve effects on a common receptor site.

Biochemical antagonism can be defined as the process by which one drug decreases the amount of another drug that is available within the body to produce an effect. This may be due to one drug's ability to decrease the absorption, increase the excretion, or alter the metabolism of the other drug. For example, phenobarbital increases the rate of metabolism of the anticoagulant warfarin through induction of hepatic drug-metabolizing enzymes (Chapter 4).

Chemical antagonism is the inhibition of a drug's action as a result of its chemical interaction with another substance. An example is the interaction in the stomach between tetracycline antibiotics and an antacid or food rich in calcium ions. Calcium ions combine with the antibiotic and reduce its absorption and thus its antibacterial effect. There are many other examples of chemical antagonism between two drugs (eg, the antibiotics gentamicin and carbenicillin chemically neutralize each other); between a drug and a fluid in which it may be diluted before administration (eg, epinephrine is inactivated in solutions containing sodium bicarbonate); or between drugs and chemicals in the devices with which they are administered (eg, nitroglycerin reacts with the polyvinylchloride used to make many intravenous bags and tubing).

The last major type of drug antagonism is **physiologic antagonism,** sometimes called **functional antagonism.** In this case two agonists act at *different receptors,* and by *different mechanisms of action,* to produce effects that counteract each other. An example is the antagonism between acetylcholine and epinephrine, both of which are physiologic regulators of heart rate (and many other body functions). Acetylcholine acts on acetylcholine receptors on heart cells to de-

Table 6–1 Selected Examples of Drugs That Do Not Act Through Stimulation of Specific Receptors

Drug Class	Example	Probable Mechanism of Drug Action
Drugs Acting Through Physical Actions on Cells		
General anesthetics	Halothane	Presumably alters physiochemical properties of nerve cell membranes in brain
Saline cathartics	Magnesium sulfate (Epsom salt)	Increases osmotic pressure in gastrointestinal tract; withdraws water into gut lumen; increases expulsion of gut contents
Osmotic diuretics	Mannitol	Increases urine production by increasing osmotic pressure of urine, reducing reabsorption of water
Drugs Acting Through Chemical Actions on Other Chemicals or on Cells		
Skin disinfectants	Alcohol	Denature proteins on bacterial cell walls
Antidotes for heavy metal poisoning	Dimercaprol, EDTA, deferoxamine	Chelates (chemically binds) heavy metal ions
Anticoagulants	Heparin	Neutralizes electrical charge on a plasma protein needed to initiate blood clotting
Antacids	Sodium bicarbonate	Chemically neutralizes acid in stomach
Drugs Acting Through Alteration of Normal Metabolic Pathways		
Anticancer drugs	5-Fluorouracil	Substitutes for uracil in synthesis of messenger RNA; leads to formation of nonfunctional proteins in, and death of, cancer cells
Antiparkinson drugs	Levodopa	Is synthesized to a neurotransmitter, dopamine, that helps alleviate symptoms of parkinsonism
Antidepressant	Isocarboxazid	Inhibits metabolic inactivation of the natural neurotransmitter norepinephrine in nerve endings

crease heart rate. Epinephrine acts on other receptors, and by a different mechanism of action increases heart rate. If the two agents are present simultaneously, their effects oppose each other, and the overall result may be no change of heart rate.

Drug Actions That Are Not Mediated by Specific Receptors

The actions of many important drugs follow the dose–response relationship described above, but do not involve specific receptors, and no specific receptor blockers are available to counteract their effects. Table 6–1 summarizes some of these nonreceptor-mediated drug actions, and gives examples of each.

Annotated Bibliography

Julien RM. *Drugs and the body.* New York: W.H. Freeman, 1988. *Dr. Julien gives an outstanding and refreshingly clear coverage of how many common classes of drugs affect us. If you have the slightest interest in your body, and the effects of drugs on it, read this book; you will enjoy and learn from it.*

Levine RR. *Pharmacology: Drug actions and reactions.* 4th ed. Boston: Little, Brown, 1990. *Dr. Levine's entire text is devoted to explaining fundamental concepts about pharmacology and the principles of drug action. Her text addresses general principles, rather than details, about specific drugs and their therapeutic uses. It explains otherwise difficult concepts in an unusually understandable way, supplementing the text with excellent diagrams and citing specific examples to explain a point. Any student wishing more information about basic pharmacologic principles is encouraged to read Dr. Levine's excellent book.*

Schwertz DW. Basic principles of pharmacologic action. *Nurs Clin North Am* 1991;26(2):245–262. *An excellent summary of not only how drugs "should" work, but also how other drugs, disease, and other patient-related factors, can affect the response to drugs, the overall therapeutic plan, and the nursing process.*

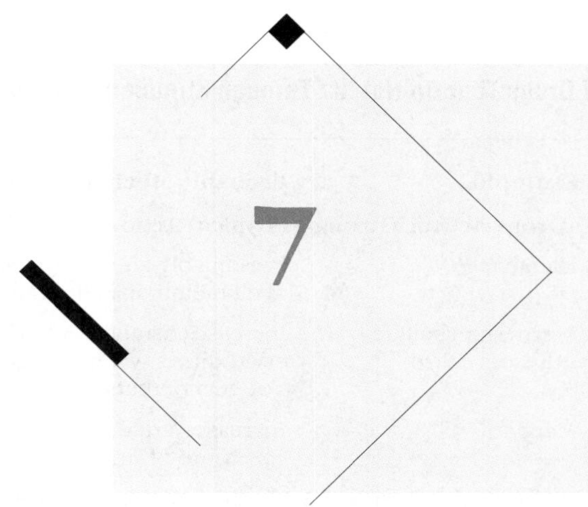

Patient-Related Factors That Affect Drug Response

In simplest terms, the effects of drugs administered to a human being are affected by two factors. One is pharmacokinetic: how absorption, distribution, metabolism, and excretion determine how much drug gets to sites of action, and how long it remains there to cause a response. The other is pharmacodynamic: how drug molecules cause a response once they reach their targets. The major assumption in Chapters 4 through 6, which covered general principles of pharmacokinetics and pharmacodynamics, was that we were dealing with "average" persons who experience average responses to usual doses of a drug. In reality (that is, in clinical practice), other factors can, and often do, alter the ways patients respond to or take drugs, and the nurse should be aware of these factors.

Since physiology, pathophysiology, and drug actions are all based on biology, it should not be surprising that many altered responses to medication have a biologic basis. However, other factors, including such things as culture, ethnicity, beliefs, and even economics, can affect not only a patient's attitudes toward illness or drug therapy but also the actual biologic response to drugs. Consideration of these nonbiologic factors is clearly important to providing optimal care in a holistic way, yet they are often overlooked.

The focus of this chapter is on major biologic and nonbiologic factors that alter drug response and drug therapy, and special circumstances in which other therapeutic goals or methods must be used. Age, perhaps the most universal and unavoidable modifier of drug responses, is discussed in the next chapter.

Biologic Factors That Affect Drug Response

Biologic factors are those that mainly, and directly, affect pharmacokinetics and pharmacodynamics. They include such things as gender, genetics, and nutrition. However, if one considers that drugs are most often used to modify a disease process, pathophysiology assumes the greatest overall importance.

Pathophysiology

The number of pathophysiologic conditions that can alter drug responses is so immense that it is impossible to cover all of them here. Likewise, there are many ways in which dysfunction can alter pharmacokinetics or pharmacodynamics. A more practical way to help understand the nature of the problem is to review the consequences of dysfunction affecting major organs or organ systems. Sometimes the actions of a particular drug are regulated most by a particular system. If that system is dysfunctional, another drug that depends more on another, more normal, system, can be used as an alternative. However, that is not always an option.

Several additional points are worth mentioning.

1. The consequences of organ system dysfunction can be unpredictable, leading to increases *or* decreases in the intensity or duration of desired therapeutic effects, side effects, or drug interactions.
2. Although the primary role of an organ or system, and its impact on drugs, may seem clear-cut, a host of secondary roles and consequences can be less obvious and are often overlooked.
3. Dysfunction of one organ or system often will be accompanied by, or can eventually lead to, dysfunction in other systems.
4. Drugs themselves can cause or intensify dysfunction of one or more organs or organ systems.
5. Finally, regardless of the drug, the dysfunction, or any laboratory tests that give information about the drug or the system, careful assessment for both desired and unwanted drug effects is crucial.

Renal Disease

As might be expected, the primary effect of renal disease is a pharmacokinetic change: altered drug excretion. The pathology may include changes in renal blood flow, changes in how well different parts of the nephron work, or both.

The severity and type of renal disease, and the dependence of a particular drug (or its metabolites) on kidney function, will affect the clinical significance of the altered drug response. Either the dose or frequency of administration of drugs that depend heavily on renal function for removal from the body must be reduced unless a suitable alternative that depends less on excretion can be substituted. One of the most common ways of assessing renal function is a laboratory test that measures serum levels of creatinine. Those values can then be used to calculate *creatinine clearance,* which is a good indicator of kidney function. Package inserts for many drugs will give recommended dosage adjustments based on specific creatinine levels. However, for most drugs the guideline is simply to reduce the dose, monitor the patient accordingly, and measure blood levels of the drug if possible.

Secondary effects of renal disease are also important. If a drug is extensively bound to plasma proteins, loss of protein into the urine can significantly increase the amount of free (active) drug in the bloodstream. This can not only increase the effect of the drug, but also change its distribution and metabolism.

Fluid retention owing to renal dysfunction can reduce the concentration of, and potentially lessen the activity of, water-soluble drugs in the bloodstream. Excessive fluid loss can do the opposite.

Since the kidneys also regulate the chemical composition of the blood, renal dysfunction and the electrolyte imbalances arising from it can cause pharmacodynamic changes. For example, hypokalemia caused by excessive renal potassium loss can greatly increase the potential toxicity of digitalis, even when digitalis blood levels are in a normal, therapeutic range.

Liver Disease

The major pharmacologic change attributable to liver dysfunction is reduced drug metabolism and the resultant increase in blood drug levels. Reduced drug metabolism can arise from dysfunction of the liver cells themselves or from decreased hepatic blood flow, and it can affect any drug that depends heavily on metabolic conversion to compounds that are less active (and potentially less toxic) or more readily excreted by the kidneys.

Hepatic dysfunction affects any highly metabolized drug, regardless of the administration route used to get the drug into the bloodstream. However, reduced hepatic function takes on added importance if a drug is given orally and depends considerably on first-pass metabolism (p. 60) to limit how much actually reaches the bloodstream. Conditions such as portasystemic shunting, in which drugs absorbed from the gut bypass the liver and enter the systemic circulation more or less directly, can magnify problems associated with drugs that depend on first-pass metabolism.

The liver is usually viewed as the major site at which chemicals, such as drugs, are broken down. However, it is also an important site for synthesis of molecules relevant to drug action. Perhaps the most important role of the liver in this regard is the synthesis of plasma proteins. In liver dysfunction, therefore, the free blood levels of drugs that are highly protein-bound can increase significantly, causing excessive or adverse effects in yet another way.

Gastrointestinal Disease

Alterations of the gastrointestinal (GI) tract have a major influence on pharmacokinetics; the main effect is impaired absorption of orally administered drugs. Changes of local pH, as from increased or decreased acid secretion in the stomach, or bicarbonate secretion in the duodenum, can affect drug ionization and therefore the ability of molecules to be absorbed. A change in gut motility, such as occurs with diarrhea or vomiting, or reduced intestinal blood flow will also impair absorption.

However, GI dysfunction does not cause only pharmacokinetic changes, nor does it affect only orally administered drugs. For example, systemic electrolyte imbalances, or generalized or specific nutritional deficiencies, can arise from altered secretion, motility, or blood flow in the GI tract. These, in turn, can significantly change the ways in which many drugs already in the bloodstream act on their cellular targets, or the ways in which the cells respond to the drugs. These are pharmacodynamic alterations that could occur regardless of the route of drug administration.

The liver and pancreas are, properly, part of the gastrointestinal system, and so still more outcomes of GI tract disease can be identified. Problems owing to liver dysfunction have been highlighted above. Since the pancreas is responsible for synthesizing and releasing enzymes and other substances responsible for digestion, hormones (eg, insulin), and other mediators with local or systemic actions, a variety of pharmacokinetic and pharmacodynamic changes of drug action could occur when pancreatic dysfunction occurs.

Cardiovascular Disease

Heart failure, which can be defined as any decreased ability of the heart to pump blood, is one of the most common cardiovascular disorders. Given the central role of the heart in supplying blood to all the organs, cardiac failure is also the condition with the greatest potential to cause altered responses to drugs.

A generalized slowing of drug distribution throughout the body caused by the heart's diminished pumping activity is not as important as it might seem. The main problem is that if the heart fails, so do the other organs. Thus, decreased renal, hepatic, and intestinal blood flow can lead to changes in all the processes ascribed to those organs, discussed above.

Nutrition

Diet composition and eating habits alter mainly the pharmacokinetics of drugs, and nutritional disease or nutritional deficiencies mainly alter drug effects.

Diet

Diet composition and eating patterns can modify drug actions. Food in the stomach or intestine may inhibit drug absorption by acting as a mechanical barrier. When a drug is taken with food, absorption may be delayed, resulting in lower peak blood levels. Delayed absorption does not mean that the drug is incompletely absorbed; rather, absorption takes longer to occur. Conversely, absorption rates may be increased in the fasting patient, resulting in a quicker response to a drug. If blood levels rise too quickly, acute side effects or toxicity may occur.

Drug absorption can also be decreased—or increased—by chemical interaction with foods or by prolonged exposure to the gastrointestinal environment. Some drugs (certain penicillins, for example) are destroyed by exposure to gastric acid. Other drugs (eg, tetracycline) interact with calcium in foods (mainly milk and milk products) to form an insoluble complex, thereby reducing, not merely slowing, absorption. Interactions with nonnutrient substances, such as fiber and pectin, are also known to slow or decrease absorption of some drugs. Food intake may enhance the absorption of other drugs.

Drug metabolism can also be affected by dietary intake. A high-protein–low-carbohydrate diet tends to promote rapid metabolism, as do vegetables such as cabbage and brussels sprouts, and charcoal broiling of foods.

Diet composition also alters rates of renal and biliary excretion. High-protein or high-fat diets may decrease biliary excretion of some drugs, while a high-fiber diet may increase excretion. Dietary electrolytes and proteins, which alter urine pH, influence drug excretion and reabsorption by the kidney.

Nutritional Disease

As may be expected, obese patients have more extensive distribution of highly lipid-soluble drugs. The alteration in distribution may also result in slowed elimination. Dieting, with rapid-loss of body fat, may release into the bloodstream highly fat-soluble drugs that had been stored in the body's fatty tissues.

Malnutrition is usually complex, with many different deficiencies occurring together. The different forms of malnutrition alter drug effects in various ways. Hypoalbuminemia occurs with most forms of malnutrition and generally increases the serum level of protein-bound drugs and the risk of overdosage. Conversely, the lack of protein binding can increase renal excretion of drugs, resulting in more rapid elimination.

Protein, mineral, and vitamin deficiencies alter enzyme activity, which alters drug metabolism (pharmacokinetics) or activity (pharmacodynamics). Hepatic drug metabolism is generally enhanced by protein-calorie malnutrition in adults, but is decreased in children. Similar differences have been found for renal excretion, with elimination times increased in protein-calorie malnourished children and decreased in undernourished adults.

Biologic Rhythms

Biologic rhythms are self-sustaining, time-dependent rises and falls in the activity of body processes. The *circadian rhythm* is a biologic rhythm that repeats itself in a cycle that lasts roughly 24 hours, affecting such things as body temperature, blood pressure, and heart and respiratory rates.

Biologic rhythms are internally controlled, but they can be altered by a variety of factors, mainly those coming from the external environment. Jet lag and staying awake all night to study for an exam are two common examples of activities that can alter the biologic clock. Biologic rhythms have the potential to alter the pharmacokinetics and pharmacodynamics of drugs, but for most medications their effect is insignificant and they are not a major factor in deciding when to administer a particular drug.

In terms of therapeutics, cyclic fluctuations in hormone levels are the most important biologic rhythm. When hormones are used as replacement therapy for a hormone deficiency, the goal is to mimic the natural rises and falls of hormone levels, so proper timing of administration is crucial. For example, insulin is given to a diabetic person before a meal so that its blood levels (and effects) will be high at the proper time, when blood glucose levels rise after eating. Corticosteroids are usually given in the morning to persons with a hypofunctioning adrenal cortex, again for the purpose of mimicking what should occur naturally.

In other cases, the goal is not to mimic natural patterns but to overcome or counteract them. The best example is the use of estrogen and progesterone as oral contraceptives. Here the intent is to create, at a specific time governed by normal biologic patterns, hormone levels that are very nonphysiologic, and also very effective in preventing conception. Even though the goal may be different from that in hormone replacement therapy, proper timing of drug administration is still critical.

Gender

For the most part, gender has little or no clinically significant effect on the fate, action, or use of most drugs. An obvious exception, of course, is the current use of hormones to prevent pregnancy, or to manage symptoms of menopause or other conditions found only in females. Another example of how gender affects drug action and use involves the treatment (or causation) of some hormone-dependent cancers. For instance, "female" hormones (estrogens and progestins) may suppress some cancers in males, yet estrogen used as replacement therapy in menopause *may* increase the risk of breast carcinoma. Conversely, androgens, which can be considered "male" hormones, can suppress some cancers found in women.

Genetics

Based on our current knowledge, genetic factors account for many instances in which a patient's response to a "usual" does of certain drugs is absent or excessive, or unusually short or very prolonged. Even rarer are genetic factors that cause a different *kind* of response, rather than a different *intensity* of response, to a certain drug. As noted in Chapter 9, these are called *idiosyncratic reactions.* They usually involve genetically determined differences in the rates of drug metabolism, or unusual changes in the metabolic pathways that convert a drug to other substances. Genetic factors that alter drug response are inherited. They may be prevalent in a relatively large subpopulation of people (eg, those of Asian or European descent), or may be more or less confined to a few individuals and their offspring.

Genetic research is one of the most promising and important areas of biomedical research. In the near future it is likely to show that there are many more hereditary factors involved in altered drug responses—and even in the occurrence of diseases that are treated with drugs—than we now appreciate.

Drug Effects as Modifiers of Drug Effects

All the information presented in this chapter and in Chapters 4, 5, and 6 can be summarized in two very simple, but very important statements:

1. Drugs affect physiology and pathophysiology.
2. Physiology and pathophysiology are the major factors that affect the actions of, and responses to, drugs.

This seems like roundabout logic, but it is absolutely true. The sentences mean that the biologic effects of one drug can, and often do, have considerable impact on the biologic responses to other drugs. (In fact, some drugs actually alter their own effects.) To carry this one step further, the more drugs administered to a patient, the greater the potential variability in drug responses—desired or not. Multidrug therapy is especially common in the elderly, who may have several diseases for which treatment with many drugs is necessary. Special considerations for the elderly (and for children) are covered in Chapter 8, which deals with age as a determinant of drug effects. General principles concerning drug–drug interactions are covered in detail in Chapter 9. But first, it is important to consider some of the equally important nonbiologic factors that affect drug action and drug use.

Psychosocial Factors That Affect Drug Response

Economic, social, cultural, intellectual, and ethnic background, as well as attitudes and health beliefs, all influence drug therapy.

Economic Factors and Resources

Drugs are one of the most cost-effective health interventions available. Some patients may associate economic cost with effectiveness—if a drug is very expensive, then it must be very effective. Conversely, an inexpensive drug may be thought of as being less effective.

In some situations, however, the cost of medications may adversely affect drug therapy. Some patients simply cannot afford to purchase a drug, or they may look at the perceived cost–benefit ratio and decide that the expense does not justify the expected benefits of therapy. The result may be to never take a drug, to discontinue a medication early, or to reduce the dosage of a medication. Generic drugs usually provide a lower-cost alternative to brand name drugs, and may be an effective way to reduce drug costs.

Attitudes Toward Medications

Attitudes develop over a long period and are based on past experiences and learning. Psychosocial, cultural, physiologic, and spiritual backgrounds interact to form a mind-set unique to each patient. Among the most influential forces in attitude development are cultural beliefs and practices. The patient's willingness and ability to adhere to therapeutic recommendations (compliance; see below) can be improved by assessing the patient's attitude and working within the patient's own framework. Response to a drug is modulated by the total person, and is not just a biologic response.

Placebo Effects

A placebo is a substance that is biologically inactive, yet can cause a response when taken by a patient. The word *placebo* means "I will please" in Latin. It is a term that recognizes the fact that the visual and verbal cues the patient receives from the provider, as well as the expectations and attitudes of the patient, can cause an effect. The administration of a tablet containing nothing but starch may calm an anxious person. Injecting nothing but a few milliliters of saline may alleviate pain in another.

The placebo effect is usually attributed to the power of suggestion, and is linked not only to the expectations and attitudes of the patient, but also to those of the person administering the drug. As such, the frequency or intensity of the placebo response is highly variable. Nevertheless, it is an important factor that modifies drug responses. Indeed, it is so important that the testing of new drugs before approval and widespread clinical use at some point includes comparisons of the new (and active) drug with a placebo.

There are several ethical and legal implications of placebo therapy for the nurse who is caring for ill patients. One is that the nurse should not administer placebos when he or she believes safe and effective active drugs can be used instead. If the nurse has any concerns about administering a placebo to a given patient, he or she should notify the prescribing physician and document the concerns and the physician's responses in writing. If the nurse believes the placebo is a reasonable and effective alternative, most legal and ethical guidelines dictate that patients (or others who are legally responsible for their care) be informed of the treatment, and that the patient's or guardian's questions are both solicited and answered honestly. Again, written documentation is important.

Such ethical and legal dilemmas concerning the use of a placebo instead of an active drug will occur during the nurse's career. (Indeed, the likelihood of such instances will increase as there is more dialogue about care for the terminally ill.) In the vast majority of situations, however, active drugs will be prescribed. Capitalize on the potential of the placebo effect to have a positive influence on drug therapy by conveying a positive and caring attitude to the patient. There may be no scientific explanation for this, but it cannot hurt.

Cultural Differences

Cultural attitudes toward illness and drug therapy vary widely. It is important for the nurse to be aware of these attitudes. Those of us who have grown up in Western cultures may be used to a certain type of medical care, but for others, things may be very different. For example, herbology (the use of herbs as medications) is an important part of Chinese and other Asian cultures, as it is for many of the Native Americans who live in this country. Many herbal remedies contain ingredients that are pharmacologically identical or similar to, or can interact with, those prescribed by Western physicians. This can set the stage for drug interactions, or toxicity, or antagonism of prescribed drug effects.

It is also common for persons to have ethnically based attitudes about when to seek health care, or from whom to seek it. For example, some Chinese persons may go to both an herbologist and a Western physician. These practitioners may prescribe the same or different medications. And it may be awkward for the patient to tell one practitioner that he or she is being treated by another who might have a different (and sometimes culturally unacceptable) therapeutic approach.

Cultural dimensions are also a part of administering medicines and patient teaching. When teaching about a medication schedule, it may not be appropriate to suggest taking a pill "three times a day with meals," since in many cultures meals are not eaten three times a day, but in smaller portions at more frequent intervals.

It is also important to consider whom to involve in the patient teaching. While most Western societies have dyad relationships, Third World societies usually have multiperson health-care networks. Because an extended and large family network is often involved in health care, and because language barriers can make communication difficult, it may be particularly important to involve several family members in teaching about medication.

Self-Medication

Many drugs or drug combinations are sold without medical supervision or prescription. The high incidence of self-medication should be of concern to health professionals. Many products claiming to alleviate common ailments can be found in most drug stores. Patients are bombarded with advertising that encourages self-medication. The selection of safe and appropriate products is sometimes influenced more by expensive advertising than by knowledge and understanding.

Many reasons for self-medication exist. Frequently, it is due to the inconvenience and cost of seeking qualified medical guidance. Other common reasons include the desire for privacy, and the inability to understand or accurately diagnose underlying medical problems so that professional care is sought.

Self-medication need not be considered a negative behavior. When done appropriately, it is desirable and is an important component of primary health care. However, the consumer needs to be educated about the basic facts and the appropriate use of over-the-counter (OTC) drugs.

It is essential that health-care providers be alert for self-medication in patients. Often the patient does not volunteer information about self-medication. Interactions between OTC drugs and prescription drugs, as well as inappropriate drug self-medication, should be identified during the nursing assessment. For example, aspirin or aspirin-containing preparations may prolong the effect of certain anticoagulants and cause serious bleeding problems. Some OTC medications, particularly cold remedies and nose drops, contain drugs that may increase blood pressure and can be dangerous for individuals who are already hypertensive.

Patients may also alter or use prescription drugs indiscriminately. They tend to discontinue disliked medications, maintain and reuse outdated medications, or "share" prescribed medications with others. All of these are potentially dangerous self-medication practices.

Compliance and Noncompliance

The extent to which a patient follows directions from a health professional is termed **compliance.** Compliance with a drug regimen refers to adherence to the prescribed dose, method of administration, dose scheduling, and any other related factors. Many things affect a patient's adherence to (compliance) or degree of deviation from (noncompliance) a drug treatment regimen.

Research indicates that at least one quarter to one half of all outpatients fail, for various reasons, to follow their prescribed drug therapy correctly. Surprisingly, factors such as gender, age, social class, education, and mental status show little consistency in affecting compliance. Noncompliance is more common when treatment regimens are complex, asymptomatic or psychiatric disorders are present, long treatment periods are required, and troublesome side effects exist. Among the factors that have been implicated by research to have an important effect on drug compliance are patient and health personnel communication, level of patient instruction, severity of illness and symptoms as assessed by the patient, fear of side effects, forgetfulness, and inconvenient dose schedule.

TRENDS AND CONTROVERSIES IN PHARMACOLOGY

Is Noncompliance a Nonissue?

A great deal of research during the 1960s and 1970s tried unsuccessfully to identify the characteristics of the "noncompliant patient." The underlying premise of the research was that caregivers needed to identify "bad" patients and convince them to take their medicine. After scores of studies, it is clear that age, sex, marital status, educational level, income, and other personal factors are not consistently associated with noncompliance. In fact, noncompliance is so widespread that it might be considered more normal than exceptional.

Because judgments about patients were often implicit in early work on compliance, the terms adherence and nonadherence were introduced as alternatives (Blackwell, 1976). While these terms are preferred by some, they don't alter the complexity and frustration—that can be experienced by patients and health care providers alike—when dealing with compliance. Today, it's clear that whichever term is used, both patients and providers share responsibilities helping to ensure that prescribed therapies are followed (Ross, 1991).

There are several possible consequences when patients do not comply with prescribed medication regimens. The obvious concern of prescribers is the possibility of a decreased therapeutic effect from the medicine that might result in unnecessary complications: a recurrence of illness; the risk of transmitting a communicable disease; or extended patient discomfort, for example. There could also be an increased rate of adverse drug reactions, especially if the patient is taking more of the drug than prescribed or he or she misses important safety directions.

Noncompliance also can lead to other problems. If a first-line drug is not taken as prescribed and the patient doesn't improve, the prescriber may increase the dose, or try a more potent drug. Either choice unnecessarily increases the patient's risk of adverse drug reactions. If this is carried even further, the patient's condition might be labeled refractory to medical treatment. Invasive diagnostic testing or surgery might be recommended.

If caregivers refrain from viewing noncompliance as a personal affront, and approach the issue objectively, the same problem-solving techniques that are used in other patient-care situations can be used. Many factors that influence compliance and noncompliance can be controlled to some extent by the doctor, nurse, or pharmacist, rather than by the patient.

If anything makes it difficult for the patient to follow a prescribed regimen, it is not likely that the drug will be taken as ordered. Working from this premise, rather than from the usual assumption of perfect compliance, focuses on the patient's perspective and makes it easier to anticipate potential problems. The easiest, most palatable dosage form usually should be the one prescribed. For example, the patient might find it easier to swallow two 300-mg tablets than one large 600-mg tablet, or he or she might prefer an orange-flavored liquid to cherry. Choices also apply to some drugs that aren't given orally. For example, a transdermal patch of a drug such as nitroglycerin might be much more convenient and pleasant to use than nitroglycerin ointment. When alternative but equally effective ways of delivering the drug are available, the patient should be given a choice. Just remember—you and other health care providers are more aware of therapeutic alternatives than are patients. Unless you familiarize yourself with those choices, and make the patient aware of them, achieving the goal of improved compliance will be harder to reach.

Perhaps most important, caregivers need to remember that the patient has a right to be noncompliant. However, noncompliance can affect the welfare of individual patients as well as public health. When compliance becomes a factor in the patient's course of therapy, good communication and an openness to whatever the patient sees as barriers to taking the medicine will help to ensure that solutions that work for both patient and prescriber can be found. It takes patients and health care providers working together to make noncompliance a nonissue.

Blackwell B: Treatment adherence. *Br J Psychiatry* 1976;129:513–531.

Ross FM: Patient compliance—whose responsibility? *Soc Sci Med* 1991;32:89–94.

Several theories have been proposed to help health-care professionals understand compliance and noncompliance. One theory states that if patients feel susceptible to illness, believe the illness to have potential serious consequences, and do not anticipate serious obstacles (such as side effects, inconvenience, or cost), they are more likely to comply with the drug regimen. Knowledge affects initial compliance, but perceived benefits are more important in determining long-term compliance.

Compliance has also been tied to the quality of

the patient–health-care provider relationship. Studies suggest that compliance is high when the health-care provider gives explicit instructions and more and clearer information and feedback. Noncompliance is the result of a problem with the patient–provider relationship. Problems may stem from differing expectations and poor communication. Communications skills are very important. Compliance will not be guaranteed just by telling patients what to do, or by saying that drug therapy will be good for them. Compliance can be enhanced, however, by an understandable presentation of information and an honest exchange of ideas between the patient and the care provider.

The patient-centered perspective assumes that patients have their own ideas about taking medications. They often do. Patients compare what they know about medication and illness with the prescribed drugs and the health-care provider's actions. Noncompliance may result when patients do not consider the treatment appropriate, or when medical regimens are not compatible with some aspect of their lives. Other patients may alter treatment regimens in an attempt to maintain control of their own medical care. Up to a point, this interest in self-care is not bad, and a patient's desire to maintain control actually can be beneficial. Patients who are genuinely concerned about their illness and treatment, and who assume some responsibility for their well-being, are likely to be more compliant (and respond better) than those who do not care.

Poor patient compliance may lead to adverse drug effects. Incorrect self-medication, inappropriate timing, underdosage, overdosage, or taking medication with or without food can all affect the results of drug therapy. The patients most at risk are those taking drugs with a narrow therapeutic index, or drugs for which the timing of the dosage is especially important.

If a patient feels that the doctor or nurse has not understood the primary complaint, or perceives the health-care provider as unfriendly, drug compliance is often reduced. Compliance is better when a patient sees the same personnel at each health-care visit.

The need for instruction, and the level of instruction needed for each drug, varies widely among patients. The best determination of appropriate instruction is made by thorough patient assessment. The need for instruction is based on several factors, including the patient's level of education, language difficulties, perceptions, and compliance with previous treatment regimens. Repeated and consistent instruction is helpful. Written instructions reinforce verbal instructions, and allow the patient to review the instructions at a later time. Specific instruction is important to compliance. If a dose should be taken at specific times, then that fact should be clearly stated (eg, "at 7 AM, 3 PM, and 11 PM" rather than "three times a day").

An acute disease or one with significant symptoms usually motivates patients to comply with drug therapy. The level of compliance drops as the duration of therapy increases or as symptoms disappear. As a rule, the longer a patient has been asymptomatic, the greater the temptation to reduce compliance. Prophylaxis (prevention) and long-term therapy are associated with the greatest risk for gradually decreased compliance.

Another reason for noncompliance is fear or dislike of side effects. For example, a hypertensive man may find that his antihypertensive medication causes impotence. Rather than accept this side effect he may stop taking the medication. Even though a patient may fear an adverse drug reaction, that concern may be withheld from the health-care provider. A thorough nursing assessment should bring out reasons for noncompliance, and the nurse may then suggest that the patient confer with the physician for an alternative treatment that will not cause the same effect. All drug therapy involves a balance between benefit and risk, and it cannot be assumed that all patients willingly accept risk. A patient may fear a particular undesirable effect, and elect not to take the drug or to undertreat himself or herself. The nurse must assess what levels of information the patient needs, wants, and can understand about possible side effects and provide a nonjudgmental atmosphere for patient teaching and discussion.

Forgetfulness may seem like an all-too-obvious reason for failing to take a medication appropriately, yet it is a common one, and one for which the nurse can provide assistance. The number of missed doses increases as the number of doses and medications increase. Numerous aids are available to help the patient remember to take medications. This is particularly important for the geriatric patient who may be taking several medications daily.

Complex therapy is hard to follow; impractical dosage regimens should be avoided if possible. A medication schedule that does not follow the patient's own schedule is not likely to be followed closely. Administration times should be adjusted as much as possible for each patient, with the drug regimen tailored to the patient's daily schedule, as long as the adjustments do not significantly hinder the desired outcomes of therapy.

Dependence

The term **drug dependence** has become commonly used in our society, and "drug dependant" is often used as a negative label. It is important for the nurse to realize that dependence on a drug is not always bad. Indeed, one should understand that many drug therapies were developed because most patients depend on them—psychologically and physiologically—for safe and effective relief of the signs and symptoms of illness. Drugs become one of the most effective, economic, safe, and acceptable means to provide wellness. In fact, most patients depend on drug therapy to maintain and prolong a productive life that would not be possible without medication. Circumstances in which drug administration (or self-administration) results in unwanted dependency will be discussed in Chapter 28.

Nursing Considerations in Special Circumstances

Pregnancy and Lactation

Pregnant and lactating women should avoid unnecessary drug use. Minor ailments should be treated with nonpharmacologic methods if possible. When drugs are used, those drugs with the least expected adverse effects should be used and the risk–benefit ratio carefully considered. Drug therapy during pregnancy necessitates close supervision. Patient education includes informed consent and explanation of possible effects of the drug on the fetus or nursing child.

No woman of childbearing age should ever be given a drug without first determining whether she is pregnant. A fundamental concept for the nurse to remember when administering a drug to a pregnant woman is that the drug will be administered to two patients, the adult and the fetus.

Several factors influence the extent to which a drug will cross the placental barrier into the fetal circulation. Drug factors that increase the rate of diffusion into fetal circulation are low molecular weight, low protein binding, high lipid solubility, and a low degree of ionization. High maternal concentrations and increased length of therapy all increase the fetal drug levels.

The effects of drugs on the fetus are variable and not completely understood. Gestational age is important in determining susceptibility to adverse effects of drug exposure. Drug transfer across the placenta is probably greatest in late pregnancy, although the fetus is most susceptible to damage during the early stages of development (first trimester). A great concern with drug therapy is that the drug will cause structural defects (teratogenesis) or impairment of normal fetal growth and development. Thalidomide is a tragic example of a drug, formerly given during pregnancy, that was later found to cause defective limb formation.

Some drugs administered chronically during pregnancy, such as narcotics or barbiturates, can lead to neonatal physiologic dependence and withdrawal symptoms. Systemic analgesics and sedatives given during the late stages of labor may cause neonatal cardiovascular and respiratory depression, and they may also delay or prolong labor.

Because of the newborn's immature physiologic systems, drugs may have a prolonged effect. Giving the mother large doses of drugs such as diazepam shortly before delivery may result in the presence of pharmacologically significant levels of the drug and its active metabolites in the neonate for up to a week after birth.

A lactating woman may also pass drugs to the nursing child through the breast milk. The same factors that influence maternal–placental transfer of drugs affect transfer of drugs into the milk. The degree of neonatal exposure is related to the concentration of drug in the milk and the amount of milk consumed.

The nurse should consider several factors related to drug therapy for mothers who wish to nurse their infants. One is to ensure that drug use is really necessary. If so, then it is important to learn whether alternative drugs might be equally effective for the mother but less likely to harm the infant.

Timing drug administration with respect to breastfeeding is also important. Feeding the child just before taking a medication, for example, can help the mother limit the child's exposure to drug. Assessing the child for expected drug effects (eg, drowsinesss or poor feeding habits when the mother is taking a central nervous system depressant) is, of course, important. The therapeutic outcome will be improved by fostering the mother's cooperation and understanding of the potential problems. The nurse may also have to serve as a liaison between the mother's physician and the pediatrician.

Surgery

The effect of surgery on drug responses has only recently been considered. Many patients are not allowed to take anything by mouth (NPO) during the 12 hours before surgery and for several hours or days after. Patients are often allowed to take oral medications with sips of water on the morning of surgery, or an alternate route of administration may be used. Gastric absorption of oral medications may be enhanced in these fasting patients.

Most medications that have been administered before surgery are continued to avoid rebound or withdrawal effects intraoperatively or during the immediate postoperative period. All members of the patient's health-care team must be aware of *all* drugs the patient has recently received.

Psychiatric Settings

In most situations psychiatric drug therapy is not used as a substitute for, but as an enhancement of, appropriate psychotherapy. The risk of overmedication exists in the treatment of any disorder, but it may be more common in the treatment of psychiatric disorders. Before drugs are used, nursing measures should be employed for the patient with altered perceptions, behavior, sleep patterns, or anxiety. Routine use of sedative-hypnotics and mood-altering drugs ordered as needed (prn) must be periodically evaluated to avoid excessive and unnecessary medication.

Chronic use of mood-altering drugs may lead to tolerance or other unwanted effects. Careful assessment is needed to identify which effects are present. Depressed or disturbed patients should be closely monitored for suicide attempts following initiation of therapy. The danger of suicide is increased as a patient's depressive state is lessened, and energy is increased, by drug therapy.

Many psychiatric patients also have coexisting medical disorders that are being treated with medications. Interactions with psychiatric drugs are common and may result in exacerbation of the medical problems, either by drug interactions or by a direct effect of psychotropic medications. For example, some of the antipsychotic and antidepressant drugs may lead to urinary retention, an important consideration for elderly men with prostatic hypertrophy, or may increase the risk of serious harm in persons who have glaucoma.

Education is very important for both the patient and the family. Medication must be taken as prescribed, and abrupt withdrawal or dosage changes must be avoided. Family members can help monitor the patient's medication regimens. The patient may experience altered states of reality, confusion, manipulative behavior, or other behavior disturbances and may be unable to comply with the medical therapy.

The effect of some psychotropic medications may not be immediately evident; weeks or months may be required to develop and maintain therapeutic effects. It is important that the patient not become discouraged and discontinue treatment.

Emergency Situations

Life-threatening situations require prompt, aggressive intervention. Assessment must be brief but thorough. Even in its briefest form, the assessment should include obtaining information about drug allergies, current medications, and preexisting medical conditions. If the patient is unconscious or obtunded, assessment may be limited to objective data; subjective data in such cases may be gathered from the patient's family and friends, if available. The presence of a badge, bracelet, or card identifying allergies, drug therapy, or significant medical history should be ascertained. If the emergency is a poisoning, the time, amount, and specific toxin involved should be determined as accurately as possible. Immediate goals are to stabilize and maintain vital functions and minimize damage. Emergencies are also a time of acute psychologic stress for the patient; the nurse must always remember to treat the whole patient, not just a physiologic system.

In emergency situations drugs are most commonly administered by intravenous bolus or infusion for rapid effect and to avoid problems with delayed or otherwise altered absorption from other routes. Mixing and administering emergency medications must be done with care and strict adherence to principles of correct drug administration to avoid potentially catastrophic errors owing to overdose or interactions.

Cancer

Caring for the patient with cancer presents many challenges to the nurse. Frequently, many factors that alter drug response are present. In addition to other preexisting diseases, cancer affects the normal physiologic functioning of many body systems. The area involved by the cancer will provide the nurse with an indication of what to expect.

Drugs or other therapies for cancer may alter drug response more than the cancer itself. Toxicities are associated with both antineoplastic drugs and radiation therapy. It is the toxic effect on the major organ systems that alters the pharmacokinetics and subsequently the drug response. Many of the drugs used in cancer treatment are highly toxic, and adverse effects can develop at any time during therapy, even when doses are within therapeutic ranges. For example, the nausea and vomiting caused by many antineoplastic agents may lead to fluid, electrolyte, and nutritional imbalances that can affect both pharmacodynamics and pharmacokinetics.

The diagnosis and subsequent treatment of cancer will evoke a wide range of psychologic responses in patients and their families. The various stages of denial, grief, and acceptance, as well as the economic burden of therapy, all affect patient attitudes and compliance with drug therapy.

Annotated Bibliography

American Academy of Pediatrics Committee on Drugs. Transfer of drugs and other chemicals into human milk. *Pediatrics* 1989; 84(5):924–936. *Contains many tables that can be consulted quickly for information about potential effects of drugs ingested by infants through breast milk, plus general advice and information. A must-see article for the pediatric nurse.*

Berlin CM Jr. Drugs and chemicals: Exposure of the nursing mother. *Pediatr Clin North Am* 1989;36(5):1089–1097. *Provides practical information to help enable nursing mothers who need medication to nurse safely.*

Conrad P. The meaning of medications: Another look at compliance. *Soc Sci Med* 1985;20(1):29–37. *Presents an alternative, patient-centered approach to managing medications, using data from 80 in-depth interviews of people with epilepsy. This approach focuses on the meanings of medication in patients everyday lives and looks at why people take their medications, as well as why they do not.*

Diamond R. Drugs and the quality of life: The patient's point of view. *J Clin Psych* 1985;46:5(Sec 2):29–35. *Addresses the issue of quality of life of patients taking long-term medication. Social functioning, acceptance of dose, compliance or lack of compliance, and the relative benefits of medication are some of the factors that contribute to treatment goals.*

Gardner M, Hurd PD, Slack M. Effect of information organization on recall of medication instructions. *J Clin Pharm Ther* 1990; 15(1):13–19. *This is the outcome of a study of how presenting drug-related information to pharmacy students affects proper knowledge recall. The results are important to all health-care providers: present the information in an organized understandable way, and recall will be enhanced.*

Gibbs S, Waters WE, George CF. The benefits of prescriptions information leaflets. *Br J Clin Pharmacol* 1989;27(6):723–739 and 28(3):345–351. *Package inserts and other prescription information leaflets can have a dramatic impact on patient knowledge and compliance. If the nurse becomes the primary communicator of information, it is essential for him or her to condense, simplify, and explain this written knowledge.*

Hill RF, Fortenberyy D, Stein HF. Culture in clinical medicine. *South Med J* 1990;83(9):1071–1080. *An exceptionally well written review of what culture should mean to, and how it should be taken into account by, health-care providers. This is a "don't miss" article for readers interested in the subject.*

Kuwaki T. *Chinese herbal therapy: A guide to its principles and practice.* Long Beach, CA: Oriental Healing Arts Institute, 1990. *This is a therapeutic manual written for practitioners of traditional Chinese herbal medicine (and its Japanese counterpart, Kampo). But it is as an invaluable "prototype" reference for any nursing student or nurse who wishes to understand the importance of cultural beliefs as a factor that modifies the patient's attitudes to Western medicine, regardless of the patient's ethnicity.*

Lawrence RA. Breastfeeding and medical disease. *Med Clin North Am* 1989; 73(3):583–603. *This article discusses the key considerations in managing the lactating woman with an illness for which the therapy includes drugs that are excreted in breast milk.*

Lund VE, Frank DI. Helping the medicine go down: Nurse's and patients' perceptions about medication compliance. *J Psychosoc Nurs Ment Health Serv* 1991;29(7):6–9. *A short but instructive insight into why patients do not comply with therapy, and how nurses view such noncompliance.*

Macleod SM, Soldin SJ. Determinants of drug disposition in man. *Clin Biochem* 1986;19:67–71. *This article reviews some of the important determinants of variation in drug disposition, such as age, gender, body weight, diet, environmental influences, drug–protein interactions, compliance, drug–drug interactions, endogenous substances, disease states, circadian variation, and genetics.*

Nice FJ. Breastfeeding and medications: An update (Part I). *J Pract Nurs* 1990;40(2):39–52. *An excellent self-instructional program for the nurse who needs to know about the impact of drug therapy on breast-feeding.*

Patient teaching. *Nurs Clin North Am* 1989;24(3):583–693. *This is an entire issue containing many must-read articles for students and practitioners who wish to learn how patient teaching—and all its ramifications—is and will continue to be an important consideration in optimal drug therapy.*

Peach H. Trends in self-prescribing and attitudes to self-medication. *Practitioner* 1983;227:1609–1613. *Sources of information about self-prescribing are discussed, and the major studies of general practitioners' and patients' attitudes to self-medication are reviewed.*

Rost K, Roter D, Bertakis K, Quill T. Physician-patient familiarity and patient recall of medication changes: The Collaborative Study Group of the SIGM Task Force and the Doctor and Patient. *Fam Med* 1990; 22(6):453–457. *An insightful discussion of how patients' familiarity with their health-care providers, as well as the amount and detail of therapy-related information provided to them, can affect understanding of and compliance with drug therapy.*

Ruffalo RL, Garabedian-Ruffalo SM, Pawlson LG. Patient compliance. *Am Fam Physician* 1985; 31(6):93–100. *The complex, multifactorial nature of compliance is discussed, as well as compliance-improving strategies based on behavioral therapy.*

Smith CH, Bidlack WR. Dietary concerns associated with the use of medications. *J Am Dietetic Assoc* 1984;84:901–914. *A research-based review of the interactions between drugs and various components in the diet, this paper covers the effect of drugs on nutritional related factors such as appetite, taste acuity, and GI function.*

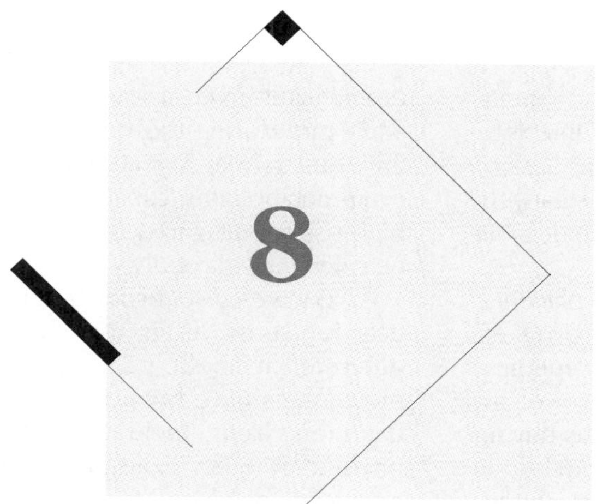

Age as a Modifier of Drug Response

Many factors can significantly alter a person's response to drugs. Indeed, even drugs can alter the response to drugs. However, by using a wellness-oriented lifestyle, and with lots of luck, we can avoid or at least minimize our exposure to most modifying factors. There are two factors over which we have no control, however. One is gender, although in general that has little clinically significant impact on responses to most drugs. The other is age, and its associated physiologic and pathophysiologic characteristics. Age has significant effects on drug responses, and it is the focus of this chapter.

It will soon become apparent, especially from reading the section of this chapter devoted to the elderly, that simultaneous diseases of organs or organ systems have considerable impact on drug responses and drug therapy. Those changes make it essential for the nurse to pay special attention to therapy at each step of the nursing process. Although certain illnesses that alter drug responses may be more common in the elderly, they are not found only in elders. As a result, much of the information presented here applies to patients of all ages. In the previous chapter you saw that many variables, unrelated to age, can affect pharmacotherapy and drug responses. The age-related and age-unrelated factors can, and usually do, go hand-in-hand, so it is important to view them as integrated, not as separate or mutually exclusive.

The behavior of drugs in neonates, infants and children, and older adults may be considerably different from that in the young adult, and so these age groups are the focus of this chapter. Because pregnancy can occur over a large range of maternal ages—and so it is less "age"-related—it will be discussed in the next chapter.

Neonates

Variable drug actions occur in neonates because of the biologic characteristics of newborns, including their small body mass, low body fat content, high body water volume, and greater membrane permeability of the skin and blood–brain barrier. The physiologic instability of premature infants also requires special consideration in drug therapy.

Physiology of Neonates

Absorption

In newborns, prolonged gastric transit time, variable gastric pH, and low levels of intestinal flora and enzyme function affect absorption when medications are given by mouth. Low peripheral perfusion rates and immature heat regulating mechanisms may also interfere with absorption. In contrast, topical medications are absorbed more quickly through the newborn's relatively thin skin barrier, so that the risk of drug toxicity is greater in these patients.

Absorption can also occur through the placenta, and so newborns should be evaluated for drug effects whenever the mother has received any medication. Drugs given to the mother for pain control or inhibition of premature labor can pass to the fetus during labor. In addition, drugs prescribed for the mother as part of her own long-term care, such as antihypertensives or hypoglycemic agents, are absorbed in utero and affect the newborn.

Distribution

The unique nature of newborn physiology has significant effects on drug distribution. Newborns have a low concentration of plasma proteins and a diminished albumin binding capacity, resulting in a decreased total plasma protein binding capacity. This decreased binding capacity can be responsible for some serious adverse drug effects. For example, plasma proteins can bind with bilirubin. Drugs that are highly protein bound can displace the bilirubin and may thereby lead to brain damage from kernicterus, as a result of hyperbilirubinemia. In addition, immature glial cell development, especially evident among premature infants, permits greater permeability of the blood–brain barrier. This allows both drugs and bilirubin rapid access to the central nervous system.

The volume of distribution within neonatal body compartments differs greatly from the adult. Total body water amounts to 70% to 80% of body weight in premature and newborn infants, compared with adult values of 50% to 55%. Extracellular fluid is about 40% of body weight, which is roughly twice the adult value. The increased body water content coupled with the low plasma binding results in an expanded volume of distribution for water-soluble drugs. A larger relative dose of such drugs may be necessary to produce the desired therapeutic effect. Conversely, the lower level of body fat in neonates may necessitate giving relatively lower doses of lipid-soluble drugs.

Metabolism

Hepatic drug-metabolizing enzymes are immature in the newborn, and are especially ineffective in the premature neonate. After birth, metabolic capacity may rise dramatically from a low of one fifth to one third the adult rate during the first weeks to more than double the adult rate at 3 years of age. Because of their poor drug-metabolizing capabilities, newborn infants are at high risk for drug toxicity; therefore, drug dosages must be calculated carefully.

Neonates also produce different metabolic products for some drugs than do adults, suggesting that different metabolic pathways may be present. Unique metabolites have been found in newborns for several common drugs, including chlorpromazine and theophylline. Another example is phenobarbital, a barbiturate commonly used for its anticonvulsant and sedative properties. Phenobarbital induces the production of an enzyme that lowers serum bilirubin levels. Newborns typically lack the enzyme and so frequently experience hyperbilirubinemia.

Excretion

Renal function is significantly decreased in neonates. As a result, neonates excrete drugs more slowly. Newborns have a diminished ability to concentrate urine and a lower urinary pH, which also affects excretion of some compounds. Renal function approaches adult levels at the end of the first year of life.

Infants and Children

A number of physiologic factors influence drug administration in infants and children. Progressive biologic maturity and growth stabilizes the body's response to drugs until drug response eventually becomes identical to that of the adult. As the child grows older body mass increases, body fat content changes, and body water volume decreases, all of which can influence drug absorption, distribution, metabolism, and excretion. In addition, anatomic barriers, such as the skin and the blood–brain barrier, become more effective as the infant matures. Rapid growth spurts during childhood and puberty may also affect drug response.

Physiologic Changes in Infants and Children

Absorption

Gastric acidity in children does not begin to approach adult values until about 2 or 3 years of age. This early relative lack of gastric acid contributes to exaggerated drug absorption so that, for example, oral benzyl penicillin (which at older ages is inactivated by gastric acid) is well absorbed in infants. Gastric emptying rate reaches adult levels at about 6 to 8 months of age. Barriers such as the skin and the blood–brain barrier become more effective as the infant grows, making the child less vulnerable to drug toxicity.

Distribution

Protein binding of drugs reaches adult levels by 1 year of age. Children continue to have a high total body water content until about 2 years of age. Thus, children younger than 2 taking highly water-soluble drugs may require larger doses than older children need.

Metabolism

Metabolic rates in infants are higher than adult levels until 2 to 3 years of age; they decline to adult rates by puberty. Therapeutic drug dosages relative to body weight may be greater for children than for adults. For example, dosages for a drug such as theophylline, frequently used to treat asthma in children, should be individualized for each child because of individual metabolic variations. Individualized treatment is achieved by monitoring the child's plasma concentrations of the drug. As the child matures, hepatic enzymes should effectively metabolize most drugs. However, interference with normal metabolism is a side effect of some drugs that can have serious consequences for children.

Excretion

Mature renal and hepatic function is not reached until 6 to 12 months of age. Until then, repeat doses of drugs should be given cautiously. Dosages of drugs normally excreted largely unchanged by the kidney, such as digoxin and gentamicin, should be calculated carefully to avoid toxicity. In older infants and children, effective excretion of drug products helps prevent drug effects from lasting too long.

Nursing Implications for Drug Treatment of Neonates, Infants, and Children

In pediatric nursing practice the nurse is responsible not only for knowing the biologic distinctions that affect pharmacokinetics in children, but also for being acquainted with common drug therapies. Specific pediatric pathology can influence drug utilization in children as well. Table 8–1 summarizes pediatric physiologic characteristics and their consequences. Other special considerations include drug dosage, administration, side effects, and drug misuse in pediatric patients.

Table 8–1 Physiologic Characteristics of Infants and Their Consequences

Characteristic	Consequence
High total body water volume	Expanded distribution, diminished blood levels of water-soluble drugs
Low body fat	Increased blood levels of lipid-soluble drugs
Increased membrane permeability, especially skin and blood–brain	Enhanced topical absorption; drugs can enter CNS rapidly
Relative lack of gastric acid	Exaggerated absorption of drugs that are partially inactivated by gastric acid, or drugs that are normally ionized at low pH
Immature body temperature regulation	May dehydrate quickly, thereby elevating blood concentrations of drug
Immature kidney or liver function	Delayed excretion or metabolism of certain drugs

Dosage

Accurate dosage selection is critical in infants and children since they do not have the mature physiologic mechanisms to compensate for errors that can result in drug overdose, toxicity, and death. For this reason, adult doses usually cannot be given to young children. Recommended pediatric drug dosages are available for many drugs, but other dosages must be extrapolated from the adult dosage. Table 8–2 presents four methods for calculating pediatric drug dosages. The first three methods are based on modification of adult dosages. The fourth method, using body surface area (BSA), is based on the surface area correlation with the basal metabolic rate. To calculate the dosage using BSA, the BSA is determined from a nomogram, such as the one shown in Figure 8–1.

None of the methods described in Table 8–2 can exactly individualize dosage, since age, weight, and BSA are only some of the factors involved in drug responses, but they do provide a reasonable relative modification of the adult dose for children. The methods of Clark,

Table 8–2 | Methods of Calculating Pediatric Doses

Clark's Rule
(for children 2 years old or younger)

$$\text{Child's dose} = \frac{\text{child's weight in pounds}}{\text{150 pounds}} \times \text{adult dose}$$

Fried's Rule
(for children 1 year old or younger)

$$\text{Child's dose} = \frac{\text{child's age in months}}{\text{150 months}} \times \text{adult dose}$$

Young's Rule
(for children 2 years old or older)

$$\text{Child's dose} = \frac{\text{child's age in years}}{\text{child's age in years} + 12} \times \text{adult dose}$$

Body Surface Area
(value for body surface area obtained from nomogram in Fig. 8–1)

$$\text{Child's dose} = \frac{\text{body surface area (m}^2\text{)}}{1.7} \times \text{adult dose}$$

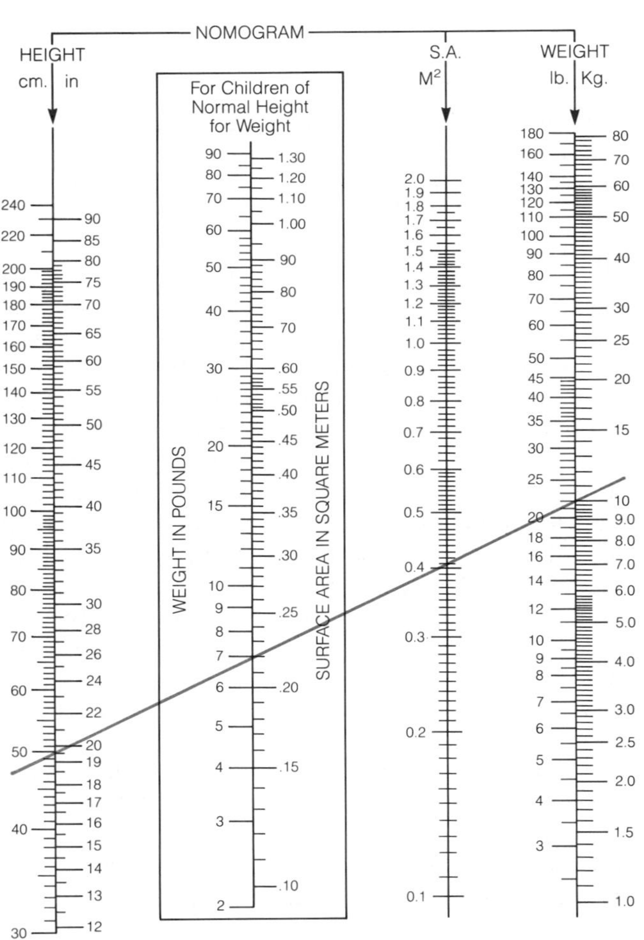

Fried, and Young are referred to as *fixed-dose rules* that assume the pediatric dosage consistently parallels the "average" adult dosage. Fried's and Young's rules are based on age, and so they do not discriminate differences for children who are small or large for their age. Clark's rule provides a dose that is based on body weight. However, none of these fixed-dose rules consider the unique physiology of neonates and infants that can affect pharmacokinetics.

Calculation of the appropriate drug dosage should also depend on the nature of the drug. As indicated previously, certain drugs may not be excreted effectively in infants because of their relative physiologic immaturity. In such cases, size is not as important a factor as physiology. Calculating dosage based on BSA is done in an effort to individualize drug dosages based on the correlation of metabolism and BSA, rather than on size or age alone. Reliability of this method depends on the accuracy with which the BSA is estimated or calculated; it can be used for patients of any size.

Administration

The administration of drugs to pediatric patients requires special nursing consideration. It is not unusual for a child to resist administration of a drug. Spilling or spitting the medicine can affect the accuracy of the dosage. However, knowledge about growth and development and experience in working with children can eliminate most dosage inaccuracies and struggles. The following list provides some nursing guidelines that are useful in the successful administration of medications to children.

1. Be honest (it will hurt; medicine is NOT candy).
2. Allow reasonable choices (color of Band-Aid, flavor of juice).
3. Assure the child that crying is okay.
4. Tell the child how long the procedure will hurt (count 1–2–3).
5. Offer comfort measures (handholding, pacifier).
6. Use age-appropriate words.

Figure 8–1

Nomogram with estimated body surface area. Draw a straight line between the child's height (on the left) and the child's weight (on the right); (see example). The point at which the line intersects the surface area (S.A.) is the estimated BSA. (**Source:** Modified from data of Boyd E, by West CD. In: Behrman RE, Vaughan VC, eds. *Nelson Textbook of Pediatrics.* 13th ed. Philadelphia: W.B. Saunders, 1987. Reprinted with the permission of the copyright owner.)

7. Explain the procedure briefly, and keep the time between explanation and administration at a minimum.
8. Prepare medication in advance.
9. Keep needles and syringes out of sight.
10. Consider methods to make a drug more palatable (eg, mask the taste by diluting the drug with food or drink, if not contraindicated).
11. Solicit parent's help.
12. Act smoothly and quickly; expertise is accomplished only through intent and practice.
13. Hold the child by cradling the head in your arms and holding arms and hands with one of yours while you administer oral medication with your other hand.

Side Effects

Adverse drug reactions can occur in children as a result of individual sensitivity or toxicity. In addition to the primary drug(s), medications also often contain other ingredients that may cause adverse effects. For example, many medications contain alcohol. Some theophylline preparations used in the treatment of childhood asthma contain up to 20% alcohol. In some cases, a child undergoing treatment with theophylline could receive the alcohol equivalent of several alcoholic drinks. This can lead to central nervous system (CNS) depression, drug interactions, and other problems. If combined with other drugs, this CNS depression may seriously harm the child.

Drug Misuse in the Pediatric Patient

Parents or guardians are most often responsible for administering medication to infants and young children. A parent's stress or fatigue from caring for a sick child may contribute to administration error. Management of drug therapy requires attention, coordination, and some understanding of the drug being given. In many cases, young or disadvantaged parents do not have the experience to ask appropriate questions about a drug to clarify their understanding of the administration instructions. Common causes of drug misuse in pediatric patients include the following.

1. Multiple medication dispensers (father, mother, babysitter), resulting in the risk of repeat or missed doses.
2. Use of incorrect prescriptions (from previous illness or another child with similar symptoms).
3. Discontinuance of medication as soon as symptoms are alleviated (particularly problematic with antibiotic and anticonvulsant therapy).
4. Accidental ingestion (medications are a common source of poisoning in childhood).
5. Baby's ingestion through breast milk of drugs taken by a lactating mother.
6. Measurement errors (considerable variance exists in the understanding of a term like "teaspoonful").
7. Misinterpretation of route of administration (eardrops may be "for" the ear or "in" the ear).
8. Spitting or spilling of medication by a resistant child, leaving parents uncertain about how much drug was actually ingested.
9. Recognition of side effects is complicated by children's lack of language and inability to recognize, understand, and communicate symptoms.
10. The belief that "if a little is good, more is better."

One solution to these potential administration problems is education. Parents should be given precise and, preferably, written administration instructions for children. If there is any indication that the parent has not understood, then the nurse should demonstrate the proper technique and have the parent perform a return demonstration. Follow-up by telephone or through a public health nurse can help assure that the parent accurately implements the medication regimen.

Older Adults

Since 1900, the number of elderly people (65 and older) in our society has grown seven times faster than the rest of the population. The elderly account for about 12 to 13% of our population today and are projected to account for well more than that by the year 2000. One of the ramifications of this rapid increase is an increase in the use of health-care services by the elderly. For example, recent evidence indicates that the number of hospital days for patients aged 85 and over is greater than for all children aged 15 and younger, even though the older adults currently are outnumbered 2 to 1 by the younger patients. Older adults use a disproportionate amount of health-care services, including prescription drugs.

Polypharmacy, the prescribing of many drugs at one time, is common in older adults. As the number and complexity of illnesses increase with age, the complexity of drug treatment also increases. Patients may receive medications from several different physicians, and there is no guarantee that each prescriber is aware of what the other is doing. Drug–drug interactions, therefore, have a major role in the adverse drug responses of older adults.

In 1972 older Americans received 22% of all prescriptions. By now that percentage has grown to over

SPOTLIGHT ON NURSING RESEARCH

Administration of over-the-counter (OTC) medications is a significant self-care practice for older adults. In order to increase understanding of factors that prompt their use, this study examined the relationship between the use of OTC medications and a series of mood, social, health, and demographic variables. The nurse investigator interviewed 186 adult volunteers 65 to 99 years of age. Participants lived in the community and managed their own medications. In addition to data obtained during semi-structured interviews, mood and social variables were measured by asking subjects to complete the Profile of Mood States, an accepted tool that measures anxiety and depression; and the Emotional Bondedness Scale, a scale that evaluates qualities of social relationships.

On average, subjects experienced 4 chronic illnesses, took 2.47 different types of prescription medication, and gave generally good, subjective ratings of their health. In contrast, subjects averaged 4.62 types of OTC medication. However, these drugs were used infrequently. Most subjects (58%) selected the term "not often" to describe their administration. Only 14% indicated that they used OTCs "very often," and 28% reported occasional use.

Based on previous work, the investigator postulated that the occurrence of both physical symptoms and mood disorders, such as anxiety or depression, would predict the use of OTC medications. In this study, a greater number of reported symptoms predicted increases in both the number of medications administered and the frequency of their use. Younger age, less emotional bondedness, higher income, and living alone also predicted greater use of OTC drugs. Interestingly, neither anxiety nor depression was associated with the frequency or number of medications used. In the present work, the total number of symptoms reported was the most influential factor examined. However, this variable accounted for only 6.7% of the variance in OTC medication use.

Studies of human behavior, such as self-administration of OTC medication, can be very complex. Certainly, this study demonstrates that it is difficult to predict the use of these medications among older adults. It also indicates that factors other than specific symptoms determine medication use. These observations point out the need for additional research about self-medication practices using OTCs. They also highlight the importance of obtaining complete medication histories that include information about the administration of nonprescription drugs, particularly in older adults taking several prescription medications.

Conn VS: Older adults: Factors that predict the use of over-the-counter medication. *J Adv Nurs* 1991;16:1190–1196.

30%, when both prescription and OTC drugs are considered. This rapid escalation in use reflects not only real growth in this area but also increased attention by the health-care community to issues of the elderly. Older adults take about three times the amount of drugs taken by people under 65, and it is estimated that approximately 20% of these patients' out-of-pocket health expenses are for drugs.

On the average, elders living in the community receive from three to five drugs each day. Those who live in nursing homes or similar provided-care settings average about eight per day, but almost a third receive from eight to 14; some receive many more.

High on the list of the most commonly prescribed drugs are those used to treat cardiovascular disorders (eg, hypertension, heart failure), CNS disorders (eg, depression, dementia, psychosis), and pain and inflammation. Nonprescription drugs that are often prescribed or self-prescribed include those affecting the gastrointestinal (GI) tract (antacids, laxatives, cathartics), and analgesic and antiinflammatory drugs that can be identical or very similar to the prescribed agents.

To say that properly managing therapy with so many drugs is "difficult" simply does not give adequate emphasis to the problem. In too many cases, even when the only drugs taken are prescribed drugs, therapy falls far short of the goal of causing less harm than good.

Pharmacokinetic Changes in Older Adults

As a person grows older, drug absorption, distribution, metabolism, and excretion can be altered through the combined influences of age-related physiologic changes, disease, nutrition, and drug therapy. The major pharmacokinetic changes are explained in the following discussion and summarized in Table 8–3. All of them help explain why, in most cases, drug doses should be re-

Table 8–3 Physiologic Characteristics in the Elderly and Their Consequences

Characteristic	Consequence
Increased gastric pH	Decreased absorption of drugs that are normally nonionized at low pH
Increased body fat	Decreased blood levels of fat-soluble drugs
Decreased body water	Increased blood levels of water-soluble drugs
Decreased serum albumin	Increased unbound drug, leading to increased drug activity
Decreased cardiac output	Decreased drug metabolism and excretion
Decreased renal blood flow	Decreased drug excretion
Decreased splanchnic blood flow	Decreased absorption of drugs given orally; decreased metabolism, excretion, or both
Decreased liver mass and hepatic blood flow	Decreased drug metabolism, especially first pass

duced in elderly persons, and why especially careful monitoring of therapy is necessary.

When thinking about how pharmacokinetic changes in the elderly (or any other patient) might necessitate changes in drug therapy, it is important to think beyond the obvious. It may be obvious, for example, that a patient will (and sometimes must) receive a drug that depends greatly on hepatic metabolism (or renal excretion) as a way to terminate its effects in the body, even if that same patient has liver (or kidney) disease. What is not so obvious, but is critically important to remember, is that most drugs depend on the interrelated functions of a variety of organs for their entry into, and elimination from, the body.

Moreover—and this appears to be especially true for the elderly—although a particular disease may appear to alter the function of mainly one organ (eg, the liver), other organs, and their functions, can be affected too. A good example of this is heart failure, a common condition in the elderly. The heart does not absorb, metabolize, or excrete drugs. But because it is responsible for delivering blood to the key drug absorptive, metabolizing, and excreting organs, heart dysfunction can cause a host of pharmacokinetic changes that complicate therapy. Likewise, drugs that exert an effect on a particular organ can also have an impact on pharmacokinetic processes carried out by other organs. Other common age-associated conditions that can have a widespread impact on pharmacokinetics include dehydration, malnutrition, hyper- or hypotension, diabetes, and pulmonary disease.

Absorption

Of the four pharmacokinetic factors that govern the fate and actions of drugs, absorption seems to be least affected in older adults. Gastric pH, which affects the ionization and diffusibility of drugs, tends to increase because of decreased gastric acid secretion. There are also decreases in gut motility, surface area, and blood flow. These changes are more likely caused by disease, nutritional status, and drug therapy than by simple age-related physiologic factors. Overall, neither the rate of drug absorption from the gut, nor the amount of a dose that is absorbed, is changed much. However, as noted below, significant age-associated decreases in hepatic metabolism can make it appear as if greater amounts of some drugs have been absorbed.

Distribution

The lean body mass of an older adult decreases by 25 to 30%. Body water decreases, and body fat increases in proportion to total body weight. Plasma concentrations of water-soluble drugs are increased because the drugs are distributed throughout a smaller relative volume of water. Plasma concentrations of lipid-soluble drugs are decreased because of distribution into a relatively greater amount of fat.

In addition, serum albumin levels usually decrease in later years. Since many drugs tend to bind to albumin, the decreased number of binding sites will lead to a proportionately higher number of unbound and therefore active molecules in the circulation. As a result, greater and potentially adverse effects may occur unless the dose is reduced appropriately. Multiple drug therapies, common in the older adult, may result in competitive displacement of some drugs from protein binding sites and thereby increase free serum concentrations.

Metabolism

Three main factors contribute to age-associated decreases in drug metabolism, mainly in the liver: decreased activity of the liver's drug metabolizing enzymes; decreased hepatic blood flow, which is responsible for delivering drugs to their site of metabolism; and decreased liver mass. Disease, altered nutritional status, and drug therapy seem to affect hepatic enzyme activity and blood flow the most.

Decreased liver function has a particularly great impact on orally administered drugs that ordinarily undergo extensive first-pass hepatic metabolism. Overall, reduced metabolism can increase the amount of some drugs that enter the bloodstream. It can simultaneously decrease the rate at which drugs appear to be removed from the blood as the result of chemical breakdown. In view of this, diminishing liver function is one more reason for advising that drug doses be reduced, and monitored more carefully, in elders.

Excretion

About two out of every three older adults have some clinically significant age-related renal dysfunction. The major changes seem to involve reduced glomerular filtration and, to a lesser extent, tubular secretion. Both processes are important for transferring drugs or their metabolites into the urine.

Renal status is usually assessed as the patient's creatinine clearance, which can be approximated from measurements of plasma creatinine levels. Such measurements are a common part of blood tests given to most patients, so the values should be looked for in the patient's chart. Package inserts for some drugs give guidelines about how to modify the dose depending on the creatinine level or clearance value. The nurse should refer to these instructions when double-checking the prescribed dose. Those guidelines do not replace the need for careful assessment of the actual drug response.

In summary, it is fair to say that there is great variability in the older adult's response to drugs. Many factors and complex interactions influence drug response and make prediction of alterations difficult. As a general principle, one should expect an increased and prolonged drug effect in the older adult. Careful evaluation and frequent monitoring of drug therapy are always needed.

Pharmacodynamic Changes in Older Adults

The paragraphs above discussed altered drug responses in the elderly because of pharmacokinetic changes. For example, an unusually heightened or prolonged response to a particular drug could be explained in terms of increased or prolonged blood levels owing to decreased metabolism or excretion. However, there is also evidence that, compared with younger persons, the elderly experience greater (or lesser) responses to a particular dose of some drugs even when the plasma concentration of free (active) drug is the same. That is, the changed response intensity is not caused by too much (or too little) drug at active sites, but by increased (or decreased) responses of the cells to the drug molecules that are there. This is a pharmacodynamic alteration of drug response.

Much less is known about pharmacodynamic changes than about pharmacokinetic alterations, in part because the pharmacodynamic changes are harder to measure. Nevertheless, some of what is known can be helpful when adjusting drug dosages for the elderly patient, anticipating altered and sometimes unwanted effects, and trying to understand why these changes make the patient more or less "sensitive" to a drug. What follows is a brief overview of how some of these changes are thought to come about, with examples of each.

Receptor or Other Cellular Changes

Decreased responses to some drugs may be caused by an age-related decrease in the number of cell receptors with which a drug must interact. This has been used to explain, for example, a relatively weaker ability of drugs like epinephrine (adrenalin) to stimulate the heart, and a relatively weaker response to drugs that block those receptors. In addition, age can bring about changes in the cell's chemical processes that are needed to translate the binding of a drug with its receptors into a biologic response.

Reflex or Homeostatic Changes

Drugs acting on one organ or system sometimes trigger reflexes aimed at maintaining, more or less, the status quo. However, in the elderly some of these compensatory processes can be impaired. This sort of control is particularly important, and common, in the cardiovascular system. For example, some antihypertensive drugs can cause an abrupt fall in blood pressure when the patient stands up suddenly—a phenomenon called *orthostatic hypotension*. Normally the autonomic nervous system responds almost instantaneously to constrict blood vessels in the legs. Without this reflex, blood can pool in the legs, and the brain could be deprived of blood long enough to cause dizziness, fainting, a fall, and serious injury. In the elderly, however, the protective reflexes seem to be diminished, and so the risks are increased.

Nutritional Changes

Nutritional deficiencies can account for some altered drug responses in the elderly. For example, warfarin, one of the most common oral drugs used to prevent abnormal blood clotting, works in the liver by inhibiting the synthesis of blood clotting factors that depend on vitamin K. An inadequate intake of vitamin K–containing foods (eg, green leafy vegetables; see Chapter 61) would intensify the anticoagulant's effects, with potentially dangerous consequences.

It is important for the nurse to realize that a patient need not be in a general state of malnourishment, since a deficiency (or excess) of just one nutrient (eg, a vitamin) can have effects on the responses to specific drugs. It is also important to assess for factors, age-related and otherwise, that could affect nutritional status. Things to be looked for as possible problems include chronic diarrhea, dehydration, diminished appetite or taste, and difficulties with chewing or swallowing. Some of these problems can be caused by age, disease, psychologic factors (eg, depression), and even by therapy with certain drugs. It is even important for the nurse to consider economic factors, which could affect a patient's ability to buy the foods that make up a proper, balanced diet.

Nursing Implications for Drug Treatment of Older Adults

Side Effects

The consequences of diseases encountered by the elderly, and of the administration of drugs used to treat them, are too numerous to discuss separately. However, it is possible to make some generalizations about the drug-induced side effects that are most likely to occur and be bothersome, since some of them can be caused by several of the drug groups commonly given to the elderly. It is also important to note that without proper recognition and management (Table 8–4), drug side effects can become so intense and disturbing that they outweigh the desired therapeutic benefits, or cause the patient to stop taking medications altogether, and therefore reduce the overall quality of life.

Antimuscarinic Effects

The antimuscarinic effects (effects caused by blocking the interaction between acetylcholine and its receptors) of many drugs constitute a significant concern for the elderly. Drugs having antimuscarinic properties that are commonly used by the elderly include drugs that dilate the pupil (mydriatics), drugs used to treat the symptoms of colds and hay fever (antihistamines), and drugs for certain kinds of mental illness (antidepressants and antipsychotic drugs). Antimuscarinic effects can worsen

Table 8–4 Common Side Effects Affecting Older Adults, and Appropriate Nursing Interventions

Side Effects	Nursing Intervention
Ataxia, confusion, dizziness, sedation	Offer, recruit assistance with activities for daily living (including drug administration); ensure patient avoids activities made dangerous by altered CNS status
Blurred vision	Reassure that blurred vision is a temporary effect of many drugs; encourage avoiding activities made dangerous by impaired vision; often responds to a change in drug, or reduced dose(s) of current drug(s)
Constipation	Give laxatives as ordered and provide diet with appropriate roughage
Dry mouth	Provide frequent sips of water and hard, sugarless candy or sugarless gum; lubricants may help dentures fit better
Eye pain	Instruct the older adult to report eye pain immediately as it may indicate exacerbation of undiagnosed glaucoma
Nasal congestion	Over-the-counter nasal decongestants may be suggested; however, OTC drugs can interact with many prescribed drugs, so consult the physician about their use
Orthostatic hypotension	Instruct the older adult to get out of bed slowly, to sit on the edge of the bed for a short while, and to rise slowly
	Observe closely to determine if a change of drug might be appropriate
Urinary hesitancy	Provide running water, privacy; run warm water over perineum; evaluate men for enlarged prostate; often responds to a change in drug, or reduced dose(s) of current drug(s)
Urinary retention, bladder distention	Give fluids; encourage frequent voiding; evaluate men for enlarged prostate; catheterize if necessary

glaucoma; prostate, bowel, and bladder problems; and hypotension.

Drugs in this category are introduced in Chapter 13.

Hypotension

As noted above, several age-associated pharmacokinetic and pharmacodynamic changes occur in the cardiovascular system. These can contribute to a prolonged, excessive lowering of blood pressure, or acute but significant (and dangerous) posture-related hypotension. This problem is caused not only by drugs given specifically to lower blood pressure (Chapter 33), but also by others that can lower blood pressure as a side effect. Examples include drugs used to treat insomnia and other sleep disorders, anxiety, depression, psychosis, parkinsonism, seizure disorders, pain, and even some manifestations of common allergies. And all these drugs have CNS depressant actions that are capable of causing other relatively common and problematic side effects for the elderly.

Sedation, Confusion, and Ataxia

The most common side effects caused by drugs with CNS depressant activity are sedation (drowsiness), confusion and disorientation, and ataxia (an impairment of coordination and balance). Some drugs, notably some of the benzodiazepines (Chapter 22), which are considered to be the preferred agents for anxiety and sleep disorders, can also produce short-term memory loss (amnesia) or "hangover," depending on their onsets and durations of action.

Besides the obvious social drawbacks of being drowsy, confused, or uncoordinated, there are some real and serious dangers, such as those posed by driving a car, operating dangerous machinery, or even walking, in an impaired state. The problems caused by prescription drugs and many OTC medications that depress the CNS can be aggravated by consuming even small amounts of alcohol, by hypotension or dehydration, and by other factors presenting themselves in the elderly person.

Another risk imposed by CNS depressants is their ability to mask or mimic CNS changes that could be valuable in recognizing or diagnosing underlying disorders such as stroke, parkinsonism, Alzheimer's disease, and dementia.

Compliance and Noncompliance

Medication compliance and noncompliance are important considerations in drug therapy for older adults, but they are not problems unique to them. It appears that, on the average, elderly persons are no less compliant with medications than younger persons. However, for elders some causes of noncompliance may be more important or more common than they are for others, and these causes should be assessed for when trying to optimize drug therapy.

1. Polypharmacy, a leading cause of adverse drug effects in the elderly, also makes the medication plan inherently difficult to comply with. This includes use of both prescription drugs, which may be ordered by several physicians (with the potential for duplication or unrecognized interactions), and self-prescribed drugs. The obvious difficulty for the patient is knowing which medications to take; and when, not only with regard to the time of day but also in terms of meals, which might interfere with drug absorption.
2. The physiologic changes that accompany aging and illness can cause such problems as forgetfulness, confusion, or anorexia, which can lead to noncompliance despite the best intent to take medications as directed.
3. Special senses, physical strength, and dexterity may be impaired. Auditory problems may make it difficult to hear advice about therapy. Visual impairments make it difficult to read written directions or labels on medication containers, or to identify the shape, size, or color of a medication. Altered taste (and smell) may make it difficult to distinguish one liquid medication from another that is packaged in a similar container and looks alike in other ways. Conditions such as arthritis can make it difficult to open medication containers, most of which have child-resistant caps.
4. Habits, practices, and social or cultural beliefs held for many years, which previously kept the patient quite well, may limit the patient's willingness to comply with therapy. Some of these factors may include the use of nonprescription drugs or other remedies, or certain diets, that can have an influence on drug responses or drug taking. Such knowledge of "myself, the way I was for years," can make taking medications, or tolerating the side effects they impose, no more acceptable than the illness.
5. Personal loss or grief, especially of recent onset, can be a disincentive to taking medications.
6. Financial considerations may make it difficult for the elderly person to decide whether purchasing medications takes priority over other necessities of life. It can also influence a decision to self-medicate

with cheaper nonprescription drugs instead of those that are prescribed.

7. Whether because of financial reasons, a period of symptom relief, or an episode of unpleasant side effects, medications may go unused and be saved until the patient feels the need to take them again. Some medications may become outdated during this time, losing some or all of their activity by the time they are taken again.

Many of the approaches that foster compliance and assess for noncompliance in any patient should be applied to the elderly. In addition, some of the unique causes of noncompliance in elders should receive special attention. An inability to hear instructions clearly should never be a major cause of noncompliance, since clearly written instructions should always be provided, and if possible should be provided to another adult (friend or family member) who might share in managing the therapy. Instructions written in large type can help some patients. Prescriptions can be written to specify closures on medication containers that are easier to open, or the patient can be advised to ask the pharmacist to do this. A host of commercially available or home-made devices that organize medications or remind the users of when to take them can be recommended.

Given the prevalence of polypharmacy for elders, it is also important for the nurse to obtain a thorough medication history, inquiring about duplicate or interacting drugs that might be prescribed by several different physicians; and about nonprescription drug use, including which medications are taken, how often, and why the patient perceived the need for them. In some cases, the nurse can identify alternative combination drug products that would allow simultaneous administration of two medicines at once; or other alternatives with longer durations of action, which would reduce the frequency with which the drug must be taken. Communication of this information between the nurse and prescribing physician becomes an important part of care.

Nursing interventions can also gain insight into the appropriateness of dosages. Reviewing laboratory test results for drug levels or indicators of impaired organ function is useful, if not essential. However, lab test results should never take the place of assessing for objective evidence of desired drug effects (eg, symptom relief), unwanted side effects and interactions, and insight into the patient's subjective responses to medication and disease. The nurse should not lose sight of the possibility that if noncompliance goes undetected as the cause of an inadequate drug response, the prescriber may assume that the drug truly is not working, and that higher doses, or still other drugs, should be administered.

Giving the patient instructions on how to be compliant is important. What often becomes more important, however, is to learn why a patient is noncompliant, and then to work with the patient to find acceptable solutions. This can only be done with meaningful, two-way communication between health-care providers and recipients.

In summary, the nurse's goals in administering drugs to elderly patients are no different than those set for any patient: maximize the benefits, minimize the risks, and do more good than harm. However, reciting the golden rule for administering drugs to the elderly, "start low, go slow," is not enough. Because of the many interactions between age-related physiology, illness, and psychosocial needs and beliefs, reaching the therapeutic goal may be difficult and challenging. Optimum yet compassionate therapy can be achieved only by an understanding of these unique age-related traits, a fundamental knowledge of drug action, and a holistic approach to care.

Annotated Bibliography

Berlin CM Jr. Advances in pediatric pharmacology and toxicology. *Adv Pediatr* 1989;36:431–459. *This comprehensive review identifies important recent developments in drug therapy for children, explains why they are important, and starts us thinking about what to expect in the near future.*

Boreus LO. *Principles of pediatric pharmacology.* New York: Churchill Livingstone, 1982:179–193. *In addition to discussions of drugs, the text covers factors influencing pediatric drug compliance and methods of improving it. Key concepts still apply.*

Cooper JW. Reviewing geriatric concerns with commonly used drugs. *Geriatrics* 1989;44(12):79–86. *Excellent for its focused summaries concerning appropriate use of individual drugs and drug groups that are widely administered to, or self-prescribed by, the elderly.*

Diamond R. Drugs and the quality of life: The patient's point of view. *J Clin Psych* 1985;46:5(Sec 2):29–35. *This article addresses the issue of quality of life of patients taking long-term medication. Social functioning, acceptance of dose, compliance or lack of compliance, and the relative benefits of medication are some of the factors that contribute to treatment goals. The content will never be out of date.*

Fonner CJ, Rushton CH, Fletcher AB. Preparation for neonatal emergencies: A neonatal emergency medication sheet. *Pediatr Nurs* 1989;15(5):527–530. *This article provides valuable advice for all nurses who are likely to be dealing with medical emergencies in neonates, and managing them with drugs.*

Guyon G. Pharmacokinetic considerations in neonatal drug therapy. *Neonatal Network* 1989;7(5):9–12. *A concise presentation of how understanding pharmacokinetic changes in the neonate can help the nurse plan, implement, and assess drug therapy for these patients.*

Harper CM, Newton PA, Walsh JR. Drug-induced illness in the elderly. *Postgrad Med* 1989;86(2):245–256. *Iatrogenic adverse drug ef-*

fects in the elderly are often reversible and preventable, but not without careful assessment for them.

Jacknowitz A, Fischer RG. Inactive ingredients in the pediatric population. *Pediatr Nurs* 1987;13(2):125. *This article provides a summary of the inactive ingredients found in prescription and OTC medications, and their potential effects on the pediatric population.*

Kick E. Patient teaching for elders. *Nurs Clin North AM* 1989; 24(3):681–686. *This article dispels myths about the inability of elders to learn, and so helps the nurse be a more effective teacher, whether about drugs or other issues.*

Lamy PP. Nonprescription drugs and the elderly. *Am Fam Phys* 1989; 39(6):175–179. *Worth reading not only for its excellent summary of the risks, benefits, and extent of OTC drug use by the elderly, but also for concise tables dealing with common OTC drugs, health-food store items, and nutrients that can affect prescribed drug therapy.*

Lamy PP. Pharmacotherapeutics in the elderly. *Md Med J* 1989;38(2): 144–148. *Adding a new drug therapy necessitates careful reassessment of the appropriateness and need for what is already prescribed. Communication and agreement between providers and recipients is also an important part of treatment.*

Lamy PP, ed. Clinical pharmacology. *Clin Geriatr Med* 1990;6(2): 1–457. *Fifteen contemporary, well-written articles cover both general topics related to drug action and drug therapy and specific topics including common age-related disorders and drug groups used by the elderly. Arguably the single best source for comprehensive coverage of drug therapy in the elderly.*

Leary PM. Adverse reactions in children: Special considerations in prevention and management. *Drug Safety* 1991;6(3):171–182. *Although adverse drug effects in children occur infrequently, they are nevertheless important. The author identifies common drugs associated with untoward effects, and basic interventions for when they occur; and stresses the need for practitioners to be familiar with the use and risks of drugs in children, the need to keep therapy as short as possible, and the importance of parental involvement and knowledge in the identification and further prevention of adverse effects.*

LeSage J. Polypharmacy in geriatric patients. *Nurs Clin North Am* 1991;26(2):273–290. *This article concisely summarizes information on the possible causes, consequences, and areas for intervention, with respect to multiple drug use.*

Litteral J. What are the clinically important drug-nutrient interactions? *Pediatr Nurs* 1990;16(6):594–596. *A short but useful summary of drug–nutrient interactions, some often overlooked, that are of special importance to children.*

Macdonald JB. The role of drugs in falls in the elderly. *Clin Geriatr Med* 1985;1(3):621–636. *This paper gives good insight into how multiple drugs and multiple diseases add up to increase the risk of a common cause of morbidity in the elderly.*

O'Brien JG, Kursch JE. "Healthy" prescribing for the elderly: How to minimize adverse drug effects and prevent "dementia in a bottle." *Postgrad Med* 1987;82(6):147–151, 154, 156. *A refreshingly holistic approach to drug therapy in the elderly, this article stresses the need for individualizing drug therapy, becoming familiar with the actions of a few drugs in a particular class, and using nondrug therapies as an aid to medications to help get the patient well.*

Roberts J, Turner N. Pharmacodynamic basis for altered drug action in the elderly. *Clin Geriatr Med* 1988;4(1):127–150. *A comprehensive review of how altered actions of drugs with their cellular targets, rather than pharmacokinetic changes, can modify drug responses in the elderly.*

Roe DA. Drug and nutrient interactions in the elderly diabetic. *Drug Nutr Interact* 1988;5(4):195–203. *Although this article focuses on nutrition, diabetes, and antidiabetic therapy, it contains a wealth of information that applies to therapy with a host of drugs, and in other disease states.*

Stewart RB, Caranasos GJ. Medication compliance in the elderly. *Med Clin North Am* 1989;73(6):1551–1563. *An excellent summary of why elders may be noncompliant, and how the problems can be overcome. Providing adequate written and verbal instructions is not enough; "exhibiting a genuine concern to patients . . . is the first step to improve compliance."*

Stolley JM, Buckwalter KC, Fjordbak B, Bush S. Iatrogenesis in the elderly: Drug-related problems. *J Gerontol Nurs* 1991;17(9): 12–17. *Thorough drug histories, simplifying medications, educating patients and care providers, and using nondrug measures can go a long way toward recognizing, preventing, or alleviating unwanted drug effects.*

Sutnick MR. Dietary guidance for the elderly. *Clin Geriatr Med* 1988;4(1):193–202. *This concise review of the subject addresses the roles of individual nutrients and the importance of body weight control, and gives useful advice on dietary assessment and counselling for the elderly.*

Tesfa A. Drug therapy in elderly patients: Diagnosis of drug-related problems. *Recent Adv Nurs* 1989;23:45–52. *This excellent article makes a strong case for the need for extra monitoring and evaluation of older patients receiving drugs, and offers insight into how approaches to drug therapy may, if not must, change in the future.*

Wallace DE, Watanabe AS. Drug effects in geriatric patients. *Drug Intell Clin Pharm* 1977;11:597–603. *Arranged in tabular format according to major drug classes, this article cites the potential effects of aging on drug responses and possible underlying mechanisms of adverse or undesired drug responses, and provides useful precautions to guard against untoward effects.*

Warner A. Drug use in the neonate: Interrelationships of pharmacokinetics, toxicity, and biochemical maturity. *Clin Chem* 1986; 32(5):721–727. *This article reviews neonatal pharmacokinetic processes with reference to some of the reported toxic reactions to drugs and drug additives, and discusses potential biochemical maturity markers as an approach to improving efficacy of drug therapy.*

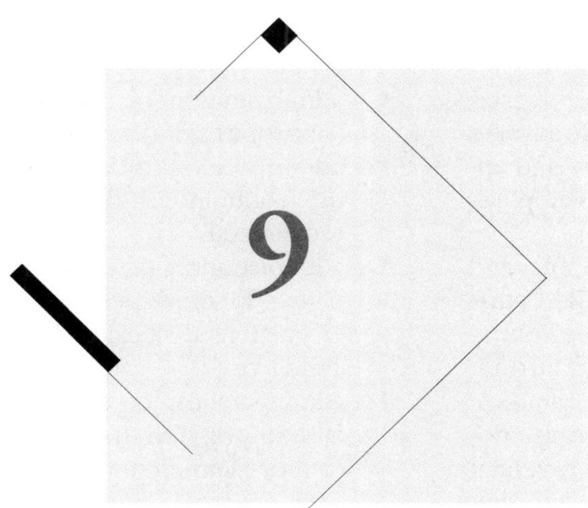

Adverse Drug Effects

An adverse drug effect is an unintended and undesirable response to the administration of one or more drugs. Few, if any, drugs are truly free of adverse effects, and although a particular drug may be safe for most patients, it may not be safe for all patients. Adverse drug effects result from complex interactions between the drug, the patient, and factors related to the patient's environment.

The manifestations of an adverse drug response may be so subtle that they can be detected only with sensitive laboratory tests; they may develop gradually, be predictable, or cause little more than minor discomfort to the patient. Others may be more obvious, develop quickly, be very unpredictable, or cause a serious or fatal outcome.

Adverse drug responses cause an estimated 300,000 hospitalizations each year. However, adverse drug responses are not a problem affecting persons only outside the hospital setting: as many as 30% of all patients will develop an adverse response to drug therapy while they are in the hospital. As a result, it is imperative that the nurse be continually alert for the possible development of adverse reactions to any drug administered to any patient.

In general, drugs cause one or more primary effects, which are the desired effects for which the drug is given. However, they also usually cause one or more secondary effects, which account for the unwanted or adverse effects. These secondary effects may be extensions of the drug's primary effect, or they may be another response caused as part of the body's attempts to compensate for the primary drug action. For example, the desired primary effect of most antihypertensive drugs is an overall lowering of blood pressure. However, a related and unwanted effect of many antihypertensive drugs is a significant fall of blood pressure, accompanied by fainting, when the patient stands rapidly. In addition, the body may attempt to compensate for reduced blood pressure by triggering processes to restore blood pressure. Such responses include increased heart rate and retention of sodium and water by the kidneys. These common responses may be considered secondary and undesired responses to antihypertensive therapy with certain drugs.

By understanding the actions of a drug, the nurse can predict many of its adverse effects. The antihypertensive drug effects noted above are examples of predictable adverse responses; another is the respiratory depression caused by the administration of a narcotic.

Although it is relatively easy to predict adverse responses to certain drugs, it is not as easy to predict which patients will develop them, or how severe the consequences may be. This provides another reason why the nurse must assess the patient for adverse effects, and be prepared to take any necessary and appropriate actions should an adverse effect develop, regardless of the drug or the patient.

Factors predisposing patients to predictable and usually serious adverse drug responses are called **contraindications** to the use of the drug. *Absolute* contraindications are those conditions under which a drug should never be administered; *relative* contraindications are those conditions under which the drug's potential benefits are expected to outweigh the potential risks. There may be no clear-cut line of distinction between a contraindicated drug and a safe and effective drug, and special circumstances may necessitate the administration of a contraindicated drug. No drug is contraindicated when a patient has a life-threatening disease or other problem for which giving the drug is the only life-saving measure.

Basis for Adverse Drug Effects

While the number and form of adverse drug reactions are virtually limitless, there are three major causes of adverse reactions: patient-related factors, iatrogenic factors, and pharmacologic factors.

Patient-Related Factors

The risk and severity of an adverse response to a drug is not due solely to the drug itself. As discussed in the previous chapter, individual physiologic, pharmacokinetic, and behavioral variability have considerable influence on a drug's effects. Some of the factors contributing to this variability include consumption of alcohol, cigarette smoking, substance abuse, preexisting disease states, genetically determined enzyme differences, and interactions with prescription and self-prescribed drugs. Within limits, knowledge of this variability can help either to predict adverse responses, and thus avoid them, or identify their causes if they do occur. Certain patient-related factors may lead to unique or unusual adverse drug responses, as discussed in Chapter 7.

Poor compliance is an important patient-related factor that increases the risk of adverse drug effects. Poor compliance includes inappropriate timing of administration, underdosage, overdosage, or taking medication improperly in relation to meals.

Drug misuse is a related consideration, particularly with self-prescribing and administration of nonprescription drugs. Examples of drug misuse include

- administration of a drug for the wrong purpose (improper self-diagnosis);
- administration of a drug in situations in which the contraindications are misunderstood or not recognized;
- administration of drugs to a particular individual by two or more persons, each unaware of the other's actions (for example, parental medication of a child); or
- administration of excessive doses based on the false impression that a bigger dose will bring faster or more complete relief of symptoms.

All these behaviors contribute to the development of adverse drug responses. The patients at greatest risk are those taking drugs with a narrow therapeutic index, patients taking drugs for which precise timing of the dose is important, or patients with an underlying medical condition that is likely to be aggravated by a particular drug.

Iatrogenic Factors

Adverse drug effects that are induced by the prescriber or other health-care provider are called **iatrogenic** effects. They are often the result of errors in drug therapy. Among the iatrogenic factors contributing to adverse reactions are improper diagnosis and prescribing and errors in dosage calculation, drug preparation, dispensing, and administration. Medication errors, such as giving a dose orally rather than intravenously or giving the drug to the wrong patient, fall into this category.

It is important to avoid a common misconception—namely, that all adverse iatrogenic effects arise because of carelessness, outright errors, or other therapeutic "mistakes." In many cases a variety of "correct" drugs or other therapies might benefit a particular patient, yet despite the best clinical judgment and skill any of the treatment approaches may cause unwanted outcomes. Nevertheless, it cannot be overly stressed that every time a drug is administered the "five rights" of medication administration must be observed (see Chapters 1 and 3): the right drug, the right dose, the right route of administration, the right patient, and the right time. Patient education and assessment for the correct use of self-administered medication is also an important nursing function.

There are five specific nursing responsibilities related to medication errors:

1. Assess and detect errors in drug therapy.
2. Report and document any errors detected.

3. Monitor the patient for adverse effects.
4. Take corrective measures to prevent or minimize adverse effects.
5. Seek to eliminate the cause of the medication error.

It is also essential that medications be prescribed and prepared correctly. Physicians, pharmacists, and nurses must collaborate in a system of checks and balances to ensure that drugs are used appropriately and safely. Every medication order or preparation should be double-checked for accuracy and appropriateness. It is far easier and safer to prevent most iatrogenic adverse drug effects than it is to treat them.

Pharmacologic Factors

Adverse reactions are often thought of as undesirably increased drug effects; however, they also include inhibition or total absence of effect. The adverse effects of a drug may actually be part of its normal action. For example, atropine, which both increases heart rate and reduces secretions, may be given to increase a patient's heart rate. The dry mouth it produces may be viewed as an undesirable or adverse effect. Conversely, atropine may be administered to reduce secretions, in which case the tachycardia it causes may be considered an adverse effect for some patients.

The use of multiple drugs is a major source of untoward drug effects. Many drugs that have the potential to interact adversely may be used in combination for an optimal therapeutic response. As the number of drugs administered to a patient increases, so does the likelihood of an adverse reaction (or interaction) occurring. For example, a patient being treated for congestive heart failure may be prescribed digoxin and the diuretic furosemide. A side effect of furosemide is the loss of potassium from the bloodstream. This, in turn, may enhance the effect of digoxin and possibly lead to the development of serious or fatal cardiac arrhythmias.

Adverse Effects Caused by Administration of a Single Drug

Adverse drug effects that result from the administration of a single drug include such reactions as drug allergy; idiosyncrasy; cumulative effects; tolerance and tachyphylaxis; dependence; toxicity and tissue damage; and carcinogenic, mutagenic, or teratogenic effects. Some adverse effects manifest themselves after only one dose; others may take weeks, months, or years of repeated administration to develop.

Drug Allergy

The patient's immune system may affect the response to medication. An *allergy* is an immune response involving an antigen–antibody reaction. Many drugs are foreign substances that can act as antigens, activating the immune system to form antibodies against the drug. If the drug is given again at a later time, the antibodies now present in the blood combine with the medication, and a systemic reaction occurs.

The manifestations of allergic drug reactions are numerous and include the full spectrum from immediate to delayed allergic responses. Skin reactions may range from a mild rash to exfoliative dermatitis. Vascular responses range from urticaria and angioedema to severe arteritis. Fever, rhinitis, bronchospasm, and anaphylactic shock are other familiar allergic responses that medications can precipitate.

The way in which antigen–antibody reactions produce their adverse effects differs according to the type of reaction. Some involve only the destruction of red blood cells (hemolysis). Others, such as bronchospasm and urticaria, involve the release of histamine, prostaglandins, serotonin, and kinins from mast cells and basophils.

An allergic reaction is highly specific to a particular causative agent and usually occurs only after prior exposure to an antigen. Since the reaction does not usually occur on the initial exposure to a drug, the patient may react unexpectedly to doses of the medication given at a later time. Sometimes persons with no known history of receiving a drug develop an allergic reaction on their first exposure to it. The response may be the result of prior environmental exposure to a related chemical that stimulated antibody production.

The potential for an allergic response may remain intact virtually forever after initial exposure. Extremely small quantities of a medication are all that are needed to provoke the reaction, and the severity of the reaction does not always relate to the dose of drug or the route of administration. Patients with a history of multiple allergies are more likely than others to develop a medication allergy. The nurse must be alert to the symptoms of an allergic response in any patient receiving a medication.

Idiosyncratic Reactions

For most patients, a given dose of a particular drug usually causes a known and predictable effect, with only slight individual variability. However, some patients respond in a highly unusual and often unpredictable way. This type of response, called an **idiosyncratic** response, usually represents a genetically determined abnormal susceptibility to a chemical. It often involves alterations in drug metabolism. The genetic alteration, and the unusual drug response it causes, often has familial or racial characteristics that are transmitted to the offspring.

Idiosyncrasy often explains unusual responses such as extreme sensitivity to very low doses of a drug, abnormally prolonged drug effects, marked resistance to even large doses of a drug, or the appearance of unusual or novel drug responses that are rarely seen in other patients.

Cumulative Effects

A *cumulative* effect is the progressively increasing response to repeated doses of a drug that occurs when the rate of drug entry into the body exceeds the rate of metabolism or excretion. As the concentration of a drug within the body rises, toxic symptoms may occur. Occasionally, a large "loading" dose of a medication is administered to achieve a desired concentration within the body quickly, followed by a lower "maintenance" dose to maintain the desired constant level of drug. The daily maintenance dose must be equal to the daily loss. If it is higher, toxicity may develop from accumulation of the drug in body tissues.

Patients with a decreased ability to metabolize or excrete a drug, such as patients with decreased renal or hepatic function, are especially prone to the cumulative effects of repeated doses. Accumulation of a drug in the body can also result from one medication interfering with the body's ability to metabolize or excrete other drugs. This is, therefore, a drug–drug interaction.

Tolerance

Tolerance is the phenomenon in which the response to a particular dose of a drug given repeatedly becomes less intense over time. To overcome tolerance, an increased dose of the drug is needed to cause a response equal in intensity to the response produced before tolerance developed. In some situations tolerance can be considered an adverse drug response because it may cause inadequate therapeutic results unless appropriate dosage increases are made.

Tolerance generally occurs with prolonged and repeated administration of a drug, but may occur after only one or two doses. The special term **tachyphylaxis** is used for such rapidly-developing tolerance. Tolerance most frequently occurs in response to drugs (depressants or stimulants) that affect the central nervous system, but the phenomenon can apply to a wide variety of drugs. The degree of tolerance that develops in response to a particular drug varies from person to person. Chronic use of alcohol, for example, may cause the development of such tolerance that the individual may experience little effect after drinking amounts of alcoholic beverage that would seriously impair a person who has not developed tolerance to this substance.

The phenomenon of **cross-tolerance** may also develop. In cross-tolerance, the individual becomes tolerant to actions of other drugs that cause similar effects in a similar way. Thus, the alcohol-tolerant individual will be tolerant to the action of barbiturates, and therefore may require doses that are much greater than normal to cause therapeutically desired sedation or sleep.

In terms of adverse drug responses, the fact that tolerance does not develop uniformly to all actions of a given drug is perhaps more important than the diminished therapeutic action. In some cases, tolerance develops to a side effect of a drug, such as nausea, sedation, or stimulation, while the primary therapeutic response is unaffected. In other cases, the reverse may be true. For example, although a patient may develop tolerance to the therapeutically desirable sedative or sleep-inducing effects of a barbiturate, no comparable tolerance develops simultaneously to the ability of these drugs to cause fatal respiratory depression. As a result, increasing the dose to regain the desired effect may have potentially fatal consequences.

There are three main types of drug tolerance: pharmacokinetic (dispositional), pharmacodynamic, and behavioral.

Pharmacokinetic Tolerance

Pharmacokinetic (dispositional) tolerance results from changes in the patient that result in reduced concentrations of drug at the site of drug action. This is frequently due to increased metabolism. The most common mechanism of pharmacokinetic tolerance is enzyme induction, in which a drug induces increased enzyme formation to metabolize a drug more rapidly. A more detailed discussion of enzyme induction is found in Chapter 4.

Pharmacodynamic Tolerance

Pharmacodynamic tolerance results from adaptive or compensatory changes within the body that result in a decreased effect of drugs on their cellular targets, even though ample amounts of drug molecules may be present. Another cause involves compensatory changes of one body system to counteract the effects of a drug on another system. Pharmacodynamic tolerance is often seen as a response to antihypertensive medications. Certain of these agents reduce blood pressure transiently, but compensatory changes within the body (tachycardia, fluid and sodium retention, vasoconstriction) lead to a return toward pretreatment blood pressure levels. Combination drug therapy is often used to blunt the adaptive changes of pharmacodynamic tolerance.

Behavioral Tolerance

Behavioral tolerance is a diminished response to one or more effects as a result of behavioral or other central nervous system adaptations. In essence, the patient "learns" to compensate for a drug effect and learns to function under the drug's influence. Behavioral tolerance is most commonly seen in response to drugs that affect the central nervous system and alter behavior.

Dependence

Dependence may be defined as the need for continued administration of drug to prevent the appearance of a characteristic withdrawal syndrome that involves either physiologic or psychologic signs and symptoms (or both). Dependence often develops in response to abuse of drugs with actions in the central nervous system, such as alcohol and other sedatives, narcotics, and stimulants (see Unit 4). Dependence may also occur with drugs affecting other body systems, and with drugs administered properly for therapeutic purposes. Like tolerance, drug dependence may develop after only days of repeated drug administration, or it may take months to occur, depending on the drug, the dosage, and various patient-related factors.

In **physical dependence,** repeated exposure to the drug causes the body to adapt through physiologic changes until it reaches a point where it can only function normally in the presence of the drug. Withdrawal symptoms associated with physical dependence generally are characterized by *rebound,* or a response opposite to the initial drug effect. For example, amphetamines act to alleviate fatigue and elevate mood. Amphetamine withdrawal is manifested by fatigue and depression.

Psychologic dependence may be found to some degree with any drug that affects the central nervous system. Some patients develop such a strong desire for a drug effect that they feel they cannot function without the drug. Dependence is more than a habit; it is a compulsion to take the drug. Lifestyles may be altered, and great risks taken, to continue using a drug.

Systemic and Local Toxicity

A *toxic* reaction may be thought of as poisoning. Any drug can be considered toxic if it is administered in an unsuitable manner or in sufficient (usually excessive) amounts. Drug toxicity is frequently an extension—due to overdosage, a cumulative effect of drug administration, or abnormal sensitivity—of the drug's desired therapeutic effect.

Toxicity is not always related to high concentrations or an "overdose" of a drug, however. The nurse should be aware of the possibility of a toxic reaction even when a drug is taken in therapeutic doses.

The spectrum of toxic effects is broad and variable. It can involve localized effects on a particular tissue, or can affect an organ, an organ system, or the entire organism. The toxic effect of a drug may be reversible, as in the gastrointestinal upset caused by some drugs, or permanent, as in the hearing damage that can result from aminoglycoside antibiotic use.

Most toxic effects from drugs occur within a short time after administration. However, some require months to develop (for example, aplastic anemia caused by the antibiotic chloramphenicol), while others may not be seen until decades later (for example, drug-induced cancers).

Tissue damage resulting from drugs, another form of toxicity, can be either local or systemic, according to the drug's site(s) of action. Local effects are those that occur at the site where the drug first comes into contact with the body. Damage to the oral and gastrointestinal mucosa caused by ingestion of a caustic substance, and gastric ulcers caused by the irritant effects of aspirin, are examples of drug-induced local tissue damage.

As with systemic toxicity, localized toxicity can be reversible or irreversible. It depends on the drug, the dose, the duration of exposure to the damaging substance, and the regenerative capacity of the affected cells. Drug-induced damage to the skin or mucosa lining the gastrointestinal tract is often completely reversible, for example, in contrast to the potentially irreversible damage to neural tissues, which have minimal regenerative capacity.

Carcinogenesis

A few drugs are known to have, or are suspected of having, the ability to induce cancer or predispose patients to the disease. The determination of a drug's carcinogenic potential is conducted with animal studies and extrapolated to human beings. The complex nature of many cancers, and a long latency period from exposure to development of malignancy, make the determination of carcinogenesis difficult. Highly carcinogenic drugs are never released for patient use; however, the carcinogenic potential of a medication may not be known until after it has been used clinically for a considerable time. Some anticancer drugs may themselves be carcinogenic under certain circumstances. Tobacco, nitrites, herbicides, hair dyes, asbestos, and certain food colorings are among the many agents known or strongly thought to be carcinogenic.

Mutagenesis

Some drugs have the ability to cause chromosomal changes that result in a permanent alteration of genetic structure. The genetic change appears in the offspring, transferred through the chromosomes of either the sperm or ova. This is particularly true of some toxins and antineoplastic agents.

Teratogenesis

Teratogenesis is the production of physical defects in the fetus during development. In general, the most critical time for organ formation is the first trimester of pregnancy. This is also the time at which drug administration to the pregnant woman poses the greatest risk of fetal malformations. Although relatively few drugs are known definitely to cause congenital birth defects, even fewer are known to be virtually free of this risk. Drugs undergoing approval for human use must be tested for teratogenic potential in animals, but the example provided by the thalidomide tragedy attests to the fact that animal studies may not apply to human beings.

Since it is difficult to determine the true teratogenic potential of drugs in human beings, it is best to assume that most drugs on the market have not been proved safe for administration during pregnancy, and to avoid their use unless the potential benefits to the mother clearly outweigh the possible risks to the fetus.

In an effort to balance the need to administer drugs to a pregnant woman and the potential for adverse fetal effects, the FDA has established five categories for the use of drugs in pregnancy (Table 9–1). The classifications are based on data obtained from animal studies and, when available, from controlled human studies. The manufacturer's package insert and information in the *Physicians' Desk Reference* indicate the category for a given drug.

Table 9–1 Food and Drug Administration Pregnancy Categories

Category	
A	No risk to the fetus based on acceptable and controlled studies in pregnant women
B	No evidence of risk to humans, either based on positive findings in animals but negative findings in human trials, or negative findings in animal studies and the absence of any adequate data from human trials
C	A potential risk, usually because there is no data from human studies, and animal studies show adverse effects or no studies have been conducted. Drugs with a pregnancy category C rating may be used when potential benefits outweigh potential risks to the fetus
D	Evidence of fetal harm based on data obtained either from investigational studies or data collected after the drug has been approved and used in pregnant women. Drugs in pregnancy category D may also be used during pregnancy if there is a favorable benefit to risk ratio
X	The drug is contraindicated during pregnancy; the potential risks clearly outweigh any real or anticipated benefits

Adverse Effects Caused by Administration of More Than One Drug

Dangerous *interactions* may occur when two or more drugs are used simultaneously, or when drugs are combined with certain foods. One drug may alter the intensity of the pharmacologic effects of another drug given concurrently. The net result may be an enhanced, diminished, or in another way altered effect of one or both drugs.

Although these drug–drug interactions are being discussed here within the context of adverse drug effects, some drug interactions may be therapeutically useful. Many drug preparations contain a combination of two or more drugs simply because the combination provides a more desirable effect than is possible with a single drug. Effects caused by the administration of more than one drug may be additive, summative, synergistic, potentiative, or antagonistic.

SPOTLIGHT ON NURSING RESEARCH

The advent of multilumen catheters for intravenous infusion has been particularly important for critically ill patients with needs for long-term, reliable venous access. These catheters reduce risks of contamination and infection associated with repeated venipuncture and multiple catheter insertion sites. They also permit incompatible drugs to be infused simultaneously. This study examined whether the infusion of incompatible drugs from separate lumens of multilumen catheters would result in adverse reactions, such as precipitation. The authors acknowledge that there are no published reports of patient problems occurring as a result of this practice, but they also point out that clinical sequelae of adverse incompatibility reactions would be difficult to identify, particularly in critically ill patients.

Because phenytoin undergoes a rapid, visible precipitation when mixed with total parenteral nutrition (TPN), the simultaneous administration of these two agents was studied using an in vitro flow system to simulate infusion into large central veins. Two types of catheters were evaluated: a double-lumen, silicone rubber catheter with adjacent infusion orifices; and a triple-lumen, polyurethane catheter with offset and staggered infusion orifices. Video recordings were made to examine stream interactions, and circulating fluid was assayed for phenytoin concentration.

Simultaneous infusion of phenytoin and TPN through separate lumens of the double-lumen catheter produced a visible, white cloud in all cases (n=10) due to phenytoin precipitation. Phenytoin crystals were generally 5–10 by 25–50 μm in size, but crystals of millimeter size were occasionally dislodged from the buildup of precipitate at the catheter tip. Precipitate was not observed when either phenytoin or TPN was administered alone through one lumen of the catheter. Simultaneous infusion of phenytoin and TPN infusion through different ports of the triple-lumen catheter did not produce visible precipitation (n=8).

Assays indicated that when phenytoin was infused with TPN through a double-lumen catheter, on average, 6% of the phenytoin administered was lost to precipitation. There was only a 1% loss when phenytoin was infused with TPN through a triple-lumen catheter. As noted in the study, these results suggest that precipitation may not produce a critical loss in the amount of phenytoin administered. However, the investigators believe that the precipitate observed is clinically significant, citing evidence that drug particulates may cause pain during injection and may increase risks of thrombophlebitis and emboli.

The findings suggest that double-lumen catheters with adjacent orifices allow greater interaction between simultaneously infused drugs as compared to triple-lumen catheters with staggered end holes for infusion. These observations have relevance for the evaluation of catheter designs. Moreover, this in vitro study demonstrates the basis for potential problems with the use of double-lumen catheters that may be clinically important when very rapid drug interactions can occur, as in the case of phenytoin and TPN.

Collins JL, Lutz RJ: In vitro study of simultaneous infusion of incompatible drugs in multilumen catheters. *Heart & Lung* 1991; 20:271–277.

Addition and Summation

Additive effects occur when two drugs with the same mechanism of action are taken; the result is equal to the sum of the responses to each drug (that is, 1 + 1 = 2). Simple additive effects can be seen with trisulfapyrimidine, a mixture of three sulfonamide antibiotics. Each of these drugs, if given alone in large doses, may form damaging crystals in the kidney tubule when the antibiotic is excreted in the urine. The overall blood levels and antimicrobial effects of the antibiotic combination are about the same as would be produced by giving the same total dose of only one of the antibiotics, since the antimicrobial actions of each agent are additive. However, because each individual agent is present in a relatively low concentration, the risk of urinary crystal formation, and resulting renal damage, is reduced.

Summation occurs when two drugs cause the same overt effect but not necessarily by the same mechanism of action. The resulting effect is still the sum of the individual effects of each drug (1 + 1 = 2).

Synergy

Synergistic effects occur when two drugs used together have a greater combined effect than the sum of the separate actions of each. Each drug used alone produces an effect, but when given in combination the intensity of the effect is greater than the sum of effects (1 + 1 = 3). An example of a common synergistic effect is that produced when alcohol is taken with sedative-hypnotic medications. If certain medications are taken together, even in moderate doses, the synergistic effect may result in a very serious outcome because of an excessive effect.

Potentiation

Potentiation occurs when one drug, completely lacking an observable effect if given alone, causes a measurable response in the presence of another (0 + 1 = 2). An example of this is the interaction of tyramine (found in some wines, cheese, and fish) and monoamine oxidase inhibitors. Tyramine alone has no effect, but when a patient taking a monoamine oxidase inhibitor ingests even a small amount of tyramine, severe and possibly fatal hypertension may occur.

Antagonism

Antagonism occurs when a combination of drugs results in an effect less than that produced when either drug is administered alone (2 + 2 = 3). Like the situation with addition, synergism, and potentiation, antagonism between two or more drugs can be beneficial or adverse, depending on the situation. The general adverse effect caused by drug antagonism is a diminished therapeutic response. One major form of antagonism, called *biochemical* or *pharmacokinetic antagonism,* involves the ability of one drug to alter the absorption, distribution, metabolism, or excretion of another (see Chapter 4). Other forms of antagonism include *pharmacologic* (or pharmacodynamic) *antagonism,* in which one drug interferes with the ability of another to react with its cell receptor sites; *biochemical antagonism,* in which two drugs that are chemically incompatible react with one another to neutralize or otherwise reduce the effects of one or both; and *physiologic* or *functional antagonism,* in which two drugs act on different structures, through different processes, to cause counteracting effects. These forms of antagonism were discussed in Chapter 6.

Nursing Implications of Adverse Drug Effects

Diagnosis of High Risk Situations and Possible and Actual Alterations Related to Adverse Drug Effects

Nursing diagnoses related to adverse drug effects are varied. The diagnostic statement is developed from the data acquired during the patient assessment, and identifies any undesirable responses the patient experiences during drug therapy. It would be an error, however, to assume that all unexpected symptoms are adverse drug reactions. Many alterations would occur even without drug therapy. Consequently, the nurse must accurately assess the basis of any potential or actual alteration to determine whether complaints such as gastrointestinal upset, drowsiness, skin rashes, itching, or headache are the result of the disease process or the drug therapy.

Each nursing diagnosis represents either an actual, high risk, or possible problem for the patient, the family, or both. The diagnosis statement includes both the condition that will respond to nursing care and the related factors influencing the condition (but not necessarily its cause). The diagnostic conclusions help to determine priorities for care, and provide direction to the nursing activities.

When administering medications to patients, the nurse might develop nursing diagnoses similar to the following:

- Knowledge deficit related to insufficient instruction about correct administration of insulin
- Noncompliance related to feminizing effects (in men) of estrogen therapy
- Ineffective individual coping related to need for lifelong drug replacement therapy with Addison's disease
- Fluid volume excess related to sodium and water retention with hydrocortisone therapy
- Body image disturbance related to hirsutism, in women, with testosterone therapy
- Sleep pattern disturbance related to insomnia with levothyroxine therapy
- High risk for injury related to ataxia with anticonvulsant therapy

Nursing diagnoses approved by the North American Nursing Diagnosis Association (NANDA) are included throughout this book, and serve as the basis for planning and implementing nursing care during drug therapy.

Nursing interventions related to high-risk situations or actual or possible adverse drug reactions often include strategies to prevent complications (eg, taking thyroid hormone supplements before breakfast to prevent insomnia), measures to ensure safe administration of medications (eg, rotating injection sites to prevent lipodystrophies with insulin), teaching to increase knowledge (eg, signs and symptoms of desired and adverse drug effects), and activities to resolve physical and psychologic effects (eg, sodium restriction with glucocorticoids, reassurance that hirsutism will resolve after drug therapy has been completed).

TRENDS AND CONTROVERSIES IN PHARMACOLOGY

Are Any Side Effects "Insignificant?"

Many frequently occurring drug side effects are regarded as insignificant, and traditionally are low on the practitioner's list of priorities. But when considering side effects such as dry mouth, blurred vision, anorexia, constipation, changes in libido, depression, dizziness, or lethargy, it might be asked to whom these effects are insignificant: to the patient or to the caregiver?

To add insult to injury, many clinicians have a different attitude toward side effects in a 30-year-old man than in a 70-year-old. A young adult is expected to be in generally good health, and physicians tend to be more aggressive in manipulating young patients' drug regimens to attain the best results with the fewest side effects. With an older patient, however, doctors and nurses are conditioned to accept so many complaints as "typical" of old age that these problems are seen as unavoidable.

While the cardiovascular changes of aging may predispose some patients to dizziness, slowed gastrointestinal tract motility may result in constipation, and life changes may contribute to depression, drugs can do these things, too. Do not accept drug-induced changes as unmanageable or, worse, unavoidable in old age.

Another bad habit some professionals have is to ignore physical complaints in patients with mental disability, as though that point eliminates the need for attention to anything else. The fact that "she has Alzheimer's" or "he's mentally retarded" is no reason to sentence the person to a wide range of physical discomforts from drugs.

Anyone who has ever had to live with drugs and their side effects knows that even minor discomforts, when they occur regularly, can leave a person feeling very unwell from day to day. This can eventually change the individual's perception of his or her state of health, and that will have further detrimental effects on physical and mental well-being as time goes by.

Some "insignificant" side effects do increase morbidity. Dry mouth, untreated, can lead to dental caries, oral infections, poor denture fit. Dizziness can result in falls. Anorexia may lead to weight loss, malnutrition, and slowed healing. Constipation can progress to impaction or paralytic ileus.

Even if there were some guarantee that side effects would never escalate into other problems, is it fair to ignore the patient's discomfort? Lower doses, alternate drug therapy, or specific therapeutic measures can offset or totally eliminate many side effects. In some cases, nondrug therapy is the alternative of choice.

Planning and Intervention in Special Situations

Allergic Reactions

The first nursing intervention related to allergic reactions involves prevention. Assessment should include the patient's and family's history of allergies as well as prior exposure and response to drugs. All patients who are unable to communicate clearly should be checked for an identification card or tag indicating the presence of a drug allergy. Allergies should be recorded on the patient's chart and on the identification bracelet. Following recognition of an allergy history, the nurse should assess for a knowledge deficit relating to the allergy and institute patient teaching.

A drug must never be administered without checking first for drug allergies and concurrent drug use. Nurses should be aware of all drugs contained in combination preparations and the possibility of cross-sensitivity between drugs. After administering a drug, the nurse should observe the patient for signs of an allergic or anaphylactic response. Anaphylaxis requires prompt and aggressive emergency treatment. At the first sign of an allergic reaction, drug administration should be stopped, the physician notified, and appropriate treatment begun. Drugs used to treat allergic reactions include epinephrine, antihistamines, adrenocorticosteroids, aminophylline, and oxygen.

Tolerance

The major nursing goals for administering drugs to which tolerance develops center on knowing whether tolerance develops toward the desired (therapeutic) response, side effects and adverse responses, or both. If the therapeutic response is likely to diminish with time, nursing measures should focus on periodic assessment of the major signs and symptoms characteristic of the condition for which the drug was given, and on changes of other body systems, caused by drug administration, that might be activated to compensate for the drug's actions. This assessment is necessary to notify the physician so that increased drug doses may be ordered if needed.

If tolerance is expected to develop for side effects or other adverse drug responses, especially if they cause alterations of the patient's physical or emotional comfort, the patient should be advised of this possibility. Such education allays undue fear, helps the patient identify positive goals along the path to recovery, encourages compliance with the medication plan, and provides a measure of reassurance that the health-care team is both knowledgeable about and interested in the patient's well-being.

Regardless of whether tolerance develops to therapeutic or untoward effects, and especially if apparent tolerance occurs when it is not expected, nursing measures should include assessment of the possibility that the diminished response to a drug is caused by noncompliance. If expected tolerance does not develop, assessment of the underlying causes is also indicated.

Dependence

Treatment of the drug-dependent patient presents many challenges to the nurse, particularly if dependence is induced by persons self-administering substances of abuse. The word *drug-dependent* may conjure up various stereotypes and images that the nurse must overcome to provide nonjudgmental care. Each drug-dependent patient has a complex set of disturbances involving both psychologic and physiologic systems, all of which must be addressed when providing nursing care. The nurse must also be aware of the potential risks of inducing physical or psychologic dependence as a result of drug administration for therapeutic purposes, and should be able to make some meaningful statement to the patient or family about those risks.

Nursing priorities include assessing the drug-dependent patient's level of physical and social impairment, coping abilities, skills, and resources. Although a necessary part of nursing care is understanding the pharmacology of drugs on which a person is dependent, such understanding is not sufficient to ensure proper treatment and support. Drug abuse and dependence are often perpetuated in a cycle based on psychologic, social, environmental, and personal factors, all of which reinforce and maintain drug usage differently for each patient. Therefore, the nursing history of drug use and abuse should include information that might give insight into factors that contribute to the development and persistence of abuse.

Nursing care during treatment and withdrawal also requires attention to physical and psychologic changes, and the appropriate supportive measures for each. Once acute withdrawal is complete, major nursing goals are promotion of wellness, continued emotional support, education, and rehabilitation. These and other aspects of care of the drug-dependent individual are discussed more fully in Chapter 28.

Poisoning

The treatment of poisoning must be prompt and, if possible, specific. Supportive management is combined with specific treatment once the poison has been identified. Assessment is aimed at identifying the specific poison as well as the time and amount of ingestion or exposure. Most poison control centers can be contacted by telephone 24 hours a day to assist with identification of specific poisons and their treatment. Appendix C gives more information about recognizing and treating poisonings.

Drug-Induced Tissue Damage or Toxicity

Nursing goals for drug administration should include attempts to avoid or minimize tissue damage, whether caused by local contact of an irritating drug with tissues at the site of administration or by systemic toxic effects. This goal can be accomplished in many ways. For example, irritating drugs, particularly those that are given orally, may be diluted or given with another substance. Nursing strategies may include administration of the drug with a compatible food or beverage; taking precautions to ensure that the patient swallows a solid dosage form (tablet or capsule) whole, without chewing; advising the patient to sip a liquid medication through a straw if the drug is damaging to the teeth; or rinsing the mouth thoroughly after administration of an irritating liquid.

The most general nursing strategy with parenteral drug administration involves selecting the proper route of administration, and then ensuring that the injection is given with proper technique. For example, if a drug must be injected into skin or muscle repeatedly, rotating injection sites can reduce the trauma that otherwise might occur if only one site were used. If large volumes of a drug must be injected, or an irritating drug must be injected frequently, the dose can be divided and given in two or more sites, the site can be massaged after injection, or cool or warm towels can be applied to the injection site (depending on the drug).

If intravenous administration is selected and the drug is irritating to the lining of the blood vessels, the drug should be administered through a large or central vein, with precautions taken to ensure that the catheter or needle is in proper position and not likely to move out of place. In this instance also, and depending on the drug, nursing strategies to reduce tissue irritation might include diluting the drug, administering it into a free-flowing intravenous line, or altering the speed of injection.

In any case, it is essential for the nurse to ensure that any diluents, or other fluids given with a drug are chemically compatible. The nurse should always assess the status of the injection site, the proper placement of the needle, and, for intravenous administration, the patency of the needle, catheter, and vessel before, during, and after administration.

Drug toxicity or other kinds of adverse responses may be more difficult to prevent or detect. The nurse needs a thorough knowledge of the characteristics of toxicity or adverse responses to a particular drug: how these untoward responses relate to the therapeutic dose of the drug or the duration of drug administration; which patients are most at risk, whether from the concurrent use of other drugs or the numerous patient-related factors; and what are the signs and symptoms of developing toxicity.

Recognizing the signs of systemic adverse responses to drugs may or may not be easy. In some cases, as when giving a drug that might alter heart rate, blood pressure, or gastrointestinal tract motility, it may be easy to detect untoward primary or second-ary responses, since they can be readily assessed with simple methods.

In other cases, particularly when the potential target of a drug's adverse actions cannot be assessed directly, the nurse's observation skills and knowledge of drug effects must be integrated with knowledge of physiology, pathophysiology, or biochemistry. Thus, the nurse administering a drug that might cause hepatotoxicity must assess the patient for signs and symptoms such as jaundice, abnormal urine color, or abdominal discomfort. Administering a drug that might cause blood dyscrasias necessitates assessment for sore throat, fever, epistaxis, or petechiae, all of which reflect the status of the blood-forming and immune systems.

The nurse's knowledge and assessment skills must also be communicated to the patient in an understandable way, as part of the teaching plan, so the patient can assume an active role in evaluating adverse drug responses.

Annotated Bibliography

Azzarello J. Reviewing your patient's medication regimen: A systematic approach. *Home Healthcare Nurse* 1989;7(6):24–26. *This short paper gives many useful tips to help ensure that medications do more good than harm, and to help you have a clearer understanding of your patient's overall therapy.*

Bowes WA Jr. The effect of medications on the lactating mother and her infant. *Clin Obstet Gynecol* 1980;23(4):1073–1080. *When the mother is breast-feeding, the nursing infant is also a target of adverse drug effects. This short paper describes how to evaluate an infant that becomes ill or fails to thrive, and what steps can be taken to eliminate the problem.*

Cook MC, Taren DL. Nutritional implications of medication use and misuse in elderly. J Fla Med Assoc 1990;77(6):606–613. *Not only medication-related considerations, but also nutritional and socioeconomic factors, should be addressed to identify and assess elderly patients' responses to drugs, and to help improve their quality of life.*

Hussar DA. Drug interactions. *Nursing '86* 1986;16:34–39. *A review of pharmacokinetic and pharmacodynamic drug interactions, with commonly encountered examples.*

Jick H. Adverse drug reactions: The magnitude of the problem. *J Allergy Clin Immunol* 1984;74(4, Pt 2):555–557. *A report of quantitative information on the clinical use and adverse effects of drugs. Reviews in-hospital and out-of-hospital morbidity and mortality from adverse drug reactions.*

Kuehm SL, Doyle MJ. Medication errors: 1977 to 1978. Experience in medical malpractice claims. NJ Med 1990;87(1):27–34. *A review of malpractice claims—unquestionably one of the potential consequences of iatrongenic adverse drug effects—revealed that "predominant categories" of problems included disregarding allergies to specific drugs; prescribing drugs without due consideration of the medical history; failing to adequately monitor therapy with certain drugs; and errors in prescription writing. Since the nurse is part of the health-care checks and balance system, and also a potential target of legal action, this paper is worth reading.*

Lamy PP. Adverse drug effects. *Clin Geriatr Med* 1990;6(2):293–307. *This expert provides unique insight into how age, polypharmacy, and medication errors made by both patients and caregivers can lead to a greater frequency of adverse drug effects in elders—and how such incidents can be reduced.*

Mathews KP. Clinical spectrum of allergic and pseudoallergic drug reactions. *J Allergy Clin Immunol* 1984;74(4, Pt 2):558–566. *An in-depth presentation of adverse drug reactions, both those based on immune mechanisms and pseudoallergic reactions that have similar clinical manifestations but do not involve antigen–antibody reaction.*

Royal Melbourne Hospital Pharmacy Department. Drug interactions. *Aust Nurses J* 1985;15:58–59. *Drug interactions of clinical significance are discussed with regard to mechanism of action.*

Stolley JM, Buckwalter KC, Fjordbak B, Bush S. Iatrogenesis in the elderly: Drug-related problems. *J Gerontol Nurs* 1991;17(9): 12–17. *This paper stresses the values of good history-taking, education (of both patients and care providers), and nursing measures, to help prevent, recognize, and manage iatrogenic adverse effects in the elderly.*

Tesfa A. Drug therapy in elderly patients: Diagnosis of drug-related problems. *Recent Adv Nurs* 1989;23:45–52. *A valuable discussion of the general problem, along with useful comments on how, with drugs and nondrug measures, nurses and other health-care providers can minimize adverse drug effects in the elderly.*

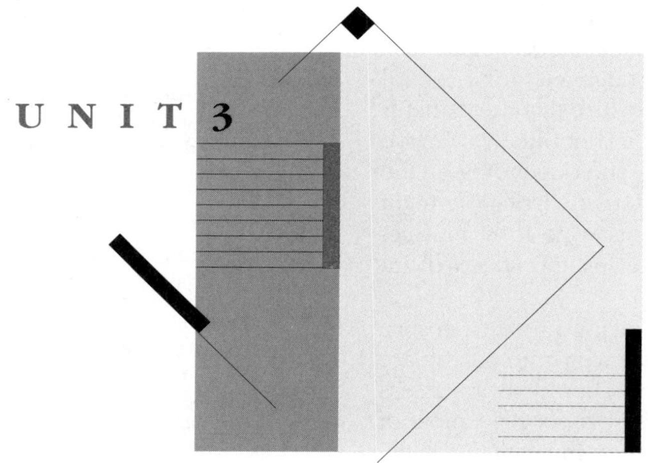

UNIT 3

Drugs That Affect the Autonomic and Somatic Nervous Systems

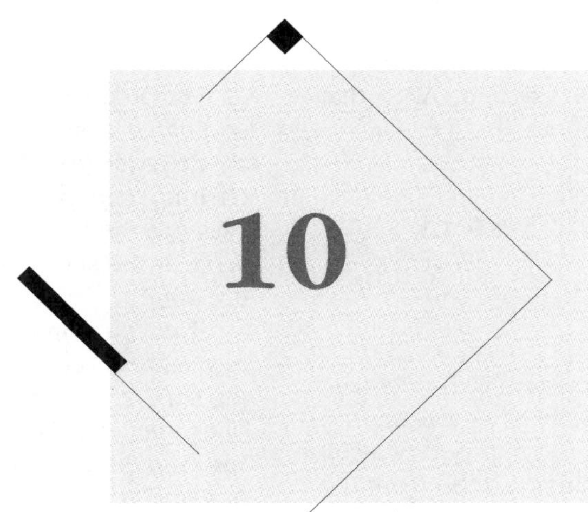

Structure and Function of the Autonomic Nervous System

Nurses must have a solid understanding of the nervous systems to understand physiology, pathophysiology, and the proper use of many drugs. This unit focuses on one part of the nervous system, the *autonomic nervous system.* In health and disease, the autonomic nervous system regulates and integrates the activities of virtually all the organ systems, and does so involuntarily—without the will or desire of the individual. When the activity of one organ system changes, the autonomic nervous system can automatically cause changes in the activity of others.

Many drugs are given specifically to increase or decrease autonomic influences on an organ or organ system. Many others are administered for purposes that, at first glance, do not seem to affect the autonomic nervous system, yet have the potential to do so. Often, the adverse effects caused by drugs that affect the autonomic nervous system, or the structures it controls can be more important than the desired effects for which the drug is given.

Anatomic Divisions of the Nervous System

Because of the complexity of the nervous system, its anatomic structures are usually considered in terms of two principal divisions, the *central nervous system (CNS)* and the *peripheral nervous system.* The CNS consists of the brain and spinal cord; it is responsible for monitoring, interpreting, and processing incoming sensory information and then transmitting signals that modify body activity based on that input. The CNS is discussed in Chapter 18.

The peripheral nervous system consists of all neural structures located outside the CNS. These structures include spinal and cranial nerves, ganglia (groups of nerve cell bodies) associated with these nerves, and sensory receptors. The peripheral nerves link all parts of the body with the CNS. Nerves that carry information from the periphery to the CNS are called **afferent** nerves, and nerves that carry information from the CNS to target structures (effectors) in the periphery are called **efferent** nerves.

The peripheral nervous system has two major subdivisions: the **somatic** nervous system, which controls skeletal muscle (voluntary movement), and the **autonomic** nervous system, which controls smooth muscle, cardiac muscle, and certain glands (involuntary functions). It is the autonomic nervous system (ANS) that maintains homeostasis within the body.

Fundamentals of Nervous System Structure and Function

Neurons

The structural unit of the nervous system is the *neuron,* or nerve cell. Figure 10–1 illustrates a typical neuron and its components. Each neuron is composed of a cell body and one or more processes that extend from the cell body. Nerve cell bodies are found in the CNS, and outside the CNS in peripheral **ganglia.** Within the CNS neuron processes form *tracts.* Outside the CNS such fiber bundles form the *peripheral nerves.*

There are two types of nerve cell processes: *dendrites* and *axons.* Dendrites conduct nerve impulses toward the cell body; axons conduct nerve impulses away from the cell body. The outer membranes of dendrites contain areas (receptors) that are receptive to chemicals that bind with the neurotransmitter chemicals released by adjacent axons. The synthesis, storage, and release of neurotransmitters occur either at the axonal nerve ending or at sites along the length of the axon known as **varicosities.** Although some nerves release their chemical mediators at the specialized varicosities, it is easier to think of all axons as having nerve endings that serve as the site of mediator release, as depicted in Figure 10–1.

Neurotransmitters enable the neurons to communicate with, and change the activity of, target cells. In doing so, the transmitter causes a characteristic response. The target of neurotransmitter action is called the **effector.** The effector can be another nerve cell or a muscle or gland cell.

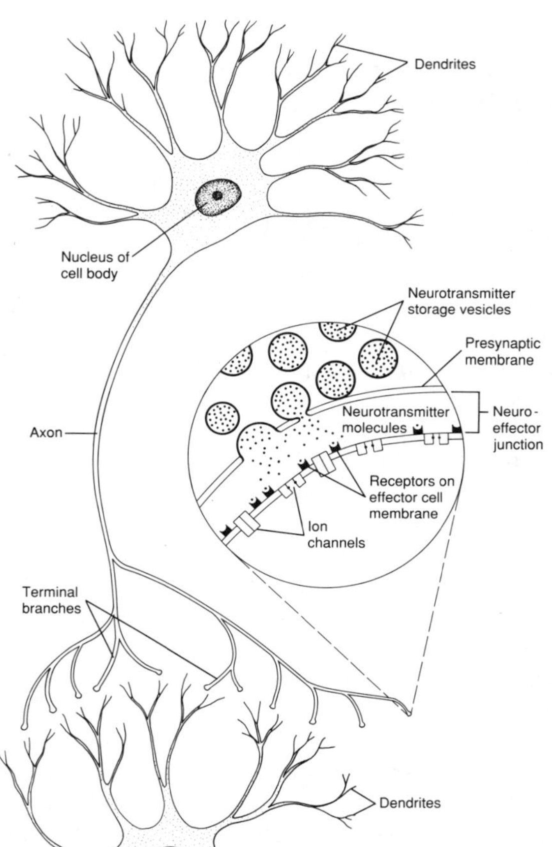

Figure 10–1

The structure of a typical neuron and a neuroeffector junction. **Inset.** Enlarged view of junction, showing neurotransmitter storage vesicles ("synaptic vesicles") in presynaptic nerve ending, some of which are emptying their contents into the junctional space as the nerve is stimulated; and receptors and ion channels on dendrites of postsynaptic (effector) cell. A similar arrangement is found when a nerve communicates with a muscle or gland cell, rather than with another nerve.

The Nerve Impulse

The plasma membrane of neurons is highly specialized to

1. Respond to a stimulus (usually provided by a neurotransmitter)
2. Generate and transmit an electrical impulse when adequately stimulated
3. Release neurotransmitters to communicate with other cells.

All these responses require almost instantaneous changes in the permeability of a neuron's membrane. Many drugs interfere with neuron function or responsiveness by altering one or more of these membrane characteristics; frequently, membrane permeability to sodium or potassium is changed. Figure 10–2 provides a brief review of how neurons stimulate other neurons and conduct impulses along the axon.

Synaptic Transmission

The nerve ending, although very close to the membrane of the effector cell with which it communicates, does not actually touch the membrane. A fluid-filled gap separates the two, across which the neurotransmitter diffuses to activate the target cell chemically. When a nerve communicates with another nerve, this gap is

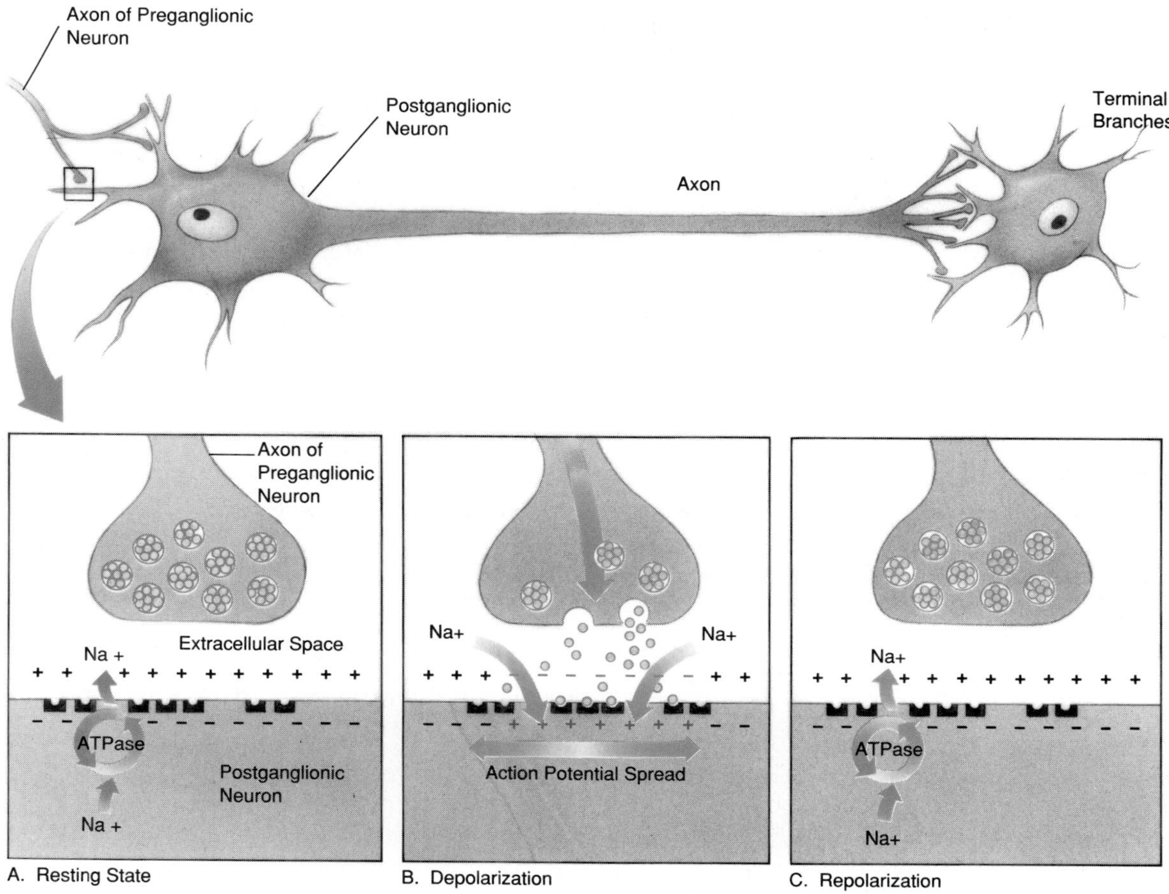

Figure 10–2

Chemical transmission from nerve to nerve, as in an autonomic ganglion.

A. Resting State. The postsynaptic cell's membrane is electrically charged ("polarized"; + charges outside, − charges inside) because of its permeability characteristics and the actions of the enzyme adenosine triphosphatase (ATPase) to "pump" sodium (Na^+) to the outside.
B. Depolarization. Activation of the presynaptic nerve releases neurotransmitter, which diffuses across the synapse and combines with its receptors on the postsynaptic membrane. The postsynaptic cell depolarizes as Na^+ rushes in. An action potential spreads down the postganglionic cell's axon, where its neurotransmitter will be released to stimulate muscle or gland cells.
C. Repolarization. Activation of the presynaptic nerve, and release of its neurotransmitter, stop. The postganglionic cell repolarizes by changing its permeability characteristics and by pumping out Na^+ once again. Both nerves, as well as the muscle or gland cells at the end of the pathway, return to their resting states.

called the *synaptic cleft.* The neuron located before (proximal to) the cleft is the *presynaptic neuron;* the neuron with which it communicates (distal to the cleft) is the *postsynaptic neuron.* When a nerve communicates with another type of cell, the general term describing the communication site is the **neuroeffector junction.** The term *neuromuscular junction* refers to the site at which a nerve releases its neurotransmitter to affect a muscle cell. Stimulation of the effector cell is a chemical event.

Neurotransmitters

Neurotransmitters do far more than simply link neurons to other neurons, muscles, or glands, to cause a response. The *type* of response that occurs is affected too. It is determined by the chemical makeup of the neurotransmitter, the specific receptor type with which it interacts, and the type of effector cell on which the receptor is found. In addition, the amount of neurotransmitter that is released affects the *intensity* of the

Table 10–1 Comparison of Anatomy, Neurotransmitters, and Target Cells of the Autonomic Nervous System

	Parasympathetic	Sympathetic
	Preganglionic Nerves	
Cell body origin	Cranial and sacral regions of spinal cord	Thoracic and lumbar region of spinal cord
Transmitter released (fiber type)	ACh (cholinergic nerve)	ACh (cholinergic nerve)
Termination of transmitter activity	Enzymatic hydrolysis by AChE	Enzymatic hydrolysis by AChE
Target of action (effectors)	Postganglionic parasympathetic nerve	Postganglionic sympathetic nerve or adrenal medulla
Ratio of preganglionic to postganglionic nerves	Usually one-to-one	Diffuse (axons synapse with many postganglionic neurons)
Effect on postganglionic nerve	Stimulation (depolarization of nerve)	Stimulation
	Postganglionic Nerves	
Receptor type stimulated by preganglionic nerve	Nicotinic (cholinergic)	Nicotinic (cholinergic)
Cell body origin	Parasympathetic ganglion in or near target structure	Sympathetic ganglion, usually near spinal cord, far from target structure*
Transmitter released (fiber type)	ACh (cholinergic)	Norepinephrine (adrenergic)*
Termination of transmitter activity	Metabolism by AChE	Reuptake into nerve ending
Target of action (effectors)	Smooth muscle, cardiac muscle, some glands	Smooth muscle, cardiac muscle, some glands
Receptor types on effectors	Muscarinic (cholinergic)	α, β (adrenergic)
Action on effector	Stimulation or inhibition, depending on effector location	Stimulation or inhibition, depending on effector location and receptor subtype involved

Key: ACh = acetylcholine; AChE = acetylcholinesterase.
*Cells of the adrenal medulla are functionally equivalent to postganglionic sympathetic nerves. When their receptors are stimulated by preganglionic sympathetic nerves, they release epinephrine into the bloodstream.

response. In general, the amount released is determined by the amount of transmitter that has been synthesized and stored, and by how intensely the nerve is stimulated. For each neurotransmitter unique processes affect how it is synthesized, stored, released, and inactivated, and how it interacts with its receptors. Each of these processes provides many points at which drugs can modify synaptic transmission; or mimic, intensify, or block the activity of neurotransmitters to stimulate their effectors.

Most neurons synthesize and release only one neurotransmitter, but they may respond to more than one neurotransmitter, as may the cells they affect. Moreover, a neuron may release from its axons a neurotransmitter different from the one that activated its dendrites. This is the case with the postganglionic neurons of the sympathetic nervous system (described later), which respond to one neurotransmitter (acetylcholine) but release another (norepinephrine).

Table 10–1 provides a review of the peripheral autonomic nervous system's two major neurotransmitters, acetylcholine and norepinephrine, including such information as which nerves they are found in; how their effects are stopped, physiologically; and on what types of receptors they act. Drugs that are chemically similar or identical to the natural neurotransmitters have important therapeutic uses, as do other drugs that can alter the effects of neurotransmitters.

The Autonomic Nervous System

The ANS includes important structures in the brain and spinal cord. However, it is most often discussed in terms of the structure and activity of its peripheral efferent fibers, which carry impulses from the CNS to effector organs. The ANS has two structural and functional divisions, the *parasympathetic* and the *sympathetic*. Each efferent pathway contains two neurons. The preganglionic nerve originates in the spinal cord and communicates through a parasympathetic or sympathetic ganglion with a postganglionic nerve that extends to an effector—cardiac muscle, smooth muscle, or a gland. Figure 10–3 shows a diagram of typical efferent pathways in

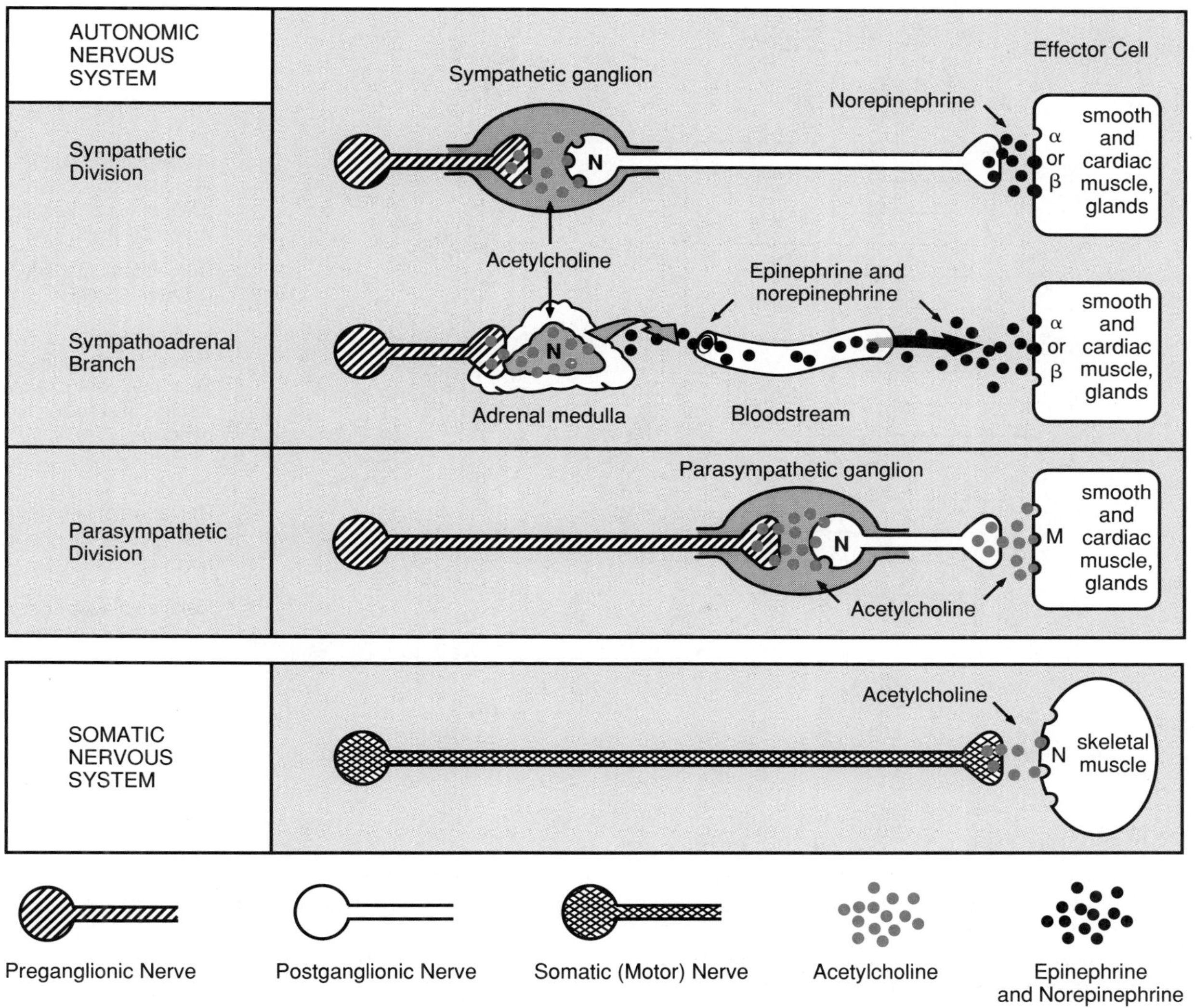

Figure 10–3

Organization of the peripheral nervous system into the autonomic (sympathetic and parasympathetic) and somatic nervous systems. *All preganglionic autonomic nerves,* and the *somatic motor nerves,* release acetylcholine (ACh) as the neurotransmitter (ie, they are **cholinergic**). The ACh they release acts on the **nicotinic** (N) subtype of cholinergic receptor, found either on postganglionic sympathetic or parasympathetic nerve cells, cells of the adrenal medulla, or skeletal muscle cells (in the somatic system). Postganglionic sympathetic nerves are called **adrenergic** because they release norepinephrine, which acts on α or β receptors on their muscle (smooth or cardiac) or gland cell targets. In the sympathoadrenal branch, the chemical message is carried through the blood by epinephrine and some norepinephrine. In the parasympathetic branch, both the preganglionic and postganglionic nerves are cholinergic. However, ACh released by the postganglionic parasympathetic nerves acts on a different subtype of cholinergic receptor, called **muscarinic** (M), found on smooth muscle, cardiac muscle, and glands. The following chapters in this unit discuss in more detail these nerves, neurotransmitters, and actions.

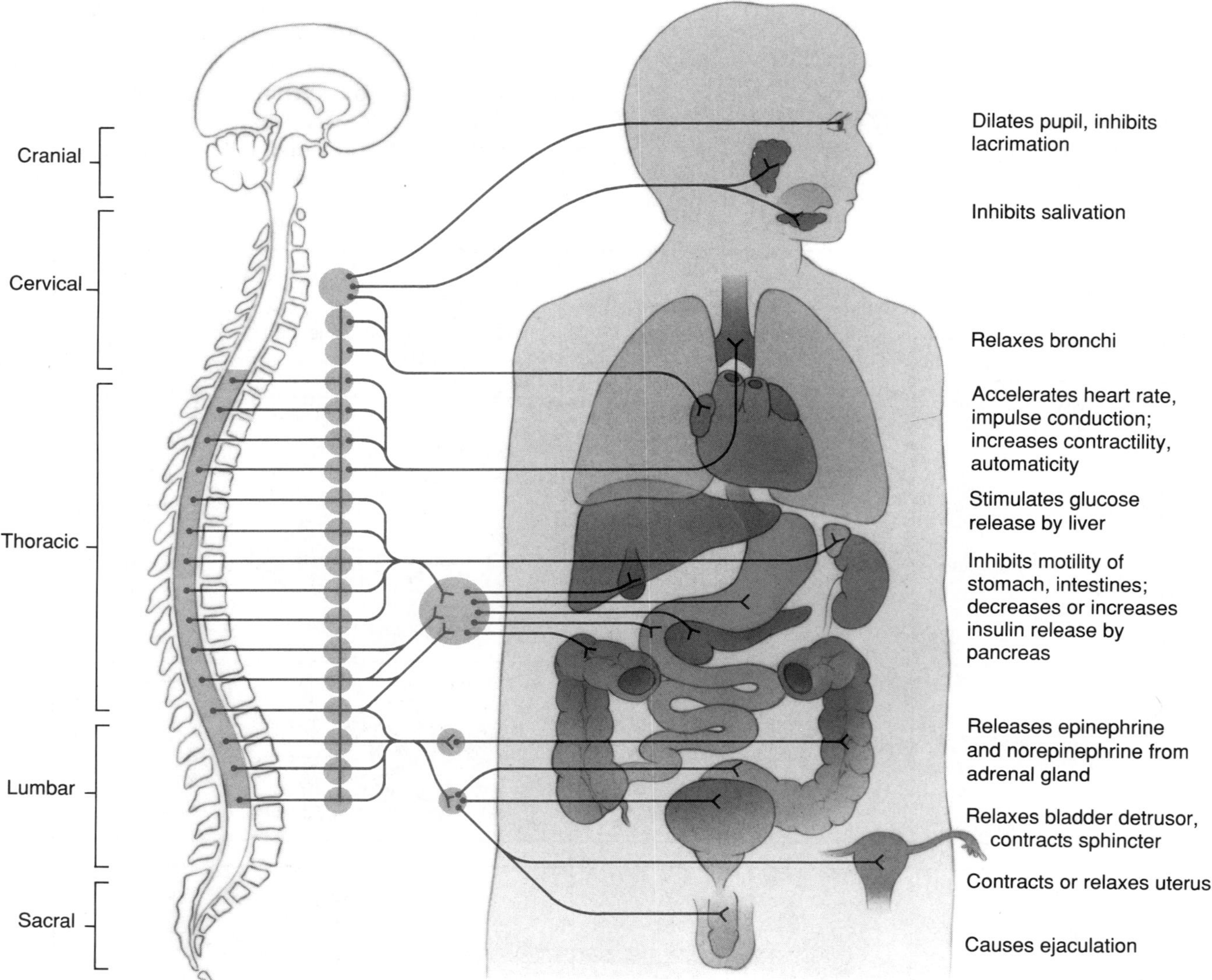

Figure 10–4A

The autonomic nervous system, sympathetic division. Autonomic pathways contain two neurons in series, but the arrangements and positions of the junctions between the presynaptic and postsynaptic cells differ. Preganglionic sympathetic nerves emerge from the thoracic and lumbar regions of the spinal cord. They have relatively short axons that interact with cell bodies of post-ganglionic sympathetic neurons in ganglia located near the spinal cord. The long axons of the postsynaptic cells leave the ganglia and travel to target organs. The adrenal medulla is, functionally, similar to a sympathetic ganglion.

the parasympathetic and sympathetic nervous systems, indicating the general anatomic arrangement and the major neurotransmitters. An efferent pathway in the somatic nervous system, which controls voluntary activity of skeletal muscle, is shown for comparison.

Roles of the Parasympathetic and Sympathetic Divisions

Usually, both branches of the ANS innervate a common effector organ, although the branches cause antagonistic (opposite) effects (Fig. 10–4). This is the concept of *dual innervation.*

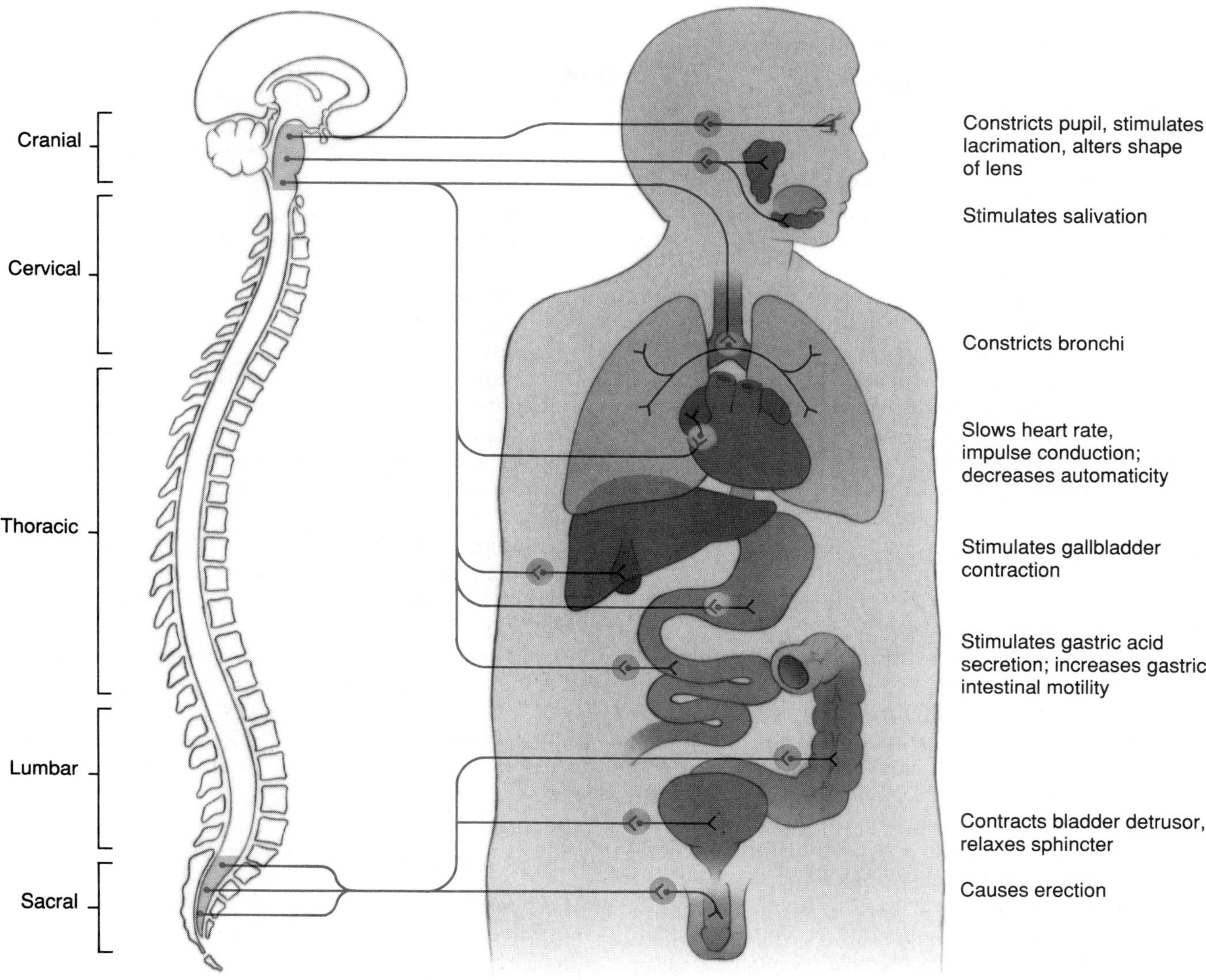

Figure 10–4B

The autonomic nervous system, parasympathetic division. Parasympathetic nerves originate in some of the cranial nerves and the sacral region of the spinal cord. Axons of the preganglionic parasympathetic nerves are much longer than those in the sympathetic division. Their synaptic connection with postganglionic parasympathetic nerves, in parasympathetic ganglia, occurs at or near the target organ.

Each branch of the ANS serves a unique role in maintaining body homeostasis. The parasympathetic branch is primarily concerned with conserving body energy, ensuring that digestion and waste elimination occur as necessary, and maintaining other vital activities at levels requiring minimal expenditure of energy.

The sympathetic branch is often referred to as the "fight or flight" system. Its function is to provide optimal conditions for appropriate responses in threatening situations. The sympathetic division is responsible for changes such as dilating the bronchi to increase oxygen delivery to the blood and other body cells, constricting blood vessels to increase blood pressure and shunt blood to vital organs, and increasing the heart rate to meet the heightened needs of all body organs. Metabolic changes needed to provide additional energy, such as mobilization of fat from adipose tissue and glucose from the liver, are also mediated by the sympathetic division. Unnecessary activities, such as motility of the gastrointestinal (GI) and urinary tracts, are reduced.

The two branches of the ANS do not act separately; rather, they have a dynamic antagonism. Slight changes in the activity of one or the other system are made continuously, and often simultaneously, in response to changing needs of the body. The opposing influences of these two systems on a given effector allow more precise control of an effector's activity than could be achieved if it were innervated by only a single system. However, the two divisions do not have equal (but opposite) control of their target organs. Rather, certain functions are controlled primarily by one division or the other. For example, the sympathetic branch provides the major control of blood pressure, whereas the parasympathetic branch exerts the major influences on the organs of the digestive and urinary tracts.

The Parasympathetic Division

The parasympathetic division (see Table 10–1) is often referred to as the *craniosacral division* because its preganglionic nerve cell bodies originate in the cranial and sacral regions of the spinal cord. In general, a single preganglionic parasympathetic neuron affects a single postganglionic neuron. This arrangement affords the parasympathetic division localized control over the organs that it serves. The preganglionic and postganglionic parasympathetic nerves are **cholinergic;** that is, they synthesize and release acetylcholine (ACh). Acetylcholine released from the preganglionic nerve stimulates the postganglionic neuron by interacting with a specific subclass of cholinergic receptor called a **nicotinic** receptor. The postganglionic neuron, once stimulated, releases ACh at the neuroeffector junction, leading to a change in the effector cell's function. The cholinergic receptor found on effector cells innervated by postganglionic parasympathetic nerves are of the **muscarinic** subclass.

Although all effectors innervated by the parasympathetic nervous system have muscarinic receptors, the kind of response (stimulation or inhibition) produced by ACh depends on the particular effector cell. For example, activation of the parasympathetic nerves to the heart causes an inhibitory response: a reduction in the heart rate. In contrast, parasympathetic effects on the smooth muscles in the airways cause an excitatory response: muscle contraction.

Several major groups of drugs alter parasympathetic nervous system activity or its influence on the function of its target organs. Drugs that mimic the effects produced naturally by ACh are called *cholinergic* drugs. Some interact directly with the muscarinic receptors on the target organs. They are called *muscarinic agonists* or **parasympathomimetic** drugs, and are discussed in Chapter 11. Others, although not capable of directly stimulating the ACh receptors, nevertheless cause important pharmacologic effects by inhibiting the normal metabolic inactivation of the neurotransmitter, thus causing an intensified response. These *acetylcholinesterase inhibitors* are discussed in Chapter 12.

Other drugs produce effects that make it appear as if the activity of the parasympathetic nervous system were reduced (Table 10–2). Atropine and related drugs, called **antimuscarinics, anticholinergics,** or **parasympatholytics,** block the ability of ACh and parasympathomimetic drugs to bind to and activate the muscarinic receptors on effector cells innervated by parasympathetic nerves. These drugs are discussed in Chapter 13.

Curare (tubocurarine) and its derivatives prevent ACh from binding to its nicotinic receptors, particularly those on skeletal muscle. This neuromuscular blocking drug, and others, is discussed in Chapter 17. The poison botulinum toxin (which causes the signs and symptoms of botulism due to food poisoning) prevents the release of ACh from *all* cholinergic nerves. In doing so it prevents *all* responses mediated by this critical neurotransmitter in the central, autonomic, and somatic nervous systems.

The Sympathetic Division

The sympathetic division (see Table 10–1) of the ANS is referred to as the *thoracolumbar division,* because the preganglionic nerves originate in the thoracic and lumbar regions of the spinal cord. It innervates all the organs or structures innervated by the parasympathetic branch.

As in the parasympathetic division, all preganglionic sympathetic nerves are cholinergic. That is, like their parasympathetic counterparts, they release ACh when stimulated, thus activating nicotinic receptors on postganglionic nerve cells. The pattern of preganglionic fiber distribution in the sympathetic division differs from that in the parasympathetic division. A single preganglionic sympathetic fiber may communicate with many postganglionic sympathetic nerves. This allows more widespread control than occurs with parasympathetic activation.

The majority of postganglionic sympathetic nerves are classified as **adrenergic,** meaning that they synthesize and release *norepinephrine* (noradrenaline), the

Table 10–2 Ways in Which Drugs Can Modify the Activity of the ANS or Its Target Structures

	Parasympathetic	Sympathetic
Ways to Increase Activity or Effects		**Agent**
Stimulate postganglionic cells directly	Nicotine (Chapter 16)	Nicotine (Chapter 16)
Release neurotransmitter from nerve in way other than *via* normal nerve stimulation	—	Mixed-acting sympathomimetics (ephedrine) or indirect-acting sympathomimetics (tyramine) (Chapter 14)
Inhibit metabolic inactivation of neurotransmitter	Acetylcholinesterase inhibitors (neostigmine; Chapter 12)	—
Enhance synthesis of neurotransmitter	—	Levodopa (Chapter 25)
Block reuptake of neurotransmitter; normal termination of its biologic activity	—	Cocaine (Chapter 14); tricyclic antidepressants (Chapter 24)
Mimic effects of neurotransmitter via a similar drug	Parasympathomimetics (bethanechol; Chapter 11)	Sympathomimetics (α- and β-adrenergic agonists, eg, epinephrine; Chapter 14)
Ways to Decrease Activity or Effects		
Block ability of preganglionic nerves to stimulate postganglionic nerves	Trimethaphan, nicotine (Chapter 16)	Trimethaphan, nicotine (Chapter 16)
Alter neurotransmitter synthesis	—	Form "false neurotransmitter" (methyldopa; Chapter 33)
Deplete neurotransmitter from nerve endings	—	Catecholamine depletors (reserpine; Chapter 33)
Inhibit release of neurotransmitter from nerve	Botulinum toxin (Chapter 17)	Bretylium (Chapter 30); monoamine oxidase inhibitors (Chapter 24)
Block neurotransmitter receptors on peripheral target cells	Muscarinic-receptor blockers (atropine; Chapter 13); nicotinic receptor blockers (tubocurarine; Chapter 17)	α-adrenergic receptor blockers (phentolamine; Chapter 15); β-adrenergic receptor blockers (propranolol; Chapter 15)

Key: — No common or clinically available agent is available to cause this effect.

agonist for receptors on effector cells. Thus, postganglionic sympathetic nerves respond to one chemical and release another.

Some preganglionic sympathetic fibers innervate cells in the adrenal medulla, which serves the same function as a sympathetic ganglion. When the adrenal medullary cells are stimulated they release *epinephrine* (adrenaline) and a small amount of norepinephrine into the bloodstream. This subdivision of the sympathetic nervous system is sometimes called the *sympathoadrenal branch*.

The effects of norepinephrine and epinephrine on their target cells are mediated by three major subtypes of adrenergic receptors: alpha$_1$ (α_1), beta$_1$ (β_1), and beta$_2$ (β_2). Norepinephrine, because of its chemical structure, affects only those cells bearing α_1- and β_1-adrenergic receptors, whereas epinephrine is an agonist for all three receptor subtypes. (A fourth subclass of receptor, called α_2, is found on the postganglionic sympathetic nerve ending. These receptors provide a negative feedback to inhibit norepinephrine release from the nerve.) Beta$_1$-adrenergic receptors are found mainly in the heart, whereas α_1- and β_2-adrenergic receptors are found on many sympathetic target organs. The different locations of these receptors on various structures, combined with their ability to respond differently to drugs, allow administration of drugs that specifically stimulate or block these receptors and the responses they mediate.

Effects similar to those caused by stimulation of the sympathetic nervous system can be produced by adrenergic agonists, or **sympathomimetic** drugs, that mimic some or all of the effects of norepinephrine or epinephrine. One way to classify these agonists is according to how they produce their effects on target cells:

- those that stimulate only postsynaptic receptors (**direct-acting** agonists; eg, phenylephrine, isoproterenol);
- those that act only by releasing norepinephrine from sympathetic nerves (**indirect-acting** agonists; eg, amphetamines);
- those that act both by stimulating receptors directly and by releasing norepinephrine (**mixed-acting** agonists; eg, ephedrine).

A second way to classify these drugs is according to whether they stimulate only α receptors, only β receptors, or both. Still other sympathomimetic drugs, including the popular drug of abuse, cocaine, act by interfering with reuptake of released norepinephrine into the nerve ending. These drugs are discussed in Chapter 14.

Drugs that inhibit the effects of sympathetic stimulation on target organs are called **sympatholytic** drugs. Most sympatholytics act by specifically blocking α receptors (eg, phentolamine), β receptors (eg, propranolol), or their subtypes. These agents, which can also be called *adrenergic receptor blockers,* are discussed in Chapter 15.

Still other drugs can alter the control that sympathetic nerves exert on their targets, but do so in other ways. For example, some drugs deplete norepinephrine from the adrenergic nerve endings, so little or no neurotransmitter is available for release when the nerve is stimulated. Others do not affect neurotransmitter stores directly, but prevent release of the transmitter. Table 10–2 gives examples of some of the ways drugs can alter sympathetic nervous system activity, and provides cross-references to chapters in which more information can be found.

Implications of Autonomic Nervous System Activity and Autonomic Drugs

Most of the chapters in this unit discuss in detail drugs that alter the activities of the autonomic nervous divisions and the structures they control. The continuous and generally antagonistic control that the parasympathetic and sympathetic nervous systems have over their effectors, and the availability of many drugs to mimic or antagonize the effects of a particular system, provide many ways to modify the activity of target structures that are under autonomic control (see Table 10–2). For example, parasympathetic influences on a particular structure can be intensified by administering an agonist that mimics parasympathetic nervous system stimulation, or by giving a drug that inhibits the opposing sympathetic influences (Fig. 10–5). Since effectors controlled by the

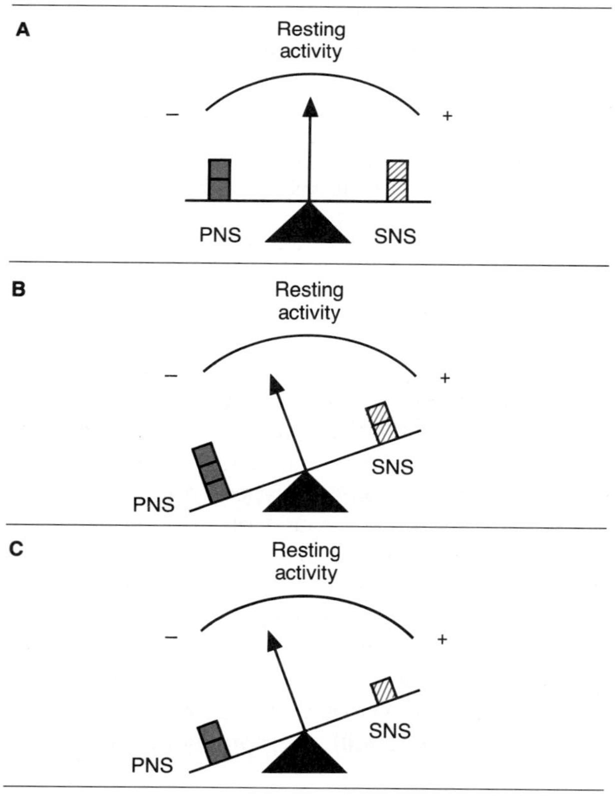

Figure 10–5

A. The resting activity of most organs is maintained by opposing influences of the parasympathetic nervous system (PNS) and its peripheral neurotransmitter acetylcholine (■), and the sympathetic nervous system (SNS) *via* norepinephrine and epinephrine (▨). **B.** One approach to altering the resting state is to increase the influence of one of the branches of the ANS. In this example, it could be done by administering a parasympathomimetic drug, which would stimulate peripheral receptors for acetylcholine. **C.** Another way to cause the same effect is to inhibit the influence of a branch of the ANS. In this example, it could be accomplished by giving a drug that blocks receptors for norepinephrine or epinephrine.

ANS have specific subtypes of receptors for neurotransmitters, even more selective effects can be achieved by administering the appropriate agonist or antagonist.

Unfortunately, few autonomic drugs behave absolutely selectively. Drugs cited as having a particular major effect on one part of the ANS may produce equally important and potentially adverse secondary effects, or they may trigger important reflexes in which the ANS attempts to compensate for (overcome) their actions. Moreover, many drugs, although not classified as autonomic agents, nevertheless cause significant effects that resemble those produced by the drugs discussed in the following chapters. Such effects must always be considered when these drugs are given to a patient. Overall, the widespread effects on the body of the ANS make the administration of drugs that affect it challenging for the nurse.

PROTOTYPE

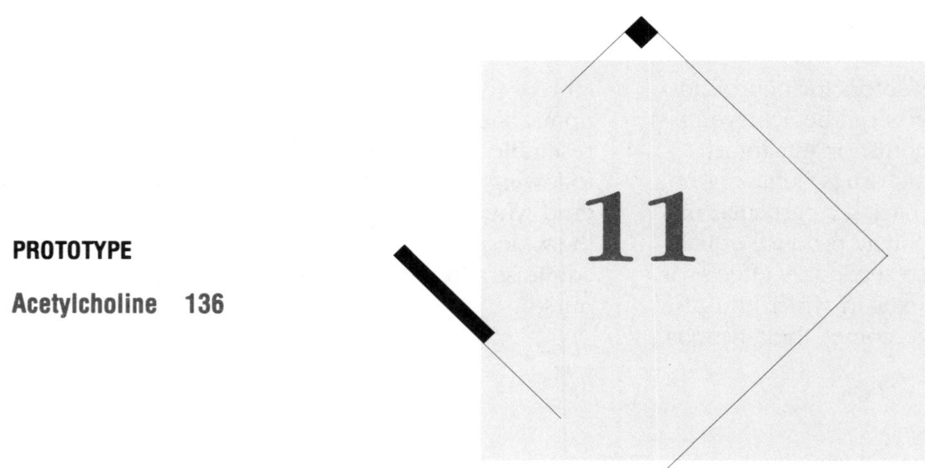

Parasympathomimetic Drugs

General Characteristics of Parasympathomimetic Drugs

Acetylcholine (ACh) is an important neurotransmitter in the autonomic, central, and somatic nervous systems. In general, any drug that shares most or all of the actions of ACh can be called a *cholinergic drug*. They can also be called *cholinergic agonists* because, like ACh itself, they stimulate specific cholinergic receptors on target cells. Those receptors are classified as either muscarinic or nicotinic, depending on where they are located (that is, what the target, or effector, cell is) and on what specific drugs block the effector cell's responses to ACh. Acetylcholine stimulates both muscarinic and nicotinic receptors. Other cholinergic drugs act mainly on one subtype of cholinergic receptor, and have little or no effect on the other. Therefore, the term "cholinergic" is not very meaningful, because it does not indicate the specific receptors where the drug in question acts.

The term *parasympathomimetic drug* refers only to those drugs that act like ACh in its role as the neurotransmitter released from postganglionic parasympathetic nerves. The term implies that these drugs *mimic* the effects of parasympathetic stimulation on the activity of smooth muscle, cardiac muscle, and certain glands. Since these structures respond to ACh through stimulation of muscarinic receptors, the drugs may also be called *muscarinic agonists*. By definition, muscarinic receptors are receptors that are stimulated by ACh (or an ACh-like agonist), and are specifically blocked by atropine or an atropine-like agent. This relationship is shown in Figure 11–1. Note that the chemical mediators of the sympathetic nervous system, norepinephrine and epinephrine, have no direct effect on ACh receptors.

Influencing Parasympathetic Nervous System Activity

Sometimes it is necessary to increase the activity of a body system that is regulated by the parasympathetic nervous system. For example, it may be necessary to constrict the pupil of the eye, slow the heart, or stimulate the urinary bladder to empty. There are several ways to do this. Since the sympathetic and parasympathetic nervous systems generally have opposing actions, these effects could be produced by inhibiting sympathetic nervous system activity (Chapter 15). However,

Major reference tables appear beginning on p. 147.

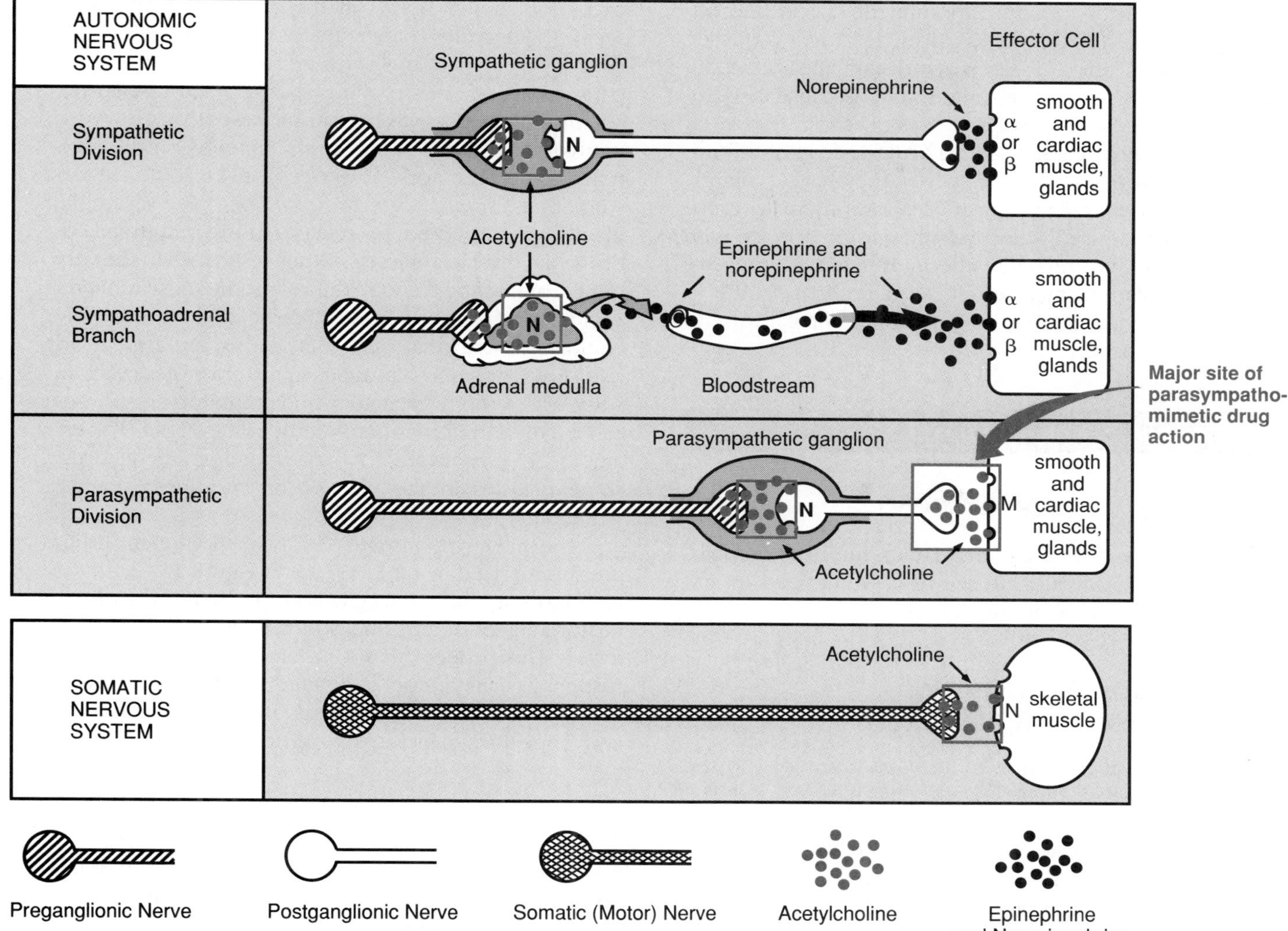

Figure 11–1

Parasympathomimetic drugs stimulate mainly muscarinic receptors (M) for acetylcholine (ACh), which are located on structures innervated by the postganglionic parasympathetic nerves. High doses of parasympathomimetic drugs, or therapeutic doses of carbachol, may stimulate nicotinic (N) receptors for ACh, which are found on postganglionic nerve cell bodies, the adrenal medulla, and on skeletal muscle (smaller green boxes).

this approach may cause undesirable effects in addition to unmasking parasympathetic activity. Another approach is to administer a drug that inhibits the activity of acetylcholinesterase (AChE), the enzyme that metabolically inactivates ACh. This would allow levels of released ACh to build up, producing longer and more intense stimulation of ACh receptors. This approach also has limitations. Acetylcholinesterase inhibitors prevent the breakdown of ACh wherever ACh is released, and in doing so they activate nicotinic, as well as muscarinic, receptors. A variety of unwanted effects on autonomic ganglia, the adrenal medulla, and skeletal muscle would occur. A third way to increase the apparent activity of the parasympathetic nervous system or cause parasympathomimetic effects is to give a parasympathomimetic drug—a specific muscarinic agonist. That approach is the topic of this chapter.

Acetylcholine is discussed as the prototype "drug." Although ACh clearly has the ability to stimulate nicotinic receptors, the discussion that follows emphasizes its muscarinic or parasympathomimetic effects. Interestingly, ACh has limited use as a drug because it is quickly metabolized before it can reach distant sites of action. It works as a neurotransmitter only because it is released from nerves right at its sites of action.

The parasympathomimetic drugs used clinically are like ACh in many ways. However, they have a slightly different chemical makeup that allows them to cause mainly the desired, selective, muscarinic actions, with no (or minimal) nicotinic effects. In addition, they are more resistant to metabolic inactivation than is ACh itself, so they have a longer and therefore clinically useful duration of action.

PROTOTYPE

Acetylcholine

Acetylcholine chloride (MIOCHOL), the drug, is pharmacologically identical to the ACh synthesized in and released by all cholinergic nerves.

Absorption, Distribution, Metabolism, and Excretion

The acetate and choline molecules that make up the ACh molecule are linked together by an ester bond. The bond can be broken easily by a process called *hydrolysis*. When ACh is taken orally, it is hydrolyzed by gastric acid, leaving virtually no drug to be absorbed. This applies to all the parasympathomimetic drugs except bethanechol. When given parenterally, ACh is hydrolyzed almost immediately by AChE, which is abundant in the bloodstream. Acetylcholinesterase does not metabolize other ACh-like esters well, so it is also called true, or specific, cholinesterase. If systemic effects of ACh were needed, very high doses would have to be given rapidly to overcome this rapid breakdown by AChE. The other parasympathomimetic drugs are metabolized by other plasma enzymes called *nonspecific cholinesterases* or *pseudocholinesterases*. In general, they are inactivated more slowly, which enables them to produce useful pharmacologic effects when given by various routes and administered at sites far away from their potential sites of action.

Pharmacologic Effects

The major effects caused by parasympathomimetic drugs are identical to those caused by stimulating the parasympathetic nervous system. (There is one important exception, noted below in the cardiovascular effects section.) Regardless of whether a parasympathomimetic drug is given, or ACh is released from a postganglionic parasympathetic nerve, the response results when the chemical interacts with muscarinic receptors. However, the type of response that occurs depends on the location of the receptors. Some responses could be described as *stimulatory* or *excitatory*. For example, glands are triggered to release more secretions, or bronchial muscle contracts. Other responses to the very same drug, acting through the very same muscarinic receptor subtype—but in a different target structure—could be described as *inhibitory*. For example, the heart rate slows, or smooth muscles in the arterioles relax. In some cases, both excitatory and inhibitory responses can occur in different parts of the same organ. For example, in response to a parasympathomimetic drug, some muscles in the bladder or intestines contract, while others relax.

The major responses to parasympathomimetic drugs are summarized in Table 11–1 and Figure 11–2. All the responses are inhibited (blocked) by the muscarinic receptor antagonist atropine, which is discussed in Chapter 13. This property is so important that a muscarinic response (or receptor) is defined as one that is caused (or activated) by ACh or a parasympathomimetic drug, and is specifically blocked by atropine.

Ocular Effects

Acetylcholine contracts the iris sphincter muscle of the eye (Fig. 11–3), causing the pupil to become smaller. This is called **miosis.** Effective doses of a parasympathomimetic drug may overcome influences of the sympathetic nervous system that dilate the pupil for good vision in dim light. Acetylcholine contracts the ciliary muscle of the eye (see Fig. 11–3), which controls the shape of the lens. Ciliary muscle contraction allows the lens to become fatter, enabling the eye to focus on nearby objects.

Cardiovascular Effects

The major effects of ACh are variable changes in blood pressure and heart rate. The responses vary because the drug causes both direct and indirect, or reflex, effects that tend to counteract one another. The direct effect of a drug is the effect that it produces on a particular cell or organ, independent of any compensatory processes that might be triggered as a result of its actions. Reflexes occur, in general, because the autonomic nervous system (ANS) likes to maintain the status quo: if a drug

Table 11–1 Responses of Major Effector Organs to Pharmacologic Doses of Parasympathomimetic Drugs (Muscarinic Agonists)

Organ	Response*
Eye	
Iris, sphincter muscle	Contracted, causing miosis
Ciliary muscle	Contracted for near vision
Lacrimal gland secretion	Increased
Respiratory system	
Bronchial smooth muscle tone	Increased (contraction)
Mucus gland secretion	Increased (thin, watery)
Heart	
Force of contraction	Slightly decreased
Rate	Decreased
Automaticity	Decreased
Impulse conduction	Decreased
Arterioles	Dilation†
Gastrointestinal tract	
Motility	Increased (contraction)
Sphincters	Relaxed
Gastric acid secretion	Increased
Salivary gland secretion	Increased
Overall	Increased motility
Skin	
Sweat gland secretion	Increased
Urinary bladder	
Detrusor	Contracted
Trigone, sphincter	Relaxed
Overall	Increased urination
Penis	Erection

*All of these responses are mediated by muscarinic receptors. Therefore, by definition they are all blocked by atropine. Compare them with the responses caused by atropine (Table 13-1, p 169) and you will see that they are opposites of one another.

†Parasympathomimetic drugs will dilate arterioles and reduce blood pressure; the effect is blocked by atropine. However, arterioles are not innervated by the parasympathetic nervous system, so stimulation of parasympathetic nerves will not cause dilation.

affects a function controlled by the ANS, the indirect effects will try to overcome that effect.

Acetylcholine (that is, parasympathomimetic drugs) directly relax smooth muscle in the arterioles, causing vasodilation. This is the only situation where there is a difference between effects caused by natural parasympathetic nerve stimulation and effects caused by the administration of a parasympathomimetic drug. Arterioles are not innervated by the parasympathetic nervous system, and so they do not dilate in response to nerve stimulation. But they do have muscarinic receptors, and will dilate when a parasympathomimetic drug is administered.

Blood pressure does not fall much when usual doses of parasympathomimetic drugs are given because the reduced pressure triggers the baroreceptor reflex, which leads to increased sympathetic nervous system activity, including vasoconstriction, that attempts to counteract the pressure fall. Very high doses of a parasympathomimetic drug must be given to lower blood pressure significantly.

Acetylcholine that is released from the major parasympathetic nerve supply to the heart, the vagus nerve, *directly* slows heart rate through an action on the pacemaker cells in the sinoatrial node. The direct effects of other parasympathomimetic agents on heart rate are identical. This fall of heart rate is called a negative **chronotropic** effect, or **bradycardia.** However, when *low doses* of ACh or a parasympathomimetic drug are given systemically, they may actually increase the heart rate slightly (**tachycardia,** or a positive chronotropic effect). The increased heart rate is solely an *indirect* effect mediated by the baroreceptor reflex and sympathetic nervous system activation. High doses of ACh or a parasympathomimetic drug overcome the baroreceptor reflex, so heart rate almost always falls.

Acetylcholine directly slows the conduction rate of electrical impulses through the atrioventricular (AV) node, which is the major electrical link that coordinates contraction of the atria and ventricles. Very high doses of ACh or another parasympathomimetic agent can cause partial or even complete AV block, and possibly cardiac arrest.

The parasympathetic nervous system has a minor role in directly regulating the heart's force of contraction. The direct effect of parasympathomimetic drugs, or parasympathetic stimulation, is a slight decrease of ventricular force (a negative **inotropic** effect).

Respiratory Effects

Acetylcholine and related parasympathomimetics stimulate bronchial smooth muscle contraction. Mucous glands in the respiratory tract are stimulated to secrete large amounts of thin, watery mucus.

Gastrointestinal Effects

Acetylcholine increases the tone and motility of the gastrointestinal (GI) tract by contracting smooth muscles in the stomach and intestinal walls. It simultaneously relaxes the various sphincters in the GI tract. Acetylcho-

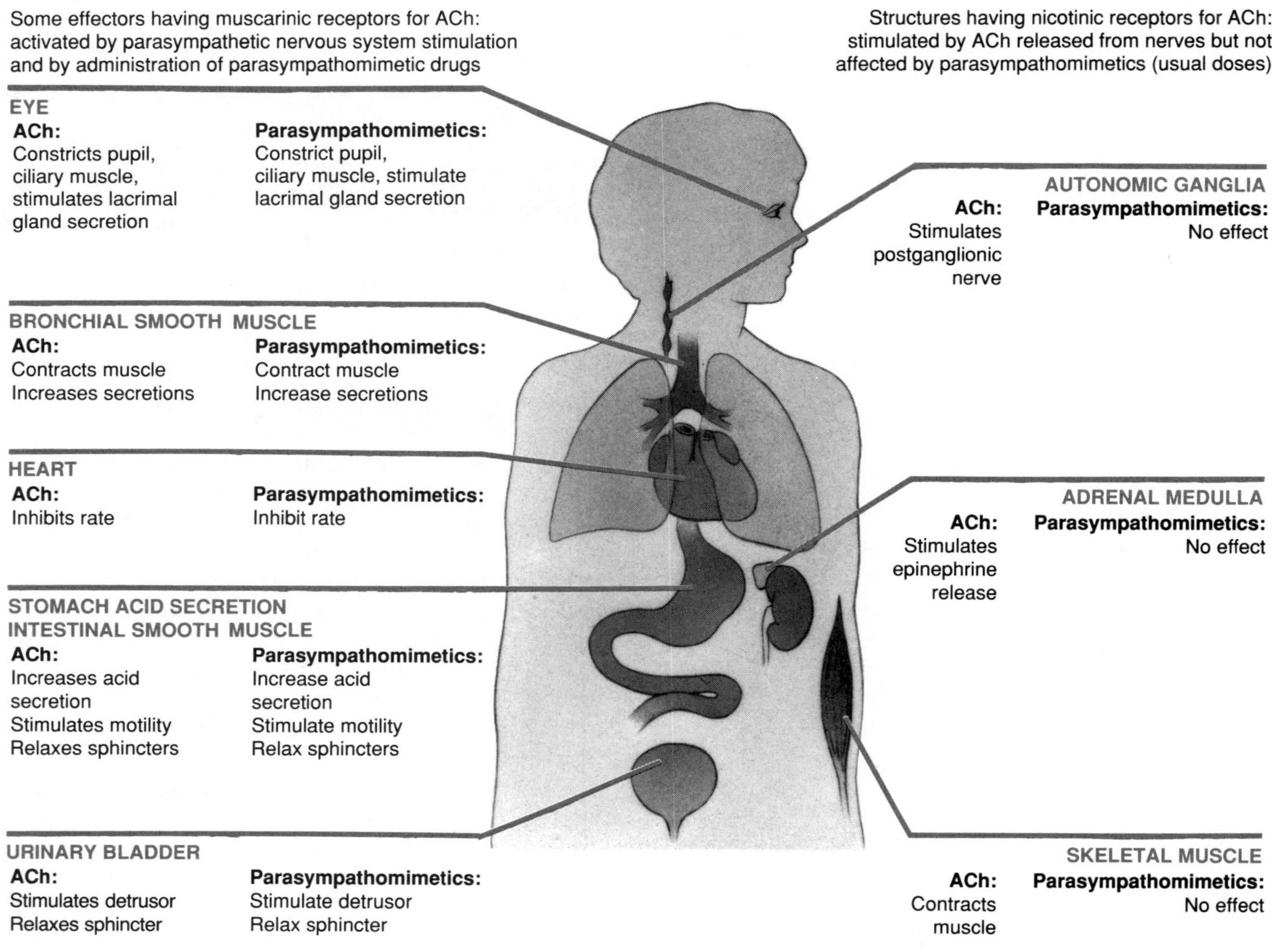

Figure 11–2

Major peripheral organs that are innervated by the parasympathetic nervous system and are affected by parasympathomimetic drugs such as bethanechol and pilocarpine. Note that the effects of acetylcholine (ACh) released from nerves supplying these structures are identical to those caused by parasympathomimetic drugs. Bethanechol and pilocarpine do not stimulate nicotinic receptors (autonomic ganglia, adrenal medulla, skeletal muscle) as well as ACh.

line stimulates parietal cells in the stomach to secrete acid, and other glands elsewhere in the GI tract to secrete mucus or saliva. The overall result is facilitation of digestion and defecation. Profuse salivation (**sialorrhea**) may occur.

Genitourinary Effects

Acetylcholine contracts the detrusor muscle of the urinary bladder. (The detrusor is the muscle you "push down on" when you try to urinate quickly.) Acetylcholine simultaneously increases the tone of the ureters, and relaxes the bladder's sphincter muscles. The overall effect is increased **micturition** (urination). Parasympathomimetic drugs do not affect urine production.

Acetylcholine also contracts uterine smooth muscle.

Sweat and Lacrimal Glands Effects

Acetylcholine and the parasympathomimetic drugs stimulate secretory activity of sweat and lacrimal glands, leading to **diaphoresis** (sweating) and lacrimation.

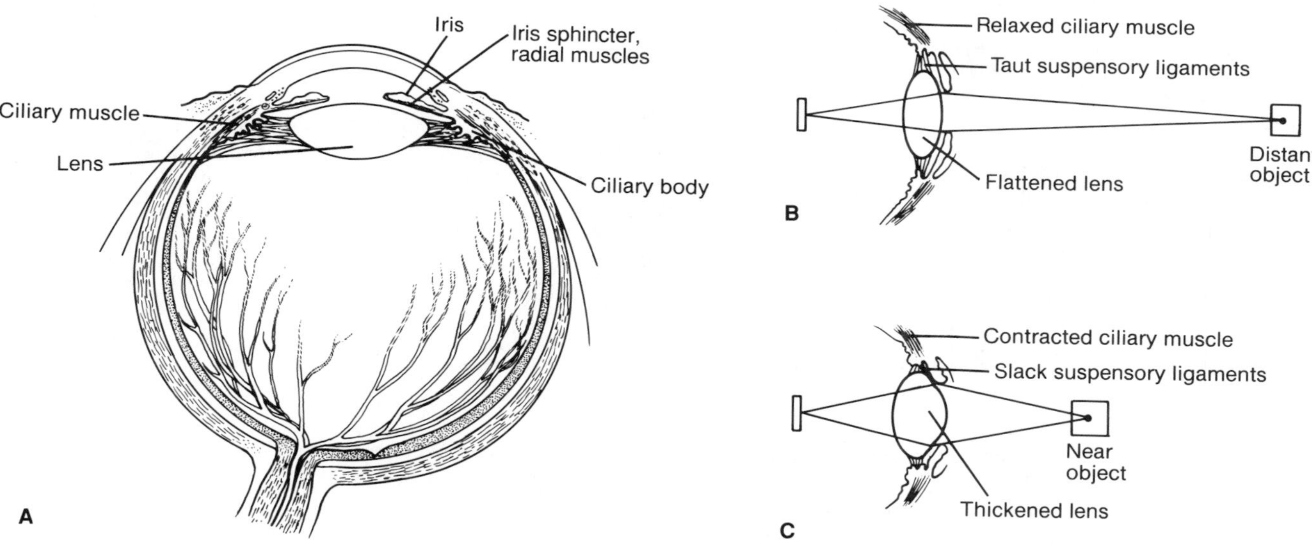

Figure 11–3

A. Eye structures involved in parasympathetic control of the shape of the lens and the size of the pupil. These responses are blocked by antimuscarinic drugs (eg, atropine).

B. In the absence of parasympathetic tone, the ciliary muscle relaxes, putting tension on suspensory ligaments attached to the lens. The lens flattens, focusing the eye on distant objects. Opposing sympathetic influences cause the pupil iris to dilate (mydriasis; not shown).

C. In the presence of parasympathetic tone, the ciliary muscle contracts, the suspensory ligaments become slack, and the lens thickens to focus on nearby objects (accommodation). The pupil also constricts (miosis).

(*Source:* Modified from Vander AJ, Sherman JH, Luciano DS. *Human Physiology: The Mechanisms of Body Function.* 5th ed. New York: McGraw-Hill, 1990.)

Clinical Indications and Administration

In theory, ACh can produce the desired clinical effects on organ systems for which other parasympathomimetics are preferred. In practice, ACh has few clinical uses, as discussed above. Acetylcholine itself is mainly used to manage glaucoma and related eye disorders, for which it is applied topically to the eye. Other parasympathomimetic drugs are also administered topically for their effects on the eye, or are given by mouth or injection for effects on the urinary tract. Dosages and routes of administration are summarized in Table 11–C.

Uses for Eye Disorders

Acetylcholine (MIOCHOL), and the related drugs carbachol and pilocarpine, are the preferred drugs for initial treatment of chronic open-angle glaucoma (also called simple or wide-angle glaucoma; see Fig. 11–4) and acute glaucoma. The therapeutic goal is to reduce elevated intraocular pressure. Topical ACh may be used intraoperatively to reduce intraocular pressure and to cause miosis, which facilitates such surgical procedures as cataract removal.

Chronic open-angle glaucoma, the most common form of glaucoma, is believed to be caused by slow degeneration of the trabeculae in the anterior chamber of the eye. These pore-like structures may collapse, thereby preventing the drainage of aqueous humor needed to prevent intraocular pressure from rising. Parasympathomimetic drugs cause miosis and contract the ciliary muscle, which stretches or realigns the trabecular pores so that aqueous humor can drain.

Acute *angle-closure* or *narrow-angle glaucoma* has other causes. In this disease, dilation of the pupil causes the iris to fold back like a curtain in the angle of the anterior chamber. The folded iris blocks aqueous humor drainage through Schlemm's canal, causing intraocular pressure to rise quickly. The rise in pressure is accompanied by sharp pain, and there is a risk of imminent blindness. The miotic effect of a parasympa-

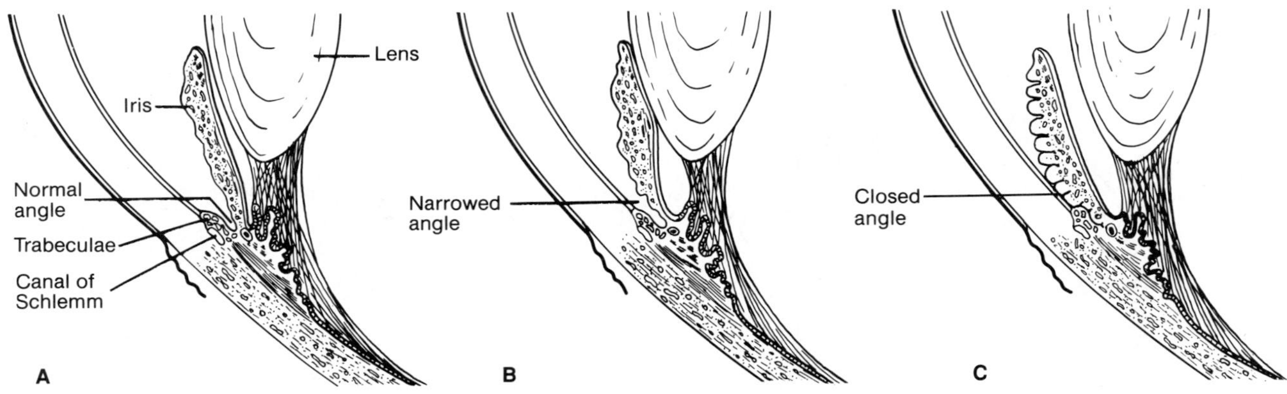

Figure 11–4

A. In the normal eye anterior chamber fluid (aqueous humor) drains through the trabeculae and canal of Schlemm.
B. In narrow-angle (angle-closure) glaucoma, the angle is narrowed, drainage is diminished, and intraocular pressure can rise.
C. If a mydriatic (pupil-dilating) drug is administered, the iris can fold back into the angle like a pleated curtain and block fluid outflow completely, triggering an acute attack. Drugs that cause miosis (pupil constriction), including parasympathomimetics and AChE inhibitors (see Chapter 12) are used to manage some cases of narrow-angle glaucoma. They unfold the "curtain" and help keep the drainage pathway open. By contracting the ciliary muscle they may also help keep the trabeculae aligned and open.
(*Source:* Modified from Ames SW, Kneisl KR. *Essentials of Adult Health Nursing.* Menlo Park, CA: Addison-Wesley, 1988, p 1169.)

thomimetic drug alleviates the blockage. Regardless of the type of glaucoma, the desired effect of any parasympathomimetic drug is a reduction of intraocular pressure, without generalized parasympathomimetic side effects on other body structures.

Acetylcholine's miotic effects last only for about 10 minutes when it is applied topically, so the drug is used mainly in acute situations. (The related drug pilocarpine has the longest duration of action, and so is preferred for long-term therapy.) Patients with severe or refractory glaucoma may need to take other drugs as well, including the AChE inhibitors, which are discussed in the next chapter; sympathomimetics, which may reduce formation of aqueous humor; carbonic anhydrase inhibitors, which also decrease aqueous humor formation; and osmotic agents such as mannitol.

NURSING IMPLICATIONS

Teach patients with glaucoma the proper technique for administering ocular medications (Appendix A), and have them demonstrate it to you. Persons administering these drugs should wash their hands first to reduce the risk of eye infection, and again after administration to avoid accidental contact of contaminated fingers with the mouth, nose, or eye. If ophthalmic drops are used, have the patient apply gentle finger pressure to the lacrimal sac for a couple of minutes after drug application to decrease the chance of drainage into the nasal mucosa and possibly into the systemic circulation. Keeping the eyelid closed for a couple of minutes after administration also increases the local effects of the drug.

Instruct patients not to miss scheduled periodic eye examinations and measurement of intraocular pressure. Weekly examinations are usually indicated during the early stages of therapy. Caution patients that failure to take their medication may cause permanent eye damage or blindness. Identify drugs, particularly drugs that dilate the pupil, that patients with glaucoma should avoid. These include antimuscarinics and other drugs with atropine-like activity (eg, antihistamines) and sympathomimetics, which are found in many over-the-counter (OTC) cold, hay fever, and allergy remedies.

Uses for Urinary or Gastrointestinal Tract Disorders

Although stimulation of the parasympathetic nervous system and the release of ACh will affect the GI and urinary tracts, ACh is not used therapeutically for this purpose. When such effects are needed, the related drug bethanechol is used instead.

Side Effects, Adverse Reactions, and Contraindications

The most important side effects of ACh itself, and of *all* parasympathomimetic drugs, are the result of their expected actions on the eye and the cardiovascular, respiratory, GI, and genitourinary systems (Table 11–S). Most can be predicted from the previous discussions.

Any side effect can be produced by any parasympathomimetic drug, regardless of the route of administration. The risk of severe, generalized side effects is generally greatest with bethanechol, which can be given parenterally. The side effects from topically administered parasympathomimetics such as ACh are usually more localized and annoying than widespread and dangerous, provided recommended doses and administration techniques are used. Nevertheless, although only a drop of a miotic agent placed on the eye may be needed to produce desired effects for glaucoma, this small amount has caused fatal responses in some patients for whom parasympathomimetics are contraindicated.

Most of the severe side effects or adverse responses due to excessive doses can be treated with atropine, the specific antidote for ACh. Atropine is discussed in Chapter 13.

Ocular Side Effects

Ocular side effects include excessive lacrimation, myopia due to drug effects on the ciliary muscle, reduced vision in dim light as a result of miosis, and brow pain. Headache may also occur. These side effects are most likely to be caused by parasympathomimetics applied topically to the eye. All topical ACh-like miotics are contraindicated in patients with corneal abrasions, acute iritis, or other ocular hypersensitivity reactions.

NURSING IMPLICATIONS

It is best to start miotic therapy in the evening, so that ocular side effects have lessened by morning. Advise patients of the expected side effects, and instruct them to notify their physician if side effects become prolonged or severe, or if they interfere with daily activities. Patients should avoid dangerous tasks requiring good visual acuity. Advise patients to notify their physician at once if eye pain develops or worsens during glaucoma therapy.

The risk of side effects or adverse effects from topical medications can be minimized greatly by using proper administration techniques and following dosage guidelines.

Cardiovascular Side Effects

Parasympathomimetic drugs can decrease blood pressure and trigger reflex tachycardia. Dizziness or lightheadedness may occur as the result of inadequate cerebral blood flow. Flushing of the skin, accompanied by diaphoresis, may be a sign of marked vasodilation. Cerebral artery dilation may cause headache. These side effects are more likely to occur with bethanechol, especially when injected, than with the topically administered drugs.

Regardless of which parasympathomimetic is used, or its route of administration, hypotension and tachycardia are particularly dangerous for patients with preexisting hypotension, bradycardia, or coronary insufficiency (as from coronary artery disease). Reduced blood pressure, combined with an increased heart rate, can reduce myocardial blood flow, increase myocardial oxygen demands, and cause angina pectoris, a symptom of a severe imbalance in oxygen supply and demand. Parasympathomimetic drugs may aggravate tachycardia that commonly accompanies hyperthyroidism, and may increase the risk of atrial fibrillation. Bethanechol, in particular, is contraindicated in persons at risk for these conditions because the drug is given systemically.

NURSING IMPLICATIONS

Monitor blood pressure, heart rate, and peripheral and apical pulses periodically during parasympathomimetic treatment.

Respiratory Side Effects

Any parasympathomimetic drug can produce severe bronchospasm and respiratory distress in asthmatics, for whom *all parasympathomimetic drugs are contraindicated.* A single drop of a topical parasympathomimetic miotic can result in death from bronchospasm. The asthmatic person's bronchial smooth muscle is so sensitive to parasympathomimetic stimulation that one of the related agents, methacholine (p 144), is used to help diagnose asthma.

NURSING IMPLICATIONS

Listen for lung sounds that may indicate bronchoconstriction or excessive secretions, and have patients report wheezing or dyspnea at once. Respiratory difficulty may indicate undiagnosed asthma or other related pulmonary disorders. If it occurs, do not administer subse-

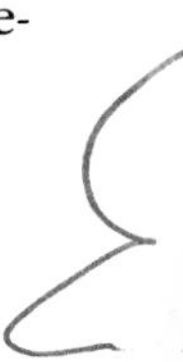

quent parasympathomimetic doses, notify the physician, and be prepared to administer the bronchodilator epinephrine, plus oxygen, at once. Advise patients who are self-administering any parasympathomimetic drug to seek professional evaluation at once if respiratory difficulty occurs, and to withhold further drug doses.

Gastrointestinal and Genitourinary Side Effects

Annoying GI side effects caused by any parasympathomimetic drug include nausea, vomiting, abdominal pain, cramping, diarrhea, excessive salivation, and urinary frequency or urgency. The ability of parasympathomimetic drugs to stimulate the GI and urinary tracts can be dangerous for patients with mechanical obstruction or weakened musculature in these sites. Intense gut or bladder stimulation could cause tearing and necessitate emergency surgery. Because they stimulate gastric acid secretion, parasympathomimetic drugs, and bethanechol in particular, are contraindicated in persons with peptic ulcer disease.

◆ Use During Pregnancy and Lactation

There have been few reports of problems following the use of parasympathomimetic drugs (other than bethanechol) in pregnant or breast-feeding women. Nevertheless, routine use should be avoided during pregnancy or breast-feeding, especially if the drug is given systemically.

◆ Use in the Elderly

The elderly may have age-related disorders, such as glaucoma or atonic bladder, for which a parasympathomimetic drug might be indicated. However, other common age-related disorders, may contraindicate their use.

Interactions with Other Drugs

Few major interactions occur between parasympathomimetic drugs and other agents (Table 11–I). Interactions are most likely to occur when bethanechol is used, because it is given systemically. Acetylcholinesterase inhibitors (eg, neostigmine; Chapter 12) prolong and intensify the actions of some parasympathomimetic drugs. Such a drug combination may be used therapeutically for patients with glaucoma who do not respond well to topical parasympathomimetics alone, but it requires careful dosage adjustments based on the clinical response and the development of systemic side effects.

Parasympathomimetics may cause excessive hypotension if administered to patients taking any antihypertensive drug. The combination need not be avoided, but blood pressure should be monitored accordingly, especially when changing the patient's medications.

Because parasympathomimetic drugs are muscarinic-receptor agonists, their effects can be antagonized partially or blocked completely by muscarinic antagonists like atropine. This explains why atropine is used to manage adverse reactions to a parasympathomimetic, particularly those due to an overdose. Other commonly used groups of drugs, including antipsychotic agents, antidepressants, some antiparkinson drugs, and antihistamines (see Table 13–2, p 174), cause appreciable antimuscarinic actions that can antagonize the desired therapeutic actions of a parasympathomimetic drug.

The ability of parasympathomimetic drugs to cause reflex tachycardia may potentiate the cardiac-stimulating actions of thyroid hormone supplements, which are often used to treat hypothyroidism. The risk of atrial fibrillation may also increase, although the risk of this interaction is low if proper dosages of the interactants are used. However, if the patient is taking excessive doses of thyroid hormone, and has developed what amounts to a hyperthyroid state, the interaction may become clinically important.

NURSING IMPLICATIONS

Obtain a thorough medication history from all patients, including use of OTC medications. Interactions with a nonprescription drug with anticholinergic activity could explain why usual doses of a parasympathomimetic drug fail to produce their anticipated actions.

Overdose and Toxicity

Signs and Symptoms

The expected pharmacologic and side effects caused by parasympathomimetic drugs predict what would happen if mild-to-moderate overdoses were taken (see Tables 11–1 and 11–S). Initial symptoms include abdominal discomfort, salivation, flushed skin, sweating, nausea, and vomiting. Ocular changes such as miosis, myopia, and excessive lacrimation occur. As blood levels of the drug rise, intense cramping, profuse diarrhea, urination, hypotension, bradycardia, and severe bronchoconstriction may occur. The effects of an overdose may not be limited to peripheral structures. Central nervous system changes may develop, including restlessness, confusion, severe anxiety, and, eventually, seizures.

At very high doses all parasympathomimetic drugs lose their selectivity as agonists for only muscarinic receptors, and signs of nicotinic receptor stimulation appear. These include stimulation of all autonomic ganglia (sympathetic and parasympathetic), leading to bizarre and often unpredictable changes in blood pressure, heart rate, and heart rhythm; and stimulation of skeletal muscle, resulting in tremor, twitching, or more intense contractions. Death may result from either cardiovascular collapse (hypotension and cardiac arrest) or asphyxia from severe bronchoconstriction, if seizures do not cause death first.

Treatment

Because most signs and symptoms of overdose reflect excessive muscarinic effects, the muscarinic-receptor blocker atropine is the preferred (and logical) antidote. The typical atropine dose, 0.6 to 0.8 mg given subcutaneously (SC), is usually effective. Atropine acts specifically at muscarinic receptors to block the effects of ACh or any other parasympathomimetic drug. It should always be readily available whenever a parasympathomimetic drug is given, especially when the drug is given parenterally. (See Chapter 13 for more information about atropine.)

If bradycardia, hypotension, or bronchoconstriction are severe, epinephrine may also be needed. Continuous monitoring and support of cardiovascular and respiratory functions are essential. It may be necessary to administer fluids and electrolytes parenterally to correct those lost through the skin, GI tract, and urine. Fluid intake and output must be monitored closely.

Mushroom Poisoning

Many years ago muscarinic receptors were given their name because they were stimulated by the alkaloid muscarine, which can be isolated from a common species of mushroom, *Amanita muscaria.* The effects of muscarine are identical to those caused by ACh, acting on smooth and cardiac muscle and glands. *Amanita muscaria* contains very small amounts of muscarine, but other species of mushrooms that are abundant in North America, and are often eaten accidentally, including species of *Clitocybe* and *Inocybe,* contain large amounts of the alkaloid. These mushrooms usually cause intense parasympathomimetic effects within an hour of ingestion, and some cases have been fatal. Atropine is the specific antidote.

Related Drugs

Only a few parasympathomimetic drugs are used clinically. Their doses are noted in Table 11–C.

Bethanechol

Bethanechol (URECHOLINE) is the only parasympathomimetic drug that is effective when taken orally. A sterile solution is available for SC injection. Bethanechol stimulates the bladder and GI tract well, and when given at recommended doses to otherwise normal persons, its cardiovascular effects are slight. The drug has practically no ability to stimulate nicotinic receptors—the ACh receptors found in autonomic glanglia and on skeletal muscle cells. A small amount of bethanechol is excreted in breast milk.

Bethanechol is indicated for the management of acute functional urinary retention (ie, retention not due to a mechanical obstruction to urine outflow). This situation may arise when the urinary bladder becomes hypoactive after surgery or childbirth, or in disorders involving inadequate neural stimulation of the bladder. The desired response is an increase of urine output and a return of normal spontaneous bladder activity, at which time bethanechol administration (especially by injection) should be stopped. Patients recovering from surgical repair of the urinary bladder or GI tract should not be given bethanechol or other parasympathomimetics routinely, since stimulation of these structures may cause physical damage. Bethanechol has been used to alleviate postoperative paralytic ileus, but this use is declining.

NURSING IMPLICATIONS

Bethanechol administration, combined with frequent, scheduled toileting and a muscle relaxant, can restore a degree of continence to elderly incontinent persons, thereby preventing skin excoriation, reducing the frequency of urinary tract infections, and improving morale, self-respect, and overall life quality.

When bethanechol is given SC, administer it 1 hour before or 2 hours after meals to reduce the risk of nausea, vomiting, or cramping. Never inject the drug intramuscularly or intravenously, which would increase the risk of severe and widespread muscarinic side effects. Stay with the patient for 10 minutes after giving the first dose to monitor the response. Have atropine readily available for injection to counteract excessive systemic side effects. Never give bethanechol to induce diuresis if urinary tract obstruction is suspected. Carefully monitor fluid intake and output. Monitor bowel sounds, and palpate the abdomen periodically. Inspect the urine and stool for signs of blood, which may indicate urinary or GI tract bleeding, and report positive findings to the physician at once.

Advise the patient to expect a sudden need to urinate, and possibly to defecate. Have a urinal or bedpan available for nonambulatory patients. If urine output does not increase within about 15 to 30 minutes after administering a usual dose of bethanechol, notify the physician at once, withhold further drug, and be prepared to catheterize the bladder. If the first dose does not increase urine output, do not administer more bethanechol until urinary tract obstruction can be ruled out. Failure to heed this precaution may lead to rupture of the bladder, ureters, or urethra.

Check blood pressure, heart rate, and pulse regularly in hospitalized patients receiving bethanechol. Monitor the electrocardiogram (ECG) if heart rhythm disturbances are suspected or likely to occur. Take precautions to guard ambulatory patients against syncope or falls due to hypotension. Assess for flushed skin or a feeling of warmth, which may indicate that an excessive dose was given.

◆ Use During Pregnancy and Lactation

Double-check orders calling for administration of bethanechol to pregnant women, since it may cause uterine contraction and premature delivery. Bethanechol is excreted in breast milk, and breastfeeding should be discontinued temporarily during treatment.

Carbachol

Carbachol is less selective as a parasympathomimetic agent than any of the other drugs discussed in this chapter except ACh itself. That is, it also exerts nicotinic stimulating effects. Like bethanechol, carbachol stimulates the GI tract and urinary bladder well, but its clinically useful effects are on the iris and ciliary muscle.

Carbachol is marketed as an ophthalmic solution (ISOPTO CARBACHOL) for topical use to reduce intraocular pressure in patients with glaucoma. Long-term use is generally reserved for patients with glaucoma who have not responded to pilocarpine or other therapies. Miosis occurs in about 2 minutes and lasts 4 to 8 hours.

A sterile preparation of carbachol (MIOSTAT) is available for injection into the anterior chamber of the eye during eye surgery.

The ability of carbachol to stimulate nicotinic receptors may cause undesirable effects that are less likely to occur with the more selective parasympathomimetics. Topical application may cause involuntary twitching of the skeletal muscle of the eyelids (blepharospasm). Skeletal muscle twitching elsewhere may also occur if sufficient drug is absorbed systemically. Stimulation of autonomic ganglia may occur, causing a variety of cardiovascular changes. Using proper doses and administration techniques minimizes these problems.

NURSING IMPLICATIONS

Patients receiving carbachol may complain of headache, eye and brow pain, and conjunctival congestion. Administer analgesics as ordered, and dim room lights to reduce eye and vision distress.

Methacholine

Methacholine (PROVOCHOLINE) is used to diagnose bronchial hyperresponsiveness in persons suspected of having asthma, but who do not have clinically apparent symptoms that make diagnosis more clear-cut. This use capitalizes on the fact that the bronchi in asthmatic patients are extremely sensitive to bronchoconstriction caused by muscarinic agents. The drug is prepared, usually by the hospital pharmacy, in a series of concentrations that are administered by inhalation. Baseline pulmonary function is measured in response to saline inhalation, and tests are repeated following administration of successively higher methacholine doses. Test changes indicating bronchoconstriction occur in asthmatic patients at lower methacoline concentrations than are needed to cause the same effects in patients without asthma.

NURSING IMPLICATIONS

Methacholine should never be administered to a patient known to have asthma, and should be given only by a physician trained in its safe and proper use. Atropine, other emergency drugs, oxygen, and means to support ventilation must be readily available whenever the drug is given.

Pilocarpine

Pilocarpine, a selective muscarinic agonist, is used as a topical miotic. It can be used chronically, to lower intraocular pressure in patients with glaucoma; or acutely, to hasten the recovery of normal vision after eye exams during which drugs that paralyze accommodation and dilate the pupil were given. Standard pilocarpine ophthalmic solutions are marketed under several trade names (eg, ISOPTO CARPINE), and come in a wide range of strengths (0.25–10%) so the dose per drop can be adjusted to the patient's needs. Most patients will respond to the 4% solution, or less.

With the pilocarpine solutions that are most often used, miosis starts almost immediately and intraocular pressure usually remains reduced for about 4 hours. For long-term therapy, the use of pilocarpine would require administration six times a day, which can be inconvenient. To overcome this problem, sustained-release ocular delivery systems for pilocarpine (OCUSERT PILO-20 and OCUSERT PILO-40) were developed. These small, oval-shaped devices are inserted into the cul-de-sac of the eye. They release a constant amount of drug around the clock for 1 week, at which time they are replaced with a new system. The ocular delivery systems are not suitable when immediate and relatively intense effects are needed, such as during an acute glaucoma attack, because they release the drug too slowly. Standard pilocarpine drops should be on-hand for these instances.

Initial administration of pilocarpine, whether by drops or the delivery system, may cause temporary severe myopia, lacrimation, brow pain, or headache. The delivery system may irritate the cornea or cause ciliary spasm.

NURSING IMPLICATIONS

Review with the patient the manufacturer's instructions for inserting and removing the pilocarpine delivery system. Have the patient demonstrate proper technique. Advise patients to check the eye periodically, especially before retiring at night and upon awakening, to ensure that the system has not fallen out of place. Advise patients not to use a damaged delivery system, which could release the drug too quickly and cause both local and systemic side effects.

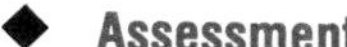

SUMMARY OF NURSING IMPLICATIONS

◆ Assessment

Assess the patient for the presence of contraindications (eg, prior allergic reactions, asthma, peptic ulcer disease, heart disease, parkinsonism, seizure disorders) before initiating parasympathomimetic drug therapy.

Recognize the signs and symptoms of excessive parasympathomimetic activity (eg, bradycardia, bronchoconstriction, diarrhea, cramps, flushing, sweating, involuntary micturition) or reflex sympathetic responses (eg, tachycardia, increased blood pressure).

◆ Nursing Diagnoses

Altered urinary elimination related to involuntary micturition.

Diarrhea related to drug effects.

Pain related to headache.

Sensory/perceptual alterations related to visual disturbances.

Ineffective breathing pattern related to wheezing and bronchoconstriction.

Ineffective airway clearance related to increased mucus secretions.

Knowledge deficit related to drug regimen.

Noncompliance related to negative consequences of drug therapy (eg, flushing, sweating).

◆ Planning/Implementation

Have atropine sulfate readily available for use if toxicity due to parasympathomimetic drug develops.

Keep life-support equipment on standby when giving parasympathomimetics parenterally.

Administer bethanechol, whether orally or subcutaneously, on an empty stomach (before meals).

Have a bedpan and urinal available.

Provide privacy for the patient.

Monitor urine output.

Provide a cool, darkened environment if eye discomfort or skin flushing develops.

◆ Patient and Family Teaching

Instruct the patient regarding drug effects, doses, and signs and symptoms of adverse effects that should be reported immediately (eg, abdominal pain that might indicate urinary or GI tract obstruction; wheezing or dyspnea).

Teach correct technique for instilling gel or solution; good hand-washing; light finger pressure on lacrimal sac for 1 minute after instillation.

◆ Evaluation

The patient/family will:

Experience desired drug effects (eg, bowel sounds, voiding, decreased ocular pain).

Determine that no adverse cardiovascular, GI, or respiratory effects are present.

Demonstrate proper administration of medication to reduce systemic absorption.

Ensure that no injury due to visual disturbances occurs, and refrain from activities requiring visual acuity in dim light.

Annotated Bibliography*

Davidson M, Stern RG, Bierer LM, et al. Cholinergic strategies in the treatment of Alzheimer's disease. *Acta Psychiatr Scand* [Suppl] 1991;366:47–51. *Alzheimer's disease, one of the most devastating disorders in the elderly, seems to involve deficiencies in cholinergic nerve or receptor activity in the central nervous system. This short paper tells us what to expect in terms of new therapies involving parasympathomimetics and AChE inhibitors, and why current treatment strategies do not seem to be working optimally.*

McCallum RW. Gastric emptying in gastroesophageal reflux and the therapeutic role of prokinetic agents. *Gastroenterol Clin North Am* 1990;19(3):551–564. *This article focuses mainly on bethanechol and other motility-stimulating agents (some experimental) in the management of gastroesophageal reflux.*

Reynolds JC. Prokinetic agents: A key in the future of gastroenterology. *Gastroenterol Clin North Am* 1989;18(2):437–457. *This article identifies the current values and uses of motility-stimulating drugs such as bethanechol, as well as the limitations that newer agents will have to overcome.*

Ruoff HJ, Fladung B, Demol P, Weihrauch TR. Gastrointestinal receptors and drugs in motility disorders. *Digestion* 1991;48(1):1–17. *A valuable review of how receptors for several types of drugs—parasympathomimetic, adrenergic, and others—can be used as pharmacologic targets for therapy of common GI motility disorders.*

*Also see the bibliography for Chapter 12, which lists other articles dealing with glaucoma therapy using other types of "cholinergic" drugs—the AChE inhibitors.

Table 11–C | Clinical Uses and Administration of Major Parasympathomimetic Drugs

AGENT	CLINICAL USES	DOSAGE AND ROUTE OF ADMINISTRATION
PROTOTYPE		
Acetylcholine		
(MIOCHOL)	Acute miosis (eg, during surgery), usually to reduce intraocular pressure in glaucoma	Topical: 0.5–2 mL instilled into the conjunctival sac; reconstitute drug immediately before use
RELATED DRUGS		
Bethanechol		
(URECHOLINE)	Management of functional urinary retention, hypoactive bladder	Oral: 10–50 mg bid–qid on empty stomach (1 hr before or 2 hr after meals)
(URECHOLINE INJECTION)	Prompt treatment of functional urinary retention	SC: 2.5–5 mg q 15–30 min as needed until normal bladder activity is restored, or up to 4 doses maximum
Carbachol		
(ISOPTO CARBACHOL, others)	Treatment of glaucoma, particularly if not responsive to pilocarpine	Topical: 1 or 2 drops of solution (ranging from 0.75%–3%) instilled into each affected eye qid
(MIOSTAT)	Production of acute miosis, reduction of intraocular pressure	Intraocular: Inject small amount (not > 0.5 mL) of sterile 0.01% solution into anterior chamber of anesthetized eye (for use by physician only)
Methacholine		
(PROVOCHOLINE)	Diagnosis of airway hyperreactivity in persons with suspected asthma	Inhalation: While monitoring pulmonary function, administer 5 breaths (by nebulizer) of solutions containing 25 μg/mL to 25 mg/mL (for use by physician only)
Pilocarpine		
(ISOPTO CARPINE, others)	Treatment of glaucoma, especially long-term	Topical: Usually 1 drop of solution (0.5%–4%) in each affected eye, repeated up to 6 times daily; solutions stronger than 0.4% seldom needed
(OCUSERT, PILO-20, PILO-40)	Long-term treatment of glaucoma	Insert delivery system into cul-de-sac of affected eye each week

Table 11–S | Major Side Effects and Contraindications of Parasympathomimetic Drugs*

BODY SYSTEM/ Side Effect	CONTRAINDICATION/ PRECAUTION	COMMENTS AND NURSING IMPLICATIONS
CENTRAL NERVOUS SYSTEM		
Dizziness, lightheadedness	Cerebrovascular disease	May be caused by hypotension from excessive dose; check blood pressure, heart rate, notify physician if abnormally low
Parkinsonian neuromuscular symptoms (tremor, rigidity, bradykinesias)	Parkinson's disease	Discontinue drug administration if symptoms develop, notify physician
EYE		
Myopia (nearsightedness), miosis		Caution patient against engaging in tasks that require distant vision or vision in dim light
Excessive lacrimation; eyelid twitching (blepharospasm)		Reduced dosage may be required if severe
RESPIRATORY		
Bronchoconstriction, wheezing, bronchospasm, increased mucus secretion in respiratory tract	Asthma, chronic obstructive lung disease	History or presence of asthma or obstructive lung disease is important contraindication for use of systemic *or* topical parasympathomimetics; assess for wheezing, other breathing difficulty, which might indicate undiagnosed pulmonary disease and/or excessive drug dose
CARDIOVASCULAR		
Tachycardia or bradycardia; arrhythmia	Bradycardia, partial or complete heart block; tachycardia; hyperthyroidism	Slight reflex tachycardia (triggered by hypotension) is expected with injected bethanechol, acceptable for otherwise healthy patients; poses arrhythmia risk in hyperthyroid patients (avoid use); bradycardia usually indicates overdose; any significant heart rate change with ophthalmic parasympathomimetic usually indicates excessive systemic absorption, excessive dose, and/or poor administration technique
Hypotension	Hypotension, vasomotor instability; ischemic heart disease	Most likely caused by parenteral bethanechol; hypotension caused by any parasympathomimetic generally indicates excessive dose
GASTROINTESTINAL		
Nausea, vomiting, diarrhea; cramping, retching; belching; gastritis; excessive salivation	Obstruction, weakness or inflammation of gut; recent gut surgery (eg, resection); peptic ulcer disease	Administer bethanechol on an empty stomach to reduce symptoms; abdominal pain may indicate gut obstruction, bloody stool may indicate bleeding; notify physician if any symptoms are severe or prolonged
SKIN		
Flushed, hot skin; diaphoresis		May indicate overdose

(*continued*)

Table 11–S **Major Side Effects and Contraindications of Parasympathomimetic Drugs*** **(*Continued*)**

BODY SYSTEM/ Side Effect	CONTRAINDICATION/ PRECAUTION	COMMENTS AND NURSING IMPLICATIONS
GENITOURINARY		
Urinary frequency; excessive urination	Obstruction, weakness, or inflammation of urinary tract	Bethanechol, given for urinary retention, should cause urination in 30–60 min; if not, notify physician, withhold additional doses until patient is evaluated, be prepared to catheterize bladder; palpate abdomen to assess bladder fullness; report pain or bloody urine; monitor fluid intake and output of hospitalized patients
Uterine pain, cramping	Pregnancy (caution)	Avoid drug use, particularly systemically (eg, bethanechol), in pregnant or nursing mothers; weigh potential adverse fetal effects (poorly documented) against benefits to mother

*Recommended doses of topically applied (ocular) parasympathomimetics are not likely to cause significant side effects unless proper administration techniques are not used; bethanechol (given systemically) is apt to affect all body systems listed. Carbachol is most likely to cause nicotinic stimulation (eg, skeletal muscle activation).

Table 11–I **Major Interactions Between Parasympathomimetic Drugs and Other Agents**

AGENT	RESULT OF INTERACTION	COMMENTS AND NURSING IMPLICATIONS
Acetylcholinesterase inhibitors (eg, neostigmine, physostigmine; Chapter 12)	Increased, prolonged effects of parasympathomimetic drug (both therapeutic and side effects)	Parasympathomimetics and AChE inhibitors may be combined for refractory glaucoma; this increases risk of systemic or ocular side effects, so close monitoring is required
Antimuscarinics (atropine, others listed at right; see also Chapter 13)	Decreased effectiveness of parasympathomimetic drug	If therapeutic doses of parasympathomimetic fail to control symptoms, check medication history to determine whether drugs with antimuscarinic activity (eg, antidepressants, antihistamines, antipsychotics) that antagonize parasympathomimetic action are being taken also

PROTOTYPE

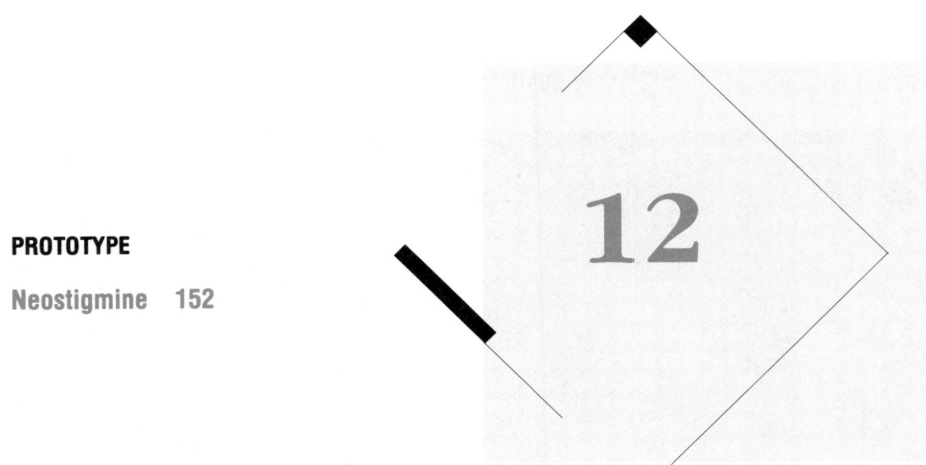

Acetylcholinesterase Inhibitors

Acetylcholine (ACh) is an important neurotransmitter in the peripheral nervous systems (Fig. 12–1). Almost instantaneously after its release from a nerve and its reaction with its cellular targets, ACh is metabolically inactivated by the enzyme acetylcholinesterase (AChE), which promptly stops the actions of the neurotransmitter on its target cells. This chapter discusses chemicals that inhibit AChE, thereby providing a way to prolong and intensify the actions of ACh. Most of these chemicals have therapeutic uses, but a few are used as poisons—both for insects and, in the setting of chemical warfare, for human beings. The prototype of the clinically useful AChE inhibitors is neostigmine.

General Characteristics of Acetylcholinesterase Inhibitors

All drugs classified as AChE inhibitors have basically similar mechanisms of action. However, the individual agents have chemical differences that affect their potency, onsets and durations of action, and ability to reach certain parts of the body. Most of the clinically useful AChE inhibitors do not readily cross the blood–brain barrier to enter the central nervous system (CNS), or enter autonomic ganglia. As a result, their effects occur mainly in the periphery. They are used mainly for their effects on skeletal muscle, particularly for managing myasthenia gravis, and for restoring skeletal muscle function that has been intentionally paralyzed for surgery or other medical reasons. Lesser uses are to cause parasympathomimetic effects on key structures, mainly the eye, gut, and bladder (see Table 12–C).

Neostigmine, the prototype and oldest member of the group, is the traditional AChE inhibitor used for long-term therapy in which either skeletal muscle-stimulating or parasympathomimetic effects are the goal. The properties of most other AChE inhibitors make them more suitable than the prototype in certain circumstances, which are discussed below.

The information given thus far states that AChE inhibitors cause cholinergic (ACh-like) effects, some of which mimic those caused by parasympathetic nervous system stimulation (ie, parasympathomimetic or muscarinic effects). Since other parasympathomimetic drugs are available (Chapter 11), as is ACh itself, you might wonder why AChE inhibitors are used at all. The answers were given in Chapter 11. To summarize:

Major reference tables appear beginning on p. 163.

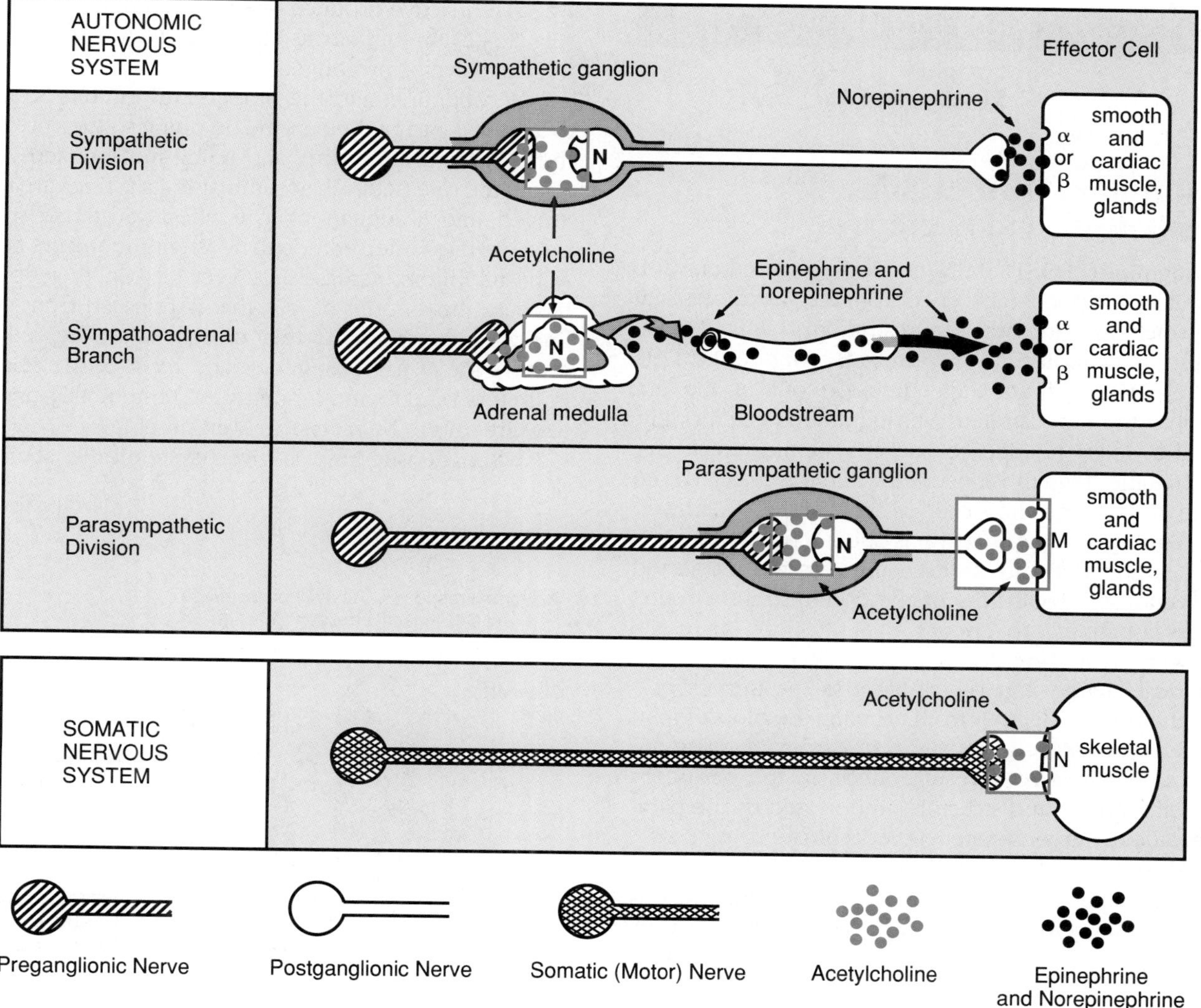

Figure 12–1

Acetylcholinesterase inhibitors theoretically act wherever ACh is released (green boxes): at somatic nerves innervating skeletal muscle; at all preganglionic nerves in the autonomic nervous system; and at postganglionic parasympathetic nerves. Both nicotinic (N) and muscarinic (M) effects occur indirectly due to the inhibitors. The actions of neostigmine and most related AChE inhibitors are limited to peripheral structures. Physostigmine enters the brain easily, so peripheral, ganglionic, and central effects occur.

- Parasympathomimetic drugs (eg, bethanechol) stimulate only the muscarinic ACh receptors, so they are not suitable when the goal is to stimulate skeletal muscle, which involves nicotinic receptors.
- Acetylcholine is metabolized so quickly that it is not suitable when longlasting effects are needed. This limitation could be overcome, theoretically, by injecting large amounts of ACh fast enough and for long enough periods to overcome its quick breakdown by AChE. But that is impractical in most cases. In contrast, the AChE inhibitors have longer durations of action, and so can cause prolonged build-up and increased activity of the ACh that is constantly being released from cholinergic nerves.

PROTOTYPE

Neostigmine

Absorption, Distribution, Metabolism, and Excretion

Neostigmine (PROSTIGMIN) and most of the other AChE inhibitors are poorly absorbed from the gastrointestinal (GI) tract following oral administration. That is because most of their molecules are ionized, owing to local pH (p 52), which limits their diffusion out of the gut and into the bloodstream. Neostigmine is given orally, but the doses needed to cause systemic effects are much higher than those needed when it is injected (see Table 12–C), and the onset of action is much slower. Neostigmine's onset of action is about 1 hour when it is given orally, but only about 5 minutes when injected intravenously. Regardless of the administration route, effects last about 2 to 4 hours.

With neostigmine and most of its related drugs, electrical charge and other chemical properties prevent the drug molecules from crossing the blood–brain barrier and entering the CNS, and from entering autonomic ganglia. As a result, effects in the periphery (skeletal muscle and structures innervated by the parasympathetic nervous system) predominate.

Most of an absorbed dose is metabolically inactivated in the liver and blood plasma. The metabolites, as well as unmetabolized drug, are excreted in the urine.

Pharmacologic Effects

Acetylcholine released from a cholinergic nerve diffuses across the neuroeffector junction to stimulate its effectors—muscle cells, gland cells, or other nerve cells, depending on the anatomic site. The effector cell membrane contains not only the receptors on which ACh acts, but also AChE. For an instant the ACh stimulates its receptors, causing an effect. Then it binds to the nearby AChE molecules and is quickly broken down (hydrolyzed) to inactive products—acetate, choline, and water (Fig. 12–2). In this way its effects are kept from becoming excessive or prolonged.

Neostigmine, and the other AChE inhibitors, bind to a critical part of the enzyme. In doing so they prevent the ACh from interacting and being metabolized. As a result, the released ACh accumulates, its actions are prolonged, and it appears as if its effects on target structures are intensified. Although neostigmine and the other AChE inhibitors increase the effects of ACh, they do not increase the amount of ACh that is released from cholinergic nerves, nor do they directly stimulate cell receptors for ACh. Neostigmine and most of the related inhibitors bind to and inhibit AChE temporarily, and so they are said to be *reversible* AChE inhibitors.

When neostigmine is given systemically, at usual

A. Normal response: Acetylcholinesterase (AChE) inactivates acetylcholine

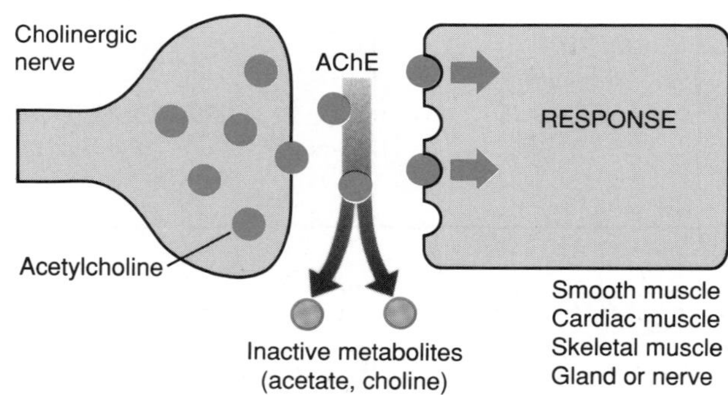

$$CH_3\overset{O}{\overset{\|}{C}}\text{-O-}CH_2\text{-}CH_2\text{-}\underset{CH_3}{\overset{CH_3}{N}}\text{-}CH_3 \xrightarrow{\text{Acetyl-cholinesterase}} CH_3\text{-}\overset{O}{\overset{\|}{C}}\text{-}\bar{O} + HO\text{-}CH_2\text{-}CH_2\text{-}\underset{CH_3}{\overset{CH_3}{N}}\text{-}CH_3$$

Acetylcholine (Active) — Acetate (Inactive) + Choline (Inactive)

B. Response in presence of AChE inhibitor

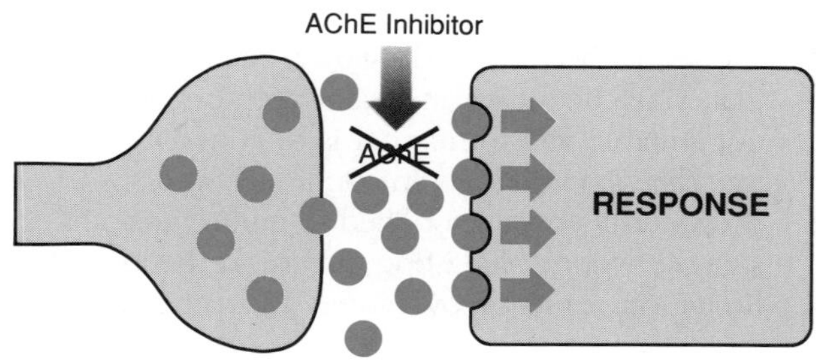

Figure 12–2

A. Acetylcholine released from any cholinergic nerve diffuses across the synaptic cleft to stimulate muscles, glands, or other nerves. It is quickly metabolized by AChE. **B.** Acetylcholinesterase inhibitors reduce inactivation of ACh. More neurotransmitter is present in the synaptic cleft, so its actions are prolonged and intensified, leading to an increased response.

doses, its major effects are on skeletal muscle and on structures innervated by the parasympathetic nervous system. Although effects at these sites will be discussed separately, and they involve different subtypes of cholinergic receptors, it is important to understand that *they usually occur simultaneously.*

Skeletal Muscle Effects

Acetylcholinesterase inhibitors increase the actions of ACh released from the motor nerves that innervate skeletal muscle. Skeletal muscle contractile activity increases through stimulation of *nicotinic* receptors on the muscle cells. This is a clinically useful effect in conditions, such as myasthenia gravis, that are characterized by skeletal muscle weakness. High doses of AChE inhibitors can cause excessive and prolonged skeletal muscle stimulation, which leads to muscle fatigue or paralysis.

Autonomic Nervous System (Parasympathomimetic or Muscarinic) Effects

In the presence of neostigmine, inhibited breakdown of ACh released by postganglionic parasympathetic nerves produces the typical parasympathomimetic effects discussed in Chapter 11. The major effects include:

- constriction of the pupil of the eye (miosis);
- decreased heart rate, automaticity, and electrical impulse conduction rates;
- increased tone and motility of the GI tract, relaxation of sphincters, and increased gastric acid secretion;
- stimulation of the urinary bladder detrusor muscle and relaxation of the sphincter;
- bronchoconstriction and increased mucus secretion in the respiratory tract; and
- increased activity of sweat and lacrimal glands.

The parasympathomimetic effects caused by neostigmine are not different from those caused by parasympathomimetic drugs such as bethanechol, but the manner in which the effects are produced differs.

Effects on Autonomic Ganglia and the Adrenal Medulla

Therapeutic doses of neostigmine and most of the other clinically useful AChE inhibitors do not diffuse well into the parasympathetic and sympathetic ganglia, or to the sites at which preganglionic sympathetic nerves innervate the adrenal medulla. However, ganglionic effects are possible with very high doses of these agents, and certainly will occur upon exposure to the AChE inhibitors used specifically as poisons (p 160).

The major outcome of inhibiting ACh breakdown in the autonomic ganglia is a simultaneous increase in stimulation of both the sympathetic and parasympathetic nervous systems, as well as the structures they control. Since these two divisions of the autonomic nervous system (ANS) usually exert opposite effects on their target structures, stimulating both at the same time would be expected to cause effects that cancel one another out. In reality, the outcome is very unpredictable, and it is usually detrimental.

Clinical Indications and Administration

Most AChE inhibitors are used for their skeletal muscle–stimulating effect or for causing parasympathomimetic effects on the eye, gut, or bladder (Table 12–C). Since these effects can occur simultaneously, when the therapeutic goal is skeletal muscle stimulation parasympathomimetic effects are side effects. The converse is also true; when AChE inhibitors are given for parasympathomimetic actions, skeletal muscle stimulation is a potential side effect.

Because skeletal muscle stimulation involves the nicotinic subtype of ACh receptor, and parasympathomimetic effects are mediated by the muscarinic subtype, the latter can be minimized or prevented altogether by administering a muscarinic receptor blocker such as atropine (Chapter 11). This is often done clinically.

One AChE inhibitor, physostigmine, is used only as an antidote for poisoning with anticholinergic (antimuscarinic) drugs. This potentially life-saving drug is discussed on page 159.

Uses in Myasthenia Gravis

Myasthenia gravis is a progressive, debilitating neuromuscular disease with symptoms thought to be caused by inadequate stimulation of skeletal muscle by ACh released from motor nerves. It appears to be an autoimmune disease that renders the nicotinic receptors on skeletal muscle cells less responsive to stimulation by ACh. By increasing the availability of ACh, the AChE inhibitor helps overcome decreased receptor responsiveness to the transmitter. The therapeutic goal is to improve skeletal muscle function. Parasympathomimetic (muscarinic) effects that may also occur are unwanted.

Signs and Symptoms

The early signs and symptoms of myasthenia gravis may be subtle. Droopy eyelids (ptosis) or muscle fatigue after even mild exercise may occur. Early in the disease, muscle strength recovers after resting. Later, abrupt episodes of muscle weakness may cause the patient to falter or stumble while walking, or to drop an object held in the hands. As the disease progresses, muscle weakness becomes more severe, and even frequent rest periods fail to restore strength. Eventually, muscle weakness may make impossible daily activities as essential as walking or eating. When the diaphragm and intercostal muscles lose function, death occurs owing to ventilatory failure, unless mechanical ventilation or drug therapy is instituted.

Diagnosis

Several sophisticated neurologic and pathologic tests help diagnose myasthenia gravis, but a traditional pharmacologic test is still used. Although neostigmine is valuable for treating myasthenia gravis, a related AChE inhibitor, edrophonium, given intravenously, is preferred for diagnosis. Edrophonium has a fast onset of action that allows prompt diagnosis, and a short duration of action that limits the duration of potential adverse effects. (See the section on edrophonium, below, for more details on its use and side effects.) The principle behind the test is simple. By increasing the availability of ACh, the inhibitor will restore muscle strength if the patient has myasthenia gravis. If the diagnosis is confirmed with edrophonium, a long-acting orally effective AChE inhibitor such as neostigmine can be used for continued treatment.

NURSING IMPLICATIONS

Side effects from the diagnostic use of edrophonium usually do not last long, nor are they likely to be severe unless there is a contraindication for any AChE inhibitor. Nevertheless, atropine (to block unwanted parasympathomimetic effects) and respiratory assist devices should be available to manage severe reactions. Atropine, given intravenously, may be used as a premedication to inhibit unwanted muscarinic responses, but careful monitoring of the patient's responses is still essential.

Treatment

Oral neostigmine bromide (PROSTIGMIN) is one of the AChE inhibitors suitable for management of myasthenia gravis. The desired therapeutic response is improvement in the patient's muscle strength, based on the ability to walk or use other limbs without excessive fatigue. The average daily dose is 150 mg (10 15-mg tablets), given in divided doses throughout the day. Adjusting the dosage properly can minimize undesirable muscarinic side effects. If they do occur, they can be managed by adjunctive therapy with atropine, which does not inhibit the desired nicotinic actions of an AChE inhibitor on skeletal muscle.

If myasthenic symptoms are severe and acute, intramuscular (IM) or subcutaneous (SC) administration of neostigmine methylsulfate (PROSTIGMIN) may be indicated. Parenteral administration increases the risk of muscarinic side effects, and so the patient is usually premedicated with atropine.

Many myasthenic patients can be controlled well with AChE inhibitors alone. Patients who do not respond well may need other drugs, including corticosteroids or other immunosuppressants (see Annotated Bibliography). Planned exercise and physical therapy programs are valuable nondrug therapies for most patients. Advanced or refractory myasthenia gravis may require other nondrug therapies, including surgical removal of the thymus gland, which participates in the autoimmune response.

Fifteen to twenty percent of treated patients will have a temporary spontaneous remission. These individuals will usually require a decreased maintenance dose of the AChE inhibitor until the disease progresses again. Thus, close monitoring of the course of the disease and the response to drug therapy are essential.

NURSING IMPLICATIONS

Determining the effective dose and how often the medication must be taken is a trial-and-error process that requires careful nursing assessment. Encourage the patient or a responsible family member to record medication intake and both objective and subjective responses to therapy. These individuals should be taught to recognize, record, and report both desired and unwanted effects.

Since some AChE inhibitors used to treat myasthenia gravis require administration many times during the day, and since many tablets may be required, the nurse should help patients devise ways to comply with the drug regimen. Stress the need for periodic assessment by the physician to optimize treatment.

Advise myasthenic patients to avoid excessive physical or emotional stress, either of which may worsen symptoms and require at least temporary dosage in-

Table 12–1 Expected Responses to the Edrophonium Test to Diagnose Adequate Therapy, Myasthenic Crisis, and Cholinergic Crisis in Patients with Myasthenia Gravis

Response to Edrophonium Test	Myasthenic Response	Normal Response*	Cholinergic Response†
Muscle strength (ptosis, diplopia, dysphagia, respiration, limb strength)‡	Increased	No change	Decreased
Muscle fasciculations (eye, face, limbs)	Absent	Present or absent	Present or absent
Muscarinic side effects (lacrimation, diaphoresis, salivation, abdominal cramps, diarrhea, micturition, vomiting)	Absent	Slight	Severe

*"Normal" indicates the anticipated response in a patient who does not have myasthenia gravis; it may also be observed if edrophonium is given to a myasthenic patient in whom therapy is optimal and stabilized.
†The cholinergic response to a test dose of edrophonium occurs in myasthenic patients who are being overtreated with AChE inhibitors.
‡Increased muscle strength caused by edrophonium indicates either underlying (undiagnosed) myasthenia gravis or an inadequate acetylcholinesterase dosage in patients with diagnosed myasthenia.

Source: Adapted from Olin BR, ed. *Drug Facts and Comparisons*. Facts and Comparisons Inc, 1992, p 724.

creases. Physical illness or surgery also increase dosage requirements. All patients with myasthenia gravis should wear a MedicAlert bracelet (or similar identification) at all times, and carry the name and dosage of the medication they are taking.

Some patients experience dysphagia due to weakness of pharyngeal muscles. Having the patient take the medication 30 to 60 minutes before meals may increase muscle strength needed for chewing and swallowing. If dysphagia interferes with swallowing tablets, AChE inhibitors dispensed as a syrup may be preferred. If dysphagia is most severe on awakening, sustained-acting preparations of AChE inhibitors may be preferred.

The Myasthenic Crisis and the Cholinergic Crisis: Too Little or Too Much Cholinesterase Inhibitor?

Muscle weakness may return during AChE inhibitor therapy. If the disease progresses, the current AChE inhibitor dose may be too low. Weakness may also occur if the patient forgets to take his or her medication as prescribed, or the prescribed dose is too low. If muscle weakness becomes severe owing to causes such as these, the patient is said to have a *myasthenic crisis*. It is caused by levels of ACh that are insufficient to stimulate skeletal muscle.

Muscle weakness may also occur if the patient's AChE inhibitor dose is too high. Aside from accidental administration of excessive doses, this situation may occur when the disease remits spontaneously and the maintenance dose is not reduced accordingly. In these "overdose" situations, weakness is due to excessive muscle stimulation and eventual fatigue due to too much ACh. If the symptoms are severe it is called a *cholinergic crisis*.

When muscle weakness develops during AChE inhibitor therapy, it is essential to determine whether the problem reflects a myasthenic crisis or a cholinergic crisis, since this affects subsequent treatment. There are several ways to make the differential diagnosis. One is to review carefully the patient's record of medication intake, daily activities, muscle strength, and side effects. Obviously, this is not useful if the patient keeps poor records, which is very common.

Excessive muscarinic side effects, or skeletal muscle weakness that becomes worse an hour after the patient takes an AChE inhibitor, are good clues that the problem is a cholinergic crisis. However, muscarinic side effects may be masked if the patient is also taking an antimuscarinic drug.

If a differential diagnosis cannot be made from clinical evidence, intravenous (IV) edrophonium may be used, similar to the way in which it is used for initial diagnosis. If edrophonium increases muscle strength (Table 12–1), weakness was due to a myasthenic crisis. This would usually indicate the need for increased maintenance doses of neostigmine or a similar drug. If edrophonium causes further muscle weakness, the problem usually indicates a cholinergic crisis, which warrants a decreased maintenance dose of the AChE inhibitor.

Postoperative Reversal of Neuromuscular Blockade

Neuromuscular blocking drugs, such as tubocurarine, are routinely used to relax or paralyze skeletal muscle during surgery. In doing so, they cause respiratory depression or paralysis by preventing stimulation of the diaphragm and intercostal muscles.

Tubocurarine and related drugs paralyze skeletal muscle by competitively blocking nicotinic ACh receptors on skeletal muscle. Postoperative administration of an AChE inhibitor overcomes blockade and restores muscle function by making more ACh available. Neostigmine methylsulfate, given by slow IV injection, can be used. The objective is to restore and maintain spontaneous ventilation. Atropine is almost always given as a pretreatment to prevent unwanted muscarinic stimulation. Nursing implications for reversal of neuromuscular blockade are discussed in Chapter 17.

Management of Postoperative Bladder or Gut Distention

Neostigmine methylsulfate, given IM or SC, can be used to increase the tone of the GI or urinary tracts, as after abdominal surgery. If treatment for a day or two is anticipated, the patient can be switched to oral neostigmine bromide (see Table 12–C) to avoid repeated injections. As noted below, and discussed for the similar use of the parasympathomimetic drug bethanechol (Chapter 11), gut and urinary tract obstruction must first be ruled out.

NURSING IMPLICATIONS

Nursing interventions used when an AChE inhibitor is given to stimulate the bladder or GI tract are the same as those used when parasympathomimetic drugs are given (see pp 140, 142). Do not give these drugs when gut or urinary tract obstruction is suspected; and be prepared to intervene, as by catheterizing the bladder, when usual doses fail to cause the expected responses within 30 to 60 minutes after administration.

Treatment of Alzheimer's Disease

There is much evidence that the memory loss that is a hallmark of Alzheimer's disease, a devastating and currently untreatable neurologic disorder, involves an inability of certain parts of the brain to synthesize adequate amounts of ACh. Thus, pharmacologic research is focusing on the use of AChE inhibitors to preserve what little ACh *is* being made, so it is better able to exert its role as a CNS neurotransmitter. The approach is analogous to using AChE inhibitors for their effects in the somatic nervous system to manage myasthenia gravis.

Currently only one drug, tacrine (to be marketed as COGNEX), is close to being approved in the United States as an aid in the management of Alzheimer's disease. The drug seems to work best when administered with lecithin, a substance that helps synthesize more ACh in the brain.

Side Effects, Adverse Reactions, and Contraindications

Side effects of the AChE inhibitors involve the ANS, skeletal muscle, and the CNS (Table 12–S). They can be predicted from the pharmacologic effects noted above.

Common peripheral muscarinic (autonomic) effects of neostigmine and related agents are similar to those noted for parasympathomimetic drugs (see Chapter 11). They include abdominal pain or cramping, diarrhea, and possibly nausea and vomiting; bradycardia; wheezing or more severe bronchoconstriction; and profuse secretion of saliva, mucus, sweat, and tears. Ocular side effects such as miosis and excessive lacrimation are most likely to occur with topically administered AChE inhibitors, but may occur with any inhibitor by any route of administration.

Nicotinic side effects are mainly seen in skeletal muscle, and include initial twitching or tremor, possibly leading to weakness, fatigue, and paralysis.

All AChE inhibitors, regardless of the route of administration or clinical indication, are contraindicated in patients with GI or urinary tract obstruction, uveitis, or acute angle-closure glaucoma. Cholinesterase inhibitors, even those given topically on the eye, are generally contraindicated in patients with asthma or obstructive pulmonary diseases. These individuals are unusually sensitive to ACh, and may suffer fatal bronchoconstriction or bronchospasm. The ability of AChE inhibitors to increase gastric acid secretion requires careful use of these drugs in patients with peptic ulcer disease.

NURSING IMPLICATIONS

Myasthenic patients taking any AChE inhibitor, for any purpose or by any administration route, should be educated about side effects, particularly those that require a physician's prompt attention. Precise reports of side effects should be part of their daily records.

Use During Pregnancy and Lactation

The safety of the AChE inhibitors in pregnancy has not been clearly established. In general, they should be used only when the potential benefits to the mother outweigh possible risks to the fetus. Uterine irritability and premature labor may occur with IV use of these drugs. It is not known whether neostigmine is excreted in human milk, or if serious side effects occur in nursing infants. The importance of the drug to the mother will influence the decision whether to discontinue nursing or discontinue the drug.

Use in Children

The same precautions noted for adults apply to children. Acetylcholinesterase inhibitors may be indicated for newborns of mothers with myasthenia gravis.

Use in the Elderly

A variety of age-related conditions involving structures and body systems affected by AChE inhibitors may increase the frequency or intensity of side effects in the elderly. Dosage reductions may be indicated, even with topically administered products, and close monitoring of responses is important regardless of the drug or administration route. Acetylcholinesterase inhibitors may cause arthralgia, which may be confused with osteoarthritis.

Interactions with Other Drugs

Acetylcholinesterase inhibitors interact with other drugs that affect the actions of ACh, particularly those acting on skeletal muscle (Table 12–I). These interactions are particularly important for patients with myasthenia gravis.

As mentioned, neostigmine can be used after surgery to antagonize the effects of tubocurarine and related nondepolarizing neuromuscular blocking agents. Neostigmine and other AChE inhibitors intensify the actions of succinylcholine, a neuromuscular blocker that paralyzes skeletal muscle in a manner not too different from the actions of ACh itself (Chapter 17, p 269). The interaction between an AChE inhibitor and succinylcholine is potentially serious: intense and prolonged paralysis of skeletal muscle may occur. Paralysis of ventilatory muscles is most dangerous, but it can be managed easily by mechanical ventilation as long as needed.

Many other drugs suppress ACh release from nerves, or depress the ability of muscles to respond to ACh. They include some general anesthetics, local anesthetics, antihistamines, some cardiac antiarrhythmics (especially disopyramide, procainamide, and quinidine), most antipsychotic drugs, and the aminoglycoside antibiotics (eg, gentamicin, neomycin, streptomycin, kanamycin). The dose of an AChE inhibitor usually needs to be selected carefully when the patient is receiving one of these interactants.

Overdose and Toxicity

There are two major causes of poisoning from AChE inhibitors. One involves accidental overdosing with therapeutic agents; the other involves poisoning with organophosphate insecticides or chemical warfare agents. Although the onset and duration of toxicity vary depending on the causative agent, the signs and symptoms are basically the same. The management of overdoses, however, depends in part on whether the cause was a reversible inhibitor (which includes most of the clinically used agents) or one with irreversible actions. This discussion focuses on management of overdoses of reversible inhibitors.

Signs and Symptoms

The signs and symptoms of AChE inhibitor overdose involve ANS, CNS, and peripheral skeletal muscle changes that are similar to those seen in a cholinergic crisis, or when intense side effects occur. These responses have been discussed above.

However, very high doses of an AChE inhibitor may also stimulate all autonomic ganglia (sympathetic and parasympathetic), as well as epinephrine release from the adrenal medulla, so that further and often unpredictable changes, especially of cardiovascular function, are likely to occur. The autonomic effects are accompanied by skeletal muscle tremor or fasciculation, followed by paralysis. Respiratory paralysis is the most common cause of death.

Treatment

In addition to standard therapy for drug overdose (eg, induced emesis, gastric lavage; see Appendix C), IV atropine sulfate will need to be given, possibly in large doses. However, atropine reverses only the muscarinic effects of AChE inhibitors, not the nicotinic effects that involve skeletal muscle or autonomic ganglia. This is important, since the major cause of death—respiratory dysfunction—is a problem involving skeletal muscle. Atropine will help normalize the cardiovascular system and the GI and urinary tracts, and will dilate the bronchi and suppress excessive secretions, thus making the patient more comfortable.

Generally, nothing is done for ventilatory paralysis except to maintain a patent airway and support ventilation for as long as needed. Careful monitoring and normalization of vital signs are essential.

NURSING IMPLICATIONS

Anticipate profuse diarrhea, urination, diaphoresis, and possible vomiting; keep the patient as clean and comfortable as possible.

Related Drugs

Demecarium, Echothiophate, and Isoflurophate

Demecarium (HUMORSOL), echothiophate iodide (PHOSPHOLINE), and isoflurophate (FLOROPRYL) are long-acting, topically effective AChE inhibitors. They are indicated for the treatment of several eye disorders for which neostigmine is not used. Their dosages are noted in Table 12–C.

Glaucoma

Cholinesterase inhibitors lower intraocular pressure, particularly in patients with chronic open-angle glaucoma and some cases of chronic or subacute angle-closure glaucoma. Initial treatment usually involves a topical parasympathomimetic drug like pilocarpine (see Chapter 11). When this proves inadequate, topical AChE inhibitors are often added to the treatment regimen, or are used in place of a parasympathomimetic. Acetylcholinesterase inhibitors contract the radial muscles of the eye and cause miosis, which facilitates drainage of aqueous humor and a lowering of interocular pressure.

Strabismus and Esotropia

Topical AChE inhibitors can be used to diagnose or treat strabismus, a condition in which the field of view of each eye differs. One common form of strabismus in children is esotropia (known more commonly as cross-eye), in which the ocular fields converge abnormally. Cholinesterase inhibitors affect smooth muscles that control accommodation, and extraorbital striated muscles that rotate the eye, leading to improved vision.

Reversal of Mydriatic and Cycloplegic Drug Actions

To facilitate some eye examinations, antimuscarinic (atropine-like) drugs are often applied to the eye to dilate the pupil (produce mydriasis) and paralyze accommodation. Once the examination has been completed, a short-acting AChE inhibitor may be applied to overcome mydriasis and restore the ability of the eye to focus normally.

NURSING IMPLICATIONS

Review with patients the drug manufacturer's instructions for proper use and storage.

Teach proper aseptic administration techniques to reduce infection. This includes thorough hand-washing, avoiding contact of the medication dispenser with the eye or skin, and keeping the dispenser clean and capped. Apply mild finger pressure to the inner canthus of the eye(s) for about 2 minutes after applying the drug, to enhance local effects and reduce systemic drug absorption and resulting side effects. Any person administering these drugs should avoid prolonged drug contact with the skin. Seal medication containers tightly after use to avoid inactivation and contamination.

Side Effects of Topically Applied Acetylcholinesterase Inhibitors

Although AChE inhibitors may produce adverse muscarinic or nicotinic effects in any part of the body, therapeutic doses of the topically applied drugs most often cause ocular problems. Annoying or painful spasm of the ciliary muscle, uncontrolled eyelid twitching (blepharospasm), and headache may occur. Conjunctivitis, ocular congestion ("blood-shot" eyes), excessive lacrimation, and myopia may also occur. Long-term use may lead to the development of cysts on the iris, or cataracts. Uveitis and acute angle-closure glaucoma contraindicate use of these drugs.

If possible, AChE inhibitors used for ophthalmic disorders should be discontinued 2 weeks before surgery, to prevent interaction with anesthetic agents or adjuncts. The disorder for which the drug was prescribed may worsen during this time, so close, frequent monitoring is required. Alternative drug therapies may be indicated.

General management of poisoning due the irreversible inhibitors echothiophate and isoflurophate follows guidelines noted for neostigmine. Additional measures noted for organophosphate insecticides may apply.

NURSING IMPLICATIONS

Patients with glaucoma who are receiving AChE inhibitors for the first time should remain in the physician's office for about 4 hours for periodic measurements of intraocular pressure. Advise patients that failure to take their medication as directed may lead to blindness. Encourage periodic follow-up examinations to evaluate effects of therapy, adjust doses, and detect adverse responses. Caution patients that miosis may interfere with night vision, and to avoid tasks requiring acute night vision. Advise them that administration of these drugs at bedtime may minimize visual disturbances. Instruct patients to report severe or persistent side effects at once, especially intense ocular pain suggesting an acute glaucoma attack. Closely monitor for adverse pulmonary effects. Even a single dose of a topical AChE inhibitor may cause serious or fatal bronchospasm in an asthmatic patient.

Edrophonium

Edrophonium chloride (TENSILON) is an injectable AChE inhibitor that is used when rapid but brief effects are wanted. Responses occur in less than 1 minute when the drug is given intravenously (preferred), and within 10 minutes after IM injection (used when venous access cannot be obtained). Effects last less than 30 minutes, regardless of the injection route.

Edrophonium was mentioned above (pp 154–155) as the preferred drug to aid in the diagnosis of myasthenia gravis and to make the differential diagnosis of myasthenic and cholinergic crises. Those are its major uses.

Another use is for postoperative reversal of muscle paralysis caused intentionally by curare-like neuromuscular blockers. However, other AChE inhibitors with longer durations of action are used more often.

Edrophonium has also been used to treat episodes of paroxysmal atrial tachycardia. The AChE inhibitor causes a build-up of ACh at the sinoatrial node, which slows the rapid atrial rate. Unfortunately, the accumulation of ACh elsewhere causes a host of unwanted parasympathomimetic and skeletal muscle side effects. As a result, other drugs (see p 201, and Chapter 30) are usually preferred for treating this cardiac disorder.

Physostigmine

Physostigmine salicylate (ANTILIRIUM) has only one approved use, but it is an important one. It is indicated for adjunctive management of poisoning from atropine or the many other drugs with intense antimuscarinic activity (see Chapter 13). These overdoses are common and potentially fatal. Antimuscarinic drugs competitively block muscarinic ACh receptors, and at high doses they essentially inactivate the entire parasympathetic nervous system. Tachycardia, constipation, urinary retention, mydriasis, and marked absence of secretions are some of the common signs and symptoms of atropine poisoning. If the antimuscarinic dose was very high, a variety of CNS effects can also occur, including high fever, delirium, hallucinations, and seizures, often leading to death.

Physostigmine is the only AChE inhibitor that penetrates the CNS well enough to overcome the dangerous central effects. The drug is given by slow IV injection or by the IM route. Very high doses (see Table 12–C) may be needed for severe anticholinergic poisoning. Physostigmine's actions last about 90 minutes, so repeated doses are required until the patient's condition improves. Other adjunctive symptomatic and supportive measures are also needed. Physostigmine should not be given to atropine-poisoned children unless the child is likely to die without it.

Pyridostigmine

Pyridostigmine bromide (MESTINON) is indicated for oral treatment of myasthenia gravis. Some clinicians consider it the preferred drug for this disease. Pyrostigmine is available in several oral forms: regular tablets, syrup, and sustained-release (MESTINON TIMESPAN) tablets. The syrup is well suited for patients who have difficulty swallowing tablets, and should be recommended if dysphagia is present.

The onset of action of regular tablets or syrup is about 60 minutes, and the duration of action is between 3 and 6 hours. Either of these preparations requires frequent administration during the day. The drug in sustained-release tablets is absorbed erratically and incompletely, and so therapy should be started with other oral forms. However, sustained-release tablets have several advantages over other drugs or oral formulations: once- or twice-daily administration, which allows patients to sleep uninterrupted, without having to take medication during the night; and less morning dysphagia.

Pyridostigmine is less likely to cause unpleasant GI side effects than equally effective doses of neostigmine.

Pyridostigmine (as MESTINON INJECTION or REGONOL) can be injected intravenously (after atropine pretreatment) to reverse postoperative neuromuscular blockade. The onset of action is less than 5 minutes, and effects last about 3 hours. The drug also can be given intramuscularly or by slow IV administration to treat symptoms of acute myasthenia gravis. Effects appear in 5 to 15 minutes, and last about 3 hours.

Organophosphate Insecticides and "Nerve Gases"

Organophosphate insecticides such as *parathion* are long-lasting AChE inhibitors frequently used in agriculture. These agents are often stored in large quantities in concentrated form, and are sprayed over large areas. Amounts of the poison sufficient to cause intoxication may be carried with the wind to distant places. Pharmacologically related to the organophosphate insecticides are some nerve gases, such as *soman* and *sarin,* developed for chemical warfare.

The liquid and vapor forms of all these chemicals are absorbed quickly through the skin and mucous membranes, producing a host of toxic signs and symptoms (Table 12–2). Death may occur within minutes of exposure.

These agents (as well as the clinically useful drugs echothiophate and isoflurophate) combine with AChE molecules, permanently inhibiting the enzyme's ability to metabolize ACh. The effects can be overcome only after the body has had time to synthesize new, active AChE molecules. Unfortunately, death occurs first, unless prompt and proper treatment is given.

Atropine is always given to reverse the toxic muscarinic effects of these agents, but it must be administered for long periods, and it does nothing to overcome the underlying cause of the symptoms. Another drug, pralidoxime chloride (PROTOPAM), is used adjunctively.

Pralidoxime reacts chemically with the AChE inhibitor, leaving the enzyme free to metabolize ACh. It has no atropine-like activity, nor any other clinical use. After atropine premedication, stabilization, and support of vital signs, pralidoxime is given by slow IV infusion over about 30 minutes. The dose can be repeated in 1 hour if symptoms such as muscle weakness persist, after which time the patient is placed on oral pralidoxime until all signs of poisoning have disappeared. As pralidoxime reactivates AChE, and ACh levels in synapses fall, side effects due to the atropine may appear.

Table 12–2 Signs and Symptoms of Poisoning with Organophosphate Insecticides or Nerve Gases Containing AChE Inhibitors*

Parasympathomimetic (due to peripheral muscarinic receptor stimulation)
- Bronchoconstriction, excessive mucus secretion
- Excessive, uncontrolled diarrhea, vomiting
- Urinary incontinence
- Bradycardia, hypotension
- Excessive sweating (diaphoresis) and lacrimation
- Miosis, myopia

Sympathomimetic (due to nicotinic receptor stimulation of sympathetic ganglia, adrenal gland)
- Tachycardia, arrhythmias, hypertension

Skeletal muscle (due to nicotinic receptor stimulation on skeletal muscle cells)
- Fasciculations
- Tremor
- Weakness
- Paralysis
- Respiratory arrest (paralysis of diaphragm, intercostal muscles)

Central nervous system (probably due to nicotinic receptor stimulation in brain)
- Confusion
- Seizures
- Coma
- Stimulation, then depression of cardiovascular, respiratory centers

*Note that many of these effects are similar to the side effects or adverse effects of high doses of AChE inhibitors used clinically.

NURSING IMPLICATIONS

Advise any individual working with organophosphate insecticides to avoid direct contact with liquids, dusts, or sprays; to wear approved protective clothing and respirators; to decontaminate their clothing properly; and to store and use the material safely to avoid the spread of poison to others. All persons who transport or provide immediate care to an individual who has been exposed to an organophosphate insecticide should wear full protective clothing and respirator masks. Decontamination, isolation, and disposal procedures for clothing and excrement are summarized in Appendix C.

Pralidoxime must be given as soon after cholinesterase inhibitor exposure as possible; it is not likely to work well when given more than 2 days after poisoning. Anticipate antimuscarinic side effects to occur as AChE activity is restored. The use of pralidoxime or atropine does not lessen the need for frequent and careful nursing assessment, or the need for other drugs that may be required to manage other signs or symptoms of toxicity. Contact a regional poison center for assistance with treating this emergency.

SUMMARY OF NURSING IMPLICATIONS

◆ Assessment

Review history for presence of conditions that contraindicate treatment with AChE inhibitors (eg, acute angle-closure glaucoma, asthma, urinary or GI tract obstruction, peptic ulcer disease, pheochromocytoma).

Recognize symptoms of a myasthenic crisis (increased ptosis; difficulty ambulating, chewing, swallowing, coughing; respiratory difficulty; increased pulse and blood pressure).

Recognize symptoms of a cholinergic crisis (cramps, diarrhea, sweating, bronchospasm, muscle fasciculations).

Assess the patient's functional ability to perform activities of daily living.

Establish baseline data: vital signs, bowel sounds, abdominal distention, intake, and output.

◆ Nursing Diagnoses

Ineffective breathing pattern related to myasthenia gravis or drug toxicity.

Self-care deficit related to inadequate drug control of muscle weakness.

Ineffective individual coping related to chronic illness (myasthenia gravis or glaucoma).

High risk for injury related to disease or drug effects.

◆ Planning/Implementation

Develop a treatment regimen with the patient to control effectively signs and symptoms.

Prepare ventilatory support devices and antidote (atropine).

Prepare for bladder catheterization if AChE inhibitor administration is unsuccessful in treating urinary retention.

Administer AChE inhibitors as needed to prevent muscle weakness from myasthenia gravis.

Monitor respiratory, cardiac, GI, and urinary tract status for signs of toxicity.

Ensure that all other cholinergics are discontinued before administering AChE inhibitor.

Give neostigmine on an empty stomach for best absorption, with food or milk if GI upset occurs.

◆ Patient and Family Teaching

Teach the patient/family to recognize myasthenic and cholinergic crises; when to notify the physician; methods to ensure regular medication dosages; importance of recording desired and adverse responses to drug; possible drug interactions.

Teach patients using topical agents for glaucoma proper administration of medication; importance of reporting severe or persistent side effects; the need for follow-up eye examinations to measure intraocular pressure.

◆ Evaluation

The patient/family will:

Comply with drug regimen to prevent blindness from glaucoma or impaired mobility or respiratory failure from myasthenia gravis.

Determine that no complications (eg, respiratory depression, muscle weakness, hypotension, dizziness, acute ocular pain) are present.

Be knowledgeable regarding disease process, drug effects (desired and untoward), administration schedule.

Continue active role in family and community; maintain self-esteem; cope with chronic illness.

Perform activities of daily living.

Return for follow-up examinations as indicated.

Annotated Bibliography

Bienfang DC, Kelly LD, Nicholson DH, Nussenblatt RB. Ophthalmology. *N Engl J Med* 1990;323(14):956–967. *A contemporary, understandable general review on ophthalmic disorders and ophthalmic drug therapies.*

Chipps E. Myasthenia gravis: The patient in crisis. *Crit Care Nurse* 1991;11(7):18–26. *An excellent look at the acute myasthenic crisis from the viewpoint of nurses caring for such critically ill patients.*

Everitt DE, Avorn J. Systemic effects of medications used to treat glaucoma. *Ann Intern Med* 1990;112(2):120–125. *Given the prevalence of glaucoma and the potential for topical glaucoma drugs to cause serious systemic effects or drug interactions, nurses dealing with these patients and drugs will find this article worth reading. It provides special insight into the care of elderly patients, who may present with multiple diseases and many drugs used to treat each of them.*

Finley JE, Pascuzzi RM. Rational therapy of myasthenia gravis. *Semin Neurol* 1990;10(1):70–82. *A well-written, contemporary review of how AChE inhibitors and many other pharmacologic and nondrug therapies are used to optimize treatment of this common neuromuscular disorder.*

Gerber SL, Cantor LB, Brater DC. Systemic drug interactions with topical glaucoma medications. *Surv Ophthalmol* 1990;35(3):205–218. *Package inserts (and pharmacology texts) warn that ocular drugs given topically can cause extraocular interactions with other medications given systemically—and they are thought to be particularly important for the elderly. This paper reviews the clinical basis for these interactions and effects, and finds that warnings for some of them may be unsupported by much clinical data.*

Goldberg I. Glaucoma—diagnostic hints. *Aust Fam Physician* 1991;20 (2):150–151, 154–162. *This article discusses simple measures to use in the early diagnosis of this potentially disabling condition.*

Havard CW, Fonseca V. New treatment approaches to myasthenia gravis. *Drugs* 1990;39(1):66–73. *Excellent coverage of not only the expected aspects of myasthenia gravis therapy, but also the genetic linkage, which should be of special interest to nurses whose myasthenic patients are women who are, or wish to be, pregnant.*

Hurvitz LM, Kaufman PL, Robin AL, Weinreb RN, Crawford K, Shaw B. New developments in the drug treatment of glaucoma. *Drugs* 1991;41(4):514–532. *Identifies not only what new drugs (or new formulations of old drugs) are likely to be available soon, but also explains problems associated with many of the current yet usually effective medications.*

Linton DM, Philcox D. Myasthenia gravis. *Dis Mon* 1990;36(11):593–637. *Long, but current and comprehensive, this article provides excellent overviews of the underlying pathophysiology, therapy (drug, surgical, and other), and prognosis of myasthenia gravis.*

Plauche WC. Myasthenia gravis in mothers and their newborns. *Clin Obstet Gynecol* 1991;34(1):82–99. *Myasthenia gravis and its treatments cause added and serious concerns when the patient is pregnant. This article reviews the risks and gives valuable insight into both pharmacologic and nondrug therapies that can reduce morbidity and mortality.*

Schwartz B. Current concepts in ophthalmology: The glaucomas. *N Engl J Med* 1978;299(4):182–184. *The causes and pathophysiologic characteristics of the various glaucomatous diseases are very confusing, as are the drug therapies. This short paper does an excellent job of explaining them. New drug treatments have been developed since this paper was published, but the basics of action, uses, and hazards for prototype agents still apply.*

Table 12–C | Clinical Uses and Administration of Major Acetylcholinesterase Inhibitors

AGENT	CLINICAL USES	DOSAGE AND ROUTE OF ADMINISTRATION
PROTOTYPE		
Neostigmine bromide (PROSTIGMIN)	Treatment of myasthenia gravis	Oral: Usually 150 mg/d (range 15–375 mg/d) administered at intervals based on symptom severity and daily fluctuations
Neostigmine methylsulfate (PROSTIGMIN INJECTION)	Rapid treatment of acute myasthenic symptoms	IM or SC: Usually 0.5 mg for rapid control of symptoms; switch to oral therapy when feasible
	Prevention of postoperative bladder distention, urinary retention	IM or SC: 0.25 mg as soon as possible postoperatively and q4h–q6h thereafter for 2–3 days
	Treatment of postoperative bladder distention	IM or SC: 0.5 mg as needed
	Treatment of postoperative urinary retention	IM or SC: 0.5 mg; after bladder is emptied continue 0.5-mg injections q3h for at least 5 injections
	Postoperative reversal of muscle paralysis induced with nondepolarizing neuromuscular blockers	IV: 0.5–2 mg (slowly); pretreat with 0.6–1.2 mg atropine (IV) to prevent parasympathomimetic side effects
RELATED DRUGS		
Demecarium bromide (HUMORSOL)	Topical miotic for glaucoma	Topical: 1 drop (children) or 2 drops (adults) of 0.125% solution to affected eye; maintenance doses: 1–2 drops twice a week to 1–2 drops twice daily; some patients may need the 0.25% solution
	Strabismus, esotropia	Topical: Usually 1 drop (0.125% solution) qd in each eye for 2 weeks, then 1 drop qod for 2–3 weeks; re-evaluate and adjust dose every 4–12 weeks; stop drug if patient requires more than 1 drop qod after 4 months of treatment
Echothiophate iodide (PHOSPHOLINE)	Glaucoma unresponsive to pilocarpine or other antiglaucoma drugs	Topical: Initially 1 drop of 0.03% solution instilled twice daily (bedtime and morning)
	Accommodative esotropia	Topical: Diagnosis: 1 drop of 0.125% solution in each eye at bedtime for 2–3 weeks. Treatment: Adjust diagnostic dose for best response
Edrophonium chloride (TENSILON)	Differential diagnosis of myasthenia gravis	IV: Adults: Inject 2 mg over 15–30 seconds; observe patient for 45 sec; inject additional 8 mg only if patient experiences no muscarinic side effects, twitching, or further reduction of weakness. Children up to 75 lbs: 1 mg initially, then up to an additional 4 mg if no response is seen; actual doses depend on age, weight
		IM (for patients with inaccessible veins): Adults: 10 mg. Children <75 lbs: 2 mg. Children >75 lbs: 5 mg
	Differential diagnosis of myasthenic, cholinergic crises	IV: Usually 1–2 mg, with careful monitoring of patient's response

(*continued*)

Table 12–C Clinical Uses and Administration of Major Acetylcholinesterase Inhibitors (*Continued*)

AGENT	CLINICAL USES	DOSAGE AND ROUTE OF ADMINISTRATION
RELATED DRUGS		
Isoflurophate (FLOROPRYL)	Glaucoma	Topical: 1/4-in. strip of 0.025% ointment in affected eye q8h–q72h
	Strabismus	Topical: No more than 1/4-in. strip into eye at night for 2 weeks
	Uncomplicated esotropia	Topical: No more than 1/4-in. strip every night for 2 weeks; reduce dose to 1/4 in. or less applied from every other night to once a week, for up to 2 months
Physostigmine Salicylate (ANTILIRIUM)	Treatment of poisoning with atropine, other anticholinergic/antimuscarinic drugs	IM: Adults: 0.5–2 mg; repeat doses up to 4 mg each every 30–60 min as necessary, more often for life-threatening signs, symptoms (arrhythmias, seizures, coma). Children: Usually 0.02 mg/kg; do not exceed 2 mg total
		IV: Adults: Usually 0.5–1 mg, given no faster than 1 mg/min. Children: 0.02 mg/kg, given no faster than 0.5 mg/min; repeat adult or pediatric doses at intervals noted for IM administration
Pralidoxime chloride (PROTOPAM)	Antidote for organophosphate poisoning	IV: Adults: Usually 1–2 g in 100 mL sterile saline, infused over 15–30 min; repeat in 1 hr if symptoms not improved; give atropine (2–4 mg, IV) with initial pralidoxime dose; switch to oral pralidoxime when symptoms improve. Children: Initially 20–40 mg/kg/dose; administer same way as for adults
		Oral: 1–3 g every 5 h for at least 5 doses
	Antidote for overdoses of clinically used cholinesterase inhibitors	IV: Initial dose as above; follow with 250 mg every 5 min until symptoms improve
Pyridostigmine bromide (MESTINON)	Treatment of myasthenia gravis	Oral: Syrup or regular tablets: 600 mg/d in divided doses according to fluctuation of symptoms throughout day. Long-acting tablets: Usually 1–3 tablets (180 mg each) once or twice daily; doses of long-acting drug should be at least 6 hr apart
(MESTINON, REGONOL)	Treatment of myasthenia gravis, particularly acute symptoms	IM or very slow IV: Usually 2 mg or 1/30th the patient's usual oral dose
	Postoperative reversal of muscle paralysis induced with nondepolarizing neuromuscular blockers	IV: 10–20 mg (slowly); pretreat with 0.6–1.2 mg atropine (IV) to prevent parasympathomimetic side effects

Table 12–S Major Side Effects and Contraindications of Acetylcholinesterase Inhibitors

BODY SYSTEM/ Side Effect	CONTRAINDICATION/ PRECAUTION	COMMENTS AND NURSING IMPLICATIONS
EYE Twitching of the eyelids (blepharospasm); stinging, burning, lacrimation; myopia; impaired vision due to cysts on iris	Acute inflammation of uvea; narrow-angle glaucoma; inflammation of iris, ciliary body	Monitor patients receiving topical AChE inhibitors for ocular irritation, lacrimation; have patient report severe eye pain at once (may indicate acute angle-closure glaucoma); encourage periodic eye exams to help adjust dosage, detect adverse responses; intraocular pressure should be monitored periodically for at least the first 4 hr after initial AChE inhibitor administration
RESPIRATORY Bronchoconstriction, wheezing, bronchospasm, increased mucus secretion	Asthma; known or likely cholinergic crisis	Be prepared for excessive respiratory secretions, severe bronchoconstriction when administering any AChE inhibitor to patient with suspected cholinergic crisis; have drugs, facilities for support of respiration readily available
CARDIOVASCULAR Bradycardia, possible hypotension	Bradycardia	Monitor heart rate, BP; heart rate and contractility may be seriously depressed in myasthenic patients receiving excessive doses of AChE inhibitors, especially if respiration is inadequate
GASTROINTESTINAL Cramping; diarrhea or vomiting; dyspepsia	Peptic ulcer disease; gut obstruction	Mild dyspepsia may be relieved by administering oral AChE inhibitors with meals or milk; notify physician if side effects are prolonged, severe; anticholinergics may be administered to reduce this muscarinic side effect; anticipate inserting rectal tube if AChE inhibitor is used to manage postoperative abdominal distention, gut atony
GENITOURINARY Excessive or involuntary micturition	Urinary tract obstruction	Notify physician if urinary problems occur in outpatients; dosage adjustment or anticholinergic drugs may be indicated; if AChE inhibitor is used for postoperative urinary retention or bladder distention, notify physician if voiding does not occur within 1 hr of administration; anticipate need to catheterize bladder
NEUROMUSCULAR Muscle tremor, fasciculations, fatigue	Cholinergic crisis	Muscle fasciculations in nonmyasthenic patients may indicate overdose or, with topical preparations, inadequate measures to reduce systemic absorption; teach proper administration technique; also see Table 12–1

Table 12–I Major Interactions Between Acetylcholinesterase Inhibitors and Other Agents

AGENT	RESULT OF INTERACTION	COMMENTS AND NURSING IMPLICATIONS
Aminoglycoside antibiotics (amikacin, gentamicin, kanamycin, neomycin, streptomycin, tobramycin; Chapter 56)	Increased muscle weakness in myasthenic patients	May cause slight neuromuscular blockade, reduce muscle function in myasthenic patients; other classes of antibiotics should be used when possible; interaction need not be avoided, but frequent assessment of muscle tone and respiration, increased dose of AChE inhibitor, may be needed
Anesthetics, general or local (Chapters 19, 20)	Depressed skeletal muscle activation	Increased doses of AChE inhibitor may be required; use caution, monitor response closely
Antiarrhythmics (disopyramide, quinidine, procainamide; Chapter 30)	See anesthetics, above	See anesthetics, above
Atropine, other antimuscarinics (Chapter 13)	Antagonism of all muscarinic effects of AChE inhibitor	Antimuscarinics are often used to control muscarinic side effects of AChE inhibitors, but may mask signs of a cholinergic crisis
Neuromuscular blockers (Chapter 17)		
Nondepolarizing type (tubocurarine, metocurine, pancuronium, others)	Antagonism of neuromuscular blockade	Interaction is used clinically to reverse muscle paralysis postoperatively; pretreatment with IV atropine necessary to prevent parasympathomimetic effects; effects of curare-like drugs may be reduced if given to patient taking AChE inhibitor
Depolarizing type (succinylcholine)	Intensified, prolonged respiratory depression; apnea	Increased ACh availability caused by AChE inhibitor intensifies succinylcholine effect; avoid simultaneous administration; if unavoidable, make sure patient is well oxygenated, breathing is supported until spontaneous respiration returns; continue close monitoring to detect return of respiratory depression, apnea

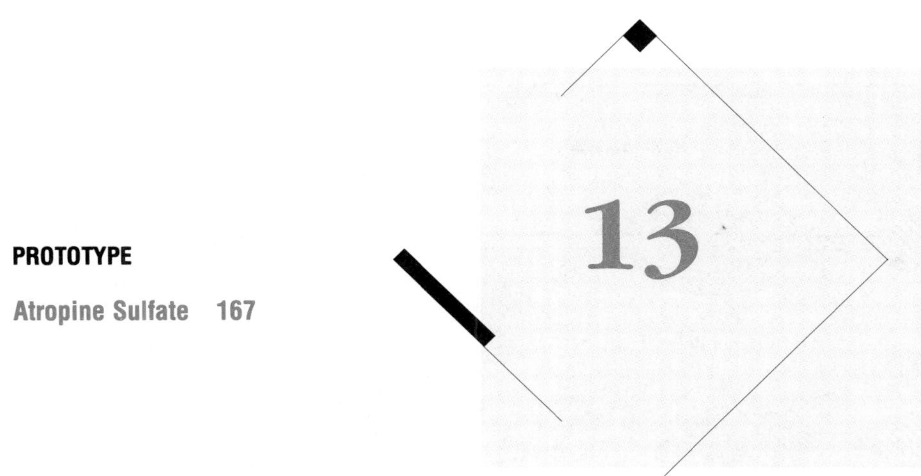

Antimuscarinic Drugs

General Characteristics of Antimuscarinic Drugs

The drugs discussed in this chapter can be classified or named in several ways, and in many cases the terms are used synonymously. These drugs antagonize the effects of acetylcholine (ACh) and other parasympathomimetic drugs (Chapter 12) on all the structures that are controlled by the parasympathetic nervous system. Because they interrupt (break, or lyse) parasympathetic control, they can be called *parasympatholytic* agents. Since they block some of the effects of ACh, they can also be called *anticholinergic* drugs. However, since therapeutic doses of these agents act mainly on the muscarinic subtype of ACh receptor, which is found on smooth muscle, cardiac muscle, and some glands, a better term is *antimuscarinic* drug. This is the term we will use throughout the book.

The antimuscarinic drugs cause diverse effects, not only on peripheral structures under parasympathetic control, but also in the central nervous system (CNS). This property provides these drugs with several important therapeutic uses, and also contributes to many side effects for which there are some common contraindications.

Major reference tables appear beginning on p. 182.

Atropine sulfate is the prototype, but many other drugs have atropine-like actions. Some are specifically classified as antimuscarinics. However, many drugs belonging to other drug classes cause significant antimuscarinic actions. Understanding the major effects of the prototype will help you to predict the beneficial and unwanted responses to any drug with antimuscarinic activity, and will help you to understand the implications of administering these drugs to your patients.

PROTOTYPE

Atropine Sulfate

Atropine sulfate is an alkaloid isolated from a common plant, *Atropa belladonna* (deadly nightshade). Atropine and several other related antimuscarinic drugs are also called *belladonna alkaloids.*

Absorption, Distribution, Metabolism, and Excretion

Atropine is readily absorbed from the gastrointestinal (GI) tract and all parenteral administration sites. Atropine and several other antimuscarinics are also fre-

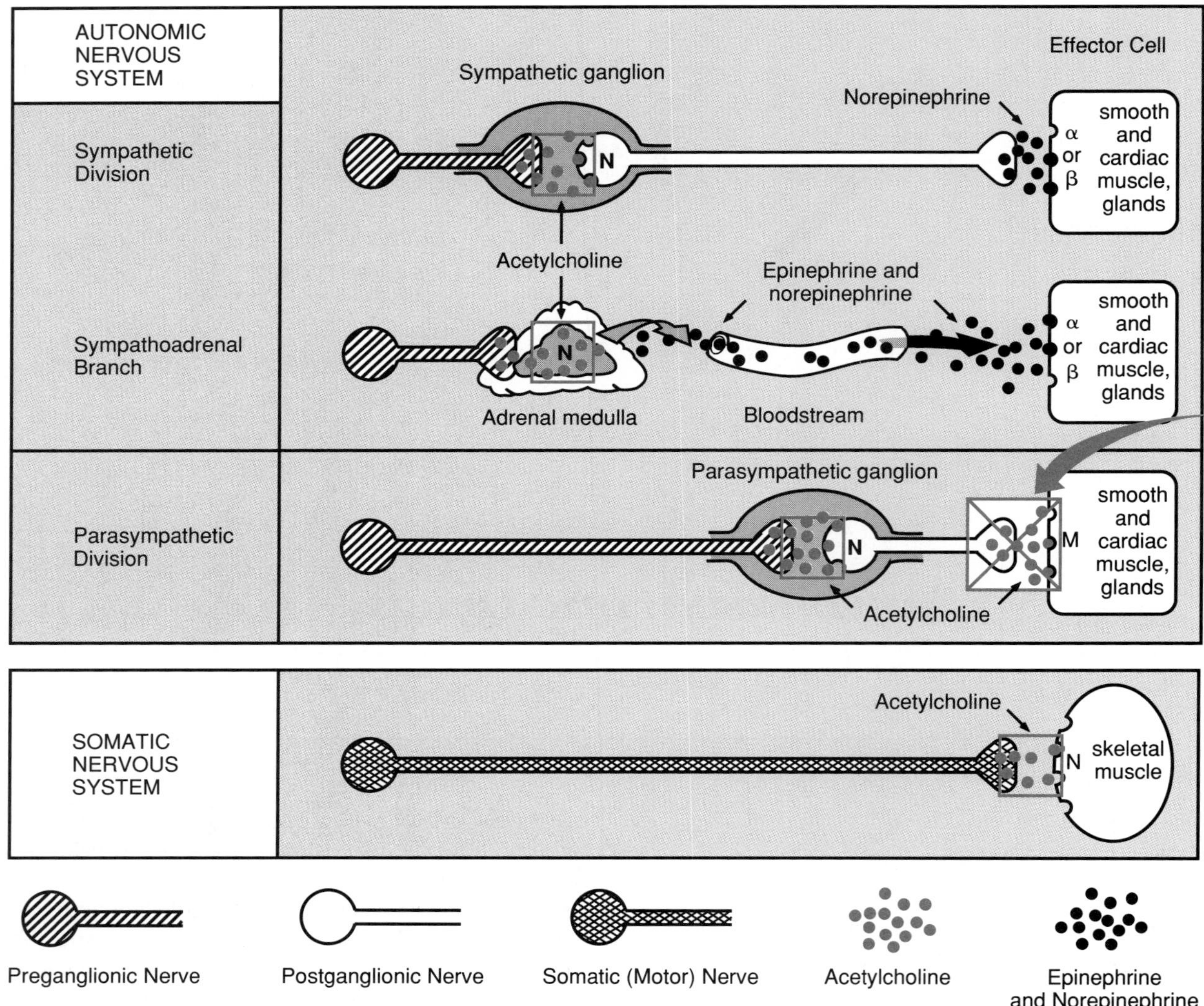

Figure 13–1

Atropine, the prototype antimuscarinic drug, mainly blocks the peripheral muscarinic (M) receptors (large green box). The effects produced are equivalent to blocking parasympathomimetic influences on peripheral structures—a parasympatholytic effect. Note that these are the same sites that are stimulated by parasympathomimetic drugs (see Chapter 11).

High doses of antimuscarinic drugs, or therapeutic doses of glycopyrrolate given parenterally, may also block ACh effects on nicotinic (N) receptors in autonomic ganglia, the adrenal medulla, and on skeletal muscle (small green boxes).

quently applied topically, primarily to the eye, and can be absorbed well enough to cause systemic effects.

Atropine is distributed throughout the body. It crosses the blood–brain barrier and enters the CNS easily. It crosses the placental barrier and enters breast milk. Most of the atropine in the bloodstream is metabolized in the liver. The intensity and duration of antimuscarinic drug effects are increased when liver function is impaired.

Peak effects of atropine occur 1 to 2 hours after oral administration. Most effects last 4 to 6 hours, but some ocular effects may last up to a week. Other antimuscarinic drugs have very different onsets and durations of action.

Pharmacologic Effects

Atropine and other antimuscarinic drugs act by blocking the effects of ACh and other parasympathomimetic drugs on the *muscarinic* subtype of cholinergic receptor (Fig. 13–1). (To be precise, they *allow* effects to occur, rather than cause new ones.) This specificity is so important that the muscarinic receptor is defined as one that is stimulated by ACh or a related drug and is *blocked by atropine.* Blockade of muscarinic receptors by antimuscarinic drugs is competitive (surmountable), which means that it can be overcome by making more agonist available. This can be done, for example, by administering a parasympathomimetic drug (Chapter 11) or an acetylcholinesterase (AChE) inhibitor (Chapter 12).

Recall from Chapter 10 that muscarinic receptors are found mainly on peripheral structures innervated by postganglionic parasympathetic nerves: smooth muscle, cardiac muscle, and certain glands (salivary, mucous, gastric, lacriminal, and sweat). Some are also found in the CNS. Muscarinic receptors differ from the nicotinic receptors found in autonomic ganglia and on skeletal muscle, which are stimulated by ACh but are not blocked by atropine.

Antimuscarinic drugs have no direct effects on the interactions of sympathetic neurotransmitters or sympathomimetic drugs (Chapter 14) with their receptors.

Table 13–1 summarizes the major effects of antimuscarinic drugs on body systems controlled by the parasympathetic nervous system. In general, their effects are the opposite of those caused by parasympathomimetic drugs or parasympathetic nerve stimulation. Most of the structures listed in Table 13–1 are also innervated by sympathetic nerves. Because of the opposing effects of these two branches of the autonomic nervous system (ANS), when effective doses of an antimuscarinic drug are given and parasympathetic influences are blocked, the remaining responses reflect the unopposed or unmasked sympathetic influences.

Table 13–1 Responses of Major Effector Organs to Pharmacologic Doses of Antimuscarinic Drugs*

Organ	Response
Eye	
Iris, sphincter muscle	Relaxed, causing mydriasis
Ciliary muscle	Relaxed, paralyzing accommodation (enabling distance vision only)
Lacrimal gland secretion	Decreased
Respiratory system	
Bronchial smooth muscle tone	Increased
Mucus gland secretion	Decreased (thickened)
Heart	
Force of contraction	Increased (very slight)
Rate	Increased
Automaticity	Increased
Impulse conduction	Increased
Arterioles	None (arterioles are not innervated by parasympathetic nerves; vasodilator response to exogenous ACh or other parasympathomimetics is blocked; see text)
Gastrointestinal tract	
Motility	Decreased (relaxation)
Sphincters	Contracted
Gastric acid secretion	Decreased
Salivary gland secretion	Decreased
Overall	Decreased motility
Skin	
Sweat gland secretion	Decreased
Urinary bladder	
Detrusor	Relaxed
Trigone, sphincter	Contracted
Overall	Decreased urination
Penis	Impaired erection (slight)

*Compare these responses with the responses caused by muscarinic-receptor agonists (Table 11–1, p 137) and you will see that they are opposites of one another.

Ocular Effects

Atropine blocks the pupil-constricting (*miotic*) effects of ACh on the iris sphincter muscle. Thus, atropine dilates the pupil to produce **mydriasis.** Atropine also blocks the ability of ACh to contract the ciliary muscle, which is the primary way the lens changes shape to focus on nearby objects (accommodation). Paralysis of accommodation is called **cycloplegia.** Distant objects appear clear and sharp, while nearby objects appear blurred. These effects occur even with very low doses of atropine.

Cardiovascular Effects

Atropine antagonizes the ability of ACh to act on the sinoatrial node to slow heart rate. In theory, atropine increases heart rate, but this is seldom seen in human beings unless high doses of atropine are given. When given parenterally, atropine often causes a paradoxical *decrease* of heart rate, presumably owing to an effect of the drug in the CNS. By antagonizing the effects of ACh on various regions of the heart, atropine improves or speeds electrical impulse conduction through the heart.

Therapeutic doses of atropine do not have a significant effect on cardiac contractility, since the parasympathetic nervous system is not a major regulator of this function. Likewise, atropine does not have a significant effect on blood pressure, since most blood vessels are not innervated by the parasympathetic nervous system, and therefore not under continual influence of ACh. However, antimuscarinic drugs can block the vasodilator effects of injected ACh or other parasympathomimetic drugs.

Gastrointestinal Effects

Very low doses of atropine antagonize the ability of ACh to stimulate salivary gland secretion. The result, dry mouth (**xerostomia**), is common. Relatively high doses of atropine inhibit gastric (hydrochloric) acid and pepsin secretion. By blocking the actions of ACh on muscles of the GI tract, atropine decreases gut motility and increases the tone of the various sphincters. The overall result resembles constipation if the drug's effect is great.

Genitourinary Effects

Urination occurs when ACh contracts the bladder's detrusor muscle and relaxes the trigone and sphincter. By preventing this, atropine impairs micturition.

Antimuscarinic drugs block the ability of the parasympathetic nervous system to contract the smooth muscles responsible for penile erection. However, the effect seldom occurs when therapeutic doses are given.

Respiratory Effects

Atropine antagonizes the ability of ACh to stimulate mucus secretion in the respiratory tract and to contract tracheal and bronchial smooth muscle. Mucus secretions diminish and thicken, and bronchodilation occurs.

Central Nervous System Effects

Therapeutic doses of atropine usually produce no obvious CNS effects in most adults, even though the drug crosses the blood–brain barrier. However, very young or old patients may experience some CNS effects after receiving low doses of atropine. Depending on the individual, the central actions (usually sedation) may be beneficial or adverse. Higher doses of atropine, and therapeutic doses of some related drugs, frequently affect the brain. Scopolamine, for example, usually causes significant sedation in addition to its peripheral effects. The extent to which sedation is due to blockade of muscarinic receptors in the CNS is not clear.

Another clinically useful central effect of most antimuscarinics, and of scopolamine in particular, is suppression of nausea and vomiting (an *antiemetic* effect).

Clinical Indications and Administration

Specific doses and routes of administration for atropine and other major antimuscarinic drugs are summarized in Table 13–C1. Doses for antimuscarinics with more limited uses are given in Table 13–C2. Be aware that patients who are very young, very old, or debilitated will require doses lower than those given below and in the tables. Many antimuscarinic drugs are not recommended for pediatric use.

Uses for Eye Disorders

Some antimuscarinic drugs, administered topically on the eye, are commonly used for their mydriatic and cycloplegic effects, as might be needed for an eye examination. Mydriasis opens the pupil for a full view of internal eye structures, and cycloplegia, which prevents the lens from changing shape, aids the examiner in measuring refraction, to help prescribe proper corrective lenses.

The cycloplegic effect of topical atropine may last for 3 or 4 days, and mydriasis may last for a week. Since this is much longer than is needed to conduct an eye examination, antimuscarinic drugs with relatively short durations of actions (cyclopentolate, tropicamide; Table 13–C2) are generally used instead. If necessary, recovery from the ocular effects of a long-acting antimuscarinic can be hastened by administering a parasympathomimetic drug (eg, pilocarpine).

Topical antimuscarinics can be used to manage inflammation of the iris and uveal tract (uveitis). Long-acting drugs (atropine, homatropine, and scopolamine) are preferred.

NURSING IMPLICATIONS

Antimuscarinic drugs used for ophthalmic effects are usually instilled into the conjunctival sac to localize the drug's effect as much as possible. The patient may need to have the medication applied anywhere from 30 minutes to 24 hours before the examination, depending on the drug. The time to onset and peak action of the selected agent must be known, so that maximum effects occur at the time of examination.

Proper methods of eye drop administration ensure correct dosage and reduce the amount of drug that can be absorbed systemically, thereby minimizing systemic effects. The general technique is discussed in Appendix A. If the patient will be self-administering the medication, the nurse should teach the proper technique and ensure that the patient can perform it correctly.

Ophthalmic ointments are less likely than eye drops to be absorbed systemically. Ointments are generally preferred for individuals who have difficulty self-administering ocular medications (for example, some elderly patients), or for whom proper administration of drops is inherently difficult, such as small children.

Glaucoma, the major ocular contraindication to antimuscarinic drugs, must be ruled out before giving any antimuscarinic drug. All patients receiving antimuscarinics, especially in the eye, should be monitored for several hours afterward for eye pain, which could indicate underlying glaucoma. These issues, and related nursing implications, are discussed in a following section.

Uses for the Cardiovascular System

Acute myocardial infarction, a variety of chronic cardiac diseases, and many drugs, can cause bradycardia—an excessively slow heart rate. Bradycardia is often accompanied by decreased electrical impulse conduction rates from the atria to the ventricles via the atrioventricular (AV) node. Consequences range from hypotension and syncope to complete circulatory collapse and cardiac arrest.

These rate and conduction problems are often mediated by excessive tone of the vagus nerve, the major parasympathetic nerve to the heart's pacemaker, the sinoatrial (SA) node, and to the AV node. Drugs that mimic the cardiac-stimulating effects of the sympathetic nervous system (sympathomimetics; Chapter 14) can be administered acutely to normalize rate and conduction, but often parenteral atropine (0.4–0.5 mg, preferably IV) is used instead, to block the unwanted cardiac-depressant parasympathetic effects.

Antimuscarinics and sympathomimetics are seldom used in contemporary therapy for long-term management of bradycardia or decreased AV conduction; surgically implanted pacemakers are used more often instead.

NURSING IMPLICATIONS

Measure vital signs, especially heart rate, peripheral pulses, and blood pressure, in all patients before giving any antimuscarinic drug parenterally. Closely monitor all patients for several minutes after giving an antimuscarinic. Anticipate additional cardiac slowing in the first 1 to 2 minutes after parenteral (especially IV) administration of atropine.

Uses for Gastrointestinal Tract Disorders

More antimuscarinic drugs are approved for GI tract uses than for any other purpose. They have been used for years to inhibit gastric acid secretion, which plays a role in the pathophysiology of peptic ulcer disease; and to inhibit excessive motility or spasm of the gut, as occurs in "irritable bowel syndrome." Tables 13–C1 and 13–C2 list some of these drugs, along with their dosages. Most of them are synthetic agents, with structures that are claimed to localize their effects in the GI tract, thereby causing fewer systemic side effects than might occur with atropine, for example. However, typical atropine-like side effects certainly can occur.

Today, however, the use of any currently approved antimuscarinic drug for peptic ulcer disease is rarely warranted, and basically the same applies to their use in gut hypermotility disorders. Many other classes of drugs that are more effective are available. Most of them cause fewer side effects and drug interactions, have fewer contraindicating conditions, and do more than simply alleviate symptoms. (One antimuscarinic, pirenzipine, is *very* selective for inhibiting gastric acid secretion, and it is used in other countries for peptic ulcer disease. It will probably be approved in the United States soon. Interestingly, most clinical studies show that pirenzipine is no more effective than the nonantimuscarinic alternatives.) Preferred drugs for managing peptic ulcer disease are discussed in Chapter 40, and those for managing gut hypermotility disorders in Chapters 41 and 42.

Antimuscarinic drugs are also used occasionally to decrease gut motility to facilitate radiologic diagnosis of some GI diseases, and to manage biliary tract spasm (for which they are given with narcotics for pain relief).

NURSING IMPLICATIONS

Question orders that call for the use of an antimuscarinic drug to treat an acute or chronic GI disorder, unless you can be sure that safer and usually more effective drugs were tried first and were ineffective. If the antimuscarinic is used, assess bowel sounds, the amount and quality of the feces, and the frequency of defecation. Monitor periodically during therapy to help detect constipation or paralytic ileus, which are adverse drug-induced effects. Be aware that doses of antimuscarinic drugs needed to affect the GI tract are likely to cause effects on other body systems, and monitor accordingly, especially if the patient is elderly. Oral dosage forms should be taken 20 to 30 minutes before a meal to avoid reduced absorption caused by food.

Uses for Urinary Tract Disorders

Some drugs with antimuscarinic activity are used to treat neurogenic bladder disease, a condition in which increased sensitivity of the bladder to parasympathetic influences causes urinary frequency or incontinence. Antimuscarinics can also be used to manage bladder spasm or incontinence due to other causes, such as enuresis in children.

NURSING IMPLICATIONS

Monitor urine output in hospitalized patients receiving an antimuscarinic drug, to detect both beneficial effects (reduction of hesitancy or frequency) and adverse responses. All patients, but especially older males who may have prostatic hypertrophy, should be advised to report immediately any obvious difficulty in urinating or decreases of urine output. Encourage the patient to void before taking an antimuscarinic drug.

Uses in Anesthesiology and Surgery

Antimuscarinic drugs have several important uses in the setting of surgery and anesthesia. Understanding these uses is important not only for surgical nurses, but also for nurses caring for patients before and after surgery.

Injectable atropine, or the related drugs glycopyrrolate or scopolamine, are used as premedications before general anesthesia. They help reduce airway secretions during surgery, but their major role is to prevent the often intense reflex slowing of the heart that occurs during induction of general anesthesia and intubation of the airway. They can also be given during surgery to manage bradycardia. Scopolamine has other properties that make it a useful preanesthetic medication: it makes the patient drowsy and less anxious, and tends to cause some amnesia, which is one goal of general anesthesia (p 303).

The preoperative or intraoperative use of antimuscarinics is potentially dangerous. Some of the inhaled anesthetics used in modern anesthesia "sensitize" the heart to the stimulating effects of epinephrine and norepinephrine. By blocking opposing parasympathetic effects, an antimuscarinic can increase the risk of tachycardia and arrhythmias.

Antimuscarinic drugs have another important use in the surgery/anesthesia setting. Many surgical patients are not only anesthetized, but also given a drug that intentionally paralyzes skeletal muscles for the duration of the operation. The paralyzing drugs, called *neuromuscular blockers* (Chapter 17), prevent ACh from stimulating the skeletal muscle via the nicotinic receptors. As noted in the previous chapter, when surgery is complete an AChE inhibitor (eg, neostigmine) is given to reactivate skeletal muscle so the patient can breathe voluntarily. Given alone, an AChE inhibitor will cause a build-up of ACh at the somatic motor nerve endings, leading to the desired skeletal muscle effects; and at postganglionic parasympathetic nerve endings, causing a host of potentially unwanted muscarinic effects. Giving an antimuscarinic drug just before the AChE inhibitor prevents the unwanted parasympathomimetic effects, but does not interfere with the desired skeletal muscle (nicotinic) actions. Atropine and glycopyrrolate are used for this purpose.

NURSING IMPLICATIONS

Patients who will receive antimuscarinic premedication before surgery should be told to expect drowsiness and visual changes that require staying in bed. Raise the bed's side rails for safety. Anticipate that any antimuscarinic drug given before, during, or at the end of surgery will continue for several hours to exert effects on virtually all body systems that are under autonomic control; monitor accordingly.

Management of Excessive or Unwanted Muscarinic Effects of Parasympathomimetic Drugs and Acetylcholinergic Inhibitors

Excessive doses of parasympathomimetic drugs (eg, bethanechol) or AChE inhibitors (eg, neostigmine) cause adverse responses that resemble stimulation of the entire parasympathetic nervous system. Unwanted muscarinic side effects may also occur when therapeutic doses of AChE inhibitors are given to treat myasthenia gravis, or to reverse neuromuscular blockade postoperatively. Atropine antagonizes these responses. In fact, atropine should always be available for injection whenever parasympathomimetic or AChE-inhibitor drugs are given parenterally.

Antidote for Muscarine (Mushroom) Poisoning

Accidental poisoning with some species of wild mushroom (such as *Clitocybe* and *Inocybe;* see Chapter 11) is relatively common in some parts of the country. These fungi contain muscarine and other powerful muscarinic alkaloids that can cause serious poisoning. Major signs and symptoms are identical to those noted for parasympathomimetic drug overdoses. Autonomic problems may be accompanied by bizarre CNS changes such as confusion, disorientation, and hallucinations. Since atropine is a specific muscarinic receptor blocker, it is the antidote of choice for these poisonings. Doses of 1 to 2 mg (IV or SC) may need to be administered repeatedly, and frequently, to relieve the toxic symptoms.

Management of Motion Sickness

As a group, drugs that cause atropine-like actions in the CNS effectively prevent motion sickness and the resulting nausea and vomiting. They are much less effective for treating motion-sickness symptoms that have already developed. Scopolamine seems to work best. Many other prescription and nonprescription drugs used for motion sickness (see Chapter 42) may cause significant antimuscarinic side effects.

Other Clinical Indications

Management of the Common Cold and Seasonal Allergies

Belladonna alkaloids, scopolamine, and antihistamines that have atropine-like actions dry mucus secretions in the upper respiratory tract. These agents are found in both prescription and over-the-counter (OTC) medications used to relieve symptoms of the common cold or seasonal allergies (hay fever), such as runny nose (**rhinorrhea**) and watery eyes.

Although the doses found in nonprescription medications are generally low, and some may be subtherapeutic, they nevertheless can produce typical atropine-like side effects. They should not be taken by individuals for whom atropine is contraindicated. (Chapter 14 and Appendix B discuss other cold and allergy products that may be more effective and potentially safer than oral antimuscarinics.)

Treatment of Acute Asthma and Emphysema

Atropine solutions, given by inhalation with a **nebulizer,** are often used to help stop acute asthma attacks. The related drug ipratropium (ATROVENT) is given by inhalation for emphysema. These drugs work by blocking ACh-mediated bronchoconstriction. They are discussed more in Chapter 38. At this point it is more important to note that *systemic administration of any drug with appreciable antimuscarinic activity is generally contraindicated in persons with asthma.* The explanation is given in the respiratory side effects section.

Parkinsonism

Some antimuscarinic drugs with prominent actions in the CNS are routinely used to manage parkinsonism and some parkinsonian side effects of drugs used to treat schizophrenia. The pathophysiology of parkinsonism (which provides the rationale for antimuscarinic drug use), the specific drugs that are used, and the desired outcomes of therapy are discussed in Chapter 25. At this point it is necessary only to remember that this special group of antimuscarinics shares all the contraindications noted for atropine.

Side Effects, Adverse Reactions, and Contraindications

For many patients, the side effects and adverse responses of antimuscarinic drugs can be more important than the beneficial effects for which they are given. The outcomes of these unwanted responses can range from mild and merely annoying to outright dangerous. Although the focus of this chapter is on the prototype, atropine, remember the following points when planning and assessing therapy and teaching patients about medications:

- Unwanted effects generally are caused by blockade of muscarinic receptors in the peripheral parasympathetic nervous system, but some involve CNS effects.
- Adverse effects are most likely to occur with systemic administration, but agents that are given topically (eg, on the eye) can cause problems too.
- Any of the drugs called antimuscarinic (anticholinergic, or atropine-like) agents (ie, those in Tables 13–C1 and 13–C2) share the key properties noted for atropine.
- Many widely used drug classes, and drugs within a class, share atropine's side effects, contraindications, and interactions. Some are prescription medications; others are OTC products meant for self-prescribing—which is usually done without consulting a knowledgeable health-care provider first. Their generic names, trade names, pharmaco-

logic classifications, or uses (see Table 13–2) rarely give any clue that these drugs can exert significant atropine-like actions—as well as other actions they may possess. Thus, the uninformed practitioner who prescribes or administers them, or the person who self-medicates with them, may not realize that possibly serious consequences can occur.

If you understand the pharmacology of atropine, you should be able to understand how and why many of the other drugs with atropine-like activity can cause problems. Table 13–5 summarizes the key side effects and contraindications.

Ocular Side Effects

Cycloplegia and **photophobia** ("day-blindness") due to mydriasis, are very common visual side effects. Corneal irritation may result from diminished lacrimation.

Table 13–2 Major Drug Groups That Cause Antimuscarinic Side Effects and Share Contraindications Noted for Atropine

Drug Group	Example
Antianxiety agents (some benzodiazepines) (Chapter 22)	Diazepam (VALIUM)
Antiarrhythmics (some) (Chapter 30)	Disopyramide (NORPACE)
Antidepressants, tricyclics (most) (Chapter 24)	Imipramine (TOFRANIL)
Antihistamines* (H_1-receptor antagonists, most) (Chapter 51)	Diphenhydramine (BENADRYL)
Antiparkinson drugs (classified as "centrally acting anticholinergics") (Chapter 25)	Benztropine (COGENTIN) Trihexyphenidyl (ARTANE)
Antipsychotics: phenothiazines, and butyrophenones (Chapter 23)	Chlorpromazine (THORAZINE) Haloperidol (HALDOL)
Sedative/hypnotics (some) (Chapter 22)	Glutethimide (DORIDEN) Methyprylon (NOLUDAR) Scopolamine

*Drug or drug group likely to be found in many nonprescription cough, cold, allergy, and sleep-aid products.

Note: The terms *anticholinergic, atropine-like, antimuscarinic,* and *parasympatholytic* are considered synonymous.

The visual disturbances are generally more annoying than dangerous, and some can (and usually should) be treated with nondrug measures (see below). However, poor vision may interfere with the safety of tasks requiring good visual acuity, and so they should be avoided if they pose a danger.

Dilation of the pupil not only contributes to photophobia, but also can obstruct the normal outflow of aqueous humor from the anterior chamber of the eye, elevating intraocular pressure (see p 140 and Fig. 11–4). Glaucoma is an *absolute contraindication* to the use of any drug with atropine-like activity. Giving any drug with antimuscarinic activity to a person with glaucoma can precipitate an extremely painful acute attack that could lead to blindness. Development of ocular pain during the course of therapy with any drug may indicate undiagnosed glaucoma. It is a medical emergency that demands immediate discontinuation of antimuscarinic therapy (at least temporarily) and assessment by a physician.

Gastrointestinal Side Effects

Dry mouth (**xerostomia**) is the *most common* side effect produced by therapeutic doses of drugs with antimuscarinic activity. This problem is usually more annoying than dangerous, and can usually be managed with simple nondrug interventions. Prolonged or severe xerostomia may lead to dysphagia, choking on food, and an inability to eat, resulting in weight loss.

Constipation is another side effect. Antimuscarinics should be administered with care, if at all, to any patient with low GI tract motility (which is common in elderly or debilitated patients, and occurs frequently after abdominal surgery), or to patients with diminished bowel sounds. Paralytic ileus, the most serious adverse response affecting the GI tract, may develop. Paralytic ileus contraindicates the use of any drug with antimuscarinic activity.

Other contraindications include severe ulcerative colitis, toxic megacolon, and GI obstruction or weakness of the gut musculature; accumulation of food or feces in the gut as a result of reduced motility can cause rupture, hemorrhage, and peritonitis.

Genitourinary Side Effects

Urinary hesitancy, urinary retention, or overflow urinary incontinence may be caused by antimuscarinic effects on the bladder and other parts of the urinary tract. Antimuscarinics are contraindicated in patients with prostatic hypertrophy (most elderly males should be suspected of having this) or other conditions that restrict normal urine flow. An antimuscarinic drug may cause acute urinary retention or bladder distention leading to damage of the bladder, ureters, or kidneys.

Exocrine Gland Side Effects

Diminished sweat gland secretions, which normally help cool the body, may raise body temperature and cause fever or heat stroke. The risk of fever is increased in patients who engage in strenuous work or live in warm environments. Facial flushing should be considered as a sign of potential toxicity in adults. Localized skin flushing is common in children taking even therapeutic doses of antimuscarinic drugs, and it is not a reliable indicator of adverse reactions in children.

Respiratory Side Effects

For most patients, drugs with antimuscarinic activity do not cause important respiratory side effects. Their ability to decrease and dry mucus secretions in the airways is actually of some value when they are used for mild symptoms (eg, runny nose) of hay fever or the common cold.

The situation is much different if the patient has asthma, in whom systemically administered antimuscarinics do something good, and something that is potentially very bad. They beneficially relax bronchial smooth muscle, and so dilate the bronchi. However, patients with asthma tend to secrete large amounts of mucus, and have difficulty clearing those secretions from the lower respiratory tree. Antimuscarinics thicken the mucus so much that it tends to build up, mechanically narrowing the airway passages and plugging-up some altogether. The reduced airflow caused by mucus plugging outweighs the increase caused by bronchodilation. In general, systemic administration of drugs with antimuscarinic activity is contraindicated for persons with asthma. The accepted use of *inhaled* antimuscarinics for acute asthma and chronic emphysema is discussed in Chapter 37.

Cardiovascular Side Effects

Patients who have abnormally high heart rates (tachycardia) or other tachyarrhythmias should be given atropine and related drugs cautiously, if at all, to avoid further increases of heart rate. The precaution applies to hyperthyroid patients, who generally have sinus tachycardia, and to persons receiving a general anesthetic that sensitizes the heart to sympathetic influences or sympathomimetic drugs. Since increasing the heart rate increases the oxygen demands of the heart, atropine may precipitate an attack of angina pectoris in patients with coronary artery disease.

Skeletal Muscle Side Effects

Antimuscarinic drugs may be prescribed for persons with myasthenia gravis who are being treated with AChE inhibitors (Chapter 12). The goal is to block only the unwanted parasympathomimetic effects of the inhibitor (eg, GI or cardiovascular effects). Usual doses of most atropine-like drugs do that, but if the dose is too high they start to block the nicotinic ACh receptors on skeletal muscle also. The increased muscle weakness or decreased exercise tolerance is often mistaken as evidence of an inadequate dose of the AChE inhibitor (rather than too much antimuscarinic drug), and the prescriber may incorrectly increase it.

There is another potential concern for these patients. The appearance of widespread or severe muscarinic side effects during AChE inhibitor therapy is one good clue that its dose is too high. If the patient is also taking an antimuscarinic drug, those important clues will be masked.

Central Nervous System Side Effects

Antimuscarinics, especially scopolamine, can produce enough drowsiness to impair judgment, motor skills, and coordination. Paradoxical excitement may occur in some patients, especially elderly or debilitated persons. These CNS side effects are intensified by other CNS depressants, including alcohol. The risks to the patient are compounded by visual disturbances.

NURSING IMPLICATIONS

Given the diversity of drugs with antimuscarinic actions, and the many side effects that can occur, providing therapy that is effective, safe, and tolerable to the patient can be challenging to the nurse. The task can be made somewhat easier by:

- learning the major classes of drugs, both prescription and OTC, that have antimuscarinic activity;
- identifying the related side effects that could affect most patients;
- assessing each patient individually, before and during therapy, to help differentiate between side effects that are likely to pose real dangers (and might contraindicate drug use) and those likely to be annoying but not necessarily hazardous;

- preventing, recognizing, and managing side effects or adverse responses; and
- communicating the necessary information to the patient, especially if he or she will be treated on an outpatient basis and will be self-medicating.

As noted above, and summarized in Table 13–S, virtually every major body system can be a target of antimuscarinic side effects. For most of these systems, *objective* indicators of side effects may occur—things that can be measured (heart rate and blood pressure, fluid intake/output, etc), felt (eg, fullness of the abdomen), seen (eg, flushed skin, pupil size or lack of response to light), or heard (eg, lung or bowel sounds).

However, no matter how complete, objective assessment alone will not detect the many *subjective* but nevertheless important side effects that can occur—including the two that are most common, dry mouth and blurred vision. The nurse should ask about key side effects explicitly, and not rely on patients to volunteer the information. Some side effects that may seem inconsequential to the caregiver can actually pose serious problems for some patients. For example, blurred vision, combined with sedation or ataxia, can increase the risk of a fall. Dry mouth can make chewing and swallowing solid foods difficult, and over the long run could lead to decreased food intake, nutritional deficiencies, and aggravation of the decreased gut motility that is also a direct side effect of an antimuscarinic drug.

Nondrug interventions (Table 13–S) can alleviate many side effects. They are usually effective, and almost always should be tried before using other drugs to counteract them. Frequent sips of water can reduce annoying dry mouth; maintaining adequate bulk and fluid in the diet can reduce the risk of constipation or paralytic ileus; wearing sunglasses can reduce distress from photophobia. Therefore, in addition to advising patients about the side effects, advise them of acceptable ways to deal with them. There may be no easy way to deal with some side effects, such as blurred vision, other than to have the patient use appropriate cautions and modify their lifestyle as necessary.

Be sure to use the same precautions noted for atropine when administering any medication that causes antimuscarinic effects.

◆ Use During Pregnancy and Lactation

No good information is available about the safety of using typical antimuscarinic drugs (eg, atropine, scopolamine) during pregnancy or lactation. The best advice is to avoid them (especially during the first trimester of pregnancy) unless maternal benefits are expected to outweigh potential dangers to the fetus, and proper monitoring can be provided. Issues related to the use of other drug classes that have strong atropine-like activity, such as antihistamines, antidepressants, and antipsychotic drugs, are covered in Chapters 51, 24, and 23, respectively.

◆ Use in Children

Children are, in general, more sensitive to antimuscarinic drugs and their side effects. Virtually all the indications for using these drugs in adults apply to children. However, most children are exposed to antimuscarinics in the form of antihistamines (Chapter 51), found in OTC medications for relief of cold, flu, or allergy symptoms. Advise parents or guardians to follow all label instructions and warnings precisely. Children with recurrent respiratory symptoms should be evaluated for asthma, the most common chronic pediatric respiratory disorder, for which systemic antimuscarinics are contraindicated. Parents or guardians of children with diagnosed asthma should be explicitly advised to avoid the use of OTC medications for respiratory symptoms, unless directed to use them by a physician. The *Handbook of Nonprescription Drugs,* published periodically by the American Pharmaceutical Association, is the best source of information about these and other OTC medications (ingredients, uses, etc).

The treatment of nocturnal enuresis (nighttime bedwetting), which often involves the drug imipramine (see Chapter 24), is another situation in which children may be exposed to medications with significant antimuscarinic side effects.

◆ Use in the Elderly

Side effects caused by antimuscarinic drugs can be particularly bothersome, and potentially dangerous, for the elderly (Table 13–S). A decreased ability to metabolize or excrete these medications is only one reason why older adults appear to be more sensitive to their effects. A factor that is perhaps more important is the prevalence of age-related conditions that would relatively or absolutely contraindicate antimuscarinic use.

Impaired cognition, gait, balance, psychomotor skills, vision, and function of the GI and urinary systems are more common in the elderly. Any of these age-associated changes can be intensified by similar effects caused by antimuscarinic drugs. Indeed, because many antimuscarinic side effects mimic age-associated physiologic and pathophysiologic changes, the clinician may not know whether a certain sign or symptom is or is not drug-induced. If it is incorrectly assumed that a change is caused by age or illness, still more drugs (some with anticholinergic activity) may be prescribed, inappropriately, to treat them. Thus, a thorough drug history is essential, and when the patient is receiving many drugs from several physicians, the burden of sifting through all the information may fall upon the nurse.

The guidelines noted earlier about assessing for side effects, managing them, and teaching patients are perhaps more important for elders than they are for any other individuals. The use of nondrug measures to prevent or manage side effects takes on added importance if the patient's medication list is already long.

Finally, all elderly patients should be screened for glaucoma before administering any antimuscarinic (or other pupil-dilating) drug. Males should also be screened for prostatic hypertrophy before treatment starts, owing to the risk of causing acute urinary retention. Although glaucoma or prostatic hypertrophy may not be found in the pretreatment exam, the nurse still needs to be continually alert for related or other adverse effects after treatment begins.

Interactions with Other Drugs

Interactions between antimuscarinic drugs and other medications (Table 13–I) may occur regardless of the dose of the interactants or the duration of therapy, and can involve either prescription or OTC medications.

Because so many prescription and OTC drugs or drug classes have antimuscarinic activity, and because they are used for so many different purposes, it should not be surprising that one of the most common types of interaction involves the combined use of two or more antimuscarinics. The outcome can range anywhere from added discomfort to outright toxicity. Combined administration should be avoided, but often that is not possible. Thus, it is important to use the lowest effective dose of each medication, and to perform frequent and close assessment of the patient's responses to help with the dosage adjustments.

Interactions with other drugs that appear to have clinical significance (Table 13–I) include:

- antagonism of the desired effects of the major antipsychotic drugs, the phenothiazines, plus additive CNS depression and peripheral antimuscarinic effects;
- more complete absorption, and potentially excessive or toxic effects, of some slowly absorbed oral dosage forms of digoxin, which currently is the most widely used drug for treating heart failure;
- opposed effects of drugs such as metoclopramide, which are used to increase gut motility; and
- reduced absorption of orally administered antimuscarinics when ingested along with antacids.

There are other interactions that are thought to have less general impact on therapy. Nevertheless, the nurse should always assess the patient more closely when antimuscarinics are administered with

- *other drugs that cause one or more effects that are similar in kind, but differ in how they are produced.* This is how narcotics (eg, morphine) and antimuscarinics can interact to decrease motility of the GI and urinary tracts. The interaction can be desirable if dosages are adjusted properly, excessive if they are not. Another example is the administration of antimuscarinics, which unmask sympathetic stimulation of most organs, along with true sympathomimetic drugs (Chapter 14). In particular, the cardiovascular effects of this interaction (excessive stimulation of heart rate and contractility) can become very important for some patients.
- *other drugs that cause opposite pharmacologic effects, especially on structures that are affected by ACh.* An example is the ability of antimuscarinic drugs to counteract the effects of cholinergic drugs (ie, parasympathomimetics or AChE inhibitors). Giving drugs with opposite effects may seem illogical, but this type of interaction does provide the rationale for using atropine as an antidote for cholinergic drug overdoses (or vice versa); or using an antimuscarinic drug to block unwanted parasympathomimetic effects in patients with myasthenia gravis being treated with an AChE inhibitor. Another example would be the interaction of antimuscarinics, which dilate the pupil of the eye, with other drugs that constrict it. Here, too, the clinical significance of the interaction depends on the situation. If the interactants are given intentionally, as to reverse pupil dilation after an eye exam, the interaction is desirable. On the other hand, if the patient has glaucoma (for example) and is being treated with a miotic drug, the mydriasis caused by administration of an antimuscarinic would be unwanted and potentially dangerous.

NURSING IMPLICATIONS

The medication history should include specific questions about the use of potential OTC drug interactants. Patient teaching should include specific comments, supplemented with a written list, about OTC interactants that should be avoided. Since patients are not likely to bring in the ingredients list from the package of their OTC medications, use the latest edition of *Drug Facts and Comparisons* to help you get this information.

Overdose and Toxicity

Overdoses of antimuscarinic drugs are common, mainly because of the widespread availability and use of many drugs with atropine-like activity. The signs and symptoms of overdose—called the *anticholinergic or antimuscarinic syndrome*—are usually so characteristic that they are easy to recognize. Most antimuscarinic drugs cause similar responses. Unique aspects of toxicity caused by other drugs with antimuscarinic activity (antidepressants, antipsychotics, and so on) are discussed in their respective chapters.

Signs and Symptoms

Mild to moderate overdoses, whether chronic or acute, primarily affect peripheral structures. Dry mouth, blurred vision, and photophobia, which occur with therapeutic doses, become more intense and bothersome. Decreased defecation and urination may develop, but the patient may not detect them readily. Heart rate may decrease first, and then rise. The patient's skin becomes dry and warm owing to inhibited sweating, which also reduces heat loss via perspiration and elevates body temperature. The face, neck, and upper arms may become flushed (the so-called "atropine flush"), presumably owing to reflex blood vessel dilation in response to increased body temperature. (Skin flushing is a reliable indicator of atropine toxicity in adults, but not in children, who may become flushed after taking therapeutic doses. The presence of a rash and flushing together is a better indicator of a poisoned child than flushing alone.) The combined effects of dry mouth and decreased sweating often make the patient quite thirsty, but lack of salivary secretions may make drinking or eating difficult. Antimuscarinics that affect the CNS intensely, such as scopolamine, antidepressants, antihistamines, antiparkinson drugs, and antipsychotics, usually cause added drowsiness or sedation.

As blood levels rise, the peripheral effects become more intense, and CNS signs and symptoms become prominent. The patient starts to fit the classic description of atropine poisoning:

- dry as a bone: sweat, salivary, and respiratory secretions are inhibited;
- red as a beet: the atropine flush becomes more intense and generalized;
- blind as a bat: paralysis of accommodation and mydriasis significantly interfere with vision;
- hot as a furnace: decreased cutaneous heat loss, but continued or increased generation of body heat, causes a profound fever and, potentially, seizures (rectal temperatures in severely poisoned children have exceeded 109°F [47°C]); and
- mad as a hatter: confusion, agitation, slurred speech, disorientation, hallucinations, and delirium develop.

Physical examination reveals tachycardia and palpitations; clear lungs; an absence of bowel sounds; an inability to defecate or urinate, even though the bowel or bladder may be full; and marked muscle weakness. Eventually, the patient becomes comatose, and has seizures either before or after lapsing into the coma. Death is usually caused by respiratory failure and shock. Aggressive therapy is needed to save a seriously poisoned patient.

Treatment

If the overdose was due to an orally administered antimuscarinic drug, standard first-aid measures (Appendix C) should be started to prevent further drug absorption. Regardless of how the overdose occurred, vital signs should be measured and normalized. Baseline values are essential for comparison with changes caused by subsequent treatment. Use sponge baths or a hypothermia blanket, not an antipyretic drug such as aspirin, to reduce body temperature. It may be necessary to insert a bladder catheter to relieve pressure and to collect urine for accurate monitoring of fluid output. Parenteral fluids may be needed to restore blood pressure. The patient should be placed in a dim, quiet environment, and should be subjected to no more external stimulation than is necessary for monitoring vital signs and providing treatment.

The AChE inhibitor physostigmine (ANTILIRIUM; Chapter 12) is a specific and effective antidote for severe antimuscarinic drug overdoses. It is given intravenously. Physostigmine is the *only* cholinesterase inhibitor that works not only in the periphery but also crosses the blood–brain barrier well enough to reverse the dangerous CNS effects of antimuscarinic drugs.

Physostigmine usually causes an obvious increase of

salivation or sweating, the appearance of bowel sounds, normalization of heart rate, normalization of behavior and orientation, and cessation of seizures.

Physostigmine has a relatively short duration of action compared with most antimuscarinic drugs, so it may have to be administered several times during the course of treatment. Physostigmine must be injected slowly; rapid injection may cause seizures or profound bradycardia or heart block. Physostigmine causes its own untoward effects, so it should be used only for serious poisoning accompanied by seizures or dangerously psychotic behavior.

Physostigmine is useful for life-threatening overdoses of any drug that causes intense atropine-like effects.

Other anticonvulsants should generally be avoided, since physostigmine is a more specific and effective treatment. The major drug for treatment of acute seizures, diazepam (VALIUM; Chapter 22), may be used cautiously. However, it also causes antimuscarinic effects. Barbiturates and other anticonvulsants should be avoided because they may further depress consciousness, blood pressure, and respiration.

NURSING IMPLICATIONS

Be especially alert for signs and symptoms of toxicity, especially in small children or the elderly. Advise parents that the atropine flush, unaccompanied by other significant changes, does not necessarily indicate pediatric overdose. Conversely, the lack of flushed skin in a child does not necessarily indicate safe blood levels of an antimuscarinic drug, so other signs or symptoms should be looked for. Any signs of intoxication should be reported immediately, offending drugs should be discontinued, thorough examination *at a hospital* should be encouraged, and necessary supportive or treatment measures should be started at once.

Related Drugs

The major related drugs share most of the actions, and all the side effects and contraindications, noted for atropine. However, there are some important differences. Table 13–C1 shows their indications, dosages, and routes of administration.

Glycopyrrolate

Orally administered glycopyrrolate (ROBINUL) is indicated for adjunctive management of peptic ulcer disease, but other classes of antiulcer drugs are used much more often (Chapter 40). However, injectable glycopyrrolate is still an important drug for surgery-related uses: as a preanesthetic medication, to manage intraoperative bradycardia, and to prevent muscarinic side effects upon reversal of neuromuscular blockade with AChE inhibitors.

Be aware that the parenteral dosage form of glycopyrrolate is not compatible with many drugs and intravenous fluids that are commonly given to the surgical patient. In general, avoid mixing glycopyrrolate with other drugs in the same syringe. Always check the package insert first.

Unlike many other antimuscarinics (eg, scopolamine), glycopyrrolate does not enter the CNS well. Thus, therapeutic and side effects mainly involve structures innervated by the parasympathetic nervous system. However, unlike most other related drugs, at high doses glycopyrrolate can also block nicotinic ACh receptors, which are found in autonomic ganglia and on skeletal muscle. The major consequence of ganglionic blockade is orthostatic hypotension, which may make ambulatory patients prone to fainting or a fall if they stand up too quickly. The skeletal muscle effects usually involve muscle weakness, and they require that glycopyrrolate be used with extreme caution in patients with myasthenia gravis.

Propantheline Bromide

Propantheline (PRO-BANTHĪNE) is an antimuscarinic drug that, at recommended doses, is said to preferentially reduce gastric acid secretion and GI motility. Nevertheless, the drug may cause atropine-like peripheral side effects elsewhere. Propantheline's only approved indication is as adjunctive therapy of peptic ulcer disease. Propantheline is not indicated for pediatric use.

Scopolamine Hydrobromide

Scopolamine, also called hyoscine, produces considerably more sedation and control of motion sickness than atropine when therapeutic doses are given. It is used as

- an antispasmodic for the GI or urinary tracts;
- a preoperative sedative;
- a topical miotic;
- an agent to manage upper respiratory tract secretions due to seasonal allergies and related disorders; and
- prophylaxis or therapy for motion sickness.

Until recently, scopolamine was used frequently in obstetrics, in combination with the narcotics morphine or meperidine, to produce prepartum analgesia and amnesia ("twilight sleep"). This practice has been largely abandoned, mainly because postpartum drowsiness and amnesia were excessive and prolonged, and other drugs are more effective and safer.

In addition to oral, parenteral, and topical ophthalmic solutions and ointments, scopolamine is available in a transdermal drug delivery system (TRANSDERM-SCŌP) that is an effective, convenient, and commonly used means to prevent symptoms of motion sickness. Scopolamine is contained in a patch that is applied to the skin behind one ear. It delivers a constant, controlled dose for 3 days. The patch should be applied 4 hours before the anticipated start of travel. Scopolamine, even as a patch, should not be used in any patient for whom atropine is contraindicated.

Miscellaneous Drugs

The many other antimuscarinic drugs are used primarily for ocular or GI indications. They are listed in Table 13–C2. Those used for ophthalmology differ from atropine mainly in onsets and durations of action. The drugs indicated for peptic ulcer disease and gut spasm are not prescribed often, because more effective alternatives are available (Chapter 40).

Many antimuscarinics are found in drug combinations that contain more than one belladonna alkaloid (for example, atropine plus scopolamine plus hyoscyamine), or with other antiemetics or sedatives, such as alcohol or phenobarbital. Many authorities question whether combination products are safer or more effective than one containing an antimuscarinic alone. Mild sedation may benefit certain patients with GI disorders, but the additives may increase the risk of side effects and drug interactions. Alcohol is contraindicated in peptic ulcer disease. Alcohol, and especially phenobarbital, stimulates the liver's ability to metabolize many other drugs, which can lead to significant drug interactions. If a multiple-drug combination is prescribed, particularly close observation is necessary to identify undesirable responses.

SUMMARY OF NURSING IMPLICATIONS

◆ Assessment

Assess patients for preexisting conditions that are aggravated by the antimuscarinics: angle-closure glaucoma; history of cardiovascular disease (angina, hypertension, tachycardia, hyperthyroidism, congestive heart failure); GI conditions (constipation, bowel obstruction, paralytic ileus); urologic problems (primary retention, prostatic hypertrophy); pulmonary diseases (asthma, chronic obstructive lung disease); and pregnancy.

Obtain baseline cardiovascular vital signs before administering an antimuscarinic drug systemically.

Assess patients for muscle weakness or unusual exercise-induced fatigue, which may indicate undiagnosed myasthenia gravis; notify the physician.

Inquire specifically about the use of offending drugs that might contribute to their symptoms when assessing asthmatic patients.

Recommend that all elderly patients be screened for glaucoma before starting therapy, and periodically thereafter.

Assess for signs of atropine overdose; adverse reactions are more common in children and elderly.

◆ Nursing Diagnoses

High risk for injury related to visual changes (blurred vision, photophobia).

Noncompliance related to disturbing side effects (dry mouth, gut, and bladder changes).

Altered urinary elimination related to side effects: retention and hesitancy.

Constipation related to drug side effects.

Altered thought processes related to age, drug effects: confusion, disorientation.

Sexual dysfunction related to adverse drug effects.

◆ Planning/Implementation

Monitor vital signs for several minutes after giving an antimuscarinic, especially when it is given parenterally; report significant changes and withhold subsequent doses until advised by physician.

Monitor for eye pain and instruct patient to report pain immediately. It may indicate undiagnosed glaucoma, which could lead to blindness.

Monitor urine output, bowel regularity, bowel sounds, and vital signs of hospitalized patients. Changes will be more common in elderly patients.

Recognize both peripheral and CNS signs and symptoms of antimuscarinic drug intoxication: absence of secretions; flushed, dry skin; fever; altered mental state. Intoxication is more common with parenteral administration.

Check drug doses carefully; slight errors can result in toxicity.

Give oral dosage forms 30 minutes before meals to increase absorption.

Advise patient to suck on hard sugarless candies, chew sugarless gum, or sip water if dry mouth occurs.

Suggest sunglasses to reduce distress of photophobia.

Caution patient to avoid physical stress or prolonged exposure to heat.

◆ Patient and Family Teaching

Instruct patient to recognize and report signs of heat prostration, blurred vision, chest pain, allergic reactions.

Alert patient to possible drowsiness and impaired coordination, which can interfere with simple activities, work, and driving.

Advise patients to avoid OTC medications that contain drugs that produce additive antimuscarinic actions (eg, antihistamines).

Instruct parents or guardians that children are particularly susceptible to slight overdoses of antimuscarinic drugs. Advise them that the atropine flush is not a reliable indicator of toxicity in children.

Provide sexual counseling and refer as needed for problems related to drug-induced sexual dysfunction.

◆ Evaluation

The patient/family will:

Verbalize understanding of limitations on activities such as driving.

Comply with treatment regimen: take medication as prescribed.

Anticipate side effects and notify nurse or physician for evaluation and possible dosage adjustment.

Ensure that recommended measures are effective to relieve common side effects (eg, dry mouth, photophobia, bowel and bladder alterations).

Maintain optimal level of emotional and physical functioning: no confusion, able to continue self-care.

Annotated Bibliography

Bailey LD Jr., Stewart WR Jr., McCallum RW. New directions in the irritable bowel syndrome. *Gastroenterol Clin North Am* 1991;20 (2):335–349. *Irritable bowel syndrome (IBS) is a term that encompasses a host of GI disorders. This paper discusses the effectiveness and limitations of current therapies, and the need for newer drugs, as the pathophysiology of IBS becomes better understood.*

Borzyskowski M, Mundy AR. The management of the neuropathic bladder in childhood. *Pediatr Nephrol* 1988;2(1):56–66. *This paper focuses on what the author describes as "realistic" approaches to treatment of this disorder, which can involve drugs, surgery, and help from the patient.*

Peters NL. Snipping the thread of life: Antimuscarinic side effects of medications in the elderly. *Arch Intern Med* 1989;149:2414–2420. *If you read no other paper on the subject, and even if your patient is not elderly, read this comprehensive but very understandable article.*

Ruoff JH, Fladung B, Demol P, Weihrauch TR. Gastrointestinal receptors and drugs in motility disorders. *Digestion* 1991;48(1):1–17. *A good overview of the functions of ACh receptors in the GI tract, particularly with respect to drug therapy for some common GI disorders.*

Sourander LB. Treatment of urinary incontinence: The place of drugs. *Gerontology* 1990;36(Suppl. 2):19–26. *The author stresses the need for a better understanding of the pathophysiology of incontinence, establishing an effective drug treatment plan, and considering the importance of nondrug interventions as aids to drug therapy.*

Staskin DR, Wein AJ, Andersson KE. Urinary incontinence: Classification and pharmacological therapy. *Ciba Found Symp* 1990;151: 289–306; discussion 306–317. *A valuable look at causes and current therapies for incontinence, and some of the uncertainties about clinical studies used to evaluate drugs for bladder dysfunction.*

Stockbrugger RW: Antimuscarinic drugs. *Methods Find Exp Clin Pharmacol* 1989;11(Suppl 1):79–86. *Reviews current antimuscarinic drugs, and what new drugs to expect as we learn more about subtypes of muscarinic receptors, especially for their actions in the GI tract.*

Table 13–C1 Clinical Uses and Administration of Major Antimuscarinic Drugs

AGENT	CLINICAL USES	DOSAGE AND ROUTE OF ADMINISTRATION
PROTOTYPE		
Atropine sulfate	Preanesthetic medication; intraoperative bradycardia (parenteral); therapy of spastic gut disorders; therapy of ureteral or biliary colic	Oral or IM: Adults: 0.4–0.6 mg, repeated in 4–6 h as needed. Children: 7–16 lbs, 0.1 mg; 17–24 lbs, 0.15 mg; 24–40 lbs, 0.2 mg; 40–65 lbs, 0.3 mg; 65–90 lbs, 0.4 mg; over 90 lbs, give adult dose; may be used concomitantly with morphine for ureteral, biliary colic
	Prevention of muscarinic side effects when reversing neuromuscular blockade postoperatively with AChE inhibitor	IV (or IM or SC): 0.6–1.2 mg, given several minutes before or simultaneous with administration of neostigmine or pyridostigmine; use separate syringes for the two drugs
	Antidote for muscarine poisoning (see Chapter 11)	IV (or SC for situations not immediately life threatening): Adults: 1–2 mg, depending on severity of symptoms; repeat every 5–60 min as needed. Children: Usually 50 μg/kg repeated every 10–30 min
(ISOPTO-ATROPINE)	Mydriasis, cycloplegia, for eye examinations (eg, refraction)	Topical: Adults: Instill 1 drop into eye twice daily for 1–2 days before exam. Children: Instill 1–2 drops (0.5% solution only) twice daily for 1–3 days before exam and 1 hr before exam
	Treatment of uveitis	Topical: Adults: Instill 1 or 2 drops into eye(s) up to qid. Children: 1 or 2 drops of 0.5% solution up to tid.
RELATED DRUGS		
Glycopyrrolate		
(ROBINUL, ROBINUL FORTE)	Adjunctive therapy of peptic ulcer disease	Oral: Adults, children > 12: Initially 1 mg (1 ROBINUL tablet) tid or 2 mg bid–tid; maintenance dose usually 1 or 2 mg bid; ROBINUL FORTE (2 mg per tablet): Usually 1 tablet bid or tid
(ROBINUL INJECTABLE)		IM or IV: Adults only: Usually 0.1 or 0.2 mg as single dose or repeated at 4-hr intervals as needed, up to 4 daily doses, for prompt control of acid secretion; switch to oral form as soon as possible
	Preanesthetic medication to reduce secretions	IM: Adults: 2 μg/lb of body weight 30-60 min before induction. Children: As for adults; children less than 2 may require 4 μg/lb of weight
	Intraoperative treatment of vagally mediated bradycardia	IV: Adults: 0.1 mg, repeated as needed at 2–3 min intervals based on heart rate. Children: 2 μg/lb, not to exceed total of 100 μg
	Prevention of muscarinic side effects when reversing neuromuscular blockade with AChE inhibitor (see atropine, above)	IV: Adults: 200 μg for each 1 mg of neostigmine or 5 mg of pyridostigmine
Propantheline bromide		
(PRO-BANTHĪNE)	Adjunctive therapy of peptic ulcer disease	Oral: Usually 15 mg taken 30 min before meals and 30 mg at bedtime; 7.5 mg for mild symptoms, geriatric or light-weight patients

(continued)

Table 13–C1 Clinical Uses and Administration of Major Antimuscarinic Drugs (*Continued*)

AGENT	CLINICAL USES	DOSAGE AND ROUTE OF ADMINISTRATION
Scopolamine hydrobromide (also called *hyoscine hydrobromide*)	Treatment of irritable bowel syndrome, diverticulitis; preanesthetic medication as for atropine; management of postencephalitic parkinsonism	IM, SC, or IV (after suitable dilution): Adults: 0.3–0.6 mg. Children: 6 μg/kg, maximum 0.3 mg total
(TRANSDERM-SCŌP)	Prophylaxis of motion sickness	Topical: Apply one patch at least 4 but no more than 12 hr before anticipated travel; replace patch after 3 days if more prolonged effects are needed
(ISOPTO-HYOSCINE)	Mydriasis, cycloplegia for eye examinations	Topical: Instill 1 or 2 drops into eye(s) up to 4 qid

Table 13–C2 Clinical Uses and Administration of Miscellaneous Antimuscarinic Drugs

AGENT	CLINICAL USES	DOSAGE AND ROUTE OF ADMINISTRATION
Belladonna alkaloid mixtures (various products)	Adjunctive therapy of peptic ulcer disease, irritable bowel syndrome	Oral or Sublingual: 0.25–0.5 mg tid (actual dose depends on product) SC: 0.25–0.5 mg qd or bid
Clidinium bromide		
(QUARZAN; LIBRAX)	Adjunctive therapy of peptic ulcer disease	Oral: Most adults: 2.5 or 5 mg before meals and at bedtime. Elderly persons: 2.5 mg with meals only
Cyclopentolate		
(CYCLOGYL)	Mydriasis, cycloplegia for eye examinations	Topical: Adults: Instill 1 drop of 1% or 2% solution into eye(s), repeat in 5 min. Children: Usually 1 drop of 0.5%–2% solution, followed 5 min later by 1 drop of 0.5% or 1% solution if needed; treatment on day before exam usually not needed for children
Dicyclomine		
(BENTYL)	Antispasmodic, for irritable bowel syndrome (irritable, spastic colon; mucous colitis)	Oral: Initially 20 mg with meals and at bedtime; increase to 40 mg qid if necessary and tolerated by patient; normally should not be administered for more than 2 weeks IM: Usually 20 mg qid, with switch to oral therapy as soon as possible
Homatropine hydrobromide		
(ISOPTO-HOMATROPINE, others)	Mydriasis, cycloplegia for eye examinations	Topical: Instill 1 or 2 drops of 2% solution immediately before exam, repeat in 5–10 min if necessary
	Treatment of uveitis	Topical: Instill 1 or 2 drops every 3–4 hr

(*continued*)

Table 13–C2 **Clinical Uses and Administration of Miscellaneous Antimuscarinic Drugs (*Continued*)**

AGENT	CLINICAL USES	DOSAGE AND ROUTE OF ADMINISTRATION
L-Hyoscyamine sulfate		
(LEVSIN, LEVSINEX TIMECAPS)	Adjunctive therapy of peptic ulcer disease, irritable bowel syndrome	Oral: Adults: 0.125–0.25 mg tid-qid. Children: See manufacturer's recommendation; doses, preferred formulation vary considerably according to age; TIMECAPS (adults only): 1 or 2 capsules every 12 hr
(LEVSIN INJECTION)	Severe GI symptoms in above conditions	SC, IM, or IV: Usually 0.25–0.5 mg bid to qid
	Preanesthetic medication	SC, IM, or IV: Usually 5 μg/kg body weight, given 30–60 min before anesthesia induction or at time of administration of preanesthetic narcotics, sedatives
	Treatment of intraoperative bradycardia; adjunct to reversal of neuromuscular blockade after surgery	IV: 0.3–0.6 mg for each 0.5–2 mg of neostigmine
Isopropamide		
(DARBID; in COMBID)	Adjunctive therapy of peptic ulcer disease	Oral: 5 mg q12h (Note: COMBID, also indicated for irritable bowel syndrome, contains prochlorperazine)
Methantheline bromide		
(BANTHINE)	Adjunctive therapy of peptic ulcer disease	Oral: 50 or 100 mg q6h
Oxybutynin		
(DITROPAN)	Symptomatic relief of bladder instability (eg, urgency, frequency, functional incontinence)	Oral: Adults: 5 mg bid-tid; Children: 5 mg bid
Tropicamide		
(MYDRIACYL)	Mydriasis, cycloplegia for eye examinations	Topical: Instill 1–2 drops of 0.5% or 1% solution into eye(s) immediately before exam; repeat in 5 min if necessary

Table 13–S | Major Side Effects and Contraindications of Antimuscarinic Drugs

BODY SYSTEM/ Side Effect	CONTRAINDICATION/ PRECAUTION	COMMENTS AND NURSING IMPLICATIONS
CENTRAL NERVOUS SYSTEM		
Drowsiness, sedation, ataxia		Sedation is expected response with systemically administered scopolamine; if significant or accompanied by ataxia or visual impairments, have patient remain in bed or assist ambulation until effect diminishes; when seen with other antimuscarinics, may indicate excessive dose; notify physician
Excitement, agitation (paradoxical effect at therapeutic doses)		Paradoxical response is expected, particularly in elderly, debilitated, or very young patients; observe, orient patient and protect from falls; notify physician, use reduced doses of drug; delirium or hallucinations usually indicate toxicity
EYE	Glaucoma	Encourage elderly patients to be screened for glaucoma before administration; recommend sunglasses to reduce discomfort from photophobia, avoidance of tasks made dangerous by cycloplegia (very common), artificial tears for eye irritation from reduced lacrimation; advise patient about expected duration of side effects, and to notify physician at once if eye pain, indicating possible glaucoma, develops
Mydriasis and photophobia; cycloplegia, impaired distant vision; ocular irritation due to decreased lacrimation		
RESPIRATORY	Asthma	Systemic antimuscarinics may excessively dry mucus in respiratory tract, cause mucus plugging; avoid oral or parenteral use of any drug with atropine-like activity; inhaled atropine may be acceptable for selected asthma patients (see text)
Wheezing, breathing difficulty, mucus plugging		
CARDIOVASCULAR	Tachycardia; tachyarrhythmia; ischemic heart disease; hyperthyroidism	Periodically monitor heart rate, rhythm, peripheral pulse rate and quality, BP, especially in hospitalized patients receiving parenteral antimuscarinics; ECG advisable for high-risk patients; discontinue drug, notify physician if rate or rhythm disturbances develop
Tachycardia, tachyarrhythmias; paradoxical bradycardia (usually after parenteral administration)		
Hypotension (especially parenteral glycopyrrolate)	Hypotension, shock	May reflect ganglionic (nicotinic) blockade by glycopyrrolate; less likely with other antimuscarinics; do not repeat same dose until physician is notified of pressure fall
GASTROINTESTINAL	Obstruction, weakness, severe inflammation or recent gut surgery; hypomotility of gut	Monitor amount, quality of stool in hospitalized patients; advise outpatients to report at once constipation, difficult defecation, which may develop into paralytic ileus; encourage adequate food/fluid intake to hydrate stool; recommend dietary changes (bran, other bulk-forming foods) or bulk-forming laxatives to reduce constipation not modified well by dietary changes; encourage patients to defecate when urge develops
Decreased bowel motility, possible constipation, abdominal distention; dry stool, painful defecation; paralytic ileus		
Dry mouth, possible dysphagia		Recommend frequent sips of water, sucking hard sugarless candy, artificial saliva for this most common side effect; inquire about dysphagia that may be severe enough to cause choking on food, inadequate food instake

(continued)

Table 13–S **Major Side Effects and Contraindications of Antimuscarinic Drugs (*Continued*)**

BODY SYSTEM/ Side Effect	CONTRAINDICATION/ PRECAUTION	COMMENTS AND NURSING IMPLICATIONS
SKIN Flushed, warm skin; rash		Flushing may indicate overdose, but in absence of rash, other side effects, is not reliable indicator of toxicity in children; assess patients for other indicators of excessive doses, including fever, and withhold further doses if overdose is suspected
Dry skin, reduced heat loss via skin	Fever	Inhibited sweating reduces heat loss through skin, leads to fever; check temperature, other signs of possible atropine toxicity, but also eliminate other causes of fever (eg, infection); reduce temperature with sponge baths, etc, notify physician, withhold subsequent antimuscarinic doses, be prepared to give physostigmine if seizure develops
GENITOURINARY Difficult micturition, urinary retention, bladder or abdominal distention; possible bladder or renal infection due to urine reflux into renal pelvis	Obstruction, weakness, severe inflammation of urinary tract; recent urologic surgery	Monitor fluid intake, urine output in hospitalized patients, palpate bladder periodically to assess for fullness; be prepared to catheterize if acute retention occurs; advise patients to report difficult or diminished urination; encourage appropriate fluid intake, voiding when the urge occurs
NEUROMUSCULAR Muscle weakness	Myasthenia gravis	Muscle weakness, caused by nicotinic receptor blockade, is more likely with parenteral glycopyrrolate; marked muscle weakness with therapeutic dose of any antimuscarinic may indicate undiagnosed myasthenia gravis; notify physician for further evaluation

Table 13–1 | Major Interactions Between Antimuscarinics and Other Agents

AGENT	RESULT OF INTERACTION	COMMENTS AND NURSING IMPLICATIONS
Interactions with Other Major Drug Groups Having Antimuscarinic Activity		
Antidepressants, tricyclic; antihistamines (H_1-receptor antagonists); antiparkinson drugs (centrally acting antimuscarinics); antipsychotics; anxiolytics, sedatives/hypnotics; *see Table 13-2*	Increased intensity of antimuscarinic side effects, CNS depression	All these drugs cause additive antimuscarinic actions; some also cause additive CNS depression; avoid combined administration or reduce doses of each used if interaction is unavoidable; monitor closely for both peripheral and central signs of drug action
Other Interactions		
Amantadine (Chapters 25, 57)	Increased antimuscarinic side effects	Mechanism unknown; monitor responses closely, use lowest effective doses of both agents
Antacids, antidiarrheals (Chapters 40, 41)	Decreased absorption, effectiveness of antimuscarinic	Do not administer concurrently; space drug administration by about 2 hr if possible; antacid–antimuscarinic interaction is common, since both are indicated for treatment of peptic ulcer disease
Antipsychotics (phenothiazines; Chapter 23)	Reduced control of psychosis symptoms	Avoid interaction if possible; monitor for loss of symptom control (mechanism unknown); also expect, assess for additive antimuscarinic and CNS depressant effects
Digoxin (Chapter 31)	Increased digoxin absorption, risk of toxicity	Digoxin tablets and oral elixir are incompletely absorbed, yet cause desired response with proper dosages; reduced gut motility in presence of antimuscarinic can increase amount of digoxin absorbed, possibly causing excessive (toxic) effects; avoid interaction; if unavoidable, notify physician (digoxin dose should be reduced), monitor carefully; digoxin "liquid in capsule" formulation is absorbed almost completely and not affected by antimuscarinics, is preferred if combined use is necessary; see Table 31–2

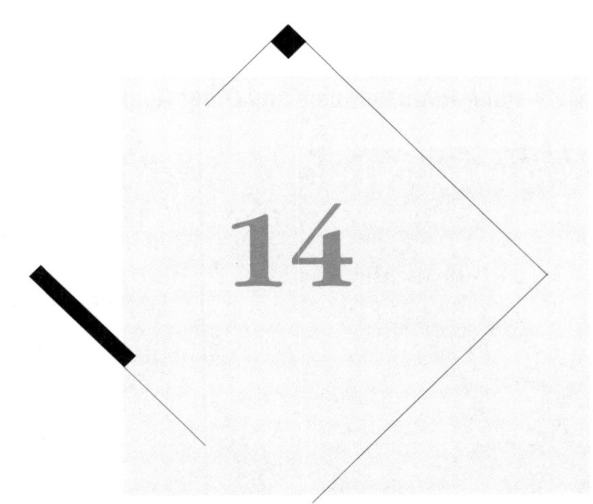

PROTOTYPES

Sympathomimetic Drugs

This chapter discusses drugs, called *sympathomimetics,* that mediate the actions of the sympathetic nervous system or affect structures controlled by it. It starts with a general introduction to the topic and a brief review of adrenergic receptor subtypes and the effects they mediate. The rest of the chapter is divided into five major parts. Parts I through III discuss three major classes of sympathomimetic drugs that are grouped according to the unique ways in which they cause their effects. The content is important not only to understanding the therapeutic uses of these medications, but also to understanding how the sympathetic nervous system works through the chemicals that it releases. Part IV is a short section that discusses selected drugs that cause effects that look as if the sympathetic nervous system were being stimulated. Those drugs can have dramatic effects on your patients' responses to sympathomimetics. Part V, another short section, focuses on sympathomimetics found in common and widely used—and misused—over-the-counter (OTC) medications, with an emphasis on their proper uses and potential dangers.

General Characteristics of Sympathomimetic Drugs

Sympathetic nervous system activity is mediated by norepinephrine released from adrenergic nerves, and by epinephrine released from the adrenal medulla. Sympathomimetic drugs produce effects that mimic one or more of the effects produced by these mediators. Other terms used to describe sympathomimetic drugs include *adrenergic drugs, adrenergic agonists,* and *sympathomimetic amines.* Epinephrine, norepinephrine, and several other sympathomimetic drugs are also classified as **catecholamines** because of their chemical structures.

Ways to Produce Sympathomimetic Effects

Sympathomimetic drugs can be classified according to how they cause their effects: *direct-acting sympathomimetics, mixed-acting sympathomimetics,* and *indirect-acting sympathomimetics.* The direct-acting sympathomimetics can be classified further according to the specific adrenergic receptor type(s) they stimulate—alpha (α) or beta (β). Each group has its own prototype drug.

Major reference tables appear beginning on p 215.

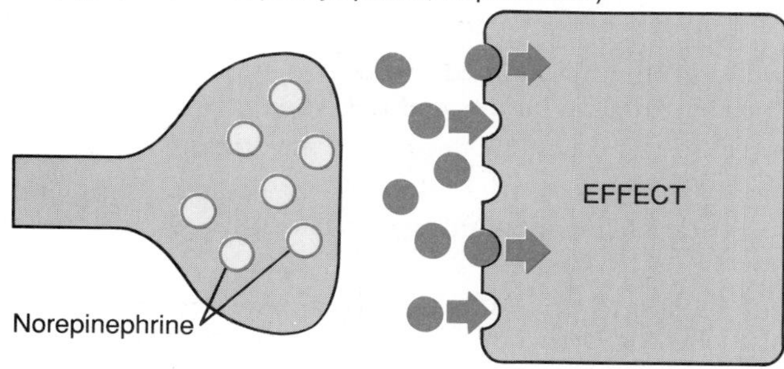

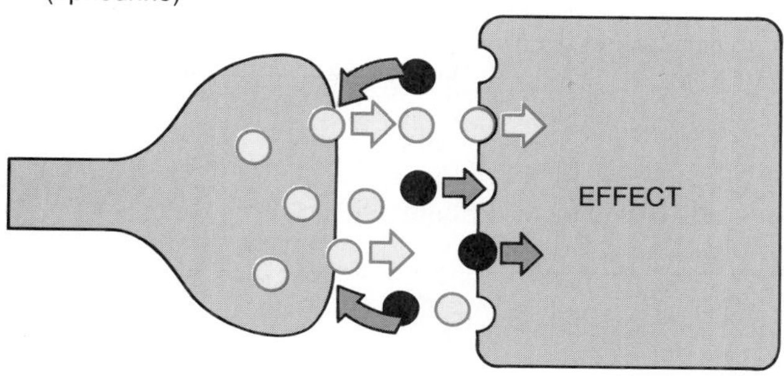

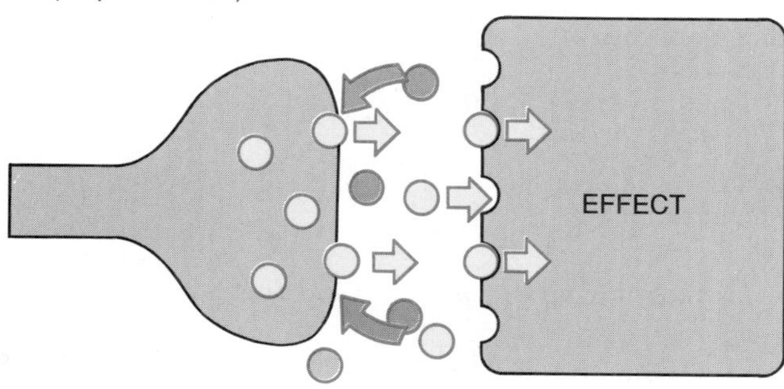

Figure 14–1

Sympathomimetic drugs act in one of three ways:
A. Direct-acting sympathomimetics cause their effects only by interacting directly with receptors on the effectors. The response depends on the agonist's specificity (α and/or β) and the receptor types found on effector cell.
B. Mixed-acting sympathomimetics act directly on target cell receptors, *and* simultaneously release norepinephrine from adrenergic nerves, which also acts on the effectors. Depending on the sympathomimetic, the responses can resemble the responses caused by epinephrine or norepinephrine.
C. Indirect-acting sympathomimetics work *only* by entering the nerve and releasing norepinephrine, which then stimulates the receptors. Drugs that prevent indirect-acting sympathomimetics from entering the nerve ending (eg, tricyclic antidepressants) completely abolish their activity.

- A direct-acting sympathomimetic drug acts *directly* as an agonist on one or more adrenergic receptor subtypes (Fig. 14–1A). The endogenous sympathetic mediators, epinephrine and norepinephrine, and most of the important sympathomimetic drugs, act in this way.
- Mixed-acting sympathomimetic drugs not only stimulate adrenergic receptors directly, but also cause sympathetic nerve endings to release norepinephrine (Fig. 14–1B). Ephedrine is an example of a mixed-acting sympathomimetic.
- Indirect-acting sympathomimetic drugs act *only* by releasing norepinephrine from sympathetic nerves, and have no direct effect on effector cell receptors (Fig. 14–1C). An example of an indirect-acting sympathomimetic is amphetamine.

Adrenergic Receptor Subtypes

Recall from Chapter 10 that adrenergic receptors are classified as either α or β. The receptor type is defined by the agonists that stimulate it, as well as by its reaction to certain blocking agents (Table 14–1). Sympathomimetic drugs may stimulate α-adrenergic receptors, β-adrenergic receptors, or both.

Alpha-Adrenergic Receptors

An α-adrenergic receptor can be defined as one that is stimulated by an α agonist such as phenylephrine, is specifically blocked by an antagonist such as phentolamine, and is not affected by drugs having *only* β agonist or antagonist activity. There are two major subtypes of α receptors, α_1 and α_2.

Alpha$_1$-adrenergic receptors are found mainly on postsynaptic target cells (effector cells) innervated by the sympathetic nervous system. They mediate the various sympathetic responses listed in Table 14–2.

Alpha$_2$-adrenergic receptors are found mainly on presynaptic adrenergic nerve endings. When stimulated by an appropriate drug, α_2 receptors inhibit the release of norepinephrine from the nerve. The α_2 receptor is the physiologic feedback regulator of norepinephrine release from adrenergic nerves.

Table 14–1 **Adrenergic Receptors: Major Subtypes, Locations, and Functions**

Receptor	Location	Major Function When Stimulated by Endogenous Mediator or Appropriate Pharmacologic Agonist
α_1	Postsynaptic on effector cell	Mediates typical α responses on effectors (eg, mydriasis, vasoconstriction)
α_2*	Presynaptic on adrenergic nerve varicosity (nerve ending)	Provides feedback inhibition of further norepinephrine release from adrenergic nerve
β_1	Postsynaptic on effector cell (mainly in heart)	Mainly mediates cardiac stimulation (rate, contractile force, automaticity, impulse conduction rates through atrial, ventricular, nodal tissue); also lipolysis by fat cells, renin release by kidney
β_2	Postsynaptic on effector cell (other than heart)	Mediates most β responses on effectors other than heart (bronchodilation, vasodilation, relaxation of pregnant uterus, glycogenolysis)

*There are also α_2 receptors on vascular smooth muscle cells located away from the typical sympathetic neuro-effector junction. These postsynaptic α_2 receptors may mediate vasoconstriction caused by α agonists administered as drugs; they do not mediate vasoconstriction due to normal sympathetic nervous system stimulation.

Table 14–2 **Responses of Major Effector Organs to Sympathomimetic Drugs (α or β Agonists)**

Organ	Receptor Type	Response
Eye		
Iris, dilator muscle	α	Contracted, causing mydriasis
Respiratory system		
Bronchial smooth muscle tone	β_2	Decreased (relaxation)
Mucus secretions	α	Decreased (thickened)
Heart		
Force of contraction	β_1	Increased
Rate	β_1	Increased
Automaticity	β_1	Increased
Impulse conduction	β_1	Increased
Arterioles and large veins	α β_2	Constriction Dilation
Metabolic effects		
Fat cells	β_1	Increased lipolysis
Skeletal muscle, liver	β_2	Glycogen breakdown
Pancreas	β_2	Increased insulin release
Gastrointestinal tract		
Motility	α, β_2	Decreased
Sphincters	α	Contracted
Overall		Decreased tone, motility
Urinary bladder		
Detrusor	β_2	Relaxation
Trigone, sphincter	α	Contraction
Overall		Decreased urination
Kidney		
Renin secretion	β_1	Increased
Skin		
Pilomotor muscles	α	Contraction
Uterus		
Nonpregnant	β_2	Relaxation
Pregnant	α	Contraction
Male sex organs	α	Ejaculation

Beta-Adrenergic Receptors

A β-adrenergic receptor can be defined as a receptor that is stimulated by an agonist such as isoproterenol, is specifically blocked by an antagonist such as propranolol, and is not affected by drugs having *only* α agonist or antagonist activity. The major responses mediated by β receptors are summarized in Table 14–2.

Like α receptors, the most important β receptors can be classified as β_1 or β_2. Both types of β receptors are found postsynaptically, on effector cells. Beta$_1$-adrenergic receptors are found mainly in the heart, while β_2 receptors are found in most other organs and tissues (see Table 14–2).

Selectivity of Sympathomimetic Drugs

Sympathomimetic drugs differ in terms of how selective they are for stimulating one or more kinds of adrenergic receptor (Fig. 14–2). At one extreme is epinephrine, the least selective agonist because it stimulates *all* α and *all* β receptors. Norepinephrine, which stimulates all α receptors but only β_1 receptors, is slightly more selective.

Only synthetic direct-acting sympathomimetics are even more selective in terms of the receptor type they stimulate. Phenylephrine stimulates only α receptors, whereas isoproterenol and related agents stimulate only β receptors. Some sympathomimetics are so selective that under certain conditions they stimulate only one subtype of α or β receptor. The chemical structures of these drugs are similar in many ways, but their slight structural differences are enough to cause dramatic differences in the kinds of receptors they can stimulate and, therefore, the effects they produce.

Knowing the selectivity of a sympathomimetic drug for adrenergic receptors, and the location of those receptors, helps predict the responses that occur when the drug is given to a patient. It also helps predict the responses to specific adrenergic receptor blockers (see Chapter 15).

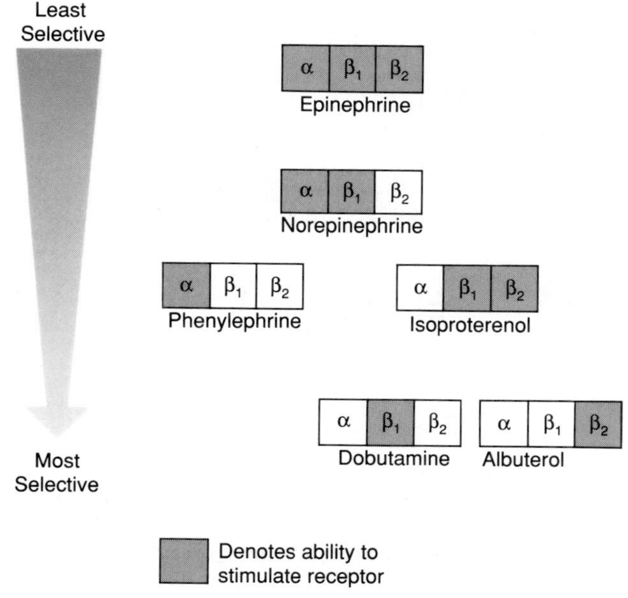

Figure 14–2

Receptor-stimulating abilities of the major direct-acting sympathomimetics. The diversity of the pharmacologic profiles, ranging from epinephrine (which is not at all selective), to highly selective agents such as dobutamine and albuterol, affect the actions, uses, and side effects of these drugs.

I. Direct-Acting Sympathomimetics

Most sympathomimetic drugs are direct-acting agonists for adrenergic receptors. They range from being totally nonselective (they stimulate all α and all β receptors), to highly selective and able to stimulate only one subtype of α or β receptor. The following discussion begins by considering the least selective agonist, epinephrine. Once you have learned about it, it will be easier to understand the effects of other sympathomimetics.

PROTOTYPE

Epinephrine

The drug epinephrine (ADRENALIN; called adrenaline or arterenol in Europe) is identical to the epinephrine that is synthesized in the adrenal medulla. It is the only major sympathomimetic drug that stimulates all adrenergic receptors (see Fig. 14–2).

Absorption, Distribution, Metabolism, and Excretion

The catecholamine structure of epinephrine affects its absorption, distribution, metabolism, and excretion. Since the body treats other catecholamines (norepinephrine, isoproterenol, dopamine, and dobutamine) in a similar manner, these properties will be discussed only once.

Epinephrine is inactivated by gastric acid, and so it must be given parenterally or, when the goal is to cause local effects, topically. When epinephrine is injected, its effects appear within minutes. Once the drug enters the bloodstream it is metabolized mainly by two enzymes, catechol-O-methyl-transferase (COMT) and monoamine oxidase (MAO). Rapid metabolism accounts for epinephrine's relatively short duration of action, and the need to give repeated doses (or special formulations) to prolong its effects.

Epinephrine's metabolites are much less active than epinephrine itself, and most are excreted in the urine. Urinary levels of these metabolites can be measured and used to diagnose diseases in which epinephrine synthesis or metabolism is abnormal. One such condition is pheochromocytoma, a tumor (usually of the adrenal medulla) that produces excessive amounts of epinephrine and norepinephrine. Epinephrine and other catecholamines do not cross the blood–brain barrier and enter the central nervous system (CNS) well unless very high doses are given.

Pharmacologic Effects

Epinephrine produces all the major effects seen when the entire sympathetic nervous system is stimulated (see Table 14–2).

Cardiovascular Effects

Typical cardiovascular responses to an intravenous (IV) injection of an "average" dose of epinephrine are shown in Figure 14–3. (Effects of other major sympathomimetics are shown for comparison.) Epinephrine *directly* stimulates myocardial beta$_1$ receptors, thus increasing

- the force of cardiac contraction (a positive *inotropic* effect),
- heart rate (a positive *chronotropic* effect),
- the rate of electrical impulse conduction through the heart (a positive *dromotropic* effect), and
- the heart's ability to generate electrical impulses (*automaticity*).

Epinephrine constricts arterioles in the skin, mucous membranes, and mesentery. This vasoconstriction, which is mediated by α receptors, causes systolic blood pressure to rise slightly. Simultaneous cardiac stimulation increases systolic pressure further. Epinephrine dilates larger arterioles, such as those in skeletal muscle. Vasodilation is mediated by β_2 receptors, and it causes diastolic pressure to fall slightly. The overall effect is a modest increase of mean (average) blood pressure and of the pulse pressure (systolic minus diastolic). Total peripheral resistance, which reflects both peripheral vasoconstriction and vasodilation, falls slightly. This re-

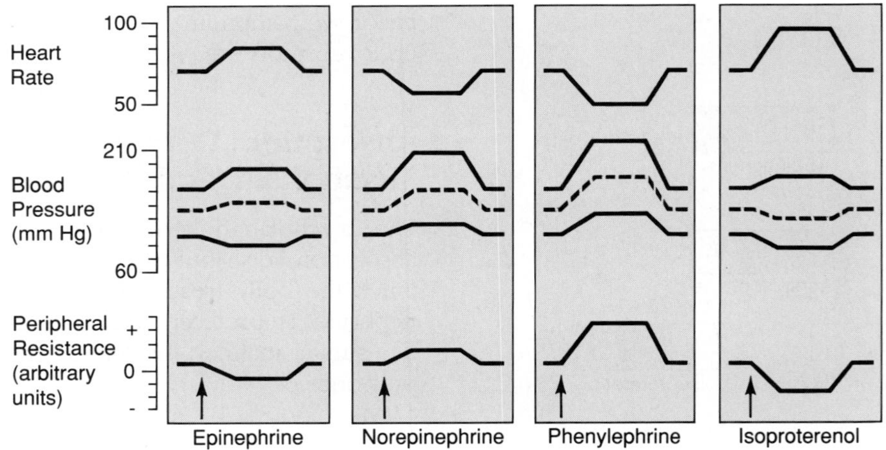

Figure 14–3

Typical cardiovascular responses to IV injection (at arrows) of single "effective" dose of major adrenergic agonists: epinephrine (α, β_1, β_2), norepinephrine (α, β_1), phenylephrine (α), and isoproterenol (β_1, β_2). Changes of blood pressure and peripheral resistance (which reflect a balance between vasodilation and vasoconstriction) are mainly *direct* effects of agonists. Heart rate responses reflect mainly direct effects of epinephrine or *reflex* changes triggered via the baroreceptors in response to changes of mean blood pressure (dashed lines) with norepinephrine, phenylephrine; isoproterenol has additive direct and reflex changes.

sponse indicates that at this dose vasodilation outweighs vasoconstriction.

Whether blood pressure or heart rate falls or rises in a particular patient, or whether the change is small or great, depends on the dose of epinephrine, its route of administration, and how fast it is given. For example, very large doses of epinephrine injected quickly raise blood pressure considerably, and can actually trigger reflex bradycardia via the baroreceptors.

The vascular effects of epinephrine, combined with its great ability to increase heart rate and contractile force, usually increase cardiac output. Cardiac output is defined as heart rate multiplied by stroke volume, which is the amount of blood pumped by the heart each time it beats. In general, if a drug increases heart rate and contractile force, and dilates some blood vessels (decreases peripheral resistance), it will increase cardiac output.

Epinephrine stimulates β_1 receptors on cells in the kidney's juxtaglomerular apparatus to release renin. Renin release indirectly increases the release of aldosterone and the formation of angiotensin II, both of which further elevate blood pressure through their effects on the kidneys and blood vessels. Activation of the renin–angiotensin system, and its pathophysiologic role in heart failure and hypertension, are discussed in Chapters 31 and 33.

Respiratory Effects

Epinephrine is a powerful and physiologically important bronchodilator. Bronchial smooth muscle relaxation is mediated by β_2 receptors. Bronchodilation is most evident and clinically useful in the presence of bronchoconstriction caused by diseases such as asthma, for which epinephrine's ability to reduce histamine release from mast cells also becomes important.

Epinephrine is an effective *decongestant.* It reduces the amount of secretions produced by mucous glands, and makes the secretions more viscous. This is due to epinephrine's ability to constrict small arterioles in the respiratory tract mucosa.

Ocular Effects

Epinephrine dilates the pupil of the eye by stimulating (contracting) the iris dilator muscle. The effect, called **mydriasis,** is mediated by α receptors. Epinephrine also reduces the formation of aqueous humor that fills the anterior chamber of the eye, facilitates drainage of aqueous humor out of the anterior chamber, and decongests the conjunctiva.

Gastrointestinal and Genitourinary Effects

Epinephrine relaxes the smooth muscles that control gastrointestinal (GI) tract tone and motility. These inhibitory effects are mediated by both α and β_2 receptors. (This is one of the few instances in which both types of adrenergic receptors mediate the same response in the same organ.) Epinephrine stimulates α receptors to contract (close) sphincters in the GI tract. The overall effect is decreased activity of the GI tract.

Epinephrine's effects on smooth muscles of the urinary tract parallel those on the GI tract. For example, the detrusor muscle that compresses the bladder is relaxed (β_2), while the tone of the sphincter and the ureters is increased (α).

The smooth muscle of the uterus responds to epinephrine in a way that is regulated by hormonal influences, such as those due to pregnancy. Beta$_2$-adrenergic receptors predominate in the nonpregnant uterus, and the uterus relaxes when they are stimulated. Epinephrine relaxes the nonpregnant uterus. Alpha-adrenergic receptors predominate during pregnancy and its associated hormonal changes. In pregnancy, and especially near term, epinephrine contracts the uterus. Drugs that act only as β agonists will, however, relax the pregnant uterus, indicating that some β receptors remain.

Endocrine and Metabolic Effects

Epinephrine has important effects on fat and carbohydrate metabolism. It acts through α receptors to break down complex fats (lipolysis) from fat cells, thereby increasing blood free fatty acid levels. By stimulating α and β_2 receptors in the liver, epinephrine increases the breakdown of glycogen to glucose (glycogenolysis), causing blood glucose levels to rise. Epinephrine has variable direct and indirect effects on pancreatic insulin release.

Dermal Effects

Epinephrine, through its actions on α receptors in the skin, causes piloerection ("goose flesh") and localized stimulation of sweat glands, particularly on the palms of the hands (so-called adrenergic sweating). These effects, as well as many of the cardiovascular effects such as increased heart rate and force, are obvious signs of epinephrine's actions in the "fight or flight" response to stress.

Clinical Indications and Administration

Epinephrine is used as a bronchodilator or cardiac stimulant, as a vasoconstrictor, as an ophthalmic decongestant, and to treat hypoglycemia. Its major clinical uses and doses are summarized in Table 14–C1. There are several different preparations of epinephrine, each suited for a particular use and route of administration. General nursing implications concerning epinephrine administration are found on page 195.

Uses for the Respiratory System

Epinephrine solution, usually injected subcutaneously, causes prompt but relatively brief bronchodilation that can abort severe, acute asthma attacks. Injectable products such as SUS-PHRINE, which contains epinephrine as both a solution and a slowly dissolving suspension, provide more longlasting effects in emergencies. Epinephrine suspension must be given only by subcutaneous (SC) injection. Epinephrine can also be given by inhalation, and is available in pressurized cannisters that deliver a fixed amount ("metered dose") of the drug when activated. This dosage form, which is convenient for self-administration, has been used for management of chronic asthma symptoms.

Epinephrine is clearly an effective bronchodilator, but *nowadays there is rarely a good reason to use it for asthma or related pulmonary disorders,* whether acutely or chronically. That is because the drug not only dilates the bronchi (a desirable β_2-mediated effect), but also causes many unwanted and potentially dangerous effects, particularly on the heart (β_1 stimulation) and blood vessels (α-mediated vasoconstriction). Drugs called "selective" β_2-adrenergic agonists are almost always preferred. They are discussed on pages 205 to 206. Chapter 38 gives a more complete discussion of asthma therapy.

Management of Acute Hypersensitivity Reactions and Anaphylaxis

Epinephrine is the drug of choice for managing severe and potentially fatal allergic (**anaphylactic**) reactions to drugs, insect or animal venoms, and some foods. The preferred administration route is SC injection. The major problems in anaphylaxis include severe bronchospasm and profound hypotension, caused by the release of histamine and other bronchoconstrictor and vasodilating mediators from immunologically activated mast cells. Epinephrine acts as a physiologic antagonist of these mediators, dilating the bronchi and constricting arterioles to raise blood pressure; it also stabilizes the mast cells, reducing further mediator release.

NURSING IMPLICATIONS

Single-dose epinephrine injection devices (eg, EPIPEN) may be prescribed for patients who are likely to develop anaphylaxis when stung by venomous insects, for example. Patients should understand and be able to demonstrate proper administration techniques before they are given such a product for use. Teach patients to carry the medication with them at all times. Teach desired injection sites (the thigh and the deltoid muscle), sites to avoid (the buttocks), and the need to massage the site gently after injection to enhance drug absorption. Caution them that the self-administration device is for first aid only; that they should seek immediate emergency medical care if stung, even if they experience relief from the self-injected drug.

Uses for the Cardiovascular System

Epinephrine solution is used to restore cardiovascular function in patients who have suffered a cardiac arrest. It is not given to restart the heart, as many people believe, but to increase blood pressure, which facilitates blood flow to the vital organs. In the absence of a heart beat, epinephrine will work only if external or internal cardiac compressions are being delivered, so cardiopulmonary resuscitation (CPR) is a crucial adjunct to the drug. The preferred administration route is IV injection. If a patent vein cannot be found, squirting the drug down the airway is the next best choice, since the drug can be absorbed through mucous membranes in the airways. Epinephrine can also be injected directly into the heart (intracardially).

Another cardiovascular use is prophylaxis or treatment of syncope due to Stokes–Adams syndrome, a cardiac disorder in which patients experience periods of complete atrioventricular (AV) block, ventricular standstill, or fibrillation (see also the section on isoproterenol).

Epinephrine solutions can be applied topically on mucous membranes or cut skin to produce hemostasis, as during surgery. Hemostasis is the result of epinephrine's vasoconstrictor activity.

Adjunctive Use in Local Anesthetics

Epinephrine is a common ingredient in some formulations of local anesthetics that are used for spinal anesthesia, and for more localized pain control in many surgical or dental procedures. Epinephrine is included for its local vasoconstrictor activity: when injected with the anesthetic it constricts nearby arterioles, reduces blood flow to the injection site, and keeps the blood from washing the anesthetic away from the desired site of action into the systemic circulation. More information about the use (and misuse) and dosages of epinephrine and other vasoconstrictors with local anesthetics is given in Chapter 19.

Uses for Eye Disorders

Epinephrine, administered topically in the form of drops, has several important uses in ophthalmology. It is used as a mydriatic drug to facilitate examination of the eye. It is also useful for treating some patients with chronic open-angle glaucoma, the type of glaucoma in which outflow of aqueous humor is not blocked by the iris. Epinephrine lowers intraocular pressure mainly by increasing aqueous humor outflow. (As noted below, epinephrine is contraindicated in patients with acute angle-closure glaucoma.) Epinephrine can also be applied topically to the eye to provide corneal decongestion or to control hemorrhage.

NURSING IMPLICATIONS

If two or more topical ophthalmic medications are prescribed, instruct the patient to space the administration of each by 10 minutes or so. The conjunctival sac cannot hold large amounts of drug, and administering several at once will probably cause loss of some medication. See Appendix A for general information about techniques for eyedrop administration and related nursing implications.

General Nursing Implications for Administration of Epinephrine

The general precautions noted for epinephrine apply to most other sympathomimetics. The drug is available in a wide range of strengths, from weak to concentrated, for specific uses. Before injecting epinephrine by any route, double-check the label for concentration and expiration date, and inspect the drug. Fresh solutions of epinephrine and other sympathomimetics should be clear and colorless. They become oxidized and inactivated shortly after exposure to light or air, and their color usually changes to brown or pink. Store the product in its original container, protected from light, and do not open the container or dilute the solution until you are ready to use it. Oxidized or outdated solutions should be discarded immediately.

If the epinephrine solution must be diluted before use, consult the manufacturer's recommendations for diluents first. In general, epinephrine and other sympathomimetic solutions should not be diluted in or mixed with alkaline solutions (for example, sodium bicarbonate) or plain saline because they will oxidize promptly. Solutions containing dextrose (glucose) are preferred; dextrose slows the oxidation of epinephrine and most other sympathomimetics.

Do not add epinephrine or other sympathomimetics directly to blood or plasma infusions. Ensure that only the sterile *solution* is given intravenously. Use proper technique (aspiration before injection, massaging the injection site) when injecting these drugs subcutaneously. Accidental IV injection of an epinephrine suspension can cause cerebrovascular hemorrhage from a sharp rise in blood pressure, or myocardial infarction or arrhythmias from excessive cardiac stimulation. Drug particles from the suspension can also block small vessels. If epinephrine injections must be given repeatedly (especially SC), rotate injection sites to avoid tissue irritation or necrosis due to local vasoconstriction.

Side Effects, Adverse Reactions, and Contraindications

Epinephrine can produce side effects in virtually any patient who receives the drug, regardless of its route of administration. Because this drug can stimulate all α and β receptors, it can cause all the side effects noted in Table 14–S. Patients who are unusually sensitive to epinephrine and other sympathomimetics are noted below. *There is absolutely no contraindication to using epinephrine for treating cardiac arrest, anaphylaxis, or status asthmaticus.* In these emergencies, possible adverse responses are trivial compared with the likely consequences of not using the drug: death.

Cardiovascular Side Effects

The most serious side effects of epinephrine are due to cardiovascular stimulation. They are particularly dangerous for patients with a history of hypertension or cardiac diseases such as arrhythmias, myocardial infarction, or angina pectoris. Hyperthyroid patients are also more sensitive, since high thyroid hormone levels cause additive cardiovascular stimulation.

High doses of epinephrine significantly elevate blood pressure in all patients. Even slight increases of blood pressure may be dangerous for hypertensive patients. Important signs or symptoms of hypertension include severe headache, blanching of the skin (vasoconstriction directs blood flow away from the surface of the skin, so it looks pale), diaphoresis, tightness of the chest, and vomiting. Severe hypertension may rupture blood vessels, particularly if the patient already has an aneurysm. Intracranial bleeding and stroke are important concerns; patients who have suffered a stroke should be treated cautiously with epinephrine.

Epinephrine and other sympathomimetics with cardiac stimulating or vasoconstrictor actions may cause myocardial **ischemia** and its major symptom, angina pectoris. Ischemia and angina develop when myocardial oxygen demands, which reflect the amount of work the heart must perform, exceed myocardial oxygen supply. Oxygen demand increases because epinephrine significantly increases both heart rate and contractility. These effects may not be accompanied by a sufficient increase of coronary blood flow to provide an adequate supply of oxygen. A myocardial infarction (heart attack) is liable to occur if the patient has ischemic heart disease such as coronary atherosclerosis.

Epinephrine may cause tachycardia or other cardiac tachyarrhythmias. Myocardial ischemia induced by sympathomimetics also increases the risk and potential danger of arrhythmias. Some general anesthetic agents, such as halothane (FLUOTHANE; see Chapter 20), sensitize the heart to the arrhythmia-producing effects of epinephrine (see Table 14–I).

NURSING IMPLICATIONS

Monitor vital signs closely for at least 3 to 5 minutes, or until they stabilize, after injecting epinephrine.

Ocular Side Effects

Epinephrine is contraindicated in patients with *narrow-angle* (angle-closure) glaucoma because mydriasis further restricts flow of aqueous humor out of the anterior chamber, causing pressure to rise. This adverse response is shared by all other drugs that cause mydriasis, including all α agonists and antimuscarinics (atropine-like drugs; see Chapter 13).

NURSING IMPLICATIONS

If a patient taking any drug with mydriatic activity reports eye pain, the physician should be notified, and the patient's intraocular pressure measured, at once. Pain may indicate an acute glaucoma attack, a medical emergency that can lead to permanent blindness if not treated immediately.

Endocrine and Metabolic Side Effects

The ability of epinephrine to elevate blood glucose and insulin levels may cause problems for diabetics, and so it should be used cautiously in these patients. This problem is shared by most other sympathomimetic drugs, including those available OTC (see page 211).

NURSING IMPLICATIONS

Monitor blood sugar levels closely, regardless of which sympathomimetic drug is given. Advise diabetic patients about OTC products that should be avoided unless prior approval has been obtained.

Central Nervous System Side Effects

Anxiety, nervousness or uneasiness, and muscle tremor are relatively common side effects, even when low doses of epinephrine are given. Severe CNS side effects may indicate overdose.

NURSING IMPLICATIONS

If a patient reports sudden uneasiness that was not present before administration of any sympathomimetic, vital signs should be checked at once, and the dose of drug should be rechecked as soon as possible. Central side effects not due to epinephrine overdoses can usually be managed by allowing the patient to rest quietly and by offering reassurance. Advise patients receiving epinephrine to avoid other stimulants such as caffeine and nicotine.

◆ Use During Pregnancy and Lactation

There are no adequate and well-controlled studies to provide conclusive evidence either for or against the use of epinephrine in pregnancy. As noted above, epinephrine should never be withheld for treating life-threatening conditions.

◆ Use in Children

The primary use of epinephrine in pediatrics is for treating severe allergic reactions. Children are more sensitive to sympathomimetics than young adults. Dosages are given in Table 14–C1.

◆ Use in the Elderly

Geriatric patients are particularly sensitive to all sympathomimetics. They cannot tolerate sudden changes of blood pressure; increased heart rate and contractility may precipitate angina in persons with coronary artery disease, which is prevalent in this population. The elderly usually require lower doses than those given to middle-aged adults, as well as closer monitoring of drug effects.

Interactions with Other Drugs

Many drugs interact with epinephrine and most other sympathomimetics (see Table 14–1). Most of the important interactions involve aggravation of cardiovascular problems such as hypertension, myocardial ischemia, and arrhythmias.

Some interactions are important because they show how the body adapts to changes of normal sympathetic tone. Reserpine, an antihypertensive drug that *depletes* norepinephrine from adrenergic nerve endings, reduces the overall level of sympathetic tone. When any direct-acting sympathomimetic is given to someone taking reserpine, the response is more intense than would be expected from the dose. This occurs because the adrenergic receptors, chronically deprived of normal stimulation because of the catecholamine depletor, become "supersensitive." The implication is that if sympathomimetic drug effects must be produced in persons taking catecholamine depletors, very low doses of the sympathomimetic must be given to avoid potentially dangerous hypertension, cardiac stimulation, or both.

Conversely, if a person is chronically exposed to high levels of sympathomimetic stimulation, their receptors seem to become subsensitive, and tolerance develops to the effects of sympathomimetic drugs.

NURSING IMPLICATIONS

Many drug interactions involving sympathomimetics should be avoided. If they cannot, sympathomimetic doses must be adjusted carefully to avoid untoward responses. Adverse responses in which sympathomimetic effects are intensified are managed in much the same way as epinephrine overdoses. Regardless of the type of interaction, or the drugs involved, problems can be minimized by obtaining a thorough drug history, adjusting doses accordingly, and closely monitoring the patient's responses.

Overdose and Toxicity

The most serious consequences of epinephrine overdose are cardiovascular: hypertension, possibly leading to stroke or acute pulmonary edema; and tachycardia, possibly leading to myocardial ischemia or arrhythmias.

Rapidly acting parenteral vasodilators (eg, nitroprusside) can be used to lower blood pressure. Antiarrhythmic drugs such as lidocaine should be given as needed. Since the cardiovascular effects of epinephrine overdoses involve excessive stimulation of both α- and β-adrenergic receptors, injection of a combined α- and β-blocking drug such as labetalol may be used if there are no major contraindications.

An α-blocker (eg, phentolamine) should not be used alone: blood pressure will fall, but there is a great risk of causing arrhythmias or myocardial infarction as heart rate reflexly increases. Likewise, a β-blocker (eg, propranolol) should never be used as the sole treatment: it will cause blood pressure to rise even more, for a while, as β-mediated vasodilation is inhibited and the more important α-mediated vasoconstriction is left unopposed. Thereafter, the weakened β-blocked heart will no longer be able to pump against the high arterial pressure, and acute heart failure and pulmonary edema can occur. In general, avoid using any drug with β-blocking activity if the patient has a history of asthma or obstructive pulmonary disease.

NURSING IMPLICATIONS

The actual interventions used for the patient will depend greatly on information provided to the physician by the nurse: carefully and frequently assessing vital signs, the electrocardiogram (ECG), and neurologic status; identifying alterations that seem to pose the greatest immediate risk to the patient; and giving information about underlying conditions that pose a special risk to the patient, whether from the overdose or interventions used to manage it. Keep the patient calm and administer oxygen.

Related Drugs

Dipivefrin

Dipivefrin hydrochloride (PROPINE) is a topical ophthalmic agent that is used only for lowering intraocular pressure in the treatment of chronic open-angle glaucoma. It is interesting because it is a **prodrug**—one that is inactive until it is administered and metabolized. Dipivefrin readily diffuses into the eye and is metabolized locally to epinephrine. Like epinephrine, its major ocular contraindication is narrow-angle glaucoma.

Levonordefrin

Levonordefrin (NEO-COBEFRIN) is used exclusively in dentistry as a vasoconstrictor additive to some local anesthetics. Refer to dental therapeutics texts for further discussions of this agent.

NOREPINEPHRINE

Norepinephrine, the naturally occurring sympathetic neurotransmitter, is identical to synthetic norepinephrine (LEVOPHED; called levarterenol or noradrenaline in Europe). The only chemical difference between norepinephrine and epinephrine is the absence of a methyl group on norepinephrine. However, this slight difference greatly changes its effects. Because of norepinephrine's important physiologic roles, it will be described in more depth than would ordinarily be used for prototype-related agents.

Absorption, Distribution, Metabolism, and Excretion

The features of absorption, distribution, and excretion noted for epinephrine generally apply to norepinephrine. Monoamine oxidase located in the sympathetic nerve ending metabolizes norepinephrine, thereby regulating the amount of transmitter that is stored and released when the nerve is stimulated.

Pharmacologic Effects

Norepinephrine is an agonist for α and β_1 receptors, and so causes all the direct effects that those receptors mediate (see Table 14–2). The drug causes *no* β_2 receptor stimulation. Most of the α-mediated effects caused by norepinephrine on structures outside the cardiovascular system are weak in comparison with those caused by epinephrine, and they are seldom clinically useful. The most important effects of norepinephrine involve direct effects on the blood vessels and heart, and simultaneous indirect (autonomic reflex) effects triggered by the direct actions.

The typical response to an IV injection of norepinephrine is shown in Figure 14–3. Like epinephrine, norepinephrine constricts some arterioles by stimulating vascular α receptors, so systolic pressure rises. However, since norepinephrine has no β_2 activity, and so cannot dilate some peripheral blood vessels, vasoconstriction is unopposed. As a result, diastolic and mean arterial pressures also rise, leading to an increase of total peripheral resistance. Thus, norepinephrine always causes a **vasopressor** ("pressor") response.

The direct effects of norepinephrine on the heart are identical to those of epinephrine: increased rate, force, impulse conduction, and automaticity, all of which are mediated by β_1 receptors. However, increased blood pressure activates the baroreceptor reflex, which decreases sympathetic tone to the heart and simultaneously increases parasympathetic tone. This reflex effect outweighs the direct cardiac-stimulating effects, so bradycardia usually occurs.

Although norepinephrine stimulates cardiac contractility, when given to a normal person its ability to increase peripheral resistance and reflexly to slow heart rate allows cardiac output to rise only slightly. Norepinephrine usually increases cardiac output if given to a hypotensive patient. Very high doses may decrease cardiac output by causing excessive increases of peripheral resistance and marked bradycardia.

Clinical Indications and Administration

Norepinephrine has few uses. It is mainly used for its cardiovascular effects in the management of certain forms of acute hypotension or cardiovascular collapse (shock). The drug is given intravenously; dosages are noted in Table 14–C1. However, with a better understanding of the pathophysiology of the different forms of shock, and with the availability of other drugs that affect the heart and vasculature in a more desirable way, norepinephrine is seldom used anymore.

Norepinephrine can be used to counteract acute hypotension caused by drugs that cause excessive vasodilation, but in many cases selective vasoconstrictors (eg, the agonist phenylephrine) are preferred. It is used to manage cardiogenic shock, which is cardiovascular collapse caused by acute heart failure, as may occur following a heart attack. However, in that condition, the sympathetic nervous system is usually already maximally activated, causing intense vasoconstriction and cardiac stimulation in an attempt to help force blood through the vital organs. Norepinephrine can do more harm than good by stimulating the oxygen-deprived heart even more (possibly worsening arrhythmias and cell death); and by intensifying the already intense vasoconstriction, reducing vital organ blood flow further. Other drugs that stimulate the heart more efficiently (eg, dobutamine, amrinone), and cause less peripheral vasoconstriction, are usually preferred.

Similarly, norepinephrine and other drugs with vasoconstrictor actions are not proper treatment for hypotension caused by blood loss vasculature (hemorrhagic or hypovolemic shock). In this condition, as in cardiogenic shock, the sympathetic nervous system is already activated to elevate blood pressure, and causing more vasoconstriction by administering a sympathomimetic drug could do much more harm than good. The initial treatment of choice is cautious IV fluid or blood replacement.

NURSING IMPLICATIONS

Guidelines for preparing epinephrine solutions apply also to norepinephrine. Use a calibrated pump to regulate the infusion rate precisely. Vital signs, including blood pressure and heart rate, and an ECG, should be monitored every 2 to 5 minutes until the desired blood pressure is reached and periodically thereafter so that the dose can be adjusted as needed.

Direct and continuous measurement of arterial and venous pressure, with appropriate catheters, is preferred to methods such as a cuff and sphygmomanometer. Some institutions have policies that specify requirements for administration and monitoring; check first.

If very high doses of norepinephrine are needed to obtain the desired blood pressure, check for blood or fluid loss as possible causes of the hypotension. Cautious IV fluid therapy may help restore blood pressure and reduce the need for excessive doses of norepinephrine. Avoid abrupt discontinuation of norepinephrine or other vasopressor infusions; it is liable to cause acute cardiac failure and hypotension.

Side Effects, Adverse Reactions, and Contraindications

Most of the side effects and contraindications for norepinephrine are similar to those for epinephrine (see Table 14–C1). However, norepinephrine is much more likely to cause bradycardia or hypertension. Norepinephrine's potent vasoconstrictor actions, which are not balanced by vasodilation, lead to an additional adverse response: tissue necrosis due to extravasation. Although norepinephrine has few clinical uses, the problems discussed in the next section are very important when it is used, and *they apply to the IV use of any drug that has powerful vasoconstrictor activity.*

Norepinephrine Extravasation

If proper IV infusion techniques and patient monitoring are not used when giving norepinephrine (or any other potent vasoconstrictor), the drug can seep out of the vein and diffuse into the surrounding tissues. This process is called **extravasation**. When it occurs, norepinephrine exerts its vasoconstrictor activity and drastically reduces or even stops both the infusion and blood flow to the tissue. This produces local ischemia that may cause the affected tissue, or tissue distal to the extravasated site, to become necrotic or gangrenous. Such tissue damage has necessitated limb amputation. Decreased blood flow also favors the development of thrombi and emboli.

Norepinephrine extravasation is easy to recognize. The rate of the infusion slows or stops; the skin surrounding the needle or catheter insertion site becomes hard, pale, or otherwise discolored; the extremity beyond the administration site becomes noticeably cold because circulation is poor; and the patient may report numbness or tingling (paresthesias) of the affected limb. Distal pulses in the affected limb become weak or absent.

Treatment of Extravasation

The problems from norepinephrine extravasation are the result of its ability to stimulate α receptors in blood vessels. This effect can be inhibited by administering the α blocker phentolamine. As soon as extravasation is recognized the vasoconstrictor infusion should be stopped. Phentolamine should be injected liberally into the subcutaneous tissues at several places around the affected area. This alone often restores blood flow, but phentolamine's effects can be increased by gently applying warm moist towels to the tissues. Some clinicians add 5 to 10 mg of phentolamine to the norepinephrine infusion solution to prevent local vasoconstriction if extravasation should occur. This dose of α blocker is sufficient to prevent local vasoconstriction and the problems of extravasation, but does not block norepinephrine's systemic pressor or cardiac-stimulating actions.

NURSING IMPLICATIONS

Proper administration technique and frequent patient monitoring are the best ways to prevent vasoconstrictor extravasation. Infusion into a central vein is preferred. Otherwise, use the largest vein that can be reached conveniently. Avoid leg veins, especially in geriatric patients who are apt to have preexisting peripheral vascular disease that could retard drug infusion and increase the risk of extravasation or thrombosis. Use a long IV catheter so the drug enters the bloodstream at some distance from where the needle penetrated the skin and vein. Check flow through the infusion line periodically, and observe for the signs of extravasation noted above. If norepinephrine is given into a peripheral vein, the skin over the vein may become blanched, but other signs of extravasation may not appear. If this occurs discontinue the infusion and restart it elsewhere.

Interactions with Other Drugs

The major drug interactions involving norepinephrine, and ways to manage them, are similar to those for epinephrine (see Table 14–1).

Overdose and Toxicity

Hypertension and marked bradycardia are the most common and dangerous consequences of norepinephrine overdose. Phentolamine, an α-blocker, can be given to lower blood pressure. It should reflexly normalize heart rate also. A β blocker may be needed if excessive cardiac stimulation persists.

Direct-Acting Sympathomimetics with More Selective Activity

In many clinical situations it is desirable to stimulate only α or β receptors. Since epinephrine and norepinephrine do not act selectively, other direct-acting sympathomimetics with more limited agonist activity have been developed.

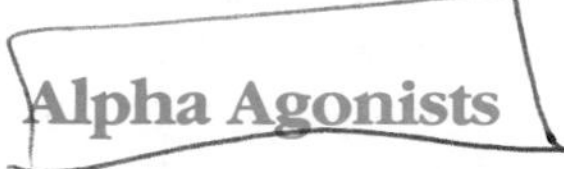

Alpha Agonists

PROTOTYPE

Phenylephrine

Phenylephrine (NEO-SYNEPHRINE) is the prototype. It is often called a "pure" α agonist, meaning that it has no effect on β receptors (see Fig. 14–2).

Absorption, Distribution, Metabolism, and Excretion

Phenylephrine is absorbed from the gut, but so erratically that the drug is rarely given orally. Instead, it is given by injection or by topical administration. Phenylephrine is not a catecholamine, and so is not metabolized by COMT (the enzyme that helps break down epinephrine, for example). Monoamine oxidase activity in the liver is the major pathway for metabolizing phenylephrine. However, phenylephrine metabolism is slow enough that effects from a single SC injection last about an hour, compared with durations of only a few minutes for epinephrine or norepinephrine solution given the same way.

Pharmacologic Effects

The major effects of phenylephrine reflect its direct stimulation of postsynaptic α receptors. (Phenylephrine weakly causes norepinephrine release from adrenergic nerves, so some texts classify it as a mixed-acting sympathomimetic [see ephedrine p 207]. However, this effect contributes so little to the drug's overall actions, particularly when reasonable doses are given, that phenylephrine is considered here as a direct-acting agonist with no β-mediated effects.)

Cardiovascular Effects

Like norepinephrine, phenylephrine causes both direct and reflex cardiovascular effects. The most important direct effect is constriction of arterioles. The drug causes no vasodilation. When given systemically, phenylephrine elevates both systolic and diastolic blood pressures (a pressor response; see Fig. 14–3). Phenylephrine has no direct effect on cardiac rate, force, automaticity, or impulse conduction, all of which are mediated by β receptors. However, the pressor response activates the baroreceptor reflex and causes the heart rate to slow. Vasoconstriction and reflex bradycardia reduce cardiac output.

Other Useful Effects

Phenylephrine constricts the fine arterioles in the eye and the mucosa of the upper respiratory tract, producing a decongestant action. Mucus and lacrimal secretions decrease. The decongestant action can occur with low doses of phenylephrine that do not significantly increase blood pressure. Phenylephrine dilates the pupil of the eye.

Clinical Indications and Administration

The clinical uses for phenylephrine are summarized in Table 14–C1. Most of them relate in one way or another to the drug's vasoconstrictor actions. Phenylephrine is given by injection or by topical administration.

Uses for the Cardiovascular System

Management of Hypotension

Phenylephrine is preferred over norepinephrine for managing acute hypotension, particularly that which is caused by drugs that cause vasodilation. For example, it can be used intraoperatively to prevent or reverse the low blood pressure that is often caused by local anesthetics, given for spinal anesthesia, which can also inhibit sympathetic nerves controlling blood vessel tone in the lower extremities. Being a pure α agonist, phenylephrine is also a preferred antidote for overdoses of α-blocking drugs. Depending on the situation, phenylephrine can be given subcutaneously or intramuscularly, but IV infusion gives the best control of blood pressure.

Since phenylephrine lacks cardiac-stimulating activity (and actually can cause cardiac depression via the baroreceptors), it is not a suitable substitute for norepinephrine or related drugs when hypotension is caused or accompanied by cardiac depression, such as in acute heart failure. And, for reasons noted above for norepinephrine, phenylephrine should not be used to manage hypotension caused by hypovolemia.

Prolongation of Local Anesthetic Activity

Like epinephrine, phenylephrine can be used to prolong the action of local anesthetics injected intraspinally or by infiltration of the skin or mucous membranes.

Management of Paroxysmal Atrial Tachycardia

Phenylephrine, injected intravenously, provides one way to terminate paroxysmal atrial tachycardia (PAT). It is an arrhythmia in which episodes of very rapid atrial contractions may progress to more dangerous ventricular arrhythmias. Phenylephrine actually works indirectly in this situation: the direct response to its injection is a rise of blood pressure, which then triggers the baroreceptor reflex. It is the sudden and relatively intense increase of cardiac-slowing parasympathetic tone, and the simultaneous decrease of opposing sympathetic influences, that often stops the arrhythmia.

The increased blood pressure that phenylephrine must cause to stop PAT can be dangerous for some patients. There are alternative drugs to stop the arrhythmia, including the rapidly acting acetylcholinesterase inhibitor edrophonium, and some antiarrhythmic agents such as the β-adrenergic blocker propanolol.

Uses for Eye Disorders

Phenylephrine is used extensively in ophthalmology and ophthalmic surgery for its mydriatic, decongestant, and hemostatic actions. Sterile ophthalmic solutions containing 0.12% to 10% phenylephrine are used topically to diagnose or treat various eye disorders (Table 14–C1). Since phenylephrine does not paralyze accommodation, which is often necessary for some eye examinations or operations, atropine or a related antimuscarinic drug (see Chapter 13) may be used adjunctively.

NURSING IMPLICATIONS

Ophthalmic solutions of phenylephrine often cause eye pain and irritation. Before administering this drug, determine whether the physician has ordered a topical local anesthetic, which should be applied first. Also make sure that narrow-angle glaucoma, a contraindication, has been ruled out.

Uses for the Respiratory System

Phenylephrine is a nasal decongestant ingredient in OTC remedies used to relieve upper respiratory tract symptoms of the common cold, sinusitis, hay fever, and similar disorders. Until recently, several orally administered products contained the drug, often in combination with other drugs such as antihistamines (H_1 blockers; Chapter 51) or analgesics/antipyretics (eg, aspirin, acetaminophen; Chapter 52). However, owing to poor oral absorption, and the presence of doses that often were subtherapeutic, very few OTC drugs containing phenylephrine are left on the market, and none are available by prescription. Phenylephrine is still an important ingredient in many nasal decongestant drops and sprays. Nursing implications for the use of OTC products containing phenylephrine and other sympathomimetics are discussed later in this chapter.

Side Effects, Adverse Reactions, and Contraindications

Cardiovascular Side Effects

Hypertension and all of its consequences are the most serious adverse responses to phenylephrine and other α agonists (see Table 14–S). Hypertension is most likely to occur when phenylephrine is injected, but significant increases of blood pressure may occur regardless of the route of administration. Even OTC products containing relatively low doses of the drug should be avoided by individuals with hypertension, except when recommended by a physician.

Reflex bradycardia is usually slight and harmless unless phenylephrine is injected. However, reflexly decreased heart rate and electrical impulse conduction may be dangerous for a patient who already has a very slow heart rate or partial heart block; complete heart block or cardiac arrest may occur. Like norepinephrine, phenylephrine and other α agonists should be used cautiously in patients with peripheral vascular diseases. Precautions for guarding against and managing norepinephrine extravasation apply also to phenylephrine and related drugs.

Ocular Side Effects

Phenylephrine is prescribed for some patients with open-angle glaucoma because it reduces intraocular pressure. However, its mydriatic action can reduce outflow of aqueous humor and increase intraocular pressure if the patient has narrow-angle glaucoma, for which α agonists are absolutely contraindicated. Since angle-closure may occur in a patient being treated for open-angle glaucoma, it is essential that intraocular pressure be measured frequently and that the patient be instructed to notify the physician at once if eye pain develops.

Metabolic Side Effects

The ability of α agonists to inhibit insulin release may cause problems for diabetic patients. This is a greater problem if the diabetic patient self-administers large doses of OTC sympathomimetics (eg, decongestants) without supervision.

Genitourinary Side Effects

Drugs with α agonist activity, through their ability to increase bladder sphincter tone, may pose some risk of acute urinary retention in males with prostatic hypertrophy. Some patients may experience urinary difficulty or pain.

Central Nervous System Side Effects

Signs of mild CNS stimulation may occur, even with recommended doses of phenylephrine. More intense signs should be considered as possible indicators of overdose or idiosyncratic reactions.

General Nursing Implications for Side Effects of Phenylephrine

The availability without prescription of phenylephrine and similar drugs increases the risk of adverse effects or misuse in the presence of contraindications. Many side effects can be avoided by carefully considering a patient's history before giving phenylephrine or a related drug. Assessment for side effects is generally the same as noted for norepinephrine; emphasis should be placed on the most serious adverse signs and symptoms: eye pain of glaucoma, hypertension, bradycardia, altered blood glucose levels, and changes of bladder function. Insomnia, due to mild CNS stimulation, can be avoided by administering the drug well before bedtime. It is important to identify high-risk patients and teach them which drugs to avoid or to use only on a physician's order.

◆ Use During Pregnancy and Lactation

It is not known whether phenylephrine causes fetal harm, but it should probably be avoided, especially during the first trimester. Inappropriate use of phenylephrine or other vasoconstrictors may aggravate pregnancy-associated hypertension, perhaps to a dangerous level.

If phenylephrine is used during labor, either as an additive to local anesthesia or to correct hypotension, and the mother is also receiving an oxytocic drug (which may elevate blood pressure) to stimulate labor, monitor blood pressure carefully. The combination may cause severe hypertension, and possibly a cerebral hemorrhage. There is no conclusive evidence about the risks of phenylephrine use by women who are breast-feeding their infants.

◆ Use in Children

Pediatric use of phenylephrine is generally limited to treatment of hypotension during spinal anesthesia, upper respiratory tract congestion, and certain ophthalmic disorders. Doses must be measured carefully (Table 14–C1). Over-the-counter products made specifically for pediatric use should be used. Topical ophthalmic products containing phenylephrine should not be used for infants.

◆ Use in the Elderly

The major age-related concerns include the prevalence of cardiovascular disease and narrow-angle glaucoma, both of which can be aggravated even with the use of topical phenylephrine or other α agonists. A thorough physical examination should be done before these drugs are administered to elders. Owing to the prevalence of prostatic hypertrophy, and the potential ability of α agonists to reduce bladder function, elderly males should be monitored closely for urinary difficulty.

Interactions with Other Drugs

The major drug interactions involving phenylephrine are listed in Table 14–I. Most are similar to those described for epinephrine and norepinephrine.

Overdose and Toxicity

Hypertension with reflex bradycardia is the most serious and common problem caused by α agonist overdoses. The specific antidote is the α blocker phentolamine, which will lower blood pressure and simultaneously alleviate reflex bradycardia. Regardless of the patient, the dose, or the indication, phentolamine should always be readily available whenever phenylephrine is to be injected.

Related Drugs

Methoxamine

Methoxamine (VASOXYL) is used as a vasopressor for acute hypotension. It is given intravenously for prompt effects, or intramuscularly when longer effects are desired.

Naphazoline, Oxymetazoline, Tetrahydrozoline, Xylometazoline

These α agonists are found in OTC or prescription cough, cold, allergy, or ophthalmic decongestant products. They are discussed later in the section on sympathomimetics in OTC drugs. Dosages are summarized in Table 14–C1.

Selective Alpha$_2$-Adrenergic Agonists

A few drugs selectively stimulate the α_2 receptors. The most useful of these agents act mainly on the α_2 receptors in cardiovascular control centers of the *central* nervous system, leading to decreased sympathetic outflow to the periphery. The most important response is reduced blood pressure, and so the "centrally acting α_2 agonists" are used as antihypertensive drugs. Clonidine (CATAPRES) is the prototype; it is discussed in Chapter 33.

A clonidine derivative, apraclonidine (IOPIDINE), is a topical ophthalmic drug. It reduces intraocular pressure (in a way that is not fully understood), but is not used for glaucoma, like other sympathomimetics. Its only indication is for preventing sudden rises of intraocular pressure that often occur in response to laser surgery of the eye (see Table 14–C1).

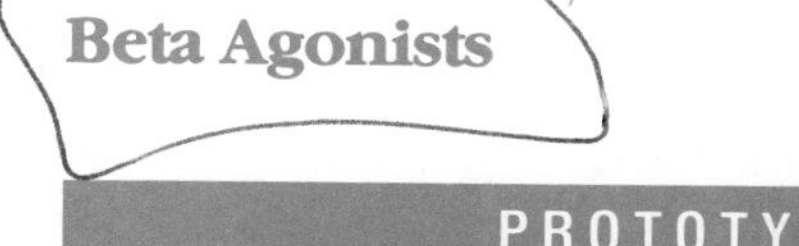

Beta Agonists

PROTOTYPE

Isoproterenol

Drugs that stimulate only β receptors are used mainly to stimulate the heart or dilate the bronchi. Isoproterenol (ISUPREL), the prototype, stimulates both β_1 and β_2 receptors. It has no effect on α receptors (see Fig. 14–2).

Absorption, Distribution, Metabolism, and Excretion

Isoproterenol is a catecholamine. Its pharmacokinetics are similar to those discussed for epinephrine.

Pharmacologic Effects

The major effects of isoproterenol (see Table 14–2) are on the cardiovascular and respiratory systems, and on carbohydrate and lipid metabolism.

Cardiovascular Effects

Isoproterenol is a vasodilator. Its effect is greatest in the mesentery and large arterioles found in skeletal muscle. Vasodilation reduces diastolic blood pressure and peripheral resistance (a depressor response; see Fig. 14–3). Isoproterenol does not constrict any blood vessels because it lacks α-agonist activity.

Isoproterenol directly increases cardiac contractile force, rate, electrical impulse conduction, and automaticity. Increased heart rate and contractile force may increase systolic pressure slightly, but mean arterial pressure usually drops because of the greater fall of diastolic pressure. Heart rate increases considerably because isoproterenol stimulates the heart both directly and by way of the baroreceptor response triggered by decreased blood pressure. Overall, isoproterenol increases cardiac output by increasing heart rate and contractility and by decreasing peripheral resistance.

Respiratory and Other Effects

Isoproterenol is an excellent bronchodilator. Metabolic effects include increased blood levels of glucose, insulin, and free fatty acids. Isoproterenol stimulates renin release from the kidney.

Clinical Indications and Administration

Isoproterenol is used mainly for cardiovascular and respiratory disorders (see Table 14–C1).

Uses for the Cardiovascular System

Isoproterenol, usually given by IV infusion, can be used to manage cardiogenic shock. The drug's ability to both stimulate the heart and dilate peripheral blood vessels gives it an advantage over norepinephrine, for example, which can reduce peripheral blood flow because of its unwanted α-mediated vasoconstrictor activity. Even so, isoproterenol's use for this indication has fallen considerably with the availability of newer and more selective drugs such as dobutamine and dopamine.

Isoproterenol remains an important drug for managing cardiac arrhythmias that seem to be due to inadequate sympathetic stimulation of the heart. These include sinus bradycardia, carotid sinus hypersensitivity, and Stokes–Adams syndrome. In carotid sinus hypersensitivity the baroreceptors act as if blood pressure is too high, triggering reflex cardiac slowing that could involve merely sinus bradycardia, or complete AV block, which is more serious. Stokes–Adams syndrome involves episodes of abrupt hypotension and fainting caused by AV block, ventricular tachycardia, or fibrillation. Isoproterenol is usually given intravenously for acute and life-threatening arrhythmias. It has also been given sublingually (tablets placed under the tongue) for long-term management of some of these rhythm disorders. (Isoproterenol sublingual tablets must not be swallowed; the drug is a catecholamine and so is inactivated by gastric acid.)

Uses for the Respiratory System

For many years, isoproterenol was the most important drug for managing asthma and other respiratory disorders (other than anaphylaxis) in which bronchoconstriction posed a major problem. Parenteral, inhaled, and sublingual dosage forms all were used, the choice depending on the severity of the bronchoconstriction. Isoproterenol is still indicated for these purposes, but it is used much less frequently now that other drugs with more selective actions on the β_2 receptors that mediate bronchoconstriction, and have somewhat lesser effects on the cardiac (β_1) receptors, are available.

Side Effects, Adverse Reactions, and Contraindications

Like most sympathomimetic drugs (see Table 14–S), doses of isoproterenol that are even slightly higher than normal, or usual doses administered to sensitive patients (eg, children, the elderly) may produce signs of CNS stimulation and muscle tremor. More serious adverse responses include tachycardia or tachyarrhythmias, and the potential development or worsening of angina pectoris in patients with coronary artery disease or hyperthyroidism. Isoproterenol shares epinephrine's ability to cause hyperglycemia and related problems for diabetic patients. Isoproterenol accelerates maternal and fetal heart rates. When used near term, it and other β agonists may relax the uterus and prolong labor. Nursing implications noted for most other sympathomimetics, particularly epinephrine, apply.

Interactions with Other Drugs

The major interactions between isoproterenol and other drugs are similar to those noted for epinephrine (see Table 14–I). Interactions causing hypertension are uncommon because isoproterenol lacks vasoconstrictor activity.

Overdose and Toxicity

Most of the problems caused by overdoses of isoproterenol and other β agonists can be managed by *cautious* administration of a β blocker (see Chapter 15). As noted for overdoses of epinephrine, the so-called cardioselective β blockers are preferred if the patient has asthma or obstructive pulmonary disease.

Related Drugs

Nylidrin and Isoxsuprine

The other nonselective β-adrenergic agonists, nylidrin (ARLIDIN) and isoxsuprine (VASODILAN), are used mainly as vasodilators to manage peripheral vascular diseases in which there is poor blood flow to the extremities, such as Raynaud's disease, arteriosclerosis obliterans, gangrene, and frostbite. The same side effects, contraindications, drug–drug interactions, and general precautions noted for isoproterenol apply.

Selective Beta$_1$ Agonists

Dobutamine and dopamine, when given at therapeutic doses, preferentially stimulate β_1 receptors, so cardiac stimulation is the major effect. They are catecholamines, and so their metabolic fates are similar to those noted for epinephrine. They are given by IV infusion. Both drugs have a rapid onset of action and a short duration of action. These properties allow their doses to be titrated precisely as the patient's needs change, and permit rapid recovery from excessive effects from overdoses. This is important, because the drugs are potent, with only slight dose changes causing large effects. Dobutamine and dopamine increase cardiac output and so are used to treat acute heart failure, whether due to sudden worsening of chronic heart failure or to cardiac surgery. This topic is discussed more fully in Chapter 31.

Dobutamine

Dobutamine (DOBUTREX) mainly stimulates cardiac contractile force (a positive inotropic effect), with less change of heart rate than dopamine or isoproterenol causes. The dose (see Table 14–C1) is based on the patient's vital signs before and during drug administration. High doses may cause tachycardia or arrhythmias.

Dopamine

Dopamine is a naturally occurring catecholamine. It functions as a neurotransmitter, particularly in parts of the CNS where it acts on specific dopamine receptors. Synthetic dopamine (INTROPIN) can be used instead of dobutamine as a cardiac stimulant for acute heart failure. It is administered in a similar way.

Low therapeutic doses of dopamine behave much like dobutamine, as a selective cardiac stimulant. The drug also dilates some blood vessels, especially those in the mesentery and kidneys, which may reflect stimulation of either β_2 or dopamine receptors. The overall result is increased cardiac output and peripheral blood flow.

High doses of dopamine may cause arrhythmias. They also cause the adrenergic nerves to release norepinephrine (which explains why some texts classify dopamine as a mixed-acting sympathomimetic). Norepinephrine release due to high doses of dopamine causes peripheral vasoconstriction and decreased perfusion of peripheral organs, particularly the kidneys. It is clearly an unwanted response.

NURSING IMPLICATIONS

Guidelines for storage and dilution of epinephrine apply also to dobutamine and dopamine. If dopamine extravasates it can cause local tissue necrosis. The relevant precautions noted for norepinephrine apply. Because of the potency and rapid actions of these drugs, vital signs must be checked constantly.

Selective Beta$_2$ Agonists

Albuterol and Others

Asthma and emphysema are common chronic pulmonary disorders that benefit from the bronchodilator (β_2) effects of isoproterenol. However, many patients with pulmonary disease have no cardiovascular disorders that would benefit from isoproterenol's ability to also stimulate β_1 receptors. Many other patients have cardiovascular disease, or metabolic disorders such as diabetes, that actually could be made considerably worse by isoproterenol, especially if given long-term to manage chronic lung disease. Research eventually led to the development of several sympathomimetics that are *relatively* selective for the β_2 receptors. The first one approved for use in the United States was albuterol (see below).

This class of drugs has an interesting history that teaches an important lesson. When the drugs were being developed and studied in isolated lung and heart preparations, it was found that they dilated the bronchi just as well as isoproterenol, but they caused much less cardiac stimulation. The hope was that these agents would serve as "selective bronchodilators" and be quite free of many unwanted effects caused by isoproterenol.

However, once these drugs were given to human beings, and enough data were collected to characterize their effects more completely, it was found that *prefer-*

ential β_2-stimulating effects occur only when they are given in low doses and by inhalation, which somewhat confines their actions to the respiratory passages. However, when these drugs are given orally or by injection, or when high doses are given by any route, they cause all the β-mediated cardiovascular and metabolic effects that isoproterenol causes.

Understanding this dose- and route-dependent limitation is critically important, because these drugs have been given with the false assumption that they are totally selective β_2 agonists (or totally selective bronchodilators), and so they will cause no unwanted (or even dangerous) cardiovascular or metabolic side effects. (Even if these drugs were "pure" β_2 agonists, they would dilate some peripheral blood vessels and trigger reflex tachycardia, increase blood glucose levels, and so on.)

Nevertheless, oral, inhaled, and parenteral dosage forms of these drugs were eventually approved and marketed. They have become the preferred agents for causing acute or chronic bronchodilation, regardless of whether the patient has or does not have cardiovascular or metabolic disorders.

Albuterol (PROVENTIL; VENTOLIN) and metaproterenol (ALUPENT; METAPREL) are administered either orally or by inhalation, Terbutaline (BRETHINE; BRICANYL) is given either orally, by inhalation, or by SC injection. Bitolerol (TORNALATE), isoetharine (BRONKOMETER; BRONKOSOL), and pirbuterol (MAXAIR) are administered only by inhalation. Their doses are given in Table 14–C1. The inhalers are designed so that two puffs provide the usual recommended dose. Tolerance to bronchodilation may develop with continued use.

NURSING IMPLICATIONS

There are several key points for the nurse to remember about these important drugs:

1. Regardless of how they are classified, anticipate that these medications can cause all the side effects noted for isoproterenol.
2. Many persons using these drugs will be using other antiasthma drugs that can potentiate CNS and cardiovascular stimulation caused by the sympathomimetic (see isoproterenol). This is another reason close monitoring of pertinent vital signs is essential.
3. All interventions concerning isoproterenol's side effects, contraindications, overdoses, and drug interactions apply also to selective β_2 agonists.
4. Overdoses or interactions are treated as noted for isoproterenol. Be aware, however, that virtually every patient receiving one of the selective β_2 agonists has a pulmonary disorder that could be aggravated by administering a β blocker, the drug of choice for β agonist overdose. Extreme caution must be used, therefore.

More specific information and advice concerning the use of albuterol and similar bronchodilators are found in Chapter 38, which deals specifically with asthma therapy. However, it is important to note here that these drugs should be avoided, if possible, during later stages of pregnancy. The reason will become apparent in the following discussion of ritodrine, a drug with a similar pharmacologic profile, but a very different clinical use.

Ritodrine

Ritodrine (YUTOPAR) is also classified as a relatively selective β_2 agonist. However, it is used only for its effects on the uterus. It relaxes the pregnant uterus and is given to suppress premature labor. Once premature labor has been diagnosed an IV infusion of ritodrine is usually begun. Results obtained from monitoring maternal vital signs, uterine contractions, and fetal heart rate are used to adjust the dose. The ritodrine infusion is usually continued for about 12 hours after uterine contractions stop. Oral therapy is started about 30 minutes before IV administration is stopped, and is continued until it is safe to allow labor to progress.

With oral use, and especially with IV use, excessive stimulation of both maternal or fetal circulatory systems may occur. This reflects activation of both β_1 and β_2 receptors by the drug. For the mother, palpitations and chest pain, possibly reflecting angina pectoris, are key signs of excessive cardiac stimulation. A heart rate over 140 beats per minute that does not return quickly to lower levels when the infusion rate is reduced often predicts developing maternal pulmonary edema; deaths have occurred. Assess closely.

NURSING IMPLICATIONS

Place the mother in the left lateral recumbent position throughout IV ritodrine administration to minimize the risk of hypotension. Monitor fluid intake and output and both maternal and fetal vital signs. Avoid overhydration, which increases the risk of pulmonary edema. Ritodrine administration should be stopped at once if pulmonary edema is suspected.

II. Mixed-Acting Sympathomimetics

Mixed-acting sympathomimetics derived their name because their effects are due to a mixture of two main actions (see Fig. 14–1B): they directly stimulate all α and all β adrenergic receptors, much like epinephrine, and they work indirectly by releasing norepinephrine from adrenergic nerve endings. The prototype is ephedrine. This plant-derived drug has been used for thousands of years, but its value has declined considerably with the development of more effective and more selective sympathomimetics.

PROTOTYPE

Ephedrine

Absorption, Distribution, Metabolism, and Excretion

Ephedrine and the other mixed-acting sympathomimetics are not catecholamines, and so they are not inactivated by gastric acid and can be given orally. Other formulations of ephedrine are administered topically or parenterally. Ephedrine is excreted unchanged by the kidneys.

As a group, mixed-acting sympathomimetics have chemical structures that enable them to enter the CNS much better than the direct-acting sympathomimetics discussed above.

Pharmocologic Effects

Ephedrine causes virtually all the peripheral sympathomimetic effects caused by epinephrine. When the drug is injected, the effects are somewhat more similar to those caused by norepinephrine, especially in terms of cardiovascular effects, of which vasoconstriction and cardiac stimulation predominate. Collectively, ephedrine's peripheral effects are generally weaker in intensity than those caused by epinephrine or norepinephrine, but are more longlasting.

Systemic administration of usual doses of ephedrine or other mixed-acting sympathomimetics generally causes mild CNS stimulation. Responses include slightly increased wakefulness or alertness (called an **analeptic** effect), and increased resistance to fatigue. Appetite may be suppressed also (an **anorexigenic** effect). With continued administration, tolerance develops to many of the peripheral and CNS effects because repeated doses deplete some of the norepinephrine content of nerves, which is an important part of the drug's actions. Higher doses must be given to overcome tolerance and restore the response intensity.

Clinical Indications and Administration

Mixed-acting sympathomimetics have several clinical uses (Table 14–C2). However, in nearly every case in which ephedrine can be used, especially for long-term effects that require a prescription medication, alternative drugs are preferred. That is mainly because ephedrine and other mixed-acting sympathomimetics cause relatively weak effects; cannot selectively stimulate one type of adrenergic receptor without affecting others (and so cause side effects that can be unwanted or frankly dangerous for some patients); tend to cause CNS stimulation even though such effects are not needed; and lose much of their activity, owing to tolerance, with continued use.

Bronchodilation

Before the availability of orally effective β_2 agonists such as albuterol, ephedrine was the major drug used for long-term management of asthma. Because of the limitations noted in the previous paragraph, ephedrine is seldom used anymore; it is found in only a few OTC products. It is still available as an injectable solution for acute bronchospasm, but is rarely used.

Nasal Decongestion

Ephedrine is found in a few topically administered products used to alleviate nasal decongestion. Other mixed-acting sympathomimetics, given orally or topically, are used more commonly.

Management of Acute Hypotension

Ephedrine, given by SC or slow IV injection, is indicated for managing acute hypotension, particularly that which is caused by drugs. The related agents mephentermine and metaraminol (see below), or a direct-acting α agonist such as phenylephrine, is usually used instead.

Other Uses

Ephedrine is used as an adjunct to the management of myasthenia gravis. It seems to increase the release of acetylcholine at the neuromuscular junction. It is also used for its analeptic actions to manage narcolepsy, but other sympathomimetics with greater CNS-stimulating activity, such as the amphetamines, are used more frequently. Ephedrine's weak appetite-suppressant effect is not used clinically.

Side Effects, Adverse Reactions, and Contraindications

The autonomic side effects noted for epinephrine (Table 14–S) apply to ephedrine, other mixed-acting sympathomimetics, and to the indirect-acting sympathomimetics (eg, amphetamine) that are discussed shortly. Central nervous system stimulation can also be considered a side effect. Contraindications for epinephrine also apply. Even nonprescription products containing relatively small amounts of mixed-acting sympathomimetics can cause significant problems for persons with contraindicating conditions that are quite prevalent (eg, glaucoma, diabetes, hypertension).

An important contraindication to the use of any mixed-acting (or indirect-acting) sympathomimetic is *pheochromocytoma,* which is a rare but potentially deadly tumor of the adrenal medulla or other tissues that make large amounts of epinephrine and norepinephrine. The tumor releases the catecholamines into the bloodstream, causing such problems as hypertension and tachycardia. By abruptly releasing even more catecholamines from the tumor, mixed-acting sympathomimetics can cause a hypertensive crisis (and possibly stroke), myocardial infarction, or cardiac arrhythmias.

Interactions with Other Drugs

Mixed-acting sympathomimetics participate in most of the drug–drug interactions noted for epinephrine (Table 14–I) Drugs such as reserpine, which deplete some norepinephrine from adrenergic nerves, will reduce the effectiveness of mixed-acting sympathomimetics, because their actions depend in part on norepinephrine release.

The ability of mixed-acting sympathomimetics to cause catecholamine release can lead to a drug interaction that, though uncommon, is one of the most dangerous drug interactions known to occur. It involves the interaction between mixed-acting (or indirect-acting) sympathomimetics with monoamine oxidase (MAO) inhibitors, which are occasionally used to treat psychiatric depression (see Chapter 24) that does not respond to safer drugs.

Monoamine oxidase is an enzyme found in adrenergic nerve endings, where it helps to regulate the amount of norepinephrine in the nerve ending by metabolically inactivating some of the neurotransmitter that is not stored in synaptic vesicles. When MAO is inhibited, norepinephrine levels in the nerve build up. When a mixed-acting sympathomimetic is given, the extra amount of norepinephrine is released (see Fig. 24–2, p 427). The resulting sympathomimetic responses are greater than normal, and can be dangerous or even life-threatening for some patients.

Monoamine oxidase is also found in the gut and liver. It has an important role in the metabolism of many orally administered sympathomimetics, including ephedrine, as they are being absorbed. Normally, the effects caused by the oral sympathomimetic are due to only the relatively small amount of unmetabolized drug that reaches the systemic circulation. When MAO is inhibited, more drug reaches the circulation, and excessive effects can occur.

NURSING IMPLICATIONS

The interaction between MAO inhibitors and mixed- or indirect-acting sympathomimetics can be fatal. Patients taking an MAO inhibitor should be thoroughly educated to avoid the use of drugs, even those available OTC, that have mixed- or indirect-acting sympathomimetic activity. If sympathomimetic therapy is essential, the MAO inhibitor should be discontinued at least 2 weeks before starting treatment.

Overdose and Toxicity

Overdoses of mixed-acting sympathomimetics mainly involve norepinephrine-like cardiovascular changes plus CNS signs and symptoms that can range from erratic or confused behavior to delirium, hallucinations, or seizures. Central nervous system changes also may cause stimulation of ventilation.

The overdose usually occurs by the oral route, so standard first-aid measures to limit further drug absorption (ie, induced emesis as permitted by the patient's condition; see Appendix C) should be tried first. Thereafter, treatment is symptomatic and supportive, guided by frequent assessment of the patient's vital signs. As noted for epinephrine overdoses, vasodilators may be indicated to lower blood pressure, and combined therapy with both α and β blockers may be helpful.

Monitoring the agitated patient, and protecting them from self-harm, is important. Otherwise, excessive CNS stimulation is best left untreated unless seizures occur, in which case anticonvulsant therapy becomes important. Some clinicians administer CNS depressants to counteract CNS stimulation, but this is dangerous because often the drug-induced depression becomes more of a problem than the prior stimulation. Administration of urinary acidifiers such as ammonium chloride will increase ephedrine excretion, but most poison centers no longer recommend this.

Related Drugs

Two related mixed-acting sympathomimetics are available only by prescription. Two others are found in many OTC products.

Mephentermine and Metaraminol

Mephentermine (WYAMINE) and metaraminol (ARAMINE) are used to manage acute hypotension. Metaraminol acts almost exclusively as a vasoconstrictor (α agonist). Mephentermine constricts most arterioles, but also dilates others, through β_2 responses, and so may cause less of a reduction in blood flow to vital organs. The drugs are generally given by IM injection to prevent hypotension (as before giving a spinal anesthetic), and by IV injection or infusion (depending on the urgency of the situation) for treating hypotension. Dosages for SC injection are listed in the package inserts, but this route is seldom used because local tissue irritation can occur, and because drugs injected subcutaneously are slowly and unreliably absorbed if the patient is already hypotensive.

Mephentermine or metaraminol should not be mixed with other drugs in the same syringe, or administered in the same IV line that is being used to deliver other medications.

Phenylpropanolamine and Pseudoephedrine

Phenylpropanolamine (often abbreviated "PPA") and pseudoephedrine (eg, SUDAFED) are the mixed-acting sympathomimetics found in most OTC nasal decongestants and cold/allergy remedies. They are discussed at the end of the chapter in the section devoted to the use of these nonprescription remedies. Typical dosages are noted in Table 14–C2.

III. Indirect-Acting Sympathomimetics

By definition, drugs classified as indirect-acting sympathomimetics exert their effects *only* by releasing endogenous catecholamines—mainly norepinephrine from adrenergic nerves (see Fig. 14–1C); and, to a lesser extent, epinephrine from the adrenal medulla. Unlike ephedrine and other mixed-acting sympathomimetics, they do not have even weak direct actions on adrenergic receptors. The prototype *class* of indirect-acting sympathomimetics is the amphetamines.

PROTOTYPE

Amphetamines

Amphetamines are sympathomimetic drugs that exert powerful CNS-stimulating actions. The CNS stimulation provides the main reason for their use, and their widespread abuse. Like addictive drugs such as morphine, amphetamines are classified as Schedule II substances under the federal Controlled Substances Act.

What follows is a short overview of the general pharmacologic properties, and peripheral autonomic effects, of mixed-acting sympathomimetics, focusing on amphetamines. More inforamtion is found in Chapter 27, which deals with CNS stimulants, and in Chapter 28, which is devoted to the more general issues of substance abuse.

Pharmacologic Effects

Because amphetamines act mainly by releasing norepinephrine, their peripheral autonomic effects are very similar to those of norepinephrine itself. They increase blood pressure; increase or decrease heart rate, depending on how much the baroreceptor reflex is activated by blood pressure changes; decongest mucous membranes; dilate the pupil of the eye; and cause several effects on glucose and fat metabolism.

More importantly, they enter the CNS well, causing stimulatory effects that are much more intense than those caused by other sympathomimetics, and that provide the major reason these drugs are abused.

Tolerance develops to the peripheral and CNS effects. It occurs quickly, often after only one or two doses. This rapidly developing tolerance to drug action is called **tachyphylaxis.** A major cause of tolerance to amphetamines relates to their mechanism of action: they release norepinephrine from nerves, and if the interval between one dose and the next is too short, there is inadequate time for the nerves to replenish their neurotransmitter stores, and so the intensity of the response diminishes.

Clinical Indications and Administration

Amphetamines are no longer approved for use for their peripheral sympathomimetic effects. Their indications all relate to their effects in the CNS (see Chapter 27). They include management of narcolepsy, in which their general CNS stimulating effects are helpful; treatment of attention deficit disorder in children, in which these drugs exert a paradoxical "depressant" effect on psychomotor activity; and adjunctive treatment of life-threatening obesity, for which their profound appetite-suppressant (anorexigenic) effects are of some value. Federal, state, and institutional laws and policies place tight controls on the use, prescribing, and dispensing of amphetamines.

Side Effects, Contraindications, Drug Interactions, and Toxicity

Because of how amphetamines work, their peripheral autonomic side effects, related contraindications, drug–drug interactions, and signs and symptoms of toxicity are basically identical to those noted for the direct-acting agonists epinephrine and norepinephrine, and for the mixed-acting sympathomimetic ephedrine. Cardiovascular problems, especially hypertension, usually are the most important and most dangerous concerns involving the peripheral nervous system. In addition, excessive CNS stimulation becomes problematic; seizures are a potential consequence of overdoses. See Chapter 27 for more details about these issues and their management.

Related Agent

Tyramine

Tyramine, derived from the common amino acid tyrosine, is rarely used as a drug. This indirect-acting sympathomimetic has much toxicologic importance, however. Tyramine is abundant in dairy products (aged or strong cheeses, yogurt); some fruits and vegetables (avocados, bananas, figs, raisins, fava beans); alcoholic beverages (dark beers, chianti, and sherry wines); liver, salami, sausage, and similar highly processed meats; pickled herring; and most breads prepared with yeast.

The tyramine content of these foods and beverages is too low to cause sympathomimetic effects in normal individuals. That is because tyramine, a monoamine, is metabolically inactivated by MAO as it is absorbed from the gut. However, in persons taking MAO inhibitors, enough unmetabolized tyramine can reach the systemic circulation that sympathomimetic effects will occur. Since MAO inhibitors increase the amount of norepinephrine stored in the nerve ending, and because tyramine will suddenly increase that excess neurotransmitter, dangerous or even life-threatening episodes of hypertension and cardiac stimulation will occur.

IV. Other Drugs That Cause or Intensify Sympathomimetic Effects

There are other clinically important ways by which drugs produce or intensify sympathomimetic effects. Each is discussed briefly here.

Interference with Norepinephrine Reuptake

Cocaine, and a group of drugs called tricyclic antidepressants, interfere with the reuptake of norepinephrine released from adrenergic nerves. They block the neuronal "amine pump," the major way that the activity of released norepinephrine is stopped.

Cocaine

Cocaine, one of the most well-known drugs of abuse, produces marked centrally mediated euphoric effects plus important peripheral sympathomimetic actions. These effects are largely the result of inhibition of norepinephrine reuptake in the periphery and in the CNS. In the presence of cocaine, norepinephrine released by normal nerve activity accumulates in the neuroeffector junction, thus intensifying its effects. Since norepinephrine is an α and β_1 agonist, cocaine heightens only the responses mediated by those receptors. Cocaine also intensifies the responses produced by injected norepinephrine and dopamine, since these catecholamines are handled in part by reuptake into nerves.

Cocaine also blocks the uptake of drugs that must enter the nerve to exert their effects. For example, it reduces the actions of mixed-acting sympathomimetics such as ephedrine. Ephedrine's actions are not completely abolished because it can still stimulate adrenergic receptors directly, although weakly. Cocaine completely abolishes responses to indirect-acting sympathomimetics, such as amphetamines.

Cocaine acts directly as a potent vasoconstrictor and local anesthetic. These actions are discussed more fully in Chapter 19. Although the peripheral effects of cocaine are interesting and often important, it is best known as a CNS stimulant, which has earned it the dubious honor of being a major drug of abuse. Its CNS actions and abuse characteristics are discussed in Chapters 27 and 28.

Tricyclic Antidepressants

Imipramine and several related drugs called *tricyclic antidepressants* are first-line agents for treating psychiatric depression. Among their pharmacologic effects is the ability to block norepinephrine reuptake, as described for cocaine. Therefore, tricyclic antidepressants potentiate the sympathetic responses to normal adrenergic nerve stimulation, reduce the effects of ephedrine and other mixed-acting sympathomimetics, and abolish the effects of cocaine. Other aspects of antidepressant pharmacology are presented in Chapter 24.

Interference with Feedback Regulation of Norepinephrine Release

Yohimbine is an unusual drug that is seldom used clinically. It selectively *blocks* the presynaptic α_2 receptor that, when stimulated, normally stops norepinephrine release from adrenergic nerves. In the presence of yohimbine, norepinephrine release continues longer than normal, so sympathomimetic effects are intensified.

Miscellaneous Drugs That Cause Norepinephrine Release

Bretylium, a drug used to treat cardiac arrhythmias (see Chapter 30), initially releases norepinephrine from adrenergic nerves, causing a sympathomimetic effect. Guanethidine, a rarely used antihypertensive drug, does the same when it is first given. Interestingly, once the sympathomimetic effects have passed these drugs actually cause long-term suppression of sympathetic nerve activity (a sympatholytic effect).

V. Sympathomimetics Used in Over-the-Counter Medications

Sympathomimetics with α-adrenergic agonist activity are found in the hundreds of asthma, appetite-suppressant, cough, cold, allergy, and nasal and ophthalmic decongestant remedies that are available without prescription. Table 14–3 lists some major product categories and the sympathomimetics they contain. The direct-acting α agonists include phenylephrine, naphazoline, oxymetazoline, tetrahydrozoline, and xylometazoline. (Miscellaneous sympathomimetics with α-agonist activity, such as propylhexedrine and levodesoxyephedrine, are found in a small number of in-

Table 14–3 Sympathomimetic Drugs in Some Major Over-the-Counter Product Groups

Product Group*	Ephedrine	Epinephrine	Naphazoline	Oxymetazoline	Phenylephrine	Phenylpropanolamine	Pseudoephedrine	Tetrahydrozoline	Xylometazoline
Antitussives					X	X	X		
Appetite suppressants						X			
Asthma aerosols (inhaled)		X							
Asthma bronchodilators	X								
Cold and allergy combinations					X†	X	X		
Nasal decongestants (topical)	X†		X†	X	X				X†
Ophthalmic decongestants (topical)			X	X	X			X	

*Products are given orally unless noted otherwise. Oral bronchodilators for asthma and cold/allergy products often contain other drugs that may add to symptom relief, may cause other side effects, or have other contraindications: for example, theophylline (Chapter 38) in oral asthma remedies; antihistamines and/or analgesics-antipyretics (Chapters 51 and 52) in cold and allergy products. Some sympathomimetics not found in OTC products may be available in prescription medications.

†Drug is found in very few OTC medications within this product group.

haled nasal decongestant OTC products. They will not be discussed further.) The common mixed-acting sympathomimetics used in OTC products are phenylpropanolamine and pseudoephedrine.

Medications containing any of these products are intended for short-term relief of minor symptoms. In general, their side effects, contraindications, and drug interactions are similar to those noted for their respective prototypes, phenylephrine and ephedrine.

Oxymetazoline and Xylometazoline

Oxymetazoline and xylometazoline are ingredients in several OTC nasal decongestant sprays and mists. They have a longer duration of action than phenylephrine, and so they need to be administered only once or twice a day. This has theoretical advantages, as noted below.

The use of nasal decongestant sprays or drops, regardless of their ingredients, should be limited to a few days of treatment. Chronic use of excessive doses may produce drug-induced nasal irritation or inflammation (**rhinitis medicamentosa**). These products should not be used if the patient already has rhinitis.

A more serious problem of improper nasal decongestant use is *rebound nasal congestion*. Initial doses of the product may produce desired symptomatic relief, but if the patient continues to use the drug for more than a couple of days in a row more severe congestion occurs as the effects of each dose wear off. This favors habitual use and the need to exceed recommended doses, thereby increasing the risk of adverse systemic effects and damage to the nasal mucosa.

Naphazoline and Tetrahydrozoline

Naphazoline and tetrahydrozoline are found in several topical ophthalmic decongestants marketed to alleviate ocular symptoms of hay fever or other mild allergies. Unlike other α agonists, high doses of naphazoline produce CNS depression, rather than stimulation. Precautions that apply to the use of prescription ocular products apply to the OTC agents as well.

Phenylpropanolamine

Phenylpropanolamine (PPA) is the most common decongestant ingredient in OTC *oral* medications marketed for symptomatic relief of nasal stuffiness or rhinorrhea due to the common cold and mild respiratory tract allergies. It is also found in some cough remedies, and a few prescription medications for relief of cold and allergy symptoms.

Phenylpropanolamine has a weak anorexigenic action, and so is the active ingredient in most OTC weight-reduction aids. There is disagreement over whether these products, when combined with a proper diet, are better than diet alone to help individuals lose weight. Obviously, a supervised diet, with exercise, is safer than drugs for patients with diseases that contraindicate sympathomimetic drug use, or persons taking drugs that interact with sympathomimetics. Many people believe that a larger dose will increase relief of cold symptoms, or make weight loss faster or easier; usually all it does is increase the risk of adverse effects.

Pseudoephedrine

Pseudoephedrine (SUDAFED) is used orally as a decongestant for symptomatic relief of the common cold or seasonal allergies. Like phenylpropanolamine, pseudoephedrine is found in many OTC products. It has no obvious therapeutic advantages over ephedrine, and is often more expensive.

General Nursing Implications for OTC Cold and Allergy Preparations

There are many OTC oral and topically applied products available for people who do not wish to suffer even minor distress from symptoms of the common cold, allergies, or flu. Each product is advertised to have some unique property that helps it relieve symptoms faster or better than a competing product, or ingredients that enable it to alleviate many symptoms at once. There are so many products with claims of superiority that even experienced health-care professionals find it difficult to recommend (or purchase for personal use) one product over another. What follows is information that can help you use or recommend such medications wisely. Drugs that are discussed in other chapters are cross-referenced.

1. Identify the symptom(s) for which relief is sought.
2. Identify all the drugs in the product so drug actions can be matched with symptoms to be treated, and so the use of drugs that are contraindicated (whether because of disease or potential interactions) can be avoided. Don't use a "shotgun" approach. Common ingredients include:
    - sympathomimetics: found in nearly all orally administered and topical products; they act solely, but often effectively, as decongestants; most products are more alike, rather than different, with respect to having a sympathomimetic as an ingredient

- antihistamines: in many oral products (Chapter 51); dry secretions through antimuscarinic actions, cause typical atropine-like side effects; are generally irrational when symptoms are not caused by allergy; can cause significant CNS depression, and so are common ingredients in products advertised for night-time relief; have risk of excessive CNS depression, drug interactions
- cough suppressants (antitussives; Chapter 21): useful for cough, needless otherwise
- alcohol (Chapter 22): has no known effect on cold or allergy symptoms, is more important because of added CNS depression, potential for drug interactions
- analgesics/antipyretics (Chapter 52): useful if mild aches and pains, or fever, are present, needless otherwise; aspirin is contraindicated for many patients (eg, those with asthma), interacts with many other drugs; acetaminophen has potential for liver, renal damage with long-term high-dose use

3. Keep current in terms of products and their ingredients. Manufacturers may reformulate their products by adding, deleting, or substituting an ingredient, but they may not always change the product name. These changes may not be included in the most recent reference books available to you (eg, the *PDR for Nonprescription Drugs; Drug Facts & Comparisons*). When in doubt, check with a pharmacist.
4. Use topical products (eg, nasal drops or sprays) instead of oral products when mucous membrane congestion is the major symptom to be relieved.
   - drops and sprays help localize effects to the desired sites of action, thereby minimizing (but not eliminating) unwanted or dangerous systemic effects. In addition, topical products usually contain only one active ingredient, a sympathomimetic, thereby reducing the number of side effects, drug interactions, and risks owing to contraindications. Relatively few oral products contain only one ingredient, but it is worth looking for one if only one desired effect is needed.
   - When selecting nasal drops or sprays, pick one with a long-acting ingredient (eg, oxymetazoline or xylometazoline) to minimize such problems as rebound nasal congestion that are more common with short-acting drugs.
5. Use products specifically labeled for pediatric use when treating a child. Use nasal drops for very small children and infants, as it is very difficult to give the proper dosage of nasal sprays. Get advice from a physician if the child is less than 2 years old.
6. Follow all label guidelines concerning dosage and duration of therapy; and warnings related to adverse effects or contraindications. Explain the information to patients who may be unable to read or understand them, or who may be unaware or unsure of contraindicating medical conditions or the use of interacting drugs. Avoid the false yet common belief that if the recommended dose is good, twice the dose is twice as good.
7. Be aware that symptoms of the common cold are self-limiting; they are likely to disappear in spite of drug therapy, not because of it. Weigh the anticipated benefits of taking a medication against the potential risks.
8. Interpret advertising claims and slogans with knowledge, objectivity, and a grain of skepticism. Products advertised to relieve a long list of symptoms usually contain a relatively long list of ingredients—each with one or more potential contraindications, side effects, and so on. Products that "won't interfere with sleep" tend to cause drowsiness or sleepiness, and can cause significant problems with daytime activities. Conversely, other products that "won't make you sleepy" often cause unpleasant jitteriness during waking hours, and could interfere with sleep if taken late in the day.
9. Shop wisely. In general, brand name products are more expensive, but not more effective, than store-brand medications with the same ingredients.

SUMMARY OF NURSING IMPLICATIONS

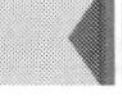

Assessment

Before initiating sympathomimetic drug therapy, ensure that no underlying conditions are present to contraindicate drug use (eg, arrhythmias, hypertension, narrow-angle glaucoma, hyperthyroidism, prostatic hypertrophy).

Take a medication history, noting current use of drugs that may interact with sympathomimetic agents.

Note the patient's baseline physical assessment, to recognize desired and untoward effects of drug therapy.

Nursing Diagnoses

Decreased cardiac output related to drug intolerance.

Altered peripheral tissue perfusion related to vasoconstriction.

Impaired tissue integrity related to extravasation of vasoconstrictor drug.

Sensory/perceptual alterations related to drug side effects: insomnia, dizziness.

Urinary retention related to bladder sphincter spasm.

Knowledge deficit regarding drug regimen: potential drug abuse.

◆ Planning/Implementation

Administer the medication safely; check for appropriate route of administration and drug concentration.

Monitor closely for signs of cardiovascular problems, particularly with IV administration; document the ECG; determine patient's normal blood pressure.

Provide a restful, quiet environment to promote sleep; reduce noise; modify group care as needed to provide rest periods; limit visitors; administer drugs well before bedtime.

Check IV sites regularly for signs of infiltration, extravasation (eg, blanched, hard, cold, discolored skin); use infusion pump to ensure accurate drug delivery rate; secure IV site when moving patient.

Regularly check stock of drugs for color, clarity of solutions, expiration dates.

Maintain adequate fluid intake and output; check for bladder distention; have patient void before taking drug if there is a history of prostatic hypertrophy.

Be familiar with drugs used in emergency treatments and overdoses; have life-support equipment and antidotes readily available.

Support and encourage patient when side effects occur; explain effects of drug.

◆ Patient and Family Teaching

Instruct patient on: self-administration of medications; avoiding OTC drugs, particularly cold remedies and diet pills; problems associated with rebound drug effects and dependence; importance of reporting difficult voiding, chest pain, difficult breathing, or headache; precautions to take when side effects occur (avoid driving if anxious or excited; use sunglasses for photophobia; sit down and rest if palpitations occur).

◆ Evaluation

The patient/family will:

Experience no adverse cardiac or respiratory effects: rate and rhythm normal; blood pressure normal; airway is unobstructed (no wheezing or dyspnea).

Comply with drug regimen; take medication as prescribed; ensure that side effects are absent or tolerable.

Be knowledgeable regarding safe administration, potential side effects, and drug interactions to avoid.

Ensure that no injuries associated with drug therapy occur (eg, falls while ambulating; tissue necrosis); habituation does not occur.

Return for routine follow-up; receive adequate outpatient care.

Annotated Bibliography

Brodde OE. Beta- and alpha-adrenoceptor-agonists and -antagonists in chronic heart failure. *Basic Res Cardiol* 1990;85 (Suppl. 1):57–66. *A valuable article for students wishing more information about how α and β receptors, and drugs that affect them, play a role in heart failure.*

Brown CG, Werman HA. Adrenergic agonists during cardiopulmonary resuscitation. *Resuscitation* 1990;19(1):1–16. *In CPR, is too little epinephrine used too late? This interesting article addresses this and other questions about the current and future roles of sympathomimetics in managing cardiac arrest, for which survival statistics are grim.*

Chatterjee K, De Marco T. Central and peripheral adrenergic receptor agonists in heart failure. *Eur Heart J* 1989;10(Suppl. B):55–63. *A worthwhile overview of how central and peripheral adrenergic receptors play a part in the pathophysiology and treatment of heart failure.*

Dei Cas L, Metra M, Visioli O. Clinical pharmacology of inodilators. *J Cardiovasc Pharmacol* 1989;14(Suppl. 8):S60–71. *A good review of how drugs that both stimulate the heart and dilate the peripheral vasculature can have an important role in the management of heart failure.*

Handbook of Nonprescription Drugs. 9th ed. American Pharmaceutical Association, Washington, DC, 1990. *Your single most valuable reference for easy-to-find information about OTC drugs—uses, limitations, ingredients, dosages. Chapters most related to sympathomimetics include those on Cold and Allergy Products (by Bryant and Lombardi, Ch. 8); Asthma Products (Kelly and Lindley, Ch. 9); and Ophthalmics (Gourley, Ch. 20). The minichapter by Veerman and Mardadis (Appendix B) gives valuable information about pediatric products.*

Hurvitz LM, Kaufman PL, Robin AL, Weinreb RN, Crawford K, Shaw B. New developments in the drug treatment of glaucoma. *Drugs* 1991;41(4):514–532. *A thorough but thoroughly readable summary of current and future drug therapies—with sympathetic agents and others—for this common eye disorder.*

McAuliffe-Curtin D, Buckley C. Review of alpha adrenoceptor function in the eye. *Eye* 1989;3(Pt. 4):472–476. *Summarizes the roles of α-receptors, and drugs that affect them, in the management of chronic simple glaucoma.*

Smith CV. Reversing acute intrapartum fetal distress using tocolytic drugs. *Clin Obstet Gynecol* 1991;34(2):352–359. *A worthwhile article for those interested in more information about the use of uterine-relaxing (tocolytic) drugs in the management of premature labor and fetal distress.*

Table 14–C1 Clinical Uses and Administration of Major Direct-Acting Sympathomimetic Drugs

AGENT	CLINICAL USES	DOSAGE AND ROUTE OF ADMINISTRATION
Nonselective (Alpha and Beta) Agonists		
PROTOTYPE		
Epinephrine		
(ADRENALIN CHLORIDE)	Treatment of broncho-constriction, anaphylaxis	SC (preferred) or IM: Adults: 0.3–0.5 mg, depending on symptom severity. Children ≤ 12: 0.01 mg/kg (0.3 mg/m^2 body surface area) up to 0.5 mg maximum
	Cardiac resuscitation	IV or Intracardiac: Dilute 0.5–1 mg with 10 mL sterile normal saline and inject after starting CPR
	Adjunct to spinal anesthesia (prevention, control of hypotension)	Various routes for spinal anesthesia: Add 0.2–0.4 mg to anesthetic
	Prolongation of local (cutaneous) anesthesia	Infiltration: Use concentrations of 1:100,000 (0.01 mg/mL)–1:20,000 (0.05 mg/mL)
(EPIPEN, EPIPEN JR)	Bronchoconstriction, as for regular epinephrine (for self-administration by patient)	SC: EPIPEN (for adults) delivers 0.3 mg; EPIPEN JR (for children) delivers 0.15 mg
(SUS-PHRINE) (sustained-acting suspension)	More prolonged broncho-dilation than with regular epinephrine, as for acute asthma, anaphylaxis	SC: Adults: 0.5–1.5 mg given not more than q6h. Children 1 month–12 years: 0.025 mg/kg; maximum dose for children < 30 kg is 0.75 mg
(BRONKAID; MEDIHALER-EPI; PRIMATENE; VAPONEFRIN)	Management of infrequent mild wheezing or bronchoconstriction, as in asthma	Inhaler: For adults and responsible children > 6: 1 puff of metered-dose inhaler as needed, not to exceed 1 puff q3–4h or 5 puffs per day
(EPIFRIN; EPINAL; EPITRATE; EPPY/N; GLAUCON)	Ophthalmic decongestion, hemorrhage control, mydriasis, reduction of intraocular pressure	Topical: Dilute to 1:10,000 (0.1 mg/mL)–1:1,000 (1 mg/mL) and apply to eye(s)
RELATED DRUGS		
Dipivefrin hydrochloride		
(PROPINE)	Chronic open-angle glaucoma	Topical: 1 drop q12h
Norepinephrine bitartrate		
(LEVOPHED)	Treatment of acute hypotension; adjunctive treatment of cardiac arrest	IV: Initially infuse at 8–12 μg/min, adjust to maintain systolic BP between 80–100 mm Hg (usually 2–4 μg/min); limit infusion rate to 2 μg/min for children. (Note: if patient was hypertensive before event, raise systolic BP to no more than 40 mm Hg less than previous systolic BP.)
Selective Alpha Agonists		
PROTOTYPE		
Phenylephrine hydrochloride		
(NEO-SYNEPHRINE)	Management of mild-to-moderate hypotension	SC, IM: 2–5 mg (0.2–0.5 mL of 1% solution) IV: 0.2 mg, repeating at intervals of no more than 10–15 min if needed
	Management of severe hypotension	IV infusion: Initially 100–180 μg/min, then 40–60 μg/min based on vital signs when patient stabilizes

(continued)

Table 14–C1 Clinical Uses and Administration of Major Direct-Acting Sympathomimetic Drugs (*Continued*)

AGENT	CLINICAL USES	DOSAGE AND ROUTE OF ADMINISTRATION
	Management of paroxysmal atrial or supraventricular tachycardia, hypotensive emergencies	IV injection: Use doses noted for mild-to-moderate hypotension but give by direct IV injection; do not exceed initial dose of 0.5 mg
	Adjunct to spinal anesthesia: prevention, treatment of hypotension	SC or IM: 2–3 mg given 3–4 min before injecting anesthetic for preventing hypotension IV: 0.1–0.2 mg to treat hypotension
	Prolongation of spinal anesthetic action	Various spinal routes: Add 2–5 mg to desired anesthetic solution
	Prolongation of local (cutaneous) anesthesia	Infiltration: Add 1 mg to every 20 mL of anesthetic solution
	Ophthalmic decongestion, mydriasis	Topical: Anesthetize cornea, then apply 1 drop of 10% solution; repeat after 1 hr if needed
	Uveitis; prevention, treatment of iris adhesions (synechiae)	Topical: Apply 1 drop of 2.5% or 10% solution; repeat as necessary; use adjunctively with anticholinergics, hot compresses
	Treatment of open-angle glaucoma	Topical: 1 drop of 2.5% or 10% solution on each eye; use with anticholinergics; repeat as needed
	Ocular examinations: retinal observation, measurement of refractive errors	Topical: 1 drop of 2.5% solution; use with anticholinergic for cycloplegia when needed (as for determining refractive errors of lens)
	Preoperative mydriasis	Topical: Apply 1 drop of 2.5% or 10% solution 30–60 min before eye surgery
	Diagnosis of angle-closure glaucoma	Topical: Measure intraocular pressure, then apply 2.5% solution; 3–5 mm Hg pressure rise may indicate angle closure
	Minor eye irritation	Topical: 1–2 drops of 0.12% solution bid–qid
	Nasal decongestion	Topical: Adults: 1 or 2 sprays of 0.25% (or 0.5% or 1% for resistant cases) solution q4h; children > 6: 1 or 2 sprays of 0.25% solution q3–4h; children 2–6: 1 drop of 0.125% or 0.2% solution q2–4h
RELATED DRUGS		
Methoxamine (VASOXYL)	Treatment of acute (eg, intraoperative) hypotension	IV: 3–5 mg IM: 10–20 mg
Naphazoline (various products)	Nasal decongestion	Topical: Adults, children ≥ 12: 2 drops of 0.05% solution q3h
	Ocular vasoconstriction/decongestion	Topical: 1 or 2 drops (strengths from 0.012%–0.1%) q3–4h
Oxymetazoline (various products)	Nasal decongestion	Topical: Adults, children ≥ 6: 2 or 3 drops or sprays of 0.05% solution AM and PM; children 2–5: 2 or 3 drops or sprays of 0.025% solution AM and PM
	Ocular irritation	Topical: 1 or 2 drops of 0.025% solution q6h
Tetrahydrozoline (various products)	Nasal decongestion	Topical: Adults, children ≥ 6: 2–4 drops of 0.1% solution q3h; children 2–6: 2 or 3 drops of 0.05% solution q4–6h
	Ocular decongestion	Topical: 1 or 2 drops of 0.05% solution bid–qid

(continued)

Table 14–C1 Clinical Uses and Administration of Major Direct-Acting Sympathomimetic Drugs (*Continued*)

AGENT	CLINICAL USES	DOSAGE AND ROUTE OF ADMINISTRATION
Xylometazoline (various products)	Nasal decongestion	Topical: Adults, children ≥ 12: 2 or 3 drops or sprays of 0.1% solution q8–10h; children 2–12: 2 or 3 drops of 0.05% solution q8–10h
	Nonselective Beta ($Beta_1$ and $Beta_2$) Agonists	
PROTOTYPE		
Isoproterenol		
(ISUPREL)	Acute heart failure	IV infusion: Initially 0.5–5 μg/min, then adjust according to vital signs
	Adjunctive treatment of cardiac arrest, certain cardiac arrhythmias (eg, AV block, Stokes–Adams syndrome)	IV injection: Initially 0.02–0.06 mg (1–3 mL), followed by repeated doses of 0.01–0.2 mg (0.5–10 mL) as needed IV infusion: 5 μg/min IM: Initially 0.2 mg followed by 0.02–1 mg as needed SC: Initially 0.2 mg followed by 0.15–0.2 mg as needed Intracardiac: 0.02 mg (for cardiac arrest only)
	Management of intraoperative bronchospasm	IV: Initially 0.01–0.02 mg (0.5–1 mL); repeat as needed
(ISUPREL GLOSSETS)	Management of chronic syncope, as in Stokes–Adams syndrome	Sublingual: 10 or 15 mg as needed
	Management of chronic bronchoconstriction, as in asthma	Sublingual: Adults: Usually 10 mg, no more than 60 mg/day. Children: Usually 5 or 10 mg as for adults, not to exceed 30 mg/day
(ISUPREL, MEDIHALER-ISO)	Management of bronchospasm in asthma, chronic obstructive pulmonary disease (COPD)	Inhalation: Adults: One or two puffs of metered-dose inhaler; repeat up to 6 times a day depending on severity of symptoms Hand nebulizer: Adults or children: Usually 5–15 deep inhalations of a nebulized 1:200 (5 mg/mL) solution (adults), 1:200 (5 mg/mL) solution (children)
RELATED DRUGS		
Ethylnorepinephrine		
(BRONKEPHRINE)	Management of acute bronchospasm	SC or IM: Adults: 1–2 mg repeated as needed. Children: 0.2–1 mg depending on age, weight
Isoxsuprine hydrochloride		
(VASODILAN)	Management of cerebrovascular insufficiency, peripheral vascular disease	Oral: 10 or 20 mg tid or qid
Nylidrin hydrochloride		
(ARLIDIN)	Management of peripheral vascular disease, ischemic disorders of inner ear	Oral: 3–12 mg tid or qid

(continued)

Table 14–C1 Clinical Uses and Administration of Major Direct-Acting Sympathomimetic Drugs (*Continued*)

AGENT	CLINICAL USES	DOSAGE AND ROUTE OF ADMINISTRATION
"Selective" Beta$_2$ Agonists		
Dobutamine		
(DOBUTREX)	Management of acute heart failure	IV: Infuse 2.5–10 μg/kg body weight/min (more or less depending on vital signs)
Dopamine hydrochloride		
(INTROPIN)	Management of acute heart failure	IV: Infuse at initial rate of 2–5 μg/kg/min, increasing to about 20 μg/kg min if needed
Albuterol sulfate		
(PROVENTIL; VENTOLIN)	Bronchodilation in asthma, other forms of COPD	Inhalation: Adults, children > 12: 1 to 2 puffs of metered-dose inhaler; repeat q4–6h Oral: Adults, children > 12: 2–4 mg tid–qid; maximum 8 mg qid if necessary. Children 6–14: 2 mg tid–qid; children 2–6: 0.1 mg/kg (or 2 mg, whichever is less) 3 tid
Bitolterol mesylate		
(TORNALATE)	Bronchodilation, as for albuterol	Inhalation: Adults, children > 12: 2 puffs of metered-dose inhaler q8h
Isoetharine mesylate or hydrochloride		
(BRONKOMETER, BRONKOSOL)	Bronchodilation, as for albuterol	Inhalation: metered-dose inhaler: Adults: 1 or 2 puffs no more often than q4h Hand nebulizer or intermittent positive-pressure breathing (IPPB) apparatus: see package insert
Metaproterenol sulfate		
(ALUPENT, METAPREL)	Bronchodilation, as for albuterol	Inhalation: Adults only: 3 puffs of metered-dose inhaler q3–4h as needed; maximum 12 puffs per day Hand nebulizer: 10 inhalations of undiluted 5% solution no more often than q4h IPPB devices: 0.3 mL tid or qid Oral: Tablets: Adults: 20 mg tid or qid. Children 6–9 years or < 60 lbs: 10 mg tid or qid; > 9 years or > 60 lbs: 20 mg tid or qid Syrup: Adults, children > 6 or > 60 lbs: same dosage as for tablets; children < 6: approx. 1.3–2.6 mg/kg/d in divided doses (use syrup only)
Pirbuterol		
(MAXAIR)	Bronchodilation, as for albuterol	Inhalation: Adults, children > 12: 2 puffs of metered-dose inhaler 4–6qh (up to 12 inhalations/day maximum)
Ritodrine hydrochloride		
(YUTOPAR)	Suppression of premature uterine contractions (premature labor)	IV: Infuse initially at 100 μg/min, increasing gradually to 150–350 μg/min based on monitoring of uterine activity, maternal and fetal vital signs; continue up to 12 hr, switch to oral route if longer treatment needed Oral: 10 mg q2h for first 24 hr; maintenance dose is 10 to 20 mg q4–6h; begin first oral dose 30 min before stopping IV

(continued)

Table 14–C1 | Clinical Uses and Administration of Major Direct-Acting Sympathomimetic Drugs (*Continued*)

AGENT	CLINICAL USES	DOSAGE AND ROUTE OF ADMINISTRATION
Terbutaline Sulfate		
(BRETHINE, BRICANYL)	Brochodilation, as for albuterol	Oral: Adults: 2.5–5 mg 6qh during waking hours (not to exceed 15 mg in any 24-hr period). Children 12–15: 2.5 mg tid
	Immediate bronchodilation for acute bronchospasm	SC: 0.25 mg, repeated if improvement not seen in 15–30 min (not to exceed 0.5 mg per 4-hr period)
(BRETHAIRE)	Bronchodilation, as for albuterol	Inhalation: Adults, children > 12: 2 puffs of metered dose inhaler q4–6h

Table 14–C2 | Clinical Uses and Administration of Major Mixed-Acting Sympathomimetic Drugs

AGENT	CLINICAL USES	DOSAGE AND ROUTE OF ADMINISTRATION
PROTOTYPE		
Ephedrine (in various proprietary products)	Symptomatic relief of mild asthma, seasonal allergies	Oral: Adults: 25 or 50 mg initially, then 25 mg q4h. Children 6–12: one-half adult dose or 3 mg/kg/day in divided doses
	Treatment of hypotension, shock	SC: 15–50 mg IV: 20 mg injected slowly
RELATED DRUGS		
Mephentermine		
(WYAMINE)	Treatment of hypotension, shock (including drug induced)	IV: 30–45 mg; additional 30-mg doses if needed
	Prevention of hypotension due to spinal anesthesia	IM: 30–45 mg 10–20 min before giving anesthetic; 15 mg in obstetric patients
Metaraminol		
(ARAMINE)	Treatment of hypotension, shock	IV: Infuse 15–100 mg in 250–500 mL saline or D_5W slowly to reach and maintain desired blood pressure; for severe shock inject 0.5–5 mg directly, followed by infusion of 0.5–1 mg/mL or more of appropriate parenteral solution
	Prevention of hypotension due to spinal anesthesia	IM or SC: 2–10 mg 10–20 min before giving anesthetic
Phenylpropanolamine (in various proprietary products)	Symptomatic relief of nasal congestion from the common cold, rhinitis, sinusitis, or seasonal allergies	Oral: Adults: 25 mg q4h (150 mg/24 hr maximum). Children 6 to < 12: 12.5 mg q4h (75 mg/24 hr maximum). Children 2 to < 6: 6.25 mg q4h (37.5 mg/24 hr maximum)
Pseudoephedrine		
(SUDAFED, others)	Symptomatic relief of nasal, eustachian tube congestion	Oral: Adults: 60 mg q4h (240 mg/24 hr maximum). Children 6 to < 12: 30 mg q4h (120 mg/24 hr maximum). Children 2 to < 6: 15 mg q4h (60 mg/24 hr maximum)

Table 14–S | Major Side Effects and Contraindications of Sympathomimetic Drugs

BODY SYSTEM/ Side Effect	CONTRAINDICATION/ PRECAUTION	COMMENTS AND NURSING IMPLICATIONS
Major Side Effects of Sympathomimetics with Alpha Agonist Activity		
EYE Mydriasis, photophobia	Narrow-angle glaucoma	Mydriasis from topical sympathomimetics used for ocular exam usually lasts 6 hr or less; advise patient to wear sunglasses until pupils can constrict adequately; advise patient to report ocular pain at once, since this may indicate undiagnosed glaucoma
METABOLIC Hypoglycemia	Poorly controlled diabetes mellitus	Monitor blood glucose levels frequently in patients with poorly controlled diabetes, anticipate change in antidiabetic drug therapy; discourage use of OTC sympathomimetics by diabetic patient unless under physician's supervision
CARDIOVASCULAR Heart	Severe bradycardia, heart block	Most likely with pure α agonists (eg, phenylephrine)
Reflex bradycardia		
Anginal pain, myocardial ischemia, infarction	Coronary artery disease; recent myocardial infarction	α Agonists may cause coronary vasoconstriction, myocardial ischemia, infarction; of greater concern with drugs that also increase heart rate (eg, epinephrine)
Arterioles		
Hypertension, headache	Hypertension, history of stroke	Advise hypertensive patients to avoid taking any drug with α-agonist activity except on physician's advice; check BP before, periodically after administering α agonist to any patient; notify physician at once if patient reports headache, visual disturbances, or shows signs of stroke (eg, slurred speech, paresis)
Reduced extremity blood flow, thrombosis	Peripheral vascular diseases (eg, Buerger's disease, Raynaud's disease)	Drugs with α-agonist activity, especially if given systemically, may reduce blood flow to limbs; advise patient to report paresthesias; monitor skin color, temperature; notify physician, be prepared to administer α blocker (eg, phentolamine) if extremity blood flow is reduced appreciably
Tissue ischemia, necrosis, gangrene from extravasation		When α agonists (including dopamine) must be infused, use large or central vein; periodically check skin color, temperature, speed of solution inflow; if signs of extravasation occur, discontinue infusion, restart elsewhere if needed; apply warm compresses to affected area, inject α blocker (phentolamine) liberally around affected area, monitor BP
GENITOURINARY Urinary hesitancy, retention	Cautious use in elderly males with prostatic hypertrophy	Incidence of problems generally low, but requires careful monitoring in high-risk patients; report difficulty or pain in urination, abdominal distention
Uterine pain, especially during menstruation; premature or excessive uterine contractions at or near term	Cautious use during pregnancy	α Receptors predominate in pregnant uterus, mediate uterine contraction; use cautiously near term; may cause dysmenorrhea at other times

(continued)

Table 14–S | **Major Side Effects and Contraindications of Sympathomimetic Drugs (*Continued*)**

BODY SYSTEM/ Side Effect	CONTRAINDICATION/ PRECAUTION	COMMENTS AND NURSING IMPLICATIONS
Major Side Effects of Sympathomimetics with Beta-Agonist Activity		
METABOLIC Hyperglycemia	Poorly controlled diabetes mellitus (unless β agonist given for emergency treatment, eg, cardiac failure, acute and severe bronchoconstriction)	β Agonists (and to some extent α agonists) increase hepatic glycogenolysis; monitor blood glucose levels, antidiabetic drug requirements if β agonists must be given; drugs also having α-agonist activity (eg, epinephrine, mixed-acting sympathomimetics) may complicate problem by increasing release of insulin from pancreas
CARDIOVASCULAR Heart		
Tachycardia, palpitations, anginal pain	Tachycardia, tachyarrhythmias, ischemic heart disease	β Agonists, regardless of selectivity, may directly or reflexly stimulate heart rate; unless absolutely necessary (eg, acute bronchoconstriction), avoid or use reduced doses of β agonists if heart rate is above 100/min or there are signs of arrhythmias (eg, premature atrial, ventricular contractions) in the absence of heart block; monitor cardiac vital signs, including ECG, when giving β agonists parenterally or by any route to high-risk patients
Blood vessels		
Hypotension	Hypotension not due to cardiac failure	β Agonists are vasodilators; avoid systemic administration or inhalation of high doses in hypotensive patients; β agonists may improve blood pressure if hypotension is due to cardiac failure
GENITOURINARY Delay, prolongation of normal labor	Preterm labor (unless needed for management of medical emergency)	Uterine-relaxant effect of β agonists provides reason for use of ritodrine for preterm labor; use late in normal pregnancy may prolong parturition, should be avoided unless absolutely necessary
Additional Side Effects, Contraindications, for Mixed- or Indirect-Acting Sympathomimetics		
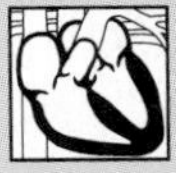 **CARDIOVASCULAR** Hypertensive crisis, excessive cardiac stimulation, stroke	Pheochromocytoma	Interaction due to ability of these sympathomimetics to release massive amounts of catecholamines that may be present in tumor; response may occur abruptly, is potentially fatal; provide pheochromocytoma patients with list of drugs, tyramine-containing foods to avoid, stress importance of precautions; assess for headache, palpitations, other indications that patient may have ingested contraindicated drug

Table 14–1 **Major Interactions Between Sympathomimetics and Other Agents**

AGENT	RESULT OF INTERACTION	COMMENTS AND NURSING IMPLICATIONS
Major Interactions Involving Epinephrine, Norepinephrine, and Most Other Sympathomimetics		
α-Methyldopa (Chapter 33)	Increased risk of hypertension, poor control of blood pressure	α-Methyldopa, a centrally acting antihypertensive, forms a metabolite (α-methylnorepinephrine) that is a weak vasopressor; vasopressor actions of direct- and mixed-acting sympathomimetics may be additive; avoid sympathomimetic use; if unavoidable, initial sympathomimetic dose may need to be as low as 1/10–1/5 usual dose; monitor blood pressure closely, be prepared to lower elevated blood pressure with α blocker (eg, phentolamine)
Antidepressants (tricyclics; Chapter 24)	Increased risk of arrhythmias, tachycardia, hypertension	Tricyclic antidepressants block neuronal reuptake of norepinephrine, some other direct-acting sympathomimetics, thereby potentiating their effects, particularly cardiac and blood vessel stimulation; actions of mixed-acting sympathomimetics are also intensified; antidepressants' atropine-like action may contribute to tachycardia; avoid interaction or use lowest effective sympathomimetic dose; interaction less likely to occur with doxepin; monitor vital signs closely; see Atropine, below
Aminophylline	See Theophylline, below	
Antihistamines (H_1 blockers; eg, diphenhydramine; Chapter 51)	Risk of tachycardia	See Atropine, below
Atropine, other drugs with antimuscarinic activity (eg, antidepressants, antihistamines, antipsychotics; Table 13–2, p 174)	Risk of tachycardia, arrhythmias	Drugs with antimuscarinic actions block bradycardic effects of parasympathetic nervous system, may potentiate tachycardia and increased cardiac impulse conduction by drugs that directly or reflexly stimulate heart (eg, epinephrine, pure β agonists); not usually necessary to avoid interaction unless tachycardia already present; monitor heart rate closely
β Blockers (eg, propranolol, others; Chapter 15)	Increased chance of severe hypertension, bradycardia, arrhythmias, heart failure	β Blockers leave vasoconstrictor effects of drugs with α-agonist activity unopposed, leading to marked BP rise; reflex cardiac slowing may be intensified; avoid interaction; risk of hypertension, but not of bradycardia, may be reduced by use of cardioselective β blocker (eg, atenolol, metoprolol)
Digitalis glycosides (digoxin; Chapter 31)	Increased chance of ventricular arrhythmias	High or toxic doses of digitalis may increase ventricular automaticity that is potentiated by β agonist
Halothane, most other inhalational general anesthetics (Chapter 20)	Increased chance of ventricular arrhythmias, fibrillation	Halothane sensitizes heart to catecholamines; arrhythmia risk increased by high BP, hypoxia, increased blood carbon dioxide levels
Insulin, oral hypoglycemic (antidiabetic) drugs (Chapter 46)	Hyperglycemia, difficulty maintaining stable blood glucose levels	Sympathomimetics may elevate blood glucose levels, reducing requirements for insulin, other antidiabetic drugs; avoid interaction if possible; monitor blood glucose levels periodically, especially in poorly controlled diabetics
Methylxanthines	See Theophylline, below	
Oxytocin, vasopressin (Chapter 49)	Increased chance of hypertension	These drugs elevate blood pressure; effects may be additive with sympathomimetic drug

(continued)

Table 14–I | Major Interactions Between Sympathomimetics and Other Agents (*Continued*)

AGENT	RESULT OF INTERACTION	COMMENTS AND NURSING IMPLICATIONS
Theophylline, aminophylline, other methylxanthines (Chapter 38)	Increased risk of excessive cardiac or CNS stimulation	Theophylline, aminophylline, and other methylxanthines (see Chapter 38) are often combined with β agonists for synergistic bronchodilator effects; synergistically stimulate heart and CNS; if combined therapy is used, monitor for tachycardia, palpitations, anxiety
Thyroid hormones (Chapter 47)	Increased sympathomimetic effects, especially on heart	Thyroid hormone produces catecholamine-like effects; avoid combined use
Additional or Special Interactions Involving Mixed- or Indirect-Acting Sympathomimetics		
Antidepressants, tricyclics (Chapter 24)	Abolished effects of indirect-acting sympathomimetics; reduced intensity of response to mixed-acting sympathomimetics	Antidepressants block ability of indirect- or mixed-acting sympathomimetics to enter adrenergic nerve endings, release norepinephrine; direct-acting sympathomimetics should be used, but at reduced doses, if sympathomimetic effects are needed
Monoamine oxidase inhibitors (Chapter 24)	Risk of severe or fatal hypertensive crisis, stroke	Avoidance of interaction is essential; discontinue MAO inhibitor at least 2 weeks before administering sympathomimetic
Additional Interactions Involving Dopamine		
Monoamine oxidase inhibitors (Chapter 24)	See entry under Mixed-Acting Sympathomimetics, above	Use dopamine cautiously, since it may release norepinephrine
Phenytoin (Chapter 26)	Severe hypotension, bradycardia, seizures	Interaction has been fatal; monitor closely; may need to discontinue phenytoin, use other anticonvulsants

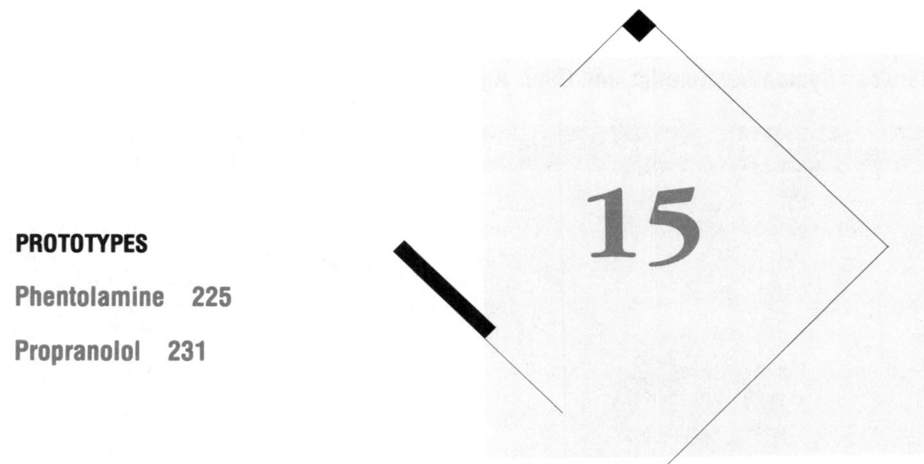

PROTOTYPES

Adrenergic-Receptor Blocking Drugs

General Characteristics of Adrenergic-Receptor Blocking Drugs

Adrenergic-receptor blockers are pharmacologic antagonists of the sympathomimetic agonists discussed in Chapter 14. They can also be called *sympatholytic* drugs to indicate that they lyse (break) sympathetic influences throughout the body. Most adrenergic blockers are competitive antagonists: their effects can be overcome by increasing the dose of an appropriate agonist. Adrenergic blockers do not occur naturally in the body.

Recall that adrenergic agonists are classified according to whether they stimulate α receptors, β receptors, or both. The blockers are classified in a similar way, as α blockers or β blockers. Most blockers block only one receptor subtype, α or β. Just as some sympathomimetic agonists selectively stimulate one subtype of α or β receptor (1 or 2), some antagonists have the same selectivity.

Giving an adrenergic blocker is the most common way to suppress specific and usually undesirable effects caused by excessive stimulation of adrenergic receptors, as can result from disease or from high doses of sympathomimetic drugs. Less common but nevertheless clinically important ways to cause sympatholytic effects exist, as discussed briefly at the end of the chapter.

Predicting the Effects of an Adrenergic Blocker

Understanding how the autonomic nervous system (ANS) regulates a particular organ or structure helps predict the response produced by a particular blocker (Table 15–1). Recall that many effectors are innervated by both the sympathetic and parasympathetic nervous systems. Each branch is more or less continuously active, and each generally produces opposite effects on a given target organ.

Giving a drug that blocks responses mediated by the sympathetic nervous system causes effects that appear as if the parasympathetic branch were activated. For example, bronchodilation is mediated by the effects of epinephrine on β receptors of smooth muscle; the parasympathetic neurotransmitter acetylcholine (ACh) constricts the bronchi. Therefore, a β blocker causes (or, more correctly, unmasks or allows) parasympathetic influences to predominate, and bronchoconstriction occurs. In a few places, control of an effector is

Major reference tables appear beginning on p. 243.

Table 15–1 Responses of Major Effector Organs to Pharmacologic Doses of Alpha or Beta Blockers

Structure	Receptor Type	Response to Appropriate Blocker*
Eye		
Iris, pupil size	α	Miosis
Respiratory system		
Bronchial smooth muscle tone	β_2	Increased (constriction)
Mucus secretions	α	Increased (thin)
Heart		
Force of contraction	β_1	Decreased
Rate	β_1	Decreased
Automaticity	β_1	Decreased
Impulse conduction	β_1	Decreased
Arterioles	α	Dilation
	β_2	Constriction
Large veins	α	Dilation
	β_2	Constriction
Metabolic effects		
Fat cells	α, β_1	Decreased lipolysis
Skeletal muscle, liver	α, β_2	Decreased glycogen breakdown
Pancreas	α	Increased insulin release
	β_2	Decreased insulin release
Exocrine glands	α	Increased secretions (eg, saliva, lacrimal fluid, mucus)
Gastrointestinal tract		
Motility	α, β_2	Increased } Slight
Sphincters	α	Relaxed } Slight
Overall activity		Increased } Slight
Kidney		
Renin secretion	β_1	Decreased
Urinary bladder		
Detrusor	β_2	Constriction } Slight
Trigone, sphincter	α	Relaxation } Slight
Overall activity		Increased } Slight
Uterus		
Nonpregnant	β_2	Contraction
Pregnant	α	Relaxation
Penis	α	Impaired ejaculation

*Most of these responses reflect an unmasking of opposing parasympathetic influences on the named structures.

balanced by opposing effects of α- and β-adrenergic receptors. For example, some arterioles have both α receptors that cause vasoconstriction when stimulated, and β receptors that cause vasodilation when activated. Blocking the β receptors could unmask the effects mediated by α receptors, and if a drug such as epinephrine were present, vasoconstriction would occur and blood pressure would rise.

With only one exception (see labetalol, p 240), α blockers block only α receptors; they do not block β receptors. The reverse is true for β blockers. Likewise, adrenergic blockers do not block receptors for other transmitters, hormones, or drugs. For example, α or β blockers do not block ACh or histamine receptors.

Although the direct effects of adrenergic blockers at most sites are generally quite predictable, cardiovascular responses are not so straightforward. (This was also the case for adrenergic agonists, which were discussed in the previous chapter.) Cardiovascular responses reflect not only direct effects of an adrenergic blocker but also important reflex effects that occur when, for example, blood pressure is changed. Virtually all the reflex effects that occur involve the baroreceptor reflex. The discussions that follow indicate both the direct effects and any reflex changes that are apt to occur in response to an adrenergic blocker. When assessing patients who will receive one of these drugs, monitoring both the direct and reflex responses is critically important.

Alpha-Adrenergic Blockers

Alpha blockers block all the effects of phenylephrine or other "pure" α agonists; some effects of epinephrine, which stimulates both α and β receptors; and no effects of isoproterenol or other "pure" β agonists. Phentolamine (REGITINE) is the prototype.

PROTOTYPE

Phentolamine

Absorption, Distribution, Metabolism, and Excretion

Phentolamine is absorbed from the gastrointestinal (GI) tract but is excreted so rapidly by the kidneys that it is hard to achieve therapeutic blood levels when it is given orally. Therefore, it is given only parenterally.

Pharmacologic Effects

Phentolamine blocks both α_1 and α_2 receptors. The α_1 receptors, found postsynaptically on effectors, mediate responses such as vasoconstriction and mydriasis. When they are blocked, the opposite effects occur. The α_2 receptors occur mainly presynaptically on adrenergic nerve endings. Stimulation of α_2 receptors inhibits norepinephrine release from the activated nerve. By blocking these receptors, phentolamine increases norepinephrine release.

Cardiovascular Effects

The most important effects of phentolamine and related α blockers are on the cardiovascular system.

Effects on Blood Pressure

By blocking α receptors that are being stimulated almost continually by epinephrine and norepinephrine, phentolamine dilates arterioles. Blood pressure and total peripheral resistance fall. How much the blood pressure falls depends on the level of sympathetic "tone" when the drug is given. In a normal, recumbent person, in whom sympathetic tone is low, blood pressure falls very little, if at all. When sympathetic tone is high, as when the person stands, exercises, or has received a large dose of vasoconstrictor (α-stimulating) drug, the blood pressure fall is much greater.

Phentolamine's ability to lower blood pressure is very pronounced when a person stands up. The act of standing quickly triggers reflexes that activate the sympathetic nervous system, causing vasoconstriction to prevent blood from pooling in the legs. In the presence of phentolamine, the sympathetic reflex is activated but blood vessels cannot constrict because their α receptors are blocked. Blood pools in the legs, blood pressure falls rapidly, and blood flow to the brain decreases. When this happens, the patient becomes dizzy and lightheaded, and may faint. The same hypotensive effect occurs when a person remains standing, without moving, for a long time. The general phenomenon effect is called postural or **orthostatic hypotension.**

Indirect (Reflex) Effects on the Heart

Phentolamine does not directly affect sympathetic control of the major aspects of heart function; that is the role of β_1 receptors. However, by lowering blood pressure phentolamine activates the baroreceptor reflex and sympathetic nerve activity, indirectly increasing heart rate and contractility. Since phentolamine blocks presynaptic α receptors (α_2), it removes the physiologic "feedback inhibition" of norepinephrine release. The increased amounts of released norepinephrine further increase cardiac stimulation.

The overall cardiovascular response to usual doses of phentolamine is, therefore, increased cardiac output owing to peripheral vasodilation and reflex increases of heart rate and contractility.

Other Effects

Other direct effects produced by α blockers include miosis, increased lacrimation and mucus secretion in the upper respiratory tract, and increased gastric acid secretion and GI motility, all of which reflect unmasking of opposing parasympathetic effects on the target organs. Alpha blockers also impair ejaculation. None of these actions are clinically useful; they all account for side effects.

Clinical Indications and Administration

Phentolamine is used mainly for its effects on blood vessels. The drug's major clinical indications are listed in Table 15–C1. Intravenous (IV) injection and infusion are the preferred routes of administration for most uses, since intramuscular (IM) injections are painful. Phentolamine is injected subcutaneously only to manage vasoconstrictor extravasation.

Treatment and Diagnosis of Pheochromocytoma

Phentolamine is used to control acute episodes of hypertension in patients with a pheochromocytoma—an uncommon but serious tumor that secretes large amounts of epinephrine and norepinephrine. The drug has a more important role during surgery to remove a pheochromocytoma, when the surgeon's handling and cutting of the tumor release large amounts of catecholamines into the bloodstream. Phentolamine prevents blood pressure from rising too high, which otherwise might cause a stroke. Treatment of the pheochromocytoma patient, whether acutely or chronically, involves the adjunctive use of β-adrenergic blockers, as discussed later. Because of phentolamine's short duration of action and because it must be administered by injection, it is not used for long-term management of pheochromocytoma.

In the past, phentolamine was commonly used to diagnose pheochromocytoma. In the "phentolamine test," the drug is injected (IV or, preferably, IM) into a patient who is lying quietly. If blood pressure quickly and significantly drops, there is a good chance that the patient has a pheochromocytoma. Little if any change of blood pressure would occur in a normal individual. However, the test is dangerous, since it may cause severe hypotension and marked reflex tachycardia. Pheochromocytoma is usually diagnosed with much safer chemical tests of blood and urinary catecholamine levels, so the phentolamine test is not used often.

NURSING IMPLICATIONS

Have patients who will receive phentolamine for diagnosis of a pheochromocytoma lie quietly for at least half an hour before drug administration, and check blood pressure several times to ensure that it has stabilized. Once the physician gives the drug, record blood pressure every 30 seconds to 2 minutes for at least 5 minutes, and then every 5 to 10 minutes thereafter for at least half an hour. Notify the physician at once if pressure falls excessively or if any side effects or adverse responses occur. To guard against orthostatic hypotension, have the patient avoid ambulating for 30 to 60 minutes after the test.

Treatment and Prevention of Vasoconstrictor Extravasation

Phentolamine is the drug of choice for treating extravasation of vasoconstrictors. The drug, diluted in sterile isotonic saline, is infiltrated liberally around subcutaneous (SC) tissues in the affected area.

NURSING IMPLICATIONS

When using phentolamine to treat vasoconstrictor extravasation, apply warm moist towels to the area to increase blood flow and enhance the drug's actions. It is essential to give phentolamine as soon as vasoconstrictor extravasation is recognized. Repeated injections may be needed until local blood flow improves. Check peripheral pulses and skin temperature at and distal to the extravasation site to assess the effectiveness of interventions, and ask the patient whether signs of vascular insufficiency, such as paresthesias, are declining.

Adjunctive Treatment of Cardiogenic Shock

Phentolamine is occasionally infused intravenously along with norepinephrine to increase cardiac output in acute heart failure, as might occur after heart surgery. (This combination is often called "L & R," for LEVOPHED and REGITINE, by critical-care professionals who use it.) The α blocker prevents norepinephrine's vasoconstrictor effect, leaves its β_1 cardiac-stimulating effect unopposed, and allows norepinephrine to act like a "pure" β_1 agonist such as dobutamine. The heart is stimulated, peripheral resistance falls, cardiac output improves, and problems of extravasation are reduced. Preferred drugs for treating acute heart failure are discussed in Chapter 31.

Treatment of Peripheral Vascular Disorders

Phentolamine is used to treat acute symptoms of peripheral vascular diseases when blood flow to the extremities is reduced so much that tissue ischemia, necrosis, or gangrene can occur. These conditions include some kinds of scleroderma, Raynaud's disease, frostbite, and other conditions in which excessive sympathetic nerve activity seems to be the main cause of the problem. The orally effective α blocker phenoxybenzamine is used for long-term therapy. Vascular disorders such as atherosclerosis or thrombotic disease, in which peripheral blood vessels are physically blocked, do not respond well to α blockers.

Treatment of Hypertension Resulting from Vasoconstrictor Drug Overdoses

Intravenous phentolamine is usually the preferred treatment for hypertensive emergencies caused by vasoconstrictor drugs such as phenylephrine and norepinephrine.

Role of Alpha Blockers in Essential Hypertension

Alpha blockers such as phentolamine are not very useful for treating essential hypertension, the most common form of high blood pressure. They desirably lower blood pressure, but they also cause excessive and undesirable reflex tachycardia. As noted on page 231 and explained in more detail in Chapter 33, selective α_1 blockers such as prazosin are preferred for treating essential hypertension.

Side Effects, Adverse Reactions, and Contraindications

Cardiovascular Side Effects

The cardiovascular actions of phentolamine and other α blockers cause most of their important side effects (Table 15–S1). Orthostatic hypotension is common, even with "usual" doses, and it is both disturbing and potentially dangerous. High doses of α blockers cause hypotension and tachycardia in normal patients. Drugs with α-blocking activity are more likely to produce orthostatic hypotension than any other group of drugs. Reflex cardiac stimulation resulting from reduced blood pressure can also be intense and dangerous, since it greatly increases the heart's workload and oxygen requirements. Cardiac stimulation with hypotension can cause myocardial ischemia that may lead to angina pectoris or myocardial infarction, especially if the patient has coronary artery disease. Therefore, most α blockers are relatively contraindicated in patients with a history of cardiac disease. Alpha blockers are also contraindicated in patients who have recently experienced a stroke. Although brain damage can be caused or worsened by excessively high blood pressure, excessive hypotension is also dangerous; it reduces cerebral blood flow and can increase the size of a brain infarction.

Problems Caused by "Parasympathetic Predominance"

Alpha blockers upset the normal balance between α-mediated sympathetic responses and the opposing parasympathetic influences, causing a syndrome known as "parasympathetic predominance." The syndrome is of most concern with long-term α blocker treatment. Signs and symptoms involving the GI tract include diarrhea and increased gastric acid secretion, which contribute to GI upset. Alpha blockers, particularly when used chronically, can cause or worsen peptic ulcer disease, which generally contraindicates their long-term use. Excessive salivation is also an expected side effect. Other signs include excessive lacrimation, and increased production of thin, watery mucus that causes nasal stuffiness or congestion. Miosis may prevent good vision in dim light.

Ejaculatory Failure in Males

Alpha blockers inhibit ejaculation. This is seldom a problem with acute administration of phentolamine, but is an important cause of noncompliance with long-term α-blocker therapy.

NURSING IMPLICATIONS

Because phentolamine is given only by injection for relatively short-term effects in nonambulatory patients, nursing measures related to its side effects are primarily limited to acute monitoring of cardiovascular status and its consequences. Monitoring should focus on objective indicators such as heart rate, rhythm, and blood pressure; and related indicators (eg, skin color and temperature, level of consciousness, urine output). Obtain baseline measurements for comparison with those taken after drug administration. The frequency of monitoring after drug injection depends mainly on the acuity of the patient's condition. When phentolamine is used to treat a hypertensive emergency, for example, continuous monitoring is needed until the patient stabilizes and there is good reason to believe that no sudden or dramatic changes are likely to occur.

Many more side effects become problematic with long-term oral administration of related α blockers, and they require more nursing interventions. This is discussed on pages 229–230.

◆ Use During Pregnancy and Lactation

Phentolamine, or other α blockers, are not suitable drugs for managing chronic or acute hypertension during pregnancy. Preferred drugs are discussed in Chapter 33. The safe use of phentolamine in lactating women has not been established. The potential risks and benefits to the mother and child must be assessed.

◆ Use in Children

The uses of phentolamine in children, and the related precautions, are generally the same as those noted for adults.

◆ Use in the Elderly

Elderly persons do not tolerate sudden changes of blood pressure or heart rate as well as younger persons do. Orthostatic hypotension is a particular problem, especially when accompanied by cerebrovascular disease, which is common in the elderly. Monitoring should focus on cardiovascular changes, the adequacy of tissue perfusion, and the patient's alertness, orientation, and overall level of consciousness.

Interactions with Other Drugs

The only specific interactions with α blockers involve the α agonists that might be used to overcome overdoses. Otherwise, the interactions are of a more general nature, and are primarily important for ambulatory patients taking orally effective α blockers. Interactions mainly involve other drugs (Table 15–11) that further lower blood pressure (eg, most other antihypertensive drugs, and alcohol), or increase heart rate further (sympathomimetics with β agonist activity; antimuscarinic agents). Interactions with β agonists, including epinephrine and all the sympathomimetic bronchodilators, can be particularly dangerous. Those drugs will increase heart rate both directly (via stimulation of β_1 receptors on the heart) and indirectly (via the baroreceptor reflex that is triggered when they lower blood pressure through β_2-mediated vasodilation).

NURSING IMPLICATIONS

If interactants must be given, periodically check heart rate and rhythm, blood pressure, and signs of adequate peripheral and cerebral blood flow. Provide patients with written lists of drugs to avoid, including nonprescription agents.

Overdose and Toxicity

The most important consequences of α blocker overdose are severe hypotension and reflex cardiac stimulation, both of which may lead to shock, arrhythmias, angina, and myocardial infarction. The preferred treatment for mild responses is careful IV fluid administration. Otherwise, injection of a selective α agonist (phenylephrine or methoxamine) is indicated. Increasing blood pressure, whether by giving fluid or drugs, reflexly decreases heart rate. Norepinephrine is an acceptable but less suitable second choice. Although it stimulates α receptors to overcome vasodilation, its cardiac stimulating action may increase heart rate further. *Never* use epinephrine, for reasons noted above in the drug interaction section.

NURSING IMPLICATIONS

Place the patient in a supine, head-low position to maintain cerebral blood flow. Monitor IV infusion rates carefully, and use a drug infusion pump if one is available. The same interventions for managing excessive cardiovascular side effects apply to management of overdoses.

Related Drugs

Two agents, phenoxybenzamine and tolazoline, as well as several drugs in a group called ergot alkaloids, block all the α-adrenergic receptors.

Phenoxybenzamine

Unlike phentolamine, phenoxybenzamine (DIBENZYLINE) blocks α receptors in a noncompetitive (nonsurmountable) fashion. Phenoxybenzamine is given orally and has a much longer duration of action than phentolamine. These properties make phenoxybenzamine useful for treating chronic disorders such as pheochromocytoma or peripheral vascular disease, where parenteral therapy is impractical. In cases of pheochromocytoma, adjunctive therapy with β blockers is often needed to control tachycardia and increased renin release, both of which are triggered by reduced blood pressure. As noted in Chapter 33, other α blockers are used more often.

Phenoxybenzamine causes all the side effects noted for acute administration of phentolamine, but other problems develop with long-term therapy. Prolonged blood pressure reduction can increase plasma renin, aldosterone, and angiotensin II levels, leading to salt and water retention and a counteracting of the blood pressure–lowering effect. The risks of edema and heart failure increase. Long-term therapy can cause prolonged GI upset and diarrhea, as well as excessive lacrimation and nasal stuffiness. Increased acid secretion intensifies the risk of ulcers, and antiulcer therapy may be needed. In males, prolonged sexual dysfunction may be a cause of unwillingness to take the drug as directed, if at all.

Phenoxybenzamine overdoses may be more difficult to treat than phentolamine overdoses, since phenoxybenzamine is a noncompetitive blocker with long-lasting effects. As a result, giving α agonists to overcome excessive hypotension may not work well. Administration of parenteral fluids often works.

NURSING IMPLICATIONS

Advise patients taking phenoxybenzamine that several weeks of therapy may be required for its desired effects to occur. Improvement in patients with pheochromocytoma is assessed as reductions of heart rate and blood pressure and fewer episodes of diaphoresis. For the patient with peripheral vascular disease, improvement is assessed as decreased paresthesias and exercise-induced fatigue, and improved skin color and temperature.

Patients taking phenoxybenzamine eventually will be treated as outpatients, and immediate care for the side effects that almost certainly will occur will not be readily available. Thus, it is important to advise them of the key side effects, to give them proper instructions that will help prevent or minimize the unwanted drug actions, and to advise them that with continued therapy some of the side effects may become less disturbing. Nondrug interventions are preferred, and are usually very effective.

A most important concern relates to preventing orthostatic hypotension and its many potential consequences: syncope, falls, and potentially a stroke; and even angina caused by myocardial ischemia as blood pressure suddenly falls and the heart accelerates. Instruct patients to sit and then stand up very slowly, and to use a steady object such as a chair or bed for support when they stand. Assist them with standing and walking during the early stages of treatment. Advise them to expect lightheadedness when they stand up, or stand too long in one place without moving; and that if they become lightheaded or unsteady they should immediately lie down or sit and assume a head-low position. Many patients benefit from elastic stockings, which help keep blood from pooling in the legs, but they should be fitted properly to ensure that they do not interfere with blood flow. Advise patients that if problems owing to hypotension persist after several weeks of therapy, or if they become severe at any time, they should contact their physician at once.

Giving phenoxybenzamine with milk or foods will reduce GI upset. However, notify the physician at once if severe GI pain, epigastric distress, or tarry stools develop, since these may indicate peptic ulcers caused or worsened by the drug. Dietary changes should be tried first to alleviate diarrhea. The patient should report severe diarrhea at once, since serious fluid and electrolyte imbalances may aggravate hypotension. Antimuscarinic drugs, even those in over-the-counter (OTC) products, should be avoided for relief of common side effects such as nasal stuffiness or excessive lacrimation. The antimuscarinics may provide symptomatic relief, but can aggravate tachycardia or counteract the α blocker's desired effects. Advise patients that poor vision in dim light makes tasks such as operating a motor vehicle after dark dangerous. Males should be advised to expect sexual dysfunction, and should be cautioned that discontinuing the medication to alleviate the problem could hinder therapy of a potentially serious disorder.

Phenoxybenzamine is mutagenic and must not be given to pregnant women, especially during the first trimester. The drug is excreted in breast milk, and so breast-feeding is contraindicated during treatment.

Ergot Alkaloids

During the Middle Ages epidemics known as Holy Fire or St. Anthony's Fire swept Europe. The disorder caused spontaneous abortions, in utero fetal death, burning and numbness of the extremities, and gangrene severe enough that affected limbs turned hard and black and eventually fell off the body without bleeding. Hundreds of years later the disease was traced to a variety of naturally occurring chemicals, called *ergot alkaloids,* produced by a fungus growing on contaminated food grains (rye and wheat). Three groups of ergot alkaloids were eventually isolated and studied. They all produce, to varying degrees, three major effects (Table 15–2): *uterine*

Table 15–2 Major Groups of Ergot Alkaloids, Representative Agents, and Pharmacologic Activities

Alkaloid Group	Alkaloids	Proprietary Name(s)	Relative Pharmacologic Activities	Major Therapeutic Use
Ergotamine	Ergotamine	BELLERGAL, CAFERGOT, ERGOMAR, ERGOSTAT, WIGRAINE	vasoconstrictor $\geq$ oxytocic $>$ α blockade	Migraine headache
Ergonovine	Ergonovine Methylergonovine	ERGOTRATE METHERGINE	oxytocic $\gg$ vasoconstrictor; no α blockade	Prevention, treatment of postpartum bleeding (see Chapter 49)
Ergotoxine*	Ergocornine Ergocristine Ergocryptine	CIRCANOL, DEAPRIL, HYDERGINE	α blockade $\gg$ vasoconstrictor $>$ oxytocic	Idiopathic dementia or other decline of mental skills in patients $>$ 60 years

Key: $>$, greater than; $\geq$, greater than or equal to; $\gg$ much greater than.

*All three of the alkaloids, after chemical modification, are present in products called ergoloid mesylates.

stimulation (oxytocic effects), *vasoconstriction* that is not mediated by α receptors, and *α-receptor blockade.*

One group of ergot alkaloids, to which *methylergonovine* belongs, causes potent oxytocic effects and is used to control postpartum uterine hemorrhage.

The second group, exemplified by *ergotamine,* has potent vasoconstrictor activity. Ergotamine is used to manage migraine headaches, presumably because it prevents painful, pulsating dilation of the cerebral arteries.

The third group is the *ergotoxines.* It contains three major alkaloids that, after being chemically modified (by the pharmaceutical firm), act mainly as α blockers. A mixture of these three modified alkaloids is referred to as *ergoloid mesylates.* Their α-blocking activity is used mainly to dilate cerebral blood vessels and increase cerebral blood flow, which can relieve symptoms of age-related or **idiopathic** (cause unknown) declines of mental function in the elderly. Ergoloid mesylates are usually taken sublingually. Three to four weeks of therapy are usually required before symptomatic improvement appears. Long-term use of sublingual preparations may cause buccal (oral) irritation and swelling. Tablets that are swallowed may cause GI distress.

NURSING IMPLICATIONS

Nursing implications for therapy with ergoloid mesylates are similar to those noted for phenoxybenzamine. Also focus on potential buccal side effects: soothing mouthwashes may alleviate oral discomfort from the sublingual dosage forms. Be aware that ergoloid mesylates may aggravate symptoms of psychosis in persons with a history of psychosis, and so are contraindicated for them. Also, they are not indicated when altered mental status can be traced to specific drugs or diseases (eg, parkinsonism, Alzheimer's disease, or tumors).

Drugs That Block Only One Subclass of Alpha Receptor

Doxazosin, Prazosin, and Terazosin

Doxazosin (CARDURA), prazosin (MINIPRESS), and terazosin (HYTRIN) differ from other α blockers in that they block only α_1 receptors. They are orally effective drugs that are used to manage essential hypertension. Their ability to block only postsynaptic α receptors reduces the severity of cardiac stimulation that always occurs with drugs such as phentolamine. Since these drugs leave α_2 (presynaptic) receptors unblocked, released norepinephrine can exert its inhibitory effect on further neurotransmitter release. These drugs, their dosages, and related nursing implications, are discussed in more detail in Chapter 33.

Beta-Adrenergic Blockers

There are many important drugs that block only β-adrenergic receptors (Table 15–C2 and 15–3). They are used much more often than their α-blocking counterparts. Propranolol hydrochloride (INDERAL) is the prototype.

PROTOTYPE

Propranolol

Propranolol is classified as a nonselective β blocker because it blocks all β_1 and β_2 receptors. It has more approved uses than any other β blocker (see Table 15–3). Some of the related drugs have unique properties that may be more desirable in certain clinical situations.

Absorption, Distribution, Metabolism, and Excretion

Propranolol is absorbed well from the GI tract, so it is often given orally. Signs of β blockade appear approximately 30 minutes after oral administration, and peak effects occur in 1 to about 3 hours. Food does not significantly affect the absorption of propranolol or most other β blockers.

Propranolol is almost completely metabolized in the liver, and its metabolites are excreted by the kidneys. The metabolites are not active as β blockers. Propranolol undergoes considerable "first-pass" metabolism (p 60) when given orally: initial doses are metabolized so completely by the liver that little active drug is left to reach the systemic circulation. With repeated administration, however, the liver's enzymes become saturated with the drug, and less drug becomes inactivated. This fact has important implications. If rapid effects are needed, propranolol must be given by injection. The great dependence on liver metabolism also means that propanolol's effects will be significantly increased and prolonged in persons with liver disease, and will be either increased or decreased by other drugs that inhibit or stimulate the liver's drug-metabo-

Table 15–3 | Special Properties and Approved Uses of Beta-Adrenergic Blockers

PROPERTY	Acebutolol	Atenolol	Betaxolol	Carteolol	Esmolol	Labetalol	Levobunolol	Metipranolol	Metoprolol	Nadolol	Penbutolol	Pindolol	Propranolol	Timolol
Nonselective				X		X	X	X		X	X	X	X	X
"Cardioselective"	X	X	X		X				X					
ISA				X		X					X	X		
α-Blockade						X								
APPROVED USES														
Hypertension	X	X	X	X		X							X	X
Angina pectoris		X							X	X			X	
Arrhythmias*	X				X								X	
Post-MI cardioprotection		X							X				X	X
Pheochromocytoma													X	
Hypertrophic Subaortic Stenosis													X	
Migraine prophylaxis													X	
Essential Tremor													X	
Glaucoma			X	X			X	X						X

Key: ISA = intrinsic sympathomimetic activity; X = has property or use.

*Arrhythmias for which marked β-blockers are indicated vary with the drug but generally involve catecholamine-mediated arrhythmias (eg, supraventricular, sinus, and ventricular tachycardias). Only topical formulations of β-blockers are approved for glaucoma.

lizing enzymes. Propranolol's usual half-life is 4 to 6 hours.

Propranolol is very lipid soluble, so it enters the central nervous system (CNS) well. It crosses the placenta, and is excreted in breast milk.

Most other β blockers differ from propranolol in terms of how much they depend on hepatic metabolism or renal excretion for termination of their activity. They also have different lipid solubilities, which affects their ability to act in the CNS.

Pharmacologic Effects

Propranolol competitively blocks all sympathetic responses that are mediated by β-adrenergic receptors (see Table 15–1). Therefore, it blocks all the effects of isoproterenol, the β-mediated effects of epinephrine and norepinephrine, and none of the effects of phenylephrine. By blocking some sympathetic responses, β blockers may unmask certain signs of parasympathetic activity, even though the drugs do not affect ACh receptors.

Virtually every pharmacologic effect discussed below can be clinically useful for many patients with a variety of illnesses. For other patients these same effects can be very dangerous.

Cardiovascular Effects

By blocking the β_1 receptors in the heart, propranolol decreases heart rate, force of contraction, automaticity, and the rate of electrical impulse transmission through the heart muscle and its specialized conducting tissues. These effects reduce myocardial work and oxygen demand, and may reduce cardiac output. Importantly, β blockade prevents the reflex tachycardia that occurs whenever blood pressure falls.

Beta blockers *usually* lower blood pressure in hypertensive people. This *antihypertensive* effect, which is clinically useful, occurs because of reduced cardiac contractility and heart rate; reduced renin release from the kidney, which lowers angiotensin II levels; and some ill-defined effect in the CNS that reduces sympathetic outflow, so that vasoconstriction and cardiac stimulation decrease. The uncommon but nevertheless important instances in which β blockers can increase blood pressure are discussed later.

Beta blockers may reduce coronary blood flow and the delivery of oxygen and nutrients to the heart muscle. This presumably occurs because β blockade in the coronary arteries leaves α-mediated vasoconstrictor responses to norepinephrine and epinephrine unopposed. Coronary blood flow may fall also because of reduced blood pressure, the major driving force for blood flow through the coronary arteries. Theoretically, this reduced oxygen delivery could cause cardiac ischemia and its major symptom, angina pectoris. However, the ability of β blockers to reduce myocardial oxygen supply is usually outweighed by their ability to reduce the heart's oxygen demand, which is determined by heart rate and contractility. As is discussed briefly here and in more detail in Chapter 34, β blockers are actually very useful *anti*anginal drugs.

Propranolol produces membrane-stabilizing or local anesthetic-like effects on the heart. This action, combined with its ability to block β receptors, contributes to the drug's antiarrhythmic activity.

Respiratory Effects

Propranolol antagonizes the bronchodilator effects of circulating epinephrine on β_2 receptors in bronchial smooth muscle, and unmasks the bronchoconstrictor effects of ACh released by parasympathetic nerves.

Metabolic Effects

Beta agonists increase the release of fat from adipose tissue, glucose production by the liver and skeletal muscle, and insulin release from the pancreas. Propanolol antagonizes these effects, resulting in reduced blood levels of free fatty acids, glucose, and insulin. Beta blockers will also slow the recovery of blood glucose levels toward normal when an episode of hypoglycemia occurs, as occurs after fasting or the administration of antidiabetic drugs (eg, insulin) in excessive dosages.

Genitourinary Effects

Smooth muscle in the nonpregnant uterus contains abundant β_2 receptors, which mediate uterine relaxation. Propranolol may thus cause uterine contraction.

Other Effects

Propranolol decreases aqueous humor formation in the eye, and reduces intraocular pressure, in some patients with glaucoma. It acts in the CNS to reduce anxiety and cause sedation. It is not known how these effects occur.

Clinical Indications and Administration

Propranolol hydrochloride is usually used for its cardiovascular effects. It can be given orally or parenterally. A long-acting oral preparation (INDERAL-LA) is available. Doses are shown in Table 15–C2.

NURSING IMPLICATIONS

For all indications, the dose of propranolol may vary considerably from those shown in the table. Since propranolol depends on hepatic metabolism to terminate its activity, dosages will have to be adjusted whenever liver function is altered, as by age, disease, or other drugs. For example the "average adult dose" may need to be reduced by 75% or so in patients with severely impaired hepatic function. Alternatively, very high doses may be needed to manage some severe symptoms.

Treatment of Essential Hypertension

Propranolol and all other orally effective β blockers have important roles in the long-term treatment of essential hypertension, the most common type of high blood pressure. The mechanisms for this effect were noted earlier. Beta blockers are particularly effective when high blood pressure appears to involve excessive sympathetic activity, as in cases of hypertension plus tachycardia, or is accompanied by high plasma renin levels.

Beta blockers alone may control *mild* hypertension well, which is desirable because their side effects are usually infrequent and mild compared with those of most other antihypertensive agents. Hypertension is also treated with β blockers in combination with other antihypertensive drugs that cause reflex tachycardia as a side effect. Adjunctive use of a β blocker keeps heart rate at more normal and tolerable levels. Some antihypertensive agents also increase renin release, which would counteract lowered blood pressure. This, too, can be controlled by concurrent use of a β blocker. The antihypertensive effects of β blockers are additive to those of other classes of antihypertensive drugs. The use of β blockers with other antihypertensive drugs (particularly diuretics) is so common that **fixed-dose combinations** are widely used. For example, INDERIDE contains propranolol and the diuretic hydrochlorothiazide. The use and misuse of these combinations are discussed more fully in Chapter 33.

Treatment of Angina Pectoris

Propranolol, and a few other orally effective β blockers, are indicated for managing angina pectoris—chest pain that is a symptom of myocardial ischemia. Ischemia occurs when the heart's oxygen demands exceed its supply of oxygenated blood. Ischemia and anginal pain often occur because of coronary artery disease such as atherosclerosis. When the patient is resting, blood flow through diseased vessels may be enough to satisfy the heart's oxygen requirements. However, during stressful situations, such as exercise, sympathetic stimulation of the heart increases oxygen demands; the narrowed vessels may be unable to deliver an adequate supply of oxygenated blood, and anginal pain is liable to occur.

Beta blockers alleviate angina and ischemia associated with coronary artery disease by reducing heart rate and contractility, both of which lower the heart's oxygen demands. The drugs can be used alone to treat angina, especially angina that occurs with exercise. They may also be indicated as adjuncts to antianginal therapy with other drugs, such as nitroglycerin (Chapter 34). Nitroglycerin lowers blood pressure, triggers reflex tachycardia, and increases the heart's oxygen demands, thus counteracting its desired antianginal effects. When combined with a drug like nitroglycerin, a β blocker prevents tachycardia and adds its own antianginal effects—reduction of heart rate and contractility.

Beta blockers may increase the frequency or severity of anginal attacks in some patients (see the section on side effects). This often indicates that the underlying cause of angina is coronary artery spasm.

Treatment of Cardiac Arrhythmias

Propranolol is used to control cardiac arrhythmias that are caused mainly by excessive sympathetic stimulation. This includes atrial or ventricular tachycardia as caused by β-agonist overdoses, hyperthyroidism, and general anesthetics such as halothane that "sensitize" the heart to catecholamines. The drug is given orally for long-term treatment, or by slow IV injection for acute or life-threatening rhythm disturbances.

Treatment of Pheochromocytoma

Alpha-adrenergic blockers are sometimes used to lower high blood pressure caused by a pheochromocytoma. However, they do not alleviate excessive cardiac stimulation. In fact, giving only an α blocker causes considerably *more* cardiac stimulation because the blood pressure fall triggers reflex tachycardia, which may lead to angina or arrhythmias. Reflex cardiac stimulation is blocked by giving propranolol.

Although both α and β blockers are indicated, the sequence of administration is critical: the α blocker *must* be given first. If a β blocker is the first or only drug administered, blood pressure will rise, often dramatically. This occurs because peripheral vasodilation, mediated by β_2 receptors, is blocked. Only α-mediated vasoconstriction will occur. Heart rate and contractility will fall because of the *direct* cardiac depressant effects of the β blocker, combined with intense *reflex* slowing of the heart as the baroreceptors respond to increased blood pressure. The slowly beating, weakened heart may be unable to pump blood effectively against the very high arterial pressure, and the patient may experience acute and possibly fatal heart failure or cardiac arrest.

Treatment of Hypertrophic Subaortic Stenosis

Hypertrophic subaortic stenosis is a cardiac disorder in which the ventricle and interventricular septum just below the aortic root are thickened enough to partly block the outflow of blood from the left ventricle. As the patient ages the ventricle enlarges (hypertrophies) in an attempt to generate more force to pump blood past the blockage. The heart's oxygen demands increase as the workload increases, but oxygen supply may not keep pace. Angina pectoris and other clinical findings (such as murmurs) usually occur. Small doses of propranolol may help decrease cardiac work so that oxygen demands and anginal symptoms fall. High doses may depress the heart too much, leading to heart failure.

Prophylaxis of Common Migraine Headache

About 10% of the population experience some form of severe headache known as *migraine*. Patients with frequent migraine attacks generally require drug therapy, and many of them respond well to the prophylactic use of propranolol. The drug decreases the frequency and severity of attacks. Propranolol probably acts by blocking dilation of cerebral blood vessels, which causes headache, at least during part of the attack. Propranolol is not very effective for treating an ongoing headache; other drugs, such as ergotamine (p 230), are usually used instead.

Adjunctive Management of Hyperthyroidism

Common signs and symptoms of hyperthyroidism include tachycardia, muscle tremor, and anxiety. Propranolol can be used to relieve these symptoms, acutely or chronically. However, it does not specifically antagonize the effects of thyroid hormone, nor does it reduce thyroid hormone levels in the blood, so the patient will still be "hyperthyroid." Propranolol can be used adjunctively with antithyroid drugs (see Chapter 47). Propranolol is also useful for controlling tachycardia and arrhythmias before or during thyroidectomy.

"Cardioprotection": Prevention of Recurrent Myocardial Infarction and Sudden Cardiac Death

Administration of propranolol to patients who have recently suffered their first myocardial infarction (heart attack) reduces early postinfarction mortality, controls arrhythmias, and improves cardiac output during the recovery period. Long-term β blocker treatment also reduces the risk of reinfarction and arrhythmias that causes sudden cardiac death. Several other β blockers are also approved for this use. Beta blockers should not be used if the heart attack has destroyed so much cardiac tissue that cardiogenic shock occurs.

Treatment of Glaucoma

Beta blockers, administered topically on the eye, are used to reduce intraocular pressure in some patients with glaucoma. Propranolol, the prototype, is not used for this purpose; the related drugs that have this indication are identified below and in Table 15–1.

Management of Essential Tremor

Propranolol is approved for relieving hereditary or familial essential tremor, a form of skeletal muscle tremor that usually is confined to the upper extremities. Propranolol and other β blockers are not indicated for other causes of tremor, such as parkinsonism.

NURSING IMPLICATIONS

Oral β blockers can be administered with or shortly after meals, but they should be taken at a consistent time each day with respect to meals. Expect the need to reduce doses when the patient has liver dysfunction. Dosage adjustments needed because of drug–drug interactions are noted below.

Monitor the electrocardiogram (ECG) continuously when administering any IV β blocker, or when giving the drug to any person with arrhythmias. If large doses are required or the patient is severely ill, monitor systemic and pulmonary venous and arterial pressures also.

Side Effects, Adverse Reactions, and Contraindications

For most patients, β blockers usually produce few side effects; those that do occur are generally mild. However, if the patient has severe cardiac disease, respiratory disease, or diabetes mellitus, any β blocker could be dangerous. Systemic therapy poses the greatest risks. Even topical administration of β blockers (as for glaucoma) can cause serious or fatal responses in high-risk patients. Side effects of β blockade are summarized in Table 15–S2. In general, all side effects are treated by gradually reducing the β blocker dosage.

Cardiovascular Side Effects

Systemically administered β blockers, even at usual therapeutic doses, tend to slow heart rate slightly in all patients. However, the most common side effect is a decreased ability of heart rate to increase upon exercise, which can decrease the patient's exercise tolerance.

High doses of any β blocker can decrease heart function enough to produce heart failure or cardiac arrest. However, even "ordinary" doses can cause bradycardia, hypotension, heart failure, cardiogenic shock, or cardiac arrest if heart function is already impaired. Beta blockers are relatively or absolutely contraindicated if the patient has sinus bradycardia (heart rate less than about 50 beats per minute), heart block greater than first degree (a P–R interval longer than about 200 msec), systolic blood pressure lower than 100 mm Hg, or any sign of heart failure or cardiogenic shock. Included in this list of contraindicating conditions is Wolff–Parkinson–White (WPW) syndrome, a disorder in which the patient experiences periods of atrioventricular block that could be made worse by even small doses of β blockers.

Although β blockers are indicated for managing exercise-induced angina, some patients taking these drugs may experience an increased frequency or severity of anginal attacks. This usually indicates a form of angina pectoris known as variant, vasospastic, or Prinzmetal's angina. It is caused by coronary artery spasm (constriction) when β blockade leaves unopposed the α mediated vasoconstrictor influences of epinephrine and norepinephrine. Beta blockers are therefore contraindicated for persons with vasospastic angina. Chest pain that begins or increases in severity during β-blocker therapy may indicate underlying vasospastic angina.

Unmasked vasoconstriction caused by β blockers may reduce blood flow to the mesentery, brain, or extremities in patients with vascular disease. Signs of vascular insufficiency depend on what vessels are affected.

Although β blockers usually lower blood pressure in hypertensive patients, in some patients they may increase pressure. This usually indicates that circulating epinephrine levels are unusually high, and often suggests underlying pheochromocytoma. Blood pressure rises because β blockade in the systemic circulation unmasks α-mediated vasoconstriction. The dangers of β blockade alone for the pheochromocytoma patient were noted earlier.

Respiratory Side Effects

Administration of most β blockers to a patient with asthma or obstructive pulmonary disease (eg, emphysema) may cause bronchoconstriction. Some individuals may experience only wheezing, but others may experience bronchospasm severe enough to cause asphyxia and death. Death from respiratory problems has occurred even after topical ocular application of small doses of a β blocker for glaucoma. Therefore, β blockers are generally contraindicated in patients with asthma or emphysema. Blockade of bronchodilation contributes to reduced exercise tolerance in most patients.

Metabolic Side Effects

Beta blockers should be used with extreme care in patients with diabetes mellitus. This is particularly true for drugs such as propranolol, which block β_2 receptors. Beta blockers not only cause hypoglycemia, but they also remove one of the important physiologic signals that a diabetic patient may use to detect hypoglycemia—tachycardia. Overall, the consequences of giving a β blocker to a diabetic patient could range from very mild (fainting) to very serious (hypoglycemic coma). Even in the absence of severe hypoglycemia, and regardless of whether or how the diabetic person is treated, β blockers make it difficult to stabilize blood sugar levels. The β blockers that are relatively specific for β_1 receptors (p 240) seem to be preferred for diabetic patients because they are somewhat less likely to alter blood glucose levels.

Beta blockers can mask responses such as tachycardia that occur if a patient receives excessive or toxic doses of thyroid hormone supplements, as used to treat hypothyroidism. Likewise, β blockade can mask signs of severe hyperthyroidism, as caused by a thyroid tumor. Beta blockers should therefore be used with care in any of these individuals. Lastly, abrupt withdrawal of β blocker therapy in hyperthyroid patients is liable to produce a severe hyperthyroid crisis (thyroid storm), resulting in excessive cardiac stimulation, angina, infarction, or fatal arrhythmias.

Central Nervous System Side Effects

Drowsiness is the most common CNS side effect of β blockers, particularly propranolol, which is very lipid soluble and enters the CNS easily. Problems owing to CNS depression usually become less with continued treatment. The degree of drowsiness is dose-dependent.

Other Side Effects

Some β blockers cause GI cramps, muscle cramps, pruritus, or skin rashes, but these side effects are rare.

NURSING IMPLICATIONS

Always rule out the major contraindicating conditions before administering any β blocker: heart failure or bradycardia, asthma or related obstructive lung diseases, and diabetes. Withhold further doses of β blockers, and notify the physician at once, if any of the following occur.

- Heart rate or blood pressure falls markedly and suddenly after the previous dose was given
- Blood pressure rises suddenly or markedly
- Anginal pain appears or worsens
- Signs of worsening heart failure appear (eg, edema, weight gain)
- Cardiac rhythm changes in an unwanted way
- Respiratory difficulty occurs (wheezing or dyspnea, especially at night or during exercise)
- Evidence of hypoglycemia or thyrotoxicosis is apparent
- Signs and symptoms of vascular insufficiency appear

Monitor all patients periodically for weight gain and edema that might indicate developing or worsening heart failure. Use extra caution if the patient is also receiving digitalis or has impairments of automaticity or impulse conduction (for example, Wolff–Parkinson–White syndrome).

Encourage patients to monitor their pulse, heart rhythm, and blood pressure, and to observe for signs of the side effects or adverse responses noted above. Virtually all of these responses require immediate notification of the physician and follow-up assessment.

If a patient receiving a β blocker wishes to exercise or participate in sports, and no contraindicating medical condition exists, discuss with the patient and physician problems related to reduced exercise tolerance. Changes of drug therapy (for example, use of β blockers with special properties) or modification of physical activity may be indicated.

Advise diabetic patients who must take a β blocker to follow recommended dietary and drug therapy closely, and to assess carefully their response to physical activity. Teach them that diaphoresis, hunger, or the sudden onset of fatigue or irritability, rather than tachycardia, should be used as an indication of hypoglycemia. Blood glucose levels should be checked more often than usual if the patient receives any β blocker. Foods and beverages rich in rapidly absorbed sugar, or special glucose supplements, should be readily available to treat hypoglycemia.

Encourage hyperthyroid patients, or hypothyroid patients taking thyroid supplements, to have periodic blood tests and physical examinations to detect excessive thyroid hormone levels or potential thyrotoxicosis that may be masked by β blockers.

Caution patients that drowsiness or fatigue may be expected during the first stages of β blocker therapy. Caution them to refrain from activities requiring unimpaired mental acuity, such as operating a motor vehicle or dangerous machinery, until tolerance develops. Notify the physician if prolonged or excessive drowsiness occurs, or if the patient becomes emotionally depressed.

◆ Use During Pregnancy and Lactation

Manufacturers do not recommend giving β blockers during pregnancy. However, many disorders for which β blockers are indicated (angina, hypertension, arrhythmias) are potentially dangerous to the mother or fetus if left untreated. In these situations, β blocker therapy can be continued as long as maternal and fetal responses are monitored closely. The use of β blockers for pregnancy-associated hypertension is discussed in Chapter 33. Women who become pregnant while taking β blockers should be advised to notify their physician at once. Propranolol administration does not rule out breastfeeding, but the nursing infant should be assessed for potential unwanted effects.

◆ Use in Children

Children are more sensitive than young adults to side effects caused by β blockers. Blood levels may accumulate in very young children with immature hepatic function, even when doses are given according to body weight. When assessing responses to β blockers, be aware that childrens' normal heart rates and blood pressures differ from young adults. Also be aware of the higher prevalence of asthma in children.

◆ Use in the Elderly

Beta blockers are commonly used in the elderly to treat hypertension, angina, and cardiac arrhythmias. The effectiveness of these drugs in the elderly may be less than in younger adults. Doses must be reduced to account for declining hepatic or renal function, concomitant therapy with interacting drugs, and lesser tolerance of side effects. Assessment for side effects should focus on the development or worsening of heart failure, respiratory difficulty, and diabetes. Elderly patients are also more likely than young adults to have conditions that require very cautious drug use and monitoring, including heart failure, renal or hepatic impairment, diabetes, peripheral or cerebral vascular disease, or obstructive lung disease. Other medical conditions are likely to be treated with potential drug interactants—another reason for careful monitoring of β blocker therapy.

Discontinuing Beta Blocker Therapy

For a variety of reasons, long-term therapy with β blockers may need to be discontinued, at least temporarily. However, although no hard rule dictates *when* to stop treatment, there is a rule about *how* to stop it. Unless the situation is an emergency, if a β blocker has been administered systemically for more than a week or so the dose should be tapered gradually. *Abruptly stopping therapy is extremely dangerous because it poses a great risk of excessive cardiac stimulation.* If the patient was receiving a β blocker for hypertension, blood pressure can abruptly rise to higher than pretreatment levels, causing a hypertensive episode and, potentially, a stroke. If the indication was for management of angina, or the patient had undiagnosed ischemic heart disease, the sudden stop of therapy could cause myocardial infarction. If the indication was arrhythmia therapy, serious arrhythmias are liable to develop upon withdrawal. These responses are thought to occur because β receptors become supersensitive to epinephrine and norepinephrine during prolonged β blockade. When β blocker therapy is stopped suddenly, the receptors overrespond to even usual levels of catecholamines, causing unusually intense responses.

NURSING IMPLICATIONS

Never discontinue a β blocker abruptly unless doing so would prevent a medical emergency, and the patient can be monitored in a hospital for potential adverse responses. Question medication orders calling for abrupt discontinuation. Whenever possible, gradually decrease the dose of the β blocker over a period of at least 1 to 2 weeks. Instruct your patients about the potential dangers of stopping therapy on their own, and monitor blood pressure and heart rate frequently during withdrawal.

Interactions with Other Drugs

Beta-adrenergic blockers participate in many important drug–drug interactions. They are summarized in Table 15–12, along with cross-references to chapters in which the interactants are discussed in more detail. Interactions involving the prototype, propranolol, are the most studied.

The most important interaction to avoid, if at all possible, involves the parenteral administration of epinephrine to persons taking β blockers. The outcome can be a severe hypertensive crisis accompanied by profound bradycardia, with the potential for cardiac failure or arrest. In this situation epinephrine acts essentially as a pure α agonist, constricting blood vessels and triggering reflex bradycardia that adds to the bradycardia caused by the β blocker. It may be impossible to avoid the interaction if epinephrine is being used as an emergency drug, as to manage anaphylaxis (for which epinephrine is the drug of choice) or β blocker overdoses (for which it is not). In these and other situations, extreme caution and very careful monitoring are essential. The nurse should also be aware that any other drug with α-agonist activity, including some that are available OTC and can be self-prescribed (eg, phenylephrine or phenylpropanolamine), can cause a similar problem.

Other interactions involve drugs that add to the cardiac depression caused by β blockers (eg, digoxin and verapamil; and parenteral administration of lidocaine and phenytoin); and those that either stimulate or inhibit β blocker metabolism (eg, alcohol, barbiturates, cimetidine, oral phenytoin, and even the nicotine in tobacco smoke). Interactions involving altered metabolism affect mainly propranolol and the related drug metoprolol because they depend the most on the liver for terminating their activity. Many of these interactions need not be avoided, but proper monitoring for desired and adverse responses, and careful instructions to the patient, are crucial for making combined therapy safe and effective.

NURSING IMPLICATIONS

Give the patient a written list of medications that are likely to interact with the β blocker. Include OTC drugs. When interacting drugs are added to β blocker therapy, doses of one or both agents may need to be changed. The patient's responses to the modified treatment must be followed closely until they stabilize. Smoking counteracts many of the desired cardiovascular effects of β blockers; encourage smokers to quit.

Overdose and Toxicity

Managing true overdoses of β blockers, or severe adverse reactions to any dose of these drugs administered to persons with one or more contraindicating conditions, requires careful assessment so that the most important problems can be identified and corrected first. In many cases, more than one problem can place the patient at risk, and that situation can affect the treatment. If a true overdose occurred, and it was caused by oral dosage forms, standard first-aid measures to reduce further drug absorption are indicated (see Appendix C).

Common problems affect the heart: bradycardia, decreased cardiac contractility, and varying degrees of atrioventricular (AV) block. Collectively, one or more of these problems often cause hypotension also and could lead to acute heart failure or cardiac arrest. The first thing to do is place the patient in the supine position, head-low, to maintain cerebral blood flow. The antimuscarinic drug atropine, given intravenously, is usually administered first so that the cardiac-depressant influences of the parasympathetic nervous system are blocked. Atropine should increase heart rate and contractility, which should indirectly help normalize blood pressure. If one or two doses of atropine do not work, a β agonist such as dopamine or dobutamine can be given, but relatively large doses probably will be needed to overcome β blockade. With epinephrine or norepinephrine, α-receptor–mediated vasoconstriction will predominate, increasing blood pressure but doing relatively less to support the heart. Glucagon (see Chapter 46), a drug that can increase cardiac function even in the presence of β blockade, is often effective when other measures fail.

Atropine will do little or nothing to counteract the bronchoconstriction or hypoglycemia that are of special concern for persons with asthma or diabetes, respectively. Anticipate the use of IV β agonists, or the unrelated bronchodilator aminophylline (and oxygen), to manage bronchoconstriction. Intravenous infusions of glucose usually are indicated to manage hypoglycemia.

NURSING IMPLICATIONS

Drugs for treating β blocker overdoses should be readily available whenever a β blocker is injected or given to a seriously ill patient. Careful assessment of vital signs helps direct treatment and the patient's response to it.

Maintain a patent IV route for giving drugs and for withdrawing blood samples. Invasive monitoring of cardiovascular status is often required.

Never administer drugs with only α-agonist activity (eg, phenylephrine) to counteract hypotension. They will increase blood pressure, but will reflexly add to cardiac depression, making matters worse. Question orders for giving a digitalis preparation. These are well known as stimulants of cardiac contractility, but they also decrease electrical impulse conduction through the AV node, and greatly increase the risk of heart block. Likewise, avoid giving IV fluids, which can overload the work capacity of the depressed heart and also cause heart failure.

Related Drugs

Most of the related drugs are nonselective β_1 and β_2 blockers, just like propranolol. However, a few have one or more special properties. The list of approved β blockers is so long (and growing) that you should consult the package insert for more details about a particular agent. However, some general comments about the major similarities and differences of the related drugs, compared with the prototype, should help sort out the information.

- The other β blockers depend on hepatic metabolism, or renal excretion of the unmetabolized drug, to different degrees. For example, propranolol itself, and the related drug metoprolol, depend almost completely on the liver to metabolize them to inactive substances. In contrast, nearly all of the related drug nadolol is eliminated in the urine without prior metabolism. Thus, dosage reductions may be required for some of the drugs given to patients with impaired hepatic or renal function, of if an interacting drug that affects the liver or kidney is to be used. In some cases, rather than adjusting dosages it may be better to use a different β blocker.
- Most β blockers are formulated for oral administration, and all of those orally effective drugs are indicated for managing angina pectoris and essential hypertension; some are marketed as fixed-dose combinations with diuretics (Chapter 33) for added antihypertensive effects. Some β blockers are available in parenteral or topical formulations, in addition to or instead of oral dosage forms, with special uses approved for each. No β blocker has all the uses for which propranolol is approved.
- These drugs differ in potency, so typical dosages (Table 15–C2) differ.
- If a patient does not respond adequately to one β blocker, given for a particular indication, they probably will not respond better to an alternative that has the same indication. The only difference is likely to be in terms of side effects, and even here the drug-related differences may be slight.
- Some orally effective β blockers have longer durations of action and so are suitable for once-daily administration. That property may be an asset to compliance for some patients, but a longer duration of therapeutic effects is necessarily accompanied by a longer duration of adverse effects, if they should occur because of overdose or drug interactions.
- Most β blockers enter the CNS less well than propranolol, and so they may be preferred if CNS side effects, such as sedation, become a problem.
- If a given β blocker is contraindicated for a particular patient, assume that all other β blockers will be also. Some of these agents have special properties (see below) that can *reduce* certain side effects for certain patients, but they do not eliminate the risks altogether.
- Adverse effects can occur regardless of the administration route. Systemic administration obviously poses the greatest risk, the proper monitoring devices and emergency drugs should always be available when any β blocker is to be injected. However, serious responses can occur with the topical administration of ophthalmic β blockers for glaucoma. For example, deaths have been reported after administering just one drop (usually the "right" dose) of some ophthalmic preparations to patients with severe pulmonary disease.
- Overdoses, toxicity, or drug–drug interactions are generally the same as for propranolol, and are managed the same way.

Special Properties of Some β-Adrenergic Blockers

A few β blockers have a property called ***intrinsic sympathomimetic activity*** (ISA); several are classified as "cardioselective"; and one β blocker also blocks α-adrenergic receptors. Each property is caused by a unique chemical structure of the drug, which gives it theoretic or actual advantages, for some patients, over alternatives that do not share the property.

Intrinsic Sympathomimetic Activity

Carteolol (CARTROL), penbutolol (LEVATOL), and pindolol (VISKEN) are three nonselective β blockers that have ISA. (Another drug with ISA is mentioned in the next paragraph.) Intrinsic sympathomimetic activity means that when sympathetic tone throughout the body is relatively low, such as at rest, these drugs weakly *stimulate* β receptors. In doing so, they cause less depression of resting heart rate and contractility and blood glucose levels, and less bronchoconstriction, than β blockers without ISA. However, when sympathetic tone rises, as during exercise, these drugs effectively block the stimulating effects of epinephrine and norepinephrine. The alternative drugs with ISA, which are approved for oral therapy of essential hypertension, might therefore be chosen over a β blocker without ISA for patients in whom slight resting bradycardia, bronchoconstriction, or hypoglycemia poses a problem. Nevertheless, they still share all the contraindications noted for the prototype, and so nursing assessment is no less of a challenge.

"Cardioselectivity"

All the drugs described so far block both β_1- and β_2-adrenergic receptors. However, when β blockers are used for their cardiovascular effects (hypertension, angina, arrhythmias), as most of them are, only blockade of the β_1 receptors is necessary. Blocking β_2 receptors, as in the lungs, liver, or peripheral vasculature, is unnecessary. For patients who also have pulmonary disorders or diabetes, β_2 blockade is clearly unwanted, if not dangerous. To overcome this limitation somewhat, pharmaceutical manufacturers have developed newer agents with structures that exert greatest blocking activity on the β_1 receptors. They include acebutolol (SECTRAL; which also has ISA), atenolol (TENORMIN), betaxolol (KERLONE is the oral dosage form; BETOPTIC is the topical ophthalmic preparation for glaucoma), esmolol (BREVIBLOC; available only for IV use), and metoprolol (LOPRESSOR). Their uses are summarized in Figure 15–1; dosages are in Table 15–C2.

The term *cardioselectivity* is misleading. It has been incorrectly interpreted to mean that drugs with this property block *only* the β receptors found in the heart—the β_1 receptors—and that these drugs have absolutely no ability to block β_2 receptors. What the term really means is that when low doses of a cardioselective β blocker are given (or when blood levels are low), these drugs *mainly* block β_1 receptors, such as those in the heart. By comparison, their effects on β_2 receptors is weak, but those receptors are, nevertheless, partially blocked.

More importantly, when blood levels of these drugs become too high (whether because of actual overdose, because dosage adjustments to compensate for diminished metabolism or excretion are not properly made, or because the patient is unusually sensitive to one of these agents), these drugs work just as well as a nonselective blocker (eg, propranolol) to block all the β receptors. (The situation is analogous to the "selective" β_1 agonist bronchodilators, such as albuterol, as discussed in Chapter 14: they mainly stimulate β_1 receptors under certain conditions, but can stimulate all β receptors well in others.)

Cardioselectivity usually makes these drugs a better choice than a nonselective β blocker for patients with *mild* pulmonary disease or diabetes. However, they are not without risk for these patients; they are not absolutely safe; and they should not be used for patients in whom any β blocker would be absolutely contraindicated. Thus, once again, it is prudent to use for these drugs all the nursing measures that would be used for the prototype, propranolol.

Alpha Blockade

One currently approved β blocker, labetalol (NORMODYNE, TRANDATE) differs from all other β blockers because it also has some *α-adrenergic blocking activity*. Thus, it can lower blood pressure not only in the way that all other β blockers do, but also by inhibiting vasoconstriction in the peripheral vasculature. Its only use is for management of hypertension (long-term, with the oral dosage forms, or acutely with a parenteral formulation). Labetalol is not cardioselective and does not have ISA. Precautions for its use are the same as those noted for propranolol.

Other Drugs That Cause Sympatholytic Effects

Several other drugs have effects that make it appear as if the activity of the entire sympathetic nervous system is decreased. However, none of these sympatholytic agents act by blocking adrenergic receptors, as do all the other drugs discussed in this chapter. These drug examples are given here not just because they are pharmacologically interesting, but because some of them are commonly used. The drugs are discussed in more detail in other chapters. At this point simply try to appreciate that there are many ways to inhibit the activity of structures controlled by the sympathetic nervous system.

- *Reserpine,* the related antihypertensive drugs guanabenz and guanadrel (Chapter 33), and a seldom-used antihypertensive, guanethidine, deplete norepinephrine from adrenergic nerve endings. When the nerves are stimulated, there is less neurotransmitter to be released, and so the resulting sympathomimetic effects are decreased.

- *Clonidine* and α-methyldopa are also antihypertensive drugs (Chapter 33). They are α-adrenergic *agonists* that act mainly in the brain's cardiovascular control centers to reduce activity of all the sympathetic nerves (reduced "sympathetic outflow"). Clonidine also acts peripherally to stimulate the presynaptic α_2 receptors found on adrenergic nerve endings.
- *Bretylium,* an antiarrhythmic drug (Chapter 30), acts as if it seals off the adrenergic nerve endings. Even though the nerve endings contain norepinephrine, when the nerve is stimulated the neurotransmitter is not released.

SUMMARY OF NURSING IMPLICATIONS

◆ Assessment

Review patient's history for presence of underlying medical conditions that contraindicate therapy with an α or β blocker (chronic obstructive lung disease, particularly asthma; overt cardiac failure, hypotension, or heart block; diabetes).

Identify drugs from the medication history that require cautious concurrent use because of potential drug interactions (monoamine oxidase inhibitors, catecholamine depletors, insulin, many OTC drugs, cimetidine if receiving propranolol).

Establish baseline data before initiating drug therapy: cardiovascular, respiratory, and mental status; laboratory tests to indicate organ function or disorders such as diabetes, liver disease.

◆ Nursing Diagnoses

Decreased cardiac output related to orthostatic hypotension (α blockers) or heart disease (β blockers).

Sexual dysfunction related to drug therapy (primarily α blockers).

Altered cerebral or peripheral tissue perfusion related to vasoconstriction, disease (α or β blockers).

Impaired gas exchange related to bronchoconstriction (β blockers).

Altered nutrition: less than body requirements related to hypoglycemia (β blockers).

Sensory/perceptual alterations: dizziness related to drug therapy (α or β blockers).

Noncompliance related to undesirable drug effects or inadequate understanding of drug regimen (α or β blockers).

Fatigue related to drug effects (α or β blockers).

◆ Planning/Implementation

Prepare and administer medication safely, at the same time each day.

Administer α blocker before β blocker if used together for initial treatment of a pheochromocytoma.

Monitor vital signs for indications of detrimental responses to drug therapy, such as cardiac failure, bronchoconstriction, or inadequate tissue perfusion.

Control unnecessary environmental stress, as drug therapy can inhibit adaptive responses.

Assist patient with activity and ambulation to prevent injury associated with dizziness, drowsiness.

Reassure and encourage patient when dealing with distressing side effects (eg, sexual dysfunction, GI distress, fatigue), and advise that side effects may disappear or diminish with continued drug use.

◆ Patient and Family Teaching

Instruct the patient and family in the following: the desired and side effects of drugs; the importance of never abruptly discontinuing drug; potential drug interactions, including avoidance of OTC preparations without physician approval; stress-management techniques; when to notify physician (ie, signs of heart failure, hypotension, breathing difficulty); how to avoid postural (orthostatic) hypotension; the importance of taking the drug with or shortly after meals at the same time each day to decrease GI distress (phenoxybenzamine) and increase absorption; and how to take pulse.

◆ Evaluation

The patient/family will:

Achieve desired therapeutic effects (eg, normotensive; anginal pain relieved; regular cardiac rhythm; tissue integrity maintained; normal activity resumed).

Comply with drug regimen as prescribed; continue drug even with side effects that are annoying but not dangerous (eg, nasal stuffiness, miosis, sexual dysfunction).

Experience minimal to no serious side effects (respiratory difficulty, heart failure or rhythm disturbances, hypoglycemia); laboratory values remain within normal limits.

Be knowledgeable regarding safe administration and management of drug therapy.

Annotated Bibliography

Note: The following articles apply to general uses of adrenergic blockers, or uses that are not discussed elsewhere. See the annotated bibliographies of other chapters for papers dealing with the use of these drugs for patients with arrhythmias (Chapter 30), hypertension (Chapter 33), and angina (Chapter 34).

Blanchard DG, Ross J Jr. Hypertrophic cardiomyopathy: Prognosis with medical or surgical therapy. *Clin Cardiol* 1991;14(1):11–19. *Beta blockers relieve symptoms, but do not appear to affect long-term survival. This article discusses the role of adrenergic blockers, other drug classes, and surgical intervention, in the management of patients with cardiomyopathy.*

Buckley MM, Goa KL, Clissold SP. Ocular betaxolol: A review of its pharmacological properties, and therapeutic efficacy in glaucoma and ocular hypertension. *Drugs* 1990;40(1):75–90. *An interesting article that will help you understand how a topical formulation of this cardioselective β blocker is used for ocular effects, and why such a drug might have advantages over other β blockers.*

Cooper JW. Reviewing geriatric concerns with commonly used drugs. *Geriatrics* 1989;44:79–86. *Covering many therapeutic agents used often in elders, this short article also gives good advice about the use of β blockers.*

Frishman WH, Lazar EJ, Gorodokin G. Pharmacokinetic optimisation of therapy with beta-adrenergic blocking agents. *Clin Pharmacokinet* 1991;20(4):311–318. *Valuable for readers wishing more information on how altered hepatic metabolism or renal excretion—including that which is affected by age, race, and habits such as smoking—can alter the distribution, actions, and elimination of β blockers.*

Gerber SL, Cantor LB, Brater DC. Systemic drug interactions with topical glaucoma medications. *Surv Ophthalmol* 1990;35(3):205–218. *Topical antiglaucoma drugs, including β blockers, are absorbed systemically. The related adverse effects are prominently displayed in package insert warnings. Yet, are they clinically important? This article addresses that issue.*

Gordon NF, Duncan JJ. Effect of beta-blockers on exercise physiology: Implications for exercise training. *Med Sci Sports Exerc* 1991;23(6):668–676. *Beta blockers, like other drugs, are used to help patients maintain a normal lifestyle. If exercise is one of your patient's interests, and a β blocker is one of his or her drugs, this article can aid in your planning, assessment, and teaching.*

Grisanti JM. Raynaud's phenomenon. *Am Fam Physician* 1990;41(1):134–142. *An overview of how α-adrenergic blockers, newer drugs, and nondrug therapies can help manage patients with this peripheral vascular disease.*

Hansson L. Review of state-of-the-art beta-blocker therapy. *Am J Cardiol* 1991;67(10):43B–46B. *A short and interesting look at what β blocker therapy has already accomplished, and what future goals remain to be realized with them.*

Jaillon P. Relevance of intrinsic sympathomimetic activity for beta blockers. *Am J Cardiol* 1990;66(9):21C–23C. *A brief but informative review of the potential advantages of β blockers with ISA.*

Nash DT. Alpha-adrenergic blockers: Mechanism of action, blood pressure control, and effects on lipoprotein metabolism. *Clin Cardiol* 1990;13(11):764–772. *Worth reading now because this article discusses how both α- and β-adrenergic receptors play a role in hypertension, and how some of their blockers play a role in its therapy.*

Opie LH. Required beta blocker profile in the elderly. *Cardiovasc Drugs Ther* 1991;4(Suppl. 6):1273–1280. *Problems with β-blocker therapy in your elderly patient? Consult this short article for why the problems may have arisen, and what you might suggest to overcome them.*

Polansky JR. Beta-adrenergic therapy for glaucoma. *Int Ophthalmol Clin* 1990;30(3):219–229. *A good summary of how β-receptor drugs, both agonists and antagonists, fit into the therapy of glaucoma.*

van Zwieten PA. Comparative properties of various beta-blockers, with an outlook to the future. *Clin Physiol Biochem* 1990;8(Suppl. 2):18–27. *There's more to consider than β blockade. This article summarizes the clinical importance of other properties: cardioselectivity, ISA, the ability to block α receptors also, duration of action, and more.*

Walling AD. Drug prophylaxis for migraine headaches. *Am Fam Physician* 1990;42(2):425–432. *A well-written article about the use of β blockers, and many other drug classes, in the prevention of disabling migraine headaches.*

Table 15–C1 | Clinical Uses and Administration of Major Alpha-Adrenergic Receptor Blocking Drugs

AGENT	CLINICAL USES	DOSAGE AND ROUTE OF ADMINISTRATION
	Alpha$_1$ and Alpha$_2$ Receptor Blockers	
PROTOTYPE		
Phentolamine		
(REGITINE)	Control of hypertensive episodes in pheochromocytoma	IV (preferred) or IM: 5 mg for adults, 1 mg for children, repeated as necessary to lower BP
	Diagnosis of pheochromocytoma	IM (preferred) or IV: 5 mg for adults, 1 mg for children; BP drop ≥ 35 mm Hg systolic or ≥ 25 mm Hg diastolic usually indicates pheochromocytoma
	Treatment of extravasation of vasoconstrictor (eg, norepinephrine)	SC: Dilute 5–10 mg in 10 mL sterile isotonic saline, infiltrate liberally around area of extravasation; usually not effective if given > 12 hr after incident, best given immediately
	Prevention of norepinephrine extravasation	IV: Add 10 mg to each liter of norepinephrine infusion
RELATED DRUGS		
Ergoloid mesylates (dihydroergocristine, dihydroergocryptine, dihydroergocornine)		
(CIRCANOL, DEAPRIL-ST, HYDERGINE)	Symptomatic treatment of idiopathic mental deterioration in elderly patients with probable cerebrovascular insufficiency	Sublingual or oral: Usually 1 mg (contains 0.33 mg of each component) tid
Phenoxybenzamine		
(DIBENZYLINE)	Treatment (short- or long-term) of episodes of hypertension or sweating in pheochromocytoma patients	Oral: 10 mg bid; increase to 20–40 mg bid or tid if side effects (eg, orthostatic hypotension) are minimal; usually used adjunctively with β-blocker to control reflex tachycardia
Tolazoline		
(PRISCOLINE)	Treatment of pulmonary hypertension in newborns who fail to respond to other therapies (eg, oxygen, mechanical ventilation)	IV (into scalp vein): Initially infuse at 1–2 mg/kg/hr, then continue at 1–2 mg/kg/hr as needed

Table 15–S1 Major Side Effects and Contraindications of Alpha-Adrenergic Receptor Blocking Drugs

BODY SYSTEM Side Effect	CONTRAINDICATION/ PRECAUTION	COMMENTS AND NURSING IMPLICATIONS
EYE		
Miosis, impaired dilation of iris in dim light		If night vision is poor, caution patient against operating motor vehicle after dark
Excessive lacrimation		Consult physician if side effects bothersome to patient; physician may recommend topical ophthalmic decongestants; caution patient against self-prescribing decongestants, particularly systemic (orally administered) agents
UPPER RESPIRATORY		
Excessive, thin mucus secretions; rhinorrhea		Consult physician; comments noted for excessive lacrimation apply
CARDIOVASCULAR		
Hypotension, particularly orthostatic	Hypotension; coronary, cerebral vascular insufficiency (ie, angina, MI, stroke); peripheral vascular insufficiency due to causes other than those for which α blockers are indicated	Measure BP before and periodically after administering α blocker; BP must be measured at ½–3 min intervals for at least 15 min if phentolamine used for pheochromocytoma diagnosis; observe for signs, symptoms of inadequate blood flow to heart (eg, angina), brain (dizziness), extremities (skin color, temperature); instruct ambulatory patients to sit, stand slowly, assume head-low seated position if dizziness occurs
Reflex tachycardia	Tachycardia; tachyarrhythmias; history of ischemic heart disease (eg, angina)	Measure heart rate, assess rhythm, withhold α blocker if tachycardia or arrhythmias present; notify physician if patient complains of anginal pain; physician may prescribe β blocker to control heart rate, particularly if patient has pheochromocytoma
Aggravation of heart failure, edema		Reduced BP increases plasma renin, aldosterone levels, leading to salt, water retention; monitor weight periodically as index of edema and assess for other signs of heart failure
GASTROINTESTINAL		
Dyspepsia; abdominal pain	Active or recent peptic ulcer	Report severe abdominal pain, tarry stools that may indicate bleeding ulcer
Diarrhea		Notify physician if diarrhea is frequent or severe
GENITOURINARY		
Inhibited ejaculation		May be unavoidable; advise patient to weigh potential benefits of α blocker therapy with impaired sexual performance against persistence of disorder for which α blocker was prescribed; erection is not affected

Table 15–I1 Major Interactions Between Alpha-Adrenergic Receptor Blocking Drugs and Other Agents*

AGENT	RESULT OF INTERACTION	COMMENTS AND NURSING IMPLICATIONS
Alcohol	Added hypotensive effect	Alcohol is a vasodilator; encourage patient to moderate or discontinue alcohol use
Antihypertensive drugs (all; see Chapter 33)	Added hypotensive effect; added tachycardia (with antihypertensives other than β-blockers)	Avoid combined use if possible, otherwise monitor accordingly
Antimuscarinic drugs (all; Chapter 13)	Increased risk or severity of tachycardia	Monitor accordingly if combined therapy is essential; teach patient about OTC drugs with antimuscarinic activity that should be avoided; see Table 13–I
Epinephrine, other sympathomimetics with β-agonist activity, including all sympathomimetic bronchodilators (Chapter 14, Chapter 38)	Increased risk or severity of tachycardia	Monitor accordingly; drugs with both α- and β-agonist activity will act as "pure" β agonists in presence of α blockade

*Interactions are of most concern in ambulatory patients (eg, those taking phenoxybenzamine).

Table 15–C2 Clinical Uses and Administration of Beta-Adrenergic Receptor Blocking Drugs*

AGENT	CLINICAL USES	DOSAGE AND ROUTE OF ADMINISTRATION
Nonselective Beta-Adrenergic Blockers		
PROTOTYPE		
Propranolol		
(INDERAL; INDERAL-LA)	Hypertension	Oral: 40 mg bid or one 80-mg long-acting capsule (INDERAL-LA) once daily; gradually increase to 120–240 mg/d in divided doses (long-acting capsules once daily) until pressure controlled adequately; ordinarily do not exceed 640 mg/d; reduce dose when used with other antihypertensive drugs.
	Angina pectoris	Oral: 80–320 mg/d in 2, 3, or 4 divided doses (or one 80-mg long-acting capsule once daily); gradually increase to 160–320 mg/d as needed
	Tachyarrhythmias	Oral: 10–30 mg, tid or qid; long-acting preparation not recommended
	Life-threatening or anesthesia-induced arrhythmias	IV: 0.5–3 mg, given no faster than 1 mg/min; give second dose after 2 min if necessary, further doses no more often than every 4 hr
	Hypertrophic subaortic stenosis	Oral: 20–40 mg tid or qid (or one 80-mg or 160-mg long-acting capsule once daily)
	Preoperative adjunctive management of pheochromocytoma	Oral: 20 mg tid; start 3 days before surgery; use with, give after α blocker; long-acting preparation not recommended
	Long-term adjunctive therapy of pheochromocytoma	Oral: 20 mg tid; use with α blocker; long-acting preparation not recommended

(continued)

Table 15–C2 Clinical Uses and Administration of Beta-Adrenergic Receptor Blocking Drugs* (*Continued*)

AGENT	CLINICAL USES	DOSAGE AND ROUTE OF ADMINISTRATION
	Prophylaxis of migraine headache	Oral: 40 mg bid (or one 80-mg long-acting capsule once daily); maintenance dose 160–240 mg/d (divided doses for regular tablets, single dose of long-acting capsule)
	Prevention of sudden cardiac death after myocardial infarction in patients with stable hemodynamics	Oral: 180–240 mg/d in 2 or 3 divided doses; long-acting preparation not indicated
	Symptomatic relief of familial or hereditary essential skeletal muscle tremor	Oral: 40 mg bid; optimal daily dose is approximately 120 mg in divided doses (long-acting preparation not indicated)
RELATED DRUGS		
Carteolol		
(CARTROL)	Hypertension	Oral: Initially 2.5 mg once daily; maintenance dose 2.5–5 mg once daily
(OCUPRESS)	Chronic open-angle glaucoma, ocular hypertension	Topical: 1 drop of 1% solution twice daily
Levobunolol		
(BETAGAN)	Chronic open-angle glaucoma, ocular hypertension	Topical: 1 drop of 0.5% solution daily
Metipranolol		
(OPTIPRANOLOL)	Ocular hypertension, glaucoma	Topical: 1 drop of 0.3% solution bid
Nadolol		
(CORGARD)	Angina or hypertension	Oral: 40 mg once daily; can be increased in increments of 40–80 mg up to maintenance dose of 40–240 mg/d (angina) or 40–320 mg/d (hypertension); usual maintenance dose is 40–80 mg
Penbutolol		
(LEVATOL)	Hypertension	Oral: 20 mg once daily
Pindolol		
(VISKEN)	Hypertension	Oral: 5 mg twice daily; if satisfactory response not seen in 3–4 weeks increase by 10 mg/d up to maximum of 60 mg/d (in 2 divided doses)
Timolol		
(BLOCADREN)	Hypertension	Oral: 10 mg twice daily; maintenance dose usually 10–20 mg bid, up to maximum of 30 mg bid
	Prevention of sudden cardiac death after myocardial infarction	Oral: 10 mg bid
(TIMOPTIC)	Glaucoma	Topical: 1 drop of 0.25% solution q12h; 12-h, reduce to 1 drop per day when intraocular pressure is controlled; may use 0.5% solution if lower dose ineffective

(continued)

Table 15–C2 Clinical Uses and Administration of Beta-Adrenergic Receptor Blocking Drugs* (*Continued*)

AGENT	CLINICAL USES	DOSAGE AND ROUTE OF ADMINISTRATION
"Cardioselective" ($Beta_1$) Beta Blockers		
Acebutolol		
(SECTRAL)	Hypertension	Oral: 400 mg once daily or 200 mg bid; maintenance doses usually 400–800 mg/d in single or divided doses
	Premature ventricular contractions	Oral: 200 mg bid; maintenance dose 300–600 mg bid
Atenolol		
(TENORMIN)	Hypertension	Oral: 50 mg/d up to maximum of 100 mg/d
	Angina pectoris	Oral: 50 mg once daily; if necessary increase after 1 week to 100 mg/d (200 mg may be needed)
Betaxolol		
(BETOPTIC)	Glaucoma	Topical: 1 drop (0.5% solution) bid
(KERLONE)	Hypertension	Oral: 10 mg once daily; maintenance dose up to 20 mg once daily
Esmolol		
(BREVIBLOC)	Treatment of supraventricular tachycardia, sinus tachycardia, atrial flutter or fibrillation	IV: Give loading dose of 500 μg/kg/min for 1 min, decrease to 50 μg/kg/min; most arrhythmias respond to 50–200 μg/kg/min
Metoprolol		
(LOPRESSOR)	Hypertension, angina pectoris	Oral: 50 mg bid (may be preferred for hypertension) or 100 mg once daily (preferred for angina); increase at weekly intervals as needed; usual maintenance dose 100 mg bid, may be as high as 450 mg/d in divided doses
	Prevention of sudden cardiac death after myocardial infarction	IV: 5 mg, followed by two more doses at 2-min intervals; begin oral doses 15 min later Oral: 50 mg q6h for 48 hours; maintenance doses 100 mg bid for at least 3 months, preferably for 1–3 years to reduce chance of reinfarction
(TOPROL XL)	Hypertension Angina pectoris	Oral: 50–100 mg once daily Oral: 100 mg once daily
Mixed Beta and Alpha Blocker		
Labetalol		
(NORMODYNE, TRANDATE)	Hypertension	Oral: 100 mg twice daily; increase gradually to maintenance dose of 200–400 mg bid, up to maximum of 2400 mg/d in divided doses for severe hypertension
	Hypertensive episodes	IV: 20 mg or 0.25% mg/kg, whichever is less, injected over 2 min; if needed give additional 40- or 80-mg doses at 10-min intervals up to cumulative dose of 300 mg; alternatively, infuse at 2 mg/min

*See Chapter 33 for dosages of antihypertensive products containing a beta blocker and a diuretic.

Table 15–S2 Major Side Effects and Contraindications of Beta-Adrenergic Receptor Blocking Drugs

BODY SYSTEM Side Effect	CONTRAINDICATION/ PRECAUTION	COMMENTS AND NURSING IMPLICATIONS
CENTRAL NERVOUS SYSTEM		
Dizziness, drowsiness, fatigue, altered sleep (insomnia, nightmares)	Questionable neurologic status (relative contraindication)	Most common with propranolol, which enters CNS readily; intensity tends to diminish with continued drug use; advise patient to avoid tasks made dangerous by drowsiness, and to report intense responses to nurse or physician; dizziness may indicate hypotension, regardless of β blocker used
ENDOCRINE		
Hypoglycemia; delayed recovery from hypoglycemia	Labile, poorly controlled, or drug-dependent diabetes mellitus	If β-blocker therapy essential, cardioselective agents usually are preferred; encourage compliance with diabetes treatment regimen, close monitoring of blood glucose levels; advise that diaphoresis, thirst, and hunger are better indications of hypoglycemia than tachycardia
Masking of hyperthyroidism, thyrotoxicosis		Beta blockers, routinely used to prevent tachycardia in hyperthyroid patients, impair early diagnosis of thyrotoxicosis. Monitor serum thyroid hormone levels periodically, ensure patient receives lowest effective doses of thyroid supplements, β blockers.
RESPIRATORY		
Wheezing, dyspnea, bronchospasm, laryngospasm	Asthma, emphysema, bronchitis, other forms of chronic obstructive pulmonary disease	All β blockers contraindicated for severe obstructive pulmonary disease; cardioselective agents preferred if β blocker is essential, closer monitoring is critical; have patient report breathing difficulty at once
CARDIOVASCULAR		
Bradycardia, progressive heart block, asystole	Sinus bradycardia; heart rate < 50/min; heart block > first degree	Evaluate cardiovascular status closely before and after giving β blocker; dizziness, drowsiness may indicate excessive cardiovascular effects; anticipate need to give IV atropine for bradycardia or heart block, especially if β blocker is to be given by IV route
Reduced exercise tolerance		Less common, problematic, with β blockers having ISA
Hypotension, shock	Systolic blood pressure < 100 mm Hg	Check BP before and after giving β blocker, especially parenterally; if excessive hypotension occurs, place patient in supine, head-low position; anticipate need for atropine (IV)—restoring heart rate and contractility usually restores BP
Precipitation, worsening of heart failure	Moderate-to-severe heart failure; cardiogenic shock	Assess closely for signs, symptoms of heart failure if β blocker must be given; teach patient to monitor body weight, report fatigue or breathing difficulty that may indicate worsening of condition; dopamine, dobutamine, or glucagon preferred for treating acute heart failure in β-blocked patient; avoid digitalis, which increases risk of AV block
Increased frequency or severity of anginal attacks	Vasospastic (Prinzmetal's or variant) angina	Caused by unmasking of α-mediated vasoconstriction in coronary arteries; β blockers, used alone, suitable only for chronic stable (exercise-induced) angina; advise patient to report side effect at once
Increased BP in hypertensive patient		May indicate pheochromocytoma; notify physician

Table 15–12 **Major Interactions Between Beta-Adrenergic Receptor Blocking Drugs and Other Agents***

AGENT	RESULT OF INTERACTION	COMMENTS AND NURSING IMPLICATIONS
Alcohol (Chapter 22)	Increased CNS depression, increased or decreased β-blocker action	Have patient moderate alcohol use; acute high-dose alcohol ingestion lowers BP, inhibits metabolism of β blockers (propranolol, metoprolol); low-dose alcohol intake stimulates metabolism
Antiinflammatory drugs, non-steroidal (Chapter 52)	Decreased antihypertensive effect of β blockers	Occurs with both prescription and OTC agents (ie, ibuprofen; ADVIL, NUPRIN); combined use should be under physician's supervision; interactants inhibit synthesis of prostaglandins that seem to play role in all β blockers' antihypertensive effects
Antipsychotic drugs (eg, chlorpromazine; Chapter 23)	Increased actions, side effects, of one or both interactants	Monitor accordingly; may need to decrease dose of one or both drugs
Antithyroid drugs, oral (Chapter 47)	Decreased metabolism, increased effects, of β blockers; masking of tachycardia if hyperthyroidism occurs	Starting therapy of hyperthyroidism reduces metabolic-stimulating effects of excess thyroid hormone levels, slows propranolol (and metoprolol) metabolism; monitor closely, reduced β-blocker dose may be needed
Barbiturates (eg, phenobarbital, Chapter 22)	Reduced blood levels, effects, of β blockers	May occur rapidly with start of combined therapy; barbiturates stimulate hepatic metabolism, affects mainly propranolol, metoprolol; monitor accordingly
Cimetidine (Chapter 40)	Increased blood levels, actions, side effects of β blocker or cimetidine	Interactants inhibit hepatic metabolism of one another; less likely to occur with cimetidine alternatives, β blockers other than propranolol, metoprolol; monitor accordingly if these interactants must be given
Digoxin (Chapter 31)	Increased risk of AV block, potential cardiac arrest	Must avoid using β blockers to manage most digoxin-induced arrhythmias, using digoxin for stimulating heart in β-blocker overdoses; both drugs exert powerful inhibitory effects on electrical impulse conduction through AV node
Epinephrine (Chapter 14)	Sudden, severe hypertension, reflex bradycardia	Avoid interaction if at all possible; occurs because β-blocker–mediated vasodilation is abolished, leaving interactant's α-mediated vasoconstriction unopposed; treatment of anaphylaxis (for which epinephrine is drug of choice) becomes problematic; involves *all* β blockers, *all* sympathomimetics with α-agonist activity (including OTCs, eg, phenylpropanolamine), although intensity of response may be less with other sympathomimet-
Insulin, other antidiabetic drugs (Chapter 46)	Prolonged hypoglycemia, delayed recovery from hypoglycemia; masking of hypoglycemia symptom (tachycardia)	Avoid combined use if possible; may need to lower dose of insulin or other hypoglycemic drug if problematic; less likely to be severe or problematic if β blocker is cardioselective or has ISA; teach patient to rely on other indicators of hypoglycemia (eg, diaphoresis)
Lidocaine (Chapters 19, 30)	Increased cardiac depression	Occurs rapidly; avoid rapid IV bolus injections, follow lidocaine infusion guidelines closely; lidocaine and β blockers are both cardiac depressants; propranolol slows lidocaine's hepatic inactivation
Phenytoin (Chapter 26)	Decreased β-blocker effects (with long-term therapy)	Mechanism, outcomes, nursing implications identical to those for barbiturates, above
	Increased cardiac depression (acute)	IV bolus administration of phenytoin (as for arrhythmias, seizures) causes added cardiac depression; inject slowly, monitor accordingly

(continued)

Table 15–12 Major Interactions Between Beta-Adrenergic Receptor Blocking Drugs and Other Agents* (*Continued*)

AGENT	RESULT OF INTERACTION	COMMENTS AND NURSING IMPLICATIONS
Rifampin (Chapter 57)	Decreased β-blocker effects	May occur rapidly with onset of combined therapy; interactant stimulates hepatic metabolism, mainly affects propranolol, metoprolol
Theophylline (and aminophylline; Chapter 38)	Increased risk of theophylline toxicity; reduced effectiveness of theophylline as bronchodilator, reduced cardiovascular effects of β blocker	Avoid combination, use cardioselective agent if β blocker is essential; interactants have opposing effects on bronchi, heart; propranolol also inhibits metabolic inactivation of theophylline
Tobacco smoke (nicotine; Chapter 16)	Decrease or antagonism of all desired β-blocker effects	Nicotine in tobacco smoke stimulates sympathetic nervous system, stimulates β-blocker metabolism; directly triggers bronchoconstriction; encourage patient to stop smoking; monitor drug responses closely if patient quits, as β-blocker doses may need to be reduced
Verapamil (Chapters 33, 34)	Increased risk of cardiac depression, AV block	Additive effects may occur rapidly with start of combined therapy; probably affects all β blockers, all administration routes, including topical; monitor closely if interaction unavoidable

*Unless noted otherwise, interactions apply to all β-adrenergic blockers, and clearly apply to the prototype, propranolol. Interactions that involve altered β-blocker metabolism apply mainly to propranolol and metoprolol because they depend the most on hepatic metabolism for termination of their effects.

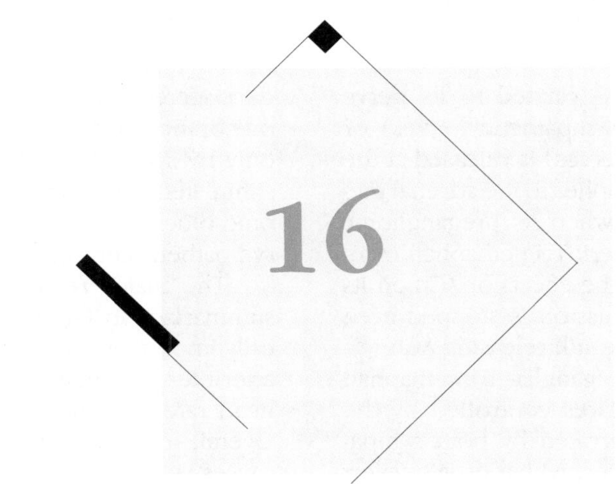

Ganglionic Blockers and Stimulants

General Characteristics of Ganglionic Blockers and Stimulants

Smooth muscle, cardiac muscle, and glands that are innervated by the autonomic nervous system (ANS) are linked to their regulatory centers in the central nervous system (CNS) by sympathetic and parasympathetic *ganglia.* Ganglia are the critical anatomic sites of chemical transmission between preganglionic and postganglionic nerves. Drugs that inhibit this process are called *ganglionic blockers;* those that mimic it are *ganglionic stimulants.* Because of their crucial site of action, these drugs can affect the activity of virtually all structures controlled by the ANS.

Major reference tables appear beginning on p. 260.

Ganglionic Blockers

PROTOTYPE

Trimethaphan

Absorption, Distribution, Metabolism, and Excretion

Trimethaphan (ARFONAD) is supplied as the camphorsulfonate (camsylate) salt. It is poorly absorbed from the gastrointestinal (GI) tract, and is given only by slow intravenous (IV) infusion. Its effects appear in 2 or 3 minutes and last about 10 minutes after the infusion is stopped. An infusion must be used because effects from a single injection are too brief, since the drug is eliminated rapidly. Trimethaphan is partly metabolized by plasma esterases (pseudocholinesterases); the rest is eliminated unchanged.

Pharmacologic Effects

Recall that preganglionic nerve endings release acetylcholine (ACh), which stimulates nicotinic receptors on the postganglionic nerve. The postganglionic nerve depolarizes, an action potential is carried to its nerve ending, and either ACh (parasympathetic nerves) or norepinephrine (sympathetic nerves) is released at the final target. The same process applies to the adrenal medulla: it releases epinephrine when its preganglionic sympathetic nerves are stimulated. Trimethaphan competitively antagonizes (blocks) the effects of ACh on its receptors, so ganglionic transmission is stopped even though preganglionic nerves are still releasing ACh.

By blocking all autonomic ganglia, trimethaphan affects the activity of all structures controlled by the ANS. Many structures are innervated by both sympathetic and parasympathetic nerves, which usually exert opposite but unequal actions. When a ganglionic blocker is given, it appears as if the nervous system branch with the greatest resting influence is affected most. Each structure operates at its own resting level. For example, salivary glands are under greater resting control by the parasympathetic nervous system, which normally increases secretions. Ganglionic blockers therefore reduce secretions. Some structures are controlled by only one branch of the ANS. Arterioles, which are innervated only by sympathetic nerves and which constrict when stimulated, are an example. In the presence of a ganglionic blocker, arterioles dilate because they lose their sympathetic control.

Table 16–1 Responses to Autonomic Ganglionic Blockade*

Structure	Response
Effectors Mainly Under Parasympathetic Tone at Rest	
Eye	
Iris dilator muscle	Mydriasis
Ciliary muscle	Cycloplegia
Heart	
Sinoatrial node	Tachycardia
Exocrine glands	
Mucus	Decreased secretions
Salivary	Decreased secretions
Sweat	Decreased secretions
Gastrointestinal tract	Decreased tone, motility (constipation)
Urinary bladder	Decreased micturition (urinary retention)
Effectors Mainly Under Sympathetic Tone at Rest	
Ventricular myocardium	Decreased force of contraction
Arterioles and veins	Dilation, reduced blood pressure and venous return

*All these are expected effects; all except moderate reductions of blood pressure are considered to be side effects or adverse responses in most patients.

The major responses to ganglionic blockers are summarized in Table 16–1. The most obvious and clinically important effects are on the cardiovascular system: arterioles and veins dilate, lowering blood pressure; heart rate increases; and cardiac contractile force falls. Overall, cardiac output increases. Trimethaphan also causes release of histamine, which is a vasodilator, cardiac-stimulating substance found in mast cells throughout the body (Chapter 36). This effect, which is not caused by blocking the autonomic ganglia, nevertheless contributes to the cardiovascular changes caused by ganglionic blockade. In most cases, the effects of ganglionic blockade on other organs and organ systems are unwanted, and so they will be discussed in the section on side effects.

It is important to note that key reflexes that depend on a functionally intact ANS will no longer operate when the ganglia are blocked. The baroreceptor reflex, which normally increases heart rate when blood pressure falls (or slows the rate when pressure rises), is abolished. Likewise, pupillary responses to light—dilation in dim light, constriction in bright light—are also absent.

Clinical Indications and Administration

Trimethaphan has few clinical indications (Table 16–C), and all of them make use of the drug's ability to dilate blood vessels and lower blood pressure. The drug is given by IV infusion, with doses adjusted to provide the desired intensity of effect. For each indication, the parenteral drug nitroprusside sodium is usually used instead. Chapter 33 addresses the actions and uses of antihypertensive drugs in general.

Controlled Hypotension During Surgery

Trimethaphan can be used to cause controlled hypotension during certain types of surgery. This effect reduces tissue swelling, which is a particular problem in surgery of the brain, spinal cord, and eye. It also reduces bleeding, which is valuable in cosmetic surgery.

Management of Hypertensive Crises

Trimethaphan can be used to lower blood pressure in hypertensive emergencies, in which stroke is a common complication. However, this drug is far from ideal. It will lower blood pressure, but it also blocks autonomic reflexes that are assessed as an important part of the neurologic evaluation.

Management of Hypertension plus Aortic Aneurysms

Hypertension complicated by an aortic aneurysm is fairly common, and is always a medical emergency. An aneurysm is a balloon-like weakening of the blood vessel wall. High blood pressure, and pressure pulsations with each heart beat, can cause it to rupture. Death occurs in seconds. Trimethaphan beneficially lowers blood pressure, and also reduces the large pressure pulses associated with each heart beat. Indeed, it is the only single drug that can do this, and so it may be a preferred agent in this setting. However, other drug combinations can also cause the same effects, and they are usually used instead.

Adjunctive Therapy of Acute Pulmonary Edema

Trimethaphan is indicated for emergency treatment of acute pulmonary edema. It reduces blood pressure and venous return to the heart, which alleviates congestion (edema) in the pulmonary circulation. Here, too, nitroprusside is almost always used instead.

NURSING IMPLICATIONS

Trimethaphan is usually prepared as a 1 mg/mL solution in 5% dextrose. Administer the drug with an infusion pump for precise control of the dose and, therefore, the response. Do not use standard IV drip chambers unless a pump is not available. Give trimethaphan through an indwelling IV catheter. Monitor vital signs every minute or two until blood pressure and heart rate stabilize, every 5 minutes during the remainder of drug administration, and for about 10 minutes after the infusion is stopped. Patients who were hypertensive before receiving trimethaphan (or any other antihypertensive drug) cannot tolerate sudden or large falls of blood pressure. Therefore, the nurse should try to learn the patient's usual predrug blood pressure range before administering trimethaphan.

Side Effects, Adverse Reactions, and Contraindications

Ganglionic blockers produce many side effects. Few, other than hypotension and impairment of autonomic reflexes, cause significant problems when trimethaphan is used because the drug is given acutely under controlled conditions to nonambulatory patients and its actions disappear quickly. Side effects, related contraindications, and relevant nursing implications are summarized in Table 16–S.

Excessive hypotension, assessed as the supine blood pressure, is the most important side effect. Ganglionic blockers are therefore contraindicated for any patient at great risk of excessive or uncontrolled hypotension. This includes patients who are in, or are at imminent risk of being in, hypovolemic or cardiogenic shock or stroke; and persons with atherosclerotic or diabetic lesions of blood vessels in major organs (brain, heart, kidney). These precautions apply to virtually all hypotensive drugs.

Ganglionic blockade prevents cardiovascular reflexes that are normally triggered to prevent orthostatic or hypotension. This is not a problem with trimethaphan, since patients receiving the drug are not ambulatory when the drug is given. However, it is a significant problem with the related drug mecamylamine.

A definite side effect of ganglionic blockade is the prevention of autonomic reflexes that are important for evaluating a patient's neurologic status, as when a stroke is suspected. For example, the pupils will be dilated, but it will be impossible to tell whether this is simply the expected response to the drug or a sign of brain damage. Pupillary constriction (miosis) in response to light, an autonomic reflex, is also inhibited. In summary, trimethaphan is contraindicated for patients with head injury, stroke, or most other causes of brain damage or dysfunction.

Trimethaphan is contraindicated for persons with asthma and chronic obstructive pulmonary disease (COPD) because it is liable to trigger severe bronchospasm. This adverse effect is caused mainly by the drug's ability to release histamine, a bronchoconstrictor, rather than by its ganglionic blocking actions.

NURSING IMPLICATIONS

If hypotension occurs, place the patient in a modified Trendelenburg position (head down, feet up), and slow or stop drug infusion at once. This usually restores blood pressure quickly.

◆ Use During Pregnancy and Lactation

The major pregnancy-related danger of ganglionic blockers is maternal hypotension, which can significantly decrease placental blood flow and harm the fetus. Women taking the orally effective related drug mecamylamine should be discouraged from breast-feeding their infants. It is highly unlikely that a woman receiving trimethaphan will be able to give breast-feedings.

◆ Use in Children

Trimethaphan is not indicated for children under 12 years old.

◆ Use in the Elderly

Trimethaphan must be used cautiously in elderly patients, who are less tolerant of any sudden or large blood pressure change. Excessive hypotension can aggravate arteriosclerosis and cardiac, renal, hepatic, or cerebrovascular disease, which are common in this population. Ganglionic blockers may cause urinary retention, particularly in men with prostatic hypertrophy. Risks from hypotension and urine retention are more problematic with long-term use of mecamylamine, but precautions still apply to trimethaphan.

Interactions with Other Drugs

The hypotensive effect of ganglionic blockers is potentiated by other drugs that lower blood pressure, including other antihypertensive drugs, general anesthetics, and alcohol. Trimethaphan intensifies and prolongs neuromuscular blockade caused by succinylcholine, and perhaps neuromuscular blockade caused by tubocurarine and related drugs. These agents are frequently used during surgery, a time when trimethaphan is used. Major interactions are summarized in Table 16–I.

NURSING IMPLICATIONS

If the patient has received trimethaphan and a neuromuscular blocker, anticipate the need for more prolonged mechanical support of ventilation and longer postoperative observation to ensure adequate recovery of spontaneous ventilation.

Overdoses and Toxicity

The major concern from overdoses is excessive hypotension and its related adverse effects. Measures to deal with it were discussed earlier.

Related Drug

Mecamylamine

Mecamylamine (INVERSINE) is an orally effective ganglionic blocker that is indicated for therapy of moderately severe to severe essential hypertension and uncomplicated cases of malignant hypertension. It is rarely used, however, because many other antihypertensive drugs are equally effective, cause fewer side effects, and have fewer contraindications. They are discussed in Chapter 33. Low doses should be used initially (see Table 16–C) and maintenance doses reached gradually to guard against side effects. In general, the optimal dose is one that just causes the appearance of mild postural or orthostatic hypotension.

Since mecamylamine is used chronically in ambulatory patients, sometimes in a poorly supervised outpatient setting, the risk of side effects noted for trimethaphan is increased. Orthostatic hypotension is a common problem. Upon standing, reflexes normally cause vasoconstriction, which prevents pooling of blood in the legs. With ganglionic blockade, there is no reflex, so dizziness, fainting, and falls are likely. The use of other drugs, especially alcohol, increases the risk of hypotension and its problems.

Side effects outside the cardiovascular system also become important with long-term use of mecamylamine. Mydriasis can increase intraocular pressure; glaucoma is the related contraindication. Reduced lacrimal secretions may favor ocular irritation. Decreased gut motility may cause constipation or paralytic ileus, and so the presence of disorders in which gut motility is reduced generally contraindicate mecamylamine therapy. Prolonged decreases of bladder activity can cause urinary hesitancy or retention; prostatic hypertrophy is the major related contraindication. Diminished sweating may cause fever, especially in hot environ ments. Both erection and ejaculation will be impaired in males.

If side effects or drug interactions occur, the dose should be reduced gradually if possible. Rapid decreases, or abruptly stopping administration, can cause blood pressure to rise above predrug levels quickly. The risk of stroke or acute heart failure is high. When used along with most other hypertensive agents, reduced doses of mecamylamine and the other agent(s) are indicated.

Overdoses of mecamylamine cause hypotension and its expected consequences. Cardiovascular collapse may occur. Other signs and symptoms include nausea, vomiting, constipation or paralytic ileus, urinary retention, and blurred vision. Mecamylamine readily crosses the blood–brain barrier and can cause anxiety, tremor, choreiform movements, and seizures. Overdoses are treated as noted for trimethaphan, with the use of anticonvulsants if needed.

NURSING IMPLICATIONS

Anticipate that adverse responses and drug interactions caused by mecamylamine will be more frequent than noted for trimethaphan. Therefore, more nursing interventions, including patient teaching, will be required. Administer mecamylamine after meals for more gradual absorption, to avoid sudden falls of blood pressure, and to achieve more stable blood pressure control. Morning doses should be small to avoid more pronounced daytime effects.

Monitor blood pressure in all positions (supine, sitting, standing), but use pressure changes after standing to help assess the effective dose. Instruct the patient to get up slowly from a supine or sitting position to avoid postural hypotension, and to assume a seated, head-low position if dizziness occurs. Assisted ambulation may be needed. Notify the physician if these measures fail to work. Advise patients to avoid hot environments, exercise, and alcohol intake, which increase the risk and severity of hypotension. Assess for changes of bowel or bladder habits, eye pain, and difficulty with breathing. It is important to discuss the potential risks of discontinuing mecamylamine therapy abruptly.

◆ Use During Pregnancy and Lactation

The risks of hypotension during pregnancy, noted for trimethaphan, apply also to mecamylamine. The drug should be used during pregnancy only when absolutely needed for a serious maternal condition. It should never be used for expected blood pressure increases during normal pregnancy, and should not be used for more serious hypertension unless other drugs have been tried first (see Chapter 33). Mecamylamine is excreted in breast milk and may cause all of its side effects in a nursing infant. Breastfeeding should therefore be discouraged.

◆ Use in the Elderly

The increased incidence of contraindicating conditions in the elderly, plus the increased use of interacting drugs, require extra caution and observation for these persons.

Ganglionic Stimulant

PROTOTYPE

Nicotine

Nicotine is a potent, naturally occurring alkaloid isolated from tobacco leaf and found in tobacco smoke. It is the substance for which the nicotinic subtype of ACh receptor was named. Nicotine has only one therapeutic use: to curb habitual cigarette smoking. Nicotine is also one of the most toxic drugs known.

Absorption, Distribution, Metabolism, and Excretion

Nicotine is quickly absorbed through mucous membranes. About two thirds of the nicotine in tobacco smoke is absorbed through the oral mucosa, and if a smoker inhales, nearly all the nicotine will be absorbed. Nicotine is quickly metabolized, but not fast enough to prevent the drug's marked effects. Nicotine and its metabolites are excreted in urine and maternal milk. Urinary excretion decreases when the urine is alkaline.

Pharmacologic Effects and Side Effects

Nicotine is both a nicotinic receptor stimulant and an inhibitor. At low concentrations, it mimics the effects of ACh by stimulating receptors on the sympathetic *and* parasympathetic postganglionic cells, and on adrenal medullary cells; at skeletal muscle; and at cholinergic synapses in parts of the brain and spinal cord. With repeated exposure to these low concentrations, as might occur with continued smoking, tolerance seems to develop and the intensity of the responses diminishes.

At high concentrations, nicotine causes excessive and prolonged cell depolarization, and so the cells are no longer able to function normally. In the ganglia, for example, transmission between preganglionic and postganglionic nerves is blocked, in much the same way that trimethaphan causes this response. Skeletal muscle fatigues and becomes paralyzed.

None of the pharmacologic effects of nicotine can be considered desirable in the usual sense. Therefore, expected responses and side effects are considered together. Tolerance to some effects develops with continued nicotine administration (habitual smoking).

Peripheral Effects Caused by Actions on Autonomic Ganglia

The peripheral autonomic effects caused by low, ganglionic-stimulating amounts of nicotine are basically the opposite of those caused by usual doses of a ganglionic blocker (see Table 16–1). They reflect simultaneous activation of both the parasympathetic and sympathetic branches of the ANS, with effects of the "predominant" branch on a particular structure being the most apparent.

The most important changes involve the cardiovascular system, and include vasoconstriction and increases of heart rate and contractile force. Nicotine may also make the myocardium more irritable or sensitive to arrhythmias caused by catecholamines.

Tolerance to the cardiovascular effects develops slowly. Tachycardia and hypertension, although less severe than initially, usually continue with continued smoking. Continued sympathomimetic effects from nicotine in tobacco smoke have been cited as contributing to the worsening of hypertension and peripheral vascular diseases, as well as to the heart, brain, or kidney damage in patients with atherosclerosis or diabetes.

The GI and urinary tracts, as well as exocrine glands, are normally under major control by the parasympathetic nervous system. Thus, ganglionic stimulation intensifies the parasympathomimetic influences on these structures, causing such effects as pupillary constriction; increased secretions from mucus, salivary, and sweat glands; and potential diarrhea and urination owing to stimulation of GI and urinary tract motility, and relaxation of sphincters. Gastric acid secretion also increases. The bronchi may constrict because of parasympathetic influences, and because of irritation by smoke, if that is the route of nicotine administration. While none of these effects are desirable for anyone (as was true for the cardiovascular effects), some of them become especially important (and potentially dangerous) for persons with certain diseases. For example, bronchoconstriction and increased mucus secretion are greater risks for persons with asthma or other pulmonary diseases; increased gastric acid secretion can worsen ulcers; and so on.

Skeletal Muscle Effects

Nicotine stimulates the nicotinic receptors that activate skeletal muscle. Muscle tremor or twitching may occur.

Central Nervous System Effects

Nicotine may be the only major ingredient in tobacco that leads to habitual smoking. Although the act of smoking itself is a behavior that fosters the habit, true pharmacologic effects also are involved.

Low doses of nicotine can cause an "arousal effect" that includes subjective feelings of increased mental acuity or performance; and some ill-defined "tranquilizing" effect at other times. These effects may motivate some people to keep smoking. Nausea and vomiting are common, especially with initial exposure. Nicotine also stimulates respiration. With repeated exposure to the drug, tolerance develops to some of the CNS effects.

NURSING IMPLICATIONS

Teach about the dangers of nicotine from tobacco smoke, especially if they have cardiovascular or respiratory problems or peptic ulcer disease.

◆ Use During Pregnancy and Lactation

Women who smoke during pregnancy have a greater risk of placental insufficiency and delivering an infant with low birth weight. Nicotine passes freely into breast milk and may cause potentially serious adverse effects in the infant.

◆ Use in Children

Children are unusually sensitive to all effects of nicotine. Tobacco smoking may cause immediate and long-term adverse effects on growth and health.

◆ Use in the Elderly

Most common age-related disorders, particularly those involving the cardiopulmonary system, increase the risk of adverse effects due to nicotine.

Clinical Indications, Side Effects, and Contraindications

The only approved use for nicotine is as an aid to help adult cigarette smokers stop smoking. Used as an adjunct to behavioral modifications, nicotine provides the smoker with some of the objective and subjective effects of the chemical, but without all the adverse effects caused by smoke and the many substances in it. For most patients, with continued use the desire to smoke will diminish or stop altogether.

There are two pharmaceutic formulations of nicotine, both available only by prescription. One is a sugar-free, flavored gum, which contains 2 mg of nicotine per piece, bound to a resin that helps release it slowly. This product is marketed as NICORETTE. The user chews one piece of gum slowly each time the urge to smoke arises. The average smoker needs about a dozen pieces of gum each day. The daily limit is 30 pieces, used for no more than 3 months. The gum has some drawbacks. Nausea is relatively common, even for habitual smokers. The nicotine in the gum may also cause oral lesions. Other problems relate to the act of chewing itself. They can include jaw problems, which may be a limitation for persons with weak temperomandibular joints; and other problems for persons who wear dentures or other oral appliances. There is also a potential risk of adverse effects in children who equate this gum with candy, but the bitter taste usually curbs excessive or repeated use.

Newer formulations, marketed as HABITROL, NICODERM, and PROSTEP, contain nicotine in an adhesive-backed skin patch. These transdermal delivery systems release the nicotine slowly through the skin into the bloodstream, providing a more constant effect than can be achieved with the gum. One patch is applied to a hairless area of skin on the upper body, and replaced with a fresh patch each day. Skin irritation, which can be caused by either the active drug or the patch itself, is fairly common with this product. Usually, however, it is not severe. Nevertheless, the user should be instructed to rotate application sites frequently so that a given area of skin is not exposed to the patch frequently or for too long. The patches are available in three "strengths"; usually patches containing the highest amount of nicotine are used first, and the dose is gradually reduced as the patient's desire to continue smoking diminishes.

No nicotine product should be used by pregnant women. Ideally women of childbearing age should be given a pregnancy test before starting nicotine substitution therapy. Other absolute or relative contraindications are conditions in which nicotine, whether administered via smoke or one of these products, can cause added problems. They include a history of coronary artery disease (eg, angina or recent myocardial infarction), hypertension, arrhythmias, or pheochromocytoma; peptic ulcer disease; and hyperthyroidism or diabetes mellitus.

NURSING IMPLICATIONS

Nicotine-containing products are not cure-alls. They will not work well unless the user wants to stop smoking. Importantly, they should be used in combination with behavior-modifying therapies, tailored to the needs of the individual in a way that maximizes compliance and reinforces the desire to break a pharmacologic addiction and a behavioral habit. The values and limitations of these products, their proper use, and the need for nonpharmacologic support must be stressed to and understood by the patient. A thorough health and medication history should be obtained before a patient is started on one of these products, so that contraindicating conditions can be detected.

Additional nursing measures that should be used include assessing for oral lesions or other related problems in persons using nicotine gum; and checking for skin irritation caused by the transdermal product. All patients should be advised that, on withdrawal from smoking or nicotine use, they are likely to gain weight and be restless. These discomforts usually subside in a few weeks if abstinence is maintained. Women who are using these products should be advised to notify their physician at once if they become pregnant.

Acute Nicotine Poisoning

Lethal doses of nicotine, about 60 mg for an adult, cause death in a few minutes. Less than half that dose can cause serious illness or death in children. Early symptoms of poisoning can be predicted from the previous discussion of adverse reactions. The poisoned individual becomes extremely nauseated; he or she vomits, defecates, salivates, and sweats profusely. Skeletal muscles are initially stimulated, then quickly fatigue. Heart rate and blood pressure rise initially, then soon fall. Respiratory stimulation and then depression occur. Respiratory collapse, cardiovascular collapse, and seizures may all contribute to death.

Lethal nicotine poisoning was more common when concentrated solutions of the drug were available in insecticides or products used to euthanize animals. Today, nicotine intoxication occurs mainly from ingestion or excessive smoking of tobacco products by children. Little information is available about poisoning from nicotine gum.

Most cases of poisoning from tobacco or nicotine gum are very unpleasant but rarely fatal. A child experimenting with smoking usually experiences such severe distress from smoking one or two cigarettes that he or she will refrain from smoking more unless peer pressure is overwhelming. Eating tobacco is a common cause of childhood poisoning, but tobacco in the stomach delays gastric emptying, so that absorption of nicotine in the small intestine is slowed and usually causes vomiting that expels the substance.

Nicotine poisoning is treated symptomatically. If intoxication is due to ingestion of a tobacco product or nicotine-containing gum, and the patient has intact gag reflexes, vomiting should be induced with syrup of ipecac, even if vomiting occurred spontaneously. Other interventions, such as gastric lavage and administration of activated charcoal, should be used to adsorb and remove any remaining drug. Oxygen and ventilatory assistance are used to keep blood gases near normal, and blood pressure and heart rate are supported with autonomic drugs selected according to vital signs.

Nicotine gum is contraindicated during pregnancy.

NURSING IMPLICATIONS

Always recommend prompt evaluation and treatment of possible nicotine poisoning in a hospital. Avoid giving any alkaline substance, such as antacids or milk, to relieve gastric discomfort. These substances will increase nicotine absorption and possibly make the poisoning worse.

Interactions with Other Drugs

Nicotine, and perhaps other substances that are also found in tobacco smoke, can stimulate the liver's drug-metabolizing enzyme systems. This can result in an increased rate of metabolism of many other drugs that are metabolized in the liver, thereby lowering their blood levels and their effects.

Probably the most well established and clinically important interaction of this type involves nicotine (whether inhaled in smoke or administered as a drug) and the methylxanthine bronchodilators (theophylline is the prototype; see Chapter 38) that are widely used to manage asthma and obstructive pulmonary disease. Thus, dosage adjustments to compensate for the interaction usually are needed. Patients who take these bronchodilators and continue to smoke, for example, may need daily theophylline dosages that are 50% higher than those needed for symptom control in otherwise identical nonsmokers. (Smoking also causes obvious adverse pulmonary effects on the respiratory disorders for which the bronchodilators were prescribed in the first place.) Since the liver's metabolic rates will fall toward normal as the person reduces or stops their nicotine intake (or smoking), dosages of drugs such as theophylline will have to be decreased to compensate for the loss of the interaction, and to prevent potential toxicity.

SUMMARY OF NURSING IMPLICATIONS 

◆ Assessment

Review past history for known contraindications to drug therapy (coronary artery disease, renal failure, peptic ulcer disease, diabetes, chronic obstructive lung disease or asthma, Addison's disease).

Note current medications, recognizing the potentiating effect of direct vasodilators and diuretics on actions of ganglionic blockers.

Determine normal blood pressure as a basis for evaluating drug effectiveness.

Record pulse and respirations before starting drug therapy, to help predict side effects.

◆ Nursing Diagnoses

Knowledge deficit related to drug therapy: dosage, schedule, side effects.

Decreased cardiac output related to drug side effects: altered heart rate, blood pressure.

Altered tissue perfusion related to blood pressure changes.

Altered oral mucous membranes related to nicotine gum; altered skin integrity related to transdermal nicotine.

Constipation or diarrhea related to drug side effects.

Sexual dysfunction related to impotence from ganglionic blockers.

Impaired gas exchange related to bronchoconstriction (ganglionic blockers) or increased respiratory secretions (nicotine gum).

High risk for injury related to orthostatic hypotension, dizziness, syncope.

◆ Planning/Implementation

Administer trimethaphan slowly and in gradually increasing amounts until desired blood pressure is achieved; use an infusion pump.

Monitor blood pressure frequently while administering ganglionic blocker.

Have emergency equipment available in case cardiovascular or cerebrovascular problems occur.

Provide encouragement and support during drug therapy; allow patient or client to verbalize frustrations and concerns (sexual dysfunction with ganglionic blockers; quitting smoking); refer for counseling if needed.

◆ Patient and Family Teaching

Instruct patient or client regarding diagnosis, drug therapy, doses, expected outcomes, and side effects, particularly those that must be reported.

Teach patient or client proper technique for chewing nicotine gum to enhance effects and minimize gastric and oral irritation or jaw pain.

◆ Evaluation

The patient/family will:

Achieve blood pressure control (normotensive) with ganglionic blockers.

Experience minimal side effects; control postural or orthostatic blood pressure changes; resolve sexual dysfunction.

Cope with drug effects; comply with regimen; keep follow-up appointments.

Annotated Bibliography

Daughton DM, Heatley SA, Prendergast JJ, et al. Effect of transdermal nicotine delivery as an adjunct to low-intervention smoking cessation therapy: A randomized, placebo-controlled, double-blind study. *Arch Intern Med* 1991;151(4):749–752. *Nicotine-containing skin patches, whether worn 24 hours a day or during waking hours only, significantly improved the outcome of a stop-smoking program, and significantly reduced tobacco withdrawal symptoms.*

Ray O., Ksir C. Nicotine. In: *Drugs, society, and human behavior.* 5th ed. St. Louis: C. V. Mosby, 1990:190–214. *Extensively referenced and easy to read, this chapter summarizes the pharmacologic effects of nicotine, and reviews aspects of smoking and its adverse health and social effects. Other chapters in this book discuss effects and abuse of other important drug groups.*

Table 16–C | Clinical Uses and Administration of Ganglionic Blockers and Nicotine

AGENT	CLINICAL USES	DOSAGE AND ROUTE OF ADMINISTRATION
	Ganglionic Blockers	
PROTOTYPE		
Trimethaphan camsylate (ARFONAD)	Production of controlled intraoperative hypotension	IV: Adults: Infuse at 3–4 mg/min (1 mg/mL) until desired BP is reached; use infusion pump, indwelling IV catheter. Children ≥ 12: Dilute as above, infuse at 50–150 μg/kg/min
	Emergency treatment of hypertensive episodes, adjunctive therapy of acute pulmonary edema	See above
RELATED DRUG		
Mecamylamine (INVERSINE)	Treatment of moderately severe to severe essential hypertension	Oral: Average maintenance dose is 25 mg/d in 3 divided doses; give smaller portion of divided dose in AM; adequate dose based on onset of mild postural or orthostatic hypotension; for adults only
	Treatment of uncomplicated cases of malignant hypertension	
	Ganglionic Stimulant	
PROTOTYPE		
Nicotine (NICORETTE)	Adjunctive aid to behavioral therapy, abstinence, to help adults quit cigarette smoking	Chew 1 piece of gum slowly and intermittently upon urge to smoke; average daily dose is 10–12 pieces
(HABITROL, NICODERM, PROSTEP)	As for NICORETTE GUM	Apply one transdermal therapeutic patch to clean, dry, intact area of skin, replace with fresh patch q24h

Table 16–S | Major Side Effects and Contraindications of Ganglionic Blockers and Nicotine

BODY SYSTEM/ Side Effect	CONTRAINDICATION/ PRECAUTION	COMMENTS AND NURSING IMPLICATIONS
	Ganglionic Blockers	
CENTRAL NERVOUS SYSTEM Anxiety, agitation, tremor, seizures	Questionable or impaired neurologic status	
EYE Mydriasis, photophobia; cycloplegia	Glaucoma	Problems greatest with chronic mecamylamine therapy; monitor intraocular pressure, especially in the elderly; advise patient to report eye pain at once; teach nondrug ways to deal with photophobia (eg, sunglasses), avoidance of tasks made dangerous by poor visual acuity
Ocular dryness, irritation		Recommend artificial tears (eg, LACRIL) to alleviate irritation
RESPIRATORY Wheezing, dyspnea, bronchospasm	Asthma, COPD	Advise patient to report respiratory difficulty at once; may indicate bronchoconstriction or heart failure
CARDIOVASCULAR Excessive hypotension (supine)	Ischemic vascular disease of major organs, extremities; diabetes, hypercortisolism due to Addison's disease, corticosteroid therapy	Usually related to overdose or drug interaction; monitor for signs of major organ ischemia (eg, ECG, urine output, mental function); notify physician; reduced dose of blocker and/or interacting drug may be needed
Orthostatic/postural hypotension	Cerebrovascular disease; diabetes, hypercortisolism	Most likely to occur during mecamylamine therapy in outpatients; mild hypotension indicates therapeutic dose; if excessive (eg, syncope, falls occur), notify physician; recommend support hose; ensure adequate hydration via fluid intake; salt intake as permitted by BP, avoidance of hot environments and vigorous exercise
Tachycardia, arrhythmias, anginal pain, heart failure	Ischemic heart disease, history of arrhythmias, infarction	Monitor heart rate, rhythm; notify physician if palpitations, tachycardia, signs of heart failure develop; is more problematic with mecamylamine
GASTROINTESTINAL Constipation, paralytic ileus	Prior constipation, risk of paralytic ileus (ie, GI surgery); gut obstruction	Recommend nondrug interventions: increased intake of bulky foods, nonalcoholic beverages, exercise as permitted by health; avoid laxatives unless directed by physician; advise patient to notify physician at once if sudden bowel changes, abdominal pain occur; risk greatest with long-term mecamylamine therapy
SKIN Flushing, fever due to reduced cutaneous heat loss via perspiration		Advise patient to avoid strenuous exercise in hot environment; wear clothing appropriate for environment; report fever at once

(continued)

Table 16–S Major Side Effects and Contraindications of Ganglionic Blockers and Nicotine (*Continued*)

BODY SYSTEM/ Side Effect	CONTRAINDICATION/ PRECAUTION	COMMENTS AND NURSING IMPLICATIONS
	Ganglionic Blockers	
GENITOURINARY Urinary hesitancy, retention	Prostatic hypertrophy, obstructive bladder disease	Advise patient to report sudden or marked changes in ability to urinate, lower abdominal pain; risk greatest with long-term mecamylamine therapy
Failure of erection, ejaculation in males		Applies to long-term mecamylamine therapy for hypertension; notify physician if side effect interferes with compliance; reappraisal of therapy, substitution of alternative antihypertensive drugs may be indicated
	Ganglionic Stimulant: Nicotine	
CENTRAL NERVOUS SYSTEM Agitation, tremors; seizures with toxic doses	History of seizure disorders	Discourage smoking; if side effects caused by nicotine gum or patch, reduce dose, notify physician
RESPIRATORY Bronchoconstriction	Asthma	Stress the need to stop smoking; if patient is taking theophylline or a related bronchodilator (eg, aminophylline), monitor clinical response and blood levels, since nicotine can lower blood levels; anticipate need for higher-than-usual theophylline doses for smokers, and the need to reduce the daily dose when smoking or nicotine therapy is stopped
CARDIOVASCULAR Tachycardia, palpitations, arrhythmias	Arrhythmias, tachycardia, hyperthyroidism	Discourage smoking, avoid use of nicotine in patients with these and other cardiovascular disorders
Hypertension	Hypertension, pheochromocytoma	Avoid smoking, nicotine use, either of which may worsen high BP or counteract antihypertensive drug actions
Hypotension		Occurs with toxic doses or in response to nicotine inhalation in nonsmokers; may cause cardiovascular collapse
GASTROINTESTINAL Diarrhea, gastric pain, worsening of peptic ulcer disease; nausea, vomiting	Active, recent, or recurrent peptic ulcer disease; chronic or severe diarrhea, obstructive bowel disease, gastroenteritis	Nicotine stimulates gastric acid secretion and gut motility; emphasize need to quit smoking; avoid nicotine therapy

Table 16–I **Major Interactions Between Ganglionic Blockers or Nicotine and Other Drugs**

AGENT	RESULT OF INTERACTION	COMMENTS AND NURSING IMPLICATIONS
Major Interactions Involving Ganglionic Blockers		
Alcohol (Chapter 22)	Increased risk of hypotension	Caution patient taking mecamylamine to avoid alcohol use
Other antihypertensive drugs (Chapter 33)	Excessive or prolonged hypotension	Hypotension can be avoided by using reduced doses and adjusting infusion rate to desired response
Succinylcholine (Chapter 17)	Prolonged or more intense muscle paralysis; apnea; recurrence of apnea after succinylcholine administration	Monitor for prolonged respiratory depression; interaction may affect other neuromuscular blockers (eg, curare)
Major Interaction Involving Nicotine		
Aminophylline, theophylline (Chapter 38)	Inadequate bronchodilation, control of COPD symptoms	Ingredients in tobacco smoke increase rate of metabolism of these bronchodilators, reduce blood levels and desired effects; to alleviate symptoms, monitor blood levels and therapeutic response during therapy; discourage smoking

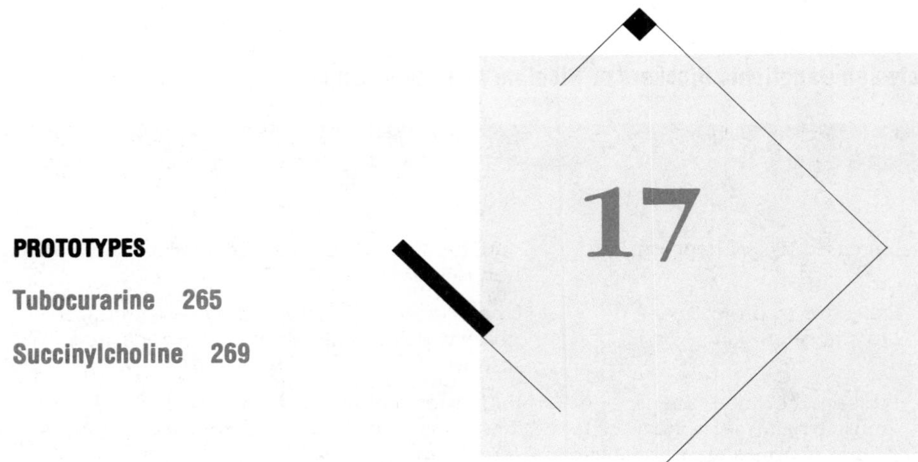

PROTOTYPES

Neuromuscular Blockers and Miscellaneous Skeletal Muscle Relaxants

General Characteristics of Neuromuscular Blockers

Several previous chapters in this unit described drugs that mimic or inhibit the actions of acetylcholine (ACh) on muscarinic receptors of smooth and cardiac muscles and certain glands. This chapter focuses mainly on drugs that affect the nicotinic receptors for ACh found on skeletal muscle.

The drugs, called *neuromuscular blockers,* are used to cause complete muscle relaxation—virtual paralysis. They fall into two major groups, *nondepolarizing* blockers and *depolarizing* blockers, based on how they affect the muscle cell.

All neuromuscular blockers paralyze skeletal muscle, share the same general indications, and have one major adverse effect—weakness or paralysis of muscles needed for spontaneous ventilation. Selection of an agent for a given patient is based on the type of procedure for which the drug will be used, the drug's duration of action, and on several special patient-related factors that could increase the risk of adverse responses to a particular blocker.

Many hospitals allow only anesthesiologists or certified nurse-anesthetists to administer these effective but potentially dangerous drugs (check institutional policies), but most nurses will be responsible for caring for patients before or after their use.

Regulation and Pharmacologic Alteration of Skeletal Muscle Activity

Motor nerves that innervate skeletal muscle release ACh, which diffuses across the neuromuscular junction, binds to nicotinic receptors on the muscle cell, and then depolarizes the cell. Eventually, the chemical message leads to muscle cell contraction. The effects of ACh are stopped rapidly when nearby acetylcholinesterase (AChE) metabolically inactivates the neurotransmitter. The muscle cell repolarizes and relaxes in preparation for another stimulus.

There are four major ways that drugs can interfere with this process to reduce or totally inhibit muscle function. Only the first two are used when selective paralysis of skeletal muscle is desired.

1. Block the nicotinic receptors on the muscle cell so they cannot be activated by ACh. The muscle cell will not depolarize, or contract. This is how nondepolarizing neuromuscular blockers such as tubocurarine work.

Major reference tables appear beginning on p. 277.

2. Give a drug that is a nicotinic receptor agonist, like ACh, but with a longer duration of action. Prolonged depolarization causes the muscle to become insensitive to further stimulation by ACh, leading to paralysis. This is basically how the depolarizing blocker succinylcholine works.
3. Inhibit the metabolism of ACh released from motor nerves by giving an AChE inhibitor. The resulting buildup of ACh would eventually cause the muscle to become insensitive. However, as noted in Chapter 12, AChE inhibitors cause ACh accumulation wherever the transmitter is released, so other (unwanted) effects—including parasympathomimetic (muscarinic) effects on smooth muscle, the heart, and glands—would occur too. The AChE inhibitors are not used to paralyze skeletal muscle, but as noted later they are routinely used to *reverse* paralysis caused by nondepolarizing blockers.
4. Inhibit the function of spinal nerves that control skeletal muscle. This is how some "centrally acting" skeletal muscle relaxants work. They are discussed briefly at the end of the chapter.

Nondepolarizing Neuromuscular Blockers

PROTOTYPE

Tubocurarine

d-Tubocurarine chloride ("curare") is the traditional prototype of a group of drugs that paralyze skeletal muscle by preventing muscle cell depolarization. The chemical was originally isolated from a plant root used for centuries by South American Indians as a dart and arrow poison for hunting. (They stored their roots in bamboo tubes, hence the name *tubo*curarine.) The related curare-like nondepolarizing blockers are atracurium, doxacurium, gallamine, metocurine, pancuronium, pipecuronium, and vecuronium.

Nursing implications that apply to the use of all neuromuscular blockers are given on page 272.

Absorption, Distribution, Metabolism, and Excretion

Tubocurarine, like all other neuromuscular blockers, is given intravenously. Tubocurarine is partly metabolized by the liver, but most of the drug is excreted by the kidneys unchanged. Therefore, the drug's duration of action is prolonged in patients with impaired renal function. Other neuromuscular blockers with different patterns of elimination may be preferred when concerns exist about the patient's ability to eliminate a particular agent.

Pharmacologic Effects

All nondepolarizing blockers competitively block the ability of ACh to bind to nicotinic receptors on skeletal muscle, thereby preventing muscle depolarization. As molecules of tubocurarine accumulate at the receptors, muscle contractility becomes progressively weaker, and within minutes the muscle is completely relaxed (flaccid) and paralyzed. Competitive blockade means that it can be overcome, and muscle activity restored quickly, by increasing the availability of the agonist, ACh. This provides the rationale for administering AChE inhibitors to reverse the actions of a nondepolarizing neuromuscular blocker when muscle paralysis is no longer wanted.

Muscle groups that are highly innervated are more sensitive to the effects of neuromuscular blockers. Muscles that control delicate movements of the face, mouth, and eye are affected first, followed by muscles of the limbs, neck, and trunk. The diaphragm and intercostal muscles, which are essential for ventilation, are the least sensitive and so are the last to be affected. Recovery of muscle function after neuromuscular blockade occurs in the reverse order, with ventilatory activity reappearing first. This sequence of paralysis and reactivation applies to all neuromuscular blockers.

Tubocurarine's main effects are on skeletal muscle nicotinic receptors, but it also weakly blocks nicotinic receptors in autonomic ganglia and causes histamine release from mast cells. Both effects are considered to be side effects, and are discussed later. Newer nondepolarizing blockers tend to cause less ganglionic blockade or histamine release. None of the neuromuscular blockers except pancuronium, given at therapeutic doses, block muscarinic receptors, and so they have no atropine-like actions or contraindications.

The neuromuscular blockers merely paralyze patients; they do not alter consciousness, or awareness or perception of pain.

Clinical Indications and Administration

Tubocurarine and all the other curare-like neuromuscular blockers are generally used whenever the goal is to cause muscle paralysis lasting for more than a few minutes. All these drugs are used for assisting tracheal intubation and for causing muscle paralysis during surgery. These uses are discussed first. Tubocurarine and several related drugs also have additional uses (Table 17–C). The drug will be given either by slow intravenous (IV) injection alone, or by IV injection followed by an infusion. The procedure used depends on the drug selected and on the desired duration of effects.

Endotracheal Intubation

Inserting an endotracheal tube triggers gag reflexes that make the procedure difficult for the caregiver and uncomfortable for the patient. These reflexes can be prevented by first administering a neuromuscular blocker. Tubocurarine and related nondepolarizing blockers, which take a few mintues to cause satisfactory muscle relaxation, are generally used when intubation is not done under emergency conditions, and when more longlasting effects after intubation are wanted. (When immediate effects are wanted, the anesthesiologist may instead use succinylcholine, a rapid- but short-acting neuromuscular blocker. In many cases, succinylcholine is given first for intubation, and muscle paralysis is continued with a curare-like drug.)

Adjunct to Surgical Anesthesia

Muscle relaxation is one goal of surgical anesthesia. It is particularly important in orthopedic surgery, in which a limb may need to be manipulated to set a fracture; or in abdominal surgery that requires wide retraction of abdominal muscles to provide good access to internal organs. General anesthetics (Chapter 20) cause some muscle relaxation, but the amount is generally inadequate for surgery unless very high doses of anesthetic are given. However, such doses may cause potentially dangerous depression of the central nervous and cardiovascular systems. The adjunctive use of a neuromuscular blocker provides excellent muscle relaxation without the need for excessive doses of anesthetic.

Tubocurarine or a related blocker is usually injected just before the first skin incision is made. The anesthesiologist or nurse-anesthetist will then help assess whether blockade is sufficient by electrically stimulating muscles or their nerve supplies. This assessment can be done periodically during surgery to determine the need for additional doses of the blocker, and after surgery to help assess the recovery of muscle activity.

The effects of curare-like blockers take anywhere from 30 minutes to several hours to disappear on their own (Table 17–1). The time depends on the drug, the dose, whether repeated dosages were given or other drugs were administered also, and on unique characteristics of each patient.

Table 17–1 Typical Neuromuscular Blocker Durations of Action*

Ultrashort (3–5 min)
- Succinylcholine (depolarizing agent)

Short (15–60 min)
- Atracurium
- Mivacurium
- Vecuronium

Intermediate (45–90 min)
- Gallamine
- Metocurine
- Pancuronium
- d-Tubocurarine

Long (> 90 min)
- Doxacurium
- Pipecuronium

*Durations vary from patient to patient. Times noted above are approximate, and assume administration of a single effective dose to patients who were also given balanced anesthesia (eg, preoperative induction agents and intraoperative anesthetics; see Chapter 20).

However, it is rare to allow such prolonged recovery once surgery is completed, since it is important to help the patient regain spontaneous ventilation quickly. Thus, muscle paralysis is usually reversed pharmacologically, by injecting an AChE inhibitor such as neostigmine, which increases ACh levels at the somatic neuromuscular junction and overcomes blockade caused by the paralyzing agent. Since AChE inhibitors also increase ACh levels at structures innervated by parasympathetic nerves, an antimuscarinic drug (atropine or glycopyrrolate; p 172) is routinely injected just before, or along with, the AChE inhibitor. This prevents unwanted parasympathomimetic effects such as bradycardia, bronchoconstriction, increased secretions, and increases of gastrointestinal (GI) and urinary tract motility.

Ventilator Control

Some seriously ill patients have a degree of spontaneous ventilation, but it may not be enough to maintain adequate blood oxygenation and pulmonary integrity. Thus, they must be placed on mechanical ventilation. However, their own respiratory drive tends to "fight" the ventilator. To counteract this, such patients are given doses of a neuromuscular blocker that is sufficient to suppress their ability to breathe, allowing the ventilator to do all the work for them. Tubocurare itself is not often used for this purpose, but several other curare-like drugs are (e.g., pancuronium). High doses of other drugs, including morphine (Chapter 21) and diazepam (Chapter 22), can also be used for this purpose, alone or in combination with a neuromuscular blocker. One advantage of these alternatives, for some patients, is their added ability to alleviate apprehension and (in the case of morphine) pain.

Adjunct to Electroconvulsive Therapy

Some patients with severe psychiatric depression that does not respond to usually effective antidepressant drugs (Chapter 24) may be given electroconvulsive therapy (ECT). Side effects of ECT, which involves administering an electrical current through the anesthetized patient's brain, include convulsions that cause intense muscle contraction and potential bone fractures or dislocations; and loss of airway patency, leading to impaired or absent ventilation and its consequences. Thus, short-acting neuromuscular blockers such as tubocurare or the related blocker metocurine are used adjunctively. These drugs facilitate inserting an endotracheal tube or oral airway, and prevent the muscle contractions that occur when the shock is given.

Diagnosis of Myasthenia Gravis

Tubocurarine is occasionally used to help make the diagnosis of myasthenia gravis when the "edrophonium test" results (Chapter 12) are inconclusive. Tubocurarine is used because myasthenic patients already have impaired skeletal muscle function, and they are unusually sensitive to neuromuscular blockers. They are given a dose of the drug so low (about one tenth the usual dose) that patients without myasthenia gravis would have little if any response to it. The myasthenic patient, however, will respond with a dramatic increase of muscle weakness.

Miscellaneous Uses

Some of the nondepolarizing neuromuscular blockers are used as adjuncts in the therapy of acute seizure disorders, such as those that might be caused by head trauma or some drugs. Anticonvulsant drugs (Chapter 26) such as diazepam are the primary therapies for seizures, but neuromuscular blockade (and ventilatory support) may be valuable for preventing widespread and intense muscle contraction and damage if the seizures cannot be controlled.

Another use of curare-like neuromuscular blockers is in the management of tetanus, a potentially fatal bacterial infection. The blockers prevent the intense muscle contracture and rigidity (tetany) that can cause a host of serious systemic problems (eg, blood electrolyte imbalances owing to muscle damage), and also aid in mechanical ventilation of the patient. Such treatment usually involves prolonged neuromuscular blockade (days or weeks), and so requires nursing care that is more intense and time-consuming than when the same drugs are administered for more acute effects, such as during surgery.

Side Effects, Adverse Reactions, and Contraindications

The most serious adverse response to *any* neuromuscular blocker (Table 17–S) is prolonged weakness or paralysis of the muscles needed for adequate spontaneous ventilation. If ventilation is impaired too much or for too long, permanent brain damage or death can occur. Ventilatory depression can be intensified and prolonged by common conditions, including debility, fever, decreased renal function (which slows excretion of most neuromuscular blockers), and electrolyte imbalances (abnormally low levels of serum calcium or potassium, or elevated serum magnesium). Electrolyte imbalances may be caused by illness or by other drugs that the patient may receive, and such drugs can cause other unwanted effects as well (see drug interactions, below). These ventilatory problems can be managed by ensuring that the patient is adequately oxygenated, and maintained on mechanical ventilation for as long as needed. If proper monitoring and support facilities are available, serious problems should not occur.

Tubocurarine tends to cause more cardiovascular changes, which usually are unwanted, than the other curare-like blockers. At high doses it can interfere with neurotransmission across the autonomic ganglia. Blockade of sympathetic ganglia inhibits peripheral vasoconstriction, causing blood pressure to fall. Blockade of parasympathetic ganglia, which happens simultaneously, increases heart rate as opposing parasympathetic tone is lost. Tubocurarine also releases histamine, a vasodilator and cardiac-stimulating substance, from mast cells (Chapter 51).

Histamine release caused by tubocurarine is potentially dangerous for other reasons. Histamine is also a powerful bronchoconstrictor that can cause serious respiratory problems if the patient has a pulmonary disorder such as asthma or emphysema, which are contraindications to tubocurarine use. Another concern, which affects far fewer people, relates to the ability of histamine to release epinephrine from the adrenal medulla. If the patient has a pheochromocytoma, a sudden and large increase of the blood epinephrine level can cause *hyper*tension and tachycardia.

◆ Use During Pregnancy and Lactation

Although little hard information is available about the risks of administering neuromuscular blockers to pregnant women, none of them should be used unless absolutely needed. One indication where they may be needed is for cesarean sections. In this instance the blocker should be administered as close as possible to actual delivery of the fetus, to minimize exposure of the infant to the drug. Long-acting related agents such as doxacurium or pipecuronium should be avoided, to keep maternal effects as short as possible.

Cesarean section is the definitive treatment for severe pregnancy-associated hypertension (preeclampsia and eclampsia), which often is managed preoperatively with magnesium salts to prevent seizures.

Be aware that elevated maternal blood magnesium levels will prolong and intensify neuromuscular blockade. Monitor ventilatory status in both mother and child.

◆ Use in Children

Nondepolarizing blockers, in doses normalized to body weight, are used for children. An infant's ability to hold the eyelids open or raise the legs can help assess the resolution of drug effects.

◆ Use in the Elderly

Age-related cardiovascular or pulmonary diseases may increase the risk of hypotension or bronchoconstriction. Elderly patients are less able to compensate quickly or effectively for changes of heart rate and blood pressure. Overall, extra close observation is required. Anticipate longer recovery times (eg, return of satisfactory spontaneous ventilation).

Interactions with Other Drugs

Many common drugs, some of them used routinely in the perioperative settings in which a curare-like neuromuscular blocker would be used, can interact (Table 17–I). The most important interactants are inhaled anesthetics (eg, enflurane, halothane; Chapter 20) and aminoglycoside antibiotics (eg, gentamicin; Chapter 56). These drugs cause neuromuscular blockade in their own right. When given shortly before, along with, or shortly after true neuromuscular blockers, the outcome usually is more intense and prolonged muscle paralysis. The most important outcome is prolonged ventilatory impairment. Sometimes the neuromuscular blocker–aminoglycoside interaction can be avoided by using other classes of antibiotics, or withholding the aminoglycoside as long as possible after recovery from surgery. However, the blocker–anesthetic interaction usually cannot be avoided, since one interactant is routinely used as an adjunct to the other. In any case, close monitoring of ventilatory status and the ready availability of mechanical ventilation devices are essential.

Most of the other interactants (see Table 17–I) also result in enhanced and prolonged muscle paralysis, so the precautions noted above apply.

NURSING IMPLICATIONS

Note all current medications on the front of the chart or anesthesia flow sheet as an alert to possible interactions. If possible, drugs that potentiate neuromuscular blockade should not be given until there is no doubt that the patient can maintain adequate unassisted ventilation. Careful monitoring is still required when they are eventually given.

Overdose and Toxicity

Prolonged apnea, and all its consequences, is the most important concern with overdoses of any neuromuscular blocker. The most immediate interventions needed are to be sure that the patient's airway is patent and that ventilation can be supported as long as needed. Once that is done, attention can be turned to assessing and correcting vital signs as needed, and reversing neuromuscular blockade with atropine pretreatment followed by injection of an AChE inhibitor.

Treatments for other changes, such as those affecting heart rate and blood pressure, will be determined by an assessment of pertinent vital signs. Bronchoconstriction, which might arise from histamine release caused by tubocurarine (and the related drug atracurium), is best managed with a sympathomimetic. The choice of bronchodilator (eg, epinephrine or a selective β-agonist) may depend on the patient's cardiovascular status.

Related Drugs

Seven other nondepolarizing neuromuscular blockers are approved for use in the United States. All of them are indicated for use as anesthesia adjuncts, and most are indicated for assisting with endotracheal intubation or for ventilator control. Virtually all the major side effects or adverse responses (notably ventilatory depression), drug–drug interactions, and precautions noted for the prototype apply to these alternatives. Major differences relate to potency; duration of action (see Table 17–1), which can be quite variable for some agents, depending on the dose and whether repeated doses were given; whether they are metabolized or excreted by the kidneys; and whether they cause other potentially important effects, especially on the cardiovascular system. These properties may make a given agent preferred, or less suitable, for certain patients.

Atracurium, Mivacurium, and Vecuronium

Atracurium (TRACRIUM), mivacurium (MIVACRON) and vecuronium (NORCURON) have shorter durations of action than tubocurarine when single doses are given and neuromuscular blockade is not pharmacologically reversed. Significant recovery of muscle function usually returns in about 30 minutes. These drugs are eliminated by hepatic metabolism. Atracurium and mivacurium are inactivated by plasma esterases, and so altered renal or hepatic function has little impact on the duration of action. They also tend to cause histamine release, as does the prototype. Vecuronium depends on hepatic metabolism, and so patients with liver dysfunction may experience more prolonged effects. Any of these drugs can cause bradycardia, which may be accompanied by hypotension.

Gallamine, Metocurine, and Pancuronium

Gallamine, metocurine, and pancuronium have durations of action that are, in general, similar to that of tubocurarine. Gallamine (FLAXEDIL) and metocurine (METUBINE) are noteworthy because they are eliminated completely by the kidneys without prior metabolism. Gallamine tends to cause some antimuscarinic (atropine-like) actions that can increase heart rate. Pancuronium (PAVULON) causes considerable antimuscarinic effects, with increases of heart rate that usually are higher than those caused by any other neuromuscular blocker. This effect, combined with the ability of many inhaled anesthetics to sensitize the heart to epinephrine and norepinephrine, can increase the risk of tachycardia or arrhythmias.

Doxacurium and Pipecuronium

Doxacurium (NUROMAX) and pipecuronium (ARDUAN) have the longest durations of action (60 to 90 minutes, or longer), and so they are indicated for operative procedures when longlasting neuromuscular blockade is anticipated. These drugs seem to cause fewer changes of heart rate or blood pressure than the other curare-like blockers, which can be an advantage for patients with unstable cardiovascular status.

Depolarizing Neuromuscular Blocker

PROTOTYPE

Succinylcholine

Succinylcholine (ANECTINE) is the only depolarizing blocker available for use in the United States. It causes neuromuscular blockade in a way that is very different from that of the drugs discussed so far. This difference is clinically important.

Absorption, Distribution, Metabolism, and Excretion

Succinylcholine, like ACh, is an ester of choline. Succinylcholine is metabolized quickly by plasma and liver pseudocholinesterases, not the specific cholinesterase (AChE) that metabolizes ACh. Quick metabolism provides succinylcholine with the shortest duration of action of all neuromuscular blockers. The drug is usually given intravenously, but can be injected intramuscularly if a suitable vein cannot be found.

Pharmacologic Effects

Like ACh, but unlike any of the nondepolarizing blockers, succinylcholine *stimulates* nicotinic receptors, primarily those found on skeletal muscle. When succinylcholine is first administered it initially depolarizes the muscle cells and causes fasciculations or, in some patients, quite intense muscle contractions. Muscle stimulation lasts about 30 seconds, and is followed by muscle paralysis as the muscle becomes unresponsive to stimulation.

Paralysis lasts only about 5 minutes after giving a single therapeutic dose. This is called Phase I block; it is *noncompetitive,* meaning that it cannot be overcome by giving an AChE inhibitor, as is commonly done to reverse the effects of a curare-like blocker. If longer paralysis is needed, supplemental doses of succinylcholine must be injected or infused.

Prolonged succinylcholine administration causes accumulation of one of its metabolites, succinylmonocholine. This substance has a relatively long duration of action, and it produces *competitive* (curare-like) blockade, called Phase II block. Many anesthesiologists consider Phase II block as an indication of overdose, not a desired response.

Therapeutic doses of succinylcholine have little effect on autonomic ganglia. However, high doses may stimulate the ganglia, leading to cardiovascular side effects. Succinylcholine causes less histamine release than tubocurarine.

Clinical Indications and Administration

The very rapid but brief action of succinylcholine makes it a useful drug for endotracheal intubation, especially when the situation is an emergency. The drug is also useful for short procedures such as ECT, cardioversion, and some diagnostic tests (eg, endoscopy, bronchoscopy). In all but extreme emergencies, the drug should be given only after the patient has been premedicated with suitable sedatives or anxiety-relieving agents, or (preferably) after they are fully anesthetized. Succinylcholine's effects cannot, and need not, be reversed pharmacologically, as is routinely done with a curare-like blocker.

When longer neuromuscular blockade is anticipated, as for surgery, the anesthesiologist or nurse-anesthetist has several options. One is to give repeated injections of succinylcholine as needed, or continue administering the drug by IV infusion. A special formulation, marketed as ANECTINE FLO-PACK, is made specifically for infusion. In many cases, however, the patient will be given an IV injection of succinylcholine first, and then intubated. In a few minutes, after the effects of succinylcholine have begun to wear-off, blockade is continued with a curare-like blocker for the duration of the procedure.

Side Effects, Adverse Reactions, and Contraindications

General Side Effects

The major concern with succinylcholine is the same as for any neuromuscular blocker: prolonged ventilatory depression owing to muscle weakness or paralysis. Succinylcholine may increase blood pressure through stimulation of sympathetic ganglia, and bradycardia through stimulation of parasympathetic ganglia. Bradycardia becomes more intense with repeated succinylcholine injections. Infants are particularly sensitive to this cardiac-slowing effect, even with single doses. Atropine can be given before or after succinylcholine is administered to help keep heart rate from falling too much.

The intense skeletal muscle contractions that occur soon after succinylcholine is injected also cause side effects, some of which are potentially serious. Most patients who receive this drug will experience muscle pain during the recovery period. However, the contractions can be so intense that bone fractures or dislocations can occur, and muscles, tendons, or ligaments may be torn. Thus, this blocker is generally contraindicated for patients who have musculoskeletal problems, including osteoporosis or trauma, that may make them particularly vulnerable to further damage.

Vigorous contraction may also cause potassium to leak from the muscle cells into the bloodstream. The resulting hyperkalemia can increase the risk of cardiac arrhythmias. The risk is intensified if the patient has suffered major burns or trauma, which can cause hyperkalemia in their own right. (Sometimes the anesthesiologist will give a nondepolarizing blocker before giving succinylcholine. This will prevent the muscle contractions.)

Succinylcholine should also be used with care, if at all, in patients who have glaucoma, ocular damage, or will be undergoing eye surgery. The drug increases intraocular pressure, and causes contractions of eye muscles that can lead to further ocular damage.

NURSING IMPLICATIONS

Advise patients to expect postprocedure muscle pain and stiffness. After recovery, apply warm towels to help alleviate pain. Administer analgesics, and encourage ambulation as ordered and permitted by the patient's condition.

Increased Sensitivity of Patients with Pseudocholinesterase Deficiency

A variety of medical conditions and drugs (see drug interactions section) can cause significant falls in the blood levels of pseudocholinesterase, the enzyme responsible for metabolically inactivating succinylcholine. These individuals are more sensitive to the blocker, and tend to experience much longer-lasting paralysis after receiving even one dose of this drug. Medical conditions associated with low pseudocholinesterase levels include severe liver disease, hypothyroidism, anemias, cancer, and malnutrition. Pseudocholinesterase levels also fall during the later stages of pregnancy, and can remain low for several days postpartum. There are also some patients (about 1 out of 3600 in the general population) who, despite being perfectly normal otherwise, have an inherited deficiency or total lack of pseudocholinesterase. Patients with medically related cholinesterase deficiencies usually can be identified before they receive succinylcholine, and so prolonged effects can be anticipated, dosages can be reduced, or other blockers can be used instead. However, a genetically determined enzyme deficiency may go undetected until after the drug has been given, and paralysis may last several hours, rather than a few minutes.

Malignant Hyperthermia

Administration of succinylcholine, usually when accompanied by general anesthesia with halothane or similar agents, may trigger a life-threatening syndrome called *malignant hyperthermia*. It involves abnormally prolonged and intense skeletal muscle contraction (contracture or rigor). It occurs because the drugs disrupt the biochemical processes that control movements of calcium ion that normally allow muscle cells to relax between contractions. Increased muscle metabolism generates considerable heat, consumes large amounts of oxygen, and releases large amounts of potassium into the blood. Body temperature rises quickly and markedly (104°F or more), and the skin may become mottled. Ventilatory patterns change dramatically. Soon after initial symptoms develop, hyperkalemia may cause tachycardia and arrhythmias, and wide swings of blood pressure. Cyanosis, severe acidosis, and cardiovascular collapse are liable to occur.

The incidence of malignant hypterthermia is about 1 in 15,000 anesthesias, but if it develops it is fatal about 80% of the time. It is most likely to occur in patients with some underlying skeletal muscle disorder (myopathy). Myopathy and the possibility of increased sensitivity to succinylcholine and halothane can be detected by preoperative muscle biopsy and measurements of certain serum enzyme levels. Unfortunately, biopsies are not done routinely. Other laboratory tests, physical characteristics of the patient, and knowledge of the patient's or family's genetic background may also help identify those at a high risk.

Treatment of malignant hyperthermia includes reducing body temperature by surface cooling or irrigation of the abdomen with chilled solutions, administration of 100% oxygen, and injection of *dantrolene sodium* (p 273).

◆ Use During Pregnancy and Lactation

Succinylcholine is frequently used as a muscle relaxant during cesarean delivery. Small amounts of the drug cross the placental barrier, but normally do not endanger the fetus. However, repeated high doses or inadequate maternal levels of pseudocholinesterase activity may cause effects in the neonate. Monitor the newborn for these changes. The effects of succinylcholine will have disappeared by the time the mother is ready to breast-feed her newborn. Therefore, other drugs the patient receives will determine whether breast-feeding is permissible.

◆ Use in Children

Succinylcholine may cause profound bradycardia or cardiac arrest in children. As in adults, it is more common following a second dose. The effect can be minimized by atropine.

◆ Use in the Elderly

Elderly patients, because of age-related disorders, are predisposed to side effects and complications. Important factors include the presence of glaucoma, impaired cardiopulmonary status, bone fragility, and concurrent use of interacting drugs.

Interactions with Other Drugs

The most important interactants with succinylcholine are drugs that prolong and intensify its effects, and so can make a relatively brief episode of ventilatory inhibition more prolonged and dangerous. Aminoglycoside antibiotics, noted earlier as drugs that cause neuromuscular blockade and can intensify the effects of curare-like blockers, interact similarly with succinylcholine. Other agents that can interact are drugs that inhibit plasma cholinesterase levels, thereby inhibiting metabolic inactivation of succinylcholine and prolonging its effects: echothiophate and other "irreversible" AChE inhibitors used topically for glaucoma; metoclopramide, a stimulant of GI motility; procaine and its derivatives, which are used as local anesthetics; quinidine, a very commonly used antiarrhythmic drug; and the ganglionic blocker/antihypertensive drug trimethaphan.

Overdose and Toxicity

Succinylcholine overdoses are managed with ventilatory support and oxygen administration. Cardiovascular problems such as bradycardia or hypotension are treated symptomatically and with appropriate drugs, such as atropine and vasopressors. The same approach applies to most drug interactions involving succinylcholine. Identify blood electrolyte abnormalities so they can be corrected.

General Nursing Implications for All Neuromuscular Blockers

The nurse has several important roles and responsibilities when caring for patients who will receive, or have just received, any neuromuscular blocker. Many of those responsibilities apply to all postoperative or critically ill patients, including those on long-term ventilator support, and are covered in most medical–surgical or intensive-care nursing texts. Look for more information in textbooks written for nurse-anesthetists and other nursing specialists.

What follows summarizes key points that apply mainly to uses or effects of the neuromuscular blockers themselves. Nearly all the important concerns are related to their ability to impair muscle function in general, and ventilation in particular. They apply regardless of which neuromuscular blocker is given; whether the procedure for which the drug is given was surgical or diagnostic; and regardless of whether the patient is kept in the operating or procedure room until the return of ventilation is considered "adequate."

- Most importantly, be sure that devices to maintain a patent airway, and some means to support ventilation mechanically, are immediately available and in working order.
- Teach patients before a procedure that until the effects of a neuromuscular blocker wear off sufficiently, they will be unable to communicate (verbally or otherwise) concerns about pain or other discomforts (including muscle pain caused by succinylcholine); after the procedure, give reassurance that you are aware of this inability.
- Be sure that preoperative medications have been administered as ordered, and in the proper sequence.
- Use typical durations of neuromuscular blocker action only as a guideline for anticipating how long ventilatory impairment may last. Use information in the patient's chart and anesthesia flowsheet (prior and recent medical and drug history; current electrolyte and blood gas data; use of anesthesia, anesthesia adjuncts, other medications) to help predict whether recovery will be unusually prolonged, or muscle impairment might occur.
- Check orders for drugs that will be administered after the procedure for potential interactions that could cause a return of inadequate muscle strength; identify potential interactants before giving the drug if there is a concern.
- Some drugs (eg, barbiturates) and alkaline IV solutions (eg, those with bicarbonate) are physically incompatible with neuromuscular blockers, yet they may need to be administered to a patient being maintained on an infusion of the blocker (as for long-term ventilator control). Ordinarily, use a separate IV infusion line for each drug, and do not mix them in the same syringe.
- Be aware that during recovery increased pain or anxiety will not trigger usual changes in ventilatory rate, depth, or pattern, which otherwise might indicate the need for supplemental pain- or anxiety-relieving drugs. Assess for changes of blood pressure and heart rate as signs of such problems.
- Do not overlook the effects of neuromuscular blockers on gag reflexes and the ability to swallow. Avoid giving medications orally (other than by nasogastric tube) until it is clearly safe to do so.
- Give due attention to the patient's overall condition and the effects of neuromuscular blockers on ventilatory status, but do not overlook potentially important or longlasting effects of other drugs that have been administered (eg, antimuscarinics that are routinely used when muscle paralysis is reversed).
- If the patient has received succinylcholine and any inhaled anesthetic, be aware that although malignant hyperthermia is rare it is often fatal: monitor body temperature, skin color, and muscle tone closely and frequently; report any sudden changes at once; and be prepared to intervene.

Other Drugs Used to Inhibit Skeletal Muscle Function

Several drugs that reduce but do not abolish skeletal muscle activity are indicated as adjuncts for the relief of chronic or acute neuromuscular disorders caused by disease or trauma (see Table 17–C). Unlike neuromuscular blockers, many of these drugs act on nervous tissue, not on the muscle itself. Nondrug measures play an important part in the management of patients receiving these medications.

Baclofen

Baclofen (LIORESAL) is an orally effective drug that probably acts by suppressing spinal reflexes involved in skeletal muscle activation. The drug is indicated for relief of muscle spasticity associated with multiple sclerosis. It may alleviate spasticity caused by spinal cord injury. Baclofen has not been proven to be effective in alleviating muscle spasms associated with stroke, cerebral palsy, or parkinsonism. It is mainly eliminated by renal excretion without prior metabolism, so reduced doses are generally indicated for patients with renal dysfunction.

Sedation is common, but baclofen may cause euphoria in some patients. Hallucinations and seizures may occur if the drug is withdrawn abruptly. Genitourinary problems, including urinary frequency, occur in about 10% of patients receiving this drug. Both the central nervous system (CNS) and urinary problems may be partly due to the neuromuscular disorder for which baclofen was given. Dermatologic reactions, including hirsutism and photosensitive or acne-like rashes, may develop.

Baclofen overdoses usually cause intense CNS depression, and may cause coma and seizures. Overdoses are treated symptomatically. Mechanical ventilation and anticonvulsant drugs may be needed for severe poisoning. Central nervous system or respiratory stimulants should not be used, since they increase the risk of seizures.

Dantrolene

Skeletal muscle contracts when its intracellular stores of calcium ion are released following depolarization. Dantrolene (DANTRIUM) acts in skeletal muscle cells to interfere with calcium release, thereby reducing muscle contraction.

Dantrolene has an essential role in the prophylaxis and treatment of malignant hyperthermia. For prophylaxis in high-risk patients, oral dantrolene can be given for 2 days before surgery, with the final dose given a few hours before operation. This will usually prevent or at least reduce the severity of hyperthermia. If fever develops during surgery, regardless of the patient's history or probable cause of elevated temperature, IV dantrolene is given immediately and topical or systemic cooling techniques are begun to keep temperature from rising further. Since untreated malignant hyperthermia is frequently fatal, there is no contraindication to the use of dantrolene for this purpose.

Dantrolene is also indicated for the management of chronic spasticity due to multiple sclerosis or spinal cord injuries. It may alleviate chronic spasticity due to stroke and cerebral palsy. The desired response, which determines the maintenance dose, depends on the goals set for each patient (for example, ability to engage in exercise, ability to walk satisfactorily with braces, and so on). Because of potentially serious adverse responses, do not exceed the maximum recommended dose, and discontinue dantrolene administration if the desired response is not achieved after about 45 days of treatment.

The most common side effect of dantrolene therapy is drowsiness. Dantrolene may cause severe diarrhea, which generally requires therapy to be discontinued until normal GI function returns. If diarrhea returns after dantrolene administration is resumed, the patient should be taken off the drug permanently. Dantrolene may aggravate asthma and other obstructive lung diseases, or heart failure. Patients with these disorders should be monitored closely if dantrolene must be used.

Hepatotoxicity, and potentially fatal hepatitis, are the most serious adverse effects of dantrolene. If hepatotoxicity occurs, it usually appears between the third and twelfth months of therapy. Dantrolene is contraindicated in patients with active liver disease, such as hepatitis or cirrhosis, unless it is being given for emergency treatment of malignant hyperthermia. All patients receiving dantrolene chronically, regardless of the dosage, should have periodic liver function tests.

Dantrolene overdoses are treated symptomatically. Respiratory and cardiovascular support may be needed.

Drugs for Acute Musculoskeletal Disorders

Several drugs are used to relieve symptoms of acute musculoskeletal disorders, including those caused by minor trauma (whiplash, muscle sprains, athletic injuries) that are accompanied by spasm and pain. Most of these drugs are given orally and are indicated for short-term use adjunctively with bedrest and a physical therapy plan individualized for each patient. Their dosages are summarized in Table 17–C. Some of these drugs are also available as fixed-dose combination products that contain aspirin to alleviate pain and inflammation. Many patients (eg, asthmatics) can experience severe adverse responses to even small dosages of aspirin, and aspirin can interact with many other drugs (see Chapter 52). Therefore, it is important to double-check the patient's health and medication history to rule out additional unwanted effects that may be caused by one of these aspirin-containing combination products. Not all clinicians agree that these drugs are efficacious. All these drugs cause CNS depression as side effects, and their effects are potentiated by other CNS depressants, including alcohol. Therefore, relevant nursing implications noted for baclofen and dantrolene apply.

Diazepam (VALIUM) is also indicated for adjunctive relief of skeletal muscle spasm. Since its major use is as an anxiety-relieving drug, however, it is discussed in Chapter 22.

Carisoprodol, Chlorzoxazone, and Cyclobenzaprine

Carisoprodol (SOMA), chlorzoxazone (PARAFLEX; PARAFON FORTE), and cyclobenzaprine (FLEXERIL) act centrally or in the spinal cord to reduce reflex neural activation of skeletal muscle.

Metaxalone, Methocarbamol, and Orphenadrine Citrate

Metaxalone (SKELAXIN), methocarbamol (ROBAXIN), and orphenadrine citrate (NORFLEX) have indications similar to carisoprodol. They probably act in a nonspecific way that causes generalized CNS depression similar to that caused by barbiturates (Chapter 22). Parenteral dosage forms of methocarbamol are indicated for more severe cases of musculoskeletal disorders, including adjunctive management of tetanus.

Cyclobenzaprine causes significant antimuscarinic effects. For this reason, it is contraindicated or should be used cautiously in patients with glaucoma, tachycardia, obstructive bowel or bladder disease (including prostatic hypertrophy), and other situations in which atropine should not be given. Nursing implications noted for atropine (Chapter 13) apply also to cyclobenzaprine.

Quinine Sulfate

Quinine sulfate (QUINAMM) is found in both prescription and over-the-counter products that are used to treat the nocturnal leg cramps that some patients experience during sleep. It appears to act by directly depressing skeletal muscle function in several ways. It shares the toxicities and drug–drug interactions identified for a chemically similar drug, the cardiac antiarrhythmic agent quinidine (Chapter 30).

NURSING IMPLICATIONS

Drug therapy with any skeletal muscle relaxant should be combined with nursing measures that facilitate desired drug effects, including optimal positioning, meticulous skin care, and pain relief if needed. These drugs should be used as adjuncts to, not as substitutes for, a prescribed program of rest and physical therapy aimed at restoring muscle function.

All of these agents have the ability to cause drowsiness, sedation, ataxia, and other signs of CNS depression. Nursing measures that are appropriate for any CNS depressant apply to these drugs. Important ones include providing assisted ambulation as needed; discouraging activities made dangerous by CNS depression (eg, driving, operating hazardous machinery); and stressing the need to avoid taking any other CNS depressants, including alcohol, without a physician's advice.

All these drugs should be used cautiously during pregnancy, and only with close prenatal monitoring. Breast-feeding should be discouraged when any of these drugs are being used.

Botulinum Toxin Type A

Botulinum toxin is a unique neuromuscular blocker that has uses much different from those of all other agents discussed in this chapter. The lethal agent in food poisoning known as botulism, it was described briefly on page 130 as a substance that inhibits ACh release from *all* cholinergic nerves in the body. (Botulinum antitoxin, a treatment for the otherwise fatal poisoning, is discussed in Chapter 54.)

Botulinum toxin Type A is now available for therapeutic uses that capitalize on its actions. Marketed as OCULINUM, it is used to cause prolonged but temporary weakening or paralysis of skeletal muscles that control rotation of the eye, or other muscles in the ocular region. This effect is useful for treating some cases of severe or refractory blepharospasm (involuntary, spasmodic eyelid twitching) and other facial muscle spasms, and some cases of strabismus (visual impairment caused by the inability of one eye to move with the other). The drug is given by injection using specialized devices that help ensure drug placement directly into the desired muscle(s), and that can actually measure the developing effects of the drug on muscle function as it is administered.

Injecting the drug into adult patients is usually done after pretreatment with local anesthetics; pediatric patients may be premedicated with oral or injectable sedatives, or given nitrous oxide inhalations during the procedure. The effects of botulinum toxin given in this way usually last 2 to 4 months (at which time retreatment may be indicated), but in some cases only a couple of treatments, combined with proper eye exercises, may cause permanent cures.

This procedure, which uses a potentially lethal drug, should be performed only by specially trained ophthalmologists. But, when done properly, treatment is effective, safe, and quite free of serious side effects (most of which are limited to the eye). Nursing responsibilities may include patient education about the treatment and the need for follow-up visits and prescribed exercises; and monitoring responses to premedications.

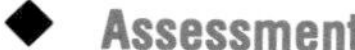

SUMMARY OF NURSING IMPLICATIONS

Assessment

Establish baseline laboratory values for factors that may alter the response to neuromuscular blockers (eg, potassium, calcium, and magnesium levels; creatinine clearance; and blood urea nitrogen levels).

Assess respiratory function for rate, depth, and adequacy (breath sounds) before drug administration.

Record routine vital signs and fluid intake and output throughout the course of drug therapy and recovery.

Complete a nursing history to include current drug regimens, past medical conditions, and allergies that may contraindicate or necessitate cautious use of neuromuscular blockers.

Nursing Diagnoses

Knowledge deficit related to drug therapy.

Fear related to muscle paralysis.

Impaired physical mobility: paralysis.

Pain related to procedures or muscle contraction (succinylcholine).

Ineffective breathing pattern related to neuromuscular blockade: inadequate ventilation or apnea.

Sensory/perceptual alteration related to centrally acting muscle relaxants.

High risk for injury related to changes in skeletal muscle strength, CNS effects of drug.

High risk for aspiration related to muscular weakness.

Planning/Implementation

Prepare for endotracheal intubation, suction, ventilatory support, and oxygen before administration of neuromuscular blockers.

Have antidote (neostigmine or pyridostigmine) available when nondepolarizing blockers are used.

Avoid mixing tubocurarine or related drugs with alkaline solutions (eg, barbiturates) to avoid precipitation.

Monitor sequence of muscle paralysis (eyelids, facial muscles, limbs, trunk, respiratory muscles) and recovery (reverse order).

Check gag reflex and swallowing before administering oral medications or food to a patient recovering from neuromuscular blockade.

Reassure patients during muscle paralysis that they are being cared for carefully: they may be alert, able to hear and see, but be unable to communicate.

Premedicate with analgesics, sedatives, or tranquilizers as ordered before and during paralysis; note changes in heart rate and blood pressure as indications for supplemental drugs.

Prevent physical and psychologic complications associated with prolonged paralysis and immobility: use optimal positioning, turn patient, control environmental noise and light, reduce pain, assess skin to prevent damage due to pressure.

Encourage patients to express fears and concerns regarding procedure; advise them about sensations, signs, and symptoms to anticipate, and about how long recovery will take.

Prepare patients who will receive succinylcholine for generalized muscle pain or stiffness; apply heat to alleviate pain, administer analgesics as necessary.

Monitor patients after surgery for signs of malignant hyperthermia when succinylcholine and an inhalation anesthetic were used; observe for muscular rigidity or tremor, mottling of skin, elevated temperature. Have dantrolene available.

Patient and Family Teaching

Instruct patients receiving skeletal muscle relaxants (baclofen, dantrolene) to avoid ingestion of CNS depressants, including alcohol. Because of possible sedation and impaired reflexes and coordination, they should avoid hazardous tasks.

Advise patients not to discontinue baclofen abruptly, as hallucinations or convulsions may occur.

Evaluation

The patient/family will:

Recover completely following paralysis; patient regains normal muscle function.

Experience minimal adverse drug effects; no prolonged respiratory depression; vital signs within normal limits.

Achieve desired level of functioning with skeletal muscle relaxant therapy.

Annotated Bibliography

Ashby D. Malignant hyperthermia: A potential crisis in the postanesthesia care unit. *J Post Anesth Nurs* 1990;5(4):279–281. *Reviews the etiology, biochemistry, and treatment of malignant hyperthermia, and presents a case study involving malignant hyperthermia in the PACU.*

Batlan DE, Zaid GJ, Johnston WC. Neuromuscular blockade in the emergency department. *J Emerg Med* 1987;5(3):225–232. *Covering a variety of topics ranging from basic pharmacologic actions to clinical use, this paper discusses the role of neuromuscular blockers in the emergency room. Although newer blockers (doxacurium and pipecuronium) are not included, the paper is still worth reading.*

Costarino AT, Polin RA. Neuromuscular relaxants in the neonate. *Clin Perinatol* 1987;14(4):965–989. *After reviewing basic actions of the neuromuscular blockers, this article explains why these drugs are among the most commonly used medications in the intensive-care nursery, and what should be looked for when caring for patients.*

Durbin CG Jr. Neuromuscular blocking agents and sedative drugs: Clinical uses and toxic effects in the critical care unit. *Crit Care Clin* 1991;7(3):489–506. *Discusses drug selection, therapeutic goal-setting, and monitoring for ICU patients receiving neuromuscular blockers.*

O'Brien DD. Review and update of neuromuscular blocking agents. *Crit Care Nurse* 1989;9(10):76–80. *A short but informative article about the use of neuromuscular blockers in the postanesthesia and intensive-care settings, from a nursing perspective.*

Smith SM, Brown HO, Toman JEP, Goodman LS. The lack of cerebral effects of *d*-tubocurarine. *Anesthesiology* 1947;8:1–14. *Dr. Smith allowed himself to receive a large dose of curare while fully conscious. Read this and you will see (and never forget) how your pharmacologically paralyzed patients feel, and why providing reassurance to them is such an important part of care.*

Table 17–C Clinical Uses and Administration of Neuromuscular Blocking Drugs and Other Drugs That Affect Skeletal Muscle Function

AGENT	CLINICAL USES	DOSAGE AND ROUTE OF ADMINISTRATION
	Neuromuscular Blockers ***Nondepolarizing Blockers***	
PROTOTYPE		
d-Tubocurarine chloride	Adjunct to anesthesia, electroconvulsive therapy, or intubation; intraoperative muscle relaxation, ventilator control, management of tetany	IV: For otherwise healthy 70-kg patient: 6–9 mg (40–60 units) at time of initial skin incision; 3–4.5 mg 3–5 min later if needed; additional 3-mg doses given at 30-min intervals as needed. Children: Reduce dose in proportion to body weight
	Diagnosis of myasthenia gravis	IV: Inject about 1 mg with close monitoring of vital signs
RELATED DRUGS		
Atracurium besylate (TRACRIUM)	Adjunct to surgical anesthesia, intubation; ventilator control	IV: Adults, children ≥ 2: 0.3–0.5 mg/kg as bolus; maintain with continuous infusion; reduce initial dose to 0.3–0.4 mg/kg, infuse slowly, if patient has questionable cardiac or pulmonary status or is at risk from histamine release; reduce initial dose by half if patient is already anesthetized with enflurane or isoflurane
Doxacurium chloride (NUROMAX)	Adjunct to anesthesia, intubation	IV: Adults: 0.05 mg/kg initially. Children: 0.03 mg/kg initially
Gallamine triethiodide (FLAXEDIL)	Adjunct to anesthesia	IV: Usually 0.5–1.0 mg/kg
Metocurine iodide (METUBINE)	Adjunct to anesthesia, ECT, intubation	IV: Adults: 0.2–0.4 mg/kg by slow injection over 30–60 sec; supplement with 0.5–1 mg as needed for prolonged effects during surgery
Mivacurium chloride (MIVACRON)	Adjunct to anesthesia, intubation	IV: Adults: 0.15 mg/kg initially, usually maintain with 6–7 μg/kg/min (based on body weight) as needed. Children 2–12 years; 0.20 mg/kg initially; maintain with ~14μg/kg/min
Pancuronium bromide (PAVULON)	Adjunct to anesthesia, intubation, ventilator control	IV: Adults, most pediatric patients: 0.04–0.1 mg/kg injection; supplement with 0.01 mg/kg as needed; may use larger initial doses (0.06–0.1 mg/kg) to shorten onset, prolong duration. Neonates: Start with no more than 0.02 mg/kg
Pipecuronium bromide (ARDUAN)	Adjunct to anesthesia, intubation	IV: Adults, children: 0.07–0.085 mg/kg initially (dose adjusted to ideal body weight for obese patients)
Vecuronium bromide (NORCURON)	Adjunct to anesthesia, intubation, ventilator control	IV: Adults, children ≥ 10: 0.08–0.1 mg/kg; for more prolonged effects, give 0.01–0.015 mg/kg 25–40 min after first dose. Children aged 1–10 require higher initial doses. Children aged 7 weeks–1 year require lower doses

(continued)

Table 17–C Clinical Uses and Administration of Neuromuscular Blocking Drugs and Other Drugs That Affect Skeletal Muscle Function (*Continued*)

AGENT	CLINICAL USES	DOSAGE AND ROUTE OF ADMINISTRATION
	Depolarizing Blocker	
PROTOTYPE AND SOLE AGENT		
Succinylcholine		
(ANECTINE)	Emergency endotracheal intubation, adjunct to ECT, short diagnostic procedures, initial preoperative muscle paralysis	IV (preferred): Adults: 0.6 mg/kg; use smaller test doses in patients with known or suspected cholinesterase deficiency. Infants, small children: 2 mg/kg initially. Older children, adolescents: 1 mg/kg initially
		IM: 3–4 mg/kg, with a maximum total dose of 150 mg
(ANECTINE, ANECTINE FLO-PACK)	Prolonged surgical muscle relaxation	IV: Give initial dose as above, supplement with smaller doses as needed, or give 2.5–4.3 mg/min as infusion for long procedures
	Other Drugs Affecting Skeletal Muscle	
Baclofen		
(LIORESAL)	Relief of spasticity of multiple sclerosis, spinal cord injury	Oral: 5 mg tid; usual maintenance dose is 10-20 mg qid
Carisoprodol		
(SOMA)	Symptomatic, adjunctive relief of acute painful musculoskeletal conditions	Oral: 350 mg tid and hs; not recommended for children younger than 12
(SOMA COMPOUND)		Oral: 1–2 tablets (also contains aspirin) qid
Chlorzoxazone		
(PARAFLEX)	See carisoprodol	Oral: Adults: 250 mg tid or qid; for severe pain, 500 mg tid or qid increasing to 750 mg tid or qid if response not adequate. Children: 125-500 mg tid or qid based on age, weight
(PARAFON-FORTE DSC)	See carisoprodol	Oral: Adults: 1 tablet qid
Cyclobenzaprine		
(FLEXERIL)	See carisoprodol	Oral: Adults: Usually 10 mg tid, not to exceed 60 mg/day; administer for no more than 2–3 weeks
Dantrolene sodium		
(DANTRIUM)	Chronic spasticity; see baclofen	Oral: Adults: Initially 25 mg daily; increase to 25 mg bid–qid as needed, up to maximum of 100 mg qid. Children: 0.5 mg/kg bid; increase up to 3 mg/kg bid–qid up to maximum of 100 mg qid
	Prophylaxis of malignant hyperthermia	Oral: Adults, children: 4–8 mg/kg/d in 3 or 4 divided doses starting 1–2 days before surgery, with final dose about 3hr preoperatively
		IV: Usually 2.5 mg/kg, starting about 75 min before anticipated anesthesia, infused over about 1 hr
	Treatment of malignant hyperthermia	IV: Adults, children: Rapidly inject minimum of 1 mg/kg as soon as symptoms appear, repeating until symptoms subside or maximum dose of 10 mg/kg is reached; repeat if symptoms reappear

(continued)

Table 17–C Clinical Uses and Administration of Neuromuscular Blocking Drugs and Other Drugs That Affect Skeletal Muscle Function (*Continued*)

AGENT	CLINICAL USES	DOSAGE AND ROUTE OF ADMINISTRATION
	Postcrisis therapy of malignant hyperthermia	Oral: 4–8 mg/kg/day in 4 divided doses (1–2 mg/kg each) for 1–3 days after development of malignant hyperthermia crisis
Metaxalone		
(SKELAXIN)	See carisoprodol	Oral: Adults or children > 12: 800 mg tid or qid
Methocarbamol		
(ROBAXIN)	See carisoprodol	Oral: Adults: 1.5 g qid, then 1.0 g qid
	Moderate-to-severe painful musculoskeletal conditions	IV or IM: Initially 1 g (moderate symptoms)–3 g (severe) per day in divided doses; do not exceed 300 mg/min when given IV; use gluteus for IM injection, do not exceed 500 mg site; do not give parenterally for > 3 consecutive days; switch to oral therapy when feasible
	Initial adjunctive therapy of tetanus	IV: Adults: 1–2 g injected (bolus) into vein, plus balance to make total of 3 g added to IV infusion; repeat every 6 hr until nasogastric tube can be inserted. Children: Minimum of 15 mg/kg initially, repeat every 6 hr as needed
	Adjunctive maintenance therapy of tetanus	Oral (nasogastric tube): Dissolve tablets in water, administer up to total daily dose of 24 g
(ROBAXISAL)	See carisoprodol	Oral: Adults, children ≥ 12: 2 tablets qid (contains aspirin)
Orphenadrine citrate		
(NORFLEX)	Adjunctive therapy of painful acute musculoskeletal conditions	Oral: 100 mg twice daily IM or IV: For moderate-to-severe symptoms, 60 mg, repeated in 12 hrs, then switch to oral therapy
(NORGESIC)	See orphenadrine	Oral: Adults: 1 or 2 tablets 3 or 4 times daily (contains aspirin and caffeine)
(NORGESIC FORTE)	See orphenadrine	Oral: Adults: ½ to 1 tablet (contains twice the dose of each agent in NORGESIC) 3 or 4 times daily
Quinine sulfate		
(QUINAMM, others)	Prevention, treatment of nocturnal recumbency leg cramps	Oral: 260–300 mg at bedtime, and after evening meal if necessary

Table 17–S Major Side Effects and Contraindications of Neuromuscular Blockers

BODY SYSTEM/ Side Effect	CONTRAINDICATION/ PRECAUTION	COMMENTS AND NURSING IMPLICATIONS
Common to All Neuromuscular Blockers		
RESPIRATORY		
Prolonged respiratory depression, apnea	Lack of means to establish, maintain patent airway, support ventilation	Duration of paralysis variable, depends on neuromuscular blocker, other drugs, patient-related characteristics; monitor frequently and closely
Bronchoconstriction	Asthma (caution)	Caused by histamine release, more common with tubocurarine, atracurium; may impair ventilation, even in intubated, ventilator-supported patient
Caused Mainly by Nondepolarizing Blockers		
CARDIOVASCULAR		
Tachycardia		Response variable, most likely to occur with gallamine (slight), pancuronium (more intense) owing to antimuscarinic effect, or with tubocurarine or atracurium because of histamine release
Hypotension		Variable, most likely to be triggered by histamine-releasers (tubocurarine, atracurium)
Caused Mainly by Succinylcholine		
EYE		
Eye pain, damage, increased intraocular pressure	Ocular surgery, trauma; history of glaucoma	Vigorous contraction of ocular muscles may damage delicate eye structures; succinylcholine increases intraocular pressure; have patient report eye pain at once, notify physician for measurement of intraocular pressure (tonometry), possible treatment
CARDIOVASCULAR		
Bradycardia	Bradycardia, heart block	Most likely to occur in neonates or patients receiving more than one succinylcholine dose during a given procedure; prevent or treat with atropine
Arrhythmias	Arrhythmias, hyperkalemia due to drugs, disease, trauma	Muscle cells depolarized by succinylcholine may release potassium in amounts sufficient to cause hyperkalemia, arrhythmias; risk increased in patients with preexisting hyperkalemia (severe trauma, burns, impaired neurologic or respiratory status); monitor ECG, have antiarrhythmic drugs available
MUSCULOSKELETAL		
Pain, soreness; bone dislocations or fractures	Trauma; predisposition to fractures (eg, osteomalacia)	Generalized muscle pain common after succinylcholine; advise patient before drug use; best managed with nondrug comfort measures (moist heat, etc)
Malignant hyperthermia	Personal or family history of malignant hyperthermia or "adverse reaction" to general anesthesia	Rare but potentially fatal; assess body temperature frequently in any patient who received succinylcholine and any inhaled anesthetic; fever may or may not be accompanied by muscle rigidity; notify physician at once of any signs, symptoms; be prepared to cool patient physically, administer dantrolene

(continued)

Table 17–S **Major Side Effects and Contraindications of Neuromuscular Blockers (*Continued*)**

BODY SYSTEM/ Side Effect	CONTRAINDICATION/ PRECAUTION	COMMENTS AND NURSING IMPLICATIONS
Key Side Effect of Dantrolene		
LIVER Liver dysfunction, failure	Active liver disease (eg, hepatitis, cirrhosis)	Check baseline liver function test results for comparison with values taken during treatment; abnormalities most likely to appear between 3 and 12 months of long-term therapy; liver dysfunction does *not* contraindicate dantrolene use for emergency management of malignant hyperthermia
Side Effect Shared by Most "Centrally-Acting" Skeletal Muscle Relaxants		
CENTRAL NERVOUS SYSTEM Drowsiness, sedation, confusion, ataxia	Questionable neurologic status	Caution patient against operating motor vehicles, dangerous machinery, or other tasks requiring unimpaired mental acuity, judgment, and coordination; advise patient to avoid alcohol, other depressant drugs

Table 17–I **Major Interactions Between Neuromuscular Blockers and Other Agents**

AGENT	RESULT OF INTERACTION	COMMENTS AND NURSING IMPLICATIONS
Major Interactions Involving Nondepolarizing Neuromusclar Blockers		
Aminoglycoside antibiotics (gentamicin, others; see Chapter 56)	Prolonged or intensified muscle paralysis (eg, prolonged apnea)	These antibiotics tend to cause neuromuscular blockade in their own right; use other classes of antibiotics if possible, otherwise anticipate and monitor for likely result of interaction
Anesthetics, inhaled (halothane, others; Chapter 20)	Prolonged or intensified muscle paralysis	Common and important, given frequent adjunctive use of neuromuscular blockers and these anesthetics; monitor accordingly
Ketamine (Chapter 20)	Prolonged or intensified muscle paralysis	Check anesthesia flowsheets and anticipate need for longer ventilatory support if ketamine was the anesthetic
Magnesium salts (Chapters 41, 61)	Prolonged or intensified muscle paralysis	Of most concern for obstetric patients who received IV magnesium for eclampsia and were delivered by cesarean section; elevated magnesium levels intensify neuromuscular blockade; monitor accordingly
Quinidine (Chapter 30)	Prolonged or intensified muscle paralysis	High doses of this common antiarrhythmic may be used before, during, or after surgery involving neuromuscular blocker; interactant depresses skeletal muscle function; anticipate interaction, monitor accordingly
Theophylline, aminophylline (Chapter 38)	Antagonism of neuromuscular blockade	Of most concern for patients on ventilator support; these interactants appear to stimulate skeletal muscle directly; monitor accordingly and report evidence of interaction at once for possible change of bronchodilator therapy

(continued)

Table 17–I **Major Interactions Between Neuromuscular Blockers and Other Agents (*Continued*)**

AGENT	RESULT OF INTERACTION	COMMENTS AND NURSING IMPLICATIONS
Major Interactions Involving Succinylcholine		
Acetylcholinesterase inhibitors (e.g., long-acting agents such as echothiophate; Chapter 12)	Prolonged or intensified muscle paralysis	Check chart; even topically applied AChE inhibitors used for glaucoma can inhibit plasma cholinesterase levels enough to inhibit succinylcholine metabolism, prolong its actions; monitor accordingly
Aminoglycoside antibiotics (Chapter 56)	Prolonged or intensified muscle paralysis	See interactions involving nondepolarizing blockers, above
Plasma cholinesterase inhibitors, other: cyclophosphamide (Chapter 59); lidocaine (Chapter 30); metoclopramide (Chapter 42); procaine (Chapter 19); quinidine (Chapter 30); trimethaphan (Chapters 16, 33)	Prolonged or intensified muscle paralysis	Can inhibit succinylcholine's metabolic inactivation; check chart; anticipate need for ventilatory support, even when succinylcholine used for brief actions (eg, intubation)
Major Interactions Involving Most Other Drugs That Affect Skeletal Muscle Function		
Sedatives, hypnotics, and related drugs, including alcohol	Increased risk of CNS depression	Virtually all drugs used to relieve muscle spasticity or treat acute musculoskeletal conditions cause drowsiness that is potentiated by other drugs that cause sedation; advise patients to avoid interactants except on the advice and supervision of a physician

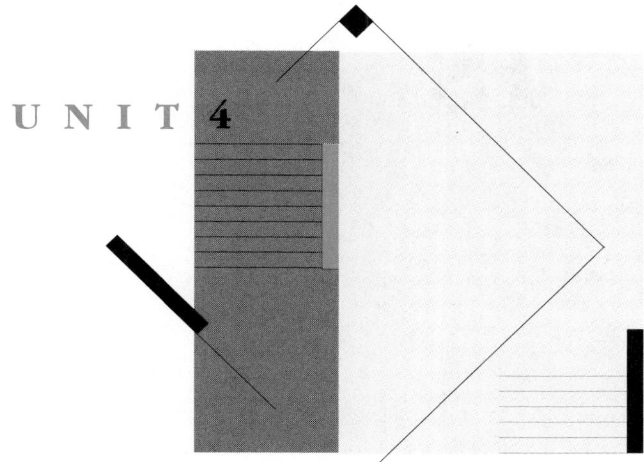

Drugs That Affect the Central Nervous System

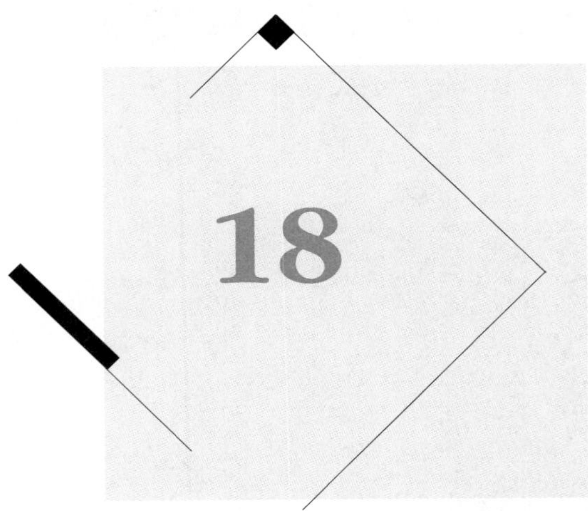

Structure and Function of the Central Nervous System

The central nervous system (CNS), composed of the brain and spinal cord, is the body's major integrating and coordinating system. Through its two major parts, the brain and the spinal cord, the CNS monitors and controls consciousness, sensory perception, motor responses; and personality, behavior, and emotion. It does so using a variety of chemical mediators and a host of complex and specialized neural pathways. These activities are common sources of dysfunction, and a variety of drugs are used for their direct effects on the CNS.

However, many drugs, whose major desired effect occurs outside the CNS, can cause important and potentially serious side effects in the CNS. Good examples are the many drugs used for their cardiovascular effects, as for the treatment of heart failure or high blood pressure. The primary consequences of these CNS side effects, such as sedation, confusion, or loss of judgment or coordination, can have important secondary effects as well: a fall, a motor vehicle accident, loss of appetite, or even an impaired ability to follow directions about how and when to take medications properly. The CNS is also the primary target of action of drugs that are widely used in our society for their mind-altering effects.

This introductory chapter begins with a brief review of the basics of CNS structure and function. It concludes with a summary of the topics presented in the rest of the unit's chapters.

Functional Anatomy of the Central Nervous System

Brain

The brain is divided into three major subdivisions: the *forebrain,* the *midbrain,* and the *hindbrain.* These subdivisions each exert control over different physiologic functions, which are summarized in Table 18–1. The cerebral hemispheres of the forebrain are divided into lobes. Each lobe also has distinct functional areas (Fig. 18–1).

Reticular Formation

The reticular formation (originally called the *reticular activating system,* or RAS) is a key target of action of drugs acting on the CNS. It is a network of neurons spread throughout the brainstem and extending up into the diencephalon. The axonal branches of these neu-

Table 18–1 Functions Regulated by the Central Nervous System

Area of Brain	Functions Controlled
Cerebral cortex (see Fig. 18-1)	Analysis (reception, integration, and organization) of input from body's sensory receptors (eg, pressure, pain, temperature) and facilitation of appropriate response (primary sensory area and somatosensory association area). Interpretation of input from the special sense organs (visual, olfactory, and auditory areas)
	Complex memory and higher intellectual activities (eg, foresight, judgment, elaboration of thought) (frontal association area)
	Conscious or voluntary movement of skeletal muscles (primary motor area), motor control of speech (Broca's area), contraction of muscles in a specific sequence for repetitious tasks (eg, typing) (premotor area)
Cerebral medulla	Impulse transfer to or from the cortical neurons
Basal ganglia (extrapyramidal system)	Locomotor activity and postural reflex integration, regulation
Corpus callosum	Communication between the left and right hemispheres
Thalamus	Sensory signal (pain, temperature, pressure) relay to cortical sensory areas for localization and interpretation
Hypothalamus	Regulation of many body functions, including body temperature, water balance, fat and carbohydrate metabolism, sleep-wake cycles, and appetite. Regulation of pituitary gland hormone release
Limbic system (visceral brain)	Regulation of visceral motor functions and emotional behavior (eg, expression of fear, sorrow, aggression, pleasure, etc) through interactions with higher cortical centers and hypothalamus. Autonomic nervous system activity modulation
Cerebral peduncles (red nucleus)	Impulse coordination between cerebellum and cerebral hemispheres for coordination of movements, sense of balance
Pons	Regulation of respiration
Medulla oblongata	Regulation of heart rate, respiratory rhythm, blood pressure, and involuntary reflexes (swallowing, vomiting)
Cerebellum	Unconscious control of skeletal muscle activity, balance, and equilibrium

rons are widely distributed, interacting with spinal cord neurons and with hypothalamic nuclei. The reticular formation exerts control over the cerebral cortex. Overall, the reticular system

- regulates consciousness and general levels of alertness;
- regulates sensory and motor activity, filtering incoming sensory information and relaying only that information requiring response from the cerebral cortex;
- modifies the rate at which spinal motor neurons stimulate the body musculature; and
- receives inhibitory signals from the cortex, processing it along with neural evidence of reduced sensory input, to provide a sleep-inducing mechanism.

Spinal Cord

The spinal cord, a continuation of the brainstem, functions as an association and communication center. It is important in spinal reflex activity, and provides sensory and motor neural pathways to and from higher nervous centers. The spinal cord gray matter, located in the center of the cord along its long (cranial to caudal) axis, contains mainly nerve cell bodies and nonmyelinated nerve fibers. The white matter that surrounds the gray matter is composed of nerve fibers bundled together to form ascending (sensory) and descending (motor) nerve tracts. The *spinothalamic* tracts are ascending sensory tracts for pain, temperature, touch, vibration, spatial position of the body, and so on. They relay impulses to the thalamus. One major descending motor

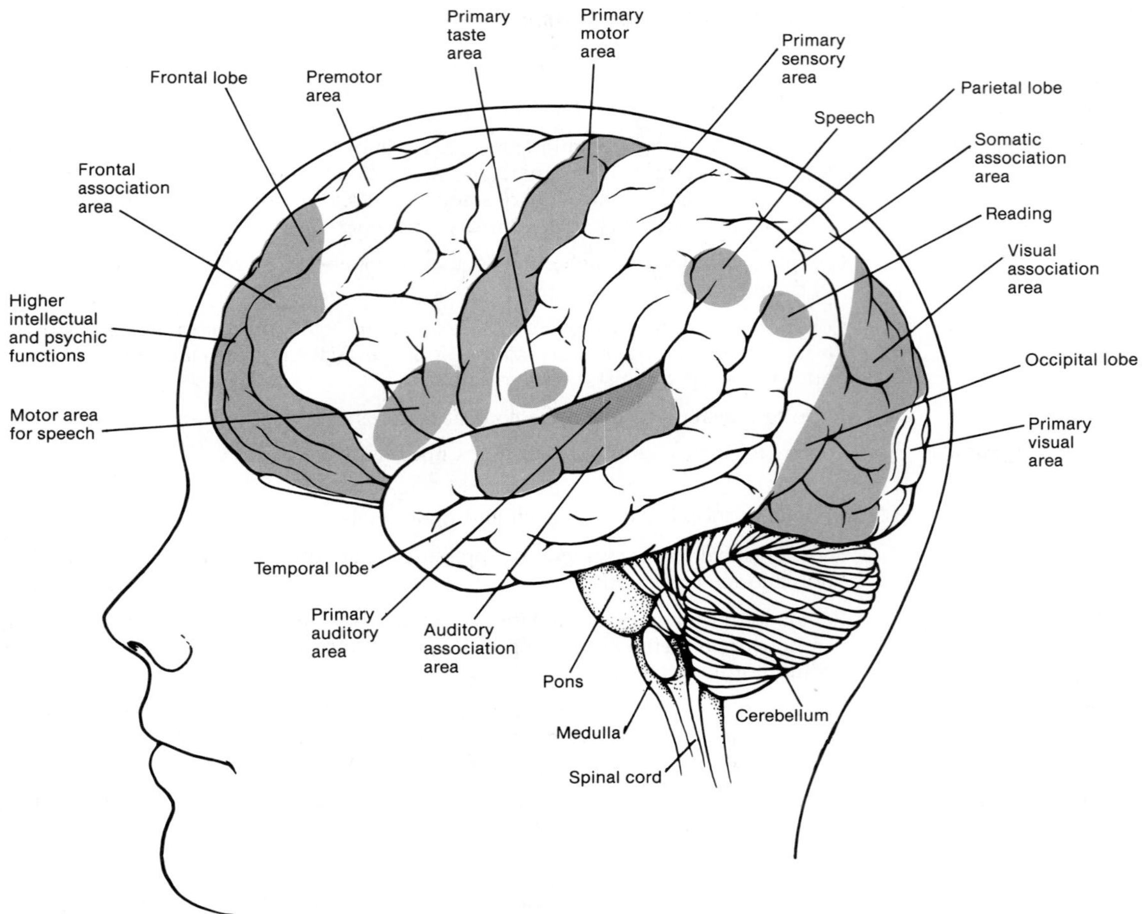

Figure 18–1

Lobes and general functional areas of the cerebral cortex (see Table 18–1 for a list of functions controlled by the cerebral cortex).

tract is the *pyramidal* (corticospinal) tract. It controls voluntary movement. Other tracts, collectively called the *extrapyramidal* tracts, integrate and modulate involuntary movement.

Chemical Transmission of Messages in the Central Nervous System

Neural activity in the CNS depends largely on a balance between the opposing effects of excitatory and inhibitory neurotransmitters and other chemicals that affect target cell receptors at particular times. (This is not very different from the way sympathetic and parasympathetic nerves in the autonomic nervous system affect their target structures. Indeed, basic principles of synaptic transmission and the roles of neurotransmitters that were reviewed in Chapter 10 generally apply to what occurs in the CNS.)

Some of the neurotransmitters identified in the previous unit as being important in the autonomic nervous system—acetylcholine and norepinephrine, for example—are important in parts of the CNS also. However, there are also many more chemicals. They are identified and described briefly in Table 18–2. Many other substances in the CNS, such as peptides (small proteins), do not fit the traditional description of a neurotransmitter, but they are important nonetheless. Many

Table 18–2 Neurotransmitters and Neuromodulators in the Central Nervous System

Mediator	Comments
Acetylcholine	Important neurotransmitter for basal nuclei, large pyramidal cells of motor cortex
Biogenic amines Histamine Serotonin Catecholamines (eg, dopamine, norepinephrine)	Increases in levels, activities, of these transmitters tend to cause cerebral stimulation; decreases tend to cause opposite effects; precise role of histamine unknown; serotonin, catcholamine deficiencies are important in etiology of psychiatric depression; dopamine excess contributes to schizophrenia, deficiency leads to parkinsonism
Amino acid neurotransmitters Glycine Gamma-aminobutyric acid (GABA) Glutamate Aspartate	Are universal cell constituents; glycine found mainly in spinal cord interneurons, as is GABA, which is also found in basal nuclei, cerebellum; both are inhibitory neurotransmitters; glutamate, found in spinal cord and cerebellum, is excitatory neurotransmitter; aspartate is probably inhibitory
Neuropeptides Gut-brain peptides Vasoactive intestinal peptide (VIP), cholecystokinin (CCK), substance P, neurotensin, enkephalins, insulin Hypothalamic-releasing factors Thyrotropin-releasing hormone (TRH), luteinizing hormone-releasing hormone (LHRH), somatostatin Pituitary peptides Adrenocorticotropin (ACTH); β-endorphin, melanocyte stimulating hormone (MSH) Miscellaneous Oxytocin, vasopressin	Not considered true neurotransmitters: have longer actions, seem to be effective at lower concentrations, may have no specific mechanism (identified) for inactivation; some have hormone-like actions; cause neuron inhibition or excitation

of these substances, some of which exert longlasting effects, are called *neuromodulators* or *neurohormones*. They are also identified in Table 18–2.

The Blood–Brain Barrier

The blood–brain barrier differs from most other parts of the CNS because it is not composed of neural tissue. Nevertheless, it is important to brain function and, in particular, to the effects of drugs on brain activity. The blood–brain barrier is a structural and functional specialization of the capillary endothelial cells that are found in all organs. Modifications of these cells restrict the ability of many drugs and other blood-borne molecules to diffuse from the circulation into the cerebrospinal fluid (CSF) and brain tissues. When the blood–brain barrier is intact, only molecules that are very lipid soluble and uncharged (nonionized), or those for which there are suitable active transport "pumps," can pass across it readily.

In general, the blood–brain barrier is beneficial in drug therapy. It allows the systemic administration of often high concentrations of many drugs for their effects outside the CNS, yet prevents appreciable entry of those drugs into the brain. As a result, it "protects" the CNS from adverse effects of many drugs. Of course, drugs that exert their major effects in the brain (eg, those discussed in this unit) have structures that allow for easy crossing of the barrier. However, the gateway provided by the blood–brain barrier can be altered by disease or other factors, of which CNS infection and inflammation are the most common and important. Increased permeability of the barrier can be either desirable or unwanted. For example, antibiotics that might normally be excluded from the CNS by an intact blood–brain barrier may now enter in larger amounts. That would be desirable when the goal is to treat a brain infection. In contrast, increased permeability can increase brain entry of drugs that normally should be excluded, thereby exposing the patient to more, or more intense, central side effects.

Special administration routes may be needed if it is essential to deliver therapeutic amounts of drug to the brain (as for managing some brain infections or cancers). These routes include intrathecal or intracerebral injections or infusions.

Physiology of the Central Nervous System

Although the CNS has a tremendous variety of functions, pharmacologic agents that affect the CNS primarily affect sensory and motor integration or emotional and intellectual integration. Therefore, only these functions are reviewed here.

Sensory and Motor Integration

Sensory Pathways

Impulses from peripheral sensory receptors convey information from the skin, viscera, and muscles to the *somatosensory cortex.* Impulses from the special sense organs (eye, taste buds, and ear) reach special sensory cortical areas located in the *occipital* and *temporal lobes.* The neural messages then are conveyed to the nearby association areas for analysis, interpretation, and activation of the motor cortex for any necessary muscle response. The fact that some sensory stimuli cause affective responses indicates that the *limbic system* is also involved. The upward flow of sensory transmission is modulated by the brainstem reticular formation. It appears that many CNS depressant drugs exert their effects by blocking transmission by the reticular neurons rather than by acting on the cerebral cortex itself. Although direct sensory pathway input still occurs, such drugs temporarily depress the consciousness-promoting activity of the reticular system.

Muscular Activity

Although some muscle activation is the result of spinal cord–mediated reflexes, voluntary muscle activity is always initiated by the pyramidal neurons of the motor cortex, which transmit impulses down the pyramidal tracts to the skeletal muscles on the opposite side of the body. Axonal collaterals from this pathway project to the basal nuclei, thalamus, and the brainstem neurons—including the reticular neurons.

Lesions of the pyramidal tract result in a recognizable reduction in the speed of voluntary muscle contraction and hypotonia (loss of function), as well as certain instances of hyperexcitability (release of functions otherwise kept in check by the descending impulses of this pathway).

The structures of the extrapyramidal system (the cerebellum, basal nuclei, and brainstem motor centers) are also important in the control and coordination of motor activity. The fibers that make up the extrapyramidal pathways are responsible for the complex adjustments needed to maintain balance, posture, and the proper degree of muscle contraction for well-controlled and smooth muscle activity.

Lesions of the basal nuclei cause characteristic involuntary movements such as tremors, chorea, and disorders in initiation of movement. Such lesions are found in a number of motor disorders, including Parkinson's disease, Huntington's disease, and Syndenham's chorea. In Parkinson's disease it has been found that a deficiency of dopamine (a neurotransmitter) is responsible for disruption of extrapyramidal system communication; therefore, replacement of this chemical is beneficial in reducing symptoms. Additionally, since acetylcholine (ACh) is a natural antagonist to dopamine's actions, antiparkinson therapy can also be aimed at antagonizing the central effects of ACh.

Excesses or deficiencies of other CNS neurotransmitters also underlie several other disorders for which pharmacologic therapy is initiated. For example, excessive activity of dopamine is thought to contribute to schizophrenia, and deficiencies of catecholamines are thought to have a role in depression. Consequently, CNS drugs that target these neurotransmitters or the structures they control may hamper the neural control mechanisms needed for smooth coordinated muscle activity. Depressant drugs and alcohol cause a loss of motor coordination, or **ataxia.** The antipsychotics may affect the extrapyramidal system, causing parkinsonian signs and symptoms.

Emotional and Intellectual Integration

Although much remains to be learned about the mechanisms involved in higher cognitive function, it is known that much of what is called "behavior" results from an interaction between the cerebral cortex and the more primitive limbic system. Drugs such as the opiates and antipsychotic drugs, in effect, prevent communication between the cortex and the limbic system and blunt emotional responses. Behavior is also influenced by the hypothalamic releasing factors and by a variety of hormones. The hypothalamic releasing factors (discussed in Chapter 44) are thought to act directly on the brain, independently of their effects on the release of anterior pituitary hormones. Specific hormone receptors have also been identified in a number of limbic structures, and these hormones are thought to be involved in long-term regulation of mood or emotional states.

The CNS Drugs

Drugs that affect mainly the CNS often have been classified, functionally, as being either CNS depressants or CNS stimulants. Although the overall effects of a particular agent may appear as if overall CNS activity is inhibited or increased, such a simple classification of the drugs is insufficient to describe their effects fully. That is true mainly because the actions of these drugs often are complex. Given the complexity of CNS structure, function, and biochemistry, that should not be surprising.

Chapter 19 discusses drugs called *local anesthetics*. Although these drugs are often given by routes that direct their actions on peripheral nerves, they eventually affect the input of unpleasant sensory information to the spinal cord and brain. And, without question, the CNS is an important site of their adverse effects. Chapter 20 discusses the important general anesthetics, which have made major surgery and other pain-causing procedures safe and tolerable. Drugs discussed in both these chapters appear to exert generalized inhibitory actions on most of the important aspects of nerve cell function.

Chapter 21 discusses drugs that prevent pain in another way, and have a great and all-too-often-seen liability for abuse—the narcotics. This is the first chapter in which you will realize that brain cells actually contain receptors for foreign substances such as morphine and heroin, and that stimulation of these receptors by such agents can profoundly affect the CNS through those effects.

Chapters 22 to 25 discuss drugs that are important in several ways:

- they cause valuable therapeutic effects in some common and disabling chronic CNS disorders;
- studies of their basic pharmacologic actions have provided valuable clues about the biochemical basis for emotion and behavior, both normal and abnormal;
- and, although these drugs are used mainly for their effects in the brain, they cause important and often serious peripheral side effects on many structures controlled by the autonomic nervous system.

Chapter 22 describes general CNS depressants that are used mainly to relieve anxiety and insomnia. Some have special uses, and many are misused, including alcohol, which fits into this category. Chapter 23 discusses drugs to treat psychoses—schizophrenia and other related psychiatric disorders. Chapter 24 presents drugs used for another common psychiatric disorder, depression, and drugs used to treat mania, which is often seen in patients with psychiatric depression. Chapter 25 gives an overview of several classes of drugs that act mainly in the brain's extrapyramidal system. They are used to alleviate symptoms of Parkinson's disease. These chapters will give you a good understanding of how altering a delicate balance between the actions of two or more neurotransmitters can have such a great impact on emotional and motor activity.

Chapter 26 discusses the actions and proper use of drugs used to treat seizure disorders, including epilepsy. Chapter 27 discusses drugs that act mainly as cerebral cortical stimulants. Their overall therapeutic uses are somewhat limited, compared with agents discussed in previous chapters, but they are important for some patient populations. Moreover, the effects of these drugs can become important to all of us when these substances are misused or abused.

The unit ends with Chapter 28, which discusses many of the general pharmacologic, social, and nursing issues related to substance abuse. Although a few abused drugs exert their major effects outside the CNS, the basic principles discussed in this chapter have broad application to the overall problems.

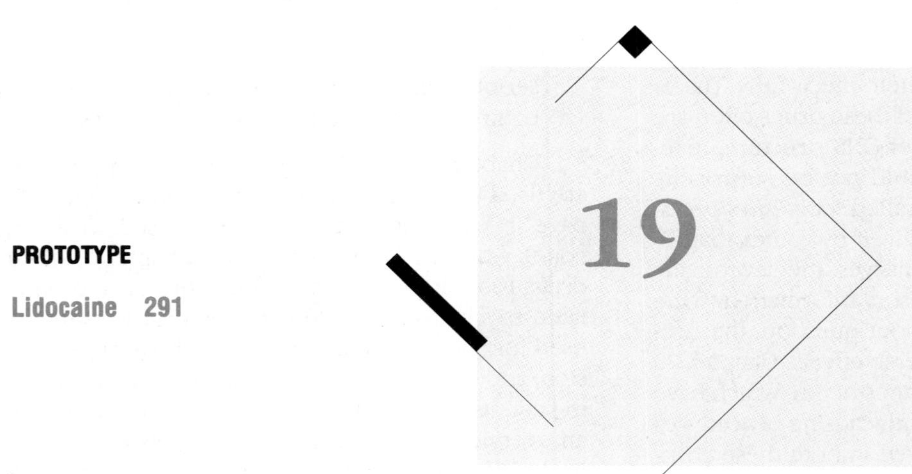

PROTOTYPE

Local Anesthetic Agents

General Characteristics of Local Anesthetics

Local anesthetic drugs are used to prevent or suppress unpleasant sensations, usually pain, in or on a discrete area of the body. They are also called *regional analgesics.* Depending on the drug that is selected, its dose, and how it is administered, local anesthetics can be used for discrete analgesic effects, such as reducing pain caused by filling dental caries, or for analgesia of larger body regions, including spinal anesthesia for abdominal surgery. Regardless of how they are used, local anesthetics suppress pain through actions on peripheral sensory nerves, without causing the sedation or unconsciousness that narcotics or general anesthetics cause. They are often used instead of general anesthetics in surgery because they alleviate pain without the risks associated with putting a patient to sleep, and usually allow quicker return to normal activity. The major local anesthetic drugs and their uses are summarized in Table 19–C.

Chemical Classes of Local Anesthetics

There are two classes of local anesthetics, based on whether the major parts of the drug molecule are linked by an *ester* or an *amide* bond. Procaine can be considered the prototype of the ester-type local anesthetics. Although it was the most effective and widely used local anesthetic years ago (and most people are familiar with its major trade name, NOVOCAIN), the drug is seldom used anymore. Lidocaine (XYLOCAINE) is the prototype amide-type local anesthetic. It can be considered the prototype of *all* local anesthetics, for reasons to be noted shortly. Major differences between lidocaine and procaine are highlighted throughout the chapter.

The chemical differences between the two classes of anesthetics do not affect how they cause their major effects, but they do determine how they are metabolized in the body, and help predict whether a patient who is at risk of a potentially fatal adverse reaction to one local anesthetic can safely receive another.

Major reference tables appear beginning on p. 301.

PROTOTYPE

Lidocaine

Absorption, Distribution, Metabolism, and Excretion

Local anesthetics are not given orally because they are inactivated by gastric acid and because that route of administration has no common use. They are injected at or near the region to be anesthetized, or are applied topically. Several of the more important parenteral administration techniques are discussed below, but regardless of which technique is used, the aim is to place the drug either near its desired site of action or at the nerve supply to that region. At the usual pH of healthy body tissues, local anesthetic molecules are in the nonionized form and can diffuse readily from their site of application to, and then into, nearby nerves. The actions of local anesthetics are dramatically reduced when they are injected into tissues with an abnormally low (acidic) pH, as discussed later.

Even though local anesthetics are rarely given systemically for analgesia, molecules of these drugs eventually reach the bloodstream. In fact, they *must* reach the bloodstream to be metabolically inactivated. How and where a local anesthetic is metabolized depends on whether it is an ester or an amide.

Metabolites of the local anesthetics are much less active than the original drug. Therefore, a local anesthetic that is metabolized quickly must be given frequently and in high doses to produce satisfactory analgesia for the time needed for most procedures. Most of the newer local anesthetics are more resistant to metabolism, which generally makes them more potent and longlasting. However, since toxicity is caused by unmetabolized local anesthetic molecules, decreased rates of inactivation increase not only potency and duration of action but also the chance of adverse effects.

Lidocaine and other amide-type local anesthetics are metabolized by hepatic drug metabolizing enzymes. Their actions are intensified and prolonged in persons with impaired hepatic function.

Pharmacologic Effects

Although local anesthetics are given mainly for their ability to suppress the activity of sensory nerves, they have the ability to suppress the activity of all excitable tissue—other nerves and smooth, cardiac, and skeletal muscle—if the concentration is sufficiently high. Effects on tissue other than sensory nerves are generally unwanted. Regardless of the tissue that is affected, local anesthetics act by diffusing through the cell membrane and then interfering with the flux of ions (mainly sodium and calcium) across cell membranes, which inhibits depolarization and the generation of an action potential. Unlike anticholinergic, neuromuscular blocking, or ganglionic blocking drugs, local anesthetics do not block specific neurotransmitter receptors.

Effects on Nerves

Sensory nerves are most sensitive to the effects of local anesthetics, and their function is inhibited first. This occurs because they have a very small diameter and lack a myelin sheath, which allows easy entry of local anesthetic into the nerve cell. Pain disappears first, followed by sensations of cold, heat, touch, and pressure. With increasing concentrations or doses, larger nerve fibers and those with myelin sheaths, including autonomic nerve fibers and motor nerves, are also inhibited. This often occurs when spinal anesthesia techniques are used. Recovery from anesthesia occurs in the reverse order: motor nerves recover first, followed by autonomic nerves and, lastly, sensory nerves. Pain is generally the last sensation to return.

Local anesthetic molecules that cross the blood–brain barrier alter the activity of nervous tissue in the central nervous system (CNS). This is almost always a manifestation of toxicity, and so will be discussed in that section.

Effects on Smooth and Cardiac Muscle

Most local anesthetics relax vascular smooth muscle and reduce blood pressure. They act on the heart to inhibit contractile force, electrical excitability, and impulse conduction. Because of this action, lidocaine and some related local anesthetics are used to control arrhythmias.

Clinical Indications and Administration

The following discussion focuses on the use of local anesthetics as regional analgesics. Lidocaine and several related drugs are also important cardiac antiarrhythmic drugs, as discussed in Chapter 30.

Lidocaine is the overall prototype and the most widely used local anesthetic because it has properties that make it almost ideal.

- It is effective whether administered topically or by any of several parenteral routes.

- It is effective even when used without supplemental drugs, such as vasoconstrictors.
- It has a prompt onset of action, yet a duration of action that is long enough to enable most surgical procedures to be completed without need for frequent drug administration.
- It has satisfactory potency—large volumes of drug need not be administered to cause desired effects.
- Its toxicity is sufficiently low that therapeutic doses are not likely to produce significant side effects or adverse responses if they are administered correctly.
- It is much less likely to cause allergic reactions than ester-type local anesthetics such as procaine.

Local Analgesia

Local anesthetics used for relief or prevention of regional pain are administered in several ways. Nursing implications that are more or less specific to particular administration routes will be noted in turn. Nursing implications that apply to most routes are presented separately.

Topical Anesthesia

Mucosal surfaces are permeable to many drugs, and they are rich in sensory nerve endings, so they can be anesthetized very easily by topical administration of anesthetic solutions, creams, ointments, or gels. Topical application is mainly used, and is usually sufficient, for procedures such as inserting a device into an orifice (for example, a urethral catheter or an endotracheal tube), or for alleviating pain caused by subsequent injections of other drugs into the tissues (for example, before injecting another local anesthetic into the gums). Local anesthetics generally are not effective when applied topically to unbroken skin, which serves as an effective barrier against diffusion of local anesthetic molecules.

NURSING IMPLICATIONS

Applying any local anesthetic to the throat may suppress the normal swallowing, cough, and gag reflexes that are necessary to prevent aspiration into the lungs of secretions, gastric juice, food, or beverages. Instruct patients who have received topical local anesthetics on the mouth or throat to avoid eating or drinking for at least 1 hour after drug administration to reduce the risk of aspiration, choking, or accidentally biting the tongue, lips, or cheek.

Topical application of a local anesthetic to mucous membranes or skin is acceptable only for short-term or infrequent use on relatively small body areas. Long-term or frequent use can cause mucosal irritation, dermatitis, or other adverse responses. Application to large areas, or to lacerated or abraded surfaces, can lead to excessive drug absorption into the bloodstream and systemic toxicity. If a local anesthetic is dispensed for self-administration, instruct patients about proper, safe use.

Infiltration Anesthesia

Subcutaneous or intradermal injection (infiltration) of local anesthetics is commonly used to suppress pain associated with suturing lacerations, making small surgical incisions, and performing some dental procedures. Infiltration anesthesia involves injecting the drug directly into the area to be anesthetized. Lidocaine solutions with concentrations between 0.5% and 1.0% (5–10 mg/mL) are generally used. To minimize the risk of toxicity the total administered dose of lidocaine should not exceed 300 mg. For small surgical wounds these doses are usually more than sufficient. However, when large areas need to be anesthetized, or when the procedure is long, such as with repair of multiple lacerations, the risk of systemic toxicity increases if more drug must be given. As discussed later, alternative administration techniques or the addition of a vasoconstrictor drug can be used to achieve the desired effect without the need for exceeding the maximum safe dose.

NURSING IMPLICATIONS

Injectable local anesthetics should be diluted and given in the smallest volume of solution capable of producing anesthesia. Very close monitoring is required with infiltration of highly vascular areas, such as the scalp or face, particularly when highly concentrated solutions or large volumes are given. Injection into these sites increases the risk of toxicity.

Regional Conduction Block Anesthesia

When the area to be anesthetized is large or difficult to reach directly, or otherwise would require many injections, a modification of infiltration anesthesia—called *regional conduction block* or *nerve block anesthesia*—can be used. The technique is also used when the site to be anesthetized is ischemic, necrotic, or encapsulated, as by a cyst. Local anesthetics will not work well when injected directly into these abnormal regions because reduced blood flow prevents the anesthetic from reaching nerves, and low tissue pH associated with necrosis prevents diffusion of drug into the nerve cell. Most techniques for regional conduction block anesthesia involve injecting the drug near the large nerve trunks or plexuses proximal to the desired surgical site. This effectively "isolates" the region from pain-sensing centers in the CNS. Solutions used for regional block analgesia are usually more concentrated (2% lidocaine) than solutions used for infiltration, and the total dose is usually lower (50 mg of lidocaine).

NURSING IMPLICATIONS

Explain the procedure for a nerve block to the patient to ensure cooperation and to reduce anxiety. An extremity receiving a nerve block must be protected: elevate it on pillows to reduce edema; position it for comfort; and pad siderails or protect the limb with pillows until sensation returns. Note the color and temperature of the affected extremity every 15 to 30 minutes.

Spinal and Epidural Anesthesia

Spinal and epidural anesthesia, which are variations of regional block techniques, are often used to suppress pain in the abdomen, pubic region, or legs. For spinal anesthesia (subarachnoid block) relatively small amounts of local anesthetic are injected beneath the dura in the spinal fluid of the lower lumbar region. The injection sites are well below the tip of the spinal cord, and the drug acts mainly on spinal nerve roots passing through this area. Spinal anesthesia not only affects sensory nerves, but is also likely to affect autonomic and motor nerves. Because autonomic fibers are affected, blood pressure may fall. The blood pressure decrease is usually slight and can be controlled without other drugs by carefully positioning the patient. Anesthesia begins in only a few minutes. It can be maintained for several hours by selecting a drug with an appropriate duration of action or by occasionally infusing small volumes of drug into the injection site.

The area of the body that is anesthetized can be controlled by adjusting the composition of the local anesthetic solution and by positioning the patient. For low spinal anesthesia the anesthetic solution is made *hyperbaric*—denser than spinal fluid—by adding glucose, and the patient can be laid flat. For higher levels of anesthesia solutions that are less dense than spinal fluid (*hypobaric*) may be used, and the patient is often placed in the Trendelenburg position. However, this practice increases the risk of drug reaching higher regions of the CNS, such as the medulla, where respiration may be affected, and of severe postanesthesia headache.

Epidural (peridural) anesthesia is achieved by injecting the drug into the epidural (extradural) space, located in the spinal canal between the bone and dura mater, usually in the lower lumbar region. The technique is often used in obstetrics, orthopedic surgery, and other surgical procedures involving the lower half of the body. One advantage of this technique is that the drug presumably has less access to the spinal cord and, therefore, to higher regions of the CNS such as the brain respiratory centers. Since the dura is not penetrated, the risk of headache is low. Caudal anesthesia is a variation of epidural anesthetic technique.

NURSING IMPLICATIONS

Headache after spinal anesthesia occurs as a result of leakage of cerebrospinal fluid from the puncture site. If headache occurs, having the patient lie flat and quietly in bed for 6 to 12 hours usually relieves discomfort. Adequate hydration also reduces the risk or severity of headache. The patient may be turned from side to side as long as the head is kept flat. Note the level of postoperative paralysis, observing for possible impairment of ventilation. Also monitor the patient for hypotension, tachycardia, and urinary retention. If the patient is unable to void within 8 to 12 hours, notify the physician for possible bladder catheterization.

Local anesthetics that contain preservatives (sulfites or compounds called *parabens*) should never be given by spinal, epidural, or similar injection techniques in or near the spinal cord. These additives may cause serious or permanent nerve damage.

Intravenous Regional Anesthesia

Intravenous (IV) regional anesthesia is the only major technique in which a local anesthetic is administered intravenously to suppress pain. It is used to anesthetize an entire arm or, less commonly, a leg. Blood flow to the extremity is occluded with a tourniquet, and a dilute solution of local anesthetic is injected. Some of the injected drug diffuses out of the vasculature and eventually reaches nerves. Analgesia lasts as long as the tourniquet remains in place. Since blood flow is stopped and the limb becomes ischemic, the duration of the procedure must be kept shorter than 30 to 60 minutes to avoid permanent tissue damage or ischemic pain after the procedure. The maximum recommended lidocaine dose for IV regional analgesia is 300 mg.

NURSING IMPLICATIONS

If tourniquet pressure is reduced too quickly, large and possibly toxic amounts of drug can be released into the systemic circulation. Major nursing responsibilities include close and frequent assessment for side effects and adverse responses, and assessment of limb color, temperature, and function.

Use of Vasoconstrictors in Local Anesthetics

Sympathomimetic vasoconstrictors are often added to local anesthetic solutions, particularly those that are used for infiltration or nerve block anesthesia. Epinephrine, usually at concentrations of 1:100,000 or 1:200,000 (0.01 and 0.005 mg/mL, respectively), is used most often. Vasoconstrictors are added because of their ability to act as a "chemical tourniquet," reducing blood flow to the injection site. This slows the rate of local anesthetic absorption into the bloodstream, which reduces the risk of toxicity by allowing metabolism to keep pace with rates of absorption. Vasoconstrictors also shorten the onset of local anesthetic action, increase anesthetic depth (that is, the apparent potency of the local anesthetic), and prolong anesthetic action by keeping the anesthetic localized in the vicinity of the desired nerves rather than being "washed away" by the blood. Including a vasoconstrictor may allow a single injection of a low concentration of local anesthetic to suffice, whereas repeated injections of higher anesthetic concentrations might be needed if the vasoconstrictor were not used.

NURSING IMPLICATIONS

The general contraindications and precautions concerning the use of vasoconstrictors (history of angina, arrhythmias, or ischemic heart disease; hypertension) are noted in Chapter 14. However, special precautions apply for their use in local anesthetics. Vasoconstrictors should not be used in local anesthetics given to highly vascularized areas of skin or body that have a single path for blood supply, including the fingers and toes, the ear lobes, and the penis. Administering a local anesthetic containing a vasoconstrictor to these sites may reduce blood flow enough to cause tissue ischemia and necrosis. The vasoconstrictive action is also potentially damaging to inflamed or infected tissue. Children, geriatric patients, and debilitated individuals are more sensitive to vasoconstrictors (and to local anesthetics), so doses usually need to be reduced for these persons.

General Nursing Implications for the Administration of Local Anesthetics

The major alternative to local anesthesia, general anesthesia, renders the patient unconscious and unaware of the procedure being performed, thereby alleviating much emotional stress. Since the patient receiving a local anesthetic may be sedated but awake, it is essential for the nurse to help allay fear and anxiety before and during the procedure.

Always double-check the local anesthetic container. Although they are marked and usually color-coded to indicate the concentration and ingredients, it is easy to select the wrong formulation, especially during emergencies. Check for proper concentration; the presence of preservatives, which should not be used for spinal anesthesia or administered to persons with prior allergic reactions to the preservative; and the presence of a vasoconstrictor, which could have other contraindications. Do not use solutions that are outdated, or are not clear, colorless, and precipitate-free. Never inject solutions intended for topical application. Regardless of the drug, formulation or route of administration, always record the amount of drug given (concentration and volume) and the time of administration, so that maximum safe doses are not exceeded.

Unless a local anesthetic is injected into a mucosal surface that has just been anesthetized with a topical anesthetic, the initial injection will cause minor pain (likened to a mild bee sting) until its effects develop (usually a few seconds). Inform the patient that this will occur.

Until full sensory function has returned, take precautions to prevent accidental trauma to vulnerable body regions that have been anesthetized (especially oral tissues and extremities). Affected extremities should be padded and elevated as needed. If the patient has received a local anesthetic that can affect blood pressure or lower extremity function, such as spinal anesthesia or a lower extremity nerve block, confine the patient to bed, with raised siderails, until full sensation has returned and vital signs have normalized. Assisted ambulation is required initially.

To reduce contact with the drug and the risk of allergic responses, always wear gloves when administering local anesthetics by any route.

Side Effects, Adverse Reactions, and Contraindications

The major side effects of local anesthetics, summarized in Table 19–S, involve the central nervous and cardiovascular systems. Side effects are generally slight when the drugs are used as recommended.

Common CNS side effects can be quite variable, ranging from drowsiness to excitement or agitation. Sedation is most common with low doses of lidocaine. Higher doses of lidocaine, and most doses of virtually any other local anesthetic, cause signs of central stimulation, which should be considered as a warning of impending toxicity. Impaired peripheral sensory and motor function are expected consequences of local anesthetic administration. Longlasting regional paresthesias and paralysis, which may be quite disturbing, can occur. Blockade of autonomic (sympathetic) nerves to the lower extremities can cause postural hypotension.

NURSING IMPLICATIONS

Since CNS changes may reflect toxicity, discontinue further administration of the anesthetic, at least temporarily, and review the cumulative dose administered. Temporary discontinuation of administration, combined with reassurance and orientation, usually alleviates the CNS changes, whether caused by the drug or the stress of the procedure. Anticipate that the patient will have some persistent suppression of sensory, motor, or autonomic nerve function after receiving a local anesthetic. Report prolonged sensory impairment to the physician at once. Most of the related general nursing implications, and those associated with particular administration routes, were noted earlier. To guard against orthostatic hypotension following spinal or lower-extremity nerve block anesthesia, instruct the patient to sit and stand slowly, and to lie down or assume a seated, head-low position at once if dizziness occurs. Initial assistance with ambulation is essential. Nursing implications for the use of lidocaine as an antiarrhythmic are discussed in Chapter 30.

Allergic Reactions

The only major contraindication to the use of a local anesthetic is a history of allergic reactions to that agent, to a local anesthetic that belongs to the same chemical class, or to a preservative in the anesthetic. Allergic reactions occur in about 1% of patients receiving local anesthetics. They are more commonly caused by ester-type local anesthetics such as procaine, and are rare with amides such as lidocaine. There is little or no cross-reactivity between the two major classes of local anesthetics: amide-types usually will not trigger an allergic reaction in a patient who is allergic to an ester, for example. Many allergic reactions are due to the local anesthetic drug or its metabolites, but some may be triggered by paraben, sulfite, or bisulfite preservatives, which may be included to prolong the drug's shelf life.

Like other true allergies, these reactions are immunologic (antigen–antibody) responses that activate mast cells and release a host of potent vasodilator and bronchoconstrictor substances such as histamine. Reactions usually occur within 1 to 2 minutes after the drug is administered, but some serious responses have occurred several hours later. Signs and symptoms can range from slight wheezing or "tightness of the chest" to severe or potentially fatal bronchoconstriction, hypotension, and other classic signs of anaphylaxis. Serious reactions are most likely to occur when local anesthetics are injected. But, as with any drug-induced allergy, even minute amounts of local anesthetic administered topically, as on mucous membranes, can cause a serious response.

Treatment is based on the severity of the response. The antihistamine diphenhydramine can be given orally for *mild* reactions, particularly those limited to the skin, or intramuscularly for more serious reactions. The usual oral or IM dose is 50 mg. However, diphenhydramine will not reverse bronchoconstriction or hypotension, and should not be relied on if symptoms are life-threatening. In this instance, an IV line should be established and oxygen administered by mask. Epinephrine (50–500 μg, depending on the severity of symptoms, given intravenously) should be administered at once. Cardiopulmonary resuscitation may be needed. Corticosteroids or antihistamines can be used adjunctively.

Although vasoconstrictors added to local anesthetic solutions will reduce the risk of toxicity, they will *not* reduce the risk or severity of an allergic reaction.

NURSING IMPLICATIONS

Many individuals have received a local anesthetic for dental work or repair of a skin laceration, and recall an "adverse reaction." It may have been drug-induced or may simply have been a stressful response to the situation for which the drug was given. Moreover, many people who receive these drugs refer to every local anesthetic as "novocain," despite the fact that NOVOCAIN (procaine) is seldom used. (Unfortunately, many health-care professionals call these drugs novocain when speaking with the patient or family, which often perpetuates the misinformation.) Unless the response and the cause are clearly and correctly documented in the medication history, and the information is available to you, this information is unreliable. Nevertheless, such reports must be charted and reported to the physician before administering more local anesthetic. Baseline vital signs must be recorded for comparison with changes caused by the local anesthetic, and emergency drugs and life-support systems must be readily available. Since ester-type local anesthetics are usually the cause of allergic responses, an amide should be used unless it is known with certainty that an amide was the offending drug.

◆ Use During Pregnancy and Lactation

Epidural or caudal anesthesia is commonly used during the late stages of labor. In addition to monitoring the mother, check fetal heart sounds every 5 to 15 minutes. Adverse effects such as slowed labor or the need for forceps delivery can occur. The safe use of local anesthetics during pregnancy, other than during labor, has not been established.

◆ Use in Children

Reduced doses of parenteral local anesthetics are generally recommended for children.

◆ Use in the Elderly

Prolonged effects from epidural anesthesia may occur in the elderly because of a narrowed intervertebral opening, which impairs drug distribution. Elderly individuals often have impaired cardiovascular reflexes, and so are at greater risk of postural hypotension following anesthesia of the lower body. Reduced hepatic function, also common in the elderly, may prolong the action of lidocaine and related amides. There is also a greater risk of CNS side effects, including excitement or disorientation, following the use of any local anesthetic. Age-associated cardiovascular diseases also increase the risk of adverse effects of vasoconstrictors that might be administered with a local anesthetic. Overall, close and frequent monitoring is essential when local anesthetics are used in elderly patients.

Interactions with Other Drugs

Since lidocaine and other amides are detoxified by hepatic metabolism, drugs that inhibit the liver's enzymes can increase the risk of excessive or prolonged anesthetic effects. The interactants most often cited (Table 19–I) are propranolol, the prototype β-blocker, and cimetidine, the prototype histamine H_2 receptor blocker. In practice, however, few significant drug interactions occur when local anesthetics are given for short-term effects by one of the common administration techniques used for regional anesthesia, especially if maximum recommended dosages are not exceeded. The risks of interactions are reduced even more if the solution contains a vasoconstrictor. That is because the vasoconstrictor delays entry of the anesthetic into the bloodstream, which is necessary for interactions to occur. (Of course, vasoconstrictors such as epinephrine can participate in their own interactions; see Table 14–I, p 222.) The risk of interactions increases when lidocaine is used as an antiarrhythmic drug; this very different use is discussed in Chapter 30.

Overdose and Toxicity

There are three major causes for overdose: accidental use of a solution that is too concentrated for the intended use; careless repeated administration, as may occur during a lengthy procedure or for treatment of multiple lacerations; and accidental IV injection. In any case, toxicity occurs when the ability of the liver to metabolize the drug cannot keep pace with drug entry into the bloodstream. The presence of a vasoconstrictor in a local anesthetic will reduce systemic absorption and, therefore, the risk of toxicity if proper precautions and techniques are used.

Signs and Symptoms

As with side effects, local anesthetic toxicity affects mainly the central nervous and cardiovascular systems. The early effects on the CNS depend on the particular anesthetic used. Lidocaine and mepivacaine are unique because they initially cause sedation or drowsiness and may relax the patient as blood levels rise. Virtually all other local anesthetics tend to cause signs of CNS stimulation (anxiety, uneasiness, fear, talkativeness) without prior sedation. All local anesthetics cause obvious signs of CNS stimulation as blood levels reach a toxic range. The patient may experience muscle twitching, followed soon by a massive seizure (status epilepticus) that must be treated pharmacologically to prevent death. Cardiovascular effects mainly reflect actions of local anesthetics on blood vessels and the heart. These drugs cause hypotension by relaxing vascular smooth muscle and by directly depressing heart rate, automaticity, and contractile force. Cardiovascular collapse or cardiac arrest can occur. If the local anesthetic preparation responsible for toxicity contains a vasoconstrictor, blood pressure and heart rate may not fall much, or initial hypertension may occur, followed by hypotension.

Treatment

Once the patient develops signs and symptoms that could reflect local anesthetic toxicity, the first measure is to discontinue further anesthetic administration and begin frequent, careful monitoring of vital signs. The patient should then be placed in the Trendelenburg position. This should alleviate subjective responses if the cause of the symptoms is stress associated with the procedure. In cases of true toxicity, place the patient in a supine position, give oxygen, and establish an IV line. Monitor blood pressure closely because it may change suddenly and dramatically. Monitor heart rate and rhythm with an electrocardiogram if possible. Seizures, the most common and dangerous consequence of local anesthetic toxicity, are best managed by IV administration of diazepam (VALIUM; 5–10 mg). If the cause of toxicity was a vasoconstrictor-free local anesthetic, careful administration of epinephrine or another vasopressor agent may be indicated. Cardiopulmonary resuscitation is used as needed.

NURSING IMPLICATIONS

It is relatively easy to avoid the major causes of local anesthetic overdose: Recheck the label to ensure that the proper preparation is used; keep careful records of the amount and strength of local anesthetic that is given, and the times it is administered; and use proper injection technique to avoid accidental IV administration. Psychologic responses to the stress of a dental or medical procedure can mimic some signs of local anesthetic toxicity, and it may be difficult to distinguish between the causes. Since anesthetic blood levels are seldom measured routinely, it is essential to assess the patient carefully. Emergency drugs and devices for cardiopulmonary support and monitoring must always be at hand when local anesthetics are given parenterally.

Related Amides

Bupivacaine, Etidocaine, Mepivacaine, and Prilocaine

These injectable drugs differ from lidocaine mainly in terms of potency and duration of action. They are available with or without added vasoconstrictor. Usual dosages are listed in Table 19–C.

Bupivacaine (MARCAINE) is about four times as potent as lidocaine, and has a longer duration of action—up to about 12 hours when the epinephrine-containing solution is used. Bupivacaine's prolonged action may make it more suitable than the prototype for long procedures. One of its uses is in obstetrics, in which it seems to have a lower incidence of adverse effects on the newborn. However, this drug is contraindicated for administration by paracervical block techniques in obstetrics, and the strongest bupivacaine solution, 0.75%, should not be used by any route in obstetrics. In each of these cases there have been reports of deaths, owing to cardiac arrest that could not be managed with resuscitation procedures that otherwise would have been effective. Because of similar dangers, bupivacaine should not be used for IV regional block techniques in any patient.

Etidocaine (DURANEST), also available with or without added epinephrine, is used mainly for nerve block, lumbar peridural, or caudal anesthesia techniques. It is somewhat less potent than lidocaine, but has a usual duration of action that is about 50% longer.

Mepivacaine (CARBOCAINE) formulations for medical (nondental) use contain no vasoconstrictor. The drug is administered by infiltration or by several nerve block procedures. Mepivacaine is about twice as potent as vasoconstrictor-free lidocaine, but its duration of action is almost identical to that of the prototype. The dental formulation of mepivacaine contains levonordefrin, a sympathomimetic vasoconstrictor. Mepivacaine is noteworthy because it crosses the placental barrier quite well, and so if it is given to pregnant women or used for obstetrics, the fetus or newborn should be monitored closely for potential bradycardia. The drug should also be used cautiously, at reduced dosages, in persons with renal dysfunction.

Prilocaine (CITANEST) is used almost exclusively for dental procedures.

Ester-Type Local Anesthetic

PROCAINE

Procaine (NOVOCAIN) can be considered the prototype of the ester-class of local anesthetics. The drug has been available since the early 1900s, and before the development of lidocaine it was the most widely used local anesthetic. What follows is a brief summary of its major properties. By comparing them with the properties that make lidocaine almost ideal (pp 291–292) you should see why procaine is no longer a preferred anesthetic.

Procaine, given alone, is not very potent. It has a slow onset of action, and its effects rarely last more than 30 minutes because it is metabolized rapidly in the bloodstream by plasma esterases. Unless procaine is injected with a vasoconstrictor to prolong and intensify its actions, it is difficult to achieve satisfactory analgesia, and the drug is virtually ineffective when used topically on the skin or mucous membranes. Compared with lidocaine and other amides, procaine and the related ester anesthetics also trigger allergic reactions more often. However, as noted above, many adverse reactions that patients attribute to novocain may not have been caused by procaine, or may not have been true allergic reactions at all.

Procaine has one other important and relatively unique characteristic that affects its use. It involves a relatively small number of patients who, because of a genetic deficiency of plasma esterases, do not metabolize procaine or other ester-type local anesthetics well. Because metabolism is responsible for "detoxifying" these anesthetics, such patients can experience prolonged or excessive effects of the drug unless dosages are reduced. In many cases, it is impossible to identify the esterase-deficient patients before the drug is given, so careful monitoring for adverse effects is required. However, if this genetic alteration is known, amide-type local anesthetics should be used instead.

Procaine does not participate in common and clinically significant drug interactions that are likely to occur outside the operating room setting. It and the neuromuscular blocker succinylcholine do depend on the same enzymes for metabolic inactivation, and so can compete with one another. When these drugs are administered within a short time of one another (for example, succinylcholine is given for tracheal intubation and procaine is used for spinal anesthesia), the anesthetic can prolong the ventilatory depression or apnea caused by the paralyzing agent. Monitoring for this potential interaction, and being prepared to deal with it (with ventilatory support), is all that is usually necessary.

Other Esters

Benzocaine, Chloroprocaine, Propoxycaine, and Tetracaine

Benzocaine (AMERICAINE, others) is a topical anesthetic found mainly in over-the-counter (OTC) products used to alleviate minor skin or mucous membrane discomfort (sunburn, insect bites, skin rashes, sore throats, teething pain, and so on). The minimum effective concentration is around 0.5%, although some products contain less. Although benzocaine is a comparatively weak local anesthetic, even in comparison with procaine, it has the potential to cause adverse effects. Because it is available without prescription, products containing this drug tend to be misused, especially by application to large body areas or to broken skin. The consequences of this misuse can range from mild allergic reactions, such as dermatitis, to more severe localized or systemic responses in persons who are unusually sensitive to the drug. A prescription product containing benzocaine plus a lubricant is used to anesthetize mucous membranes to facilitate insertion of catheters, nasal airways, and instruments (eg, laryngoscopes).

Chloroprocaine (NESACAINE) is an injectable drug used for various infiltration and nerve block procedures. It is metabolized faster than procaine, and so has a shorter duration of action. Because of this, some clinicians prefer it for obstetric use, since its effects on the mother and newborn usually are quite brief. The drug is not available with an added vasoconstrictor. Chloroprocaine contains a preservative, which contraindicates its use for caudal or epidural block procedures. If these anesthetic techniques are used, the preservative-free formulation (NESACAINE-MPF) must be used.

Propoxycaine is a parenteral agent used only in dental practice. It is marketed as RAVOCAINE, a product that also contains procaine and a vasoconstrictor.

Tetracaine (PONTOCAINE) is about five to 10 times as potent as procaine. Parenteral formulations of the drug are used only for spinal anesthesia. They are preservative- and vasoconstrictor-free, and some are available premixed with dextrose to increase their density, which, along with positioning of the patient, helps the anesthesiologist or anesthetist adjust the level of anesthesia. The drug is also available as a powder that can be dissolved in dextrose solution, water, or even the patient's own spinal fluid, before injection. Topical formulations are available, by prescription or OTC, for anesthetizing the skin or mucous membranes.

Miscellaneous Local Anesthetics

Several other drugs are occasionally used for local anesthesia, but they are placed in this section because they have either special actions or uses.

Cocaine

Cocaine, widely known as a CNS stimulant and drug of abuse (see Chapter 27), was actually the first local anesthetic to be used frequently in medical practice. The drug is still used for topical anesthesia of mucous membranes of the eye, nasopharynx, and the tracheobronchial tree. Cocaine is noteworthy for several reasons in addition to its popularity as an abused substance. As noted in Chapter 14, cocaine has sympathomimetic activity, and it is the only local anesthetic with this property. One consequence of this action is vasoconstriction, and so cocaine can control both pain and bleeding from cut mucosal surfaces. It can also contribute to elevations of blood pressure if large amounts are used. Cocaine should never be administered with another vasoconstrictor, regardless of the use or administration route. The sympathomimetic actions have other potential consequences. When applied to the eye, cocaine's vasoconstrictor action can dry and potentially damage the cornea, so the eye must be kept adequately irrigated. It also dilates the pupil, and so should not be administered to persons with narrow-angle glaucoma.

Diphenhydramine

Diphenhydramine (BENADRYL), the prototype antihistamine (Chapter 51) is an unusual drug because it exerts many pharmacologic effects and has approved uses for managing allergies and parkinsonism, as well as being a sleep aid. The drug also has clinically useful local anesthetic activity when it is infiltrated into the skin. Diphenhydramine is not used routinely as a local anesthetic, nor is it approved for this purpose, but the drug does have a unique therapeutic role. It is neither an amide nor an ester, and so will not cross-react with either of those agents. Thus, diphenhydramine (as a 1% injectable solution) may be used when infiltration analgesia is indicated but the patient reports a prior adverse response to one of the more traditional local anesthetics and the precise cause or nature of the reaction cannot be identified.

Butamben, Dibucaine, Pramoxine, and Dyclonine

Butamben (BUTESIN), dibucaine (NUPERCAINAL), or pramoxine (TRONOTHANE, others) are found in several OTC products used to anesthetize the skin or mucous membranes (e.g., of the anus). Dyclonine (DYCLONE) is a prescription product for anesthetizing mucous membranes of the oropharynx in preparation for endoscopy. Precautions noted above for other topical local anesthetics apply also to these drugs.

Other Techniques for Producing Local Anesthesia

Both physical and pharmacologic means can be used to relieve localized pain. Ice packs or cold compresses can be applied to a traumatized region to relieve pain. Another way to produce brief topical local anesthesia is to apply ethyl chloride. It is a volatile (and flammable) liquid that is sprayed on intact skin; it quickly evaporates and in doing so cools the area and temporarily obscures pain. Ethyl chloride is commonly used to treat muscle sprains and other athletic injuries.

More-or-less permanent local analgesia can be produced for patients with intractable pain by injecting **neurolytic** agents such as phenol or 50% solutions of ethyl alcohol. These treatments permanently destroy the nerves; they are extremely toxic and should be administered with great care.

SUMMARY OF NURSING IMPLICATIONS

◆ Assessment

Before anesthetic administration:

Review the patient's history for possible allergic or other untoward reactions to local anesthetics.

Assess the patient's emotional response to the forthcoming procedure, with the understanding that anxiety reactions may mimic signs of drug toxicity.

Determine the patient's understanding of the intended procedure.

Establish baseline vital signs as a reference for changes following drug administration; abnormalities may necessitate a change in anesthetic agent (eg, no vasoconstrictors if the patient is hypertensive).

After anesthetic administration:

Check gag reflexes, cough effectiveness, and swallowing ability (after local anesthetic administration to throat or mouth).

Determine effects and effectiveness of anesthesia: loss of sensation; level of paralysis (with spinal anesthesia); color and temperature of anesthetized limb.

Assess need for pain medication following return of sensations.

◆ Nursing Diagnoses

Knowledge deficit related to limited understanding of operative procedure and anesthetic administration.

Anxiety related to anticipated surgical and anesthesia experience.

High risk for injury related to sensory deficit following local anesthesia.

Pain related to procedure, reversal of anesthesia, or spinal headache.

Altered urinary elimination related to spinal anesthesia: retention.

Ineffective breathing pattern related to impaired ventilatory function following spinal anesthesia.

High risk for impaired skin integrity related to prolonged local anesthetic effects, constrained physical activity.

High risk for aspiration related to anesthesia of throat or mouth.

◆ Planning/Implementation

Have monitoring and life-support systems and emergency drugs available before injecting a local anesthetic.

Dilute anesthetic as ordered.

Record amount and time given to anticipate desired versus adverse effects.

Use proper swabs, syringes, and gloves when administering anesthetics to prevent skin irritation or other adverse effects.

Monitor vital signs for altered blood pressure, pulse, and respiratory depression.

Monitor closely patients receiving infiltration of anesthetics in highly vascularized areas for increased risk of side effects, toxicity.

Reassure patient that loss of sensation or movement is temporary and normal.

Raise bed rails until anesthetic effects are completely reversed.

Protect anesthetized area from injury; position for comfort and alignment.

Elevate limb following nerve block to reduce edema; note color and temperature of extremity.

Following spinal anesthesia have patient lie flat for 6 to 12 hours and ensure adequate hydration to minimize incidence of spinal headache.

Note time when sensation and mobility return; anticipate that prolonged effects will be more likely in elderly patients.

Assist with initial ambulation.

◆ Patient and Family Teaching

Teach the patient/family:

To avoid eating or drinking for at least 1 hour after receiving an anesthetic on the throat or mouth to reduce the risk of aspiration, choking, or accidental trauma to oral tissues.

Proper administration of topical local anesthetics: frequency, amount, and the need to avoid excessive or liberal application or use on cut tissues.

About sensation and movement changes following local anesthetic use.

To rest following use of a long-acting anesthetic to prevent injury to operative area.

About possible pain and discomfort when local anesthetic effect disappears.

◆ Evaluation

The patient/family will:

Regain sensory and motor function following local anesthetic use.

Experience no adverse effects from the anesthetic or its ingredients (CNS reactions, tissue trauma, headache, ventilatory impairment, allergy).

Demonstrate an ability to follow postanesthesia regimen (eg, protection of operative site, avoidance of food or drink as directed).

Verbalize a reduction in anxiety after procedure.

Annotated Bibliography

Berde CB. Pediatric postoperative pain management. *Pediatr Clin North Am* 1989;36(4):921–940. *In contrast with the article by Selbst and Henretig (below), this paper reviews effective methods to relieve pain in children following surgery.*

Brownridge P. Treatment options for the relief of pain during childbirth. *Drugs* 1991;41(1):69–80. *Valuable not only for its discussion of the actions and uses of local anesthetics in childbirth, but also for its consideration of personal and cultural factors that contribute to a woman's desire or reluctance to receive these drugs.*

Gaukroger PB. Paediatric analgesia. Which drug? Which dose? *Drugs* 1991;41(1):52–59. *A short but balanced discussion of all the pharmacologic options that should be considered for providing pain relief in children.*

Glazer S, Portenoy RK. Systemic local anesthetics in pain control. *J Pain Symptom Manage* 1991;6(1):30–39. *Reviews the pharmacology of local anesthetics and identifies the potential efficacy of some of these drugs when given by systemic routes, including oral.*

Kaye KW. Surgery using local anesthesia in the elderly. *Clin Geriatr Med* 1990;6(1):85–99. *An excellent discussion of the advantages of local anesthesia over general anesthesia for surgery in the elderly.*

Selbst SM, Henretig FM. The treatment of pain in the emergency department. *Pediatr Clin North Am* 1989;36(4):965–978. *Unique because this article addresses not only pharmacologic interventions to alleviate pain (including local anesthetics and other drugs), but also "tricks" to help alleviate fear and pain in pediatric patients. The article concludes with American Academy of Pediatrics guidelines for outpatient sedation.*

Synder BA. Regional anesthesia in the pediatric patient. *Nurse Anesth* 1990;1(1):16–20. *A succinct but valuable review of how regional analgesia is affected by unique physiologic and pharmacokinetic features of the pediatric population, and why regional analgesia should be considered more often as a valuable technique for children.*

Table 19–C | Clinical Uses and Administration of Major Local Anesthetics

AGENT	MAJOR ROUTES OF ADMINISTRATION	MAXIMUM RECOMMENDED DOSES*
PROTOTYPE AMIDE (AND OVERALL PROTOTYPE)		
Lidocaine		
(XYLOCAINE)	Topical anesthesia	0.5%–5% for skin, 2%–10% for mucous membranes
	Regional parenteral anesthesia	Infiltration: 300 mg Nerve block: 30–300 mg Spinal: 100 mg
	Control of cardiac arrhythmias	See Chapter 30
RELATED AMIDES		
Bupivacaine		
(eg, MARCAINE)	Infiltration, nerve block, epidural, or spinal anesthesia	175 mg without epinephrine; 225 mg with epinephrine
Etidocaine		
(DURANEST)	Infiltration or nerve block anesthesia	300 mg without epinephrine; 400 mg with epinephrine
Mepivacaine		
(CARBOCAINE)	Infiltration or nerve block anesthesia	400 mg
Prilocaine		
(CITANEST)	Infiltration or nerve block anesthesia	600 mg
PROTOTYPE ESTER		
Procaine		
(NOVOCAIN)	Infiltration, nerve block, or spinal anesthesia	1 g (with or without vasoconstrictor, as permitted by administration route)
RELATED ESTERS		
Benzocaine		
(AMERICAINE, others)	Topical anesthesia	0.5%–20%
Chloroprocaine		
(NESACAINE)	Infiltration, epidural, nerve block, or IV regional anesthesia	800 mg without epinephrine; 1 g with epinephrine
Tetracaine		
(PONTOCAINE)	Topical (mucous membranes of nose, throat) anesthesia	2%
	Spinal anesthesia	15 mg

*Maximum doses vary according to the patient's age and health, and the route of administration. Doses listed without a vasoconstrictor indicate that the manufacturer does not supply or recommend medical use of the drug with a vasoconstrictor.

Table 19–S **Major Side Effects of and Contraindications for Local Anesthetic Drugs**

BODY SYSTEM/ Side Effect	CONTRAINDICATION/ PRECAUTION	COMMENTS AND NURSING IMPLICATIONS
Ganglionic Blockers		
CENTRAL NERVOUS SYSTEM Dose-dependent stimulation: restlessness, anxiety	Use cautiously in patients with seizure history	Attempt to determine whether these are psychologic responses or are actually early signs of possible toxicity; record doses of and times at which local anesthetics are given
Drowsiness, sedation		Primarily occurs with therapeutic doses of mepivacaine
RESPIRATORY Wheezing, dyspnea, bronchospasm	Prior allergic reaction to any local anesthetic of same chemical class	Usually indicates allergic reaction; always obtain and chart history that is as complete as possible (cause, nature of response, date) before local anesthetic administration; consider any respiratory difficulty as sign of potential anaphylaxis and be prepared to treat as such
CARDIOVASCULAR Hypotension	Hypotension, shock	Occurs with high or toxic doses given by any route (due to direct vasodilator effects), or usual doses given for spinal anesthesia (due to altered sympathetic nerve activity); assist with early ambulation, advise patient to sit or lie down immediately if dizziness occurs; if hypotension is sudden or severe, anticipate and be prepared to treat anaphylaxis
Bradycardia	Bradycardia	Consider as an indication of potential toxicity

Table 19–I **Interactions Between Local Anesthetics and Other Agents***

AGENT	RESULT OF INTERACTION	COMMENTS AND NURSING IMPLICATIONS
Interactions Involving Lidocaine,† Other Amides		
β-Adrenergic blockers (esp. propranolol; Chapter 15)	Increased, prolonged local anesthetic effects owing to reduced local anesthetic metabolism	Assess for evidence of excessive anesthetic effects (eg, CNS stimulation, cardiac or BP depression); keep track of local anesthetic doses to ensure maximum recommended doses are not exceeded
Cimetidine (Chapter 40)	As for β-blockers, above	As for β-blockers, above; much less likely to occur with cimetidine alternatives
Interaction Involving Procaine (Other Ester-type Local Anesthetics?)		
Succinylcholine (Chapter 17)	Prolongation or return of ventilatory depression	Monitor accordingly

*See Table 14–I, pp 222–223, for interactions that may involve vasoconstrictors that can be included in local anesthetic solutions.
†Interactions are more common and clinically significant when lidocaine is used as an antiarrhythmic drug; see Chapter 30.

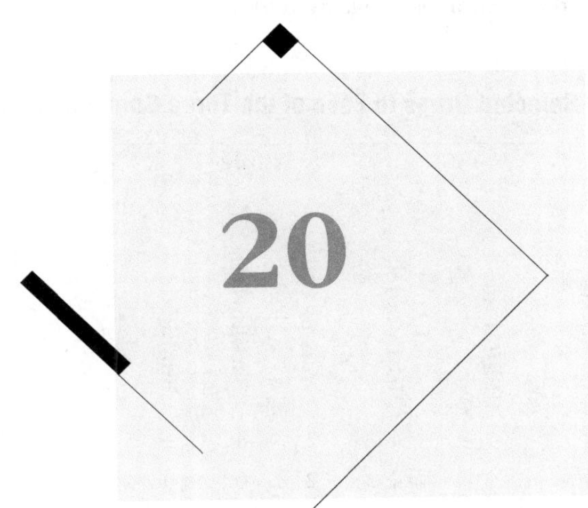

PROTOTYPE

General Anesthetic Agents

Before 1845, surgery was uncommon because of the lack of satisfactory methods for producing a state of general anesthesia. In 1845 and 1846, the analgesic effect of nitrous oxide and the anesthetic properties of both chloroform and diethyl ether were demonstrated. This led to the rapid introduction of general anesthesia into medicine, and provided the first major group of drugs to be administered by inhalation. In 1929, cyclopropane was introduced as a fourth inhalation agent. Of these four drugs, only nitrous oxide is still in clinical use today. Ether and cyclopropane are explosive, and chloroform is toxic to the liver.

The ongoing search for an inhalation anesthetic that was neither explosive nor highly toxic led to the development in 1956 of halothane (FLUOTHANE). More recently, two halogenated ethers have been introduced: enflurane (ETHRANE) and isoflurane (FORANE).

Although the toxicity of inhalation anesthetics has been greatly reduced, injectable drugs remain widely used as anesthetic supplements.

- *Muscle relaxants* allow lighter levels of general anesthesia and reduce the cardiovascular depression that can occur with high doses of inhalation agents that otherwise would be needed;
- anesthetic *narcotics* provide intense degrees of intraoperative analgesia (pain prevention);
- *benzodiazepines* serve as alternative agents for inducing anesthesia;
- *ketamine* is useful for producing amnesia and analgesia in specialized situations; and
- other injectable drugs, such as *etomidate* and *propofol,* have special properties and uses of their own.

In summary, the years since 1845 have seen a change from deep ether anesthesia to techniques using a combination of nonexplosive inhalation anesthetics and parenterally administered drugs. The general anesthetic agents used in modern clinical practice are summarized in Table 20–C.

Techniques for General Anesthesia

General anesthesia can be defined as a state of absence of awareness that consists of three components:

1. Amnesia with unconsciousness
2. Analgesia
3. Muscle relaxation

For the unconscious or anesthetized patient, analgesia is not simply a lack of pain sensation. It is defined

Major reference tables appear beginning on p. 319.

Table 20–1 The Contribution of Selected Drugs to Each of the Three Components of the State of General Anesthesia

	Halothane	Enflurane	Isoflurane	Nitrous Oxide	Barbiturates	Etomidate	Propofol	Opiates	Ketamine	Benzodiazepines	Neuromuscular Blockers
Amnesia and unconsciousness	4	4	4	2	4	4	4	1–2	4	2–3	0
Analgesia	4	4	4	2	0	0	0–1	3–4	3	0	0
Muscle relaxation	1–2	2–3	2–3	0	0	0	0	0	0	0	4

The numbers 0 to 4 refer to the relative intensity of effect induced by each agent, with 0 indicating no effect and 4 the greatest effect.
Source: From Julien RM. *Understanding Anesthesia.* Reading, MA: Addison-Wesley, 1984: 152. Reprinted with permission.

as autonomic nervous system (ANS) stability, and it is assessed by continuous monitoring of autonomic responses such as blood pressure, heart rate, pupillary dilation, and sweating. The muscle relaxation that occurs during general anesthesia is a depression of neuromuscular transmission and a loss of skeletal muscle tone that ultimately leads to muscle paralysis, providing relaxation sufficient for endotracheal intubation and intrathoracic or intraabdominal surgery. Table 20–1 outlines the relative contribution of various drugs used during general anesthesia to the three desired goals. A general anesthetic *technique* combines several drugs to produce conditions adequate for either the induction or the maintenance of general anesthesia, while enabling the use of relatively low doses of each agent.

The anesthetic technique begins with anesthesia induction, which is the process of taking a patient from the awake state to one in which surgery can be started. Ultra–short-acting *barbiturates* such as thiopental are the induction agents most widely used to provide amnesia and unconsciousness, but several alternatives can be used instead. These drugs are discussed more on pages 350 to 355.

Short-acting *narcotics* such as fentanyl cause analgesia for both induction and for the surgical procedure. Using these narcotics requires a reduction in the total dose of other induction agents, but they provide a degree of autonomic stability that is needed to conduct stressful procedures, such as tracheal intubation. Giving a narcotic for induction is particularly useful for patients with cardiac disease, in whom it is necessary to maintain stable cardiac output and blood pressure.

If muscle relaxation is desired during induction (eg, for tracheal intubation) it can be achieved by giving any of the *neuromuscular blockers* that are discussed in Chapter 17.

Following induction, the state of general anesthesia is maintained with combinations of the agents listed in Table 20–1. The choice of agent depends on physician preference, the patient's general health, patient position, and surgical requirements that might necessitate controlled ventilation or muscle relaxation. The most widely used techniques for maintaining general anesthesia use *inhalation anesthesia,* with the patient breathing a mixture of oxygen, nitrous oxide, and one of the three volatile anesthetic liquids (isoflurane, enflurane, or halothane). A patient's inability to tolerate the cardiovascular depression that can be produced by a volatile anesthetic may necessitate a reduction in its dosage and an increase in the dosage of parenterally administered supplements. It is important to note that rapid intravenous (IV) induction (usually with thiopental), together with extensive use of IV narcotics, has made traditional assessment of anesthetic depth (pupil diameter, respiratory pattern, and so on) unreliable and obsolete (despite the mention of such assessment methods in most other general pharmacology texts). Monitoring anesthetic depth today is much more technical and is primarily aimed at assessing cardiovascular and pulmonary function.

While many of the agents listed in Table 20–C can provide suitable operating conditions, the volatile anesthetic liquids remain by far the most widely used anesthetics. Such use is due to their ease of administration, rapid reversibility, controllability, and predictable amnestic effects at doses below those that cause significant cardiovascular depression. The primary disadvantages of these agents are cardiovascular depression and the lack of postoperative analgesia, both of which are minimized by the judicious use of narcotic analgesics. Limitations specific to individual agents or drug groups are discussed later in the chapter.

I. Inhalation Anesthetics

Isoflurane, enflurane, and halothane are the three inhalation anesthetics used in contemporary anesthesia practice. They are volatile liquids. (That is, they readily form vapors that can be inhaled.) Nitrous oxide, a gas with analgesic properties, is commonly used in combination with one of the volatile liquids to reduce the anesthetic requirement of the latter.

The dosage units for inhalation anesthetics and nitrous oxide are not the familiar milligrams or milliliters. Instead, dosage is calculated as the percent of the anesthetic vapor present in the gas mixture that the patient inhales. A comparison between agents is made by comparing the percentage of vapor for each compound that is needed to produce anesthesia: lower concentrations indicate greater potency. To standardize the method of comparing potencies of these agents, the term *MAC* (the *m*inimum *a*nesthetic *c*oncentration) has been coined. The MAC is defined as that concentration of anesthetic (expressed as the percent of anesthetic gas or vapor of the inhaled concentration mixed in oxygen) that prevents response to a standard painful stimulus in 50% of subjects. Key factors that alter the anesthetic dose—the MAC—include hypothermia, pregnancy, old age, and the concomitant use of other anesthetics or narcotics. The MAC for the various inhalation anesthetics, together with the effects of each agent on the heart, the lungs, and the brain, are listed in Table 20–2. Halothane is discussed as the prototype inhalation anesthetic.

Halothane

Halothane (FLUOTHANE) is a potent general anesthetic, and was the first nonflammable inhalation anesthetic developed. The MAC of halothane in oxygen is 0.78%. A concentration of 0.5% to 1.0% in a mixture of 60% to 70% nitrous oxide plus 30% to 40% oxygen causes general anesthesia for virtually all patients. Advantages of halothane include rapid onset of action and fairly

Table 20–2 Summary of Organ System Effects of Inhaled Anesthetics

	Halothane	Enflurane	Isoflurane	Nitrous Oxide
Cardiovascular effects				
Heart rate	↓	← →, ↑	↑	← →
Stroke volume	↓	← →, ↓	← →	← →
Cardiac output	↓↓	↓	← →	← →, ↓
Myocardial contractility	↓↓	↓↓	← →	↓
Myocardial O_2 consumption	↓	↓	↓	← →, ↑
Right atrial pressure	↑, ↓	↑, ↓	↑, ↓	↑
Systemic vascular resistance	↓	↓↓	↓↓↓	↑
Mean arterial pressure	↓	↓	↓	← →
Pulmonary effects				
Airway resistance	↓	↓	↓	← →
Pulmonary vascular resistance	↓	↓	↓	↑
CNS effects				
Cerebral blood flow	↑↑	↑↑	↑↑	↑
Cerebral metabolic rate	↓	↓	↓	← →, ↑
Miscellaneous				
Anesthetic potency (MAC*)	0.75%	1.68%	1.15%	105%
Percent metabolized	20%–25%	2%–5%	0.3%–0.5%	0%

Key: ↑ or ↓ = mild increase or decrease; ↑↑ or ↓↓ = moderate increase or decrease; ↓↓↓ = marked decrease; ← → = little or no change.

*MAC is defined as the minimum alveolar concentration of an anesthetic that abolishes reflex movement in 50% of subjects given a painful stimulus (eg, skin incision). MAC is reduced in hypothermia, pregnancy, old age, and by the addition of other anesthetics or narcotics.

Source: Adapted from Julien RM. *Understanding anesthesia*. Reading, MA: Addison-Wesley, 1984: 91. Reprinted with permission of the copyright owner.

rapid termination of effect, qualities that allow anesthetic depth to be easily controlled and awakening to be reasonably quick when halothane administration is discontinued. Halothane is not explosive, and is relatively nontoxic when properly used. There is, however, an unresolved problem of hepatotoxicity that has resulted in a decline in its use, favoring the increased use of enflurane and isoflurane.

Absorption, Distribution, Metabolism, and Excretion

The relationship between anesthetic solubility in blood and lipid is important to the pharmacokinetics of these drugs. It is also a concept that may be difficult to understand. Halothane, and indeed all inhaled anesthetic vapors and gases, must diffuse into the blood from the air in the alveoli. The blood then carries the drug molecules to their desired sites of action in the central nervous system (CNS), where they must diffuse out of the blood and into the lipid-rich brain tissue. It is the concentration of drug in the brain, not in the blood, that is most important for the pharmacologic effect. The blood must become "saturated" with drug before the drug can start to leave the blood and enter brain tissue and cause the onset of effects (induction). As a result, an inhaled anesthetic that is highly soluble in the blood will require a longer time to induce anesthesia than one that is less soluble in blood. Similarly, diffusion of drug molecules out of the brain tissue contributes importantly to the disappearance of effects once anesthetic administration is stopped. Therefore, anesthetics that are highly soluble in lipid will have longer durations of action because they stay in the brain longer.

Halothane is taken up rapidly in the blood following inhalation. However, because it is more soluble in blood than other inhaled anesthetics, induction with halothane takes longer than with other agents. In addition, halothane is about twice as soluble in body fat as its major alternatives, enflurane or isoflurane, so it takes longer for its effects to diminish when administration is stopped.

Approximately 70% to 80% of halothane is eliminated by the lungs; the rest undergoes hepatic metabolism. The major metabolic by-products are thought to be nontoxic. Alternate pathways of metabolism that may lead to drug-induced liver damage are discussed later.

Pharmacologic Effects

Inhaled anesthetics produce reversible depression of the CNS. The intensity of depression parallels the partial pressure of the gas or vapor in the brain. At equilibrium (such as during the maintenance of anesthesia), the alveolar concentration of inhaled anesthetics is closely correlated with the partial pressure of the anesthetic in the brain.

The mechanism by which inhaled anesthetics produce anesthesia involves an action on lipophilic (fat-rich) sites on neuronal membranes, which alters the structure of membrane proteins and disrupts membrane ion fluxes. This theory follows from the fact that anesthetic potency closely parallels lipid solubility.

Clinical Indications and Administration

The major clinical use of halothane is for the maintenance of a state of general anesthesia sufficient to allow surgery. Its potential toxicity has limited this use in favor of newer agents. However, halothane remains widely used in pediatric anesthesia because toxicity is rare in children. Halothane causes only minimal skeletal muscle relaxation. Therefore, if skeletal muscle relaxation is required to conduct certain surgical procedures, a neuromuscular blocker usually must be given also. A more detailed discussion of administration and doses is beyond the scope of this chapter; only physician anesthesiologists and nurse-anesthetists are allowed to administer the drug.

Side Effects, Adverse Reactions, and Contraindications

Halothane and the other inhaled anesthetics have widespread effects throughout the body. Since most of the effects, other than the desired state of general anesthesia, can be considered side effects, they will be discussed here. For some patients, a certain side effect may be desirable. For other patients, the effect may be potentially harmful.

Central Nervous System Side Effects

Halothane depresses all parts of the CNS, decreasing neuronal activity and simultaneously decreasing cerebral metabolic rate. Halothane, however, alters the normal relationship between cerebral metabolic rate and cerebral blood flow: neuronal activity is depressed, but cerebral blood flow is increased as a result of a direct relaxation of the smooth muscle of the cerebral blood vessels. This cerebral vasodilation increases intracranial pressure (ICP). Halothane is therefore contraindicated in patients with head injury or increased ICP due to other causes, such as brain tumors.

Cardiovascular and Renal Side Effects

Halothane causes a dose-dependent depression of the circulatory system. Heart rate and myocardial contractility fall, and so cardiac output (heart rate × stroke volume) falls by about 20% to 50%. Halothane also causes smooth muscle in the peripheral vasculature (pulmonary, systemic, and elsewhere) to relax. Reduced cardiac output, combined with vasodilation, causes arterial blood pressure to fall by 50% to 75% of preoperative levels, depending on the halothane dose. These cardiovascular effects reduce renal blood flow, and so urine output falls, often by 30% to 40% during anesthesia. Myocardial blood flow and oxygen delivery also fall. These changes would be expected to cause cardiac ischemic damage. However, myocardial damage does not occur because halothane also reduces myocardial oxygen demand.

Normally, such large falls of blood pressure would trigger the baroreceptor reflex to compensate for it, but halothane also depresses the baroreceptors, so these circulatory changes remain. The inhibited autonomic reflexes, hypotension, bradycardia, and reduced urine output can persist while the patient is in the recovery room. Therefore, anticipate and monitor for these side effects.

Although halothane depresses cardiac force and rate, it sensitizes the heart to the arrhythmia-causing effects of catecholamines (eg, epinephrine and sympathomimetic drugs like it). That is, halothane is **arrhythmogenic.** The implication is that activation of the sympathetic nervous system (eg, from stresses imposed by anesthesia or surgery), or the administration of any catecholamine that might be needed during surgery or recovery (eg, cardiac stimulants, vasopressor drugs, adrenergic bronchodilators), increases the risk of arrhythmias, which can be quite serious and require immediate intervention.

NURSING IMPLICATIONS

Carefully monitor patients recovering from halothane anesthesia for arrhythmias, especially if adrenergic cardiac stimulants, vasoconstrictors, or bronchodilators are used during or after surgery or if the patient chronically takes such medications.

Respiratory Side Effects

Halothane relaxes the bronchi, and often can reverse or prevent bronchospasm. This can make halothane useful in patients with asthma or chronic obstructive pulmonary disease. However, its use is limited because such patients may need, or may already be taking, sympathomimetic bronchodilator drugs that can also increase the risk of arrhythmias in the presence of halothane.

Uterine Side Effects

As with the pulmonary effects of halothane, effects on the uterus could be either desirable or unwanted in the obstetric setting. Halothane relaxes the uterus, which is an advantage if intrauterine manipulations are needed. After delivery, however, persistent uterine muscle relaxation can increase postpartum bleeding, and this effect can counteract the effects of oxytocic drugs (uterine stimulants such as oxytocin; Chapter 49) that are given to contract the uterus and reduce bleeding.

Skeletal Muscle Side Effects

Halothane, and all the other volatile liquid anesthetics, can trigger an uncontrolled hypermetabolic reaction in skeletal muscle when used in combination with the neuromuscular blocker succinylcholine. As noted in Chapter 17, this rare but often fatal syndrome, called ***malignant hyperthermia,*** usually occurs in genetically predisposed persons. It is characterized by profound fever and metabolic acidosis caused by intense skeletal muscle contraction, and can develop quickly, often without warning. The pathophysiology and treatment of malignant hyperthermia are discussed in Chapter 17.

Hepatic Side Effects

For most patients, halothane causes no adverse effects on the liver. However, the drug has been implicated in rare cases of hepatic toxicity, presumably caused by metabolism of the drug to reactive by-products that damage liver cells. This probably occurs in no more than 1 out of 10,000 to 20,000 patients receiving the drug. An even smaller number of patients develop hepatic necrosis. These adverse hepatic reactions seem to be related to obesity and middle age; they have not been reported in children receiving this drug.

NURSING IMPLICATIONS

While the choice of anesthetic remains the anesthesiologist's responsibility, operating and recovery room nurses need to be familiar with complications of halothane anesthesia.

Halothane-induced sensitization of the heart to epinephrine and other catecholamines limits the total dose of epinephrine-containing local anesthetic solution that can be used during and shortly after surgery. Close attention must be paid to the amounts of such drugs that are used and to the time intervals between their administration. Electrocardiographic monitoring is recommended.

The nursing staff in the operating and recovery rooms must be aware of the role of halothane in malignant hyperthermia, as well as its symptoms and the protocol for its treatment (see Chapter 17). Necessary components for treatment and resuscitation, including an ample supply of dantrolene, a fully equipped resuscitation cart (including cardioversion equipment), cooling blankets, and ice packs, should be readily available.

The peripheral vasodilating effect of halothane predisposes the patient to significant loss of body heat. Thus, vigorous attempts should be made to assist the patient with the maintenance of body temperature to protect against unnecessary heat loss.

Carefully monitor for hypotension, bradycardia, and depressed ventilation.

Finally, report any postoperative alterations in liver function or signs of liver failure immediately.

Interactions with Other Drugs

Drug interactions involving halothane are common. Interactions involving catecholamines, which may lead to potentially serious arrhythmias, were mentioned earlier. Frequent causes of this interaction include bronchodilators or vasopressors (whether administered alone to support or elevate blood pressure, or as components of local anesthetics that are often given for local pain relief). Other agents that interact through increasing sympathetic influences include the tricyclic antidepressants and cocaine. Patients receiving these drugs should be anesthetized with agents other than halothane whenever possible. The cardiac depressant effects of halothane are potentiated by other cardiac depressants, particularly quinidine (and perhaps most other antiarrhythmic drugs), β-adrenergic blockers, and calcium-channel blockers. Narcotic analgesics potentiate the respiratory depressant effects of halothane. Halothane potentiates the actions of nondepolarizing neuromuscular blockers (tubocurarine and related agents) and ganglionic blockers.

NURSING IMPLICATIONS

If the use of interacting drugs cannot be avoided (for example, use of sympathomimetics to control intraoperative hypotension or bronchospasm), or alternatives to halothane cannot be used, the lowest effective dose of the interactant must be used. This dose is usually lower than the safe dose for a person who has not been anesthetized with halothane. For example, patients anesthetized with halothane should receive no more than 1.5 μg of epinephrine per kilogram of body weight. Carefully assess for, and be prepared to deal with, the likely adverse consequences of interactions involving drugs the patient is currently receiving or those that might be used in common emergencies, such as hypotension, arrhythmias, or bronchospasm. Try to obtain a complete history of substance abuse. Drugs such as alcohol, narcotics, and cocaine or amphetamines (both of which are sympathomimetics) can cause serious effects during anesthesia if their presence is unknown and unaccounted for.

Overdose and Toxicity

Halothane overdoses usually present as excessive cardiac depression with reduced cardiac output and hypotension. This can reduce organ perfusion and cause severe tissue ischemia. Respiratory depression caused by halothane potentiates toxicity. Both the vasodilatory effects and the respiratory acidosis produced by halothane increase ICP. Overdosage necessitates cessation of drug administration and ventilation with pure oxygen.

More commonly observed toxicities include cardiac arrhythmias, shivering, nausea, and emesis. The severe toxic reactions, hepatic necrosis and malignant hyperthermia, were discussed above.

Related Drugs

The other widely used inhalational anesthetics are enflurane, isoflurane, and nitrous oxide. Table 20–2 compares some of their key properties with those of halothane. Nitrous oxide is a gas. Enflurane and isoflurane are, like halothane, volatile liquids, but they are less toxic than the prototype and possess most of the characteristics considered essential for an ideal anesthetic.

Three other inhaled anesthetics are available. Methoxyflurane (PENTHRANE) is a volatile liquid. It is extensively metabolized to fluoride, which is potentially nephrotoxic. Methoxyflurane is seldom used, and only in special circumstances when profound or prolonged anesthesia is not anticipated. Cyclopropane and ethylene are highly explosive gases, and so are rarely used. These drugs will not be discussed further.

Enflurane

Enflurane (ETHRANE) is one of two halogenated ether anesthetics in clinical use (the other is isoflurane). Enflurane is approximately half as potent as halothane; its MAC is 1.68%. Although enflurane is similar to halothane in many respects, it differs in others. These comparisons follow.

Enflurane's solubility in both blood and fat is intermediate between that of halothane and isoflurane. Thus, induction and emergence are relatively fast—faster than with halothane and slower than with isoflurane. Varying the enflurane concentration in the inspired gas mixture gives smooth and fairly rapid changes in the anesthetic depth. Roughly 95% to 98% of the administered dose is eliminated unchanged by the lungs.

Enflurane, like halothane, decreases blood pressure. However, with enflurane the major cause is peripheral vasodilation, not depression of cardiac contractility. Owing to decreased blood pressure, enflurane can reduce renal blood flow and urine production, but IV fluid infusion usually restores urine output. Overall, however, the drug can decrease cardiac output, and the effect can be particularly significant, and unwanted, in patients with cardiac disease. Enflurane either does not change heart rate, or increases it; bradycardia is uncommon. The drug is less arrhythmogenic than halothane.

Enflurane causes dose-dependent depression of respiration, and to an extent greater than that seen with halothane at comparable levels of anesthesia (ie, at comparable MACs). Tidal volume, the amount of air entering or leaving the lungs during a single breath, is significantly decreased. The drug also depresses the respiratory center's response to decreased blood oxygen levels and increased carbon dioxide levels, which normally stimulate ventilation as a protective reflex. As a result, the anesthesiologist usually needs to control the patient's ventilation. Of course, if a neuromuscular blocker is also given, ventilation *must* be controlled.

Enflurane relaxes uterine smooth muscle in the same way as halothane, and so the same precautions apply to its use in a pregnant woman at term.

Enflurane is a better skeletal muscle relaxant than halothane, but the effect usually is not sufficient for surgery inside the major body cavities, and so neuromuscular blockers are still important adjuncts in many cases. However, neuromuscular blocker doses lower than those generally needed during halothane-based anesthesia are usually sufficient when enflurane is used.

One unique effect of enflurane anesthesia is the production of electroencephalogram (EEG) patterns that resemble those seen in patients with epilepsy. Whether enflurane is a convulsant drug is still being debated, but much clinical experience with this anesthetic has shown that it can be used safely for most patients, without undue concern about triggering seizures, unless the dose is too high. Nevertheless, caution dictates that other agents should be used if the person to be anesthetized has a seizure disorder. Like halothane, enflurane reduces cerebral metabolic and oxygen consumption rates, dilates cerebral blood vessels, and increases both cerebral blood flow and ICP.

There have been a few isolated reports of liver damage caused by enflurane, but hepatic necrosis has not been reported, even when the drug has been given to patients suffering from severe hypoxia.

Isoflurane

Isoflurane (FORANE), which is structurally related to enflurane, has become the most widely used anesthetic vapor because of several key properties. Its low blood solubility gives very rapid anesthesia induction and recovery, and facilitates control of anesthesia depth. Nearly all the drug (>99.5%) is excreted unchanged via the lungs. Because there is so little formation of metabolites, which are thought to contribute to the liver or kidney damage halothane and enflurane can cause, the risk of damage to these organs is significantly reduced when isoflurane is used.

Compared with halothane and enflurane, isoflurane causes the least cardiac depression but the most peripheral vasodilation. It also dilates the coronary arteries and reduces cardiac work. Whether these effects are good or bad for patients with ischemic heart disease is debatable. Overall, however, isoflurane maintains cardiac output well. Importantly, it is less arrhythmogenic than halothane or enflurane. And, when the dose is kept below 0.5% MAC and the patient is hyperventilated, isoflurane causes little increase in ICP, making it a good anesthetic for patients undergoing intracranial surgery. Neuromuscular blockers may be needed as adjuncts to provide adequate skeletal muscle relaxation for patients undergoing surgery of major body cavities.

NURSING IMPLICATIONS

The rapid pulmonary elimination of isoflurane means that patients awaken quite rapidly following termination of anesthesia, thus experiencing surgical discomfort early in the recovery period. Intraoperative administration of opiate narcotics can help moderate such discomfort. However, in most institutions, narcotics are administered intravenously in the recovery room for rapid control of pain. (Intramuscularly administered narcotics are not preferred for pain control in the immediate postoperative period because of their delayed onset of action.) Standing orders for IV narcotic administration by recovery room nurses are advised.

The lack of systemic toxicity and the rapid elimination of isoflurane imply that most drug-induced complications (such as hypotension or respiratory depression) will occur in the operating room during surgery and are not usually of major concern postoperatively.

Nitrous Oxide

Nitrous oxide ("laughing gas") is a colorless, odorless, tasteless gas. It is the most widely used anesthetic in clinical practice, despite the fact that, when used alone, it cannot predictably produce general anesthesia. Rather, its mild analgesic and amnestic properties make it a useful supplement to other, more potent anesthetics.

General Properties, Uses, and Effects

Nitrous oxide is relatively insoluble in blood or fat. Thus, the blood and brain become rapidly saturated: patients lose consciousness quickly when drug administration starts, and regain consciousness quickly when it stops. Nitrous oxide is excreted unchanged by the lungs, with little or none of it being metabolized first.

Usual concentrations of nitrous oxide, 65% to 70%, administered with 30% to 35% oxygen, can cause unconsciousness in most patients. However, muscle relaxation, autonomic stability, and amnesia are inadequate unless narcotics or volatile anesthetics are given also. Thus, the usual inhaled anesthetic mixture contains 65% to 70% nitrous oxide, 30% to 35% oxygen, and 0.5% to 2% halothane, enflurane, or isoflurane (the amount depending on the MAC of the volatile liquid, the patient's age and physical status, and whether narcotics are used also). Neuromuscular blockers will also be needed if skeletal muscle relaxation is necessary.

Nitrous oxide has mixed effects on the cardiovascular system. It mildly depresses heart rate, contractility, and cardiac output, which tends to lower blood pressure, but pressure seldom falls much because the drug also causes weak sympathomimetic effects, including an increase of peripheral vascular resistance. Including nitrous oxide in the inhaled gas mixture reduces the dose of a voltaile liquid anesthetic that would otherwise be needed, and so reduces the amount of cardiac depression that the latter drugs otherwise might cause. However, in patients who have coronary artery disease and preexisting myocardial dysfunction, nitrous oxide can cause enough added cardiac depression to become clinically significant.

Nitrous oxide increases cerebral blood flow. It can also increase ICP, but the increases are usually modest and can be reduced by also giving the patients a benzodiazepine or barbiturate (see midazolam, thiopental, below). Other drugs and anesthesia techniques can be used when nitrous oxide is given to patients undergoing intracranial surgery.

In other regards, nitrous oxide appears to be relatively benign. It exerts little or no effect on the uterus, and therefore can be used safely in obstetrics. It exerts no significant, acute effects on the respiratory, renal, or hepatic systems. As noted in the next section, however, the drug may cause problems for health-care providers who are chronically exposed to it in their occupational environment.

Toxicity from Chronic Exposure

There has been concern about the long-term health effects from occupational exposure to trace amounts of nitrous oxide. Operating room personnel and many surgeons, dentists, and dental assistants are at risk of significant exposure to the gas. One concern relates to the ability of nitrous oxide to lower levels of methionine synthetase, an enzyme that is essential for the synthesis of vitamin B_{12}, which is important for normal nerve function. Some individuals exposed to this gas for prolonged periods have developed neurologic symptoms consistent with vitamin B_{12} deficiency. These abnormalities tend to improve slowly when chronic exposure to the gas is discontinued.

There have also been reports that chronic exposure to nitrous oxide can cause gene mutations, cancer, or birth defects (**mutagenic, carcinogenic,** and **teratogenic** effects, respectively). A reasonable and current interpretation of the data, which are conflicting, is that nitrous oxide (and the other inhaled anesthetics) are not mutagenic or carcinogenic. Their teratogenic potential is less clear. Retrospective studies have reported increased rates of spontaneous abortion in female operating room and dental personnel, and occasionally in wives of male personnel. A cause-and-effect relationship has not been demonstrated, and ongoing studies indicate that adverse effects, if any, occur at a much lower frequency than was once feared. Indeed, more recent reports in both the anesthesia and the occupational medicine literature indicate that occupational exposure to trace amounts of nitrous oxide does not pose a significant health risk.

Further research is needed to evaluate the potential toxicity of inhalation anesthetics. Nevertheless, anesthesiologists and operating room personnel should work to minimize the levels of gases in the operating room by carefully evaluating the integrity of scavenging systems and gas connecters.

NURSING IMPLICATIONS

Nitrous oxide is usually administered at high concentration (up to 75% of the inhaled gas mixture). This practice, combined with very rapid elimination, places the patient at risk for transient postanesthetic hypoxia. Such hypoxia can be minimized by administering supplemental oxygen for about 5 minutes after surgery.

Experimental Agents

Enflurane and isoflurane are excellent anesthetics, but there is an ongoing search for even better drugs. Two agents that are currently under investigation are desflurane and sevoflurane. Of the two, desflurane seems to be the most promising. Both drugs are volatile liquids, but they have physical or chemical properties that will require some modification of the anesthesia machines that are currently used.

Desflurane differs from isoflurane only by the presence of a fluorine atom instead of a chlorine atom. Its blood:gas solubility ratio is very close to that of nitrous oxide, so anesthesia induction and recovery are very quick, and anesthesia depth can be controlled easily. These properties make desflurane an advantageous agent when rapid awakening is desirable, as in outpatient anesthesia settings. Cardiovascular and respiratory effects are similar to those of isoflurane. Desflurane is eliminated by the lungs almost completely unchanged, so the risk of organ damage from metabolites appears to be low; organ toxicity has not been reported.

Sevoflurane also provides rapid awakening from anesthesia. It, however, is significantly metabolized, and raises serum fluoride concentrations. Although this may lead to renal or hepatic toxicity, problems have not yet been reported.

II. Parenteral Agents

Several general anesthetic agents are administered parenterally. They can be loosely grouped according to use. Barbiturates (primarily thiopental), benzodiazepines (mainly midazolam), and two unrelated drugs, ketamine and etomidate, are used solely for induction of general anesthesia. The others are used for both induction and maintenance of anesthesia: narcotics (mainly fentanyl); and propofol, which is used for induction and maintenance of anesthesia for relatively short procedures in outpatients.

Barbiturate Induction Agents

Thiopental (PENTOTHAL), methohexital (BREVITAL), and thiamylal (SURITAL) are classified as ultra–short-acting barbiturates. They are given intravenously either to induce general anesthesia that will be maintained with other drugs, or to produce brief periods of unconsciousness. The three drugs are so similar that only thiopental is discussed here. Only aspects related to anesthesia induction will be summarized. Basic pharmacologic properties of the barbiturates are discussed in Chapter 22.

Thiopental

Thiopental, like the other induction barbiturates, is very soluble in lipid. Consciousness is lost 10 to 15 seconds after a single IV injection. This is the time needed for the drug to travel from the injection site to the brain, where the drug is rapidly taken up. Unconsciousness lasts several minutes. The intensity of CNS depression decreases progressively until consciousness returns, in about 10 to 20 minutes. The duration of action is brief because the drug quickly diffuses out of the brain and redistributes to other tissues, such as muscle, fat, and bone. Thiopental is eventually cleared from the body by hepatic metabolism and by renal excretion of the metabolites. This process, which has a half-life of 4 to 6 hours, accounts for the delay in psychomotor recovery after anesthesia.

The major pharmacologic effect of the induction barbiturates is a dose-dependent depression of CNS activity. Unlike the volatile anesthetics, the barbiturates reduce cerebral blood flow, ICP, and cerebral metabolic rate (Table 20–3). These properties make thiopental useful in intracranial surgery and possibly in protecting injured brain tissue in patients with acute ICP increases, such as after head injury.

Barbiturates have no analgesic effects. If pain is present, the lack of analgesia plus drug-induced intoxication can cause agitation and disorientation. This occurs most frequently at the end of surgery, when patients are in the early stages of recovery and may be experiencing both pain and disorientation.

Induction doses of thiopental may cause adverse cardiovascular effects, including myocardial depression and decreased cardiac output, stroke volume, and peripheral vascular resistance. While normal induction doses might be tolerated by a healthy patient, profound and sudden hypotension and even cardiovascular col-

Table 20–3 **Summary of Organ System Effects of Intravenous Anesthetics**

	Barbiturates	Benzo-diazepines	Narcotics	Ketamine	Etomidate
Cardiovascular effects					
Myocardial contractility	↓	←→	0	↑	←→
Cardiac output	↓	←→	0	↑	←→
Mean arterial pressure and systemic vascular resistance	↓	←→	0	↑	←→
Pulmonary effects					
Respiratory rate	←→	←→	↓↓	←→	←→
Tidal volume and minute ventilation	↓↓	↓	↓ or ↓↓	←→	←→
CO_2 sensitivity	↓	←→	↓↓	←→	←→
CNS effects					
Cerebral blood flow	↓↓	↓	←→	↑↑	↓
Cerebral metabolic rate	↓↓	↓	←→	↑	↓
Analgesia	0	0	↑↑	↑↑	0
Intracranial pressure	↓↓	←→	←→	↑↑	↓

Key: 0 = no change; ↑ or ↓ = mild increase or decrease; ↑↑ or ↓↓ = marked increase or decrease; ←→ = little or no change.

Source: Adapted from Julien RM. *Understanding Anesthesia*. Reading, MA: Addison-Wesley, 1984:100. Reprinted with permission.

lapse might occur in patients with cardiac or vascular disease, in hypovolemic patients, or in the elderly.

Another side effect of ultra–short-acting barbiturates is respiratory depression; apnea is common.

Intravenous administration of thiopental to asthmatic patients or others who are allergic to it has been reported to induce bronchospasm, so it should be used with caution in these individuals.

Complications of Induction Barbiturates

Complications most frequently involve the cardiovascular and respiratory depression noted above. Less frequent but potentially serious complications include anaphylaxis, venous irritation, gangrene or loss of a limb because of accidental intraarterial injection, and precipitation of an attack of porphyria. Porphyria, or a history of it, contraindicates barbiturate use.

NURSING IMPLICATIONS

Disorientation and lack of analgesia can cause a state of drunken agitation following termination of anesthesia and surgery when a barbiturate has been used. Nurses working in the recovery room should be particularly alert to the potential for self-injury in such patients (especially children and young adults), and institute appropriate precautions. The long elimination half-life of thiopental produces significant psychomotor dysfunction for 24 to 30 hours after anesthesia. Patients and their families must be educated to avoid motor vehicle operation or the performance of psychomotor tasks for at least that time following anesthesia. Since more and more patients are undergoing surgery in ambulatory care (outpatient) facilities and are discharged within a few hours of surgery (within one half-life of thiopental), close observation and education are particularly important.

Benzodiazepine Induction Agent

Midazolam

Midazolam (VERSED) is one of three benzodiazepines available in parenteral formulation, and it is of particular use in anesthesia. (The other two, diazepam and lorazepam, are of limited use in anesthesia because of poor water solubility, slower onsets of action, and longer half-lives.) The pharmacologic properties of midazolam related to its use in anesthesia are discussed here.

Sedation and amnesia characterize the primary actions and clinical uses of midazolam. Upon injection, this water-soluble drug is transformed into a more lipid-soluble substance that rapidly penetrates the blood–brain barrier, inducing unconsciousness in about 45 to 90 seconds. Because it is administered as an aqueous solution, it is nonirritating to the veins; one can thus minimize the pain and phlebitis that can follow diazepam injection.

Midazolam is rapidly distributed throughout the body, and is metabolized in the liver; it has an elimination half-life of about 2 hours. However, when compared with the induction barbiturates, the onset of unconsciousness is slower and recovery times are longer. Therefore, midazolam will not likely replace thiopental as a "routine" induction agent for healthy surgical patients.

The effects of midazolam on the CNS resemble those of the induction barbiturates: it acts as a CNS depressant and an amnestic, and it reduces neuronal activity, cerebral blood flow, and ICP; however, it lacks analgesic effects (see Table 20–3).

Cardiovascular effects of midazolam are *usually* relatively minor. It is therefore useful as an induction agent in seriously ill patients with cardiovascular disease. Effects on the lungs, liver, kidneys, skeletal muscle, and smooth muscle are relatively benign. Midazolam is used both as a preanesthetic medication and as an intraoperative sedative and amnestic.

The IV use of midazolam is not without complications. Since its introduction to clinical use in 1987, the drug has been associated with several dozen deaths, and many episodes of nonfatal respiratory and cardiovascular depression. These adverse responses occurred mainly when the drug was administered for "conscious sedation" (also called amnestic sedation)—a situation in which sedation and amnesia are desirable for patients undergoing uncomfortable procedures such as endoscopy. Patients in these situations benefit from the wanted actions of the drug, but the potential hypoxia, hypotension, and respiratory depression that can also occur must be avoided. Once these unwanted episodes were recognized, earlier recommended dosage schedules were drastically reduced. Nevertheless, close monitoring (physical and electronic) is mandatory, and appropriate personnel, drugs, and equipment for emergency resuscitation must be readily available.

NURSING IMPLICATIONS

Nurses are often responsible for giving midazolam, and for monitoring the patient during the procedures for which it is given. Even low doses may cause sleep, respiratory depression, and apnea. Therefore, the following guidelines are important:

- give an initial dose of no more than 2 mg total, regardless of body weight, to normal healthy adults;
- reduce doses to 1 mg or less for elderly or debilitated patients, or those also medicated with other CNS depressants or narcotics;
- never give the drug as an IV bolus. Infuse it over at least 2 minutes, and use larger volumes of a more dilute solution (1 mg/mL or less) rather than small volumes of more concentrated solutions, to help avoid giving the drug too fast;
- be aware that some patients respond to even lower doses than those recommended. Therefore,
- assess the patient's response as the drug is going in, and stop the infusion when the desired effect, such as the onset of slurred speech, begins; and
- always wait at least 2 minutes before giving more, so you can assess the full effect of the first dose.

All patients receiving midazolam for conscious sedation should remain responsive to verbal stimulation. Giving supplemental oxygen and monitoring peripheral tissue oxygenation (several easy-to-use devices are available) are strongly urged.

The various CNS effects, combined with the lack of analgesic effects, can cause disorientation and behavioral excitement, which can mimic or be potentiated by hypoxia. Individuals caring for patients given parenteral benzodiazepines need to be skilled in managing obtunded patients. Needless injuries and fatalities have resulted from underestimating the problems that midazolam can cause.

Other Intravenous Induction Agents

Ketamine

Ketamine (KETALAR) is a *dissociative* anesthetic agent that is chemically related to phencyclidine (PCP, or "angel dust"), a psychomimetic drug noted for its ability to cause hallucinations (Chapter 28).

Ketamine's onset of action is within 30 to 60 seconds after IV injection, and about 3 to 8 minutes after intramuscular (IM) injection. The elimination half-life, which parallels the duration of action and the recovery from drug effects, is about 3 hours. Recovery will be prolonged if ketamine is used adjunctively with barbiturates, benzodiazepines, or narcotics.

Ketamine causes powerful analgesic and amnestic effects. At usual analgesic and amnestic doses (about

1 mg/kg) it induces a behavioral state in which the patient appears "dissociated" from the environment. Patients may appear to be awake, with open eyes, but they have spontaneous, involuntary movements. The drug also can induce hallucinations—a **psychotomimetic** effect—although not as often as the related drug phencyclidine. Many of the postoperative psychotomimetic complications from ketamine are probably caused by overdosage. The incidence of these effects can be reduced by concomitant administration of a benzodiazepine such as midazolam.

Ketamine leaves autonomic reflexes intact, and it usually activates the sympathetic nervous system by causing catecholamine release, which increases peripheral vascular resistance and heart rate. Sympathetic stimulation also masks the drug's direct cardiac-depressant effects. Ketamine stimulates respiratory rate, dilates the bronchi, and increases skeletal muscle tone.

Ketamine is not a desirable agent for routine use in anesthesia. However, it is extremely useful in specific situations, including:

- High-risk surgical patients, especially those who are hypovolemic or hypotensive (because it activates the sympathetic nervous system).
- Pediatric patients, in whom IV induction of anesthesia may be difficult (the drug is given intramuscularly to these patients).
- Asthmatic patients (because of its bronchodilating properties).
- Burn patients, as an amnestic and analgesic during debridement, painful dressing changes, or skin grafting procedures.
- Occasionally for brief surgical or diagnostic procedures where untoward cardiovascular or respiratory depression is undesirable.

If skeletal muscle relaxation is needed, a neuromuscular blocker must be given adjunctively because ketamine has no skeletal muscle relaxant actions.

There are also situations in which ketamine should be avoided, whether because of underlying medical problems or because of the use of interacting drugs. Ketamine increases cerebral blood flow and ICP, and should not be used during anesthesia for neurosurgical procedures. Its sympathomimetic effects make it undesirable for patients with coronary artery disease or poorly controlled hypertension. They also necessitate cautious use of other drugs that raise blood pressure. Ketamine probably should be avoided during alcohol withdrawal and during intoxication with psychotomimetic drugs.

NURSING IMPLICATIONS

Patients must be closely observed postoperatively for signs of hallucinations, delusions, or disorientation. A quiet wake-up period, and avoidance of excessive stimulation, may lessen side effects. Do not leave the patient unattended if side effects occur. The drug's potent analgesic effect predisposes patients to painless self-abuse, so they must be protected from themselves during the recovery period. Calmly reassure patients and reorient them to the surroundings.

Etomidate

Etomidate (AMIDATE) is an induction anesthetic that differs chemically from the barbiturates and benzodiazepines. Given intravenously, unconsciousness occurs within 1 minute and lasts about 5 minutes; the patient usually awakens fully in about 7 to 14 minutes. The drug is rapidly metabolized in the liver and plasma. Although the elimination half-life is about 4 hours, clinical effects are usually minimal after about 1 to 1.5 hours.

Etomidate lacks analgesic or muscle relaxing properties, and can cause myoclonus on injection. Thus, concomitant use of a neuromuscular blocker such as succinylcholine is frequently required, especially if endotracheal intubation will follow. Unlike the barbiturates, etomidate causes only slight depression of subcortical structures, so cardiovascular and respiratory depression is mild. The relative lack of cardiovascular effects, and the brief duration of action, make etomidate useful for inducing anesthesia in high-risk patients or patients for whom prolonged effects of benzodiazepines are unwanted or must be avoided, such as those undergoing a brief procedure.

In addition to myoclonus, pain on injection is the most common side effect of etomidate. The drug's ability to cause adrenal suppression may be the major limitation of its clinical usefulness.

NURSING IMPLICATIONS

Anticipate that patients will awaken rapidly and be left without residual analgesia. If they have undergone a painful surgical procedure or manipulation, postoperative analgesia may be required; IV narcotics are most effective.

Intravenous Drugs Used for Anesthesia Induction and Maintenance

There are three anesthetic narcotics intended primarily for use during the perioperative period. Fentanyl (SUBLIMAZE) can be considered the prototype. Its two derivatives are alfentanyl (ALFENTA) and sufentanil (SUFENTA). All three are synthetic narcotics and resemble morphine pharmacologically (see Chapter 21). Only those aspects relating particularly to anesthesia will be discussed here. These drugs are useful in anesthesia because they are relatively short acting and provide autonomic stability by blunting the sympathetic response to painful stimuli, thus providing intense analgesia for surgery.

All three agents are much more potent analgesics than morphine, but at equivalent analgesic doses they cause the same degree of respiratory depression. Anesthetic doses of these drugs produce a relatively stress-free state characterized by minimal cardiovascular changes and reduced sympathetic nervous system activation. When given before surgery, any of these drugs will ease the physiologic stresses imposed by laryngoscopy, intubation, and skin incisions. These drugs are also useful for debilitated patients who do not tolerate most inhalation anesthetics well.

Fentanyl

Fentanyl (SUBLIMAZE) has about 50 to 80 times the analgesic potency of morphine. Administered intravenously, fentanyl has a rapid onset and a brief duration of action (45 minutes to 1 hour).

Fentanyl causes analgesia plus varying degrees of sedation and mood changes, intense respiratory depression, and mental clouding. Respiratory rate is depressed much more than tidal volume. Indeed, in spontaneously breathing patients, respiratory rate can be used as an index of the degree of the respiratory depression induced by this agent. Respiratory depression occurs because this drug decreases the responsiveness of the respiratory centers in the brainstem to increasing levels of carbon dioxide in arterial blood.

Like other narcotics, fentanyl depresses cough reflexes. Postoperatively, this may be detrimental since it may reduce the patient's ability to clear secretions.

Fentanyl produces either no change or slight decreases in cerebral blood flow, cerebral metabolic rate, and ICP.

Narcotics, even in the high doses used in certain anesthetic techniques, produce little effect on the cardiovascular system in supine patients. However, when mixed with nitrous oxide, significant cardiovascular depression can occur.

Fentanyl is indicated for management of acute pain (as might occur with certain surgical or diagnostic procedures), as an analgesic supplement for regional or general anesthesia, or as the primary anesthetic agent in special procedures. It is widely used for the induction and maintenance of anesthesia in patients with cardiovascular disease and with peripheral vascular-, carotid-, or coronary-occlusive disease. Some reduction in peripheral vascular resistance may occur; it can be minimized by maintaining the patient in the supine position, by preloading the patient with fluid, and by judicious use of vasoconstrictors. Fentanyl can also be used for postoperative analgesia, but its short duration of action necessitates frequent administration, which makes it inconvenient to use.

The normal adult dose of fentanyl is in the range of 1 to 5 μg/kg, but doses as high as 25 to 100 μg/kg have been administered for cardiac surgery. Advantages of high-dose narcotic anesthesia include "stress-free" anesthesia, reduced levels of circulating catecholamines, and cardiovascular stability. Postoperative ventilatory support is frequently needed following high-dose narcotic anesthesia.

There are two other dosage forms of fentanyl. One is an injectable preparation, marketed as INNOVAR, in which fentanyl is combined with the major tranquilizer droperidol. This product, which causes *neuroleptanalgesia*—analgesia plus amnesia in a patient who otherwise appears conscious—is given before some surgical or diagnostic procedures. The other formulation, marketed as DURAGESIC, contains fentanyl alone. The drug is contained in a transdermal delivery system that is applied to the skin, releasing a constant rate of fentanyl into the bloodstream. It is used solely as an analgesic to manage chronic pain (eg, that associated with cancer) in patients who require a narcotic. This use is discussed more fully in Chapter 21.

NURSING IMPLICATIONS

Postoperative ventilatory depression is the most important complication of parenteral fentanyl use; the nurse must closely monitor respiratory rate. Since this drug also depresses cough reflexes, it can interfere with the patient's ability to clear secretions. Therefore, the patient must be encouraged to breathe deeply and cough to avoid mucous plugging of the alveoli.

The narcotic antagonist naloxone (NARCAN; see Chapter 21) effectively reverses respiratory depression caused by fentanyl and other narcotics. This effect is clinically useful. However, naloxone also blocks the analgesic effect of narcotics, and so hampers postoperative pain relief. In addition, the short half-life of naloxone predisposes to "renarcotization" as the antagonistic effect dissipates and respiratory depression recurs. Monitor the patient appropriately.

Anesthetic narcotics, especially fentanyl and some closely related, illicitly manufactured derivatives ("designer drugs"), are frequently abused, both by medical personnel and street users. Medical personnel must be particularly aware of the attractions of parenteral narcotics, and be alert to anyone who might be drawn to their use. When fentanyl is injected, respiratory arrest can occur and is frequently fatal unless rapidly treated.

Alfentanyl

Alfentanyl (ALFENTA) has only one quarter the potency of fentanyl. Its duration of action is about one third to one half as long (about 5 to 15 minutes), so alfentanyl is considered an ultra–short-acting narcotic. Alfentanyl is frequently administered by continuous IV infusion to maintain a persistent action. Even though alfentanyl has a very brief duration of action, termination of its clinical effect is much slower owing to slow redistribution from the brain to muscle and fat. Repeated doses can exert more prolonged effects as storage depots become saturated with drug and blood levels of the drug increase. Following anesthesia with alfentanyl, the nurse should be alert for signs of respiratory depression and be prepared to treat it appropriately.

Sufentanil

Sufentanil (SUFENTA) is five to ten times more potent than fentanyl, has a similar duration of action, and causes significantly more sedation. It is used as an analgesic adjunct for maintenance of balanced anesthesia. Sufentanil is cleared from the brain and bloodstream more quickly than fentanyl, which usually allows more rapid postoperative recovery.

Nonnarcotic Anesthetic

Propofol

Propofol (DIPRIVAN) is a new IV drug that is chemically unrelated to all other anesthetics, and it is gaining widespread use in outpatient settings. It is a sedative-hypnotic, like the barbiturates. Propofol is injected intravenously to induce anesthesia. It has mild analgesic actions, and blunts the autonomic–hemodynamic responses that usually occur upon intubation. Given by IV infusion, or by intermittent IV injection, propofol also can be used to maintain general anesthesia in conjunction with other drugs.

Propofol induces unconsciousness within 1 minute of injection. Its effects are also brief. If propofol is not used with other, longer acting drugs, the patient regains consciousness in several minutes, often appearing remarkably alert and free of usual side effects from anesthesia. It is safe for use in patients with porphyria (for whom barbiturates are contraindicated) or a susceptibility to malignant hyperthermia (which contraindicates the use of halothane and related inhaled drugs).

Propofol does have some limitations. Intravenous injections can be painful. Pain can be reduced by injecting the drug into a large vein, or by IV injection of a local anesthetic first. Propofol should be used cautiously in patients with ischemic coronary or peripheral vascular disease, especially if it is used along with nitrous oxide or narcotics. Depression of cardiac contractility, blood pressure, and respiration (including apnea) can occur. Hypotension may be a particular problem in the elderly.

SUMMARY OF NURSING IMPLICATIONS

◆ Assessment

Review patient and family history for prior untoward effects of anesthesia (eg, malignant hyperthermia, which is genetically linked).

Complete a nursing history, including personal health habits (eg, smoking, alcohol abuse), allergies, and concurrent conditions or diseases that can influence choice of anesthesia.

Identify any prescription or over-the-counter drugs taken within 72 hours of surgery that may cause a drug–drug interaction during anesthesia.

Assess physiologic and psychologic status and routine laboratory results preoperatively; establish baseline vital signs.

◆ Nursing Diagnoses

Fear related to need for surgery, possible death, or general anesthesia.

Knowledge deficit related to surgical procedure and anesthetic process.

Decreased cardiac output related to anesthetic side effects.

Pain related to surgical procedure or manipulation.

High risk for injury related to disorientation and self-abuse (ketamine anesthesia).

Sensory/perceptual alterations: Kinesthetic related to effects of general anesthesia.

Altered urinary elimination (retention or inadequate) related to anesthetic drug effects.

High risk for aspiration related to vomiting following anesthesia.

Ineffective airway clearance related to depressed cough reflex.

Ineffective breathing pattern related to ventilatory depression.

Impaired swallowing related to anesthetic effects.

◆ Planning/Implementation

Monitor the electrocardiogram for bradycardia and other cardiac arrhythmias, particularly during ketamine use.

Observe for signs and symptoms of malignant hyperthermia during use of certain inhalation anesthetics (eg, halothane).

Prepare for treatment of malignant hyperthermia: measures to support vital functions (resuscitation, dantrolene sodium), and reduce body temperature (cooling blanket, ice packs).

Measure urine output periodically to determine anesthetic effect on renal function.

Monitor vital signs carefully for signs of hypotension, bradycardia, and depressed ventilation.

Position patient on side postoperatively, if possible, to prevent aspiration if vomiting occurs; have suctioning equipment available.

Medicate for pain as ordered; patient may require only one quarter to one half ordered dose of analgesic initially.

Administer supplemental oxygen, particularly following use of nitrous oxide, to prevent hypoxia.

Keep side rails up and protect patient from injury if agitation occurs.

Provide quiet environment for patients recovering from ketamine administration.

Provide humidification (mist mask) to reduce throat irritation following tracheal intubation during general anesthesia.

Encourage frequent coughing and deep breathing to prevent pulmonary complications following general anesthesia.

◆ Patient and Family Teaching

Teach the patient/family:

About anticipated surgery; answer questions about anesthesia and surgery; teach effective coughing and deep breathing preoperatively.

About activity, diet, or medications, verbally and in writing.

To avoid operating motor vehicles or performing psychomotor tasks for at least 24 to 30 hours following barbiturate anesthesia.

◆ Evaluation

The patient/family will:

Recover completely from general anesthesia; regain consciousness; be oriented; have stable vital signs.

Verbalize positive feelings about the surgical and anesthetic experience.

Cough and deep breathe effectively; have breath sounds present and clear bilaterally.

Experience no complications of general anesthesia (eg, respiratory complications, renal insufficiency, cardiac irregularities, nausea, vomiting).

Achieve relief from postoperative pain.

Annotated Bibliography

Becker LC. Is isoflurane dangerous for the patient with coronary artery disease? *Anesthesiology* 1987;66:259–261. *An important discussion of the effects of this drug on cardiac function.*

Bonica J. *The management of pain. 2nd ed.* Philadelphia: Lea & Febiger, 1990. *A two-volume update of a classic text.*

Cheng EY, Nimphius N, Kampine JP. Anesthetic drugs and emergency departments. *Anesth Analg* 1992;74:272–275. *Many drugs commonly given by anesthesiologists in the operating room are given in other settings (eg, emergency departments), where adequate care and monitoring might not be available, and the physician may not have the expertise to use the drug in an optimally safe way. Since you may face this situation yourself, the information here can be very helpful.*

Erickson HA, Kallan AJB. Hospitalization for miscarriage and delivery outcome among Swedish nurses working in operating rooms 1973–1978. *Anesth Analg* 1985;64:981–988. *A comprehensive study of the potentially toxic effects of anesthetics on exposed female workers. The effects were by and large benign.*

Julien RM. *Understanding anesthesia.* Reading, MA: Addison–Wesley, 1984. *A basic introduction to anesthesia written at an elementary level. Intended primarily for those who desire an overview of anesthesiology and an appreciation of its scope of practice. A valuable resource for all nurses involved in perioperative patient care.*

Miller RD, ed. *Anesthesia.* 3rd ed. New York: Churchill Livingstone, 1990. *A two-volume treatise of anesthetic practice. Perhaps the most thorough, in-depth treatment of anesthesiology currently available.*

Stoelting RK. *Pharmacology and physiology in anesthetic practice.* 2nd ed. Philadelphia: J.B. Lippincott, 1991.

Stoelting RK, Miller RD. *Basics of anesthesia.* 2nd ed. New York: 1989. Churchill Livingstone, 1989.

Waugman WR, Foster SD. New advances in anesthesia. *Nurs Clin North Am* 1991;26(2):451–461. *Discusses recent, important pharmacologic advances in anesthesia (including neuromuscular blockers and induction agents), and why they are important to nurses.*

Wood M, Wood AJJ. *Drugs and Anesthesia.* 2nd ed. Baltimore: Williams & Wilkins, 1990. *An update of a popular, readable anesthetic pharmacology text.*

Table 20–C **Clinical Uses and Administration of Major General Anesthetic Agents and Other CNS Drugs Used During General Anesthesia**

AGENT	CLINICAL USES	DOSAGE AND ROUTE OF ADMINISTRATION
Inhalation Agents		
PROTOTYPE		
Halothane (FLUOTHANE)	Maintenance of general anesthesia	0.4%–2.0% as component of inhaled anesthetic mixture
Enflurane (ETHRANE)	Same as halothane	1.0%–2.5% as component of inhaled anesthetic mixture
Isoflurane (FORANE)	Same as halothane	1.0%–3.0% as component of inhaled anesthetic mixture
Nitrous oxide	Supplement to inhaled volatile anesthetics	30%–70% as component of inhaled anesthetic (maintain minimum oxygen concentration of 30%)
	Inhaled analgesic and amnestic for conscious sedation procedures	
Parenteral Induction Agents		
Etomidate (AMIDATE)	Induction of general anesthesia	IV: Usually 0.3 mg/kg
Ketamine (KETALAR)	Induction of general anesthesia	IV: 1–4.5 mg/kg IM: 6.5–13 mg/kg
	Amnestic, analgesic sedation	IV: 0.2–0.5 mg/kg
	Maintenance of intraoperative amnesia	IV: 0.5–1.0 mg/kg/hr
Methohexital (BREVITAL)	Induction of general anesthesia	IV: 1–2 mg/kg Rectal: 15–25 mg/kg
	Maintenance of anesthesia, supplement to anesthesia	Induce as above, repeat 20–40 mg doses every 4–7 min as needed, or give 0.2% solution (in 5% dextrose solution or 0.9% sodium chloride) by continuous infusion (approximately 1 drop/sec)
Midazolam (VERSED)	Induction of general anesthesia	IV: 0.1–0.25 mg/kg
	Preanesthetic medication	IM: 0.05–0.08 mg/kg
	Amnestic sedation	IV: 0.035 mg/kg incrementally to a maximum total of 3.5–5 mg
Propofol (DIPRIVAN)	Induction of general anesthesia	IV: 2.0–2.5 mg/kg
	Maintenance of anesthesia	IV: 0.1–0.2 mg/kg/min

(continued)

Table 20–C Clinical Uses and Administration of Major General Anesthetic Agents and Other CNS Drugs Used During General Anesthesia (*Continued*)

AGENT	CLINICAL USES	DOSAGE AND ROUTE OF ADMINISTRATION
Thiamylal		
(SURITAL)	Induction of general anesthesia	IV: 2–5 μg/kg, with doses reduced as with thiopental
	Maintenance of anesthesia	Induce as above, repeat 25–50 mg doses by intermittent injection as needed, or infuse 0.3% solution slowly (eg, 1 drop/sec)
Thiopental		
(PENTOTHAL)	Induction of general anesthesia	IV: 2–6 mg/kg, with doses reduced in elderly and debilitated patients and in those with cardiovascular disease or instability
	Sole anesthetic for short (<15 min) operative procedures	Induce as above, give repeated 25–50 mg doses as needed, or give IV drip of 0.2% or 0.4% solution at rate needed to maintain desired level of anesthesia
Parenteral Anesthetic Narcotics		
Alfentanyl		
(ALFENTA)	Anesthesia induction	IV: 130–245 μg/kg over 3 min, followed by infusion of 0.5–1.5 μg/kg/min or use of inhalation general anesthetic
	Analgesic adjunct to anesthesia with barbiturate/nitrous oxide/oxygen for short surgical procedures	IV: 8–50 μg/kg over 3 min, followed by incremental injections of 3–5 μg/kg, up to total of 8–75 μg/kg; induction, incremental maintenance, and total dose depend on expected duration of anesthesia, use of assisted ventilation, etc
	Adjunct to anesthesia/analgesia with nitrous oxide/oxygen (for procedures lasting more than 45 min)	IV; Induce with 50–75 μg/kg; maintain with continuous infusion of 0.5–3.0 μg/kg/min
Fentanyl		
(SUBLIMAZE)	Intraoperative analgesia	IV: 1–5 μg/kg, up to 50–100 μg/kg for cardiac surgery
	Postoperative pain relief	IM: 50–100 μg, repeated in 1–2 hr
	Anesthetic premedication	IM: 50–100 μg 30–60 min before surgery
	Adjunct to general anesthesia	IM: 2–20 μg/kg (or give IV slowly over 1–2 min). Children 2–12: 2–3 μg/kg
	Adjunct to regional anesthesia/analgesia (incl. maintenance after induction with fentanyl)	IM: 50–100 μg (or give IV slowly over 1–2 min)
	Anesthesia (with oxygen and muscle relaxant)	IV: 50–100 μg/kg as needed (doses of 20–50 μg/kg may be used along with nitrous oxide/oxygen
Fentanyl plus droperidol		
(INNOVAR)	Preoperative tranquilizer/analgesic	IM: Adults: 0.5–2 mL 45–60 min before operative or diagnostic procedure. Children: 0.25 mL/20 lb body weight

(continued)

Table 20–C | **Clinical Uses and Administration of Major General Anesthetic Agents and Other CNS Drugs Used During General Anesthesia (*Continued*)**

AGENT	CLINICAL USES	DOSAGE AND ROUTE OF ADMINISTRATION
	Induction of general anesthesia	Slow IV: Adults: 1 mL/20–25 lb body weight. Children <12: 0.25 mL/20 lb body weight. *Note:* Maintain anesthesia with fentanyl alone (SUBLIMAZE)
Sufentanil (SUFENTA)	Anesthesia (with oxygen and muscle relaxant) during special cardiac, neurosurgical procedures	IV: 8–30 μg/kg, supplemented with oxygen and muscle relaxant drug (see fentanyl)
	Anesthetic supplement	IV: Up to 8 μg/kg, based on the doses of other anesthetics or analgesics

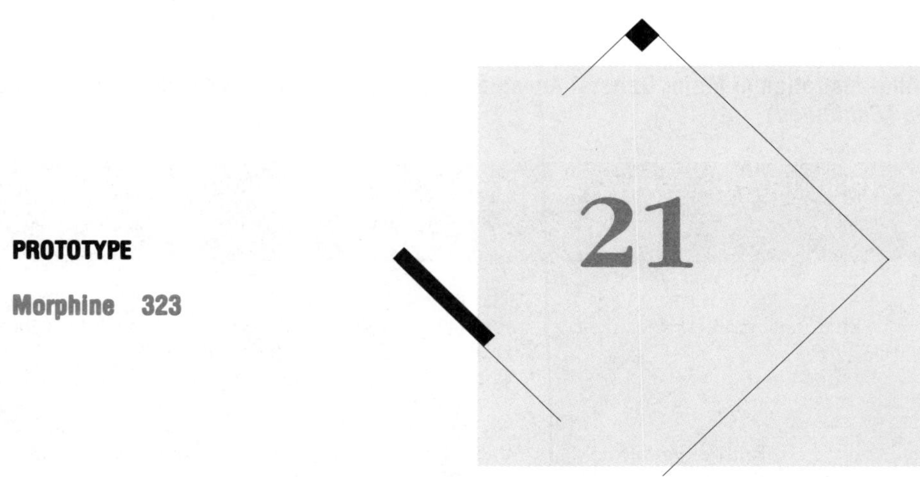

PROTOTYPE

21 Narcotic Analgesics and Their Antagonists

Analgesic drugs prevent or relieve pain. The drugs discussed in this chapter are classified as **narcotic** analgesics because they can also cause stupor or insensibility (narcosis), and their use is controlled by stringent laws. They are also classified as **opiates** because they are chemically related to morphine and codeine, the major alkaloids of the opium poppy (*Papaver somniferum*). Most of the opiates have the same major pharmacologic actions, clinical uses, and potential for abuse as morphine, the prototype. Opiates with special uses and drugs that antagonize the effects of opiates are discussed at the end of the chapter.

I. Morphine, Endogenous Morphine-Like Proteins, and Opiate Receptors

Most of the actions of morphine are due to its ability to act as an agonist for—that is, to stimulate—specific opiate receptors, the two most important of which are called mu (μ) and kappa (κ).

Opiate receptors were discovered in the late 1970s. Years before, receptors for epinephrine and acetylcholine (ACh) were found, but that was not a surprise because they were known to be important chemicals found naturally within the body. But why should the body have receptors for substances thought to occur only in poppies? More research showed that the brain and spinal cord contained a small protein (a peptide) that had morphine-like properties, including the ability to inhibit nerve signals that participated in the pain response. This peptide was called *enkephalin*. Other work found an enkephalin-like substance that was eventually named β-endorphin. It was part of a bigger molecule located in, and released by, the pituitary gland along with adrenocorticotropic hormone (ACTH), which has an important role in the body's response to severe stress, such as that triggered by pain.

Much more is now known about opiate receptors and the naturally occurring substances and drugs that stimulate or block them. It is known, for example, that pain relief caused by acupuncture involves the release of endorphins, and that this effect can be blocked by naloxone, a specific narcotic receptor blocker that has some important clinical uses based upon its ability to block the effects of morphine, heroin, and drugs like them. More recent experiments suggest that endogenous opiates (or deficiencies of them) are important not only to the response to pain and stress, but also

Major reference tables appear beginning on p 340.

to opiate addiction and, possibly, to other psychiatric disorders.

General Characteristics of Pure Narcotic Agonist Analgesics

Morphine is the prototype of all the narcotic analgesics. Although many of the other agents are more or less potent than morphine, and some produce relatively specific clinically useful effects, all the opiates share several common properties, each of which will be discussed in more detail later.

1. They act *only* as agonists on specific opiate receptors, and their effects are blocked by antagonists such as naloxone.
2. With few exceptions, they produce greater analgesia than can be produced by even high doses of nonnarcotic analgesics such as aspirin.
3. When given at doses that cause equal analgesic effects, they cause equivalent degrees of respiratory depression, a major side effect. As a result, they share common contraindications related to respiratory depression.
4. Most cause drowsiness and are able to interact with other central nervous system (CNS) depressants.
5. Tolerance develops to many of the major effects with repeated drug administration, and when tolerance develops to one opiate it develops to others. Likewise, they can cause physical dependence and are prone to abuse.
6. They cause most of the other side effects and adverse responses, and participate in other important drug–drug interactions, that are described for morphine.

PROTOTYPE

Morphine

Morphine is the standard against which all other narcotics are compared. It is often the first drug selected to control severe pain.

Absorption, Distribution, Metabolism, and Excretion

Morphine is absorbed erratically from the gastrointestinal (GI) tract, and it undergoes significant first-pass hepatic metabolism when given by this route. Morphine is distributed throughout the body, and sufficient amounts cross the blood–brain barrier to account for most of its pharmacologic effects. Morphine has a plasma half-life of about 3 hours, which is due mainly to its nearly complete metabolism in the liver. Morphine crosses the placental barrier well, and is excreted in maternal milk.

Pharmacologic Effects

Morphine causes diverse pharmacologic effects, many of which occur in the brain, through its effects on opiate receptors. The major effects are summarized in Table 21–1. The specific opiate receptor blocker naloxone will prevent or reverse most of these effects.

Central Nervous System Effects

Morphine depresses the CNS, but, unlike drugs such as alcohol or barbiturates, it does not cause uniform depression throughout the major brain structures.

Analgesia

Morphine effectively relieves severe pain, particularly dull, chronic pain, regardless of its cause or anatomic source. Analgesia is due to the drug's effects in the CNS and spinal cord. Thus, morphine differs from drugs such as aspirin that act peripherally and are effective mainly for relief of mild-to-moderate musculoskeletal pain owing to inflammation. Morphine not only alleviates pain but also alters the perception of pain, so that discomfort is less distressing or more tolerable. This subjective response is clinically beneficial. Tolerance develops to the analgesic effect, so that higher drug doses may be needed if prolonged and adequate pain relief is a clinical goal.

Other Subjective Responses

Most individuals who receive usual doses of morphine become drowsy, lethargic, and apathetic about their surroundings or condition. In the presence of pain, analgesia plus the subjective responses can allow rest or restful sleep. Typical doses usually do not cause sleep. Some individuals become paradoxically excited or excessively aroused after receiving morphine.

Morphine alters mood. Many patients, particularly those suffering from pain, become slightly euphoric. This is due partly to relief of discomfort. However, giving morphine to a pain-free individual may cause either euphoria (which contributes to the abuse of morphine and related drugs) or dysphoria—unpleasant responses such as anxiety, fear, or generalized uneasiness.

Table 21–1 Major Pharmacologic Effects of Morphine*

Organ or System Affected	Response and Comments
Central nervous system	Analgesia; sedation; drowsiness; ataxia; euphoria or dysphoria; impaired reflexes, coordination; dizziness, syncope; nausea, vomiting (increased, especially with low initial doses in ambulatory patients, suppressed with higher doses)
Eye	Miosis
Endocrine and metabolic	Increased pituitary release of ACTH, antidiuretic hormone, prolactin (and possibly growth hormone); decreased release of luteinizing hormone, thyrotropin
Respiratory	Decreased respiratory rate, depth (including tidal volume); bronchoconstriction (normally slight; due to histamine release)
Cardiovascular	Slight reduction of blood pressure, heart rate (partly due to central inhibition of autonomic control over circulation; histamine release may be involved)
Gastrointestinal	Increased tone of antrum of stomach; increased tone, decreased propulsive movements of intestines; increased tone of anal sphincter; increased tone of gallbladder, bile ducts; increased gallbladder pressure (biliary spasm not common with therapeutic doses of morphine)
Skin	Flushing, warmth, especially on face, neck, upper thorax (mainly due to histamine release)
Genitourinary	Increased tone of detrusor, bladder sphincter, ureter; slight decrease of uterine muscle tone

*Depending on the dose and the person to whom it is given, some of the effects may be desired or may be considered as side effects or adverse responses. Other opiates generally cause most of these effects, but the intensity may vary.

Respiratory Effects

Therapeutic doses of morphine usually cause respiratory depression. Low doses mainly depress respiratory depth, while higher doses also depress rate. This effect is due both to the drug's actions on the brain's medullary respiratory control center and to the drug's ability to suppress the medulla's response to blood carbon dioxide levels. Normally, a rise of blood carbon dioxide levels, as occurs when ventilation is suppressed, triggers the respiratory drive. Morphine inhibits this essential protective response. Increased blood carbon dioxide levels also elevate cerebrospinal fluid and intracranial pressures. Morphine's ability to release histamine, which causes bronchoconstriction, is another potentially adverse effect on ventilation.

The time to maximum respiratory depression varies with the route of administration, ranging from about 5 minutes after intravenous (IV) injection to an hour or more after intramuscular (IM) injection. Respiration usually returns to normal within 7 hours after a single analgesic dose is given.

Tolerance develops to respiratory depression. A person who has developed tolerance may experience only slight effects after receiving doses that could cause serious or fatal respiratory depression in a nontolerant person.

Morphine also acts in the medulla to suppress cough reflexes.

Emetic Effects

Initial administration of morphine stimulates the brain's chemoreceptor trigger zone (CTZ), or vomiting center. It also sensitizes the inner ear's vestibular apparatus, which contributes to nausea, especially in ambulatory individuals. Continued morphine administration, or administration of higher doses, suppresses the CTZ, and nausea and vomiting are less likely to occur. The morphine derivative *apomorphine* has such marked and selective ability to stimulate the CTZ that it is used primarily as an emetic.

Ocular Effects

Morphine causes miosis through a central effect on autonomic nerves that control pupil size. The iris is constricted even in very dim light, and will dilate only when so much drug has been taken that life-threatening respiratory depression and cerebral oxygen deprivation (anoxia) develop. The presence of miosis (pinpoint pupils) in long-term narcotic abusers, who have developed tolerance to many other opiate effects, indicates that tolerance does not develop to miosis.

Gastrointestinal Effects

Morphine increases smooth muscle tone in various parts of the GI tract. Major effects include reduced intestinal propulsive movements and peristalsis, and increased tone of the rectal sphincter. The overall effect is constipation. Morphine also causes spasm of the gallbladder and the biliary ducts, leading to increased biliary tract pressure.

Genitourinary Effects

The spasmogenic effects of morphine on smooth muscle of the bladder and ureters are similar to those that occur in the GI tract. Therapeutic doses generally increase the tone and amplitude of contraction of the ureter, especially the lower portion. The tone of the bladder's detrusor muscle and sphincter is increased. The actions on the bladder musculature, combined with diminished urine production through effects on blood pressure and renal blood flow, diminish the sensation of a full bladder and the desire and ability to void. Analgesic doses of morphine slightly depress uterine muscle and may prolong labor.

Cardiovascular Effects

Therapeutic doses of morphine cause few major changes in cardiovascular function, particularly in recumbent patients with relatively normal cardiovascular status. Blood pressure may fall slightly owing to a central effect that reduces sympathetic tone to veins and arterioles and releases histamine, a vasodilator. Postural hypotension in the standing individual may be especially problematic, however. Large doses of morphine, given acutely, reduce cardiac work by decreasing venous return and arterial pressure (afterload). This action is used therapeutically for patients with acute heart failure and pulmonary edema.

Morphine may cause flushing of the upper trunk, arms, neck, and face. This reflects vasodilation caused by histamine release, which is abundant in the skin in these areas.

Endocrine and Metabolic Effects

Morphine slightly elevates blood glucose levels. It does so by stimulating epinephrine release from the adrenal medulla, which in turn increases glycogen breakdown from liver and skeletal muscle.

Clinical Indications and Administration

The clinical uses and administration of morphine and the related opiates are summarized in Table 21–C1.

Analgesia

Morphine is used to control moderate to severe pain. Several administration routes can be used.

Oral and Rectal Administration

Oral therapy can be used when parenteral administration is not needed. Morphine is available in immediate-release tablets and oral solutions, which are usually given every 4 hours; and in controlled-release (slow-release) formulations (MS CONTIN, ROXANOL SR), to be given every 8 hours. Analgesic therapy ordinarily should not be started with oral dosage forms (and especially with the slow-release preparations) owing to their relatively slow onset of action, especially with initial doses. Because the drug is absorbed incompletely, and much of the first dose is metabolically inactivated in the liver owing to the first-pass effect, peak effects may require up to 2 hours to develop. These factors usually require that initial oral dosages (10–30 mg) be higher than those needed when morphine is injected. With continued administration, as blood levels stabilize, oral dosages come closer to those given by IM injection (eg, 10 mg). Overall, if oral therapy is planned, it is best to begin with parenteral administration to get blood levels into an effective range quickly.

Morphine can be instilled into the rectum, but this route is seldom used.

NURSING IMPLICATIONS

Oral solutions of morphine may be diluted in juice or another palatable beverage. Standard morphine tablets may be crushed and mixed with food if the patient has trouble swallowing. Sustained-acting tablets must be swallowed whole, and they should not be relied on for initial pain relief.

Parenteral Administration

Morphine can be given by all the major injection routes. Usual dosages are listed in Table 21–C1. The actual dose needed to keep a patient relatively pain-free and comfortable depends on the severity of pain and the patient's perception of it. For example, some patients in severe pain may require initial doses 50% of 100% higher than "usual." Larger doses will also be needed if the patient develops tolerance as the result of prolonged use. These and related issues, such as the potential development of dependence, are considered in separate Nursing Implications sections.

Table 21–2 Time to Onset and Peak Action, Duration of Action, and Equivalent Analgesic Doses of Selected Narcotic Analgesics*

	Onset (min)	Peak (hr)	Duration (hr)	Equianalgesic Dose (mg)	
				IM	Oral
Morphine	15–60	0.5–1	3–7	10	60†
Codeine	10–30	0.5–1	4–6	120	200
Hydromorphone	15–30	0.5–1	4–5	1.5	7.5
Meperidine	10–45	0.5–1	2–4	75	300
Methadone	30–60	0.5–1	4–6‡	10	20
Oxymorphone	5–10	0.5–1	3–6	1	—
Propoxyphene (oral)	30–60	2–2.5	4–6	—	130

*Data for all drugs, except propoxyphene, reflect IM injection.

†When morphine is administered repeatedly by mouth, much lower oral doses (eg, 15–25 mg) may eventually provide analgesia equivalent to 10 mg of morphine given IM.

‡With continued administration methadone's half-life and duration will be prolonged further.

Source: Adapted from *Drug Facts and Comparisons.* St. Louis, Facts and Comparisons, Inc., 1992.

With IM injection, analgesia begins in about 20 minutes and lasts 3 to 7 hours (Table 21–2). The onset of action is somewhat slower with subcutaneous (SC) injection, but the typical dose, 10 mg (for a 70-kg patient), is the same. Almost immediate pain control and subjective relief of anxiety can be achieved with IV administration. The effects are short-lived, so more prolonged pain control can be achieved by continuing with an IV infusion of the drug or by switching to other parenteral routes. Epidural infusions or intrathecal injections can be used for special circumstances (eg, intraoperatively) or for prolonged pain control.

NURSING IMPLICATIONS

Over the long run, giving narcotics at regular intervals provides better analgesia and comfort, with lower total doses, than when administration is delayed (as on a "prn" schedule) until pain becomes intolerable. Giving a proper dose of the drug 30 to 60 minutes before a planned pain-provoking activity, such as ambulation or dressing changes, also provides a better effect with less drug. A patient's complaint that pain has become unbearable before the next scheduled dose often means that the prior dose was inadequate or not timed properly. And, when the next dose is given in these instances, a much higher dose may be needed to restore adequate comfort. Such wide fluctuations in blood levels give not only wide swings in symptom relief, but also periods of greater side effects such as respiratory or generalized CNS depression.

Some patients, for a variety of valid reasons, may not wish to receive narcotics, especially by periodic injections. Some will not verbalize the need for these drugs, perhaps out of fear of becoming addicted, even though they are in pain or discomfort. Other patients, because of physical or drug-induced conditions, may not be able to express the need for more pain control. Lack of adequate analgesia not only causes discomfort but also can interfere with recovery if, for example, the patient cannot ambulate, cough or breathe deeply to clear secretions, or simply rest.

Many drawbacks associated with intermittent narcotic injection can be overcome by using a continuous drug infusion, including those that are controlled, in part, by the patient.

Patient-Controlled Analgesia

One of the most significant advances in pain control using narcotics is the development of patient-controlled analgesia (PCA). It is suitable for many patients—pediatric patients included—with postoperative pain, trauma-caused pain, or chronic pain from diseases such as cancer. This technique provides analgesic effects that are much more acceptable to patients, and to nursing personnel, than those that can be achieved with intermittent narcotic injections, whether given on a scheduled or as-needed basis. Overall, proper analgesic use, especially by PCA, facilitates recovery and can shorten the hospital stay.

Patient-controlled analgesia is based on the pharmacologic principle that giving small narcotic doses fre-

SPOTLIGHT ON NURSING RESEARCH

Patients provide the best source of information about the pain they are experiencing. When nurses and other health professionals rely on their own observations and judgments to evaluate patients' pain, they often underestimate severity, leading to inadequate pain management. Furthermore, lack of consistent documentation frequently hampers coordinated pain control efforts.

In this study, nurses teamed up with a clinical pharmacist to test the hypothesis that the use of standardized documentation tools would improve patients' pain control, as evidenced by lower pain intensity ratings. The investigators employed a 0 to 10 numerical rating scale to evaluate the intensity of pain in a documented problem of pain. Data collection occurred at random times for three consecutive days.

Consenting subjects were asked to rate the intensity of their pain at the time of questioning ("now" pain) and to rate the "worst," "least," and "average" pain experienced during the previous 24 hours. Following data collection from 23 control subjects, brief inservice and written instructions were used to introduce a patient assessment tool and pain flow sheet to the nursing staff. Pain ratings were then obtained from 20 treatment group subjects.

The patient assessment tool was originally developed by Meinhart (1983),[1] and the pain flow sheet was designed by McMillan et al. (1988).[2] In the present study, the original tools were used with only minor modifications. The assessment tool evaluated affective, cognitive, behavioral, and sensory components of a patient's pain, and was to be completed as an initial pain assessment. The pain flow sheet was to be completed at least once each shift. This form documented pharmacologic and nonpharmacologic interventions for pain and also included the patient's evaluation of pain using the numerical rating scale.

On day 1, "now" pain ratings were significantly higher in treatment as compared to control group subjects; no other differences were observed. By day 3, however, subjects in treatment group tended to report a lower intensity of "now" pain and rated their "average" pain as significantly lower than that experienced by the control group. When compared with the control group, a significantly greater number of treatment group subjects reported a reduction in "now" and "average" pain ratings from day 1 to day 3. These results are only indicative of pain control outcomes using the pain flow sheet, since poststudy review revealed that use of the patient assessment tool was inconsistent.

As hypothesized, the findings of this study support the use of a standardized pain flow sheet to improve pain control, in agreement with other research. The authors suggest that the need for duplicate charting may have hindered use of the patient assessment tool. Although based on a small convenience sample, a strength of this work is related to the selection of valid, previously tested documentation tools. Within institutions, small studies may be essential to acquire staff support for the implementation of standardized documentation, to document the feasibility of this approach, and to justify the inclusion of these forms in patients' permanent medical records.

[1]Meinhart NT, McCaffery M: *Pain: A Nursing Approach to Assessment and Analysis.* Norwalk, CT: Appleton-Century-Crofts, 1983.

[2]McMillian SC et al.: A validity and reliability study of two tools for assessing and managing pain. *Oncol Nurs Forum* 1988;15:735–741.

Faries JE, Mills DS, Goldsmith KW, Phillips KD, Orr J: Systematic pain records and their impact on pain control a pilot study. *Cancer Nurs* 1991;14:306–313.

quently (or continuously) provides better and more stable pain control (from steadier blood levels of the drug) than less frequent injections of larger doses. Although PCA systems differ somewhat, each consists of an electronically controlled infusion pump that connects a drug reservoir (usually containing morphine or the related drug meperidine; p 334) to an indwelling catheter, usually in a peripheral vein. Like most infusion pumps, the pump on a PCA apparatus is set to give a constant, low-dose infusion of the drug. However, these systems are also attached to a switch that the patient can activate, triggering the infusion of a small but nevertheless effective bolus of drug when needed. Nursing or medical personnel preset the pump so the amount of drug that is infused continuously, the amount given when the patient activates the switch, and the total amount administered over a specified time (eg, 1 hour), cannot exceed a certain limit. Thus, patients can exert some control over their own analgesic therapy: they can trigger an additional dose as soon as increased pain is sensed (or in anticipation of a painful procedure, such as ambulation or a dressing change), without having to

SPOTLIGHT ON NURSING RESEARCH

Self-report measures are accepted as a valid method of pain assessment for adults. In children, the usefulness of this type of pain assessment has been controversial. However, there is increasing recognition that children can communicate about their pain in meaningful ways. Such communication is essential for effective pain treatment.

The "Oucher" scale is a self-report instrument that has been shown to provide an effective measure of pain intensity in preschool and young school-age children. The scale used for children 3 to 7 years of age consists of six photographs of a 4-year-old European-American boy. These photographs are arranged in a manner to show increasing levels of pain through facial expressions. To use the scale, the children select the picture most closely illustrating what he or she "hurts like."

The Oucher scale is a tested, easy-to-use tool, but validation of the instrument has not included culturally diverse populations. This study focused on the development of measures to assist young Hispanic and African-American children to communicate about pain. The authors' initial objective was to test the Oucher scale with African-American and Hispanic children. However, it was decided that this approach would not address concerns about the instrument's cultural relevance and sensitivity. Therefore, alternative Oucher scales for both Hispanic and African-American children were developed using a conceptual framework derived from Orem's Self-Care Theory of Nursing.[1]

African-American and Hispanic adults, as well as 3- to 7-year-old children, participated in instrumental development. Informed consent was obtained from both children and their parents. Interviews were used to determine children's understanding of the concept of "pain" or "hurt." Photographs of facial expressions were taken of one Hispanic child and three African-American children when the children were experiencing pain and at times when they were pain-free. Like the Oucher, the final scales contained six photographs that ranged from expressions of "no hurt at all" to "the biggest hurt you could ever have." Adults limited the initial series of 40 to 60 photographs of each child to a set of 18 photographs that were then sorted by children of the same ethnic group. To evaluate children's developmental capability to understand the concept of photographic sorting, they were asked to perform a simple task: put six equilateral triangles of varying sizes in an order from smallest to largest. Only data from children who were able to complete the task successfully were included in the ranking analysis used to create the final scales.

Following instrument development, the content validity of the scales was examined by a second group of African-American (n=143) and Hispanic (n=112) children. The children were asked to select the picture showing "no hurt at all" and to place it at the bottom of a "sticky board."

The selected picture showing "the biggest hurt you could ever have" was placed at the top of the board, and then the next illustration of "the biggest hurt" was chosen from the remaining pictures until all were used. There was a strong measure of within-group agreement on the order of the photographs for both groups when children were able to complete the geometric task successfully. However, the instrument was not found to be a valid measure of pain intensity for the 15% of children from each group that were unable to perform this task.

The authors note that the accurate assessment of pain in children has clear implications for pain relief. This study demonstrates that African-American and Hispanic children as young as 3 years old can make and communicate judgments about pain. Moreover, the findings suggest that a brief, geometric task may be useful in determining the ability of a child to assess and to communicate his or her pain using Oucher type scales.

While additional validity testing is warranted, this study makes a significant contribution to nursing practice and research through the development of a valid, culturally appropriate tool for pain assessment in children.

[1]Orem DE: *Nursing: Concepts of practice.* 4th ed. New York: Mosby, 1991.

Villarruel AM, Denyes MJ: Pain assessment in children: Theoretical and empirical validity. *Adv Nurs Sci* 1991;14(2):32–41.

wait for a nurse to administer the drug; yet, because of a "lock-out" feature on the pump, they cannot overdose themselves. The pumps can also be set to give a higher continuous infusion dose at night, so sleep is less likely to be interrupted by pain. Epidural narcotic administration via PCA is also becoming more common.

NURSING IMPLICATIONS

Explain to the patient how PCA works. If the patient is to undergo a procedure (eg, surgery), and PCA is likely to be used afterward, do your initial teaching beforehand, then review your instructions and answer other questions afterward. Key points of patient teaching include what the apparatus does, and how the patient will operate it; it is important to allay concerns that an accidental overdose might occur if the patient activates the machine too often. Advise patients that activating the switch will trigger drug delivery, but that it may take 5 to 10 minutes for them to sense the full effect, and advise them before the start of a pain-provoking procedure so they can time the bolus properly.

Other Uses

Adjunct to Mechanical Ventilation

Many patients who require mechanically assisted or supported ventilation have enough respiratory drive to "fight" the ventilator. Curare-like neuromuscular blockers or high doses of diazepam are often used to overcome the drive, but they do not provide analgesia, which may also be needed. Relatively high IM or IV doses of morphine (≥20 mg) may be given. As long as ventilation is supported properly and vital signs are kept normal, few problems result from this practice. This is another instance in which morphine-induced respiratory depression is desirable.

Adjunctive Therapy of Acute Cardiac Failure and Pulmonary Edema

Morphine (2–4 mg given IV as needed) plays an important part in the emergency management of acute heart failure and the pulmonary edema that often accompanies it. In this situation morphine

- reduces afterload and venous return to the heart, which reduces the heart's workload and lessens congestion in the pulmonary circulation;
- relieves anxiety; and
- helps convert rapid, inefficient, and distressing breathing efforts to slower, less laborious, and more efficient breathing, which improves oxygen and carbon dioxide exchange.

NURSING IMPLICATIONS

Since morphine causes adverse respiratory effects, pay close attention to the patient's blood gases and vital signs during this medical emergency.

Adjunct to Anesthesia, Special Anesthesia

Analgesic doses of morphine can be used as a preanesthetic medication. Very high doses (1 mg/kg IV) can be used as a special anesthetic agent, particularly for cardiac surgery and some neurosurgical procedures in which the physiologic stresses caused by other general anesthetics must be avoided. (Anesthetic doses are higher than doses that otherwise would cause fatal respiratory depression, but the patient's ventilation and cardiovascular status are supported.) The use of injectable narcotics specifically indicated for anesthesia (alfentanyl, fentanyl, sufentanil) is discussed in Chapter 20.

Management of Diarrhea and Cough

Morphine can be used to control diarrhea or to suppress cough. However, morphine's potentially serious effects limit its routine use for these purposes. Related drugs with selective antidiarrheal or antitussive activity are usually preferred; they are discussed below.

Side Effects, Adverse Reactions, and Contraindications

Many of the pharmacologic effects of morphine may be considered as side effects in some patients. Some may be unavoidable, even when therapeutic doses are given. They are summarized in Table 21–S.

Nausea, vomiting, and *hypotension* are relatively common side effects, especially in ambulatory patients. Because morphine can lower blood pressure and interfere with some important cardiovascular reflexes, it is generally contraindicated in patients with shock or bradycardia.

Biliary spasm, constipation, and *urinary retention* may occur. Gallbladder and biliary tract spasm may cause intense pain in persons with gallstones or pancreatitis, for whom morphine is usually contraindicated. In some patients morphine's ability to stimulate the urinary bladder's detrusor muscle outweighs its ability to increase sphincter tone, and so urinary urgency could occur. However, the drug's CNS effects usually dull perception of a full bladder or bowel, so urinary retention and constipation are more common.

Respiratory depression is the most dangerous consequence of acute morphine administration. It may cause serious alterations of blood gases and brain oxygenation if the patient's ventilatory status is not monitored and managed properly. As noted earlier, respiratory depression is likely to be greatest after parenteral administration, particularly in patients who have not developed tolerance through prior narcotic use. Morphine is therefore generally contraindicated for most patients who are not on ventilators and who have poor pulmonary function (unless caused by acute pulmonary edema), including patients with emphysema or asthma. Many asthmatic patients are at added risk from morphine's ability to cause histamine release and intense bronchoconstriction.

Other important contraindications related to respiratory depression include closed head injury or recent brain surgery. In either case, increased intracranial pressure, cerebral vasodilation, and hypotension can aggravate brain damage. These effects, combined with sedation, confusion, alterations of subjective responses, and suppression of some reflexes, can severely hamper evaluation of the patient's neurologic status.

Impaired hepatic function prolongs morphine's duration of action and can intensify its effects. The drug is relatively contraindicated in patients with severe hepatic failure, including persons with alcohol-induced hepatic damage. In the presence of lesser degrees of hepatic dysfunction, it may be necessary to reduce the dose or prolong the dosage interval.

True allergic reactions to morphine are rare. The skin rashes or flushing that sometimes occur usually are reflections of histamine release.

NURSING IMPLICATIONS

All the organ systems that are affected by the opiates should be monitored closely. A physician should be notified and drug administration delayed if

- the patient appears excessively sedated or confused;
- respiration is shallow or respiratory rate is less than 12 per minute;
- there is evidence or suspicion of neurologic impairment owing to any undiagnosed cause; or
- heart rate or blood pressure is low.

If the patient's condition permits it, periodic changes of position and respiratory therapy will help guard against possible atelectasis and poor ventilation.

Since nausea, vomiting, and postural hypotension are more likely to occur or be severe in ambulatory patients, the best intervention is to have the patient return to bed if these problems arise. Protect patients from falls by raising bed rails, assisting with ambulation, and so on.

Monitor fluid intake and output in hospitalized patients to help detect constipation and urinary retention, and encourage fluid and fiber intake as permitted by the patient's overall condition to minimize these problems. Encourage patients to urinate every 4 hours or so, and palpate the lower abdomen periodically to determine whether the bowel or bladder is full.

Tolerance and Physical Dependence

According to federal law morphine and many other narcotic analgesics noted in this chapter are classified as Schedule II drugs, an indication of their high potential for abuse, mainly for euphoric effects. With continued administration, **tolerance** and **physical dependence** can occur.

Tolerance is a general term indicating that through one or more processes associated with repeated drug administration, the body adapts to the presence of the drug. Higher doses are then required to produce a given response. For narcotics, analgesia, euphoria, and respiratory depression are probably the most important effects to which tolerance develops. Narcotic analgesics also participate in a phenomenon called *cross-tolerance:* If a person becomes tolerant to the actions of one opiate, he or she will also be tolerant to the actions of others. Tolerance to the euphoric effects explains why individuals addicted to opiates often require very high doses to continue deriving satisfaction; tolerance to respiratory depression explains why they are not killed by drug doses that would be lethal for a nontolerant person.

Physical dependence is a condition in which sufficient levels of drug must be continuously present to maintain the person's current biochemical, physiologic, or psychologic status, even though it may be altered from what is normal for a drug-free person. If physical dependence occurs, a withdrawal syndrome develops when drug administration is stopped, inadequate doses are taken, or a narcotic antagonist is administered. Withdrawal signs and symptoms are discussed in the next section. The opiates also cause **cross-dependence:** If a person who is physically dependent on one opiate takes appropriate doses of another, the withdrawal syndrome will not occur.

NURSING IMPLICATIONS

If a switch from one narcotic to another is ordered, be aware that higher-than-usual doses of the new drug will be necessary if the patient has developed tolerance.

There is excessive concern about the development of physical dependence to morphine and related drugs used for valid indications. The true incidence of physical dependence is under 1% for patients receiving narcotics for fewer than 10 days, and the risk of addiction (craving the drug after the pain is gone) is even less. Although some degree of tolerance usually develops when narcotics are administered for pain, many more patients will require progressively lower doses as the causes of pain subside. Advise patients and their families of this low risk to allay concerns, and identify the problems that may arise if the patient is undermedicated. However, if the patient is receiving adequate analgesic doses, but frequently requests narcotics, review the history and medication record for indications of prior abuse, and assess for anxiety or true alterations of comfort that may cause excessive requests. For patients with severe, terminal pain, providing comfort and the ability to interact meaningfully with others is the primary concern. Although such patients may require very high narcotic doses, and physical dependence may develop, concerns over these issues should not prevent administration of any narcotic dose that is needed.

Withdrawal

Narcotic withdrawal is distressing. But, unlike the situation with barbiturate or alcohol withdrawal (see Chapter 22), it is rarely if ever fatal, even without treatment. The major signs and symptoms appear as a reversal of many of morphine's pharmacologic effects, and resemble a severe case of influenza. Respiration, blood pressure, and body temperature rise. Muscle aches develop and the patient complains of being cold and extremely uncomfortable. Nausea; vomiting; profuse diarrhea, lacrimation, and sweating; and significant piloerection ("goose flesh") occur. Many of these signs reflect increased activity of the autonomic nervous system. Anxiety and insomnia occur.

The severity of withdrawal depends on the degree of tolerance that has developed, which in turn depends on the drug, its dosage, and how long it has been taken. The speed with which withdrawal occurs, and its duration, depends on the duration of action of the drug responsible for dependence. For example, withdrawal from morphine will appear sooner and be more intense, and have a shorter duration, than withdrawal from a long-acting narcotic such as methadone. This is one reason why methadone is used to treat physical dependence and to wean individuals from narcotics.

NURSING IMPLICATIONS

Be able to recognize the early signs and symptoms of withdrawal. Focus nursing care on monitoring and supporting vital signs and fluid and electrolyte balance, and on supporting psychologic responses. Institute appropriate measures to prevent self-inflicted injury to the patient.

◆ Use During Pregnancy and Lactation

Babies born to mothers who are physically dependent on opiates have a high risk of being physically dependent, and may undergo withdrawal after delivery. Some may also require administration of the narcotic antagonist, naloxone, to restore normal respiration. It is essential to stress to women the need to avoid taking narcotics (and virtually all other drugs except as ordered by a physician) during pregnancy.

Morphine should not be given routinely for analgesia during childbirth, since it may prolong labor by inhibiting uterine contractions, and cause respiratory depression in the newborn. Narcotics with shorter actions (see Table 21–C1) are preferred. Regardless of the narcotic selected, to avoid delayed parturition and neonatal respiratory depression, give the drug only after uterine contractions have become regular. Fetal vital signs and ventilation must be checked and normalized at once.

◆ Use in Children

Morphine doses are based on body weight. Children usually receive 0.1 to 0.2 mg/kg per dose, with a maximum of 15 mg.

◆ Use in the Elderly

Elderly patients should be given reduced doses to avoid excessive sedation, confusion, a "detached" feeling, respiratory depression, and hypotension. Interventions such as positioning, careful handling of injured tissues, application of heat or cold, relief of pressure, and nondrug measures to alleviate stress and anxiety and promote relaxation can help reduce analgesic requirements. Elderly patients are at greater risk of urinary retention and constipation; standard nondrug measures should be implemented to prevent or treat these conditions.

Interactions with Other Drugs

The narcotic analgesics interact with all other drugs that also cause CNS depression (Table 21–I). The potential outcome is excessive CNS depression and any of its consequences; the greatest risk is excessive respiratory depression. Cimetidine (Chapter 40), one of the most widely used antiulcer drugs, may also intensify the CNS depressant effects of morphine and most other narcotics. This interaction is thought to occur because cimetidine inhibits the hepatic metabolism of the opiates, thereby increasing their blood levels and effects.

Interactions Owing to Incompatibilities

Injectable formulations of morphine and other narcotics may interact physically or chemically if they are mixed with other injectable drugs. These medication *incompatibilities* are most likely to occur in pre- and postoperative settings, in which alleviating pain and other common responses to surgery are important goals. The result of these interactions usually is the inactivation of one or both medications, so that their effects are reduced or eliminated. In other cases, however, drugs may precipitate; injecting precipitated chemicals into a vein is dangerous, and potentially fatal.

Examples of incompatible drugs include most barbiturates, which might be used to cause added sedation; anxiety-relieving drugs such as diazepam; atropine, which might be used to reduce airway secretions or control cardiovascular changes; drugs such as hydroxyzine, used to control nausea and vomiting; anticonvulsants such as phenytoin; and the injectable anticoagulant heparin.

Whether one drug is (in)compatible with another depends not only on the actual medications, but also on how and when they are mixed and administered. Some drugs may be incompatible when mixed together, in relatively dilute concentrations, in an IV fluid that is to be infused; some react when they eventually mix if they are infused through a common "Y-site" on an IV setup; and others are incompatible if mixed in the same syringe, which might be done if they are to be injected directly (eg, by the IM route). Some incompatibilities are easy to spot: there may be a color change or the appearance of cloudiness in an IV bag or syringe. However, others occur without any obvious sign.

The time during which drugs are in contact with one another before administration is also important. For example, many injectable drugs that are listed as "compatible" with another when mixed in the same syringe (see Appendix Table D–1) are compatible for only 15 minutes or so. That means that they must be given within that time. Other medications are instantaneously incompatible, and cannot be mixed together no matter how soon thereafter you give them.

NURSING IMPLICATIONS

It is not necessary to memorize the various drug–drug incompatibilities, but it is important to know the general concept. If it is your responsibility to mix two injectable drugs, always check a current information source (eg, package inserts or a knowledgeable pharmacy professional in your facility) before mixing and injecting two or more drugs.

It is often necessary to administer morphine with some of its interactants. The patient's respiratory, cardiac, and general neurologic status must be followed closely. Reduced doses of the narcotic, the interactant, or both, are often needed to reduce the chance of excessive effects. If severe CNS depression occurs, reduce the doses of one or all interactants. The narcotic antagonist naloxone may need to be given, and assisted ventilation may be needed; have these ready to use. In general, whenever a narcotic is given, alone or with other drugs, anticipate excessive respiratory depression and have the means to deal with it readily available.

Become familiar with the parenteral drugs that are physically incompatible with morphine. If there is any doubt, use separate syringes for each.

Overdose and Toxicity

Signs and Symptoms

Four times the usual analgesic dose of any narcotic analgesic (eg, 40 mg of IM morphine), given parenterally to a nontolerant person, is usually lethal unless treatment is begun promptly. Pinpoint pupils and varying degrees of depressed respiration, consciousness, and blood pressure indicate overdoses with most opiates. Respiratory depression is the most serious consequence. Cheyne–Stokes respiration develops, followed by respiratory arrest and cerebral or brainstem anoxia. As respiration and brain oxygenation progressively decline, inhibited function of cardiovascular control centers in the CNS lead to hypotension and possible cardiovascular collapse. The pupils will remain small and almost completely unresponsive to light until profound brain damage has occurred, at which time they will become fixed and dilated.

Treatment

Treatment is generally straightforward. Injection of the antagonist naloxone usually restores both CNS and cardiovascular function. Mechanical support of ventilation is almost always required until naloxone's effects appear and the patient can maintain adequate spontaneous ventilation. Parenteral fluids or sympathomimetics may be necessary to support cardiovascular status further. The important use of naloxone for both treatment and diagnosis of narcotic overdoses is discussed later.

Related Drugs

Several other drugs (see Table 21–C1) are pharmacologically related to morphine. Most are classified as ***pure narcotic agonists,*** meaning that they produce the main pharmacologic effects noted for morphine.

Morphine-Like Pure Narcotic Agonists

Most drugs discussed in this section, and others listed in Table 21–C1, are used mainly as analgesics; some have special uses that do not depend on analgesic activity. They are either semisynthetic morphine derivatives or are completely synthetic. Most of these drugs share the general properties of all opiates, which were noted in the beginning of the chapter. Some differ in terms of analgesic potency (milligrams needed to cause equivalent analgesia), but they are as effective as morphine for relieving severe pain. Table 21–2 lists doses equivalent to a 10-mg dose of morphine, along with typical onsets and durations of action. Others are less efficacious, and are indicated only for relief of relatively mild or moderate pain.

Codeine

Codeine (methylmorphine) is the only legal narcotic analgesic other than morphine that is isolated from the opium poppy. Codeine phosphate can be given orally or injected intramuscularly or subcutaneously; codeine sulfate is given only orally. Codeine has about one tenth the analgesic potency of morphine, and is generally used for mild-to-moderate pain. Analgesic doses of codeine cause less respiratory depression and less intracranial pressure increases than morphine, and so it is often a preferred analgesic for patients with head injury or slightly impaired neurologic status. If high doses are given to any patient in an inappropriate attempt to relieve severe pain, codeine may cause more sedation, constipation, and orthostatic hypotension than a proper morphine dose.

Codeine has about five times the analgesic potency of aspirin or acetaminophen, and it is often administered with one of these nonnarcotic pain relievers. The combination seems to provide analgesia superior to that which can be provided by even high doses of any of the drugs given alone. Proprietary mixtures of codeine with aspirin or acetaminophen are classified as Schedule III agents.

Codeine is also widely used as an antitussive (see Table 21–C1 for dosages).

NURSING IMPLICATIONS

Oral codeine often causes nausea or GI upset. Giving the drug with food may reduce distress.

Fentanyl

Fentanyl (as SUBLIMAZE), a potent morphine-like analgesic, has been available for years as an IV anesthetic (Chapter 20, pp 315–316). The drug is also available in a transdermal delivery system that is marketed as DURAGESIC. It is indicated for long-term pain control, such as for patients with chronic or terminal cancer pain. The transdermal delivery system is basically an adhesive "patch" that contains the drug. Applied to the skin, it releases the fentanyl gradually but steadily through the skin and into the bloodstream over its life, 72 hours, at which time the patch is replaced. This route bypasses the first-pass metabolism that would inactivate oral fentanyl, and makes repeated injection or continuous IV infusion (a major drawback for long-term therapy) unnecessary.

NURSING IMPLICATIONS

Transdermal fentanyl offers ease of dosing, consistent effects, and convenience, for chronic pain control. All this can be a boon to patients and caregivers. However, like other narcotics administered by other routes, transdermal fentanyl may cause all the side effects, adverse reactions, and drug interactions noted for morphine. Potential problems are more likely to occur in the elderly—the patients most likely to receive DURAGESIC. The transdermal route itself entails special considerations. The patch releases the drug slowly, and so is unsuitable for initial analgesic therapy or for management of episodes of increased pain. (This general principle applies to other transdermally delivered drugs, such as clonidine and nitroglycerin.) Therefore, other analgesics, given at proper dosages and by more rapidly acting injectable routes, will be needed for coverage. With combined narcotic administration in these instances, it is essential to assess closely and frequently for narcotic–narcotic interactions (particularly respiratory depression), which are best prevented by reducing the dose of the injected drug. Removal of the patch in the event of adverse effects or interactions—one proper action—requires at least 12 hours of close monitoring while the drug slowly clears from the body. The narcotic antagonist naloxone can be used for intense, acute adverse effects or narcotic interactions.

Heroin

Heroin is diacetyl morphine. This slight chemical difference makes heroin more lipid soluble than morphine, allowing faster entry into the brain, especially when it is injected intravenously. This rapid CNS effect, and the resulting euphoria, accounts for the popularity of heroin as a drug of abuse. Once the drug reaches the brain it is eventually converted into morphine, which causes all the pharmacologic effects.

In some countries, heroin is a legal drug that is used as an analgesic, even though it is no more effective than other narcotics, such as morphine, when they are given in adequate doses. In the United States, heroin is classified as a Schedule I drug. That means it has no medical use, and its manufacture, importation, or possession is illegal.

Hydromorphone

Hydromorphone (DILAUDID) is approximately five to ten times as potent as morphine sulfate, but the drug has a similar onset and duration of action. Oral, parenteral, and rectal dosage forms are available. The drug is indicated for moderate-to-severe pain. It is one of the most soluble narcotic analgesics, so it is often preferred for patients who require large IV narcotic doses but cannot tolerate the large volumes of parenteral solutions needed to give other narcotics. Oral hydromorphone is also indicated for management of cough, but codeine is used much more frequently. Hydromorphone is a popular drug of abuse on the street and among health-care professionals.

NURSING IMPLICATIONS

A concentrated preparation of hydromorphone (DILAUDID HP) is available. It contains 10 mg/mL of drug, compared with the 1 to 4 mg/mL found in other injectable preparations. Although DILAUDID HP is packaged differently, it is important to double-check the label before administration to avoid a potentially serious overdose.

Meperidine

Meperidine (DEMEROL) is used for analgesia, as a preoperative medication, and as an anesthetic supplement. Meperidine has approximately the same potency as morphine, and a somewhat shorter duration of action. It causes less fetal respiratory depression than most other narcotics, and so is more suitable for obstetric analgesia. Meperidine is available combined with the major tranquilizer promethazine as the proprietary product MEPERGAN; it is used as a preoperative sedative/analgesic.

Meperidine causes less urinary retention, constipation, and antitussive activity than morphine. Unlike most other narcotic analgesics, therapeutic doses of meperidine may cause mydriasis, and so it should be administered with caution (or avoided) in patients with glaucoma.

Toxic doses of meperidine cause not only morphine-like respiratory depression but also signs of cortical stimulation: muscle twitches or tremors, hyperreflexia, agitation, increased responsiveness to external stimuli, hallucinations, and seizures. The meperidine derivative propoxyphene (DARVON, DARVOCET) causes similar toxic responses.

Meperidine participates in two important drug–drug interactions that do not involve morphine or most other injectable narcotics. Both are serious and should be avoided. The most serious interaction involves monoamine oxidase (MAO) inhibitors, a class of antidepressants (see Chapter 24). The outcome is severe CNS stimulation and seizures that may progress quickly to coma and respiratory arrest. This interaction may occur even if meperidine is given to a patient who has stopped taking a MAO inhibitor several weeks before. The other interaction involves phenothiazine antipsychotic drugs (Chapter 23), which are widely used. The outcome is an acute episode of excessive sedation and hypotension.

NURSING IMPLICATIONS

Have patients take syrups containing meperidine with a full glass of water to minimize a local anesthetic effect in the mouth. Subcutaneous injections are painful and not recommended.

If meperidine is used in labor and delivery, avoid

giving the drug until uterine contractions have become regular. Monitor the newborn closely for respiratory depression.

Withhold meperidine administration, and notify the physician, if the patient shows signs of significant CNS stimulation from the previous dose, or it caused ocular pain that could indicate a glaucoma attack. If a meperidine overdose occurs, allow the patient to rest quietly during monitoring, and avoid disruptive visual and auditory stimuli.

Methadone

Methadone (DOLOPHINE), which has analgesic potency equivalent to morphine, has the longest duration of action of any narcotic. Its plasma half-life is initially about 24 hours, and may become longer after repeated administration. The drug is used as an analgesic for relief of severe pain, particularly when pain is chronic and sedation will benefit the patient. Since the drug has such a long half-life, and several days are needed for its blood levels and analgesic effects to stabilize, analgesic therapy is begun with shorter-acting narcotics, which are then tapered as methadone's effects develop. Methadone is unsuitable as a prepartum analgesic because of its ability to cause significant and longlasting fetal respiratory depression.

Methadone, usually given orally, is a primary therapy for detoxification or temporary maintenance treatment of narcotic addiction. Detoxification therapy is based on the concept of substituting one addicting narcotic (methadone) for another (such as heroin). Then, under close daily supervision, the methadone dosage is gradually reduced to produce withdrawal. Since methadone has a long duration of action, withdrawal is mild, gradual, and more tolerable.

NURSING IMPLICATIONS

By law, methadone detoxification therapy must last no more than 21 consecutive days. Such treatment for addiction lasting more than 21 consecutive days is considered maintenance therapy. Methadone maintenance or detoxification therapy can be done only in approved, supervised centers. Methadone can be given as an analgesic for as long as it is medically justified.

The person responsible for dispensing methadone to outpatients should witness ingestion of the drug to prevent the possibility of hoarding or sale to others. Anticipate that withdrawal symptoms will begin 36 to 72 hours after detoxification treatment is begun and will last 10 to 14 days.

Opiates and Opiate Derivatives Used Mainly for Managing Diarrhea

Diphenoxylate (in LOMOTIL, which also contains atropine) and loperamide (IMODIUM) are meperidine derivatives used exclusively as antidiarrheal drugs. They have no useful analgesic action and a relatively low abuse potential. However, overdoses may cause significant morphine-like CNS and respiratory depression. Another common opiate antidiarrheal is paregoric (camphorated tincture of opium). Paregoric contains 0.4% opium (equivalent to 0.04% morphine). It should not be confused with plain opium tincture, which contains 10% opium (1% morphine); accidentally giving opium tincture instead of paregoric is liable to cause serious toxicity. Antidiarrheal drugs, and related nursing implications, are discussed in Chapter 41.

Opiates and Opiate Derivatives Used for Managing Cough

The use of codeine and hydromorphone as cough suppressants was noted earlier. They, and the related drug hydrocodone (HYCODAN; see Table 21–C1), are clearly effective, but they pose some risk of typical morphine-like side effects and have a relatively high abuse potential.

Dextromethorphan, which is chemically related to the opiates, has antitussive activity and few of the other beneficial or deleterious properties of the other drugs. It causes no analgesia or euphoria, very little sedation, and has no abuse potential, yet its antitussive activity is equivalent to codeine. It is not classified as a narcotic. Dextromethorphan is found in many over-the-counter (OTC) cough and cold products. It is used for symptomatic relief of coughs that frequently accompany the common cold.

NURSING IMPLICATIONS

Antitussive drugs are most appropriately used to suppress nonproductive cough, particularly when coughing interferes with wound healing, comfort, or sleep. However, in many instances cough is beneficial, especially when it is productive. Antitussive agents can be prescribed with expectorants or mucus-thinning drugs to help remove secretions from the respiratory tract.

When permissible, keeping the patient well hydrated by oral fluid intake (1 to 2 liters of water daily) will help thin and remove respiratory secretions.

Opiates Used for Anesthesia

The uses of narcotics in the setting of general anesthesia were discussed in Chapter 20. The drugs are alfentanyl (ALFENTA), fentanyl (SUBLIMAZE, also an ingredient in INNOVAR), and sufentanyl (SUFENTA). Fentanyl is also used as an analgesic. The parenteral dosage form, owing to its very short duration of action that necessitates frequent administration, is relatively unsuitable for managing all but relatively brief episodes of pain. Transdermal fentanyl (DURAGESIC), used for chronic pain control, was discussed above.

Opiate Derivatives Used as Peripheral Vasodilators

Papaverine (eg, PAVABID) and ethaverine (ETHATAB, others) are alkaloids isolated from the opium poppy. They have no narcotic activity, or uses or abuse potential typically associated with morphine. They are vasodilators used to relieve peripheral, cerebral, or coronary vasospasm; ethaverine has also been used as a GI or genitourinary antispasmodic. There is no objective evidence that these drugs are effective in these conditions, and they have the potential to cause adverse effects. Nothing more will be said about these drugs; consult package inserts if your patient is receiving one of them.

II. Mixed Narcotic Agonist-Antagonists

Five drugs (see Table 21–C2 for dosages) are classified as mixed narcotic agonist-antagonists, and are indicated mainly for the relief of mild-to-moderate pain: buprenorphine (BUPRENEX), butorphanol (STADOL), dezocine (DALGAN), nalbuphine (NUBAIN), and pentazocine (TALWIN). This mixed agonist-antagonist classification means that, under some circumstances, these drugs stimulate opiate receptors. However, they also block the ability of the pure narcotic agonists (eg, morphine) to interact with and stimulate those same receptors.

What this means in clinical use is that when one of these drugs is given at proper doses to a patient who has received no other narcotic, it causes the desired analgesia. This is how these drugs *should* be used. (Additionally, they can cause all the other unwanted effects noted for morphine, so these should be assessed for also.) However, when any mixed agonist-antagonist is given to a patient who is already receiving morphine or a pure narcotic agonist, it will antagonize the effects of the other drug. In this instance, it counteracts analgesia, and can induce withdrawal if the patient is physically dependent on another opiate. This is how these mixed-acting drugs should *not* be used.

Of the five drugs, pentazocine is noteworthy for several reasons that relate to its formulations. Pentazocine is available alone or in fixed-dose combinations with either acetaminophen (marketed as TALACEN) or aspirin (TALWIN Compound). Another product, TALWIN NX, contains pentazocine plus the narcotic *antagonist* naloxone. This orally administered product seems to be an illogical drug combination, but it is not. It was formulated to reduce the potential for abuse. The amount of naloxone in the product is so low that when the tablet is ingested—the proper administration route—so little of the antagonist reaches the bloodstream that it does essentially nothing. However, when the product is dissolved so it can be injected intravenously, as a narcotics abuser may do, the amount of naloxone is sufficient to block pentazocine's euphoric effect, thereby curtailing further use of this product. If the abuser is physically dependent on opiates, this practice may get enough of the antagonist into the bloodstream to induce withdrawal.

All the desired and unwanted effects of the mixed narcotic agonist-antagonists are prevented or reversed by pure narcotic antagonists such as naloxone, which are discussed in the next section.

NURSING IMPLICATIONS

Never administer any mixed narcotic agonist-antagonist to persons already receiving a pure agonist narcotic. Doing so will cause return or intensification of pain. Similarly, do not give them to persons known to be physically dependent on a narcotic, since withdrawal may occur.

III. Pure Narcotic Antagonists

Naloxone and naltrexone (Table 21–C2) are classified as pure narcotic antagonists; they specifically block opiate receptors and inhibit or reverse (competitively antagonize) the effects produced by agonists such as morphine and most of the drugs discussed thus far in the chapter. Naloxone and naltrexone have no actions as narcotic agonists; they do not cause analgesia, respiratory depression, or virtually any other effect when given to a drug-free patient or a person who has taken another class of drugs. The antagonists are used to counteract undesirable opiate-induced respiratory depression, but they will also antagonize the beneficial analgesic effects of opiates if the patient has underlying pain.

Naloxone

Naloxone (NARCAN) is a short-acting, parenteral narcotic antagonist. It is used acutely to antagonize opiate-induced respiratory depression, whether caused by excessive doses that were given therapeutically or by a self-administered overdose. It is an important and often-used emergency drug.

When naloxone is given to reverse postoperative respiratory depression following therapeutic narcotic administration, the usual dose is 0.1 or 0.2 mg given intravenously. Additional doses can be given until spontaneous respiration improves sufficiently and alertness returns. The dose can be repeated every 1 to 3 hours as needed. The major concerns with using naloxone in this way are administration of excessive doses that would inhibit narcotic-induced analgesia, and the gradual reappearance of respiratory depression as the antagonist's short-lived effects wear off.

To manage a known or suspected narcotic overdose, 0.4 to 2 mg of naloxone is given intravenously (IM or SC routes can be used if IV administration is not possible). The dose can be repeated at 2- to 3-minute intervals. If ventilatory status does not improve after one or two doses, the overdose is probably not due to a narcotic. If spontaneous respiration returns, a narcotic was involved. The patient is then monitored and supported as necessary, and naloxone administration is repeated every 1 to 3 hours until there is little doubt that effective spontaneous ventilation will be maintained.

NURSING IMPLICATIONS

Naloxone is not a substitute for cardiopulmonary resuscitation when emergency support of circulation or ventilation is indicated. It is only a potentially useful emergency drug. Always remember that it will not improve ventilation or other aspects of CNS depression caused by drugs other than narcotics. Since naloxone's duration of action is much shorter than that of most narcotic analgesics, be prepared to give repeated naloxone doses until enough of the agonist has been metabolized or excreted that respiratory depression does not return. The patient must be monitored closely until danger has passed, yet assessed for adequate pain relief if a narcotic was given therapeutically. Be prepared for the rapid development of a withdrawal syndrome if a narcotic antagonist is given to a patient who is physically dependent on a narcotic. Should this occur, close monitoring may be all that is needed, since naloxone's short action will allow withdrawal symptoms to subside. Be aware, however, that respiratory depression may return.

Naltrexone

Naltrexone (TREXAN) is a long-acting, orally effective narcotic antagonist. Its longer duration of action makes it more convenient than naloxone when long-term effects are needed. However, naltrexone does not work quickly enough to be useful for initial treatment of narcotic overdoses. Naloxone is given during the acute respiratory crisis. If withdrawal does not occur, naltrexone therapy is started until the patient recovers fully.

Naltrexone is used in supervised programs to prevent readdiction in narcotic addicts. The patient is usually given a drug-free period lasting 7 to 10 days, and then given a test dose of naloxone to ensure that no withdrawal syndrome occurs. If there is no evidence of withdrawal, oral naltrexone therapy can be started. If the patient takes naltrexone as ordered, there will be no euphoria (the major cause of abuse) if the patient takes a narcotic.

NURSING IMPLICATIONS

Successful treatment of addiction with naltrexone requires that the patient be highly motivated to abstain from opiates; the antagonist does not curb the abuser's craving for narcotics. Psychologic counseling and emotional support are essential components of naltrexone therapy. Recommend that persons taking naltrexone carry identification indicating their drug treatment, so that health-care providers will be aware of it if an emergency arises.

SUMMARY OF NURSING IMPLICATIONS

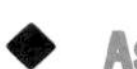

Assessment

Review past and current history for contraindications to narcotic analgesics (eg, closed head injury, gallbladder disease).

Identify previous reactions to narcotics and concurrent drug therapy requiring cautious use of narcotics (eg, other CNS depressants).

Establish baseline vital signs (respirations, pulse, blood pressure), physical assessment data (bowel elimination, urinary frequency), and laboratory values (liver and renal function).

Assess for adequacy of pain control; frequent requests or requests for larger doses may reflect actual pain, history of prior narcotic use or abuse, or improper drug administration; review history and medication record.

◆ Nursing Diagnoses

Pain related to disease, surgical procedure, or fear of addiction.

Constipation related to narcotic effects.

Ineffective individual coping related to pain; potential for drug dependence.

Altered nutrition: less than body requirements related to nausea from drug therapy.

Ineffective breathing pattern related to respiratory depression from narcotic.

Knowledge deficit related to medication regimen.

High risk for injury related to narcotic side effects.

Ineffective airway clearance related to cough suppression with narcotic.

Sensory/perceptual alteration related to medication effects (eg, dizziness).

Urinary retention related to morphine administration.

◆ Planning/Implementation

Withhold narcotics when cause of pain is unknown.

Anticipate need for pain medication (note clues) to prevent agitation and the need for higher and more frequent doses.

Administer doses at regular intervals; use nondrug measures to increase patient comfort and reduce dose.

Avoid giving narcotics to obstetric patients before active labor begins unless directed otherwise; prepare to deal with postpartum fetal respiratory depression.

Know the major parenteral drugs that should not be mixed in the same syringe with narcotics.

Monitor for excessive respiratory depression; withhold drug if respiratory rate below 12/min, irregular, or shallow; notify physician.

Have narcotic antagonists or respiratory assistance available when giving a narcotic.

Monitor blood pressure and heart rate; notify physician if unacceptably low, withhold drug; lower dose may be indicated.

Encourage patient to rest if nausea, dizziness, or hypotension occurs; protect from falls (side rails up).

Measure fluid intake and output to detect urinary retention or constipation; encourage patient to urinate every 4 hours; palpate bladder; report abdominal pain or discomfort associated with defecation or urination.

Encourage coughing and deep breathing; reposition to improve ventilation and atelectasis.

Observe closely for signs of excessive sedation if receiving other CNS depressants or cimetidine, or if a neuromuscular blocker was used; avoid concurrent use of meperidine and MAO inhibitors or phenothiazines.

Recognize signs of narcotic overdose (respiratory depression, excessive sedation, pinpoint pupils); prepare for naloxone administration and cardiopulmonary resuscitation.

Give antitussive drugs or narcotics to patients with productive cough only when it is severe, interferes with sleep, or causes damage to wounds.

◆ Patient and Family Teaching

Teach the patient/family:

That proper administration of narcotics is not likely to cause dependence or addiction.

Proper use of PCA apparatus; operation, avoiding accidental overdose, timing for optimum effects.

To take pain medication before severe pain develops.

To take medication with food if GI upset occurs.

To avoid driving, operating machinery, or performing dangerous tasks if drowsiness, dizziness, or visual changes occur.

To report adverse effects to nurse or physician (constipation, urinary retention, rash, changes in behavior).

To refrain from taking narcotics and to seek psychiatric or drug counseling when taking naltrexone.

◆ Evaluation

The patient/family will:

Report relief from pain; achieve therapeutic level of drug; not develop dependence or tolerance.

Demonstrate knowledge of alternate methods of pain relief (eg, relaxation techniques, positioning).

Experience no adverse drug effects (eg, respiratory depression, constipation, urinary retention); have normal bowel and bladder function; experience no nausea and vomiting.

Resume optimal activity level and self-care ability.

Verbalize awareness of community resources and need for counseling about chemical dependence.

Annotated Bibliography

Berde CB. Pediatric postoperative pain management. *Pediatr Clin North Am* 1989;36(4):921–940. *Reviews effective methods to relieve pain in children after surgery, discusses "major barriers to treatment," and considers narcotic administration routes that are less painful than intermittent injections.*

Brownridge P. Treatment options for the relief of pain during childbirth. *Drugs* 1991;41(1):69–80. *An excellent review of trends, techniques, and drugs for pain relief in the contemporary obstetrics setting.*

Burckhardt CS. Chronic pain. *Nurs Clin North Am* 1990;25(4): 863–870. *Despite increased knowledge about psychologic and physiologic factors that contribute to the etiology of chronic pain, more is needed when it comes to assessing and treating it adequately. This article discusses a comprehensive, holistic approach to the problem and the patient.*

Choiniere M, Melzack R, Girard N, Rondeau J, Paquin M-J. Comparisons between patients' and nurses' assessment of pain and medication efficacy in severe burn injuries. *Pain* 1990;40:143–152. *This study showed some important disparities between patients' and nurses' assessments of pain. The article concludes with four recommendations related to nursing assessment, planning, and implementation and the need for more education for patients and care providers; and a consideration of other forms of pharmacotherapy that involve less nursing intervention but adequate, individualized patient care.*

Donovan MI. Acute pain relief. *Nurs Clin North Am* 1990;25(4): 851–861. *Stresses the need for nurses to develop more knowledge about pain and pain relief; to be assertive in seeking effective analgesic therapies; and to assume a greater responsibility in gaining adequate pain control for their patients.*

Egbert AM. Help for the hurting elderly: Safe use of drugs to relieve pain. *Postgrad Med* 1991;89(4):217–222, 225, 228. *Explains how age-related factors affect the pharmacokinetics and pharmacodynamics of analgesics, and how these factors can affect the choice and use of pain-relieving drugs.*

Egbert AM, Parks LH, Short LM, Burnett ML. Randomized trial of postoperative patient-controlled analgesia vs. intramuscular narcotics in frail elderly men. *Arch Intern Med* 1990;150:1897–1903. *Assesses the pros and cons of PCA versus traditional parenteral narcotic therapy and other alternatives. PCA significantly improved pain control without causing added sedation, and reduced postoperative confusion and serious pulmonary complications.*

Eland JM. Pain in children. *Nurs Clin North Am* 1990;25(4):871–874. *Valuable for its discussions of pharmacologic interventions for managing pain in children; misconceptions or myths about pediatric pain; the need to manage pain; and ways to assess pain and pain relief.*

Enck RE. Pain control in the ambulatory elderly. *Geriatrics* 1991;46 (3):49–53, 57–58, 60. *Reviews principles of the etiology, assessment, and management of pain, and explains when and why nonopioids may be preferred to narcotic analgesics.*

Foley KM, et al. Management of cancer pain. *Cancer* 1989;63(11; Suppl):2257–2386. *Eighteen articles from a symposium on the subject. Topics range from basic pharmacology to contemporary issues on epidemiology, assessment, psychiatric and surgical interventions, and consideration of the patient's quality of life. Noteworthy is the article by Inturrisi (pp 2308–2320) dealing with an overview of drug therapy and the "three step analgesic ladder."*

Gorman E, Warfield CA. The opioid-dependent patient with acute pain. *Hosp Pract* 1987;22(11):113–120. *Gives useful advice about alleviating severe pain in narcotic-dependent patients.*

Gureno MA, Reisinger CL. Patient controlled analgesia for the young pediatric patient. *Pediatr Nurs* 1991;17(3):251–254. *This study found that PCA was a successful pain control method for children 3 years of age and older, and led to the implementation of new pain management policies and practices.*

Mooney NE. Pain management in the orthopedic patient. *Nurs Clin North Am* 1991;26(1):73–87. *A valuable discussion of the assessment and management of pain, using both pharmacologic and nonpharmacologic methods, in orthopedic patients.*

Slack J, Faut-Callahan M. Pain management. *Nurs Clin North Am* 1991;26(2):463–476. *A good overview of the theoretical and practical aspects of pain and pain management, with an emphasis on the important role of nurses.*

Stevens B. Development and testing of a pediatric pain management sheet. *Pediatr Nurs* 1990;16(6):543–548. *The author developed and pretested a useful flow sheet to give the care provider a "simple means of documenting the child's pain experience." "... nurses who implemented [it] had patients who were in less pain, were assessed more frequently..." and received more adequate narcotic analgesic therapy.*

Wall RT III. Use of analgesics in the elderly. *Clin Geriatr Med* 1990;6(2):345–364. *A balanced review of the topic, covering both narcotic and nonnarcotic analgesics and nondrug therapies. "State-of-the-art analgesic care is not widespread [because of] barriers ... in knowledge, skills, and attitudes among health care providers." The author addresses this issue and discusses narcotic, nonnarcotic, and nondrug approaches to optimize pain management in elders.*

Weis OF, Sriwatanakul K, Alloza JL, Weintraub M, Lasagna L. Attitudes of patients, housestaff, and nurses toward postoperative analgesic care. *Anesth Analg* 1983;62:70–74. *Surprisingly few practitioners felt that complete pain relief is a goal of postoperative care, and many felt that pain and distress are acceptable and should be relieved only when it peaks and becomes unacceptable. The cause? Lack of proper education about narcotics. Worthwhile reading despite its publication date.*

Wilkie DJ. Cancer pain management: State-of-the-art nursing care. *Nurs Clin North Am* 1990;25(2):331–343. *An excellent review of a holistic approach to managing cancer pain and cancer patients.*

Table 21–C1 **Clinical Uses and Administration of Major Narcotic Analgesics and Related Pure Narcotic Agonists**

AGENT	CLINICAL USES	DOSAGE AND ROUTE OF ADMINISTRATION
PROTOTYPE		
Morphine sulfate	Relief of moderate-to-severe pain	IM or SC: Adults: Usually 10 mg q4h–q6h. Children: 0.1–0.2 mg/kg per dose up to 15 mg maximum
		IV: Initial bolus of 4 mg (2–10 mg/70 kg body weight), given ≤1 mg/min, then adjust, based on response; may give total daily dose as IV drip with morphine diluted in 5% D_5W to concentration of 0.5–1 mg/mL; give initial bolus injection (1–5 mg) before starting drip to control pain quickly
		Epidural: 5 mg initially, with repeated doses of 1–2 mg prn; can give as continuous drip of 2–4 mg/24 h (not to exceed 10 mg/24 hr)
		Intrathecal: Usually 0.2–1mg
	Adjunctive therapy of acute congestive heart failure, pulmonary edema, dyspnea	IV: Usually 2–4 mg, repeated prn
	Ventilator control	IM or IV: Usually 20 mg q4h prn
	Special anesthesia	IV: 1 mg/kg body weight, infused at a rate of 5–10 mg/min
(ROXANOL, ROXANOL-100)	Relief of moderate-to-severe pain	Oral: Usually 10–30 mg of liquid or immediate-release tablets q4h–q5h; usually 30 mg q8h of sustained-release tablets (eg, ROXANOL SR)
		Rectal: 10–20 mg q4h
RELATED DRUGS		
Alfentanyl		
(ALFENTA)	Anesthesia	See Chapter 20
Codeine	Relief of mild-to-moderate pain	Oral, SC, or IM: Adults: Usually 15–60 mg qid. Children: 0.5 mg/kg q4h-q6h
	Relief of cough	Oral: Adults: Usually 10–20 mg q4h–q6h, not exceeding 120 mg/24hr. Children 6–12; 5–10 mg q4h–q6h, not exceeding 60 mg/24h. Children 2–6: 2.5–5 mg q4h-q6h, not exceeding 30 mg/24 hr
Dextromethorphan		
(BENYLIN DM, ROMILAR CF, others)	Relief of cough	Oral: Adults: 10–20 mg q4h or 30 mg q6h–q8h. Children 6–12: 5–10 mg q4h or 15 mg; 2–6: 2.5–5 mg q4h or 7.5 mg q6h–q8h
Fentanyl		
(SUBLIMAZE)	Anesthesia, anesthesia adjunct	See Chapter 20
(DURAGESIC)	Relief of moderate-to-severe pain	Transdermal: Apply 1 patch to skin q72h
Hydrocodone plus homatropine		
(HYCODAN)	Relief of cough	Oral: Adults: 5 mg q4h–q6h (eg, after meals and at bedtime).

(continued)

Table 21–C1 **Clinical Uses and Administration of Major Narcotic Analgesics and Related Pure Narcotic Agonists (*Continued*)**

AGENT	CLINICAL USES	DOSAGE AND ROUTE OF ADMINISTRATION
RELATED DRUGS		
Hydrocodone plus acetaminophen		
(ZYDONE)	Management of moderate to moderately severe pain	Oral: Adults: Usually 1 or 2 capsules (depending on severity of pain) q6h; capsules contain 500 mg acetaminophen and 5 mg hydrocodone
Hydromorphone		
(DILAUDID)	Relief of moderate-to-severe pain	IM or SC: 1–2 mg q4h–q6h (or give IV over 2–3 min)
		Oral: 2 mg q4h–q6h
		Rectal: 1 suppository (3 mg) q6h–q8h
	Relief of cough	Oral: 1 mg q3h–q4h
Levorphanol		
(LEVO-DROMORAN)	Relief of moderate-to-severe pain; preanesthetic medication	Oral, SC: Usually 2 mg, repeated in 4–6 hr if needed (may be given with 0.2 mg levallorphan to reduce respiratory depression)
Meperidine		
(DEMEROL)	Relief of moderate-to-severe pain	Oral, IM, or SC: Adults: 50–150 mg q3h–q4h. Children: 1–1.8 mg/kg.
	Obstetric analgesia	IM: 50–100 mg when pain and labor become regular, repeated in 1–3 hr as needed
	Anesthetic supplement	IV: Slowly inject 10 mg/mL or infuse 1 mg/mL until desired degree of analgesia and sedation is obtained
Meperidine plus promethazine		
(MEPERGAN)	Preoperative sedation/analgesia	Note: Each mL of MEPERGAN contains 25 mg of meperidine and 25 mg of promethazine
		IM: Adults: 1–2 mL q3h–q4h prn. Children <12; 0.2 mL/10 lb of body weight (may be given IV, but not SC)
Methadone		
(DOLOPHINE)	Relief of severe pain, especially if chronic or terminal	IM or Oral: 2.5–10 mg q3h–q4h (may be given SC)
	Detoxification treatment of narcotic addiction; treatment of acute narcotic withdrawal	IM or Oral: Initially 15–20 mg (may need to use more based on degree of narcotic tolerance); stabilize patient for 2–3 d, then reduce dose by 10%–20% per day
Opium, powdered		
(B AND O SUPPRETTES)	Relief of moderate-to-severe pain due to ureteral spasm	Rectal: 1 suppository (contains 30 to 60 mg powdered opium plus belladonna extract) once or twice a day
Opium alkaloids		
(PANTOPON)	Relief of severe pain	IM or SC: Usually 5–20 mg q4h–q5h

(continued)

Table 21–C1 Clinical Uses and Administration of Major Narcotic Analgesics and Related Pure Narcotic Agonists (*Continued*)

AGENT	CLINICAL USES	DOSAGE AND ROUTE OF ADMINISTRATION
RELATED DRUGS		
Opium tincture		
(laudanum)	Antidiarrheal	Oral: Adults: 0.3–1 mL up to qid (each mL contains 1% morphine; do not confuse with camphorated opium tincture)
Opium tincture, camphorated		
(paregoric, PAREPECTOLIN)	Antidiarrheal	Oral: Adults: 5–10 mL after every loose stool (not exceeding 4 doses/d). Children: 0.25–0.5 mL/kg body weight (each mL contains 0.04% morphine)
Oxycodone		
(ROXICODONE)	Relief of moderate-to-severe pain	Oral: Adults: Usually 5 mg q6h (some proprietary products contain oxycodone with aspirin or acetaminophen)
Oxymorphone		
(NUMORPHAN)	Relief of moderate-to-severe pain	SC or IM: 1–1.5 mg q4h–q6h IV: 0.5 mg q4h–q6h Rectal: 5 mg q4h–q6h
	Obstetric analgesia	IM: 0.5–1 mg once labor and pain become regular
Propoxyphene HCl		
(DARVON)	Relief of mild-to-moderate pain	Oral: 32–65 mg q4h, not to exceed 390 mg/d (also available with acetaminophen or aspirin plus caffeine)
Propoxyphene napsylate		
(DARVON–N)	Relief of mild-to-moderate pain	Oral: 50–100 mg q4h, not to exceed 600 mg/d (also available with aspirin or acetaminophen)
Sufentanil		
(SUFENTA)	Anesthesia	See Chapter 20

Table 21–S **Major Side Effects of and Contraindications for Morphine and Most Other Narcotic Analgesics**

BODY SYSTEM/ Side Effect	CONTRAINDICATION/ PRECAUTION	COMMENTS AND NURSING IMPLICATIONS
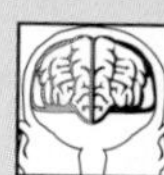 **CENTRAL NERVOUS SYSTEM** Sedation; drowsiness; ataxia; euphoria or dysphoria; impaired reflexes, coordination; dizziness, syncope; nausea, vomiting	Impaired neurologic status; head trauma or brain surgery (agents such as codeine may be acceptable in some situations); cautious use in chronic alcoholics; acute intoxication with alcohol, other CNS depressants, and during delirium tremens	If possible, withhold narcotic administration to patients with impaired neurologic status until cause can be determined and closed-head injury can be ruled out; caution ambulatory patients to avoid tasks (eg, driving, operating hazardous machinery) made dangerous by CNS depression, impaired coordination, etc; caution against self-administration of interacting CNS depressants (Table 21-I); dizziness, nausea, vomiting best managed by having patient lie down; assist with ambulation as needed; tolerance develops to most CNS side effects with continued use
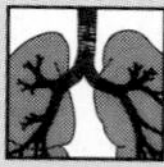 **RESPIRATORY** Decreased rate or depth of respiration; Kussmaul or Cheyne-Stokes respiration; apnea	Severely impaired respiratory function; no access to mechanical ventilatory support; cautious use with asthma, emphysema, other pulmonary disorders; delirium tremens	Monitor respiratory status closely and often, especially with parenteral (IM, IV, epidural) narcotic use; always have naloxone readily available to counteract excessive effects; report labored or shallow breathing, ventilatory rates <10/min at once, withhold additional doses until problem can be diagnosed or corrected; assess skin, mucous membrane color as indicator of blood oxygenation, use oximeter or direct blood gas measurements if possible and indicated by patient's condition; decreased ventilation and increased blood carbon dioxide levels increase intracranial pressure and alter preexisting brain damage or swelling, if present; tolerance to respiratory depression develops with continued use
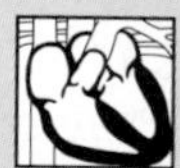 **CARDIOVASCULAR** Hypotension, bradycardia	Preexisting hypotension, hypovolemia, bradycardia	Avoid narcotic use in most forms of shock unless IV access and other means to support circulation are established
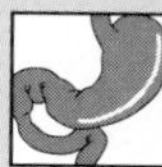 **GASTROINTESTINAL** Constipation, abdominal obstruction; paralytic ileus; aggravation of anorectal disorders	Preexisting constipation, obstruction, ileus	Most common side effect, constipation, is often dose-dependent, related to diet and hydration status, level of physical activity; may be aggravated by drug effects that lessen sensation of full bowel; best handled initially by dietary measures (adequate intake of fluid, bulk-forming foods); consult physician before recommending laxatives, stool softeners; monitor stool frequency, amount, consistency, report significant changes from patient's norm; little tolerance develops with continued narcotic administration
Abdominal pain; rupture of gallbladder, bile ducts	Use cautiously in patients with cholecystitis, biliary tract obstruction	Report pain for further evaluation
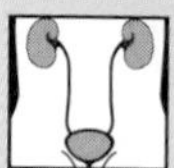 **URINARY** Urinary retention; infrequent or difficult urination; possible urinary urgency	Use cautiously in patients with prostatic hypertrophy	Encourage regular voiding, adequate fluid intake; monitor fluid intake, output
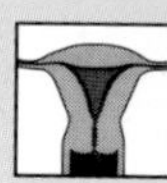 **UTERUS** Decreased uterine contractility, prolonged labor	Avoid use before development of rhythmic uterine contractions	When given during labor closely monitor uterine contractions, fetal heart rate; short-acting narcotics (eg, meperidine, pentazocine) are preferred, produce less postpartum fetal respiratory depression

Table 21–I Major Interactions Between Opiates and Other Agents

AGENT	RESULT OF INTERACTION	COMMENTS AND NURSING IMPLICATIONS
Interactions Involving Most Narcotic Analgesics		
Cimetidine (Chapter 40)	Excessive generalized CNS depression, potential for excessive ventilatory depression	Cimetidine appears to reduce hepatic metabolism of most narcotics; use reduced narcotic doses, monitor accordingly, if interaction is unavoidable; newer cimetidine alternatives (eg, ranitidine) are less likely to interact
CNS depressants (other): alcohol, other sedative-hypnotics and anxiety-relieving drugs (Chapter 22); most antipsychotics (Chapter 23), antidepressants (Chapter 24); centrally acting antiparkinson drugs (eg, benztropine, Chapter 25); antihistamines (eg, diphenhydramine; Chapter 38); many antihypertensive drugs (eg, β-blockers, clonidine; Chapter 33)	Excessive CNS depression, potential for excessive ventilatory depression	Use reduced dosages of prescribed interactants and monitor accordingly if interaction is unavoidable; give outpatients proper instructions about which OTC medications to avoid or use only upon advice of a physician
Mixed agonist-antagonist narcotics (Table 21-C2)	Reduced analgesic effects	Avoid combined use with pure narcotic analgesics (morphine-like drugs)
Interactions Affecting Mainly Meperidine		
Monoamine oxidase (MAO) inhibitor antidepressants (Chapter 24)	Acute, intense CNS stimulation, potential seizures; eventual coma, respiratory depression, arrest	Essential to avoid interaction; separate administration of these agents by at least 2 weeks; use alternative narcotics (eg, morphine) for pain control
Phenothiazine antipsychotics (eg, chlorpromazine; Chapter 23)	Acute CNS depression, hypotension	Avoid interaction; use other narcotics

Table 21–C2 **Clinical Uses and Administration of Mixed Narcotic Agonists-Antagonists**

AGENT	CLINICAL USES	DOSAGE AND ROUTE OF ADMINISTRATION
Buprenorphine		
(BUPRENEX)	Relief of moderate-to-severe pain	IM or slow IV injection: Adults, children >13: 0.3 mg q6h
Butorphanol		
(STADOL)	Relief of moderate-to-severe pain; preoperative/preanesthetic medication; supplement to anesthesia	IM: 2 mg initially, then 1–4 mg q3h–q4h prn IV: 1 mg initially and prn (dose may range from 0.5–2 mg)
Dezocine		
(DALGAN)	Relief of mild-to-moderate pain	IV: Adults: 2.5–10 mg q2h–q4h IM: 5–20 mg q3h–6h (up to 120 mg) maximum; not recommended for children <18 years
Nalbuphine		
(NUBAIN)	Relief of moderate-to-severe pain; obstetric analgesia; supplement to surgical anesthesia	SC, IM, or IV: 10 mg prn q3h–q6h (not to exceed 20 mg per dose or 160 mg/24 hr)
Pentazocine		
(TALWIN)	Relief of moderate-to-severe pain; preoperative or preanesthetic adjunct; surgical anesthetic supplement	IM or IV: 30 mg q3h–q4h (not to exceed, per dose, 60 mg IM or SC, 30 mg IV, or a total of 360 mg/d by any route); SC may be used but is painful, may cause tissue damage; rotate injection sites.
	Obstetric analgesia	IM: 30 mg single dose after regular labor begins, repeated no more than twice at 2–3 hr intervals IV: 20 mg, as for IM
Pentazocine plus acetaminophen		
(TALACEN)	Relief of mild-to-moderate pain	Oral: Usually 1 tablet (contains 25 mg pentazocine and 650 mg acetaminophen) q4h, up to 6 tablets a day
Pentazocine plus aspirin		
(TALWIN Compound)	Relief of mild-to-moderate pain	Oral: 2 tablets (each contains 12.5 mg pentazocine and 325 mg aspirin) tid or qid
Pentazocine plus naloxone		
(TALWIN NX)	Relief of moderate-to-severe pain	Oral: Adults: 1 tablet (contains 50 mg pentazocine and 0.5 mg naloxone) q3h–q4h, up to 12 tablets per day maximum
Naloxone		
(NARCAN)	Treatment of postoperative respiratory depression due to narcotics	IV: 0.1–0.2 mg, repeated until desired degree of spontaneous respiration, alertness is restored
	Treatment of known or suspected narcotic overdoses	IV: 0.4–2 mg, repeated several times at 2–3-min intervals (may give IM or SC if IV route not available)
Naltrexone		
(TREXAN)	Narcotic detoxification, prevention of readdiction to narcotics	Oral: Initially 25 mg; if no withdrawal signs appear maintain on 50 mg/d, 100 mg qod, or 150 mg every third day

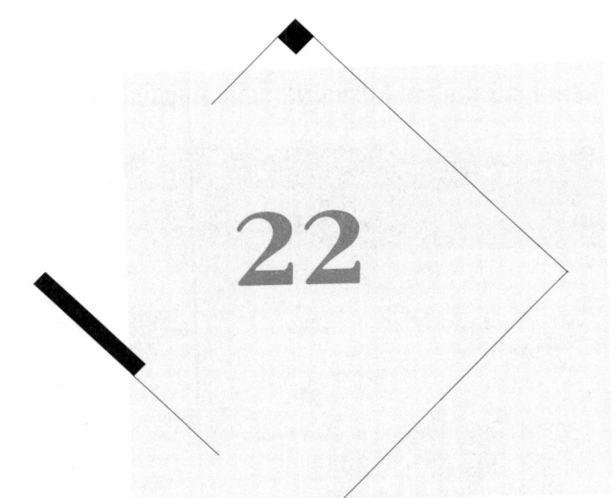

PROTOTYPES

Sedatives, Hypnotics, and Anxiolytics

This chapter discusses drugs that cause what might be described as generalized, dose-dependent depression of the brain. They are widely used to cause an overall calming or *sedative* effect; to alleviate anxiety—an *anxiolytic* effect; or to facilitate or cause sleep—a *hypnotic* effect. Some drugs also have special uses, such as the management of seizure disorders or the induction of anesthesia. Because of their central nervous system (CNS) depressant effects, and the consequences of that action, many of these drugs are widely abused.

The chapter is organized into four major parts. The first covers drugs that, because of their chemical structure, are called *barbiturates.* The prototype is phenobarbital. Barbiturates are the oldest of the prescription CNS depressants, but their use is declining as newer agents are developed. However, they are still important drugs. The second section discusses drugs that are classified chemically as *benzodiazepines.* The prototype, diazepam, and several related drugs, have some therapeutic advantages over the barbiturates. As a result, they are more widely used. The third section identifies and briefly discusses miscellaneous sedatives and hypnotics. The chapter ends with a discussion of ethyl alcohol.

Major reference tables appear beginning on p 369.

I. Barbiturates

General Characteristics of Barbiturates

All the barbiturates have the potential to cause similar pharmacologic effects owing to their ability to depress the CNS and other body systems. They cause similar side effects, have similar contraindications, and essentially participate in the same drug–drug interactions. Indeed, many of the properties to be described for the barbiturates, and the nursing implications related to them, apply to virtually any drug that causes CNS depression.

The barbiturates have a chemical structure that is similar to a substance called *barbituric acid.* However, the individual drugs have unique structural differences that affect their pharmacokinetics (absorption, distribution, metabolism, and excretion). These differences affect the actions of a particular agent, and also affect the choice of one barbiturate over another when the goal is to cause a certain therapeutic action.

PROTOTYPE

Phenobarbital

The prototype, phenobarbital (originally marketed as LUMINAL), has been used as a drug for decades. It still has some important uses.

Absorption, Distribution, Metabolism, and Excretion

Most of the barbiturates, including the prototype, are absorbed well from the gastrointestinal (GI) tract and are given orally. These oral formulations are in a chemical form known as the *free acid.* The sodium salts of these and other barbiturates are injectable dosage forms. They are usually given intravenously, but intramuscular (IM) injections are occasionally given. The barbiturates are distributed into all the body tissues, cross the placental barrier, and are excreted in breast milk.

One of the most important chemical properties of the individual barbiturates is lipid solubility. It affects the speed with which a barbiturate diffuses into the CNS, its major site of action, and the speed with which it leaves the CNS. Thus, it affects both the time to onset of drug action and the duration of action. This property is clinically important when selecting a particular barbiturate for a particular use. Chemical structure and lipid solubility also determine the extent to which a particular barbiturate depends on renal excretion or hepatic metabolism for elimination from the body, which can have important implications for certain patients with liver or kidney disease.

Table 22–1 and Figure 22–1 compare and contrast properties and uses of the major barbiturates. They show a general and progressive relationship between the drugs' lipid solubility and their actions and fates in the body. Of the commonly used barbiturates, phenobarbital is the least lipid soluble. It has a slow onset of action because it diffuses into the brain slowly; and a long duration of action because it leaves the brain slowly. It is used when relatively mild but longlasting CNS depression is the therapeutic goal. And, although most of the phenobarbital in the bloodstream is metabolized by the liver, some of the drug is excreted unchanged by the kidneys. Renal excretion of phenobarbital depends on the pH of the urine. In normally acidic urine most of the phenobarbital molecules are in the nonionized, or electrically uncharged, form. Thus, once they are filtered into the kidneys they can easily diffuse back into the bloodstream, which partly accounts for the drug's long half-life. However, if the urine is made more alkaline, such as by administering sodium bicarbonate to the patient, the increased pH shifts the phenobarbital molecules into the electrically charged, or less diffusible, form. These molecules do not diffuse back into the bloodstream, and so are excreted in the urine. The ability to increase phenobarbital excretion by alkalinizing the urine is important; it may be necessary when the patient's phenobarbital blood levels are too high, as might occur with an overdose. This is discussed more fully on page 63.

The other barbiturates—amobarbital, pentobarbital, secobarbital, and thiopental—are listed in the order of increasing lipid solubility. Compared with phenobarbital they have progressively faster onsets of action but shorter durations of action. Thiopental (PEN-

Table 22–1 Pharmacokinetic Comparison of Major Barbiturates*

Drug	Relative Onset of Action	Peak Effect (hr)	Relative Duration of Action	Average Half-Life (hr)
Phenobarbital	Slow (>60 min)	10–12	Long	80
Amobarbital	Moderate (45 min)	6–8	Intermediate	25
Pentobarbital	Rapid (10–15 min)	3–4	Short	20–50
Secobarbital	Rapid (10–15 min)	3–4	Short	25
Thiopental (IV)	Ultra–fast (<1 min)	0.25	Ultra–short	3–8

*Values for all drugs, except thiopental, are for oral administration. Onsets and durations of action may vary considerably. Higher or lower doses than those indicated may have to be given, depending on the patient's age, renal and hepatic status, intensity of the desired response, and the overall degree of CNS stimulation when the drug is given.

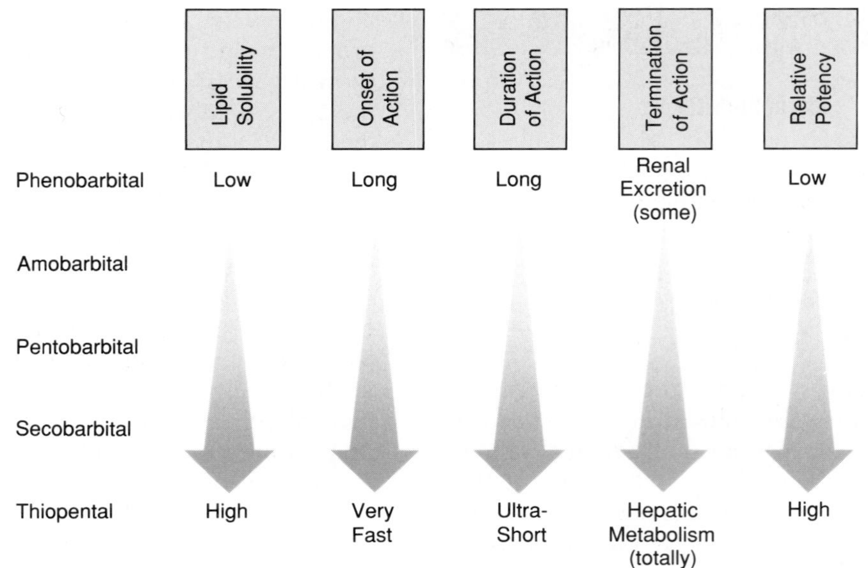

Figure 22–1

General relationships between the lipid solubility of barbiturates and their time-courses of action, potency, and dependency on renal excretion or hepatic metabolism. The greater the lipid solubility, the faster the drug enters and then leaves the CNS (faster onset, shorter duration of action), the greater the drug's dependence on hepatic metabolism, and, in general, the greater the CNS depressant potency. These relationships do not apply as well to the benzodiazepines.

TOTHAL) is the most lipid soluble of all these drugs. It enters and depresses the brain almost instantaneously when it is given intravenously, its major administration route. However, its duration of action is very short because it diffuses out of the CNS and distributes to other tissues very quickly. Thus, thiopental is used mainly when intense but brief CNS depression is desired. Thiopental is eliminated from the body solely by hepatic metabolism.

Induction of Drug-Metabolizing Enzymes by Barbiturates

With repeated administration, the barbiturates induce (stimulate) the liver cells to synthesize more of the enzymes that are responsible for metabolizing the barbiturates themselves, plus virtually any other drugs that are metabolized by the liver. This effect can lower blood levels of metabolized drugs, and shorten their plasma half-lives. Overall, it is a cause of some common and clinically significant drug–drug interactions; it partly explains why tolerance develops to many effects of the barbiturates when they are administered repeatedly; and it is one reason why drugs that do not induce the liver enzymes (eg, benzodiazepines, discussed below) are often preferred to a barbiturate.

Pharmacologic Effects

Central Nervous System Depression

The most obvious effect of barbiturates is CNS depression. The way in which the effect occurs is not known with certainty. It may involve generalized changes in nerve metabolism, or may involve the ability of these drugs to increase the activity of "inhibitory neurotransmitters" that are released by some nerve cells. The intensity of the response is dose-dependent. It can range from very subtle or mild sedation with very low doses, to sleep, anesthesia, coma, and death with progressively higher doses. With repeated barbiturate administration, tolerance develops to the CNS depressant effects.

Barbiturates act rather uniformly throughout the brain, but the reticular system seems to be particularly sensitive to even low doses of these drugs. That system controls activity of the cerebral cortex and serves as an activating or arousal system that helps maintain wakefulness. Other brain pathways, such as those responsible for the perception of and response to pain, are much less sensitive to barbiturates.

Effects on Sleep

Low (sedative) doses of barbiturates may relieve anxiety, cause relaxation, and facilitate or *allow* sleep. Higher (hypnotic) doses *produce* sleep that resembles natural sleep in many ways: heart rate, blood pressure, and respiratory rate and depth fall slightly, and the patient can be aroused easily. However, hypnotic doses of barbiturates depress the time spent in rapid eye movement (REM) sleep, when many dreams occur. Depressed REM sleep time leads to some important side effects.

Anticonvulsant Effects

Low doses of phenobarbital and a few other barbiturates have "selective" anticonvulsant activity: they can inhibit abnormal brain electrical activity responsible for seizures without causing marked sedation. All barbiturates have anticonvulsant activity at high doses.

Paradoxical Central Nervous System Stimulation

Very low doses of barbiturates can cause paradoxical excitement, disorientation, or agitation. The effect, which is almost always unwanted in the clinical situation (and so can become an important side effect), resembles the "high" caused by an alcoholic beverage. It does not occur because the barbiturates (or alcohol) actually stimulate any part of the brain. Instead, "stimulation" is thought to be caused by the ability of such low drug doses to selectively depress inhibitory nerve pathways in the brain (Fig. 22–2). This unmasks the opposing effects of stimulatory nerve pathways or transmitters. With higher dosages, all nerve pathways are depressed.

Effects on Pain

Unlike morphine and other narcotics, barbiturates do not cause selective analgesic effects. They alleviate pain only when such large doses have been given that the patient is anesthetized or near coma, when virtually all parts of the CNS are profoundly depressed. Low (sedative) barbiturate doses actually appear to increase the sensation of pain, causing what has been called a *hyperalgesic effect.*

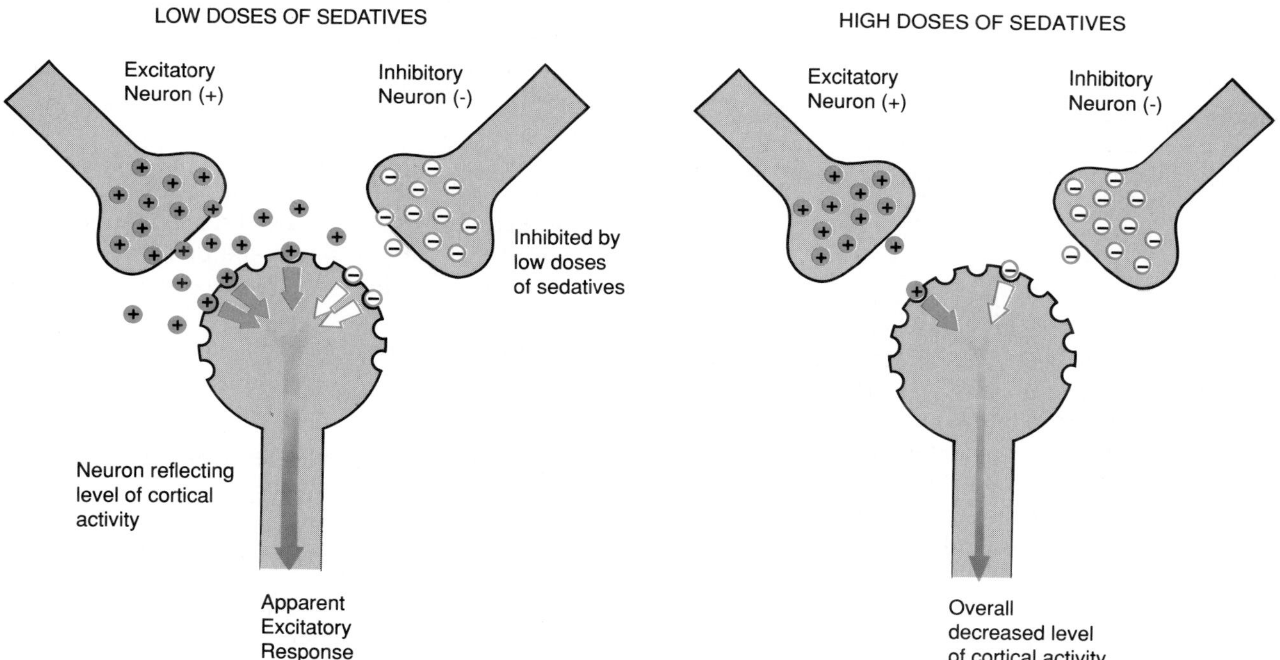

Figure 22–2

Model to help explain paradoxical CNS "stimulation" by low doses of barbiturates, alcohol, and most other general CNS depressants. Consider the overall level of CNS activity as a balance between opposing effects of nerves that release excitatory neurotransmitters (+) and nerves that release inhibitory transmitters (−). Inhibitory nerves seem to be more sensitive to the effects of CNS depressants, and are inhibited at low drug brain levels. It now appears as if the overall system is activated because excitatory nerve influences predominate (left). At higher dosages, all nerves are depressed, and overall CNS activity appears depressed (right).

Effects on Other Organ Systems

Therapeutic doses of barbiturates cause minimal effects on other organ systems. Very high doses directly depress the heart and blood vessels, causing bradycardia and hypotension. Toxic doses markedly depress all nerve and muscle tissues.

Clinical Indications and Administration

In theory, if the barbiturate dose is adjusted correctly, any degree of CNS depression ranging from sedation to anesthesia can be produced. However, the unique pharmacokinetic properties of each barbiturate make some more suitable than others for a particular use (Table 22–C1). In general, long-acting barbiturates are mainly used for long-term effects (daytime sedation or chronic treatment of seizures), and short-acting ones are used for immediate but brief effects (sleep or anesthesia). Barbiturates are still important drugs, but their side effects and drug interactions, described later, account for their declining use.

Sedation

Phenobarbital may be used to produce slight but relatively long-lasting sedation. Anxiety symptoms, if present, may be reduced as well. Unlike the benzodiazepines, barbiturates lack "selective" antianxiety activity.

Hypnosis

Tripling the sedative dose induces sleep (a hypnotic effect). This might be indicated for persons with insomnia or to prepare a patient for anesthesia. Phenobarbital is seldom used as a hypnotic because its slow onset of action delays sleep induction, and its prolonged effects cause drowsiness that can carry through into the following day. Barbiturates with faster onsets and shorter durations (see the section on related drugs) are used instead.

Management of Chronic or Acute Seizures

Phenobarbital can be used alone or with other anticonvulsant drugs to manage certain chronic seizure disorders. Unlike barbiturate use for sedation, anxiety, or hypnosis, long-term use for chronic seizure disorders is acceptable and often necessary. Phenobarbital or an ultra–short-acting barbiturate may be injected intravenously to terminate acute generalized seizures, such as status epilepticus. However, diazepam, given intravenously, is preferred for this use. Anticonvulsant drug therapy is discussed more fully in Chapter 26.

Anesthesia

The ultra–short-acting barbiturates (thiamylal, thiopental, and methohexital), given parenterally, are used for inducing profound CNS depression needed for anesthesia.

NURSING IMPLICATIONS

Virtually all sedatives or hypnotics, including barbiturates, are intended for short-term use (treatment of chronic seizure disorders is an exception). Longer use will result in the development of tolerance and an increased risk of dependence. Patients who require hypnotics for more than about 2 weeks, or anxiety-relieving drugs for more than about a month, should be encouraged to obtain thorough medical and psychologic examinations to diagnose the underlying cause and possibly to find adjunctive or alternative therapies.

If both barbiturates and narcotics are given as preoperative medications, use reduced doses of both to reduce the chance of excessive or prolonged respiratory or cardiovascular depression. Since barbiturates lack analgesic action and may intensify the patient's perception of pain, do not rely on them for postoperative pain control. Barbiturates should be discontinued as soon as possible after surgery so that full doses of narcotics can be given with less risk of excessive effects or interactions.

Barbiturates are chemically incompatible with most other drugs. Do not mix them in the same syringe.

Side Effects, Adverse Reactions, and Contraindications

Central Nervous System Side Effects

Overall, the most important side effects (Table 22–S1) of barbiturates relate to their CNS depressant effects. Most of them are also caused by other drug classes discussed in this chapter. Some problems occur during therapy, while others occur when therapy is stopped.

Excessive or prolonged sedation is the most common side effect. It is usually dose-dependent, and of most concern when it interferes with normal daytime activities. The effect is called a ***hangover*** if the daytime CNS depression was caused by effects of a drug taken specifically for nighttime (hypnotic) effects. (Unlike the hangover caused by drinking too much alcohol, that associated with barbiturates and other CNS depressants is not accompanied by headache or gastrointestinal upset.) Sedation, and the potential for ataxia, are not simply annoying; they can be dangerous owing to the risk of falls or other injuries that could result when the impaired person tries to perform tasks that require a clear head and intact reflexes and motor skills.

The use of barbiturate hypnotics can cause depression of REM sleep. Its signs and symptoms include restless sleep, early awakening, and anxiousness or irritability during the following day. This is a major problem associated with the use of barbiturates, but not of the more widely used benzodiazepines that are discussed in the next section.

Paradoxical excitement and confusion are potential side effects, and they seem to be particularly problematic when low doses of a general CNS depressant are given to children, the elderly, or debilitated patients.

Two side effects can occur when therapy with a barbiturate or another general CNS depressant is stopped suddenly. One is *rebound insomnia:* it involves increased sleeplessness (more awake time at night), even when compared with the patient's pretreatment sleep problems. The other can be called *rebound anxiety:* it involves increased anxiety when administration of a CNS depressant used to relieve daytime anxiety or to cause daytime sedation is stopped.

Respiratory and Cardiovascular Side Effects

Problems affecting the respiratory and cardiovascular systems are usually slight unless barbiturate dosages are high, the drug is injected, or the patient has preexisting and significant pulmonary or cardiovascular disease. Rapid intravenous (IV) injection of a barbiturate, as to stop seizures or induce anesthesia, can cause laryngospasm and hypotension. Slowing the injection rate (no more than 60 mg/min) is usually all that is needed to minimize these problems.

Nutritional and Metabolic Side Effects

Long-term barbiturate administration can stimulate the breakdown of vitamins K and D in the liver, and cause deficiencies of these vitamins if the problem is not prevented (preferred) or corrected by giving vitamin supplements. Vitamin K plays a crucial role in the synthesis of blood-clotting factors; a deficiency increases the risk of excessive bleeding tendencies. It is a potential problem for any patient receiving barbiturates chronically, but is most important for pregnant women who take phenobarbital chronically for seizures. (This is discussed more fully in the section on pregnancy and lactation.) Vitamin D deficiencies can interfere with normal calcium absorption and metabolism. The major related problems include osteomalacia and osteoporosis, and the resulting increase of bone fragility.

A history of porphyria is an absolute contraindication to the use of any barbiturate for any purpose. Porphyria is a rare inherited metabolic disorder caused by excessive hepatic synthesis of chemicals called *porphyrins,* which are eventually used to synthesize heme proteins (eg, hemoglobin). Barbiturates stimulate porphyrin synthesis even more. The most serious consequence of this effect is nerve lesions in the periphery and brain. These lesions are painful, disabling, and potentially permanent or fatal.

Other Side Effects

Injectable formulations of barbiturates are very alkaline and can cause pain and tissue damage at the injection site. For this reason, IM injections should be given deeply and only when necessary, and subcutaneous (SC) injections should be avoided. Although IV injection is preferred, pain, phlebitis, and thrombosis can occur with this route. Accidental intraarterial injection must be avoided by using proper injection techniques, as it is liable to cause arterial spasm and significantly reduce blood flow to structures distal to the injection site.

Patients with a history of any serious adverse response to barbiturates should not receive these drugs again.

NURSING IMPLICATIONS

For most patients, nursing measures should focus on CNS side effects and all its potential consequences, especially disorientation, ataxia, falls, and other physical risks associated with drowsiness or impaired coordination and judgment. Anticipate paradoxical CNS stimulation in elderly patients and children, especially during the start of therapy. Explicitly advise patients to avoid potentially dangerous tasks, including driving a car. Careful assessment is important not only during CNS depressant therapy, but also after it has been stopped.

Tolerance and Physical Dependence

Repeated barbiturate administration produces tolerance, physical dependence, and psychologic dependence. Most barbiturates are classified as Schedule II or

Schedule III agents because of their abuse potential. Patterns and symptoms of barbiturate dependence are similar to those seen with chronic alcoholism, and may involve cyclic use of CNS stimulants. Like the narcotics, barbiturates cause cross-tolerance: persons tolerant to one barbiturate will be tolerant to all others.

Tolerance to barbiturates develops for two main reasons.

1. By inducing the hepatic drug-metabolizing enzymes, the drug's blood level and half-life fall. A diminished effect occurs unless the dose is increased to compensate. This phenomenon is called *drug disposition tolerance.*
2. With continued administration, the CNS somehow adapts, becoming less sensitive to the drug's depressant effects. This has been called *functional tolerance.*

Significant tolerance develops to the sedative and hypnotic effects, but only slight tolerance develops to the lethal effects. This narrowing between therapeutic and lethal doses (that is, a decreased margin of safety) increases the risk of fatal overdoses. Adaptation of the CNS also contributes to physical dependence—the need for continued drug administration to maintain the physiologic status quo and prevent the development of a withdrawal syndrome. Again, like the narcotics, cross-dependence to barbiturates occurs: if a person has become dependent on one barbiturate, another can be substituted and withdrawal will not occur if the proper dose is given.

Withdrawal Signs and Symptoms

The intensity of withdrawal symptoms depends on the degree of tolerance that has developed, which is related to the dose of barbiturate, and on the length of administration. Both the intensity and duration of withdrawal also depend on the duration of action of the drug that was used. Withdrawal from a long-acting barbiturate such as phenobarbital is often prolonged, gradual, and mild. In contrast, withdrawal is more intense, but of shorter duration, with short-acting barbiturates.

Mild barbiturate withdrawal symptoms include disturbed sleep, insomnia, and anxiety. Severe withdrawal also causes delirium, muscle tremor or twitching, and generalized seizures (status epilepticus). Signs of severe, uncontrolled withdrawal from a barbiturate are often more intense than those seen during alcohol withdrawal, and are clearly more dangerous than narcotic withdrawal: barbiturate withdrawal can be fatal.

If barbiturate tolerance or dependence occurs, the dose should be reduced gradually (by about 10% per day) under a physician's supervision to reduce withdrawal severity. It is common to substitute appropriate doses of phenobarbital before weaning if dependence is due to a shorter-acting barbiturate. This prolongs withdrawal and reduces the intensity of symptoms. The patient is then gradually weaned from the phenobarbital. If severe symptoms occur during early withdrawal, they can be managed with parenteral phenobarbital.

NURSING IMPLICATIONS

Little can be done to prevent individuals from seeking prescriptions for CNS depressants from several physicians, and from refusing to reveal information about drug abuse. However, the abuse potential can be minimized if the nurse attempts to ensure that general medical and legal guidelines are followed—duration of therapy, number of doses dispensed, refills, no sharing of drugs, avoiding other CNS-active drugs, and so on.

If dependence on any CNS depressant occurs, careful nursing assessment, including monitoring of both physical and psychologic changes, is essential once drug use is stopped. During this time, and especially during obvious withdrawal, the patient's environment should be as free as possible from disturbing influences; continual support and reassurance should be provided.

◆ Use During Pregnancy and Lactation

Caution pregnant women against taking barbiturates during pregnancy, unless the drugs are needed to control seizures. Advise all women to consult a physician immediately if they become pregnant during barbiturate treatment. If sufficiently high doses are taken during early pregnancy, fetal malformations or death may occur. Chronic barbiturate use during late pregnancy may cause physical dependence and withdrawal in the newborn, which may require temporary phenobarbital administration to the infant to suppress symptoms. Even acute use near term or during labor may suppress uterine contractions, prolong labor, and cause fetal CNS or respiratory depression.

Long-term barbiturate administration, particularly during the last trimester, may cause fetal deficiencies of vitamin K–dependent clotting factors, which predisposes the newborn to excessive bleeding or hemorrhage. If barbiturate therapy must be continued during pregnancy, the mother should receive supplemental vitamin K (phytonadione) start-

TRENDS AND CONTROVERSIES IN PHARMACOLOGY

◆ *Drug-Related Mental Changes*

Mental changes are possible whenever drugs are taken. It is not uncommon for drugs to cause confusion, disorientation, agitation, psychosis, or depression, especially in very young, elderly, or debilitated patients.

There are several mechanisms by which drugs can affect mental function (Wolanin and Phillips, 1981; Palmieri, 1991). Any drug that lowers blood pressure or reduces cardiac output can decrease cerebral blood flow and thereby compromise brain function. The patient's symptoms may be continuous or sporadic, or they may be most pronounced with position changes. Problems in carrying on a conversation, disorientation, and dizziness may be evident.

Drugs that can depress the respiratory center, such as narcotics, can cause lethargy, memory deficits, perceptual problems, or delusions.

Hypoglycemia from insulin or oral antidiabetic drugs can cause nervousness, irritability, apprehension, and difficulty in concentrating. Marijuana, in addition to its direct effects on brain function, may also cause blood sugar changes in some people. Mental changes that are brought about by low blood sugar are relatively easy to pinpoint, as symptoms are quickly relieved by the administration of glucose.

Fluid or electrolyte imbalance from diuretics, for example, or chronic alcohol use can cause confusion and other mental changes.

Some drugs, such as the anticholinergics, may alter the levels of chemicals in the brain and cause disorientation, impaired memory, or agitation. This may also be the general mechanism by which estrogens, adrenal corticosteroids, and many antihypertensive lead to mental depression.

The patients at highest risk for drug-induced mental changes are people who are debilitated or malnourished, have impaired renal or hepatic function, are taking many different drugs, or are very young or very old. Head trauma or central nervous system infection also contribute to an increased risk.

Mental changes may be acute and dramatic or slow and subtle. In older patients, the first sign of an adverse reaction to any drug is often some type of mental impairment. Unfortunately, society is quick to attribute confusion, agitation, disorientation, or personality changes to "old age" when in fact these problems may be drug-induced. It is important to remember that many adverse effects are dose-related and that elderly patients often should receive lower dosages than younger patients to obtain the same therapeutic effect (Thomas, 1988).

Confusion is a rather generic term that means different things to different people. Is the person lethargic? Disoriented? Inappropriate in conversation? Agitated? Hallucinating? Is there a pattern to the mental changes? Do the changes occur only at night? Only when drug effects might be peaking? Only after prn drugs have been administered? The more detailed the description of the patient's behavior, the greater the likelihood that a cause of the symptoms can be identified.

Palmieri DT: Clearing up the confusion: Adverse effects of medications in the elderly. *J Ger Nurs* 1991;17(10):32–35.

Thomas D: Assessment and management of agitation in the elderly. *Geriatrics* 1988; 43(6):45–53.

Wolanin MO, Phillips LR: *Confusion: Prevention and Care.* Mosby 1981; 156–158.

ing about 1 month before anticipated delivery, as should the infant upon delivery. This precaution applies to many anticonvulsant drugs, and is discussed in Chapter 26. The concentration of some barbiturates in maternal milk may be close to that in maternal blood. Nursing infants may ingest enough drug to experience sedation, lethargy, poor feeding habits, weight loss, and altered liver function. Some authorities believe that actual risks to the nursing infant are relatively low if maternal drug doses are kept low, if the child can be nursed just before the next scheduled drug dose, and if the child's response is monitored closely.

◆ Use in Children

The major use of barbiturates in children is for treatment of chronic seizure disorders (see Chapter 26 for related implications). Regardless of the use or drug, the child's response to a CNS depressant is variable. Signs of paradoxical CNS stimulation are common during early therapy.

◆ Use in the Elderly

Excessive sedation, dizziness, weakness, unsteadiness, impaired judgment, paradoxical excitement, and confusion are more common side effects in the elderly. These responses may also be due to an underlying physical or mental illness, so careful assessment to determine the cause is important. In most instances, especially when problems such as anxiety or insomnia do not pose a physical or emotional threat, nondrug therapies are preferred: exercise, other planned and relaxing physical or social activities, and so on. Always consider that elderly patients are relatively less tolerant of most drug-induced effects, and are likely to have other conditions requiring therapy with potentially interacting drugs. These concerns apply to all sedative, hypnotic, and anxiety-relieving drugs. Alternatives to the barbiturates, particularly the benzodiazepines, are usually preferred.

Interactions with Other Drugs

Barbiturates, and virtually all other drugs that cause CNS depression (regardless of their chemical class or use), interact to cause additive or greater degrees of CNS depression. When possible, combined use of these interactants should be avoided. If the interaction is unavoidable, reduced doses of each drug are usually indicated, and extra close monitoring of the response (and perhaps of drug levels in the blood) is essential.

The ability of barbiturates to stimulate the liver's drug metabolizing enzymes can shorten the half-life and reduce the effects of most other drugs that depend on hepatic metabolism. This theoretically applies to a long list of drugs, but is most important for many corticosteroids, doxycycline, oral contraceptives, quinidine, some tetracyclines, theophylline, valproic acid, and oral anticoagulants (Table 22–I1). Monoamine oxidase (MAO) inhibitors and valproic acid inhibit barbiturate metabolism, and may cause intense CNS depression if the barbiturate dose is not reduced.

NURSING IMPLICATIONS

When adding a barbiturate to therapy with an interactant, the interactant's dose may have to be increased to maintain therapeutic blood levels. When a barbiturate is discontinued during multidrug therapy, the interactant's dose may have to be reduced to prevent its blood level from climbing once hepatic enzymes are no longer stimulated. Responses to all interactants should be noted frequently. Anticipate the potential need for drawing blood for analysis of drug levels during combined therapy.

Overdose and Toxicity

Barbiturate overdoses are relatively common, especially in outpatients. Often they involve simultaneous use of other CNS depressants, including alcohol. Depending on the barbiturate, its dose, and the types and amounts of other drugs involved, signs of intoxication may range from excessive sedation to respiratory depression, cardiovascular collapse, coma, and death.

There is no antidote for barbiturate overdose. Treatment is purely supportive and symptomatic. Since diminished consciousness and gag reflexes are common with CNS depressant overdoses, induced emesis is frequently contraindicated (see Appendix C). Gastric lavage becomes the major approach to reducing further drug absorption. The primary concern is to maintain adequate ventilation by inserting an airway, giving oxygen, and assisting ventilation as needed. Vital signs should be monitored closely, and parenteral fluids should be given for dehydration or shock. If the patient has good renal function, a diuretic such as mannitol (Chapter 32) can be injected to increase renal excretion. Parenteral administration of sodium bicarbonate may correct acidosis caused by respiratory depression. It also alkalinizes the urine and increases phenobarbital excretion, but is not likely to increase elimination of most other barbiturates. Hemodialysis may be needed for life-threatening intoxication. Stimulants should never be used, as they may cause seizures or excessive cardiovascular stimulation.

NURSING IMPLICATIONS

Barbiturate overdoses may mimic the effects of head trauma, stroke, diabetic coma, or postseizure depression. Obtain as much patient-related history as possible to help make the proper diagnosis so proper treatment can be started before the results of blood tests for drug levels are available.

Drug automatism ("automatic" drug-taking) has been cited as a cause of overdose with barbiturates and other sedatives or hypnotics, especially in elderly or debilitated outpatients. These persons may take a recommended bedtime dose of drug, become confused and unable to remember whether they took the medication, and take another dose. This cycle may be repeated several times, leading to an overdose. If you cannot depend on the patient to take the correct dose, recruit a responsible person to administer the drug.

Related Drugs

Other barbiturates are listed in Table 22–C1. Their pharmacologic actions are identical to those noted for the prototype. In general, their onsets and durations of action determine their use.

Amobarbital, Pentobarbital, and Secobarbital

Pentobarbital (NEMBUTAL) and secobarbital (SECONAL) are short-acting barbiturates that are used mainly as hypnotics for persons who have trouble falling asleep but usually sleep uninterrupted. Amobarbital (AMYTAL), which has a somewhat longer duration of action, is sometimes prescribed for persons who wake frequently during the night.

Mephobarbital and Metharbital

Mephobarbital (MEBARAL) and metharbital (GEMONIL), two very-long-acting barbiturates, are used only for managing seizure disorders (see Chapter 26). Their actions are virtually identical to the prototype.

Thiamylal, Thiopental, and Methohexital

Thiamylal (SURITAL), thiopental (PENTOTHAL), and methohexital (BREVITAL) are ultra–short-acting barbiturates that are given only parenterally, mainly for anesthesia-related uses (see Chapter 20). Thiopental is also used in psychiatry for narcoanalysis and narcosynthesis. In these procedures enough of the drug is administered to make the patient drowsy and briefly confused, but still awake. Soon the patient reaches a state of consciousness in which suppressed thoughts can be verbalized in response to questions by the physician. This technique can provide important insight into underlying psychiatric problems. Thiopental gained its popular name "truth serum" because of this use.

II. Benzodiazepines

Studies in the 1950s showed that a group of chemicals, called *benzodiazepines,* calmed agitated animals without causing ataxia or sleep. Since then, many related compounds with several important clinical indications (Table 22–C2) have become available. Diazepam (VALIUM) is the prototype. In recent years it has been the most frequently prescribed drug in the United States.

General Characteristics of Benzodiazepines

One way to characterize the benzodiazepines is to compare and contrast them with barbiturates. These two classes of drugs are chemically different, but agents in both groups can be used for the same clinical indications. As was true for barbiturates, the onset and duration of action of a particular benzodiazepine will affect its use. For example, a benzodiazepine with a short duration of action would be better suited for use as a hypnotic than as a daytime sedative or anxiety-relieving medication. However, with the benzodiazepines there is no neat or predictable relationship between onset and duration of action, as is true for barbiturates. The primary pharmacologic effect, CNS depression, and the side effects related to that action, are also similar for drugs in the two classes.

PROTOTYPE

Diazepam

Absorption, Distribution, Metabolism, and Excretion

Diazepam can be given orally or by injection. The drug distributes widely throughout the body, and enters the CNS well. The drug, and its metabolites, cross the placental barrier and are excreted in breast milk at levels that come close to those in maternal blood.

When only a single dose of diazepam is given, or when diazepam therapy is first started, the drug's CNS depressant effects appear within minutes (depending on the administration route) and last less than a day. However, when administration is continued, as is often done when the drug is used to manage anxiety, the effects are prolonged considerably. That is because some of diazepam's many metabolites are active CNS depressants, and some have half-lives that are much longer than that of diazepam itself (Fig. 22–3). When administration is continued, there is a tendency for these long-acting metabolites to accumulate in the bloodstream and brain, which can lead to excessive and prolonged effects that usually are unwanted.

Many of the other benzodiazepines (identified in the Related Drugs section) also are metabolized, and some form the same active metabolites. Indeed, some of the metabolites have been synthesized in the laboratory and are themselves available as drugs. The

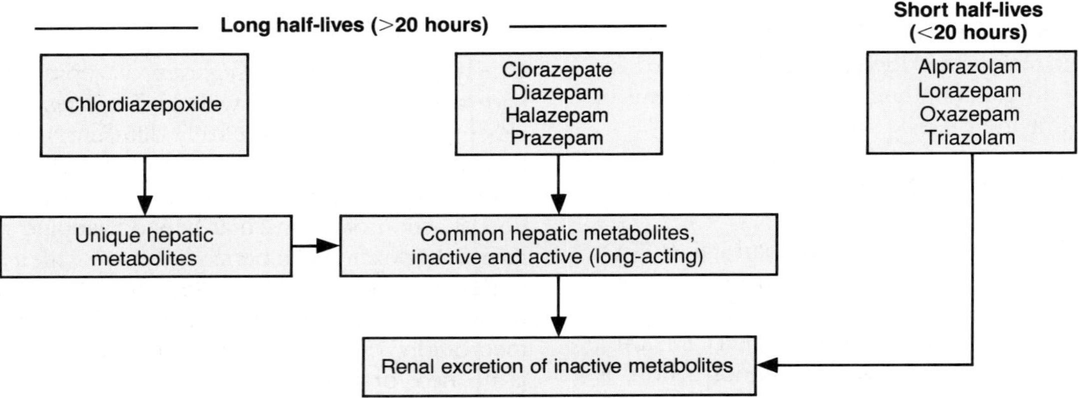

Figure 22–3

Different benzodiazepine anxiolytics may be converted to the same metabolite(s), some of which are biologically active and have durations of action that are much longer than those of the drugs that formed them. One metabolite, oxazepam, is itself available as a drug. Durations of action have no bearing on whether the onset of action is relatively slow or fast. Most benzodiazepine hypnotics (not shown here; see Table 22–C2) mainly form inactive metabolites or are excreted unchanged, and have half-lives shorter than those shown for alprazolam and others.

metabolites of a particular benzodiazepine may have longer or shorter half-lives than the parent (original) drug; and those metabolites may be pharmacologically active as CNS depressants, or may be inactive. Some benzodiazepines have very fast onsets of action, caused mainly by the effects of the unmetabolized drug that was given to the patient; plus very long durations of action caused by the metabolites. Others have slow onsets of action and brief durations of action.

In summary, the predictable pharmacokinetic relationships that described the barbiturates (slow onset, long duration; fast onset, short duration) simply do not apply to benzodiazepines. In theory, this allows the clinician to pick a particular benzodiazepine with pharmacokinetic properties that are closest to the patient's individual needs.

NURSING IMPLICATIONS

You will learn more about the onsets and durations of action of the individual benzodiazepines as you gain more clinical experience with them. At this point it is more important simply to (1) be aware of the lack of relationship between a benzodiazepine's onset and duration of action; and (2) understand that these properties, and the dependence of a particular agent on hepatic metabolism or renal excretion, can have a bearing on whether a particular drug might be more or less suitable than another for a certain patient.

Pharmacologic Effects

Low doses of most benzodiazepines alleviate anxiety or agitation, sometimes without causing barbiturate-like sedation. Higher doses cause sedation, sleep, or anesthesia. Diazepam and some related benzodiazepines have clinically useful anticonvulsant actions, and central or spinal actions that inhibit abnormal activation of skeletal muscle. Many of these effects may be due to the drug's ability to increase activity or release of the inhibitory neurotransmitter gamma-aminobutyric acid (GABA) in parts of the CNS, where benzodiazepine receptors have been found.

Clinical Indications and Administration

There are three reasons why benzodiazepines are usually preferred to a barbiturate or to any other drug that shares the same approved uses.

1. They have a much greater margin of safety.
2. They are less likely to interact with other drugs.
3. They are less likely to cause physical dependence.

The indications for diazepam, and the usual dosages, are summarized in Table 22–C2.

Uses for Anxiety Disorders

Diazepam and many related drugs are indicated for short-term relief of anxiety symptoms. These drugs are best used for acute anxiety accompanied by apprehension, frequent overreactivity to simple life situations, excessive autonomic activity (diarrhea, diaphoresis), and muscular tension. No anxiolytic drug should be prescribed for mild and infrequent anxiety resulting from ordinary life stresses to which most individuals can adapt or cope, nor should they be used for more than 4 months at a time. Benzodiazepines are useful adjuncts to relieving anxiety accompanying medical problems such as peptic ulcer disease, angina, or hypertension. However, they should not be used instead of the drugs indicated for these conditions.

Benzodiazepines have been called "minor tranquilizers," but they are not suitable substitutes for antipsychotic drugs (Chapter 23) for severe psychiatric disorders, nor for antidepressants (Chapter 24) in persons with true psychiatric depression. However, benzodiazepines may be useful adjuncts to antidepressant drug therapy for persons with depressive illness accompanied by severe anxiety. New studies are showing the efficacy of benzodiazepines for patients who suffer from panic disorders.

Hypnosis

The sedative and anxiety-relieving effects of diazepam can facilitate sleep, and doses that are sufficiently high can cause sleep. Diazepam itself is not indicated as a hypnotic; other benzodiazepines are, however. Sleep induced by a benzodiazepine is similar to that caused by a barbiturate hypnotic in terms of the rather natural changes of cardiovascular and respiratory function. One important difference between the two groups of drugs, however, is that benzodiazepines do not suppress REM sleep. This is an advantage, especially if a hypnotic must be given for more than a couple of nights in a row. However, the benzodiazepine hypnotics lose some of their effectiveness, and tend to cause barbiturate-like effects that can carry over into waking hours, after about 4 weeks of consecutive use. Continued use after this time is seldom justified for the typical patient with common insomnia, regardless of what class of hypnotic drug is being administered.

Uses for Musculoskeletal Disorders

Diazepam is approved for relief of mild muscle spasm resulting from minor trauma or athletic injuries. It can be given orally or parenterally. It theoretically acts centrally to reduce motor nerve impulses to skeletal muscle. Diazepam is also indicated for managing spasticity associated with spinal cord injuries or tetanus.

Benzodiazepines may be no more effective for mild and acute musculoskeletal conditions than antiinflammatory drugs such as aspirin (Chapter 52), bed rest, and local application of heat. However, sedation and anxiety-relief may benefit some patients.

Management of Acute and Chronic Seizure Disorders

Diazepam, injected intravenously, is a drug of choice for treating status epilepticus. Because of diazepam's short initial duration of action, repeated injections may be needed for recurrent seizures. Oral diazepam may be used for long-term treatment of epilepsy or other recurrent seizure disorders, but other classes of anticonvulsant drugs are used much more often (Chapter 26).

Management of Acute Alcohol Withdrawal

Diazepam is an effective drug for managing signs and symptoms of acute alcohol withdrawal. It alleviates seizures, hyperactivity, and anxiety. Unlike other drugs used for this purpose, including barbiturates and paraldehyde, diazepam is much less likely to cause respiratory and cardiovascular depression. Many centers specializing in management of alcohol withdrawal initially give a relatively large oral or IV dose, followed by smaller repeated doses until sedation develops and other withdrawal symptoms diminish. Oral therapy can then be started if effects are still needed. With repeated administration, the long half-lives of diazepam's active metabolites provide a gradual, smooth recovery.

Sedation, Anxiety Relief, Amnesia for Surgical or Diagnostic Procedures

Diazepam, and some of the other benzodiazepines, are used as premedications for surgery or medical or diagnostic procedures such as cardioversion or endoscopy. They are usually given by injection for this purpose, with the preferred route (IV or IM) depending on the drug and the situation. Anxiety relief, sedation, or sleep (depending on the dose) are clearly advantageous in these situations, and they can also be achieved with barbiturates. However, the benzodiazepines cause another effect, not shared by barbiturates, that is clearly an advantage to the patient about to undergo a physically or emotionally stressful procedure. It is called *anterograde amnesia*. It can be defined as a loss of memory about events that occur shortly after the drug is given. As noted below, this amnesia-causing effect is also a side effect of some of the benzodiazepines used for other purposes, such as the management of insomnia.

NURSING IMPLICATIONS

Most nursing measures noted for the administration and use of barbiturates apply also to benzodiazepines. Be aware that IM injections of diazepam are painful and may cause phlebitis. Diazepam and other benzodiazepines are chemically incompatible with most other drugs; do not mix them in the same syringe. The IV route is most reliable. Give diazepam no faster than 5 mg/min; if an infusion set is used inject as close to the insertion site as possible.

Side Effects, Adverse Reactions, and Contraindications

Most of the CNS, cardiovascular, and respiratory side effects caused by benzodiazepines are similar to those described for phenobarbital and the other barbiturates (see Table 22–S1). The intensity and duration of the side effects depend on the drug (especially its half-life and the half-lives of its active metabolites), the dose, and patient-related factors such as age and overall health. Tolerance to CNS depressant effects seems to develop with continued use.

Although benzodiazepines have some important advantages over barbiturates for most uses, they can cause some unique and important problems (Table 22–S2). High oral doses of diazepam, or usual injected doses, can cause antimuscarinic (atropine-like) side effects, including dry mouth, mydriasis, and blurred vision. The pupil-dilating effect necessitates cautious use in persons with narrow-angle glaucoma, a common disorder in elderly persons and one for which antimuscarinic drugs are contraindicated.

Benzodiazepines indicated for use as hypnotics cause less REM sleep depression, and so are generally preferred. Even so, rebound insomnia can still be a problem when therapy is stopped. More importantly, perhaps, are the growing number of reports that short-acting benzodiazepine hypnotics can cause a relatively high incidence of confusion, amnesia, bizarre behavior, agitation, and hallucinations. Most of the information about these potentially serious effects has focused on the related drug triazolam (HALCION), which became a very widely used hypnotic soon after it was approved for use. These adverse reports have caused drug-regulating agencies in some countries to ban the use of triazolam altogether; in others, such as the United States, stronger label warnings and guidelines for reduced dosages (especially important for the elderly patient) have been imposed.

Benzodiazepines do not stimulate hepatic drug-metabolizing enzymes. Therefore, problems related to porphyria or vitamin K or D deficiencies, described for phenobarbital, do not occur.

NURSING IMPLICATIONS

All nursing implications that apply to the CNS side effects of phenobarbital apply to diazepam. Additional nursing implications specific for diazepam's antimuscarinic side effects are the same as for atropine (see pp 173–176).

◆ Use During Pregnancy and Lactation

Benzodiazepines have the potential to cause fetal deformities when administered to pregnant women during the first trimester. Thus, these drugs should not be used for such indications as managing anxiety or insomnia unless it is absolutely necessary. Women taking these drugs should be instructed to notify their physician at once if they become pregnant.

Benzodiazepines and their metabolites are excreted in breast milk, and can potentially cause the same effects as noted for barbiturates in nursing infants. However, some clinicians report few problems in breast-fed neonates when low dosages of benzodiazepines are used, and a feeding is started and finished just before a drug dose is taken.

◆ Use in Children

Children exhibit variable responses to benzodiazepines, just as they do to barbiturates, and the lowest effective dose should be used. Do not give IV diazepam to children less than 30 days old unless it is to treat status epilepticus.

◆ Use in the Elderly

Elderly persons are, in general, much more sensitive to the side effects of benzodiazepines than younger persons, including children. Age-related changes in liver or renal function can affect the selection of a particular benzodiazepine for them, and changes in CNS status can affect the response to any of these drugs. Problems owing to confusion, ataxia, and the more unusual responses associated with drugs such as triazolam, are more common and potentially more disruptive and dangerous. Maintenance doses, and especially initial doses, should be lower than those recommended for adults.

Also be aware that elderly persons are more likely to have underlying medical conditions (eg, glaucoma, prostatic hypertrophy) that can be aggravated by diazepam's antimuscarinic effects.

Tolerance, Dependence, and Abuse

Long-term benzodiazepine administration for anxiety relief or management of insomnia can cause psychologic dependence. And, contrary to earlier beliefs, physical dependence does occur, as evidenced by the physiologic signs and symptoms of withdrawal on abrupt discontinuation. In most cases, they resemble the rebound insomnia and anxiety described for barbiturates. These problems seem to be more common with benzodiazepines having short durations of action. They can be minimized by keeping the duration of therapy as short as possible, and by discontinuing the drug gradually, tapering the dose.

NURSING IMPLICATIONS

Benzodiazepines are popular drugs of abuse, often in combination with alcohol and other depressants. Patients seeking easy relief from anxiety often ask for prescriptions, even specifying the brand name product they would like. Some physicians are quite willing to comply, since benzodiazepines are perceived as very safe and not all physicians agree that dependence may occur. Nevertheless, nursing guidelines noted for the barbiturates clearly apply to the benzodiazepines.

Interactions with Other Drugs

Benzodiazepines interact with all other CNS depressants to cause additive (or greater) CNS depressant effects. Alcohol is probably the most common interactant. Other interactants (Table 22–I2) include mainly drugs that can inhibit the hepatic metabolism of diazepam and several other benzodiazepines, with the potential outcome being excessive sedation or impaired psychomotor function.

The benzodiazepines do not cause barbiturate-like stimulation of the hepatic enzyme systems. As a result, they do not speed the metabolic rates of other drugs that depend on liver metabolism for their removal from the body.

Overdose and Toxicity

Unlike barbiturates, the benzodiazepines have an extremely high margin of safety. Massive doses of diazepam, taken alone, may cause serious depression of the central nervous, respiratory, and cardiovascular systems, but there have been few proven deaths. However, the simultaneous use of even low doses of any other CNS depressant, including alcohol, dramatically increases the risk of fatality. Coma may occur, and respiratory arrest and cardiovascular collapse are the major causes of death in these combined overdoses.

Symptomatic, supportive care to maintain adequate ventilatory and cardiovascular/renal status is the main way to manage benzodiazepine overdoses. For many years the acetylcholinesterase inhibitor physostigmine (ANTILIRIUM; Chapter 12) has been used as an adjunct to the management of life-threatening benzodiazepine overdoses. Recently, however, a specific and very effective benzodiazepine receptor blocker, flumazenil (MAZICON), has been approved. As described in more detail below, flumazenil has become a first-line drug for diagnosing benzodiazepine overdoses. Although it may make the diagnosis and management of benzodiazepine overdoses easier, and it helps the patient recover more quickly, it does not replace the need for proper assessment and other forms of treatment.

Related Drugs

There are now over a dozen orally effective benzodiazepines, in addition to diazepam, that are approved for use in the United States (see Table 22–C2). About half of them are indicated mainly for short-term relief of anxiety symptoms. The rest are indicated as hypnotics. Some of these drugs, plus a few other injectable benzodiazepines, have additional uses such as the management of seizures, or as a preanesthetic medication.

In general, no one benzodiazepine anxiolytic (or hypnotic) drug stands out as being clearly more effective, advantageous, or safe than another. Overall, drug–drug interactions and side effects (with the possible exception of the behavioral and amnesia-causing effects thought to occur with triazolam), are similar among the alternatives.

Ideally, then, the choice of a particular agent should be based on the best match between

- the pharmacokinetic properties of the individual drug (eg, onset and duration of action, dependence on hepatic metabolism, and the plasma half-lives of the metabolites or parent drug); and
- the needs and characteristics of the individual patient (eg, symptom severity and time-course; liver or renal status; age, and overall health).

As noted above, the pharmacokinetic properties of these drugs can vary widely, with fast onsets not necessarily being associated with short durations of effect. Cost may also be a factor, as some benzodiazepines are much more expensive than others. Regardless of the drug that is used, it is important to

- start therapy with lower-than-usual doses for elderly or debilitated patients;
- monitor the actual responses of *all* patients, focusing on CNS responses, but not ignoring other potential effects; and
- avoid use of these drugs as anxiolytics or hypnotics continuously for times beyond those ordinarily recommended.

NURSING IMPLICATIONS

Benzodiazepines are, for the most part, the most ideal group of anxiolytics and hypnotics currently available. However, new ones are being developed and will be approved for use. Like all the benzodiazepines that came before them, there will be claims of therapeutic superiority or properties that are in some way better suited for certain (or most) patients. As a result, they are likely to be widely prescribed, and misprescribed. If the future repeats the past, anticipate that with increased or widespread clinical use following approval, unexpected problems are likely to be found. Some drugs may be removed from the market; others may remain, but with tighter controls and regulations imposed on their use, dose, or dispensing.

FLUMAZENIL: A Benzodiazepine Antagonist

Flumazenil (MAZICON) selectively blocks benzodiazepine receptors. In doing so it reduces or completely eliminates the effects of any benzodiazepine that may have been administered before or after. Given the widespread medical use of benzodiazepines, and their frequent involvement in overdoses, flumazenil represents a major therapeutic breakthrough.

Flumazenil's effects are very specific. It does not block receptors, or reverse or prevent responses to, other antagonists—eg, catecholamines, acetylcholine, or narcotics. Flumazenil has no direct CNS stimulating effects of its own. Thus, it will not cause effects when given to a patient who has received no other drugs, and it will not reverse the depressant effects of drugs such as barbiturates or alcohol, which do not work through specific receptor sites. Finally, flumazenil does not speed the metabolism or excretion of benzodiazepines; it merely blocks their effects.

Flumazenil has two major uses the capitalize on its specific benzodiazepine receptor-blocking activity. For both, the drug is given intravenously. Small doses, given repeatedly as needed (see Table 22-C2), are preferred to giving a single large dose. If the patient is likely to respond to the drug, effects should be seen within 30 to 60 seconds.

Reversal of Intended Benzodiazepine Effects

One main use of flumazenil is to reverse the CNS depressant effects of benzodiazepines that are administered to patients intentionally. This includes the use of benzodiazepines for conscious sedation and amnesia before or during diagnostic or surgical procedures, and the use of benzodiazepines as part of a multidrug anesthesia regimen. Flumazenil will hasten the patient's recovery to a more awake, alert state. Flumazenil blocks only those effects caused by a benzodiazepine, so it will not change the actions of other drugs that may also have been administered.

Flumazenil is an important adjunctive drug for patients who will remain hospitalized after a procedure for which a benzodiazepine is given. It is perhaps more valuable for outpatient procedures because it will allow the patient to leave for home in a more awake state.

Diagnostic Aid and Antidote for Benzodiazepine Overdoses

The second main use of flumazenil is to help diagnose and then manage overdoses that involve benzodiazepines. Assume that a patient presents with CNS depression (and perhaps ventilatory depression also) due to a drug overdose of unknown cause. If injecting one or two recommended doses of flumazenil increases the level of consciousness or ventilatory status within a few minutes, then one can assume that a benzodiazepine was involved. Repeated doses of flumazenil can then be given during the recovery period, as needed, while the body eliminates the benzodiazepine by metabolism or excretion. During that time it is still essential to maintain a patent airway, to support ventilation and other vital signs, and to monitor the patient appropriately.

Nurses and other care providers should know how to interpret the presence or absence of responses to flumazenil in drug overdose situations. A response to flumazenil means that one or more benzodiazepines have been taken, but it does not rule out the possibility that other drugs may also have been taken. Care will still be required, and blood toxicology tests are still indicated. Flumazenil may not work as well as expected, or at all, if the overdose victim has also taken very large doses of other classes of CNS or respiratory depressant drugs. For example, if the patient has also consumed large amounts of alcohol, or barbiturates, or narcotics, these other drugs may exert such intense CNS depressant effects that blocking just the effects of the benzodiazepine might do little to improve the patient's condition. Further evaluation and treatment are also necessary here. One intervention in overdoses of unknown cause will almost certainly involve administering the specific narcotic blocker, naloxone (NARCAN), to help determine whether a narcotic was involved. (See the section on narcotic antagonists, on pages 336 to 337, to see how similar their actions and uses are to those just described for flumazenil.)

Precautions and Potential Dangers with Flumazenil Use

There are potential risks associated with the administration of flumazenil. Most of them apply whether the patient has received a benzodiazepine for therapeutic purposes or as part of an overdose.

Return of Sedation and Ventilatory Depression

Flumazenil has a relatively short duration of action compared with those of many of the benzodiazepines. Thus, when the effects of flumazenil wear off, the depressant effects of a benzodiazepine that is still circulating in the bloodstream may reappear. This requires close monitoring and support and, possibly, the administration of more flumazenil. Patients who had poor ventilatory function before benzodiazepine and flumazenil administration will require especially close monitoring to ensure adequate ventilation. They may require ventilatory support.

Precautions are also important even when benzodiazepines with relatively short durations of action have been used. For example, when midazolam is used for an outpatient procedure, and then flumazenil is given before discharge, the patient may leave the facility relatively alert but he or she may redevelop drowsiness or ataxia several hours later. Thus, it is important to advise patients and others who will be caring for them of this possibility. They should not drive, or engage in other hazardous activities, until they are fully recovered.

Benzodiazepine Withdrawal

Quickly and effectively reversing benzodiazepine actions with flumazenil may bring on signs and symptoms of benzodiazepine withdrawal in persons who are physically dependent on them. As described on page 359, these responses could include anxiety, irritability, insomnia, or even seizures. The type and severity of these responses will depend on the benzodiazepine that has been given, its dose, how long it has been administered prior to flumazenil use, and the indication(s) for benzodiazepine administration. The risks for persons who have received a benzodiazepine for only a couple of days prior are low.

Seizures

Seizures are particularly dangerous responses to flumazenil if the patient has a history of seizure disorders, is taking anticonvulsant drugs, or has overdosed with seizure-causing medications. The benzodiazepine receptors that flumazenil blocks are the same receptors that are normally stimulated by the neurotransmitter, GABA (see p. 356, above). Among other things, GABA's inhibitory actions help keep abnormal brain electrical activity in check. When GABA receptors are blocked, seizures may occur in susceptible patients. The risks are greater in patients who are currently taking an anticonvulsant medication.

The risks of seizures after flumazenil administration are probably greatest in patients who have overdoses of seizure-causing drugs. The antidepressants are probably the most important in this regard, because they may be prescribed for persons who are also taking benzodiazepines, and they are relatively common ingredients in suicide attempts involving multiple drug overdoses. Patients who overdose on benzodiazepines and antidepressants together may not experience seizures because the benzodiazepines help to inhibit seizure development. However, when benzodiazepine effects are blocked by flumazenil, the seizure-causing effects of the antidepressant may be unmasked. Deaths have occurred in this way.

Flumazenil may also increase the risk of cardiac arrhythmias in susceptible patients.

NURSING IMPLICATIONS

Flumazenil can be mixed with or added to D_5W, lactated Ringer's, or normal saline if needed. Do not mix it with other fluids or other drugs, including naloxone that might be used to assess for narcotic overdoses. Discard any flumazenil that has been removed from its original container and not used within 24 hours.

◆ Use During Pregnancy and Lactation

Flumazenil can be used as an antidote in emergencies involving excessive benzodiazepine effects, but only if it is felt that not using it poses a greater risk to the mother. Otherwise, flumazenil should not be given to pregnant women, and it should not be used routinely to reverse usual effects of benzodiazepines that might be given during pregnancy or labor and delivery.

◆ Use in Children

There is no information about the potential adverse effects of flumazenil in children, but use of the drug is not recommended.

◆ Use in the Elderly

No special precautions or dosage adjustments are needed for elderly patients.

III. Nonbarbiturate, Nonbenzodiazepine Hypnotics and Sedatives

Several other drugs, which are not chemically classified as either barbiturates or benzodiazepines, are approved for use as sedatives or hypnotics. Their indications and dosages are summarized in Table 22–C3. All of them share the general CNS-depressant side effects and contraindications noted for the barbiturates and benzodiazepines. However, some of them cause additional and unique side effects or drug interactions, or have other properties that can be important for certain patients. That information is summarized in Table 22–S3.

Overall, very few of these miscellaneous sedatives and hypnotics have any advantage over a benzodiazepine with the same approved indication. Possible exceptions are hydroxyzine (VISTARIL) and diphenhydramine (BENADRYL). These drugs, which are available in both oral and parenteral dosage forms, are classified as histamine-receptor blockers (antihistamines). (Diphenhydramine is the prototype of the antihistamines, and is discussed in more detail in Chapter 51.) They cause dose-dependent sedation, which is therapeutically useful in its own right. However, they also suppress nausea and vomiting, which makes them useful for preventing postoperative emesis (hydroxyzine) or motion sickness (diphenhydramine), especially when the sedative effect is helpful too. The antihistamines, and diphenhydramine in particular, cause intense antimuscarinic (atropine-like) side effects, and share the contraindications noted for atropine (p 185).

Nonprescription Products with Sedative Ingredients

Over-the-counter (OTC) products marketed specifically as sleep aids contain one of three sedating antihistamines: doxylamine, diphenhydramine, or pyrilamine. An antihistamine is also the usual sedative ingredient in combination-drug remedies marketed to relieve mild pain, inflammation, or fever, and advertised for nighttime ("PM") use. They are also found in many OTC products used for upper-respiratory-tract symptoms or cough remedies, some of which are advertised as being better suited for use at bedtime. Some OTC medications in these and other product categories contain alcohol as the sedative ingredient.

NURSING IMPLICATIONS

The recommended (label) dosages of CNS depressants in OTC products are generally in a therapeutic range—they are capable of causing the claimed desired effects. More importantly, they are clearly sufficient to cause side effects, to pose risks to patients who have a contraindicating condition, and to interact with other drugs the patient may be taking. Patients who self-administer these and other OTC drugs often do so without the advice or knowledge of a health-care provider. Therefore, it is essential to consider these medications in history-taking, assessment, and evaluation.

IV. Ethyl Alcohol

Ethanol (ethyl alcohol; "alcohol"), a general CNS depressant, has limited therapeutic uses. It is the most widely abused CNS depressant; it can cause serious medical and social problems, and interacts with many other drugs.

Absorption, Distribution, Metabolism, and Excretion

Ethanol is rapidly absorbed from the gastrointestinal (GI) tract. The presence of food in the gut, especially food rich in milk products or fat, slows absorption. Ethanol is distributed throughout the body and readily enters the CNS, where it exerts its most obvious effects. It crosses the placenta and enters the fetal circulation. Alcohol quickly enters maternal milk, where its concentration may be as high as 95% of maternal blood concentrations.

Ethanol is metabolized in the liver. The enzyme alcohol dehydrogenase first converts it to acetaldehyde, which is toxic in high concentrations. However, aldehyde dehydrogenase quickly metabolizes acetaldehyde to acetate, which is nontoxic and is further metabolized like other carbohydrates. Aldehyde dehydrogenase is inhibited by the drug disulfiram, discussed at the end of this section.

Unlike many drugs, the rate of ethanol metabolism is not always directly related to the blood ethanol concentration. The average adult can metabolize no more than about 10 mL of ethanol per hour, which is somewhat less than the amount of alcohol in 12 oz of beer, 4 oz of wine (10%–12% alcohol), or a shot (1.5 oz) of 80-proof (40% alcohol) liquor. Increasing intoxication occurs if alcohol is consumed faster than it is metabolized. Small amounts of ethanol are eliminated in the urine and expired air. The alcohol concentration in expired air is almost always about 0.05% of the blood concentration. This explains why law enforcement officials use breath tests to estimate a driver's blood alcohol level.

Acute ethanol ingestion inhibits the liver's drug-metabolizing enzyme systems; chronic ingestion stimulates them, much like phenobarbital does. Both effects contribute to important drug–drug interactions. Enzyme stimulation by chronic ethanol consumption also contributes to tolerance.

Pharmacologic Effects

Central Nervous System Effects

Alcohol depresses the CNS much like the barbiturates do. Low doses often cause paradoxical stimulation, excitement, or emotional lability. Higher doses cause obvious sedation; loss of balance, coordination, and judgment; impaired gait; and other characteristics generally associated with an intoxicated person. All doses of ethanol slow motor reflexes, but sensitive tests may be needed to detect this effect when small amounts of alcohol have been ingested. Blood alcohol concentrations over 450 to 550 mg% (450–550 mg/100 mL) may cause coma and death. The relationship between blood ethanol concentration and effect is summarized in Table 22–2.

Table 22–2 Relationship Between Alcohol Consumption, Blood Alcohol Levels, and Degree of Central Nervous System Impairment*

Blood Level (mg/100 mL blood)	Anticipated Effect on Central Nervous System
<30	Reflexes, sensory function generally intact, but subtle changes can be detected with sensitive tests; legally safe for driving
30–50	Greater impairment of judgment, reflexes, and coordination; alterations of sensory perception; changes are enough to alter driving skills but not enough to be illegal in United States; this blood level occurs (in average adult) after consuming the equivalent of two ounces of 86-proof spirits, 8 ounces of wine, or two 12-ounce bottles of beer
50–150	Judgment, reflexes, and coordination usually impaired measurably; blood levels over 50 or 100 mg/100 mL are usually sufficient for charge of legally impaired driving when accompanied by other evidence; the equivalent of 6 ounces of 86-proof spirits, drunk quickly, is enough to produce a blood level of 150 mg/100 mL
150–400	Moderate-to-severe intoxication, deteriorating judgment, reflexes, and coordination; aggressive behavior often develops, followed by progression to lethargy, sedation
400–600	Severe intoxication; individual usually sleeps and arousal is difficult; blood levels of approximately 500 mg/100 mL or more are liable to produce coma and death

*Values given are approximate, and reflect alcohol consumption, cumulative blood levels, and response of otherwise healthy average adults (60–70 kg). Body weight and lean body mass have important effects on the response. Legal limits for driving, and classifications of impaired motor vehicle operation, vary among the states.

Effects on Other Organ Systems

Modest doses of ethanol do not significantly affect respiration, heart rate, or blood pressure. Alcohol weakly dilates peripheral (cutaneous) blood vessels, leading to warm, pink skin; this can increase heat loss through the skin and lower body temperature. Alcohol stimulates gastric blood flow and acid secretion, and irritates the GI tract. It also increases urine output. The diuresis is due in part to the large volumes of water that are often consumed with alcohol, and to inhibition of antidiuretic hormone release in the CNS.

Clinical Indications and Administration

Ethanol has only a few recognized medical uses. A glass of wine before dinner, for example, may stimulate appetite; an afternoon drink may alleviate simple anxiety. Some studies suggest that modest ethanol consumption reduces the risk of some cardiovascular diseases. Ethanol can be given as a slow IV infusion to delay preterm labor, through its inhibitory effects on uterine tone. However, the sympathomimetic uterine relaxant ritodrine (YUTOPAR, Chapters 14 and 49) is generally preferred because it does not cause fetal CNS depression. Intravenous administration of ethanol is the preferred treatment for poisoning with methyl alcohol (methanol; wood alcohol). When given for this purpose the liver preferentially metabolizes ethyl alcohol, which reduces metabolism of methyl alcohol to its very toxic product formaldehyde.

There are several indications for topical administration of ethanol on the skin. It is a solvent for chemicals and plant irritants, such as those causing poison ivy: thoroughly washing the skin with ethanol soon after contact can prevent a rash or reduce its severity. High concentrations of ethanol (about 70%) can be used as a topical disinfectant, and to prevent decubiti in bedridden patients. However, ethanol dries the skin, leading to itching, caking, and an increased risk of abrasions. Other approaches are generally preferred. Ethanol, when applied to the skin, evaporates quickly. This cooling action can be used to help lower body temperature in a febrile patient.

NURSING IMPLICATIONS

Isopropyl alcohol (rubbing alcohol) is usually used instead of ethyl alcohol for topical use on intact skin. Isopropyl and methyl alcohol must never be injected or ingested; they are very poisonous.

Side Effects, Adverse Reactions, and Contraindications

There is no good proof that infrequent consumption of small amounts of ethanol has adverse effects on healthy nonpregnant adults. Without question, excessive or inappropriate use of this drug can cause a host of medical, social, legal, and economic problems, as discussed in Chapter 28.

The most common and important side effects of ethanol ingestion are due to CNS depression, as described for barbiturates, but other important concerns exist (Table 22–S4). Acute ingestion of alcohol, at any dose, causes gastric irritation. Long-term, high-dose intake can cause ulcers. The risk of serious GI hemorrhage in the ulcer patient who is a chronic high-dose alcohol user is increased by ethanol's ability to decrease synthesis of hepatic blood-clotting factors.

Chronic high-dose ethanol intake irreversibly damages the liver, heart, and brain. Altered hepatic metabolism of natural foodstuffs leads to accumulation of fatty deposits in the liver and to cirrhosis. Organ damage and malnutrition are likely to occur if an individual ingests large amounts of alcohol at the expense of a well-balanced diet; alcohol provides ample calories but no vitamins and few proteins. Nutritional deficiency may cause myocarditis, cardiomegaly, heart failure, and brain damage. Brain dysfunction is often seen first as a loss of short-term memory. Altered sleep patterns, similar to those produced by barbiturates, often occur.

Chronic ethanol intake by males can produce gynecomastia, impotence, and sterility. These adverse effects result in part from increased hepatic breakdown of testosterone plus inhibited testosterone synthesis.

NURSING IMPLICATIONS

Ethanol is a common ingredient in many liquid drug formulations. The amount of added alcohol varies considerably, but even recommended doses of some products may be sufficient to cause sedation or interactions with other drugs. These products should be avoided when the effects of alcohol are unwanted.

Tolerance, Dependence, and Withdrawal

Repeated alcohol intake leads to tolerance, physical dependence, and a withdrawal syndrome when administration is stopped. Mild withdrawal is usually accompanied by sleep disorders, daytime anxiety, and agitation. Diazepam, administered under close supervision, may be useful to reduce mild withdrawal symptoms. In cases of severe dependence, withdrawal is liable to cause hallucinations, psychosis, or fatal seizures. Antipsychotic drugs may be indicated for psychiatric responses. Parenteral therapy with diazepam or other emergency anticonvulsants is essential if seizures occur. Delirium tremens ("DTs"), the most life-threatening manifestation of alcohol withdrawal, is characterized by all of the above symptoms and signs plus the risk of cardiovascular collapse and cerebral edema. In addition to the drugs noted above, administration of sympathomimetics and other emergency drugs may be needed to prevent death.

NURSING IMPLICATIONS

Patients undergoing alcohol withdrawal are often extremely agitated and easily provoked, even by routine measurements of vital signs, feeding, and bathing. Continual reassurance of the patient is essential. Monitor them closely, and do not leave them alone if possible. Keep the room well lighted at night if DTs occur. Avoid physical restraints. If vomiting is likely to occur, position the patient on his or her side to prevent aspiration of vomitus.

Care of the alcoholic patient can be complex and discouraging. Anticipate altered liver function, which may cause other disorders, alter responses to drugs, and affect nutritional state. Addressing nutritional needs is as important as meeting psychologic and medical needs. Patients should be encouraged to eat a nutritious diet high in protein, calories, and B-complex vitamins.

◆ Use During Pregnancy and Lactation

Alcohol ingestion during pregnancy is a great and valid concern. Most authorities recommend minimal alcohol consumption during pregnancy, especially during the first trimester, and some recommend total abstinence during pregnancy. The greatest risk is the *fetal alcohol syndrome,* characterized by inhibited in utero and postpartum growth and development, learning, and acquisition of motor skills. Women who consume high amounts of alcohol, even periodically, should be discouraged from breast-feeding. An occasional alcoholic beverage consumed by a nursing mother may cause some pharmacologic effects in the nursing infant, but there is no good evidence of harm.

◆ Use in Children

Recommend that parents wishing to give an OTC cough or cold remedy to their child choose an alcohol-free product. Recommended doses of OTC products with alcohol do not contain enough alcohol to suppress cough but do contain enough to cause unwanted CNS effects.

◆ Use in the Elderly

An occasional drink of alcohol, particularly before meals, may improve appetite. Be aware, however, that even modest amounts of alcohol may aggravate common age-related conditions such as confusion or diabetes mellitus, or interact with drugs commonly given to elderly patients. Assess for age-related mental or physical conditions that may contribute to ethanol abuse in the elderly.

Interactions with Other Drugs

Alcohol intensifies the central actions of virtually all other CNS depressants, and participates in several other important interactions (Table 22–13). The combined effects may make it difficult for the person to perceive or appreciate the degree of impairment or its potential dangers. The combination of chloral hydrate and ethanol (known in old movies as "knock-out drops" or a "Mickey Finn") is especially interesting and dangerous. Alcohol stimulates the metabolism of chloral hydrate to the more potent CNS depressant trichloroethanol. Trichloroethanol, in turn, inhibits ethanol's metabolic inactivation. The result is profound CNS depression. Alcohol apparently lowers the minimum lethal blood level for propoxyphene; most fatal propoxyphene overdoses involve alcohol consumption.

Alcohol hypoglycemia caused by oral antidiabetic/hypoglycemic drugs; and gastric irritation from aspirin and other nonsteroidal antiinflammatory drugs. Although aspirin is a popular hangover remedy, frequent aspirin use after alcohol intake increases the risk of ulcer formation or bleeding. Advise people to avoid this potentially serious interaction.

Disulfiram causes severe adverse responses (described later) when ethanol is ingested. Other drugs, including some cephalosporin antibiotics (cefamandole, cefoperazone, cefotetan, moxalactam), oral hypoglycemics, and metronidazole cause disulfiram-like interactions.

Overdose and Toxicity

Acute ethanol overdoses can be fatal owing to barbiturate-like depression of the CNS and respiratory and cardiovascular systems. Gastrointestinal bleeding or hemorrhage may occur. The drug's ability to promote heat loss may also cause fatal hypothermia in cold environments. Although acute intoxication with ethanol alone can be fatal, most deaths are due to combined ingestion with other depressants. Treatment is symptomatic and supportive.

Disulfiram

Disulfiram (ANTABUSE) inhibits the enzyme aldehyde dehydrogenase, causing ethanol metabolism to stop at the production of acetaldehyde. When acetaldehyde accumulates it causes unpleasant and potentially dangerous adverse responses. Disulfiram is used adjunctively (with counseling and other nondrug measures) to help consenting alcoholics stop drinking completely. The unpleasant responses that occur when alcohol is consumed during disulfiram therapy are used to reinforce the desire to remain sober. Disulfiram therapy is usually started with a single 500-mg dose, preferably taken at night to prevent sedation from interfering with daytime activities. This dose is taken for 1 or 2 weeks, and then is usually reduced for maintenance therapy to an average daily dose of 250 mg. The daily dose should never exceed 500 mg. Disulfiram therapy alone is not a cure for alcohol abuse.

The disulfiram–alcohol interaction usually lasts about 1 hour, although it may last longer if blood alcohol levels are sufficiently high. The intensity of the response depends on the blood level of acetaldehyde, which depends on the blood alcohol level. Common signs and symptoms include diaphoresis and flushing of the upper extremities, neck, and face; throbbing headache; nausea and profuse vomiting; palpitations; tightness of the chest and dyspnea; tremor; weakness; and an overall feeling of being very ill. Severe responses include arrhythmias, myocardial infarction, acute cardiac failure, seizures, coma, and death. Treatment with oxygen, vasopressors, antiarrhythmics, and anticonvulsants may be needed.

Because of the potential seriousness of the response, disulfiram should be used with extreme caution in patients with severe cardiovascular disease, hepatic disease (including alcohol-induced cirrhosis), hypothyroidism, and renal disease. Disulfiram should not be given during pregnancy.

NURSING IMPLICATIONS

Disulfiram therapy should be voluntary. The drug should not be given to patients who wish to continue drinking, even in moderation, or to persons who cannot be trusted to remain abstinent. Disulfiram should *never* be given to an intoxicated person or a person who has consumed alcohol in the past 2 weeks. It was once common for physicians to administer a small amount of ethanol to patients after a week or two of therapy so they would experience and "appreciate" the deterrent effect of the adverse response. This practice is potentially dangerous.

Advise patients and their families to avoid common causes of accidental but potentially serious interactions: foods prepared with alcohol; alcohol-containing drugs (including many OTC drugs); some mouthwashes; and toiletries such as after-shave lotions or colognes. Advise patients to carry or wear appropriate identification indicating their use of disulfiram. Identify and stress the value of alcohol abuse programs and other support measures. Stress that disulfiram alone is not a cure for alcohol abuse.

SUMMARY OF NURSING IMPLICATIONS

◆ Assessment

Determine patient's level of anxiety and usual methods of coping (eg, use of drugs, alcohol, smoking).

Complete nursing history to include sleeping patterns and history of medications that may be potential interactants.

Identify current abilities to manage activities of daily living if anxiety is present.

Establish baseline physical assessment data before administering medications.

◆ Nursing Diagnoses

Sleep pattern disturbance related to [specific patient problem].

Ineffective breathing pattern related to CNS depression following drug administration.

High risk for injury related to drug side effects (confusion, dizziness, ataxia).

Knowledge deficit related to prescribed drug regimen.

Ineffective individual coping related to anxiety; high risk for drug abuse.

Sensory/perceptual alterations (specify type) related to drug side effects.

◆ Planning/Implementation

Have patient remain in bed following the initial dose of a hypnotic.

Monitor patient's response to medication; assist with walking; protect from falls.

Monitor respirations every 5 to 15 minutes following IV administration; have resuscitation equipment available; naloxone ineffective for respiratory depression caused by barbiturates, benzodiazepines, and all other non-narcotics.

Observe elderly, very young, or debilitated patients for paradoxical stimulation, excitement, or confusion; raise side rails.

Reduce dose of other depressant drugs (ie, narcotics) when given with sedatives, to reduce risk of excessive CNS, respiratory, or cardiovascular depression.

Do not rely on barbiturates or benzodiazepines for pain relief.

Use careful technique for injecting barbiturates: sedatives are alkaline and can cause tissue necrosis with extravasation. Avoid intraarterial injection, which may cause arterial spasm or thrombosis.

Give IM injections in a large muscle; limit volume to 5 mL per injection site; rotate sites.

Recognize signs and symptoms of porphyria: skin rash, abdominal pain, or muscle weakness or pain.

Do not give barbiturates to pregnant women; fetal damage can occur.

Observe patient for signs of withdrawal when discontinuing sedatives, hypnotics, or anxiolytics (eg, increased anxiety, insomnia, irritability, delirium, seizures); notify physician.

If overdose occurs, change patient's position frequently, monitor breath sounds, and check body temperature to detect infection and prevent decubiti.

Give paraldehyde in ample amounts of ice-cold juice or other beverage to minimize poor taste and mouth irritation; keep patient's room well ventilated to reduce offensive odor from breath; frequent use of air freshener is advised.

Closely observe patient undergoing withdrawal or detoxification; taking vital signs, feeding, or bathing may agitate patient.

◆ Patient and Family Teaching

Teach the patient/family:

To seek thorough medical and psychologic evaluation when hypnotic use extends past 2 weeks.

To avoid operating dangerous machinery, driving, or engaging in tasks requiring good reflexes, coordination, and unaltered thought until medication effects can be determined.

To use other or additional forms of contraception if taking steroidal preparations and barbiturates; notify physician immediately if pregnancy is suspected.

To have family administer medications to elderly or debilitated patients who are confused easily or unable to self-administer proper doses.

That hypnotics should not be kept at bedside or any other quickly accessible place.

About signs of excessive antimuscarinic side effects, from diazepam particularly; to report ocular pain at once, other visual disturbances, or changes in normal gut or bladder function (eg, constipation, urinary retention).

To avoid alcohol completely if pregnant; explain potential risk of fetal alcohol syndrome.

To avoid alcohol when taking sedatives or CNS depressants.

To avoid use of aspirin or other nonsteroidal anti-inflammatory drugs for symptomatic relief of alcohol hangover; recommend acetaminophen.

To seek proper supportive therapy; provide list of local agencies or individuals specializing in abuse problems; involve family.

◆ Evaluation

The patient/family will:

Report adequate rest.

Use sleeping (hypnotic) aids appropriately.

Report any dizziness or unsteadiness during activities; verbalize need for assistance.

Achieve optimal activity level without incidence.

Demonstrate ability to follow prescribed regimen; take medication as ordered.

Verbalize reduction in anxiety.

Identify effective and ineffective (eg, use of alcohol, drugs) coping patterns; avoid drug abuse.

Experience no adverse drug effects.

Annotated Bibliography

Balter MB, Uhlenhuth EH. The beneficial and adverse effects of hypnotics. *J Clin Psychiatry* 1991;52(Suppl.):16–23. *An interesting summary of how patients viewed their responses, good and bad, to prescription hypnotics and OTC sleep aids.*

Cooper JW. Reviewing geriatric concerns with commonly used drugs. *Geriatrics* 1989;44(12):79–86. *Covering many therapeutic agents used often in elders, this short article also gives good advice about the use of hypnotics and anxiolytics.*

Dubovsky SL. Generalized anxiety disorder: New concepts and psychopharmacologic therapies. *J Clin Psychiatry* 1990;51(Suppl.): 3–10. *Useful not only for its overview of drug therapy for anxiety, but also for its holistic approach to the problem: the values of careful assessment for medical illnesses that can aggravate anxiety; withdrawal of all unnecessary medications (including unneeded CNS depressants) and caffeine; structured relaxation techniques; and psychotherapy.*

Gerbino PP. Complications of alcohol use combined with drug therapy in the elderly. *J Am Geriatr Soc* 1982;30(11 Suppl.):

S88–S93. *Despite its publication date, this is a timeless article on how chronic alcohol ingestion can impair drug therapy, cause potentially serious drug interactions, and compromise overall adherence to an otherwise well-planned treatment program.*

Gorman JM, Papp LA. Chronic anxiety: Deciding the length of treatment. *J Clin Psychiatry* 1990;51(Suppl.):11–15. *One guiding rule for anxiety therapy is to use the lowest effective dose for the shortest possible time. This article discusses when bending the rule may be needed, but stresses that the other general rule—make the benefits outweigh the risks—must still be followed through careful drug selection and frequent evaluation of treatment.*

Macdonald JB. The role of drugs in falls in the elderly. *Clin Geriatr Med* 1985;1(3):621–636. *Still a valuable article on an important and often overlooked cause of morbidity and mortality in elders. It focuses on barbiturates, but discusses other drugs; and shows how polypharmacy and the presence of multiple diseases compounds the risk of serious drug-related falls.*

Nakra BR, Grossberg GT. Peck B. Insomnia in the elderly. *Am Fam Physician* 1991;43(2):477–483. *This well-written article discusses the most common sleep disorder in the elderly, identifies pros and cons of various therapeutic options, and considers the values and limitations of nondrug therapies.*

Pasnau RO, Bystritsky A. Importance of treating anxiety in the elderly ill patient. *Psychiatr Med* 1990;8(3):163–173. *While there may be valid reasons to keep the number of drugs given to elders at a minimum, in some cases therapy of disorders such as anxiety can be both necessary and safe if certain precautions are taken.*

Prinz PN, Vitiello MV, Raskind MA, Thorpy MJ. Geriatrics: Sleep disorders and aging. *N Engl J. Med* 1990;323(8):520–526. *An excellent article dealing with age-related sleep disorders, covering both etiology and treatment.*

Salzman C. Anxiety in the elderly: Treatment strategies. *J Clin Psychiatry* 1990;51(Suppl.):18–21. (See also discussion on pp 29–32.) *Discusses management of simple anxiety and anxiety accompanied by depression. Discusses the benzodiazepines in general, but also considers important pharmacokinetic and pharmacodynamic properties of individual benzodiazepines that can affect their selection and the patient's responses to them, especially regarding side effects.*

Teboul E, Chouinard G. A guide to benzodiazepine selection. Part II: Clinical aspects. *Can J Psychiatry* 1991;36(1):62–73. *Valuable coverage of how the onsets and durations of benzodiazepine action can be used to help select a preferred drug for a particular use and patient. Discusses other issues, including treatment of the elderly and suspected drug abusers; and special properties of some benzodiazepines.*

Wysowski DK, Barash D. Adverse behavioral reactions attributed to triazolam in the Food and Drug Administration's Spontaneous Reporting System. *Arch Intern Med* 1991;151(10):2003–2008. *After reading this you may begin wondering how one of these benzodiazepines got to be the most widely prescribed hypnotic in the world. You will also learn why it is important to report adverse effects caused by drugs.*

Table 22–C1 Clinical Uses and Administration of Major Barbiturates

AGENT	CLINICAL USES	DOSAGE AND ROUTE OF ADMINISTRATION
PROTOTYPE		
Phenobarbital		
(LUMINAL)	Sedation	Oral: Adults: 15–30 mg, bid–qid. Children: 2 mg/kg/24 hr in divided doses
	Hypnosis	Oral: Adults: 100–320 mg hs
	Management of seizure disorders	Oral: Adults: 50–100 mg bid or tid or hs. Children: 15–50 mg bid or tid (or 3–5 mg/kg/d in three divided doses or as single bedtime dose)
RELATED DRUGS		
Amobarbital		
(AMYTAL)	Sedation	Oral: 30–50 mg bid or tid
	Hypnosis	Oral: 100–200 mg hs
	Preanesthetic sedation	Oral: 200 mg 1–2 hr before surgery
	Obstetric sedative	Oral: 200–400 mg, repeated prn at 1–3 hr intervals up to total of 1 g
	Control of chronic seizures	Oral: 65 mg bid–qid
	Control of acute seizures	IM or IV (preferred): 65–500 mg, up to 1 g maximum
Aprobarbital		
(ALURATE)	Sedation	Oral: 40 mg tid
	Hypnosis	Oral: 40–80 mg hs for mild insomnia, 80–160 mg for pronounced insomnia
Butabarbital		
(BUTISOL)	Sedation	Oral: Adults: 15–30 mg tid or qid. Children: 7.5–30 mg, depending on age, weight, etc
	Hypnosis	Oral: 50–100 mg hs
	Preoperative medication	Oral: 50–100 mg 60–90 min before surgery
Butalbital		
(in FIORICET, FIORINAL)	Sedation in presence of musculoskeletal pain, headache	Oral: 50 mg tid–qid (available as proprietary drug mixture with caffeine, analgesic)
Mephobarbital		
(MEBARAL)	Seizures (see Chapter 26)	
Metharbital		
(GEMONIL)	Seizures (see Chapter 26)	
Methohexital		
(BREVITAL)	Induction, maintenance of general anesthesia	See Chapter 20, Table 20–C

(continued)

Table 22–C1 Clinical Uses and Administration of Major Barbiturates (*Continued*)

AGENT	CLINICAL USES	DOSAGE AND ROUTE OF ADMINISTRATION
Pentobarbital (NEMBUTAL)	Sedation	Oral: Adults: 20 mg tid or qid. Children: 2–6 mg/kg/24 hr in divided doses, depending on age, weight, desired degree of sedation, up to 100 mg maximum (usually 8–30 mg per dose)
	Hypnosis	Oral: Adults: 100 mg hs. Children: No recommended dose; twice sedative dose usually effective. Rectal: Adults: one 120-mg or 200-mg suppository hs. Children 12–14 years (80–110 lb): 60 or 120 mg; 5–12 years (40–80 lb): 60 mg; 1–4 years (20–40 lb): 30 or 60 mg; 2 months–1 year (10–20 lb): 30 mg
	Preoperative medication	IM: Adults: 150–200 mg (in 5 mL or less volume). Children: 2–6 mg/kg up to 100 mg maximum IV: Adults: Usually 100 mg for average 70-kg patient (use only when IM administration not possible or very rapid effects are needed)
Secobarbital (SECONAL)	Hypnosis	Oral: 100 mg hs (adults only)
	Preoperative medication	Oral: Adults: 200–300 mg 1–2 hr before surgery. Children: 2-6 mg/kg, up to 100 mg maximum
Talbutal (LOTUSATE)	Hypnosis	Oral: 120 mg 15–30 min before bedtime
Thiamylal (SURITAL)	Induction, maintenance of general anesthesia	See Chapter 20, Table 20-C
Thiopental (PENTOTHAL)	Induction of anesthesia	See Chapter 20, Table 20-C
	Treatment of acute seizures (eg, drug-induced)	IV: Usually 75–125 mg immediately; seizures from local anesthetic overdoses may require 125–250 mg; repeat prn

Table 22–S1 Major Side Effects and Contraindications for Barbiturates and Most Other CNS Depressants

BODY SYSTEM/ Side Effect	CONTRAINDICATION/ PRECAUTION	COMMENTS AND NURSING IMPLICATIONS
CENTRAL NERVOUS SYSTEM		
Dose-dependent depression (drowsiness, ataxia, leading to sleep, coma, death)	Impaired consciousness, undiagnosed neurologic disorders, history of drug abuse	Observe all patients closely during initial barbiturate administration; take precautions to prevent falls; encourage patient to remain in bed after taking hypnotic doses; observe for signs of confusion, ataxia, excessive depression; advise patients to avoid alcohol, other sedatives (including OTC) unless specifically prescribed by physician
Paradoxical excitement		Most common in elderly or debilitated patients; observe for signs of agitation, confusion; take precautions to prevent harm to patient
METABOLIC		
Increased porphyrin synthesis	Porphyria (active or history of) is absolute contraindication	Monitor patient for fever, abdominal or muscle pain, paralysis that might indicate undiagnosed porphyria; applies to barbiturates, most CNS depressants other than benzodiazepines
RESPIRATORY		
Sleep-like slowing of respiration with therapeutic doses	Severely impaired ventilation	
Cough, laryngospasm		Occurs with rapid IV injection of barbiturates, as during anesthesia induction; give small test dose, inject slowly, have facilities for intubation, oxygen administration ready
CARDIOVASCULAR		
Sleep-like decreases of heart rate, blood pressure with therapeutic doses	Severe cardiovascular disease; shock	Monitor heart rate, blood pressure, when barbiturates are given parenterally or when given to elderly or debilitated patients

Table 22–I1 Major Interactions Involving Barbiturates and Most Other CNS Depressants

AGENT	RESULT OF INTERACTION	COMMENTS AND NURSING IMPLICATIONS
Interactions Common to All General CNS Depressants		
All other CNS depressants, including alcohol; anticonvulsants; antidepressants; antihistamines; antipsychotics; centrally acting anticholinergics used for parkinsonism; centrally acting antihypertensives; narcotics; other sedative/hypnotics and anxiolytics	Increased sedation, loss of coordination, judgment, reflexes; increased risk of serious overdose	Caution patients against consuming other CNS depressants, including alcohol and OTC medications, unless recommended or approved by physician
Interactions Involving Barbiturates		
Corticosteroids (Chapter 45)	Decreased steroid actions	Due to increased steroid metabolism; most likely to occur with high doses of barbiturates; monitor steroid responses; if necessary, increase steroid dose or use benzodiazepines instead
Doxycycline (Chapter 56)	Decreased doxycycline activity (antibiotic effect)	Due to increased doxycycline metabolism; other tetracyclines apparently do not interact, are preferred
Oral contraceptives (Chapter 49)	Failure of contraception; spotting; breakthrough bleeding	Due to increased steroid metabolism; increasing dose of ethynyl estradiol in contraceptive may restore efficacy, suppress breakthrough bleeding, etc. Advise patients to seek medical evaluation at once if pregnancy occurs, as barbiturates are contraindicated; recommend other forms of contraception (eg, diaphragm, spermicides, condom). Fluid retention caused by oral contraceptives may lower seizure threshold in seizure-prone patients who may be receiving a barbiturate
Quinidine (Chapter 30)	Reduced antiarrhythmic effect of quinidine	Due to increased quinidine metabolism, monitor ECG closely; physician should increase quinidine dose with start of barbiturate therapy, decrease quinidine dose when barbiturates are discontinued
Theophylline (Chapter 38)	Reduced bronchodilator effect of theophylline; poor control of asthma, COPD; wheezing, bronchoconstriction, dyspnea	Barbiturates may increase theophylline elimination by 30%–40%; physician may cautiously increase theophylline dose and monitor theophylline blood levels; monitor CNS status closely for signs of stimulation if this is done; dyphylline, which is not metabolized, does not interact and may be preferred
Valproic acid (Chapter 26)	Increased sedation due to barbiturate accumulation; poor seizure control	Monitor patient closely for excessive sedation or poor seizure control; valproic acid inhibits barbiturate metabolism; barbiturates stimulate valproic acid metabolism; reducing barbiturate dose by 30%–75% may be necessary
Warfarin, other oral anticoagulants (Chapter 35)	Inadequate anticoagulation *or* excessive bleeding, hemorrhage	Monitor patient closely for signs of inadequate or excessive blood clotting; monitor prothrombin time periodically; barbiturates increase metabolism of oral anticoagulants, may lead to increased clotting; alternatively, barbiturates suppress clotting factor synthesis, may potentiate anticoagulant drug action

Table 22–C2 Clinical Uses and Administration of Major Benzodiazepines and Their Antagonist

AGENT	CLINICAL USES	DOSAGE AND ROUTE OF ADMINISTRATION
PROTOTYPE		
Diazepam (VALIUM)	Management of anxiety	Oral: Adults: 2–10 mg tid–qid. Children: 1–2.5 mg taken as for adults; reduce dose in geriatric or debilitated patients to 2–2.5 mg qd or bid, increasing as needed and tolerated. IM or IV: 2–5 mg, repeated in 3–4 hr intervals for moderate anxiety; 5–10 mg for severe anxiety
	Acute alcohol withdrawal	Oral: 10 mg tid or qid for first day, reduced thereafter to 5 mg tid or qid prn. IM or IV: 10 mg initially, then 5–10 mg every 3–4 hr if needed; switch to oral therapy as needed
	Adjunctive therapy of chronic seizure disorders	Oral: 2–10 mg bid–qid
	Emergency treatment of status epilepticus, recurrent seizures	IV: Adults: 5–10 mg, repeated at 10–15-min intervals, up to total of 30 mg, given as slow injection. Children >5 years: 1 mg every 2–5 min, repeated in 2–4 hr as needed; infants >30 days, children <5 years: 0.2–0.5 mg as for older children, up to total dose of 5 mg
	Adjunctive therapy of skeletal muscle spasm	Oral: 2–10 mg 2 bid–tid IM or IV: 5–10 mg initially, repeated in 3–4 hr prn
	Tetanus	IM or IV: Children >5 years: 5–10 mg, repeated every 3–4 hr; infants >30 days old, children <5 years: 1–2 mg, repeated as above
	Relief of apprehension prior to electric cardioversion	IV: 5–15 mg 5–10 min before procedure
	Relief of apprehension prior to endoscopy	IV: Usually 10–20 mg shortly before procedure (reduce dose if narcotics also used); may give 5–10 mg IM 30 min before procedure when IV route not feasible
	Relief of preoperative anxiety	IM (preferred route): 10 mg
RELATED DRUGS		
Alprazolam (XANAX)	Management of anxiety	Oral: Usually 0.25–0.5 mg tid, up to maximum of 4 mg/d in divided doses. Elderly or debilitated patients: Usually 0.25 mg bid or tid
Chlordiazepoxide (LIBRIUM)	Management of anxiety, including preoperative and that associated with alcohol withdrawal	Oral: Adults: 5 or 10 mg tid or qid for mild-to-moderate anxiety (or for preoperative anxiety, given day before surgery); 20 or 25 mg tid or qid for severe anxiety. Debilitated or geriatric patients: 5 mg bid–qid. Children >6 years: 5 mg bid–qid (or 10 mg bid–tid)

(continued)

Table 22–C2 **Clinical Uses and Administration of Major Benzodiazepines and Their Antagonist (*Continued*)**

AGENT	CLINICAL USES	DOSAGE AND ROUTE OF ADMINISTRATION
	Management of acute alcohol withdrawal and associated anxiety, agitation	IM or IV: 50–100 mg, repeated in 2–4 hr prn until agitation subsides; may give same dose orally, but not preferred for this indication, maximum daily dose should be ≤300 mg
	Preoperative relief of anxiety	IM: 50–100 mg 1hr before surgery (also see oral dose above)
Chlordiazepoxide plus amitriptyline		
(LIMBITROL)	Treatment of psychiatric depression accompanied by anxiety	Oral: 3 or 4 tablets per day; LIMBITROL contains either 5 mg chlordiazepoxide + 12.5 amitriptyline (for mild-to-moderate symptoms) or 10 mg and 25 mg, respectively (for moderate-to-severe symptoms); best to give majority of daily dose at bedtime; some patients may require higher doses or dosing at bedtime only
Chlordiazepoxide plus esterified estrogens		
(MENRIUM)	Management of anxiety, tension, vasomotor complaints due to menopause	Oral: 3 tablets per day; MENRIUM preparations contain 5 or 10 mg chlordiazepoxide and 0.2–0.4 mg esterified estrogens
Clorazepate dipotassium		
(TRANXENE, TRANXENE-SD)	Management of anxiety	Oral: Immediate-release product: Adults: 15 mg hs or bid, or 7.5 mg tid or qid. Elderly or debilitated patients: initially 7.5–15 mg/d in two divided doses. TRANXENE-SD (sustained action; not for starting therapy): one 22.5-mg tablet replaces 3 daily 7.5-mg tablets of immediate-release product, or one 11.25-mg tablet instead of lower daily doses
	Adjunctive therapy of chronic seizure disorders	Adults, children >12 years: 7.5 mg tid, increasing as needed by not more than 7.5 mg/week and not exceeding total daily dose of 90 mg. Children 9–12 years: 7.5 mg bid, increasing weekly as needed up to maximum daily dose of 60 mg
	Relief of acute alcohol withdrawal symptoms	Oral: First day: 30 mg initially, then 30–60 mg for remainder of day in divided doses (remaining daily doses should be divided in 3 daily portions); second day: 45–90 mg; third day: 22.5–45 mg; fourth day: 15–30 mg, gradually decreasing thereafter to 7.5–15 mg/d and discontinuing when patient is stable.
Estazolam		
(PRO-SOM)	Hypnosis for short-term management of insomnia	Oral: Adults: 1 mg hs (0.5–1 mg for elderly)
Flurazepam		
(DALMANE)	Hypnosis	Oral: Patients >15 years: 30 mg hs. Elderly or debilitated patients: 15 mg hs

(continued)

Table 22–C2 Clinical Uses and Administration of Major Benzodiazepines and Their Antagonist (*Continued*)

AGENT	CLINICAL USES	DOSAGE AND ROUTE OF ADMINISTRATION
Halazepam		
(PAXIPAM)	Management of anxiety	Oral: Usually 20–40 mg tid or qid; adjust to optimal dose (80–160 mg/d in 3 or 4 divided doses); recommended starting dose for debilitated patients or patients >70 years is 20 mg qd or bid
Lorazepam		
(ATIVAN)	Management of anxiety, anxiety associated with depressive symptoms	Oral: Usually 1–2 mg bid or tid (up to 10 mg/d in divided doses). Elderly or debilitated patients: usually 1–2 mg/d in divided doses
	Hypnosis when insomnia is due to anxiety	Oral: 2–4 mg hs
	Preanesthetic medication, especially when relief of anxiety and decreased recall (amnesia) are desired	IM: 0.05 mg/kg (up to 4 mg total) given at least 2 hr before surgery IV: 0.044 mg/kg (up to 2 mg total) given 15–20 min before surgery
Midazolam		
(VERSED)	Preanesthetic/prediagnostic medication	IM: For preoperative use, 0.05–0.08 mg/kg IV: 0.1–0.15 mg/kg, or up to 0.2 mg/kg; maintenance doses usually 25% of initial dose; reduce dose by 25%–30% if narcotics are used adjunctively
	Induction of general anesthesia	See Chapter 20, Table 20–C
Oxazepam		
(SERAX)	Management of anxiety	Oral: Adults, children >12 years: 10–15 mg tid or qid for mild-to-moderate anxiety; 15–30 mg tid or qid for severe anxiety; limit initial doses to 10 mg tid for elderly
	Management of acute alcohol intoxication with anxiety, related symptoms on withdrawal	Oral: 15–30 mg tid or qid
Prazepam		
(CENTRAX)	Management of anxiety	Oral: Usually 10 mg tid with subsequent adjustments to total daily dose of 20–60 mg/d. Elderly or debilitated patients: initially 5 mg bid–tid
Quazepam		
(DORAL)	Management of anxiety	Oral: Adults: 7.5–15 mg initially
Temazepam	Hypnosis	
(RESTORIL)		Oral: Patients >18 years: 30 mg hs. Elderly or debilitated patients: 15 mg hs
Triazolam		
(HALCION)	Hypnosis	Oral: Usually 0.125–0.5 mg hs. Elderly or debilitated patients: 0.125 or 0.25 mg hs

(continued)

Table 22–C2 Clinical Uses and Administration of Major Benzodiazepines and Their Antagonist (*Continued*)

AGENT	CLINICAL USES	DOSAGE AND ROUTE OF ADMINISTRATION
	Benzodine Antagonist	
Flumazenil (MAZICON)	Reversal of conscious sedation, general anesthesia effects due to benzodiazepines	IV: Infuse 0.2 mg over 15 sec; assess response for 45 sec, give additional 0.2 mg doses at 60 sec intervals if needed, but do not exceed 1 mg total; for long-acting benzodiazepines, may repeat 0.2–1 mg dose at 20 min intervals; do not give >3 mg in any 60 min period
	Management of known/ suspected benzodiazepine overdose	IV: Infuse 0.2 mg over 30 sec; if level of consciousness does not improve in 30 sec, give 0.3 mg more over 30 sec; may give additional 0.5 mg doses at intervals up to total of 3 mg

Table 22–S2 Major Side Effects and Contraindications for Benzodiazepines

BODY SYSTEM/ Side Effect	CONTRAINDICATION/ PRECAUTION	COMMENTS AND NURSING IMPLICATIONS
CENTRAL NERVOUS SYSTEM See barbiturates, Table 22–S1		
EYE Photophobia due to mydriasis; blurred vision due to cycloplegia	Glaucoma	Due to antimuscarinic (atropine-like) action; applies to diazepam, probably most other benzodiazepines, especially when high doses are used, or drug is injected; (see Table 13–S for complete description of antimuscarinic side effects, nursing implications)
MOUTH Dry mouth		
RESPIRATORY See barbiturates, Table 22–S1		
CARDIOVASCULAR See barbiturates, Table 22–S1		
GASTROINTESTINAL Constipation	Diminished gut motility; paralytic ileus; constipation	
GENITOURINARY Urinary retention	Prostatic hypertrophy	

Table 22–I2 | Major Interactions Between Benzodiazepines and Other Agents

AGENT	RESULT OF INTERACTION	COMMENTS AND NURSING IMPLICATIONS
All other CNS depressants	See Table 22-I1	
Cimetidine (Chapter 40)	Increased, prolonged CNS depression	Cimetidine may increase diazepam's oral absorption, inhibit metabolism, prolong half-life; probably applies to alprazolam, chlordiazepoxide, triazolam; less likely with lorazepam, oxazepam, temazepam, or when ranitidine or famotidine is used instead of cimetidine; if interaction unavoidable, monitor responses closely
Isoniazid (Chapter 57)	Increased benzodiazepine effects	Isoniazid inhibits benzodiazepine metabolism
Rifampin (Chapter 57)	Reduced benzodiazepine effects	Rifampin stimulates benzodiazepine metabolism

Table 22–C3 | Clinical Uses and Administration of Other CNS Depressants

AGENT	CLINICAL USES	DOSAGE AND ROUTE OF ADMINISTRATION
Buspirone		
(BuSpar)	Management of anxiety	Oral: 5 mg tid to start, increase to 60 mg/d maximum, in divided doses
Chloral hydrate		
(NOCTEC)	Hypnosis for insomnia or as preoperative medication	Oral: 0.5–1 g 15–30 min before bedtime or 1/2 hr before surgery. Children: 50 mg/kg, up to maximum 1 g
	Sedation	Oral: Adults: 250 mg tid, after meals, not exceeding 2 g for single dose or total daily dose. Children: 25 mg/kg but not exceeding 0.5 g
Chlormezanone		
(TRANCOPAL)	Management of anxiety	Oral: Adults: 100–200 mg tid–qid. Children 5–12 years: 50–100 mg tid or qid
Diphenhydramine		
(BENADRYL)	Nighttime sleep aid	Oral: Adults: 50 mg hs
	Allergy symptoms; motion sickness; parkinsonism	See Table 51–C
Ethchlorvynol		
(PLACIDYL)	Hypnosis	Oral: Usually 500 mg hs; 750–1000 mg for severe insomnia

(continued)

Table 22–C3 **Clinical Uses and Administration of Other CNS Depressants (*Continued*)**

AGENT	CLINICAL USES	DOSAGE AND ROUTE OF ADMINISTRATION
Hydroxyzine		
(ATARAX, VISTARIL)	Management of anxiety	Oral: Adults: 50–100 mg qid. Children <6 years: 50 mg/d in divided doses; >6 years: 50–100 mg/d in divided doses
	Sedation for acute psychiatric emergencies (including alcoholism)	IM: 50–100 mg immediately, repeated every 4–6 hr prn
	Pre- or postoperative medication (for sedation, emesis control)	Oral: Adults: 50–100 mg. Children: 0.6 mg/kg IM: Adults: 25–100 mg. Children: 1.1 mg/kg
	Allergies; emesis control	See Table 51–C
Meprobamate		
(EQUANIL, MILTOWN)	Management of anxiety	Oral: Adults: Usually 400 mg tid or qid, or 600 mg bid. Children 6–12 years: 100–200 mg bid or tid
(MEPROSPAN) (sustained-acting meprobamate preparation)	See meprobamate	Oral: Adults: 1 or 2 400-mg capsules in AM and hs. Children 6–12 years: one 200-mg capsule in AM and hs
Meprobamate plus aspirin		
(EQUIGESIC)	Treatment of short-term anxiety accompanied by musculoskeletal pain	Oral: 1 or 2 tablets tid or qid
Meprobamate plus benactyzine		
(DEPROL)	Depression accompanied by anxiety	Oral: 1 tablet tid or qid
Meprobamate plus conjugated estrogens (PMB 200, 400)	Management of anxiety associated with menopause	Oral: One tablet of either strength tid
Meprobamate plus tridihexethyl		
(PATHIBAMATE)	Management of irritable bowel syndrome accompanied by anxiety	Oral: One tablet tid with meals and 2 tablets hs (2 PATHIBAMATE-200 tablets may be taken at the above times if greater anticholinergic action is needed)
Paraldehyde		
(PARAL)	Sedation, hypnosis, especially due to alcohol withdrawal	Oral or Rectal: Adults: 4–8 mL (1g/mL) for hypnosis, 5–10 mL for sedation. Children: 0.3 mL/kg for hypnosis, 0.15 mL/kg for sedation (IM also)
	Acute alcohol withdrawal, seizures due to tetanus, eclampsia, status epilepticus, drug poisoning	IM: 5 mL IV (not preferred): 3–5 mL
Propiomazine		
(LARGON)	Sedation before, during surgery, during labor	IM or IV: Adults: Usually 20 mg. Children: Usually 1.1 mg/kg

Table 22–S3 Unique Side Effects, Contraindications, or Other Properties of Selected Miscellaneous CNS Depressants

AGENT	SIDE EFFECT OR OTHER PROPERTY	COMMENTS AND NURSING IMPLICATIONS
Chloral hydrate (NOCTEC)	Epigastric distress is common	Contraindicated in peptic ulcer disease; otherwise, administer with milk or food to reduce GI distress Profound alcohol interaction (see Table 22–13)
Diphenhydramine (BENADRYL)	Causes often-intense antimuscarinic (atropine-like) side effects (eg, dry mouth, blurred vision) Has useful antiemetic actions Available as OTC sleep aid	Avoid use whenever atropine itself is contraindicated: glaucoma, prostatic hypertrophy, etc (see Table 13–S; see Chapter 51 for other properties)
Meprobamate (EQUANIL, MILTOWN)		Of all miscellaneous CNS depressants, is most like phenobarbital in terms of actions, uses, side effects, etc
Paraldehyde (PARAL)	Has very unpleasant taste (oral administration)	Administer oral liquids well diluted in iced juice or milk
	Very offensive breath odor (any administration route)	Ventilate room, use air freshener, patient may be unaware of breath odor
	Anorectal irritation (rectal administration)	Avoid rectal administration if patient has anorectal disease, including hemorrhoids; always dilute drug with at least 2 volumes of olive oil or suitable alternative
	Vascular pain, irritation (IV administration)	Dilute with several volumes 0.9% sodium chloride before injecting
	Decomposes to potentially toxic substances (all dosage forms)	Follow storage guidelines, discard if there is odor of vinegar (acetic acid)
	Incompatible with plastics, forms potentially toxic products (all dosage forms)	Never mix, measure, or administer with plastic containers, syringes

Table 22–13 **Major Interactions Between Alcohol and Other Agents**

AGENT	RESULT OF INTERACTION	COMMENTS AND NURSING IMPLICATIONS
Aspirin, other nonsteroidal anti-inflammatory drugs (Chapter 52)	Increased gastric irritation, risk of hemorrhage	Avoid concomitant use; advise patients to use acetaminophen cautiously, and to avoid aspirin and other nonsteroidal drugs for management of hangovers due to alcohol
	Increased risk of bleeding	Avoid interaction; aspirin and related drugs inhibit platelet aggregation, chronic alcohol use inhibits hepatic synthesis of clotting factors
Cephalosporin antibiotics (Chapter 56)	Disulfiram-like reaction within 48–72 hr after cefamandole, cefoperazone, cefotetan, moxalactam	Advise patients not to take alcohol for 48–72 hr after cephalosporin therapy (or for several days before, if possible)
Chloral hydrate	Profound CNS depression	Avoid interaction: chloral hydrate has been called "knock-out drops" when used as alcohol additive to sedate unsuspecting victims; combination is called "Mickey Finn"; interactant slows alcohol's metabolic inactivation, alcohol stimulates metabolism of chloral hydrate to more powerful CNS depressant
Chlorpromazine, other phenothiazines (Chapter 23)	Possible increase of extrapyramidal (parkinsonian) side effects; likely increase of sedation	Monitor accordingly
Chlorpropamide, other oral antidiabetic drugs (Chapter 46)	Risk of excessive hypoglycemia	Alcohol reduces blood glucose levels, potentiates oral antidiabetic drug effect; avoid alcohol use or monitor blood glucose levels closely; may occur with tolbutamide, less likely to occur with glyburide, glipizide
Cimetidine (Chapter 40)	Increased CNS depression	Cimetidine may increase alcohol absorption; since cimetidine is indicated for peptic ulcer disease, for which alcohol is contraindicated, alcohol use should be avoided
Diazepam, other benzodiazepines	Excessive CNS depression	
Disulfiram	Severe headache, palpitations, tachycardia, diaphoresis, etc (see p 366)	Avoid interaction; caution patients against ingesting foods, drugs made with alcohol, use of topical alcohol-containing products
Metronidazole (Chapter 57)	Disulfiram-like reaction	Avoid concomitant use; monitor
Phenytoin (Chapter 26)	Decreased duration, intensity of phenytoin's anticonvulsant activity	Discontinuation of ethanol administration after long-term use increases phenytoin clearance; monitor phenytoin levels, anticonvulsant response closely in patients who take alcohol chronically; avoid interaction if possible
Propoxyphene (Chapter 21)	Increased risk of severe CNS depression, death	Alcohol somehow lowers the lethal blood level of propoxyphene; advise patients to avoid combined use

Table 22–S4 **Additional Side Effects of and Contraindications for Alcohol**

BODY SYSTEM / Side Effect	CONTRAINDICATION/ PRECAUTION	COMMENTS AND NURSING IMPLICATIONS
CENTRAL NERVOUS SYSTEM		
See barbiturates, Table 22–S1; chronic high-dose use may suppress short-term memory, permanently destroy neural tissue		Assess for patterns of alcohol abuse; inquire about memory lapses, blackouts, impaired job performance, etc
METABOLIC OR ENDOCRINE		
Accumulation of fat, protein in liver; cirrhosis; altered clotting factor synthesis; hypoglycemia	Severe liver disease; diabetes mellitus	
Gynecomastia, impotence in males due to reduced testosterone synthesis		
Malnutrition with chronic alcoholism		Stress to alcohol abusers and families the need for a balanced diet and the need to reduce alcohol consumption
CARDIOVASCULAR		
See barbiturates, Table 22–S1; chronic high-dose use may produce cardiomyopathy, heart failure		
RENAL		
Increased urine output, dehydration	Dehydration; diabetes insipidus or mellitus	

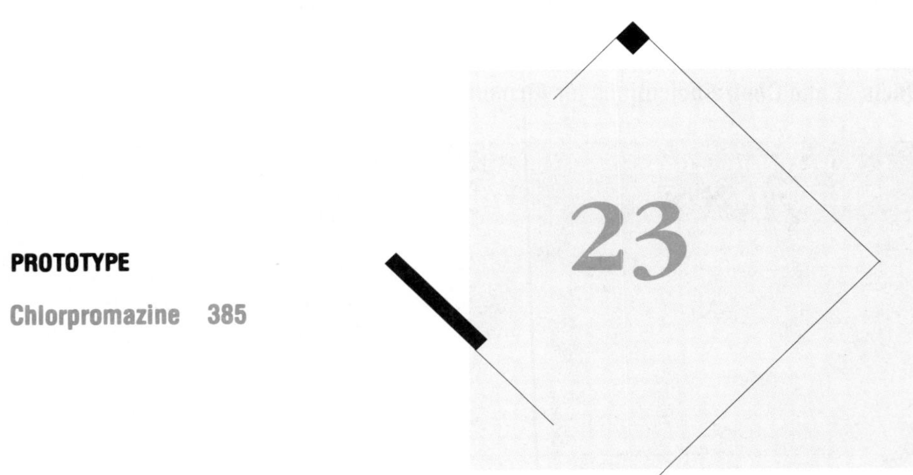

PROTOTYPE

Chlorpromazine 385

Antipsychotic Drugs

Hundreds of thousands of Americans suffer from psychosis, a disintegrative life pattern that interferes with the ordinary demands of life. Before the introduction of antipsychotic drugs these individuals were hospitalized under often poor or cruel conditions. Some were subjected to inappropriate treatments (eg, lobotomy or electroconvulsive therapy) as clinicians desperately sought to find effective treatment forms. These treatments rarely restored productive function. Contemporary drug therapy, combined with psychotherapy, has accomplished many of the goals unattained with prior treatments.

Schizophrenia

Schizophrenia, one of the major forms of psychosis, is not a single disease, but a group of psychiatric alterations. Its classic symptoms are discussed here in terms of the effects of antipsychotic drugs on them. The causes and classification of mental illness, including schizophrenia, have been debated for years, and reviewing these issues is beyond the scope of this text. (The reader is referred to the *Diagnostic and Statistical Manual of Mental Disorders* (DSM-III-R) of the American Psychiatric Association for further information on the classification of schizophrenia.) The current belief is that schizophrenia reflects interactions between psychosocial and biologic factors. Studies of antipsychotic drug actions have provided considerable insight into understanding some of the biologic factors that seem to cause schizophrenia.

General Characteristics of Antipsychotic Drugs

The prototype antipsychotic drug, chlorpromazine (THORAZINE), has been available since the late 1940s. Antipsychotics have also been called *major tranquilizers, ataractics* (drugs that produce calmness or serenity), or *neuroleptics* (since they can produce symptoms resembling certain nervous system disorders).

Antipsychotic Drug Classes Based on Chemical Structure

All antipsychotic drugs fall into one of seven major chemical classes. The prototype, chlorpromazine, is chemically classified as a phenothiazine. It will be discussed extensively. Other antipsychotics, belonging to the phe-

Major reference tables appear beginning on p. 404.

nothiazine group or to other chemical classes, will be discussed briefly. All these drugs reduce signs and symptoms of psychiatric disorders such as schizophrenia, but they differ in terms of structure, which affects their potency; their time-course of action; the type, intensity, and frequency of side effects; and special clinical uses. The major groups of antipsychotic drugs, representative drugs in each, and their important characteristics are summarized in Table 23–1.

Antipsychotic Drug Classes Based on Potency

Antipsychotic drugs can be classified according to potency—the dose needed to produce a given degree of antipsychotic action. Chlorpromazine is the standard for comparison, even though it is one of the least potent. As shown in Table 23–2, potencies vary considerably from drug to drug. Despite chlorpromazine's low potency, it is clearly effective for treating psychosis; it also has other important actions and uses that will be discussed later. And it seems that for antipsychotic drugs, potency has implications for the types and intensities of side effects that are likely to occur, not simply implications for how large a dose must be administered. This too will be discussed later.

Selecting an Antipsychotic Drug

Although many antipsychotic drugs are available, none stands out as being superior, overall, to another. However, for a variety of reasons a given patient may respond better or quicker to one drug, or to a drug in a particular chemical class, than to another. Selecting the best drug for a given situation and patient is an important step in therapy. The selection is usually based on the physician's experiences and preferences, the patient's mental history (the nature and possible causes of symptoms), responses to prior antipsychotic drug therapy (if a given drug was effective for a patient when used before, it will probably be effective if therapy must be restarted), and assessment of the risk of drug-induced side effects.

Symptoms Modified by Antipsychotic Drug Therapy

Patients are given antipsychotic drugs for specific reasons. They may be objective (the patient's behavior prevents normal social interactions), subjective (the patient reports psychotic symptoms and desires relief), or both. The symptoms become the yardstick by which to measure the effectiveness or ineffectiveness of an antipsychotic drug. Antipsychotic drugs have variable but important abilities to alleviate symptoms reflecting disorders of ***perception, thought, activity, consciousness, social interactions,*** and ***affect,*** whether the symptoms are due to schizophrenia, mania, or organic mental disorder (OMD). The symptoms, and the effects of antipsychotic drugs on them, are described in Table 23–3.

PROTOTYPE

Chlorpromazine

Absorption, Distribution, Metabolism, and Excretion

When chlorpromazine is taken orally, only about one third is absorbed. However, absorption is rapid, whether the drug is given orally, rectally, or parenterally. Sedation or a tranquilizing effect occurs within 60 minutes after an oral or rectal dose, and within 10 minutes after injection. Antipsychotic actions take much longer to develop. Since chlorpromazine accumulates in fatty tissues and is slowly released from these storage sites, traces of the drug and its metabolites can be detected in the urine many months after therapy has stopped. This accounts for the continued therapeutic effect seen in some patients who quit taking this medication.

Chlorpromazine is almost completely bound (95%–98%) to plasma protein. The drug undergoes extensive first-pass hepatic metabolism, and dozens of metabolites are formed. The metabolites undergo extensive enterohepatic recirculation and are eventually excreted in the urine. Less than 1% of the drug is excreted unchanged by the kidneys. The usual plasma half-life is about 30 hours; it is prolonged by impaired hepatic function. The long half-life accounts in part for the relatively long time required for blood levels to reach a steady-state or plateau (4–7 days), and for the slow onset of a full antipsychotic action (6 weeks or longer).

NURSING IMPLICATIONS

Some studies comparing generic and brand-name oral dosage forms of the same antipsychotic drug have shown large differences in bioavailability and in the actual amount of active drug per unit dose. These factors could contribute to accidental underdosing or overdosing when a patient is switched from one to the other. Check with the physician and pharmacist if the specific product ordered cannot be given.

Table 23–1 | Chemical Classes of Antipsychotic Drugs, Representative Drugs, and Their Major Properties

Drugs	Major Properties
Phenothiazines *Aliphatics* Chlorpromazine* (THORAZINE) Promazine (SPARINE) Trifluopromazine (VESPRIN)	Rapid onset of action; marked sedative properties (tolerance develops); moderate risk of extrapyramidal side effects; greater risk of atropine-like side effects
Piperidines Mesoridazine (SERENTIL) Thioridazine (MELLARIL)	Variable onset: less sedating than chlorpromazine; less likely to cause extrapyramidal side effects
Piperazines Fluphenazine (PROLIXIN, PERMITIL) Perphenazine (TRILAFON) Prochlorperazine (COMPAZINE) Trifluoperazine (STELAZINE)	Variable onset, duration, some with very long (>1 week) durations; sedation, atropine-like actions usually slight; potent antipsychotic action; greatest risk of extrapyramidal side effects; good antiemetic activity
Butyrophenone Haloperidol (HALDOL)	Potent, prompt antipsychotic actions; less sedating than phenothiazines at equivalent antipsychotic doses; less likely to produce severe atropine-like side effects; extrapyramidal side effects may be marked and occur shortly after treatment starts; good alternative for patients resistant or allergic to phenothiazines
Dibenzodiazepine Clozapine (CLOZARIL)	For patients refractory to other antipsychotics: low incidence of extrapyramidal symptoms, similar to thioridazine in anticholinergic effects; major concern is high incidence of agranulocytosis
Dibenzoxapine Loxapine (LOXITANE)	Similar to chlorpromazine
Dihydroindolone Molindone (MOBAN)	Similar to haloperidol
Diphenylbutylpiperidine Pimozide (ORAP)	Similar to haloperidol
Thioxanthenes Chlorprothixene (TARACTAN) Thiothixene (NAVANE)	Similar to chlorpromazine

*Chlorpromazine is considered the prototype of all antipsychotic drugs.

Table 23–2 | Daily Dose Ranges and Relative Potencies of Selected Antipsychotic Drugs

Generic Name	Proprietary Name	Usual Daily Dose Range for Adult Inpatients (mg)	Relative Potency*
Chlorpromazine	**THORAZINE**	**300-800**	**1**
Chlorprothixene	TARACTAN	75–600	1
Clozapine	CLOZARIL	300–900	2
Fluphenazine	PROLIXIN, PERMITIL	0.5–40	50
Haloperidol	HALDOL	1–15	50
Loxapine	LOXITANE	20–250	10
Molindone	MOBAN	15–225	10
Perphenazine	TRILAFON	12–64	10
Thioridazine	MELLARIL	150–800	1
Thiothixene	NAVANE	8–30	20
Trifluoperazine	STELAZINE	2–40	20

*Chlorpromazine is the prototype and the standard for comparison with other drugs; chlorpromazine = 1.

Source: Adapted from *Drug Facts & Comparisons*, 1992:265.

Table 23–3 Major Symptoms of Schizophrenia and Their Modification by Antipsychotic Drugs

Symptoms	Comments
Disorders of perception Hallucinations (usually auditory; may be visual) Delusions (somatic, grandiose, religious, etc) Illusions Paranoia	Patient's acceptance that these are altered perceptions, different from reality, is a positive therapeutic response
Disorders of thought Flights of ideas Retardation Blocking Introspection Ambivalence Loose associations Poverty of speech	Improved clarity of thought due to treatment may alleviate such secondary problems as insomnia
Disorders of activity Psychomotor agitation Catatonia	Rapid induction of neuroleptic syndrome by antipsychotic drugs often desirable
Disorders of consciousness Confusion Incoherent speech Clouding Generalized feelings of "going crazy"	Are anxiety-provoking; confusion may be most compromising to patient, but also most responsive to antipsychotic drugs
Disorders of social interactions Decreased attention to appearance, social amenities (introspection; autism) Inadequate or inappropriate communication Hostility Withdrawal	Secondary problems further remove patient from others; antipsychotics help redirect attention, energy, toward others; psychotherapy most helpful when these are improved
Disorders of affect Inappropriate, unusual responses to situations Flattened or blunted affect Ambivalence Overreactive, labile, or otherwise inappropriate affective responses	May be treated only with antidepressants when not accompanied by schizophrenic symptoms; when accompanied by schizophrenic symptoms, are very responsive to antipsychotic drugs

Pharmacologic Effects

The major use of chlorpromazine and related drugs is to manage psychiatric disorders, which implies that their major site of action is in the central nervous system (CNS). However, they affect a host of other body systems. Some of the effects are unwanted, some are clinically desirable, and many are unrelated to their actions as antipsychotic agents in the CNS.

Central Nervous System Effects

Sedation and Antipsychotic Actions

Chlorpromazine rather quickly produces a **neuroleptic syndrome**, characterized by sedation, emotional quieting, psychomotor slowing, and affective indifference. The patient may still be aware of situations that had caused unusual sadness, anger, or fright, but is less distressed by them. Relief of subjective distress, combined with sedation and psychomotor slowing, reduces the risk of self-harm or harm to others, and makes the patient more receptive to psychotherapy.

Antipsychotic drugs generally depress the CNS, but less than comparable doses of alcohol, barbiturates, or other sedative-hypnotic agents. This is particularly true when high doses are given. With continued administration, tolerance to some of these effects, particularly sedation, usually occurs.

When antipsychotic drug concentrations in the CNS reach effective levels, a true **antipsychotic** effect develops. It is characterized by normalization of thought, mood, and behavior. Sedation need not occur for antipsychotic actions to occur.

The exact site and mechanism of action of the phenothiazines are not known. Their sedative and antipsychotic actions are probably due to blockade of dopamine receptors in the brain's limbic system, the major system that regulates emotions. Dopamine appears to be an important neurotransmitter in this system. (As noted later, blockade of dopamine receptors by antipsychotic agents also accounts for some of their adverse responses.) The ability of antipsychotic drugs to block dopamine receptors and alleviate symptoms of schizophrenia suggests that excessive dopamine activity has a crucial role in the development of schizophrenic symptoms. This concept is supported by studies showing that drugs that increase brain dopamine levels, such as the amphetamines, can produce schizophrenic symptoms. In fact, in emergency medicine it is often difficult to distinguish amphetamine-induced paranoid psychosis from acute paranoia due to schizophrenia.

Antiemetic Actions

The chemoreceptor trigger zone, located in the medulla oblongata, is the major regulator of the sensations of nausea and vomiting. These sensations are provoked by

SPOTLIGHT ON NURSING RESEARCH

This research effort looked at the cost:benefit ratio of antipsychotic therapy by asking the recipients of neuroleptic treatment to respond to important questions regarding these drugs. The author provides the reader with a foundation for inquisitiveness by suggesting that nurses are the most involved health-care professionals in the administration of psychotropic drugs. While the physician may write the order from a distance, the nurse actually gives the medication, assures compliance, and monitors for efficacy or side effects. When adverse responses occur, the nurse is most closely associated with these negative consequences.

The author questioned 132 schizophrenia sufferers to ascertain their views on medication. Contrary to popular myths, most revealed a favorable view of neuroleptic agents. "Clients seemed to understand the fine balance between costs and benefits better than many health-care professionals imagine."

In response to the question "What do you find useful in helping you cope with your illness?", 31% of the respondents replied "medication." Only family support ranked higher. To the question "Which single factor do you think has helped your recovery most?", 30% mentioned their "medication." No other single factor rated as high a response. In response to the question "Which single factor do you think has hindered your recovery most?", only 14% of the patients pointed to neuroleptic drugs, suggesting absence of response-set bias. The author suggests the last question vindicates the use of long-term antipsychotic therapy.

This research indicates that among this small sample of patients with schizophrenia, most recognize the benefits of antipsychotic drug therapy even while experiencing negative reactions. As one individual remarked, "They're by no means ideal (due to side effects), but knowing by experience a life without these drugs is horrific, I have to count my blessings."

The significance of this information is best summarized by the author: "Because nurses spend more time communicating with clients than physicians, they are ideally placed to find out how patients perceive neuroleptic therapy, and to provide information, advice, and counseling support."

Chapman T: The nurse's role in neuroleptic medications. *J Psychosoc Nurs Ment Health Surv* 1991;29:6–8.

stimulation of dopamine receptors, whether by disease or by such drugs as morphine. By blocking these receptors, the phenothiazines suppress nausea or vomiting.

Hypothalamic and Pituitary Effects

Dopamine helps regulate function of the pituitary gland and hypothalamus. Therapeutic doses of chlorpromazine and related drugs affect the pituitary, eventually increasing prolactin release into the blood. This can cause certain endocrine side effects, which are noted later. In the hypothalamus, dopamine helps regulate body temperature. That process can also be altered by antipsychotic drugs.

Peripheral Autonomic and Antihistaminic Effects

All the antipsychotic drugs can block peripheral muscarinic acetylcholine (ACh) receptors, α-adrenergic receptors, and histamine (H_1) receptors. Some of these actions can be used therapeutically for some nonpsychiatric patients, but when the drugs are administered for psychoses they often cause disturbing side effects. The ability to block these peripheral receptors varies from drug to drug, and depends, of course, on the dose. Chlorpromazine causes moderate anticholinergic (antimuscarinic or atropine-like) and α-adrenergic blocking effects.

Clinical Indications and Administration

Management of Schizophrenia and Related Psychiatric Disorders

The major clinical uses for antipsychotic drugs are to treat schizophrenia, psychotic symptoms related to OMD, and the manic phase of manic-depressive illness (Table 23–C). Approximately 85% of all chronic, hospitalized schizophrenic patients receive antipsychotic drugs. When adequate doses are used and psychotherapy is provided, about 95% of them show some degree of improvement within 6 to 8 weeks after starting therapy.

Dosage Forms

In psychiatric settings, the route of antipsychotic drug administration is important. Most antipsychotic drugs are available for oral or parenteral use. The dosage form that is selected depends on a variety of factors.

Oral

All major antipsychotic drugs are available as tablets or capsules, and many are available as liquid concentrates or suspensions. Tablets and capsules are most convenient to administer, but least suitable when compliance problems exist. Some patients refuse to take any drug initially because they feel that doing so is an admission of illness. Others claim unpleasant subjective responses to the drugs, and become reluctant to take them after a while. Noncompliant patients may "cheek" a tablet (place it in the side of the mouth). The desired therapeutic goal depends on the patient's actually receiving proper doses regularly for long periods of time. If noncompliance is not detected, it will also be impossible to assess for true drug effects. A needless switch to an alternative drug might result. Therefore, liquid concentrates or suspensions, which cannot be cheeked easily, may be preferred for some hospitalized patients suspected of being noncompliant with solid dosage forms. Liquids are also useful for patients who, because of physical problems, cannot swallow tablets or capsules.

NURSING IMPLICATIONS

It is essential for the nurse to ascertain that the drug has been swallowed. Family members or other responsible individuals should be recruited to help maintain compliance by outpatients.

Liquid drug concentrates should be diluted with at least 60 mL of some pleasant-tasting beverage, soup, or pudding to mask the drug's taste. Most nonalcoholic beverages are acceptable for chlorpromazine and most related drugs. (An exception is the related phenothiazine, fluphenazine hydrochloride.) Phenothiazine concentrates should be stored, tightly capped, in containers that protect them from light. They should be diluted for use immediately before administration.

Parenteral

Antipsychotic drugs can be injected intramuscularly to acutely agitated or combative patients; to patients with poor drug absorptive capacity as a result of gastrointestinal (GI) disease or concomitant use of other drugs that interfere with drug absorption (antacids, laxatives); and to patients who pose a significant compliance problem with oral medications. When used to manage acute symptoms, psychosedation usually occurs within 10 minutes of injection. Oral therapy should be started once symptoms are controlled (1 or 2 days for severely agitated or manic hospitalized patients). Long-term daily parenteral therapy is generally impractical and undesirable. Longer-acting drugs, such as fluphenazine decanoate or haloperidol decanoate, which can be injected every 2 to 4 weeks, can be used in this instance. Regardless of the drug used, some adverse responses or side effects are likely to occur more quickly or be more intense when antipsychotics are injected. Intravenous (IV) administration is not recommended, mainly because of the risk of potentially severe CNS depression or cardiovascular side effects.

NURSING IMPLICATIONS

Parenteral antipsychotics should be given by deep intramuscular (IM) injection, preferably in the upper outer quadrant of the buttocks or the mid-lateral thigh. Avoid other sites to reduce discomfort from drug-induced irritation. The syringe and needle (21-gauge is often recommended) should be completely dry, since moisture causes most antipsychotic drug solutions to become cloudy. Parenteral solutions of most antipsychotics can be diluted with sterile saline or a 2% solution of procaine (assuming the patient has no allergy to the local anesthetic) to reduce injection-site pain. Always aspirate before injecting to avoid accidental IV administration. Frequent contact with antipsychotic solutions (or suppositories) may cause dermatitis, so precautions, such as the use of rubber gloves, should be taken.

Try to ensure that the patient lies quietly after the injection, and monitor closely for side effects and adverse responses for at least half an hour after giving the injection, especially if the patient has received an interacting CNS depressant or cardiovascular drug.

Rectal

Chlorpromazine suppositories are used primarily for children and adults who cannot take oral medications (for example, those who are vomiting profusely) and for whom parenteral administration is not desired.

Other Psychiatric or Neurologic Uses

Chlorpromazine and some of the other antipsychotic drugs can be used to manage excessive anxiety, tension, or agitation in discharged psychiatric patients. They can

SPOTLIGHT ON NURSING RESEARCH

Nurses' abilities to demonstrate the efficacy of their practice have become increasingly important in today's world of rising health care costs. Without the objective support that can be obtained through research, selected programs may be eliminated. This study provides an example of how a clinical study can be used to document the effectiveness of a specific nursing intervention.

Fluphenazine injections are often administered to schizophrenic patients who are unable to assume responsibility for taking oral antipsychotic medication on a regular basis. The confusion, paranoia, memory deficits, or other manifestations of the illness make an oral regimen impractical for some patients. However, injectable medications cannot guarantee successful control of the disorder if patients do not return to the clinic for regular injections.

This nurse-physician team hypothesized that a nursing intervention group would reduce hospitalizations of outpatients receiving fluphenazine injections. Groups were designed to provide a "homebase" for patients, along with regular medication administration and surveillance, information about drug effects and side effects, and group work to improve such symptoms as apathy, social withdrawal, hallucinations, decreased activities of daily living, and lack of interaction skills.

Twenty-nine male veterans receiving depot fluphenazine (PROLIXIN DECANOATE) for treatment of various types of schizophrenia were studied. The men were divided into four groups and each man attended hourly sessions that met twice a week, weekly, biweekly, or monthly, depending on individual medication and social support needs. Ranging from 24 to 70 years of age, most subjects lived with a parent or grandparent and attended "PROLIXIN groups" as a long-term treatment modality. Members remained in these groups from 12 to 57 months, with an average attendance of 46.9 months.

The investigators compared the number and length of psychiatric admissions for each group member before and after initiation of the nurse-run groups. It was important to evaluate both variables, because an intervention could potentially decrease the number of patient admissions but increase the number of days hospitalized.

The results of the study were startling. The mean number of admissions was 2.6 before group treatment versus 1.0 after treatment. The mean *total* (cumulative) length of admissions was 133.7 days before compared to 30.8 days following initiation of the nursing treatment. The mean *average* length of each admission was 71.4 days before treatment and 13.2 after treatment. Together, these findings clearly document the success of the nursing intervention.

Interestingly, the range of group members' fluphenazine doses increased over the course of group treatment. This observation suggests that group treatment increased attention to the individualization of drug dosage. Furthermore, target symptoms observed by the nurse-investigator improved in many patients. As she notes, during the first two years of group sessions she did all the talking. In the third year, group members began talking to her. During the fourth year, they began speaking, very tentatively, with each other. In the fifth year, a few members were even getting together in the canteen for coffee.

In addition to noting improvement in patient outcomes, the authors emphasize the cost-effectiveness of depot fluphenazine and group therapy. They were able to combine therapy with medication administration and surveillance for seven veterans over a one hour period. Individually treated patients would not only miss the benefits of group therapy, they would take longer to treat—an average of 15 to 30 minutes for each patients. In this study the long-term nature of both the nursing intervention and patient outcomes illustrate the importance of allowing enough time to measure the impact of clinical interventions.

Selender JM, Miller WC: Prolixin groups. *J Psych Nurs* 1985;23(11): 16–20.

also be used, for a limited time (12 weeks or less), for nonpsychotic patients who do not respond adequately to anxiolytic drugs such as the benzodiazepines. Antipsychotic drugs are often used to manage short-term psychoses that may occur in disoriented, acutely ill hospitalized patients, particularly those who have experienced severe trauma or undergone major surgery ("ICU-itis"). Therapy usually lasts only a couple of days, a time that may be sufficient for the development of side effects. Chlorpromazine can be used, but the related drug haloperidol is often preferred. Antidepressant drugs (discussed in the next chapter) are generally used for severe depressive illness. However, when depression is accompanied by agitation or psychosis, phenothiazines might be used adjunctively. The related drug perphenazine is often used in this way. Antipsychotic drugs may be used in the initial treatment of the manic phase of manic-depressive illness, for which lithium (also discussed in the next chapter) is the major drug treatment. Theoretically, the prompt psychosedative effects of the antipsychotic drug may provide temporary relief until the antimanic effects of lithium develop—about 7 to 10 days. However, the combination should be used cautiously because of a potentially severe interaction between lithium and antipsychotic drugs. Additionally, the antiemetic effects of the antipsychotics can mask nausea and vomiting, which are early signs of lithium toxicity.

Other Uses

Drugs classified as or chemically related to antipsychotic agents have a few uses that are unrelated to their ability to treat psychoses (see Table 23–C for most of these uses). Chlorpromazine has more of these indications than related agents, but alternatives may be preferred for specific uses.

Side Effects, Adverse Reactions, and Contraindications

Antipsychotic drugs cause many side effects and adverse responses (Table 23–S). The most common and important involve the peripheral autonomic nervous system (antimuscarinic, antiadrenergic effects) and the extrapyramidal system of the CNS. It appears that chlorpromazine and other "low-potency" phenothiazines pose a higher risk of autonomic side effects. The "high-potency" antipsychotics (fluphenazine or haloperidol, for example) seem to pose a greater risk of extrapyramidal side effects. This relationship between potency and the incidence and type of side effects is controversial, but it is a convenient approach for the student and is accepted by many practitioners. The relative frequencies and intensities of major side effects caused by alternative antipsychotic drugs are summarized for quick comparison in Table 23–4.

Peripheral Antimuscarinic Side Effects

All antipsychotic drugs can produce the same side effects noted for atropine, and are due to the same action: blockade of acetylcholine's actions on peripheral muscarinic receptors (see Chapter 13 for additional details). Some are simply mild and annoying, but others may be intense and dangerous, particularly with parenteral use. The most common side effects are dry mouth, blurred vision caused by cycloplegia, and photophobia caused by mydriasis. Increased intraocular pressure, as well as tachycardia, constipation, and urinary frequency, hesitancy, or retention are more clearly dangerous for persons with glaucoma, cardiovascular disease, prostatic hypertrophy, or any other condition that contraindicates the use of atropine. In essence, all contraindications for atropine apply to antipsychotics, except in the case of a psychiatric emergency.

Table 23–4 Relative Frequency of Side Effects Caused by Selected Antipsychotic Drugs

Drug Group, Example	Antimuscarinic Side Effects	Orthostatic Pyramidal tension	Extrapyramidal Side Effects	Sedation
Phenothiazines				
Chlorpromazine	++	+++	++	+++
Fluphenazine	+	+	+++	+
Thioridazine	+++	+++	+	+++
Nonphenothiazines				
Clozapine	+++	+++	+	+++
Loxapine	+	++	+++	++
Haloperidol	+	+	+++	+
Molindone	+	+	++	+
Thiothixene	+	+	+++	+

Key: + = infrequent occurrence; ++ = occasional occurrence; +++ = frequent occurrence.

Source: Adapted from *Drug Facts & Comparisons,* 1992:265.

NURSING IMPLICATIONS

All aspects of the nursing process that apply to the side effects, adverse responses, and contraindications for atropine (see Chapter 13) apply also to the antipsychotics. As with atropine, mild or innocuous problems tend to become less disturbing with time and are best handled with nondrug measures. Be aware that the risks of some severe responses, such as acute urinary retention and the need for immediate bladder catheterization, are potentially great, particularly in hospitalized patients.

Gastrointestinal upset caused by orally administered antipsychotics is not an antimuscarinic side effect. It can be prevented or reduced by having the patient take the medication with meals. If antacids are ordered, they should not be administered less than 1 hour before or 2 hours after giving the antipsychotic, to avoid significant reductions in drug absorption.

Antiadrenergic Side Effects

Because most antipsychotic drugs block peripheral α-adrenergic receptors, they cause side effects similar to phentolamine (see Chapter 15). As with antimuscarinic effects, antiadrenergic side effects are more likely to be produced by one of the low-potency phenothiazines and by parenteral administration. The most clinically significant manifestation of α-blockade is hypotension, particularly orthostatic hypotension. Hypotension usually causes tachycardia, triggered reflexly by decreased blood pressure and intensified by atropine-like cardiac stimulation. Although they are generally mild, and subside after a few weeks of treatment, orthostatic hypotension and tachycardia can be sufficiently intense and frequent to cause injury due to a fall. This is of special concern in the elderly. Prolonged or excessive cardiovascular effects can also lead to edema, weight gain, and heart failure in susceptible patients. Sudden death owing to acute heart failure or arrhythmias has occurred. Overall, the cardiovascular effects generally contraindicate antipsychotic drug use for patients with severe hypotension, heart failure, or a history of arrhythmias. If initial parenteral doses of an antipsychotic cause such effects as unacceptable degrees of hypotension, additional doses should be withheld.

Antimuscarinic side effects tend to dry secretions in the respiratory tract, but α-blocking actions could predominate and cause nasal congestion or stuffiness. Alpha blockade may also cause ejaculatory failure in males, contributing to noncompliance. It may be difficult to determine whether this problem is due to the drug or the underlying psychiatric disorder.

NURSING IMPLICATIONS

All nursing measures that apply to phentolamine apply to the antipsychotics. (See Chapter 15, pp 225–230.) If possible, monitor pulse and blood pressure (supine, sitting, and standing) of hospitalized patients before and periodically after each dose. Heart rate and pressures should also be checked closely at each outpatient visit. Assess for signs of heart failure, especially in physically ill or older patients. Obtain a baseline electrocardiogram (ECG) in patients considered to be at risk of cardiac side effects, for comparison with others obtained periodically during treatment.

It is essential to minimize problems of orthostatic hypotension. Instruct patients to sit for a couple of minutes before attempting to rise slowly; to support themselves with a bed, chair, or table; and to assume a seated, head-low position at once if lightheadedness occurs. Monitor and assist ambulation as needed. Elastic stockings may help reduce dizziness resulting from pooling of blood in the legs. If hypotension persists, notify the physician; a medication change or dosage adjustment may be indicated. Severe hypotension with fainting and possible injury may occur if patients taking antipsychotic drugs, especially patients just starting therapy, step into a hot shower. Take precautions against this, and advise patients and their families of the danger.

If nasal congestion or stuffiness is problematic, notify the physician. Discourage use of over-the-counter (OTC) decongestants or other remedies that might seem appropriate. These medications, regardless of their ingredients, can cause unpredictable and possibly serious interactions.

If male sexual performance is impaired, suggest that the patient attempt intercourse in a relaxed, stress-free atmosphere.

Extrapyramidal Side Effects

Extrapyramidal side effects are a group of symptoms, often involving abnormal involuntary movement disorders, that are often caused by antipsychotic drugs. They reflect a chemical imbalance in the extrapyramidal system of the brain. This system controls skeletal muscle movements, tone, and postural reflexes by maintaining a proper balance between the opposing effects of two neurotransmitters, dopamine and ACh. Imbalances and related symptoms may occur if an antipsychotic's ability to block dopamine receptors leaves the effects of ACh relatively unopposed. (Recall that blockade of dopamine receptors in the CNS accounts for the ability of antipsychotics to alleviate symptoms of psychosis.) Other symptoms occur when the antimuscarinic actions of the antipsychotics predominate, leading to a relative "excess" of dopamine activity. Some extrapyramidal side effects are easily recognized by others (objective), but some can be sensed only by the patient (subjective). The risks of extrapyramidal side effects are relatively low with chlorpromazine and other "low-potency" antipsychotic drugs, and high with "high-potency" antipsychotics such as haloperidol. Theoretically, the prominent antimuscarinic property of chlorpromazine "treats" the neurotransmitter imbalance before it occurs. For *all* antipsychotics, however, these adverse responses are among the most important and most difficult to manage.

Akathisia and Other Dysphoric Responses

Akathisias are dysphoric (unpleasant) subjective responses to antipsychotic drugs: they are sensed only by the patient, and cannot be seen. Akathisias are extremely common, accounting for about 50% of all extrapyramidal symptoms, and contribute more to noncompliance than any other antipsychotic drug side effect. They usually develop within a few months after starting therapy, and are most common among patients 30 to 60 years old. Akathisias are often characterized by an uncontrollable urge to move (although other extrapyramidal side effects may make doing so difficult). The patient may report feeling jittery, uneasy, or having considerable "nervous energy." Akathisias may lead to feelings of personal failure, humiliation, lack of self-worth, or inadequacy. Unenlightened health-care staff often mistake akathisias, which are drug-induced, as symptoms of schizophrenia.

Other dysphoric responses include patients' reports that their medications make them feel worse, that they are "allergic" to them, or that they are unbearably uncomfortable, regardless of where they are or what they are doing. A reduced dose of antipsychotic drug, and possibly starting antimuscarinic–antiparkinson drugs, may help. Dysphoric responses often lead to refusal to take oral medications, so parenteral therapy may be required.

Parkinsonism

Antipsychotic drugs can produce involuntary muscle disorders that resemble many signs and symptoms of Parkinson's disease (see Chapter 25). Drug-induced parkinsonism usually occurs during the first 3 months of therapy, affects about one third of patients, and is most common among patients under 40. The symptoms reflect diminished activity of dopamine, and excessive effects of ACh, in the extrapyramidal system. Noncompliance may occur if the patient becomes aware of or embarrassed by the symptoms. Antipsychotic drugs are generally contraindicated for persons with parkinsonian symptoms.

Dystonias, Dyskinesias, and Akinesias

These reactions can cause great emotional discomfort and potential physical harm for many persons taking antipsychotic drugs. They, too, may reflect excessive activity of dopamine in the extrapyramidal system. Dystonias (literally, disordered muscle tonicity), which may appear within days of starting treatment, often cause rigidity in muscles controlling posture or gait. Ocular involvement (frequent blinking, twitching, or closure of the eyelids [blepharospasm]) may occur and can become annoying. The most frightening ocular complication is an *oculogyric crisis,* in which tonic spasm of muscles controlling eyeball movement causes the eyes to roll back. The patient may become panic-struck when this occurs. Dystonic reactions may continue up to 48 hours after the offending drug has been discontinued.

Dyskinesia refers to any abnormal voluntary skeletal muscle movement. Dyskinesias may be seen as incomplete, fragmented ("jerky"), slow, or absent action of small or large muscle groups. Bradykinesia and akinesia refer to slow or absent muscle activities, respectively. The patient's facial appearance often provides a clue that dyskinesias are developing: face muscles are motionless, the face loses expression, the eyes stare without blinking, and the patient may appear dazed yet be completely lucid (hence the term *mask-like facies*). Mild bradykinesias may appear as a behavioral state characterized by few gestures, reduced spontaneity of speech or action, and apathy. They are difficult to distinguish from some of the negative symptoms of chronic schizophrenia, such as apathy, withdrawal, blunted affect, or not caring. Often they cause an inability to begin and then to stop muscle activity normally, whether it involves muscles needed to walk, talk, or to perform other simple tasks. Many patients are aware of and report the bradykinesias, and some develop depression that complicates the original psychiatric problem. Some patients may also develop drug-induced postpsychotic depression, with many symptoms that resemble bradykinesias.

Tardive Dyskinesia

Tardive dyskinesias are the most serious drug-induced extrapyramidal side effect. The term *tardive* implies that the symptoms develop late during antipsychotic drug therapy—sometimes after months or years of treatment. However, depending on the drug (they are more likely

Table 23–5 Signs, Symptoms, and Potential Complications of Tardive Dyskinesias Based on Muscle Groups Affected

Musculature and Effect	Complications	Musculature and Effect	Complications
Ocular Blepharospasm (eyelid twitching) Blinking Facial Grimaces Tics		Neck Retrocollis (spasmodic movement of the head backward) Torticollis (twisting movement of the head, often to side)	
Oral Cheek puffing Lip smacking Pouting Puckering Sucking	Inability to wear dentures, eat, drink, swallow safely or adequately	Trunk Diaphragmatic movements Pelvic thrusting or rotation Rocking Shoulder shrugging	Impaired breathing; impaired posture, gait, possible falls
Jaw Chewing Lateral jaw movements	Loosening of temperomandibular joint; pain, fractures	Limbs Ankle flexion, rotation Ballistic movements (thrusting of the limbs) Choreoathetoid finger movement Foot tapping Toe movement Wrist flexion or torsion	Impaired posture, gait, possible falls
Tongue Choreoathetoid tongue movements (continual, rapid or slow, writhing movements) Tongue protrusion		Miscellaneous signs Generalized rigidity Myoclonic jerks	
Pharyngeal Clonic soft palate movements Involuntary swallowing Abnormal sounds due to above		**Overall consequences, complications** Weight loss due to constant movement Inability to carry out daily living tasks Psychologic reactions ranging from embarrassment to suicide	

to occur with "high-potency" antipsychotics), the dosage, and patient-related factors, they may occur sooner. Any antipsychotic drug or dosage can produce them, and the underlying psychiatric cause for which the drug was prescribed does not affect the risk. The overall incidence is about 10% to 20%, but may be as high as 40% in some outpatient populations and 60% in chronically hospitalized patients.

Tardive dyskinesias and their complications cause significant emotional and physical problems sufficient to interfere with daily life and health. Table 23–5 lists some of the muscle groups that can be affected, and the potential secondary consequences to the patient. The involuntary movements are generally coordinated, rhythmic, and stereotyped; fluctuate in severity over time; and disappear with sleep. They can also be induced or intensified by emotional arousal or by asking the patient to perform certain physical tasks. They usually affect the muscles of the mouth and face, but are not limited to those sites. The patient may develop difficulty writing, and penmanship often changes dramatically, from large but shaky to very small (micrographia). Indeed, these characteristics are useful aids to help the nurse assess the development of dyskinesias. Many of the diagnostic procedures are part of the AIMS (Abnormal Involuntary Movement Scale) test, which helps evaluate the presence and severity of tardive dyskinesia.

Paradoxically, although antipsychotics can cause tardive dyskinesias, they may also suppress or mask their clinical signs. The danger is that although the biochemical processes that cause tardive dyskinesias may have occurred and developed to the point that they are irreversible and not responsive to drug treatment, the ability to diagnose them is drastically reduced.

Therapeutic Guidelines

The following guidelines help increase the likelihood of therapeutic success, yet decrease the chance of serious adverse responses such as tardive dyskinesias. Question medication orders when these guidelines are not followed.

1. Antipsychotic drugs should not be used for nonapproved indications. They are not appropriate, for example, for relief of simple anxiety. Similarly, antipsychotics indicated only for managing schizophrenia should not be used to treat nonpsychiatric symptoms such as emesis.
2. Antipsychotic drug use and doses should be limited in certain patient populations. For example, elderly patients (particularly women) or patients with brain damage are at greater risk of tardive dyskinesias.
3. The lowest effective daily dose should always be used during maintenance therapy, since there appears to be a relationship between the dose and extrapyramidal side effects. Excessive sedation may also interfere with participation in psychotherapy or with interpersonal relations. Importantly, geriatric patients may have reduced liver function that will require reduced doses compared with a younger adult with the same psychiatric symptoms.
4. Patients should be given periodic "drug holidays," during which drug treatment is suspended temporarily. Many patients can tolerate periodically skipping weekend doses without sacrificing control of psychiatric symptoms. The drug holidays must be planned by the physician, not the patient.
5. Patients should be weaned gradually from the drug after 1 year of continuous drug therapy. This allows assessment of the need for continued therapy, and helps detect the development of tardive dyskinesias, the symptoms of which may have been masked during treatment.

If tardive dyskinesias are suspected at any time, notify the physician at once. Ideally, the physician will reduce the dose and reevaluate the patient. Alternatives include discontinuing antipsychotic drug therapy altogether (which may not be possible) or switching to another agent.

Antiparkinson drugs (Chapter 25) may be prescribed to treat some extrapyramidal side effects, but they do not help tardive dyskinesias. They may not only mask some cardinal extrapyramidal signs but also can potentiate the antimuscarinic side effects of the antipsychotics. Antiparkinson drug administration for drug-induced parkinsonism should stop after 90 days. Controversies concerning the use of antiparkinson drugs for prophylaxis of drug-induced extrapyramidal side effects are discussed in Chapter 25.

NURSING IMPLICATIONS

Every effort must be made to assess the patient to detect extrapyramidal side effects as early as possible. The diagnostic clues described above can be seen or provoked by the skilled nurse, and it is easy for the nurse to perform the AIMS test. Early assessment and intervention can help prevent this severe, debilitating, and irreversible adverse drug response. If extrapyramidal reactions occur, the patient or family may become upset. Offer reassurance and indicate that interventions such as reducing the drug dose will usually help.

Neuroleptic Malignant Syndrome

The neuroleptic malignant syndrome is a combination of extrapyramidal symptoms, hyperthermia, and various autonomic disturbances. It is an underdiagnosed adverse response to antipsychotic drugs. It occurs in as many as 1% of patients taking antipsychotic drugs; of this number, 20% to 30% may die. There is no reliable patient-related characteristic that will predict its development. However, it is more likely to occur with high-potency phenothiazines and haloperidol. The syndrome appears to be an idiosyncrasy, since it may occur after administration of therapeutic doses of antipsychotic drugs, with blood levels of the drug well below the toxic range.

Symptoms may develop within hours after starting antipsychotic drug therapy, or months may pass until they occur. They include muscular rigidity and tremor, impaired ventilation, muteness, altered consciousness, and autonomic hyperactivity (tachycardia, diaphoresis). Body temperatures as high as 42.2°C (108°F) have been reported. Several of the symptoms are similar to those caused by malignant hyperthermia, heat stroke, and lethal catatonia. Therefore, early assessment and careful differential diagnosis are imperative for proper treatment.

NURSING IMPLICATIONS

Monitor closely for neuromuscular and autonomic signs, check body temperature frequently, and keep the patient adequately hydrated. Notify the physician at once if any clue of the syndrome occurs. Particularly close monitoring is indicated for patients taking both antipsychotics and lithium, a combination that seems to increase the risk of the neuroleptic malignant syndrome.

If neuroleptic malignant syndrome develops, antipsychotic drug therapy should be discontinued at once. Elevated body temperature is best managed with antipyretic drugs and physical means such as ice packs and cooling blankets. Parenteral fluids may be indicated for dehydration. Rigidity of the mouth and throat musculature may interfere with the ability to eat or drink; respiratory muscle rigidity may make breathing difficult and inadequate. Measures to ensure adequate hydration, nutritional status, and ventilation are likely to be necessary.

Sedation and Reduced Seizure Thresholds

Therapeutic doses of most antipsychotic drugs cause some degree of sedation. Tolerance to this effect usually develops. Until then, patients should be advised to avoid operating motor vehicles or dangerous machinery, or performing tasks that require mental acuity. If the patient's condition permits, a single dose of antipsychotic drug given at bedtime may help alleviate daytime sedation. Intense sedation, especially if prolonged, is not desirable unless the patient is extremely hyperactive or combative.

Antipsychotic drugs lower the seizure threshold, and should not be administered to comatose patients or those with head injuries or suspected brain tumors unless absolutely necessary. Extreme care must be used if they are given to persons with a history of seizures. Likewise, they should not be given during acute withdrawal from opiates, barbiturates, or alcohol. However, antipsychotics may have some value in managing psychoses associated with chronic alcoholism. As noted earlier, chlorpromazine is particularly useful for managing amphetamine-induced psychoses.

Endocrine or Metabolic Side Effects

Drug-induced interference with regulation of hormone secretion in the CNS can be a significant problem. Increased serum prolactin levels often cause amenorrhea and galactorrhea in women taking antipsychotics. (Amenorrhea may also be caused by the underlying psychiatric disorder.) Gynecomastia may occur in any patient; in males, particularly, it may contribute to noncompliance or frank refusal to take the drug. Phenothiazines may cause false-positive pregnancy tests (pseudopregnancy).

Chlorpromazine can inhibit insulin release and impair glucose tolerance. This is a particular problem for prediabetic or diabetic patients. Phenothiazine-induced hyperglycemia may contribute to excessive appetite, weight gain, and thirst in some patients. Switching to another antipsychotic drug such as haloperidol may alleviate this problem, but could cause others.

NURSING IMPLICATIONS

Monitor blood and urine glucose levels closely in diabetic or prediabetic patients, and assess for adequate antidiabetic drug therapy. Exercise and diet may help limit weight gain. Severe or disturbing endocrine problems may necessitate decreasing the dose or switching drugs.

Abnormal Skin Pigmentation

Phenothiazines may cause blue-gray skin discoloration that is intensified on exposure to sunlight. It is most likely to occur with high-dose, long-term treatment, but can be caused by any antipsychotic drug or dosage. Excessive pigmentation of the cornea and lens of the eye may also occur.

NURSING IMPLICATIONS

Advise patients to cover exposed areas of the skin to minimize the photosensitive reaction. Do not place immobilized patients in direct sunlight. Advise patients to report visual disturbances. Periodic eye examinations are important.

Altered Regulation, Perception of Temperature

Initial administration of antipsychotic drugs, especially parenterally, may elevate body temperature. With continued use, the patient may become either hypothermic or hyperthermic because of both central (eg, hypothalamic) and peripheral autonomic (eg, diminished heat loss via sweating) drug effects. However, other drug-induced CNS effects may make the patient unaware of or unconcerned about potentially dangerous changes of body temperature. Fatal hypothermia and heat stroke have occurred.

NURSING IMPLICATIONS

It is important to ensure that the patient is not subjected to extremes of heat or cold, that he or she avoid vigorous exercise in hot environments, and that clothing is appropriate for the environment.

Hypersensitivity and Allergy

Antipsychotic drugs, particularly phenothiazines, may cause hepatitis and jaundice. It is presumably a hypersensitivity reaction that occurs regardless of the dose. It affects about 4% of patients, and usually occurs between 2 and 4 weeks after starting therapy. The consequences are generally mild if detected early enough.

Blood dyscrasias resulting from bone marrow suppression include leukocytosis, leukopenia, eosinophilia and, rarely, fatal agranulocytosis. They may occur suddenly, typically between the end of the first and the start of the fourth month of treatment. Elderly, debilitated women seem to be at greatest risk.

Allergic reactions (hives, bronchoconstriction, fever, or laryngeal edema) may occur. They may be caused by the antipsychotic drug itself, or by tartrazine dye that is found in oral dosage forms of some of these drugs.

NURSING IMPLICATIONS

Notify the physician at once if there is any indication of a hypersensitivity or allergic reaction. Do not rely on pruritus, otherwise a diagnostic clue, as a warning of impending hepatitis; the antipruritic/antihistaminic effect of the phenothiazines can mask this symptom. Sudden fever, sore throat, or flu- or cold-like symptoms should be reported at once, since they may indicate a blood dyscrasia. Blood tests should be performed immediately, and antipsychotic therapy should be stopped if they are positive. If detected early, discontinuing therapy or switching to a drug in a different class usually eliminates symptoms. If a patient has experienced any hypersensitivity or allergic reaction, question medication orders calling for resumed therapy with the offending drug or one belonging to the same chemical class or phenothiazine subclass.

Tolerance and Physical Dependence

Antipsychotic drugs are not addicting in the sense applied to drugs such as narcotics. With continued use tolerance to effects such as sedation often occurs, and there is generally cross-tolerance between classes and subclasses of the antipsychotic drugs. Long-term high-dose antipsychotic drug therapy also causes physical dependence, since a withdrawal syndrome may occur on abrupt discontinuation of therapy, or when the physician attempts to switch from high doses of one potent antipsychotic drug to another. Withdrawal is characterized by ***withdrawal-emergent dyskinesias*** that are often indistinguishable from tardive dyskinesias. Other acute extrapyramidal reactions, hypotension, and autonomic manifestations may develop. They are thought to occur because dopamine-rich regions of the brain that have been suppressed by antipsychotic drugs become supersensitive to dopamine, and excessive activity occurs once the antagonist is no longer present in adequate amounts.

NURSING IMPLICATIONS

Because antipsychotic therapy involves long-term administration of a mind-altering drug, patients or their family may become concerned about addiction. If so, discuss the treatment plan to allay such concerns. Unless there is a critical reason to do so (eg, blood dyscrasias occur), antipsychotic drugs should not be withdrawn abruptly. Advise patients and their families about this.

◆ Use During Pregnancy and Lactation

The safety of chlorpromazine and other drugs discussed in this chapter during pregnancy has not been established. Use at this time is generally contraindicated. Antipsychotics in the piperazine class are absolutely contraindicated regardless of the reason for which they would be used. Caution women taking any antipsychotic against conception, and recommend effective contraceptive drugs or devices. If conception occurs or is suspected, notify the physician at once. With true pregnancy, antipsychotic drug therapy should be discontinued unless potential benefits to the mother outweigh possible fetal risks. If antipsychotic therapy must be continued, every attempt should be made to discontinue the drug approximately 2 weeks before anticipated delivery. Extrapyramidal side effects, hyperreflexia, and jaundice are relatively common in newborns of women taking antipsychotics during pregnancy. Many of the antipsychotics are excreted in breast milk, so bottle-feeding should be encouraged.

◆ Use in Children

Although antipsychotic drugs are generally not recommended for children under 12 years old, chlorpromazine can be used over the age of 6 months if necessary. Children with illnesses such as chickenpox, measles, gastroenteritis, or dehydration are more susceptible to adverse neuromuscular reactions, particularly dystonias.

◆ Use in the Elderly

As noted above, elderly patients are more likely to experience extrapyramidal and autonomic reactions, such as orthostatic hypotension, and are much less tolerant of them than younger persons. Expected age-related factors are likely to alter drug elimination rates and cause mental changes that complicate assessment of adverse central effects that may be either drug- or age-related. In addition, elderly patients are likely to have other conditions that contraindicate antipsychotic drug use or increase the risk of drug interactions.

Interactions with Other Drugs

Antipsychotic drugs interact adversely with many other therapeutic agents (Table 23–I). Most interactions have been demonstrated with chlorpromazine, but it is assumed that other antipsychotic drugs will interact also, unless noted otherwise. Antipsychotic drugs potentiate the actions of all other CNS depressants, so care must be taken when these drugs are given concomitantly. It may be necessary to reduce the dose of an interacting CNS depressant by 50% to 75% to avoid excessive depression.

NURSING IMPLICATIONS

Be sure your teaching about drug interactions includes mention of alcohol and nonprescription medications—especially those with CNS depressant or stimulant actions, or those affecting the GI tract. Ideally, no other drugs or medications should be taken without a physician's prior approval and dosage recommendations.

Assess closely for drowsiness, dizziness, or faintness in patients known to be or suspected of taking other CNS depressants.

Overdose and Toxicity

Signs and Symptoms

Antipsychotic drug overdoses are fairly common, but rarely fatal if no other drugs were also taken. The major signs of overdose include progressive increases of CNS depression (including coma), hypotension, and extrapyramidal reactions. Other responses include agitation or restlessness, seizures, fever, pronounced antimuscarinic symptoms, and arrhythmias. Combined overdose with most other drugs, especially other CNS depressants, increases the severity of symptoms.

Treatment

Treatment is symptomatic and supportive. Gastric lavage may help if performed shortly after ingestion of tablets or capsules. Vomiting ordinarily should not be induced since dystonias of the head and neck, impaired cough reflexes, and possible seizures increase the risk of aspiration. Moderate degrees of CNS depression need not be treated. Severe depression may respond to an amphetamine, but there is a risk of seizures. Amphetamines or antimuscarinic–antiparkinson drugs (benztropine, trihexyphenidyl, diphenhydramine) may help overcome severe extrapyramidal reactions. Norepinephrine or phenylephrine are preferred for restoring excessively low blood pressure. Epinephrine should be avoided; since antipsychotics block α receptors, epinephrine will act like a "pure" β agonist and could lower blood pressure further.

Related Drugs

Table 23–C lists the major antipsychotic drugs, their uses, and dosages. The actual dose that will be given must reflect the severity of symptoms and other unique factors such as age, general health, and so on. For example, patients with mild symptoms, geriatric patients, and most outpatients usually do not require and should not receive the high doses that may be indicated for a young adult with severe symptoms who requires close in-hospital monitoring. The minimal therapeutic dose of chlorpromazine for psychotic patients is 300 to 400 mg per day, given in two or three divided doses. Equivalent doses of other antipsychotic drugs can be calculated from the information given in Tables 23–2 and 23–C. The decision to use or switch to an alternative agent often depends heavily on nursing assessment of the patient's response. Keep three principles in mind when assessing the response for a possible drug change.

1. It is impossible to evaluate a drug's potential therapeutic value if the patient is not taking it as ordered.
2. The drug currently being used should be given a fair trial (typically 3 to 6 weeks).
3. If the drug must be changed, the new agent should be taken from a different chemical class (or subclass of the phenothiazines), thus allowing the patient to profit from inherent differences between classes (see Table 23–1).

NURSING IMPLICATIONS

Several studies have shown that patient education or various reinforcing programs (including stern warnings about adverse consequences of noncompliance) do little to improve compliance. Good rapport between the nurse and patient, which includes providing emotional support and the opportunity for the patient to discuss the situation openly, seems to be more effective than most other strategies.

Patients or their families may wish an end to psychiatric symptoms yet not desire antipsychotic drug therapy. The nurse's advice as a patient advocate may be sought. There is a potential conflict between quickly alleviating symptoms of schizophrenia, with the possible risk of overmedicating the patient, and administering very low doses, which may be subtherapeutic. Both are equally undesirable and not in the patient's best interests. The nurse must understand the conflict and explain alternatives to the patient and family. By monitoring the patient's responses to drug therapy, and by providing appropriate nondrug interventions to support the patient and others, the nurse can help optimize the acceptability of therapy and its outcome.

Another common concern arises because inpatients often compare their medications and dosages. One patient may take twice the dose of the same drug another may take and wonder if his or her mental disorder is twice as severe. When this occurs the nurse should explain the major patient-related factors that affect the dose.

Antipsychotic drugs provide useful and desired actions, but they do so at the risk of numerous side effects and adverse responses, some of which are devastating and irreversible. All patients have the right to be advised of both the potential benefits and risks. Nevertheless, too much information, or information provided carelessly, can cause excessive anxiety and concerns about physical and psychiatric symptoms. Teaching patients about potential problems must be weighed against the risk of presenting a gloomy image, fear, or apprehension. Nurses should provide information in a discrete way that uses their psychotherapeutic interactive skills and is least likely to worsen the patient's psychiatric state. Although compliance with prescribed drug treatments should be encouraged, because it is an essential component of treatment, be vigilant and prepared to intervene if complications threaten the patient's welfare.

Related Phenothiazine Antipsychotic Drugs

Major general properties of the three phenothiazine subclasses, and drugs in each, are summarized in Table 23–1. The following section highlights the groups, and briefly discusses special properties of individual agents. Drugs such as promethazine (PHENERGAN) and trimeprazine (TEMARIL), which are phenothiazines in the chemical sense, are used exclusively for nonpsychiatric indications such as management of emesis or pruritus. They are not discussed in this chapter.

Aliphatics: Chlorpromazine, Promazine, and Trifluopromazine

Promazine (SPARINE), and particularly trifluopromazine (VESPRIN), are similar in most regards to the prototype chlorpromazine. These two drugs are not commonly prescribed. Promazine is considered to be the least effective of all antipsychotic agents.

Piperazines: Fluphenazine, Perphenazine, Prochlorperazine, and Trifluoperazine

Piperazines are potent antipsychotic agents. They pose the greatest risk of extrapyramidal side effects, but cause the least sedation. They are absolutely contraindicated during pregnancy owing to a great risk of birth defects.

Fluphenazine is the most potent phenothiazine. The decanoate salt (PROLIXIN DECANOATE), given parenterally, is unique because of its very long duration of action, enabling administration once every 2 to 4 weeks. It is therefore suitable for patients who are not compliant with oral medications, or for others who have difficulty taking other antipsychotics on a daily basis. Fluphenazine hydrochloride (PERMITIL, PROLIXIN) has a duration of action comparable to chlorpromazine. Oral concentrates of this drug should not be mixed in or given with beverages containing pectins (apple juice), tannins (tea, some other fruit beverages), or caffeine (tea, coffee, colas, and some other soft drinks), because they can chemically interact.

Perphenazine (TRILAFON) is often used in conjunction with antidepressants for patients with psychosis plus severe depressive illness. It can be prescribed separately or as a fixed-dose combination with amitriptyline (TRIAVIL). Perphenazine and prochlorperazine (COMPAZINE) are also used as antiemetics.

Piperidines: Mesoridazine, and Thioridazine

The piperidine drugs are generally less sedating and less likely to cause extrapyramidal side effects than chlorpromazine. Very low doses of thioridazine (MELLARIL) appear to be well suited for short-term relief of a variety of signs and symptoms of what has been described as *senile dementia*.

Nonphenothiazine Antipsychotic Drugs

Nonphenothiazines, particularly haloperidol, are often the first antipsychotics ordered for acute psychosis. The nonphenothiazines share the same general side effects, adverse responses, contraindications, and drug interactions as chlorpromazine, although their incidence or severity may differ. The major properties of the nonphenothiazines are summarized in Table 23–1; potencies, relative to chlorpromazine, are noted in Table 23–2; dosages and specific uses are summarized in Table 23–C; and comparisons of the frequency of side effects are noted in Table 23–4. Starting doses usually should be at or near the lowest recommended dose, and increased only gradually as needed, based on the patient's response.

Chlorprothixene and Thiothixene

Chlorprothixene (TARACTAN) and thiothixene (NAVANE) are classified as *thioxanthenes*. Oral and IM dosage forms of each are available. Chlorprothixene's actions closely resemble those of chlorpromazine, but chlorprothixene is slightly more potent. Thiothixene acts much like the piperazine-type phenothiazines (eg, trifluoperazine). It is about 20 times as potent as chlorpromazine. Side effects of these drugs are similar to those of the related phenothiazines: a relatively great incidence of sedation, hypotension, and antimuscarinic effects. The risk of extrapyramidal side effects is less than with a drug such as haloperidol.

Clozapine

Clozapine (CLOZARIL), a *dibenzodiazepine*, is a unique antipsychotic drug. It was approved for use in the United States in early 1990. It is used for treating psychosis in patients who do not respond adequately to more traditional antipsychotic drugs, including the prototype, chlorpromazine (approximately 10%–20% of the treated population). It can also be used for the additional 20% to 30% of patients who relapse within a year of traditional treatment. In these situations, clozapine often alleviates symptoms when other drugs have failed to do so.

Clozapine should not be used as a starting drug because of the seriousness of one side effect, agranulocytosis. This may seem surprising when one compares the similarities between clozapine and the other antipsychotics. In general, these drugs would be equally efficacious if used to begin therapy. Moreover, several side effects of clozapine and the others are similar in frequency or intensity, including autonomic (eg, antimuscarinic) side effects. They usually appear at the start of treatment and are dose-dependent. This characteristic explains in part the need to start clozapine therapy at a low dose (see Table 23–C). In addition, like other antipsychotics, clozapine reduces the seizure threshold in a dose-dependent fashion, and can cause seizures. The incidence may be higher with clozapine than with alternatives.

Clozapine has one major advantage over other antipsychotics. Like the others, clozapine blocks dopamine receptors in the brain's limbic system. That effect accounts for the antipsychotic action. In contrast with the alternatives, however, clozapine does not block dopamine receptors in the extrapyramidal system (the brain's striatum) very well. As a result, clozapine causes far fewer extrapyramidal side effects.

As noted above the major property of clozapine that restricts its use to refractory psychosis is a risk of bone marrow depression which may lead to agranulocytosis. The overall incidence of this blood dyscrasia with clozapine is 1% to 2%. That is not a small number, considering the total number of patients who receive antipsychotic drugs, and it is higher than the incidence with alternatives. Importantly, the mortality rate from clozapine-associated agranulocytosis is thought to be as high as 30%. In early clinical trials, agranulocytosis usually occurred during the first 6 months of therapy and developed gradually. However, it has occurred earlier or progressed more quickly in some patients; and it may not be dose-dependent. The drug-monitoring procedures discussed in the nursing implications section have reduced the incidence of agranulocytosis dramatically.

NURSING IMPLICATIONS

Owing to the risk of agranulocytosis, clozapine's manufacturer imposed specific and strict requirements to minimize the risks and optimize safe therapy by detecting the blood dyscrasia early. The manufacturer also established a central registry to monitor initial and continued use of the drug for every patient. Some key points are (1) baseline blood tests (white cell count and differential) showing normal values (eg, WBC >3500/μL) must be done before dispensing the drug to start therapy. (2) Only 1 week's supply of drug can be dispensed at a time. (3) Blood tests must be repeated weekly, be within stated limits, and be reported to the registry system, in order for the next week's dose to be authorized for dispensing. (4) Further medication with the drug will stop, at least temporarily, if blood tests are abnormal. (5) All patients with abnormal blood tests during clozapine therapy must be monitored for at least 4 weeks after the drug is discontinued.

Institutions with responsibility for physicians and pharmacy services can apply to participate in this program. Individual physicians or pharmacies may do so

TRENDS AND CONTROVERSIES IN PHARMACOLOGY

The Clozapine "Catch"

Clozapine has been described as "the first truly new antipsychotic drug introduced in the last 40 years" (Buch, 1992). Yet this truly new drug was patented almost 30 years ago. Its development was placed on the back burner after it became evident that the drug caused an unacceptably high (1–2%) incidence of agranulocytosis, a potentially lethal complication. In early clinical trials, about one-third of patients with clozapine-induced agranulocytosis died.

The reintroduction of clozapine and its approval by the FDA marked recognition that it provides an alternative for the treatment of severely ill schizophrenic patients who fail to respond to conventional antipsychotic drugs, such as chlorpromazine. The availability of therapeutic alternatives is critically important, since experience indicates that about 10 to 20% of schizophrenic patients show little benefit from previously available antipsychotic drugs. In addition, clozapine provides an option for patients who develop the problem of tardive dyskinesia during treatment.

The symptoms of tardive dyskinesia are seen in as many as 40% of the patients taking conventional drugs and can be disabling. They have not been observed in patients treated with clozapine, although the drug may cause mild extrapyramidal symptoms. Furthermore, clozapine has a lower incidence of hyperprolactinemia and related side effects when compared with other antipsychotics. Like most of these drugs, however, clozapine has some side effects that are generally dose-related, including atropine-like symptoms and seizures. But, in contrast to other side effects, the occurrence of agranulocytosis is greater with clozapine than with other antipsychotics, and the incidence may not be dose-related. At present, it is not clear which persons are at risk, although there is some evidence suggesting that risks may be increased in women and in people of Jewish or Finnish descent, probably due to genetic factors.

Because of the potential benefits of clozapine therapy, the FDA approved marketing the drug in the United States in 1990. But to deal with the possible hazards of therapy, there was a catch—*no normal white cell or granulocyte count, no drug.* To enforce this guideline, clozapine's manufacturer set up a unique system that required weekly blood samples for monitoring patients' white blood cell counts by a specific, contracted laboratory. If baseline values were not normal, treatment would not start; and if they became abnormal during treatment, the supply of the medication would stop.

Essentially, this approach removed therapeutic decision-making from primary health care providers and took away from local pharmacies the responsibility for dispensing the drug. In addition, the decision to use a single laboratory engendered concerns regarding inconvenience, duplication of effort (since patients continued to have blood counts performed by local hospitals and physicians), and expense (about $9,000 each year). Not surprisingly, mandated procedures stimulated a great deal of controversy. And experience with clozapine raised questions about legislated guidelines in drug delivery that could deprive patients who lacked effective therapeutic alternatives of an effective treatment.

There is a need to weigh the benefits of any type of drug therapy against side effects or possible adverse reactions. Associated costs and acceptability to patients must also be considered in treatment decisions. In the case of clozapine, the manufacturer took unique steps to ensure that potentially fatal consequences of agranulocytosis would be minimized. Policies have loosened somewhat. Today, the drug is available through physicians, pharmacies, and health care facilities that are registered with the manufacturer and have agreed to follow specific guidelines for monitoring blood counts and protecting at-risk patients. The costs of clozapine and required monitoring remain very high, which may preclude treatment for some individuals. Cautious use of this drug certainly seems warranted—just as caution is needed for every drug. Yet one must wonder whether restrictive guidelines to "protect" some patients actually deprives others of an effective treatment for which there are no alternatives.

Buch DL: Clozapine: A novel antipsychotic. *Am Fam Physician* 1992;45:795–799.

Baldessarini RJ, Frankenburg FR: Clozapine a novel antipsychotic agent. *N Engl J Med* 1991;324:746–754.

also. In either case, they must certify, in writing, that the above guidelines (and others) will be followed faithfully. If the manufacturer accepts the application, therapy may begin.

Become familiar with the monitoring system if your patient is taking clozapine. Review for them the potential values and goals of the protocol and the weekly follow-ups that are part of it. The system may seem excessive and inconvenient; it is controversial; and it is clearly expensive (roughly $4000 per year). However this drug has the potential to alleviate disabling symptoms when others cannot.

Focus on monitoring blood test data, but do not overlook assessment for other potential side effects (eg, antimuscarinic), adverse reactions (eg, seizures), and all drug interactions noted for chlorpromazine.

Haloperidol

Haloperidol (HALDOL) belongs to the *butyrophenone* class. The drug is absorbed well from the GI tract. Like fluphenazine, it is about 50 times more potent than chlorpromazine. The drug is available in tablets or as a liquid concentrate for oral administration, or as a sterile liquid for IM injection. Effects from a single dose of these preparations last 2 to 3 days.

Haloperidol is prescribed for psychosis more than any other nonphenothiazine, particularly in pediatric psychiatry and for alleviating acute symptoms of psychosis in critical-care settings. Another indication is treatment of Gilles de la Tourette's disease (maladie des tics), for which it is more effective than the phenothiazines.

The decanoate salt of haloperidol has a very long duration of action. It is given only by IM injection, usually at 4-week intervals. This preparation is often preferred for maintenance therapy of psychosis or Tourette's disease, which usually requires long-term treatment. Candidates for haloperidol decanoate maintenance therapy should be stabilized first on oral haloperidol, which reduces the risk of an unexpected, excessive, and very longlasting response that might occur if the decanoate were given first. The usual starting dose of haloperidol decanoate is 10 to 15 times greater than the previous daily dose of oral haloperidol. Regular oral or parenteral dosage forms of haloperidol can be used to supplement the decanoate salt for dosage adjustments, as when symptoms periodically worsen.

Haloperidol poses a relatively high risk of extrapyramidal side effects, and it should not be given to patients prone to developing parkinsonism. However, it has less antimuscarinic, hypotensive, and sedative actions than most phenothiazines, so haloperidol is often preferred when these side effects must be minimized.

Loxapine

Loxapine (LOXITANE), a *dibenzoxapine,* is chemically distinct from the other major antipsychotic drug classes. Orally administered loxapine (capsules or oral concentrates) is absorbed well from the GI tract. A parenteral preparation for IM use is also available. Loxapine oral concentrate should be mixed with a citrus juice shortly before the patient takes it, to mask the unpleasant taste. Loxapine has about 10 times the antipsychotic potency of chlorpromazine. Extrapyramidal side effects occur in approximately 20% of patients receiving the drug. Sedation, occurring about 30 minutes after administration and lasting about 12 hours, is also relatively common. Both extrapyramidal side effects and sedation are most common during the first few days of loxapine therapy, or when doses are increased. Antimuscarinic side effects and hypotension are not frequent and usually are not severe.

Molindone

Molindone (MOBAN) is classified as a *dihydroindolone.* It is absorbed well from the GI tract, and is given only orally. It is extensively metabolized in the liver. Molindone is about 10 times as potent as chlorpromazine. No parenteral dosage forms are available. Molindone is used only to treat symptoms of psychosis. It causes considerable initial drowsiness, to which tolerance develops with continued administration. Drowsiness is a major reason why dosage adjustments must be made no more often than every 3 to 4 days. Molindone has been reported to cause heavy menstruation in previously amenorrheic women. Otherwise its side effects are similar to piperazine-type phenothiazines (eg, trifluoperazine). Molindone tablets contain calcium ions, which can interfere with the absorption of tetracycline antibiotics or phenytoin. Molindone concentrate contains metabisulfite, which may cause severe allergic reactions in some patients, particularly those with a history of asthma.

Pimozide

Pimozide (ORAP), a *diphenylbutylpiperidine,* is an orally effective neuroleptic drug that is indicated only for managing severe motor or vocal tics in patients with Tourette's disease, or tics that have failed to respond to therapy with other drugs indicated for this disorder. It is not indicated for psychosis or schizophrenia. Despite its limited use pimozide may cause all the CNS and peripheral side effects noted for haloperidol.

 SUMMARY OF NURSING IMPLICATIONS 

◆ Assessment

Establish baseline vital signs, laboratory studies (and ECG if ordered), which provide an indication of side effects, or allergic or hypersensitivity reactions (eg, hepatitis, blood dyscrasias).

Assess physiologic and psychologic status before therapy to help determine dosage needs and assess later progress.

Recognize early signs of tardive dyskinesia; use AIMS test.

Identify concurrent conditions that may be aggravated by antipsychotic drug use (eg, glaucoma, diabetes).

Determine family members' abilities to understand patient's condition and assist with therapy.

Complete nursing history to include level of anxiety, presence of symptoms of psychosis, and unpredictable behavior.

◆ Nursing Diagnoses

Knowledge deficit related to drug therapy purposes and effects.

High risk for injury related to adverse drug effects (eg, postural hypotension, agitation).

Noncompliance related to adverse physiologic responses to drug (hypotension, impotence, dyskinesias, akathisia, etc).

Sensory/perceptual alteration related to drug effects (eg, blurred vision, akathisia, dyskinesia).

Constipation related to drug therapy.

Urinary retention related to adverse drug effects.

◆ Planning/Implementation

Ensure that the drug has been taken; observe ingestion and check mouth and cheek.

Give drug as ordered: liquid form in at least 60 mL (2 oz) of compatible beverage to mask taste; dilute concentrate and give immediately; take with food to minimize GI upset; give IM injection into upper outer quadrant or mid-lateral thigh; aspirate before injecting; use gloves when handling solutions or suppositories to prevent skin irritation.

Check BP (supine, sitting, standing) and pulse before and after each dose; observe for side effects, especially those related to the central and autonomic nervous systems (eg, sedation, aggression, hypotension).

Prevent falls associated with postural hypotension; have patient sit on side of bed before rising; assume head-low position if dizziness occurs; wear elastic stockings; avoid hot showers.

Offer comfort measures for dry mouth: chewing gum, hard candies, lip balm.

Monitor urinary output; check inactive patients, older males, or patients on high doses for bladder distention.

Record bowel movements daily.

Assist with ambulation if blurred vision present; dim room lights for photosensitivity.

Monitor for indications of neuroleptic malignant syndrome; notify physician immediately if clinical signs present: muscle rigidity, fever, depressed neurologic status; ensure adequate hydration, nutrition, and ventilation.

Protect patient from exposure to extreme heat or cold; provide appropriate clothing for environment.

Recognize impending hypersensitivity or allergy: pruritus or jaundice with hepatitis; flu or cold-like symptoms, evidence of bleeding, with blood dyscrasia.

Observe and document involuntary movements: body part(s) involved, intensity and duration of movements.

◆ Patient and Family Teaching

Teach the patient/family:

About potentially beneficial and deleterious consequences; however, such information must be weighed against creating fear or undue apprehension; use psychotherapeutic skills to give information in discrete way.

To comply with drug treatment; family should be observant of untoward drug responses and report them immediately.

To avoid activities requiring clear vision for a few weeks (blurred vision usually normalizes); to report ocular pain immediately.

About the importance of exercise, fluids and fiber in diet in case constipation occurs.

To watch for signs or symptoms of heart failure: weight gain, dyspnea, distended neck veins, tachycardia.

About possible impaired male sexual performance; relaxed, stress-free atmosphere may help.

To avoid conception; women should practice effective contraception; phenothiazines may cause false-positive pregnancy tests.

To avoid exposure to sunlight; keep skin covered, but with clothing appropriate to environment.

That addiction is not a concern.

◆ Evaluation

The patient/family will:

Demonstrate ability to follow prescribed regimen; take medication as ordered; participate in agreed-on plan of care.

Avoid physical injury; report any dizziness; verbalize need for assistance.

Verbalize reduction in anxiety.

Demonstrate ability to adapt to physiologic changes; recognize that deficits are most likely temporary.

Experience minimal or no adverse drug effects (eg, constipation, urinary retention, sexual impairment).

Identify effective coping patterns to use or acknowledge inability to accept situation.

Achieve improved mental status (eg, appropriate responses and behavior).

Annotated Bibliography

Andreasen NC, Olsen S. Negative vs positive schizophrenia. *Arch Gen Psychiatry* 1982;39:789–794. *Nancy Andreasen, a leading authority in the field of schizophrenia, provides one of the early reviews on the criteria for looking at schizophrenia from a positive framework. This framework allows the nurse to incorporate patient behaviors that can be observed in everyday assessment-gathering and then formulate reasonable care goals based on that assessment data. Andreasen's 1984 book,* The Broken Brain, *is another excellent resource.*

Arana GW, Goff DC. Baldessarini RJ, Keepers GA. Efficacy of anticholinergic prophylaxis for neuroleptic-induced acute dystonia. *Am J Psychiatry* 1988;145:993–996. *A brief but well-written review of clinical studies that address the risks and benefits of prophylaxis of antipsychotic drug-induced motor disorders.*

Blumenreich P, Lippmann S, Bacani-Oropilla T. Violent patients: Are you prepared to deal with them? *Postgrad Med* 1991;90:201–206. *The sound advice in this article may pay off in many ways if you are faced with an aggressive and potentially dangerous patient. Both pharmacologic and nondrug measures are discussed.*

Glod CA. Psychopharmacology and clinical practice. *Nurs Clin North Am* 1991;26:375–399. *A unique view on how pharmacotherapy for psychiatric disorders, and the clinical outcomes, can be varied, sometimes unpredictable, and full of pitfalls.*

Haller E, Binder RL. Clozapine and seizures. *Am J Psychiatry* 1990; 147:1069–1071. *The manufacturer of CLOZARIL reports a 5% prevalence of seizures with doses of 600 to 900 mg per day. Haller and Binder outline six recommendations to decrease the incidence.*

Harvis KA. Care plan approach to dementia. *Geriatr Nurs* 1990;11: 76–80. *An important article for nurses working with patients with dementia.*

Johnson DAW. Pharmacological treatment of patients with schizophrenia: Past and present problems and potential future therapy. *Drugs* 1990;39:481a–488a. *A useful review of drug treatment of schizophrenia. The author covers important topics such as treatment of relapse, drug holidays, "microdose" regimens, and the concomitant use of antiparkinson and antidepressant drugs with antipsychotics. Johnson concludes with an appeal for newer drugs that have a more selective action on receptors responsible for symptoms.*

Kelleher KJ, Hohman AA, Larson DB. Prescription of psychotropics to children in office-based practice. *Am J Dis Child* 1989;143: 855–859. *This is the first research effort to report the extent of psychotropic drug prescription to children on an outpatient basis. The authors found considerable deviation between actual prescribing practices and standards of care recommended for children treated with psychotropic drugs, including gaps in follow-up and concurrent psychotherapy.*

Keltner NL, Folks DG. Clozapine: Miracle or Mirage? *Perspect Psychiatr Care* 1991;27:35–36. *Keltner and Folks write a quarterly "Psychopharmacology Update" column in this nursing journal. The columns provide important information and key insights into current issues in psychopharmacology. This article on clozapine uses a question-and-answer approach to address key concerns about this relatively new drug.*

Mallett P. Anticholinergic drugs in psychiatry. *Int J Clin Pharmacol Res* 1989;4:261–271. *An interesting overview of the role drugs with atropine-like activity play in the management of diverse psychiatric disorders.*

Miller LJ. Clinical strategies for the use of psychotropic drugs during pregnancy. *Psychiatr Med* 1991;9:275–298. *A current and important review of maternal and fetal risks arising from the use of psychoactive drugs during pregnancy, and treatment strategies designed to minimize the risks. A must-read article for nurses working in this area.*

Richelson E. Neuroleptic affinities for human brain receptors and their use in predicting adverse effects. *J Clin Psychiatry* 1984;45:331–336. *This article discusses the affinity of antipsychotics for specific receptors, and relates this to therapeutic and undesirable clinical responses. Since the efficacy of neuroleptics appears to be equal, the information presented in this paper may help the physician minimize the often unequal adverse effects. One of the most useful papers to help understand drug selection rationales.*

Rifkin A, Doddi S, Basawaraj K, Borenstein M, Wachpress M. Dosage of haloperidol for schizophrenia. *Arch Gen Psychiatry* 1991;48: 166–170. *Antipsychotic drug dosages for schizophrenic patients often are taken for granted. These researchers wanted to find out about the efficacy of "routine" haloperidol dosages. Eighty-seven newly admitted patients were placed on 10, 30, or 80 mg per day. The lowest dose was just as effective as the higher doses.*

Wood KA, Harris MJ, Morreale A, Rizos AL. Drug-induced psychosis and depression in the elderly. *Psychiatr Clin North Am* 1988;11: 167–193. *Long but worth reading, this article reviews the major drug groups that can cause psychosis in elders, and gives advice about how to minimize actual problems.*

Table 23–C | **Clinical Uses and Administration of Major Antipsychotic Drugs**

AGENT	CLINICAL USES	DOSAGE AND ROUTE OF ADMINISTRATION
PROTOTYPE		
Chlorpromazine (THORAZINE) (aliphatic phenothiazine)	Psychosis	Oral: Adults: 10 mg tid or qid or 25 mg bid or tid (most outpatients); for more severe symptoms in outpatients, 25 mg tid, increased after 1 or 2 days by 20–50 mg and again at semiweekly intervals as needed. Maintenance doses 200–800 mg/d in divided doses, with 1000 mg/d (maximum) possibly needed for severely ill hospitalized patients. Children: 0.25 mg/lb body weight q6h–q8h (0.5 mg/lb rectally); gradually increase to 50–100 mg/d for severely ill hospitalized children
	Acutely agitated, manic, or disturbed patients requiring immediate treatment	IM: Adults: initially 25 mg, repeated in 1 hr as needed; switch to oral dose (25–50 mg tid) when possible. Children: 0.25 mg/lb q6h–q8h prn; maximum daily doses: 2–5 years, 40 mg; 5–12 yrs, 75 mg, unless not controlled otherwise
	Excessive anxiety, tension, agitation (eg, discharged mental patients)	Oral: (Adults only): See doses for psychosis, above. Continue optimum dose for 2 weeks, taper to average of 200 mg/d
	Nonpsychotic anxiety	Oral: (Adults only): Divided doses of ≤100 mg/d for no more than 12 weeks IM: 25 mg, repeat in 1 hr if needed, followed by switch to oral therapy
	Nausea and vomiting (not surgery-related)	Oral: Adults: 10–25 mg q4h–q6h prn. Children: 0.25 mg/lb q4h–q6h prn Rectal: Adults: 50 or 100 mg (one-half or one suppository) q6h–q8h prn. Children: 0.5 mg/lb every 8 h IM: Adults: 25 mg, repeat or increase to 50 mg q3h–q4h prn until vomiting stops or blood pressure falls. Children: 0.25 mg/lb q6h–q8h
	Preoperative, postoperative control of nausea, vomiting	Oral: Adults: Preoperative: 25–50 mg 2–3 hr before surgery. Postoperative: 10–25 mg q4h–q6h prn. Children: 0.25 mg/lb 2–3 hr preoperatively and/or at 4–6-hr intervals postoperatively IM: Adults: Preoperative: 12.5–25 mg 1–2 hr before surgery. Intraoperative for severe acute nausea and vomiting: 12.5 mg at 0.5-hr intervals prn if blood pressure acceptable. Postoperative: 12.5–25 mg repeated in 1 hr if needed and permitted by blood pressure. Children: 0.25 mg/lb 1–2 hr preoperatively: 0.125 mg/lb intraoperatively; 0.25 mg/lb postoperatively, repeat in 1 hr if needed and permitted by blood pressure IV: Adults: 2 mg at 2-min intervals during surgery for intractable nausea and vomiting, not exceeding 25 mg total. Children: 1 mg at 2-min intervals, not exceeding total IM dose recommended above
	Acute intermittent porphyria	Oral: Adults: 25–50 mg tid or qid IM: 25 mg tid or qid until oral therapy possible

(continued)

Table 23–C Clinical Uses and Administration of Major Antipsychotic Drugs (*Continued*)

AGENT	CLINICAL USES	DOSAGE AND ROUTE OF ADMINISTRATION
	Tetanus	IM: Adults: 25–50 mg tid or qid (usually adjunctively with barbiturates). Children: 0.25 mg/lb tid or qid IV: Adults: 25–50 mg, diluted to at least 1 mg/mL and given no faster than 1 mg/min. Children: Same as IM dose, given no faster than 0.5 mg/min
RELATED DRUGS		
Chlorprothixene (TARACTAN) (thioxanthene; nonphenothiazine)	Psychosis	Oral: Adults: 25–50 mg tid or qid; maintenance ordinarily <600 mg/d in divided doses. Children >6 years: 10–25 mg tid or qid IM: Adults, children 12 and older: 25–50 mg up to tid or qid
Clozapine (CLOZARIL) (dibenzodiazepine)	Treatment-resistant schizophrenia	Oral: Adults: Initially 25 mg qid or bid; increase by 25–50 mg/d until reaching 300–450 mg/d by end of second week. Make further adjustments only at weekly or twice-weekly intervals, in increments no greater than 100 mg; typical maintenance dosage 300–900 mg/d. Safety for children under 16 not established
Fluphenazine HCl (PROLIXIN) (piperazine phenothiazine)	Psychosis	Oral: (Adults only): Initially 0.5–10 mg/d in 3 or 4 divided doses. Severely disturbed patients may require to 40 mg/d. Maintenance: Adjust to lowest effective dose, usually 1–5 mg/d (in evening). Geriatric patients: 1–2.5 mg/d initially; use lowest effective maintenance dose. Children: Not recommended
Fluphenazine decanoate (PROLIXIN DECANOATE)	Long-term management of chronic schizophrenia, other patients requiring parenteral therapy	IM: 12.5–25 mg initially and repeated every 2–4 weeks for maintenance
Haloperidol (HALDOL) (butyrophenone, nonphenothiazine)	Psychosis in adults or children, Tourette's disease in adults	Oral: Adults: Initially 0.5–2 mg (moderate symptoms or geriatric patients) or 3–5 mg (severe symptoms or chronic or resistant patients) bid or tid. Maintenance doses usually <100 mg/d in divided doses. Children: 0.05–0.15 mg/kg/d; daily doses >6 mg/d not likely to be more effective
	Prompt control of psychotic symptoms (eg, agitation) in patients with moderate-to-severe symptoms	IM: Adults: Initially 2–5 mg; repeat every 1–8 hr depending on severity, response of symptoms
	Nonpsychotic behavior in disturbed or hyperactive children	Oral: 0.05–0.075 mg/kg/d

(*continued*)

Table 23–C | **Clinical Uses and Administration of Major Antipsychotic Drugs (*Continued*)**

AGENT	CLINICAL USES	DOSAGE AND ROUTE OF ADMINISTRATION
RELATED DRUGS		
Haloperidol decanoate		
(HALDOL DECANOATE)	Long-term therapy of psychosis	IM: Initially 10–15 times the previous oral haloperidol dose, not to exceed 100 mg every 4 weeks; monthly maintenance doses should not exceed 300 mg; inject no more than 3 mL (150 mg) per site
Loxapine		
(LOXITANE)	Psychosis	Oral: Adults only: Initially 10 mg bid; 25 mg bid may be needed for severe symptoms. Maintenance dose: Increase initial dose rapidly over first week to 30–50 mg bid; do not exceed 250 mg/d
(dibenzoxapine, nonphenothiazine)		IM: 12.5-50 mg q4h-q6h prn; switch to oral therapy within 5 days if possible
Mesoridazine		
(SERENTIL)	Psychosis	Oral: Adults only: Initially 50 mg tid. Maintenance 100-400 mg/d in divided doses
(piperidine phenothiazine)	Severe anxiety, tension of severe psychoneurotic disorders	Oral: Initially 10 mg tid. Maintenance 30–150 mg/d (may be in divided doses)
	Psychoses of chronic alcoholism	Oral: Initially 25 mg bid. Maintenance 50–200 mg/d in divided doses
	Behavioral problems of mental deficiency, OMD	Oral: Initially 25 mg tid. Maintenance 75–300 mg/d in divided doses
	All indications requiring prompt treatment	IM: 25 mg initially, repeat in 30–60 min as needed. Optimum daily dose 25–200 mg
Molindone		
(MOBAN)	Psychosis	Oral: Adults, children >12 years: Initially 50–75 mg/d, increase in 3 or 4 days to 100 mg/d. Maintenance dose increased or decreased to 5–15 mg (mild symptoms) or 10–25 mg (moderate symptoms) tid or qid; severe symptoms may require up to 225 mg/d (eg, 75 mg tid). Use lower dose range for elderly or debilitated patients
(dihydroindolone, nonphenothiazine)		
Perphenazine		
(TRILAFON)	Psychosis	Oral (regular 2–16 mg tablets, 8-mg repeat-action tablets, concentrate): Adults, children >12 years: nonhospitalized, moderately disturbed patients: 4–8 mg tid or 1 or 2 repeat-action tablets bid, re-duced as soon as possible to lowest effective dose. Hospitalized patients: 8–16-mg tablets bid-qid or 1–4 repeat-action tablets bid, not to exceed 64 mg/d
(piperazine phenothiazine)		IM: Adults: 5 (or 10) mg q6h prn. Children over 12 years may receive the lowest limit of adult dosage

(*continued*)

Table 23–C Clinical Uses and Administration of Major Antipsychotic Drugs (*Continued*)

AGENT	CLINICAL USES	DOSAGE AND ROUTE OF ADMINISTRATION
RELATED DRUGS		
	Severe nausea and vomiting in adults	Oral: 8-16 mg/d in divided doses (24 mg/d sometimes needed) IM: 5 or 10 mg IV: For intractable vomiting, hiccoughs, or intraoperative wretching dilute parenteral solution to 0.5 mg/mL with sterile normal saline, give no more than 1 mg every 1–2 min; do not exceed 5 mg total
Pimozide (ORAP) (diphenylbutylpiperidine, nonphenothiazine)	Treatment of motor and vocal tics of Tourette's disease in patients not responding to other appropriate drugs	Oral: Adults, children >12 years: Initially 1 or 2 mg/d in 2 divided doses; maintenance dose is lesser of 0.2 mg/kg/d or 10 mg/d; daily dose should not exceed lesser of 0.2 mg/kg or 10 mg
Prochlorperazine (COMPAZINE) (piperazine phenothiazine)	Psychosis	Oral: Adult: Intially 5 or 10 mg tid or qid; maintenance usually 50–75 mg/d (100–150 mg/d for severe symptoms). Children (oral or rectal) 2–12 years: 2.5 mg bid or tid; maximum daily dose <20 mg for ages 2–5, <25 mg for ages 6–12 IM: Adults: Initially 10–20 mg q2h–q4h (or 4qh–6qh if prolonged treatment anticipated). Children <12 years: 0.06 mg/lb body weight
	Nonpsychotic anxiety in adults	Oral: Usually 5 mg tid or qid or 15-mg timed-release capsule in morning or 10-mg timed-release capsule (q12h)
	Severe nausea and vomiting (other than related to surgery)	Oral: Adults: 5 or 10 mg tid or qid; timed-release capsules, see dose for nonpsychotic anxiety, above. Children (oral or rectal): 20-29 lbs: 2.5 mg qd or bid (maximum 7.5 mg/d); 30-39 lbs: 2.5 mg bid or tid (maximum 10 mg/d); 40-85 lbs: 2.5 mg tid or 5 mg bid (maximum 15 mg/d) Rectal: Adults: 25 mg bid
	Severe nausea and vomiting due to surgery (adults only)	IM: 5–10 mg 1–2 hr before inducing anesthesia or during or after surgery (1 repeat dose allowed) IV: Single slow injection of 5–10 mg 15–30 min before induction, or during or after surgery; or slow infusion of 20 mg, diluted in at least 1 L of IV fluid, 15–30 min before induction
Promazine (SPARINE) (aliphatic phenothiazine)	Psychosis	IM: Adults, children12 years: Initially 50–150 mg, depending on degree of excitation, age; if not effective repeat in 30 min up to total of 300 mg; maintenance doses of 10–200 mg given at 4–6 hr intervals if needed

(*continued*)

Table 23–C | **Clinical Uses and Administration of Major Antipsychotic Drugs (*Continued*)**

AGENT	CLINICAL USES	DOSAGE AND ROUTE OF ADMINISTRATION
RELATED DRUGS		
Thioridazine		
(MELLARIL) (piperidine phenothiazine)	Psychosis	Oral: Adults: Initially 50–100 mg tid; increase gradually to maximum of 800 mg/d, reduce when symptoms controlled to 200–800 mg/d in 2–4 divided doses. Children 2–12 years: 0.5–3 mg/kg/d (25 mg bid or tid for severely disturbed or psychotic children); do not exceed 3 mg/kg/d
	Short-term (<12 week) treatment of moderate to marked depression plus anxiety, anxious depression, tension, sleep disturbances, fears in geriatric patients	Adults: Usually 25 mg tid (range 10 mg bid–qid to 50 mg tid or qid); lower limit preferred for geriatric patients.
Thiothixene		
(NAVANE) (thioxanthene nonphenothiazine)	Psychosis	Oral: Adults, children >12 years: Initially 2 mg tid or 5 mg bid (severe symptoms); optimum maintenance dose 20–30 mg/d; maximum effective dose 60 mg/d. Once-a-day therapy may suffice for some patients IM: Adults, children >12 years: 4 mg bid–qid (usual range 16–20 mg/d, not to exceed 30 mg/d)
Trifluoperazine		
(STELAZINE) (piperazine phenothiazine)	Psychosis	Oral: Adults:: 2–5 mg bid, optimum maintenance dose 15–20 mg/d. Children 6–12 years, hospitalized or closely supervised: 1 mg qd or bid, increased to maintenance usually not exeeding 15 mg/d IM: Adults: 1–2 mg q4–6h as needed (total daily dose should rarely exceed 10 mg). Children: 1 mg qd
	Nonpsychotic anxiety	Oral: Adults only: 1–2 mg bid. Maximum of 6 mg/d for no more than 12 weeks

Table 23–S | **Major Side Effects of and Contraindications for Antipsychotic Drugs**

BODY SYSTEM/ Side Effect	CONTRAINDICATION/ PRECAUTION	COMMENTS AND NURSING IMPLICATIONS
CENTRAL NERVOUS SYSTEM		
Parkinsonism	History of parkinsonism	Monitor for cardinal signs (tremor, rigidity, etc; see text); notify physician for possible prescription of antiparkinson drugs, change of antipsychotic drug or dose
Akathisias		Reassure patient who reports jitteriness and "excess energy," and attempt to differentiate from agitation; may be alleviated with antiparkinson drugs; anticipate change of drug or dose, start of parenteral therapy for patients who become noncompliant due to adverse subjective response to antipsychotic medication.
Dystonias		Notify physician for possible prescription of antiparkinson drugs
Tardive dyskinesias		Carefully observe movements, gait, handwriting; consult physician about use of periodic drug holidays; consult when antiparkinson drugs, which may mask dyskinesias, are given for more than 90 days
Oculogyric crisis		Give ordered antihistamine or antimuscarinic at once, notify physician immediately if one is not ordered; reassure patient; remove emotionally arousing stimuli; anticipate reduced dose of antipsychotic drug
Seizures	History of seizure disorders (caution)	Antipsychotics lower seizure threshold; overall incidence about 1% in antipsychotic drug–treated patients, is dose-dependent; apparently more frequent with clozapine; EEG must be normal to use clozapine doses >600 mg/d; monitor *all* patients accordingly; use suitable anticonvulsants (eg, IV diazepam, Chapter 26) to stop acute seizures
EYE		
Blurred vision (cycloplegia or paraylsis of accommodation)		Advise patient to avoid tasks requiring visual acuity until tolerance develops (typically in a few weeks)
Ocular pain, photophobia, mydriasis	Narrow-angle glaucoma	Have patient report acute eye pain at once; may indicate acute glaucoma attack; photophobia may be helped by having patient wear sunglasses
Impaired vision		Excessive antipsychotic drug doses may cause melanin deposits on cornea; recommend periodic ophthalmic examinations for patients taking high doses chronically
ENDOCRINE		
Hyperglycemia	Severe or poorly controlled diabetes mellitus	Monitor blood glucose levels, insulin or hypoglycemic drug requirements of diabetic patients
Intolerance of extreme heat, cold; possible heat stroke or fatal hypothermia		Advise patients to avoid exposure to excessively cold or hot environments, avoid physical stress in hot weather, dress appropriately for environmental temperature

(continued)

Table 23–S | Major Side Effects and Contraindications for Antipsychotic Drugs *(Continued)*

BODY SYSTEM/ Side Effect	CONTRAINDICATION/ PRECAUTION	COMMENTS AND NURSING IMPLICATIONS
RESPIRATORY		
Nasal congestion		Notify physician if severe; decongestants should be taken only with physician's advice
Wheezing, dyspnea	Severe bronchial asthma, emphysema	Reduce dose or change drug if severe; may be due to atropine-like thickening of mucus in respiratory passages
CARDIOVASCULAR		
Hypotension, especially orthostatic, leading to dizziness, syncope	Prior hypotension, history of syncope, cerebrovascular disease (eg, stroke), coronary artery disease	Advise patient to get out of bed or chair slowly, dangle feet from bed for several minutes before standing; assist unsteady patients with walking; instruct patient to assume sitting, head-low position if dizzy; syncope likely to occur due to hypotension; monitor BP before each dose when patient is hospitalized; consult physician before giving increased or parenteral doses of antipsychotic drugs if BP is excessively low; may require reduced dose of antipsychotic, change of drug; most likely to occur with high doses of low-potency antipsychotics or in elderly or debilitated patients
Tachycardia, irregular pulse, arrhythmias	History of cardiac disease (arrhythmias, angina, coronary atherosclerosis)	Usually a reflex triggered by fall of blood pressure; best prevented by interventions noted for hypotension, above; obtain baseline and subsequent ECG in high-risk patients (see above)
GASTROINTESTINAL		
Dry mouth		Have patient suck hard sugarless candy, chew gum, or rinse mouth frequently with water; an atropine-like side effect
Constipation	Preexisting constipation, obstructive or paralytic gut disorder	Encourage exercise, added dietary fiber, water intake; use laxatives only upon advice of physician; report hard, painful, or infrequent stools (or any sudden change from predrug bowel pattern); an atropine-like side effect
Jaundice, abdominal pain	Prior hypersensitivity to drug	Notify physician at once: may indicate serious hepatotoxic hypersensitivity reaction to drug; make sure patient does not receive same drug that previously caused hepatotoxicity
SKIN		
Blue-gray skin rash		Is photosensitive, not likely to be severe unless maximum recommended doses are exceeded; have patient wear protective clothing appropriate for environment

(continued)

Table 23–S **Major Side Effects and Contraindications for Antipsychotic Drugs *(Continued)***

BODY SYSTEM/ Side Effect	CONTRAINDICATION/ PRECAUTION	COMMENTS AND NURSING IMPLICATIONS
GENITOURINARY Urinary retention	Prostatic hypertrophy or obstructive uropathy	Report, monitor for, decreased urine output, abdominal (bladder) distention; encourage frequent voiding; be prepared for bladder catheterization of susceptible hospitalized patients, especially older males or those taking high doses of antipsychotics; an atropine-like side effect
Urinary hesitancy		Recommend privacy; warm water run over perineum may facilitate voiding
Galactorrhea		Recommend bra pads, changed frequently to reduce chance of infection; due to increased prolactin release
Gynecomastia		Affects males and females; may require discontinuing, switching from offending drug
Impaired ejaculation		Important cause of noncompliance by males; encourage support from spouse, intercourse at nonstressful times; may be caused by drug or underlying psychiatric disorder, and difficult to determine which
Amenorrhea		May be caused by drug or underlying disorder; may be alleviated partly by encouraging exercise
	Pregnancy	Advise women to notify physician at once if conception occurs, as antipsychotics may be embryotoxic; if antipsychotics are continued during pregnancy, attempt to wean dose 2 weeks before anticipated delivery, expect adverse neurologic effects in newborn

Table 23–I | **Major Interactions Between Antipsychotics and Other Agents**

AGENT	RESULT OF INTERACTION	COMMENTS AND NURSING IMPLICATIONS
Alcohol (Chapter 22)	Increased CNS depression; increased extrapyramidal side effects	Avoid interaction if possible; caution patients about OTC medications containing alcohol that should be avoided; see CNS depressants, below
Amphetamines (Chapter 27)	Decreased antipsychotic actions	Normally avoid combined use; amphetamines and most antipsychotic drugs seem to have mutually antagonistic CNS actions (which explains use of amphetamines for treating severe antipsychotic drug overdoses)
Antacids (magnesium and aluminum products) (Chapter 40)	Possible decreased antipsychotic effect	Discourage excessive or unsupervised antacid use; administer antipsychotic drugs with food to reduce GI upset, or give antacid 1 hr before or 2 hr after giving oral antipsychotic; interaction may occur because antacid interferes with absorption of antipsychotic from GI tract
Antimuscarinics (atropine, H_1-type antihistamines, antidepressants, etc) (Chapter 13)	Increased risk of excessive atropine-like side effects or toxicity	Discourage unsupervised use of these drugs; monitor for pertinent signs (constipation, blurred vision, fever, etc)
Benztropine	Possible decreased antipsychotic effect, increased risk or severity of peripheral antimuscarinic side effects, masking of extrapyramidal side effects, onset of tardive dyskinesias	Monitor pertinent patient responses closely, evaluate for poor control of psychosis, excessive anticholinergic actions; onset of tardive dyskinesias may be more difficult to detect; limit use of benztropine as directed (see text and Chapter 24); interaction may also apply to trihexyphenidyl; see antimuscarinics, above
CNS depressants (barbiturates, antihistamines, antianxiety or antidepressant drugs, etc) (Chapter 22)	Risk of increased sedation, more severe CNS depression	Monitor patient closely for excessive sedation, etc; see alcohol, above
Diazoxide (Chapter 33)	Possible severe hyperglycemia, prediabetic coma	Most likely to occur with oral diazoxide therapy; monitor blood glucose levels closely if combined drug administration is planned, especially for diabetic or prediabetic patients
Lithium (Chapter 24)	Poor control of psychosis with combined therapy	Avoid interaction if possible, monitor patient responses and lithium levels carefully if unavoidable; lithium may cause 20%–70% decrease in blood levels of chlorpromazine
	Masked signs of lithium toxicity	See above; most antipsychotic drugs mask nausea and vomiting, which are early signs of lithium intoxication
	Neurotoxicity: confusion, delirium, seizures, encephalopathy	Monitor pertinent CNS signs closely if combined therapy needed; reaction most likely to occur during early combined therapy with therapeutic doses of each agent; most likely to occur, be severe with haloperidol, thioridazine
Meperidine, morphine (Chapter 21)	Increased risk of severe CNS depression, respiratory depression, hypotension	Monitor relevant vital signs closely when combined drug therapy is required
Propranolol (Chapter 15)	Increased effects of either or both drugs	Monitor responses to both drugs closely; monitor propranolol blood levels if needed. Propranolol blood levels are initially decreased considerably by first-pass hepatic metabolism (Chapter 4); this metabolism is inhibited by chlorpromazine. Atenolol, nadolol, pindolol, timolol (Chapter 15) depend less on first-pass metabolism, may be preferred if combined drug therapy is needed

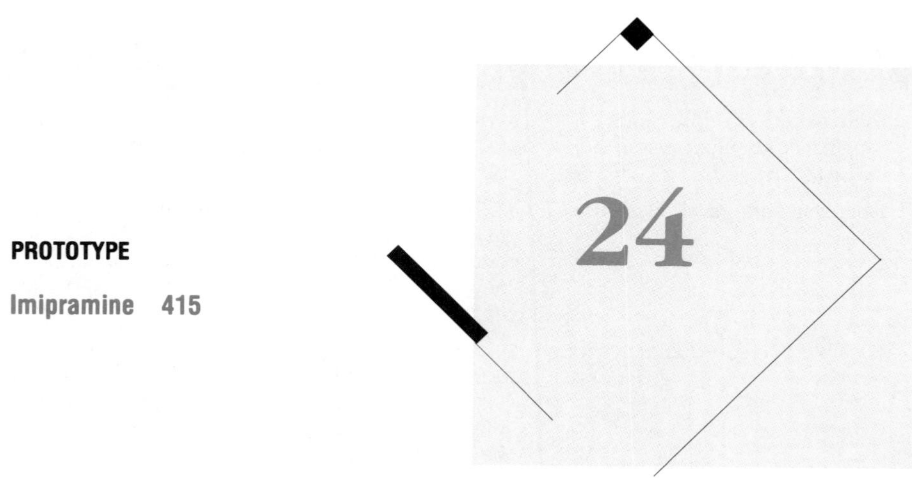

PROTOTYPE

Drugs for the Treatment of Depression and Mania

Affective disorders are disorders of mood characterized by either extreme depression (dysphoria), extreme elation (euphoria; mania), or both. This chapter begins with a brief overview of affective disorders, focusing on depression and its probable causes, before introducing the two major classes of antidepressant drugs: *tricyclic antidepressants* (and related agents), and *monoamine oxidase inhibitors*. The antimanic drug, lithium, is discussed at the end of the chapter.

Depression

Everyone periodically feels sadness, guilt, or other symptoms of depression (Table 24–1) in response to personal loss or failure. Such feelings are normal and usually self-limiting—and most people are able to withstand the vicissitudes of life and carry on normally. Antidepressant drugs are seldom used for such short-lived episodes. However, when an identifiable stressor has overwhelmed a person's ability to cope with it, and symptoms persist beyond "normal," antidepressants may be needed. Some form of depression that would benefit from treatment affects approximately 15% of all adults during any given year. The lifetime incidence is about twice as high in women (about 23%) as in men. Table 24–2 presents an overview of depression types and preferred treatments.

Table 24–1 Typical Symptoms of Depression

Common	Others
Apathy	Fatigue
Sadness	Thoughts of death
Sleep disturbances (insomnia and/or hypersomnia)	Decreased libido
Hopelessness	Ruminations of inadequacy
Helplessness	Psychomotor agitation
Worthlessness	Private verbal beratings of self
Guilt	Spontaneous crying without apparent cause

Neurochemical Theory of Depression

Studies of many drugs acting in the brain revealed a pattern that provided a reasonable explanation of how endogenous (nonreactive) depression might arise, and

Major reference tables appear beginning on p. 435.

Table 24–2 | Overview of Depression Types and Preferred Treatments

Type of Depression	Special Characteristics	Preferred Treatments
Endogenous (neurochemical; lacks specific stressor; most likely caused by an imbalance or deficiency of neurotransmitters)	Decreased energy; avolition; anhedonia (inability to derive pleasure from life); diurnal variation of symptoms, usually worse in morning; lack of response to environmental changes (does not find humor in anything); vegetative signs (sleeping, eating disorders)	Best treated with tricyclic and related antidepressants; MAO inhibitors may be useful
Reactive (reaction to a loss)	Anxiety, tension, and decreased appetite; able to respond to environmental change (eg, laughs at something funny); symptoms usually self-limiting	Antidepressants usually not used because of self-limiting nature; antianxiety drugs, or hypnotics for insomnia, may be helpful but may cause dependency, hinder dealing with underlying problems, and so may be countertherapeutic
Dysthymia (neurotic, characterologic; a lifestyle depression that lacks specific stressors)	Poor interpersonal relation skills; unhappy with life (eg, job, position, family); dissatisfied with many things (eg, fault-finding, chronic complaining) but refuses to accept blame; preoccupied with loss or injustices, feels "short-changed" by life; emotionally labile, often weeps; feels demanding, irritable, angry, dependent, anxious, and hypochondriacal; able to respond to environmental changes	Psychotherapy is primary treatment; tricyclic antidepressants occasionally prescribed
Melancholia (involutional)	Usually occurs after the age of 45; characterized by more somatic symptoms, hypochondriasis, insomnia, and anorexia than other depressions; somatic or nihilistic delusions may occur; anhedonia common; lifting of depression, even momentarily, is rare	Tricyclic antidepressants, related drugs, often used; agitated form is helped most by antidepressants; electroconvulsive therapy may be very effective
Manic depression	Mood swings encompassing both depressive and manic symptoms are common; high-energy symptoms common during manic phase: flight of ideas, insomnia, hyperactivity, grandiosity, intense irritability, denial of illness, labile affect, manipulativeness, assaultive behavior	Lithium is drug of choice
Drug-induced	Characteristics depend largely on causative agent(s); may be relatively common with some antihypertensives (clonidine, methyldopa, propranolol, reserpine, and similar drugs); benzodiazepines, corticosteroids, general CNS depressants, overtranquilization with antipsychotic drugs	Identify offending drugs; discontinue if medically permissible

how some drugs alleviate its symptoms. The cause seems to involve a chemical imbalance between, or deficiency of, one or several brain neurotransmitters (biogenic amines): norepinephrine, serotonin, and perhaps dopamine. For example, reserpine depletes brain levels of these transmitters, thereby reducing the chemical message between nerves, and causes depression in some patients. In contrast, a common effect, improved mood, is produced by drugs with such diverse CNS effects as the ability to:

1. stimulate the release of neurotransmitters (amphetamines);
2. inhibit transmitter breakdown (MAO inhibitors); or
3. intensify neurotransmitter action by blocking transmitter reuptake into nerve endings (tricyclic antidepressants).

New evidence suggests that β-adrenergic receptors may also be involved in depression: chronic administration of antidepressants may reduce the sensitivity or down-regulate β_1 and α_2 receptors while upregulating α_1 receptors. This view does help explain why the mere increase in norepinephrine or serotonin levels (which occurs soon after initiating therapy) does not produce an antidepressant effect. The change in receptor sensitivity corresponds more closely with clinical improvement. At this point in our understanding, it is safe to say that there is no single view that satisfactorily explains the effectiveness of antidepressant drugs.

Selection of an Antidepressant

The drugs used to treat depression before the availability of modern agents often were no more effective than no treatment at all. Contemporary drugs, used for appropriate forms of depression, cause remission of symptoms in about 85% of treated patients.

Tricyclic antidepressants are usually selected first. Although no tricyclic appears to be more effective than the prototype, imipramine, some may produce their effects slightly faster. Their slightly different potencies usually are not clinically important. However, and importantly, they differ in their ability to cause side effects (Table 24–3). Routes of administration may also be a factor. All antidepressants are available as tablets or capsules for oral administration, which is the most common route. If an oral liquid formulation is needed, the choice is limited to nortriptyline. If parenteral administration is necessary, the choice is limited to imipramine and amitriptyline.

Laboratory tests, which are seldom performed routinely, may help guide initial selection of an antidepressant drug. The tests measure levels of the key biogenic amines or their metabolites in the urine or cerebrospinal fluid. The results may indicate whether a deficiency exists of a particular neurotransmitter, so that an antidepressant with a preferential ability to affect it might be tried first (see Table 24–3). For example, antidepressants that are chemically referred to as *secondary amines* (amoxapine, desipramine, nortriptyline, and protriptyline) primarily increase norepinephrine availability in the central nervous system (CNS). *Tertiary amines* (imipramine, amitriptyline, doxepin, and trimipramine) seem to have a greater effect on serotonin. Some of the very new drugs, exemplified by fluoxetine, appear to exert selective effects on serotonin. They are discussed at the end of the related drugs section. If a drug belonging to one subclass proves to be ineffective

Table 24–3 Pharmacologic Profiles and Half-Lives of Tricyclic Antidepressants and Related Drugs

Antidepressant	Antimuscarinic Effect	Antianxiety Effect	Sedative Effect	Serotonin Potentiation	Norepinephrine Potentiation	Half Life (hr)
Imipramine	2x	2x	2x	4x	2x	11–25
Amitryptyline	4x	5x	4x	4x	2x	31–46
Amoxapine	3x	2x	2x	2x	3x	8
Bupropion	2x	0	2x	0/1x	0/1x	8–24
Clomipramine	3x	1x	3x	5x	2x	19–37
Desipramine	1x	1x	1x	2x	4x	12–24
Doxepin	2x	3x	3x	2x	1x	8–24
Fluoxetine	1x	0	0/1x	5x	1x	7–9 d
Maprotiline	2x	3x	2x	0/1x	3x	21–25
Nortriptyline	2x	1x	2x	3x	2x	18–44
Protriptyline	3x	0	1x	2x	4x	67–89
Trazodone	1x	4x	2x	3x	0	4–9
Trimipramine	2x	3x	3x	1x	1x	7–30

Key: x = relative intensity of effect; 0 = none.

Source: Adapted from *Drug Facts & Comparisons*, 1992:262k.

after a trial period (often 1 month), a drug in another subclass might be tried instead.

I. Tricyclic Antidepressants

The tricyclic antidepressants derived their name because, chemically, the drug molecule contains three hydrocarbon rings. The prototype tricyclic is imipramine (TOFRANIL). Indeed, this drug has properties that make it the prototype for several antidepressants that are not, chemically, tricyclics.

PROTOTYPE

Imipramine

Absorption, Distribution, Metabolism, and Excretion

Imipramine and related antidepressants are absorbed well from the gastrointestinal (GI) tract. After oral administration, peak plasma concentrations occur within 3 to 4 hours. The drug is highly bound to plasma proteins (90% to 95%), and so its effects are due to a very small fraction of free drug molecules. Imipramine is metabolized in the liver to many other compounds, some of which have antidepressant properties and are, themselves, available as drugs. Most antidepressant metabolites are excreted in the urine.

Imipramine's normal plasma half-life is 24 hours. This value is prolonged, often considerably, in the elderly, younger patients with immature drug metabolizing enzyme systems, or any person with diminished liver function from such causes as drugs or diseases. Other potential alterations that prolong the half-life include decreased plasma protein levels, which increase the amount of unbound drug in the blood; and decreased total body water content, which may further elevate serum concentrations of these water-soluble drugs. These factors are common in the elderly.

Pharmacologic Effects

Imipramine and related drugs affect depressive symptoms through actions on brain neurotransmitters. They also have important peripheral actions, some of which are unrelated to their antidepressant effects and are often unwanted. Imipramine ranks high in terms of its ability to produce both desired central effects and unwanted peripheral actions (see Table 24–3).

Central Effects

Antidepressant Action

The actions of norepinephrine, serotonin, and dopamine, released from their nerves, are normally terminated by an "amine pump," which causes reuptake of the transmitter molecules into the nerve ending (Fig. 24–1A). Imipramine and related antidepressants inhibit reuptake (Fig. 24–1B), thereby increasing the amount of neurotransmitter available to stimulate postsynaptic receptors, and prolonging their stimulatory action. This has been cited as the major mechanism of tricyclic antidepressant action. However, although these antidepressants block reuptake quickly, *it usually takes 2 to 4 weeks for signs of depression relief to occur.* Furthermore, since some antidepressants seem to lack any effect on neurotransmitter reuptake, other effects may contribute to their antidepressant action.

Sedation

Antidepressant drugs cause sedation soon after administration. Sedation may be intense initially, especially with tertiary tricyclic antidepressants such as imipramine, but the intensity usually decreases with continued treatment. (Interestingly, some antidepressants, such as protriptyline, do not cause appreciable sedation and may actually cause insomnia from CNS stimulation.) Sedation is clearly not the cause of antidepressant action, since barbiturates and other sedatives with general CNS depressant actions do not alleviate depression, and may actually worsen it.

Improved Appetite

Antidepressant drugs improve appetite, perhaps as a secondary response to an overall improvement of mood.

Peripheral Effects

Tricyclic antidepressants block reuptake of norepinephrine into peripheral adrenergic (sympathetic) nerves, which makes it appear as if structures controlled by the sympathetic nervous system are being stimulated more. Cardiovascular responses, such as tachycardia, are the most obvious. The peripheral sympathomimetic actions are, without question, unwanted when these drugs are used as typical antidepressants. Therefore, they will be discussed later as side effects.

Antidepressants block peripheral muscarinic acetylcholine (ACh) receptors found on structures innervated by the parasympathetic nervous system. The effects are similar to those caused by atropine. The antimuscarinic

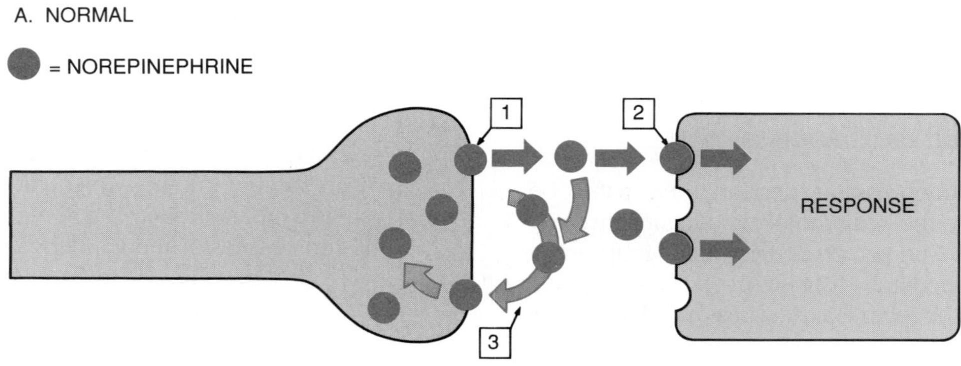

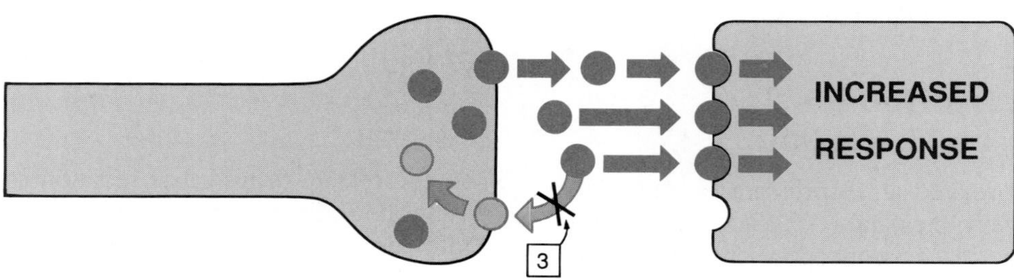

Figure 24–1

Neurotransmission in the CNS and general action of tricyclic antidepressants. Normal nerve activation (**A**) releases neurotransmitter (1), which interacts with postsnyaptic receptors (2) and then undergoes reuptake into nerve by an "amine pump" (3). Tricyclic antidepressants (**B**) block reuptake; neurotransmitter stays in the vicinity of receptors, causing greater or more prolonged stimulation of target cell. In the CNS, this corrects an apparent neurotransmitter imbalance and reduces depression symptoms. Antidepressants have different abilities to affect nerves that release norepinephrine, dopamine, or serotonin as the transmitter (see Table 24–3).

action can be used therapeutically for some nonpsychiatric indications (for example, childhood enuresis). More often, like the peripheral sympathomimetic actions, antimuscarinic actions account for frequent and disturbing side effects.

Clinical Indications and Administration

Depression

Imipramine and other related antidepressants (Table 24–C1) are used almost exclusively to treat depression, including major depression and depression associated with psychotic disorders (schizophrenia; manic-depressive illness), organic mental syndrome, and some physical illnesses. Other indications include the management of anxiety associated with alcoholism, involutional depression (melancholia), and manic-depressive disorder. Antidepressants are not indicated as preventive therapy for depression.

Depression in the Elderly

Depression and dysphoria are common in older persons. Some studies have indicated that as many as 15% of elderly people may be suffering from depression and could benefit from intervention. Furthermore, many older patients who become confused or apathetic are diagnosed as having dementia, when in fact the symptoms they are exhibiting stem from depression. In view of the respective prognoses, it is important to recognize and treat depression in the elderly.

A biologic explanation for depression among the elderly rests on the understanding that monoamine oxidase activity increases with age, thus diminishing the levels of biogenic amines. When coupled with the increase in losses sustained by an older person, it is not difficult to comprehend the extent of depression among the older age group.

Finally, depression and dementia are not mutually exclusive, and depression superimposed upon a chronic dementia can only make the care of that individual more difficult. Most patients with dementia are hospitalized because of behaviors (eg, agitation, insomnia, and apathy) that are symptoms of depression, and not for cognitive deficits. Thus, treating these individuals with antidepressants may be the key to keeping them in their homes longer.

Other Psychiatric Indications

Imipramine has been used successfully to treat phobic attacks, particularly agoraphobia (fear of being alone in large open spaces or in public). Tricyclic antidepressants may also counteract some adverse effects of amphetamine overdoses.

Nonpsychiatric Uses

Imipramine is indicated for childhood enuresis (nocturnal bedwetting). Its beneficial effects are probably due to antimuscarinic actions on the bladder. The drug loses effectiveness with long-term use for this purpose.

Unapproved Uses

Imipramine and several other antidepressants have been used to treat a variety of other disorders and symptoms, including intractable pain, peripheral neuritis and neuralgia, attention deficit disorders, and some forms of migraine headaches and sleep apnea. No dosages are recommended here for these unapproved uses.

NURSING IMPLICATIONS

Be sure to inform patients about the "lag period" between the start of therapy and the time when a clinical effect begins to appear—3 weeks or more for many of the tricyclics. This information helps prevent discouragement over apparently slow progress.

Side Effects, Adverse Reactions, and Contraindications

Central and peripheral autonomic side effects are common, particularly with imipramine. Their consequences range from disturbing, but innocuous, to dangerous (Table 24–S1; see also Table 24–3).

Peripheral Autonomic Side Effects

Antimuscarinic (atropine-like) side effects may be prominent and pose major limitations to therapy with imipramine and related drugs. The common side effects include dry mouth, blurred vision, diminished lacrimation, and photophobia owing to mydriasis. Other less common but expected antimuscarinic side effects may occur: decreased gut and bladder function, tachycardia, and diminished heat loss via perspiration. The related contraindications and precautions for atropine (Chapter 13, Table 13–S) apply to a tricyclic antidepressant. As noted later, they are particularly important for the elderly.

Cardiovascular responses are serious hazards of therapeutic antidepressant doses. Orthostatic hypotension is common. Tachycardia is also common and potentially severe because several drug-induced effects contribute to it: a reflex increase of heart rate triggered by hypotension; atropine-like effects on the sinoatrial node, which unmasks sympathetic influences; and prolonged and excessive direct cardiac stimulation by blockade of norepinephrine reuptake into the heart's sympathetic nerve supply. Tachycardia plus reduced blood pressure may cause, prolong, or intensify attacks of angina pectoris, and may cause myocardial infarction. Other adverse responses are arrhythmias (conduction defects, heart block), congestive heart failure resulting from prolonged and excessive cardiac stimulation, and stroke. Hyperthyroidism or therapy with thyroid hormones increases the risk of arrhythmias. Imipramine and most other antidepressants should therefore be used with caution in patients with a history of any cardiovascular disorder. They are contraindicated during the acute recovery phase following myocardial infarction.

NURSING IMPLICATIONS

Educate patients to expect the many peripheral autonomic side effects, and help them discriminate between those that are simply annoying, such as dry mouth, and those that are potentially dangerous, such as ocular pain of glaucoma owing to mydriasis. Use and recommend nondrug interventions to alleviate side effects whenever possible. Virtually every nursing measure that applies to persons taking atropine should be used for patients taking tricyclic antidepressants. Nursing implications for the most common side effects are reviewed in Table 24–S1.

Central Nervous System Side Effects

Sedation is very common. It is most intense during early therapy, and tends to decrease after about three weeks of treatment. Sedation can be beneficial for patients with depression complicated by insomnia or anxiety. For any patient, however, sedation can pose dangers from common daily activities such as driving or operating hazardous machinery.

Anxiety, insomnia, nightmares, ataxia, tremors, and seizures may occur. Nightmares are particularly troublesome, and some patients who have longed for sleep dread it because of them. Antidepressants lower the seizure threshold, so patients with a history of seizure disorders, or persons receiving electroconvulsive therapy (ECT), are at increased risk. Imipramine bears some structural resemblance to chlorpromazine and related phenothiazines, and has occasionally caused extrapyramidal reactions that are typical with antipsychotic drug therapy. Imipramine may exacerbate psychotic symptoms in persons with schizophrenia and manic-depressive disorder. Confusion, disorientation, delusions, agitation, and hallucinations are related symptoms found in antidepressant-induced delirium. These usually occur when serum antidepressant levels are elevated, but may occur at therapeutic levels.

Suicidal tendencies are relatively common in depressed persons. Tricyclics and other antidepressants increase the patient's energy for committing suicide, often by antidepressant or multiple-drug overdoses. Antidepressants may be prescribed for these individuals, but added precautions must be taken.

NURSING IMPLICATIONS

Caution patients about the dangers of driving or operating hazardous machinery. Be aware of factors that increase the risk of antidepressant-induced delirium: high serum antidepressant levels, organic mental disorder (OMD), and concomitant antipsychotic drug administration. If a patient experiences antidepressant-induced delirium, discontinue the drug by gradually reducing the dosage over several days. Careful monitoring is essential during this time. Observe for signs of acute psychosis in depressed psychotic patients who receive imipramine, and for the development of mania in persons with manic-depressive disorder. Important supportive measures include reassuring the patient that symptoms will decrease when the offending medication is withdrawn. Monitor patients with a history of seizure disorders closely.

It is essential to take precautions against suicide. The history should include information about prior suicide attempts and substance abuse, which might increase the risk of accidental overdose. Check to be sure that outpatient prescriptions are for a limited number of doses and refills, which may further lower the risk of intentional overdose. Drug hoarding and self-administered overdoses occur in the hospital, so it is important to ensure that the patient has swallowed the medication. Frequent informal patient interviews, the use of rating scales for suicidal tendencies, and assessment of the frequency with which prescriptions are refilled, may also help. Forthright questions, such as asking whether the patient is thinking about self-harm, will not increase the risk of suicide. Family members should be asked to report any evidence of potential suicidal tendencies in the patient.

Advise patients and family members that antidepressants are not addicting.

Other Side Effects

Bone marrow depression, leading to thrombocytopenia or eosinophilia, may occur. Fatal agranulocytosis is rare. Gastrointestinal disturbances include nausea, vomiting, and diarrhea; altered liver function, sometimes with jaundice; parotid gland swelling; black tongue; and weight gain or weight loss due to increased appetite or drug-induced anorexia, respectively. Endocrine side effects include testicular swelling and impotence in males; galactorrhea in females; and, in either sex, gynecomastia and increases or decreases of libido. Allergic reactions include skin rashes, petechiae, and urticaria.

NURSING IMPLICATIONS

Be alert for signs of hepatic reactions, including jaundice, rashes, nausea, anorexia, and abdominal pain. Abnormal bruising or bleeding, fever, sore throat, malaise, or other flu-like symptoms may reflect blood dyscrasias. Complete blood counts should be obtained before antidepressant therapy is begun and periodically thereafter. If there is any indication of a potentially serious adverse reaction, the drug should be withheld temporarily, the physician notified at once, and a complete physical examination performed.

Other General Contraindications and Precautions

In addition to specific contraindications related to key autonomic or central effects, there are other general contraindications for imipramine and related antidepressants.

- The presence of severe renal or hepatic impairment, which may elevate antidepressant blood levels.
- Concomitant use of monoamine oxidase (MAO) inhibitors (see below).
- The presence of known allergy to antidepressants or their ingredients.

Be aware that oral doxepin (ADAPIN only; not SINEQUAN), desipramine, and imipramine contain tartrazine dye (FD&C Yellow No. 5), which has triggered adverse reactions ranging from hives to bronchoconstriction, hypotension, and full anaphylactoid responses in persons who are allergic to it. Assess for this allergy when completing the history.

Antidepressants may be given, but extra caution is indicated, for patients who consume alcohol, which may cause excessive CNS depression; will be undergoing elective surgery, which usually requires gradual reduction of antidepressant doses several days preoperatively; and will be undergoing ECT, which increases the risk of seizures.

Use During Pregnancy and Lactation

Tricyclic antidepressants and related drugs cross the placental barrier and are excreted in breast milk. The safe use of these drugs during pregnancy or lactation has not been established, so they should be used only if the potential benefit to the mother is likely to outweigh the risks to the fetus or infant.

Use in Children

Imipramine is used in children mainly for treating nighttime enuresis. Common adverse reactions include nervousness, sleep disorders, tiredness, and mild GI disturbances. Children are reported to be more sensitive than adults to acute overdoses of this drug. Therefore, imipramine should be used only in children over 6 years of age, and only as a temporary adjunctive measure. Imipramine pamoate (TOFRANIL-PM) should never be given to children because of the potential for overdose: the smallest available unit dose of this drug is 75 mg, which is too much for a child.

Use in the Elderly

Drug doses for the elderly should be small initially, and increased slowly while the patient is monitored for desired and untoward responses. Use of a single bedtime dose may help alleviate daytime side effects, but may cause problems if the patient gets up during the night. The risk of all adverse effects involving the central and peripheral autonomic nervous systems are significantly greater in the elderly. Major factors contributing to this include the pharmacokinetic factors noted above (diminished hepatic function; reduced plasma protein levels and body water content); the prevalence of contraindicating or complicating physical and mental disorders, and drugs used to treat them; and a diminished physiologic ability to adapt to or compensate for drug-induced effects such as hypotension, tachycardia, and altered bowel and bladder function. If there are extra concerns about cardiovascular side effects, the related drug doxepin (SINEQUAN) may be preferred because it has the lowest incidence of related side effects. Ideally, all elderly patients should be screened for glaucoma before starting antidepressant therapy. Nortriptyline, yet another antidepressant, seems to be the best overall antidepressant for use in the elderly.

Interactions with Other Drugs

Imipramine and all the tricyclic (or tricyclic-like) antidepressants interact with a variety of other drugs (Table 24–11). The most common important interactions involve simultaneous use of other drugs that also cause CNS depression or antimuscarinic effects. The usual outcome is additive or greater intensification of these side effects, usually to an unwanted degree; outright toxicity may occur.

Two other interactants include MAO inhibitors and guanethidine. The interaction with MAO inhibitors, which are also used as antidepressants (see below), can cause an intense antimuscarinic poison syndrome (fever, seizures) plus a potentially fatal hypertensive episode. It must be avoided by not administering these two classes of antidepressants within 2 weeks of one another. The interaction with guanethidine (Chapter 33), an antihypertensive drug, involves antagonism of the antihypertensive drug's actions, leading to poor blood pressure control. It occurs because the antidepressants block the uptake of guanethidine into adrenergic nerve endings, the drug's site of action. (This is similar to the way in which antidepressants block reuptake of norepinephrine into these nerves.) The interaction should be avoided. Fortunately, MAO inhibitors and guanethidine are seldom used anymore, but since both are still on the market the possibility of encountering patients who are at risk is real.

NURSING IMPLICATIONS

The more common interactants with imipramine and its related agents are not only prescribed agents but also nonprescription drugs, including alcohol and antihistamines (eg, diphenhydramine; Chapter 51). Therefore, a thorough review of over-the-counter (OTC) medication use, and proper patient education to avoid use of interacting OTC agents, is important.

Overdose and Toxicity

Antidepressants are frequently used in suicide attempts by patients whom they are meant to help. The margin between therapeutic and lethal doses is small; only 10 to 30 times the daily dose can be fatal, and even less may be required if interacting drugs are ingested simultaneously. The incidence and severity of adverse responses are not necessarily related to plasma levels of the offending drug. A given drug level is likely to cause more serious responses in very young, old, or debilitated persons, or in persons taking other medications that cause additive CNS-depressant or antimuscarinic effects. Likewise, blood levels do not necessarily predict the onset of symptoms, or how quickly they may progress. Any overdose should be considered as potentially fatal.

Signs and Symptoms

Both peripheral and central effects occur with tricyclic antidepressant overdoses. Many signs and symptoms are like those caused by overdoses of sedative-antimuscarinic drugs, such as scopolamine. Peripheral symptoms include tachycardia, severe hypotension (and possible shock), mydriasis, and either diaphoresis or inhibited sweating. The cardiovascular changes can occur suddenly and cause acute heart failure or arrhythmias. Diarrhea may occur early after ingestion of acute overdoses, but when overdoses are taken chronically or initial diarrhea has subsided, constipation develops. Urinary retention is common. Centrally mediated changes such as muscle rigidity, hyperactive reflexes, and choreiform movements are likely. Other central effects range from sedation, ataxia, and agitation to stupor, coma, respiratory depression, and seizures (especially with the related drugs amoxapine and maprotiline).

Treatment

All patients, even those with only suspected antidepressant overdoses, should be admitted to the hospital for monitoring and anticipated treatment. If the overdose is recent and the patient is alert, induced vomiting and gastric lavage with activated charcoal should be used to prevent further drug absorption. Blood pressure, heart rate and rhythm, and respiration must be monitored closely. A patent airway and adequate gas exchange must be maintained. All patients should receive an initial electrocardiogram (ECG). If any abnormalities are detected, continuous monitoring for at least 72 hours is necessary. Relapses, particularly involving cardiac arrhythmias, have occurred after apparent "recovery" from overdoses. Digitalis, administered to counteract heart failure, may cause or worsen conduction defects and arrhythmias.

Stimulant drugs should never be administered to counteract sedation. Seizures are controlled best with intravenous (IV) diazepam. High fever can be alleviated by frequent use of sponge baths. One adjunct for severe antidepressant poisoning is physostigmine (ANTILIRIUM), the acetylcholinesterase inhibitor that is also the antidote for poisoning with atropine and most other antimuscarinic drugs (see Table 12-C, p 164 for dosages). Its effectiveness in antidepressant overdoses supports the idea that antimuscarinic problems are important. Physostigmine's duration of action is much shorter than that of most antidepressants, so repeated doses will usually be needed.

NURSING IMPLICATIONS

Implementing precautions to detect and guard against suicide attempts, as noted above, are very important. Since children are more sensitive to overdoses than adults, precautions should be taken to prevent accidental (and suicidal) overdoses and to detect them early. Adult patients should be advised to keep their antidepressant medication out of reach of children. Other precautionary and educational measures are necessary for both the patient and the family. The nurse's proximity to the patient offers a good opportunity to provide this information.

Related Drugs

Imipramine hydrochloride, the prototype, is widely used. Other drugs with similar structures have similar actions, and they participate in the same drug–drug interactions. Side effects are the same, but the intensities vary from drug to drug (see Table 24–3). Some of the drugs described below do not have imipramine's tricyclic structure. However, their most important pharmacologic properties are so similar to those of the prototype that they are presented here as related drugs.

Regardless of the drug that is selected, reduced doses are indicated for elderly patients and are recommended for outpatients who cannot be supervised and assessed frequently. The dosages of related drugs are summarized in Table 24–C1.

Amitriptyline

Amitriptyline (ELAVIL, ENDEP) is a popular tricyclic. Compared with most other antidepressants, amitriptyline causes more antimuscarinic side effects. It is the most sedating anti-depressant. The sedative effects are particularly suited for patients with agitated involutional depression; however, the same action makes amitriptyline less than ideal for the elderly. If amitriptyline is selected, in addition to using low initial doses it may be advisable to give the entire dose, or a major fraction of it, at bedtime to minimize daytime sedation. Amitriptyline is also available in a parenteral formulation, and as an oral, fixed-dose combination with perphenazine, an antipsychotic drug (marketed as TRIAVIL and ETRAFON).

Amoxapine

Amoxapine (ASENDIN) is not, chemically, a tricyclic compound. It is classified as a dibenzoxazepine, a metabolite of the antipsychotic drug loxapine. Because of its similarity to antipsychotics, amoxapine may cause extrapyramidal side effects. Its antimuscarinic and sedative effects are similar in severity and incidence to those caused by imipramine. Amoxapine has a more rapid onset of action than the tricyclics (4 to 7 days vs. 3 weeks or more), and it may cause fewer cardiovascular side effects. It is not recommended for children under 16 years of age.

Bupropion

Bupropion (WELLBUTRIN) is chemically unrelated to the other antidepressants. The drug's mechanism of action is not known for certain; however, it does not inhibit reuptake of norepinephrine or serotonin, as do the tricyclics; nor does it inhibit MAO, as do the drugs discussed on page 423. Nevertheless, bupropion is effective. Although most side effects of this drug are generally similar to those caused by imipramine, the incidence of seizures during bupropion therapy may be as much as four times higher than the incidence when more traditional agents are used; monitor accordingly. The risk of seizures appears to be dose-dependent, and can be minimized by not exceeding a total daily dose of 450 mg; dividing the dosage over the day, giving no more than 150 mg at one time; and making dosage increases gradual. Otherwise, this drug has a very high margin of safety, a valuable property if overdoses occur.

Clomipramine

Clomipramine, marketed as ANAFRANIL, is relatively new to the American market. It is chemically similar to imipramine, but it is used exclusively for treating obsessive-compulsive disorder (OCD), a complex and disabling ritualistic behavior syndrome that affects an estimated one (or more) out of 100 persons in our society. Clomipramine is the only tricyclic with this indication. An estimated 70% of patients with OCD who are treated with this drug experience some symptom relief. The drug's true mechanism of action is not known. However, it is thought that its ability to block serotonin reuptake somehow weakens obsessive thoughts and enhances the patient's will to resist ritualistic behaviors. General side effects, drug interactions, and related precautions noted for imipramine apply also to clomipramine.

Desipramine

Desipramine (NORPRAMIN, PERTOFRANE) is a naturally occurring metabolite of imipramine. Compared with imipramine it causes a lower incidence of antimuscarinic, cardiovascular, and sedative side effects. Some authorities claim that it is the preferred antidepressant for elderly patients. Desipramine has become the most widely prescribed antidepressant for adults. It is not recommended for children. Oral desipramine contains tartrazine dye (FD&C Yellow No. 5).

Doxepin

Doxepin (ADAPIN, SINEQUAN) causes more sedation than most antidepressants. Overall the drug causes a low incidence of cardiovascular problems and is preferred for patients with a cardiac history. Doxepin relieves anxiety soon after therapy is started, but the onset of true antidepressant actions takes several weeks to develop. Doxepin is not recommended for children under age 12. ADAPIN contains tartrazine dye.

Imipramine Pamoate

Imipramine pamoate (TOFRANIL-PM) is equivalent to imipramine hydrochloride on a milligram-for-milligram basis. It is used for depression, like the hydrochloride, but it is given as a single bedtime dose. Imipramine pamoate should not be given to children because the minimum unit dose available, 75 mg, is too high for children.

Maprotiline

Maprotiline (LUDIOMIL) is a *tetracyclic* antidepressant. Despite its different chemical structure, it is similar in many ways to the tricyclics. It causes about the same incidence and severity of antimuscarinic side effects and sedation as imipramine. Therapeutic effects can be seen in 3 to 7 days. Maprotiline has been associated with seizures at therapeutic doses. It is not recommended for patients less than 18 years old.

Nortriptyline

Nortriptyline (AVENTYL, PAMELOR) is a metabolite of amitriptyline. Next to desipramine, it causes the fewest sedative and antimuscarinic side effects, and is least likely to cause hypotension. These properties make it useful and perhaps the best tolerated antidepressant for elderly patients. Nortriptyline is not recommended for children.

Protriptyline

Protriptyline (VIVACTIL), a tricyclic, is noteworthy because it lacks sedative or anxiolytic properties. In fact, it has activating properties that make it especially suitable for withdrawn or anergic patients or patients who sleep too much. The onset of antidepressant activity may occur in as little as 1 week. Therapy should be started, or initial increased doses given, in the morning. This reduces the risk of insomnia. The safety and effectiveness of protriptyline for children has not been established.

Trazodone

Trazodone (DESYREL) differs chemically from other antidepressants. Its use is increasing because of its virtual lack of atropine-like side effects and a low incidence of orthostatic hypotension. Some studies have also shown that trazodone produces few adverse cardiac effects, but there is no agreement on this point. Trazodone increases intraocular pressure less than most related antidepressants, but persons at risk of glaucoma still require periodic ophthalmic assessment. Trazodone should be taken soon after the patient ingests a light meal, which increases drug absorption by about 20%. Taking the drug on an empty stomach or under fasting conditions reduces absorption and increases the risk of dizziness or lightheadedness.

A unique adverse response to trazodone is priapism. Men taking this drug should be instructed emphatically to report prolonged or inappropriate penile erection at once; drug discontinuation will be necessary. About one in three patients with trazodone-induced priapism has required surgical intervention, and in several permanent impairment of erectile function caused impotence.

Trimipramine

Trimipramine (SURMONTIL) is similar to imipramine. It is very sedating and causes moderate anticholinergic side effects. It is not recommended for use in children.

Selective Serotonin Reuptake Inhibitors

Fluoxetine and Sertraline

Fluoxetine (PROZAC), and sertraline (ZOLOFT) differ from imipramine and all the other related drugs because of their unique mechanism of action. They are selective serotonin reuptake inhibitors (SSRIs), having little significant effect on dopamine- or norepinephrine-containing nerves. Overall, the SSRIs are being studied extensively in the hope that they will prove to be more effective than the other antidepressants. Their selective actions on serotonin may also provide new clues about the biochemical basis of such disorders as depression.

These drugs have relatively long half-lives, owing in part to the formation of active metabolites. For example, fluoxetine itself has a half-life of about 72 hours, but some of its metabolites have a half-life of around 1 week. The half life of sertraline is about 26 hours. These pharmacokinetic properties allow once-daily dosing, but stable blood levels and clinical effects will appear slowly, and dose-related side effects tend to be longlasting even when the dose is decreased or the drug is discontinued altogether.

Based on current information, these drugs may be no better than imipramine or the other agents discussed in the related drugs section when used to begin depression therapy for the typical patient. However, they may prove to be more effective for patients who are refractory to imipramine and imipramine-like agents, or who cannot tolerate the tricyclics for one reason or another.

Fluoxetine is both approved and in clinical use as this is being written. It tends to cause fewer and milder autonomic and CNS depressant side effects than imipramine and most of the other antidepressants discussed in the related drugs section. Its major side effects are anxiety, insomnia, and skin rash (about a 15% incidence for the latter). It is an expensive drug costing about $1.50 per tablet. Fluoxetine allegedly has a greater incidence of adverse behavioral reactions directed toward one's self (including suicide attempts) and others (aggressive, combative, or homicidal tendencies). This is discussed further in the nursing implications section below.

Sertraline is the newest SSRI to be approved for managing depression. Other anticipated uses will probably include management of OCD and, perhaps, panic disorders. Sertraline has a side effect profile similar to fluoxetine however it may have an advantage due to a reduced half-life and cost. A new SSRI, fluvoxamine (FLOXYFRAL), is similar to both fluoxetine and sertraline, but is not currently approved for treating depression.

NURSING IMPLICATIONS

Fluoxetine has received more attention in the lay press than most other drugs. When it was introduced to the U.S. market in the early 1990s it was heralded as a major breakthrough because of its ability to relieve symptoms when other drugs could not. Other attributes made the drug attractive to the medical community: its novel mechanism of action (as an SSRI), its convenient once-daily dosing schedule, and its relatively good overall side-effects profile. Once fluoxetine gained widespread use, however, there was a growing number of reports of suicides and homicides attributed (rightly or wrongly) to the drug. Over 50 law suits related to these adverse effects have been filed against the drug's manufacturer. (As noted above, suicidal thoughts and behaviors can be brought on by any antidepressant.)

There is not enough data to make a fair judgment about fluoxetine's risks, nor to say whether similar problems are likely to be caused by sertraline or other SSRIs that might be marketed. Nevertheless, it is important for the nurse to assess for suicidal, aggressive, or psychotic behaviors in patients taking these drugs—just as it is important to do so when other antidepressants are used. Monitor for these behavioral changes, but do not overlook assessment for any of the potential CNS or peripheral side effects that were noted for the prototype, imipramine. With proper monitoring, these drugs should be considered both effective and safe for use.

II. Monoamine Oxidase Inhibitors

Monoamine oxidase inhibitors are the second major class of antidepressants. The available agents are isocarboxazid (MARPLAN), phenelzine (NARDIL), and tranylcypromine (PARNATE). There is no prototype, and so in most cases they will be discussed as a group.

The history of these drugs is interesting. They were originally used to manage tuberculosis. Patients who received them often experienced two side effects: CNS stimulation and mood elevation, and hypotension. This led to further study, and actual clinical use, for managing depression and hypertension.

The MAO inhibitors are no longer used to treat high blood pressure, and they now have limited use as antidepressants. That is not because these drugs are ineffective; they are very effective in these regards. Rather, it is because in comparison with virtually any alternative drug they cause more intense side effects and can participate in potentially fatal interactions with drugs and some common foods. Although MAO inhibitors are not used widely, and they are certainly not first-line antidepressant drugs, there are patients who receive these medications and are at risk of serious unwanted responses if therapy is not managed and assessed properly. What follows is a brief overview that relates the actions of these drugs to the desired and unwanted effects they cause.

Absorption, Distribution, Metabolism, and Excretion

The MAO inhibitors are given orally. They are absorbed well from the GI tract and metabolized in the liver. The metabolites are excreted in the urine.

Pharmacologic Effects

Monoamine oxidase is important in the CNS and elsewhere in the body. It is a major enzyme responsible for metabolically inactivating norepinephrine, dopamine, and serotonin—all of which are neurotransmitters that are, chemically, monoamines.

There are actually two forms or subtypes of the enzyme. One is called MAO-B because it is located in parts of the brain. The other, MAO-A, is found elsewhere—especially in the GI tract and liver, and in peripheral adrenergic nerves. Isocarboxazid, phenelzine, and tranylcypromine inhibit both MAO-A and MAO-B. (As you will see in Chapter 25, newer drugs that selectively inhibit MAO-B are becoming available and have advantages over the drugs discussed here because of their primary CNS action.)

Central Nervous System Effects

As noted earlier in the chapter, depression symptoms are thought to be due to a deficiency of norepinephrine, dopamine, and serotonin in parts of the brain. By inhibiting the enzyme that normally breaks down these neurotransmitters, MAO inhibitors seem to increase (or restore) the amount of chemical mediators in the nerve ending. When the nerve is depolarized, the neurotransmitter is released. Overall, then, in the brain the MAO inhibitors appear to normalize the neurotransmitter deficiency, and in doing so they tend to normalize depressed behavior.

Peripheral Sympathetic Nervous System Effects

Up to a point, MAO inhibitors cause the same effects in peripheral adrenergic (postganglionic sympathetic) nerves as they do in the brain: they tend to build up norepinephrine levels in the nerve ending by inhibiting norepinephrine breakdown. However, the MAO inhibitors also tend to "uncouple" the signal between nerve depolarization and the normal result of it, norepinephrine release. That is, it appears as if these nerves have an extra supply of norepinephrine, but the amount that gets released is much less than normal.

The overall effect appears as if sympathetic control of all the peripheral structures is reduced. The most obvious effect is reduced vasoconstriction, which in turn reduces blood pressure. It is the major reason why MAO inhibitors were used to treat high blood pressure, and it is also a major side effect when they are used to treat depression.

Gastrointestinal Effects

Monoamine oxidase is an important enzyme in the GI tract. It is there to metabolically inactivate a variety of drugs and chemicals that have a suitable chemical structure. Monoamine oxidase inhibitors, therefore, inhibit the breakdown of these substances. The enzyme is also abundant in the wall of the intestines. There it partially metabolizes some orally administered drugs and chemicals as they are being absorbed into the bloodstream. When MAO is inhibited, greater amounts of these substances escape inactivation in the gut, and they can cause increased effects once they reach the bloodstream. As will be noted soon, the combined effects of MAO inhibitors at sympathetic nerve endings and in the gut account for some of the key and very serious drug interactions.

Clinical Indications and Administration

Except in rare instances, MAO inhibitors are used only to treat refractory depression—depression symptoms that have not responded to usually effective doses of tricyclics (or other somewhat related antidepressants), psychotherapy, electroconvulsive therapy (ECT), or combinations of these preferred approaches (Table 24–C2).

There is some evidence, or at least some impression, that these drugs may be more effective than the alternatives for certain types of depression, such as atypical depressions accompanied by significant symptoms of hypersomnia, excessive anxiety, or chronic anxiety. However, that is controversial, and further discussion is beyond the scope of this book. In addition, some psychiatrists feel that MAO inhibitors are underprescribed because of undue or excessive fears about their side effects and drug interactions.

There also appears to be some differences between the three MAO inhibitors in their time-course and intensity of effects and side effects. For example, isocarboxazid appears to be the least effective, overall, and its antidepressant effects usually take about a month to appear. Phenelzine, which also has a slow onset of action, appears to be the most effective overall. Tranylcypromine has an earlier onset of action (about 10 days), and appears to be most effective for severe reactive or endogenous depression. However, it also tends to cause significant CNS stimulation.

NURSING IMPLICATIONS

Regardless of possible differences between the MAO inhibitors, the nurse should be aware that:

- The MAO inhibitors discussed above are not first-line agents for treating depression.
- They should be prescribed only by physicians (psychiatrists) who are thoroughly familiar with the potential risks associated with these agents.
- Owing to the risks, therapy should be started in a hospital so that facilities to assess for and treat adverse responses are available.
- Patients who cannot be trusted to understand the potential risks and dangers of these drugs, and to avoid common causes of problems, usually are not good candidates for these drugs. Thus, thorough and adequate patient teaching becomes critically important.
- And, as with tricyclics, patients and their families should be aware that it may take several weeks before symptom improvement appears.

Side Effects, Adverse Reactions, and Contraindications

Table 24–S2 summarizes the key side effects and related contraindications of these drugs. Those that usually are most important and common involve the central nervous and cardiovascular systems.

Central Nervous System Side Effects

Signs of CNS depression (eg, drowsiness) can occur, but more often than not the side effects reflect CNS stimulation in one form or another. The manifestations range from anxiety or insomnia to acute schizophrenic reactions. Mild symptoms of mania (hypomania) are the most common psychiatric side effects. The related contraindication is schizophrenia, which may not always be diagnosed before MAO inhibitor therapy is started. The MAO inhibitors also lower the seizure threshold, and so are contraindicated for persons with a history of seizure disorders.

Cardiovascular Side Effects

The decreased ability of peripheral sympathetic nerves to release their stores of norepinephrine leads to what looks like a "down-regulation" of the sympathetic nervous system. Cardiovascular side effects are the most important: hypotension (especially orthostatic) and decreases of heart rate and contractility. If they occur and become severe or intolerable, MAO therapy may need to be stopped, at least temporarily. The key related contraindications are preexisting hypotension or cardiac depression; and disorders that can be made worse by these problems, such as a history of ischemic heart or brain disease (eg, a history of myocardial infarction or stroke).

Other Side Effects

Many side effects are similar to those caused by tricyclic antidepressants. They include antimuscarinic side effects (dry mouth, blurred vision, and constipation), alterations of blood glucose levels, skin rashes, and blood dyscrasias. Hepatotoxicity is a potential adverse response. Hepatic dysfunction, or evidence of it (eg, jaundice) contraindicates MAO inhibitor use.

NURSING IMPLICATIONS

Nursing measures described for imipramine's side effects apply to the same side effects caused by MAO inhibitors. Monitor frequently and closely, as unwanted reactions can occur and may appear before the desired antidepressant effects develop. Be aware that owing to the long duration of effects, side effects may be longlasting, even when the dose is lowered or MAO inhibitor therapy is stopped altogether. Also be aware that abrupt discontinuation of MAO inhibitor therapy, regardless of the reason, can cause severe agitation, hallucinations, or worsening of depression symptoms.

◆ Use During Pregnancy and Lactation

The MAO inhibitors should be used during pregnancy and lactation only when the potential therapeutic benefits to the mother outweigh the risks to the fetus or child.

◆ Use in Children

Persons less than 16 years old should not receive MAO inhibitors.

◆ Use in the Elderly

The prevalence of cardiovascular disease greatly increases the risk of MAO inhibitor therapy in the elderly. The most serious dangers are excessive hypotension as an extension of the expected drug response, and severe hypertension through drug or food interactions. Tranylcypromine causes side effects that usually are so severe that the drug cannot be tolerated by the elderly. It is contraindicated for patients over 60 years old.

Interactions with Other Drugs

It should be obvious that MAO inhibitors cannot be used properly without the patient meeting certain criteria and the health-care team being able to provide proper monitoring and teaching. Almost completely, these concerns (and the reluctance of many physicians to use these drugs at all) relate to the adverse consequences of drug–drug interactions. Interactions involving MAO inhibitors are, in some important ways, different from interactions between other classes of drugs (even other classes of antidepressants). Those involving MAO inhibitors

- often are very serious or even life-threatening;
- do not require large doses of interacting substances to cause a serious response to occur;
- involve a host of drugs, including many OTC medications;
- can be triggered by the drugs most likely to be given to depressed patients before they are switched to an MAO inhibitor;
- can be caused simply by eating the wrong food or drinking the wrong beverage;
- usually are "must avoid," rather than "avoid if possible," interactions.

Table 24–12 lists the major interacting drugs and drug classes, the consequences of their interactions with MAO inhibitors, and related nursing implications. The most important interactions involve sympathomimetics.

Interactions Involving Sympathomimetics

Certain classes of sympathomimetic drugs interact with MAO inhibitors to cause an acute, severe, and sometimes fatal hypertensive crisis. These are the mixed-acting sympathomimetics, which act in part by releasing norepinephrine from adrenergic nerve endings; and the indirect-acting sympathomimetics, which act totally through norepinephrine release (see Chapter 14). Mixed-acting sympathomimetics include pseudoephedrine and phenylpropanolamine, which are common ingredients in OTC decongestants and weight-loss remedies. High doses of dopamine, which is used as a cardiac stimulant, and levodopa, an antiparkinson drug that is metabolized to dopamine, also release norepinephrine and interact with MAO inhibitors. Amphetamine is an example of an indirect-acting sympathomimetic drug. Another example is tyramine, which is not a typical drug but a substance found in a variety of foods and beverages (Table 24–4).

How the interaction occurs is pictured in Figure 24–2, and summarized here. Recall that MAO inhibitors act in peripheral adrenergic nerve endings to cause a build-up of norepinephrine. The MAO inhibitors also prevent norepinephrine release in response to *normal* nerve activity. However, they *do not* prevent the mixed- and indirect-acting sympathomimetics from causing release. Thus, when the sympathomimetic is administered it can, and will, release this extra supply of norepinephrine. An intense response occurs.

The MAO inhibitors increase the likelihood of the interaction in another way. For example, the tyramine normally ingested in food or drink rarely causes any sympathomimetic effects because the nutrient is metabolically inactivated by MAO in the gut; very little reaches the circulation. However, when MAO is inhibited tyramine is not metabolized, and it can reach pharmacologically effective levels in the bloodstream. Thus, tyramine is better able to cause its sympathomimetic effects, and they are intensified further by the presence of more norepinephrine in the nerve endings.

If an interaction of this type occurs, the goal is to quickly but safely lower blood pressure. This is often done by administering the emergency vasodilator drug nitroprusside (Chapter 33). Other approaches include giving the α-adrenergic blocker phentolamine (REGITINE), which specifically counteracts the excessive vasoconstriction caused by norepinephrine; or chlorpromazine, which also has α-blocking activity. Regardless, providing symptomatic, supportive care based on frequent assessment of vital signs is essential.

Table 24–4 | Tyramine-Rich Foods and Beverages

Dairy products
- Cheese; aged and strong varieties
- Sour cream
- Yogurt

Fruits and vegetables
- Avocados
- Bananas
- Fava beans
- Canned figs
- Raisins

Meats
- Liver
- Pickled herring
- Salami
- Sausage
- Tenderized meat

Alcoholic beverages
- Beer
- Chianti and sherry wine

Other foods, beverages
- Caffeine (coffees, colas, teas)
- Chocolate
- Licorice
- Soy sauce
- Yeast

Other Interactions

Several other drugs, noted in Table 24–12, interact. The interaction usually involves the ability of an MAO inhibitor to (1) inhibit the metabolism of the interactant; (2) cause similar and therefore additive effects; or (3) interact through both of these mechanisms.

The very serious interaction with imipramine and related antidepressants was mentioned above. Additional interactants are insulin and oral antidiabetic drugs (excessive hypoglycemia); other drugs with antimuscarinic activity (excessive atropine-like side effects or a true antimuscarinic syndrome); antihypertensive drugs (excessive hypotension and its consequences); and other CNS depressants (excessive CNS depression). Being CNS depressants, narcotics can interact with MAO inhibitors. However, most narcotics can be administered to persons taking MAO inhibitors (morphine is preferred) provided narcotic doses are kept low and the patient's responses are monitored adequately. One exception is

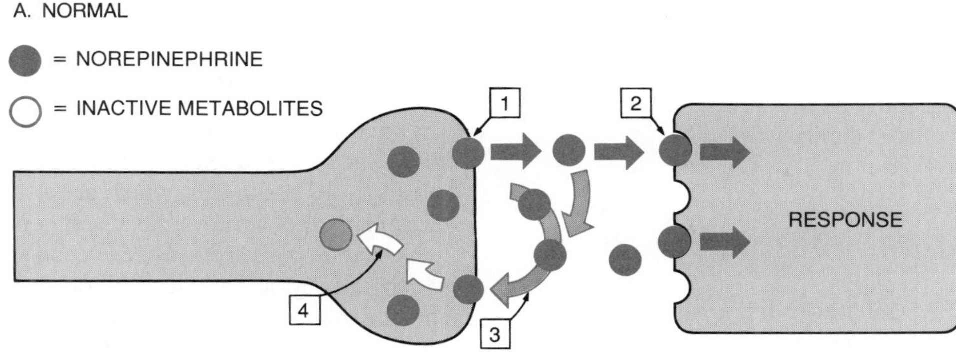

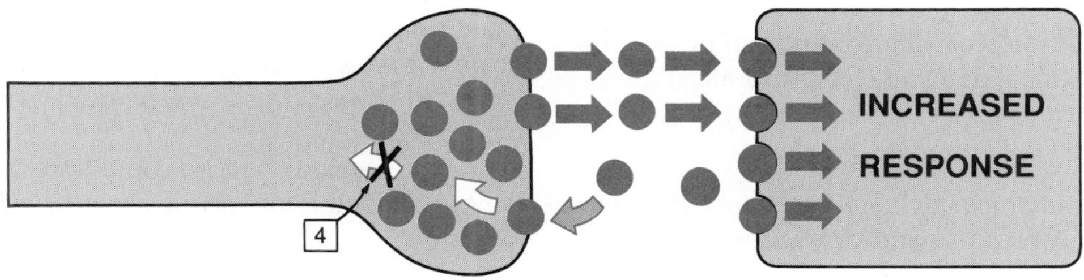

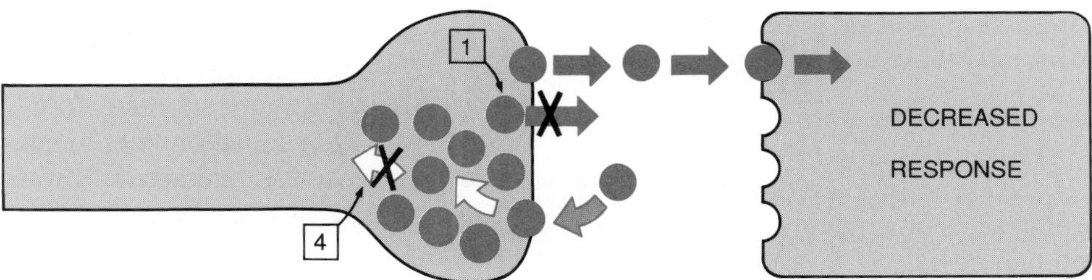

Figure 24–2

Central and peripheral actions of MAO inhibitors. Steps 1, 2, and 3 show same processes as described in Figure 24–1: norepinephrine release, activation of target cell, and reuptake. Step 4 represents metabolic inactivation of norepinephrine by MAO.

A. Normal nerve.

B. MAO effects in the CNS. Less neurotransmitter is metabolized, and neurotransmitter levels rise; this increased amount is released upon nerve stimulation, causing heightened effect that is thought to reduce depression symptoms.

C. Effects in peripheral adrenergic nerves. MAO inhibitors increase neuronal norepinephrine levels as in the CNS, but also block norepinephrine release upon normal nerve stimulation. This contributes to such side effects as vasodilation (reduced blood pressure). Mixed- and indirect-acting sympathomimetics are dangerous interactants because they can abruptly release this extra neurotransmitter, causing intense and potentially fatal responses (eg, hypertensive crisis).

meperidine (DEMEROL); it can cause a rapidly appearing, serious toxic syndrome characterized by profound CNS depression or coma; seizures; respiratory depression; and hypertension. The meperidine-like drug propoxyphene may interact similarly.

NURSING IMPLICATIONS

Remember that MAO inhibitors and many of their interacting drugs have long plasma half-lives, so a serious and quickly appearing response may occur even if therapy with one of these drugs has been discontinued for a couple of days. Space the administration of interactants by at least 1 week—2 if possible. This is especially true for the must-avoid interactants:

- mixed- and indirect-acting sympathomimetics (including levodopa, dopamine, and tyramine);
- imipramine and similar antidepressants; and
- meperidine.

Since many interacting drugs (eg, alcohol, antihistamines) are available OTC, and interaction is bound to occur unless the patient is taught to avoid them, and the advice is followed. The same applies to foods and beverages that are rich in tyramine.

The dangers from hypertension caused by prescription and nonprescription sympathomimetics, as well as from very common foods, cannot be overstated. Three elements of nursing assessment and intervention are required for patients taking these drugs.

1. Routinely monitor blood pressure.
2. Since blood pressure checks alone may not be adequate, be prepared (and prepare others) to assess for early warning signs of a hypertensive crisis (eg, flushing, chest tightness).
3. Provide explicit instructions about, and a written list of, interacting drugs, foods, and beverages.

Some psychiatrists prescribe a small supply of chlorpromazine for their MAO inhibitor–treated patients to take, as an initial first-aid measure if a throbbing headache occurs. If chlorpromazine is prescribed, it is essential to ensure that the patient is capable of recognizing the major signs and can be trusted to take the drug as directed. Chlorpromazine gives only temporary or incomplete relief from hypertension, and it may cause intense anticholinergic interactions with the MAO inhibitor. Therefore, patients who actually take this drug for a possible crisis should be instructed to notify their physician at once.

Overdose and Toxicity

Signs and Symptoms

The toxic or lethal dose of most MAO inhibitors is only about six to ten times the daily therapeutic dose. The most serious responses, which are dose-dependent, affect mainly the cardiovascular and central nervous systems. The major cardiovascular change is hypotension, which can seriously reduce blood flow to (cause ischemia in) all the vital organs. The heart and brain are most important because they are most sensitive to ischemia. Myocardial ischemia can lead to a heart attack. Cerebral ischemia, depending on its severity, can cause problems ranging from drowsiness, dizziness, or confusion, to coma and stroke. Chest pain or headache may also present as signs of inadequate blood supply to the heart and brain. Some patients also become irritable, and seizures may occur. Body temperature often rises dramatically in severe overdoses. Acute urinary retention has been reported.

The scenario is more complicated, and treatment is more difficult if interacting drugs have been taken also.

Treatment

Since MAO inhibitors are taken orally, initial treatment involves standard first-aid measures (eg, gastric lavage) that would be used for any oral overdose. And, as with other overdoses, symptomatic supportive care is the norm, based on stabilizing altered vital signs. Normalizing blood pressure usually comes first. It must be done with a direct-acting vasopressor (eg, norepinephrine), never with the sympathomimetic drugs identified in the previous section as interactants. Invasive monitoring of cardiovascular status, and having continual IV access, is essential. Seizures are treated with IV diazepam. Fever is managed with nondrug measures such as cooling the patient with cool water or a hypothermia blanket.

III. Lithium

Lithium is a naturally occurring element. Chemically, it is similar to sodium, but sufficient differences exist to give lithium unique biologic properties and usefulness for treating the manic phase of manic-depressive illness (bipolar disorder). Lithium chloride was used in the 1940s as a salt (sodium chloride) substitute for patients with heart failure or hypertension, but its use was banned after reports of fatal lithium poisoning. Around the same time, experiments showed, quite accidentally, that lithium calmed animals. The first report describing the therapeutic effects of lithium in manic-depressive psychosis appeared in 1949.

For various medical and financial reasons lithium was not used again in the United States until 20 years later. Since then, this cheap, naturally occurring salt has helped thousands of persons with mania lead more normal and productive lives. Lithium remains the drug of choice for treating manic-depressive illness, but as many as 30% of patients treated in the manic phase of bipolar illness do not respond to the drug, or are intolerant of it. Thus, there is an active search for more effective alternatives. See the article by Keltner and Folks, cited in the Annotated Bibliography for this chapter, for more information.

Absorption, Distribution, Metabolism, and Excretion

Lithium, which is given orally, is absorbed quickly and well. Blood levels peak in 1 to 3 hours. It is distributed throughout the body, and over 95% is excreted, without prior metabolism, by the kidneys. Lithium's plasma half-life is about 24 hours in normal individuals, but is prolonged in patients with impaired renal function. For example, the plasma half-life in many healthy elderly patients is about 36 hours, and dosage reductions of about 50% are indicated to prevent drug accumulation.

Lithium's absorption, distribution, and excretion are closely linked to those of sodium. Reduced dietary sodium intake, or increased sodium loss (as through excessive sweating, diarrhea, or drugs), prolong lithium's half-life and can cause dangerously high blood levels if the lithium dose is not reduced or a normal sodium balance regained. In contrast, excessive sodium intake or reduced sodium loss increases lithium excretion, reduces lithium blood levels, and antagonizes the drug's therapeutic actions.

Pharmacologic Effects

Small amounts of lithium ion substitute for sodium ion, an essential regulator of nerve function. It inhibits nerve metabolism, alters neuronal reuptake of norepinephrine, serotonin, and dopamine, and reduces neurotransmitter release. In manic patients, mood is normalized. Lithium's ability to alter the activity of sodium as a regulator of function in other organs accounts for many of the drug's side effects.

Clinical Indications and Administration

Lithium is indicated for the treatment and prophylaxis of the manic phase of manic-depressive illness (Table 24–C3). It decreases both the severity and number of manic episodes. Lithium is effective in about 80% of cases. Although lithium blood levels peak within hours after administration, clinical effectiveness does not appear for 1 to 2 weeks. Lithium beneficially affects the depressed phase of manic-depressive illness. Present evidence suggests the drug is not effective in endogenous depression without mania.

Lithium carbonate (ESKALITH; LITHANE) is available as tablets or capsules; lithium citrate (CIBALITH-S) is a liquid. A timed-release form of lithium carbonate (LITHOBID) is available for twice-daily use, which may reduce compliance problems. LITHOBID is indicated only for maintenance therapy to replace immediate-acting dosage forms, not for initial treatment.

The lithium dose is based on both the clinical response to the drug and measurements of serum lithium levels. The typical dose for acute mania, 1,800 mg per day in divided doses, usually achieves a desired blood level between 1.0 and 1.5 mEq/L. Maintenance doses are adjusted to maintain a blood level between 0.6 and 1.2 mEq/L. Persons with impaired renal function need reduced doses.

NURSING IMPLICATIONS

Advise patients or their families of the lag period after the onset of therapy. Anticipate initial simultaneous use of an antipsychotic drug to decrease agitation quickly in persons with severe, acute mania, and the need to taper its dosage as the effects of lithium develop. Be aware that the lithium–antipsychotic combination poses some risks. This is noted in the drug interactions section, below.

Side Effects, Adverse Reactions, and Contraindications

Lithium's side effects (Table 24–S3) cause major compliance problems, and potential dangers, for some patients. Since a close relationship exists between sodium and lithium blood levels and drug effects, sodium intake and loss have important roles in the development of side effects and toxicity. Unfortunately, sodium balance is affected by such common factors as diet and excessive sweating. The true dangers reflect the drug's extraordinarily low margin of safety: side effects or possible low-level toxicity may occur at lithium levels between 0.6 and 1.5 mEq/L, the therapeutic range. Toxic blood levels are 1.5 to 2.0 mEq/L or more.

Side effects often involve the GI tract first, usually during the first few weeks of treatment. They include nausea, dry mouth, diarrhea, and thirst. Other common side effects include drowsiness, mild hand tremor, polyuria, weight gain, a bloated feeling, sleeplessness, and lightheadedness. These early effects occur with therapeutic blood levels, and should disappear after about the sixth week of therapy if blood levels do not rise. Their severity increases with increasing blood levels. Weight gain, an unpleasant metallic taste, altered taste of some foods, headache, pruritus, and edema of the hands and ankles are side effects that are unrelated to lithium blood levels.

Lithium affects thyroid function and may cause or worsen hypothyroidism. Thyroid hormone replacement therapy may be indicated for symptomatic hypothyroidism.

Lithium is generally contraindicated in patients with significant renal or cardiovascular disease, severe debilitation or dehydration, or sodium depletion.

NURSING IMPLICATIONS

Lithium's low therapeutic index and its dependence on blood sodium levels necessitate blood chemistry measurements before starting treatment and frequently for several weeks thereafter. High-risk patients may require daily blood tests. Once the patient is stabilized, monthly blood tests are usually adequate. Blood samples should be drawn when lithium levels are likely to be at their lowest level (8 to 12 hours after the last dose or immediately before the first morning dose).

Consistent dietary sodium intake should be a primary goal. Provide the patient and family members with a list of foods that are rich in sodium, and discourage excessive use of table salt and salt substitutes, which may cause hyponatremia. Advise persons responsible for preparing the patient's meals not to increase or decrease salt content dramatically. It may be useful to consult a dietitian to plan a diet and provide relevant information. If the patient has a cardiovascular disease in which sodium restriction or diuretic (sodium-wasting) drugs are indicated, consult with all physicians involved to ensure that neither antimanic nor cardiac therapy is compromised. Some knowledgeable patients are aware of the relationship between sodium intake and such cardiovascular problems as edema, which is apt to occur during lithium therapy. Caution them strongly against reducing their sodium intake unless it is known to be excessive.

Prepare patients for expected side effects, and identify those that should disappear gradually. Likewise, identify side effects that require immediate notification of the physician: vomiting, severe tremor, sedation, muscle weakness, and vertigo. Give lithium with meals to help reduce nausea, and encourage the patient to drink 2.5 to 3 L of water each day. This should alleviate dry mouth and polydipsia, and help maintain normal fluid balance. Be aware, however, that excessive water intake or urine output may alter serum sodium and lithium levels adversely.

Hand tremors or drowsiness may hinder simple tasks such as driving, operating machinery, or even writing. Since many patients experiencing these side effects are easily agitated, it is important to calm and reassure them. Ankle edema is best managed by elevating the feet. Exercise programs may be helpful, but the patient's activity should be monitored to prevent excessive sweating, sodium loss, and aggravation of side effects or toxicity. If excessive sweating or diarrhea occurs, extra fluid and sodium intake should be provided, using lithium and sodium blood levels as a guideline. Help the patient develop a consistent but tolerable exercise program with an appropriate amount of rest.

Periodic thyroid function tests may be ordered, since edema, weight gain, and lethargy may be due either to the lithium or to thyroid suppression. Explain the reason for such tests.

Obtain information about cardiac and renal disease when taking a nursing history of manic-depressive patients who will receive lithium. If any contraindication exists, withhold lithium unless a psychiatric emergency that is deemed life-threatening exists.

◆ Use During Pregnancy and Lactation

Lithium, a suspected teratogen, crosses the placental barrier and is excreted in breast milk. It should not be used during pregnancy (especially the first trimester). Breast-feeding should be avoided.

◆ Use in Children

There is no information about the safety and effectiveness of lithium for children under 12 years of age.

◆ Use in the Elderly

All precautions noted for younger adults apply to the elderly. Anticipate the need for reduced dosages to account for decreased renal function. Extra careful monitoring is needed because of the prevalence of altered diet and fluid intake, and common age-related diseases and the use of interacting drugs to treat them.

Interactions with Other Drugs

Table 24–13 summarizes the drugs that interact with lithium. Usually, the most important interactions involve drugs that alter serum lithium levels and upset the slight distinction between subtherapeutic, effective, and potentially toxic serum lithium levels.

Of all the interactants, diuretics are the most important. All the commonly used diuretics are indicated for managing high blood pressure or edema (eg, that associated with heart failure); and, like lithium itself, they are usually used on a long-term basis, increasing the eventual risk of an interaction. Diuretics increase renal sodium excretion and indirectly decrease lithium excretion. Through this effect, previously safe and effective lithium doses can lead to toxic blood levels. To magnify the problem, patients receiving diuretics are often placed on low-sodium diets, and take table salt substitutes, which lower serum sodium levels and increase lithium levels further. Nonsteroidal antiinflammatory drugs, particularly indomethacin, may also elevate lithium levels.

A variety of drugs can decrease lithium levels and counteract its effects. They include commonly ingested substances such as caffeine, alcohol, and antacids. Acetazolamide interacts in this way also. It is a diuretic, but is seldom used for that purpose. Instead, the interaction with lithium is most likely to arise during the more common use of acetazolamide as an anticonvulsant or to manage glaucoma (see Chapters 26 and 32). The cause is acetazolamide's ability to aklalinize the urine, which increases lithium excretion.

Several other interactions do not involve drug-induced changes of lithium levels, but they are important nonetheless, especially in the psychiatric population. Lithium can reduce chlorpromazine blood levels; in turn, chlorpromazine can mask nausea, which is a sign of lithium toxicity. When used with another important antipsychotic, haloperidol, there is a risk of neurotoxicity. The potential outcome is serious enough that the lithium–haloperidol combination is best avoided.

The most important acute interaction involves neuromuscular blocking drugs, which are usually administered as part of the premedication plan for electroconvulsive therapy. Lithium can prolong the respiratory depression caused by these blockers.

NURSING IMPLICATIONS

Lithium can be used with most of its interactants, but this usually requires adjustments of the lithium dose. Combined use always requires closer monitoring of the therapeutic responses, and is best done with more frequent monitoring of serum lithium levels to guide dosage adjustments. Use extra care to ensure that dietary sodium intake is regulated properly, since some of the interactants affect the body's sodium handling. Stress the importance of avoiding or limiting the intake of alcohol, which tends to be abused by persons with manic-depressive illness.

Overdose and Toxicity

Lithium's low margin of safety is noted above. Toxicity seldom develops at lithium levels below about 1.5 mEq/L, but individuals who are unusually sensitive to the drug, including many elderly patients, may show symptoms. Intoxication is usually insidious and may be provoked by common conditions that affect fluid and electrolyte balance: dietary or drug-induced decreases of salt intake, dehydration, and vomiting or diarrhea.

Signs and Symptoms

When lithium serum levels are between 1.5 and 2 mEq/L, diarrhea, vomiting, drowsiness, muscle weakness, and some loss of coordination can occur. Levels of 2 mEq/L and above can cause ataxia, giddiness, tinnitus, blurred vision, and a large output of dilute urine that may cause hypotension and dehydration. Restlessness, slurred speech, confusion, mental and motor retardation, or sleepiness may occur. Serum levels above 3 mEq/L are very dangerous and affect many organs. Important cardiovascular changes include arrhythmias and irregular pulses, hypotension, and, potentially, circulatory and respiratory collapse. Choreoathetoid muscle movements, muscle hyperirritability, and exaggerated deep tendon reflexes may occur. Profound overdoses may cause stupor, coma, and seizures. Death can be caused by any combination of the major symptoms, but it is usually related to impaired ventilation.

Treatment

There is no pharmacologic antidote for lithium poisoning. Aside from reducing further lithium absorption, the general treatment involves hastening its excretion and normalizing blood sodium levels. In many cases discontinuing lithium administration and providing supportive nursing and medical care are sufficient. Gastric lavage may help, but care must be taken to avoid altering serum electrolyte levels further. Drugs that reduce lithium excretion, particularly oral diuretics and nonsteroidal antiinflammatory agents, should be discontinued if possible. If serum lithium levels are below about 2.5 mEq/L, normal saline infusions may be sufficient to provide enough volume to normalize blood pressure, and to provide enough sodium to counteract lithium's effects and enhance its excretion. Two nontraditional diuretics may help enhance lithium excretion: mannitol, through its action to increase urine production; and acetazolamide, through its ability to alkalinize the urine. Increased urine production will necessitate giving parenteral fluids having the proper volume and composition (based on laboratory data) to prevent hypovolemia and undesired electrolyte changes. Hemodialysis may be indicated, particularly if other interventions fail to reduce lithium levels to about 1 mEq/L after a day or so of treatment.

NURSING IMPLICATIONS

Drowsiness, nausea, and diarrhea may be either expected early side effects of lithium treatment or indicators of toxicity. It is essential to use careful observation and assessment, and not merely blood lithium levels, to help diagnose toxicity and guide treatment.

SUMMARY OF NURSING IMPLICATIONS

◆ Assessment

Establish baseline assessment data, to recognize adverse drug effects (eg, liver enzymes, vital signs, renal function, mental status, speech pattern, affect, weight).

Assess for signs or symptoms indicating noncompliance, including missed doses or cessation of treatment, or poor therapeutic response.

Observe for major symptoms of depression: apathy, sadness, sleep disturbances, hopelessness, guilt, decreased libido, verbal beratings of self, and spontaneous crying.

Review history for conditions that may be aggravated by tricyclic antidepressants (eg, glaucoma, cardiovascular disease, GI conditions, urologic conditions, seizures, pregnancy).

Identify conditions from history that may be aggravated by MAO inhibitors (eg, hepatic and renal disease, cardiovascular and cerebrovascular disease, hypoglycemia, seizure disorder).

Recognize side effects or toxic reactions; assess for onset and duration.

◆ Nursing Diagnoses

Noncompliance related to negative perception of drug treatment.

Knowledge deficit related to purpose of drug therapy.

High risk for injury related to impaired behavior pattern (suicide risk) and drug side effects (hypotension, ataxia).

Sensory/perceptual alteration related to drug effects: visual changes, dizziness, drowsiness.

Altered nutrition: less than body requirements related to nausea, vomiting, loss of appetite.

Decreased cardiac output related to arrhythmias and tachycardia from drug therapy.

Altered thought processes related to flight of ideas, distractibility, and lack of judgment associated with affective disorder.

Anxiety, panic level, related to bipolar disorder.

Urinary retention related to drug side effects.

Constipation related to adverse drug effects.

◆ Planning/Implementation

Provide reassurance and emotional support to deal with problems and stigmas; include family members when permissible and acceptable to patient.

Monitor for "cheeking" or hoarding; may indicate plan for suicide attempt.

Check drug dosages carefully; slight overdose may cause serious toxicity.

Monitor for suicidal thought content or behavior; suicidal tendencies may be greater as antidepressants increase energy or motivation.

Monitor vital signs: pulse rate and blood pressure in supine, sitting, and standing positions; withhold tricyclic antidepressants if symptomatic hypotension, tachycardia, or arrhythmias occur; recognize signs of high blood pressure due to interactions involving MAO inhibitors (rubbing of chest, sweating, dilated pupils).

Give most tricyclic antidepressants in single bedtime dose to decrease perception of annoying side effects.

Observe for early signs of toxicity: antidepressants (drowsiness, tachycardia, mydriasis, hypotension, agitation, vomiting, confusion, fever, restlessness, sweating); MAO inhibitors (dizziness, vertigo, fatigue); lithium (diarrhea, vomiting, drowsiness, muscle weakness, ataxia, giddiness, polyuria); discontinue drug and notify physician.

Discontinue drug and notify physician if CNS overstimulation causes psychiatric responses such as hypomania, acute schizophrenia, or delirium.

Withhold MAO inhibitors or tricyclic antidepressants if symptoms of hepatotoxicity (jaundice, rashes, nausea, abdominal pain) or blood dyscrasias (fever, sore throat, malaise, "flu") develop.

Observe diabetic patients carefully to detect hypoglycemia or potentiation of insulin action.

Monitor serum lithium levels to determine drug effectiveness and need for dosage change, and to avoid serious adverse reactions; draw blood 8 to 12 hours after last dose or immediately before morning dose.

Weigh patient weekly; maintain weight chart; report unusual weight gain (particularly with lithium).

◆ Patient and Family Teaching

Teach the patient/family:

That drugs used for affective disorders have a lag period up to 1 month; discouragement can be expected.

About the importance of adhering to a prescribed medication regimen; discourage increasing dose to hasten or increase response.

To avoid OTC drugs, particularly those containing sympathomimetics or antimuscarinics, for patients taking tricyclic antidepressants or MAO inhibitors, sodium bicarbonate or antacids with lithium, alcohol with any of the above; serious interactions may occur; provide list of drugs to avoid.

About acceptable ways to deal with anticipated minor side effects: dry mouth (hard candies, small sips of water, mouth rinse); visual disturbances (sunglasses, artificial tears, assistance with ambulation); constipation (bulk-forming foods, increased water intake); urinary retention (privacy during toilet use, running warm water over perineum, adequate fluids); decreased perspiration (appropriate clothing, avoid unnecessary exercise); orthostatic hypotension (slow positional changes, avoid hot baths/showers); drowsiness (take larger dose at bedtime with physician approval, avoid operating motor vehicle).

That discontinuing tricyclic antidepressants without physician's advice may result in muscarinic rebound (nausea, vomiting, insomnia); discontinuing MAO inhibitors may cause severe agitation, hallucinations, or worsening of depression.

About drugs, foods (high in tyramine), and beverages that interact with MAO inhibitors; provide list.

To report throbbing headache, palpitations, neck stiffness, nausea, vomiting, tachycardia or bradycardia, or sweating immediately.

To take lithium with meals to reduce nausea; however, eat about same time each day to maintain serum levels.

About the need for adequate sodium to maintain lithium blood levels and response; depleted sodium will lead to excessive lithium effects, and increased sodium to decreased lithium levels.

To drink 10 to 12 8-oz glasses of water a day.

About the need for dietary consistency; to notify physician before initiating diet or exercise program or therapy with other drugs.

◆ Evaluation

The patient/family will:

Achieve desired therapeutic serum level of drug.

Participate in agreed-on plan of care.

Comply with postdischarge laboratory appointments for serum level evaluation.

Participate in activities of daily living and decision-making; express interest in diversions and recreation; show concern for appearance.

Verbalize need for counseling and physical activity in conjunction with drug therapy.

Experience minimal to no adverse drug effects; have stable vital signs; experience no GI distress.

Reach level of behavioral stability; have less anxiety; sleep better; talk, walk less.

Annotated Bibliography

Abraham IL, Neese JB, Westerman PS. Depression. Nursing implications of a clinical and social problem. *Nurs Clin North Am* 1991;26:527–544. *An excellent contemporary review of the social, economic, and personal impact of depression and its many treatment options.*

Brasfield KH. Practical psychopharmacologic considerations in depression. *Nurs Clin North Am* 1991;26:651–663. *Discusses how characteristics of individual antidepressants should be matched to unique patient-related characteristics; how and when blood level measurements are useful therapeutic guides; and which drug interactions can pose problems.*

Dubovsky SL. Understanding and treating depression in anxious patients. *J Clin Psychiatry* 1990;51(Suppl.):3–8. (See also discussion on pp 14–17.) *A short but useful review of how the coexistence of anxiety and depression can complicate diagnosis, drug selection, and therapeutic monitoring.*

James W, Lippman S. Bupropion: Overview and prescribing guidelines in depression. *South Med J* 1991;84:222–224. *A concise but valuable review of this antidepressant.*

Keltner NL, Folks DG. Alternatives to lithium in the treatment of bipolar disorder. *Perspect Psych Care* 1991;27:36–37. *Keltner and Folks have an ongoing "Psychopharmacology Update" column in this journal. This article discusses carbamazepine and valproic acid as alternatives to lithium for treating patients with bipolar disorder.*

Miller LJ. Clinical strategies for the use of psychotropic drugs during pregnancy. *Psychiatr Med* 1991;9:275–298. *An invaluable discussion of the topic, focusing on not only antidepressants, but also drugs used for schizophrenia, parkinsonism, and anxiety.*

Neese JB. Depression in the general hospital. *Nurs Clin North Am* 1991;26:613–622. *The frequency of depression combined with medical illness poses a great challenge to nurses. This article reviews the common findings in and successful drug and non-drug interventions for these patients.*

Pary R, Tobias C, Lippman S. Fluoxetine: Prescribing guidelines for the newest antidepressant. *South Med J* 1989;82:1005–1009. *This article provides a concise and objective view of a drug that has been a recent focus of controversy, criticism, and lawsuits.*

Potter WZ, Rudorfer MV, Manji H. The pharmacologic treatment of depression. *N Engl J Med* 1991;325:633–642. An excellent, contemporary review of depression symptoms and classification; diagnoses as predictors of the response to treatment; and pharmacotherapy and other treatment approaches. Well-designed tables help you get the needed information quickly.

Rudorfer MV, Potter WZ. Antidepressants: A comparative review of the clinical pharmacology and therapeutic use of the "newer" versus the "older" drugs. *Drugs* 1989;37:713–738. *A thorough review and update of new antidepressants, and a summary of limitations of the older agents. This paper should whet the appetite of students considering psychiatric nursing as a career.*

Smoyak SA. Victims and villains. *J Psychosoc Nurs Ment Health Serv* 1991;29:3. *A blistering editorial that takes dead aim at the sensationalization of fluoxetine by the mass media. Worth reading to help appreciate a complex issue in psychiatry today.*

Steiner D, Marcopulos B. Depression in the elderly. Characteristics and clinical management. *Nurs Clin North Am* 1991;26:585–600. *Whether your elderly depressed patient is living in the community, is institutionalized, or has a concomitant medical illness, careful evaluation and treatment is necessary. These issues are discussed, with an emphasis on the important roles of nurses.*

Watsky EJ, Salzman C. Psychotropic drug interactions. *Hosp Comm Psychiatry* 1991;42:247–256. *Summarizes and categorizes psychotropic drug interactions according to severity and clinical significance. Useful also for the antipsychotic drugs discussed in Chapter 23.*

Whitley GG. Ritualistic behavior: Breaking the cycle. *J Psychosoc Nurs Ment Health Serv* 1991;20:31–35. *A useful discussion of obsessive-compulsive disorder and the use of drugs such as clomipramine to manage it.*

Wood KA, Harris MJ, Morreale A, Rizos AL. Drug-induced psychosis and depression in the elderly. *Psychiatr Clin North Am* 1988;11:167–193. *Given the prevalence of polypharmacy in the elderly, this article about drugs that can cause psychiatric disorders in older individuals is especially worth reading.*

Table 24–C1 Clinical Uses and Administration of Tricyclic Antidepressants and Related Drugs

AGENT	CLINICAL USES	DOSAGE AND ROUTE OF ADMINISTRATION
PROTOTYPE		
Imipramine (TOFRANIL)	Endogenous depression and other depression	Oral: Adults: 100 mg/d to start for hospitalized patients; usual maintenance dose 50–150 mg/d. Elderly and adolescents: 10 mg tid or qid to start, usually should not exceed 100 mg/d IM: Adults: 25 mg bid–qid until oral form can be used
	Childhood enuresis	Oral: Children >6 years: 25 mg/d 1 hr before bedtime to start; after 1 wk increase to 50 mg/d (6–12 years), and to 75 mg (>12 years) if needed. Do not exceed 2.5 mg/kg/d
Imipramine pamoate (TOFRANIL-PM)	Depression, especially endogenous depression	Oral: Adults: 75 mg/hs; 200 mg/d, if needed; usual maintenance dose 75–150 mg/d (some patients require divided dose). Elderly, adolescents: Since the lowest unit dosage is 75 mg, imipramine pamoate is *not* usually prescribed for these age
RELATED DRUGS		
Amitriptyline (ELAVIL, ENDEP)	Depression, especially endogenous depression	Oral: Adults: 25 mg tid to start, followed by increase in late-afternoon or bedtime dose to total of 150 mg/d in divided doses, if needed. Maintenance: 50–100 mg hs. Elderly and adolescents: 10 mg tid plus 20 mg hs may be sufficient. Not recommended for children <12 years IM: Adults: 20–30 mg qid to start; replace with oral form as soon as possible
Amoxapine (ASENDIN)	Endogenous depression, depression accompanied by anxiety or agitation, dysthymia or reactive depressions	Oral: Adults: 50 mg bid or tid to start, followed, if tolerated, by increase at end of first week to 100 mg tid, if tolerated; usual maintenance dose 200–300 mg/d given in a single bedtime dose. Elderly: Start with 25 mg bid or tid; if no intolerance noted may increase to 50 mg bid or tid by end of first week; usually 100–150 mg/d is sufficient. Not recommended for children <16 years
Bupropion (WELLBUTRIN)	Depression	Oral: Adults: 100 mg in AM and 100 mg in PM, to start. Based on response may be increased to 100 mg tid up to a maximum of 450 mg/d. Not recommended for children <18 years

(continued)

Table 24–C1 Clinical Uses and Administration of Tricyclic Antidepressants and Related Drugs (*Continued*)

AGENT	CLINICAL USES	DOSAGE AND ROUTE OF ADMINISTRATION
Clomipramine (ANAFRANIL)	Obsessive-compulsive disorder	Oral: Adults: Begin with 25 mg/d, slowly increase to 100 mg/d by 2 weeks. Maximum is 250 mg/d in divided doses. After titration a single bedtime dose can be used to minimize daytime sleepiness. Children and adolescents: Begin with 25 mg/d, gradually increase during first 2 weeks, as tolerated, to daily maximum of 3 mg/kg or 100 mg, whichever is smaller. Maximum daily dosage is 3 mg/kg or 200 mg, whichever is smaller. After titration, one bedtime can be used
Desipramine (NORPRAMIN, PERTOFRANE)	Depression, especially endogenous depression	Oral: Adults Start with 25 mg tid, increase gradually to 200 mg/d total. Do not exceed 300 mg/d. Maintenance usually 100-200 mg hs or in divided doses. Elderly and adolescents: Usually 25 mg qd–qid. Start at lower dose, increase according to tolerance and clinical response. Do not exceed 150 mg/d in these age groups. Not recommended for children
Doxepin (ADAPIN, SINEQUAN)	Depression and anxiety associated with involutional depression or manic-depressive disorder. Depression and/or anxiety associated with neurosis, alcoholism, or organic disease. Neurotic (dysthymic) symptoms that respond to doxepin include anxiety, tension, somatic symptoms, sleep disturbances, guilt, anergia, fear, apprehension, and worry	Oral: Adults: Start with 25 mg tid. Usual optimal dose is 25–50 mg tid. May increase to 300 mg/d. Emotional symptoms accompanied by organic disease may be controlled by 25 mg qd or bid. Once-per-day dose should not exceed 150 mg. The 150-mg capsule strength intended for maintenance therapy only. Elderly: No specific dosage instructions exist. Adjust carefully based on patient's condition. Not recommended for children
Fluoxetine (PROZAC)	Depression	Oral: Adults: Usually 20 mg each morning. Give bid (morning and noon) for daily doses >20 mg, but not to exceed 80 mg/d maximum. Elderly: No differences in response noted between elderly and younger patients. Safety not established for children or adolescents

(continued)

Table 24–C1 Clinical Uses and Administration of Tricyclic Antidepressants and Related Drugs (*Continued*)

AGENT	CLINICAL USES	DOSAGE AND ROUTE OF ADMINISTRATION
Maprotiline (LUDIOMIL)	Endogenous depression, dysthymia, depressive phase of manic-depression, anxiety associated with depression	Oral: Adults: Outpatients (mild-to-moderate depression) start with 75 mg/d in single or divided doses for 2 weeks, increase in 25-mg increments to 150 mg/d, in single or divided doses if needed. For more severely depressed (hospitalized) patients start with 100–150 mg/d in single or divided doses, if needed and tolerated, increase to 225 mg/d. Do not exceed 225 mg/d. Maintenance dose: 75–150 mg in single or divided doses. Elderly: Initially 25 mg daily; 50–75 mg in single or divided doses usually satisfactory for maintenance. Not recommended for children <18 years
Nortriptyline (AVENTYL, PAMELOR)	Depression, especially endogenous depression	Oral: Adults: Start with low doses; 25 mg tid or qid or 75–100 mg hs. Maintenance dose should be lowest effective dose. Doses above 150 mg/d are not recommended. Elderly and adolescents 30–50 mg/d in divided doses or all at bedtime. Not recommended for children
Protriptyline (VIVACTIL)	Depression, especially in withdrawn and anergic patients	Oral: Adults: Start with 5–10 mg tid–qid. Increase to 60 mg/d, if necessary. Elderly and adolescents: Start with 5 mg tid. In the elderly, monitor cardiovascular system closely if dose exceeds 20 mg/d. Not recommended for children
Sertraline (ZOLOFT)	Depression	Oral: Adults: Dose is 50–200 mg qd
Trazodone (DESYREL)	Depression, especially endogenous depression	Oral: Adults: Start with 50 mg tid. Increase by 50 mg/d every 3 or 4 days. Maximum outpatient dosage is 400 mg/d; maximum for inpatients is 600 mg/d. Once response is adequate, reduce to lowest effective dose. Elderly: No specific dosage instructions. Not recommended for children <18 years
Trimipramine (SURMONTIL)	Depression, especially endogenous depression	Oral: Adults: For hospitalized patients, start with 100 mg/d in divided doses, gradually increase to 50 mg qid, if needed; maximum daily dose for hospitalized patients is 250–300 mg. For outpatients, initially 75 mg/d in divided doses, increased to 150 mg/d; should not exceed 200 mg; maintenance dose 50–150 mg/d; may be given as single bedtime does. Elderly and adolescents: Start with 50 mg/d, increase to 100 mg/d, if needed. Not recommended for children

Table 24–S1 **Major Side Effects of and Contraindications for Tricyclic Antidepressants and Related Drugs**

BODY SYSTEM/ Side Effect	CONTRAINDICATION/ PRECAUTION	COMMENTS AND NURSING IMPLICATIONS
CENTRAL NERVOUS SYSTEM		
Sedation, ataxia		Instruct patients to avoid performing tasks that require sharp mental or motor skills; advise that alcohol and other sedatives enhance CNS depression. Daytime sedation can be minimized if drug is given at bedtime. Sedation usually subsides in 3 weeks
Confusion, delirium	Concomitant antipsychotic use is associated with delirium	Be aware of risk factors associated with tricyclic-induced delirium. Confused patients may require supervision of all activities. Monitor nighttime behavior of confused patients, as confusion worsens at night. Withhold drug if delirium occurs
EYE		
Blurred vision; photophobia		Antimuscarinic side effect. Instruct patient to wear sunglasses out of doors, be cautious with tasks (eg, driving), in which good vision is required; assist elderly patients in ambulation if needed
Obstruction of normal aqueous humor outflow; increased intraocular pressure	Glaucoma	Antimuscarinic side effect. Instruct patient to report ocular pain immediately; acute pain may indicate undiagnosed glaucoma
Decreased lacrimation		Antimuscarinic side effect. Recommend artificial tears to reduce irritation
CARDIOVASCULAR		
Hypotension, especially orthostatic		Instruct patient to rise slowly from sitting or lying positions, and to sit on the side of the bed for 2 full minutes upon awakening. Instruct patients to avoid standing in one place too long and taking hot baths or showers. Elderly patients may need assistance
Arrhythmias, tachycardia, palpitations	Congestive heart failure, myocardial infarction, tachycardia, conduction defects, hyperthyroidism	Record vital signs daily or more often if ordered; observe for adverse reactions; if patient is experiencing tachycardia withhold the drug and seek medical evaluation
GASTROINTESTINAL		
Dry mouth		Antimuscarinic side effect. Recommend sugarless hard candies, sips of water. Good oral care is important, especially after eating
Constipation (decreased gut motility)	Chronic constipation, paralytic ileus, intestinal obstruction	Manage mild constipation first with dietary changes: increased fluids and bulk-forming foods. Monitor intake and output. Elderly and debilitated patients are at higher risk. Examine abdomen for distention and tenderness, auscultate bowel sounds
SWEAT GLANDS		
Decreased sweating	Unnecessary vigorous exercise	Instruct patient to be cautious about strenuous work, particularly in hot weather, and to wear loose, light clothing. Patient may need to change clothing, bedding more often than normal. Help patient plan leisure activities

(continued)

Table 24–S1 Major Side Effects of and Contraindications for Tricyclic Antidepressants and Related Drugs (*Continued*)

BODY SYSTEM/ Side Effect	CONTRAINDICATION/ PRECAUTION	COMMENTS AND NURSING IMPLICATIONS
GENITOURINARY		
Urinary retention, hesitancy	Urinary retention, prostatic hypertrophy (older males)	Antimuscarinic side effect. Monitor urinary output, check for bladder distention. Instruct, encourage patient to respond to the need to urinate (sometimes depressed individuals will "put off" urinating). Instruct patient to notify care provider about pain in bladder area, distention, or feeling of incomplete urination. Privacy and running warm water over the perineum may help

Table 24–I1 Major Interactions Between Tricyclic Antidepressants and Related Drugs and Other Agents

AGENT	RESULT OF INTERACTION	COMMENTS AND NURSING IMPLICATIONS
Anticoagulants, oral (Chapter 35)	Excessive anticoagulation, potential excessive bleeding, hemorrhage	Probably reflects decreased anticoagulation metabolism, develops gradually upon combined use; assess for bruising, bleeding, anticipate need for closer monitoring of coagulation profiles, reduced anticoagulant dose
Antihistamines (Chapter 51).	See antimuscarinic drugs, below	
Antihypertensive drugs, all (Chapter 33)	Excessive hypotension, especially orthostatic	Combined use is common, should be supervised and monitored closely, frequent checks of supine, standing BP and heart rate are essential
Antimuscarinic (atropine-like) drugs, all (see Chapter 13 and Table 13–1 for list)	Excessive CNS depression and peripheral atropine-like side effects; atropine poison syndrome	Avoid if possible; teach patient to avoid OTC drugs (eg, antihistamines) that may interact; monitor for signs of combined use
Climetidine (Chapter 40)	Intensified CNS and peripheral antidepressant side effects	Interactant reduces antidepressant metabolism, increases blood levels; avoid interaction or monitor closely, interaction presumably less likely with cimetidine alternatives (ranitidine, famotidine)
Clonidine (Chapter 33)	Reduced clonidine antihypertensive effects; hypertension	Tricyclics block central antihypertensive action of clonidine, other centrally acting antihypertensives; BP rise may be sudden, severe; avoid interaction
CNS depressants, all	Excessive CNS depression	Avoid interaction unless combined use is supervised by physician and can be monitored appropriately, discourage use of alcohol, other OTC drugs with sedative properties
Fluoxetine (this chapter)	Intensified antidepressant side effects	Interaction likely, given rational switch to fluoxetine in patients refractory to more traditional antidepressants; signs of interaction may not occur for 1 week to 1 month; avoid simultaneous use of fluoxetine with other antidepressants
Guanethidine (Chapter 33)	Reduced antihypertensive effects of interactant	BP rise may be gradual but significant, fortunately is uncommon owing to infrequent use of guanethidine; avoid interaction

(continued)

Table 24–I1 Major Interactions Between Tricyclic Antidepressants and Related Drugs and Other Agents (*Continued*)

AGENT	RESULT OF INTERACTION	COMMENTS AND NURSING IMPLICATIONS
Monoamine oxidase inhibitors (this chapter)	Sudden, intense CNS and peripheral atropine-like side effects; potential antimuscarinic poison syndrome	Avoid combined use; if switch between these antidepressants is planned, should stop therapy with one agent 1–2 weeks before starting with other
Thyroid hormone supplements (Chapter 47)	Tachycardia, palpitations, anginal pain, potential arrhythmias	Monitor cardiovascular status closely during combined use

Table 24–C2 Clinical Uses and Administration of MAO Inhibitors

AGENT	CLINICAL USES	DOSAGE AND ROUTE OF ADMINISTRATION
Isocarboxazid (MARPLAN)	Depression refractory to tricyclic antidepressants and ECT therapy	Oral: Adults: Start with 30 mg/d in single or divided doses. As soon as clinical improvement is observed, reduce to 10–20 mg/d or less for maintenance. If no response within 3 or 4 weeks then isocarboxazid is unlikely to benefit. Not recommended for elderly or children <16 years
Phenelzine (NARDIL)	Refractory depression, especially neurotic (dysthymia) typical or nonendogenous depression	Oral: Adults: Start with 15 mg tid, followed by a rapid increase to 60–90 mg/d until maximum benefit is achieved; then reduce over several weeks to as low as 15 mg/d or 15 mg qod. Response may not be apparent until 60 mg/d has been given for 4 weeks or more. Not recommended for children <16 years
Tranylcypromine (PARNATE)	Major refractory depression in hospitalized or closely supervised patients	Oral: Adults: Start with 10 mg in AM and 10 mg in afternoon for 2 weeks; if necessary, increase to 20 mg in AM and 10 mg in afternoon for 1 week. If no improvement noted by this time, further administration is unlikely to help. Maintenance: 10 mg qd or bid. Contraindicated in people >60 years

Table 24–S2 **Major Side Effects of and Contraindications for MAO Inhibitors**

BODY SYSTEM/ Side Effect	CONTRAINDICATION/ PRECAUTION	COMMENTS AND NURSING IMPLICATIONS
CENTRAL NERVOUS SYSTEM Overstimulation such as agitation, hypomania, acute schizophrenic reactions	Quiescent schizophrenia, undiagnosed manic-depressive illness	Withhold next dose pending further evaluation by physician
EYE Blurred vision		See tricyclic antidepressants, Table 24–S1
CARDIOVASCULAR Hypotension	Hypotension	Monitor BP frequently; use interventions mentioned in Table 24–S1 to prevent injuries from falls
GASTROINTESTINAL Dry mouth, constipation		See tricyclic antidepressants, Table 24–S1

Table 24–I2 **Major Interations Between MAO Inhibitors and Other Agents**

AGENT	RESULT OF INTERACTION	COMMENTS AND NURSING IMPLICATIONS
Antidepressants (all agents in other classes)	Syndrome reflecting atropine poisoning	Avoid interaction; see text and Table 24-I1
Antidiabetic drugs (insulin and oral antidiabetics; Chapter 46)	Hypoglycemia	MAO inhibitors increase insulin release, inhibit metabolism of oral agents; symptoms may appear gradually; if interaction is unavoidable, monitor responses and blood glucose levels with extra care, anticipate need for reduced antidiabetic drug dosages
Antihistamines (Chapter 51)	See antimuscarinic drugs, below	
Antihypertensive drugs (Chapter 33)	Excessive hypotension, especially orthostatic	Additive effects; avoid, or monitor BP closely if unavoidable; anticipate need to reduce dosage of one or both interactants
Antimuscarinic (atropine-like) drugs, all (see Chapter 13 and Table 13–1 for list)	Excessive antimuscarinic side effects, potential antimuscarinic poisoning syndrome	Avoid if possible; may be due to impaired metabolism of interactant by MAO inhibitor; teach patient to avoid OTC drugs (eg, antihistamines) that have antimuscarinic actions
CNS depressants	Excessive CNS depression	Additive effect; avoid if possible, discourage unsupervised use of OTC sedatives, especially alcohol
Meperidine (Chapter 21)	Profound CNS stimulation, then depression, coma, possible death	Avoid interaction; morphine is preferred narcotic for patients taking MAO inhibitors
Sympathomimetics, mixed- and indirect-acting (catecholamine releasers; see text and Chapter 14); dopamine and levodopa	Hypertension, hypertensive crisis, stroke	Must avoid; occurs quickly, may be preceded by headache, palpitations; triggered by many OTC drugs (eg, decongestants, weight-loss aids) and by tyramine-containing foods (Table 24–4); explicit, understandable patient teaching, compliance, are essential

Table 24–C3 | Clinical Use and Administration of Lithium

AGENT	CLINICAL USES	DOSAGE AND ROUTE OF ADMINISTRATION
Lithium (CIBALITH, ESKALITH, LITHOBID, LITHONATE)	Manic episodes of manic-depressive illness	Oral: Adults: For acute episodes, 600 mg of immediate-acting product tid. Maintenance and prophylactic dose: 900-1200 mg/d. Sustained-acting product (LITHOBID) may be substituted for maintenance after initial stabilization on immediate-acting form; administer twice daily. Elderly: Elderly patients often respond to reduced dosage. Not recommended for children <12 years

Table 24–S3 | Side Effects of and Contraindications for Lithium

BODY SYSTEM/ Side Effect	CONTRAINDICATION/ PRECAUTION	COMMENTS AND NURSING IMPLICATIONS
CENTRAL NERVOUS SYSTEM		
Confusion, restlessness, sleeplessness Sedation		Instruct patient and family about signs of lithium toxicity. Withhold lithium and notify the physician if severe side effects occur
EYE		
Blurred vision		
CARDIOVASCULAR		
Arrhythmias, tachycardia, palpitations		
GASTROINTESTINAL		
Dry mouth, constipation		See tricyclic antidepressants
Nausea		Can be reduced by taking lithium with meals
Thirst		Instruct the patient to drink 10–12 8-oz glasses of water a day
Diarrhea		Monitor closely; depletion of electrolytes can cause higher serum lithium levels
Weight gain		Maintain daily weight record; the nurse may need to consult with a dietitian. Evaluate for hypothyroidism as possible cause

Table 24–13 Major Interactions Between Lithium and Other Drugs

AGENT	RESULT OF INTERACTION	COMMENTS AND NURSING IMPLICATIONS
Acetazolamide (Chapter 32)	Reduced serum lithium levels, poor symptom control	Interactant is commonly used for seizure disorders, glaucoma, so interaction may be unavoidable; check medication history carefully, encourage patient to share full medication history with other prescribing physicians (eg, neurologists, ophthalmologists) so that noninteracting drugs might be used instead
Alcohol (Chapter 22)	Reduced serum lithium levels, poor symptom control	Discourage alcohol intake, assess for noncompliance
Antipsychotic drugs (eg, chlorpromazine, Chapter 23; see haloperidol, below)	Decreased blood levels, effects, of antipsychotics; masking of nausea, a key indicator of lithium toxicity	Monitor for both outcomes of interaction; check serum lithium levels more closely
Diuretics (thiazides, high-ceiling, potassium-sparing; Chapter 32) and salt (sodium chloride) substitutes	Increased lithium levels, increased risk of side effects, potential toxicity	Anticipate need to reduce lithium dose during combined therapy, more frequent evaluation of clinical responses, serum lithium measurements, are important; need to maintain adequate dietary sodium intake takes on added importance; is an important and common interaction
Haloperidol (Chapter 23)	Potential neurotoxicity	Avoid interaction
Indomethacin (Chapter 52)	Increased lithium blood levels, effects	As for diuretics, above; not known whether other nonsteroidal antiinflammatory drugs (including aspirin) interact similarly
Neuromuscular blockers (Chapter 17)	Prolonged ventilatory depression, apnea, caused by neuromuscular ventilation	Anticipate result of interaction, need for more prolonged support of ventilation; no drug or dose changes are needed for this acute effect
Theophylline (also aminophylline; Chapter 38)	Decreased lithium blood levels, effects	Monitor accordingly, anticipate need for cautious increase of lithium dose during combined therapy, interaction with caffeine, which is pharmacologically similar to theophylline, is not established fully

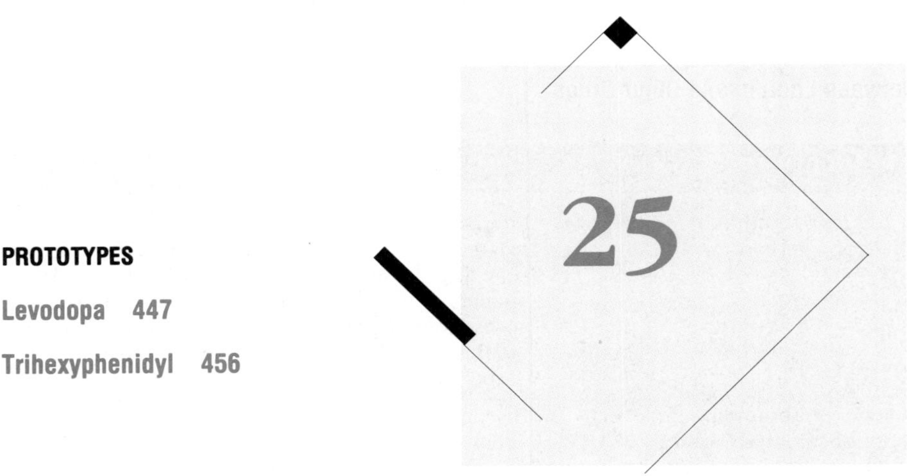

PROTOTYPES

25

Antiparkinson Agents

Parkinsonism is a progressive, chronic, degenerative disorder involving brain regions that control such activities as posture, balance, and locomotion. It afflicts over one million Americans. (The terms *Parkinson's disease, paralysis agitans,* and *shaking palsy* are traditionally used when the cause is unknown. This book uses the general term *parkinsonism* for all cases.) This chapter emphasizes drug therapy. The causes, symptoms, and diagnosis are summarized to help understand the basis for drug therapy. However, details about these topics, and nursing roles related to them, are beyond the scope of this book.

Causes of Parkinsonism

Many patients who develop parkinsonism are age 40 or older, so natural age-related processes may be involved, but the precise cause is not always known. That is, the disease is often *idiopathic.* Identifiable causes that are not age-related include brain disease or injury (tumors, trauma, encephalitis, cerebrovascular disease) and exposure to environmental toxins such as carbon monoxide or manganese. Drug-induced parkinsonism is relatively common, and is one of the most serious adverse responses to antipsychotic agents (Chapter 23). Several cases of severe, abrupt, and apparently irreversible parkinsonism have been traced to "designer drugs" that contain a neurotoxic contaminant, MPTP. Parkinsonism is not heritable or contagious.

The Biochemistry of Parkinsonism

Regardless of the cause, involuntary movement disorders seen in parkinsonism reflect an imbalance between inhibitory effects of the neurotransmitter dopamine and opposing stimulatory effects of acetylcholine (ACh) in the brain's extrapyramidal system and basal ganglia, such that the actions of ACh predominate (Fig. 25–1). In many cases, dopaminergic nerves degenerate or their neurotransmitter stores are depleted. In parkinsonism caused by antipsychotic drugs, dopaminergic neurons are normal, but dopamine receptors on target cells are pharmacologically blocked. (Recall that blockade of dopamine receptors accounts for the desired actions of antipsychotic drugs.)

Major reference tables appear beginning on p. 464.

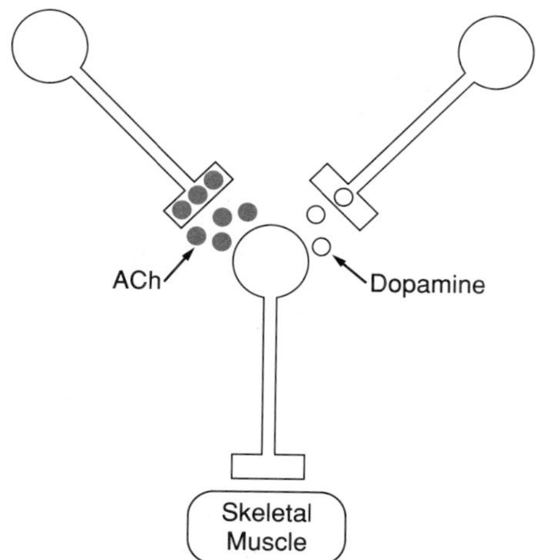

Drug Interventions

A. Dopaminergic
- –increase dopamine synthesis: *levodopa*
- –inhibit dopamine breakdown in nerves: *selegiline*
- –release more dopamine from nerves: *amantadine*
- –stimulate dopamine receptors directly with dopamine agonist: *bromocriptine*

B. Antimuscarinic
- –block muscarinic ACh receptors: *trihexyphenidyl*

Figure 25–1

Model of parkinsonism: biochemical basis and treatment approaches. Signs and symptoms reflect an imbalance between opposing effects of muscarinic and dopaminergic neurons in extrapyramidal system, which eventually controls involuntary skeletal muscle activity. It appears as if dopamine's effects are reduced. Most drug interventions affect the dopamine side in one way or another (prototypes shown in italics); alternatively, or adjunctively, centrally acting antimuscarinic drugs can be used to reduce effects of ACh.

Primary Symptoms

Early symptoms of parkinsonism include fatigue or muscle weakness. Initially, it may go unrecognized because the symptoms are not bothersome, or are so nonspecific that they could reflect many other disorders, or even excessive physical exertion. As the disorder progresses, three primary diagnostic symptoms develop: *rigidity, tremor,* and *bradykinesia.* Depending on the patient and the stage of parkinsonism, some primary symptoms may be apparent at rest. Others are induced or intensified by physical activity or procedures used in the neurologic assessment. The patient may be aware of some symptoms but not of others.

Rigidity involves increased muscle tone ("hypertonicity"). It occurs at rest, but increases when the muscles are moved. Extending the patient's arm, for example, reveals increasing resistance, sometimes smooth and sometimes ratchet-like ("cogwheel rigidity"), but not the sudden loss of resistance that occurs with spasticity. Rigidity of the back and neck muscles contributes to the stooped-over posture often seen in parkinsonism.

Tremor involves repetitive muscle activity that is best seen during rest. It usually begins in the hands and can be detected in about 75% of individuals with parkinsonism. Tremor can also affect muscles in the head and neck ("head bobbing" is common), tongue, and legs. Resting tremors are most responsive to treatment with the drugs noted in this chapter. Tremors brought on by activating maneuvers are more resistant to treatment.

Bradykinesias (literally, slow movements) present as difficulty in initiating and then stopping voluntary movements, and performing movements slowly. Bradykinesias or akinesias (lack of movement) also cause many normal movements to be absent. Patients appear as if they are apathetic and slow moving. Bradykinesias and akinesias are the most disabling of the primary symptoms.

The primary symptoms often make it difficult for patients to maintain their balance while standing or after changing position, and often affect gait (use of short, shuffling steps; lack of noticeable arm swing). These problems may cause the patient to fall. Other simple but essential activities of daily living also may become affected.

Secondary Symptoms

The primary symptoms cause or contribute to secondary physical symptoms that reflect impaired activity of other body muscle groups. Bradykinesia or rigidity of throat and mouth musculature can cause speech impairments, drooling, and dysphagia, eventually leading to eating impairments and problems such as weight loss, nutritional problems, and, especially in elderly patients, constipation. Altered thoracic muscle activity can impair

TRENDS AND CONTROVERSIES IN PHARMACOLOGY

Caring for the Elderly Patient with Parkinsonism

One of the unfortunate facts of pharmacologic treatment of elderly parkinsonian patients is that some symptoms are drug-resistant. For instance, imbalance and postural instability, bladder dysfunction, constipation, speech difficulties, and psychologic problems (all bothersome at any age) become major concerns in the elderly. Postural imbalance is the cause of many falls, and falls are an important cause of death in elderly patients. Constipation and bladder dysfunction are not uncommon problems among older people in general, but when muscle function is compromised by parkinsonism, what might be annoying to the "normal" older person can become a serious health problem. Drugs that increase bladder motility are often not helpful, and long-term use of laxatives raises other health concerns. Speech problems cause communication difficulties and may cause all but the most motivated caregiver "not to bother." Simply put, a number of parkinsonian symptoms can continue unabated even in "successful" treatment, and those symptoms are related to health and safety issues. Nurses should be aware and be prepared to intervene to help the patient compensate for lost abilities and functions.

"High tech without high touch" is a real problem for elderly patients with this illness. While physicians routinely rely upon drug therapy as their primary avenue for helping the parkinsonism patient, the patients themselves want and need more.Patients have led productive, meaningful lives, and may still be doing so when they first seek help for this illness. To become an object of pharmacologic "experimentation" is unsettling and a source of undignified irritation. Hence, working with elderly parkinsonism patients requires a sensitivity to psychosocial needs, a willingness to go beyond pharmacologic interventions, and an understanding that most of these patients are not suffering from significant cognitive disability (ie, they understand what is going on and should not be "talked down to"). Supporting dignity and respect are major nondrug health-care issues that must be incorporated into the care plan.

Clough CG. Parkinson's disease: Management. *Lancet* 1991; 337:1324-1327.

breathing; bladder involvement may cause urgency, frequency, prolonged urination, or dribbling; and lower extremity involvement may favor edema. Bradykinesias, rigidity, and tremor may also cause handwriting to become small (micrographia) and difficult to read. Many of these physical symptoms can be helped by antiparkinson drugs plus the adjunctive nondrug measures summarized on page 460.

Secondary emotional problems, ranging from embarrassment to severe depression, may occur before or in response to altered motor function. Depression contributes to altered sleep patterns and, in many patients, impaired sexual desire or performance. Depression, sometimes accompanied by anxiety or agitation, may become so severe that treating it is a greater priority than treating the motor dysfunction. Antidepressant drugs may alleviate some physical symptoms of parkinsonism, and antiparkinson drugs often alleviate depression. Behavior resembling senility may develop, especially in older patients with advanced parkinsonism, but it is not an inevitable outcome (see the box "Caring for the Elderly Person with Parkinsonism").

Diagnosis

Only a thorough neurologic examination, combined with a complete physical examination to detect other disorders that mimic parkinsonism, can confirm the diagnosis. Many rating scales that consider the location, kinds, and severity of physical symptoms, and the degree to which they affect daily living activities, are used in the evaluation. More definitive tests are being developed to detect parkinsonism in its early stages.

NURSING IMPLICATIONS

Assessment should include a thorough check of the drug history to help identify causes. It is essential to assess vital signs and look for evidence of the primary and secondary physical and emotional symptoms noted earlier. Symptoms affecting posture, gait, balance, facial expression, speech, and handwriting are particularly easy to assess. They should be evaluated as completely as possible during rest and activity with the various maneuvers described in other texts. Baseline assessment is

Table 25–1 | Antiparkinson Drug Summary

Drug	Stage of Disease	Major Mechanism of Action	Target Symptoms
Levodopa (DOPAR, LARODOPA)	All	Increases synthesis of dopamine in the brain	All
Carbidopa (in SINEMET)	All for which levodopa is used	Blocks peripheral conversion of levodopa; spares levodopa for conversion to dopamine in brain	As for levodopa
Amantadine (SYMMETREL)	Mild to moderate	Releases dopamine in CNS	All
Bromocriptine (PARLODEL)	All, but especially when high levodopa doses are needed	Directly stimulates dopamine receptors	All
Antimuscarinics	Mild to moderate; adjunctively with levodopa for advanced stages	Blocks acetylcholine receptors	Rigidity, tremors, and drooling
Selegiline (ELDEPRYL)	Used when response to levodopa-carbidopa begins to deteriorate	Inhibits MAO type B	All

Source: Adapted from *Parkinson's Disease Handbook*. New York, American Parkinson Disease Association.

essential for later assessment of the effects of drug therapy.

Treatment Rationale

Drug therapy attempts to restore the imbalance in the extrapyramidal system between dopamine and ACh (see Fig. 25–1). This is accomplished by administering drugs that either (1) increase the relative activity of dopamine (dopaminergic drugs) or (2) decrease the effects of ACh (antimuscarinic drugs) in the central nervous system (CNS). No drug cures the disease; antiparkinson drugs only relieve some of the major symptoms, and are best used with appropriate physical therapy and psychosocial support and counseling. A prototype drug in each group is discussed in detail. Table 25–1 summarizes the major drugs and their key properties.

NURSING IMPLICATIONS

Regardless of the drug or drugs used, any antiparkinson agent may beneficially affect some symptoms but worsen others. Understand that the effects of these drugs can mimic, cause, or worsen other physical or psychologic disorders, particularly those common in elderly individuals. Stress to the patient and family the importance of physical therapy and emotional support or counseling.

I. Dopaminergic Agents

Since parkinsonian symptoms are due to a relative deficiency of dopamine, dopamine itself would appear to be an ideal treatment. However, dopamine itself is *not* very effective. Alternative approaches are used, including administration of

- levodopa, the metabolic precursor of dopamine,
- amantadine, which releases dopamine from dopaminergic neurons,
- bromocriptine, which causes central dopamine-like agonist actions, or
- selegiline, which inhibits the metabolic inactivation of dopamine inside nerves.

All four drugs are orally effective.

PROTOTYPE

Levodopa

Levodopa (DOPAR, LARODOPA), the drug, is identical to the naturally occurring chemical dihydroxyphenylalanine (DOPA). DOPA is formed within the body from the dietary amino acids phenylalanine and tyrosine. Through the actions of the enzyme DOPA decarboxylase, DOPA is converted to dopamine as part of the natural catecholamine synthesis pathway. Dopamine, in

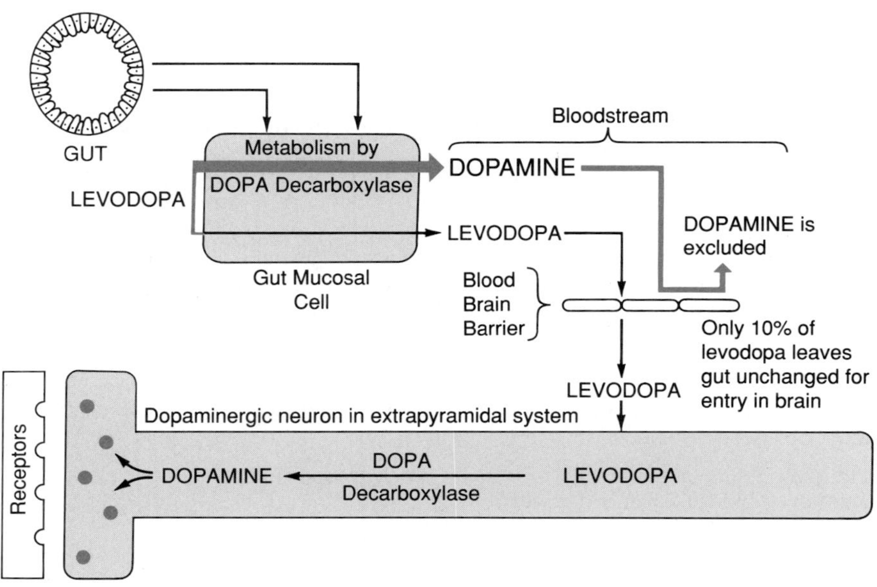

Figure 25–2

Fates of orally administered levodopa. Most levodopa (equivalent to DOPA, dihydroxyphenylalanine) is enzymatically converted in the periphery to dopamine. Dopamine cannot cross the blood–brain barrier to reach the desired target of antiparkinson action in the extrapyramidal system. The majority of the administered dose is ineffective. Increasing the levodopa dose to increase the amount that eventually reaches the CNS increases peripheral side effects.

turn, can be metabolized further to norepinephrine and epinephrine, mainly in peripheral adrenergic nerves and in the adrenal medulla.

Absorption, Distribution, Metabolism, and Excretion

Levodopa can be given orally. However, before it reaches the bloodstream about 90% of the drug is metabolized to dopamine in the gastrointestinal (GI) tract, which has an abundant supply of DOPA decarboxylase (Fig. 25–2). Dopamine does not cross the blood–brain barrier well, so the vast majority of administered levodopa is "wasted" by peripheral conversion to a chemical that cannot reach the CNS. Only a small amount of unchanged levodopa, about 10% of the administered dose, crosses the blood–brain barrier for eventual synthesis of dopamine. Unfortunately, this amount may be insufficient to cause therapeutic effects, especially if the patient has moderate or severe parkinsonian symptoms. This problem could be overcome by giving very large doses of levodopa, but that would also affect dopamine levels in the periphery, leading to significant sympathomimetic side effects. As noted later, the simultaneous use of carbidopa is a better way to overcome the problem.

Pharmacologic Effects

Levodopa entering the CNS is taken up by dopaminergic nerves and metabolized, through actions of DOPA decarboxylase, to dopamine. This often restores the dopamine–ACh imbalance and reduces symptoms.

Clinical Indications and Administration

Levodopa is used for all causes of parkinsonism except those that are drug-induced. It can be used for all stages of disease (mild to advanced), and favorably influences all major symptoms (see Table 25–1). To reduce the risk of side effects, the dosage (Table 25–C) must be individualized, and increases should be gradual.

Symptomatic relief of tremor and rigidity usually starts to develop in about 3 weeks, but some patients may experience a "lag period," with no significant improvement, lasting 3 to 6 months. Improved mood and a sense of well-being may be the first effects to appear. The optimal response to levodopa rarely lasts more than a few years. Thereafter, continued levodopa administration leads to large daily variations in the drug's ability to suppress symptoms of parkinsonism. Eventu-

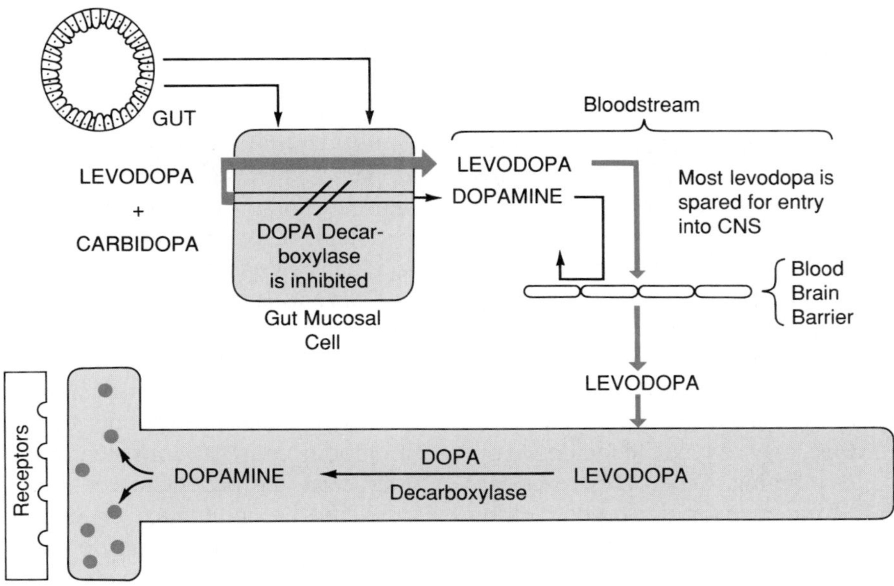

Figure 25–3

The effect of administering levodopa with carbidopa. Carbidopa, which is combined with levodopa in SINEMET, inhibits DOPA decarboxylase in the gut, thereby reducing peripheral conversion of levodopa to dopamine. More unmetabolized levodopa is spared for entry into the CNS, where it can exert its beneficial effects after being converted to dopamine. Vitamin B_6 (pyridoxine) does the opposite: it stimulates peripheral metabolism of levodopa, counteracts the therapeutic effect.

ally, a more general reduction in its effectiveness occurs. These problems are discussed later.

Levodopa plus Carbidopa

A relatively common way to enhance the therapeutic effects of levodopa without having to increase the dosage greatly is to administer it with carbidopa. Carbidopa alone has no beneficial effects in patients with parkinsonism. The drug inhibits DOPA decarboxylase in the GI tract (Fig. 25–3), thereby sparing a large amount of administered levodopa from metabolic conversion to dopamine before it can cross the blood–brain barrier. In the U.S., carbidopa is typically administered as part of a fixed-dose combination with levodopa, marketed as SINEMET. The product comes in several strengths (for example, SINEMET 10/100 contains 10 mg of carbidopa and 100 mg of levodopa) to help optimize therapy for each patient. Tablets of different strengths can be used to adjust the dosage further. The correct dose of SINEMET should contain only about 25% of the amount of plain levodopa administered the previous day. SINEMET may control parkinsonian symptoms better and with lower doses of levodopa than would otherwise be needed. A carbidopa-only product (LODOSYN) is available directly from the manufacturer for those few patients who require individual titration.

NURSING IMPLICATIONS

Advise patients and their families about levodopa's delayed onset of action. Stress the need for patients to resume daily activities as soon as possible, but to do so gradually and as permitted by their overall physical condition and drug-induced side effects. If the patient is to be switched from plain levodopa to SINEMET, discontinue the levodopa at least 8 hours before starting SINEMET. This will help avoid or minimize sudden and intense effects caused by increased peripheral dopamine levels.

Side Effects, Adverse Reactions, and Contraindications

Levodopa and the other dopaminergic agents cause not only similar therapeutic effects, but also many similar central and peripheral side effects and adverse responses. Common features are discussed here and summarized in Table 25–S. Untoward responses unique to individual agents are noted separately.

The side effects and adverse reactions to levodopa are caused both by the drug itself and by its initial conversion to dopamine and further metabolism to norepinephrine and epinephrine. Nausea and vomiting are among the most common untoward responses. They are due in part to direct drug effects on the GI tract, although dopamine's ability to stimulate the brain's chemoreceptor trigger zone is important. Anorexia may develop for the same reason. Although most patients taking levodopa develop these responses early in therapy, tolerance usually occurs after several weeks. Concurrent administration of carbidopa, by allowing a reduced dose of levodopa, may reduce the incidence or severity of nausea and vomiting. Other CNS reactions include choreiform movements (rapid, irregular, jerky involuntary movements), ataxia, hand tremors, insomnia, nightmares, anxiety, agitation, suicidal depression, or psychosis. (As noted in the previous chapter, increased activity of dopamine in parts of the CNS is thought to be a major contributor to the development of schizophrenia. This may explain why dopaminergic drugs may cause or worsen psychotic behavior if they are given to someone with a history of similar mental disorders.) Some of these adverse responses, particularly the involuntary movements, are likely to occur in most patients taking levodopa for a year or so.

Peripheral side effects caused by levodopa or its metabolite, dopamine, are also important and relatively common. The major cardiovascular side effect is hypotension (usually orthostatic), owing to peripheral vasodilation. This, in turn, may cause headache, dizziness, syncope, and reflex tachycardia. Dopamine stimulates the heart directly. Tolerance usually develops to orthostatic hypotension. The cardiovascular effects necessitate caution when administering these drugs to patients with a history of myocardial infarction, ischemic heart disease, arrhythmias, or hyperthyroidism. Pheochromocytoma is an important contraindication because dopamine, formed from levodopa, acts as a mixed-acting sympathomimetic. As such, it can release massive amounts of catecholamines from the tumor, which could cause a serious or fatal hypertensive crisis.

Bizarre breathing patterns, somehow caused by levodopa, may contribute to respiratory problems. Dopaminergic drugs cause mydriasis and so are contraindicated in patients with narrow-angle glaucoma. Gastrointestinal side effects include dry mouth, dysphagia, and constipation, and an increased risk of GI bleeding in patients with peptic ulcer disease (also a relative contraindication). Any dopaminergic drug can cause urinary retention or hesitancy. Levodopa (and SINEMET) can discolor and darken the urine, sweat, or saliva.

A most serious response, caused by abrupt discontinuation of levodopa therapy, is the *neuroleptic malignant syndrome*. It is due to a rapid fall in brain dopamine levels and is characterized by high fever and muscle rigidity (parkinsonian crisis). To minimize this problem, levodopa doses should always be reduced gradually when possible.

Levodopa may increase levels of blood urea nitrogen (BUN), lactate dehydrogenase (LDH), transaminases (AST, ALT), bilirubin, and alkaline phosphatase, reflecting renal or hepatic damage. The drug may reduce white blood cell counts, hematocrit, and blood hemoglobin content. Consistently low white cell counts may make the patient susceptible to infection, and necessitate discontinuance of levodopa. Levodopa interferes with several diagnostic tests. It may give falsely high levels of plasma protein-bound iodine, plasma or urinary uric acid, and urinary protein; depending on the test used, urinary glucose or catecholamine metabolite tests may be falsely positive or negative.

NURSING IMPLICATIONS

Monitoring for side effects and alterations of laboratory test results is as important as assessing for desired drug effects. Advise patients about the side effects that are most likely to occur, and those likely to diminish as tolerance develops. Instruct them to notify the physician if side effects become severe or do not decline with time, which may necessitate reducing the dose or discontinuing the drug. Patients with a history of cardiovascular diseases or hyperthyroidism should be monitored closely for blood pressure changes and heart rate or rhythm disturbances. It is best to monitor the electrocardiogram (ECG) when therapy is started in a high-risk patient. All patients should be instructed to report at once palpitations, irregular pulses, dizziness (especially upon standing), and other undesirable changes. Patients who experience lightheadedness should be advised to stand slowly and support themselves as needed to guard against a fall. Inpatients may require assistance with walking. Elastic support stockings may help reduce postural changes of blood pressure.

Blurred vision, combined with hypotension, dizziness, tremor, confusion, or faintness, can become dangers for such normal tasks as walking and standing, and great risks if the patient attempts to operate a motor vehicle or machinery. Recommend that outpatients modify their environment to remove hazards such as throw rugs and poor lighting, and to avoid tasks that require good vision, coordination, and mental clearness. Recommend sunglasses to relieve discomfort from photophobia. Patients with open-angle glaucoma may receive levodopa, but periodic assessment is necessary; pretreatment screening for glaucoma is advised for elderly patients. All patients should be instructed to report sudden eye pain at once, since it may indicate an acute glaucoma attack.

Levodopa is best taken between meals, but may be taken with meals to alleviate GI upset and nausea. However, food (particularly protein-rich food) can significantly interfere with levodopa absorption. Inquire about abdominal pain, and assess for evidence of blood in the stool (tests for occult blood; black, tarry stools). Instruct patients to report any sign of potential peptic ulcer disease or urinary retention to the physician at once.

Pay particular attention to patients' eating habits and nutritional status, especially during early therapy. Although antiparkinson drugs may improve appetite by alleviating anorexia, depression, or dysphagia, other drug-induced problems (dry mouth or nausea) may counteract the benefits. Dry mouth, dysphagia, and related problems are best handled by recommending the use of hard, sugarless candies, or frequent sips of water. Advise patients that discoloration of the urine or secretions is no cause for concern.

Assess mental status and behavior periodically to guard against the development or worsening of psychosis or depression. If involuntary movement disorders occur the patient should be thoroughly evaluated at once by the physician to determine whether they reflect worsening of parkinsonism, are drug-induced, or are the result of abrupt discontinuation of therapy.

◆ Use During Pregnancy and Lactation

The safety of levodopa (or SINEMET) in pregnant women has not been established. Use is recommended only when potential benefits outweigh potential dangers to the mother and child. Breastfeeding should be discouraged during therapy with any antiparkinson drug.

◆ Use in Children

The safety of levodopa or other antiparkinson drugs for children under the age of 12 years has not been established.

◆ Use in the Elderly

The elderly are not only more likely to require antiparkinson treatment, but also are more likely to have other conditions that contraindicate or complicate therapy, to be taking interacting drugs, and to be less tolerant of most drug-induced side effects and adverse responses.

Problems Associated with Long-Term Levodopa Use

Although levodopa effectively controls tremor, rigidity, and bradykinesias, after several years of successful and continuous therapy about half of treated patients develop other major problems.

1. Abnormal involuntary movements (dyskinesias).
2. *End of dose failure.* As therapy continues, the length of time during which a given dose of levodopa controls symptoms progressively decreases, and symptoms recur before the next scheduled dose is taken. This problem can be alleviated somewhat by administering the daily dose in smaller increments more frequently during the day, but eventually this approach also fails. Increasing the daily dose may hasten the development of abnormal involuntary movements and the appearance of the "on-off phenomenon."
3. *On-off phenomenon.* Large fluctuations in the control of parkinsonian symptoms develop from day to day or even during a given day. The patient may be relatively symptom-free for several hours, and then develop severe involuntary movements, drooling, or other symptoms within a matter of minutes, lasting for up to a few hours. The phenomenon may be triggered by emotional stress or may be related to fluctuations in levodopa or dopamine levels in the blood or brain. As with end-of-dose failure, more frequent administration of levodopa is usually helpful, but only temporarily.
4. *Secondary levodopa failure.* After 2 to 5 years of levodopa treatment, its overall effectiveness may be lost, as evidenced by poor control of tremor, rigidity, and bradykinesias. Although better control could be regained by increasing the dose, this also increases the risk of side effects or adverse responses.

When one or more of these problems develop, adjunctive drugs such as bromocriptine usually must be added to the treatment plan.

NURSING IMPLICATIONS

Careful assessment of the patient who has been taking levodopa for several years can help distinguish between worsening of symptoms caused by disease progression and characteristic loss of drug effectiveness. Try to determine whether symptom control is lost gradually or abruptly, when symptoms appear in relation to the next dose, and whether they are triggered or worsened by external factors such as physical or emotional stress. Persons responsible for the patient's care should be consulted to help obtain this information, and should be encouraged to keep a daily log of the patient's responses, especially if drug effectiveness seems to be diminishing.

Interactions with Other Drugs

Interactions between levodopa and other drugs are summarized in Table 25–I. They apply whether levodopa is administered with or without carbidopa. The most serious interactions involve monoamine oxidase (MAO) inhibitors—those used to treat depression (Chapter 24), and selegiline, which is indicated for parkinsonism (see below). The potential outcome of the interaction is an acute hypertensive episode, and possibly a stroke. It occurs because dopamine can release large amounts of norepinephrine from peripheral adrenergic nerves.

Vitamin B_6 (pyridoxine) is another important interactant. The actions of this vitamin are essentially the opposite of those of carbidopa: it stimulates the enzyme DOPA decarboxylase in the gut, thereby stimulating the peripheral conversion of levodopa to dopamine. In doing so it reduces the amount of unmetabolized levodopa that can enter the CNS; the antiparkinson effects of levodopa are reduced. Vitamin B_6 is found naturally in many foods (avocados, lentils, lima beans), it is found in vitamin-supplemented foods (eg, breakfast cereals), and is a common ingredient in multivitamin supplements. The amounts of vitamin B_6 in any of these sources may be enough to counteract good control of parkinsonian symptoms. Results of the interaction may appear quickly.

Simultaneous administration of phenytoin, a common anticonvulsant (Chapter 26), can also counteract levodopa's effects. The cause of the interaction is not known.

NURSING IMPLICATIONS

Interactions between levodopa and prescription drugs can be avoided or recognized by obtaining a complete medication history, by providing patients with written lists of drugs or foods to avoid, and by assessing for pertinent and expected signs of interactions so that therapy can be modified as needed. The dangerous interaction with MAO inhibitors must be avoided. Problems involving vitamin B_6 may be more difficult to avoid. Eating habits and nutritional status may be impaired enough to require intervention, whether by a physician or by a patient who self-prescribes vitamin supplements. Instruct patients specifically against taking medications or foods supplemented with B_6. The pyridoxine-free vitamin supplement LAROBEC, formulated specifically for patients taking levodopa, should be used instead.

Overdose and Toxicity

Levodopa overdoses can cause any of the adverse responses already discussed. Blepharospasm (spasmodic twitching of the eyelids) and peripheral muscle twitching may be early signs of toxicity. Hypotension and cardiac arrhythmias are likely to be the most dangerous manifestations of toxicity, and may need therapy with appropriate drugs or parenteral fluids. The ECG and pertinent vital signs must be monitored continuously and corrected as needed until the patient's condition improves and stabilizes. Standard first-aid interventions to reduce drug absorption (see Appendix C) are used during initial treatment of overdoses.

Other Dopaminergic Drugs

Amantadine

Amantadine (SYMMETREL) is an antiviral drug that is useful in parkinsonism. Although it is less effective than levodopa when used alone, it is often the first drug prescribed for mild parkinsonism. Unlike levodopa, amantadine is useful for managing drug-induced parkinsonism.

Absorption, Distribution, Metabolism, and Excretion

Amantadine is absorbed well from the GI tract. Peak plasma levels occur about 4 hours after administration, and the half-life is 18 to 24 hours. Amantadine is eliminated by renal excretion without prior metabolism. Acidifying the urine hastens its elimination.

NURSING IMPLICATIONS

Renal function should be assessed before starting amantadine therapy and periodically thereafter. Impaired renal function may require reduced dosages.

Pharmacologic Effects

Amantadine alleviates parkinsonian symptoms by releasing dopamine from CNS neurons that have not yet degenerated. It may also slow the reuptake of released dopamine into nerves, thus intensifying stimulation of postsynaptic cells. Since its effectiveness depends on residual dopamine, amantadine is less effective in advanced stages of parkinsonism. Its effectiveness can be improved by concurrent administration of levodopa, which increases brain dopamine levels. Amantadine causes some antimuscarinic effects, and they contribute to its beneficial actions.

Clinical Indications and Administration

Amantadine is used as an antiviral drug to treat or prevent influenza A infections (Chapter 57). It can be used as the sole drug treatment for parkinsonism, or it can be used in combination with other drugs, particularly levodopa. It is effective for most cases of parkinsonism, including those that are drug-induced. Amantadine can alleviate all major symptoms (see Table 25–1). The usual daily dose is 200 mg (see Table 25–C). Patients with idiopathic Parkinson's disease may need higher doses than patients with drug-induced parkinsonism. Combining amantadine with other antiparkinson drugs usually hastens and improves therapeutic effectiveness at reduced doses of each agent, thereby reducing the risk or severity of side effects from each agent. With levodopa in particular, combined treatment dramatically shortens the onset of symptomatic relief, from weeks or months with levodopa alone to only a few days. When amantadine is added to the therapy of patients already taking levodopa, it appears to level daily fluctuations in the response, and it may restore levodopa's effectiveness in patients who require reduced doses because of side effects. Amantadine therapy should never be discontinued abruptly, since acute worsening of symptoms or an acute parkinsonian crisis may result.

NURSING IMPLICATIONS

Question orders for large amantadine doses when the drug is added to therapy with other antiparkinson drugs, or when initial therapy involves two agents. Monitor responses to amantadine closely, and assess for a return or worsening of extrapyramidal symptoms after a few months of therapy, which requires further evaluation by the physician and possible dosage adjustments or the use of other drugs. Be aware that discontinuing amantadine therapy for several weeks may restore the drug's effectiveness; however, this should be done gradually. Stress the need for patients to continue taking the drug as directed. Inquire about difficulty swallowing the amantadine capsules, which are large. If this occurs, amantadine syrup may be substituted. Give divided doses when the total daily dose is 300 mg or more.

Side Effects, Adverse Reactions, and Contraindications

Drowsiness and confusion are the most common central side effects of amantadine (see Table 25–S). More serious responses include frank depression and possible psychosis (delusions, hallucinations). Amantadine lowers the brain's seizure threshold and may cause seizures in patients with a history of seizures. Peripheral side effects include blurred vision (which complicates problems owing to drowsiness or confusion), orthostatic hypotension, and urinary retention. The drug has been reported to cause or worsen congestive heart failure.

A unique side effect of amantadine is *livedo reticularis,* a dermatologic reaction in which the skin becomes mottled and purple-colored, and localized edema develops. Livedo reticularis is more noticeable when the patient is standing or exposed to cold. It is reversible within 2 to 6 weeks after discontinuation of amantadine, but ceasing amantadine therapy generally is not necessary. The only absolute contraindication to amantadine use is allergy or hypersensitivity to it.

NURSING IMPLICATIONS

Orthostatic hypotension, combined with amantadine's unpredictable effectiveness, necessitates instructing the patient to resume normal activities gradually and carefully. In addition to the precautions noted for levodopa, also observe for signs of peripheral edema, livedo reticularis, and signs of generalized edema or dyspnea that could indicate congestive heart failure. These changes, as well as any indication of a lowered seizure threshold, should be reported to the physician at once.

Interactions with Other Drugs

Amantadine participates in one general interaction (see Table 25–I): It potentiates the atropine-like actions of other drugs with antimuscarinic properties, including other antimuscarinic–antiparkinson drugs and antipsychotics. (Theoretically, the interaction is less likely to be severe with antipsychotics such as haloperidol, which has minimal antimuscarinic activity, than with drugs such as chlorpromazine.) The interaction could lead to a syndrome of antimuscarinic poisoning (pp 178–179). Reducing the dose of either interactant usually reduces the incidence and severity of the problems.

NURSING IMPLICATIONS

None of the interactions must be avoided; however, increased vigilance is required in elderly patients, who are less tolerant of their results, or when the interaction involves other drugs with atropine-like activity. Specifically advise patients not to take over-the-counter (OTC) drugs with atropine-like activity (including antihistamines and most other cough, cold, and allergy remedies) unless approved by their physician.

Overdose and Toxicity

Symptoms of amantadine overdose include acute urinary retention, arrhythmias, hypotension, hyperactivity, seizures, or acute toxic psychosis (disorientation, confusion, and visual hallucinations, which may develop early). Standard first-aid measures to reduce further drug absorption are appropriate (see Appendix C) as permitted by the patient's condition. If the patient has good cardiac and renal status, force large amounts of orally administered fluid; IV fluid administration may be necessary. Urinary acidification with drugs such as ammonium chloride to hasten renal excretion of amantadine is controversial. Since amantadine depends on renal elimination, but urinary retention may occur, bladder catheterization may be required. No specific antidote to amantadine exists, but physostigmine, the drug of choice for treating atropine poisoning, has been reported to reverse many adverse CNS responses to overdoses. Anticonvulsant, antiarrhythmic, or vasopressor drugs may be given as needed.

Bromocriptine

Bromocriptine (PARLODEL) is a dopaminergic drug with interesting uses in neurology and endocrinology.

Absorption, Distribution, Metabolism, and Excretion

Bromocriptine is not absorbed well from the GI tract, but therapeutic blood levels can be reached with continued administration. Most of the absorbed drug is metabolized in the liver, and the metabolites are excreted in the feces.

Pharmacologic Effects

Bromocriptine acts as a dopamine-like agonist to stimulate dopamine receptors directly, particularly in the pituitary gland and extrapyramidal system. Unlike the drugs discussed so far, it neither stimulates dopamine synthesis nor causes dopamine release.

Relatively low blood concentrations of bromocriptine mimic the effects of dopamine to inhibit prolactin release from the anterior pituitary gland. Bromocriptine does not significantly affect pituitary release of other hormones in normal individuals, but it dramatically lowers blood levels of growth hormone in patients with acromegaly. Higher blood levels of bromocriptine stimulate dopaminergic receptors in the substantia nigra, and in doing so may help correct the dopamine–ACh imbalance in parkinsonism.

Clinical Indications and Administration

The prolactin-reducing actions of bromocriptine are used clinically to treat amenorrhea, galactorrhea, and female infertility, and to suppress lactation. It is also used to manage acromegaly caused by pituitary tumors. These uses are discussed in Chapter 44.

When used for parkinsonism, the drug alleviates the major symptoms (see Table 25–1). It is often used adjunctively with levodopa, particularly when high doses of levodopa are needed, when side effects such as dyskinesias develop, or when levodopa loses its effectiveness. Bromocriptine smooths the daily response to levodopa, and reduces the severity of the "on-off" and "end-of-dose" phenomena. To reduce the risk of side effects and adverse responses, bromocriptine doses must be started as low as possible (see Table 25–C). The dose can be increased at 2- to 4-week intervals if needed. Assessment should be performed at least biweekly during early therapy. If the patient is already taking levodopa, the levodopa dose should not be changed for 2 to 4 weeks after starting bromocriptine.

Bromocriptine has been used to treat neuroleptic malignant syndrome. This is not an approved indication.

Side Effects, Adverse Reactions, and Contraindications

Bromocriptine produces or intensifies many side effects noted for levodopa (see Table 25–S). Hypotension is common. For example, about 30% of patients receiving relatively low doses of bromocriptine for postpartum suppression of lactation experience hypotension severe enough to cause dizziness or fainting; doses used for parkinsonism are generally much higher. Therefore, the drug should not be given to patients with unstable blood pressure or cardiac function, and should be used cautiously (if at all) if the patient has any form of ischemic vascular disease.

Bromocriptine may cause such mental disturbances as anxiety, depression, confusion, or hallucinations. Interference with daytime activities can be reduced by taking the drug at night or by reducing the dose. Nevertheless, problems may be so severe or persistent that complete discontinuation of bromocriptine use is necessary. Long-term treatment (6 to 36 months) has been associated with pulmonary problems (infiltration, effusion) that slowly resolve after drug withdrawal.

By lowering serum prolactin levels bromocriptine may mask signs of a pituitary tumor. Therefore, it should be used cautiously, and only after a thorough diagnostic work-up, if a tumor is suspected. The drug is contraindicated during pregnancy. Although this contraindication applies to all other antiparkinson drugs, it is particularly relevant to bromocriptine, which increases fertility and the chance of conception. Bromocriptine is chemically related to some of the ergot alkaloids (Chapter 15), and should not be administered to individuals for whom ergot drugs are contraindicated.

NURSING IMPLICATIONS

Precautions noted for levodopa apply also to bromocriptine. If side effects are caught early enough, reducing the bromocriptine dose may be all that is needed. Strongly advise women to avoid conception during therapy. Bromocriptine interferes with the effectiveness of oral contraceptives, so the nurse should provide counseling about effective alternative methods. Instruct women to advise their physician at once if they suspect pregnancy. Bromocriptine should not be given postpartum to women who are undecided about whether to breast-feed their infant, because lactation may be suppressed until the next pregnancy.

Interactions with Other Drugs

Drug interactions that involve bromocriptine (Table 25–I) generally are mild and not clinically significant as long as the prescriber is aware of them and modifies dosages of one or more of the interactants accordingly. Combined use of bromocriptine with other antihypertensive drugs can cause excessive hypotension. Bromocriptine and antipsychotic drugs may interact to reduce each other's therapeutic effects (since bromocriptine stimulates dopamine receptors and antipsychotics block them). There is also some evidence that this antiparkinson drug, owing to its endocrine effects, can antagonize the effects of oral contraceptives. Since pregnancy contraindicates bromocriptine use, additional or other contraceptive measures should be used.

Overdose and Toxicity

Bromocriptine overdoses intensify the adverse reactions already discussed. There is no specific antidote. Treatment involves symptomatic, supportive care and immediate discontinuation of drug administration.

Pergolide

Pergolide (PERMAX) is a newer dopamine receptor agonist. It is pharmacologically similar to bromocriptine in most respects, and is 10 to 1000 times more potent. It is used as an adjunct to levodopa and carbidopa, tending to reduce the fluctuating response that often develops with levodopa. Hypotension (especially orthostatic) and a variety of CNS disturbances (including hallucinations) are among the more common and potentially dangerous side effects of this drug.

Selegiline

Selegiline (ELDEPRYL) has a mechanism of action that differs from all the other dopaminergic antiparkinson drugs. At therapeutic doses (see Table 25–C) it acts as a selective inhibitor of the brain form of monoamine oxidase (MAO-B). Through this action it inhibits metabolic inactivation of dopamine in dopamine-containing neurons, and increases the amount of dopamine available for release and activation of target neurons in the extrapyramidal system. The drug's metabolites, amphetamine and methamphetamine, may also contribute to the relief of some parkinsonian symptoms. These drug effects are thought to relieve symptoms of parkinsonism. However, other properties of the drug may actually halt the progression of the disease, causing a protective effect against further degeneration. If this proves true, selegiline or other drugs like it may offer a considerable therapeutic advantage over alternative agents that clearly do little beyond reducing symptoms.

Selegiline is used as an adjunct to levodopa and carbidopa, particularly in patients who have responded poorly to the latter drugs. The drug has not proven to be effective when used as the sole agent for treating parkinsonism.

Nausea, dizziness, lightheadedness, and fainting are the most common side effects. Otherwise, the side-effect profile is similar to that of levodopa.

When selegiline is administered at doses above the recommended 10 mg per day maximum, the drug appears to lose its selectivity for inhibiting MAO-B. Thus, it can act nonselectively and also inhibit the other major form of MAO (MAO-A), which is found in the gut and peripheral sympathetic nervous system (see Chapter 24, which discusses the use of nonselective MAO inhibitors—isocarboxazid, phenelzine, and tranylcypromine—as antidepressants). Consequences of this dose-related, generalized MAO inhibition include a greater incidence of hypotension (Table 24–I2), and a much greater risk of potentially serious or life-threatening acute hypertensive responses owing to interactions with mixed- and indirect-acting sympathomimetics, including levodopa and dietary tyramine (Table 24–4). Patients being treated with selegiline should not receive meperidine if a narcotic analgesic must be given.

Overdoses of selegiline are likely to present in the same way as those of nonspecific MAO inhibitors, and are treated in the same way.

NURSING IMPLICATIONS

Although selegiline acts mainly as an MAO inhibitor in the brain when therapeutic doses are given, assume that the drug has the potential to inhibit MAO throughout the body. Assume that all nursing implications noted for side effects and drug–drug interactions noted for the MAO inhibitor-antidepressants apply to this antiparkinson drug. See Chapter 24 for more information.

II. Centrally Acting Antimuscarinic Agents

Synthetic antimuscarinic (atropine-like) drugs with relatively high activity in the CNS are used more often than dopaminergic drugs for initial treatment of early parkinsonism and for drug-induced extrapyramidal reactions. These agents help restore the brain's dopamine–ACh imbalance in a manner different from those of the drugs discussed so far.

PROTOTYPE

Trihexyphenidyl

Absorption, Distribution, Metabolism, and Excretion

Trihexyphenidyl and the related drugs are usually given orally. They have a duration of action of 4 to 6 hours, and are excreted by the kidneys.

Pharmacologic Effects

Trihexyphenidyl and related antimuscarinic drugs act in the brain to inhibit the actions of ACh on key excitatory nerve pathways. They do so by competitively blocking the ability of ACh to stimulate its receptors. They may also inhibit reuptake and storage of dopamine into dopaminergic nerves. Both effects restore the dopamine–ACh balance and reduce parkinsonian signs and symptoms. Trihexyphenidyl is effective regardless of whether symptoms are caused by disease (degeneration of dopaminergic nerves) or drugs. Although trihexyphenidyl and related drugs are classified as centrally acting, they can produce all of the peripheral antimuscarinic effects noted for atropine (Chapter 13).

Clinical Indications and Administration

Trihexyphenidyl (ARTANE) can be used alone as a starting drug for treating early, mild parkinsonism. More often, it is added later as an adjunct to dopaminergic drugs, particularly levodopa, for moderate to advanced symptoms. As with other antiparkinson drug combinations, this approach often provides better control with lower doses and fewer side effects from each. Nevertheless, side effects are very troublesome for some patients, and appropriate dosages are not always achieved easily. Trihexyphenidyl can also be used to prevent or treat extrapyramidal reactions caused by antipsychotic drugs. Regardless of the indication, therapy should be started with low doses that are increased gradually to minimize adverse reactions. These drugs usually alleviate rigidity and tremor well, but they are not very effective for alleviating bradykinesias and problems of balance or walking. Dosage schedules are summarized in Table 25–C. The drug is available as immediate-acting tablets, an elixir, or as a sustained-release preparation (ARTANE SEQUELS).

Parkinsonism

Whether trihexyphenidyl is used as initial treatment or is added to other therapy, the usual starting dose is 1 mg per day of an immediate-acting preparation. Gradual increases can be made every 3 to 5 days, based on the response. The usual daily dose is 3 to 6 mg. When added to levodopa therapy, the daily dose of each drug may eventually need to be reduced.

Drug-Induced Extrapyramidal Reactions

When trihexyphenidyl is used to treat extrapyramidal side effects, as caused by antipsychotic drugs, the same initial dose (1 mg) is used, but doses can be increased by 1 mg every few hours, up to a maximum of 15 mg per day. The dosage of the offending antipsychotic drug should be reduced or the drug should be temporarily withheld when starting trihexyphenidyl treatment. It may be possible to discontinue trihexyphenidyl after the extrapyramidal reactions have been controlled. Oral trihexyphenidyl does not act rapidly enough to control acute dystonic reactions such as oculogyric crisis or severe torticollis. These situations may require parenteral administration of benztropine or biperiden (see later section on related drugs).

NURSING IMPLICATIONS

Daily trihexyphenidyl maintenance doses of 10 mg or more may be divided and given four times a day, with meals and at bedtime, to decrease adverse reactions and daytime drowsiness. ARTANE SEQUELS, indicated only for maintenance therapy, can be substituted on a milligram-for-milligram basis for regular trihexyphenidyl tablets or elixir and given once daily or every 12 hours as needed. If patients have difficulty swallowing trihexyphenidyl tablets or elixir and given once or every 12 hours as needed. If patients have difficulty swallowing trihexyphenidyl tablets or SEQUELS, notify the physician and suggest that they be switched to the elixir.

Regardless of the indication for a centrally acting antimuscarinic, frequent nursing assessment is necessary to guide therapy. If one of these drugs is used to treat acute untoward reactions to antipsychotic drugs, the desired antipsychotic actions may be inhibited or lost. Dose adjustments, through careful nursing assessment, can reduce this risk.

Controversies About Antimuscarinic Prophylaxis of Drug-Induced Extrapyramidal Side Effects

There is little argument about using centrally acting antimuscarinics to treat extrapyramidal side effects caused by antipsychotic drugs. However, their prophylactic use is controversial.

Several arguments are used to support prophylactic use.

1. Antiparkinson agents are particularly effective for preventing drug-induced akinesias, which often are not detected early enough or are misdiagnosed as listlessness related to underlying mental illness. Prophylactic use would save the patient from being the victim of poor assessment skills.
2. Antiparkinson agents would prevent frightening acute dystonic reactions.
3. Since extrapyramidal reactions are a major reason for noncompliance with antipsychotic drug therapy, prophylactic use of antiparkinson drugs would facilitate compliance.

There are also several arguments against prophylactic use.

1. Only a few patients (5%–15%) develop extrapyramidal reactions.
2. Antiparkinson drugs cause additional side effects, some of which may be dangerous or annoying enough to cause noncompliance.
3. Antiparkinson drugs mask the development of tardive dyskinesias which, if not detected and treated early enough, may be irreversible and devastating.
4. Antiparkinson drugs are an extra cost to the patient or the insurer.

Most psychiatrists believe that the disadvantages or risks of prophylactic antimuscarinic therapy usually outweigh the advantages, and so do not prescribe these agents in this way. Teenage males are an exception. They have a very high rate of drug-induced extrapyramidal reactions, and centrally acting antimuscarinics are often given prophylactically to this group.

NURSING IMPLICATIONS

Correct assessment of the psychotic patient is imperative to help make the proper diagnosis, thereby aiding use of the proper drug and avoidance of an inappropriate one. For example, acute dystonic disorders that are treatable with centrally acting antimuscarinics can be mistaken for some bizarre psychotic manifestation for which an antipsychotic drug might be indicated. Since very high daily doses of centrally acting antimuscarinics may be ordered initially for acute drug-induced reactions, be sure to verify the order if there is doubt about either the dose or the diagnosis.

Side Effects, Adverse Reactions, and Contraindications

Compared with other antiparkinson drugs, antimuscarinics are most likely to cause distressing and potentially dangerous side effects. The "central" action of trihexyphenidyl and related drugs is only relative, so all side effects caused by atropine, and the related contraindications and nursing implications, apply (see Table 13–S). Only those of particular relevance to the parkinsonian or psychiatric patient are emphasized here.

Side effects involving the CNS can cause psychiatric disturbances such as marked confusion, agitation, or disturbed behavior, particularly in patients with cerebral atherosclerosis (one cause of parkinsonism) or idiosyncratic reactions to other centrally acting drugs. Memory loss (often misdiagnosed as senility in the elderly patient) may occur in schizophrenic patients treated with trihexyphenidyl. Muscle weakness, drowsiness, delusions, and hallucinations can occur. Trihexyphenidyl often produces euphoria or improved mood, which may be desirable for some parkinsonian patients but not for those in whom agitation or uneasiness occurs. (In contrast, benztropine often produces sedation that may benefit some patients but be undesirable for others.)

Common peripheral atropine-like side effects occur in 30% to 50% of patients taking trihexyphenidyl. In addition to the drug itself, factors such as age, altered diet, and diminished physical activity—more prevalent in persons being treated for parkinsonism or drug-induced extrapyramidal reactions than in other individuals—contribute to their increased incidence and severity. For example, diminished food intake and physical activity increase the risk of constipation or paralytic ileus; there is an increased risk of urinary retention, especially in elderly males; and the risk of an acute glaucoma attack is greater in the elderly, as is the risk of confusion or falls. In contrast, decreased salivary secretions that are generally considered undesirable in most other instances may be beneficial for parkinsonian patients. Hypotension and skin rashes may occur, but they are not common. Some side effects often diminish with continued therapy, but others may require reducing the dosage.

NURSING IMPLICATIONS

All nursing implications noted for atropine apply to trihexyphenidyl and related drugs (see Chapter 13, pp 180–181). In addition to careful assessment of physical responses, mental status should be assessed frequently and carefully. Increasing antimuscarinic doses slowly helps minimize side effects. If common problems such as blurred vision, dry mouth, constipation, and bladder problems occur, try to relieve them with nondrug measures. Some side effects simply require reassuring the patient, and having the patient take necessary precautions, limit certain activities, and wait for tolerance to develop. Be aware that significant constipation, urinary retention, or eye pain may indicate serious underlying problems that require prompt evaluation by a physician. Psychiatric disturbances also require immediate notification. Often, problems can be resolved by discontinuing the offending drug for a few days and then resuming treatment at a lower dose.

Interactions with Other Drugs

Trihexyphenidyl and the other centrally acting antimuscarinic drugs can interact with any other antimuscarinic agents (prescription or OTC; Table 24–I) that might be administered also. The outcome varies. However, it usually involves increased and potentially distressing (or dangerous) atropine-like side effects, owing to additive actions of these drugs in the CNS and in the peripheral autonomic nervous system. When the interactant is an antipsychotic drug (eg, haloperidol, chlorpromazine, or other phenothiazines), the outcome can also include antagonism of the antipsychotic drug's therapeutic effects, actual worsening of schizophrenia symptoms, and the potential development of tardive dyskinesias (especially with haloperidol). Signs and symptoms of these interactions may take several days to appear after combined therapy is started.

The sedative effects of centrally acting antimuscarinics are intensified by alcohol and other general CNS depressants. If combined administration is necessary, frequent assessment is essential. Antacids and antidiarrheal drugs decrease the absorption and effectiveness of trihexyphenidyl and related drugs given orally.

NURSING IMPLICATIONS

Obtaining a careful history will help avoid or predict drug interactions. It is equally important to educate patients about prescription and OTC interactants that should be avoided. Individuals who cannot limit their intake of alcohol or other depressants should be observed closely. Problems owing to concurrent use of antacids or antidiarrheals can be reduced by giving them 1 to 2 hours before or after antimuscarinic administration. Patients should self-medicate with these drugs only on the advice of a physician.

Overdose and Toxicity

Signs and symptoms of overdoses with trihexyphenidyl and related drugs, or of interactions with other antimuscarinics, resemble those caused by overdoses of atropine or scopolamine (see Chapter 13). All the central and peripheral responses noted earlier as side effects are intensified. Central signs and symptoms can range from confusion, excitement, delirium, and hallucinations to profound sedation and coma. Fatal seizures (status epilepticus) may develop, often due to high fever that is characteristic of atropine poisoning.

General treatment involves standard first-aid measures to reduce further absorption, and monitoring and normalization of all vital signs. Special aspects of treatment are similar to those used for atropine or scopolamine poisoning, including the need for reducing body temperature (with physical means such as ice packs or a hypothermia blanket), treatment of seizures with parenteral diazepam, and the use of the "atropine antidote" physostigmine (ANTILIRIUM) for life-threatening cases.

NURSING IMPLICATIONS

When overdoses occur in outpatients for whom a centrally acting antimuscarinic drug is prescribed, anticipate and be prepared to treat a multiple-drug overdose. Often such overdoses involve other drugs with intense CNS-depressant activity, including alcohol. To help reduce the risk of accidental or suicidal overdose in outpatients with diminished mental status or prior psychiatric disorders, try to recruit another individual who will be responsible for administering the drug to the patient. Children are particularly susceptible to even slight overdoses of antimuscarinic drugs, so it is essential to instruct persons given these medications to keep them well out of a child's reach.

Related Drugs

Benztropine and biperiden, classified as centrally acting antimuscarinics, may be used instead of trihexyphenidyl.

Benztropine

Benztropine (COGENTIN) is used as adjunctive therapy (with levodopa-containing drugs) to treat most forms of parkinsonism, including postencephalitic parkinsonism. It may also be used to treat drug-induced extrapyramidal disorders and dystonias and as prophylaxis for recurrent or transient drug-induced extrapyramidal reactions. Benztropine dosages are summarized in Table 25–C. The drug is usually given orally. A parenteral dosage form, given intramuscularly, is used for psychotic patients who cannot comply with oral therapy and for patients suffering from a severe, acute, drug-induced dystonic reaction. Oral therapy should be started when the patient's condition stabilizes after intramuscular (IM) use.

Benztropine belongs to a different chemical class than trihexyphenidyl, and so may prove to be effective for some patients who fail to respond adequately to the prototype. It causes greater and more longlasting muscle relaxation and sedation than trihexyphenidyl. The sedative effect may be desirable for patients who do not require or cannot tolerate the euphoric effect often caused by trihexyphenidyl, or for parkinsonian patients with insomnia. In contrast, this drug's sedative effects may interfere with daily activities or complicate proper mental assessment. The sedative effects will be more prominent in overdoses or drug interactions. Otherwise, benztropine should be considered equivalent to trihexyphenidyl in terms of peripheral and behavioral side effects, toxicity, overdoses, and the related nursing implications.

Biperiden

Biperiden (AKINETON) is used adjunctively for all forms of parkinsonism, including drug-induced extrapyramidal side effects. It is chemically related to trihexyphenidyl, and so is not likely to be effective for patients who do not respond well to trihexyphenidyl. Biperiden is usually given orally, but a parenteral dosage form, given intramuscularly or intravenously, can be used for acute drug-induced extrapyramidal symptoms. Dosages are noted in Table 25–C.

Other Drugs Used for Parkinsonism

In selected patients, several other drugs may be used instead of or in addition to the primary therapies noted thus far. Some are classified as antispasmodics or antihistaminics, but probably exert beneficial effects because of their central antimuscarinic actions. All of them should be considered equivalent to atropine or scopolamine in terms of side effects, contraindications, drug–drug interactions, and toxicities. The usual dosages for these drugs are listed in Table 25–C.

Diphenhydramine

Diphenhydramine (BENADRYL), the prototype antihistamine (H_1 receptor antagonist), is indicated for the management of most forms of parkinsonism. It causes atropine-like effects and appears to inhibit dopamine reuptake. Diphenhydramine is well suited for use alone to manage parkinsonism in elderly patients who cannot tolerate more potent antimuscarinic drugs. The drug can also be used adjunctively with the traditional centrally acting antimuscarinics, enabling management of symptoms with relatively low doses of each drug. Oral administration is generally used, but diphenhydramine can be given parenterally for prompt control of severe symptoms. Diphenhydramine's sedative and peripheral autonomic actions and side effects vary in intensity from patient to patient. More details about the pharmacology and uses of diphenhydramine are noted in Chapter 51.

Ethopropazine

Ethopropazine (PARSIDOL) is a phenothiazine derivative with marked antimuscarinic activity. Ethopropazine is noteworthy because most other phenothiazines worsen parkinsonism (Chapter 23), and it does not. It is indicated for adjunctive therapy of parkinsonism, including drug-induced parkinsonism.

Procyclidine

Procyclidine (KEMADRIN) is used as adjunctive therapy for all types of parkinsonism and drug-induced extrapyramidal disorders. It has atropine-like activity as well as appreciable antispasmodic effects on smooth muscle. Procyclidine appears to be particularly effective for alleviating rigidity and sialorrhea (excessive salivation) in parkinsonism, including drug-induced parkinsonism. It is not as effective for relieving tremor, and may actually increase tremor during early therapy. Procyclidine dosages are noted in Table 25–C. If the drug is added to therapy with other antiparkinson drugs, their dosages should be reduced gradually when procyclidine administration is started.

Table 25–2 Daily Living Tips for Patients with Parkinsonism

The following daily living tips, most of which are recommended by the American Parkinson Disease Association, may help the person with parkinsonism (see Annotated Bibliography).

1. Tremors of the arms and hands lead to many frustrations. They can best be managed by pressing the elbow of the affected arm against the body to stabilize the upper arm. The desired activity should then be performed as quickly as possible.
2. Dressing is a problem for many patients with parkinsonism. Suggest that patients wear loose, lightweight clothing. Garments that close in front, and those that fasten with VELCRO rather than buttons or zippers, may be preferable. If stiffness affects one side of the body more than the other, recommend that the patient put on or remove garments from that side first. Slip-on shoes or shoes that fasten with elastic laces or VELCRO may be preferable to standard laced shoes, and a long-handled shoe horn may be helpful. Avoid high-heeled shoes or other styles that make walking difficult since poor posture, gait, and balance are common but dangerous problems.
3. To prevent bathing accidents, instruct patients to place a no-slip rubber mat in the tub, install grab-bars, and remove glass tub or shower doors; a shower chair may be helpful. Soap can be retrieved easier during bathing if it is attached to a rope and placed in a convenient place in the bath or shower.
4. Walking is often hazardous for patients with parkinsonism because they tend to walk on the balls of their feet with their heels raised, which causes them to shuffle at faster and faster speeds. To discourage shuffling, teach patients to stop walking; place their feet at least 8 inches apart; correct their posture; think about taking a large step, and take a step by bringing their foot up higher in a "marching fashion."
5. Turning can also cause falls. Teach patients to walk into the turn, never pivoting on one foot.
6. If patients have difficulty getting out of bed because of nighttime stiffness and rigidity, recommend that they lie on their side close to the edge of the bed and drop their legs over the edge while pushing down with their elbow on the bed and with their opposite hand.

Adjunctive Therapies

Drugs are only a part of the multifaceted therapy of parkinsonism. Important nondrug therapies include psychologic counseling (including special support groups), physical therapy (ideally planned and supervised by a physical therapist), and speech therapy. Collectively, these adjuncts help improve muscle function, foster greater independence in daily living activities, and provide important psychologic benefits that might allow reduced drug dosages or the need for fewer drugs. Advice presented in Table 25–2 should be given to parkinsonian patients and their families. Most patients will ask whether they can continue to operate a motor vehicle and continue their jobs. Having to stop these activities may be particularly distressing to the parkinsonian patient. Whether the patient can perform these tasks depends on limitations imposed not only by the underlying disorder but also by prescribed drugs.

Nutritional status is an important concern for many persons with parkinsonism. There is no ideal diet for these individuals. However, some evidence exists that protein-rich foods increase the severity or fluctuations of rigidity and bradykinesias, particularly during levodopa therapy. If these problems occur, dietary changes may help without having to change otherwise effective therapy.

SUMMARY OF NURSING IMPLICATIONS

Assessment

Gather baseline neurologic data (eg, severity of tremors, rigidity, ability to initiate movement) as basis for care plan and evaluation of treatment effectiveness.

Assess for manifestations of primary symptoms of parkinsonism (eg, alterations in gait or posture, abnormal facial expressions, difficulty in getting in or out of bed, or inability to initiate or stop movement or perform activities of daily living).

Assess for changes in communication skills (slow or slurred speech, micrographia or other penmanship changes).

Complete nursing history to include sleep patterns (eg, awakening at night, nightmares, vivid dreams).

Determine mental status: depression, low self-esteem, suicidal ideation owing to progressively deteriorating physical condition.

Review history for major conditions aggravated by most antiparkinson drugs (glaucoma, cardiovascular disease, GI disorders, urologic conditions, pulmonary disease).

Complete baseline physical assessment of all systems; drugs can alter liver, kidneys, and blood components.

Screen for glaucoma before starting antimuscarinic therapy in elderly.

Determine availability of family or friends for drug-taking supervision if needed.

Nursing Diagnoses

Knowledge deficit related to disease progression, treatment regimen, and antiparkinson drug effects.

Ineffective individual coping related to diagnosis of Parkinson's disease.

Self-esteem disturbance related to loss of function from disease.

High risk for injury related to disease and drug side effects.

Sensory/perceptual alteration related to adverse CNS effects.

Self-care deficit related to nervous system disorder.

Sleep pattern disturbance related to disease or medication use.

Impaired physical mobility related to muscle dysfunction.

Constipation related to disease or drug therapy.

Altered nutrition: less than body requirements related to disease progression or ineffective drug therapy.

Noncompliance related to negative side effects of prescribed treatment.

Planning/Implementation

Make referrals for physical, occupational, or speech therapy as special problems arise; plan for interdisciplinary health team conference.

Use nondrug measures to promote sleep and reduce stiffness (eg, provide quiet room and moderate daytime exercise or physical therapy, turn frequently during night).

Anticipate diminished desire and ability to eat: dysfunction of mouth, throat musculature may cause annoying, embarrassing, or dangerous problems (eg, inadequate chewing, excessive salivation, dysphagia, impaired gag reflex).

Weigh regularly to monitor nutritional status; appetite and eating may improve with drug therapy, or worsen due to drug side effects.

Increase daily intake of bulk-forming foods and water (2500 to 3000 mL per day), and encourage exercise to prevent or relieve constipation.

Monitor closely fluid intake and output of elderly males, inactive patients, or those with advanced symptoms; report sudden or marked changes of bladder habits.

Provide encouragement that therapies will alleviate many symptoms if treatment is followed; advise of a lag period of days to months as appropriate for drug(s) prescribed.

Observe for antiparkinson drug side effects; inquire about and respect subjective complaints.

Give drug(s) with meals if nausea and vomiting occur; avoid high-protein foods, which can reduce absorption and interfere with levodopa response.

Apply elastic stockings to reduce problems owing to orthostatic hypotension.

Monitor blood pressure regularly, particularly during dose adjustment.

Withhold drug and notify physician when eye pain, blepharospasm, psychotic symptoms, or other symptoms of toxicity appear.

Check dosages carefully; even slight errors can result in toxicity.

Discontinue levodopa 8 hours before switching to levodopa–carbidopa combination.

Monitor for abdominal pain and occult blood with levodopa; report signs of GI bleeding; peptic ulcer disease can reoccur.

Monitor for relevant signs of untoward interactions with antihypertensives and antipsychotics particularly; do not give levodopa and MAO inhibitors concurrently to avoid severe hypertensive crisis or atropine poisoning.

Observe for signs indicative of impending seizures with amantadine.

If dysphagia is present, swallowing large amantadine capsules may be difficult; notify physician: alternatives (eg, amantadine syrup) may be prescribed.

Monitor for unique reaction to amantadine (mottled, edematous, purple-colored skin) indicative of livedo reticularis; notify physician.

Avoid giving amantadine with other antimuscarinic drugs; a syndrome resembling atropine poisoning may occur.

◆ Patient and Family Teaching

Teach the patient/family:

That changes in communication skills are common and may diminish with treatment; suggest massaging to relax patient's facial and neck muscles to improve speaking.

To report sudden or marked changes of bowel or bladder function immediately.

About the importance of becoming involved in a parkinsonism support group.

To wear sunglasses when out-of-doors if photophobia is present; to report eye pain immediately as it may indicate glaucoma.

To avoid driving, ambulation, and reading with blurred vision; to notify physician if side effect persists after several weeks.

To rise slowly and use support when standing and when walking initially to prevent falls caused by orthostatic hypotension and lightheadedness; have patient/family rid environment of hazards that might contribute to falling.

That levodopa may darken or discolor urine, sweat, or saliva, and is not a cause for concern.

That vitamin B_6 (pyridoxine) counteracts beneficial effects of levodopa; to avoid OTC vitamins, B_6-supplemented foods, or B_6-rich foods.

To practice contraception with methods other than birth control pills if taking bromocriptine; notify physician if pregnancy occurs or is suspected.

To avoid strenuous exercises in hot weather, and wear light, loose clothing if anhidrosis (lack of sweating) is a problem.

About OTC drugs to avoid; provide list.

To keep drugs out of reach of children.

◆ Evaluation

The patient/family will:

Experience relief from parkinsonian symptoms (eg, decreased rigidity, tremor, and bradykinesia).

Perform activities of daily living with increased independence.

Cope effectively with diagnosis and limitations; seek personal and family support.

Achieve optimal activity level without injury.

Increase strength, endurance, and mobility.

Report adequate rest; sleep through the night.

Report passage of stool of usual consistency.

Demonstrate ability to follow treatment regimen; take medication as prescribed; recognize and report side effects.

Annotated Bibliography

Agid Y. Parkinson's disease: Pathophysiology. *Lancet* 1991;337: 1321–1323. *"Idiopathic Parkinson's disease is the only neurodegenerative disorder in which symptoms can be successfully treated long term." Agid begins with this comment and then provides a brief but powerful review of the pathologic features of this disease.*

Boodhoo JA, Sandler M. Anticholinergic antiparkinsonian drugs in psychiatry. *Br J Hosp Med* 1991;46:167–169. *Concisely reviews the practical use and side effects of centrally acting antimuscarinics for managing drug-induced extrapyramidal disorders.*

Clough CG. Parkinson's disease: Management. *Lancet* 1991;337: 1324–1327. *A good review of basic management issues: treatment failures, extents of cognitive decline, resistant symptoms, psychosocial difficulties, and pharmacologic pros and cons.*

de Roin S, Winters S. Amantadine hydrochloride: Current and new uses. *J Neurosci Nurs* 1990;22:322–325. *Reviews actions and therapeutic uses of this interesting drug.*

Koller WC, Hubble JP. Levodopa therapy in Parkinson's disease. *Neurology* 1990;40(Suppl. 3):40–47. *Summarizes why and when this traditional drug remains an important first-line agent. A synopsis of discussion questions (pp 47–49) provides added valuable insight.*

Langtry HD, Clissold SP. Pergolide: A review of its pharmacological properties and therapeutic potential in Parkinson's disease.

Drugs 1990;39:491–506. *A comprehensive review of this dopamine agonist: pharmacologic properties, results of clinical trials; adverse effects; and dosage recommendations. Citing over 90 references, the authors provide a meaningful resource for students, particularly those who are interested in geriatric nursing.*

Lavin MR, Rifkin A. Prophylactic antiparkinson drug use. *J Clin Pharmacol* 1991;31:763–768, 769–777. *This two-part article reviews controversies surrounding the use and later discontinuation of antiparkinson drugs for preventing antipsychotic-induced extrapyramidal side effects. After analyzing the benefit-risk balance, the authors conclude that most patients taking neuroleptic drugs would benefit from prophylactic and maintenance antiparkinson drug therapy.*

Madeley P, Hulley JL, Wildgust H, Mindham RHS. Parkinson's disease and driving ability. *J Neurol Neurosurg Psychiatry* 1990;53: 580–582. *At what point should a patient with parkinsonism not be allowed to drive? The authors found that individuals who scored as "moderately disabled" should be carefully considered before driving privileges are granted.*

Parkinson's Disease Handbook: A Guide for Patients and Their Families. New York: American Parkinson Disease Association. *An excellent resource for patients, families, and health-care professionals who need to refresh their knowledge on the subject. The handbook covers all dimensions of the disease, providing information on symptoms, drugs, support groups, and so on. Single copies are available free of charge; call 1–800–223–APDA for information.*

Peters NL. Snipping the thread of life: Antimuscarinic side effects in the elderly. Arch Intern Med 1989;149:2414–2420. *Without question, your single best source for easily understood, practical information (and review) about how atropine-like drugs (including those used for parkinsonism, and all others with which they interact) can have a devastating but preventable impact on the elderly.*

Robertson DR, George CF. Drug therapy for Parkinson's disease in the elderly. *Br Med Bull* 1990;46:124–146. *A comprehensive but worth-reading review of age-related factors in managing parkinsonism: altered drug actions and pharmacokinetics; problems in diagnosis and therapeutic management; and the need for a "multidisciplinary approach . . . to help the patient and . . . caregiver . . . cope with fundamental disabilities."*

Siris SG. Pharmacological treatment of substance-abusing schizophrenic patients. *Schizophr Bull* 1990;16:111–122. *In addition to discussing the potential values of antiparkinson drugs, the author gives an excellent overview of clinical dilemmas that arise when the patient is diagnosed with both schizophrenia and substance abuse.*

Table 25–C | Clinical Uses and Administration of Major Antiparkinson Agents

AGENT	CLINICAL USES	DOSAGE AND ROUTE OF ADMINISTRATION
Dopaminergic Drugs		
PROTOTYPE		
Levodopa (DOPAR, LARODOPA)	Parkinsonism, except drug-induced	Oral: Adults: Initially 0.5–1 g/d in 2 or more divided doses (with food); follow by increases every 3–7 d of up to 0.75 g/d as tolerated, until desired response occurs. Dose should rarely exceed 8 g/d without close supervision. Not recommended for children under 12
RELATED DRUGS		
Carbidopa/levodopa (SINEMET)	Parkinsonism	Oral: Adults: Initially 1 SINEMET 25/100 tablet tid, followed, if needed, by increases of 1 tablet qd or qod, up to 6 tablets/d. If SINEMET 10/100 is used, start with 1 tablet tid or qid, followed, if needed, by increases of 1 tablet qd or qod up to 2 tablets qid. Not recommended for children under 18
(SINEMET CR)	Parkinsonism	Oral: Adults: Replace immediate-acting SINEMET with from 1 tablet SINEMET CR (controlled-release) bid to up to 5 tablets/d in 3 or more divided doses, based on current levodopa dose; not for initial therapy
Amantadine (SYMMETREL)	Parkinsonism	Oral: Adults: 100 mg bid to start; increase if necessary up to 400 mg/d in divided doses. Maintain close supervision if daily dose ≥300 mg
	Drug-induced extrapyramidal reactions	Oral: Adults: 100 mg bid to start, followed, if necessary, by up to 300 mg/d in divided doses
	Prophylaxis, treatment of influenza A respiratory illness	See Chapter 57
Bromocriptine (PARLODEL)	Parkinsonism	Oral: Adults: 1.25 mg bid, with meals, to start; if necessary, increase by 2.5 mg/d every 14–28 days (up to 100 mg/d); maintain the dosage of levodopa, if possible, until maximum therapeutic response is achieved. Assess every 2 weeks to ensure lowest effective dose is used. Not recommended for children under 15.
	Treatment of amenorrhea, galactorrhea, female infertility associated with hyperprolactinemia; prevention of physiological lactation	See Chapter 44
Pergolide (PERMAX)	Adjunctive treatment of parkinsonism	Oral: Adults: 0.05 mg for first 2 days. Increase by 0.1–0.15 mg/d every 3 days for 12 days, then by 0.25 mg/d every 3 days until optimal dosage is achieved. Typical dose is 1 mg tid

(continued)

Table 25–C | **Clinical Uses and Administration of Major Antiparkinson Agents (*Continued*)**

AGENT	CLINICAL USES	DOSAGE AND ROUTE OF ADMINISTRATION
RELATED DRUGS		
Selegiline		
(ELDEPRYL)	Adjunctive treatment of parkinsonism	Oral: Adults: 5 mg at breakfast and lunch. After 2 or 3 days of treatment levodopa-carbidopa can usually be reduced by 10%–30%
	Centrally Acting Antimuscarinic Drugs	
PROTOTYPE		
Tribexyphenidyl		
(ARTANE)	Parkinsonism	Oral: Adults: 1 mg/d to start; if needed, increase by 2 mg/d at 3–5-d intervals to 6–10 mg/d in divided doses at mealtime. May substitute sustained-release product (ARTANE SEQUELS) on mg-for-mg basis for some patients; administer single dose after breakfast, second dose (if needed) 12 hr later
	Drug-induced extrapyramidal reactions	Oral: Adults: 1 mg to start; if needed, after several hours increase to 15 mg/d; usual range is 5–15 mg/d. Children: Use based on physician's judgement
RELATED DRUGS		
Benztropine		
(COGENTIN)	Parkinsonism	Oral or IM: Adults: 0.5–1 mg hs to start; increase up to 4–6 mg/d if needed; usual maintenance dose is 1–2 mg/d
	Postencephalitic parkinsonism	Oral or IM: Adults: 2 mg/d to start, followed by up to 6 mg/d, if needed; usual maintenance dose1–2 mg/d
	Drug-induced extrapyramidal reactions	Oral or IM: Adults: 1–4 mg, qd or bid
	Drug-induced, acute dystonic reactions	Adults: Initially 1–2 mg IM; follow by 1–2 mg orally, bid, to prevent recurrence
	Prophylaxis of recurrent or transient drug-induced extrapyramidal reactions	Oral: Adults: 1–2 mg bid or tid prn; reassess need for continued therapy after 1–2 weeks by withdrawing drug temporarily. Not recommended for children under 3 years; use with caution in older children
Biperiden		
(AKINETON)	Parkinsonism	Oral: Adults: 2 mg tid or qid
	Drug-induced extrapyramidal reactions	Oral: Adults: 2 mg qd–tid Parenteral: 2 mg IM or IV every half hour, prn, up to 8 mg/24 hr

(continued)

Table 25–C Clinical Uses and Administration of Major Antiparkinson Agents (*Continued*)

AGENT	CLINICAL USES	DOSAGE AND ROUTE OF ADMINISTRATION
RELATED DRUGS		
Diphenhydramine (BENADRYL)	Parkinsonism; also used adjunctively with centrally acting antimuscarinics	Oral: Adults: 25–50 mg tid or qid; may be taken adjunctively with antimuscarinics Parenteral: 10–50 mg (or up to 100 mg, if needed) IM (deeply), or IV, up to 400 mg/d maximum. Children: >20 lb: Oral, IV, IM: 5 mg/d up to 300/mg maximum
Ethopropazine (PARSIDOL)	Adjunctive treatment of parkinsonism	Oral: Adults: Usually 50 mg qd or bid to start; 100–600 mg/d for maintenance
Procyclidine (KEMADRIN)	Adjunctive treatment of parkinsonism; particularly effective when rigidity and sialorrhea are present	Oral: Adults: 2.5 mg tid after meals to start; increase gradually to 5 mg tid, with additional 5-mg bedtime dose if needed
	Drug-induced extrapyramidal reactions	Oral: Adults: 2.5 mg tid after meals to start; increase by 2.5 mg/d until symptoms are relieved; usual maintenance dosage 10–20 mg/d

Table 25–S Major Side Effects of and Contraindications for Antiparkinson Drugs

BODY SYSTEM/ Side Effect	CONTRAINDICATION/ PRECAUTION	COMMENTS AND NURSING IMPLICATIONS
Levodopa		
CENTRAL NERVOUS SYSTEM Headaches, dizziness, weakness, faintness, confusion, insomnia, nightmares, hallucinations, delusions, agitation, anxiety, euphoria, fatigue, suicidal thoughts, involuntary movements		Most of these side effects are relatively common and should be treated symptomatically. Instruct patient to be careful when driving or operating hazardous machinery. Psychosis is not common; if it occurs the drug should be discontinued and restarted at a lower dosage. Evaluate mental status regularly and ask family to report personality changes. Evaluate patient's involuntary movements to determine if they are drug-induced. Elderly individuals may need drug-taking supervised by family members, others
EYE Blurred vision		Instruct patient to avoid tasks in which good vision is required
Mydriasis	Narrow-angle glaucoma	Instruct patient to report eye pain immediately
RESPIRATORY Cough, hoarseness, disturbed breathing	History of asthma, emphysema	Be cautious if patient with a history of asthma or emphysema is given these drugs

(continued)

Table 25–S | **Major Side Effects of and Contraindications for Antiparkinson Drugs (*Continued*)**

BODY SYSTEM/ Side Effect	CONTRAINDICATION/ PRECAUTION	COMMENTS AND NURSING IMPLICATIONS
	Levodopa	
CARDIOVASCULAR Orthostatic hypotension, palpitations, cardiac irregularities	Cardiovascular disease, history of MI and residual arrhythmias; patients receiving antihypertensives should be observed closely for hypotensive episodes	Advise patient to rise slowly, change positions gradually, and not to stand in one place too long. Notify physician if patient complains of palpitations. Monitor pulse and BP; if possible, patients with history of cardiovascular problems should have treatment initiated where cardiac monitoring capability is available
GASTROINTESTINAL Nausea and vomiting, dry mouth, dysphagia		Give drug with meals to decrease nausea and vomiting; however, high protein ingestion compromises effectiveness of levodopa. Dry mouth can be alleviated with sips of water, rinses, hard sugarless candy. Dysphagia may require special observation because it can make eating uncomfortable and dangerous
Bleeding	History of peptic ulcer	Notify physician if stools are darkened, occult blood is found, or patient complains of abdominal pain
Anorexia		Allow patient adequate time to eat; weigh periodically
GENITOURINARY Urinary retention and incontinence Darkened urine		Instruct patient to urinate as soon as the urge is felt. Also, advise patient to drink adequate fluids, to run water over the perineum, and to turn on tapwater to stimulate urination. Incontinence may be decreased by frequent toileting. Special underclothing can be purchased to absorb urine. Instruct patient about the possibility of darkened urine to allay fears
MUSCULOSKELETAL Choreiform movements, dystonia, ataxia, increased hand tremor, muscle twitching, blepharospasm		Muscle twitching, blepharospasm, ataxia, may be early signs of toxicity. Abnormal involuntary movements sometimes caused by prolonged use of these drugs; dosage may need to be reduced. Advise physician of musculoskeletal reactions. Caution patient concerning hazardous activities
	Amantadine	
CENTRAL NERVOUS SYSTEM Depression, psychosis, decreased concentration, insomnia, dizziness, slurred speech, ataxia	History of psychosis or uncontrolled neurosis	Psychosis requires discontinuation of drug (at least for a while). Evaluate mental status regularly and ask family to report personality changes. Advise patient that some side effects diminish as tolerance develops
Increased seizure activity	History of seizures	Observe seizure-prone patients closely; if seizure activity is believed to be probable, place patient on bedrest with padded side rails

(continued)

Table 25–S Major Side Effects of and Contraindications for Antiparkinson Drugs (*Continued*)

BODY SYSTEM/ Side Effect	CONTRAINDICATION/ PRECAUTION	COMMENTS AND NURSING IMPLICATIONS
EYE Blurred vision		Instruct patient to avoid tasks in which good vision is demanded
CARDIOVASCULAR Congestive heart failure	Congestive heart failure	Monitor BP, check for edema and fluid retention, auscultate lungs for fluid. Instruct patient to report chest heaviness and dyspnea on exertion
Orthostatic hypotension		See levodopa
Tachycardia, arrhythmias		See levodopa
GASTROINTESTINAL Anorexia, nausea, vomiting, dry mouth		See levodopa
DERMATOLOGIC Livedo reticularis		A common dermatologic side effect; observe for mottled, purple-colored skin with localized edema
Bromocriptine		
CENTRAL NERVOUS SYSTEM Headache, dizziness, fatigue, choreiform movements, confusion, hallucinations	May cause mental disturbances in patients with mild dementias	See levodopa
RESPIRATORY Shortness of breath		Instruct patient to avoid strenuous activities and to change positions gradually; monitor respiratory status.
CARDIOVASCULAR Hypotension	Ischemic heart disease, peripheral vascular disease	See levodopa; monitor blood pressure frequently and encourage rest. (Also see Chapter 44)
GASTROINTESTINAL Nausea, vomiting		See levodopa
Trihexyphenidyl and Other Centrally Acting Antimuscarinics		
See atropine, scopolamine, Table 13–S		

Table 25–I Major Interactions Between Antiparkinson Drugs and Other Agents

AGENT	RESULT OF INTERACTION	COMMENTS AND NURSING IMPLICATIONS
Interactions Involving Levodopa (with or without Carbidopa)		
Antihypertensive drugs (most; Chapter 33)	Additive hypotension, especially orthostatic	Potential interaction; monitor BP (supine, sitting, standing) frequently, report symptomatic hypotension (eg, dizziness); advise patient to stand up slowly
Antipsychotic drugs (Chapter 23)	Potential antagonism of either interactant's therapeutic actions	Monitor accordingly if combined use is essential
Monoamine oxidase inhibitors (Chapter 24), including selegiline (pp 455)	Acute hypertension, hypertensive crisis, potential stroke or death	Severe headache is often an early warning sign; emergency treatment (eg, phentolamine to lower BP) is essential; avoid combined use of nonspecific MAO inhibitors (antidepressants) altogether; do not exceed maximum recommended daily dose of selegiline (Table 25-C)
Phenytoin (Chapter 26)	Reduced control of parkinsonian symptoms	Gradual onset; monitor accordingly if interaction unavoidable; may require increased levodopa dose, decreased phenytoin dose, depending on whether seizure or parkinson control takes priority
Pyridoxine (vitamin B_6)	Dramatically reduced control of parkinsonian symptoms	Avoid interaction; provide patient with written list of foods to avoid; discourage use of multivitamin supplements without physician's approval; LAROBEC, a B_6-free product, is indicated when nutritional supplementation is needed
Interactions Involving Amantadine		
Antimuscarinic drugs, other (eg, antidepressants, antihistamines, antipsychotics; see Table 13-1, p 169)	Potential additive CNS and peripheral atropine-like side effects	Avoid interaction if possible; is important to discourage unsupervised use of OTC drugs with antimuscarinic activity (eg, allergy, cold remedies containing antihistamines); monitor accordingly if interaction is unavoidable
Interactions Involving Bromocriptine		
Antihypertensive drugs	See levodopa, above	
Contraceptives, oral (Chapter 49)	Reduced contraceptive effects, pregnancy	Potential interaction requires use of added or alternative and effective contraception methods; consequences particularly important owing to fetal risks from bromocriptine use during pregnancy; advise patient to notify physician at once if pregnancy occurs, is suspected

(continued)

Table 25–1 **Major Interactions Between Antiparkinson Drugs and Other Agents (*Continued*)**

AGENT	RESULT OF INTERACTION	COMMENTS AND NURSING IMPLICATIONS
Interactions Involving Selegiline		
Levodopa	See levodopa-MAO inhibitors, above	
Meperidine (Chapter 21)	Severe, acute CNS stimulation followed by profound depression, coma, possibly death	Avoid interaction; morphine is preferred if narcotic analgesic is indicated
Interactions Involving Trihexyphenidyl, Other Centrally Acting Antimuscarinic-Antiparkinson Drugs		
Antimuscarinic drugs, other (see amantadine, above)	Increased risk, severity of CNS, peripheral atropine-like side effects, possible antimuscarinic poisoning syndrome	Outcome of interaction usually occurs gradually; avoid interaction when possible, monitor accordingly if not, give patient explicit instructions to avoid unsupervised use of OTC drugs with antimuscarinic actions
Antipsychotics (Chapter 23)	Additive antimuscarinic side effects, reduced antipsychotic drug effectiveness, worsening of psychosis symptoms	Monitor accordingly if interaction is unavoidable; loss of schizophrenia symptom control may be particularly important with haloperidol
CNS depressants, general (eg, alcohol, barbiturates, benzodiazepines; Chapter 22)	Additive CNS depression	Avoid needless use of CNS depressants, especially alcohol; monitor accordingly otherwise; may be lesser problem with trihexyphenidyl, which causes less CNS depression than alternatives (eg, benztropine, diphenhydramine)

PROTOTYPES

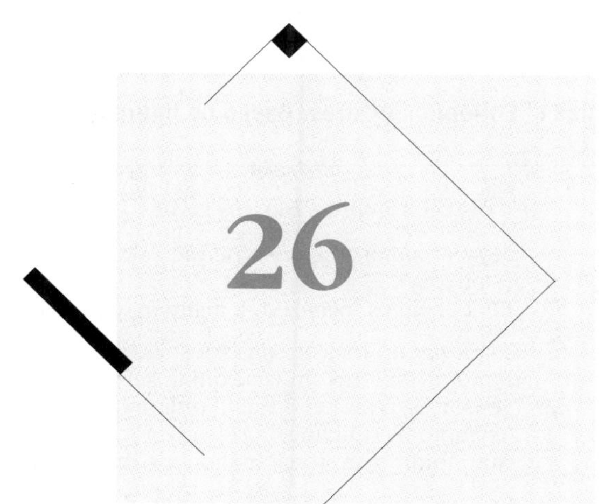

Anticonvulsant Drugs

Epilepsy is the most common disorder involving chronic seizures, or abnormal brain electrical activity. It has potentially devastating social and economic impact; fortunately, however, many *anticonvulsant* drugs exist that can treat it effectively. Some of these drugs are also useful for managing acute seizures, such as those caused by high fever or drugs.

Part I of this chapter reviews the major causes and characteristics of epileptic seizures to provide a rationale for the use and actions of anticonvulsant drugs. Part II discusses principles that apply to anticonvulsant drug therapy in general, then identifies five major groups or classes of anticonvulsant medications; several miscellaneous, but nevertheless important, anticonvulsant drugs; and drugs that have anticonvulsant actions but that are used for other purposes as well. Part III of the chapter reviews general nursing implications, including nondrug aspects of nursing care for persons with seizure disorders and the important issue of anticonvulsant therapy during pregnancy.

Major reference tables appear beginning on p. 495.

I. Epilepsy

Epilepsy is a diagnostic term used to identify a group of chronic central nervous system (CNS) disorders. All forms of epilepsy involve episodes of abnormal electrical activity (seizures) in the brain, mainly in the cerebral cortex. Seizures are self-sustaining for various periods of time, but eventually are self-limiting. Often they are accompanied by characteristic body movements (convulsions), and may involve autonomic hyperactivity and other changes. The overall incidence of epilepsy ranges from 0.5% to 2%. Brain injury, meningitis, acute alcohol ingestion, stroke, and neoplasms are relatively common causes of seizures, but most cases of epilepsy are idiopathic, meaning that the etiology is unknown. About 80% of the cases of idiopathic epilepsy begin before the age of 18.

Categories of Epileptic Seizures

There are sufficient differences between seizures to distinguish subtypes, and internationally accepted criteria have been established (Table 26–1). Each subtype has a characteristic electroencephalogram (EEG) pattern, as well as characteristic physical and neurologic signs and

Table 26–1 Major Characteristics of Epileptic Seizures, Based on International Classification

Seizure Type	Comments and Characteristics
I. Partial (focal or local)	Most common seizure type (accounts for about 70% of adults, 40% of children, with epilepsy) EEG changes localized, initially may evolve into other seizure types
A. Simple partial	Typically no loss of consciousness Motor symptoms (in jacksonian seizures) Sensory symptoms (visual, auditory, gustatory, hallucinations) and somatosensory symptoms (tingling) Autonomic symptoms (pallor, sweating, vomiting, flushing)
B. Complex partial	Consciousness impaired at onset of seizure or later, after onset of simple partial seizure
C. Partial evolving to generalized tonic-clonic	
II. Generalized	Involves symmetrical (both hemispheres) distribution of abnormal brain discharge Bilateral motor changes Consciousness may be totally impaired
	Nonconvulsive Seizures
A. Absence	Abrupt loss of consciousness, usually lasting <10 sec Usually begins in childhood, often stops spontaneously during teenage years Impairment of consciousness only (petit mal) Mild clonic component Atonic component: diminution of muscle tone Automatisms Autonomic components
B. Myoclonic	Single or multiple jerks, typically lasting 3–10 sec Sudden, brief, shock–like contractions, generalized or confined
C. Atonic	Sudden diminution of muscle tone ("drop attacks")
	Convulsive Seizures
D. Clonic	Occurs mostly in childhood Generalized convulsive seizures lacking tonic component Characterized by clonic jerks Postictal phase typically short
E. Tonic	Sustained contraction of large muscles Continuous tension of chest musculature impairs ventilation, causes pallor, more serious problems if prolonged
F. Tonic-clonic	Consciousness lost abruptly Series of muscle spasms lasting 3–5 min from onset to recovery Postictal state may last from a few minutes to about half an hour; often characterized by confusion, dizziness, sleepiness, "glazed" look
G. Status epilepticus	Could apply to any prolonged or repetitive seizure, best used to describe repetitive or fused tonic–clonic seizures A medical emergency requiring immediate drug intervention to prevent brain damage or death due to impaired ventilation Only seizure for which there is no contraindication to drug use
III. Unclassified epileptic seizures	Includes all seizures that cannot be classified whether because of inadequate or incomplete criteria, characteristics

Source: Modified from Commission on Classification and Terminology of the International League Against Epilepsy: Proposal for revised clinical and electroencephalographic classification of epileptic seizures. *Epilepsia* 1981;22:489–501.

symptoms that result from abnormal brain function. *The type of seizure, not its cause, is the major determinant of the drugs that will be selected to manage it.* More than 50% of patients with epilepsy develop more than one type of seizure disorder, and a different anticonvulsant may be needed for each. Seizures are usually classified as either partial (focal) or generalized.

Partial Seizures

Partial seizures are the most common seizure type, affecting about 67% of all adults and 40% of all children with epilepsy. Brain lesions and EEG changes are usually confined to one part of a cerebral hemisphere, but abnormal brain activity may spread through the same hemisphere or affect the other hemisphere. Partial seizures are divided into the simple and complex types. Simple partial seizures do not impair consciousness; whereas complex partial seizures, which often originate in the anterior temporal lobe, do impair consciousness. Depending on the type of partial seizure, muscle activity, sensory changes, or autonomic or psychic symptoms may predominate.

Generalized Seizures

Generalized seizures involve a symmetric distribution of abnormal brain discharges. Generalized seizures can be divided further into nonconvulsive types that mainly cause unresponsiveness and amnesia, and convulsive types that cause total impairment of consciousness and major convulsions. Absence seizures are an important subclass of nonconvulsive generalized seizures, especially in children. Absence seizures are characterized by an abrupt loss of consciousness but an absence of major or obvious muscle contractions. Absence seizures are so brief and lacking in obvious motor activity that others may be unaware that a seizure has occurred. True petit mal seizures are a type of absence seizure that is distinguished by a characteristic three-per-second spike-and-wave EEG pattern. Absence or petit mal seizures may evolve into a long-lasting tonic-clonic seizure disorder. Other forms of minor generalized seizures include myolonic and atonic seizures.

Most members of the lay public, when asked to describe an epileptic seizure, describe the dramatic generalized tonic-clonic convulsive seizure (formerly called a grand mal seizure). It is characterized by intense, repetitive tonic-clonic contractions of the entire body owing to activation of virtually all brain pathways. It may be preceded by sensory alterations (an aura) that forewarn the patient of what is to follow. The seizure may last only a few minutes, but is often followed by a longer period of postictal (postseizure) depression. Tonic-clonic seizures pose a relatively great risk of physical harm; falls, tongue lacerations, and bone and muscle damage can result from the vigorous, sustained, and repetitive muscle activity. The most serious concern in a tonic-clonic seizure is hypoxic brain damage caused by prolonged contraction of thoracic, neck, and jaw musculature, which impairs respiration and blood oxygenation. Other types of convulsive, generalized seizures are noted in Table 26–1.

Status epilepticus is a state in which several generalized convulsive seizures occur successively without intervals of restored consciousness or normal muscle activity. Status epilepticus differs from other tonic-clonic seizures because it is not self-limiting. Prolonged impairment of respiration and brain oxygenation during status epilepticus poses a great risk of permanent brain damage or death unless skilled treatment and anticonvulsant drug therapy is started at once.

II. Anticonvulsants

Anticonvulsant drugs, regardless of their precise mechanism of action or the cause of seizures, effectively suppress the start of seizures (abnormal brain electrical activity), reduce the spread of seizures to other brain regions, or both. Anticonvulsants rarely, if ever, treat the underlying cause of the seizures. Drug therapy of epilepsy is almost always essential. Even if a seizure-causing brain lesion can be removed surgically, one or more drugs will often be used both before and after the operation. Acute seizures caused by fever or drugs, for which other treatments are indicated, may also require adjunctive anticonvulsant therapy. Many different classes of drugs are used to treat seizures. Most of the anticonvulsant drugs belong to one of five major chemical classes: hydantoins; barbiturates; succinimides; benzodiazepines; and oxazolidinediones. There are also other anticonvulsants that, based on chemical properties, do not fit into one of these classes. In addition, other drugs, used mainly for other therapeutic purposes, have limited or special uses to control seizures.

Drug Selection

Complete and precise diagnosis is essential before any anticonvulsant drug is administered, since the seizure type, not the underlying cause, determines the drug of choice. Table 26–2 summarizes the usefulness of the anticonvulsants for major seizure types.

Table 26–2 Relative Value of Anticonvulsants for Major Seizure Types

			Seizure Type		
Anticonvulsant	**Tonic-clonic**	**Absence (petit mal)**	**Simple partial (focal)**	**Complex partial (psychomotor)**	**Status epilepticus**
Hydantoins					
Ethotoin	X			X	
Mephenytoin	X (R)		X (R)	X (R)	
Phenytoin	1		X	X	2
Barbiturates					
Mephobarbital	X	X			
Metharbital	X	X			
Phenobarbital	1		X	X	2 or 3
Primidone	2		X	X	
Succinimides					
Ethosuximide		1			
Methsuximide		2			
Phensuximide		X (R)			
Benzodiazepines					
Clonazepam		2			
Diazepam					1
Oxazolidinediones					
Paramethadione		X (R)			
Trimethadione		X (R)			
Others					
Acetazolamide	X	X			
Carbamazepine	2			2	
Lidocaine*					X (R)
Magnesium sulfate†					
Paraldehyde#					
Phenacemide				X (R)	
Valproic acid	1	1		X	

Key: 1 = first-choice drug; 2 = second choice drug; 3 = third choice drug; (R) = used when seizures are refractory to other drugs; X = may be used

*Last choice for refractory status epilepticus.

†Used for magnesium deficiency–related seizures.

#Used for alcohol withdrawal–related seizures.

Several drugs might be effective for a particular seizure type. The one that is actually selected for initial treatment may be no more effective than alternative or "second-line" agents, but it usually carries a significantly lower risk of causing severe adverse reactions. Regardless of the relative safety of any anticonvulsant drug, a comprehensive medical evaluation is an absolutely essential prerequisite to therapy. Another consideration in selecting an anticonvulsant, especially for persons with multiple seizure types, is whether it may help one seizure type but aggravate others. For example, phenytoin, which is the preferred drug for many patients with tonic-clonic seizures, can increase the incidence or severity of absence seizures.

General Therapeutic Goals and Dosing Strategies

There are common goals for anticonvulsant therapy, and general principles that apply to reaching them. Nevertheless, therapy must be individualized for each patient, particularly with regard to drug dosages needed to achieve and then maintain therapeutic anticonvulsant

Table 26–3 Pharmacokinetic Comparison of Selected Anticonvulsants

Agent	Time to Steady-State (days)*	Therapeutic Serum Levels	Toxic Blood Level	Half-Life (hr)*	Protein Bound
Carbamazepine	2–4	4–12 μg/mL	>12 μg/mL	12–17	76%
Clonazepam	3–7	20–80 μg/mL	>80 ng/mL	18–60	47%
Diazepam	5–8	not known	not known	20–50	99%
Ethosuximide	5–10	40–100 μg/mL	>100 μg/mL	60 (Adult)	0%
Phenobarbital	16–21	15–30 μg/mL	>40 μg/mL	80 (before increased hepatic metabolism rate is induced	40%–60%
Phenytoin	7–10	10–20 μg/mL	>20 μg/mL	7–42 (dose-dependent)	90%
Primidone†	1–5	5–12 μg/mL	>12 μg/mL	3–12	0%
Valproic acid	2–4	50–100 μg/mL	>100 μg/mL	6–16	90%

*Values assume repeated administration at usual dosage intervals.
†When primidone is administered, phenobarbital levels must also be measured.

drug blood levels (Table 26–3). The optimal therapeutic outcome is to make the patient seizure-free and fully functional without causing drug-induced side effects or adverse responses, which differ markedly among the major drugs.

Ideally, when there is no urgent need to suppress seizures, the risk of side effects can be reduced by starting therapy with the lowest effective dose of a single anticonvulsant, gradually reaching a steady therapeutic blood level. The initial dose is usually one quarter to one third of the recommended maintenance dose. This is particularly important for such drugs as carbamazepine, valproic acid, and primidone, which may cause appreciable dose-related side effects. In contrast, drugs such as phenytoin, phenobarbital, or ethosuximide are relatively free of serious side effects; initial doses may be close to maintenance doses.

If low doses of the drug of choice fail to reduce or prevent seizures, the dosage can be increased until either the desired effect or toxicity develops. If toxicity limits therapy, or seizures persist, combined therapy with low doses of two or more anticonvulsant drugs, each of which potentiates the actions of the others, may be tried. Combination therapy may permit gradual discontinuation of the first-choice drug. If there is still no improvement the patient can be switched to a different anticonvulsant—usually one that often carries a greater risk of adverse effects. This "crossover" must be planned carefully to avoid worsening of seizure activity (***breakthrough seizures***) when therapy with one anticonvulsant is stopped. Multiple-drug therapy is also necessary for the many patients who have more than one type of seizure disorder, each of which will require its own drug. Compared with the use of a high dose of only one drug, multiple-drug therapy may be effective and may reduce the risk of side effects caused by each agent. However, it increases the risk of drug interactions.

Despite careful patient evaluation and drug selection, the outcome of therapy may only be fewer or less severe seizures, and many therapeutic pitfalls may arise. Nevertheless, approximately 70% to 80% of patients benefit from proper drug treatment.

Anticonvulsant Drug Serum Concentrations

The chronic nature of epilepsy requires long-term management to make the patient free from symptoms and side effects. This is achieved by attaining and maintaining consistent (steady-state) therapeutic blood concentrations of anticonvulsant drugs with as little fluctuation as possible. Therapeutic blood levels, and the typical times needed to reach them after therapy is begun, are shown in Table 26–3. These times depend in part on the anticonvulsant's half-life (which is influenced by the individual's ability to metabolize and excrete the drug), and, to a degree, on the dosage interval. The interval between doses should not be greater than one serum half-life of the drug.

Anticonvulsant drug serum levels affect both the ability to achieve seizure control and the likelihood of causing most drug-induced side effects or toxicity. Measurements of blood levels also help the treatment team determine whether poor therapeutic responses are due to noncompliance (the major reason for a poor therapeutic outcome), or other causes such as malabsorption, rapid drug elimination, or use of the wrong drug. However, blood levels alone cannot, and should not, be used as the only means to assess the response. Some adverse responses to anticonvulsant drugs may occur regardless of the drug's blood level. Numbers on a laboratory report cannot replace careful assessment or the need for common sense.

NURSING IMPLICATIONS

There are six general rules to follow.

1. Give anticonvulsants on time to help achieve and maintain steady-state blood levels and responses.
2. Be familiar with the patient's history, including the results of pretreatment laboratory test results, before initial administration of any anticonvulsant.
3. Double-check medication orders, especially those calling for high initial doses of an anticonvulsant. Most drugs should be started at low doses and increased gradually to reach therapeutic blood concentrations.
4. Be aware that drug dosages are highly individualized. In addition to laboratory tests, rely on observation skills to assess the patient's response. Notify the physician if there are concerns.
5. If an anticonvulsant is to be discontinued, the dosage should be reduced gradually to reduce the risk of rebound seizures or status epilepticus. Regardless of the reason for discontinuation, notify all persons responsible for the patient's care at once so that closer monitoring can be started and alternative drugs prescribed. If discontinuation is required because of an allergic drug response, a chemically unrelated anticonvulsant must be used. Observe closely and frequently when treatment with the new agent is begun.
6. Draw blood for measurement of anticonvulsant levels at the proper time. Unless the patient shows signs of drug toxicity, the physician will want to know the trough level, which is the lowest blood concentration during a 24-hour period. It occurs at the end of the longest dosage interval, usually early in the morning before the patient takes the first dose and daily meal.

A. Hydantoins

Hydantoins have been considered the most effective anticonvulsants for treating tonic-clonic and complex partial seizures. Their ability to control seizures without causing sedation provided the first clue that generalized CNS depression was not necessary for anticonvulsant activity. Phenytoin (called diphenylhydantoin in older texts) is the prototype. The most common brand name is DILANTIN.

PROTOTYPE

Phenytoin

Absorption, Distribution, Metabolism, and Excretion

Phenytoin formulations available for oral administration include immediate-acting tablets, capsules, and suspensions, which cause peak blood levels to occur roughly 2 hours after administration. There are also extended-acting capsules, which are absorbed more slowly (peak blood levels occur in about 6 hours), but which cause more longlasting blood levels after each dose. Parenteral formulations can be given intramuscularly or intravenously. When phenytoin is injected intramuscularly, however, the drug is absorbed irregularly and incompletely. Indeed, giving phenytoin by intramuscular (IM) injection actually results in blood levels that are about 50% lower than if the same dose were given as an immediate-acting oral dosage form.

Phenytoin is extensively bound to plasma proteins. Nearly all the drug is eventually metabolized by the liver, and the metabolites are excreted in the urine. Thus, dosage reductions become important for persons with altered liver function. Phenytoin induces (stimulates) the liver's drug metabolizing enzyme systems. As noted below, this is a cause of some important drug interactions. Table 26–3 summarizes some of the key pharmacokinetic data.

Pharmacologic Effects

Phenytoin inhibits the spread of seizure activity, primarily in the motor cortex, and reduces the activity of brainstem centers responsible for the tonic phase of generalized tonic-clonic seizures. These effects are due to the drug's ability to normalize abnormal fluxes of sodium across nerve cell membranes during or after depolarization, which otherwise make the nerve hyperexcitable.

Phenytoin depresses cardiac electrical conduction in a similar manner, particularly in the arrhythmic heart. This action is used therapeutically, as discussed in Chapter 30.

Clinical Indications and Administration

Therapeutic anticonvulsant blood levels for phenytoin range from 10 μg/mL to around 20 μg/mL. This drug is most effective for managing tonic-clonic seizures (see Table 26–2), including those associated with neurosurgery. However, it is only a second-line agent for managing the tonic-clonic seizures that characterize status epilepticus, for which intravenous (IV) diazepam is the preferred agent. Phenytoin is less effective than most other anticonvulsants for managing simple partial seizures. Importantly, it is ineffective for managing absence seizures; in fact, it often worsens these seizures. An unrelated, approved use for phenytoin is the management of trigeminal neuralgia. Dosages and dosing protocols for these uses, and for the various dosage forms and administration routes, are summarized in Table 26–C.

NURSING IMPLICATIONS

Overall, and regardless of the reason for which phenytoin is given, differences in this drug's absorption and metabolism rates make it important to individualize the dosages for each patient, and to monitor the responses (and blood levels, if needed) frequently. The various formulations and brands can differ by as much as 90% in their bioavailabilities. Do not switch between administration routes without making dosage adjustments for bioavailability and bioequivalence. Likewise, be aware (and make your patients aware) of potentially important differences between formulations given by the same route, including those between brand-name or generic products. Advise patients who are getting prescription refills to stay with the same product and brand, and to ask the pharmacist about potential differences if the prescription is refilled with a different product.

There are other important considerations for phenytoin therapy.

With oral phenytoin dosage forms:

- Do not use extended-acting preparations to start therapy; reaching steady blood levels usually occurs too slowly.
- Shake phenytoin oral suspensions well before measuring the dose, else settling of the drug particles could lead to underdosing, and almost certainly will make it difficult to obtain consistency from dose to dose.

With all parenteral phenytoin formulations:

- Do not administer them if they are cloudy or contain a precipitate; they should be clear and slightly yellow.
- Monitor cardiovascular and respiratory status closely; this is especially important when phenytoin is given intravenously, for which electrocardiographic monitoring is recommended.
- Avoid mixing with other drugs, and check compatibilities with IV fluids. Phenytoin will precipitate in D_5W solution. This is because phenytoin is poorly soluble and is incompatible with most other drugs.
- Use a large-bore needle or catheter for IV administration, infuse over 30 to 60 minutes when possible, avoid prolonged infusions (discard 4 hours after preparation), and flush the needle or catheter with a small amount of sterile saline when administration is done. These are important measures because phenytoin is very alkaline and irritating to blood vessels.
- When switching from oral to IM phenytoin, be sure to increase the IM dose appropriately; and when returning to oral therapy, reduce the oral dose.

Side Effects, Adverse Reactions, and Contraindications

Table 26–S summarizes the side effects associated with phenytoin administration. The risk and severity generally are much greater when phenytoin is given for its usual indication: the long-term management of chronic seizure disorders.

The most common side effects caused by phenytoin reflect CNS depression, and include sluggishness, ataxia, confusion, slurred speech, and nystagmus. Overall, however, phenytoin is considered to be the least sedating anticonvulsant. Common gastrointestinal (GI) responses include constipation, nausea, and vomiting.

Some of the other key side effects affect the skin (rashes, acne, hair and gingival overgrowth), the blood and blood-forming tissues (eg, megaloblastic anemia), and the liver. Nutrient deficiencies involving folic acid and vitamins D and K are relatively common with long-term phenytoin use. They reflect the drug's ability to stimulate the hepatic metabolism of these nutrients, and may require nutritional intervention to prevent such related problems as bleeding tendencies and osteomalacia (related to deficiencies of vitamins K and D, respectively).

Skin rashes, a lupus erythematosus–like syndrome, true hepatic damage, and blood dyscrasias have been reported in persons receiving phenytoin, and may not be dose-related. Although these usually are uncommon idiosyncratic reactions, they are potentially dangerous. Thus, close monitoring is required.

Injecting phenytoin too rapidly by the IV route can cause profound CNS depression and a variety of adverse cardiovascular reactions. These usually reflect acute toxicity, and so are discussed separately, below.

There are a few specific contraindications to phenytoin use. Hypersensitivity or allergy to phenytoin or other hydantoins precludes its use. Additionally, patients with hematologic or hepatic disorders should not receive phenytoin. Because phenytoin has appreciable effects on cardiac electrical activity, it should not be given parenterally, unless unavoidable, to patients with sinus bradycardia, sinoatrial block, second- and third-degree AV block, or Stokes-Adams syndrome (periods of unconsciousness caused by episodes of heart block). There is no contraindication to using phenytoin for status epilepticus.

NURSING IMPLICATIONS

Table 26–S summarizes the key points for what should be done to prevent, detect, or manage side effects associated with phenytoin or other anticonvulsants. This is just as important as assessing for desired anticonvulsant drug actions.

The CNS-depressant side effects noted for phenytoin generally apply to all anticonvulsants, and the related nursing implication are generally the same as would apply to any CNS depressant drug (eg, barbiturates). The most important ones include making patients aware of the potential responses, and then cautioning them against participating in activities that may be made more dangerous because of impaired alertness, coordination, or vision. The common GI disturbances are best handled by advising patients to take oral phenytoin with food. They should learn to do this consistently to minimize fluctuations in the speed and amount of drug that would be absorbed if timing of drug administration with respect to meals was haphazard. Constipation is best managed with nondrug measures (increase dietary fluid and bulk intake). Laxatives are a last-choice intervention, and should be used only with the advice and supervision of a physician. Improper laxative use can interfere with the absorption and effectiveness of phenytoin (and all other anticonvulsants), and can cause or worsen a variety of medical disorders, including seizure disorders.

Although some skin rashes and blood and nutrient abnormalities are relatively common with long-term phenytoin therapy and some are relatively benign or treatable, the risk of serious reactions is real. These too must be assessed for frequently, because all require evaluation by a physician in order to decide what to do next. Blood disorders such as anemia or coagulation factor deficiencies may not be accompanied by obvious signs and symptoms (eg, fatigue, increased bruising or bleeding). Therefore, baseline blood studies are essential before therapy starts, and they should be performed at regular intervals during treatment, even if the patient appears symptom-free. Liver function studies are equally important. If liver function declines during therapy and goes undetected, dose-dependent side effects of phenytoin are almost certain to occur and be intense.

◆ Use During Pregnancy and Lactation

The use of phenytoin during pregnancy has been linked to the development of birth defects that include cleft lip and palate and cardiac malformations. However, and as noted in more detail on page 491, it is not known whether these have been caused by the drug or by maternal seizures that have not been managed adequately with anticonvulsant therapy.

It is clear, however, that children born to women who take phenytoin throughout pregnancy or near term develop clotting defects. They reflect neonatal deficiencies in vitamin K–dependent clotting factors. The bleeding tendencies put the newborn at risk of excessive bleeding or frank hemorrhage. They are usually most pronounced during the first postpartum day, and may occur despite the presence of normal maternal clotting factor levels.

To reduce this risk, vitamin K (phytonadione) should be given prophylactically to the mother starting about 1 month before delivery, and newborns should receive vitamin K shortly after delivery. Clotting studies should be performed on the infant. Repeated injections of vitamin K, concentrated clotting factors, or fresh-frozen plasma can be given for persistent clotting abnormalities. Breast-feeding during phenytoin therapy is not recommended because the drug is excreted in breast milk.

◆ Use in Children

A common and unique response to phenytoin, particularly in children, is gingival hyperplasia. It is especially problematic in young developmentally impaired patients. Unless proper precautions are taken, the gums may become tender and bleed easily, and may grow completely over the teeth. Encourage good oral hygiene, particularly thorough but gentle brushing and flossing of the teeth, to reduce the risk of gingival hyperplasia. Notify the patient's dentist about phenytoin use.

Overgrowth of body hair, coarsening of facial features, and worsening of acne can cause added physical and emotional problems for older children, many of whom already live with the stigmas and misconceptions associated with seizure disorders.

◆ Use in the Elderly

Side effects or manifestations of toxicity, particularly those involving the CNS (drowsiness, ataxia), occur earlier and may be more problematic in the elderly. Age-related declines of hepatic function may be an important factor. In addition, the prevalence of other medical or mental conditions, each of which may require therapy with a potentially interacting drug, complicates phenytoin therapy. Anticipate a greater incidence of adverse cardiovascular responses, especially arrhythmias, in elderly persons who receive phenytoin. The risks associated with IV use of this drug are increased.

Interactions with Other Drugs

Phenytoin interacts with many drugs. Even when one considers only interactions that are known or likely to occur, and excludes those that are more theoretical than based in clinical reality, the list is long (Table 26–1). Most interactions involve one drug's ability to stimulate or inhibit the hepatic metabolism of the other, leading to decreased or increased blood levels of the affected drug. In many cases, phenytoin causes the interaction by stimulating the liver's ability to metabolize (and thereby reduce the therapeutic effect of) the other drug. This applies, for example, to interactions with oral anticoagulants; oral contraceptives; corticosteroids; the immunosuppressant cyclosporine; the major antiparkinson drug levodopa; and a widely used bronchodilator, theophylline. Conversely, some drugs (of which the antiulcer drug cimetidine is the most common example) can inhibit phenytoin's metabolism, causing blood levels of the anticonvulsant to rise. The outcome can be a worsening of side effects, or the development of true toxicity.

Most of these interactions need not be avoided as long as the health-care team is aware of the potential for the interaction and its consequences, and can monitor the patient's responses and drug blood levels adequately. Indeed, some of the interactants with phenytoin are other anticonvulsants that may have to be prescribed in order to achieve optimum seizure control, whether for a patient who is refractory to a single agent, or for one who has multiple seizure types that require a different anticonvulsant for each. Examples are carbamazepine, phenacemide, phenurone, and valproic acid.

Frequent nursing assessment, and teaching the patient to report signs or symptoms of drug interactions, are critically important to help achieve safe and effective combination drug therapy.

NURSING IMPLICATIONS

Several strategies can be used to minimize problems related to interactions involving other drugs that interact with phenytoin and other anticonvulsants.

- Educate patients to be aware of the drugs they are taking, preferably by providing them with a written list. Advise them to carry this information with them, and to wear an identification bracelet (eg, MedicAlert) so that others who may care for them in an emergency can be aware of their seizure disorder and their medication plan.
- Give a written list of interacting drugs to avoid—especially over-the-counter (OTC) agents such as acetaminophen, alcohol, and other sedating medications—and encourage patients to consult their health-care provider before taking nonprescription drugs.
- Whether the interaction involves a prescription drug or an OTC agent recommended by the physician, understand (and stress to patients) the importance of consistency in the administration of these drugs (dosages, timing of doses). This is important so that somewhat predictable problems arising from the interaction will not be made unpredictable because of haphazard medication administration.
- Be aware that consequences of the interactions are likely to be greatest when the administration of one drug is started, and again when it is stopped. It is during these times that the true extent of the interaction may not have developed fully, because changing blood levels (and effects) of one drug or the other have yet to stabilize. These are also the times when it is necessary to use increased vigilance in assessing for changes in the patient's responses to the drugs, and to use more frequent blood tests to measure blood levels of one or both interactants. This information will help the physi-

cian decide whether or how to adjust drug dosages, or whether it is best to discontinue one of the interactants altogether.

- Stress the need for patients to recognize key signs of increased or decreased drug effects, and to understand the reason for more frequent blood tests and dosage changes.

Overdose and Toxicity

Some signs and symptoms of phenytoin overdoses differ in important ways from overdoses of other anticonvulsants, but treatment is similar for all of them. *There is no specific, safe, and universally effective antidote for any anticonvulsant.* Anticonvulsant overdoses are medical emergencies that require skilled assessment to guide subsequent treatment. The combined use of interacting drugs can complicate assessment and treatment of overdoses.

Signs and symptoms of phenytoin toxicity develop when blood levels reach 20 to 50 μg/mL. Two to five grams of phenytoin taken at once (or serum levels above 100 μg/mL) are lethal. Symptoms of toxicity include nystagmus, ataxia, dysarthria, tremor, slurred speech, and nausea and vomiting. Hypotension may develop, followed by circulatory and ventilatory failure, coma, and death.

Standard interventions are used to reduce further drug absorption: induced emesis (if permitted by the patient's condition), repeated gastric lavage and suctioning, and administration of activated charcoal to bind unabsorbed drug. Hemodialysis or total exchange transfusions may be indicated, particularly for severely overdosed children. Vital signs, particularly those reflecting cardiopulmonary status, must be monitored closely and corrected or supported as necessary.

Related Drugs

Ethotoin and mephenytoin are the related hydantoins. Neither is used as often as phenytoin, or is considered a first-line anticonvulsant. Their dosages are listed in Table 26–C.

Ethotoin

Ethotoin (PEGANONE) is indicated for tonic-clonic and complex partial seizures, and can be given alone or with most other anticonvulsants. Use extreme care if ethotoin is administered with phenacemide (PHENURONE). This combination may cause paranoid symptoms.

Mephenytoin

Mephenytoin (MESANTOIN) is indicated for treatment of tonic-clonic, complex partial, and simple partial seizures in patients who have not responded to phenytoin or ethotoin. It is used only for refractory cases because it is more toxic than other hydantoins, particularly with regard to a higher incidence of agranulocytosis and aplastic anemia. Mephenytoin is more sedating than the other hydantoins.

B. Long-Acting Barbiturates

Long-acting barbiturates, of which the prototype is phenobarbital, are used as sedatives in seizure-free individuals. However they are also useful as anticonvulsants. This use is the only one for which long-term administration of barbiturates is considered safe, effective, and medically acceptable. The barbiturates have been discussed in more detail in Chapter 22; only those aspects related to their use as anticonvulsants are presented here. Anticonvulsant doses are listed in Table 26–C.

Phenobarbital

Phenobarbital, the prototype barbiturate, shares the major indications noted for phenytoin. Oral phenobarbital is generally preferred to phenytoin for children because the barbiturate does not cause gingival hyperplasia. And, like phenytoin, phenobarbital has either no effect on absence seizures or worsens them. Given intravenously, phenobarbital can be used to treat various acute seizures, including status epilepticus.

Sedation and drowsiness are the most common side effects when phenobarbital is used as an oral anticonvulsant (despite its alleged selective anticonvulsant properties) in adults. Children may experience paradoxical hyperexcitability, irritability, or similar mood or behavioral changes (see p 349). Any other side effects noted for the barbiturates can also occur; all related contraindications and nursing implications apply (see Table 22–S1, p 371). However, prolonged use of phenobarbital for seizure control increases the risk of some side effects, particularly vitamin D and K deficiencies owing to the barbiturate's ability to induce the liver's drug-metabolizing enzyme system. Prophylactic vitamin supplement therapy, as noted above for phenytoin, is often needed for patients taking the barbiturate. Pregnancy-related precautions noted for phenytoin (eg, the risk of postpartum bleeding tendencies in the newborn) also apply.

The drug interactions involving phenobarbital were summarized in Table 22–I1 (p 372). Most of them occur because of the barbiturate's well-known ability to stimulate the hepatic enzymes. Although interactions with all other anticonvulsants are potentially important, the interaction between phenobarbital and valproic acid is particularly serious: valproic acid can triple phenobarbital blood levels. In this instance the interaction occurs because valproic acid inhibits phenobarbital's metabolism. The outcome can be a serious, acute episode of CNS depression. The risks are far greater than the similar interaction between valproic acid and phenytoin. Combined therapy is permissible, but therapy must be supervised with extreme care, especially when valproic acid is added to or removed from the treatment plan.

NURSING IMPLICATIONS

Avoid parenteral phenobarbital administration unless oral administration is impossible or prompt anticonvulsant effects are essential (as with status epilepticus). When it is injected, use the IV route, making sure the drug is given no faster than 60 mg/minute. This should help reduce the risks of excessive hypotension and further impairment of respiration. Careful assessment of neurologic, cardiovascular, and respiratory status is essential once the drug has been injected. Always have resuscitation equipment readily available.

Mephobarbital and Metharbital

Mephobarbital (MEBARAL) is metabolized to phenobarbital. Metharbital (GEMONIL) is metabolized to barbital, which has a duration of action that is even longer than that of phenobarbital. Both drugs share phenobarbital's use for long-term oral therpay of tonic-clonic seizures. Unlike phenobarbital, these alternatives are also suitable for managing absence seizures. Mephobarbital seems to cause less sedation than phenobarbital, and metharbital seems to cause slightly more. These drugs can be used alone, or combined (usually with phenobarbital, phenytoin, or both). When combinations are used, dosage adjustments usually must be made to account for additive CNS depressant effects and for the ability of the barbiturates to stimulate the metabolism of the other agents.

Primidone

Primidone (MYSOLINE), also an orally administered anticonvulsant, is structurally related to the barbiturates. In fact, one of its metabolites is phenobarbital, which contributes to the anticonvulsant effects caused by primidone itself. The drug can be used alone or in combination with other anticonvulsants.

Primidone is seldom used as a first-line drug when a barbiturate is indicated because it poses a greater risk of adverse responses. The most common side effects, ataxia and vertigo, are most intense when therapy is begun. They usually disappear with continued therapy, but reduced doses may be required. Occasional side effects include GI upset, nystagmus, diplopia, emotional disturbances, impotence, and morbilliform rashes. Rare cases of megaloblastic anemia occur that respond to treatment with folic acid. Primidone administration can be continued during this time. As with the barbiturates, porphyria is an absolute contraindication to primidone use.

C. Succinimides

Ethosuximide (ZARONTIN) is the prototype of a class of anticonvulsants called *succinimides*. They are chemically distinct from the hydantoins and barbiturates. Related drugs are methsuximide and phensuximide. Their clinical importance lies in their suitability for treating absence and petit mal seizures, which do not respond well to the drugs mentioned above.

PROTOTYPE

Ethosuximide

Absorption, Distribution, Metabolism, and Excretion

Ethosuximide (ZARONTIN) is absorbed well when taken orally, has a half-life of about 60 hours in adults (30 hours in children), and reaches a serum steady-state in 5 to 10 days. The drug undergoes hepatic metabolism and renal excretion.

Pharmacologic Effects

Ethosuximide decreases seizure frequency by depressing the motor cortex and by reducing CNS sensitivity to convulsive nerve stimuli. It suppresses the three-cycle-per-second spike-and-wave activity that is characteristic of petit mal seizures.

Clinical Indications and Administration

Ethosuximide (see Table 26–C) is indicated for absence seizures. Trimethadione (p 483) may be more effective, but ethosuximide is used more often because of its relatively lower toxicity. Valproic acid (p 484) is gaining popularity as the preferred drug for absence seizures and other generalized seizure disorders.

Ethosuximide can be used with other anticonvulsants to treat patients with seizures in addition to absence seizures. However, it can increase the risk of tonic-clonic seizures, so higher doses of the drug indicated for that type of seizure may be required. Administration of ethosuximide alone can increase the risk of tonic-clonic seizures in susceptible patients.

Ethosuximide's long half-life permits once-daily administration. For any patient, daily doses should be 1.5 g or less to decrease the risk of side effects and toxicity. Higher doses should be used only if the patient can be supervised closely.

Side Effects, Adverse Reactions, and Contraindications

Gastrointestinal symptoms (particularly nausea, vomiting, cramps, diarrhea, and anorexia) are the most common side effects caused by ethosuximide (see Table 26–S).

The major contraindication to the use of any succinimide, other than drug allergy, is liver or renal damage, which may be aggravated or caused by these drugs. In addition, giving ethosuximide to patients with impaired hepatic function will prolong the drug's already long half-life, increasing the risk of longlasting toxicity. Ethosuximide can be given during pregnancy if needed and if appropriate care is given. Breast-feeding should be discouraged.

NURSING IMPLICATIONS

Administer ethosuximide with meals to reduce GI distress. Emphasize the need for complete blood counts and renal and liver function tests before starting ethosuximide therapy, and at regular intervals thereafter, to help detect serious adverse responses as early as possible. Give usual precautions related to drowsiness. If depression or aggression occur, ethosuximide may need to be withdrawn gradually. Closely monitor patients with a history of tonic-clonic seizures.

Interactions with Other Drugs

The only specific drug interaction involves the ability of ethosuximide to decrease the blood levels and therapeutic effects of primidone (Table 26–I). Appropriate monitoring to help guide dosage adjustments (see the drug interactions section for phenytoin) usually is all that is needed. This is especially important when starting or stopping therapy with one of the interactants.

Overdose and Toxicity

Overdoses of succinimides intensify the GI, CNS, hematologic, and dermatologic side effects noted in Table 26–S. Ataxia, lethargy, dizziness, or sedation are often the earliest signs of an overdose. Severe reactions include myopia, vaginal bleeding, profound CNS depression, and systemic lupus erythematosus. Overdoses are treated symptomatically and supportively.

NURSING IMPLICATIONS

Advise patients who miss one dose of ethosuximide not to take a double dose to make up for it. Since ethosuximide has such a long half-life, doubling the dose is liable to increase blood levels dramatically, increasing the risk or severity of side effects or toxicity. If toxicity occurs, anticipate that symptoms, and the need for proper care, will be longlasting.

Related Drugs

Methsuximide and phensuximide are the other approved succinimides. Both share the same mechanisms of action, indications, and side effects noted for ethosuximide. They have different efficacies and risks of toxicity. Recommended dosages are noted in Table 26–S.

Methsuximide

Methsuximide (CELONTIN) is as effective as ethosuximide for treating absence seizures, but it is slightly more toxic. Therefore, methsuximide should be reserved for patients who have not responded to ethosuximide or another drug, the lowest effective dose should be used, and doses should be increased no more often than once per week.

Phensuximide

Phensuximide (MILONTIN) is thought to be slightly less effective than ethosuximide or methsuximide.

D. Benzodiazepines

The prototype benzodiazepine, diazepam (VALIUM), is perhaps the most well-known anxiolytic drug. It and a related agent, clonazepam, also have clinically useful anticonvulsant activities. See Chapter 22 for more details about diazepam, including dosages for other indications (Table 22–C2); side effects and contraindications (Table 22–S2); and drug interactions (Table 22–I2).

Diazepam

Oral diazepam is used as adjunctive treatment for several chronic seizure disorders. However, it is most well-known and wisely used as the drug of choice for status epilepticus. Single doses of 5 to 10 mg generally stop seizures in about 5 minutes in adults, and are effective about 95% of the time. (See Table 26–C for doses.)

A single IV dose of diazepam may quickly control seizures, but seizures may return as blood levels of the drug quickly drop to subtherapeutic levels. Anticipate this, since repeated doses may be required at 10- to 15-minute intervals. Usually, no more than 30 mg of diazepam should be used to treat a given episode of status epilepticus. However, since these seizures are fatal if they are not stopped, there may be no way to avoid exceeding this limit. Alternatively, some physicians may treat the patient initially with IV diazepam, then switch to an IV infusion of phenytoin or phenobarbital, either of which has a longer duration of action. Although these combinations usually will stop previously resistant seizures, they also cause an added risk of excessive respiratory and cardiovascular depression. Ventilatory depression is a particular problem with diazepam–phenobarbital combinations, and the two drugs should not be given at the same time. Be prepared to assess for these unwanted effects and to support ventilation and blood pressure as needed.

If these approaches do not work, anticipate the administration of paraldehyde (Chapter 22, p 378). As a last result, the patient will be given a neuromuscular blocker to suppress all skeletal muscle activity; intubated; and placed under general anesthesia and invasive monitoring as anticonvulsant therapies are tried.

NURSING IMPLICATIONS

When diazepam is used for status epilepticus, it is often common to administer an IV bolus injection of 50 mL of 50% glucose immediately before or after the anticonvulsant. This is done to replenish the brain's metabolic fuel, which along with oxygen has been depleted during a massive and sometimes prolonged seizure. Oxygen administration will be started as soon as possible.

Be aware that giving an IV injection to a patient experiencing intense tonic-clonic convulsions is not easy. It requires good composure and help from as many people as necessary. If IV injection is not possible, IM injections of diazepam into a large muscle are the next best choice. Have ample supplies of diazepam and other anticonvulsants, as well as the means to support blood pressure and ventilation, on hand.

There is absolutely no contraindication to the use of diazepam for managing status epilepticus.

Clonazepam

Clonazepam (KLONOPIN) is used to treat absence epilepsy, a petit mal variant epilepsy called Lennox-Gastaut, and myoclonic seizures. About one third of patients experience breakthrough seizures, which may indicate tolerance to the drug. Clonazepam can be used cautiously during pregnancy and breast-feeding. Combined administration of clonazepam and valproic acid may cause prolonged episodes of absence seizures (absence status epilepticus).

E. Oxazolidinediones

Paramethadione and Trimethadione

Trimethadione (TRIDIONE), which has been in use for nearly 50 years, is so similar to the related drug paramethadione (PARADIONE), that they will be considered together. They are basically last-choice drugs for managing absence seizures.

These drugs are quickly absorbed from the GI tract. Trimethadione is converted to an active metabolite that is excreted by the kidneys. It has a very long half-life (approximately 1 to 2 weeks), and so steady-state blood levels may not be reached for a month or more. Comparable information about paramethadione is not known, other than that the drug is extensively metabolized.

Trimethadione and paramethadione are indicated for treating refractory absence seizures. Dosages are given in Table 26–C. They are not first-line agents because they can cause serious and sometimes fatal adverse effects: hepatic and renal damage; blood dyscrasias; exfoliative dermatitis; systemic lupus erythematosus; and a myasthenia gravis–like syndrome. Less serious side effects include drowsiness (especially during initial therapy); photophobia (dose-dependent); and GI disturbances (eg, nausea, vomiting, and anorexia and associated weight loss). Acneiform rashes may also occur. In addition, these drugs are very teratogenic. Of all the anticonvulsants they pose the greatest risk to the fetus. They should be administered during pregnancy only after all other alternatives have been tried and have been proven ineffective, and only when maternal benefits are hoped to outweigh the fetal risks. Breast-feeding should be discouraged.

Trimethadione and paramethadione interact with other CNS depressants to cause added CNS depression. One specific interaction involves valproic acid, which can elevate trimethadione blood levels and increase the risks or intensity of side effects.

Therapeutic blood levels of trimethadione's active metabolite are about 700 μg/mL. Since toxic blood levels for most anticonvulsants are only slightly higher than therapeutic levels, blood levels not far above the 700 μg/mL value are likely to cause serious dose-related problems. Early manifestations of toxicity include worsening of the CNS and visual side effects noted above. Serious overdoses can cause coma. Treatment is symptomatic and supportive; alkalinizing the urine seems to speed the elimination of trimethadione's longlasting active metabolite.

NURSING IMPLICATIONS

Owing to the potentially serious adverse effects of these drugs, close supervision of patients taking them is essential. The drug should be withdrawn as quickly and safely as possible if one of the following appear: lymph node enlargement or other potential indicators of lupus; jaundice or other indicators of hepatic damage; bleeding, bruising, sore throat, or other possible signs of blood dyscrasias; and skin rashes. Although most rashes caused by these drugs usually are not serious, they can be indicators of an early stage of exfoliative dermatitis, which can be fatal. Even apparently benign rashes should be allowed to heal before resuming therapy with these drugs.

Paramethadione liquid dosage forms have a high alcohol content. They should be diluted well with a suitable beverage to mask the taste if they are to be administered to children.

F. Other Anticonvulsants

Carbamazepine, phenacemide, and valproic acid are the remaining drugs used for chronic treatment of seizures. They are listed here only because their chemical structures differ from those of the drugs mentioned earlier. Valproic acid is discussed first because it is the only one of the three that is considered a first-line anticonvulsant. The others are effective but not preferred because of a greater risk of toxicity.

Valproic Acid

Valproic acid (DEPAKENE) has a broad range of anticonvulsant activity. It is gaining acceptance as the most effective drug for generalized seizures.

Absorption, Distribution, Metabolism, and Excretion

Valproic acid, whether administered as capsules or syrup, is absorbed very quickly from the GI tract. Peak serum levels occur in less than 4 hours. Valproic acid is extensively bound to plasma proteins. It has a relatively short plasma half-life—about 6 to 16 hours. It is metabolized to at least one other compound that is excreted in the urine; otherwise, little is known about its biologic fate. The sodium salt of valproic acid (divalproex sodium; DEPAKOTE) is available in enteric-coated tablets. The coating delays drug absorption by about 1 hour.

Pharmacologic Effects

Valproic acid appears to inhibit the spread of abnormal discharges through the brain. This effect may be the result of the drug's ability to increase brain levels of GABA, an inhibitory neurotransmitter.

Clinical Indications and Administration

Valproic acid is indicated for the treatment of absence, tonic-clonic, myoclonic, and complex partial seizures (see Table 26–2). Some authorities consider it to be the drug of choice for these seizures unless the patient is pregnant. The usual starting dose is about 15 mg/kg per day for adults or children. (This low dose reduces the incidence of some annoying side effects.) The therapeutic blood level is 50 to 100 μg/mL. Since valproic acid has a relatively short half-life, steady-state blood levels are achieved best by giving the drug in three or four equal divided doses.

Side Effects, Adverse Reactions, and Contraindications

The use of valproic acid is growing because of its broad utility and its freedom from frequent serious side effects. Next to phenytoin, this anticonvulsant is least likely to cause drowsiness or sedation at therapeutic blood levels if no other anticonvulsants, particularly barbiturates, are being taken. Moderate nausea, vomiting, and diarrhea are common during early therapy, but they usually disappear and rarely require drug discontinuation. Gastrointestinal irritation is less when enteric-coated tablets are used. Approximately 10% of patients taking valproic acid chronically experience weight gain, and a few suffer from transient alopecia.

There have been a few reports of fatal hepatotoxicity during valproic acid therapy, but it is not known whether liver damage was actually caused by the drug. Nevertheless, valproic acid and its sodium salt are contraindicated in patients with hepatic disease, dysfunction, or any abnormality of liver function tests. The drugs should be used with extreme caution in patients with prior liver disorders. Hepatic dysfunction is most likely to occur during the first 6 months of valproic acid treatment, and is thought to pose a greater risk to patients taking other anticonvulsants, patients with prior hepatic dysfunction, patients with severe seizure disorders (especially if accompanied by mental retardation), and children. Therefore, liver function tests are essential before starting valproic acid therapy, and should be done regularly thereafter. If such tests indicate damage or dysfunction during treatment, valproic acid should be discontinued. Allergic and hypersensitivity reactions, although rare, contraindicate the use of valproic acid.

◆ Use During Pregnancy and Lactation

Valproic acid is one of the least suitable anticonvulsants for use in pregnancy; it should not be given during this time unless seizures fail to respond to other drugs. The drug is teratogenic, and its use during pregnancy has been linked to disabling developmental abnormalities of the CNS. If it must be used, amniocentesis should be performed before the twentieth week of gestation. If there are early indicators of adverse fetal effects, options concerning therapy and continued pregnancy should be discussed.

◆ Use in Children

Children under the age of 2 years have a greater risk of developing fatal hepatotoxicity, particularly if they are taking other anticonvulsants, have congenital metabolic disorders, or severe seizures.

◆ Use in the Elderly

Age-related declines of hepatic function, the prevalence of organic brain disease, and lesser tolerance of drug side effects on the CNS increase the risk of untoward responses in the elderly.

Interactions with Other Drugs

Several important interactions (Table 26–1) may be encountered during anticonvulsant therapy with valproic acid. Aspirin, the most commonly used antiinflammatory drug (Chapter 52), can displace the anticonvulsant from plasma protein binding sites and increase valproate blood levels and side effects. Valproic acid inhibits phenobarbital metabolism, leading to increased barbiturate blood levels. The usual response is excessive sedation, but true phenobarbital toxicity can occur. Conversely, phenobarbital can stimulate valproic acid metabolism, lowering the latter drug's blood levels and therapeutic effects. This interaction almost always necessitates careful reductions in the phenobarbital dose. A similar interaction may occur with alcohol ingestion and with combined valproic acid and carbamazepine use: reduced valproate levels and increased levels of carbamazepine. The interaction with phenytoin was noted above.

NURSING IMPLICATIONS

Given the prevalence with which aspirin and alcohol are self-administered for a variety of reasons, it is important to discourage such unsupervised use. It is not known whether other prescription or nonprescription (eg, ibuprofen) nonsteroidal antiinflammatory drugs interact, but the nurse should be aware of the possibility. Acetaminophen (eg, TYLENOL) belongs to a different drug class, and does not interact; it should be recommended for relief of mild pain or fever. General monitoring precautions apply to the other interactions. When valproic acid and phenobarbital are used together, anticipate the need for reducing the phenobarbital dose by 30% to 70%.

Overdose and Toxicity

The major concern of valproic acid overdose is profound CNS depression and possible deep coma. It is most likely to occur when valproic acid and phenobarbital are given concomitantly. Since valproic acid is absorbed so quickly, standard first-aid measures to reduce drug absorption (gastric lavage, forced emesis, and so on) are not likely to help unless they are used very soon after ingestion. (These measures may be more effective if the overdose was due to divalproex sodium, which is absorbed more slowly.) Other supportive measures directed toward respiratory and cardiovascular status are the same as noted for other anticonvulsants. Interestingly, the narcotic antagonist naloxone (NARCAN) may reverse the central depressant effects of valproic acid overdose, but it may also counteract anticonvulsant effects, leading to the recurrence of severe seizures.

Carbamazepine

Carbamazepine (TEGRETOL) is chemically related to the tricyclic antidepressants. Indeed, when carbamazepine is used for epilepsy some patients report improved mood. It is an effective anticonvulsant, but is a second-choice agent because of its toxicity.

Absorption, Distribution, Metabolism, and Excretion

Carbamazepine is slowly and incompletely absorbed from the GI tract. Taking the drug with food improves absorption. Peak serum levels occur within 4 to 5 hours after oral administration. Carbamazepine is metabolized in the liver to active metabolites that are excreted in the urine. The half-life is between 12 and 17 hours with chronic therapy.

Pharmacologic Effects

The mechanism of carbamazepine's anticonvulsant action is not known.

Clinical Indications and Administration

Carbamazepine is indicated for complex partial or tonic-clonic seizures, or multiple-seizure disorders involving both partial and tonic-clonic seizures. Absence seizures do not respond to carbamazepine. It is also indicated for relief of pain caused by trigeminal or glossopharyngeal neuralgia. It may be effective for treating affective psychosis, particularly cases that are rapidly cycling or unresponsive to lithium.

The therapeutic anticonvulsant serum level of carbamazepine is between 4 and 12 μg/mL. When used alone, the usual adult starting dose is 200 mg given twice daily. Common daily maintenance doses are between 800 and 1200 mg (the maximum recommended adult daily dose), given in three or four divided doses. Pediatric dosages are listed in Table 26–C.

NURSING IMPLICATIONS

Instruct patients to take carbamazepine with meals, since food improves its absorption. To minimize fluctuations in blood levels owing to altered absorption, encourage consistency in timing the dose with respect to meals.

Side Effects, Adverse Reactions, and Contraindications

Common side effects (Table 26–S) of carbamazepine include drowsiness, dizziness, unsteadiness, nausea, and diplopia. Blood dyscrasias, some of which have involved fatal aplastic anemia, agranulocytosis, thrombocytopenia, or leukopenia, are the most serious adverse reactions. The incidence of blood dyscrasias is low (estimated at less than 1 in 50,000), but carbamazepine is nevertheless contraindicated in persons with a history of bone marrow depression or abnormal blood counts. Other adverse reactions include activation of latent psychosis, confusion in the elderly, hepatic damage, and renal dysfunction. Rashes, diaphoresis, dyspnea, and cardiovascular changes (heart failure or hypo- or hypertension) are relatively uncommon. Patients with histories of allergy or hypersensitivity to carbamazepine or tricyclic antidepressants should not receive this anticonvulsant.

Carbamazepine should be used cautiously during pregnancy. Carbamazepine levels in breast milk may be as high as 60% of the maternal blood concentration, so breast-feeding is usually discouraged.

NURSING IMPLICATIONS

Complete blood counts and tests of renal and hepatic function should be done before and periodically during carbamazepine therapy. Significant abnormalities require immediate notification of the physician, discontinuation of the drug, and administration of other anticonvulsants to prevent seizures from reappearing. If carbamazepine therapy is stopped because of abnormal blood test results, the tests should be repeated daily to assess recovery. Frequent bone marrow aspiration and examination may be necessary. Instruct patients taking carbamazepine to notify the nurse or physician at once if signs of infection or abnormal blood clotting occur. Notify the physician if the patient experiences a reemergence of psychotic thinking or confusion. Elderly patients may require assistance with ambulation.

Interactions with Other Drugs

Carbamazepine's side effects account for its use as a second-line agent, but drug interactions (Table 26–I) can cause added problems also. The interactants include several of the anticonvulsants that have already been mentioned (phenytoin, primidone, and valproic acid), plus other drugs in several classes: antibiotics (tetracyclines and the antitubercular antibiotic isoniazid); oral anticoagulants; cimetidine, an antiulcer drug; and the psychiatric drugs haloperidol and lithium. Most of these interactions result in increased carbamazepine blood levels, which can increase the risk of side efffects or true toxicity if dosages are not adjusted properly. The interaction with tetracycline antibiotics is probably the most important one to avoid.

Overdose and Toxicity

Neuromuscular disturbances are the earliest and most pronounced signs of carbamazepine toxicity. They include muscular restlessness, twitching or other involuntary movements, exaggerated reflexes, and eventually reflex depression. Large overdoses may cause coma, convulsions, and breathing irregularity or difficulty. Cardiovascular changes are likely to be modest unless massive overdoses have been taken, in which case tachycardia, other arrhythmias, hypertension, or shock may develop. Lethal doses range from 5 g in small children to 30 g in adults.

Treatment of overdose is symptomatic and supportive. Vomiting should be induced immediately, unless contraindicated. Gastric lavage should be performed, and activated charcoal administered, as soon as possible, even if several hours have elapsed since ingestion of an overdose, and particularly if the patient has also been consuming alcohol. Cathartics may limit further carbamazepine absorption. Forced diuresis with mannitol may hasten renal excretion. Small children who are severely intoxicated may require exchange transfusions. Parenteral diazepam or phenobarbital is indicated to control acute seizures caused by a carbamazepine overdose.

NURSING IMPLICATIONS

Be prepared to intubate patients for possible respiratory difficulty or arrest, and have diazepam available for possible seizures. Elevate the patient's legs if hypotension develops. Profound hypotension or shock may require invasive monitoring of blood pressure and administration of IV fluids, plasma expanders, or a vasoconstrictor. Vital signs should be monitored closely for several days or until the patient is fully recovered.

Phenacemide

Phenacemide (PHENURONE) is an effective anticonvulsant drug that is seldom used because of its toxicity.

Absorption, Distribution, Metabolism, and Excretion

Phenacemide is well absorbed from the GI tract. It is metabolized in the liver to two inactive metabolites that are excreted in the urine. Its onset of action is between 30 and 60 minutes.

Pharmacologic Effects

Phenacemide increases the seizure threshold through an unknown mechanism.

Clinical Indications and Administration

Phenacemide is indicated for complex partial seizures, but should be prescribed only if the patient has failed to respond adequately to other, safer, drugs. The average maintenance dose is between 2 and 3 g per day, given in three equal divided doses. However, much lower doses (250–500 mg three times daily) should be used initially to reduce the risk of side effects. One half the adult dose is used for children between 5 and 10 years old. Phenacemide can be used adjunctively with other anticonvulsants.

Side Effects, Adverse Reactions, and Contraindications

Phenacemide produces severe side effects (see Table 26–S). Common GI responses include anorexia, associated weight loss, and nausea. Other common side effects are drowsiness, dizziness, weakness, and ataxia. Phenacemide can cause severe adverse psychologic responses, including personality change, aggression, suicidal tendencies, and acute psychosis, which may require discontinuation of the drug. Individuals with previous personality disorders should be treated cautiously (if at all) with this agent. The most serious adverse responses to phenacemide use include liver damage, ne-

Table 26–4 Nursing Interventions During a Seizure

Prevent injury
- Help patient lie down in safe location if seizure is imminent
- Maintain or establish adequate airway; use care in positioning head; clear oral secretions; avoid inserting airway device in mouth if teeth are clenched
- Protect head from injury, but do not restrain
- Pad siderails, if appropriate
- Anticipate need for IV anticonvulsant (eg, diazepam) administration for status epilepticus, but be aware of institutional policies concerning administration of these drugs, if not already ordered, before giving them
- Advise patient (family member, others) to avoid self–treatment of a seizure by taking another dose of a prescribed oral anticonvulsant; proper medical care is essential

Assess seizure characteristics to aid diagnosis and eventual treatment
- Convulsions: present or absent? generalized or confined to certain muscle groups or side of body?
- Consciousness: lost or not? If so, how long?
- Duration of seizure or resulting convulsive state
- Evidence of autonomic hyperactivity: diaphoresis, loss of bowel or bladder control

Identify precipitating factors
- Patient's activity at time of seizure onset (information may come from patient or witness)
- How long ago last seizure (if any) occurred
- Seizure triggers associated with onset? (see Table 26–5)
- Warning signs (auras) before onset? (Table 26–5)
- General medical condition, history, at time of seizure onset
- Medication history (prescribed, self-prescribed or self-administered drugs)

phritis, and fatal blood dyscrasias. Phenacemide should be used cautiously during pregnancy, and breast-feeding should be discouraged.

NURSING IMPLICATIONS

Advise patients to take phenacemide with meals to reduce the severity of GI distress. Take precautions appropriate for any drug that may cause sedation, blood dyscrasias, hepatotoxicity, or nephrotoxicity, and give explicit instructions about the relevant signs and symptoms that might indicate a dangerous response. Assess for significant personality changes during phenacemide therapy. Phenacemide therapy should be stopped if there is any evidence of hematologic, hepatic, or renal dysfunction.

Interactions with Other Drugs

Phenacemide, given with phenytoin or other hydantoins, can increase the blood levels and dose-related side effects of the latter. The drug also can increase the risk of excessive CNS depression when administered with other CNS depressants. Monitor closely if this drug is administered with any other drug that can cause similar toxic effects, such as hepatotoxicity or blood dyscrasias.

Overdose and Toxicity

Phenacemide overdoses often cause excitement and mania followed by drowsiness, ataxia, and coma. In addition to standard diagnostic and treatment measures, periodic tests of blood, liver, and renal function are needed during overdose treatment and recovery.

G. Other Drugs with Anticonvulsant Activity

Several drugs with other primary therapeutic indications are used alone or as adjuncts to anticonvulsant therapy. They are acetazolamide, lidocaine, magnesium sulfate, and paraldehyde. The doses of these special agents are given in Table 26–C.

Acetazolamide

Acetazolamide (DIAMOX) is a diuretic that inhibits the enzyme carbonic anhydrase. This effect alkalinizes the urine and causes mild systemic (metabolic) acidosis.

The modest reduction of blood pH seems to reduce the development of seizures in seizure-prone patients. Acetazolamide is mainly used as an adjunct to the therapy of absence, tonic-clonic, and myoclonic seizures, but it can be used alone. Acetazolamide is usually given orally, but it can be given IV or IM if needed; IM administration is painful and should be avoided if possible. Sustained-release oral dosage forms should not be used for anticonvulsant therapy.

The urinary alkalinizing activity of acetazolamide can be used adjunctively to treat overdoses of phenytoin, phenobarbital, or trimethadione, and overdoses of aspirin.

Acetazolamide may cause dizziness, drowsiness, and paresthesias. It may cause hypokalemia and an increased risk of arrhythmias in patients taking digitalis.

See Chapter 32 for more information about acetazolamide.

Lidocaine

Lidocaine (XYLOCAINE), the local anesthetic and antiarrhythmic drug (Chapters 19 and 30, pp 291–297 and 559–561), is generally considered the drug of last choice for treating status epilepticus. It is given intravenously, usually after every other anticonvulsant has failed to control seizures. The recommended doses, 50 to 100 mg injected rapidly, are liable to cause significant hypotension and cardiac depression. Paradoxically, perhaps, high doses of lidocaine can cause status epilepticus in seizure-free patients to whom it is given for other indications.

Magnesium Sulfate

Magnesium sulfate is indicated for seizures caused by very low serum magnesium levels, as may occur in eclampsia (for which it is the preferred anticonvulsant), hypothyroidism, and alcohol withdrawal or toxicity. Intramuscular injection is preferred, but IV injection or infusion may be used. Frequent administration may be required to suppress seizures and normalize serum magnesium levels.

Paraldehyde

Paraldehyde is a sedative/hypnotic drug with anticonvulsant activity. It was popular for managing seizures associated with acute alcohol withdrawal, but its use is declining as the use of other anticonvulsants has increased. Paraldehyde can be given intravenously or intramuscularly to control status epilepticus that is refractory to other drugs. Other aspects of this drug are presented in Chapter 22.

III. General Nursing Implications for Patients with Seizure Disorders

Much important information concerning drug-related aspects of patient education has been provided thus far. There are other essential aspects of nursing care. Those that do not relate specifically to drug therapy are only mentioned briefly. Anticonvulsant drug therapy during pregnancy is an important consideration that will be discussed in more detail.

Nursing Interventions During a Seizure

Several nursing actions are appropriate if a seizure should occur (Table 26–4). The most important goal is to prevent further harm to the patient, which might arise from a fall, contact with nearby objects, or impaired ventilation because of airway obstruction or unrelenting convulsions. This is not just a nursing responsibility: the appropriate first-aid information should be given to family members or other potential care providers who are likely to be around if a seizure occurs. Another goal, which is especially important when the patient's seizure is his or her first, is to assess carefully the characteristics of the seizure and the convulsions that may be caused by it. Gathering other pertinent information is important also. Here, too, patients or their family members can provide important insight if they are taught what to look for. Included in this is information concerning events that may trigger a seizure.

Seizure Triggers

The recurrence of seizures during anticonvulsant drug therapy has often been explained by saying that the drugs themselves simply are not as effective as they should be. That is not the case. It is true that seizures may recur even when the best in-hospital care is given to the patient—when the right dose of the right anticonvulsant drug is prescribed. However, for outpatients (who are the majority of treated persons with seizures), *the most common cause of recurrent seizures during therapy is noncompliance:* not taking prescribed anticonvulsant medications as directed—skipping doses, timing administration in a haphazard or careless way, and so on. Related to this is recurrent exposure of the

Table 26–5 | Possible Seizure Triggers

Pharmacologic
- Noncompliance with otherwise effective therapy—skipped or haphazardly timed doses (primary cause of recurrent seizures in outpatients)
- Use of drugs that cause seizures or lower seizure threshold
  - CNS stimulants (cocaine, amphetamines, caffeine, weight–loss aids, and other "stimulants")
  - Antidepressants, antipsychotics, certain narcotics (eg, meperidine), dopaminergic antiparkinson drugs (eg, levodopa, especially at high doses)
  - Acute/abrupt withdrawal from generalized CNS depressants (eg, alcohol, barbiturates) or from anticonvulsant drugs

Acute or chronic pathophysiologic/environmental factors (may cause or be associated with aura that can be recognized by patient)
- Fever
- Blood electrolyte or pH imbalances (eg, from excessive vomiting, diarrhea, sweating; alkalosis favors seizures)
- Hormonal changes, endocrine imbalances (including pregnancy)
- Nutritional deficiencies, starvation
- Emotional stress
- Physical stress (eg, excessive exercise, hyperventilation)
- Bright and/or flashing lights (eg, strobe lights, auto headlights)

patient to seizure "triggers": drugs and environmental factors that can cause seizures.

Quite often, seizure-prone patients will learn to recognize certain activities that may trigger a seizure. Some patients also experience an *aura*. An aura is a signal of an impending seizure: a bout of sweating or dizziness, or heightened or altered sensory information (an unusual smell, sound, or vision), for example. Indeed, some patients with recurrent seizures can interpret a particular response as a warning sign that a seizure is about to occur. It is important for the nurse to be aware of these factors. However, it is also essential that the patient, family members, and others who may have an impact on the patient's care be taught about the importance of medication compliance, avoidance of seizure triggers, and recognition of clues that a seizure is about to occur. Table 26–5 summarizes some of the key points about these issues.

Psychosocial Concerns

Employment, driving, recreation, social affairs, and even daily activities such as bathing can cause psychosocial concerns or physical dangers for individuals with seizure disorders. The acceptability of these activities, and strategies to reduce risks, must be considered individually for every patient. In general, however, the decision should be based not only on problems caused by the seizure disorder but also on responses to drug therapy, particularly those involving drowsiness, sedation, and ataxia. Even modest alcohol consumption is clearly contraindicated. Although many restrictions imposed on seizure-prone individuals may seem overly conservative, patients should be encouraged that they can lead normal, active, seizure-free lives by observing a few safety rules and by following prescribed anticonvulsant regimens.

Patient and Family Education

It is important for the nurse to help the patient, family, and community understand the patient's limitations and capabilities, and what can or cannot be done safely during drug treatment. The nurse should help dispel myths about epilepsy that have caused stereotypes, fears, and prejudices. Common myths relate to links between epilepsy and brain damage, mental retardation, or psychosis. Although controversies exist about some of these concepts, the availability of good diagnostic and treatment methods has dramatically reduced the incidence of these once-common problems.

Two other myths are that anticonvulsant drugs cure epilepsy, and that persistence of seizures despite treatment indicates a lack of effective drugs. Anticonvulsants are not cures for idiopathic epilepsy, but they usually control the symptoms effectively if the proper drug is selected and the patient complies with all pharmacologic and nondrug aspects of therapy.

Overall, counseling and encouragement are essential. In view of the most common cause for anticonvulsant drug therapy failure, noncompliance, the crucial drug-related implication is to help the patient and family understand the need to take prescribed medications as directed by the physician.

TRENDS AND CONTROVERSIES IN PHARMACOLOGY

Lifelong Drug Therapy

Persons with many types of chronic conditions, such as seizure disorders or hypertension, are told they will need to continue taking medications indefinitely—probably for the rest of their lives. Although this may indeed be the case, the presence of a chronic illness should not preclude periodic reassessment of the need for drug therapy. In addition to drug costs, adverse effects may increase with duration of treatment. For example, extended anticonvulsant therapy can cause significant patient problems—including gingival hyperplasia, osteomalacia, cerebellar degeneration, and behavior disorders. In some situations, the long-term sequelae of drug-induced changes may be unclear, as with some of the metabolic changes in glucose and lipid metabolism caused by hypertensive drugs. These types of drug-induced changes may not pose significant problems from the patient's perspective, but they should not be ignored.

While it is not usually the nurse's responsibility to start or stop medications, it is within their role as advocates to help patients avoid unnecessary and potentially hazardous therapy. Be alert to the possibility that unneeded medications may have been prescribed. Two common and inappropriate reasons for chronic anticonvulsant therapy are febrile seizures and drug-induced seizures. As another example, antihypertensive medications may be prescribed for the phenomenon of "white coat hypertension," in which blood pressure elevations are triggered by the anxiety of seeing or being examined by a physician or nurse. Patients may also initiate diet and exercise changes that alter their medication requirements.

Nurses should become familiar with suggested practices for chronic drug treatment in their clinical areas. Kandt et al. (1985) describe general parameters for discontinuing anticonvulsant therapy. Their "ideal" candidate for drug withdrawal is a child who has experienced generalized seizures only; or a person who has been seizure-free on medication for at least three years, had few seizures before the problem was controlled, has a normal neurologic examination and developmental history, and a normal EEG at the time of drug withdrawal. The "poor" candidate for drug withdrawal has partial seizures or a mixture of seizure types, has been seizure-free on medication for less than three years, had frequent and prolonged seizures before control was established, has a persistently abnormal EEG, or has evidence of neurologic dysfunction, especially congenital dysfunction.

Based on findings of a number of prospective studies, it has been suggested that antihypertensive drugs also can be stopped in *some* patients without a subsequent rise in arterial pressure, although this topic remains the subject of debate. Potential candidates include patients with mild essential hypertension with at least one of the following characteristics: young age, normal body weight, low salt intake, no alcohol consumption, low pretreatment blood pressure, successful therapy with one drug only, and no or only minimal signs of target organ damage (Schmieder et al., 1991).

Whenever drug therapy is discontinued, medications should be withdrawn slowly, and multiple-drug regimens should be discontinued one drug at a time. Nurses should help patients learn to recognize signs of problems and should emphasize the need for reevaluation, even though patients have stopped taking medication.

Kandt RS, Bickley SK, Shimp LA: Discontinuing antiepileptic therapy. *Am Fam Physician* 1985;31(4): 177-184.

Schmieder RE, Rockstroh JK, Messerli FH: Antihypertensive therapy to stop or not to stop? *JAMA* 1991;265:1566–1571.

Anticonvulsant Use During Pregnancy and Breast-Feeding

All anticonvulsant drugs enter the fetal circulation; many are teratogenic, so there is obvious reason for concern about using these drugs during pregnancy. Several studies have shown that the risk of congenital malformations (cleft palate or lip; brain, spinal cord, or cardiac abnormalities) in offspring of women with epilepsy is about twice the risk for the normal population, for whom the overall risk is generally low. However, these studies have not shown whether malformations were caused by the drug, by some manifestation of the seizure disorder, or by other factors. For all the drugs discussed in this chapter, *except* trimethadione or valproic acid, there is a 90% chance overall that a treated woman will deliver a normal child. Without question, trimethadione and valproic acid should be used during pregnancy only when absolutely essential for seizures that do not respond adequately to another drug.

Ample evidence exists about the risks to mother and fetus of discontinuing anticonvulsants and allowing seizures—even minor ones—to continue during pregnancy. Current opinion is that if seizure control *requires* the use of anticonvulsants, drug therapy should be continued. Treatment with a single anticonvulsant is preferred. It is essential to stress compliance with drug therapy, and the need for thorough periodic prenatal examinations. Anticonvulsant blood levels in the pregnant woman probably require more frequent monitoring than in nonpregnant individuals, since pregnancy shortens the half-life of some anticonvulsants, particularly phenytoin, phenobarbital, and carbamazepine. Pregnancy does not contraindicate the use of any anticonvulsant drug for status epilepticus.

If the mother has been seizure-free for several years before conception, current anticonvulsant drugs should be withdrawn (slowly), and anticonvulsant therapy should not be started in anticipation of seizures that may not occur. Relatively few women who were seizure-free before conception will develop seizures during pregnancy unless eclampsia occurs (for which magnesium sulfate is the preferred drug). About half the women with a history of epilepsy will experience no change in the frequency or severity of seizures during pregnancy. Fewer still will experience more seizures; often, however, this reflects inadequate anticonvulsant blood levels, as from poor compliance or monitoring.

Some authorities believe that breast-feeding need not be discouraged during anticonvulsant therapy unless the infant becomes lethargic or fails to feed adequately. Nevertheless, the infant should be monitored closely for the same signs of adverse responses liable to occur in the mother.

Overall, the nurse should take an active role in counseling women of childbearing age about the potential risks of anticonvulsant drug use and possible consequences of not being treated for epilepsy during pregnancy. Discuss the pros and cons of treating epilepsy knowledgeably. Acknowledge the potential increased risk of adverse fetal effects, but also note the overwhelming likelihood of bearing a normal infant if treatment is supervised and followed properly: prenatal care, periodic physical examinations and measurements of anticonvulsant levels, adequate diet and rest, and compliance with all aspects of anticonvulsant therapy.

SUMMARY OF NURSING IMPLICATIONS

◆ Assessment

Complete a nursing history that includes medication use or disorders contraindicating anticonvulsant therapy with a particular drug; drug allergies; current symptoms; history of alcohol use/abuse; emotional response to diagnosis; and current lifestyle.

Review medical history for concurrent conditions placing patient at high risk for adverse drug effects (eg, hepatic disorders, myocardial insufficiency).

Establish baseline physical assessment, laboratory, diagnostic, and neurologic data.

◆ Nursing Diagnoses

High risk for injury related to seizure activity.

Knowledge deficit related to limited understanding of disease process and prescribed treatment.

Self-esteem disturbance related to medication dependence.

Sensory/perceptual alteration related to drug side effects (eg, ataxia, confusion).

Altered thought processes related to drowsiness, lethargy, from drug therapy.

◆ Planning/Implementation

Reassure that "normal" life can be expected with regular drug therapy, avoiding drug interactions, and seeking follow-up care as instructed.

Check vital signs and neurologic parameters regularly.

Institute seizure precautions to prevent injury.

Describe seizures accurately: prior events (triggers), presence of aura, length of seizure, level of consciousness, presence of incontinence, postictal confusion, and length of recovery.

Offer consistent emotional support to minimize strains of personality change.

When giving IV anticonvulsants, respiratory or cardiovascular depression may result if injection is too rapid; monitor ECG while giving; have resuscitation equipment availabie.

Monitor for early signs of toxicity: phenobarbital (slurred speech, ataxia, respiratory and CNS depression); diazepam (ataxia, nystagmus, slurred speech, vertigo); succinimide, valproic acid, and carbamazepine (GI distress, hematopoietic reactions, liver involvement, renal impairment, CNS depression).

Observe for gingival hyperplasia with phenytoin.

If status epilepticus occurs: have resuscitation equipment available (oral airway, oxygen, suction, AMBU bag); turn on side; slightly elevate bed; keep from injury.

◆ Patient and Family Teaching

Teach the patient/family:

To report any side effects or adverse reactions (sore throat, fever, malaise, bruises, scleral jaundice, pain, tenderness over liver, fatigue, clay-colored stools).

To have periodic urinalyses to detect renal impairment; phenytoin may color urine pink, red, or reddish-brown.

To avoid driving or operating dangerous machinery; drug-induced sedation or impaired coordination may be problematic.

To rid the environment of hazards that contribute to falls, particularly for older patients.

To change position slowly to avoid falls and injury.

To practice good oral hygiene (proper brushing, flossing, regular dental check-ups) to reduce gingival hyperplasia (phenytoin).

To take drugs as prescribed.

To avoid drugs that interact with anticonvulsants; provide list; avoid alcohol.

Not to discontinue anticonvulsant therapy abruptly.

To wear a MedicAlert bracelet indicating epilepsy and medications.

That women who become or wish to become pregnant should consult a physician.

Not to switch brands, forms, or route of administration indiscriminately, as bioavailability varies with some drugs (eg, phenytoin).

To avoid aspirin unless specifically approved by physician if taking valproic acid, as bleeding time is prolonged; to report bleeding, bruises, petechiae.

◆ Evaluation

The patient/family will:

Experience control of seizure activity.

Comply with therapeutic regimen; take medications as ordered; diet; exercise.

Interact appropriately with peer group; become involved in social/school activities.

Avoid physical injury during seizure activity.

Demonstrate ability to solve problems; participate in decision-making; respond appropriately to environment.

Eat prescribed diet; take food without difficulty.

Verbalize acceptance of self; demonstrate willingness to alter lifestyle as indicated.

Experience minimal to no adverse drug effects.

Annotated Bibliography

Ballweg DD. Neonatal seizures: An overview. *Neonatal Netw* 1991; 10:15–21. *Neonatal seizures, which are often overlooked because of their subtle manifestations, can have different etiologies; prognoses; and treatments.*

Barry K, Teixeira S. The role of the nurse in the diagnostic classification and management of epileptic seizures. *J Neurosurg Nurs* 1985;15:243–249. *Discusses nursing roles in seizure management, and reviews problems caused by inadequate knowledge, improper diagnosis, and inappropriate anticonvulsants use.*

Browne TR. The pharmacokinetics of agents used to treat status epilepticus. *Neurology* 1990;40(Suppl. 2):28–32. *This should help you understand both the theories and realities of using anticonvulsants to treat status epilepticus.*

Callaghan N, Garrett A, Goggin T. Withdrawal of anticonvulsant drugs in patients free of seizures for two years: A prospective study. *N Engl J Med* 1988;318:942–946. *The authors conclude that withdrawal of anticonvulsants should be considered for treated patients who have been seizure-free for 2 years. More importantly, perhaps, they identify the types of seizures, and the drug treatments, that are associated with the best and worst outcomes.*

Cleland PG. Risk-benefit assessment of anticonvulsants in women of child-bearing potential. *Drug Safety* 1991;6:70–81. *Important reading not only for information about the actions and uses of anticonvulsants during pregnancy, but also for insight into clinical decision-making, counseling, and therapeutic monitoring.*

Cooper JW. Reviewing geriatric concerns with commonly used drugs. *Geriatrics* 1989;44:79–86. *Covering many drug classes used often in elders, this short article also gives good advice about the use of anticonvulsants.*

Dalessio JD. Seizure disorders and pregnancy. *N Engl J Med* 1985; 312:559–563. *Focuses on the various issues concerning pregnancy and tonic-clonic and partial complex seizures that become generalized; provides an important discussion of seizure therapy during pregnancy; discusses teratogenicity of anticonvulsant drugs.*

Dreifuss FE. Toxic effects of drugs used in the ICU: Anticonvulsant agents. *Crit Care Clin* 1991;7:521–532. *Well worth reading for its unique consideration of how serious medical or surgical conditions requiring intensive care and a host of drug interventions can complicate the use of anticonvulsants and increase the risk of their toxic effects.*

Dunn DW. Status epilepticus in infancy and childhood. *Neurol Clin* 1990;8:647–657. *Worth reading for its attention to how "supportive care" (nondrug measures included) can help reduce morbidity and mortality associated with this otherwise fatal convulsive state.*

Dupius RE, Miranda-Massari J. Anticonvulsants: Pharmacotherapeutic issues in the critically ill patient. *AACN Clin Issues Crit Care Nurs* 1991;2:639–656. *A must-read article for critical care nurses.*

Elwes R. Management of epilepsy. *Practitioner* 1991;235:563–668. *Summarizes aspects of diagnosis, therapeutic planning and monitoring, and problems that may arise during therapy. This article should be of interest to any nurse who deals with patients with chronic seizure disorders.*

Fishel M, Sauer S, Allen J. When you give phenytoin i.v. *RN* 1990; 53:58–59. *Helpful tips, no embellishments, about the IV use of phenytoin.*

Kiker M. Antiepileptic drugs for children: Carbamazepine and valproic acid derivatives. *J Neurosci Nurs* 1991;23:130–132. *Although this short paper focuses on two drugs, it provides valuable information to help the nurse provide long-term support, teaching, and counseling to parents of children with epilepsy.*

The overall goal is an improved medical and psychosocial outcome.

Kilpatrick CJ, Moulds RF. Anticonvulsants in pregnancy. *Med J Aust* 1991;154:199–202. *The authors review over 20 years of clinical data and make useful summaries of pregnancy- and treatment-related risks; pharmacokinetic changes during pregnancy; therapeutic strategies and monitoring; and breast-feeding issues.*

Mattson RH. Selection of drugs for the treatment of epilepsy. *Semin Neurol* 1990;10:406–413. *Makes specific recommendations for matching the anticonvulsant drug with the seizure type, yet provides insight into how therapy can (and should) be individualized to increase the likelihood of a desired outcome.*

Meador KJ, Loring DW, Allen ME, Zamrini EY, Moore EE, Abney OL, King DW. Comparative cognitive effects of carbamazepine and phenytoin in healthy adults. *Neurology* 1991;41:1537–1540. *Do anticonvulsant drugs cause cognitive deficits, and, if so, are there differences in effect among these agents? Meador et al. find insignificant differences in drug-induced cognitive impairment between carbamazepine and phenytoin; differences between drug and nondrug cognitive states have little practical impact on the patient receiving drugs.*

Nuwer MR, Browne TR, Dodson WE et al: Generic substitutions for antiepileptic drugs. *Neurology* 1990;40:1647–1651. *An excellent overview of problems that can arise with anticonvulsant drug substitution, and reasons why they can occur; especially important for patients receiving phenytoin or carbamazepine.*

Pellock JM, Willmore LJ. A rational guide to routine blood monitoring in patients receiving antiepileptic drugs. *Neurology* 1991;41:961–964. *This informative article outlines the steps needed for successful monitoring of the drug regimen of patients taking anticonvulsants.*

Pugh CB, Garnett WR. Current issues in the treatment of epilepsy. *Clin Pharm* 1991;10:335–358. *An excellent review of general principles of anticonvulsant therapy; current issues involving use and monitoring of these drugs; difficult therapeutic decisions that may have to be made; and compliance. Specifically discusses most of the anticonvulsants that are in widespread use—their pharmacokinetics, actions and indications, side effects, and drug interactions.*

Seetharam MN, Pellock JM. Risk-benefit assessment of carbamazepine in children. *Drug Safety* 1991;6:148–158. *Carbamazepine is a major antiepileptic drug for children. Reviews key points about this drug's actions, pharmacokinetics, efficacy, and adverse effects, and identifies ways to optimize its use.*

Sibai BM. Magnesium sulfate is the ideal anticonvulsant in preeclampsia-eclampsia. *Am J Obstet Gynecol* 1990;162:1141–1145. *The author makes a good case for why magnesium sulfate should be considered the best anticonvulsant in this medical emergency, and why phenytoin, which is becoming popular for this indication, is not known to be safer or more effective.*

Theodore WH. Clinical pharmacology of antiepileptic drugs: Selected topics. *Neurol Clin* 1990;8:177–191. *Covers a variety of basic principles of anticonvulsant therapy, and concludes with an example of how interactions between pharmacokinetic and pharmacodynamic aspects of drug action can help explain the clinical effects of anticonvulsants.*

Trimble MR. *The Psychoses of Epilepsy.* New York: Raven Press, 1991. *The author defines two types of relations between behavioral and seizure disorders: a "forced normalization," wherein the EEG normalizes during psychotic behavior and seizures prevent or ameliorate psychosis; and abnormal behavior as a direct seizure phenomenon. Trimble carefully and critically analyzes clinical data over 100 years. Case studies enhance this effort.*

Wallace SJ. Anti-epileptic drug monitoring: An overview. *Dev Med Child Neurol* 1990;32:923–926. *A short but valuable review of how best to monitor drug therapy of the most common neurologic disorder in children.*

Wilhlem J, Morris D, Hotham N. Epilepsy and pregnancy—a review of 98 pregnancies. *Aust N Z J Obstet Gynaecol* 1990;30:290–295. *Summarizes factors that increase the risk of seizures during pregnancy; therapeutic complications during pregnancy and delivery; and assessment of relative benefits and risks.*

Young GP. Seizures in the alcoholic patient. *Emerg Med Clin North Am* 1990;8:821–833. *Focuses on special issues related to the management of acute and chronic seizures in alcohol abusers.*

Table 26–C **Clinical Uses and Administration of Major Anticonvulsants**

AGENT	CLINICAL USES	DOSAGE AND ROUTE OF ADMINISTRATION
	Hydantoins	
PROTOTYPE		
Phenytoin		
(DILANTIN)	Tonic–clonic and complex partial seizures	Oral: Adults: 100–200 mg tid or qid. Extended form (DILANTIN KAPSEALS) given qd. Children: 4–8 mg/kg/d; children over 6 years may require minimum adult dose (300 mg)
	Status epilepticus	IV: Adults: Loading dose of 10–15 mg/kg (not >50 mg/min) followed by 100–mg maintenance dose orally or IV q6h–q8h prn. Children: 15–20 mg/kg (not >1–3 mg/kg/min)
	Prevention of seizures associated with neurosurgery	IM: Adults: 100–200 mg q4h during and after surgery
RELATED DRUGS		
Ethotoin		
(PEGANONE)	Tonic–clonic and complex partial seizures	Oral: Adult: 2000–3000 mg/d in 4–6 divided doses. Children: 500–1000 mg/d in 4–6 divided doses
Mephenytoin		
(MESANTOIN)	Tonic–clonic, simple, and complex partial seizures	Oral: Adults: 200–600 mg/d. Children: 100–400 mg/d
	Barbiturates	
Mephobarbital		
(MEBARAL)	Tonic–clonic, and absence seizures	Oral: Adults: 400–600 mg/d. Children >5 years: 32–64 mg tid or qid; <5 years: 16–32 mg
Metharbital		
(GEMONIL)	Tonic–clonic, absence myoclonic, and mixed seizures	Oral: Adults: Initially 100 mg qd–tid, adjust up to 600–800 mg/d if needed. Children: Initially 5–15 mg/kg/d; adjust to optimal level
Phenobarbital		
(LUMINAL)	Tonic–clonic, complex partial, and simple partial seizures	Oral: Adults: 50–100 mg bid or tid. Children: 3–5 mg/kg/d as single bedtime dose or in 3 divided doses
	Status epilepticus	IV: Adults: 200–320 mg, repeat after 6hr if needed. Children: 15–20 mg/kg over 10–15 min
	Daytime sedation	See Chapter 22
	Hypnosis for insomnia	See Chapter 22
Primidone		
(MYSOLINE)	Tonic–clonic, complex partial and simple partial seizures	Oral: Adults: Days 1–3, 100–125 mg hs; days 4–6, 100–125 mg bid; days 7–9, 100=125 mg tid; day 10, up to 250 mg tid or qid if needed. Children <8 years: Initially 50 mg hs, increase to 10–25 mg/kg/d in divided doses if needed; >8 years: Same as adult

(*continued*)

Table 26–C **Clinical Uses and Administration of Major Anticonvulsants (*Continued*)**

AGENT	CLINICAL USES	DOSAGE AND ROUTE OF ADMINISTRATION
	Succinimides	
PROTOTYPE		
Ethosuximide		
(ZARONTIN)	Absence seizures (petit mal)	Oral: Adults: Initially 500 mg/d, increase 250 mg/d every 4–7 days until optimal effect reached (40–100 μg/mL). Children 3–6 years: Initially 250 mg/d, increase 250 mg/d every 4–7 days (20 mg/kg/d is normal optimal dose); >6 years: same as adult
RELATED DRUGS		
Methsuximide		
(CELONTIN)	Absence seizure (petit mal)	Oral: Adults: Initially 300 mg/d, with weekly increases of 300 mg/d up to 1200 mg/d if needed. Children: Same as adult; however, changes should be in 150–mg increments
Phensuximide		
(MILONTIN)	Absence seizure (petit mal)	Oral: Adults: 500–1000 mg bid or tid (1500 mg is usual maintenance dose). Children: Same as adults
	Benzodiazepines	
Clonazepam		
(KLONOPIN)	Absence (petit mal), Lennox–Gastaut, and myoclonic seizures	Oral: Adults and children >10: Initially up to 0.5 mg tid, increasing every 3 days by 0.5–1.0 mg until optimal effect achieved; 20 mg/d is maximum dose. Children <10 years: Initially 0.01–0.03 mg/kg/d in divided doses, increasing by 0.25–0.5 mg every 3 days to 0.1–0.2 mg/kg/d in 3 divided doses
Diazepam		
(VALIUM)	Status epilepticus	IV (preferred) or IM: Adults: 5–10 mg; repeat every 10–15 min, if needed, up to total dose of 30 mg, given as a slow injection. Children >5 years: 1 mg every 2–5 min, up to 10 mg, repeated in 2–4 hr prn; >30 days to 5 years: 0.2–0.5 mg every 2–5 min, up to total dose of 5 mg
	Other uses	See Chapter 22
	Oxazolidinediones	
Paramethadione		
(PARADIONE)	Absence seizures	See Trimethadione (below)
Trimethadione		
(TRIDIONE)	Absence seizures	Oral: Adults: Initially 900 mg/d, followed by weekly increases of 300 mg/d until optimal effect is reached. Usual maintenance dose is 300–600 mg tid or qid. Children: 300–900 mg/d in 3 or 4 divided doses

(*continued*)

Table 26–C **Clinical Uses and Administration of Major Anticonvulsants (*Continued*)**

AGENT	CLINICAL USES	DOSAGE AND ROUTE OF ADMINISTRATION
Other Drugs Used as Anticonvulsants		
Carbamazepine		
(TEGRETOL)	Tonic–clonic, complex partial, and mixed seizures	Oral: Adult (>12 years): Initially 200 mg bid, with increases of 200 mg/d at weekly intervals if needed. Usual maintenance dose is 800–1200 mg/d in divided doses. Children 12–15 years should not receive more than 1000 mg/d. Children 6–12 years: Initially 100 mg bid, followed by weekly increases of 100 mg/d if needed. Usual maintenance dose is 400–800 mg/d in divided doses
	Pain associated with trigeminal neuralgia	Adults: Initially 100 mg bid, followed by increases of 100 mg q12h up to 1200 mg/d. Usual maintenance dose is 400–800 mg/d in divided doses
Phenacemide		
(PHENURONE)	Complex partial seizures	Oral: Adults: Initially 250–500 mg tid; usual maintenance dose is 2000–3000 mg/d. Children 5–10 years: One half the adult dose
Valproic acid		
(DEPAKENE)	Absence, tonic–clonic, complex partial, and myoclonic seizures	Oral: Adults: Initially 15 mg/kg/d, with weekly increases of 5–10 mg/kg/d up to 60 mg/kg/d in divided doses. Children: Same as adult
Miscellaneous Drugs with Other Major Uses, Having Anticonvulsant Activity		
Acetazolamide		
(DIAMOX)	Sole treatment or adjunct to the therapy of absence, tonic-clonic, and myoclonic seizures	Oral: Adults: Usual starting dose as adjunct: 250 mg/d. When used alone, generally 8 to 30 mg/kg/d, given in 3 or 4 divided doses IV (preferred) or IM: Adults: Dose is same as for oral administration
Lidocaine		
(XYLOCAINE)	Refractory status epilepticus	IV: Adults: Rapid injection of 1 mg/kg; if needed give 0.5 mg/kg 2 min. later; until seizure stops. When seizure stops give 30/mg/kg/min to prevent recurrences
Magnesium sulfate	Seizures due to hypomagnesemia (eg, eclampsia, hypothyroidism, alcohol withdrawal)	IM: Adults: 1–5 g of 25%–50% solution, up to 6 times/d if needed. Children: 20–40 mg/kg as 20% solution, repeated as necessary IV (if indicated): 1–4 g injected at rate not to exceed 1.5 mL/min of 10% solution. Can also infuse 4 g added to 250 mL of D_5W at rate of 3 mL/min or less
Paraldehyde	Refractory status epilepticus	IM: 5 g IV: 3–5 g

Table 26–S **Major Side Effects of and Contraindications for Anticonvulsants**

BODY SYSTEM/ Side Effect	CONTRAINDICATION/ PRECAUTION	COMMENTS AND NURSING IMPLICATIONS
Hydantoins: Phenytoin, Ethotoin, Mephenytoin		
CENTRAL NERVOUS SYSTEM Sluggishness, confusion, slurred speech	Alcohol ingestion (can increase serum phenytoin levels); hepatic or renal impairment	Elderly patients in particular should be observed as these side effects may contribute to falls and judgment mistakes that may cause injury (eg, forgetting that medication was taken or taking next dose too soon)
CARDIOVASCULAR (with IV phenytoin) Hypotension, circulatory collapse, depression of atrial and ventricular conduction, cardiac arrest	Sinus bradycardia, sinoatrial block, Adams–Stoke syndrome, second- or third-degree AV block	Do not exceed recommended IV administration rates; always monitor BP frequently
BLOOD Leukopenia, agranulocytosis	Bone marrow depression or blood dyscrasias	Assess for sore throat, fever, malaise, or bruises and instruct patient to report these; regular blood counts are essential
Megaloblastic anemia		Will usually respond to folic acid therapy
Coagulation deficits in newborn infants		Prepartum (mother) and postpartum (neonate) administration of vitamin K will prevent hemorrhage
GASTROINTESTINAL Nausea, vomiting, constipation		Give drug with meals to reduce GI side effects; diet changes and laxatives can reduce constipation
CONNECTIVE TISSUE Gingival hyperplasia, coarsening of facial features, lip enlargement, hirsutism		Dental care and meticulous oral hygiene are imperative to prevent gingival hyperplasia
SKIN Various rashes, ranging from mild measle–like (morbilliform) to very serious, such as exfoliative dermatitis and lupus erythematosus		Discontinue phenytoin and notify physician
Acne		If another drug will control seizures it should be used instead. Be sensitive to the psychologic impact of acne
Barbiturates: Phenobarbital, Mephobarbital, Metharbital, Primidone		
See Chapter 22		

(continued)

Table 26–S Major Side Effects of and Contraindications for Anticonvulsants (*Continued*)

BODY SYSTEM/ Side Effect	CONTRAINDICATION/ PRECAUTION	COMMENTS AND NURSING IMPLICATIONS
Succinimides: Ethosuximide, Methsuximide, Phensuximide		
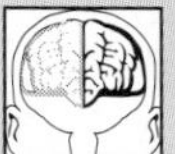 **CENTRAL NERVOUS SYSTEM** See hydantoins		
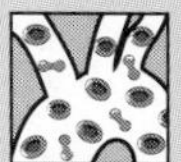 **BLOOD** See hydantoins		
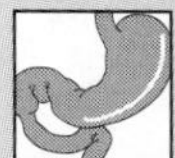 **GASTROINTESTINAL** See hydantoins		
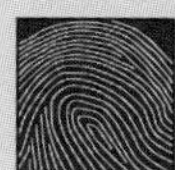 **SKIN** See hydantoins		
Benzodiazepines: Diazepam, Clonazepam		
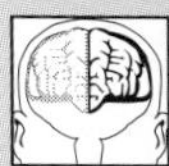 **CENTRAL NERVOUS SYSTEM** See Chapter 22, Table 22–S1	*There is no contraindication for diazepam use in status epilepticus*	
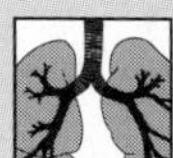 **RESPIRATORY** See Chapter 22, Table 22–S1		
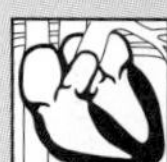 **CARDIOVASCULAR** See Chapter 22, Table 22–S1		
OTHER Antimuscarinic effects such as mydriasis, dry mouth, slight constipation, and urinary difficulty	Contraindications for atropine (see Table 13–S)	Avoid administering to patients with active narrow–angle glaucoma; observe all patients for adverse antimuscarinic effects, particularly elderly males who may have prostatic hypertrophy; advise patients to report these side effects to their physician at once. See Chapter 13 for a more complete discussion of antimuscarinic side effects

(continued)

Table 26–S | **Major Side Effects of and Contraindications for Anticonvulsants (*Continued*)**

BODY SYSTEM/ Side Effect	CONTRAINDICATION/ PRECAUTION	COMMENTS AND NURSING IMPLICATIONS
Oxazolidinediones: Paramethadione, Trimethadione		
CENTRAL NERVOUS SYSTEM See hydantoins		
BLOOD See hydantoins		Fatalities have been reported
GASTROINTESTINAL See hydantoins		
SKIN See hydantoins		Discontinue if even a mild rash occurs; contact physician
Valproic Acid		
CENTRAL NERVOUS SYSTEM Sedation (usually with combination therapy)	Impaired consciousness, undiagnosed neurologic disorder	See hydantoins
BLOOD See hydantoins		
GASTROINTESTINAL See hydantoins		
LIVER Elevated serum transaminase and LDH (dose–related) levels, hepatic failure	Liver disease	Regular liver function tests are important. Teach patient and family the signs of liver impairment; instruct patient and family to report any of these symptoms to physician or nurse

(*continued*)

Table 26–S Major Side Effects of and Contraindications for Anticonvulsants (*Continued*)

BODY SYSTEM/ Side Effect	CONTRAINDICATION/ PRECAUTION	COMMENTS AND NURSING IMPLICATIONS
Carbamazepine		
CENTRAL NERVOUS SYSTEM Dizziness, drowsiness, unsteadiness, and confusion, particularly in the elderly	Hepatic and renal impairment	Monitor accordingly
Psychosis	Latent or active psychosis	Monitor accordingly
BLOOD Aplastic anemia, leukopenia, agranulocytosis	Blood dyscrasias, bone marrow depressions caused by carbamazepine in the past	Obtain CBC before starting therapy and at weekly intervals for the first 3 months. See hydantoins for nursing implications. Fatalities have been reported
RESPIRATORY Pulmonary hypersensitivity, fever, dyspnea, pneumonitis, or pneumonia	Severe respiratory disease with impaired ventilation	Monitor respiration; observe for dyspnea, fever, and congestion notify physician if respiratory difficulties occur
CARDIOVASCULAR Congestive heart failure; aggravation of hypertension; syncope	Severe cardiovascular disease; use with caution in individuals with hypertension	Monitor heart rate and BP; assess for edema, fainting, etc.
GASTROINTESTINAL See hydantoins		
SKIN See hydantoins		
Phenacemide		
CENTRAL NERVOUS SYSTEM Dizziness, drowsiness, and ataxia	Latent or active psychosis, paranoid thinking	See hydantoins
Personality changes Suicidal ideation	Suicidal tendencies	Observe patient for personality changes; instruct family members about possible changes also but do not frighten them. Contact physician if changes do occur
BLOOD Aplastic anemia, agranulocytosis, leukopenia	Blood dyscrasias	See hydantoins. Fatalities have been reported
GASTROINTESTINAL See hydantoins		

* See Table 22–S1, p 371, for side effects of and contraindications for barbiturates.
† All side effects (excepting those relating to the skin) and contraindications are the same as those for the hydantoins.

Table 26–I | Major Interactions Between Anticonvulsants and Other Agents

AGENT	RESULT OF INTERACTION	COMMENTS AND NURSING IMPLICATIONS
General Interactions That Apply to Virtually All Anticonvulsants		
CNS depressants, others (eg, alcohol, barbiturates, narcotics, antihistamines)	Potential additive CNS depression; variable, sometimes unpredictable actions on anticonvulsant metabolism, seizure control	Actual outcome depends on class of interactant; combined use should be supervised, monitored by physician; See individual interactions, below
CNS stimulants (eg, caffeine, amphetamines, cocaine)	Physiologic antagonism of anticonvulsant actions; increased risk of seizures	Interactants have potential to cause seizures, especially at high doses; discourage use
Hydantoins: Phenytoin, Ethotoin, Mephenytoin		
Acetaminophen (Chapter 52)	Increased risk of acetaminophen hepatotoxicity with acetaminophen overdoses	Try to ascertain full medication history in overdose victims; occurs because an acetaminophen metabolite is toxic to liver; interaction not likely to be problematic if phenytoin and acetaminophen doses are kept within usual recommended ranges
Alcohol (Chapter 22)	Variable increases or decreases of phenytoin levels and effects: increased phenytoin levels, effects, with acute alcohol use; potential decreased phenytoin levels, seizure control, with chronic alcohol consumption	Occasional alcohol consumption not contraindicated, excessive use should be discouraged, necessitates closer monitoring of phenytoin levels, responses
Allopurinol (Chapter 53)	Increased phenytoin blood levels, potential excessive effects, toxicity	Monitor phenytoin levels, anticipate need to reduce dose
Amiodarone (Chapter 30)	Decreased antiarrhythmic effectiveness of amiodarone *and* decreased phenytoin metabolism with potential increased or excessive phenytoin effects, toxicity	Evidence of interaction may take weeks to appear, owing to very long half life of amiodarone; anticipate need for careful monitoring of response, drug blood levels
Anticoagulants, oral (Chapter 35)	Increased phenytoin blood levels, potential excessive effects, and increased or decreased anticoagulant effects	Monitor phenytoin levels, PTT, during combined therapy and when adding or discontinuing one of these drugs
Antineoplastic agents (eg, bleomycin, platinum compounds, methotrexate, vinblastine; Chapter 59)	Decreased phenytoin levels, reduced seizure control	Monitor blood levels, clinical response, more closely during combined therapy
Carbamazepine	Decreased carbamazepine blood levels, effectiveness; variable effects on phenytoin levels	Requires closer monitoring of blood levels of both interactants
Chloramphenicol (Chapter 56)	Increased phenytoin levels, effects, potential toxicity	Monitor blood levels of both drugs to guide dosage adjustments
Cimetidine (Chapter 40)	Increased phenytoin levels, effects; potential toxicity	Monitor phenytoin levels; cimetidine alternatives (famotidine, ranitidine) less likely to interact
Contraceptives, oral (Chapter 49)	Reduced contraceptive effectiveness, possible pregnancy	Advise use of alternative contraceptive methods during combined use and until contraceptive dose can be increased properly

(continued)

Table 26–I **Major Interactions Between Anticonvulsants and Other Agents (*Continued*)**

AGENT	RESULT OF INTERACTION	COMMENTS AND NURSING IMPLICATIONS
Corticosteroids (Chapter 45)	Decreased corticosteroid effectiveness	Monitor clinical responses during combined therapy, anticipate need to increase corticosteroid doses
Cyclosporine (Chapter 54)	Increased risk of acute organ rejection owing to reduced cyclosporine blood levels	Serious interaction; if unavoidable, monitor serum cyclosporine levels; evidence of rejection may occur within 48 hr of start of combined use
Diazoxide (oral or IV; Chapters 33, 46)	Decreased phenytoin levels, decreased effects	Monitor accordingly
Disopyramide (Chapter 30)	Decreased antiarrhythmic effect of disopyramide, increased antimuscarinic side effects	Increasing disopyramide dose to overcome interaction may cause intolerable atropine–like side effects; monitor accordingly, anticipate need to use noninteracting antiarrhythmic instead
Disulfiram (Chapter 22)	Increased phenytoin levels, risk of excessive effects, toxicity	Monitor accordingly if interaction cannot be avoided
Doxycycline (Chapter 56)	Decreased antibiotic effectiveness	Anticipate need to increase doxycycline dose; use of alternative antibiotics may be preferred
Estrogens (Chapter 49)	See contraceptives, oral, above	
Fluconazole (Chapter 57)	Increased phenytoin levels, effects; potential toxicity	Monitor anticonvulsant levels, clinical response
Folic acid (Chapter 61)	Decreased phenytoin levels, effects	Monitor anticonvulsant levels, response, especially when adding or discontinuing folate supplements
Isoniazid (Chapter 57)	Increased phenytoin levels, effects; potential toxicity	Monitor accordingly
Levodopa (Chapter 25)	Decreased levodopa levels, decreased control of parkinson's symptoms	Use combination cautiously; anticipate need to decrease phenytoin dose
Mexiletine (Chapter 30)	Decreased blood levels, antiarrhythmic effectiveness of mexiletine	Monitor blood levels, clinical effects, of both interactants
Phenacemide	Increased phenytoin levels, effects, potential toxicity	Monitor blood levels of both anticonvulsants if used together
Phenylbutazone (Chapter 52)	Increased phenytoin levels, effects, potential toxicity	Monitor accordingly; interaction may be caused by other nonsteroidal antiinflammatory drugs (eg, aspirin, ibuprofen, indomethacin)
Primidone	Increased serum primidone levels, potential excessive effects	Monitor blood levels of primidone, phenobarbital (its metabolite), and phenytoin during combined use
Rifampin (Chapter 57)	Decreased phenytoin levels, effects	Monitor accordingly
Sulfonamide antibiotics (Chapter 56)	Increased phenytoin levels, effects; potential toxicity	Monitor accordingly, especially when adding or discontinuing the antibiotic
Theophylline (Chapter 38)	Decreased seizure control by phenytoin, decreased control of pulmonary problems by theophylline	Monitor blood levels of, clinical responses to, both drugs; interaction also applies to aminophylline
Valproic acid	Increased phenytoin levels, effects; potential toxicity; *and* decreased valproic acid levels, effectiveness	Monitor blood levels of both drugs closely to help adjust dosages

(continued)

Table 26–I Major Interactions Between Anticonvulsants and Other Agents (*Continued*)

AGENT	RESULT OF INTERACTION	COMMENTS AND NURSING IMPLICATIONS
Barbiturates: Phenobarbital, Mephobarbital, Metharbital		
See Table 22–I1, p 372 and entries for other anticonvulsants in this table		
Succinimides: Ethosuximide, Methsuximide		
Primidone	Decreased levels, effects, of primidone	Monitor serum levels of, clinical responses to, primidone, phenobarbital (its metabolite), and the succinimide
Benzodiazepines: Diazepam, Clonazepam		
See Table 22–I1, and entries for other anticonvulsants in this table		
Oxazolidinediones: Paramethadione, Trimethadione		
Valproic acid	Increased trimethadione blood levels, side effects	Monitor accordingly
Valproic Acid		
Aspirin (Chapter 52)	Increased free blood levels of valproic acid, excessive effects or toxicity	Advise patients to avoid unsupervised aspirin use; combined use should be monitored (valproic acid levels) closely, especially when adding, discontinuing, aspirin; unknown whether other nonsteroidal antiinflammatory drugs interact similarly; interaction not likely to occur with acetaminophen
Barbiturates (p 372 and Chapter 22)	Increased barbiturate blood levels, excessive CNS depression	Monitor closely when adding one drug to ongoing therapy with other; similar interaction may occur with alcohol; discourage its use
Carbamazepine	Decreased valproic acid levels, decreased seizure control *and* increased carbamazepine levels, effects; possible toxicity	Monitor blood levels of, responses to, both drugs; interaction may be of slow onset and persistent, requiring closer monitoring for a month or so when adding or discontinuing one of these drugs
Phenytoin	See hydantoins	
Antibiotics, macrolides (tetracyclines, troleandomycin; Chapter 56)	Increased carbamazepine levels, potential toxicity	Avoid interaction if at all possible; excessive CNS depression can occur within a day of combined use, may require hospitalization, intensive care; other antibiotics preferred
Anticoagulants, oral (Chapter 35)	Decreased anticoagulant effect	Monitor prothrombin time more closely during combined use or when adding or discontinuing one interactant
Cimetidine (Chapter 40)	Increased carbamazepine levels, potential toxicity	Monitor during combined use; cimetidine alternatives (famotidine, ranitidine) less likely to interact
Danazol (Chapters 48, 49)	Increased carbamazepine levels, potential toxicity	Monitor accordingly

(continued)

Table 26–I Major Interactions Between Anticonvulsants and Other Agents (*Continued*)

AGENT	RESULT OF INTERACTION	COMMENTS AND NURSING IMPLICATIONS
Carbamazepine		
Haloperidol (Chapter 23)	Decreased haloperidol effects	Assess for loss of antipsychotic effect of interactant, anticipate potential need to increase its dose cautiously
Isoniazid (Chapter 57)	Increased carbamazepine levels, increased risk of isoniazid hepatotoxicity	Important to monitor blood levels of anticonvulsant, liver enzymes (eg, AST, ALT), and assess for signs of liver dysfunction (eg, jaundice, abdominal pain); avoid interaction if possible
Lithium (Chapter 24)	Syndrome of lethargy, ataxia, tremor, muscle weakness, hyperreflexia	Monitor accordingly; may occur even if blood levels of both drugs are in "therapeutic" range; may necessitate discontinuing one of the drugs
Neuromuscular blockers, curare-like (especially atracurium, pancuronium; Chapter 17)	Decreased duration, intensity of neuromuscular blockade	Monitor for reduced effectiveness, potential need to increase dose of neuromuscular blocker for adequate paralyzing effect
Phenytoin	See hydantoins	
Primidone	Decreased primidone, phenobarbital levels, increased carbamazepine levels, effects; potential toxicity	Monitor levels of, responses to, these drugs if combined use is unavoidable
Propoxyphene (Chapter 21)	Increased carbamazepine levels, effects; potential toxicity	Interaction should be avoided, as there are many more effective, noninteracting narcotic analgesics
Valproic acid	See above	
Verapamil (Chapters 33, 34)	Increased carbamazepine levels, effects; potential toxicity	Monitor accordingly; is unclear whether other calcium-channel blockers interact also
Phenacemide		
Phenytoin	See hydantoins	

PROTOTYPE

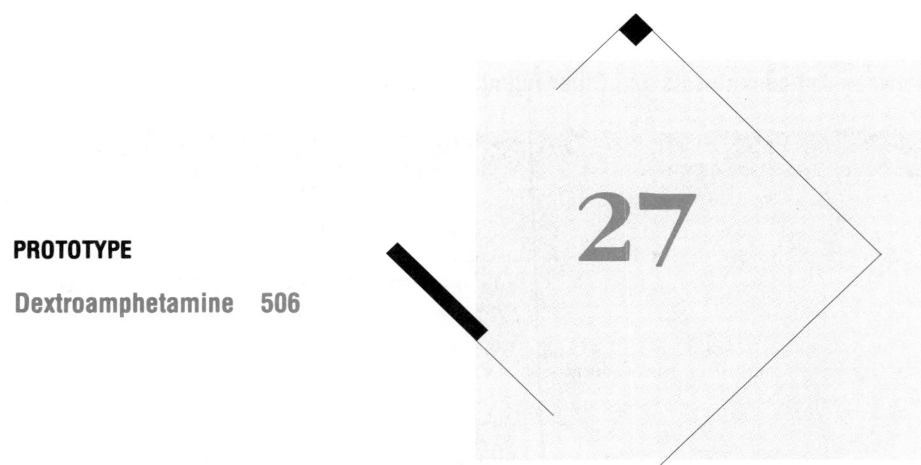

Central Nervous System Stimulants

Several therapeutically useful drugs are given to stimulate parts of the central nervous system (CNS). This chapter groups the CNS stimulants into two categories according to their major site of action in the brain. *Cerebral stimulants* primarily stimulate the cerebral cortex or cerebrum. They have several important and legitimate medical uses, as well as great potential for abuse. *Analeptics* affect mainly the brainstem, respiratory control centers in particular. They have few indications, and so are seldom used. Despite having different major sites of action, all these drugs have the ability to stimulate the entire CNS, and other body systems as well.

I. Cerebral Stimulants

The amphetamines and amphetamine **congeners** (chemical derivatives of amphetamines) are the major classes of cerebral stimulants. The amphetamines are the prototype class. Other cerebral stimulants include caffeine, methylphenidate, pemoline, and phenylpropanolamine. They are sufficiently different that they cannot be placed into one chemical class.

Amphetamines

Amphetamines were introduced in Chapter 14 as a group of sympathomimetics that have considerable ability to stimulate the CNS. Dextroamphetamine (DEXEDRINE) is considered the prototype.

PROTOTYPE

Dextroamphetamine

Absorption, Distribution, Metabolism, and Excretion

Dextroamphetamine is absorbed well from the gastrointestinal (GI) tract. Oral administration is the only legal way to give it or the related amphetamines. Dextroamphetamine is distributed throughout the body and enters the CNS easily. Both central and peripheral effects appear within 30 to 60 minutes. Effects are terminated mainly by renal excretion of unmetabolized drug, a process that is affected significantly by urine pH. When the normally acidic urine is alkalinized, dextroamphetamine molecules are uncharged and easily diffuse back

Major reference tables appear beginning on p. 519.

into the bloodstream. This slows renal elimination and prolongs the drug's serum half-life, which is normally 4 to 6 hours. Changes of amphetamine elimination resulting from urine pH changes are common and clinically important. Specific causes, and the related nursing implications, are discussed later.

Dextroamphetamine is available in immediate-acting tablets or timed-release capsules. Some other amphetamines are also available in chewable and slow-release tablets. Parenteral dosage forms are illegal in the United States.

Pharmacologic Effects

Both the central and peripheral effects of dextroamphetamine and related drugs are due mainly to their indirect-acting sympathomimetic effect: they release norepinephrine from adrenergic nerve endings. Amphetamines also slightly inhibit the reuptake of released norepinephrine into the nerve, which prolongs and intensifies the transmitter's actions.

Central Effects

Dextroamphetamine stimulates the cerebral cortex, the brainstem, and the reticular formation that links sensory tracts between the medulla and the cortex. Cortical stimulation leads to effects that are common to many of the drugs discussed in this chapter. It also contributes to the high abuse potential of these agents. Major responses include increased wakefulness, alertness, concentration, motor activity, physical performance, resistance to fatigue, improved mood, inhibited motivation and ability to sleep, and suppressed appetite (an *anorexigenic* effect). Medullary stimulation increases respiration.

At low doses amphetamines may cause paradoxic signs of CNS depression, including emotional quieting and normalization of hyperkinetic motor activity and behavior. The cause of paradoxic "depression" can be explained by considering the overall level of CNS activity as a balance between the opposing actions of inhibitory and excitatory neurons. Inhibitory neurons appear to be particularly sensitive to low concentrations of CNS stimulants. When they are stimulated, the overall effect appears as decreased CNS activity. The phenomenon parallels the way in which low doses of CNS depressants such as alcohol cause paradoxic CNS stimulation by preferentially depressing inhibitory pathways (see Fig. 22–2, p 349). In children, low doses of amphetamines may also cause apparent sedation by stimulating the immature reticular activating system, which regulates motor cortex activity. In doing so, they indirectly enable the motor cortex to respond more appropriately and selectively to external stimuli.

Irritation, depression, and fatigue develop when the stimulatory effects of an amphetamine subside. There is a strong correlation between the intensity of stimulation and pleasure on the way "up" and depression on the way "down."

Tolerance and Tachyphylaxis

Tolerance to the CNS and peripheral effects of dextroamphetamine and related agents develops quickly, often after only one or two doses. Tolerance necessitates a higher dose to maintain responses of a given intensity. Increased tolerance also develops to the lethal effects of amphetamines, such that tolerant individuals may experience only slight CNS or peripheral changes after taking doses that are hundreds of times greater than the therapeutic dose. This same high dose would easily kill an individual who has not developed amphetamine tolerance. Tolerance does ***not*** develop toward the ability of toxic amphetamine doses to cause psychosis.

One cause of tolerance is the release and eventual depletion of norepinephrine from nerve endings. After only one or two doses less norepinephrine is available for release with following doses, and so the intensity of the effect declines. Another cause of tolerance is increased elimination: By suppressing appetite, amphetamines alter the body's overall pattern of metabolism, leading to ***ketosis***. Ketone bodies are excreted into the urine. They acidify the urine and thus hasten amphetamine excretion and lower amphetamine blood levels.

Peripheral Effects

The peripheral sympathomimetic effects of amphetamines, caused by release of norepinephrine from peripheral sympathetic nerves, are discussed in Chapter 14. Therapeutic doses used for CNS effects usually cause mydriasis and slight increases of heart rate and blood pressure.

Clinical Indications and Administration

Amphetamines are used mainly as psychomotor stimulants and to treat obesity, attention deficit hyperactivity disorder, and narcolepsy. Dextroamphetamine is used most often. Dosages are summarized in Table 27–C. Amphetamines have limited use as antidepressants for persons with parkinsonism and as adjunctive therapy for a small subgroup of persons with epilepsy. They have also been evaluated as treatments for elevating mood in patients with psychiatric depression, but their benefits have been less satisfactory than expected, and are outweighed by the potential for abuse.

Obesity

Obesity contributes to many serious medical and psychologic problems. Its cause is usually simple—dietary intake of more calories than are expended through metabolism. The remedy is either to reduce caloric intake or to increase calorie utilization. It is theoretically reasonable to use drugs such as amphetamines to accomplish this, since they cause an anorexigenic effect by

- elevating mood, alleviating dysphoria that is often linked to obesity;
- suppressing brain centers that regulate feeding or provide a sensation of satiety after eating;
- diminishing senses of taste and smell that normally contribute to the sensation of hunger and the joy of eating;
- increasing motor activity to "burn" more calories; and
- suppressing repetitive behavior such as frequent eating.

Nevertheless, in practice amphetamines are only temporary measures to assist weight loss, and must be used only in that way.

Prescribing amphetamines for obesity is highly controversial because of the great risk and dangers of abuse. State and local laws have been passed because of this problem. Some clinicians consider short-term use acceptable, but only if the drugs are used to aid the effects of diet and exercise. Psychologic counseling may (and probably should) be recommended, particularly if food craving has a strong emotional basis. Most physicians agree that short-term use without dietary modification, or any chronic use for obesity, is totally unacceptable. Others believe that amphetamines should never be used unless obesity is life-threatening.

Immediate-acting formulations of anorexigenic drugs should be given 1 hour before each meal. This timing increases the chance that peak appetite suppression occurs just before or when the patient will be eating. Alternatively, timed-release capsules can be administered once daily, preferably with or after breakfast. The chance of insomnia can be reduced by taking the last dose of the day at least 6 hours before bedtime. Tolerance to the anorexigenic effect develops after several weeks of daily use. For most patients, anorexigenic drug therapy should be stopped at this time. Unless the patient continues a weight-loss program, weight may return to or exceed predrug levels after amphetamine administration is stopped.

NURSING IMPLICATIONS

Stress the need to time amphetamine doses properly, and explain the reasons for it. The evening meal may need to be eaten earlier to avoid altered sleep from late drug administration. Advise patients to swallow timed-release products whole to prevent a potentially dangerous episode of intense CNS or autonomic stimulation. Stress the need for adjunctive nondrug therapies to help reduce body weight and maintain it at a healthier level, and explain that anorexigenic agents are only temporary weight-loss aids. Monitor patients after amphetamine discontinuation for a return or increase of appetite or body weight. Be aware of the controversy about the use of amphetamines for weight loss, and understand all pertinent laws regulating their use. Question orders calling for increased amphetamine doses to restore the anorexigenic effect after tolerance occurs.

Attention Deficit Hyperactivity Disorder

Cerebral stimulants are indicated for treatment of attention deficit hyperactivity disorder (ADHD), the most common pediatric behavioral problem. The overall incidence, based on sound diagnostic criteria, is about 2% of school-age children. Boys are about twice as likely to have ADHD as girls. Characteristics of ADHD include attentional deficits, hyperactivity, abnormal motor movements (eg, poor coordination), restlessness, emotional problems (eg, low tolerance to frustration, short temper), poor interpersonal skills with peers and parents (eg, immature or bossy personality), impulsivity, and learning disability.

The related drug methylphenidate is generally the preferred drug for ADHD. However, some children respond better to amphetamines, in which case low doses of dextroamphetamine, based on the patient's age, are usually preferred (see Table 27–C). When used for ADHD, amphetamines are usually given once daily, but some children may need twice-daily dosing. Doses can be increased weekly as needed to control symptoms and compensate for tolerance. Regardless of the stimulant prescribed for ADHD, if an immediate-acting product is used it should be taken with breakfast to minimize appetite suppression and weight loss. If a second daily dose is ordered, it should be taken 4 to 6 hours later (with lunch). Once-daily use of a timed-release product may be appropriate for some patients.

Cerebral stimulants, used with psychologic counseling, benefit about 70% to 80% of children with ADHD. Improvement is assessed as increased attention skills and learning capacity, improved memory, and decreased impulsivity. These responses are accompanied by a desired and paradoxic sedative effect, discussed earlier. Cerebral stimulants do more than simply calm the child. They permit actual psychologic and emotional growth by increasing the tolerance to frustration, prolonging attention spans, stabilizing emotions, and normalizing social interactions. Relatively long-term use of amphetamines or related stimulants for ADHD is acceptable, but the patient should be reevaluated every 6 months or so. At that time the physician should attempt to discontinue drug administration gradually and determine whether further therapy is necessary. Improved behavior may persist during temporary or permanent discontinuation of the drug. Stimulants used for ADHD should be discontinued at puberty.

NURSING IMPLICATIONS

The nurse has an important role in working with children with ADHD and their parents. Stress the proper timing of stimulant administration for ADHD, and explain the reasons for it. Advise parents to weigh the child weekly, and to keep a record of the weight; height should be measured at reasonable intervals. Stress the importance of maintaining an adequate diet. If the child fails to gain weight or actually loses weight during treatment, recommend that the drug be taken right after meals. Stress ways to assess a positive response, the good potential for long-term and permanent improvement, and the importance of periodic reevaluation.

Narcolepsy

Narcolepsy is a sleep disorder in which an individual (usually an adult) is periodically overcome by a craving for sleep, or actually falls asleep. These episodes may occur many times during the day. Narcolepsy may be accompanied by cataplexy, in which muscle tone suddenly disappears, causing an abrupt fall. These events cause obvious problems in social interactions, jobs, and the safe performance of routine tasks such as driving.

Amphetamines are often effective treatments, but relatively large daily doses may be needed (see Table 27–C). Stimulants used for narcolepsy or cataplexy should be taken with meals, and no later than 6 hours before bedtime. Once-daily dosing with a sustained-release product can be used as described earlier. Chronic treatment is acceptable.

NURSING IMPLICATIONS

Caution persons with narcolepsy or cataplexy to avoid tasks that are made hazardous if sleepiness occurs. Stress the proper timing of drug administration. Recommend that patients keep a daily log of attacks so that the effectiveness of drug therapy can be assessed better.

Side Effects, Adverse Reactions, and Contraindications

The most common side effects of dextroamphetamine, and indeed of all CNS stimulants, are restlessness, dizziness, agitation, and insomnia (Table 27–S). Amphetamines can cause aggression, confusion, delusions, and hallucinations, especially in patients with a history of mental illness. True amphetamine-induced acute psychosis, another concern, is discussed later as a toxic response. Other CNS side effects include anorexia and weight loss (when used for ADHD or narcolepsy), altered libido, and impotence. Peripheral side effects involve the cardiovascular system (palpitations, tachycardia, hypertension), the GI tract (dry mouth, diarrhea or constipation, unpleasant taste), and the eye (photophobia caused by mydriasis, ocular irritation from reduced lacrimation). Ejaculatory failure may contribute to impotence in males. Abrupt withdrawal of amphetamines can cause extreme fatigue (rebound exhaustion) and psychiatric depression. Therefore, the drug should not be discontinued abruptly unless there is an overriding emergency.

A major relative contraindication to the use of amphetamines or any prescribed cerebral stimulant is a history of drug abuse. If these drugs must be prescribed, administration must be supervised closely and the responses assessed carefully. Peripheral effects contraindicate the use of amphetamines in patients with angle-closure glaucoma; such cardiovascular diseases as hypertension, angina pectoris, and tachyarrhythmias; and diabetes mellitus. Pheochromocytoma is an absolute contraindication, due to the risk of a fatal hypertensive crisis.

Amphetamine Abuse

Amphetamines and most related CNS stimulants ("uppers") are popular drugs of abuse. Some states have passed more restrictive laws. Any of these drugs, if taken chronically, can cause intense psychologic dependence and severe social dysfunctioning. Even acute use of high doses may cause personality changes or frank psychosis. Many of the stimulants are classified as Schedule II agents, like morphine and many other narcotics, in recognition of their high abuse potential. This classification imposes limits on the number of doses that can be dispensed (refills are not allowed on the same prescription form), but only partially reduces the problems of abuse.

Although the general topic of substance abuse and its management is discussed in Chapter 28, several key points about the abuse of amphetamines and other cerebral stimulants are worth summarizing here.

CNS stimulant abuse is insidious; it often develops from a desire for only short-term effects on physical or mental performance, to lose weight, or delay sleep. With adolescents, typical factors such as peer pressure often apply. Potential abusers may be anyone faced with real or perceived time-consuming obligations to perform more efficiently or faster; or anyone trying to lose weight. The drug source may be legal (a physician's prescription for the original user) or not. Since cerebral stimulants usually achieve their expected results initially, the desire to continue use is often reinforced. Unfortunately, tolerance requires the use of higher doses to maintain the desired effect, and more-frequent doses to combat depression, fatigue, and dysphoria following each dose.

If the abuser perceives the "highs" as excessive or simply unwanted, he or she may begin to consume CNS depressants. Initially these may be legal drugs, such as alcohol, but it often progresses to prescription drugs (barbiturates or benzodiazepines) obtained through legal or illegal sources. Cyclic use of stimulants and depressants often develops. Overall, the result may be impaired social interactions, financial problems, psychosis, overdoses, and suicidal or accidental death.

NURSING IMPLICATIONS

Low doses of amphetamines may be prescribed for patients with mild hypertension, but very close monitoring of blood pressure is essential. Instruct all patients, but especially the elderly, to report eye pain at once, since it may indicate an acute glaucoma attack that requires emergency treatment. Observe for both physical and behavioral signs of excessive CNS and autonomic stimulation, and try to determine whether the patient is exceeding recommended doses or becoming dependent. Also assess for key signs of abuse, including running out of medication too soon and seeking or using other CNS stimulants or depressants. Caution patients against sharing their medication, or using it for purposes other than that for which it was prescribed.

Amphetamines should be withdrawn gradually. During this time, advise patients to expect drowsiness, caution them about potential but common dangers associated with it, and discourage them from using the prescribed or other stimulant drugs. Assess for signs of depression, and take precautions to protect patients from self-inflicted injury or behavior. Patients who appear to be at great risk of self-harm should be hospitalized for observation and possible treatment.

◆ Use During Pregnancy and Lactation

Neither amphetamines nor any of the drugs discussed later should be given to pregnant women, since they may increase the risk of birth defects. Women who take these drugs should not breastfeed their infants.

◆ Use in Children

Amphetamines or related drugs such as methylphenidate (see below) currently are the most effective and widely used agents for managing ADHD, which is clearly a use in the pediatric population. However, parents or guardians should be advised to expect and to tolerate some degree of hyperactivity in the child, and to appreciate the value of nondrug therapies to help achieve treatment success. They also should be taught that the expected response to therapy is a reduction of hyperactive behavior and other manifestations of the disorder; total normalization of behavior is not a common, universal, or realistic outcome. Be sure that parents or guardians understand that they should not increase the child's dosage of CNS stimulant medication in the hope that a bigger dose will result in less hyperactivity, or better behavior or attention. More likely than not, such a dosage change will make matters worse. Persons who have prescription CNS stimulants in their home should be made aware of the abuse potential; the need to supervise therapy and time drug administration properly; and the need to keep these medications away from other persons who might wish to take them.

◆ Use in the Elderly

Elderly persons are more sensitive to all the effects of all CNS stimulants, and usually should receive dosages at the low end of the recommended adult range. Common age-related disorders such as cardiovascular disease and glaucoma predispose the elderly to adverse effects. Ideally, elderly patients should be screened for glaucoma before receiving any CNS stimulant.

Interactions with Other Drugs

The important and clinically significant interactions involving amphetamines (or most other drugs classified as CNS stimulants) are summarized in Table 27–I. Interactions between amphetamines and drugs that inhibit monoamine oxidase (MAO) inhibitors must be avoided, owing to the potential risk of a fatal outcome. Otherwise, it is usually best to avoid the other listed interactions, using alternative drugs that do not interact, when possible.

Not listed in Table 27–I are interactions of a more general nature: the ability of CNS stimulants to cause additive and potentially dangerous effects when administered with other CNS stimulants; and the ability of stimulants to counteract the central actions of drugs with CNS depressant activity.

It is also important to be aware that CNS stimulants, owing to their appetite-suppressing effects and the resulting ability to decrease food intake, can cause generalized or specific nutritional deficiencies. Altered nutritional status, in turn, can affect the actions of other drugs that may be administered to the patient. The overall issue of nutrition and drug–nutrient interactions is discussed in Chapter 61.

NURSING IMPLICATIONS

It is important to obtain a thorough medication and dietary history before the patient receives CNS stimulants. When outpatient therapy begins, it is important to stress avoidance of interacting stimulant-containing foods and beverages (eg, those containing caffeine) and over-the-counter (OTC) medications; the need to follow prescribed diets; and the values of properly timing stimulant medication administration with respect to meals. Interactions with some prescribed drugs may be unavoidable. However, if combined therapy with such drugs is known to the prescriber and others who are responsible for monitoring the patient's responses, and if the patient can be trusted to follow the prescribed treatment plan, therapeutic problems can be minimized. The greatest problems arise when CNS stimulant use is not prescribed or supervised, as with amphetamine abuse or when OTC interactants are consumed.

Overdose and Toxicity

Amphetamine overdoses are relatively common because of their widespread illegal use. Both the central and sympathetic nervous systems are affected. Toxic responses in the CNS are similar to, but more intense than, those noted as side effects. Common signs and symptoms include restlessness, tremors, exaggerated reflexes, confusion, and extreme irritability. The patient is often hyperalert, talkative, and may have been sleepless for days; paranoia, hallucinations, and violent behavior are possible. A major concern is amphetamine-induced psychosis, which is often indistinguishable from schizophrenia. Toxic doses also cause hypertension and tachyarrhythmias owing to sympathomimetic effects. Lethal doses cause profound hypertension and cerebral hemorrhage, coma, and seizures.

Amphetamine overdoses may be quickly fatal, so immediate diagnosis and treatment is essential. Emesis should be induced (as permitted by the patient's condition; see Appendix C) and other standard first-aid measures to reduce drug absorption (gastric lavage, administration of activated charcoal) should be used. Other approaches, such as forced diuresis, cathartic administration, or urinary acidification to hasten amphetamine elimination, should be used as directed by a poison-control center. Otherwise, monitor and correct vital signs as needed. The α-adrenergic blocker phentolamine, or the parenteral vasodilator nitroprusside, may be needed to lower blood pressure. Psychosis often requires parenteral administration of antipsychotic drugs such as chlorpromazine or haloperidol. Chlorpromazine also blocks α-adrenergic receptors in the periphery, which helps lower blood pressure. Seizures must be treated with a parenteral anticonvulsant, preferably intravenous (IV) diazepam.

NURSING IMPLICATIONS

Persons with suspected overdoses or adverse reactions to any CNS stimulant should be evaluated immediately in a hospital. General aspects of nursing care include assessing the patient closely so that vital signs can be normalized accordingly; interfering with further drug absorption (induced emesis, etc); attempting to identify other offending agents (stimulant overdoses often involve simultaneous depressant overdoses); reducing external stimuli as much as possible; and protecting the patient and others from harm, especially if aggressive or psychotic behavior occurs.

Related Drugs

All other amphetamines (see Table 27–C) share the central and peripheral effects and untoward responses, toxicities, and drug interactions noted for dextroamphetamine. Most share similar clinical uses. Precautions concerning the use and abuse of dextroamphetamine apply to all the others. Their possession, distribution, and use are controlled by laws. Methamphetamine (DESOXYN; known as "speed" on the street) is noteworthy because of its very high abuse potential. Abusers may dissolve methamphetamine tablets and inject the drug intravenously to experience a "rush." In doing so they expose themselves to potentially dangerous cardiovascular and psychotic reactions. Methamphetamine should be prescribed cautiously for any patient and, when prescribed, close observation and supervision is warranted. Some proprietary products contain more than one amphetamine. For example, BIPHETAMINE contains both amphetamine and dextroamphetamine; OBETROL contains equal amounts of two amphetamine and two dextroamphetamine salts.

Amphetamine Congeners Used as Anorexigenics

Several drugs (see Table 27–C) that are structurally similar to amphetamines are indicated for obesity. The congeners are used more frequently than amphetamines because they cause less euphoria and so are somewhat less likely to be abused. Benzphetamine (DIDREX), mazindol (MAZANOR, SANOREX), phenmetrazine (PRELUDIN), and phentermine (FASTIN, IONAMIN) are not dramatically different from amphetamines. The remainder have noteworthy differences that may be clinically important. Diethylpropion (TENUATE; TEPANIL) produces less cardiovascular stimulation, and so some clinicians consider it to be a safer anorexigenic for patients with mild cardiovascular problems. However, it is more likely to cause seizures in seizure-prone individuals. Fenfluramine (PONDIMIN) tends to depress the CNS and may cause psychiatric symptoms, particularly in persons who ingest alcohol acutely or chronically. Overall, fenfluramine's side effects are more severe than those of other nonamphetamine anorexigenics.

Other Cerebral Stimulants

Some cerebral stimulants are chemically unrelated to the amphetamines, and so are discussed separately.

Methylphenidate

Absorption, Distribution, Metabolism, and Excretion

Methylphenidate (RITALIN) is well absorbed from the GI tract and is distributed throughout the body. Its actions appear in about 1 hour after ingestion and last up to 6 hours. The drug is completely metabolized in the liver to inactive products that are excreted in the urine.

Pharmacologic Effects

Methylphenidate causes milder cerebral stimulating and sympathomimetic effects, but produces more intense cortical (mental) effects, than amphetamines. As with dextroamphetamine, tolerance to the CNS and peripheral effects develops with continued use.

Clinical Indications and Administration

Methylphenidate usually is the drug of choice for most children with ADHD. Methylphenidate may also be used for adults with narcolepsy. Either immediate-acting products or sustained-release tablets (RITALIN-SR) are generally acceptable for either indication. Methylphenidate is occasionally prescribed for depression, but the results have been inconclusive.

NURSING IMPLICATIONS

Most children with ADHD respond to methylphenidate. Symptomatic improvement should be seen within a few days or weeks after therapy is begun. If there are no signs of improvement after 1 month, continued methylphenidate therapy is not likely to be effective; the drug should be discontinued and alternatives evaluated. As with dextroamphetamine, the response and the need for continued drug treatment should be assessed at least every 6 months. Advise patients taking RITALIN-SR to swallow the tablet whole, not to chew it. Timing of the dose, and nursing implications related to it, are the same as those noted for treatment of ADHD or narcolepsy with dextroamphetamine.

Side Effects, Adverse Reactions, and Contraindications

The central and peripheral side effects, adverse reactions, and contraindications noted for amphetamines apply also to methylphenidate (see Table 27–S). Nervousness and insomnia are the most common side effects, particularly in children, who are also more susceptible to anorexia, weight loss, and temporary growth retardation during therapy. Methylphenidate causes anemia in some patients.

Methylphenidate is a Schedule II drug, indicating a high potential for abuse and psychologic dependence. It can cause all the severe psychologic abnormalities noted for amphetamines, including acute psychosis.

NURSING IMPLICATIONS

Virtually all the nursing implications noted for dextroamphetamine apply to methylphenidate. Patients with ADHD should be monitored closely, especially during early therapy, for paradoxical worsening of ADHD symptoms, which requires discontinuation of methylphenidate. In addition to standard periodic assessment for both desired and untoward responses (diet, weight, sleep patterns, behavioral changes, and so on), blood tests should be done to help detect anemia. Monitor for evidence of suppressed growth. Advise parents that long-term growth problems are not likely, especially after methylphenidate administration is stopped. Periodic discontinuation of methylphenidate administration reduces the problem further.

Interactions with Other Drugs

Methylphenidate generally participates in the drug interactions noted for amphetamines.

Overdose and Toxicity

Signs, symptoms, and treatment of methylphenidate overdose are the same as those noted for amphetamines, as are the related nursing implications.

Pemoline

Pemoline (CYLERT) is used exclusively for the treatment of ADHD. It is well absorbed after oral administration and has a duration of action of about 12 hours, which enables once-a-day administration (see Table 27–C). About half the absorbed dose is excreted unchanged in the urine. The rest is metabolized before excretion.

Pemoline presumably exerts its beneficial effects by increasing the storage or synthesis of dopamine, another excitatory neurotransmitter, in parts of the CNS. Beneficial effects on ADHD symptoms may not develop for 3 or 4 weeks, so parents should be advised accordingly. Pemoline causes less cerebral stimulation than any other drug used for ADHD, and peripheral sympathomimetic effects are minimal. Side effects, adverse responses, toxicity, and appropriate nursing actions are similar to those discussed for dextroamphetamine and methylphenidate. Pemoline has caused hepatic damage and dyskinesias, so ongoing assessment for signs of these problems is warranted. Pemoline's abuse potential is lower than that of most amphetamines or methylphenidate; it is classified as a Schedule IV drug.

Over-the-Counter Anorexigenics

Caffeine

Caffeine, an ingredient in coffee, tea, and numerous carbonated soft drinks, is perhaps the most widely used and abused drug. It is popular because of its CNS-stimulating action. Caffeine is also an ingredient in some OTC headache remedies, cold medications, appetite suppressants, and stimulants (Table 27–1). A related drug, theobromine, is found in cocoa and chocolate. Caffeine is related chemically to the bronchodilator drugs aminophylline and theophylline (methylxanthines; see Chapter 38). The major pharmacologic importance of caffeine is the fact that a significant number of Americans consume sufficient amounts of the drug each day to cause an anxiety-like disorder, *caffeinism*.

Absorption, Distribution, Metabolism, and Excretion

Caffeine is readily absorbed from the GI tract and has a plasma half-life of between 3 and 6 hours. The benzoate salt can be given parenterally. Caffeine is partially metabolized in the liver and excreted in the urine.

Pharmacologic Effects

Caffeine, like theophylline, stimulates the CNS and heart and relaxes smooth muscle in blood vessels and the bronchi. Vasodilation and cardiac stimulation increase renal blood flow, which may be seen as increased urine output (diuresis). Gastric acid secretion is increased. High doses stimulate respiration, vasomotor tone, and vagal tone. Caffeine's peripheral effects are weaker than those produced by theophylline. Ordinary doses of caffeine clearly produce less CNS stimulation than average doses of amphetamines. Caffeine suppresses appetite through a weak amphetamine-like action, and perhaps by elevating blood glucose levels. A certain euphoria accompanies caffeine ingestion, and it appears to be a major reason why many individuals have difficulty in breaking habitual intake of large amounts of beverages containing it.

Clinical Indications and Administration

Medical Uses

The benzoate salt of caffeine can be given intravenously or intramuscularly to manage acute circulatory failure, as a diuretic, or to counteract respiratory depression as might be caused by such CNS depressants as morphine or alcohol. Citrated caffeine can be given via nasogastric

Table 27–1 Common Sources of Caffeine

Source	Caffeine Content (approximate)
Beverages, confections	
Coffee, regular, brewed	40–180 mg/5–8 oz
Coffee, regular, instant	30–120 mg/5–8 oz
Coffee, decaffeinated, brewed or instant	1–5 mg/5–8 oz
Tea, brewed	20–110 mg/5–8 oz
Tea, instant	25–50 mg/5–8 oz
Chocolate milk	2–7 mg/5 oz
Cocoa	2–50 mg/5–8 oz
Milk chocolate	1–15 mg/oz
Bakers (unsweetened) chocolate	25–35 mg/oz
Soft drinks*	
Colas (most, sweetened or diet)	35–45 mg/12 oz
Colas (caffeine–free, sweetened or diet)	0
Dr. Pepper	40 mg/12 oz
Jolt	90 mg/12 oz
Mountain Dew	54 mg/12 oz
7-Up, Sprite, similar products	0
OTC analgesic combination products*	
Anacin, Midol, Vanquish	32 mg/tablet
Excedrin	65 mg/tablet
OTC cold combination products*	
Dristan	16 mg/tablet
OTC "stimulants"*	
Nodoz	100 mg/tablet
Vivarin	200 mg/tablet
Prescription medications	
CAFERGOT	100 mg/tablet
DARVON Compound 65	32 mg/capsule
FIORINAL	40 mg/capsule or tablet

*A selected list of brands or products in these categories. Data were obtained from product manufacturers; *Handbook of Nonprescription Drugs*, 9th ed., American Pharmaceutical Association; and *Drug Facts & Comparisons*, 1992, Facts & Comparisons, Inc.

tube as a respiratory stimulant for newborn infants. However, the drug is usually given orally. Doses up to 500 mg can be used to treat acute headaches, particularly those that are caused by therapeutic lumbar puncture. The drug presumably constricts cerebral blood vessels and prevents painful vessel pulsations. Much lower amounts of caffeine (typically 30 to 60 mg per dose) are found in some OTC headache remedies that contain a nonnarcotic analgesic also. Controversy exists over whether caffeine levels in the OTC products actually increase the ability of a true analgesic to alleviate headache.

NURSING IMPLICATIONS

Administer no more than 500 mg of caffeine parenterally at any one time. Higher doses are liable to cause excessive CNS and cardiovascular stimulation, and may eventually cause paradoxic respiratory depression. Close monitoring of blood pressure, heart rate, respiration, fluid intake and output (particularly urine output), and the level of the patient's CNS activity are essential when giving caffeine by injection. Other precautions and contraindications are noted later.

Use as a Self-Medication

Caffeine-containing beverages or OTC drugs are usually self-administered to alleviate fatigue and increase alertness (see Table 27–1 for typical caffeine contents). Brewed coffee contains between 60 and 180 mg per 5-ounce serving, and tea contains about half that amount. Colas are traditionally considered the major caffeine-containing soft drink (about 50 mg per 12-oz serving), but other carbonated beverages may contain equivalent amounts or more. Nonprescription "stimulants" contain between 100 and 200 mg per dose. When used occasionally, these small amounts of caffeine can provide some of the expected benefits. More commonly, however, caffeine is ingested habitually and in high doses. Twenty to thirty percent of the American population ingests between 500 and 600 mg of caffeine per day—four to six cups of coffee—and about 10% consume more than 1 g daily. Such continued use, without allowing the body to recover through adequate rest, leads to decreasing mental and physical performance.

Side Effects, Adverse Reactions, and Contraindications

Caffeine may overstimulate the central and sympathetic nervous systems. Common central signs, familiar to many of us, include jitteriness, restlessness, nervousness, excitement, and insomnia. Flushed face, palpitations, and diuresis are common autonomic side effects. Some persons may show signs of considerable stimulation with daily doses as low as 250 mg per day (two or three cups of brewed coffee). If a person who has not developed caffeine tolerance ingests about 1 g in a day, such CNS effects as periods of inexhaustibility, psychomotor agitation, rambling thoughts and speech, tinnitus, and hallucinations may occur. Peripheral effects include muscle twitching, tachypnea or respiratory distress, severe nausea and vomiting, and cardiac problems ranging from palpitations to arrhythmias. The effects are much milder in persons who have developed tolerance through frequent use, unless very high doses are taken.

Gastrointestinal distress can occur because caffeine irritates the gastric mucosa directly and stimulates gastric acid secretion. The drug should not be used by patients with peptic ulcer disease.

Caffeinism

Caffeinism is a syndrome caused by excessive caffeine intake. It afflicts about 10% of Americans, and is so prevalent that specific diagnostic criteria have been identified (*DSM III-R* category 305.90). Characteristics include marked anxiety, affective symptoms, and psychophysiologic complaints. Many signs and symptoms resemble manic episodes, panic disorders, or generalized anxiety disorders. Not surprisingly, many patients with caffeinism have been erroneously diagnosed as suffering from mental disorders and have been treated with psychoactive drugs. To avoid such inappropriate and possibly dangerous treatment, caffeinism must be distinguished from the other disorders it resembles. The diagnosis is confirmed if discontinuing all sources of caffeine intake causes the symptoms to resolve. When habitual caffeine use is stopped abruptly, a withdrawal syndrome may occur. It is characterized by headache, anxiety, dizziness, palpitations, and a craving for caffeine.

NURSING IMPLICATIONS

When assessing patients with anxiety symptoms, palpitations, or any of the other common possible indicators of caffeinism, specifically inquire about use of caffeine-containing beverages or drugs. If caffeinism is suspected, recommend that patients restrict or cease use of offending products, but advise them to expect the withdrawal signs and symptoms noted earlier. Teach patients the amounts of caffeine in various beverages and OTC products, and advise them that daily doses of no more than 500 mg may provide beneficial psychomotor stimulation.

Overdose and Toxicity

Doses of 10 g of caffeine taken acutely may cause all of the adverse responses noted above, plus seizures. It is virtually impossible to ingest such a dose in the form of caffeine-containing beverages (10 g is equivalent to 80 to 100 cups of coffee). However, it is relatively easy to ingest such a toxic dose in the form of caffeine-containing stimulants. Overdoses are managed symptomatically and supportively, starting with induced emesis if the patient is conscious and has no seizure activity. Parenteral administration of diazepam is indicated for seizures.

Phenylpropanolamine

Phenylpropanolamine ("PPA") is a CNS-stimulating sympathomimetic that was introduced and discussed in Chapter 14. It is the most common ingredient in nonprescription weight-loss aids, in which it may be the sole ingredient or may be combined with caffeine. The amount per capsule or tablet ranges from 25 to 75 mg. Phenylpropanolamine's sympathomimetic effects account for its more frequent use (at lower doses, usually 12.5 mg) as a decongestant in many OTC cough, cold, and allergy medications. Very high doses can produce amphetamine-like psychologic and behavioral changes. The drug's vasopressor, cardiac-stimulating, mydriatic, and hyperglycemic effects contraindicate its use in patients with cardiovascular disorders, hyperthyroidism, glaucoma, and diabetes.

NURSING IMPLICATIONS

Advise patients contemplating the use of OTC anorexigenics about their proper use, limitations, adverse responses, and potential dangers. Inform them that few if any of the OTC products are proven to be more effective than a balanced calorie-restricted diet and appropriate exercise. Encourage them to consult a physician, nutritionist, or certified fitness coordinator to learn acceptable nondrug approaches to weight loss or control. Assess for all contraindications to sympathomimetic drugs (glaucoma, cardiovascular disease, hyperthyroidism, diabetes mellitus), and discourage any patient with any of these contraindications from using an anorexigenic, particularly those containing a sympathomimetic, without prior approval from a physician.

II. Respiratory Stimulants (Analeptics)

Doxapram

Doxapram (DOPRAM) which primarily stimulates respiration, is classified as an analeptic in this text. It stimulates respiration through actions in the medullary respiratory control center and on peripheral carotid chemoreceptors, which regulate respiration by sensing blood carbon dioxide levels. Usual doses stimulate respiratory depth more than rate. High doses stimulate the entire CNS. Doxapram is given parenterally at dosages noted in Table 27–C.

Analeptics were used relatively frequently before the widespread availability of mechanical ventilators and the advances of modern pulmonary therapy. Few physicians today have heard of these drugs, and fewer still have used them. Doxapram is still approved to manage drug-induced respiratory depression (as caused by barbiturates, alcohol, or opiates), postanesthesia respiratory depression, or hypercapnia and poor ventilation caused by chronic obstructive pulmonary disease. It should be used only temporarily and when no mechanical ventilator is available. It should never be considered a primary treatment for respiratory depression, nor given to patients on a ventilator.

The adverse effects caused by doxapram may be more dangerous and difficult to treat than the condition for which it is given. The most common side effects are mild hypertension and cardiac arrhythmias caused by catecholamine release, as described for amphetamines. Doxapram is generally contraindicated in patients with high blood pressure or irregular cardiac rhythm. Catecholamine release also contraindicates its use in patients with a history of most cardiovascular diseases (stroke, coronary artery disease, arrhythmias, frank uncompensated heart failure, pheochromocytoma). Analeptics may harm, rather than help, patients with compromised respiratory function associated with pneumothorax, muscle paresis, flail chest, airway obstruction or extreme dyspnea (including that caused by acute asthma), pulmonary embolism, pulmonary fibrosis, or neuromuscular disorders. A history of seizures is another important contraindication. Doxapram overdoses may cause severe hypertension, arrhythmias, muscle hyperreflexia, and status epilepticus.

Theoretically, all of the drug interactions noted for amphetamines and other cerebral stimulants (see Table 27–I) apply to doxapram. Fortunately, since this drug usually is administered for very short periods of time to patients who are monitored closely and with emergency drugs available nearby, most interactions can be avoided, or at least recognized and treated promptly.

Central Nervous System Stimulants of Toxicologic Interest

Cocaine

Cocaine has limited medical use as a topical local anesthetic for the eye. When injected or inhaled it exerts powerful cortical stimulating activity, which contributes to its widespread abuse. Both the central and peripheral sympathomimetic effects (see Chapter 14) are due to its ability to block norepinephrine and dopamine reuptake into neurons. Hypertension, stroke, cardiac arrhythmias, and infarction are the major causes of sudden death from cocaine overdose.

Strychnine

Strychnine, which enjoyed limited clinical use years ago, is a lethal toxin that is readily absorbed after oral ingestion. It is still used as a poison for rodents and birds, and is found in adulterated street drugs; these two sources are the primary causes of strychnine poisoning. Strychnine is considered to be a powerful "stimulant," but its effects are due mainly to intense inhibitory effects on inhibitory nerve pathways in the brain and spinal cord. Shortly after ingestion strychnine causes pronounced and repeated seizures, initial respiratory stimulation, and painful and rigid extension of the trunk and extremity muscles. Even minor external stimuli may cause further seizures or periods of intense muscle activation in poisoned individuals. Death is caused by hypoxia resulting from paralysis of the medulla and strong contractions of the diaphragm that prevent inspiration. Initially, strychnine does not impair consciousness, so between seizures the victim may be quite aware that the next and potentially final seizure may develop. Overdoses are treated symptomatically and supportively. Intravenous injection of diazepam may be very effective, and mechanical support of ventilation is often needed. External stimuli should be reduced as much as possible.

SUMMARY OF NURSING IMPLICATIONS

◆ Assessment

Gather growth and development data on children prior to administering CNS stimulant therapy for comparison with treatment effects.

Complete nursing history to include seizure disorders, sleep disturbance, obesity, nervousness, depression, family history of endocrine problems, diet history, pattern of activity, and exercise.

Establish baseline physical assessment data: height, weight, bone structure, vital signs, electrocardiogram.

Inquire about use of caffeine-containing beverages or nonprescription drugs; determine usual amounts taken and response to tea, coffee, cola, or cocoa.

Review history for key contraindications to drug therapy.

Review prior drug use/abuse: indications of problems may include running out of medication too soon, attempts to obtain prescriptions from more than one physician, and use of CNS depressants (eg, excessive alcohol ingestion).

◆ Nursing Diagnoses

Sleep pattern disturbance related to drug effects or caffeine use.

Body image disturbance related to obesity.

Noncompliance related to lack of motivation, poor self-image, or negative effects of prescribed drugs.

Altered thought processes related to attention deficit hyperactivity disorder.

Altered nutrition: less than body requirements related to amphetamine abuse and anorexia.

Altered nutrition: more than body requirements related to overeating and lack of dietary control.

Sensory/perceptual alteration related to drug response (CNS stimulation or depression).

Knowledge deficit related to current drug therapy.

Altered family processes related to attention deficit hyperactivity disorder and behavior problems in child.

◆ Planning/Implementation

Administer medication at appropriate time: 1 hour before meals with obesity; early morning or with meal for ADHD or narcolepsy; not less than 6 hours before bedtime, especially with sustained-acting products.

Reassure parents that child's behavior is not willful or a result of poor parenting; that improvement may not be seen for weeks after treatment.

Provide emotional and psychologic support for child and parents.

Closely monitor cardiovascular vital signs of patients with cardiovascular disease; blood glucose in diabetics.

If overdose is suspected, monitor vital signs; be prepared to give anticonvulsants or antipsychotics.

Take precautions to protect patient from self-harm or others from injury; reduce external stimuli (noise, bright lights, unnecessary physical contact); provide reassurance; anticipate profound depression of systems initially stimulated by drug.

Do not give caffeine or related drugs to patients with peptic ulcer disease; use cautiously in patients with myocardial infarction or respiratory depression.

When giving caffeine parenterally, do not exceed the maximum dose (500 mg); have a short-acting barbiturate available to counteract excessive stimulation.

Do not administer doxapram if respirations are inadequate, airway is obstructed, patient is on ventilator, or other contraindications apply.

Mix doxapram with dextrose and water; do not use alkaline solutions.

Observe and monitor blood pressure, pulse, and body temperature closely for at least 1 hour after giving doxapram; discontinue or withhold if dyspnea or hypotension occurs; have resuscitation equipment, oxygen, and parenteral anticonvulsants readily available.

◆ Patient and Family Teaching

Teach the patient/family:

About abuse potential, without provoking fear; to use drug according to physician's direction, in prescribed doses and with periodic evaluation to reduce risk of psychologic dependence.

About dangers of sharing cerebral stimulants with others.

To prevent others from gaining access to these drugs.

To discard unused medication when drug therapy is discontinued.

To take the drug only for prescribed purposes.

To use the drug in conjunction with diet, exercise, and possible psychologic counseling for obesity.

Not to increase or otherwise alter drug therapy to hasten or improve therapeutic response.

That parent(s) should monitor child's food intake daily, and physical growth weekly.

To report weight loss, insomnia, irritability, hallucinations, worsening behavior, or adverse psychologic responses.

To keep records of narcolepsy attacks during treatment to determine improvement and possible changes in restrictions on activity.

To avoid tasks that may become hazardous if drowsiness, depression, or sleep develop suddenly.

To report ocular pain at once, as it may indicate glaucoma.

About drugs and beverages to avoid with CNS stimulants; provide list.

About alternative or additional forms of contraception, as drugs may reduce oral contraceptive effectiveness.

About the use of nonprescription anorexigenics: proper use, limitations, adverse responses, and the need for balanced low-calorie diet and exercise.

To avoid sodium bicarbonate, which alkalinizes urine and reduces amphetamine excretion, as it may cause excessive or prolonged effects.

To avoid starvation or unprescribed dietary changes that may cause ketosis, which acidifies urine and enhances amphetamine elimination.

To restrict or avoid caffeine consumption if anxiety symptoms, tachycardia, facial flushing, or other signs of caffeinism are present; warn about craving and physical and subjective symptoms.

◆ Evaluation

The patient/family will:

Demonstrate interest in appearance; lose weight.

Comply with medication regimen and weight-reduction program; return for follow-up care.

Reduce intake of caffeinated beverages.

Report adequate rest.

Identify effective coping patterns; identify sources of support.

Participate in decision-making and problem-solving; complete assignments without distraction.

Achieve normal body weight.

Report signs and symptoms of side effects; seek appropriate information as needed.

Annotated Bibliography

Anastopoulos AD, DuPaul GJ, Barkley RA. Stimulant medication and parent training therapies for attention deficit-hyperactivity disorder. *J Learn Disabil* 1991;24:210–218. *Covers drug therapy well, but also gives useful information about how teaching parenting skills can help increase the effectiveness of pharmacotherapy for ADHD.*

Appelt GD. Weight control products. In: *Handbook of Nonprescription Drugs.* 9th ed. Washington, D.C.: American Pharmaceutical Association, 1990:563–577. *The best single source for information about the use, misuse, and actions of CNS stimulants, and other important medications, as OTC weight-loss aids.*

Calis KA, Grothe DR, Elia J. Attention-deficit hyperactivity disorder. *Clin Pharm* 1990;9:632–642. *Clearly reviews epidemiology, clinical manifestations, diagnostic criteria, and clinical course of ADHD, and describes the role of drug therapy for it—focusing on dextroamphetamine, methylphenidate, and pemoline—and the values of nondrug interventions.*

Caro JP, Dombrowski SR. Sleep aid and stimulant products. In: *Handbook of Nonprescription Drugs.* 9th ed. Washington, D.C.: American Pharmaceutical Association, 1990:225–241. *The one best source of information about what your patients may be self-administering to help them go to sleep or to stay awake.*

Carpenter MA, Bodansky HJ. Drug treatment of obesity in type 2 diabetes mellitus. *Diabetic Med* 1990;7:99–104. *Given the prevalence of diabetes, and the importance of weight control, this paper should be read by nurses caring for patients with this common endocrine disorder.*

NIH consensus statement covers treatment of obesity. *Am Fam Physician* 1991;44:305–306. *A to-the-point summary of the government's position on how drug therapy of obesity should be handled.*

Ouellette EM. Legal issues in the treatment of children with attention deficit hyperactivity disorder. *J Child Neurol* 1991;6(Suppl.):S68–S75. *Not "hard core" pharmacology, but not to be overlooked if you know a child being treated with drugs for ADHD. Reading this should prompt you to review Chapter 3 of this textbook—legal issues that apply to nurses.*

Voeller KK. Clinical management of attention deficit hyperactivity disorder. *J Child Neurol* 1991;6(Suppl.):S51–S67. *A contemporary review of ADHD from a multidisciplinary viewpoint: data collection and etiology; diagnosis; management; interactions with parents and the young patient; and very informative case study reviews.*

Table 27–C Clinical Uses and Administration of Major Central Nervous System Stimulants*

AGENT	CLINICAL USES	DOSAGE AND ROUTE OF ADMINISTRATION
Cerebral Stimulants		
Amphetamines		
PROTOTYPE		
Dextroamphetamine		
(DEXEDRINE, DEXEDRINE SPANSULES) Schedule II	Obesity	Adults: Up to 30 mg/d of immediate-acting preparation in 5–10 mg divided doses 30–60 min before meals; may substitute 10- or 15-mg long-acting preparation (SPANSULE) taken in the morning if dose is appropriate
	ADHD	Children: 3–5 years: 2.5 mg qd with or immediately after meals; dosage may be raised in 2.5–mg/d increments at weekly intervals as needed; 6 years to puberty; 5 mg qd or bid, increase 5 mg/d at weekly intervals; SPANSULES may be given once-daily (in morning) if dose is appropriate. Limit daily dose of any formulation to 40 mg
	Narcolepsy	Adults: 5–60 mg/d in divided doses, or SPANSULE taken once daily. Children: 6–12 years: 5 mg qd, with weekly increases of 5 mg/d prn; >12 years: 10 mg qd, increased by 10 mg/d at weekly intervals prn. Give first dose upon awakening, additional doses at 4–6-hr intervals; SPANSULES may be substituted for once-daily administration
Other Amphetamines		
Amphetamine sulfate		
Schedule II	Obesity	Adults: 5–30 mg daily in divided doses 30–60 min before meals; 15–30 mg of sustained-release form in AM
	ADHD	Children: 3–5 years: 2.5 mg qd; daily dosage may be increased by 2.5 mg at weekly intervals; >6 years: 5 mg/d; daily dosage may be increased by 5 mg at weekly intervals. Maximum daily dose is 40 mg
	Narcolepsy	Adults: 5–60 mg daily in divided doses. Children: 6–12 years: 5 mg qd; >12 years: 10 mg qd
Amphetamine sulfate plus dextroamphetamine		
(BIPHETAMINE 12 1/2, 20) Schedule II	Obesity	Adults: 1 capsule qd, taken 10–14 hr before bedtime (BIPHETAMINE 12½ contains 6.25 mg of amphetamine and dextroamphetamine; BIPHETAMINE 20 contains 10 mg of each)
	ADHD	Children >3 years: Establish dosage with immediate–acting form of regular dextroamphetamine, substitute BIPHETAMINE accordingly for once–daily dosing: BIPHETAMINE 12½ is equivalent to 10 mg dextroamphetamine, BIPHETAMINE 20 is equivalent to 15 mg dextroamphetamine

(continued)

Table 27–C **Clinical Uses and Administration of Major Central Nervous System Stimulants* (*Continued*)**

AGENT	CLINICAL USES	DOSAGE AND ROUTE OF ADMINISTRATION
Amphetamine mixture (amphetamine sulfate plus asparate; dextroamphetamine sulfate plus saccharate)		
(OBETROL) Schedule II	Obesity	Adults: See amphetamine sulfate
Methamphetamine		
(DESOXYN, GRADUMET SR) Schedule II	Obesity	Adults: 5 mg half an hour before each meal; or one 10 or 15 mg GRADUMET tablet qd, in AM
	ADHD	Children >6 years: 5 mg qd or bid. Daily dose may be increased by 5 mg at weekly intervals. Usual effective dosage is 20–25 mg daily. One GRA-
	Amphetamine Congeners	
Benzphetamine		
(DIDREX) Schedule III	Obesity	Adults: 25–50 mg qd–tid, 1 hr before meals
Diethylpropion		
(TENUATE; TEPANIL) Schedule IV	Obesity	Adults: 25 mg tid 1 hr before meals or 75 mg of controlled–release (TENUATE DOSPAN) qd at mid-morning
Fenfluramine		
(PONDIMIN) Schedule IV	Obesity	Adults: 20 mg tid before meals. Daily dose may be increased by 20 mg at weekly intervals to maximum dose of 120 mg/d
Mazindol		
(MEZANOR; SANOREX) Schedule IV	Obesity	Adults: 1 mg tid, 1 hr before meals, or 2 mg once before lunch
Phendimetrazine		
(PLEGINE, PRELU–2, others) Schedule III	Obesity	Adults: 35 mg bid or tid, 1 hr before meals. Give the time–release form (PRELU–2) in the AM (105 mg)
Phenmetrazine		
(PRELUDIN ENDURETS) Schedule II	Obesity	Adults: 75 mg of sustained-release form (ENDURETS) qd
Phentermine		
(FASTIN) Schedule IV	Obesity	Adults: 8 mg tid or 15–37.5 qd
	Other Cerebral Stimulants	
Caffeine	Psychomotor stimulant	Adults: 100–200 mg; see Table 27–1
Caffeine citrate	Respiratory stimulation in newborns	Oral by nasogastric tube: 10 mg/kg, followed by a maintenance dose of 2.5 mg/kg/d
Caffeine sodium benzoate	Respiratory stimulation	IM or IV: Adults: 500 mg; repeat as necessary (maximum single dose is 1000 mg)

(continued)

Table 27–C Clinical Uses and Administration of Major Central Nervous System Stimulants* (*Continued*)

AGENT	CLINICAL USES	DOSAGE AND ROUTE OF ADMINISTRATION
Methylphenidate		
(RITALIN, RITALIN-SR) Schedule II	ADHD	Children >6 years: 5 mg before both breakfast and lunch; increase daily dose in 5–10-mg increments at weekly intervals. Optimal daily dose is approximately 0.3 mg/kg, should not exceed daily maximum of 60 mg regardless of body weight. Sustained-release form (RITALIN-SR) is effective for 8 hr, and can be substituted if dose corresponds
	Narcolepsy	Adults: 20–60 mg/d in divided doses 30–45 min before meals
Pemoline		
(CYLERT) Schedule IV	ADHD	Children: 37.5 mg qd in AM. Daily dose may be increased by 18.75 mg at weekly intervals to a maximum dosage of 112.5 mg/d. Usual maintenance dose 56.25–75 mg/d
Phenylpropanolamine		
(Various names)	Obesity	Adults: Follow directions on OTC package
	Analeptics	
Doxapram		
(DOPRAM)	Drug–induced respiratory depression	IV: Adults: 2 mg/kg as a single injection; repeat in 5 min, then every 1–2 hr if needed *or* 1–3 mg/min IV infusion. Maximum dose is 3 g
	Postanesthesia respiratory depression	Adults: 0.5–1 mg/kg injection repeated at 5-min intervals *or* 5 mg/min IV infusion until satisfactory response occurs; maintain at 1–3 mg/min
	COPD associated with hypercapnia	IV: Adults: 1–3 mg/min for up to 2 hr

*Except where noted, all amphetamines and amphetamine congeners are given orally.

Table 27–S **Major Side Effects of and Contraindications for CNS Stimulants**

BODY SYSTEM/ Side Effect	RELATED CONTRAINDICATION	COMMENTS AND NURSING IMPLICATIONS
Side Effects and Contraindications Common to All Cerebral Stimulants		
CENTRAL NERVOUS SYSTEM Restlessness, dizziness, insomnia, generalized overstimulation	Other sympathomimetics, caffeine, agitated states, hypersensitivity to sympathomimetic amines	Give last dose no later than 6 hr before bedtime; restlessness may require dosage reduction; children with ADHD may benefit from periodic discontinuation of drug therapy
Euphoria	History of drug abuse	Instruct about potential for dependence; monitor patient's consumption of these medications; attempt to find lowest effective dosage
Anorexia, weight loss		If drug is prescribed for ADHD or narcolepsy, advise patient to take drug with or immediately after meals; administer 1 hr before meal if prescribed for obesity. Monitor weight gain and growth in children treated for ADHD
EYE Mydriasis, photophobia	Glaucoma, especially narrow angle	When used for weight control, remind patient that it is only a short–term treatment; discuss alternate and adjunctive weight–reducing plans Monitor for, having patient report at once, sudden or intense eye pain that might indicate acute glaucoma; if it occurs, recommend immediate discontinuation of stimulant, professional evaluation; ideally have all elderly patients screened for glaucoma before use of any cerebral stimulant (prescription or OTC)
METABOLIC Hyperglycemia, worsening of diabetic signs, symptoms	Diabetes mellitus	Avoid use with diabetes mellitus, especially if severe or poorly controlled; if these drugs must be prescribed, frequent monitoring of blood glucose levels and patient's response is imperative; antidiabetic drug doses may need to be adjusted
CARDIOVASCULAR Palpitations, tachycardia, hypertension, angina, arrhythmias	Hypertension and conditions in which hypertension is a concern (eg, hyperthyroidism, cardiovascular disease, pheochromocytoma, severe tachycardia)	Monitor BP and pulse after establishing baseline parameters; question orders for more than one CNS stimulant; teach patient about OTC preparations that could cause additive effect; caffeine intake should be reduced
GASTROINTESTINAL GI upset, diarrhea		Take with meals (if appropriate) to reduce GI distress
Side Effects and Contraindications Common to Doxapram		
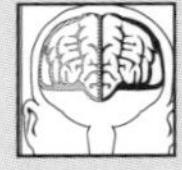 **CENTRAL NERVOUS SYSTEM** Flushing, sweating, headache, dizziness	Other sympathomimetics	Monitor patient, discontinue if patient becomes hypotensive
Convulsions	Seizure history (relative contraindication)	Have anticonvulsants, oxygen, and resuscitative equipment available

(continued)

Table 27–S | **Major Side Effects of and Contraindications for CNS Stimulants (*Continued*)**

BODY SYSTEM/ Side Effect	RELATED CONTRAINDICATION	COMMENTS AND NURSING IMPLICATIONS
RESPIRATORY Dyspnea, bronchospasm, laryngospasm, hypoventilation	Use of mechanical ventilation; compromised respiratory function due to pneumothorax, muscle paresis, flail chest, airway obstruction, or extreme dyspnea associated with acute asthma, pulmonary embolism, pulmonary fibrosis, or neuromuscular disorders (eg, myasthenia gravis)	Assess for obstructed airway; make sure that oxygen is adequate; discontinue medication if dyspnea comes on suddenly
CARDIOVASCULAR Mild hypertension, variations in heart rate, arrhythmias, chest pain, tightening in chest	Severe tachycardia, arrhythmias, hyperthyroidism, cardiac disease, uncompensated heart failure; hypertension	Monitor BP and pulse. Doxapram should not be given within 10 min of most anesthetics
GASTROINTESTINAL Nausea and vomiting		If vomiting occurs, particularly with drug-induced respiratory depression, have suction machine available

Table 27–I | **Major Interactions Between CNS Stimulants and Other Drugs**

INTERACTANT	RESULT OF INTERACTION	COMMENTS AND NURSING IMPLICATIONS
Antidiabetic (hypoglycemic) drugs (insulin, oral agents; Chapter 46)	Increased or decreased blood glucose levels, poor or inconsistent diabetes control	Avoid interaction if possible; monitor blood, urine glucose levels more closely if combined use is essential
Furazolidone (Chapter 57)	Additive central, peripheral, autonomic effects, side effects, of amphetamines	Furazolidone inhibits monoamine oxidase (see below); probably best to avoid interaction
Guanethidine (Chapter 33)	Decreased antihypertensive effect of guanethidine	Avoid interaction
Lithium (Chapter 24)	Decreased effect of one or both agents; poor control of psychiatric symptoms	Avoid interaction
Monoamine oxidase inhibitors (Chapter 24)	Acute, severe hypertensive crisis, stroke	Must avoid interaction; be sure one of the interactants has been discontinued at least 1–2 weeks before starting therapy with other agent
Sympathomimetics (Chapter 14)	Additive cardiovascular, CNS stimulation	Avoid interaction, even when sympathomimetics are in form of OTC medications (eg, decongestants)
Urinary alkalinizers (eg, sodium bicarbonate; Chapters 40, 60)	Diminished amphetamine excretion, increased blood levels, side effects or toxicity	Interaction of most concern with amphetamine overdose; still best to discourage self-prescribing of interactants (eg, baking soda) during therapy with amphetamines, related drugs

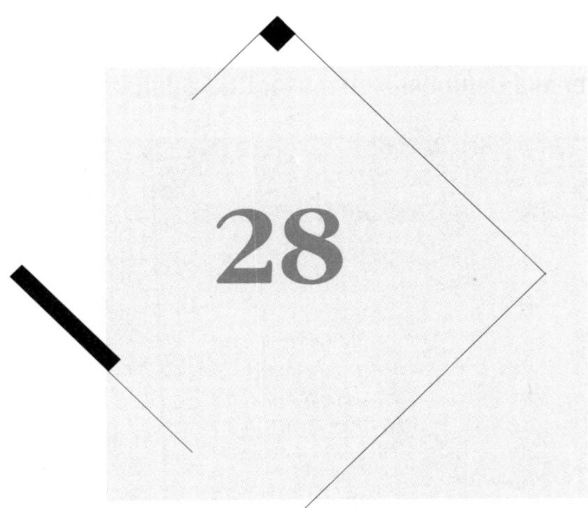

Substance Misuse and Abuse

Substance abuse and misuse generally implies the administration of any pharmacologically active agent to produce effects that are not therapeutically necessary or desirable for the individual. Most misused or abused substances have therapeutic value when given under appropriate conditions, or to individuals who need them. Others have no accepted therapeutic value and are absolutely illegal, yet they can trigger and perpetuate improper self-administration. Working definitions of some of the pertinent terms are given shortly.

Substance abuse is a multifaceted problem, with legal, social, moral, and economic implications. There are epidemiologic aspects—not only the shocking statistics on the prevalence and group-related issues of substance abuse, but also its dramatic medical impact on the user and on others (for example, the transmission of hepatitis and AIDS both to other abusers and to nonabusers). Perhaps of more direct relevance to nursing are the important psychologic and psychiatric aspects that relate to such diverse issues as motivations for abuse, recognition of the problem, and the great value of mental health care in substance abuse prevention and treatment. Many forms of substance abuse are recognized as diseases.

This chapter addresses issues pertinent to the pharmacologic aspects of substance abuse. It reviews the pharmacologic properties of drug groups, most of which have been discussed in detail elsewhere in this text, particularly in this unit. Drugs that affect the central nervous system (CNS) and its control over behavior and emotions are the most frequently abused drugs, but the abuse problem is not limited to such agents.

Most people who abuse "harder" drugs such as cocaine or heroin, abuse more than one of these substances. Some combinations of drugs have been particularly popular from time to time. Several years ago, heroin was in short supply in large metropolitan areas of the midwest, and the combination of the opiate pentazocine and the antihistamine tripelennamine (T's and Blues) was used by many who could not obtain their regular heroin. The combination of heroin and cocaine (speedball) has a reputation for being especially pleasant, and it has been reported that the pleasure of a cocaine "high" can be enhanced by drinking alcohol. This practice of combining drugs from different pharmacologic classes can make diagnosis of a drug overdose or a drug withdrawal syndrome especially difficult.

Working Definitions

Substance misuse and abuse, and such related terms as addiction, can be defined in several ways. Each definition has been hotly argued by a particular group of professionals or lay persons. The definitions of the common terms, and the substances that they encompass, change from time to time as mores, laws, and scientific data change. The applicability of a particular term such as *misuse* or *abuse* often depends on the setting in which the agent is being used. In other cases, the applicability of a term is more clear-cut. However, for most drugs—all except those for which there is no legally or medically recognized use—a spectrum exists ranging from proper use, through misuse, to abuse and addiction. (This does not mean that all, or even most, drug abuse starts with proper use of a drug. It has become recognized that drug abuse rarely begins with an appropriate prescription by a physician.) Between the extremes, it may be difficult to place a person in any one stage. Thus, the following sections provide working definitions or descriptions rather than formal definitions.

Valid Medical and Social (Recreational) Uses

Alcohol is an example of a drug with few medical uses. Alcohol is rarely prescribed medically for its diverse CNS effects, including relief of anxiety, tension, or facilitation of social interactions. Obviously, however, the drug is routinely purchased and consumed by persons legally allowed to do so. With moderate levels of consumption, recreational alcohol use in a social setting is both legal and generally held to be acceptable. That is, this pattern of use is not considered by most persons to constitute misuse.

Misuse

Misuse can be considered to have developed when there is more frequent use of a licit substance or when use of a licit substance puts the user or others at risk (as from driving while intoxicated). Using this definition, any use of tobacco would be considered misuse, since there is a health risk associated with even moderate use of tobacco. Examples of less obvious instances of drug misuse are when a person gives his or her prescription drug to friends because they "have the same problem;" or when, for a brief period of time, a person takes more of a prescribed medicine than instructed. Of course, even first-time or very infrequent use of illicit substances constitutes misuse of these drugs.

Chronic Abuse and Dependence

Chronic abuse can be considered to have occurred when the tasks of locating and taking the drug become preoccupations of the users, who are uncomfortable if they do not have their next dose conveniently at hand. Generally accepted social and economic interactions may be sacrificed for the user to obtain and take his or her drug, and drug use often continues with little regard for its potential social, medical, financial, and legal consequences.

The term *dependence* is a confusing one since it is applied to two very different processes. It refers to psychologic dependence, the condition of abuse described above where the drug has taken control of much of the user's behavior. Psychologic dependence is manifested by inappropriate drug-taking behavior. Dependence also refers to *physical* dependence, which is simply a pharmacologic result of frequent, long-term administration of any one of many drugs, only some of which are drugs of abuse. Physical dependence is easy to define since it is acknowledged to occur if, when a person suddenly stops taking a drug, a time-limited withdrawal syndrome develops. The nature of the withdrawal syndrome is specific to a particular drug class (ethanol withdrawal is much different from opioid withdrawal, for example), and it can be blocked by readministration of the drug or by administration of other drugs of that class.

An interaction between psychologic dependence and physical dependence has been suggested for decades, but few studies have attempted to clarify this interaction. Theoretically, since drug administration reverses withdrawal signs, and since withdrawal from most drugs of abuse appears to be aversive, it would seem that drug taking would have increased appeal when withdrawal signs are occurring (ie, psychologic dependence on a drug increases as physical dependence develops). The behavior of heroin addicts suggests that this is the case for these individuals. It is less clearly the case for people who abuse large amounts of alcohol or cocaine. These people take the drugs in cyclic patterns—periods of high intake are followed by periods of reduced or no intake. Frequently, withdrawal signs develop during the periods of reduced intake, but are not necessarily associated with increases in administration of these drugs.

Patients who receive large doses of dependence-producing drugs such as morphine or diazepam for relatively long periods of time to treat an underlying problem are likely to develop physical dependence on their medication. This physical dependence does not mean that psychologic dependence has developed as well. In most cases, the withdrawal signs that follow termination of long-term administration of these drugs can be attenuated by a gradual withdrawal of the medication.

The next section summarizes common drugs and drug groups that are abused. Since most of them have been discussed in other chapters, the reader is referred to the appropriate sections for more details about their actions. The information presented below is summarized in Table 28–1. Slang terms for many of the agents are listed in Table 28–2.

Drugs Affecting Mainly the Brain

Central Nervous System Depressants

As a group, the general CNS depressants are widely abused and cause both physical and psychologic dependence, as well as varying degrees of tolerance.

Alcohol

Of all the CNS depressants, alcohol is the most widely abused substance. Alcoholism or lesser degrees of problem drinking directly affect about 15 million people in the United States (estimates and criteria vary), each of whom affects the lives of many more people. There appear to be both genetic and other types of familial links to alcoholism, such that the risks increase in children of persons with the disease. Alcohol is the major cause of fatal motor vehicle accidents, and is a major cause or accompaniment of many illnesses resulting in significant morbidity (including fetal alcohol syndrome, an untoward effect on a "passive user"), hospitalizations, and mortality. It is also a significant economic burden on society.

Alcohol, barbiturate, and benzodiazepine abuse can result in development of physical dependence. The pattern of alcohol withdrawal over time is fairly constant, starting with tremors of the extremities and profuse sweating, and progressing to hallucinosis or "seeing things." The next stage is frank convulsions followed by delirium tremens (DTs), in which the person is delirious, extremely agitated, and at risk of dying from cardiovascular collapse. Of course, not all alcoholics who begin to show tremors and sweating are bound to progress to DTs and death. The severity of withdrawal depends on several factors, the most important of which are the amount of alcohol that has been consumed, the rate of consumption, and the period of time over which drinking has been heavy. Any stage of alcohol withdrawal except delirium tremens can be reversed by appropriate medication. Diazepam is commonly found to be extremely successful in attenuating alcohol withdrawal signs and calming the patient.

Treatment of alcoholism is difficult, as is treatment of drug abuse in general. Peer-support groups such as Alcoholics Anonymous have been quite successful in maintaining abstinence in recovering alcoholics. Disulfiram (ANTABUSE; Chapter 22) can be helpful in preventing alcohol consumption in the highly motivated individual.

Barbiturates and Benzodiazepines

The abuse-related aspects of barbiturates are generally similar to those noted for alcohol, as are those for barbiturate alternatives such as chloral hydrate, glutethimide, and meprobamate. Methaqualone (better known on the street as "ludes"), which was formerly available as a prescription CNS depressant and an alternative to barbiturates for some indications, has been withdrawn from the market because of its exceptionally high abuse potential. The CNS depressants are usually abused by the oral route, but some persons use parenteral routes. Barbiturates and benzodiazepines are usually abused in combination with other drugs, particularly alcohol, codeine ("Loads"), or methadone.

As noted in Chapter 22, benzodiazepines are the preferred prescription alternatives to barbiturates and related drugs for anxiety or insomnia. They are subject to abuse by individuals who have demonstrated an addictive disorder, but, with the exception of methadone-maintenance patients, who seem to have particular fondness for diazepam, most sedative abusers prefer barbiturates to benzodiazepines.

Opiates

The opiates—heroin, morphine, and related narcotics—are CNS depressants with additional actions in the brain. They cause both physical and psychologic dependence. As noted in Chapter 21, tolerance develops to many, but not all, of their diverse effects throughout the body. The preferred route of administration varies with the abuser and the availability of means to administer the drug. Many abusers prefer to inject opiates intravenously ("mainlining"), whereas others use subcutaneous injections ("skin popping") or ingest or smoke the drug, depending on the drug and the administration devices available. Parenteral narcotic abuse is a major cause of infectious disease transmission, and is also the major cause of fatal drug overdoses. Unlike the situation with alcohol or barbiturates, uncontrolled withdrawal

Table 28–1 Overview of Commonly Abused Substances

Drug or Drug Group	Tolerance	Dependence Psychologic	Dependence Physical	Comments and Nursing Implications
CNS Depressants				
Alcohol, barbiturates, related general CNS depressants (see Chapter 22)	Yes	Yes	Yes	Margin of safety narrows with habitual use, despite development of tolerance to many other effects, increasing risk of fatal overdoses: respiratory depression, asphyxia, cardiovascular collapse; uncontrolled withdrawal may be fatal, should be done gradually; anticipate nutritional deficits with long-term abusers, anticipate, assess for, cyclic use with CNS stimulants; disulfiram (ANTABUSE), available to curb alcohol abuse, is associated with medical risks from willful or accidental alcohol absorption, must be used voluntarily with close medical supervision, counseling; no known antidotes for overdose management
Benzodiazepines (see Chapter 22)	Yes	Yes	Yes	Safer for therapeutic use than barbiturates or related drugs; assumption of greater safety than alternatives may increase risk of inappropriate seeking, prescribing; risk of rebound anxiety upon withdrawal from long-term use; antidote for overdoses recenailable (flumazenil)
Opiates (see Chapter 21)	Yes	Yes	Yes	Usually abused by parenteral route, increasing risk of disease transmission through injection, blood transfusions, intercourse; popular with both medical professionals and street abusers; respiratory depression, cardiovascular collapse are usual consequences of acute overdoses; pinpoint pupils (miosis) usually accompany other signs, symptoms, in habitual users or overdose victims; ventilatory support is primary therapy for overdoses, may be assisted by use of parenteral narcotic antagonist (naloxone); oral narcotic antagonist (naltrexone) available for prevention of readdiction with supervised program of counseling for willing patients; uncontrolled withdrawal is unpleasant, not fatal
CNS Stimulants, Psychotomimetics				
Amphetemines, related CNS stimulants (methylphenidate, others; see Chapters 14, 27)	Yes	Yes	Possible	Untoward responses with either acute or habitual use reflect both CNS and peripheral (sympathomimetic) effects; tolerance develops to most effects but not to incidence of amphetamine-induced psychosis; anticipate, be prepared to treat, excessive CNS and cardiovascular stimulation during overdoses, including paranoia, aggression, psychotic manifestations, seizures, hypertension, stroke, arrhythmias; no antidote known; urinary acidification may help increase renal drug excretion; anticipate potential need to restrain patient, provide monitoring, treatment, in environment that provides minimal sensory input to patient; antipsychotic drugs, anticonvulsants, may be needed

(continued)

Table 28–1 Overview of Commonly Abused Substances (*Continued*)

Drug or Drug Group	Tolerance	Dependence Psychologic	Dependence Physical	Comments and Nursing Implications
CNS Stimulants, Psychotomimetics				
Caffeine	Yes	Yes	Slight	A common substance of abuse in many societies through intake of caffeine-containing beverages (coffee, colas, etc); abuse syndrome (caffeinism) recognized as behavioral disorder, best detected by assessing daily intake, monitoring withdrawal signs and symptoms (anxiety, irritability, etc; see Chapter 27); moderate intake safe, acceptable for most persons except those with contraindicating medical conditions such as peptic ulcer disease, seizure history, etc.
Cocaine, crack (see Chapters 14, 27)	Yes	Yes	Possible	Intense and almost immediate sympathomimetic (especially cardiovascular) and CNS-stimulating effects, the latter of which hasten prompt development of psychologic dependence; habitual cocaine use is the rule, not the exception, for most abusers; chronic abuse associated with dramatic behavioral changes; acute effects often are amphetamine-like, but may include abruptly fatal cardiovascular effects (stroke, arrhythmias), even with initial use, especially with inhaled crack; assess for nasal mucosal necrosis, other pathology such as rhinitis, with habitual users; be prepared to deal with psychotic responses with overdoses, other unusually heightened responses; crack abuse becoming epidemic because of widespread availability, initial low cost
Cannabinoids (hashish, marijuana; see Chapters 21, 42)	?	Yes	No	Abuse common in both youths and adults; no medically significant acute toxicity other than caused by behavioral changes are known; anticipate ataxia, illusions, hallucinations, other behavioral abnormalities, physical signs such as conjunctivitis, respiratory tract irritation, with acute use (usually by inhalation)
Hallucinogens (LSD, phencyclidine [PCP], dimethyltryptamine [DMT], mescaline, peyote, psilocybin, others)	?	Potential	No	Psychologic effects may be intense, rapid in onset, far outweighing physiologic effects; hallucinations, synthesesia, paranoia, delusions of grandeur, other psychotic manifestations are common; intoxicated individual often preoccupied with self; deaths are uncommon, but usually caused by behaviorally motivated factors (trying to fly off buildings, etc); flashbacks (hallucinations, dysphoria, etc) may occur weeks to months after discontinuation of hallucinogen use, particularly with LSD; great risk of neurotoxicity with contaminants in "designer drugs" (eg, MPTP, a parkinsonism-causing agent in some street drugs, including psychotomimetics, some narcotics)

(continued)

Table 28–1 Overview of Commonly Abused Substances (*Continued*)

Drug or Drug Group	Tolerance	Dependence Psychologic	Dependence Physical	Comments and Nursing Implications
CNS Stimulants, Psychotomimetics				
Tobacco (nicotine; see Chapter 16)	Yes	Yes	Probably	Use always constitutes misuse, despite perception of being acceptable recreational drug; bronchitis nearly inseparable from smoking; evidence of long-term adverse effects on nearby nonsmokers through "passive" smoke inhalation; long-term health risks such as pulmonary and cardiovascular disease, cancer, with incidence increasing with duration, amount, of smoking, age; tobacco use in form of cigarette smoking thought to be addictive; nicotine gum, transdermal patches available as adjunct to curb smoking habit
Inhalants (chloroform, ether; gasoline, lacquer, paint thinner, other petroleum distillates; carbon tetrachloride, toluene [glue]; others)	?	Yes	No	Method of administration (inhalation on gauze, in cans or bags) increases risk of hypoxia, overdose; overdoses may present in various ways, including CNS depression or stimulation, unstable cardiac, respiratory status; acute or permanent brain damage may arise; other concerns include myocardial sensitization or depression, sudden death; long-term use may be associated with brain, heart, liver damage, cancers; are popular substances of abuse in youths, persons with occupational exposure to these agents; nonfatal overdoses may present with psychic disturbances (see amphetamines), cardiovascular or pulmonary instability; no antidotes
Anabolic Steroids				
	Unknown	?	No	Most prevalent with athletes; administration usually causes desired anabolic effects, but at risk of personality disorders, male impotence, fatal liver disease; acute toxicity uncommon

from narcotics is rarely fatal. The phenomena of cross-tolerance and cross-dependence apply to the narcotics, which explains why a person who is addicted to heroin, for example, can avoid withdrawal by using sufficient doses of another narcotic such as morphine or methadone. There is no cross-tolerance or -dependence between narcotics, barbiturates, or other drug classes.

The opiates are noteworthy because they are the only group of widely abused drugs for which there is a specific antidote for management of acute overdoses (naloxone), and another that can be used on a long-term basis for prevention of readdiction (naltrexone). Methadone can also be substituted for other narcotics in maintenance or withdrawal treatments. It is used because its long duration of action provides a more prolonged but milder withdrawal syndrome when it is eventually discontinued under supervision.

Central Nervous System Stimulants

Amphetamines

Amphetamines (Chapter 27) exert powerful cerebral cortical stimulating actions and have great abuse potential. These drugs engender psychologic dependence, often soon after administration starts. Tolerance develops to most of their CNS-stimulating actions, but not to their ability to induce psychosis. This probably helps explain why psychotic behavior is a common presenting sign in persons who have taken large doses for several days. The degree of physical dependence caused by habitual amphetamine abuse is controversial. Clearly, profound CNS depression may occur on discontinuation of these drugs, but it is not clear whether this can be classified as a true, multifaceted withdrawal syndrome.

Table 28–2 Common Slang Terms for Abused Substances*

	CNS Depressants ("downers")
Barbiturates	barbs
Amobarbital	blue angels, blue birds, blue devils, blue heaven
Pentobarbital	dolls, goof balls, nimbies, yellow jackets
Secobarbital	reds, red birds, red devils, seccies, seggy
Methaqualone	love drug, lude(s), mandrake, soap, soapers (sopors)
	Opiates
Codeine	junk, schoolboy
Heroin	boy, dope, H, hard stuff, horse, joy, junk, lady Jane, Mexican mud, shit, skag, smack, stuff
Hydromorphone	D, lords
Methadone	dollies, dolls, 10-8-20
Morphine	dreamer, M, Miss Emma, monkey, morf, unkie, white stuff
	Cannabinoids
Hashish or marijuana	Acapulco gold, aunt Mary, bhang, blondie, bo, bobo, dagga, ding, doobies, dope, grass, hash, hay, hemp, J, joints, love, Mary Jane, pot, reefer, rick sticks, roach rope, stuff, tea, TJ, weed, wheat, yerba
	CNS Stimulants ("uppers")
Amphetamines	general terms: pep pills, speed, uppers, wake-ups
Amphetamine	bennies, cart wheels, football, hearts, peaches, pep pills, roses, uppers, wake-ups
Dextroamphetamine	Christmas trees, dexies, hearts, oranges
Methamphetamine	meth
Cocaine	C, coke, crack, dust, flake, gold dust, happy dust, stardust, toot
	Psychotomimetics
Dimethoxymethylamphetamine	businessman's special, DOM, STP
Lysergic acid diethylamide	acid, blue acid, hawk, heavenly blue, instant Zen, LSD, pearly gates, sugar cubes, trip, 25
Mescaline	bad seed, big chief, buttontops, cactus, half moon, mesc, mescal beans, moon, P, tops
Methylenedioxyamphetamine	love pill, MDA
Phencyclidine	angel dust, hog, PCP, peace, peace pill
Psilocybin	Mexican magic mushroom

*There are local preferences for terms, and some overlap, with a particular term being applied to different agents within a given pharmacologic class or group.

Although amphetamines are still abused, mainly by the oral route, the relative incidence has declined. Recognizing their high abuse potential, physicians have become very reluctant to prescribe amphetamines. Moreover, some locales have passed laws to restrict amphetamine prescriptions, even for the few valid medical indications. This has greatly curtailed the abuse of amphetamines obtained from licit sources. A second major reason for the decline is the increasing availability and desirability of cocaine, especially in the form of crack.

Cocaine

As with amphetamines, cocaine dependence is largely psychologic. Cocaine's onset of action is very rapid: within seconds when cocaine base is smoked, within minutes when cocaine salt is snorted. This rapid action contributes to its abuse potential. In recent history cocaine was quite expensive, and cocaine abuse was mainly associated with persons who were relatively well-off financially. Inhaling (snorting) cocaine dust, the primary route of administration, became a status symbol for a selected subpopulation. Overall, the incidence of cocaine abuse was *relatively* low until several years ago. However, a simple chemical modification of cocaine has led to the use of crack, or rock cocaine, a cheap form that, when smoked, causes an intense euphoric response that quickly and insidiously fosters development of psychologic dependence. The initial low cost of crack, the unfortunate ease of purchasing it, and the intense behavioral effects induced by it have made this substance a major drug abuse problem among people of all social classes.

The most innocent sufferers of crack addiction are babies born of mothers who used crack throughout their pregnancy. These babies are usually born prematurely, have low birth weight, a smaller head circumference, and are hyperirritable. They may require intensive neonatal care. They may also suffer developmental problems such as ADHD (see Chapter 27) that will make it more difficult for them to compete in school and throughout their lives.

Like amphetamine, cocaine is usually administered in an episodic pattern by individuals who abuse the drug on a chronic basis. During a "run" of cocaine use, the abuser may smoke or inject cocaine every hour or less throughout the day for several days. During that period, the abuser will do little else besides administer the drug. He or she will get almost no sleep and will eat little or nothing. After the run, the abuser "crashes," stops taking the drug, sleeps for 18 or more hours per day, and eats large amounts of food. He or she may also show signs of depression, which may be followed by a bout of cocaine use if the resources are available to obtain the drug.

Overall, the number of hospitalizations and sudden deaths caused by cocaine and crack has grown immensely, mainly in large urban areas but in other settings as well. Most of these deaths are believed to be caused by sudden and fatal cardiac arrhythmias that probably reflect the sympathomimetic effects of cocaine and crack.

Caffeine

Frequent ingestion of this legal CNS-stimulating substance, in the form of beverages such as coffee, tea, or soft drinks, clearly causes physiologic and psychologic dependence. The patterns of caffeine intake could properly be classified as misuse and habitual abuse. The recognized syndrome, *caffeinism,* leads to withdrawal symptoms on abrupt discontinuation by a caffeine-tolerant individual. Although caffeine intake should be avoided or curtailed by persons with certain medical disorders, for most persons there is little concern over low to moderate daily intake of this substance. More details about caffeine's actions and abuse are presented in Chapter 27.

Tobacco

Tobacco smoking is one of the most common forms of substance abuse, and is associated with habituation, dependence (mainly psychologic, but a mild withdrawal syndrome that suggests physiologic dependence can be demonstrated), and both immediate and long-term adverse health consequences. The various problems associated with smoking arise not only from the nicotine that is inhaled, but also from the inhalation of other organic substances (tars) and smoke particles. As discussed in Chapter 16, nicotine is a ganglionic stimulant and blocker that causes a host of untoward autonomic effects, particularly on the cardiovascular system. Tars are recognized carcinogens, at least with long-term or high-dose exposure, and inhalation of smoke is always associated with pulmonary inflammation and its consequence, bronchitis. Smoking is associated with an increased risk of cardiovascular and pulmonary disease, cancer, vitamin and mineral deficiencies, and such other consequences as ulcerogenesis. For the user, untoward effects of smoking increase with the amount of tobacco smoked each day, the duration of the smoking habit, age, and the presence of other risk factors, especially those involving cardiovascular disease. Cigarette smoking is rightly cited as the major risk factor, but pipe and cigar smoking, and the use of chewing tobacco, also constitute risks. With these latter forms of abuse, the incidence of oral cancer may be higher than with cigarette smoking. There is growing evidence that smoke inhalation through "passive smoking"—the inhalation by nonsmokers of environmental tobacco smoke—is not only unpleasant but also unhealthy. This has led to a ban on smoking in many public places.

The growing and justified fears over the adverse health effects of smoking, the restrictions on the ability to smoke, and the increasing feeling that smoking is no longer "trendy," have fostered the demand for aids, drugs, or other easy ways to quit smoking. The free enterprise system has responded with mass marketing of such aids, some of which have been touted as cure-alls, and few of which have proven efficacy. Currently, nicotine gum and nicotine-containing transdermal patches are approved for use to help persons quit cigarette smoking (see Chapter 16).

Cannabis

Marijuana contains the active substance delta-9-tetrahydrocannabinol (THC). Obtained mainly from the leaves and stems of the plant *Cannabis sativa,* most marijuana purchased on the street contains only about 25% to 30% of the amount of THC found in hashish, an oily substance derived from *Cannabis* resins. Marijuana is often the first illicit substance tried by school-aged children; it is the most widely used illicit agent, and it ranks only behind alcohol, tobacco, and caffeine in overall abuse frequency. Among the reasons for marijuana's popularity include its relatively low cost and the ease with which it can be grown and purchased; its known or alleged psychologic effects, including euphoria, and alterations in the senses (particularly sight and sound, which is one reason why some texts classify cannabinoids as psychotomimetics, as discussed later); enhanced creativity and sexual arousal; the ease of getting high by smoking the drug; and the relatively lesser social stigmas associated with it, compared with those associated with other illegal drugs. (In some cities in the United States possession of small amounts of marijuana is considered a misdemeanor, and offenders are given tickets much like those for motor vehicle offenses or illegal parking, often with lower fines. This is another example of the differing attitudes of what constitutes substance abuse and abused substances, even within a given overall culture.) Although the mechanism(s) of action of THC differ from those of alcohol, the behavioral impairments that occur when a person is under its influence are somewhat similar.

The use of THC is associated with mild to strong psychologic dependence. The degree of dependence depends on whether the THC is administered in the form of marijuana or hashish, and the amount and frequency of administration. There is little evidence of tolerance or physical dependence in humans. However, evidence does suggest that people who abuse "hard" drugs began their illicit drug use with marijuana. This does not mean that everyone who uses marijuana will necessarily proceed to use heroin, cocaine, or amphetamines. As with tobacco smoking, the risk of pulmonary damage is definite. It is caused not only by the active drug and smoke particles, but also by contaminants such as the insecticide paraquat, which is frequently used by law enforcement agencies in attempts to kill cannabis crops.

Psychotomimetics

Psychotomimetics are drugs that, at usual doses, alter cognition, the psyche, and sensory processes, without having marked effects on other aspects of brain function, motor function, or peripheral structures. Often their major affects are *illusions*—a distortion of one or more of the special senses (sight, hearing, taste, touch, smell)—as they respond to sensory input from the environment. Some of these agents cause *synthesesia,* in which a person may report that they can feel sounds or hear colors, for example. In other cases, the drugs will cause *hallucinations,* which can be defined as sensations for which there is no true external basis (for example, certain noises are sensed in a room that is absolutely noise-free). The overall consequence of the substance's effects may evoke many or all of the symptoms of psychosis, including aggression, depersonalized behavior, flights of grandeur, paranoia, and very labile behavior, depending on the abuser's individual response to it.

The best example of a psychotomimetic agent is lysergic acid diethylamide (LSD), which is chemically related to the ergot alkaloids. It is not known exactly how LSD acts, but evidence suggests that it acts like the neurotransmitter serotonin in certain brain pathways. The drug has been used experimentally for this purpose to probe brain neurochemical mechanisms. Much less popular than it was in the 1960s, LSD is the most potent psychotomimetic agent and is still used occasionally for its anticipated sensory-altering effects. Often, however, it causes dysphoric responses ("bad trips"). The acute physiologic effects of LSD are not dangerous. However, dysphoria and psychotic manifestations have led to deaths, mainly when the intoxicated person feels he or she can perform tasks beyond human capabilities—flying off a building or stopping a speeding locomotive, for example. LSD, and perhaps some other psychotomimetics, can cause "flashbacks." These are episodes of hallucinations, acute anxiety or panic attacks, and other dysphoric responses that may occur unexpectedly, weeks or even months after administration of the substance has stopped.

Most texts also include the amphetamine-like drugs dimethyltryptamine (DMT), dimethoxymethylamphetamine (DOM, STP), and methylenedioxyamphetamine (MDA) in the psychotomimetic drug category. They are synthetic agents, mainly synthesized in illegal laboratories specifically for sale as substances of abuse. These "designer drugs," plus others that are synthesized in illicit labs, often contain contaminants that can have devastating psychologic and physical consequences. As noted in Chapter 25, one of these contaminants is MPTP, a neurotoxin that can cause virtually immediate and permanent manifestations of parkinsonism.

Phencyclidine (PCP) is another psychotomimetic that is abused occasionally. Originally developed for special general anesthetic techniques, human use was quickly discontinued when the high incidence of post-anesthetic delirium was realized. The related drug ketamine is an approved anesthetic for human use (see Chapter 20). Phencyclidine is mainly smoked, but is also abused by oral, IV, and inhalation (snorting) routes.

Mescaline and psilocybin are natural psychotomimetic agents that exert effects overtly similar to those of LSD. Mescaline is an alkaloid extracted from the peyote cactus, which is found in northern Mexico and the southwestern regions of the United States, and has been used for religious purposes by certain groups of Indians living in those areas. Peyote refers to the dried cactus buttons, which are smoked; mescaline is the active ingredient in this substance. Psilocybin is a substance found in some mushrooms grown in the same region.

Miscellaneous Inhalants

A variety of volatile substances are inhaled for their mind-altering effects. With the exception of ether and nitrous oxide, none of these agents have been used therapeutically for their effects on the brain. Other abused inhalants include gasoline and other petroleum products (called petroleum distillates), toluene (abused mainly in the form of plastic glues), lacquer or paint thinner, trichloroethylene (often used as a degreasing agent in metal finishing), carbon tetrachloride (a common dry-cleaning agent), chloroform, freons (widely used as a refrigerant for air conditioners and freezers), and fluorocarbons (which are still used to pressurize some spray cans containing many commercial products).

The pattern of abuse of these substances indicates mainly psychologic dependence, with little or no evidence of physical dependence. The frequency with which they are abused varies greatly from person to person. All these substances carry the risk of acute toxicity during administration, mainly because of the way in which they are administered. For example, the liquids are often inhaled directly out of metal cans, or applied to gauze or paper and then inserted in a can, plastic, or paper bag. Pressurized devices often are sprayed into similar containers. This maximizes the dose of the inhaled substance (increasing its effect), but also maximizes the accumulated carbon dioxide that is exhaled and minimizes the amount of inhaled oxygen. The consequence can be hypoxia, coma, respiratory arrest, and death. Some of these agents, notably ether, sensitize the heart to the arrhythmogenic effects of catecholamines, leading to fatal arrthythmias. Others, such as trichloroethylene, depress the heart.

Even if the abuser experiences no obvious untoward effects following each abuse episode, the effects of repeated inhalation may be cumulative, leading to permanent dysfunction. There is also evidence of long-term hepatic, renal, and pulmonary toxicity, including cancer, with prolonged abuse of some of these agents.

Anabolic Steroids

Anabolic steroids (see Chapter 48) are steroid hormones with male hormone-like (androgenic) effects but with a relatively greater ability to cause protein formation and to inhibit protein breakdown (anabolic effects). They are abused, but not for their effects on the brain. Valid therapeutic uses of the anabolic steroids include management of anemias, postmenopausal osteoporosis, and promotion of weight gain after major trauma, surgery, or infections. But their ability to increase skeletal muscle mass and the physical performance of those muscles has led to the growing abuse problem, particularly among body builders, weight lifters, and athletes such as football players, in whom size and strength are considered assets. Once confined largely to professional athletes, the problem of anabolic steroid abuse has reached organized college and high school athletic programs as well as individuals wishing such effects. The potential adverse consequences include masculinization and virilization (the desired effect for most of the abusers); personality disorders and aggressiveness; and testicular atrophy, oligospermia, and impotence. The most serious concern is liver damage, which may be irreversible and can include fatal hemorrhagic liver disease or liver cancer.

Nonprescription Drugs

Alcohol, nicotine, and caffeine are the obvious examples of legal nonprescription drugs that are associated with patterns of misuse and abuse, and have the potential to cause acute and long-term adverse effects. However virtually every nonprescription drug, drug product, or drug class that is available has the potential for being misused (see Appendix B for more details).

Unless there is some serious underlying contraindicating disorder, or an interacting drug is being taken, the outcome may be no effect at all, or simply minor side effects. Nonprescription drug misuse by persons who have no other substance abuse problem is usually infrequent, not habitual. However, there are also cases of habitual over-the-counter (OTC) drug abuse, particularly for drugs with CNS effects. These include OTC sedatives (most of which contain an antihistamine) and stimulants (caffeine or sympathomimetics such as phenylpropanolamine), or sometimes both. Habitual use of these drugs need not arise from an original intent to abuse them, or even to take them for their effects on the CNS. For example, most weight-loss aids contain phenylpropanolamine. The original intent for taking the product might be simply to lose weight. However, the increased self-esteem and feeling of more energy caused by the drug's desired effects may perpetuate prolonged and clearly inappropriate use. With caffeine-containing stimulants, the initial desire may be to cram for an exam, get more housework done, and so forth. These are some of the same reasons that start and then perpetuate amphetamine abuse.

Psychologic effects of a drug usually are perceived as the major cause for habitual use, but this is not always the case. Physiologic effects are also important for some OTC drug groups. One good example is the improper use and selection of nasal decongestant sprays or drops. As noted in Chapter 14, initial administration of these drugs tends to cause the desired effect—nasal decongestion. However, when their effects wear off a rebound effect may occur—nasal congestion that may be more severe or annoying than that present before the product was administered. To overcome this, the patient may administer the drug again, perhaps in increasing doses, thus beginning a vicious cycle that is difficult to break. A similar phenomenon applies to drugs that affect bowel motility, as discussed in more detail in Chapter 41. If a person who feels constipated or has other reason to believe a laxative or cathartic drug is needed chooses the wrong drug, or administers an excessive dose, diarrhea may result and the person may then self-administer an antidiarrheal agent. In turn, the antidiarrheal drug may be effective, the patient perceives constipation again, and so administers another dose of a laxative. Another vicious cycle begins. In the case of gastrointestinal drugs, the outcome may be not only habitual use, but also long-term gut damage. One manifestation of this is a loss of spontaneous (physiologic) control over bowel motility, such that continued drug administration is necessary. In the broadest sense, this reflects a form of physical dependence, and it is caused by drugs that have virtually no effect on the brain.

NURSING IMPLICATIONS

All nurses are prepared to manage drug overdose and withdrawal symptoms. However, the treatment of drug abuse is sufficiently difficult that only psychological counselors and physicians and nurses trained to recognize and handle the wide variety of patients with this problem should attempt their comprehensive care. Some of the treatment difficulties include denial (particularly by alcoholic patients and teenage drug abusers), extreme manipulative behavior, and lying about the nature of the drug abuse problem. These behaviors make even the initial step of obtaining a drug history difficult. Drug abusers may admit to their problem and indicate a desire for treatment. They are almost always ambivalent about treatment, however, since it means losing something they are extremely fond of—their drug. Successful treatment of drug abuse is rare, time-intensive, and expensive.

Overdose Emergencies

The overall goal for managing overdoses from commonly abused substances, or in substance abusers, is no different from that which applies to any other acute overdose: save the patient's life, and prevent any morbidity that might occur (for example, brain damage caused by cerebral hypoxia associated with a narcotic overdose). The general treatment approach is outlined in Appendix C; specific interventions are identified in the particular chapters discussing the abused substances.

There are at least two other important considerations to managing overdoses in substance abusers. First, with overdoses of CNS stimulants and psychotomimetics, additional harm to the patient or to caregivers by aggressive, psychotic, or suicidal behavior must be prevented. In many such cases physical restraint is required. Often, monitoring and treatment will need to be done in a setting that reduces as much as possible external stimuli to the patient, but without sacrificing the ability to provide needed care. Second, when the cause of overdose is a substance to which the victim has become physically dependent, the withdrawal syndrome (which is likely to result from administration of the narcotic antagonist naloxone to an overdosed narcotic-dependent person) must be prevented. In either case, the major goal is to provide adequate, safe, life-saving treatment.

Nonemergency Settings

One of nurses' most important functions is to watch and listen to their patients. This function takes on additional importance for hospitalized patients who are long-term users of psychoactive drugs. These patients are not necessarily drug abusers, but they are at risk of developing withdrawal signs if their medication is abruptly terminated upon hospitalization.

Benzodiazepine, barbiturate, or alcohol withdrawal

may be particularly uncomfortable, and possibly life-threatening. The possibility of withdrawal must be considered with a patient who develops tremors, severe anxiety and insomnia, and complains of strange tastes and odors, or shows profound sweating and preconvulsive signs.

Opioid withdrawal takes quite a different course, and will also differ dramatically in patients who have abused opioids as opposed to patients who have used these drugs chronically for pain. The withdrawal signs are the same: sweating, muscle cramps, and gooseflesh, but the verbal behavior may be quite different. Opioid abusers will demand pain medication, and insist that the doses and the time intervals being used are insufficient for the pain they are experiencing. The person who is not an opioid abuser, and who has received an opioid for pain, will not make these demands if he or she is no longer in pain. The dilemma for the nurse is to differentiate the opioid abuser from the patient who is actually in pain. In this case, unless opioid abuse was confirmed upon hospital admission, it is best to assume the pain is genuine, and administer pain medication in sufficient doses to promote pain relief.

Since drug abuse treatment is best accomplished by trained professionals, the nurse can be of assistance by identifying peer support groups, counselors, and other professionals or organizations that will help the patient or client become and remain drug-free, and encourage use of those resources. Substance abuse usually starts when drugs become easy alternatives to other solutions for underlying problems. Explain to substance abusers and those who care for them—both physically and emotionally—that recovery is not easy or achievable without effort, and that there is no magic cure, pharmacologic or otherwise. Use your knowledge of drug effects and substance abuse to educate others to prevent or curtail the abuse problem, and become a role model toward that end.

Impaired Nurses and Other Health-Care Providers

Although estimates vary, about 15% of nurses will abuse one or more of the drugs discussed in this chapter. Of that number, about one in five will develop some form of addiction. The basic causes of the overall abuse problem in health-care providers are generally no different from those that apply to the population at large. However, there are other predisposing factors, including job-related stresses, relatively easy access to drugs (despite measures to hinder access to and improper use of drugs), and even the false assumption that knowing something about a particular drug's actions might help pick one that is "safe" to take.

The personal and private lives of health-care providers should not be judged under a set of rules that differ from those applied to others, unless their actions affect or may affect their ability to render professional services. Such individuals clearly have a legal, professional, and moral obligation to be fully functioning in the professional setting. With nurses and physicians, as with law enforcement officials and firefighters, for example, the risks of substance abuse affect not only abusers and their families, but also many others who rely on their uncompromised skills.

There is an obligation to avoid, prevent, and report abuse of any substance that will interfere with expected responsibilities or will breach the legally defined standards of professional care. Although one goal is to prevent job loss, legal difficulty, or other personal negative outcomes, perhaps the most important goal is to give patients no less than the best care.

SUMMARY OF NURSING IMPLICATIONS

Assessment

Observe for physical and behavioral (verbal and nonverbal) cues that may be consistent with a dependency problem.

Complete a general physical assessment and nutritional history as a basis for treatment and rehabilitation decisions.

Observe for variations in laboratory results, unanticipated responses to drug therapies, and unexplained vital sign changes consistent with abuse problems.

Nursing Diagnoses

Social isolation related to chemical dependency.

High risk for injury related to withdrawal symptoms.

Altered thought processes related to drug effects.

Ineffective individual coping related to inability to manage stressors without drugs.

Planning/Implementation

Monitor for symptoms of withdrawal; report to physician as indicated.

Observe vital signs for indications of cardiac and respiratory depression; check at least four times daily, and more often while awake.

Give medications as ordered to minimize or suppress withdrawal effects (eg, seizures during alcohol withdrawal)

Maintain safe and quiet environment during withdrawal; reduce noise, distracting lights; institute seizure precautions; use measures to promote rest and sleep.

Offer food and fluid as indicated to promote nutrition and minimize adverse withdrawal effects (eg, hypoglycemia during alcohol recovery); record intake and output.

Reassure that symptoms will lessen as drug level diminishes; empathize with difficulty recovering from chemical dependency.

Provide orientation and diversional activities as appropriate during withdrawal.

Refer to community support group depending on type of drug.

◆ Patient and Family Teaching

Teach the patient/family:

Importance of frequent attendance at support group.

Proper use of abuse deterrents (eg, disulfiram with alcohol) and signs of unpleasant effects (intense flushing, nausea, vomiting).

Caution against misuse of drug alternatives (eg, nicotine gum, methadone).

◆ Evaluation

The patient/family will:

Tolerate withdrawal symptoms; vital signs stable; oriented.

Choose to live without drugs; remain drug-free.

Experience positive social interactions; fulfill responsibilities as family member and/or employee.

Identify professional and community resources to assist with effective coping.

Annotated Bibliography

Brewer C. Combining pharmacological antagonists and behavioural psychotherapy in treating addictions: Why it is effective but unpopular. *Br J Psychiatry* 1990;157:34–40. *A thought-provoking discussion of why an effective pharmacologic approach for managing drug abuse (disulfiram for alcohol abuse) is so seldom used, and why misperceptions about this specific intervention can affect acceptance and use of other treatments for other abused substances.*

Cook JS, Fontaine KL. *Essentials of Mental Health Nursing*. 2nd ed. Menlo Park, CA: Addison-Wesley, 1990. *Addresses the generalist's role in dealing with psychosocial problems by focusing on basic concepts of psychiatric nursing, rather than the multitude of theories necessary for assuming a specialist's role. Contains valuable chapters dealing specifically with substance abuse.*

Eells MA. Strategies for promotion of avoiding harmful substances. *Nurs Clin North Am* 1991;26(4):915–927. *The focus of this paper is not on the pharmacology of abused substances, but its content can prove valuable for nurses whose patients are substance abusers who are receiving drug interventions for their chemical dependency.*

Green P. The chemically dependent nurse. *Nurs Clin North Am* 1989;24(1):81–94. *Given the prevalence, importance, and consequences of chemical dependency among nurses (and other health-care providers), this is essential reading. It discusses issues that you will inevitably face in your professional life.*

Guthrie SK. Pharmacologic interventions for the treatment of opioid dependence and withdrawal. *DICP* 1990;24(7–8):721–734. *A useful overview of current management approaches (eg, methadone, naltrexone), plus others that are being studied for their potentially valuable effects.*

Hoegerman G, Schnoll S. Narcotic use in pregnancy. *Clin Perinatol* 1991;18(1):51–76. *Covers important aspects of a persistent problem, and discusses why current approaches to it are often vastly inadequate.*

Julien RM. *A Primer of Drug Action*. 6th ed. New York: W. H. Freeman, 1992. *Aptly described as a "concise, nontechnical guide to the actions, uses, and side effects of psychoactive drugs," this text gives more pharmacologic insight than virtually any other comparable source.*

Lindenberg CS, Alexander EM, Gendrop SC, Nencioli M, Williams DG. A review of the literature on cocaine abuse in pregnancy. *Nurs Res* 1991;40(2):69–75. *Valuable not only for its review of this important topic, but also for its critique of research methods used to obtain the data. Especially worth reading for those interested in nursing research.*

Lynch M, McKeon VA. Cocaine use during pregnancy: Research findings and clinical implications. *J Obstet Gynecol Neonatal Nurs* 1990;19(4):285–292. *Reviews the pharmacologic properties of cocaine and recent clinical research findings on cocaine use during pregnancy; discusses implications for nursing care; and identifies specific nursing interventions.*

McCaffery M, Ferrell B, O'Neil-Page E, Lester M, Ferrell B. Nurses' knowledge of opioid analgesic drugs and psychological dependence. *Cancer Nurs* 1990;13(1):21–27. *Despite a focus on narcotics, this paper demonstrates how the practitioner's lack of knowledge about drug action and use can lead to misconceptions about abuse potentials and proper clinical use.*

Peters H, Theorell CJ. Fetal and neonatal effects of maternal cocaine use. *J Obstet Gynecol Neonatal Nurs* 1991;20(2):121–126. *A concise summary of the trends of cocaine abuse by mothers, and the potential consequences of a too-common problem.*

Ray OS, Ksir, C. *Drugs, Society, and Human Behavior*. 5th ed. St. Louis: Times Mirror/Mosby College Pub., 1990. *The best source for easy-to-read information about historical, cultural, and social foundations of substance abuse, plus insight into actions of the drugs themselves.*

Taft LB, Barkin RL. Drug abuse? Use and misuse of psychotropic drugs in Alzheimer's care. *J Gerontol Nurs* 1990;16(8):4–10. *Addresses one of the most common and blatant forms of iatrogenic misuse of mind-altering drugs. Discusses nursing roles to establish and monitor treatment goals, assess the incidence and severity of side effects, and provide an environment that reduces the need for drug intervention—which can become a form of patient abuse when drugs are used as chemical restraints.*

Tucker C. Acute pain and substance abuse in surgical patients. *J Neurosci Nurs* 1990;22(6):339–349. *Discusses practitioners' knowledge deficits and misconceptions about postoperative pain management; addresses issues especially important when the patient is a substance abuser; and presents three case studies to illustrate key points.*

Wilson HS, Kneisl CR. *Psychiatric Nursing*. 3r ed. Menlo Park, CA: Addison-Wesley, 1991. *Excellent coverage of substance abuse issues from a psychiatric nursing perspective.*

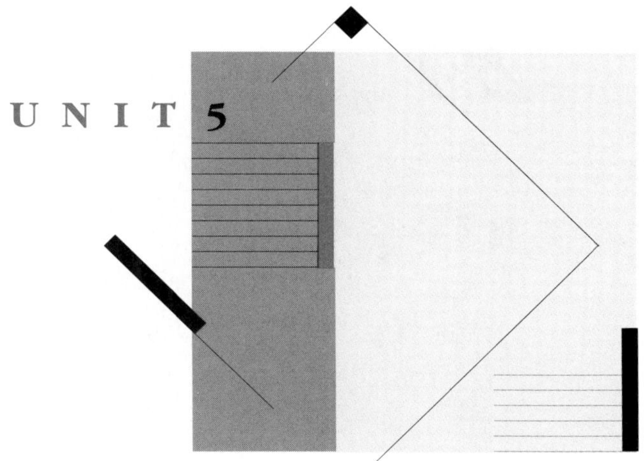

Drugs That Affect the Cardiovascular and Renal System

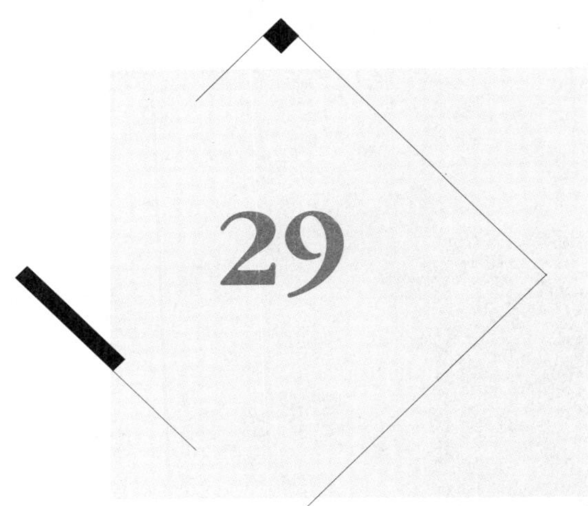

Structure and Function of the Cardiovascular and Renal Systems

The cardiovascular system is typically considered to include the heart and blood vessels, which are responsible for transporting oxygen- and nutrient-rich blood to all cells in the body. The kidneys, often considered merely as organs that rid the body of wastes, also have an essential cardiovascular role by regulating blood composition, volume, and pressure. This chapter reviews the structure, function, and interactions of these three components to provide the basis for understanding the important classes of drugs, discussed in Chapters 30 to 36, that are used to treat the *number one killer* in Western societies—cardiovascular diseases.

The Heart

The heart is a pump that simultaneously serves the pulmonary and systemic circulations. The right side of the heart pumps oxygen-poor venous blood entering its chambers into the pulmonary circulation, where gas exchange occurs. Oxygen-rich arterial blood is returned to the left side of the heart and from there is propelled into the systemic circulation, which serves the body tissues. The anatomic features of the heart are illustrated in Figure 29–1.

Coronary Circulation

The heart muscle itself (the myocardium) must receive an adequate supply of oxygenated blood for the heart to function effectively. The myocardial blood supply is provided by the right and left coronary arteries, which originate at the root of the aorta; the myocardium is drained by a number of cardiac veins that join to form the coronary sinus, the main vein of the heart.

Myocardial **ischemia** occurs when the *supply* of oxygenated blood through the coronary circulation is less than the *demands* of the heart cells for oxygen. The major symptom of cardiac ischemia is the characteristic chest pain of *angina pectoris.* There are two major causes of ischemia: decreased blood supply through the coronary arteries, and increased oxygen demand. Reduced blood supply can occur when arterial pressure, the major force driving blood through the coronary arteries, is reduced, as well as when the coronary arteries are physically obstructed, as by deposits of atherosclerotic plaques or blood cells (thrombi). The major factors leading to ischemia by increasing oxygen demand include increased heart rate and force of contraction, and elevations of blood pressure. Drugs used to treat ischemic heart disease and angina are discussed in Chapter 34.

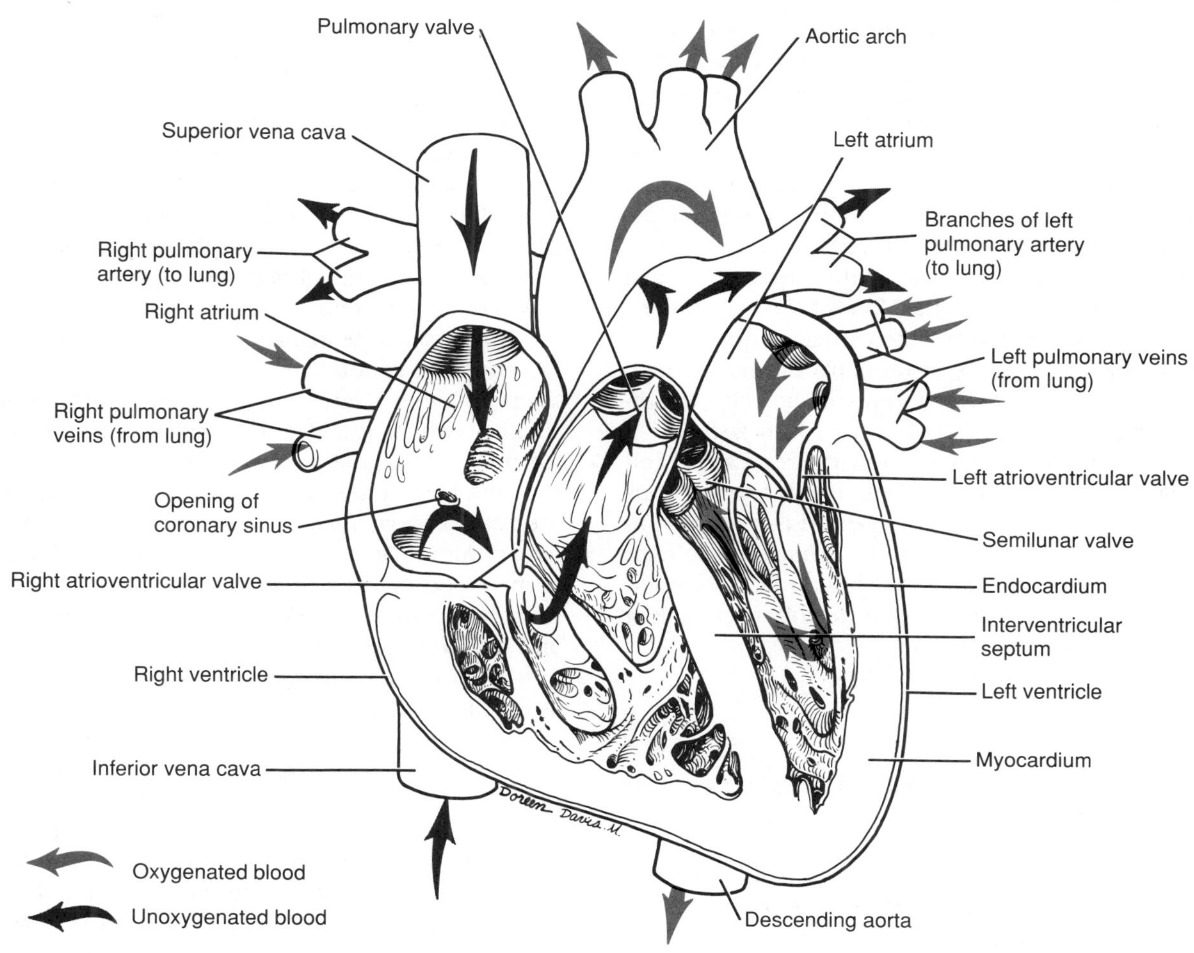

Figure 29–1

Frontal section of the heart. The arrows indicate the path of blood flow through the heart chambers, valves, and major vessels. (*Source:* Adapted from Spence AP, Mason EB. *Human Anatomy and Physiology.* 3rd ed. 1987:533. Menlo Park, CA: Benjamin/Cummings).

Conduction

The ability of cardiac muscle to contract is intrinsic; that is, it is a property of the heart muscle itself and does not depend on external nerve impulses. The impulses that direct the cells of the myocardium to contract come from the nodal and conduction systems of the heart. Before discussing the components of impulse generation and conduction, it is necessary to review the events of cardiac cell contraction.

Events of Myocardial Contraction

Like skeletal muscle, activation of cardiac muscle cells begins with electrical excitation and depolarization of the outer membrane, the sarcolemma. This step, which leads to the generation of an action potential, involves the influx of sodium and calcium ions. Depolarization is linked to actual contraction through a process called *excitation-contraction coupling.* In this process, the small amounts of calcium that enter the cell from outside trigger the release of more calcium from intracellular storage sites, the sarcoplasmic reticulum. The increased intracellular calcium level enables the two major contractile proteins of the myofilaments, actin and myosin, to use chemical energy (derived from the splitting of adenosine triphosphate [ATP]) to slide past one another. This is the actual event of contraction—the essential role of "working" myocardial cells. Any drug that increases the amount of calcium available to the contractile proteins will increase the amount of force or tension the cell can generate; that is, it will produce a positive **inotropic** effect. Such drugs, used mainly to treat chronic or acute depression of cardiac contractile force, include the digitalis glycosides and the catecholamines. They are discussed in Chapter 31.

Once contraction is complete, other processes take over to ready the cell for the next contraction. Calcium is pumped back into storage, thereby stopping the actin–myosin interaction. The cell repolarizes, primarily through activity of an enzyme in the sarcolemma that uses ATP to pump sodium back out of the cell. The action potential generated by one cardiac cell travels directly to adjacent cells by movements of ions through the intercalated disks, which join cardiac cells. Neighboring cells are then activated in an orderly fashion.

During much of repolarization, the myocardial cell is partially or completely resistant, or *refractory,* to further stimulation. This refractory period is critically important because it prevents both premature cellular activation, which could dangerously alter heart rate and rhythm, and sustained contraction (tetanization), which could also be fatal.

The Conduction System

Although the electrical and contractile properties of an individual myocardial cell are important, the most important property is the ability of all cells throughout the heart to contract as a coordinated unit. This is accomplished by the nodal and conduction systems, composed of a relatively small number of cells that are specialized in terms of their electrical activity, rather than their ability to contract. Cells in these systems have, to varying degrees, the following general properties.

1. Automaticity: the ability to initiate their own activity through spontaneous depolarization.
2. Rhythmicity: regularity of depolarization rates.
3. Conduction: the ability to transmit impulses from cell to cell at appropriate rates.
4. Refractoriness: the resistance to premature cell activation.

When any component of this system fails to operate properly, or when other heart cells that normally do not fire spontaneously do so, irregularities of heart rate and rhythm (arrhythmias, or dysrhythmias) occur. Drugs to treat such disturbances, the antiarrhythmic agents, are discussed in Chapter 30.

The components of the nodal and conduction systems are illustrated in Figure 29–2. Their activity can be monitored with an electrocardiogram (ECG; Fig. 29–3), which is a measure of changes in cardiac electrical activity (depolarization and repolarization) detected with electrodes placed on the limbs and chest. In a healthy heart, the size, duration, shape, and timing of the ECG waves tend to be relatively constant. Changes in any of these characteristics, whether caused by normal stress or the adverse effects of drugs or disease, provide extremely useful information about the nature and location of cardiac abnormalities. Overall, the ECG is a sensitive indicator of cardiac function, and provides valuable information about the activity of the heart and its conduction system.

The normal heart beat originates in the sinoatrial (SA) node. It depolarizes spontaneously at a faster rate than any other heart region (usually 60 to 80 times a minute), which allows it to dominate and set the pace for overall heart rate and rhythm (called *normal sinus rhythm*). Heart rates greater than about 100 per minute are generally classified as *tachycardias,* and rates below 60 per minute or so are called *bradycardias.* If only rate is increased or decreased, but the impulses originate normally in the SA node, the terms *sinus tachycardia* and *sinus bradycardia* can be used.

From the SA node, impulses spread through the atrial muscle, causing atrial contraction. This corresponds to the P wave on a typical (Lead II) ECG. Once impulses have passed through the atria they converge on the atrioventricular (AV) node. The AV node is the part of the conduction system with the slowest normal rate of impulse conduction. The brief but important delay it imparts allows the atria to complete their contractions before the ventricles are activated. The time needed for an impulse to pass from the atria to the ventricles, through the AV node, is estimated from the P–R interval on the ECG. Because the AV node normally permits no more than 180 impulses per minute to reach the ventricles, it protects the ventricles from excessively high rates of activation, which would interfere with the effective expulsion of blood and severely jeopardize the entire circulatory system and the organs that it serves.

Impulses leaving the AV node pass quickly through the bundle of His, the bundle branches, and the Purkinje fibers, where they activate the ventricular myocardial cells themselves. Unlike the slow rate of impulse conduction through the AV node, the rate from the bundle of His to the ventricles is rapid. This allows for coordinated and almost simultaneous ventricular activation, needed for a strong, effective pumping action. This phase is seen on the ECG as the QRS complex.

The ability of normal ventricular muscle to originate contractions (automaticity) is not as well developed as it is in the SA node. Ventricular activation depends on the ability of the AV node to deliver activating impulses. If this ability is decreased or abolished, the ventricles become electrically isolated; they then at-

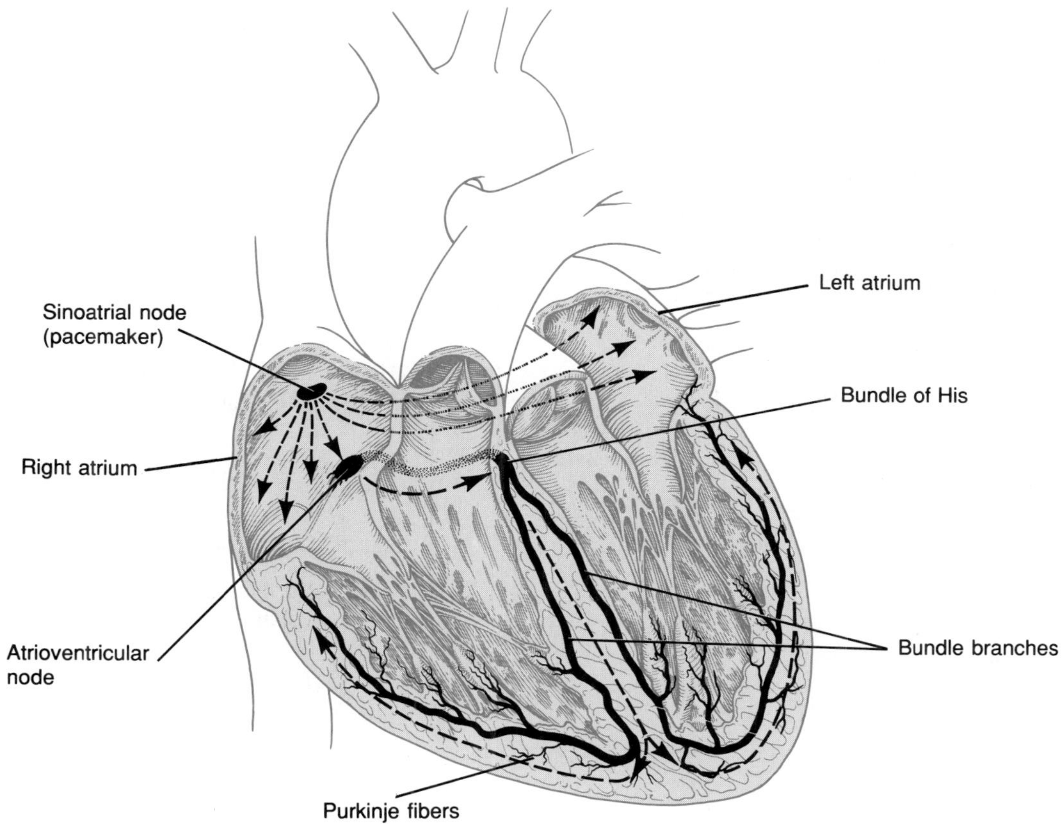

Figure 29–2

The conducting system of the heart. The dashed arrows indicate direction of depolarization from the sinoatrial node through both atria.

(*Source:* Adapted from Spence AP, Mason EB. *Human Anatomy and Physiology.* 3rd ed. 1987:542. Menlo Park, CA: Benjamin/Cummings.)

tempt to beat at their own slower rate. This condition, called *partial* or *complete heart block,* significantly reduces the ventricles' pumping actions.

The degree of partial heart block is expressed in a manner that indicates the number of P waves (or atrial contractions) that occur for each QRS complex (or ventricular contraction) arising from impulse conduction through the AV node. For example, second-degree (2:1) heart block indicates that there are two P waves for every ventricular activation. In complete heart block, no impulses arising in the atria are able to reach and activate the ventricles. If the ventricle gains the ability to generate impulses on its own, blood ejection may occur, although at a level that may not be sufficient to maintain adequate cardiac output. Alternatively, the consequence of complete heart block may be cardiac arrest. In any case, pharmaco-logic intervention or electrical pacing often is required.

The synchronous activity of the normal heart beat depends on spontaneous depolarization of the SA node and sequential triggering of other structures through the conduction of impulses along specific pathways. However, if abnormal conditions occur (as from myocardial ischemia, certain drugs, or excessive nerve influences), any region of the heart may begin firing on its own, serving as an independent, or **ectopic,** pacemaker. The heart beat becomes unsynchronized and often chaotic, leading to serious or fatal arrhythmias. The same abnormal conditions may allow impulses to travel in the wrong direction, prematurely stimulating heart regions at a time when they are supposed to be quiescent.

Autonomic Nervous System Influences

Extrinsic neural influences are not essential for heart function at rest. However, the autonomic nervous system plays an important part in enabling the heart to

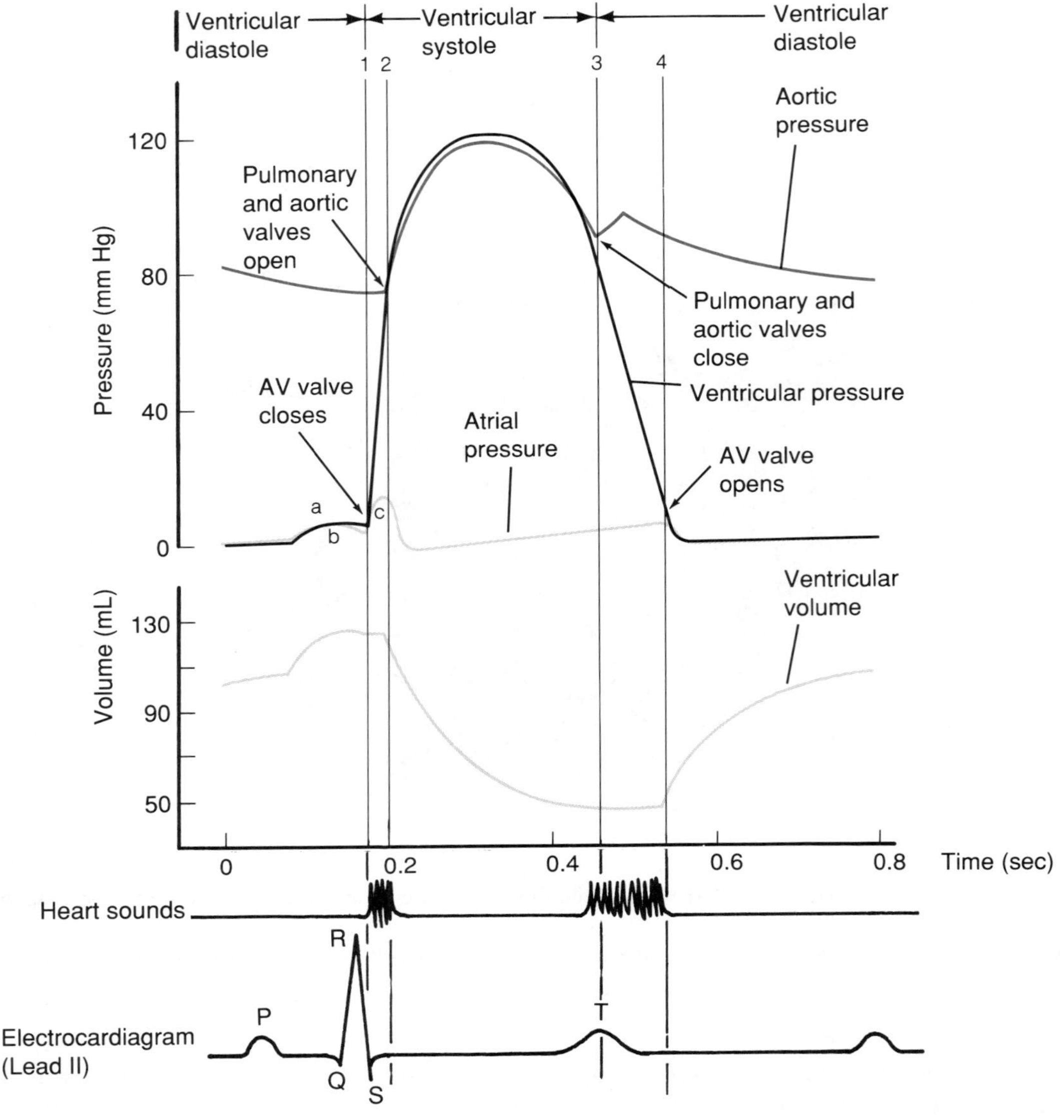

Figure 29–3

The cardiac cycle. Figure shows temporal relationships between atrial, ventricular, and aortic pressures; volume of the left ventricle as it fills and then expels blood; heart sounds; and the electrocardiogram. In this figure one cardiac cycle lasts about 800 milliseconds (0.8 sec), which corresponds to a heart rate of 75 beats per minute.

(*Source:* Adapted from Spence AP, Mason EB. *Human Anatomy and Physiology,* 3rd ed. 1987:544. Menlo Park, CA: Benjamin/Cummings.)

adapt to changing demands by regulating the electrical properties that determine rate and rhythm, and other properties affecting contractile force. Normally, the cardiac-owing effects of acetylcholine (ACh), released at the SA node by the parasympathetic nervous system, exert much greater control over resting heart rate than the opposing cardiac-accelerating influences of norepinephrine released from sympathetic nerves. Parasympathetic nerves also slow the rate of impulse conduction through the AV node. They do not innervate the ventricles, and so have no important role in regulating the force of ventricular contraction.

When stresses are imposed, parasympathetic influences decrease and sympathetic stimulation increases; heart rate rises. In addition, since sympathetic nerves also innervate the ventricular muscle, ventricular contractile force increases significantly.

The Cardiac Cycle

The cardiac cycle is equivalent to one complete heart beat, during which the two atria contract simultaneously and, as they begin to relax, the ventricles contract and then relax. The terms *systole* and *diastole* generally refer to ventricular contraction and relaxation, respectively.

Figure 29–3 illustrates the events of the cardiac cycle for the left side of the heart. The lengths of the total cardiac cycle and its individual phases are based on an average heart rate of 75 beats per minute. If the heart rate is accelerated, these periods are shortened proportionately.

The cardiac cycle can be divided into five major phases.

1. *Late diastole* is the period of atrial contraction. During this period the depolarization wave travels through the atria, causing contraction and a rise in atrial pressure, and facilitating movement of blood into the ventricles.
2. *Early systole,* the onset of ventricular contraction, begins as the depolarization wave spreads from the AV node through the ventricles. Although the ventricles are contracting, the closure of all valves prevents blood from being ejected, so this phase is also called the phase of isovolumetric contraction.
3. *Late systole* (ventricular ejection) is the time during which intraventricular pressures exceed those of the aorta and pulmonary artery. The semilunar valves are forced open and blood is expelled from the ventricles. Aortic pressure reaches its highest value during this period.
4. *Early diastole* (the rapid filling stage) occurs when the repolarization wave passes over the ventricles and the ventricles relax.
5. *Mid-diastole* (phase of slow ventricular filling) is the phase in which the heart is completely relaxed and internal pressure is low. Blood passively flows into the atria and through them into the ventricles below; the semilunar valves are closed. Approximately 80% of ventricular filling occurs during this interval. This period is followed by late diastole and the cycle begins again.

Cardiac Output, Reserve, and Failure

Cardiac Output

Cardiac output—the amount of blood ejected by the ventricles in 1 minute—is probably the best measure of how well the heart meets its obligations to provide an adequate blood supply to the body. Although the outputs of the right and left sides of the heart are equal over time, cardiac output and the factors that determine it generally refer to the main pump, the left ventricle.

Cardiac output is calculated by multiplying heart rate by stroke volume, which is the amount of blood ejected by the ventricle with each contraction. Stroke volume reflects the force or intensity of ventricular contraction. The normal resting cardiac output is about 5 liters (70 beats/min × the normal stroke volume, 70 mL = 4.9 liters). Normal cardiac output is maintained through the heart's rate–stroke volume interaction, with each factor changing (often in opposite directions) as necessary. If heart rate falls, for example, stroke volume tends to increase because the heart has more time to fill during diastole, providing more volume to be ejected with the next systole. When heart rate increases, diastolic filling time decreases, and stroke volume falls. Stress, drugs, and disease are a few of the important factors that change cardiac output through changes of heart rate, stroke volume, or both.

In addition to heart rate, three variables interact to affect stroke volume—preload, afterload, and contractility. *Preload* is the degree of ventricular stretch that exists just before contraction. The stretch is imparted mainly by the amount of blood that fills the ventricles at the end of diastole, which reflects venous return and pressure in the corresponding atrium. According to the Frank-Starling law of the heart, if other factors (heart rate, afterload, contractility) are held constant, the force of muscle contraction—or stroke volume or cardiac output—is directly proportional to the preload. Thus, if the ventricles fill with more blood, more will be ejected. However, there is a physiologic limit to the ability of increasing preload to increase stroke volume or cardiac output, and when it is exceeded cardiac output falls. This is a major cause of heart failure, as discussed later.

Afterload can be defined as the amount of tension (or force or pressure) the ventricle must develop during contraction to open the semilunar valve and expel blood. The major determinant of afterload is arterial pressure.

Contractility refers to the vigor, strength, or intensity of cardiac muscle contraction when preload and afterload are held constant. Administration of calcium ions, increased sympathetic nervous system activity, and numerous cardiac-stimulant drugs can increase contractility.

Increases of cardiac output, whether owing to increased preload, afterload, contractility, or heart rate, increase the work load and oxygen demands of the heart. This principle is critically important to the deleterious effects of high blood pressure, ischemic heart disease, and heart failure.

Cardiac Reserve and Cardiac Failure

Cardiac reserve is the heart's ability to increase its output for short periods of time, well beyond resting levels, through increases of stroke volume, heart rate, or both. Cardiac output can increase approximately fivefold (up to 30 L/min) when necessary. *Cardiac failure* is a condition in which the heart fails to meet the demands of the peripheral tissues for adequate amounts of oxygenated blood. Usually, failure implies low cardiac output because of decreased stroke volume (contractility). When demands on the heart are light and the heart is healthy, mechanisms that affect cardiac output operate normally and no symptoms appear. When the heart is diseased or compensatory mechanisms cannot adapt to additional workloads, cardiac output falls to levels insufficient to satisfy the body's requirements. When cardiac output drops too much the venous system accommodates the extra blood, and venous pressure rises. This is an attempt to increase stroke volume by increasing preload, but it eventually leads to congestion of the vital organs ("congestive heart failure").

One or more of the factors regulating cardiac output can be altered with drugs to improve the status of the failing heart. They include afterload-reducing drugs such as hydralazine and many antihypertensive agents (Chapters 31 and 33); diuretics (Chapter 32), which lower preload and afterload; and positive inotropic agents (Chapter 31), which mainly increase cardiac contractility.

The Circulation

The cardiovascular system provides not only a pump—the heart—but also a transport system for blood through the vasculature. The large arteries into which blood flows from the ventricles provide a conduit that maintains high pressure. Smaller arteries and then the arterioles, because of their variable diameter, allow precise control of pressure. The capillaries are the eventual site of gas, nutrient, and waste exchange between the tissues and the bloodstream. Blood, at much reduced pressure, eventually passes to the venules, which help the arterioles regulate intracapillary pressure, and on to the veins, which serve as blood reservoirs and channel blood back to the heart.

The structure of a typical blood vessel is illustrated in Figure 29–4. The innermost layer is composed of endothelial cells that provide a smooth lining to ensure low resistance to blood flow. The endothelium also houses the biochemical machinery that performs other functions. It has a critical role, for example, in preventing blood platelets from contacting underlying collagen, thus preventing thrombosis, a major cause of blood vessel occlusion. When the endothelium is damaged and underlying structures are exposed, the normal processes of clotting are set in motion. The endothelium is also a source of prostaglandin PGI_2 (also called *prostacyclin*), which helps dilate the vessel and maintain low resistance to blood flow.

The smooth muscle fibers of the *tunica media* (the middle layer) are kept in a constant state of tonic contraction (vasomotor tone). The fibers are innervated by sympathetic nerves that, when stimulated, constrict the vessel still more, increasing peripheral resistance and blood pressure. There is no parasympathetic innervation of peripheral blood vessels. The arterioles are the chief regulators of peripheral resistance. Arteriolar smooth muscle is responsive not only to neural regulation, but also to hormonal control, to blood oxygen and carbon dioxide tensions, and to metabolites released from the tissues.

Pulmonary arteries have substantially thinner walls than corresponding systemic arteries. Thus they offer less resistance to flow, helping to keep intravascular pressure low. Pulmonary blood flow is controlled to a lesser extent by autonomic and hormonal controls, and is more responsive to changes in blood oxygen and carbon dioxide concentrations, than the general systemic vasculature.

The structure of a typical vein differs somewhat from that of an artery. Venous lumens are generally larger to accommodate relatively large blood volumes (that is, they are *capacitance vessels*). This large capacity also helps regulate pressure within the right atrium (central venous pressure), ensuring that the pressure stays low to facilitate the return of blood to the heart, and to match venous return with cardiac output. Larger veins (but not the venae cavae) also have one-way valves, which help prevent backflow of blood.

Blood Flow

For blood to flow between two points a pressure gradient, from higher to lower pressure, is necessary. Blood flow depends on two opposing factors: peripheral resistance and arterial blood pressure.

The major factor determining peripheral resistance is the diameter of the blood vessels. As the diameter increases, resistance decreases and blood flow is im-

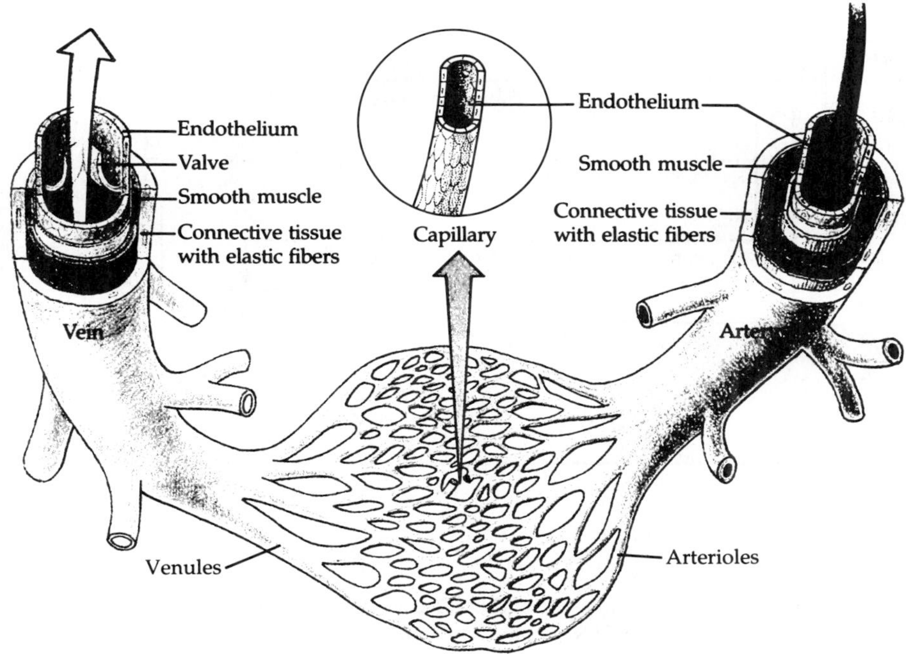

Figure 29–4

Key structures of the vasculature. Arteriolar smooth muscles constrict and relax under the influence of sympathetic nervous system activity and a variety of local (metabolic) factors. They provide the major control for peripheral resistance and blood pressure. Venules and veins, also under neural control, are a blood reservoir and conduit back to the heart. Capillaries, which lack direct constrictor or dilator control by neural influences, exchange gases, ions, nutrients, and wastes between the blood and the extravascular space. The endothelium is the site of biochemical pathways that control vascular tone and prevent adherence of blood platelets. All these structures are targets of drug action and disease processes.

(**Source:** Modified from Campbell NA. *Biology*. 1987:819. Menlo Park, CA: Benjamin/Cummings. Reprinted with permission of the copyright owner.)

proved. In vital organs, such as the heart and brain, local mechanisms (changes in oxygen or carbon dioxide levels, changes in pH) control vasodilation. In less critical body regions, sympathetic nervous system control predominates.

Blood Pressure

Blood pressure is defined as the force exerted on the wall of a blood vessel by its contained blood. Arterial pressure is the pressure that is measured most frequently. Systolic pressure is the maximum pressure reached during the peak of left ventricular ejection, and reflects the intensity of cardiac contraction. Diastolic pressure is the minimum pressure reached during a cardiac cycle, occurring just before ventricular ejection begins, and it provides some insight into overall peripheral resistance. The difference between the two pressures is the pulse pressure. Pulse pressure is increased by increases of stroke volume, the speed with which blood is ejected from the ventricle, and the stiffness of the arterial tree. It can be used to estimate what is perhaps the most important pressure measurement, ***mean*** (or average) *blood pressure,* according to the formula:

Mean arterial pressure
= diastolic pressure + ⅓ (pulse pressure).

Although blood pressure can increase or decrease beneficially in response to changing demands, significant and prolonged changes are generally adverse. Hypotension, an excessive fall of pressure, is dangerous mainly because it reduces blood flow to vital organs. This ischemia may cause permanent organ damage if hypotension lasts too long. A common cause of hypotension is reduced blood volume, as might result from dehydration or excessive bleeding.

Hypertension, an excessive increase in blood pressure, may weaken vascular walls, increasing both the risk of thrombus formation if the endothelium is damaged and the risk of rupture (aneurysm). Prolonged hy-

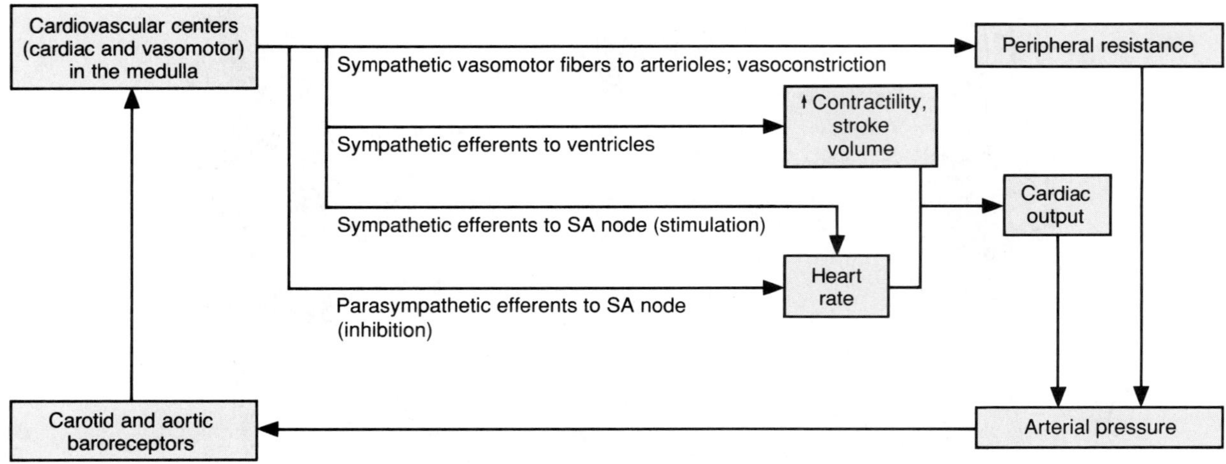

Figure 29–5

Rapidly acting neural control pathways for blood pressure and cardiac activity. Baroreceptors sense arterial pressure and trigger compensatory responses. When blood pressure falls, sympathetic activity to arterioles increases, causing vasoconstriction (increased peripheral resistance). Sympathetic cardiac stimulation also increases heart rate and stroke volume (increased cardiac output); it is accompanied by decreased parasympathetic outflow to the heart. Conversely, increased arterial pressure tends to decrease sympathetic tone to heart and vasculature.

pertension may cause secondary damage to the organs subjected to excessive pressures. Hypertension also increases afterload, which increases myocardial work and oxygen demands. With time, this may weaken the heart muscle and cause failure (hypertensive heart disease). In most cases the cause of hypertension is unknown, and the condition is called **essential hypertension.**

Regulation of Blood Pressure

Cardiovascular and renal mechanisms work together to regulate systemic blood pressure. Cardiovascular controls influence heart activity and peripheral resistance by altering the degree of constriction of the arterial bed. Renal mechanisms modify blood pressure via control of blood volume and composition (Fig. 29–5).

Cardiovascular Mechanisms in Blood Pressure Control

Reflex mechanisms provide short-term control of circulation. The most critical reflex, perhaps, is initiated by pressure sensors (baroreceptors) located in the carotid sinus and aortic arch. The baroreceptors respond to changes of mean blood pressure, transmit impulses to cardiac and vasomotor regulatory centers in the brain's medulla, and eventually alter efferent sympathetic or parasympathetic control of the heart and blood vessels. When pressure rises, the baroreceptor reflex attempts to normalize pressure by reducing vasoconstriction, cardiac contractility, and heart rate. This is accomplished mainly by decreasing sympathetic outflow. A relative increase in parasympathetic outflow to the SA node contributes to cardiac slowing. Conversely, when blood pressure falls, the baroreceptor reflex attempts to normalize blood pressure through increased sympathetic-mediated vasoconstriction, cardiac stimulation, and renal mechanisms.

Renal Mechanisms in Blood Pressure Control

Renal mechanisms provide long-term control of blood pressure via regulation of blood volume and osmolality. When blood volume or pressure is increased, the kidneys respond by excreting more salt and water in the urine. As the blood volume declines, so does blood pressure. Conversely, if blood pressure is too low, salt and water are conserved and returned to the bloodstream.

The retention or excretion of salt and water are controlled by the *renin-angiotensin II-aldosterone mechanism* (Fig. 29–6). When arterial blood pressure declines, the kidneys release renin into the blood. Renin causes

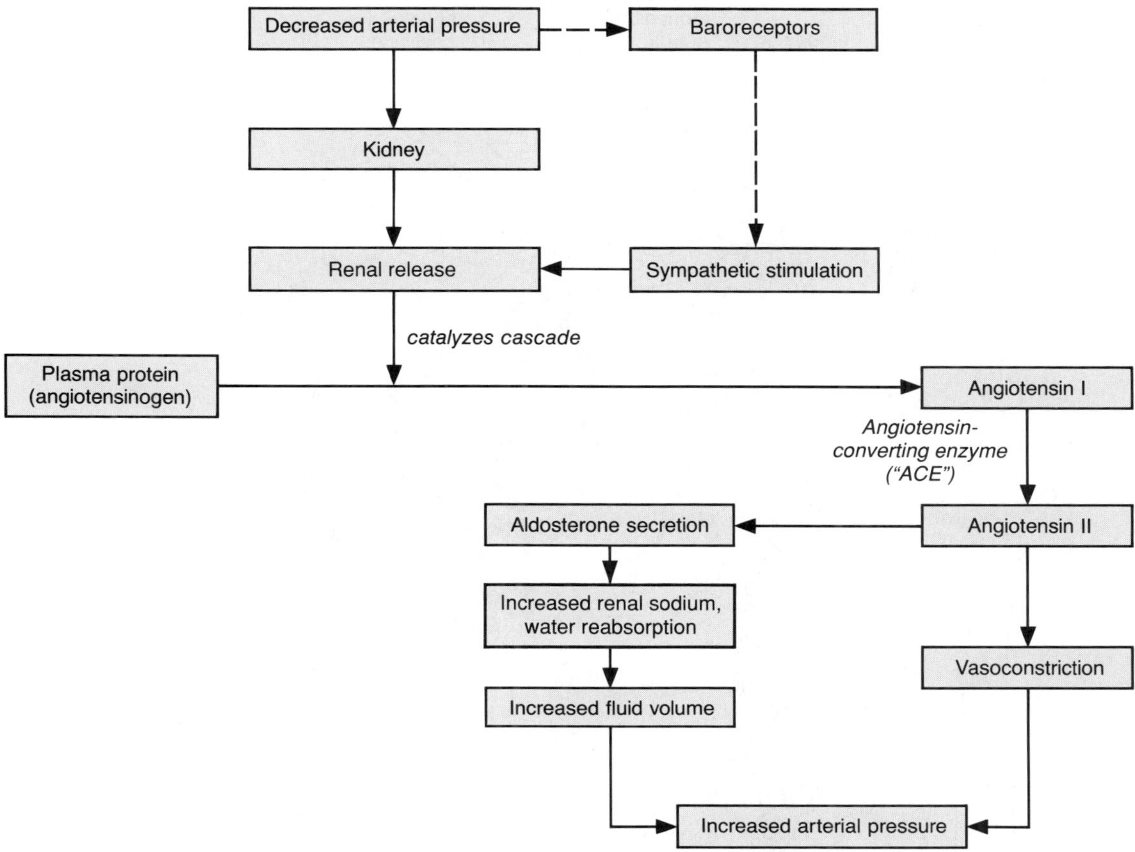

Figure 29–6

Slowly acting renal–hormonal mechanisms for blood pressure control: the renin-angiotensin II-aldosterone pathway. Note that sympathetic nervous system stimulation, part of a more rapidly acting control pathway (Fig. 29–5 and dashed lines above), also participates in this system by triggering renin release.

the appearance of angiotensin II and aldosterone in the blood. Angiotensin II causes vasoconstriction, promoting a rapid rise in systemic blood pressure. Aldosterone stimulates the kidneys to increase sodium ion reabsorption (which is accompanied by passive reabsorption of water), and to increase potassium elimination. Angiotensin II also stimulates the release of antidiuretic hormone from the hypothalamus, which also promotes water reabsorption. Excessive plasma renin levels are associated with a constant state of hypertension.

Drugs That Affect Blood Pressure Control

The many factors involved in regulating blood pressure offer a variety of targets for antihypertensive therapy, as discussed in Chapter 33. However, drugs given to lower blood pressure may trigger many of the same compensatory mechanisms that elevated pressure in the first place. As a result, more than one antihypertensive drug may be needed to interfere with the compensatory processes and achieve the therapeutic goal.

The Kidneys

The role of the kidneys in regulating blood pressure was discussed earlier. Another major physiologic role is to preserve volume and composition in the extracellular fluid. Since changes in extracellular fluid are often reflected in all the fluid compartments, the kidneys can be considered the prime regulator of fluid volume and composition throughout the body. In general, the kidneys accomplish their goals by excreting fluid (water) and substances dissolved in it (solutes, including meta-

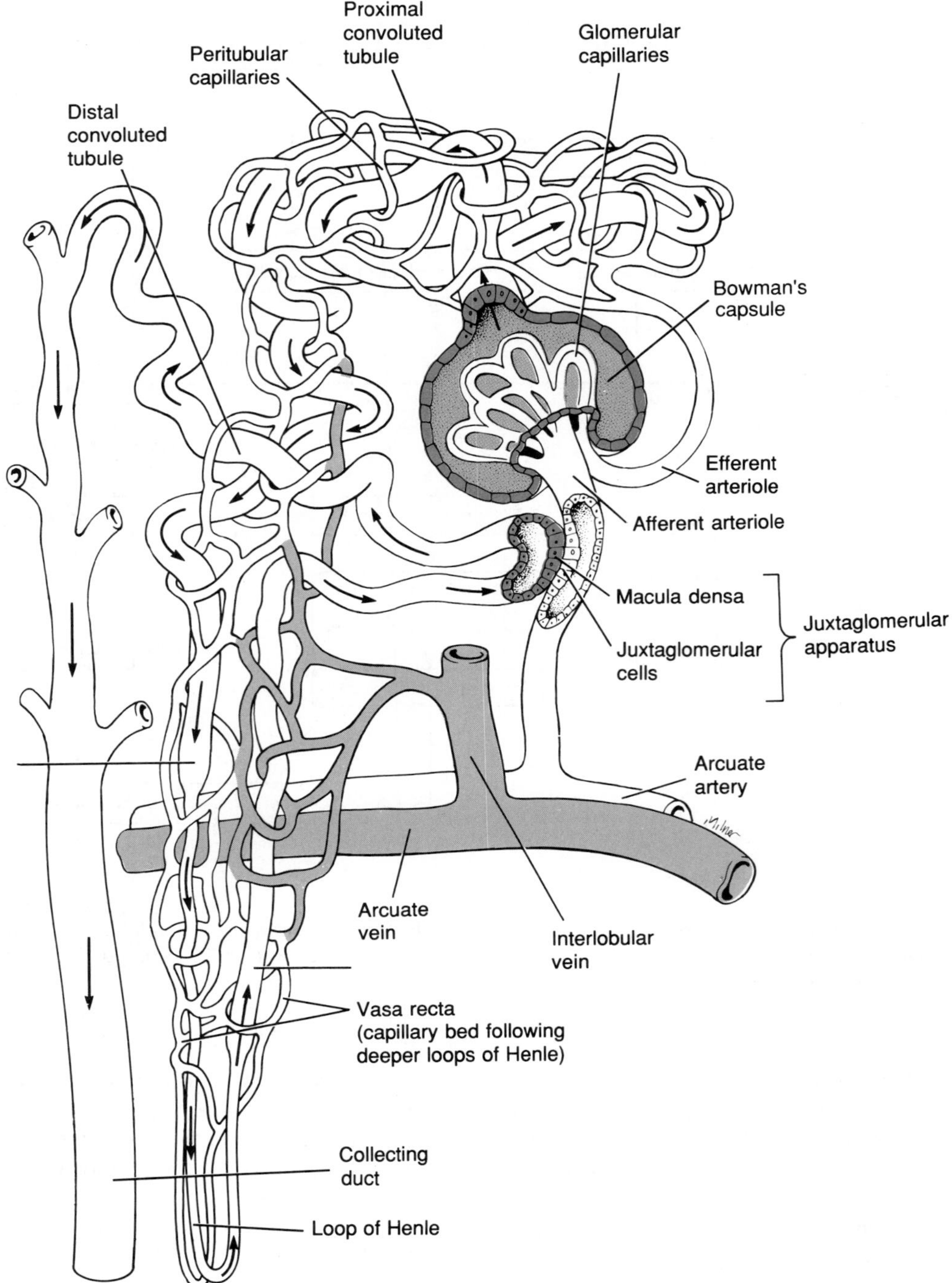

Figure 29–7

The nephron. This key structural element of the kidney helps regulate blood pressure, volume, and composition—and the cardiovascular system overall—via changes of urine volume and composition. As an ultrafiltrate of blood passes through the kidney tubules (arrows show direction of flow), urine volume and composition are changed by physical forces (eg, diffusion and osmosis); and by a variety of ion pumps, some of which are controlled by hormones (eg, aldosterone, antidiuretic hormone). Diuretic drugs (Chapter 32) play an important role in managing heart failure, edema, and hypertension through their actions on one or more parts and processes of the nephron.

bolic wastes, drugs, and toxins), and by sparing amounts of fluid and solute that are essential for body function. The source of the fluid and solute is the blood delivered to the kidneys via its arterial circulation.

The kidney uses three major processes to accomplish its roles: glomerular filtration, tubular reabsorption, and tubular secretion. Each of these processes occurs in one or more parts of the kidney's basic functional unit, the nephron, of which each kidney has about one million. A given substance delivered to the kidney may be handled by one or more of these processes as it passes through the nephron. Thus, a substance that is filtered extensively in the early parts of the nephron can be reabsorbed in later parts of the nephron so that little if any is eliminated in the urine. Diuretic drugs, discussed in Chapter 32, act mainly by altering the processes of reabsorption and secretion.

Structure and Function of the Nephron

The general structure of a nephron is illustrated in Figure 29–7. Intimately associated with each nephron are capillaries, which facilitate exchange of substances between the blood and urine. Since each region of the nephron is associated with a particular function, it is helpful to consider both aspects together.

Each nephron has a specialized and functionally important region called the juxtaglomerular apparatus. Here, some of the vascular smooth muscle cells, called *juxtaglomerular (JG) cells*, are enlarged and contain prominent renin-containing granules. The JG cells have receptors that are sensitive to blood pressure in the afferent arteriole; when pressure declines, the cells release renin. The JG cells also release renin in response to a signal from other cells, the macula densa, which are thought to sense solute concentrations.

Glomerulus

The first functional part of the nephron is the glomerulus, a ball of capillaries that is the primary site of filtration. The glomeruli form a cell- and protein-free ultrafiltrate from the blood. The ultrafiltrate passes into the first of the nephron's tubular components, Bowman's capsule. The kidneys form about 125 mL of filtrate per minute (roughly 180 liters per day), a value called the *glomerular filtration rate (GFR).* The fact that actual urine volume is far lower than 180 liters per day, and that valuable blood-borne substances such as glucose are never seen in normal urine, attests to the fact that other parts of the nephron have a great capacity to reclaim much of what was initially filtered.

Actual formation of the filtrate, and the rate of its formation (GFR), are determined by the pressure gradient between the afferent arterioles supplying the glomeruli and the efferent arterioles draining them. This, in turn, is determined mainly by systemic blood pressure. Large amounts of fluid, containing considerable amounts of needed solutes (as well as wastes), are temporarily lost from the bloodstream during filtration.

Filtration rate and pressure are maintained, despite changes in blood pressure, by autoregulation of glomerular pressure. This involves automatic changes in the resistances in the efferent and afferent arterioles. There are direct effects of blood pressure on vascular smooth muscle, as well as sympathetic influences and the actions of the renin-angiotensin II-aldosterone mechanism discussed earlier. For example, when arterial pressure rises the afferent arterioles constrict, which tends to maintain glomerular pressure at a desired lower level. When blood pressure falls the afferent arterioles dilate to accomplish the same purpose. Autoregulation maintains a relatively constant renal blood flow and GFR under most conditions, but it cannot compensate fully for great increases or decreases of blood pressure.

Proximal Tubules

Filtrate passes into the proximal tubule, which is specialized to reclaim, through the process of tubular reabsorption, much of the solute that was filtered earlier. Tubular reabsorption involves both *active transport* (dependent on metabolic energy from ATP) and *passive diffusion.* In the proximal tubule, for example, about 65% of the filtered sodium is reclaimed by active transport out of the tubule. Sodium movement causes reabsorption of water, driven by an osmotic gradient, and reabsorption of chloride ions, down an electrochemical gradient. At this site there is also appreciable reabsorption of potassium and bicarbonate, the latter of which affects both urine and blood pH.

The proximal tubule is the first major site in the nephron in which substances are actively transported into what will become urine. This process, tubular secretion, is an important pathway for the elimination of organic acids and bases, including many drugs that may not have been filtered completely in the glomerulus.

Loop of Henle

As the kidney tubules continue from the renal cortex they pass through the descending limb of the loop of Henle toward the renal medulla, into a region where the interstitial fluid becomes progressively hyperosmotic. The tubule cells in the descending limb are permeable only to water, which leaves the urine and enters the interstitium and eventually the blood. Since no ions leave the descending limb, the urine becomes concentrated.

Urine then passes into the ascending limb of Henle's loop. Here the tubule cells are impermeable to water, but they actively reabsorb chloride out of the urine; much of the remaining sodium is reabsorbed by passive diffusion. Since the urine passing through the ascending limb loses ions, but not water, it becomes more dilute once again. The most powerful diuretics act in the ascending limb to reduce the reabsorption of sodium, chloride, and water.

Distal Tubules

Urine reaching the next portion of the nephron, the distal tubule, contains only a fraction of the solute molecules found in the glomerular filtrate. What happens next depends on the availability of aldosterone. This hormone is secreted by the adrenal cortex in response to decreased blood volume or pressure, hyponatremia (a deficit of blood sodium), or hyperkalemia (increased blood potassium levels). Aldosterone stimulates sodium reabsorption from the distal tubule and stimulates potassium secretion into the urine. The process is an important way for the body to reclaim sodium and water when needed.

A recently discovered peptide "factor" acts on the distal tubule to increase the loss of sodium (a natriuretic effect) and water into the urine. It is called *atrial natriuretic factor (ANF)* because it is found in, and released from, the heart's atria. Atrial natriuretic factor may also inhibit renin and aldosterone release.

The distal tubule is an important site for regulating the pH of the urine, and consequently blood pH. When blood pH is abnormally low (that is, in acidosis), more of the bicarbonate reaching the distal tubule is reabsorbed, "new" molecules of bicarbonate are formed by the distal tubule cells and eventually released into the bloodstream, and the tubule cells secrete acid (H^+; protons) into the urine. The bicarbonate and protons arise from carbonic acid, produced through the interaction between water and carbon dioxide. The reaction is catalyzed by the enzyme *carbonic anhydrase.* When blood pH is high (alkalosis), the distal tubules reabsorb less bicarbonate from the urine, and they secrete protons into the blood.

Collecting Ducts

Urine passing from the distal tubules drains into the collecting ducts, the final opportunity for urine volume and composition to be changed. The collecting ducts pass through the increasingly higher osmotic concentrations of the medulla. Here the hormone vasopressin (antidiuretic hormone; ADH) acts to modify further urine concentration. Antidiuretic hormone is produced by the hypothalamus and stored in the posterior pituitary gland.

Receptors in the hypothalamus sense extracellular fluid solute concentration. When the body is dehydrated ADH release is high. The hormone acts on the collecting ducts to increase water reabsorption, which causes blood volume to rise, and results in excretion of a relatively small volume of concentrated urine (the antidiuretic effect). When the body is excessively hydrated, ADH release normally is low, less water is reabsorbed from the collecting ducts, and the kidneys excrete a relatively large volume of dilute urine. Drugs such as alcohol inhibit ADH release, leading to the large diuresis that is seen after ingesting that substance. Disorders such as diabetes insipidus are due to insufficient release or renal actions of ADH.

The Blood

The blood itself is an integral part of the cardiovascular system, since it is essential for delivering oxygen and nutrients to the body cells and carrying metabolic wastes to various organs for elimination. The body is endowed with several mechanisms for keeping the blood fluid, as well as others that permit it to clot in response to injury. When these processes function abnormally, serious problems, such as thrombosis and embolization, may occur, thereby adversely affecting the cardiovascular system and other vital organs. Drugs used to prevent such unwanted clotting—the anticoagulants—are discussed in Chapter 35.

Another crucial role of the blood is to carry lipids and related chemicals to all body cells, where they can be used in various ways. The lipid composition of the blood is important, especially when it is altered, since it may contribute to such serious disorders as atherosclerotic organ damage. Drugs used to regulate blood lipid composition are described in Chapter 36.

Annotated Bibliography

Abrams WB. Cardiovascular drugs in the elderly. *Chest* 1990;98:980–986. *Highly readable coverage of how aging affects the pharmacokinetics and actions of cardiovascular drugs in general, plus drug-specific comments that will help you plan and monitor therapy.*

Cooper JW. *Reviewing geriatric concerns with commonly used drugs. Geriatrics* 1989;44(12):79–86. *Covers many drug classes used often in elders, including those for cardiovascular disorders.*

Gerbino PP. Complications of alcohol use combined with drug therapy in the elderly. *J Am Geriatr Soc* 1982;30(11 Suppl.):S88–93. *Despite its publication date, this short paper highlights many interactions between cardiovascular drugs and alcohol that are still important.*

Kimm SYS, Payne GH, Lakatos E, Darby C, Sparrow A. Management of cardiovascular disease risk factors in children. *Am J Dis Child* 1990;144:967–972. *An interesting overview of how physicians in different specialties (pediatrics, general practice) perceive, diagnose, prevent, and treat cardiovascular disorders in children.*

Roe DA. Drug and nutrient interactions in elderly cardiac patients. *Drug Nutr Interact* 1988;5(4):205–212. *Important information on how nutrients and nutrition can affect cardiovascular disease and its treatment.*

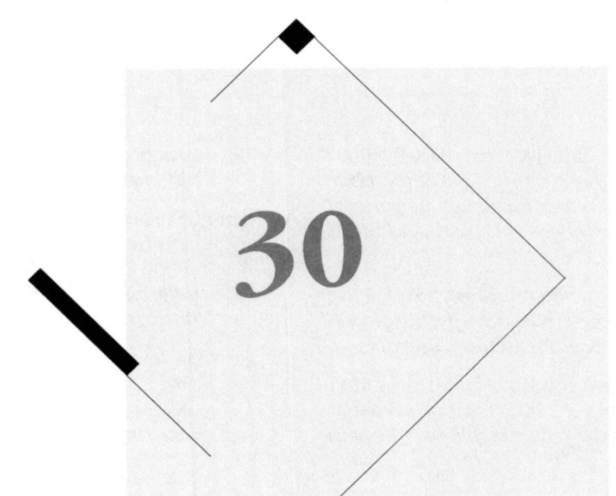

PROTOTYPES

Antiarrhythmic Drugs

Cardiac arrhythmias (sometimes called dysrhythmias) can be defined as any deviation from normal sinus rhythm and rate. Minor, brief cardiac changes occur normally during the respiratory cycle and during physical or emotional stress, and are generally harmless. However, some arrhythmias that last for more than a few moments can significantly decrease the heart's ability to pump blood adequately, leading to hypotension and decreased blood flow to vital organs. They may also progress into rhythm disorders such as ventricular fibrillation that, unless treated immediately, will be fatal within minutes. To restore normal heart rate and rhythm *antiarrhythmic drugs* must be used.

Electrophysiology of the Heart

Chapter 29 reviewed the basic electrophysiologic properties of the heart and its specialized conducting tissues. They enable each heart region to be activated by impulses passing in the proper direction (from the sinoatrial node throughout the ventricular myocardium), at the proper rate, and in the proper sequence. Arrhythmias are generated by, and manifestations of, alterations in normal electrophysiologic properties. These same electrophysiologic properties help explain why certain antiarrhythmic drugs are useful for specific indications, yet are unsuitable for others.

The important arrhythmias involve alterations of automaticity, impulse conduction, or both. Altered automaticity often arises because of electrical impulse generation at abnormal (ectopic) sites such as the atrioventricular (AV) node or the ventricular myocardium. Alterations of conduction include situations in which impulses are conducted too slowly, too quickly, or travel in the wrong direction, through a region of the heart. One important type of impaired conduction is called *reentry,* a situation in which an impulse cannot pass in the normal direction through a heart region. The impulse seeks another route around the block, reenters the conduction pathway in the wrong direction, and causes premature depolarization and contraction.

There are many causes of arrhythmias. Ischemic heart damage is probably the most common one. Others include myocardial hypertrophy (stretch of the myocardium, as often accompanies congestive heart failure), infectious diseases, anatomic heart lesions, abnormal influences of the sympathetic and parasympathetic nervous systems on the heart, and many drugs.

Major reference tables appear beginning on p. 569

Classification of Arrhythmias According to Sites of Origin or Involvement

The most common way of classifying arrhythmias clinically is based on their site of origin, which usually can be assessed using a standard 12-lead electrocardiogram (ECG). Similarly, antiarrhythmic drugs are often classified according to the types of arrhythmias that they affect best. *Supraventricular arrhythmias* are characterized by abnormal conduction in structures above the ventricles, such as the sinoatrial (SA) node or the atria themselves. Examples include sinus tachycardia (a "sinus arrhythmia"), atrial flutter, and atrial fibrillation. *Ventricular arrhythmias* originate in or involve abnormal conduction in the ventricles. Examples include premature ventricular contractions (PVCs) and ventricular fibrillation.

The atria's contractile activity does not contribute much to cardiac output if ventricular function is normal. Indeed, many patients can live quite normally with atrial arrhythmias, even atrial fibrillation, without treatment. However, atrial or other supraventricular arrhythmias often lead to devastating changes of ventricular activity. The key to this possibility is what happens at the AV node, which functions as the normal gateway for impulses into the ventricles. If AV nodal activity is suppressed considerably, ventricular rate may slow markedly or the heart may stop. Alternatively, if AV nodal activity is such that too many impulses can pass in a relatively short time, the ventricles may no longer have sufficient time to fill with and then expel blood efficiently. This inability to eject blood efficiently is the major reason why, in general, ventricular arrhythmias are much more life-threatening than others. Patients may have arrhythmias that involve both supraventricular and ventricular structures.

Antiarrhythmic Drugs

The Objectives and Mechanisms of Antiarrhythmic Drug Therapy

Antiarrhythmic drugs are given to prevent or stop any unwanted heart rate or rhythm. The ultimate goal is to preserve regular ventricular rhythm. In general, antiarrhythmic drugs act by depressing automaticity, slowing conduction rates, increasing refractoriness to premature stimulation, or by a combination of these mechanisms. They accomplish their effects mainly by altering the movement of one or more ions (sodium, potassium, calcium) across the heart cells' membranes. The essential diagnostic information provided by the ECG helps determine which antiarrhythmic drug will be used, and clearly helps assess the response to treatment.

Although antiarrhythmic drugs mainly affect electrical activity, they may affect contractile function as well. The contractile effects may be desirable outcomes of suppressing arrhythmias and restoring normal rate and rhythm, or they may be unwanted drug-induced effects. Antiarrhythmic drugs also may cause many important actions outside the heart (extracardiac effects). Most of these are undesirable or truly adverse, and they may limit the use of an otherwise effective drug for certain patients. Indeed, although one of several antiarrhythmic drugs could be used to treat a particular arrhythmia, the choice usually favors the drug with the least risk of causing adverse cardiac or extracardiac effects. This is particularly true for long-term treatment. When arrhythmias are acute and life-threatening, the importance of adverse drug-induced effects lessens in view of the potentially dire consequences of withholding treatment.

Classification of Antiarrhythmic Drugs

There is no "universal" antiarrhythmic drug, so no single prototype can be identified. Antiarrhythmic drugs are divided into four main classes, I through IV, based on their effects on cardiac electrical properties (Table 30–1). Most of the antiarrhythmics are in Class I, which is further divided into three subclasses, IA, IB, and IC. In the following sections, characteristics of each class of antiarrhythmic are discussed in turn, followed by discussions of individual drugs. When a prototype of each class or subclass can be identified easily, that agent is discussed extensively. Although drugs grouped together act in a similar way, other properties (such as onsets of action or lack of efficacy when given by certain administration routes) may determine the ultimate choice of a given agent within the group. Antiarrhythmic drugs that do not fit in the above categories are discussed at the end of the chapter.

Nursing Implications Common to All Antiarrhythmics

All antiarrhythmic drugs have the potential to worsen arrhythmias, or to cause new ones. The ECG is the only way to assess whether a drug is producing its desired actions, and a baseline (predrug) measurement is necessary to make such an evaluation. Frequent follow-up measurements are also essential.

No antiarrhythmic drug that is given by injection should be administered in a setting where adequate facilities for monitoring and support of vital functions are

Table 30–1 Classification of Antiarrhythmic Agents Based on Major Electrophysiologic Actions

Class	Agents	Electrophysiologic Effects
IA	Quinidine* Procainamide Disopyramide	Suppress automaticity by slowing spontaneous depolarization; lower electrical potential needed to trigger spontaneous depolarization; prolong action potential, thereby prolonging refractory periods so that premature stimulation is less likely to occur, especially in the ventricles
IB	Lidocaine* Mexiletine Phenytoin Tocainide	Mainly decrease action potential duration, prolong refractory period, especially in Purkinje fibers
IC	Encainide Flecainide Indecainide Moricizine Propafenone	Markedly depress automaticity by slowing spontaneous depolarization; minimal effects on action potential duration or refractory periods
II	Beta blockers (acebutolol, esmolol, propranolol*)	Suppress automaticity and impulse conduction rates by blocking catecholamine-induced electrophysiologic effects
III	Amiodarone Bretylium	Prolong action potential duration and refractory periods to exert "chemical antifibrillatory action"; have little or no effect on spontaneous depolarization
IV	Calcium-channel blockers (verapamil*)	Slow impulse conduction, prolong refractoriness, particularly in AV node

Key: * = a drug that can be readily identified as a prototype. There is no one overall prototype antiarrhythmic drug. Drugs in the same class or subclass share common electrophysiologic effects.

not immediately available. Antiarrhythmic drugs can affect other organs or organ systems. Therefore, all pertinent vital signs, not only those affecting the cardiovascular system, must be monitored closely and frequently, because there is no specific antidote for managing adverse effects of any antiarrhythmic drug.

Constant monitoring of the ECG is preferred for all hospitalized patients. Teach outpatients who will be taking antiarrhythmic drugs to measure rate and regularity of the radial pulse for a full minute. If possible, teach them to take the carotid pulse, which may be a more sensitive indicator of arrhythmias. Recommend that patients check their pulse each morning before getting out of bed, keep a written record of pulse rate and regularity, and bring this record to each office or clinic visit. Any irregularities of pulse rate or rhythm should be reported at once.

Antiarrhythmic drug therapy during pregnancy is a concern. As with any drug, antiarrhythmics should not be used during pregnancy unless the anticipated benefits to the mother outweigh the risks arising from failure to treat her arrhythmias or the possible risks to the fetus. No antiarrhythmic drug is contraindicated when it is needed to stop a potentially fatal arrhythmia, such as ventricular fibrillation. Some of the antiarrhythmics (for example, disopyramide and verapamil) are concentrated in breast milk, and breast-feeding is almost always contraindicated during therapy with these drugs. For the others, it is still best to avoid breast-feeding.

Class IA Antiarrhythmics

Antiarrhythmics in Class IA slow the rate of spontaneous depolarization of cardiac cells, which reduces automaticity; and prolong the refractory period of heart cells, making them less susceptible to premature activation by neighboring cells. Quinidine is the prototype of the Class IA antiarrhythmics. Related drugs are procainamide and disopyramide.

PROTOTYPE

Quinidine

Quinidine, one of the oldest antiarrhythmic drugs, is an alkaloid isolated from the bark of the cinchona tree. It is chemically related to quinine, an antimalarial

Table 30–2 **Comparison of Important Electrophysiologic and Hemodynamic Effects of Selected Antiarrhythmic Drugs**

	P–R Interval	Width of QRS Complex	Blood Pressure	Cardiac Output
Disopyramide	0 or ↑	0 or ↑	↑ or ↓	↑ or ↓
Lidocaine	0	0	↓	0 or ↓
Procainamide	0 or ↑	↑	↓	↓
Propranolol	0 or ↑	0 or ↑	0 or ↓	↓
Quinidine	0 or ↑	↑	↓	↓

Key: ↑ = increased or prolonged; ↓ = decreased or shortened; 0 = no appreciable change.

drug. Quinidine effectively manages many ventricular arrhythmias, but is also important for the treatment of some supraventricular rhythm disturbances. It shares some of the properties of the related Class IA drugs, especially procainamide, but has some important differences.

Absorption, Distribution, Metabolism, and Excretion

Quinidine is absorbed well from the gastrointestinal (GI) tract. About 80% of quinidine molecules in the bloodstream are bound to plasma proteins, but the drug can bind to other sites, such as skeletal muscle and the heart, very well. Most of the drug is metabolized in the liver; only a small amount is excreted unchanged by the kidneys. The usual half-life is about 3 hours.

The major quinidine salts are quinidine gluconate (DURAQUIN; QUINAGLUTE DURA-TABS [a sustained-release preparation], and a parenteral formulation), quinidine polygalacturonate (CARDIOQUIN), and quinidine sulfate (QUINORA; or the long-acting preparation, QUINIDEX EXTENTABS).

Pharmacologic Effects

A general principle in pharmacology is that most drugs cause more than one effect. Indeed, some drugs can cause opposite effects on the same target cell or system. This is clearly true for quinidine, even when one considers only its effects on the various cells that make up the heart.

Quinidine causes some effects because of its *direct* actions on heart cells; and some opposing, *indirect* effects, through its ability to interfere with control of heart function by the parasympathetic nervous system. The overall effect is, therefore, somewhat of a balance between opposite actions.

Quinidine directly depresses the excitability of most cardiac tissues: impulse conduction rates *through* the atrial and ventricular muscles are slowed, and these tissues become more refractory (resistant) to premature stimulation. This latter effect is what accounts for quinidine's ability to suppress some reentrant arrhythmias.

Simultaneously, quinidine causes some indirect effects owing to its antimuscarinic (atropine-like, or parasympathetic-blocking) actions on the heart. One of the most important indirect effects of quinidine, at usual therapeutic blood levels, is on the AV node: electrical impulse conduction rates tend to increase, indicating faster transmission of impulses *between* the atria and ventricles.

Overall, and as summarized in Table 30–2, the P–R interval is either unchanged or prolonged. The prolonged P–R interval reflects slowed impulse transmission through the atria and ventricles, but faster impulse transmission through the AV node. Quinidine's ability to widen the QRS complex is yet another indication of its ability to slow impulse conduction through the ventricles. All these effects are dose-dependent, and they provide important ways to help monitor the desired or unwanted responses to quinidine treatment.

Quinidine also causes dose-dependent depression of myocardial contractile force generation, and some peripheral vasodilator effects. As a result, cardiac output and blood pressure can fall.

Clinical Indications and Administration

Quinidine dosages for various routes and indications are listed in Table 30–C. Only immediate-acting oral dosage forms or parenteral formulations should be used to start therapy. Slow-release products are properly used only for maintenance therapy. Regardless of which route or preparation is used, the therapeutic blood level for quinidine is between 2 μg/mL and 6 μg/mL.

Quinidine is mainly used to manage supraventricular arrhythmias such as atrial flutter or fibrillation (Table 30–C). Quinidine's desired atrial effects account for its use in these conditions. However, quinidine simultaneously increases electrical impulse conduction through the AV node. This allows more impulses to reach the ventricles, which can cause serious adverse ventricular effects, including ventricular tachycardia. Thus, when quinidine therapy for atrial arrhythmias is begun (often by the IV route), the patient usually is pretreated with an injection of another drug, usually digoxin (see Chapter 31, pp 580–589). Digoxin slows AV conduction and "protects" the ventricles against further acceleration in response to the quinidine.

Currently, electrical cardioversion is used as the primary treatment of atrial flutter or fibrillation for many patients. Nevertheless, patients are often placed on oral maintenance therapy with quinidine once the arrhythmia is stopped.

Compared with many other antiarrhythmic drugs discussed in this chapter, quinidine is seldom used to manage ventricular arrhythmias. However, it can be used for paroxysmal ventricular tachycardia, provided it is not associated with complete heart block.

NURSING IMPLICATIONS

To improve absorption of oral quinidine, administer the drug at least 1 hour before or 2 hours after meals. If quinidine gluconate is given intravenously, the total dose must be given slowly, usually over 30 to 60 minutes. Because quinidine can depress cardiac contractility and blood pressure, it is essential to monitor vital signs and the ECG during initial treatment and periodically thereafter. Constant monitoring is required during intravenous (IV) administration because of the increased risk of adverse effects.

Side Effects, Adverse Reactions, and Contraindications

Side effects caused by quinidine are listed in Table 30–S, along with related contraindications and nursing implications.

The most serious unwanted effects involve quinidine's actions on the circulatory system, and they appear to be dose-dependent. They include decreased cardiac output and hypotension. The cause of hypotension is twofold. It can reflect quinidine's ability to decrease both cardiac rate and (especially) contractile force generation. Usually it is also caused by the drug's vasodilator activity, which lowers peripheral resistance and blood pressure. Patients with bradycardia, hypokalemia, or both, are at a greater risk of experiencing symptomatic hypotension (eg, syncope). There is also the potential for varying degrees of AV block (seen as a widening of the P–R interval on the ECG), impaired electrical impulse conduction through the ventricles (widening of the QRS complex), and premature ventricular contractions. Quinidine has caused ventricular fibrillation, and some cases have been fatal.

Extracardiac effects are also fairly common and important. Common GI effects include nausea, vomiting, and diarrhea. Quinidine, given in relatively high doses, is unique among all antiarrhythmic agents because of its ability to cause a side effect syndrome called *cinchonism.* Its manifestations include

- the GI side effects noted above;
- dizziness;
- **tinnitus** (ringing in the ears) or other hearing alterations; and
- visual disturbances (double-vision, altered color perception, impaired night vision).

Whether one or more of these side effects will occur in a particular patient, or how severe it will be, can be hard to predict. There is much patient-to-patient variability, even when the same drug, dose, and route are used for persons with similar arrhythmias. Indeed, some patients develop signs and symptoms of cinchonism after a single dose of quinidine. Thus, the quinidine blood level and the actual responses that occur in a given patient are the best indicators of proper dosage. It is important to note that although quinidine causes important atropine-like effects on the heart, peripheral atropine-like side effects are uncommon. As a result, quinidine does not share all the contraindications noted for atropine itself, or for the related antiarrhythmic drug disopyramide, which is discussed shortly.

Quinidine also has the potential to depress skeletal muscle contractility, and so it should be used cautiously in patients with myasthenia gravis. For any patient, the drug can stimulate the formation of platelet-destroying antibodies, leading to thrombocytopenia and the associated increased risk of bleeding. Both side effects are usually reversible upon discontinuing quinidine.

NURSING IMPLICATIONS

If oral quinidine causes GI upset, the drug may be given with food. Regardless of when the drug is given, encourage the patient to be consistent with administration time and its relation to meals. Any abnormality of pulse or other vital signs requires at least temporary discontinuation of quinidine administration at once, and immediate notification of the physician.

Use During Pregnancy and Lactation

There is little information about the effects of quinidine on the developing fetus. Potential risks and benefits should be assessed and discussed before long-term use. Quinidine is excreted in breast milk, so breast-feeding should be avoided.

Use in the Elderly

Quinidine toxicity may be more common in the elderly unless the dosage is adjusted to compensate for impaired drug elimination or advanced cardiac disease.

Interactions with Other Drugs

Many of the interactions identified for quinidine (Table 30–I) involve drugs that can stimulate quinidine's metabolism, thereby lowering blood levels to values that may be too low for effective arrhythmia control (eg, barbiturates, phenytoin, rifampin). Other interactants (eg, cimetidine) can inhibit quinidine metabolism, increasing the chance of dose-dependent adverse effects.

Most of the drugs cited as interactants can be administered with quinidine if proper monitoring for the effects of both drugs is provided. However, four drug interactions are best avoided, if possible, by using a suitable alternative to quinidine. They involve amiodarone (see p 563), oral anticoagulants, verapamil, and digitalis glycosides (digitoxin and, especially, digoxin).

The interaction with digoxin is important. It depends on the doses of the two drugs, how long they have been given to the patient, and the sequence in which they are given. As noted above, one or two small doses of digoxin are often given *before* giving quinidine to stop an atrial arrhythmia. However, a potentially serious interaction can occur if these two drugs are used in other ways. Quinidine reduces digoxin's renal excretion, and displaces digoxin from tissue binding sites. The overall result is an increase in digoxin blood levels. In practical terms, if the patient is already stabilized on digoxin, and digoxin blood levels are in the therapeutic range, starting quinidine therapy *afterwards* can cause digoxin levels to climb within a few hours to a few days into the toxic range. If the patient is already experiencing digoxin toxicity (which includes a variety of arrhythmias), and quinidine is begun, the outcome could be disastrous. The interaction can also occur with quinidine and digitoxin, which is a less-often-used digoxin alternative. However, clinical signs of the interaction may take several days to a week to appear.

NURSING IMPLICATIONS

If quinidine is to be given to a patient who is already stabilized on digoxin, the digoxin dose should be reduced several days earlier, if possible. Hypokalemia, as can be produced by the diuretics (Chapter 32) used with digoxin to treat heart failure, increases the risk of toxicity caused by quinidine, digoxin, or the two combined. Check electrolyte values first. Do not give quinidine and digoxin to patients who are hypokalemic. Never give quinidine to a patient who is experiencing digitalis toxicity.

Overdose and Toxicity

True quinidine toxicity usually occurs when blood levels are above 8 μg/mL, which is not far above the maximum therapeutic level. (That is, quinidine has a relatively low margin of safety.) Signs and symptoms include intensification of the GI side effects noted above; CNS disturbances ranging from lethargy to coma or seizures; arrhythmias that can vary from complete cardiac arrest to ventricular tachycardia or fibrillation; and hypotension owing to arrhythmias, peripheral vasodilation, and direct depression of cardiac contractility.

Oral overdoses are managed initially with the standard first-aid measures that would be used for most oral overdoses: induced emesis, gastric lavage, and administration of activated charcoal, for example (see Appendix C for more details). There is no specific antidote for quinidine's effects. However, IV administration of sodium lactate may reverse some of the adverse cardiac effects. Otherwise, care is symptomatic and supportive, based on continuous monitoring of vital signs; continuous ECG monitoring is absolutely essential.

Related Drugs

Disopyramide

Disopyramide (NORPACE) is in the same antiarrhythmic class (IA) as quinidine: their electrophysiologic effects on cardiac cells are similar. However, disopyramide differs importantly in several ways, including its clinical uses and side effects profile.

Disopyramide is available only in oral dosage forms. A slow-release formulation (NORPACE CR) is available for maintenance therapy. Disopyramide is absorbed well, reaching peak blood levels in an average of about 2 hours. About half the drug is excreted unchanged by the kidneys; nearly all the rest undergoes hepatic metabolism. Thus, either renal or hepatic dysfunction will require a reduction of the drug's usual dosage (Table 30–C).

Unlike quinidine, disopyramide is not used for atrial arrhythmias. It is used mainly for ventricular arrhythmias: ectopic or premature ventricular contractions, or bouts of ventricular tachycardia. However, disopyramide is not usually used as a first-line agent for these conditions (see lidocaine, below).

Disopyramide exerts quinidine-like antimuscarinic effects on the heart's AV node, but it also exerts common and often intense atropine-like side effects elsewhere: dry mouth occurs in about one third of patients taking this drug, and about one in 10 also experience constipation, urinary frequency or hesitancy, and blurred vision. As a result, contraindications that apply to atropine (Chapter 13, Table 13–S), including glaucoma and prostatic hypertrophy, apply also to disopyramide. These side effects may become so severe that disopyramide therapy may need to be stopped.

The cardiac-depressant effects of disopyramide can be significant. They generally contraindicate disopyramide use in patients with congestive heart failure. Nevertheless, all patients who receive this drug should be monitored for key signs and symptoms of cardiac failure.

The major interactants with disopyramide (Table 30–I) include

- most antiarrhythmics or cardiac depressants (including β-blockers and calcium-channel blockers);
- drugs that stimulate hepatic drug-metabolizing enzymes and reduce disopyramide blood levels (eg, phenytoin, barbiturates, rifampin); and
- other drugs that cause peripheral antimuscarinic side effects (see Table 13-2, p 174).

Owing to disopyramide's rapid absorption and intense cardiac effects, signs and symptoms of overdose can become serious very quickly. Cardiac effects will reflect progressive depression of electrical activity, from bradycardia and widening of the QRS complex to eventual asystole and cardiac arrest. Progressive hypotension will develop owing to suppression of cardiac electrical and contractile activity. As these cardiovascular problems develop the patient will experience increasing degrees of atropine-like side effects or toxicity. Respiratory arrest may occur.

There is no antidote for disopyramide overdose; giving symptomatic and supportive care is the norm. The priority is to support cardiac function and blood pressure with suitable drugs (eg, dopamine), fluids, or assist devices (cardiac pacing, intraaortic balloon counterpulsation) as needed.

NURSING IMPLICATIONS

In addition to taking standard precautions for the administration of antiarrhythmic drugs, it is also essential to assess closely for problems caused by disopyramide's atropine-like side effects: eye pain that may indicate an acute glaucoma attack; impaired urination or defecation; bladder or bowel distention; and diminished skeletal muscle strength or endurance, which might indicate undiagnosed myasthenia gravis. Monitor blood glucose levels periodically, especially if the patient is diabetic or prediabetic.

Not much information is available concerning the use of disopyramide during pregnancy. However, considering the possible seriousness of the arrhythmias for which it is indicated, it may be used if needed. Disopyramide is excreted in maternal milk, where drug concentrations may reach three times those found in maternal plasma. Therefore, breast-feeding should be avoided.

If disopyramide must be given to a child, he or she should be hospitalized during initial treatment and until the response stabilizes.

Procainamide

Procainamide (PRONESTYL) is chemically related to the local anesthetic drug procaine. In terms of actions on heart cells, it is similar to quinidine and disopyramide. In terms of clinical uses, it is much more like quinidine. Procainamide is available in immediate- and sustained-acting oral dosage forms (for maintenance therapy), and in parenteral formulations for intramuscular (IM) or IV use.

Procainamide is eliminated mainly by renal excretion. However, some of the drug is metabolized in the liver, through a process called *acetylation,* to an active chemical, "NAPA" (N-acetylprocainamide). The importance of this is noted below.

Procainamide shares quinidine's uses for atrial arrhythmias. Either drug can be used for these disorders, but some patients respond better to one than to another. Anticipated side effects, related contraindications, or the need to use interacting drugs, also affect the choice. Patients who will receive initial procainamide doses to stop atrial arrhythmias may need pretreatment with digoxin to keep ventricular rates in check. Unlike quinidine, procainamide is also effective for managing premature ventricular contractions or ventricular tachycardia. Dosages are summarized in Table 30–C. They should be reduced if the patient has impaired renal or liver function. Regardless of the indication, therapeutic blood levels for procainamide are between 4 μg/mL and 8 μg/mL.

Procainamide's cardiovascular side effects are similar to those of quinidine, but procainamide tends to cause less cardiac depression when the drug is given by injection, especially IV. This also favors the use of procainamide instead of quinidine when IV therapy is indicated. The most important acute response to IV injection of procainamide is hypotension, which can be severe if the drug is given too quickly. Hypotension is much less a problem with IM injection.

Procainamide does not cause cinchonism. However, it does cause some unique side effects. About one in five patients receiving procainamide for more than several months develop a reversible syndrome that resembles systemic lupus erythematosus: fever, rashes, muscle aches, and joint pain. These problems are thought to be due to unmetabolized procainamide, because the incidence appears to be higher in patients who metabolize (acetylate) the drug much slower than others. (For example, many persons of Asian descent are "rapid acetylators." They seldom develop the lupus-like syndrome in response to procainamide.)

About one out of 200 patients on long-term procainamide therapy develop agranulocytosis. The overall incidence is low, but this blood dyscrasia can be fatal if not detected early enough. Thus, in addition to frequent monitoring of the ECG and of liver and renal status, monitoring blood test results is important also.

Procainamide tends to cause fewer peripheral atropine-like side effects than quinidine. Nevertheless, it should be used cautiously if the patient is at risk from these effects. Myasthenia gravis contraindicates procainamide use also. The drug should not be administered to patients with a history of allergic reactions to procaine.

The most important interactants with procainamide (Table 30–I) are amiodarone, cimetidine, and trimethoprim. Any of these drugs can quickly increase procainamide blood levels and the risk of adverse effects. Avoid these interactions, if possible.

Procainamide has a higher margin of safety than quinidine. Toxic blood levels are roughly twice the usual maximum therapeutic value. Signs and symptoms of toxicity affect the CNS, the GI tract, and the cardiovascular system. They are quite similar to those caused by quinidine (with the exception of signs of cinchonism), and they are treated in a similar way.

NURSING IMPLICATIONS

Frequent blood tests to help detect antinuclear antibodies and blood dyscrasias are indicated for all patients who will receive procainamide on a long-term basis. Report signs or symptoms of these adverse responses at once. Pregnancy does not contraindicate the use of procainamide as an emergency drug. For long-term use, however, the potential risks and benefits must be considered, since the drug crosses the placenta. Procainamide and its metabolites are excreted in maternal milk, and so breast-feeding should be avoided. The safety and effectiveness of procainamide in children has not been established. Elderly patients, or patients with impaired renal, hepatic, or cardiac function, may experience adequate antiarrhythmic effects with lower doses or longer dose intervals.

Class IB Agents

Antiarrhythmics in Class IB decrease refractory periods, especially in Purkinje cells, but they have little effect on automaticity. Lidocaine is the prototype. Related Class IB antiarrhythmics are mexiletine, tocainide, and phenytoin.

PROTOTYPE

Lidocaine

Lidocaine (XYLOCAINE), the prototype Class IB antiarrhythmic, is the most widely used drug for the emergency management of arrhythmias. The drug is discussed in more detail in Chapter 18 in the setting of its role as the prototype local anesthetic agent. Refer to that section for more information. What follows emphasizes the drug's use for its antiarrhythmic effects, with only brief summary comments on more general properties.

Absorption, Distribution, Metabolism, and Excretion

When lidocaine is used as an antiarrhythmic it is usually given intravenously. Intramuscular injections are used less often, and common injection routes used for local anesthesia are never used when the goal is to treat arrhythmias. No oral dosage forms are available. Lidocaine is inactivated by hepatic metabolism. When liver function is normal, the half-life of a single lidocaine dose is about 30 minutes.

Pharmacologic Effects

Lidocaine's local anesthetic effects on peripheral nerves are similar to its effects on cardiac muscle and the heart's nodal and specialized conducting tissues. The drug slows depolarization, which is a key part of the action potential. When lidocaine is present at therapeutic blood levels (about 1.5–6 μg/mL), it tends to exert preferential effects on cardiac tissues that are functioning abnormally, as because of altered automaticity or electrical impulse conduction rates. It exerts a much lesser effect on normally functioning heart regions. For example, if conduction through the AV node is relatively normal, lidocaine will not enhance it (as does quinidine) or inhibit it (as do β-blockers) very much. Overall, lidocaine tends to normalize cardiac electrical activity, making the arrhythmia-causing differences between regions less different.

Lidocaine reduces cardiac contractile force, dilates peripheral blood vessels, and can depress or stimulate the CNS, in a dose-dependent way. These effects become most important when lidocaine levels enter a toxic range.

Clinical Indications and Administration

Lidocaine is generally considered to be the preferred drug for management of acute, life-threatening arrhythmias that involve or originate in the ventricles. These include ventricular tachycardia or fibrillation that may occur because of myocardial infarction, or arrhythmias caused by drugs such as digoxin (Chapter 31) and general anesthetics. Overall, lidocaine is the agent of choice for most drug-induced arrhythmias.

In most cases lidocaine is first given as an IV bolus injection to reach therapeutic blood levels quickly. This is followed by a lidocaine infusion (see Table 30–C for typical dosages) to maintain safe but effective blood levels. The ECG must be monitored when the IV route is used.

Lidocaine can be given by IM injection. However, this route should be used only in unusual circumstances, such as when no ECG monitoring is available or when venous access cannot be gained quickly enough. Regardless of whether the drug is given intravenously or intramuscularly, only vasoconstrictor-free formulations should be used; never use preparations that contain drugs such as epinephrine, which are indicated only for local anesthetic use.

Lidocaine should not be administered to control arrhythmias that are largely confined to the atria (eg, flutter or fibrillation), or arrhythmias characterized mainly by sinoatrial or AV nodal block. Lidocaine could cause more serious ventricular arrhythmias in these situations.

NURSING IMPLICATIONS

The availability of an ECG for constant monitoring of the patient's responses; other emergency drugs for control of arrhythmias, blood pressure, and possible seizures; and facilities for artificial ventilation are essential for safe and effective lidocaine use. Monitor vital signs constantly, since the effects of lidocaine appear rapidly, and toxic blood levels are not far above therapeutic levels. If possible, use an infusion pump for accurate drug delivery rates. Reserve IM administration for situations in which IV administration or ECG monitoring is not possible. The deltoid muscle is the preferred IM injection site. Injection into other muscles, such as the gluteus, may cause lidocaine blood levels to rise too high and too fast. Use proper technique to avoid accidental IV injection when IM injection is the goal.

Side Effects, Adverse Reactions, Contraindications, and Toxicity

Lidocaine has a very low margin of safety. There is not a great difference between blood levels that cause therapeutic effects, those causing mild side effects, and those associated with true toxicity. Indeed, some evidence of potentially serious toxicity may occur, in some patients, when blood levels are only one or two micrograms per milliliter over the usual therapeutic maximum. Because of this relationship, side effects and toxicity will be considered together. This relationship also underscores the need for proper monitoring of the patient throughout lidocaine therapy.

The side effects and adverse responses caused by lidocaine affect mainly the central nervous and cardiovascular systems. Therapeutic blood levels of lidocaine often cause drowsiness owing to CNS depression. Some practitioners consider this effect desirable, particularly if the patient is anxious because of a recent heart attack or surgical procedure. Other patients may experience dizziness or confusion. As blood levels rise, patients tend to become apprehensive or euphoric. With further increases, muscle tremor or twitching, visual disturbances, and numbness or tingling of the extremities (paresthesias) can occur. With true toxicity (blood levels $\geq$ 8 μg/mL), seizures, convulsions, and respiratory arrest occur.

Most patients experience side effects involving the CNS first, but cardiac and systemic cardiovascular changes eventually occur as lidocaine blood levels rise. They are apt to be seen earlier if the patient already has significant cardiovascular disease, such as heart failure. Progressive hypotension occurs owing to lidocaine's vasodilator and cardiac-depressant effects. With higher or toxic blood levels, profound hypotension, bradycardia, and eventual cardiac arrest can occur. The cardiovascular effects usually can, and should, be detected through proper monitoring of blood pressure and the ECG.

Chapter 18 identified some key contraindications for the use of lidocaine as a local anesthetic (eg, prior allergic reactions). Comments above also indicated the potential dangers of giving this drug to manage arrhythmias confined mainly to the atria. However, *if the patient is experiencing any life-threatening arrhythmia for which lidocaine is indicated, there is no contraindication to the drug's use.*

The adverse effects caused by lidocaine overdoses can progress quickly from mild to life-threatening. There is no antidote to specifically counteract the drug's effects, so early recognition of problems is essential. If toxicity occurs or is suspected, the first goal is to at least slow the IV infusion, and notify the physician immediately. With serious responses, lidocaine administration should be stopped altogether. Use standard CPR protocols as needed. Anticipate the use of anticonvulsants (eg, IV diazepam) for seizures, and the need for IV fluid or vasopressor drugs to support circulatory function. When time permits, obtain blood samples so they can be analyzed for lidocaine levels.

NURSING IMPLICATIONS

Monitor for important signs of lidocaine toxicity affecting the cardiovascular and central nervous systems. The drug's low margin of safety necessitates immediate notification of a physician, and usually an immediate reduction of the dose, if any untoward sign or symptom occurs. Prompt recognition and management of adverse reactions can prevent more serious consequences.

◆ Use During Pregnancy and Lactation

The use of lidocaine as an emergency antiarrhythmic drug is not contraindicated in pregnancy. However, breast-feeding should be discontinued if possible during prolonged administration.

◆ Use in Children

If lidocaine must be used for life-threatening arrhythmias, the recommended dose is 1 mg/kg initially, followed by an infusion of 30 μg/kg/min.

◆ Use in the Elderly

Dosage reductions may be required to compensate for reduced lidocaine elimination, particularly in patients over 60 years old. Assess closely for side effects, which may be more prevalent or severe in elderly persons.

Interactions with Other Drugs

The two most important interactants with lidocaine are propranolol and cimetidine, both of which are widely used. These drugs reduce hepatic metabolism of lidocaine, thereby increasing lidocaine blood levels and the risk of toxicity. If it is known that the patient is taking one of these interactants, the lidocaine dose and its rate of injection or infusion should be reduced. Monitor lidocaine blood levels to help with dosage adjustments during prolonged therapy. Obviously, the patient's medication history may not be known when lidocaine is used in an emergency. Some toxicity may be unavoidable, so always look for signs and symptoms.

Related Drugs

The other Class IB antiarrhythmics are mexiletine, tocainide, and phenytoin.

Mexiletine and Tocainide

Mexiletine (MEXITIL) and tocainide (TONOCARD) are orally effective antiarrhythmics. They are chemically related to lidocaine, and are used for prophylaxis of the same symptomatic ventricular arrhythmias that would be treated acutely with lidocaine. However, other orally effective drugs (eg, procainamide or β-blockers) usually should be tried before mexiletine or tocainide are turned to. Dosages are summarized in Table 30–C. Lower tocainide doses should be used for patients who have impaired renal or hepatic function. Hepatic function is the most important factor in making mexiletine dosage adjustments.

Either drug tends to cause nausea or other signs and symptoms of GI upset; lightheadedness; and tremor. Giving the drug with meals tends to reduce the problems significantly. Tocainide has caused agranulocytosis and evidence of pulmonary damage, so periodic blood tests and assessment of lung function are recommended. Otherwise, most of the precautions noted for lidocaine apply to these related drugs.

Phenytoin

Phenytoin is one of the most widely used anticonvulsant drugs (see Chapter 26, pp 476–480 for more information). It is *not approved* for use as an antiarrhythmic, but it is occasionally used for that purpose, mainly as an alternative to lidocaine (ie, a second-choice agent) to treat acute digitalis-induced arrhythmias. It is given by slow IV injection; rapid administration can cause cardiac depression, with the potential for hypotension, heart failure, or cardiac arrest. Dosages are listed in Table 30–C.

Class IC Agents

Encainide, Flecainide, Indecainide, and Propafenone

The Class IC agents reduce automaticity and electrical impulse conduction rates through the AV node and the ventricles. These properties account for the desired effects of these drugs on ventricular arrhythmias. They also account for a risk of serious or even fatal *proarrhythmic* (arrhythmia-causing or -worsening) effects, which are the most important adverse effects of these drugs.

Findings from one large clinical study (see Annotated Bibliography) showed that nearly twice as many post–myocardial infarction arrhythmia patients receiving either encainide (ENKAID) or flecainide (TAMBOCOR) experienced fatal or nonfatal cardiac arrest, associated with arrhythmias, than did patients receiving a placebo. The causes of death included bradycardia, complete heart block, and ventricular fibrillation. There is less information about risks associated with the newer drugs indecainide (DECABID; approved, not yet marketed) and propafenone (RYTHMOL), but it is wise to assume that the risks are similar for all the drugs in this class.

Because of the potential dangers, these orally effective drugs should be used only for ventricular arrhythmias that are symptomatic and are judged to pose a great risk of death without treatment—sustained ventricular tachycardia, for example. None of these drugs should be used for less severe arrhythmias (eg, occasional premature ventricular contractions). In any case, antiarrhythmic drugs in other classes should be tried first. Given the seriousness of the arrhythmias for which these drugs are indicated, treatment should start in the hospital. Dosages are listed in Table 30–C.

Dizziness, GI upset (including nausea and vomiting), headache, and visual disturbances are the most common noncardiac side effects of these drugs. The incidence and severity of these responses varies from drug to drug.

There is not much information about serious or common interactions between one of these antiarrhythmics and other drugs. The best advice is to monitor for key indicators of inadequate or excessive effects of the medications.

NURSING IMPLICATIONS

Encainide's proarrhythmic effects were, no doubt, one reason why the drug's manufacturer voluntarily withdrew it from the market. Encainide is now available only on a limited basis, upon petition to the manufacturer, for patients who started taking it before the fall of 1991. If your patient is taking one of the other Class IC agents, keep abreast of new developments; further restrictions may be placed on them also.

Miscellaneous Class I Antiarrhythmic

Moricizine

Moricizine (ETHMOZINE) is a new orally effective antiarrhythmic. It has several electrophysiologic properties shared by the Class IA antiarrhythmics. However, its actions, uses, and adverse effects are more similar to those of the Class IC antiarrhythmics just discussed. The similarities include precautions about potentially fatal proarrhythmic effects in postinfarction patients.

Class II Antiarrhythmics: Beta-Adrenergic Blockers

The β-adrenergic blockers were discussed in detail in Chapter 15. These drugs act, in part, by antagonizing the effects of catecholamines (eg, epinephrine and norepinephrine) on the heart's β_1-adrenergic receptors. Their key electrophysiologic actions include

- decreased automaticity of the SA node, the heart's normal pacemaker. This tends to cause an overall slowing of heart rate. It accounts for the use of these drugs to manage supraventricular (eg, sinus) tachycardia.
- decreased automaticity of ectopic pacemakers, especially in the ventricules. This action explains the use of some of these drugs for managing such arrhythmias as premature ventricular contractions.
- decreased impulse conduction rates through the AV node. This effect is used therapeutically to prevent unwanted increases of ventricular rates, as might occur during atrial flutter or fibrillation, or when these arrhythmias are being stopped pharmacologically.

Blockade of the β_1-adrenergic receptors also decreases cardiac contractile force.

Three β-blockers are approved for use as antiarrhythmics. Dosages and specific indications are listed in Table 30–C. Propranolol (INDERAL), the prototype, can be given orally or intravenously. Acebutolol (SECTRAL) is given orally and is indicated only for ventricular arrhythmias. Esmolol (BREVIBLOC) is given only by IV infusion. That route is necessary because esmolol has a very short half-life and duration of action, owing to rapid metabolic inactivation in the bloodstream. That property is ideal for acute use, since the desired effects usually occur quickly, and unwanted effects that might occur will not last too long once esmolol administration is stopped.

The oral β-blockers are particularly useful for long-term management of ventricular arrhythmias that occur after myocardial infarction, following initial control with a drug such as lidocaine. Indeed, long-term administration of propranolol (and some of the alternatives) has the ability to reduce arrhythmia-related mortality following a heart attack. This "cardioprotective effect" is in distinct contrast to the ability of the Class IC antiarrhythmics (eg, encainide, flecainide) to favor the development of lethal arrhythmias in recent MI patients.

The β blockers are not without adverse effects and related contraindications. These drugs can depress cardiac contractility, thereby worsening or causing heart failure; lower blood glucose levels, and delay the recovery from hypoglycemia, thereby posing an added risk to persons with diabetes; and trigger severe or fatal bronchospasm, a definite risk in patients with asthma or obstructive lung disease.

See Chapter 15 (pp 231–239) for more information on general actions, side effects, contraindications, and drug interactions. The uses of the β-blockers for managing essential hypertension and angina pectoris are discussed in Chapters 33 and 34, respectively.

Class III Antiarrhythmics

The Class III antiarrhythmics prolong the repolarization time of each action potential, and make cardiac tissue more refractory to premature stimulation. The effect is particularly great in the ventricular myocardium and in the His bundles, which are the main conduction pathways in the ventricles. The two drugs in this class, amiodarone and bretylium, share uses for serious ventricular arrhythmias that cannot be controlled with any other drugs. Aside from this, they are very different agents, and neither can be considered a prototype.

Amiodarone

Amiodarone (CORDARONE) is an orally effective antiarrhythmic with some serious side effects and unusual pharmacokinetic properties. It is not a first-line drug. It is used for life-threatening ventricular arrhythmias that cannot be controlled with other medications.

Amiodarone is absorbed reasonably well. Peak blood levels occur within a few hours after dosing, but when therapy is started it may take 3 weeks or more for clinical effects (arrhythmia control) to appear. Amiodarone and its metabolites are stored in body tissues and eliminated very slowly. The overall half-life normally is about 50 *days*—far longer than for nearly any other drug you will encounter. As a result, adverse effects that might occur can take a very long time to resolve when the drug is discontinued.

Nausea and vomiting are fairly common side effects that can be alleviated by giving the drug in divided doses. However some of the drug's other adverse effects or toxicities (see Table 30–S) are clearly more serious. As summarized in Table 30–S, they can affect the lungs, liver, neural tissue, and thyroid status. In addition, they can be longlasting or irreversible, even when therapy is stopped, because of amiodarone's long half-life.

Amiodarone's slow onset of action and long half-life also make drug interactions (Table 30–I) slow to develop, detect, and resolve. The most serious interactions involve some widely used cardiovascular drugs: oral anticoagulants; digoxin; and quinidine and procainamide.

NURSING IMPLICATIONS

The arrhythmias for which amiodarone is indicated are serious. Therefore, therapy should be started in the hospital. Patience and vigilance are important when monitoring amiodarone therapy. Waiting for the drug's desired and adverse effects to occur can be frustrating. Nevertheless, close monitoring over such a long time is precisely what is necessary when this last-resort drug is used.

NURSING IMPLICATIONS

Monitor all patients for pulmonary dysfunction (wheezing, difficulty breathing), and notify the physician at once if there are any positive signs or symptoms. Stress to the patient the need for periodic liver function and thyroid hormone studies, eye examinations, and assessment of peripheral neuromuscular activity. Assess for signs of altered thyroid function, such as weight gain or loss. Advise patients to wear clothing that covers as much skin as possible to reduce the risk or severity of photosensitive skin rashes. Closely monitor prothrombin times of patients taking warfarin or other oral anticoagulants.

Bretylium

Bretylium (BRETYLOL) is indicated for the acute treatment of life-threatening arrhythmias—ventricular fibrillation or recurrent ventricular tachycardia—that have not responded to first-line emergency interventions (lidocaine, electrical defibrillation, CPR, etc). The drug has been referred to as having specific antifibrillatory action, since it often can stop fibrillation when all other drugs have failed to do so. Bretylium is usually given by IV injection, infusion, or both; dosages are in Table 30–C.

When bretylium is first given, it *causes* norepinephrine release from adrenergic nerves, including those supplying the heart and peripheral vasculature. (This sympathomimetic effect can temporarily worsen arrhythmias.) Moments later, the drug *blocks* norepinephrine release. This is the more important and prolonged effect, and it probably accounts for the antiarrhythmia control.

In the peripheral vasculature, inhibited norepinephrine release also causes hypotension. Reduced blood pressure is the most common side effect, and it can be severe. Since patients receiving bretylium are already in the supine position, syncope that could be triggered by decreased blood pressure is not a problem. However, if the patient's systolic blood pressure falls too much below 75 mm Hg, or stays there too long, interventions to restore blood pressure (IV fluids, vasopressors) may be needed. Notify the physician if this occurs.

Nausea and vomiting are also common side effects caused by bretylium.

There are no well-documented, serious and common drug interactions that are likely to occur in patients receiving bretylium.

Class IV Antiarrhythmics

The Class IV drugs act mainly by blocking the entry of calcium ion into the cardiac cell during key parts of the action potential.

There are more than half a dozen of these *calcium-channel blockers*—also called calcium antagonists—approved for use in the United States. Only one is approved for use as an oral and parenteral antiarrhythmic: verapamil. Calcium-channel blockers are used more as antihypertensive and antianginal drugs. Because of that, what follows is only an overview of verapamil's use as an antiarrhythmic drug. Refer to Chapter 33 for more information about using calcium-channel blockers as antihypertensive agents. Chapter 34 (which deals with angina pectoris) gives more detailed comments about verapamil, the prototype of all the calcium-channel blockers.

Verapamil

Verapamil (ISOPTIN, CALAN) is available in immediate-acting and slow-release oral dosage forms, and in injectable formulations. Only the immediate-acting oral and parenteral forms are used for arrhythmias. Dosages are summarized in Table 30–C.

Verapamil depresses automaticity and impulse conduction rates, and increases the refractoriness of cardiac tissues to premature stimulation. The effects are particularly great on the SA and AV nodes. Immediate-acting oral dosage forms are used for long-term control of supraventricular arrhythmias. It is most effective for arrhythmias that involve reentry of premature electrical impulses from the ventricles, through the AV node, and back to the ventricles. Intravenous administration is used for acute therapy. (Since the approval of adenosine, discussed in the next section, the use of IV verapamil has decreased.)

Verapamil's ability to depress electrical activity in the SA and AV nodes generally is desirable. However, if the patient has nodal disease (eg, "sick sinus syndrome," which is common in the elderly), verapamil may cause excessive depression, possibly leading to conduction block. A history of nodal disease is a relative contraindication to verapamil use, and necessitates the use of smaller-than-usual dosages. Similarly, verapamil should be used cautiously, if at all, if the patient is already receiving another drug that can depress nodal tissue, especially the AV node. Digoxin and β blockers are the most important examples.

Another concern is excessive depression of cardiac contractility, and the risk of inducing heart failure. This risk is greater in persons who already have advanced heart failure; in patients with normal contractile function, but who receive IV doses that are too high or given too fast; and in patients who are receiving other cardiac depressant drugs (eg, β blockers). Giving IV verapamil too fast can also cause hypotension.

Gastrointestinal disturbances, particularly constipation, are the most common side effects associated with oral verapamil therapy. See Chapter 34 for more general information about side effects and drug interactions of verapamil and other calcium-channel blockers.

Miscellaneous Antiarrhythmics

Several drugs or drug classes have antiarrhythmic activity, but they do not fit in any of the above categories.

Adenosine

Adenosine (ADENOCARD) inhibits SA and (especially) AV nodal impulse conduction. Its major use is the acute treatment of supraventricular arrhythmias, particularly those that involve reentry to the ventricles via the AV node (see Table 30–C for doses). Adenosine has replaced IV verapamil as the preferred agent because adenosine works quickly, and side effects that might occur usually last less than a minute because the drug is cleared from the bloodstream in less than a minute by metabolism. Adenosine's cardiovascular side effects include hypotension and atrial fibrillation. Other side effects include facial flushing, sweating, headache, or dizziness, in response to vasodilation; and nausea.

Atropine

Atropine is the prototype antimuscarinic drug (Chapter 13). It exerts its cardiac effects by blocking the receptors that mediate acetylcholine's inhibitory effects on the SA and AV nodes. As an antiarrhythmic drug, atropine is used mainly to manage sinus bradycardia or AV block. Some indications include the prevention or treatment of bradycardia that occurs during surgery; bradycardia and hypotension that occurs following a heart attack; syncope that may be caused by bradycardia owing to a hyperactive carotid sinus (baroreceptor) reflex; and reversal of AV block that might occur with digitalis overdoses. The drug is usually given by IV injection; dosages are summarized in Table 30–C. See pages 167 to 179 for a complete description of atropine's actions, uses, side effects, and so on.

Digoxin

Digoxin has been mentioned in several parts of this chapter in regard to its antiarrhythmic actions. It can be used alone, or with other drugs (eg, quinidine; see above), to help control ventricular rates in patients with atrial or supraventricular arrhythmias: atrial flutter or fibrillation, and paroxysmal supraventricular tachycardia. Digoxin exerts direct and indirect (atropine-like) actions to slow impulse conduction through the AV node. This helps regulate the number of impulses that reach and activate the ventricles in a given time. (Depending on the patient, other drugs that inhibit AV nodal transmission may be used instead of digoxin—verapamil or a β blocker, for example.) Digoxin can be given intravenously for immediate effects and acute arrhythmia control, or orally for maintenance therapy or when immediate antiarrhythmic effects are not essential.

More complete information about digoxin's actions, uses, adverse effects, and drug interactions is found in Chapter 31. However, several key points should be made here, because they relate specifically to digoxin's use as an antiarrhythmic.

- Electrical cardioversion usually is the preferred treatment for atrial flutter. However, digoxin increases the heart's sensitivity to electrical shock, increasing the risk of ventricular fibrillation. If cardioversion and electrical shock are planned for a patient, cardioversion should be done first, and digoxin given later and only if needed. If the patient is already receiving digoxin (as for heart failure), and elective cardioversion of an atrial arrhythmia is planned, it is best to discontinue the digoxin about 3 days before, if possible.
- Ordinarily, do not give digoxin with other drugs that depress AV nodal conduction (eg, verapamil or a β blocker). Giving them together increases the risk of AV block. If combined therapy is essential, use reduced doses of one or both drugs.
- Digoxin may be a logical pretreatment when an atrial arrhythmia is to be managed with quinidine. However, quinidine can elevate digoxin levels and

effects in several ways, posing the risk of digoxin toxicity. Lower-than-usual doses of digoxin are indicated to minimize the risk. Quinidine should never be used to manage digoxin-induced arrhythmias, and digoxin should not be used for treating arrhythmias caused by quinidine.

Digoxin can be used to control ventricular rate in some patients with Wolff–Parkinson–White (WPW) syndrome. In this arrhythmia impulses reenter the ventricles through both a normal (AV nodal) and abnormal pathway. Digoxin will desirably reduce conduction through the AV node. However, it should not be given to patients with WPW syndrome who also have atrial fibrillation. In this instance digoxin will inhibit impulses from the atria to the ventricles via the AV node. However, it may simultaneously increase impulses through the abnormal pathway. This can trigger ventricular tachycardia or fibrillation. Quinidine, procainamide, or a β blocker are better alternatives for these patients.

Sympathomimetics

Epinephrine and isoproterenol (see Chapter 14, pp 191–197 and 203–204) have some use as antiarrhythmics. They increase automaticity of the SA node, and electrical impulse conduction through the AV node. Either drug can be used to manage Stokes–Adams syndrome, a condition in which there are episodes of AV block that cause syncope. Epinephrine can be used for acute treatment (by the IV route); isoproterenol is used mainly for long-term management (rectal or sublingual route). Parenteral epinephrine is also used as part of standard CPR protocols, along with chest compression and electrical defibrillation, to manage cardiac arrest. Ideally it is given intravenously; alternative administration routes (instillation into an endotracheal tube, or intracardiac injection) can be used when it is not possible to establish IV access.

"Pure" Vasopressors and Acetylcholinesterase Inhibitors

Drugs in two other pharmacologic classes are occasionally given for acute management of paroxysmal atrial tachycardia. They are used mainly when other interventions, such as carotid massage, fail to stop the arrhythmia. Whether one approach is used instead of another depends mainly on unique characteristics of each patient, including medical conditions that may contraindicate the use of a particular drug.

Methoxamine and phenylephrine are sympathomimetics that act mainly as vasoconstrictors. Their major use is to treat acute hypotension (see pp 200–203). However, they have some value for treating paroxysmal atrial tachycardia. When given by IV injection, they abruptly increase blood pressure and trigger the baroreceptor reflex (much like carotid massage does). That inhibits sympathetic outflow to the heart (and elsewhere) and causes intense parasympathetic activation. The acetylcholine that is released by the vagus nerve at the SA node often stops the tachycardia. Since this approach depends on the drug's ability to increase blood pressure, it should not be used for patients who are already severely hypertensive, or who are at risk of further blood pressure increases (eg, persons with a history of stroke or ischemic heart disease).

An alternative approach is to inject edrophonium, a rapidly acting acetylcholinesterase inhibitor (p 159). By inhibiting the breakdown of acetylcholine, edrophonium intensifies the cardiac-slowing effects of acetylcholine. One of the most important side effects of edrophonium is its ability to trigger severe bronchoconstriction in persons with asthma or chronic obstructive pulmonary disease. Use other approaches to stop the tachycardia for these patients.

SUMMARY OF NURSING IMPLICATIONS

◆ Assessment

Assess cardiac rhythm and rate and vital signs before initiating treatment.

Review the medication history for drugs requiring cautious concurrent use of antiarrhythmics.

Establish baseline laboratory values to recognize drug effects.

Note the presence of severe heart failure, heart block, or hypotension, which require cautious use of antiarrhythmics.

◆ Nursing Diagnoses

Decreased cardiac output related to arrhythmias.

Knowledge deficit related to antiarrhythmic drug therapy.

Altered nutrition: less than body requirements related to nausea and loss of appetite from medication.

Constipation or diarrhea related to drug effects.

Activity intolerance related to weakness and fatigue from drug therapy.

◆ Planning/Implementation

Observe ECG and vital signs for excessive drug action: depression of cardiac electrical activity (widening QRS complex); changes in heart rate (>15 beats/min above normal rate or <55 beats/min); depressed contractility; acute hypotension.

Prepare equipment for monitoring and life-support before giving a parenteral antiarrhythmic.

Administer IV lidocaine with an infusion pump whenever possible.

Observe for signs of CNS toxicity with lidocaine and its derivatives, mexiletine and tocainide: nervousness, agitation, or dizziness.

Observe for drug-induced ventricular fibrillation or hypertension initially with bretylium; thereafter, expect hypotension; notify physician if systolic pressure falls below 75 mm Hg.

With procainamide, observe for excessive cardiac depression (signs of heart failure, hypotension), AV block (excessive prolongation of the P–R interval), excessive widening of the QRS complex (0.12 sec or longer); signs of lupus-like state: skin rashes, muscle aches, flu-like symptoms.

Give quinidine with water at least 1 hour before or 2 hours after meals to improve absorption; may be taken with meals if GI upset is severe; ensure daily consistency with timing of administration.

With quinidine, monitor for signs of cinchonism, particularly visual or auditory changes (tinnitus, double vision); muscle weakness may indicate underlying myasthenia gravis.

With disopyramide, monitor for congestive heart failure, urinary retention, ocular pain; notify physician at once.

Monitor for signs of pulmonary toxicity (eg, wheezing, breathing difficulty) or hepatic dysfunction if amiodarone is used.

◆ Patient and Family Teaching

Teach the patient and family:

How to count radial pulse and the carotid pulse for 1 full minute each morning before arising; report irregularities at once.

To keep a written record of pulse rate and regularity for physician review.

The importance of follow-up blood tests as required by administered drug.

To report major or important adverse effects of administered drug.

To use nondrug measures to manage appropriate side effects (eg, frequent sips of water, or hard candies, if dry mouth is bothersome with disopyramide).

To avoid excessive exposure to sunlight, which can aggravate photosensitive drug rashes with amiodarone.

To take drugs either with or without food consistently to ensure consistent rate of absorption.

◆ Evaluation

The patient/family will:

Achieve desired therapeutic blood level of antiarrhythmic medication without serious adverse effects.

Maintain sinus rhythm; apical pulse will be regular; vital signs will be within normal limits.

Take medications as prescribed.

Annotated Bibliography

Anderson JL. Clinical implications of new studies in the treatment of benign, potentially malignant and malignant ventricular arrhythmias. *Am J Cardiol* 1990;65(4):36B–42B. *This article should be important to nurses as members of the health-care team, and advocates for patients. The basic message: antiarrhythmic drug prescribing habits need to be reassessed.*

Berns E, Naccarelli GV. Management of tachyarrhythmias after MI. *Hosp Pract [Off]* 1990;25(4):33–43. *A practical review of management of arrhythmias that occur after infarction; stresses the need to identify therapeutic end-points and to use them as a guide to therapy.*

Brown CE, Wendel GD. Cardiac arrhythmias during pregnancy. *Clin Obstet Gynecol* 1989;32(1):89–102. *Covers much of what is known about antiarrhythmic drug therapy in pregnancy, concludes that "older" drugs should be used until more is known about potential risks of using newer ones.*

Cardiac Arrhythmia Suppression Trial (CAST) Investigators. Preliminary report: Effect of encainide and flecainide on mortality in a randomized trial of arrhythmia suppression after myocardial infarction. *N Engl J Med* 1989;321:406–412. *This landmark study showed that using either of these antiarrhythmics to treat asymptomatic or mildly symptomatic post-MI arrhythmias increased the sudden death rate.*

Chan KY, Yip WC, Tay JS. Cardiovascular pharmacological therapy in children—a review. Drug therapy for cardiac arrhythmias. *J Singapore Paediatr Soc* 1989;31(1–2):14–25. *Another important summary paper for nurses dealing with pediatric arrhythmia patients; one in a series of articles covering cardiovascular disease in children.*

Garrett MM. Practical management of atrial fibrillation. *Postgrad Med* 1990;87(1):40–45, 49. *Discusses the values of cardioversion, antiarrhythmic drugs, and long-term anticoagulation for treatment of patients with this very common arrhythmia.*

Klitzner TS, Friedman WF. Cardiac arrhythmias: The role of pharmacologic intervention. *Cardiol Clin* 1989;7(2):299–318. *Of special interest to pediatric nurses, this paper relates knowledge of anatomy, electrophysiology, and basic pharmacology to the selection of antiarrhythmic drugs for children.*

Lucas WJ, Maccioli GA, Mueller RA. Advances in oral anti-arrhythmic therapy: Implications for the anaesthetist. *Can J Anaesth* 1990;37(1):94–101. *Nurse-anesthetists, as well as other nurses dealing mainly with "fresh post-op" patients, should find this well worth reading.*

Moore GP, Munter DW. Wolff-Parkinson-White syndrome: Illustrative case and brief review. *J Emerg Med* 1989;7(1):47–54. *A case study based review of WPW etiology, signs and symptoms, and therapy.*

Podrid PJ, Levine PA, Klein MP. Effect of age on antiarrhythmic drug efficacy and toxicity. *Am J Cardiol* 1989;63(11):735–739. *An important and practical paper on this very important topic.*

Pratt CM, Moye LA. The Cardiac Arrhythmia Suppression Trial: Background, interim results and implications. *Am J Cardiol* 1990; 65(4):20B–29B. *Important take-home messages from a now well-known clinical study (the CAST study), which showed unexpected risks from drugs hoped to provide significant therapeutic benefits.*

Rodriguez RD, Schocken DD. Update on sick sinus syndrome, a cardiac disorder of aging. *Geriatrics* 1990;45(1):26–30, 33–36. *Focuses on one of the most common cardiac rhythm disorders of aging, and the drugs that can worsen it.*

Singh BN. Advantages of beta blockers versus antiarrhythmic agents and calcium antagonists in secondary prevention after myocardial infarction. *Am J Cardiol* 1990;66(9):9C–20C. *Discusses drugs that can either reduce or potentially increase arrhythmia risks in heart attack survivors.*

Singh BN. Do antiarrhythmic drugs work? Some reflections on the implications of the Cardiac Arrhythmia Suppression Trial. *Clin Cardiol* 1990;13(10):725–728. *A thought-provoking discussion of how some antiarrhythmic drugs may not only "fail to work," but may also make matters worse for some patients.*

Surawicz B. Ventricular arrhythmias: Why is it so difficult to find a pharmacologic cure? *J Am Coll Cardiol* 1989;14(6):1401–1416. *Helps understand the answers to two key questions: Why isn't there a universal antiarrhythmic drug, and why do we need still more?*

Surawicz B. What determines the choice of treatment in patients with supraventricular tachycardia? *Cardiol Clin* 1990;8(3):523–533. *Unique and worth reading for its succinct, specific recommendations for antiarrhythmic therapy in patients with a variety of other medical disorders (angina, MI, CHF, pulmonary disease, diabetes, etc).*

Weiner B. Second generation antidysrhythmic agents. *Crit Care Nurs Clin North Am* 1989;1(2):417–422. *A short but worth-reading review of some of the newer antiarrhythmic agents: actions, uses, benefits, and limitations.*

Weller DM, Noone J. Mechanisms of arrhythmias: Enhanced automaticity and reentry. *Crit Care Nurse* 1989;9(5):42–67. *A good review of automaticity and reentry as causes of arrhythmias, and of the antiarrhythmic drug classes used to combat these causes.*

Wood DL. Potentially lethal ventricular arrhythmias: Minimizing the danger. *Postgrad Med* 1990;88(6):65–67, 70–71, 74. *Explains how proper drug selection and monitoring can help reduce the risks of an already serious medical problem.*

Table 30–C | **Clinical Uses and Administration of Major Antiarrhythmic Drugs***

AGENT	CLINICAL USES	DOSAGE AND ROUTE OF ADMINISTRATION
PROTOTYPE		
Acebutolol		
(SECTRAL)	Premature ventricular contractions	Oral: Initially, 200 mg bid; increase gradually as needed to 600–1200 mg/d
Adenosine		
(ADENOCARD)	Paroxysmal supraventricular tachycardia, including that associated with Wolff-Parkinson-White syndrome	IV: 6 mg as bolus (inject over 1–2 sec); if needed, repeat with 12 mg 1–2 min later; second 12-mg dose can be given if needed
Amiodarone		
(CORDARONE)	Life-threatening recurrent ventricular arrhythmias refractory to other drugs (eg, recurrent ventricular fibrillation, unstable ventricular tachycardia)	Oral: Initially, 800–1600 mg/d for 1–3 weeks; if possible, reduce to 600–800 mg/d for 1 month, maintain at 400 mg/d; give daily doses ≥ 1000 mg in two equal divided doses with meals
Bretylium		
(BRETYLOL)	Refractory ventricular fibrillation	IV: Initially, 5 mg/kg of undiluted (50 mg/mL) drug along with CPR; repeat 10 mg/kg if arrhythmia not converted, and again at 15–30-min intervals up to 30 mg/kg total. Maintenance: 5–10 mg/kg q6h or infuse 1–2 mg/kg
	Treatment, prophylaxis of recurrent ventricular tachycardia, fibrillation	IV: Dilute 1:5 with D_5W, infuse total dose of 5–10 mg/kg over 10–30 min IM: 5–10 mg/kg of undiluted drug; no more than 250 mg should be given into single injection site
Digoxin		
(LANOXIN)	Supraventricular arrhythmias; control of ventricular rate during conversion of atrial fibrillation, flutter	IV: 0.75 mg followed by 0.25 mg q4h–q6h until ventricular rate <100
Disopyramide		
(NORPACE; NORPACE CR)	PVCs, ventricular tachycardia	Oral: 150 mg of regular dosage form q6h; or 300 mg of controlled-release form q12h
Encainide		
(ENKAID)	Life-threatening symptomatic arrhythmias (eg, sustained ventricular tachycardia)	Oral: Usually 25 mg q8h; may increase, at 3- to 5-day intervals, to 35–50 mg tid (drug withdrawn from market; limited availability from manufacturer; see text)
Esmolol		
(BREVIBLOC)	Supraventricular tachycardia, sinus tachycardia, atrial flutter or fibrillation	IV: Usual dose is 500 µg/kg/min for 1 min, then decrease to 50 µg/kg/min; most arrhythmias respond to 100 µg/kg/min average
Flecainide		
(TAMBOCOR)	Life-threatening symptomatic arrhythmias (as for encainide)	Oral: Initially 100 mg q12h; maintenance dose is 50 mg q12h, maximum dose is 400 mg/d

(continued)

Table 30–C | Clinical Uses and Administration of Major Antiarrhythmic Drugs* (*Continued*)

AGENT	CLINICAL USES	DOSAGE AND ROUTE OF ADMINISTRATION
PROTOTYPE		
Idecainide (DECABID)	Severe ventricular arrhythmias deemed to be life-threatening (eg, sustained ventricular tachycardia)	Oral: Initially 50 mg q12h; if needed, increase at ≥4-day intervals to maintenance dose (75–200 mg bid)
Lidocaine (XYLOCAINE)	Ventricular tachycardia or fibrillation; arrhythmias due to anesthesia, drugs	IV: Adults: Initially, 50–100 mg bolus (about 0.7–1.4 mg/kg) at 25–50 mg/min; once arrhythmia is controlled, continue infusion of 1–4 mg/min. Children: Usually 1 mg/kg initially, followed by infusion of 30 μg/kg/min. For adults and children, switch to oral therapy with alternative as soon as possible IM: Adults: Usually 300 mg (about 4.3 mg/kg); repeat in 60 to 90 min if needed; otherwise begin IV infusion; switch to oral administration of suitable alternative as soon as possible
Mexiletine (MEXITIL)	Treatment of symptomatic ventricular tachycardia, couplets, frequent PVCs	Oral: Usually start with 200 mg q8h; after 2 or 3 days increase by 50–100 mg based on response; usual maintenance dose is 200–300 mg q8h; keep below 1200 mg/d if possible; for rapid arrhythmia control use loading dose of 400 mg, then 200 mg q8h
Moricizine (ETHMOZINE)	Severe ventricular arrhythmias deemed to be life-threatening (see encainide)	Oral: Usually 200–300 mg q8h
Phenytoin (DILANTIN)	Chronic or acute treatment of digitalis-induced arrhythmias, other arrhythmias for which lidocaine might be used	IV: Initially, 100 mg given slowly; repeat at 5–10-min intervals until arrhythmias are controlled or total dose of 1 g is given, whichever comes first Oral: Maintenance is 100 mg bid or tid
Procainamide (PRONESTYL)	Atrial fibrillation	Oral: Initially, 1.25 g followed by 1 g q4h–q6h, up to a maximum daily dose of 50 mg/kg. For long-acting preparations, begin therapy with regular procainamide, then give 1 g of long-acting product q6h
	Ventricular arrhythmias	Oral: Initially, 1 g followed by total daily dose of 50 mg/kg given as divided doses at 3-hr intervals (eg, 6 mg/kg q3h) IM: 50 mg/kg/d in 3–6 divided doses IV: 100 mg, given slowly every 5 min until arrhythmia stops; or infuse 500–600 mg over 30 min

(continued)

Table 30–C Clinical Uses and Administration of Major Antiarrhythmic Drugs* (*Continued*)

AGENT	CLINICAL USES	DOSAGE AND ROUTE OF ADMINISTRATION
PROTOTYPE		
Propafenone		
(RYTHMOL)	Severe ventricular arrhythmias deemed to be life-threatening (see encainide)	Oral: Initially 150 mg q8h; gradually increase as needed to 225 or 300 mg q8h
Propranolol		
(INDERAL)	Supraventricular arrhythmias	Oral: 20–40 mg tid or qid IV: 0.5–3 mg/kg when rapid effects are needed
Quinidine		
(CARDIOQUIN, others)	Atrial fibrillation, flutter; Wolff-Parkinson-White syndrome	Oral: Initially, 200 mg q2h up to 1 g total Maintenance dose: 200–300 q6h. Extended-acting tablets (eg, QUINIDEX EXTENTABS): Divide daily dose of regular quinidine in 2 or 3 equal doses. IV: Initially, 5–10 mg/kg given over 30–60 min; switch to oral therapy as soon as possible
Tocainide		
(TONOCARD)	As for lidocaine (not for emergency use)	Oral: Initially, 400 mg q8h; maintain with 400–600 mg tid
Verapamil		
(CALAN, ISOPTIN)	Supraventricular arrhythmias	Oral: For nondigitalized patients, usually 240–480 mg/d in 3 or 4 divided doses; for digitalized patients with chronic atrial fibrillation, 240–320 mg/d in 3 or 4 divided doses IV: 75–150 µg/kg given over 2 min; give 10 mg more 30 min later if needed

*Arranged alphabetically according to generic name.

Table 30–S Major Side Effects of and Contraindications for Antiarrhythmic Drugs*

BODY SYSTEM/ Side Effect	CONTRAINDICATION/ PRECAUTION	COMMENTS AND NURSING IMPLICATIONS
Amiodarone		
EYE Corneal deposits, impaired vision		Examine eyes, check vision, periodically
ENDOCRINE Elevation of serum thyroxine and iodine levels		Monitor thyroid function, serum thyroid hormones, and iodine periodically; assess for signs of hyper- or hypothyroidism
RESPIRATORY Progressive cough, dyspnea; pulmonary fibrosis	Poor pulmonary function	Monitor; pulmonary changes usually reversible if detected early and drug is discontinued; toxicity has been fatal
SKIN Blue-gray skin discoloration, worsened by light		Advise patient to reduce exposure to sunlight, wear suitable protective clothing
Bretylium		
CARDIOVASCULAR Hypotension with dizziness, syncope	Systolic pressure <75 mm Hg during maintenance therapy	Most common effect with maintenance therapy; monitor BP closely
Aggravation of digitalis-induced arrhythmias	Digitalis intoxication	Lidocaine is preferred for digitalis-induced arrhythmias; avoid using other antiarrhythmics
Digoxin		
CARDIOVASCULAR AV block	Heart block ≥ 2nd degree	See Chapter 31
Atrial, ventricular premature contractions		
Disopyramide		
EYE Eye pain; day-blindness	Glaucoma	Antimuscarinic actions; recommend sunglasses if bright lights cause pain; rule out glaucoma; have patient report eye pain immediately
CARDIOVASCULAR Hypotension, decreased cardiac output	Preexisting hypotension or severe heart failure	See lidocaine
Worsening of ventricular tachyarrhythmias	Atrial fibrillation, flutter	See lidocaine
GASTROINTESTINAL Dry mouth; constipation	Severe preexisting constipation	Antimuscarinic actions; sipping water, sucking hard candies may reduce problems due to dry mouth; adequate intake of fluids, bulk-forming foods may reduce problems due to constipation; have patient report sudden changes of bowel habits

(continued)

Table 30–S | **Major Side Effects of and Contraindications for Antiarrhythmic Drugs* (*Continued*)**

BODY SYSTEM/ Side Effect	CONTRAINDICATION/ PRECAUTION	COMMENTS AND NURSING IMPLICATIONS
GENITOURINARY Urinary hesitancy, retention	Prostatic hypertrophy or obstruction of GU tract	Antimuscarinic actions; monitor fluid intake, output; inquire about difficulty with urination
NEUROMUSCULAR Muscle weakness, fatigability	Myasthenia gravis	See quinidine
OTHER Nervousness; excessive hunger; weakness; thready pulse, palpitations	Poorly controlled diabetes mellitus	
Encainide, Flecainide, Indecainide, Moricizine, Propafenone		
CENTRAL NERVOUS SYSTEM Dizziness, blurred vision		Relatively common; observe patient; have patient report frequency, severity of these side effects
CARDIOVASCULAR Fatal arrhythmias; hypotension, decreased cardiac output	Recent MI, nonsymptomatic or usually innocuous arrhythmias	Monitor ECG routinely
Lidocaine, Mexiletine, Tocainide		
CENTRAL NERVOUS SYSTEM Sedation, drowsiness, paresthesias, CNS stimulation with increasing blood levels, leading to convulsions		Drowsiness common with therapeutic doses; may progress to massive convulsions; monitor neurologic status, drug blood levels; careful titration of dose reduces incidence of CNS problems
CARDIOVASCULAR Ventricular tachycardia	Atrial fibrillation or flutter (caution)	Administer cautiously to patients with atrial arrhythmias, since lidocaine has negligible effects on AV conduction at therapeutic doses
Heart block, cardiac arrest	Preexisting 2nd- or 3rd-degree heart block	High doses of lidocaine may suppress AV impulse conduction
Hypotension, decreased cardiac output	Preexisting hypotension or severe heart failure	Mainly with high doses; treatment of dangerous arrhythmias with lidocaine takes priority over problems with BP
GASTROINTESTINAL Nausea, vomiting, dyspepsia (mexiletine, tocainide)		Administer mexiletine, tocainide with meals, milk, or antacids if GI distress is severe

(continued)

Table 30–S Major Side Effects of and Contraindications for Antiarrhythmic Drugs* (*Continued*)

BODY SYSTEM/ Side Effect	CONTRAINDICATION/ PRECAUTION	COMMENTS AND NURSING IMPLICATIONS
Procainamide		
BLOOD Appearance of antinuclear antibodies; lupus-like syndrome		Baseline and subsequent periodic blood tests are indicated; assess for signs of lupus-like syndrome (arthralgia, myalgia, fever) so drug administration can be stopped if needed
CARDIOVASCULAR Prolonged AV conduction; AV block; decreased cardiac output; hypotension, syncope	Existence of any of the listed side effects	Baseline ECG and other vital signs are essential, must be closely monitored; prolonged Q–T interval is useful sign of excessive drug action
Propranolol, Other β Blockers		
CARDIOVASCULAR Bradycardia, heart block	Heart rate <40; heart block ≥2nd degree	See Chapter 15, Table 15–S
OTHER See Chapter 15, Table 15–S		
Quinidine		
CENTRAL NERVOUS SYSTEM Cinchonism: GI distress, tinnitus; visual changes (diplopia; altered color perception); dizziness		Monitor for pertinent signs; report to physician for possible dosage reduction
BLOOD Thrombocytopenia	Coagulation disorders	Monitor for signs of excessive or unusual bleeding or bruising; recommend periodic blood tests
CARDIOVASCULAR See procainamide	Digoxin-induced arrhythmias	
NEUROMUSCULAR Muscle weakness	Myasthenia gravis	Assess for weakness, fatigability that might indicate underlying disease
Verapamil: See Table 34–S, p 000		

*Drugs are listed alphabetically for ease of location.

Table 30–I **Major Interactions Between Antiarrhythmics and Other Agents***

AGENT	RESULT OF INTERACTION	COMMENTS AND NURSING IMPLICATIONS
Interactions Involving All Antiarrhythmics		
Other antiarrhythmics	Potential excessive depression of cardiac electrical activity, contractility	Combined use, when unavoidable, requires more vigilance, frequent monitoring of ECG, BP, etc; specific contraindicated combinations are noted below
Interactions Involving Amiodarone		
Anticoagulants, oral (Chapter 35)	Decreased metabolism, significantly increased effects, of anticoagulant	Potentially serious interaction that develops slowly when amiodarone is started; monitor prothrombin time more closely; may eventually necessitate reducing anticoagulant dose by as much as 50%; assess for evidence of excessive anticoagulation
Digoxin (Chapter 31)	Increased digoxin levels; potential toxicity	Serious, of slow onset as with anticoagulants; monitor digoxin levels closely; both drugs can cause similar (additive) signs of toxicity
Phenytoin (Chapter 26)	Increased phenytoin levels, effects; potential toxicity; decreased amiodarone levels, effects	Interactants alter metabolism of one another; monitor accordingly
Procainamide	See procainamide, below	
Quinidine	See quinidine, below	
Interactions Involving Disopyramide		
Hydantoins (eg, phenytoin; Chapter 26)	Increased disopyramide metabolism, decreased blood levels and effects; increased incidence or severity of antimuscarinic side effects	Monitor accordingly
Rifampin (Chapter 57)	Increased disopyramide metabolism, decreased blood levels, effects	Monitor accordingly
Interactions Involving Lidocaine		
β-Blockers (Chapter 15)	Decreased lidocaine metabolism, increased blood levels and risk of toxicity	Reduce lidocaine bolus, infusion rates; monitor lidocaine levels frequently; interaction most important with propranolol, may occur with atenolol, nadolol, pindolol
Cimetidine (Chapter 40)	As for β-blockers, above	As for β-blockers; cimetidine alternatives (famotidine, ranitidine) do not seem to interact
Succinylcholine (Chapter 17)	Prolonged neuromuscular blockade, muscle paralysis	Anticipate interaction, be prepared for longer support of ventilation
Interactions Involving Mexiletine		
Phenytoin (Chapter 26)	Decreased mexiletine effects	Monitor; see other listings for hydantoins
Theophylline, other methylxanthines (Chapter 38)	Potentially increased serum theophylline levels, toxicity	Monitor theophyline levels more closely, assess, especially for CNS stimulation

(continued)

Table 30–I Major Interactions Between Antiarrhythmics and Other Agents* (*Continued*)

AGENT	RESULT OF INTERACTION	COMMENTS AND NURSING IMPLICATIONS
Interaction Involving Moricizine		
Cimetidine (Chapter 40)	Decreased metabolism, increased blood levels, effects of moricizine	Monitor accordingly; see other interactions listing cimetidine
Interactions Involving Procainamide		
Amiodarone	Potentially marked increase of procainamide blood levels, effects, toxicity risk	Avoid interaction; otherwise, monitor clinical effects and procainamide (and metabolite) blood levels more closely
Cimetidine (Chapter 40)	Decreased procainamide metabolism; increased blood levels, effects	As for amiodarone–procainamide interaction; cimetidine alternatives presumably interact less
Trimethoprim (Chapter 57)	Decreased procainamide excretion; increased blood levels, effects	Monitor accordingly; anticipate dosage reductions
Interactions Involving Quinidine		
Amiodarone	Increased serum quinidine levels, potentially fatal arrhythmias	Effects of interaction may occur quickly; avoid if possible, monitor with extra care if not avoidable
Antacids, especially magnesium-containing products (Chapter 40)	Decreased quinidine oral absorption, blood levels, effects	Space administration of interactants by several hours; discourage patient from self-administering antacids except as ordered by physician
Anticoagulants, oral (Chapter 35)	Decreased anticoagulant metabolism, increased effect	Monitor prothrombin time, assess for signs of excessive metabolism; anticipate need for anticoagulant dosage decrease
Barbiturates (eg, phenobarbital; Chapter 22)	Increased quinidine metabolism; decreased effects	Monitor accordingly; benzodiazepine alternatives usually preferred
β-Blockers (especially propranolol, atenolol, metoprolol; Chapter 15)	Decreased metabolism, increased effects, of β-blocker	Monitor accordingly (eg, heart rate, rhythm, pulmonary function)
Cimetidine (Chapter 40)	Decreased quinidine metabolism; increased effects	Monitor quinidine blood levels, actions, more closely if interaction unavoidable; cimetidine alternatives do not appear to interact, may be preferred
Digitalis (digoxin, digitoxin; Chapter 31)	Increased digitalis blood levels, potential toxicity	Potentially serious; <3 day onset of symptoms with digoxin, about 1 week with digitoxin; avoid giving quinidine to patients stabilized on digitalis without reducing digitalis dose several days prior; never give quinidine in presence of digitalis toxicity
Hydantoins (eg, phenytoin; Chapter 26)	Increased quinidine metabolism; decreased effects	Monitor; alternative (noninteracting) anticonvulsants may be needed
Pancuronium (Chapter 17)	Increased, prolonged effects of neuromuscular blocker	Anticipate interaction and be prepared for potential need for longer ventilatory support
Rifampin (Chapter 57)	Increased quinidine metabolism; decreased effects	Avoid interaction if possible
Succinylcholine (Chapter 17)	Increased, prolonged effects of neuromuscular blocker	See pancuronium, above
Verapamil (Chapter 24)	Rapid onset of potentially severe hypotension, bradycardia, pulmonary edema, ventricular tachycardia, AV block	Avoid interaction if all possible; monitor closely; notify physician at first sign of adverse effect, be prepared to discontinue one or both drugs
Interactions Involving Verapamil:		
See Chapter 33, Table 33–I		

PROTOTYPE

Digoxin 580

Drugs for Managing Heart Failure

Heart failure can be defined as an inability of the heart to pump enough oxygen- and nutrient-containing blood to satisfy the needs of the vital organs. In short, cardiac output is too low. Failure can occur acutely, but usually progresses slowly. In some cases the heart is affected first, but in others the heart fails in response to other disorders such as longstanding hypertension or pulmonary or renal disease (Table 31–1). Heart failure can be caused by drugs, toxins, or diseases that depress the heart, or by long-term and excessive cardiac stimulation associated with drugs (eg, sympathomimetics), hormones (eg, hyperthyroidism), or mechanical heart or great vessel abnormalities (eg, valvular or aortic disease). Regardless of the cause or speed of onset, nearly all patients with heart failure eventually require drug treatment to survive.

Pathophysiology of Chronic Congestive Heart Failure

The most common form of heart failure is congestive heart failure (CHF), a state of low cardiac output that progresses over many years. When various organs sense diminished cardiac output they attempt to compensate by initiating sympathetic and hormonal reflexes aimed at improving blood flow and pressure (Fig. 31–1). These responses help correct short-term decreases of cardiac output, but over time they are often inappropriate and actually contribute to the heart's failure as a pump. The body often responds as if blood volume or blood pressure were too low, even though they may be entirely normal or actually elevated.

Sympathetic Nervous System Activation

Activation of the sympathetic nervous system is one way by which the body compensates for reduced cardiac output. Heart rate and contractile force increase via stimulation of the β_1-adrenergic receptors. Tachycardia, a sign of this, is common in many patients with CHF. Sympathetic activation also causes vasoconstriction via stimulation of α-adrenergic receptors on arterioles. This increased blood pressure normally would help to "drive" blood through the vital organs. In the patient with CHF, however, it mainly places a greater work load on the heart.

Sympathetic stimulation is a beneficial way to overcome low cardiac output, provided the heart can meet the increased work demands. The failing heart cannot

Major reference tables appear beginning on p. 595.

Table 31–1 Some Causes of Heart Failure

Primary (Originating Within the Heart)	Secondary (Originating Outside the Heart)
Aortic or valvular stenosis, valvular regurgitation	Adrenal tumors (cortical or medullary; eg, pheochromocytoma)
Cardiac depressant or stimulant drugs (eg, barbiturate overdoses, long-term antidepressant therapy, respectively)	Atherosclerosis of peripheral organs (especially kidney)
Cardiomyopathy, disease- or drug-induced (eg, adriamycin)	Hepatic disease
Congenital heart lesions	Hypertension, including pulmonary
Coronary atherosclerosis, myocardial ischemia	Hyperthyroidism
Rheumatic heart disease	Renal disease

meet such challenges for too long, however. Indeed, when cardiac stimulation and increased blood pressure persist, they actually increase the rate at which heart function deteriorates.

Excessive sympathetic cardiac simulation has some negative influences on the progression of heart failure, but the failing heart nevertheless depends on some degree of sympathetic tone to continue functioning. This dependence can be shown, quite readily, by administering a β-adrenergic blocker to a patient with CHF: the outcome can be an acute and severe worsening of heart function, with potentially fatal consequences.

Renal and Hormonal Effects

The kidneys, faced with inadequate blood flow, also attempt to compensate. They release renin, which aids in the formation of a potent vasoconstrictor, angiotensin II (A-II). Angiotensin II increases release of the hormone aldosterone, which causes the kidneys to retain more sodium and water. Increased sympathetic stimulation constricts the renal arteries, decreasing renal blood flow even further. This amplifies the unwanted cycle. Overall, these processes undesirably elevate blood volume and blood pressure, and circulatory status declines further.

Increased blood volume and water retention, combined with decreased cardiac contractility, lead to some of the cardinal signs of CHF: weight gain, edema, and ascites. Since the failing heart cannot circulate this excess volume adequately, congestion (blood stasis) develops in the capillaries and veins of various organs. Common manifestations of this include distended jugular veins, hepatomegaly owing to liver congestion, and dyspnea owing to congestion in the pulmonary circulation.

Increased blood volume also increases venous return to the heart. The ventricles fill more during diastole, which dilates the muscle and increases energy demands. Increased filling of the ventricles stretches the muscle. Through Starling's law, this increases cardiac contractility—up to a point. Thereafter, the heart can no longer expel the extra blood load, and oxygen demands that cannot be met increase further.

Another response is an increase of myocardial protein synthesis, an attempt to increase the mass of working muscle (hypertrophy). The dilated and hypertrophied heart can be seen readily on X-ray films as cardiomegaly.

This entire process contributes to a vicious cycle in which heart function declines further unless proper treatment is begun or until the patient dies.

Drug Therapy for Chronic Congestive Heart Failure

The overall objective for treating chronic heart failure is to normalize, or at least improve, cardiac output. Accomplishing this goal not only improves heart function and alleviates symptoms, but also interrupts many of the potentially harmful compensatory processes. Drugs do not cure CHF, and treatment is usually lifelong. The following list describes the specific treatment goals that can be accomplished with drugs.

1. Efficiently improve cardiac contractility to improve cardiac output. This is done with *positive inotropic drugs:* drugs that increase the force of muscle contraction—in this case, heart muscle. The positive inotropic drug used more often than any other to treat chronic CHF is digoxin, a digitalis glycoside that is discussed shortly. Sympathomimetics such as

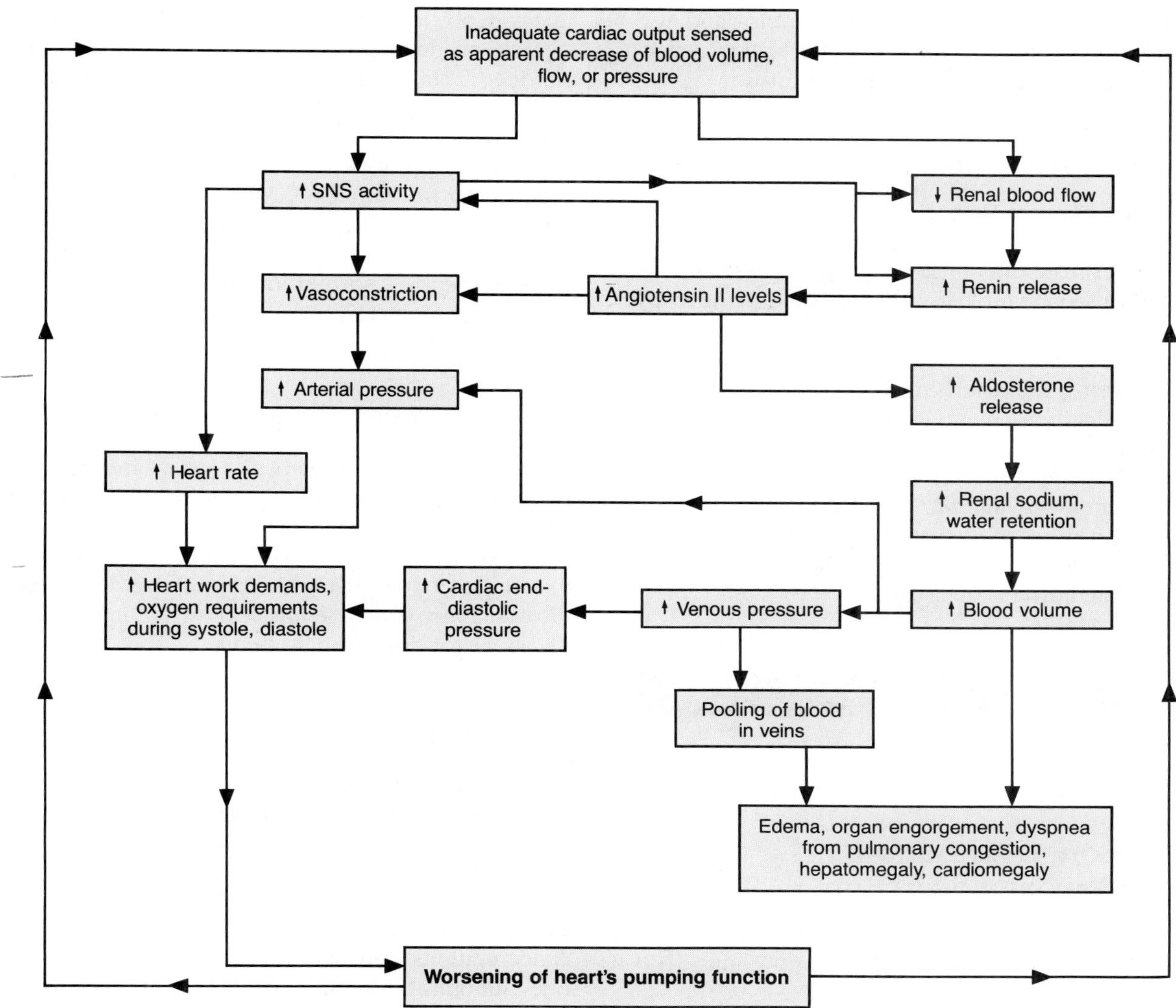

Figure 31–1

Interactive responses that contribute to CHF. When the heart loses its ability to pump adequate amounts of blood to the periphery (failure), other body systems attempt to compensate as if blood volume, flow, or pressure were reduced. A variety of responses are activated, particularly stimulation of the sympathetic nervous system and the renin-angiotensin-aldosterone system. Acutely, they may improve circulatory status. Over the long run, they contribute to signs and symptoms of heart failure and a cyclic worsening of heart function and circulatory status. Drugs used to treat heart failure—inotropic drugs (eg, digitalis), diuretics, afterload-reducing agents (eg, hydralazine), and inhibitors of angiotensin formation (captopril)—can interrupt this cycle at various points (see text).

dobutamine, and newer drugs such as amrinone, are used to treat acute heart failure.

2. Increase renal sodium and water excretion to decrease the volume and pressure of blood that the weakened heart must pump. For many patients this is accomplished with *diuretics* (Chapter 32) such as furosemide, used as an adjunct to digoxin. However, another group of drugs, called *angiotensin-converting enzyme (ACE) inhibitors,* exemplified by captopril, play an important role also.

3. Reduce in other ways the arterial pressure against which the ventricles have to pump to expel blood. This is accomplished directly by the use of *afterload-reducing drugs* such as hydralazine (pp 590, 651). (Other antihypertensive drugs can be used instead.) Drugs that improve cardiac output in

other ways (the inotropic drugs, diuretics, and ACE inhibitors) will indirectly lower afterload by reducing sympathetic nervous system stimulation.

Digitalis Glycosides

In 1785, Dr. William Withering wrote one of the most classic papers in therapeutics history. He described the use of leaves from the purple foxglove (*Digitalis*) plant to treat dropsy—better known now as CHF. In the many years since, many drugs have been isolated from the leaf, purified, and used therapeutically. These drugs share so many characteristics that they are often referred to using more general terms: *digitalis glycosides,* because their molecules contain a glucose-like sugar; *cardiac glycosides,* reflecting their primary effect on the heart; or, simply, as *digitalis.* Today, one of these drugs, digoxin, remains as the most widely used of them all. It will be considered the prototype. The only other important related drug is digitoxin.

PROTOTYPE

Digoxin

Absorption, Distribution, Metabolism, and Excretion

Digoxin is available in several dosage forms for oral or parenteral (intramuscular [IM], intravenous [IV]) administration.

The absorption of digoxin depends on the drug's pharmaceutic formulation and administration route (Table 31–2). These differences in absorption can have considerable impact on the intensity of the responses that are eventually produced. They also make it necessary to adjust dosages if dosage forms or administration routes are switched (Table 31–3).

A look at Tables 31–2 and 31–3 shows some important information about this: Oral dosage forms of digoxin are absorbed to different degrees; that is, the *bioavailabilities* are different. As little as 55% of the total dose of some digoxin tablet formulations is normally absorbed into the bloodstream. Relatively more is absorbed when the same amount (dose) is given as an elixir. And, with liquid-in-capsule formulations, nearly 100% of the administered dose is absorbed. (This is actually much more than if the same dose were given by IM injection.) There can also be clinically important differences in absorption between brand name and generic digoxin products, and even between otherwise similar products from different suppliers or manufacturers.

Once digoxin reaches the bloodstream the drug's fate is basically the same, regardless of the administration route. Most of the drug is excreted in the urine with little or no prior metabolism. A small but potentially important amount undergoes enterohepatic recirculation: active drug is concentrated in the bile, excreted in the gut, then reabsorbed into the circulation. Overall, the average plasma half-life of digoxin is about 36 hours.

NURSING IMPLICATIONS

Digoxin can be taken with or without meals. Patients with renal dysfunction usually require reduced dosages. Digitalis tablets supplied by one manufacturer may be absorbed more or less completely, faster or slower, than those of other manufacturers. These differences of bioavailability and bioequivalence have important implications for dosage adjustments.

Pharmacologic Effects

The main actions of all digitalis glycosides are increases of cardiac contractility, changes of the heart cells' electrophysiologic properties, and alterations of blood vessel tone (Table 31–4). Some of these effects are direct effects of the drug. Others are indirect, or reflexly mediated. Therapeutic effects occur with digoxin serum concentrations between 0.5 and 2.5 nanograms (ng; one-millionth of a milligram) per milliliter, provided other key laboratory data are within normal limits.

Cardiac Contractile Effects

Digoxin increases the contractile force generated by the heart cells—a positive inotropic effect. Overall, the force generated by the whole heart is increased, and cardiac output rises.

Digoxin stimulates contractility in a way that is very different from the way in which sympathomimetics (eg, norepinephrine) work, via stimulation of β_1-adrenergic receptors. For all practical purposes, digoxin's cardiac-stimulating actions have nothing at all to do with β_1-adrenergic receptors.

Digoxin's receptor is an enzyme called sodium-potassium-adenosine triphosphatase (Na, K-ATPase), which is located on the heart cell's outer membrane (the sarcolemma). When digoxin binds to the ATPase

Table 31–2 | Major Similarities and Differences Between Digoxin and Digitoxin

	Digoxin	Digitoxin
GI absorption*		
Tablets	55%–80%	90%–100%
Oral elixir, IM injection	70%–85%	NA†
Oral liquid-in-capsule	90%–100%	NA
IV injection	100%	NA
Plasma protein binding	<30%	>95%
Plasma half-life (normal)	36 hr	7 days
Major route of elimination	Renal; little or no prior metabolism	Hepatic metabolism; renal, fecal excretion of metabolites; considerable enterohepatic recirculation
"Therapeutic" serum levels	0.5–2.0 ng/mL	14–26 ng/mL
"Toxic" serum levels	>2.5 ng/mL	>35 ng/mL

*Percentage absorption may vary among products from different manufacturers, especially when oral routes are used.
†NA, not applicable.

Table 31–3 | Pharmacokinetic and Dosage Comparisons of Various Digoxin Preparations

Product	Time to Onset of Effect	Time to Peak Effect	Equivalent Dose (μg)
Regular tablet	0.5–2 hr	2–6 hr	125
Elixir	0.5–2 hr	2–6 hr	125
Liquid-in-capsule	0.5–2 hr	2–6 hr	100
IM injection	0.5–2 hr	2–6 hr	125
IV injection	5–30 min	1–4 hr	100

Table 31–4 | Major Pharmacologic Effects of Digitalis Glycosides

Direct Actions
Positive inotropy
Decreased electrical impulse conduction by SA and AV nodes
Indirect Actions
Decreased diastolic heart size, reduced wall tension
Increased renal salt and water excretion
Decreased heart rate
Decreased peripheral vasoconstriction

the enzyme's activity is inhibited. This triggers a series of steps that eventually lead to an increase in the amount of calcium ion available to trigger the contractile proteins. The greater the inhibition of ATPase, the greater the availability of calcium, and the greater the increase of contractile force. The digoxin dose, and digoxin blood levels, obviously have an impact on whether the response will be subeffective, therapeutic, or toxic. However, as noted soon, many other clinically important factors can affect digoxin's actions.

The increased contractility and cardiac output that occur in response to digoxin's direct actions lead to several beneficial indirect effects. More complete and efficient ejection of blood from the ventricles reduces diastolic heart size. This, in turn, decreases cardiac oxygen demands. Improved blood flow to the kidneys increases urine production and sodium excretion. Release or production of renin, angiotensin II, and aldosterone decrease also. Overall, these effects help reduce edema, blood volume, and blood pressure, and further ease the failing heart's work load.

Cardiac Electrophysiologic Effects

Digoxin alters the electrophysiologic properties of the heart cells and the specialized cardiac tissues that help generate and spread electrical impulses through the organ. In many ways, these electrical effects are just as important as the drug's contractile actions. Some of them occur at therapeutic doses, and are generally desirable. Others occur with higher or truly toxic doses, and are generally adverse.

Heart Rate

Heart rate is usually elevated in persons with CHF. Digoxin slows rate toward normal in one of several ways. It

- directly slows depolarization of the sinoatrial (SA) node, which is the heart's pacemaker;
- decreases sympathetic tone to the heart, and simultaneously increases parasympathetic tone. This occurs because of improved cardiac output; that is, it is an indirect electrophysiologic response that depends on digoxin's ability to increase cardiac contractility;
- increases the SA node's sensitivity to the cardiac slowing effects of acetylcholine (ACh), the parasympathetic neurotransmitter.

Automaticity

Digoxin increases automaticity of the atria and ventricles. These effects are potentially adverse, but they usually do not occur unless digoxin blood levels are too high.

Conduction Velocity

Digoxin increases the rate at which electrical impulses travel through the atria and ventricles. It simultaneously causes a dose-dependent decrease in impulse conduction rates through the atrioventricular (AV) node, which serves as the crucial electrical link between the atria and ventricles. This effect can—and should—be monitored on the electrocardiogram (ECG) as a widening of the P–R interval.

Peripheral Vascular Effects

Digoxin directly constricts some arteries and veins. However, this effect is outweighed by an opposing vasodilator effect—a decrease of peripheral resistance and of blood pressure toward more normal levels. This occurs because of digoxin's ability to increase cardiac output, which turns down sympathetic stimulation to the periphery.

Clinical Indications and Administration

Some clinicians have said that the time for digitalis has come and gone. There are probably some good reasons for making this statement. Digitalis has been around for over 200 years. The margin of safety is low. Toxicity is fairly common and potentially serious. And some of the drugs with which digitalis is usually given are the very drugs that are likely to cause toxicity. Nevertheless, digoxin is still the most widely used drug for managing chronic CHF. It is also used to manage some cardiac arrhythmias, and is occasionally used to treat acute heart failure. Typical dosages are given in Table 31–C; lower doses should be used when the patient has renal dysfunction.

Congestive Heart Failure

Digoxin alleviates symptoms of CHF, slows the progression of cardiac dysfunction, and improves the quality of life. However, it does not cure the underlying disease, and therapy may be lifelong. The drug causes a variety of desired hemodynamic effects, including a reduction of blood volume and pressure (via increased renal blood flow and urine production), but diuretics usually are given as adjuncts. If heart failure progresses to the point that digoxin and diuretics alone are not sufficient, other medications may need to be added to the treatment plan. These are discussed later in the chapter.

There are basically two ways in which digoxin therapy can be started. When the situation is not urgent, treatment can begin with oral administration, giving usual maintenance doses (125–250 μg/d) from the outset. Owing to digoxin's normal 36-hour half-life, it will take about 8 days (four to five half-lives) for the blood levels, and effects, to stabilize. This is called *gradual digitalization*.

When effects are needed more quickly, loading doses (called **digitalizing** doses) can be given initially. This can be done using oral or parenteral (preferably IV) administration routes. Treatment is then continued with maintenance doses, using the oral route when possible.

Management of Supraventricular Arrhythmias

Digoxin has antiarrhythmic activity that is useful for the management of supraventricular arrhythmias such as atrial fibrillation or flutter. The patient need not have CHF for digoxin to be used for this purpose. In these arrhythmias, the major concern is a ventricular rate that is too rapid or irregular. The impulses that activate the ventricles arise above or in the AV node, and must pass through the node before reaching the ventricles. Since digoxin depresses AV nodal conduction rates, it can slow the ventricular rate. Digoxin can be used alone, but it is more common to use it as a premedication for patients who will have supraventricular arrhythmias controlled with other antiarrhythmics, mainly quinidine or procainamide. As discussed in Chapter 30, these antiarrhythmics control atrial rate and rhythm, but simultaneously increase AV conduction; they increase the risk of excessive ventricular activation. Digoxin reduces this risk.

The nurse should be aware that drug combinations such as quinidine and digoxin are effective treatments for atrial arrhythmias. However, the most common way to stop atrial arrhythmias is to give a direct current shock to the body surface (dc cardioversion) first. As noted below, this current sensitizes the heart to the arrhythmia-causing side effects of digoxin. If, for some reason, the patient is digitalized chronically (as for CHF treatment) or acutely (in an attempt to stop the arrhythmia) before the shock is given, be prepared to deal with potentially serious ventricular arrhythmias.

NURSING IMPLICATIONS

Try to have as much information as possible before giving digoxin for the first time for any indication: baseline ECG and laboratory data; vital signs; and a thorough health and medication history. This information is important to help make dosage adjustments initially and as treatment progresses.

Therapy monitoring will involve periodic measurements of blood digoxin and electrolyte levels. Unless there is an emergency, blood samples should be drawn just before giving the next digoxin dose, and no sooner than 6 to 8 hours after the previous dose.

Become familiar with the general signs and symptoms of CHF, and the severity of those for your individual patients. Hard data (blood test results, ECGs, X-rays) clearly are important for guiding therapy. However, they do not replace the need for frequently assessing other subjective and objective clinical end-points, and seeking information from the patient about how he or she feels as treatment progresses.

It is essential to remember that although all digitalis drugs have identical mechanisms of action and similar therapeutic uses, they have different potencies and therapeutic blood levels, and they are handled differently by the body. Dosages usually need to be adjusted when switching from one digoxin formulation to another, to account for different absorption rates and extents. In general, 100 μg of IV or liquid-in-capsule digoxin is equivalent to about 125 μg of the other dosage forms or administration routes. Discourage substitution of "equivalent" digitalis products from different manufacturers without prior approval from the prescribing physician.

Encourage patients to take their digitalis at the same time each day, at a convenient time, to reduce the chance of a missed dose. Since all orally administered digitalis preparations have relatively long durations of action, it is unnecessary and unwise to administer an extra dose to make up for a missed one. Also encourage compliance with recommended low-sodium and reduced-calorie diets, which help reduce edema, body weight, and blood pressure.

Because therapeutic doses of digitalis are so small (much less than 1 mg), and even slight overdoses may cause serious toxicity, always double-check the dose before giving it. This is especially important when giving loading doses. Also double-check the name of the preparation being given: many of them are spelled or pronounced similarly.

Avoid using a rapid digitalization approach for patients who have taken a digitalis preparation within the past 2 weeks, as this may lead to toxicity. If the amount of digitalis taken during that time cannot be documented, it is best not to give more than a single daily dose. Assess responses closely for any signs of toxicity before giving the next dose.

Oral administration of digitalis is almost always preferred unless immediate drug effects are needed or the patient cannot take oral medications. Intravenous injection is the preferred parenteral route. If the IM route must be used, select a suitably large muscle, aspirate the syringe before injecting, inject deeply, massage the site well to facilitate drug absorption and reduce pain, and avoid injecting more than 500 μg into a single site. Intramuscular injections are extremely painful.

Side Effects, Adverse Reactions, and Contraindications

Side effects and adverse responses (Table 31–S) that occur during digoxin therapy can be divided into two major groups: those that affect the heart, and those that occur elsewhere (extracardiac side effects). The cardiac side effects, and the related changes in overall function of the cardiovascular system, clearly are the most important and potentially dangerous. However, some extracardiac responses may appear first; they are often easier for the patient or health-care provider to spot; and their appearance can provide good clues that more serious problems are occurring, or are apt to occur soon.

Given digoxin's narrow margin of safety, it is sometimes difficult to say whether certain unwanted responses are simply side effects, or indicators of some degree of actual drug toxicity.

Cardiac Side Effects

The most important concerns are changes of heart rate, AV nodal conduction, and overall heart rhythm. Any of these alterations can reduce cardiac output to dangerous levels.

Bradycardia, AV Block, and Arrhythmias

Patients who receive digoxin for CHF usually experience a reduction of heart rate toward normal, but excessive cardiac slowing can occur. Ventricular rates below about 60 beats per minute for adults, or 90 to 100 in children, are generally unwanted.

One of the most important and most common adverse cardiac responses to digoxin is a slowing of AV nodal conduction. This is seen on the ECG as progressive lengthening of the P–R interval. At the extreme, complete AV block and ventricular standstill may occur.

Slowing of AV nodal conduction is a risk for any patient, but more so for patients who already have some degree of preexisting AV block. For example, patients with Stokes–Adams or sick sinus syndrome may experience episodes of severe bradycardia or complete heart block. Patients with Wolff–Parkinson–White syndrome may experience ventricular tachycardia or fibrillation.

Digoxin is said to be able to cause any imaginable type of cardiac arrhythmia. However, the rhythm disorders seen most often include a combination of AV block and ventricular ectopic activity (eg, ventricular premature contractions or ventricular tachycardia). These reflect digoxin's ability to decrease nodal conduction and increase ventricular automaticity.

Extracardiac Side Effects

The key extracardiac side effects include gastrointestinal (GI) disturbances, mainly nausea, vomiting, and anorexia; and visual disturbances, often described as a green or yellow tint to white objects, or similarly colored halos around bright objects or lights (**chromatopsia**). Patients on long-term digoxin therapy may also develop gynecomastia. Presumably it occurs because of the drug's chemical structure, which resembles that of some of the sex hormones. Unlike the responses noted above, gynecomastia is not an indication of potential digoxin toxicity.

NURSING IMPLICATIONS

Many drugs cause discomforting anorexia, nausea, and vomiting as side effects. These signs and symptoms are also common accompaniments of heart disease, especially if it is not controlled well by drug therapy. However, any GI distress (or chromatopsia), regardless of the route of digoxin administration, should always be considered a warning of drug toxicity until proven otherwise. Digoxin administration should be stopped until test results are obtained. Always advise patients to report these signs and symptoms, and ask specifically about them during patient interviews. Always take the apical pulse for 1 full minute before giving any digitalis drug or preparation.

◆ Use During Pregnancy and Lactation

Digoxin crosses the placenta and is excreted in breast milk. The drug is not contraindicated during pregnancy, but monitoring fetal status is necessary. Digoxin concentrations in maternal milk may equal those in maternal blood, but the amount of drug ingested by the nursing infant is not likely to cause effects. Nevertheless, care is recommended.

◆ Use in Children

Digoxin is commonly used in pediatrics for the same indications noted for adults. The response to a given dose depends greatly on age, renal function, and body mass. Always verify the ordered dose with another nurse before administering it.

◆ Use in the Elderly

Reduced dosages are generally required to compensate for expected age-related declines of renal function, altered lean body weight, or advanced cardiac disease. These factors increase the risk of adverse effects. Digitoxin, the major related cardiac glycoside, has the lowest margin of safety in elderly patients.

Interactions with Other Drugs

Table 31–I summarizes the major drugs that are usually cited as causing clinically significant interactions with the cardiac glycosides. Also included are explanations of the likely mechanisms of the interactions; and measures the nurse can take to prevent, identify, or correct potential problems. Many of the interactions apply to digoxin; the major alternative drug, digitoxin; and those cardiac glycosides that are rarely used. (When describing these interactions, the general term *digitalis* is used to indicate that all these individual cardiac drugs are affected.) However, some interactions mainly affect digoxin, and they are more likely to cause problems with certain oral dosage forms than with others. They are listed separately.

Interactions That Involve Altered Pharmacokinetics

Most of the interactants are drugs that reduce the absorption of oral digitalis, or speed the elimination of digitalis from the body. Interactants that reduce absorption, and can lead to inadequate control of heart failure, include antacids, laxatives, and cholesterol-lowering drugs (cholestyramine, colestipol). The latter agents must be prescribed by a physician. This increases the chance that therapy can be planned and monitored properly to reduce the risk of unwanted interactions. In contrast, most antacids and laxatives are over-the-counter (OTC) drugs that are frequently self-prescribed. They are often taken in haphazard ways, in excessive dosages, or in other ways that cannot be controlled or monitored well. This drug-taking behavior is of most concern with respect to interactions with digitalis. It it is not prevented, or if information about the (mis)use of these drugs is not obtained from the patient so that therapy can be modified properly, altered responses to digitalis can cause a host of problems for both the health-care provider and the patient.

Thyroid hormone status, and drugs used to treat hyper- or hypothyroidism, also influence the pharmacokinetics and cellular actions of digitalis. Hyperthyroid patients tend to eliminate digitalis faster than patients with normal thyroid status. Their hearts also appear to be more resistant to the effects of any digitalis. In contrast, hypothyroid patients tend to eliminate digitalis slower than normal, and a given digitalis blood level tends to cause a greater-than-usual effect on their hearts. Thus, if the patient has one of these thyroid states, if already stabilized on digitalis, and if he or she is then treated with drugs to normalize thyroid status (thyroid hormones or antithyroid drugs) without adjusting the digitalis dosage, excessive or inadequate blood digitalis levels and effects can result. (Similar relationships and problems apply to thyroid hormone levels and the rate at which the related drug, digitoxin, is eliminated by hepatic metabolism.)

Quinidine is clearly an important interactant. This common antiarrhythmic drug prolongs the half-life of digitalis. The mechanism with digoxin is understood best: quinidine reduces digoxin's excretion. Regardless of the cardiac glycoside that is used, digitalis blood levels will rise unless the dose is reduced. Reductions of 30% or more may be indicated. If the patient is stabilized on digoxin, digoxin levels begin to rise almost immediately when quinidine therapy starts. It may take only a few days, or less, for toxicity to occur. It may take a week or more for signs of the quinidine–digitoxin interaction to appear. Never give quinidine to treat any arrhythmia caused by digitalis.

There are a few other drugs or drug groups that seem to have more of an effect on the pharmacokinetics of orally administered digoxin than on other glycosides or administration routes. The drugs that are used quite often, yet pose risks from interactions, include several classes of antibiotics (aminoglycosides, erythromycin, tetracyclines) and most of the anticancer drugs. See Table 31–I for a complete listing and further explanation.

Interactions Caused by Hypokalemia

The most common cause of digitalis toxicity is hypokalemia caused by adjunctive use of potassium-wasting diuretics: a high-ceiling (loop) diuretic such as furosemide, or a thiazide. Hypokalemia increases the myocardium's sensitivity to digitalis, and *even digitalis blood levels that are in the therapeutic range can cause serious or life-threatening toxicity if serum potassium levels are too low.* Use of these diuretics with digitalis is very common, if not almost routine, because they help reduce the failing heart's work load by eliminating excessive fluid and by lowering blood pressure. Use of a diuretic makes it essential to monitor serum potassium levels often, and to ensure that patients properly take potassium-sparing diuretics (eg, triamterene) or oral potassium supplements that are often prescribed also.

Thiazides and high-ceiling diuretics also cause magnesium loss into the urine. This lowering of serum magnesium levels contributes to digitalis toxicity caused by hypokalemia. Currently, however, magnesium supplements are not prescribed routinely for most CHF patients receiving both digitalis and a diuretic.

Other Drug-Induced Problems

The drugs noted above and in Table 31–I are the ones most likely to cause significant and specific interactions with a digitalis preparation. However, there are other medications that can complicate therapy of CHF in other ways. In general, these include

- drugs that *depress cardiac contractility or rate,* thereby further weakening the already-failing heart. Examples include β-adrenergic blockers (propranolol, others; Chapter 15); catecholamine-depleting antihypertensive drugs (eg, reserpine; Chapter 33); and, especially at high dosages, most local anesthetics (Chapter 19), barbiturates (Chapter 22), narcotics (Chapter 21), and antiarrhythmic drugs (Chapter 30). Of these, β-blockers clearly pose the greatest problems owing to their well-known cardiac-depressant actions and their widespread use for a host of disorders.
- drugs that *inefficiently stimulate the heart,* thereby increasing the heart's work load over the long run. Examples include all the sympathomimetics with β-adrenergic stimulating activity, including those used as bronchodilators to treat asthma or emphysema (Chapter 14); theophylline (Chapter 38); and most antidepressants (Chapter 24).
- drugs that *increase blood pressure,* increasing cardiac work in yet another way. Examples are vasoconstrictors, including oral OTC drugs used as decongestants or cold remedies (Chapter 14); and drugs that cause the body to retain salt and water (eg, systemic corticosteroids; Chapter 45).

NURSING IMPLICATIONS

Problems owing to drug–drug interactions are likely to be greater when an interactant is added to the medication plan of a patient who is already stabilized on digitalis. If a digitalis dosage adjustment is needed when adding another drug, anticipate that readjustments in the opposite direction will be needed when the interactant is discontinued.

Laboratory test results, including measurements of digitalis blood levels, serum electrolytes, and the like, are clearly essential for guiding proper therapy with interacting medications. However, they do not replace the need for careful and frequent monitoring of vital signs and other assessments aimed at determining whether the effects of digitalis are too little or too much.

Be sure medication histories include information that is as complete as possible about the use of OTC drugs (types, dosages, frequency of use, timing of dosages, etc).

Other Factors That Influence Myocardial Sensitivity to Digitalis

Many common physiologic and pathophysiologic abnormalities can alter the heart's responsiveness or sensitivity to digitalis (Table 31–5). Often, several occur at once. When one or more of these abnormalities are present, subtherapeutic or excessive (or truly toxic) responses can occur—even when the digitalis serum level is, numerically, in the "therapeutic" range. That is, what might have been the right dose of digitalis in the absence of response-modifying factors no longer is correct; the modifying factors have to be eliminated, or at least their influences reduced, or the digitalis dose must be adjusted to compensate for them.

Correcting the abnormality is preferred to merely adjusting the digitalis dosage and letting the abnormality persist. For example, if digitalis' effects are excessive because the patient is hypokalemic, hypoxic, or hypothyroid, important therapeutic goals would be to normalize blood potassium, oxygen, or thyroid hormone levels. In many cases, correcting the abnormality may be all that is needed to make the current digitalis dose the right one once again.

Without question, of most concern are alterations of the response to digitalis that suggest toxicity.

Overdose and Toxicity

Even in the reasonably well-controlled environment of the hospital, about 20% of patients receiving digitalis develop one or more signs or symptoms of toxicity. About 20% of those patients, in turn, develop serious intoxication. The risks and severity of digitalis poisoning appear to be greater in patients with more severe cardiac failure, arrhythmias, other illnesses, or trauma.

Accidental or intentional (ie, suicidal) overdoses are, of course, causes of toxicity. More often, however, the cause is an improper adjustment of the digitalis dose. That, in turn, is caused by a failure or inability of the health-care team to prevent, detect, or correct problems caused by drug interactions, the modifying factors

Table 31–5 | Other Factors That Alter Myocardial Sensitivity or Therapeutic Response to Digitalis

Factor	Comments
	Increased Sensitivity or Response to Digitalis
Hypokalemia	Occurs commonly, most likely caused by potassium-wasting diuretics, inadequate potassium supplementation; also associated with adrenal cortical tumors, severe or prolonged vomiting, diarrhea, diaphoresis
Hyperglycemia	Often caused by diabetes mellitus, especially if poorly controlled; can also cause hypokalemia
Hypercalcemia	May be caused by thiazide diuretics; associated with malignancies, renal failure, hyperparathyroidism, excessive use of oral calcium supplements, including some antacids; increases arrhythmia risks
Hypothyroidism	Caused by goiter, inadequate thyroid hormone replacement therapy after thyroidectomy, radiation therapy for thyroid cancer, overtreatment with antithyroid drugs; reduces digitalis elimination, intensifies bradycardic effects and risk of AV block
Myocardial ischemia, hypoxia	Caused by ischemic heart disease, recent MI, severe pulmonary disease; can dramatically increase risk of digitalis-induced arrhythmias
Direct-current (DC) cardioversion	Best used only as a last resort to treat arrhythmias in fully digitalized patients; if digitalis is to be used as adjunct to treatment of arrhythmias (eg, with quinidine for atrial flutter), best to use current before trying drug approaches
	Decreased Sensitivity or Response to Digitalis
Hyperkalemia	Caused by excessive or inappropriate use of potassium-containing or -retaining drugs (potassium supplements, some antibiotics, potassium-sparing diuretics); also associated with burns, trauma, infections, sepsis, uremia; antagonizes inotropic actions of digitalis, may cause arrhythmias directly
Hypocalcemia	Caused by high-ceiling diuretics, excessive laxative use, liver disease, osteomalacia, pregnancy, renal failure, sprue, and other celiac disease; reduces inotropic actions of digitalis
Hyperthyroidism	Caused by untreated or excessively treated hypothyroidism with thyroid hormone supplements

listed in the previous section (and Table 31–S), or patient noncompliance.

Signs and Symptoms

The signs and symptoms of digitalis intoxication are extensions of the side effects noted above. In most adults, the extracardiac symptoms—nausea, vomiting, anorexia, and vision changes—appear before such cardiac changes as rate and rhythm disturbances. The reverse tends to be true in children: extracardiac signs and symptoms may occur much later; they may be difficult to detect; and the young patient may not be able to report them accurately.

For all patients, cardiac changes are of most concern. Usually they include premature ventricular contractions, progressive bradycardia, and progressive slowing of AV conduction (excessive P–R interval prolongation on the ECG). Nevertheless, even if only extracardiac changes occur—and especially if several of them occur together, the safest assumption at the start is that digitalis may somehow be involved.

Assessment

The first rule to follow is not to make matters worse by giving more digitalis. If you are responsible for administering the drug, give no further doses, chart your findings and actions, and notify the physician. If the patient is self-medicating, recommend that they not take another dose, and that they seek further evaluation at once. In nearly every case, the digitalis preparation that is being given (almost always digoxin) has a half-life that is long enough that skipping one or even two doses will cause little harm, even if excessive digitalis effects are not the cause of the problems. Evaluation should be done in a hospital, where proper diagnostic and treatment facilities are available. The workup may eventually show that the patient's signs and symptoms are caused by progressive heart failure or some other medical disorder, and not by excessive digitalis effects. Nevertheless, the chance that problems could be drug-induced must be explored fully.

If the cause of the toxic signs and symptoms is a true oral overdose, standard first-aid measures (induced emesis, gastric lavage, etc) are indicated, as permitted by the patient's condition. These are described in Appendix C, and will not be discussed further here. Regardless of the potential cause, the following steps should be taken.

- Determine the patient's long-term and recent medical and medication history as best as possible. For example, whether presenting signs and symptoms were of gradual onset or came on suddenly, perhaps in response to some identifiable event, can provide helpful clues. This history-taking should not be done at the expense of further assessment and treatment, however, if the patient's condition is acute.
- Assess and then begin normalizing vital signs. This focuses on cardiovascular status, but does not exclude assessment of other body systems, such as pulmonary and renal status. These systems can be affected either by excessive drug actions or by worsening of the patient's underlying disease. Initial measurements may include only a check of the rate and quality of the pulses, and of blood pressure, but an ECG (preferably 12 lead) should be obtained as soon as possible. The ECG may reveal rhythm disturbances that appear infrequently, or that do not appear to be life-threatening. Nevertheless, it gives no indication about how high blood digoxin levels may be, or how quickly or how much the patient's condition may deteriorate.
- Check for the presence of other factors that might explain the signs and symptoms. Anticipate the need to draw a blood sample. It will be analyzed for a variety of clues about underlying problems, especially digitalis blood levels and levels of electrolytes (eg, potassium) that are likely to be altered in patients receiving digitalis along with a diuretic for CHF. Evidence of renal and hepatic function will also be looked for.

With this and other information at hand, decisions about what to do next can be made.

Treatment

Assessment can provide much information about what to do next. For example, evidence of hypoxia, which can increase the heart's sensitivity to digitalis, can be managed by oxygen administration.

Electrolytes

Often, electrolyte abnormalities such as hypokalemia are found. These should be corrected, usually by the administration of intravenous fluids formulated in such a way that they will help correct abnormalities, such as by the addition of supplemental potassium chloride and dextrose. The rate of fluid and electrolyte replenishment must be balanced in such a way that it quickly but safely corrects identified problems and helps normalize vital signs, but does not make matters worse. It is important to avoid infusing too much fluid, or infusing fluid too fast, to avoid putting added stress on the failing heart. Conversely, infusing a potassium solution that is too concentrated can irritate the blood vessels, or run the risk of stopping the heart if too much potassium-rich fluid is given too fast. Use of a central venous line is generally recommended.

Oral potassium chloride administration sometimes is acceptable if there are no life-threatening arrhythmias and the patient has good renal function.

It is important to note that although hypokalemia is a common cause of digitalis toxicity, it cannot be assumed to be the problem in every case. Thus, it is inappropriate and often dangerous to begin administering potassium, especially parenterally, until a potassium deficit is known to be present. Likewise, if the patient has signs and symptoms of severe or life-threatening digitalis toxicity, and laboratory results indicate hypokalemia, beginning treatment with oral potassium supplements or potassium-wasting drugs is improper. These slow-acting approaches should be saved until the potassium levels are corrected by parenteral routes, and the patient's overall condition has been well stabilized.

Antiarrhythmic Drugs

Antiarrhythmic drugs are often indicated (see Chapter 30). The usual goals are not only to correct the abnormalities that are likely to be seen—especially single or multiple premature ventricular contractions that can progress to ventricular tachycardia or fibrillation—but also to prevent worsening of arrhythmias or causing new ones. Lidocaine, given intravenously, is usually preferred. It will suppress ventricular ectopic beats and other abnormalities, but is not likely to cause further depression of electrical impulse conduction. Phenytoin can also be used. Some patients, who have severe bradycardia as the major cardiac abnormality, may receive atropine.

Beta-adrenergic blockers are occasionally used. They can suppress ectopic beats. However, they can also pose some risks: further slowing of heart rate; increasing degrees of AV block; and a weakening of the heart's force of contraction, which can cause increasing degrees of heart failure. In many cases, the risks of β blockade outweigh the benefits. Similar problems can occur with calcium-channel blockers (eg, verapamil). Quinidine should be used with extreme caution for digitalis-induced arrhythmias: its ability to increase serum digoxin levels (occurs quickly) or digitoxin levels (occurs more slowly, but is important nevertheless) will make matters worse.

Direct-current countershock is a standard intervention for most cases of serious ventricular arrhythmias. However, the heart of the digitalized or digitalis-toxic patient is unusually sensitive to this nondrug treatment, which can cause a worsening of arrhythmias. Countershock should be used only when other measures have failed.

Hastening Digitalis Elimination

Anticipate the use of other drugs to help eliminate excessive amounts of digitalis from the bloodstream, even if initial measures (eg, gastric lavage) have removed all unabsorbed drug from the gut. Activated charcoal, cholestyramine, or colestipol can be given orally (by nasogastric tube if necessary). These agents capitalize on the fact that a portion of digoxin (and especially digitoxin) in the bloodstream undergoes enterohepatic recirculation: they bind the digitalis that has been excreted in the gut via the bile, and prevent it from being reabsorbed into the bloodstream.

Digitalis overdoses that are thought to be life-threatening may be treated with a specific antidote, ***digoxin immune Fab*** (DIGIBIND; DIGIDOTE). The letters Fab stand for antibody fragment; the drug is a portion of an antibody, obtained from sheep, that specifically binds and thereby neutralizes digoxin (and digitoxin) in the bloodstream. It is given by IV infusion (or bolus injection when death is imminent). The dose varies, depending on the digoxin level. When digoxin immune Fab is used, the patient's condition usually improves dramatically within a couple of hours. This treatment is expensive and not readily available in all hospitals. However, all hospitals and poison control centers will have phone numbers to call and request the antidote for use.

Related Digitalis Drugs

The related drug, digitoxin, is used less than digoxin. Nevertheless, it is an important drug. The major differences between the two drugs are summarized in the next section and in Table 31–2. Digoxin, digitoxin, and the related glycoside deslanoside, share similar mechanisms of action, side effects, toxicities, and interactions with most other drugs. Dosages are listed in Table 31–C.

Digitoxin

Digitoxin is cited as the major digoxin alternative for oral therapy of CHF, but it is seldom used. These two drugs have identical mechanisms of action.

Digitoxin differs from the prototype in several ways (see Table 31–2). Among these differences are

- a much longer half-life, which gives a slower onset of action when therapy starts and more prolonged problems should toxicity from an overdose occur. Even though a parenteral dosage form of digitoxin is available, it is rarely used for acute digitalization, whether for arrhythmias or CHF, because its onset of action is too slow.
- greater binding to plasma proteins.
- elimination by hepatic metabolism, and a greater dependence on enterohepatic recirculation and the patient's liver function for making dosage adjustments. This also influences some of the drug–drug interactions in which digitoxin, but digoxin, may participate (see below).
- subtherapeutic, therapeutic, and toxic blood levels that are numerically different from those used for digoxin.

Aside from these differences, the clinical use of and nursing implications for digitoxin for CHF are much the same as the use of digoxin: diuretics are often important adjuncts; side effects (Table 31–S) and toxicities are identical in terms of signs, symptoms, and intervention; factors that increase or decrease the heart's sensitivity to digoxin do the same for digitoxin (Table 31–5); and nearly all drug–drug interactions apply to both drugs (Table 31–I).

NURSING IMPLICATIONS

Cimetidine (a widely used antiulcer drug; see Chapter 40) and, to a lesser extent propranolol (β-blockers are usually contraindicated for patients with CHF), are known for their ability to interact with a variety of drugs by inhibiting their metabolism. Alternatively, barbiturates and the long-term consumption of small amounts of alcohol can stimulate hepatic drug metabolism. Since digitoxin depends more on hepatic metabolism than does digoxin, do not overlook these potential interactants when assessing problems in adjusting digitoxin dosages for certain patients.

Deslanoside

Deslanoside (desacetyl lanatoside C; CEDILANID-D) is a cardiac glycoside available only for parenteral use. The drug has a very rapid onset of action (about 5 minutes when given intravenously). Its only indication is for emergency digitalization. It is still used occasionally for that purpose, but the same effects can be achieved almost as quickly with digoxin. Deslanoside dosages are noted in Table 31–C.

Adjuncts and Alternatives for Chronic Congestive Heart Failure

Several other drugs or drug groups are important in the management of chronic CHF. They are discussed in more detail in other chapters, since they have other major uses. These agents are presented here, in brief, to show how they fit into the overall management picture. Not all of them are approved by the FDA for heart failure therapy, but they are occasionally used nevertheless.

Afterload-Reducing Drugs

These are drugs that lower blood pressure through actions on the peripheral vasculature. In doing so they reduce the work load of the heart. Many orally effective agents are in use, but none currently is approved as a treatment for heart failure. The drugs include hydralazine (APRESOLINE; also available in parenteral dosage forms, and used for acute heart failure); α-adrenergic blockers such as prazosin (MINIPRESS; p 647); and long-acting organic nitrate vasodilators such as isosorbide dinitrate (eg, ISORDIL, SORBITRATE; p 685). Reflex tachycardia, a side effect of these drugs, can counteract the beneficial effects. It is usually dose-dependent and can be minimized with dosage adjustments. Beta-blockers can minimize reflex tachycardia also, but they are best avoided in heart failure patients.

Angiotensin-Converting Enzyme Inhibitors

These drugs, called ACE inhibitors for short, are mainly used for treating essential hypertension. They are discussed more fully in Chapter 32, which also gives their dosages. Currently, oral dosage forms of two ACE inhibitors (captopril, CAPOTEN; enalapril, VASOTEC) are approved for managing CHF. They are being prescribed earlier for CHF, especially for patients who (according to some clinical evidence) have mild CHF and hypertension and do not seem to obtain much benefit from digitalis. Depending on the patient, and the prescribing physician, an ACE inhibitor may be used alone, with a diuretic, with digitalis, or with both.

The ACE inhibitors have no direct cardiac-stimulating activity, but they do cause desirable hemodynamic changes that help the failing heart. Like more typical afterload-reducing drugs (eg, antihypertensives and organic nitrates), these agents lower blood pressure. And, like diuretics, they help manage edema and renal sodium retention. This also helps lower blood pressure and reduce cardiac work. With the ACE inhibitors, all these effects occur by their ability to interrupt the renin-angiotensin-aldosterone system (see Fig. 31–1, p 579): they reduce formation of angiotensin II, a vasoconstrictor; and reduce formation of aldosterone, a hormone that causes the kidneys to retain sodium and water and eliminate potassium. There is also evidence that some of the ACE inhibitors can actually reduce mortality in patients with severe CHF.

Diuretics

Diuretics are almost always prescribed along with digitalis for treating chronic or acute heart failure. By increasing urine production they reduce edema and blood volume, which reduces the work load of the failing heart. High-ceiling diuretics such as furosemide, rather than thiazides, are generally used because they have a higher maximum effect and the dose-response relationship can be adjusted easily and quickly. The greatest risk of using either a high-ceiling or thiazide diuretic in the digitalized patient is hypokalemia, one of the most common side effects of these drugs. Diuretics are described in more detail in Chapter 32.

Milrinone

Milrinone (PRIMACOR) is an orally effective relative of amrinone. It is being evaluated for long-term CHF therapy. Milrinone causes thrombocytopenia much less often than amrinone. However, clinical trials have also shown that long-term oral administration of this drug can increase the risk of mortality in patients with severe CHF. The future of milrinone is uncertain, but it is clear that drugs like it will soon become important in long-term CHF therapy.

Drugs for Managing Acute Heart Failure

Acute heart failure (cardiogenic shock) may occur in patients with prior heart disease. It can also occur in patients with previously good cardiac status who experience septicemia, cardiac trauma (accidental or surgical, as after open heart surgery), or overdoses of cardiac depressant drugs. When shock is due to blood loss, prompt replacement of blood or blood fluids may be all that is needed. In most other cases rapidly acting inotropic drugs are usually used.

Amrinone Lactate

Amrinone (INOCOR), a relatively new and pharmacologically unique drug, has both inotropic and afterload-reducing (vasodilator) properties. Its mechanism of action is not fully known. It does not act like digitalis, nor like sympathomimetics.

Amrinone is indicated for the short-term management of severe CHF in patients who have not responded adequately to more traditional drugs. It is not a first-line drug because it may cause several serious adverse responses. Unlike sympathomimetics, amrinone can be administered to a fully digitalized patient. The inotropic effects of amrinone and digitalis seem to be additive, yet they do not dramatically increase the risk of serious arrhythmias if serum electrolytes are within normal limits. In addition, amrinone effectively stimulates the β-blocked heart, which is another distinct therapeutic advantage for many patients.

Amrinone dosages are summarized in Table 31–C. Invasive monitoring of the response (cardiac output, pulmonary capillary wedge pressure, central venous pressure, and so on) is mandatory to help assess the response and adjust doses. Amrinone is eliminated by both renal excretion and hepatic metabolism, so the dosage may need to be reduced in patients with significant dysfunction of either system.

Short-term amrinone administration causes infrequent and generally mild side effects. Arrhythmias may occur, but they are often due to electrolyte imbalances in digitalized patients. Long-term amrinone administration may cause serious thrombocytopenia, hepatotoxicity, and hypersensitivity reactions. The appearance of any of these problems requires immediate amrinone discontinuation.

Little is known about interactions between amrinone and other drugs.

NURSING IMPLICATIONS

Like sympathomimetics (see below), which have been the mainstay of acute heart failure for years, amrinone must be diluted before use. However, amrinone's physical compatibilities differ importantly. Do not mix or dilute amrinone with, or add it to, solutions that contain dextrose (as can be done with sympathomimetics). Mix it only with sterile normal or half-normal saline. (Administration into a Y-site through which a dextrose solution is passing is acceptable.) Do not mix amrinone with furosemide; the two will precipitate immediately. Always check the package insert or ask a clinical pharmacist if you must mix or administer amrinome.

Even though amrinone is usually used for relatively short periods of time (24 hours or less), and the risks of serious adverse effects are low, predrug blood and hepatic function tests should be performed if possible. Monitor the results of subsequent tests during amrinone therapy. Significant changes, or the development of excessive bleeding, abdominal pain, or rashes may require ceasing amrinone use. Notify the physician at once if they occur.

Little is known about the safety of administering amrinone to pregnant or nursing women. It should be used only when the potential benefits outweigh potential dangers to the fetus or nursing infant.

Glucagon

Glucagon is a hormone that increases blood glucose levels in opposition to the effects of insulin (see Chapter 46). The drug also stimulates the heart in a manner that is not inhibited by β blockade. Glucagon has been used effectively to support the acutely failing, β-blocked heart, although the use is unapproved. In these settings, the drug is given intravenously (4 to 6 mg initially, followed by infusions of 4 to 12 mg/hr as needed). If glucagon is used, anticipate hyperglycemia, hypokalemia, and the added risk of arrhythmias. Anticipate hypoglycemia when glucagon administration is stopped.

Sympathomimetics

Parenterally administered sympathomimetics, specifically those that stimulate myocardial β-adrenergic (β_1 receptors) are mainly used to treat acute heart failure in patients who are not digitalized. The most commonly used agents are dobutamine (DOBUTREX) and dopamine (INTROPIN). Isoproterenol (ISUPREL) is used less often. (Norepinephrine [LEVOPHED] can also be used, but its added ability to stimulate α-adrenergic receptors in the arterioles is unwanted and requires simultaneous use of an α blocker to counteract this effect.) Since each of these drugs was discussed in detail in Chapter 14, only pertinent comments about their general use in heart failure are summarized here.

The general advantages of sympathomimetics for acute heart failure are their prompt onsets of action and their ability to stimulate the heart more vigorously than digitalis.

Sympathomimetics have several disadvantages, however. They cause considerable increases of myocardial oxygen demand when they increase contractility, and further increases if heart rate also rises. This effect is particularly unwanted if a sympathomimetic must be administered for more than a very brief time, or if the patient already has ischemic heart disease. Sympathomimetics may, in these patients, worsen ischemia (and angina pectoris) or cause infarction.

Of the individual agents, dobutamine is least likely to cause tachycardia, and so it is generally preferred. Isoproterenol almost always causes tachycardia. Dopamine increases heart rate slightly, and at high doses may cause unwanted peripheral vasoconstriction, which partially counteracts its ability to improve cardiac output. The need to administer norepinephrine with an α blocker is a cumbersome way to achieve effects that can be produced by a single drug (dobutamine), but sometimes it is the only approach that works for some patients.

A second potential disadvantage of sympathomimetics is their ability to cause arrhythmias, even when "recommended" doses are used, and especially when the patient is digitalized or has ischemic heart disease.

A third disadvantage is the speed with which the heart apparently becomes dependent on these drugs for support of function. If a parenteral sympathomimetic has been used for all but a brief period of time, abrupt drug discontinuation may cause a prompt return of impaired contractility, or worsening beyond that seen before treatment.

Lastly, the inotropic actions of all sympathomimetics are diminished in persons taking β blockers. Since β blockers are key therapies for such common cardiovascular disorders as essential hypertension or angina pectoris, and since acute heart failure may develop in these patients, the reduced efficacy of sympathomimetics is a major therapeutic limitation.

NURSING IMPLICATIONS

Monitor patients with acute heart failure closely and constantly, since their condition may change rapidly and require prompt and perhaps minute adjustment of the dosages of potent drugs. Unless life-threatening adverse responses occur, always reduce the dosage of sympathomimetic drugs gradually to reduce the risk of a return of severe heart failure.

SUMMARY OF NURSING IMPLICATIONS

Assessment

Complete baseline serum electrolyte levels and ECG for comparison during digitalis therapy.

Gather physical assessment data to include vital signs, presence of edema, urinary output, and body weight.

Assess for pharmacologic and nondrug factors (other diseases) that might increase risk of drug sensitivity to even "usual" dosages.

Assess for factors that reduce sensitivity to digitalis and would necessitate greater-than-normal dosages to achieve therapeutic response.

Review patient's current drug history for major drug–drug interactants (eg, diuretics, corticosteroids, propranolol, antacids, quinidine).

Nursing Diagnoses

Decreased cardiac output related to disease process (congestive heart failure) or adverse drug effects.

Fluid volume excess related to sodium and water retention.

Impaired gas exchange related to inadequate cardiac function and fluid in the lungs.

Knowledge deficit related to prescribed drug regimen, side effects, and possible drug interactions.

High risk for injury related to drug side effects.

Altered tissue perfusion related to inadequate cardiac function.

Planning/Implementation

Monitor electrolyte levels and ECG during the course of therapy.

Do not administer digitalis if preexisting bradycardia or heart block greater than second degree is present; patients with Wolff–Parkinson–White syndrome or atrial fibrillation may develop ventricular fibrillation with digitalis.

Obtain patient's lean body weight and consult manufacturer's tables to determine appropriateness of drug dose for each patient.

Use a deep injection site with IM digitalis; massage well following the injection; do not administer more than 500 μg into any one site.

Always double-check prescribed dose and actual dose being given; digitalis has a low margin of safety.

Changing digitalis dosage forms (eg, tablets to elixirs), routes, and possibly manufacturers' preparations may require small but important dosage adjustments.

Observe for common side effects: GI upset and anorexia; also may indicate worsening of congestive heart failure.

Give potential drug interactants at least 2 hours apart to minimize adverse effects.

Review blood test results before giving potassium supplements or potassium-sparing diuretics to digitalized patients. If parenteral potassium is indicated, give no more than 20–40 mEq/hr.

◆ Patient and Family Teaching

Teach the patient/family:

To report nausea, vomiting, anorexia, or chromatopsia immediately.

To avoid OTC preparations that may interact with digitalis (eg, antacids).

◆ Evaluation

The patient/family will:

Show signs of drug effectiveness: increased peripheral perfusion; decreased heart rate; no edema; breath sounds clear; no weight gain.

Experience minimal or no adverse drug effects: serum potassium within normal limits; no arrhythmias, complaints of colored vision, or GI distress.

Verbalize knowledge of possible drug–drug interactions and medications to avoid if not prescribed.

Return for regular medical follow-up.

Annotated Bibliography

Cody RJ. Pharmacology of angiotensin-converting enzyme inhibitors as a guide to their use in congestive heart failure. *Am J Cardiol* 1990;66(11):7D–11D. *Timely and informative, given the growing use of ACE inhibitors in CHF, and evidence that they can reduce mortality. Focuses on pharmacokinetics, which can differ dramatically from drug to drug.*

Deedwania PC. Angiotensin-converting enzyme inhibitors in congestive heart failure. *Arch Intern Med* 1990;150(9):1798–1805. *Goes beyond reviewing the overall drug class by discussing advantages and limitations of the individual agents.*

Delgizzi LJ, Ueda JN. Using inotropic and vasodilating agents in pediatric patients with cardiac disease. *AACN Clin Issues Crit Care Nurs* 1990;1(1):131–147. *Reviews developmental aspects of cardiovascular physiology and the rational use of therapeutic agents for acutely ill surgical and medical pediatric patients with cardiac disease.*

Dunbar LM. Emergency room management of congestive heart failure. *Hosp Pract* 1990;25(Suppl. 1):7–14. *This short paper should prove invaluable for nurses who will be providing first-line assessment and intervention for CHF patients.*

Fabius DB, Rein A. Intravenous amrinone therapy: Nursing implications. *Dimens Crit Care Nurs* 1990;9(6):336–342. *Essential, easy reading for critical care nurses who will be using this "inovasodilator."*

Firth BG, Yancy CW Jr. Survival in congestive heart failure: Have we made a difference? *Am J Med* 1990;88(1N):3N–8N. *Reviews some grim statistics obtained with traditional digitalis–diuretic therapy, explains why better survival may come from the use of hydralazine, organic nitrates, ACE inhibitors, and therapies yet to be evaluated.*

Francis GS. Which drug for what patient with heart failure, and when? *Cardiology* 1989;76(5):374–383. *Reviews recent clinical trials that have accounted for some trends, controversies, in the treatment of CHF; shows the growing role of ACE inhibitors, vasodilators; should help you anticipate new developments.*

Galvao M. Role of angiotensin-converting enzyme inhibitors in congestive heart failure. *Heart Lung* 1990;19(5 Pt. 1):505–511. *Compares traditional drug and nondrug therapies for CHF with new developments afforded by the ACE inhibitors.*

Haustein KO. Review: Therapeutic concepts of congestive heart failure. *Int J Clin Pharmacol Ther Toxicol* 1990;28(7):273–281. *A succinct summary of the values, limitations, and potential dangers of the drugs that can be used to treat CHF.*

Kaplan S. New drug approaches to the treatment of heart failure in infants and children. *Drugs* 1990;39(3):388–393. *A well-written overview of the causes and management of heart failure in this special population; gives valuable information to help the nurse anticipate the clinical course and complications.*

Kelly RA. Cardiac glycosides and congestive heart failure. *Am J Cardiol* 1990;65(10):10E–16E. *Focuses on controversies over the use of digitalis—alone or with adjuncts—for mild heart failure, and emphasizes clinical parameters most closely associated with toxicity.*

Kimmelstiel C, Goldberg RJ. Congestive heart failure in women: Focus on heart failure due to coronary artery disease and diabetes. *Cardiology* 1990;77(Suppl. 2):71–79. *A needed discussion of an often-overlooked topic, this focuses mainly on how infarction and diabetes affect the clinical outcome.*

Kulick DL, Rahimtoola SH. Current role of digitalis therapy in patients with congestive heart failure. *JAMA* 1991;265(22):2995–2997. *Reviews clinical data, concludes that digitalis still has an important role in CHF therapy, regardless of its limitations.*

Lang R. Medical management of chronic heart failure: Inotropic, vasodilator, or inodilator drugs? *Am Heart J* 1990;120(6 Pt. 2):1558–1564. *Reviews CHF therapy in terms of modifying the disease process, and focuses on newer drugs that have combined cardiac-stimulating and afterload-reducing properties.*

Luchi RJ, Taffet GE, Teasdale TA. Congestive heart failure in the elderly. *J Am Geriatr Soc* 1991; 39(8):810–825. *An excellent paper on CHF and its therapy in the older population.*

Matheny ML, Wolff LM. Critical dimensions of chronic care: Nursing grand rounds. *J Cardiovasc Nurs* 1990;4(3):71–88. *Interesting insight into how a nursing facility must adapt, through staff education and otherwise, to manage patients with advanced CHF.*

Nagelhout JJ. Pharmacologic treatment of heart failure. *Nurs Clin North Am* 1991;26(2):401–415. *Covers pathophysiology, therapy, and key components of the nursing process, including patient education.*

Packer M, Carver JR, Rodeheffer RJ, et al. Effect of oral milrinone on mortality in severe chronic heart failure. *N Engl J Med* 1991; 325(21):1468–1475. *Nearly 1100 patients with severe chronic CHF were treated with digoxin, diuretics, and ACE inhibitors. Half also received milrinone, an experimental oral inotropic agent that was expected to be a major breakthrough in CHF therapy. Milrinone improved hemodynamic status, but significantly increased morbidity and mortality.*

Parmley WW. Pathophysiology and current therapy of congestive heart failure. *J Am Coll Cardiol* 1989;13(4):771–785. *The focus on pathophysiology gives a better understanding of therapeutic approaches.*

Stanley R. Drug therapy of heart failure. *J Cardiovasc Nurs* 1990; 4(3):17–34. *Reviews the rationale for and clinical use of diuretics, vasodilators, and inotropes in the management of CHF.*

Vine DL. Congestive heart failure. *Am Fam Physician* 1990;42(3): 739–752. *A valuable overview of heart failure causes; diagnostic procedures; clinical findings; treatment (drug and otherwise); difficulties that should be expected and assessed for; and treatment goals.*

Table 31–C Clinical Uses and Administration of Inotropic Drugs

AGENT	CLINICAL USES	DOSAGE AND ROUTE OF ADMINISTRATION
	Digitalis Glycosides	
PROTOTYPE		
Digoxin (LANOXIN)	Congestive heart failure	*Rapid digitalization for undigitalized patient:* Adults, children >10 years: Loading dose 10–15 μg/kg of lean body weight orally (tablets or elixir) or 8–12 μg/kg IV, injected over 5 min; give half of total dose initially, rest 4–8 hr later; maintenance dose (oral tablets or elixir) 25%–35% of loading dose (on μg/kg basis) once daily. Children <10 years: Loading dose 20–60 μg/kg (tablets or elixir), depending on age, or 15–50 μg/kg IV (divided doses); maintenance dose (oral tablets or elixir) 20%–35% of loading dose, depending on age, once daily. Note: Each 100 μg of digoxin liquid-in-capsule is equivalent to 125 μg digoxin formulated as tablet or elixir; reduced dosages required for reduced creatinine clearance; IM injections painful, not recommended *Gradual digitalization:* Start with maintenance doses noted above, once daily, adjusted for drug formulation, body weight, creatinine clearance, etc (eg, 250 μg/d tablet or elixir, 200 μg/d liquid-in-capsule, for 70-kg patient with normal renal function)
	Adjunct to arrhythmia control	IV dosages somewhat higher than those used initially for CHF may be needed
RELATED DRUGS		
Deslanoside (CEDILANID-D)	Emergency digitalization for heart failure, supraventricular arrhythmias	*Emergency digitalization:* IV: 1600 μg (1.6 mg) in single or two equal divided doses IM: 1600 μg, with 800 μg in each of 2 injection sites *Rapid digitalization, loading dose technique for undigitalized patients:* IV: 600 μg followed by 400 μg, then 200 μg at 4–6 hr intervals
Digitoxin (CRYSTODIGIN)	Congestive heart failure	*Gradual digitalization:* Oral: 200 μg bid for 4 days, then 50–300 μg/d (avg 150 μg) for maintenance
	Antidote for Digitalis Intoxication	
Digoxin immune Fab (DIGIBIND)	Treatment of severe digoxin or digitoxin toxicity	IV: Usually 400 mg over 30 min through in-line 0.22 μm pore size membrane filter; inject quickly if cardiac arrest is imminent

(continued)

Table 31–C **Clinical Uses and Administration of Inotropic Drugs (*Continued*)**

AGENT	CLINICAL USES	DOSAGE AND ROUTE OF ADMINISTRATION
Sympathomimetics		
Dobutamine (DOBUTREX)	Acute heart failure	See Table 14-C
Dopamine hydrochloride (INTROPIN)	Acute heart failure	See Table 14-C
Isoproterenol (ISUPREL)	Acute heart failure	See Table 14-C
Other		
Amrinone (INOCOR)	Acute heart failure	IV: Usually dilute 1–3 mg/mL with sterile saline before use; inject 0.75 mg/kg over 2–3 min; follow with infusion of 5–10 μg/kg/min; give additional bolus injections (0.75 mg/kg) after 30 min if needed; avoid diluting in solution containing glucose; discard diluted solution after 24 hr

Table 31–S **Major Side Effects and Contraindications of Drugs Used Mainly for Heart Failure**

BODY SYSTEM/ Side Effect	CONTRAINDICATION/ PRECAUTION	COMMENTS AND NURSING IMPLICATIONS
Digitalis Glycosides		
CENTRAL NERVOUS SYSTEM Confusion, dizziness, ataxia		May indicate digitalis toxicity
EYE Chromatopsia		Consider an early sign of serious digitalis intoxication; discontinue drug
CARDIOVASCULAR Bradycardia, various degrees of heart block, including complete heart block	Preexisting bradycardia or heart block; ventricular ectopy, tachycardia	In general, do not give digitalis to patients with preexisting bradycardia, heart block, or ventricular tachycardia
Arrhythmias, various types, especially premature ventricular contractions	See above	See above; digitalis administration should be discontinued immediately if any arrhythmia not seen before drug administration is observed
GASTROINTESTINAL Nausea, vomiting, anorexia		May be sign of either underlying disease or drug intoxication; discontinue drug at least temporarily as precaution; GI distress not a good indicator of toxicity in children

(continued)

Table 31–S **Major Side Effects and Contraindications of Drugs Used Mainly for Heart Failure (*Continued*)**

BODY SYSTEM/ Side Effect	CONTRAINDICATION/ PRECAUTION	COMMENTS AND NURSING IMPLICATIONS
Amrinone		
BLOOD Thrombocytopenia		Monitor platelet counts periodically; assess for signs of impaired coagulation (excessive, abnormal bleeding, etc)
LIVER Hepatotoxicity		Monitor liver function enzymes; assess for jaundice, abdominal pain, etc

Table 31–I **Major Interactions Between Digitalis and Other Drugs**

AGENT	RESULT OF INTERACTION	COMMENTS AND NURSING IMPLICATIONS
Interactions Involving All Digitalis Drugs		
Antacids (Chapter 40)	Decreased (usual) or increased absorption, effects, of oral digitalis	Outcome, importance of interaction, depends on composition of antacid (most bind digitalis in gut, reduce absorption, effects), digitalis dosage form, timing of administration of interactants; separate administration of antacids and digitalis by as much time as feasible; discourage excessive or prolonged antacid use, especially if use not monitored by health-care provider; assess for altered digitalis responses
	Reduced control of CHF owing to sodium content of antacid	Recommend sodium-free antacids to all CHF patients who require antacids, especially chronically
Antithyroid drugs, oral (eg, propylthiouracil; Chapter 47)	Increased digitalis blood levels, effects; potential toxicity	Starting antithyroid drug therapy in a patient stabilized on digitalis decreases digitalis elimination, increases effects; monitor accordingly; anticipate need to reduce digitalis dosage to prevent toxicity
Cholestyramine (Chapter 36)	Decreased digitalis blood levels, effects	Interactant interferes with enterohepatic recirculation of digitalis, can affect oral or parenteral digitalis therapy; if cholestyramine must be used with oral digitalis, separate administration times as much as possible; monitor for reduced control of CHF signs, symptoms
Colestipol (Chapter 36)	Decreased digitalis blood levels, effects	See cholestyramine, above
Diuretics, potassium-wasting (high-ceiling, thiazides; Chapter 32)	Increased risk of digitalis toxicity, especially arrhythmias	Combined use very common, but is main cause of digitalis toxicity; interaction caused by hypokalemia and hypomagnesemia can be serious or life-threatening, even when digitalis blood levels are in therapeutic range; monitor serum K^+ and $Mg2^+$, clinical response to digitalis, often; anticipate need for adjunctive use of potassium-sparing diuretic or oral potassium supplements to prevent or treat hypokalemia

(continued)

Table 31–I **Major Interactions Between Digitalis and Other Drugs (*Continued*)**

AGENT	RESULT OF INTERACTION	COMMENTS AND NURSING IMPLICATIONS
Interactions Involving All Digitalis Drugs		
Laxatives/cathartics (Chapter 41)	Reduced digitalis absorption; increased digitalis effects, toxicity risk	Use should be supervised, kept as short as possible, administration spaced to minimize interaction; excessive electrolyte loss in stool may trigger toxicity, even if amount of digitalis absorbed is reduced
Quinidine (Chapter 30)	Increased digitalis blood levels, effects; potential toxicity	Interactant alters digitalis elimination (mechanisms for digoxin, digitoxin, differ, outcome similar); interaction of most concern, outcome appears faster (usually 3 days or less), when starting quinidine therapy in patient already stabilized on digoxin; anticipate need to reduce digitalis dose, often by 50% or more; monitor clinical responses, digitalis blood levels; *never* give quinidine to patient near or experiencing digitalis toxicity
Thyroid hormone supplements (Chapter 47)	Decreased digitalis blood levels, effects	Starting thyroid hormone supplementation in hypothyroid patient stabilized on digitalis increases digitalis elimination, reduces effects; monitor accordingly, anticipate need to increase digitalis dose cautiously
Verapamil (Chapter 34)	Increased digitalis blood levels, potential toxicity, especially risk of excessive AV nodal conduction depression, heart block	Monitor closely, focus on signs, symptoms of heart failure, P–R interval on ECG (as indicator of nodal function); assessment may indicate need to reduce digitalis dose cautiously during combined use
Interactions Involving Mainly Digoxin		
Aminoglycoside antibiotics (eg, neomycin; Chapter 56)	Potentially reduced digoxin absorption, effects	Monitor accordingly when long-term aminoglycoside therapy started in patient stabilized on digoxin; digoxin dosage may need to be increased
Amiodarone (Chapter 30)	Increased digoxin blood levels; potential toxicity	Interaction potentially serious but slow in onset owing to interactant's long half-life; anticipate need for long-term monitoring
Anticancer drugs, most (Chapter 59)	Decreased absorption of oral digoxin, decreased effects	Monitor digoxin levels, clinical responses for potential need to increase dosage; interactants thought to alter gut mucosa, reduce digoxin absorption
Bepridil (Chapter 34)	Increased digoxin blood levels, effects	Monitor responses, especially for bradycardia owing to additive depressant effects of both drugs on heart rate
Cyclosporine (Chapter 54)	Increased digoxin blood levels, risk of toxicity	Anticipate, monitor closely for signs of toxicity; be prepared to temporarily discontinue digoxin, allow blood levels, response to normalize, resume treatment with lower digoxin dosage
Erythromycin (Chapter 56)	Increased absorption of oral digoxin, increased blood levels, toxicity	Interactant inhibits gut bacteria that normally inactivate part of digoxin dose; monitor accordingly; interaction less likely to occur with digoxin capsules (normally give nearly 100% absorption) than tablets
Indomethacin (Chapter 52)	Decreased digoxin excretion, increased blood levels, effects; potential toxicity	Documented for premature infants; anticipate need to reduce digoxin dose by about half if interactant is added to stabilized patient

(continued)

Table 31–I | **Major Interactions Between Digitalis and Other Drugs (*Continued*)**

AGENT	RESULT OF INTERACTION	COMMENTS AND NURSING IMPLICATIONS
Interactions Involving Mainly Digoxin		
Metoclopramide (Chapter 42)	Decreased absorption of oral digoxin, decreased digoxin effects	Assess for inadequate digoxin effects; interactant increases gut motility, allows less time for digoxin absorption; probably less problematic for digoxin capsules (almost 100% absorbed)
Penicillamine (Chapter 52)	Decreased absorption of oral digoxin, decreased digoxin effects	Evidence of decreased digoxin effects may appear soon after starting penicillamine; assess accordingly; mechanism not certain
Propafenone (Chapter 30)	Increased digoxin effects; potential toxicity	Requires close monitoring of digoxin blood levels, clinical response to help determine need for digoxin dosage reduction
Tetracyclines (Chapter 56)	Increased absorption of oral digoxin, increased blood levels, toxicity	See erythromycin, above
Rifampin (Chapter 57)	Decreased digitoxin blood levels, effects	Interactant stimulates digitoxin metabolism; monitor blood levels, clinical response; may need to increase digitoxin dosage

PROTOTYPES

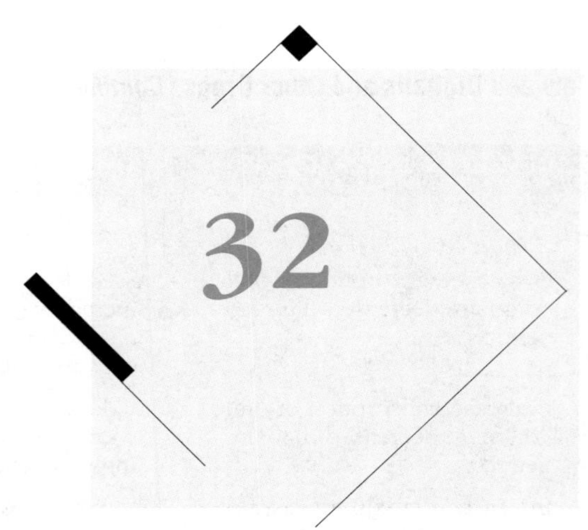

Diuretic Drugs

Diuretic drugs increase the amount of water and sodium ion that is excreted by the kidneys in the urine. These effects help rid the body of excess fluid and help lower blood pressure. They provide the rationale for using most of the common diuretics to manage edema and hypertension. The first part of this chapter discusses the major groups of orally effective diuretics—where and how they work, their uses, and the unwanted effects or potential drug interactions that are likely to occur during therapy when specific drugs are used. The second part identifies general guidelines for the optimal use of diuretics, and problems that may arise during therapy. The chapter concludes with an overview of diuretics that have limited or special uses.

I. Major Classes of Common Diuretics

There are three major classes of orally effective diuretics. Each has a prototype:

- *thiazides*—hydrochlorothiazide
- *high-ceiling diuretics*—furosemide
- *potassium-sparing diuretics*—triamterene

By definition, all these drugs exert their effects by interfering with the ability of the kidney tubules to reabsorb sodium ion. This is called a *natriuretic effect*. Since the movement of water follows the movement of sodium in many parts of the kidney tubules, increased sodium loss is accompanied by increased water loss; urine volume increases. The different diuretic classes cause these effects in different ways. Similarly, they differ in terms of how they affect renal handling of other substances, particularly potassium. The thiazides and the high-ceiling diuretics can be grouped together because they share the ability to increase potassium loss into the urine. They are *potassium-wasting*. This is a clinically important difference from the actions of drugs such as triamterene, which reduce potassium excretion and so are called *potassium-sparing*. The various diuretics also affect other ions, such as calcium; and metabolites such as glucose and uric acid.

Collectively, the similarities and differences affect the selection of a particular diuretic or diuretic class for a particular patient. They also contribute to many of the important side effects or adverse responses that may be encountered during therapy.

Major reference tables appear beginning on p. 624.

Thiazides

Hydrochlorothiazide (ESIDRIX, HYDRODIURIL, others; often abbreviated HCTZ on a patient's chart) is the prototype of a large group of diuretics. In proper chemical terminology they are called *benzothiadiazides,* but they are usually referred to simply as thiazides. Hydrochlorothiazide and all the related drugs are available as single-entity products—products that contain nothing but the diuretic agent. A few are available as fixed-dose combinations that also contain a potassium-sparing diuretic or some other type of antihypertensive drug.

PROTOTYPE

Hydrochlorothiazide

Absorption, Distribution, Metabolism, and Excretion

Hydrochlorothiazide is absorbed well from the gastrointestinal (GI) tract, and is almost always given orally. Giving the drug with food does not reduce absorption. About 60% of hydrochlorothiazide molecules in the bloodstream are bound to plasma proteins. Thiazides are excreted by the kidneys; prior metabolism is not very important. These drugs cross the placenta, enter the fetal circulation, and are excreted in maternal milk.

Pharmacologic Effects

The primary effects of thiazides, and all other diuretics for that matter, depend on their actions in the kidney tubules. By altering urine volume and composition they can eventually affect the volume and composition of the rest of the body fluids. Effects of diuretics outside the kidney can also have an impact on fluid volume and composition.

Effects on Sodium and Water

Thiazides act in the last part of the loop of Henle (Fig. 32–1), nearly into the distal tubule, to slightly inhibit ion pumps that participate in sodium and chloride reabsorption. This indirectly inhibits water reabsorption and increases urine volume slightly. Thiazides cause only modest increases of urine output—about 3 mL/min, compared with a normal value of 1 mL/min. This peak effect occurs about 5 hours after oral administration (Table 32–1). It cannot be increased much, even with very large dose increases. As a result, the thiazides are said to have a "flat" dose-response curve. Nevertheless, the modest diuretic effects of these drugs can help mobilize edema fluid and lower blood pressure.

Effects on Potassium, Magnesium, and Calcium

Therapeutic doses of thiazides increase urinary potassium and magnesium excretion, and decrease urinary calcium excretion. In doing so, they can lower serum potassium and magnesium levels, and cause serum calcium levels to rise. These effects can be clinically important, either as a desired response or an adverse effect, depending on the patient.

Effects on Uric Acid, Glucose, and Lipids

Thiazides significantly decrease renal tubular secretion of uric acid, so serum uric acid levels rise. They also inhibit pancreatic insulin release, and somehow interfere with the ability of cells throughout the body to take up glucose. As a result, they usually increase blood glucose levels. Effects on lipids are important also. Thiazides increase serum total and low-density-lipoprotein (LDL) cholesterol levels, and cause a somewhat greater increase of serum triglyceride levels. The mechanisms responsible for the effects on lipids are not fully known.

Effects on Acid–Base Balance

To varying degrees, hydrochlorothiazide and the thiazide-like diuretics increase bicarbonate loss in the urine. They do this by weakly inhibiting the enzyme *carbonic anhydrase.* In doing so they may alkalinize the urine, yet they rarely change blood pH.

Vascular Effects

Thiazides can constrict the afferent renal arterioles, which deliver blood to the glomerulus for processing into urine. This can decrease the glomerular filtration rate (GFR) and may decrease urine production under some circumstances (an antidiuretic effect). Depending on the patient, this can be beneficial or unwanted. Thiazides can also constrict the umbilical vessels and may reduce placental blood flow. The ability of these drugs to lower circulating fluid volume and blood pressure can reduce placental blood flow further.

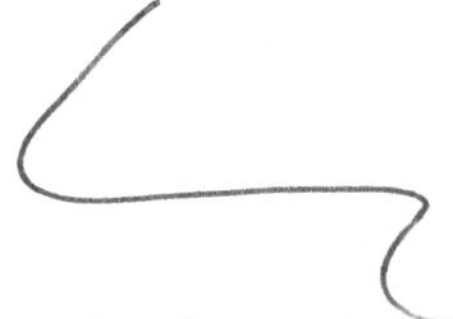

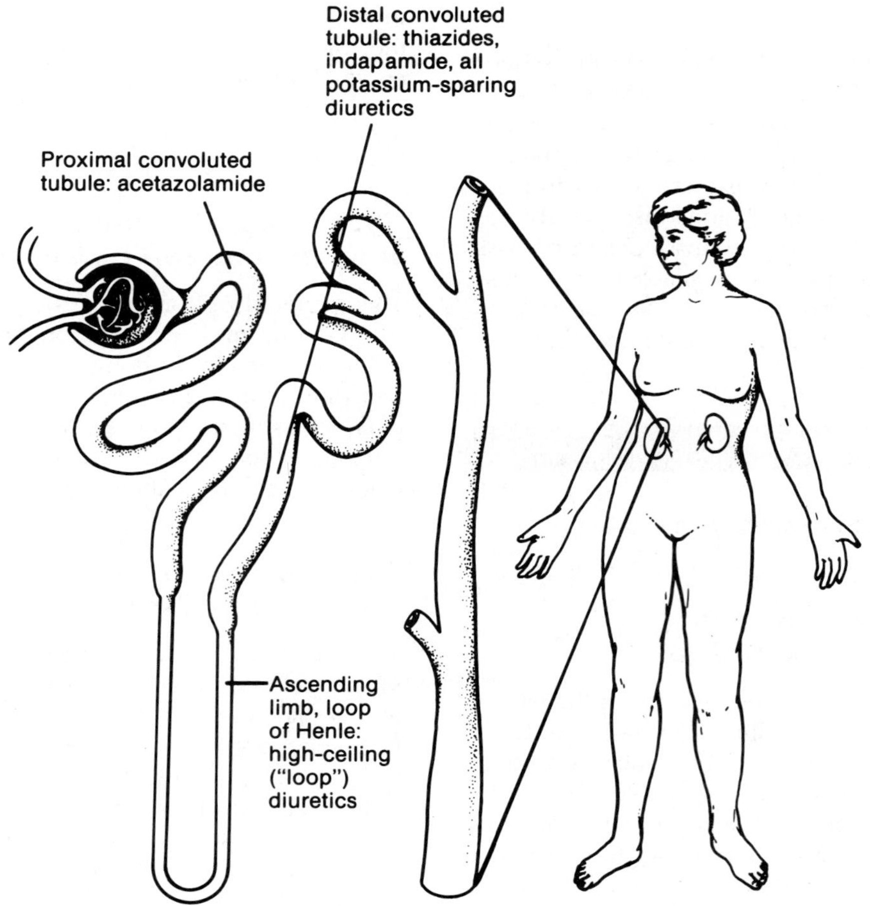

Figure 32–1

Nephron and sites of action of major orally effective diuretics.

Long-term thiazide administration, and the resulting decrease of body sodium stores, reduces the sensitivity of vascular smooth muscle to norepinephrine, the major vasoconstrictor substance in the body. This lowers total peripheral resistance and blood pressure. If blood pressure was elevated before thiazide treatment, during treatment it will often remain lower than prior levels, even after the drug's diuretic action appears to be lost.

Clinical Indications and Administration

The thiazides are mainly used to manage essential hypertension or mild chronic edema, as accompanies congestive heart failure (CHF). Table 32–2 compares the usefulness of these drugs with diuretics in other classes. Dosages are given in Table 32–C. General clinical implications for the use of thiazides and other diuretics are discussed later (pp 613–618). Those specifically related to use for heart failure or hypertension are noted in Chapters 31 and 33, respectively.

Treatment of Essential Hypertension

For years thiazides have been preferred drugs for starting therapy of mild essential hypertension. This preference is decreasing, mainly because of concerns about the unwanted ability of thiazides to raise blood levels of lipids and other metabolites. Nevertheless, although the antihypertensive actions of thiazides are modest compared with those of many other antihypertensive drugs (Chapter 33), they are clearly satisfactory for many patients with mild increases of blood pressure.

Table 32–1 | Time-Course of Action of Major Diuretics

DRUG	DIURETIC EFFECT Onset	Peak	Duration
Thiazides or Thiazide-like Diuretics (Selected Examples)			
Hydrochlorothiazide or chlorothiazide (oral)	2 hr	4 hr	6–12 hr
Chlorthalidone	2 hr	2–6 hr	24–72 hr
Metolazone	1 hr	2 hr	12–24 hr
Polythiazide	2 hr	6 hr	24–48 hr
High-Ceiling Diuretics			
Furosemide or ethacrynic acid (oral)	1 hr	1–2 hr	6–8 hr
Bumetanide (oral)	0.5–1 hr	1–2 hr	4–6 hr
Furosemide (IV)	5 min	30 min	2 hr
Bumetanide (IV)	5 min	30 min	<1 hr
Ethacrynate sodium (IV)	5 min	15–30 min	2 hr
Potassium-Sparing Diuretics			
Amiloride (oral)	2 hr	6–10 hr	24 hr
Spironolactone (oral)	1–2 days	2–3 days	2–3 days
Triamterene (oral)	2–4 hr	6–8 hr	12–16 hr

Table 32–2 | Usefulness of Diuretics in Various Medical Conditions

Indication	Thiazides and Related Diuretics	High-Ceiling Diuretics	Potassium-Sparing Diuretics
Edema-forming states (CHF, cirrhosis, nephrosis)	+	++	+*
Essential hypertension	++	+	+*
Hypercalcemia	—	++	—
Hypercalciuria	++	—	—
Diabetes insipidus	+	—	—
Renal failure	—	+	—

Key: +, useful; ++, very useful; —, not indicated.
*Usually used with one of the potassium-wasting diuretics (thiazides or high-ceiling agents).

Source: Modified from Lief PD. Appraisal and reappraisal of diuretic therapy. *Am Heart J* 1978; 96: 824–827.

Thiazides can be used alone to treat hypertension, but they also play an important adjunctive role with other classes of antihypertensive drugs. This is because (1) their antihypertensive actions are additive to those of other antihypertensive drugs; and (2) they help counteract renal sodium retention—a side effect triggered by many other antihypertensive agents. There are many proprietary antihypertensive products that contain a thiazide plus another blood pressure–lowering drug. This attests to the common adjunctive use of thiazides in treating essential hypertension.

Treatment of Edema

The ability of thiazides to increase urinary fluid output may be useful for treating mild edematous states due to disease (eg, heart failure) or water-retaining drugs (eg, corticosteroids, estrogens). However, thiazides are seldom suitable for treating more severe edema, since their peak effects often are not adequate in these situations. Likewise, their relatively slow onsets of action make them inappropriate in medical emergencies that require quick interventions for severe fluid accumulation.

Other Uses

Treatment of Hypercalciuria, Prophylaxis of Hip Fracture

The ability of thiazides to reduce renal calcium excretion is useful. These drugs can be used to treat idiopathic hypercalciuria. In this condition calcium excretion in the urine is so great that calcium stones can form and block the kidney tubules, potentially causing serious kidney damage. Hydrochlorothiazide has also been shown to reduce the incidence of hip fracture in the elderly. This may be due to its ability to increase serum calcium levels, which occurs because calcium excretion is reduced.

Management of Diabetes Insipidus

The paradoxic antidiuretic effect of hydrochlorothiazide can be used in some patients with nephrogenic diabetes insipidus. This is a form of diabetes insipidus in which antidiuretic hormone is present, but the kidneys fail to respond to it. The patient produces unusually large amounts of dilute urine each day. This **polyuria** leads to other signs and symptoms, including polydipsia (excessive thirst), dehydration, and electrolyte disturbances. Thiazides can often dramatically reduce, although not normalize, urine volume and the resulting problems.

Side Effects, Adverse Reactions, and Contraindications

Most side effects caused by thiazides are extensions of their actions on how the kidneys control water, ions, and metabolites such as uric acid, glucose, and lipids (Table 32–S). For otherwise healthy persons, these effects usually are not worrisome. For other persons the side effects may be clinically important, whether by aggravating underlying disease or by causing drug interactions. By anticipating and being prepared to deal with them, side effects need not prevent the use of these drugs. Many of the side effects noted below for the thiazides apply also to the high-ceiling diuretics, which are discussed in the next major drug section.

Sodium and Water Depletion

All diuretics have the ability to cause excessive sodium and water depletion (hyponatremia and hypovolemia, respectively). However, compared with more effective agents such as furosemide (p 608), the incidence and severity of these problems are relatively low with thiazides. This is especially true if no other diuretics are given to the patient, and measures are taken to maintain normal hydration and serum electrolyte values. Using a thiazide with another type of diuretic increases the risk of fluid and electrolyte imbalances. Such diuretic combinations are used quite often.

Polyuria is common during early diuretic therapy. Sodium and water loss may cause hypotension. This is usually orthostatic hypotension, which leads to dizziness or syncope mainly when the patient stands up abruptly. Other important signs and symptoms of hyponatremia and hypovolemia are noted in Table 32–3.

Oliguria, a significant decrease of urine production, is another potential concern. Thiazides, especially at high doses, can cause problems for patients with renal dysfunction, even that associated with aging. In the presence of renal dysfunction, continued administration of thiazides can cause further reductions of GFR and renal blood flow, which may lead to renal failure. Decreased (below baseline) urine output, increased blood urea nitrogen (BUN) levels, and increased total blood protein content (**azotemia**) are some of the signs and symptoms of this adverse effect. Patients with previously good renal function may experience reduced urine output in response to high doses of a thiazide, but this is not likely unless they are already water- and sodium-depleted.

Oliguria and, particularly, anuria, contraindicate thiazide use; continued thiazide use in these situations can cause renal failure.

Table 32–3 Common Signs and Symptoms of Electrolyte Imbalances Caused by Orally Effective Diuretics

Hypovolemia
Thirst
Oliguria
Hypotension
Dry skin and mucous membranes
Hyponatremia
Anxiety
Increased thirst
Drowsiness, confusion, stupor
Muscle weakness, twitching (convulsions if severe)
Abdominal cramping
Oliguria or anuria
Hypotension, tachycardia
Hypokalemia
Thirst
Muscle cramps or pain
Flaccid paralysis, tetany
Paralytic ileus
Cardiac arrhythmias
Lethargy, depression, irritability, confusion
Anorexia, nausea, vomiting
Hyperkalemia
Mental confusion or anxiety
Fatigue
Subjective weakness or heaviness of the extremities
Paresthesias
Dyspnea
Arrhythmias
Metabolic or Hypochloremic Alkalosis
Slow, shallow respiration (an attempt to conserve carbon dioxide)
Hypertonic muscles; tetany or convulsions
Arrhythmias

NURSING IMPLICATIONS

Azotemia may trigger a sudden onset of confusion or altered consciousness. If oliguria is due to excessive fluid loss, anticipate the need for reduced diuretic doses and oral or intravenous (IV) fluid and salt replacement to correct the deficiencies. If the patient is well hydrated or still edematous, but a thiazide proves inadequate, anticipate a switch to a more efficacious diuretic such as furosemide, and the need to investigate further the lack of response.

Hypokalemia

The potassium-wasting effect of the thiazides often can be important. *As many as half of all patients taking thiazides chronically develop hypokalemia and its related symptoms sometime during therapy.* If hypokalemia becomes severe, various neurologic, GI, muscular, and cardiac disturbances can occur (see Table 32–3). Cardiac arrhythmias are the most serious problem, and are most important for patients who are also taking digoxin or a related digitalis preparation (Chapter 31). Hypokalemia increases the risk of digitalis toxicity, yet most patients with CHF routinely take both digitalis and a potassium-wasting diuretic. Indeed, diuretic-induced hypokalemia is the most common cause of digitalis toxicity. To reduce this risk, thiazides are often used along with other drugs that counteract the potassium depletion. This is discussed on pages 611 to 613.

Hypomagnesemia

The ability of thiazides to increase urinary magnesium is seldom clinically significant for most patients. However, it can become an important problem if the patient already has magnesium deficiencies (eg, caused by chronic alcoholism or that associated with pregnancy). Hypomagnesemia, like hypokalemia, can also increase the risk of cardiac arrhythmias, especially if the patient is taking digoxin or another digitalis product.

Hypercalcemia

This side effect, caused by a thiazide's ability to reduce urinary calcium loss, can pose problems for patients with preexisting hypercalcemia, or those who are at risk for this electrolyte imbalance for other reasons.

Hyperuricemia

The ability of thiazides to increase serum uric acid levels can cause clinically significant hyperuricemia in some patients. The major outcome of this hyperuricemic effect is gout. As a result, thiazides should be used cautiously, if at all, in patients with a history of hyperuricemia or gout.

NURSING IMPLICATIONS

Patients with a history of hyperuricemia or gout generally should not receive a thiazide. However, if a thiazide is prescribed, check serum uric acid levels periodically and instruct patients to report immediately the development of gout symptoms. Allopurinol may be prescribed for these patients. It inhibits uric acid synthesis and may reduce the chance of diuretic-induced hyperuricemia. To further reduce the risk of gout, encourage patients to drink adequate amounts of water (six to eight glasses per day). With adequate diuretic therapy, this water intake should not worsen hypertension or edema.

Hyperglycemia

Thiazide-induced hyperglycemia is a concern mainly for diabetic or prediabetic patients. By altering blood glucose levels, the thiazide may necessitate a change of diet, or a change of the dose of insulin or other antidiabetic drug. Thiazide therapy usually requires increased doses of antidiabetic medications soon after diuretic therapy is started, although antidiabetic drug requirements for a few patients may decrease or remain the same. Discontinuation of thiazide administration may require another readjustment of antidiabetic therapy. Overall, thiazides must be used cautiously in diabetic or prediabetic persons.

NURSING IMPLICATIONS

Because thiazides exert a variable effect on blood glucose, blood glucose levels in diabetic or prediabetic patients should be evaluated carefully and frequently during early treatment. If possible, diuretics other than thiazides should be used for diabetics with edema or hypertension. Advise diabetic patients of possible changes of diet and drug requirements, encourage them to give extra attention to the results of at-home glucose tests, and instruct them to report at once any symptoms of hypoglycemia or hyperglycemia.

Hyperlipidemias

The ability of thiazides to elevate serum cholesterol and triglyceride levels accounts, in large part, for the reason some physicians are prescribing these drugs less often for hypertension—a disorder that often is accompanied by hyperlipidemias and atherosclerotic organ disease. For many other patients, however, such metabolic changes may be less clinically important; they can be lessened somewhat by proper diet, and can be detected early with proper monitoring.

Other Side Effects

Thiazides may cause minor GI upset. Severe GI pain, accompanied by nausea and vomiting, may indicate rare thiazide-induced pancreatitis. This is possibly an allergic reaction. In some patients the reaction may affect the liver, causing jaundice; or the bone marrow, causing blood dyscrasias (thrombocytopenia, agranulocytosis). Hives and other skin rashes may also occur. Some of these problems may be due to the sulfonamide-like structure of the thiazides. Because of the similar structures, thiazides are generally contraindicated for patients with known allergy to sulfonamide antibiotics (Chapter 56).

NURSING IMPLICATIONS

Administer thiazides with meals to reduce mild GI discomfort. Instruct patients to report at once signs of hepatic or pancreatic damage (severe abdominal pain, jaundice, urinary discoloration) or blood dyscrasias (sore throat, fever, flu-like symptoms; abnormal bruising or bleeding). These reactions are rare, but potentially dangerous.

◆ Use During Pregnancy and Lactation

Thiazides reduce edema and the increased blood pressure that may accompany pregnancy. However, they should not be given to pregnant women unless drug therapy is *absolutely necessary* and there are *no suitable alternatives* (this is seldom the case). The ability of thiazides to reduce placental blood flow may cause fetal harm. These drugs are not recommended for use by mothers who are breast-feeding their infants. See Chapter 33 for more information about the use of antihypertensive drugs during pregnancy.

◆ Use in Children

Thiazides can be used to treat edema and hypertension in children. Pediatric doses of hydrochlorothiazide are approximately 1 mg per pound of body weight per day (see (Table 32–C).

◆ Use in the Elderly

Thiazides seem to be particularly efficacious for antihypertensive therapy in the elderly. However, their metabolic and fluid-depleting side effects sometimes are problematic, and they may unexpectedly aggravate borderline renal or hepatic insufficiency. As noted before, there is also increasing interest in the use of thiazides for reducing the incidence of hip fracture in the elderly.

Interactions with Other Drugs

Diuretics participate in many drug–drug interactions. Those that are most common or clinically important are summarized and explained further in Table 32–I, along with related nursing implications. The interactions can be grouped in three ways:

- *Those that can apply to all the common orally administered diuretics,* owing to their similar effects on renal sodium and fluid handling, and on blood pressure. The key interactants are alcohol, other classes of antihypertensive drugs, laxatives and cathartics, the antimanic drug lithium, and methylxanthines such as caffeine and theophylline.
- *Those that apply to the thiazides, the high-ceiling agents, and acetazolamide,* because of their potassium-wasting actions. The important interactants are amphotericin B, digoxin and other digitalis drugs, and systemically administered corticosteroids. Interactions with digoxin are clearly the most common and clinically important, owing to the frequent concomitant use of the two groups of drugs. Magnesium loss in the urine contributes to the potentially serious problems.
- *Those that are more likely to occur with thiazides than with other classes of diuretics.* Key interactants are diazoxide and oral antidiabetic drugs such as tolbutamide, which raise or lower blood glucose levels, respectively; and probenecid, which is used to increase renal uric acid excretion. (The high-ceiling and the potassium-sparing diuretics can participate in similar interactions with these drugs. However, the frequency and severity of the interactions are thought to be less than those seen with thiazides.)

NURSING IMPLICATIONS

Thiazides can be administered with most interactants if necessary; combined use with digoxin is routine. However, it is important to anticipate the likely outcomes of interactions, and monitor for them closely and often, especially until blood levels of each agent stabilize. If adverse effects from any interaction cannot be prevented, reducing the dose of (or discontinuing) one or more agents is usually indicated.

Overdose and Toxicity

Thiazide overdoses are not likely to be serious unless other diuretics or antihypertensive drugs are coadministered, or the patient already has serious fluid or electrolyte imbalances. Major signs and symptoms include hypotension and reflex tachycardia from excessive salt and water loss. Hypokalemia may be a problem with chronic overdoses. Treatment usually involves discontinuing the diuretic and correcting blood volume and electrolytes with oral or parenteral therapy as needed. Laboratory tests are essential for guiding treatment. Standard measures to reduce drug absorption (see Appendix C) are indicated for acute overdoses.

Related Drugs

About a dozen other diuretics have pharmacologic properties similar to hydrochlorothiazide (see Table 32–C). They differ mainly in terms of doses (potency) and durations of action. Of those, chlorthalidone (HYGROTON), metolazone (DIULO, ZAROXOLYN), and quinethazone (HYDROMOX) are not, chemically, thiazides. However, some of their actions are so similar to the prototype that they can be considered equivalent. Chlorthalidone is noteworthy because its actions may last 2 to 3 days (vs about 12 hours for most others).

Indapamide

Indapamide (LOZOL) is not, chemically, a thiazide or even a thiazide-like agent. It belongs to the indolone class. Nevertheless, in terms of pharmacologic effects and clinical uses it is similar to hydrochlorothiazide in many ways. Indapamide is used as an alternative to a thiazide for managing hypertension or edema, for which its efficacy seems to be about equivalent. Dosages are listed in Table 32–C. Compared with a typical thiazide, indapamide allegedly is less likely to cause major changes of blood potassium, uric acid, glucose, or lipid levels. Nevertheless, patients at risk from these side effects require appropriate monitoring, as discussed for hydrochlorothiazide.

High-Ceiling Diuretics

This group of drugs includes the prototype, furosemide (LASIX), and two related drugs, ethacrynic acid (EDECRIN) and bumetanide (BUMEX). They are called *high-*

ceiling diuretics because their peak diuretic effects are very great. They can also be called "loop" diuretics, indicating their major site of action in the nephron—the loop of Henle (see Fig. 32–1). And, like the thiazides, they are classified as potassium-wasting.

PROTOTYPE

Furosemide

Absorption, Distribution, Metabolism, and Excretion

Furosemide is absorbed well from the GI tract, and it is often given orally. A sterile preparation is available for IM or IV injection. High-ceiling diuretics bind to plasma proteins; they are eliminated by renal excretion.

Pharmacologic Effects

Many effects of furosemide are similar in kind to those caused by thiazides, but they differ in terms of intensity.

Effects on Sodium and Water

Furosemide inhibits sodium and chloride reabsorption in the ascending limb of the loop of Henle. That is the part of the nephron where the reabsorption of these ions is the greatest, and the ability of these diuretics to inhibit these processes is considerable. Overall, compared with thiazides and virtually all other classes of common diuretics, furosemide and its related drugs

- cause a much greater peak increase of urine output;
- have a steep dose–response curve;
- often increase urine output when another class of diuretic cannot;
- cause diuresis much faster (Table 32–1); and
- are often given parenterally.

Low doses of furosemide cause a slight increase of urine output, similar to that seen with "usual" doses of a thiazide. Higher doses increase urine production much more, and it is fairly easy to titrate the dose for an optimum response. Urine outputs of 8 to 10 mL/min are common in well-hydrated or edematous patients (vs a normal rate of 1 mL/min, or 3 mL/min with a thiazide). However, the almost limitless diuretic effect also makes it easier to cause excessive fluid loss if an overdose is given.

Unlike thiazides, therapeutic doses of furosemide generally increase renal blood flow and GFR. These effects add to the diuretic responses that are caused by the drug's effects on ion transport in the kidney tubules. Therapeutic doses do not cause an antidiuretic effect. However, if the dose is too great, and hypovolemia and hypotension occur, renal blood flow, GFR, and urine output will fall.

Other Effects

Furosemide and the other high-ceiling diuretics increase renal potassium and magnesium excretion, and decrease excretion of uric acid and glucose. These effects are essentially similar to those caused by thiazides. In contrast, however, the high-ceiling diuretics increase renal calcium excretion. Effects on serum lipids do not seem to be great.

Clinical Indications and Administration

Furosemide is indicated for managing chronic edema, and for edema that accompanies acute pulmonary edema (see Tables 32–2 and 32–C). It may also be used as an alternative to a thiazide for essential hypertension. The high-ceiling diuretics are often used with other drugs, but they are not available in fixed-dose combination products.

Treatment of Edema

When the clinical goal is to manage edema, either a thiazide or a high-ceiling agent might be used. The choice is usually based on the unique needs of each patient, and on the physician's preferences. However, many physicians choose low doses of furosemide (or a related agent) over thiazides, even for mild edema, because the risks of hypokalemia, hyperuricemia, and hyperglycemia seem to be less. Additionally, if the patient does not respond to an initial low dose of a diuretic, it usually is simpler to increase the dose of a drug that was already started (i.e., a high-ceiling diuretic) than to switch from a thiazide to a high-ceiling agent. As noted earlier, the flat dose–response curve of thiazides limits their suitability when dosage increases are anticipated or needed to combat edema. In general, a high-ceiling agent is clearly preferred for managing edema caused by heart, liver, or kidney dysfunction.

A high-ceiling diuretic is clearly superior to a thiazide when the goal is to eliminate large amounts of fluid, or to do so rapidly. Their quick onset, higher peak effect, and steep dose–response relationship simply cannot be matched by other agents. In the presence of pulmonary edema, for example, prompt diuresis can quickly reduce vascular congestion, the heart's work load, and the extreme distress from breathing difficulty. For these situations, furosemide or an alternative can be given intravenously (preferred) or intramuscularly (painful). Oral administration can be started once the patient stabilizes and is able to take oral medications.

High-ceiling diuretics are also of value in managing ascites, but whether the fluid is removed pharmacologically, by syringe aspiration (paracentesis), or both, depends on the situation.

Treatment of Hypertension

High-ceiling diuretics are used less often than thiazides to treat essential hypertension, mainly because their antihypertensive efficacy is not greater and side effects such as excessive volume depletion may be more. Moreover, a high-ceiling diuretic alone is not likely to control blood pressure well in edema-free patients who have failed to respond adequately to a thiazide. When a diuretic alone is not adequate, other antihypertensive drugs (Chapter 33) usually need to be added to the therapeutic plan, or tried instead.

Furosemide or another high-ceiling diuretic can be used for hypertensive crises caused by acute fluid (blood) overload. However, in most hypertensive emergencies blood pressure is not high because of this; it is high because of excessive constriction of the peripheral blood vessels, and blood volume can be normal. In this more common situation the goal is to dilate blood vessels, not to reduce fluid levels below normal. Injecting a large dose of a powerful diuretic will quickly shift large amounts of fluid from the blood into the urine. This will lower blood pressure—often too much—and trigger reflex activation of the sympathetic nervous system. One outcome of the reflex is increased vasoconstriction, which will reduce blood flow to the vital organs even more. If furosemide is given, and then the correct antihypertensive medication is eventually administered (see nitroprusside, pp 655–656), blood pressure is liable to "bottom out." Cardiovascular collapse might occur.

Treatment of Hypercalcemia

Elevated serum calcium levels due to drugs or endocrine imbalances (eg, adrenal insufficiency, hyperparathyroidism) sometimes can be managed with furosemide.

NURSING IMPLICATIONS

Do not mix furosemide with acidic solutions. It can be mixed with isotonic saline, D_5W, or lactated Ringer's solution, for continuous IV infusion. Undiluted IV injections should not exceed 40 mg, and should be given slowly, over 2 minutes. Keep oral furosemide solutions refrigerated.

Side Effects, Adverse Reactions, and Contraindications

Many side effects caused by high-ceiling diuretics are identical to those noted for thiazides, but the risks and severity differ.

Sodium and Water Depletion, Hypotension

The greater diuretic action and steeper dose–response relationship of high-ceiling diuretics carry some risks. They increase the chance of causing excessive sodium and volume depletion, and hypotension; or changes that can occur too quickly to be tolerated well by the patient. Depressed blood pressure and volume can also lead to decreased renal function, seen as oliguria or anuria. Furosemide and related high-ceiling diuretics are contraindicated for hypotensive or anuric patients.

Urine outputs of 20 liters in a single day (roughly 44 pounds of water) have been reported when large doses of furosemide were given to grossly edematous patients. Most patients, particularly those with hepatic cirrhosis or the nephrotic syndrome, do not tolerate well these sudden and large changes of blood pressure and volume. Urine outputs of this magnitude should rarely be a goal. Unless edema is acute and life-threatening, diuresis always should be induced gradually by starting therapy with low doses.

When used too aggressively—chronically or acutely—high-ceiling diuretics can cause a syndrome called *contraction alkalosis* or *hypochloremic alkalosis.* "Contraction" implies that extracellular fluid volume (ie, blood volume) has shrunk excessively because of fluid shifts from the bloodstream into the urine. Along with the excess sodium and water loss, large amounts of chloride ion are excreted; this causes the hypochloremia. The other major anion of the blood, bicarbonate, remains in the bloodstream; this causes systemic (metabolic) alkalosis. Volume depletion, hypochloremia, and alkalosis usually occur together.

Blood pressure falls when contraction alkalosis occurs. Loss of water from the blood raises the concentration of cells and protein in the blood. This is reflected,

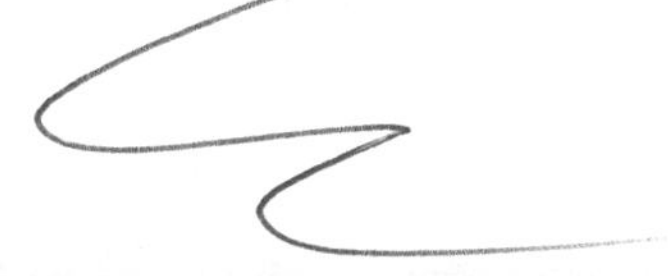

in laboratory tests, as increased hematocrit, BUN, and creatinine levels. Hemoconcentration and hypotension cause sluggish blood flow through capillaries and favors thrombosis. Characteristic signs of hypovolemic shock may occur. These events require prompt and proper measures to correct the fluid and electrolyte abnormalities, and restore blood pressure.

Hypokalemia

Chronic furosemide therapy can cause hypokalemia, even if excessive fluid loss does not occur. Furosemide may be less likely than a thiazide to cause hypokalemia when therapeutic doses are used properly, but appropriate precautions to detect or prevent it are still required. They are discussed below.

Hyperuricemia, Hyperglycemia, Hypocalcemia, and Hypomagnesemia

Furosemide inhibits uric acid excretion less than do the thiazides. However, its greater ability to cause water loss into the urine tends to concentrate uric acid in the blood. Hyperuricemic patients are therefore susceptible to a gout attack. Similarly, despite a relatively lower risk of hyperglycemia with furosemide, diabetic patients require close monitoring. The ability of furosemide and related drugs to enhance urinary calcium excretion necessitates cautious use in patients with a history of urinary calcium stones, especially if they become volume depleted and their urine volume falls because of it. Hypocalcemia is relatively uncommon. The consequences of hypomagnesemia probably are comparable to those associated with thiazides.

Hearing Impairments

High blood levels of high-ceiling diuretics, whether caused by excessive doses or by inadequate diuretic excretion, can damage the auditory nerve (ototoxicity). The hearing impairments that arise can be mild or severe, and temporary or permanent. With furosemide or the related drug bumetanide, the risks of ototoxicity are relatively low, and the auditory changes are often reversible when the drug is discontinued or its dose is reduced. The risk is greater with the related drug ethacrynic acid. Other drugs that interact to increase the risk of ototoxicity are noted below and in Table 32–I.

Other Side Effects or Adverse Responses

The high-ceiling diuretics may cause allergic reactions in patients who are allergic to sulfonamide antibiotics, because the two groups of medications have similar chemical structures. They may also cause hepatotoxicity, blood dyscrasias, or skin rashes, but these responses are also uncommon.

◆ Use During Pregnancy and Lactation

High-ceiling diuretics are rarely indicated for managing hypertension or edema associated with normal pregnancy or eclampsia/preeclampsia. Indeed, they are best avoided to prevent fetal harm caused by excessive falls of blood volume or blood pressure. Small amounts of these drugs may be excreted in breast milk. There are few reports of serious problems to nursing infants, but most physicians recommend that women taking these drugs should not breast-feed their infants.

◆ Use in Children

As with adults, oral therapy is preferred for children. Daily doses greater than 6 mg/kg are not recommended.

◆ Use in the Elderly

Elderly patients have a greater risk of excessive diuresis with circulatory collapse and, possibly, thrombosis or embolism. They are also less tolerant of rapid changes of blood pressure. Rapid or excessive diuresis often causes urinary incontinence.

Interactions with Other Drugs

High-ceiling diuretics share with the thiazides an ability to increase the risk of digoxin toxicity (owing to hypokalemia) and toxicity due to lithium (Table 32–I). The risk of hearing impairment is increased when these diuretics are administered with other ototoxic drugs, particularly the aminoglycoside antibiotics or the anticancer drug cisplatin. Finally, drugs classified as nonsteroidal antiinflammatory drugs (NSAIDs) can antagonize the diuretic effects of furosemide and related diuretics. The risks appear to be greatest with indomethacin (INDOCIN). The interaction is thought to occur because the NSAIDs inhibit the synthesis of prostaglandins, which help cause diuresis, in the kidneys.

Overdose and Toxicity

The major problems with chronic overdoses include hypotension due to excessive fluid loss, and electrolyte imbalances (eg, hyponatremia). Blood pressure and composition may need to be corrected with parenteral fluids having the proper electrolyte content. Hypotension is usually the major problem in acute overdoses. Other changes, such as hypokalemia, may not develop fully before blood pressure falls. Parenteral therapy with sodium chloride solutions may be sufficient to restore blood pressure and volume. Sympathomimetic vasoconstrictors (eg, phenylephrine, pp 200–203) may be needed for profound hypotension that does not respond to IV fluid and electrolyte infusions.

Related Drugs

Ethacrynic Acid and Bumetanide

Ethacrynic acid (EDECRIN, EDECRIN SODIUM) and bumetanide (BUMEX) are similar to furosemide in almost all ways except potency (Table 32–C). (From a clinical viewpoint, that is a trivial difference.) Either drug can be used instead of the prototype. Oral and parenteral dosage forms of each are available. Of all three high-ceiling diuretics, ethacrynic acid is thought to pose the greatest risk of ototoxicity.

Potassium-Sparing Diuretics

The diuretics discussed so far are widely used and undeniably effective, but they share the ability to cause clinically significant hypokalemia. Three *potassium-sparing diuretics,* triamterene (DYRENIUM), amiloride (MIDAMOR), and spironolactone (ALDACTONE), were developed to help minimize or prevent this problem. They decrease renal potassium excretion. However, this potassium-sparing action can create a new problem—hyperkalemia—if these drugs are not used properly.

Triamterene is the prototype. Except for potency and some pharmacokinetic properties, it is very similar to amiloride. Spironolactone has a unique mechanism of action that will be noted below.

PROTOTYPE

Triamterene

Absorption, Distribution, Metabolism, and Excretion

Triamterene is absorbed well from the GI tract. About 50% of its molecules in the bloodstream are bound to plasma protein. The drug is extensively metabolized.

Pharmacologic Effects

Triamterene slightly inhibits an ion pump in the distal tubules. This pump affects both sodium and potassium handling. Overall, sodium excretion increases and potassium loss falls. Water follows the lost sodium. The peak diuretic response to therapeutic doses, about 3 mL/min, is roughly equal to that of a thiazide; and, as with thiazides, the dose–response curve is flat. The potassium-sparing diuretics can reduce renal blood flow and GFR, but this is probably not important when patients get usual doses and have normal renal function.

Potassium-sparing diuretics do not cause major effects on blood calcium levels. Their effects on serum uric acid, glucose, and lipid levels are somewhat similar to those caused by thiazides.

Clinical Indications and Administration

The potassium-sparing diuretics are available as single-entity products or as fixed-dose combinations with hydrochlorothiazide (Table 32–4). No parenteral dosage forms are available.

Treatment of Edema and Hypertension

Potassium-sparing diuretics, used alone, are no more effective than a thiazide for lowering blood pressure or relieving edema, and they are seldom used alone for these indications. Instead, they are used much more often in combination with a potassium-wasting diuretic. This gives additive effects on sodium excretion, edema, and blood pressure; and opposing effects on potassium, which reduces the risk of hypokalemia.

Management of Hypokalemia

Potassium-sparing diuretics are used to prevent or treat mild hypokalemia, such as that due to disease (eg, hyperaldosteronism) or drugs (eg, potassium-wasting diuretics). This important topic is discussed in more detail below.

Side Effects, Adverse Reactions, and Contraindications

Sodium and Water Depletion

When used alone, potassium-sparing diuretics are not likely to cause significant water or salt loss because they are not very efficacious drugs. However, since they are

Table 32–4 Selected Fixed-Dose Combinations of Potassium-Sparing and Potassium-Wasting Diuretics*

Proprietary Name	Ingredients	How Supplied	Average Dosages
ALDACTAZIDE	25 or 50 mg spironolactone 25 or 50 mg hydroclorothiazide	tablets	Edema: up to 200 mg of each ingredient per day in single or divided doses Hypertension: 2–4 tablets/day
DYAZIDE	50 mg triamterene 25 mg hydrochlorothiazide	capsules	Edema or hypertension: 1 or 2 capsules/day or every other day
MAXZIDE	75 mg triamterene 50 mg hydrochlorothiazide	tablets	Edema or hypertension; 1 tablet/day
MODURETIC	5 mg amiloride 50 mg hydrochlorothiazide	tablets	Edema or hypertension; 1 tablet/day initially; up to 2/day maintenance

*None of these products is indicated for starting therapy for edema or hypertension. Doses of the individual drugs found in the fixed-dose combinations should first be established separately, if their doses are identical or close to those in the combination products, a switch to the combination product usually is acceptable.

Fixed-dose combinations containing a thiazide and another antihypertensive agent are listed in Chapter 33.

usually given along with a potassium-wasting diuretic, additive drug effects on sodium elimination increase the risk of hyponatremia and dehydration. Careful monitoring of the response to therapy is important.

Hyperkalemia

Excessive potassium retention (hyperkalemia; serum potassium levels ≥6.5 mEq/L) is an important side effect of any potassium-sparing diuretic. It seldom occurs, however, when the drugs are used properly to balance potassium loss caused by a potassium-wasting diuretic. The risk of hyperkalemia increases considerably when any potassium-sparing diuretic is given along with potassium-rich drugs, such as potassium penicillin, or with potassium supplements. In general, therapy with both potassium-sparing diuretics and potassium supplements should be avoided to reduce the risk of hyperkalemia. Hyperkalemia from any cause contraindicates the use of potassium-sparing diuretics.

NURSING IMPLICATIONS

If hyperkalemia develops during therapy with a potassium-sparing diuretic, the drug should be discontinued, at least temporarily. If the patient is taking other drugs that elevate potassium levels, they, too, may need to be discontinued. Patients with diabetes mellitus have a greater risk of developing hyperkalemia, complicated by metabolic acidosis, in response to potassium-sparing diuretics. If the diabetic patient develops hyperkalemia, simply discontinuing potassium-sparing diuretic therapy may not be adequate. Other measures must be taken, including careful oral or parenteral administration of glucose plus injection of a fast-acting insulin preparation, or IV infusion of sodium bicarbonate to counteract the acidosis and shift potassium from the bloodstream into the cells.

Other Side Effects

Triamterene or amiloride should not be given to patients with poor renal function or oliguria, since they may further reduce renal blood flow and GFR. Triamterene may cause a blue discoloration of the urine. This is not dangerous, and is mentioned only so that patients can be forewarned to prevent undue worry if it happens.

◆ Use During Pregnancy and Lactation

Triamterene may cross the placental barrier and enter the fetal circulation. Although no congenital effects have been reported when this drug has been given to pregnant women, routine use is inappropriate and potentially hazardous. A thiazide-like decrease of placental blood flow may also occur.

Use in Children

Potassium-sparing diuretics are generally not indicated for children.

Use in the Elderly

Hyperkalemia is more likely to occur in elderly patients if urine output is reduced. Implications related to problems other than potassium balance, noted for thiazides and high-ceiling diuretics, apply also to potassium-wasting diuretics.

Interactions with Other Drugs

Many interactions noted for other classes of diuretics apply to the potassium-sparing agents (Table 32–I). Additional important interactants include drugs or substances that elevate serum potassium levels, including some antibiotics (eg, potassium penicillin); low-salt foods (may contain higher-than-usual levels of potassium to improve taste) and salt substitutes (contain potassium chloride); and oral potassium supplements (discussed in more detail below).

Triamterene ordinarily should not be administered with the NSAID indomethacin, because renal failure is a potential outcome. The response is most likely to occur in patients with poor renal function, for whom this combination is contraindicated. However, any patient receiving triamterene and indomethacin should be monitored very closely for this potentially serious outcome.

Overdose and Toxicity

Except for the lack of hypokalemia, the signs, symptoms, and treatment of overdoses with a potassium-sparing diuretic are similar to those noted for hydrochlorothiazide.

Related Drugs

Amiloride

Amiloride (MIDAMOR), an oral diuretic, is very similar to triamterene. It is more potent: a 5 mg once-daily dose is usually adequate.

Spironolactone

Spironolactone (ALDACTONE) differs from triamterene and amiloride because it is chemically related to the hormone aldosterone. Of all the diuretics, spironolactone has the slowest onset of action (1 to 2 days for appreciable effects to occur) and the longest duration of action (about 3 days). It is extensively metabolized in the liver.

Spironolactone has a unique mechanism of action. It blocks (pharmacologically antagonizes) aldosterone receptors in the distal tubules and collecting ducts. Normally, aldosterone stimulates sodium reabsorption and potassium secretion at these sites. Spironolactone reverses these effects: sodium excretion increases, and potassium is reabsorbed and returned to the bloodstream.

Spironolactone shares the indications noted for triamterene and amiloride (Table 32–C). However, because it blocks the effects of aldosterone, it is uniquely suited for helping diagnose and treat conditions caused by excessive aldosterone production—adrenal cortical tumors, for example—or those caused by reduced aldosterone metabolism—for example, conditions involving hepatic dysfunction, as might occur with alcohol-induced liver disease.

In addition to the side effects noted for triamterene and amiloride, spironolactone's hormone-like structure can cause other side effects: gynecomastia, hirsutism, deepening of the voice, increased sweating, and oily skin, in males or females. Males may experience impotence and decreased libido; and females may develop menstrual abnormalities (eg, amenorrhea). These changes usually occur with high doses and are reversible when therapy is stopped. Breast tumors have been reported in males and females taking spironolactone, but it is not certain whether the drug caused them.

II. General Nursing Implications for Diuretic Use for Edema or Hypertension

Side effects of the drugs discussed above may limit their use or the willingness of patients to take them. With short-term use some side effects may never occur. However, most diuretics are used chronically, and treatment for common indications (congestive heart failure, essential hypertension) may be lifelong, so some side effects are unavoidable. Fortunately there are several ways to plan and monitor diuretic therapy to reduce the frequency and severity of side effects without sacrificing the desired clinical outcomes. Many of these measures are based on such clear common sense that they are often taken for granted and therefore overlooked.

Starting and Maintaining Therapy

It is relatively easy to select the right diuretic and dosage for a given patient and then start treatment. Nevertheless, sometimes the drug apparently or truly loses its effectiveness as treatment continues. This event becomes particularly important during outpatient therapy, when the frequent assessment that can be given to hospitalized patients cannot be provided.

When hypertensive or edematous patients fail to respond adequately to diuretics, it is important to identify the reason(s) before drugs are switched or the dosages of current medications are increased. For example, therapeutic failure could be due to worsening of underlying disease; failure to follow recommended diet or exercise plans; use of interacting or contraindicated drugs; or simply the patient's inability or unwillingness to comply with prescribed and otherwise proper dosages. Each problem has its own correct solution(s).

Compliance Problems

Noncompliance, especially in outpatients, can be a significant problem. Many side effects noted above are important causes of this, but they aren't the only ones. For example, the very fact that a diuretic "works" can lead to improper drug taking. Many patients taking these drugs get a good sense of how much urine they produce each day, and of how they feel. Some follow their blood pressures or weights regularly (recommend that to them). However, an obvious increase of urine output or weight loss might last only a couple of weeks after treatment starts, and the patient usually starts to feel better. Some patients interpret this as an indication that the drug has stopped working, which might lead to a self-prescribed dose increase. Others feel this means they are cured, and that drugs and physicians' visits (both expensive and inconvenient) are no longer needed; so they stop. If therapy is likely to be prolonged, tell the patient what to expect and how to respond to it.

Timing the Dose

Another avoidable cause of noncompliance is improper timing of the dose. Having to urinate at inopportune times can disrupt daytime activities or sleep. Such problems are most common during early therapy, especially before an edematous patient reaches a "dry weight"; when a high-ceiling diuretic is used; or when the patient has poor bladder control. Simple instructions about when to take the medication, tailored to the patient's lifestyle, can minimize these problems. Most patients should take their first dose of the day shortly after awakening (but timed so they are not caught off-guard while commuting to work, for example). If they must take several daily doses, the last one should be timed to avoid interrupting sleep because of the need to urinate. Some trial-and-error will be needed to find the best times, but it is worth the effort.

Values and Limitations of Salt Restriction

The beneficial actions of diuretics in edema and hypertension are due to their ability to increase sodium excretion. This can be facilitated by a low-salt diet that should be planned with the physician, a dietician, and (of course) the patient who is expected to follow it. Reduced sodium intake may permit reduced doses of diuretics, thereby reducing the risk of some side effects. However, low-sodium diets are seldom effective without drug therapy for managing chronic edema or hypertension that is more than very mild and innocuous. If your patient has a GI disorder for which antacids must be taken often (eg, peptic ulcer disease), recommend a low-sodium or sodium-free product. Discourage sodium bicarbonate (baking soda) use altogether.

Problems with Excessive Fluid and Sodium Loss

Dizziness or fainting, confusion, drowsiness, insatiable thirst or salt craving, muscle weakness, or poor skin turgor often indicate underlying hypovolemia, hyponatremia (Table 32–3), or both. These important clues are easy and important for both health-care providers and patients to recognize. Problems from sudden fluid or electrolyte loss are magnified in geriatric patients and others with decreased renal function. They may be triggered or aggravated by excessive use (abuse) of laxative/cathartic drugs, methylxanthines (eg, caffeine), or alcohol; or by severe diarrhea, vomiting, excessive physical exercise, or sweating. To help prevent or minimize these problems, recommend and encourage adequate diets that include sufficient (but not excessive) sodium and water; and discourage *excessive* exercise that leads to dehydration, and self-medication with nonprescribed interacting drugs.

Problems That Arise from Potassium Imbalances

Hypokalemia can be as dangerous as diuretic-induced hypovolemia or hyponatremia, and it is more common. Most ambulatory patients receiving a potassium-wasting diuretic develop asymptomatic hypokalemia sometime during therapy. Many of them go on to develop symptoms. Hypokalemia may occur without significant or obvious volume loss or hypotension, or alterations of other serum constituents. The problem is particularly important for patients with congestive heart failure who are receiving digoxin or another digitalis drug, because they are usually taking a potassium-wasting diuretic also. *Diuretic-induced hypokalemia is the number one cause of digitalis intoxication* (and the problems can be magnified by the magnesium deficiencies these urine-producing drugs can also cause). *Toxicity can occur at serum digitalis levels lower than those needed to cause symptoms in persons who are normokalemic.* Other diseases or drugs that cause potassium wasting make the patient even more susceptible. Therefore, it is important to know how to recognize, prevent, and treat hypokalemia.

Table 32–5 Drugs or Medical Problems That May Cause or Worsen Hypokalemia

Corticosteroid drug therapy
Excessive diarrhea, laxative abuse
Diuretic therapy (potassium-wasting agents)
Hyperaldosteronism (primary: adrenal adenoma; Cushing's disease) (secondary: impaired aldosterone metabolism, as in severe hepatic disease)
Kidney disease
Excess ingestion of licorice (contains potassium-wasting aldosterone-like substance)
Malabsorption syndrome
Excessive sweating
Ulcerative colitis

Recognizing Hypokalemia

Common early signs and symptoms include thirst, muscle weakness, lethargy, and depression (Table 32–5). Some of these indications occur when serum potassium levels fall slightly below 3.5 mEq/L (normal is 3.5–5.0 mEq/L). Symptoms increase and become more severe when potassium levels fall below 2.7 mEq/L. Muscle cramps or vomiting may occur at this point. They should be considered as signs of a severe potassium loss that may soon be followed by arrhythmias (especially in a digitalized patient), paralytic ileus, or generalized paralysis leading to respiratory arrest.

Prevention and Management

Hypokalemia can be prevented or treated in several ways, each of which has advantages and limitations. Prophylactic measures include

- dietary modifications,
- giving oral potassium supplements, *or*
- giving one of the potassium-sparing diuretics noted above.

Oral potassium supplements and potassium-sparing drugs are also useful for treating asymptomatic hypokalemia. Regardless of whether the goal is prevention or treatment, periodic measurements of serum potassium levels are important to guide therapy.

Diet

Patients taking a potassium-wasting diuretic, and who are in generally good health, may need between 20 and 150 mEq of extra potassium per day to prevent hypokalemia. Few "typical" diets provide this. There are many potassium-rich foods and beverages (Table 32–6), but some of them also contain large amounts of sodium or calories, which are unwanted. In addition, it is difficult to plan and comply with diets that provide consistent amounts of potassium from day to day, over months or years. For most patients, therefore, relying on diet alone has questionable preventive value. Dietary changes alone are also generally ineffective and inappropriate for treating patients with potassium levels close to the lower limit of normal, especially if they are taking digitalis. *Never* rely on diet alone to treat symptomatic hypokalemia; that is clearly dangerous.

Oral Potassium Supplements

Several types of prescription oral potassium supplements are available (Table 32–7). They are formulated as powders, effervescent tablets, or liquid concentrates (eg, elixirs) that are meant to be dissolved or diluted in some beverage (water, juice) before swallowing. Others are tablets or capsules meant to be swallowed. All supply standardized amounts of potassium. Therefore, they provide a reliable supplemental dose if the patient takes them as directed. The average dose of potassium to prevent hypokalemia or its recurrence is 20 mEq/d. Usually, this amount of potassium can be taken as a single daily dose. Patients who develop mild hypokalemia that requires treatment typically need anywhere from 40 to 100 mEq of extra potassium per day until potassium levels normalize. These amounts are often administered in divided doses.

Table 32–6 Potassium-Rich Foods and Beverages and Their Sodium and Calorie Contents (Approximate Values)*

	Potassium		Sodium		Calories
	mg	mEq	mg	mEq	
Beverages (per 8-oz portion)					
Apple juice, fresh	267	7	5	0.2	125
Grape juice	320	8	3	0.1	176
Grapefruit juice, fresh	400	10	5	0.2	109
Milk, whole	371	10	200	8.7	170
Orange juice, fresh	507	13	1	0.1	131
Pineapple juice, canned	374	10	3	0.1	147
Tomato juice, unsalted	615	16	615	26.7	51
Foods (per 100 g edible portion)					
Apples, sweet	116	3	1	<0.1	58
Apricots	440	11	1	<0.1	51
Bananas	420	11	1	<0.1	85
Beans, Lima	680	17	1	<0.1	123
Cantaloupe	230	6	12	0.5	30
Cauliflower	400	10	16	0.7	27
Dates, dry	790	20	1	<0.1	274
Figs, dry	780	20	34	1.5	274
Fruit cocktail, canned	160	4	5	0.2	76
Oranges	170	4	<1	<0.1	49
Peaches	160	4	<1	<0.1	46
Potatoes	410	10	3	0.1	76
Prunes	700	18	6	0.3	255
Raisins	725	18	31	1.4	289
Spinach, fresh	662	17	62	2.7	26
Tomatoes	268	7	3	0.1	22

*Patients who take potassium-wasting diuretics may require up to 100 mEq of extra potassium per day. Dietary planning, which is best done in consultation with the physician, dietician, and patient, should consider added sodium and calorie load as well. Sodium-restricted diets may allow no more than 85 mEq Na (about 4.8 grams of salt) per day; daily calorie intake may need to be limited to 2000 to 2500 calories. Thus, some potassium-rich foods may contain too much sodium or too many calories.

Most potassium supplements contain potassium chloride, which is usually preferred. If hypokalemia is accompanied by metabolic acidosis, an alkalinizing potassium salt (bicarbonate, citrate, or gluconate) should be used instead. Alkalinizing salts are contraindicated in the presence of metabolic alkalosis. *No* potassium supplement should be given routinely if the patient has oliguria or azotemia, until the underlying problem is diagnosed and corrected.

Many clinicians believe it is inappropriate to prescribe oral supplements prophylactically—that is, in anticipation of hypokalemia—unless there is good reason to suspect it is likely to occur or recur in a particular patient. Most clinicians agree that oral potassium sup-

Table 32–7 | Selected Oral Potassium Supplements*

Proprietary Name	Potassium Salt	How Supplied	Potassium per Unit	Comments
KAOCHLOR, KAOCHLOR S-F	Chloride	Liquid	20 mEq/15 mL	Contains 5% alcohol, tartrazine dye; "S-F" formulation is sugar- and tartrazine-free; dilute in several ounces of water, take after meals
KAON	Gluconate	Liquid	20 mEq/15 mL	Contains 5% alcohol; administer as for KAOCHLOR
KAON CL KAON CL-10	Chloride	Sustained-release tablets	6.7 or 10 mEq/tablet	See KAOCHLOR; contains tartrazine; sugar-coated tablets; swallow whole
KAON CL 20%	Chloride	Liquid	40 mEq/15 mL	Sugar-free; contains 5% alcohol; dilute, take with food
K-LOR	Chloride	Powder	15 or 20 mEq	See KAOCHLOR; dissolve, take after meals
KLORVESS	Chloride, bicarbonate, citrate	Effervescent tablets	20 mEq/tablet	See KAOCHLOR; sugar- and sodium-free; dissolve, sip slowly after meals
KLOTRIX	Chloride	Sustained-release tablets	10 mEq/tablet	See KAOCHLOR; swallow whole, take with meals
K-LYTE	Bicarbonate, citrate	Effervescent tablets	25 mEq/tablet	Dissolve, sip over 5–10 min after meals
K-LYTE/CL K-LYTE/CL 50	Chloride	Effervescent tablets	25 or 50 mEq/tablet	see K-LYTE
K-LYTE/CL Powder		Powder	25 mEq/scoop	See K-LYTE
K-TAB	Chloride	Sustained-release tablets	10 mEq/tablet	Swallow whole, take with meals
MICRO-K	Chloride	Sustained-release capsules	8 or 10 mEq/capsule	Swallow whole, take with meals
SLOW-K	Chloride	Sustained-release tablets	8 mEq/tablet	Swallow whole, take with meals

*Typical daily dosages for prophylaxis of hypokalemia are approximately 20 to 25 mEq of supplemental potassium. Dosages for treatment range from 40 to 100 mEq per day. General dosage guidelines and administration plans are summarized on page 615.

plements are acceptable for treating hypokalemia or preventing recurrences, but *only when symptoms are slight and potassium depletion poses no immediate health risk.*

Any oral potassium supplement can cause diarrhea. This should be evaluated thoroughly if it becomes severe or recurrent, since added fluid and electrolyte imbalances could magnify diuretic-induced problems.

Supplements formulated as powders or effervescent tablets have to be dissolved completely in water or juice before ingestion. Liquid concentrates (eg, elixirs) have to be diluted first. Few of these products taste very good, and that can hamper a patient's willingness to take them day after day. Thus, noncompliance can be a problem.

An obvious answer to the taste problem is to administer potassium as a tablet or capsule that can be swallowed. Enteric-coated potassium chloride tablets are available. The coating prevents them from dissolving in and irritating the stomach. However, when they dissolve in the duodenum they can damage the mucosa at that site instead. Manufacturers recognized these problems and developed slow-release preparations in which the salt is incorporated in a waxy matrix. This seemed to reduce the risk of ulceration, but it is not clear whether it prevents the risk altogether. Current opinion is that no enteric-coated or slow-release potassium product should be prescribed unless other measures or dosage forms have been tried first and have proven ineffective or unacceptable for a given patient. It is also important to ensure that these dosage forms are swallowed whole. Chewing them can cause not only a very unpleasant sensation in the mouth, but also severe mucosal lesions from locally high salt concentrations.

Potassium-Sparing Diuretics

Potassium-sparing diuretics, already discussed, are a common and feasible approach to treat mild hypokalemia or prevent its recurrence. One way to use them is to have the patient take a potassium-wasting diuretic on certain days, and a potassium-sparing agent on others. It is hard for many patients to keep track of that, especially if they also take several other drugs. Another approach is to have the patient take both drugs each day—either as separate medications, or, as is done more often, as a fixed-dose combination product. Combination products are convenient, but they hinder the ability to adjust the dosage of each ingredient if drug requirements change. Before prescribing them, each diuretic should be evaluated separately to ensure that the doses are right for the patient.

Severe Hypokalemia

Parenteral potassium administration is indicated if severe or symptomatic hypokalemia develops, regardless of whether the patient is taking digitalis. Frequent measurements of serum electrolyte levels and the electrocardiogram (ECG) must be used to ensure that potassium replacement is adequate but not excessive.

Hyperkalemia from the Combined Use of Potassium-Sparing Diuretics and Potassium Supplements

An easy way to cause severe hyperkalemia is to prescribe a daily potassium supplement plus a potassium-sparing diuretic. Giving such combinations is potentially dangerous, and rarely justified—especially for outpatients. If both types of drugs are ordered, the ECG and blood electrolytes must be monitored frequently. It is hard to provide this proper monitoring if the patient is not in the hospital.

Diuretic Refractoriness and Diuretic Combinations

The combined use of a potassium-wasting diuretic with a potassium-sparing agent is common, logical, and often effective. The same cannot be said for most other diuretic combinations, even though some clinicians may use them in the hope of improving upon a poor response in a patient. In general, giving two or more diuretics of the same class—two thiazides or thiazide-like agents, two high-ceiling diuretics, or two potassium-sparing drugs—will do little more than increase the risk of side effects. That is because drugs in the same class act on identical processes in the nephron. If the maximum dose of one agent does not affect kidney function well enough, giving another drug that acts in the same way will not help. In these instances, when more edema fluid has to be removed, or something must be done to prevent complete renal shut-down, the chance of success can be increased by using combinations of diuretics in different classes.

III. Miscellaneous Diuretics

Two other groups of drugs are classified as diuretics, and are used for that purpose under special circumstances: carbonic anhydrase inhibitors and osmotic agents. They are discussed briefly below. Still other drugs, notably alcohol and methylxanthines (eg, caffeine, theophylline), can cause clinically important diuresis as a side effect, and so can interact with traditional diuretics. These drugs will not be discussed further.

Carbonic Anhydrase Inhibitors

Acetazolamide (DIAMOX) was the first widely used oral diuretic. Its effects on urine output are relatively weak, so it was not effective for severe edema. Even when it was used for mild edema, its diuretic effects were short-lived and cumbersome to deal with. The drug still has limited use as a diuretic, but it is used more for other indications that depend on its major mechanism of action—the ability to inhibit the enzyme, carbonic anhydrase.

PROTOTYPE

Acetazolamide

Acetazolamide (DIAMOX) produces diuresis by inhibiting the effects of enzyme carbonic anhydrase. Although acetazolamide shares some of the uses noted for other diuretics, its unique actions make it suitable for treating glaucoma and some forms of epilepsy, for which other diuretics are worthless.

Absorption, Distribution, Metabolism, and Excretion

Acetazolamide is absorbed well from the GI tract. Peak plasma levels occur about 2 hours after administration of standard tablets, or 6 to 8 hours with the sustained-release product (DIAMOX SEQUELS). Most of the drug is excreted unchanged in the urine within 24 hours.

Pharmacologic Effects

Acetazolamide's major mechanism of action is inhibition of carbonic anhydrase. This enzyme is abundant in parts of the kidney, the eye, and the central nervous system (CNS). Carbonic anhydrase accelerates (catalyzes) the reaction between carbon dioxide and water to form carbonic acid, which then dissociates into protons (hydrogen ions) and bicarbonate ion.

Renal Effects

In the kidney, carbonic anhydrase is found mainly in proximal tubular cells. Inhibiting the enzyme here inhibits bicarbonate reabsorption. The bicarbonate lost into the urine carries sodium and water with it. The maximum increase of urine output is about 3 mL/min. Acetazolamide also increases renal potassium loss, and so it is a potassium-wasting diuretic.

The increased amount of excreted bicarbonate alkalinizes the urine. Eventually, urinary bicarbonate loss causes the blood to become acidic (ie, metabolic acidosis develops). When this occurs, continued acetazolamide administration (even at extraordinarily high doses) no longer increases urine output, but inhibition of carbonic anhydrase and systemic acidosis persist. The patient has now become **refractory** to the diuretic effect because of a systemic acid–base imbalance.

Refractoriness can be prevented or overcome by administering sodium bicarbonate. This is therapeutically awkward and, in the context of treating edema or hypertension, counterproductive. Thiazides accomplish the same goals more easily and safely.

Ocular and Central Nervous System Effects

Carbonic anhydrase levels are high in the ciliary process of the eye, where the enzyme helps synthesize aqueous humor. Acetazolamide decreases aqueous humor formation and lowers intraocular pressure. Carbonic anhydrase also has a role in synthesis of cerebrospinal fluid (CSF), and so this process is inhibited by acetazolamide. Finally, acetazolamide exerts anticonvulsant activity by a mechanism that will be noted soon. Acetazolamide's effects on the formation of aqueous humor and CSF, and its anticonvulsant actions, continue after the patient develops refractoriness to diuresis.

Clinical Indications and Administration

Acetazolamide has limited use as a diuretic for edema, and for treating chronic seizure disorders and glaucoma. It is a valuable adjunctive treatment for some drug overdoses. Dosages are noted in Table 32–C.

Treatment of Edema

Acetazolamide is occasionally used as a diuretic to manage mild edema, especially if the edema is expected to be brief. It is not a preferred diuretic for chronic edema or hypertension because its effects are self-limiting, and are accompanied by systemic acidosis. The more common diuretics do not cause these problems. Indeed, even when edema is short-lived, there is little reason to use acetazolamide instead of other diuretics.

Management of Glaucoma

Acetazolamide can be given intravenously for acute angle-closure glaucoma, which often requires emergency surgery. Lowering pressure preoperatively reduces the risk of operative complications. Oral acetazolamide is also a useful drug for chronic glaucoma. Since its therapeutic effects are due to actions in the eye, and not dependent on renal actions, long-term use is appropriate and often effective for glaucoma.

Management of Seizure Disorders

Acetazolamide is an adjunct to pharmacotherapy of some forms of epilepsy. It is particularly effective for petit mal (absence) epilepsy in children. The metabolic acidosis that develops with acetazolamide administration is thought to account for the drug's ability to supress abnormal brain electrical activity that causes or spreads seizures. With continued administration, anticonvulsant activity persists despite loss of a diuretic effect.

Drug Overdoses

Acetazolamide (usually given intravenously) can be used to manage overdoses of acidic drugs (mainly aspirin or phenobarbital), which are excreted faster in alkaline urine. Acetazolamide is usually given in a large volume of fluid along with parenteral sodium bicarbonate (which causes additional urinary alkalinization), and sometimes along with the osmotic diuretic mannitol (see below), to "force" diuresis.

Management of Hydrocephalus

Acetazolamide appears to be beneficial for some children with hydrocephalus. It works by reducing CSF formation.

NURSING IMPLICATIONS

Oral administration is preferred. If parenteral therapy is indicated, the IV route is preferred. Give no more than 500 mg over 5 minutes. Intramuscular injections of acetazolamide are very painful; avoid them.

Side Effects, Adverse Reactions, and Contraindications

Chronic acetazolamide use can cause hyponatremia, volume depletion, hypokalemia, and metabolic acidosis (Table 32–S). The first three side effects are not likely to occur unless the patient is taking other diuretics concomitantly, or there are preexisting fluid and electrolyte imbalances (which usually contraindicate acetazolamide use).

Metabolic acidosis is an expected response if treatment lasts more than a few days, owing to acetazolamide's ability to increase bicarbonate excretion. Signs and symptoms include drowsiness, anorexia, paresthesias, and increased respiratory rate (one way the body compensates to correct acidic blood pH). These are usually mild and more annoying than dangerous. However, acetazolamide should be used with extreme care in patients with poor pulmonary function (eg, emphysema). These individuals are already prone to developing respiratory acidosis, and the condition can be worsened by the drug. Preexisting acidosis contraindicates acetazolamide use.

Acetazolamide has a sulfa-like structure, and so should not be administered to patients with a history of allergic reactions to sulfonamides. Sulfonamide-like adverse reactions to acetazolamide include fever, rashes, crystalluria, and blood dyscrasias. If any of these occur, acetazolamide therapy should be stopped at once and the treatment plan should be reevaluated.

Acetazolamide may cause transient myopia.

◆ Use During Pregnancy and Lactation

Animal studies have shown that acetazolamide causes fetal malformations or death. This has not been shown in humans, but the potential risks outweigh possible benefits to the mother, especially during the first trimester. Additionally, mild benign edema of pregnancy can usually be managed well by nondrug measures. Overall, the drug should be avoided if possible.

◆ Use in the Elderly

Acetazolamide, whether used for glaucoma or other purposes, may reduce visual acuity. The elderly patient may require assistance with ambulation.

Interactions with Other Drugs

Interactions between acetazolamide and other drugs (Table 32–I) can occur regardless of the indication for which acetazolamide is given. Ordinarily, acetazolamide should not be prescribed with other diuretics, since this increases the risk of fluid and electrolyte imbalances. However, it is quite conceivable that a patient taking a diuretic prescribed by one doctor for one indication (eg, hypertension) may receive acetazolamide for glaucoma or seizures from another doctor, with an unwanted outcome. (Poor history-taking is often the cause of such preventable interactions.) Acetazolamide's ability to alkalinize the urine can decrease the renal elimination of basic drugs (eg, amphetamines), or increase excretion of acidic drugs (eg, aspirin or phenobarbital).

Related Drugs

Dichlorphenamide and Methazolamide

These drugs are indicated only for managing glaucoma. They are given orally, and are best used as adjuncts to pupil-constricting (miotic) drugs. Dosages are listed in Table 32–C. Although dichlorphenamide (DARANIDE) and methazolamide (NEPTAZANE) are not used as diuretics, diuretic effects can occur nevertheless. In addition, these agents share the same side effects, contraindications, and drug–drug interactions that were noted for acetazolamide.

Osmotic Diuretics

Osmotic diuretics, exemplified by the sugar mannitol (OSMITROL), are a special class of diuretics. They differ dramatically from all the drugs mentioned so far in terms of mechanisms of action, indications, and adverse effects. They act almost exclusively by a common physical process, osmosis.

PROTOTYPE

Mannitol

Absorption, Distribution, Metabolism, and Excretion

Mannitol is absorbed very poorly from the GI tract, so it is given intravenously. It distributes throughout the body via the bloodstream. It is confined to the bloodstream, except in the kidneys, where it undergoes glomerular filtration and eventual excretion. Mannitol is not metabolized.

Pharmacologic Effects

Mannitol increases urine production through osmotic effects in the blood and urine. When the drug is injected it increases the osmotic activity (osmolality) of the blood. This withdraws water from the extracellular space and, eventually, from cells. Water entering the blood increases blood volume and pressure. Renal blood flow and GFR increase, and these effects help increase urine production.

Once mannitol reaches the nephron, it is filtered into the urine, but it is not reabsorbed. This increases the osmolality of the urine, which inhibits reabsorption of water as urine passes through the nephron. It is yet another way that mannitol causes diuresis. (The same phenomenon accounts for the high urine outputs of diabetics who have such high blood glucose levels that glucose "spills into" the urine.) Overall, mannitol can increase urine production to 30 to 50 mL/min or more. The drug usually can maintain or increase urine production even when GFR is reduced, as in patients with acutely impaired renal function.

Osmotic withdrawal of water from cells and extracellular spaces reduces pressure in structures such as the eye and cranium. This effect is used therapeutically.

Clinical Indications and Administration

Mannitol preparations come in different concentrations, from 5 to 25 g/100 mL of fluid (ie, 5%–25%). The preparation, the dose, the volume of fluid in which it is diluted (ie, the drug concentration), and the speed with which it is given depend on the type and severity of the condition for which mannitol is being used. The drug is usually given by IV infusion, and it has the following uses:

- Preventing or treating acute renal failure. Mannitol can often maintain urine production even in the face of severe renal dysfunction. It can be given alone or with a high-ceiling diuretic.
- Treating drug overdoses. Mannitol's ability to increase urine output can facilitate the elimination of drugs that are excreted by the kidneys, and have been taken in overdose.
- Reducing intraocular pressure before or during eye surgery.
- Reducing intracranial pressure to control or reverse brain swelling before, during, or after brain surgery.
- Measuring GFR. This is a diagnostic procedure to help measure certain aspects of kidney function. Mannitol is given as a steady IV infusion. During the infusion blood and urine samples are collected, their volumes are recorded, and they are assayed for mannitol concentrations. These values are then used, along with certain mathematical formulas, to calculate the GFR.

NURSING IMPLICATIONS

Mannitol solutions often need to be diluted before use. Be sure the concentration is correct for the desired use (see package inserts or other clinical references for details). Solutions containing more than 15 g of mannitol per 100 mL (15%) may crystallize. Before you dilute or administer the drug, dissolve the crystals by warming slightly. If solutions containing 15% or more are to be infused directly, be sure to place a filter in the infusion set to prevent crystals from entering the bloodstream.

When mannitol is used for such purposes as managing drug poisonings or reducing ocular or intracranial pressure, ridding the body of excessive fluid is not the goal. Therefore, mannitol is usually diluted to a low concentration, and it is infused in relatively large volumes of parenteral solutions that contain appropriate amounts of salts and glucose. This helps replenish these substances, and needed fluids, as they are lost in the urine as part of the diuretic effect. An in-dwelling bladder catheter usually should be inserted before giving mannitol, especially by prolonged infusion.

Side Effects, Adverse Reactions, and Contraindications

The conditions for which diuretics such as thiazides and furosemide are indicated are the major side effects and contraindications for osmotic diuretics: edema, with or without heart failure, and hypertension. By increasing blood volume and pressure, mannitol can cause severe, acute heart failure, pulmonary edema, a hypertensive crisis, or stroke. The risks occur if mannitol is infused at too great a concentration, or is given too rapidly; if the patient has poor cardiac function or high blood pressure; or if renal function is so poor that a brisk diuresis does not occur soon after the drug is given. Minor but relatively common side effects include headache, chest pain, or dizziness.

NURSING IMPLICATIONS

Monitor urine output, heart rate, and blood pressure carefully. Be aware that mannitol-induced headache, chest pain, or dizziness may be signs of more severe underlying cardiovascular or neurologic problems, such as myocardial infarction or stroke.

Interactions with Other Drugs

Osmotic diuretics can increase the excretion of virtually any drug that is eliminated by the kidneys. The impact of the effect depends on how important renal excretion (without prior metabolism) is for the particular interacting drug; whether it undergoes tubular reabsorption; the dose of the osmotic agent; and the duration of its administration.

Related Drugs

Urea and Glycerol

Urea and glycerol (glycerin) are used less than mannitol. Urea can be given orally, but it has an unpleasant taste and high doses are needed to increase urine output. A sterile 30% urea solution (UREAPHIL) can be given by IV drip. It is mainly used to reduce intracranial or CSF pressure. Urea is irritating and can cause local pain, tissue necrosis, and thrombosis if it extravasates. It may dangerously elevate BUN levels, leading to coma, if given to patients with poor renal or hepatic function.

Glycerol, given orally as a 50% or 75% solution, is sometimes used to decrease intraocular pressure prior to eye surgery. These preparations are viscous and unpleasant to swallow, dry the oral mucosa because of local osmotic actions, irritate the GI tract, and often cause diarrhea. They should not be given to patients with poor renal, hepatic, or cardiac status.

 SUMMARY OF NURSING IMPLICATIONS 

◆ Assessment

Establish baseline vital signs (blood pressure, heart rate, body weight), laboratory values (Na^+, K^+), and ECG to determine drug effects.

Complete nursing history to include any weight gain, abnormal swelling of hands, feet, or around eyes, frequency of voiding, color and odor of urine, or preexisting conditions possibly contraindicating diuretic therapy (eg, renal or hepatic failure, pregnancy, gout).

Review drug history for possible interactions or altered effects during diuretic therapy (eg, lithium, digitalis, quinidine).

◆ Nursing Diagnoses

Fluid volume deficit related to increased volume and frequency of urination.

High risk for injury related to dizziness, orthostatic hypotension.

Altered urinary elimination related to increased frequency.

Altered nutrition: less than body requirements related to excessive potassium loss.

Knowledge deficit related to prescribed drug therapy.

◆ Planning/Implementation

Measure fluid intake and output and weigh daily.

Encourage compliance with special diets; report deviations from compliance; inability to follow salt-restricted or potassium-supplemented diet may require change in drug therapy.

Observe for symptoms of drug-induced hypersensitivity reactions (eg, sudden appearance of cold- or flu-like symptoms, skin rashes, severe or recurrent upper GI pain, abnormal bruising, jaundice).

Monitor patients receiving high-ceiling diuretics parenterally for signs of hypotension or hearing loss.

◆ Patient and Family Education

Teach the patient/family:

The importance of taking diuretic early in day to minimize interruption of daytime activities from increased urine output and possibly urgency.

To check weight daily, using the same scale, at the same time (preferably as soon as arising, after voiding, but before eating).

To record weight and report loss or gain of more than 3 lb in one day.

How to measure and record blood pressure each day.

To report sudden and persistent changes in volume, color, or odor of urine.

To assume a head-low, seated position if dizziness occurs; to rise slowly and dangle legs at bedside to prevent postural changes.

To expect blue coloration of urine with triamterene.

To report endocrine side effects with spironolactone: excessive body hair growth, altered menses, gynecomastia, deepening of voice, or abnormally oily skin secretions.

About the major signs of hypokalemia, hyponatremia, and dehydration (thirst, salt craving, dizziness, muscular weakness, irregular pulse); to notify physician if they occur.

To report signs or symptoms indicating altered blood glucose levels; to monitor level of urine glucose (diabetic or prediabetic patients).

To report joint inflammation, pain and immobility (hyperuricemic or gouty patients).

To monitor apical pulse for possible irregularities, and report palpitations or dizziness; periodic measurements of blood electrolytes and ECG should be performed (patients taking digitalis and a diuretic).

Warn against self-medication with over-the-counter drugs such as laxatives or cathartics (enhance potassium loss) or antacids (contain sodium), unless advised by physician.

To store tablets and capsules in tightly capped bottles, protected from light, at room temperature.

◆ Evaluation

The patient/family will:

Measure weight daily; maintain desired body weight; report no gains or losses greater than 3 lb in one day.

Show no signs of fluid retention.

Report no dizziness or faintness and avoid physical injury (no falls).

Experience no adverse drug effects (eg, hypokalemia, hypoglycemia, orthostatic hypotension, hyperuricemia).

Ingest sufficient levels of potassium-rich foods as indicated; restrict fluid and sodium in diet.

Arrange daily schedule to ensure availability of bathroom facilities during diuresis.

Comply with prescribed drug regimen.

Annoted Bibliography

Andersson OK, Gudbrandsson T, Jamerson K. Metabolic adverse effects of thiazide diuretics: The importance of normokalaemia. *J Intern Med Suppl* 1991;735:89–96. *An excellent discussion of how hypokalemia can have an important impact on other metabolic parameters (eg, altered glucose and lipid levels) and clinical responses.*

Brater DC. Use of diuretics in chronic renal insufficiency and nephrotic syndrome. *Semin Nephrol* 1988;8:333–341. *An excellent review of common and serious medical problems—pathophysiology and the basis for treatment.*

Clarke RJ. Indapamide: A diuretic of choice for the treatment of hypertension? *Am J Med Sci* 1991;301:215–220. *The author makes a good case for why this indolone diuretic is a good candidate for a first-line antihypertensive, but also identifies what questions about its use still need answering.*

Dolleris PM. Diuretic and vasopressor usage in acute renal failure: A synopsis. *Crit Care Nurs Q* 1992;14:28–31. *Given the incidence and seriousness of acute renal failure, and the importance of nursing intervention, this paper will be helpful to nurses working in this area.*

Evans JG. Diuretics for elderly patients. *J Hypertens Suppl* 1990;8:S33–S37. *When other risk factors are not present in the elderly patient, thiazides and potassium-sparing agents may be preferred to other medications for treating hypertension.*

Ferris TF. Pregnancy complicated by hypertension and renal disease. *Adv Intern Med* 1990;35:269–287. *Valuable information about the use of diuretics, and other cardiovascular medications, in this special patient population.*

Levine SD. Diuretics. *Med Clin North Am* 1989;73:271–282. *One of the better broad reviews on diuretics.*

MacLennan WJ. Update: Diuretic therapy in the elderly. *Compr Ther* 1989;15:19–24. *Short, to the point, and worth reading for recent developments.*

Mende CW. Current issues in diuretic therapy. *Hosp Pract* 1990; 25(Suppl. 1):15–21. *A practical overview of uses and problems of diuretics in common hospital and outpatient settings.*

Messner M, Brissot P. Traditional management of liver disorders. *Drugs* 1990;40(Suppl. 3):45–57. *Discusses the importance of such factors as diet and nutrition in addition to therapy with the proper diuretics.*

Tartagni F. Metabolic side effects induced by diuretic therapy: Problems and possible solutions. *Gen Pharmacol* 1988;19:45–48. *Metabolic side effects are inevitable—and important—for many patients taking diuretics. This paper offers some valuable ways to assess, prevent, and correct them.*

Ujhelyi M. Loop diuretics: A practical guide to their use and selection. *Conn Med* 1991;55:162–165. *The information provided is just what the title of this short paper states.*

Wells TG. The pharmacology and therapeutics of diuretics in the pediatric patient. *Pediatr Clin North Am* 1990;37:463–504. *An important information source if your patients are mainly children who require diuretics.*

Table 32–C | **Clinical Uses and Administration of Major Diuretics***

AGENT	CLINICAL USES	DOSAGE AND ROUTE OF ADMINISTRATION
	Thiazides or Thiazide-like Diuretics	
PROTOTYPE		
Hydrochlorothiazide		
(ESIDRIX; HYDRODIURIL; ORETIC)	Edema	Adults: 25–200 mg/d, in divided doses if total dose exceeds 100 mg/d. Children (approximately 1 mg/lb body weight): infants up to 2 years: 12.5–37.5 mg; 2–12 years: 37.5–100 mg
	Hypertension	Initially, 75 mg/d; maintenance doses 25–100 mg/d
RELATED DRUGS		
Bendroflumethiazide		
(NATURETIN)	Edema	5 mg/d up to 20 mg/d
	Hypertension	Initially, 5–20 mg/d; maintenance 2.5–15 mg/d
Benzthiazide		
(EXNA; HYDREX)	Edema	Initially, 50–200 mg/d; maintenance 50–150 mg/d
	Hypertension	25–50 mg/d
Chlorothiazide		
(DIURIL)	Edema	0.5–2 g/d in single dose or two divided doses
	Hypertension	0.5–2 g/d
	Edema or hypertension	IV: 0.5–1.0 g once or twice daily for emergency use or for patients who cannot take oral medications
Chlorthalidone		
(HYGROTON)	Edema	Initially, 50–100 mg/d; maintenance usually 100 mg/d
	Hypertension	Initially, 25 mg/d; maintenance up to 100 mg/d
Hydroflumethiazide		
(DIUCARDIN; SALURON)	Edema	25–200 mg/d
	Hypertension	50–100 mg/d, up to a maximum of 200 mg/d
Methyclothiazide		
(ENDURON)	Edema	2.5–10 mg/d
	Hypertension	2.5–5 mg/d
Metolazone		
(DIULO; ZAROXOLYN)	Edema	5–10 mg/d
	Hypertension	2.5–5 mg/d
Polythiazide		
(RENESE)	Edema	1–4 mg/d
	Hypertension	2–4 mg/d
Quinethazone		
(HYDROMOX)	Edema or hypertension	50–100 mg/d
Trichlormethiazide		
(METAHYDRIN; NAQUA)	Edema	1–4 mg/d
	Hypertension	2–4 mg/d

(continued)

Table 32–C | **Clinical Uses and Administration of Major Diuretics*** (*Continued*)

AGENT	CLINICAL USES	DOSAGE AND ROUTE OF ADMINISTRATION
Indolone		
Indapamide		
(LOZOL)	Edema or hypertension	Initially, 2.5 mg/d; increase to 5 mg/d maximum after 1 week (for edema) or after 4 weeks (for hypertension) if necessary
High-Ceiling Diuretics		
PROTOTYPE		
Furosemide		
(LASIX)	Edema	Initially, 20–80 mg as single dose; titrate in 20–40-mg increments for maintenance, up to 600 mg/d IV or IM: 20–40 mg, repeat 20-mg at 2-hr intervals prn
	Hypertension	Initially, 40 mg bid; adjust dose, add other anti-hypertensive drugs, as needed
	Hypercalcemia	120 mg/d in single or divided doses
RELATED DRUGS		
Bumetanide		
(BUMEX)	Edema	Initially, 0.5–2 mg/d as single dose, up to 10 mg if needed; manufacturer recommends alternating 3 or 4 days on drug with 1- or 2-day rest periods
		IM or IV: Initially, 0.5–1 mg; IV dose given over 1–2 min; repeat every 2–3 hr prn, do not exceed 10 mg/d
Ethacrynic acid, ethacrynate sodium		
(EDECRIN, EDECRIN SODIUM)	Edema	50–100 mg/d (ethacrynic acid), usually in divided doses
		IV: 50 mg (ethacrynate sodium) as slow injection
Potassium-Sparing Diuretics		
PROTOTYPE		
Triamterene		
(DYRENIUM)	Edema, hypertension, hypokalemia	Initially, 100 mg bid, up to 300 mg/d maximum
RELATED DRUGS		
Amiloride		
(MIDAMOR)	Edema, hypertension, hypokalemia	5 mg/d, adjunctively with potassium-wasting diuretic or other antihypertensive drug; may increase to 20 mg/d for poorly controlled hypokalemia

(continued)

Table 32–C **Clinical Uses and Administration of Major Diuretics*** (*Continued*)

AGENT	CLINICAL USES	DOSAGE AND ROUTE OF ADMINISTRATION
	Potassium-Sparing Diuretics	
RELATED DRUGS		
Spironolactone		
(ALDACTONE)	Edema	100 mg/d in single or divided doses; use with potassium-wasting diuretic if response unsatisfactory
	Hypertension	50–100 mg/d in single or divided doses; use with potassium-wasting diuretic
	Hypokalemia	25–100 mg/d
	Carbonic Anhydrase Inhibitors	
PROTOTYPE		
Acetazolamide		
(DIAMOX, DIAMOX SEQUELS)	Edema	Usually 250–375 mg in morning; intermittent dosing (2 days on drug, 1 day off) may reduce refractoriness when long-term therapy is anticipated
	Chronic open-angle glaucoma	Usually 250–1000 mg/d in divided doses if daily dose >250 mg; timed-release capsules (SEQUELS; 500 mg each) may be given twice daily
	Acute congestive (angle-closure) glaucoma	Usually 500 mg initially, then 125–250 mg q4h IV: 500 mg for prompt reduction of intraocular pressure
	Epilepsy	Usually 8–30 mg/kg in divided doses
RELATED DRUGS		
Dichlorphenamide		
(DARANIDE)	Glaucoma	100–200 mg initially, then 100 mg q12h until ocular pressure reduced adequately; maintenance 25–50 mg qd–tid
Methazolamide		
(NEPTAZANE)	Glaucoma	50–100 mg bid or tid
	Osmotic Diuretics	
PROTOTYPE		
Mannitol		
(OSMITROL)	Prevention, treatment of acute renal failure (oliguria)	IV: 50–100 g of a 5%–25% solution, given as slow infusion
	Reduction of intracranial pressure	IV: 1.5–2 g/kg body weight, as a 15%–25% solution, infused over 30–60 min
	Reduction of intraocular pressure	IV: 1.5–2 g/kg body weight, as a 20% solution, infused over 30 min
	Forced diuresis for drug overdoses	IV: Up to 200 g as slow

(continued)

Table 32–C Clinical Uses and Administration of Major Diuretics* (*Continued*)

AGENT	CLINICAL USES	DOSAGE AND ROUTE OF ADMINISTRATION
RELATED DRUGS		
Urea		
(UREAPHIL)	Reduction of intraocular or intracranial pressure	IV: 1–1.5 g/kg body weight, as a 30% solution, by slow infusion

*Unless noted otherwise, all dosages are for adults and are administered orally.

Table 32–S Major Side Effects of and Contraindications for Diuretics

BODY SYSTEM/ Side Effect	CONTRAINDICATION/ PRECAUTION	COMMENTS AND NURSING IMPLICATIONS
Most Orally Effective Diuretics		
CENTRAL NERVOUS SYSTEM Drowsiness, lethargy, confusion, anxiety		Almost always due to electrolyte imbalances (see Table 31-C); notify physician at once if mental status is altered
BLOOD Hyponatremia; dehydration; may be accompanied by hypotension, neuromuscular signs, symptoms	Salt depletion, dehydration; hypotension	Ensure adequate but not excessive intake of salt, water; periodically monitor BP, fluid intake and output; advise patient to avoid strenuous exercise; monitor for, have patient report, signs of hyponatremia or volume depletion (see Table 32-3); most likely with high-ceiling diuretics, treatment with multiple diuretics
Hyperuricemia	Severe hyperuricemia, recent history of gout	Assess for sudden onset of joint pain, inflammation, immobility, which may indicate onset of gout; symptom risk reduced with adequate hydration; incidence greatest with thiazides, high-ceiling agents
Hyperglycemia, hypoglycemia	Poorly controlled diabetes mellitus	Antidiabetic drug doses often need to be increased, may decrease or remain unchanged; check blood glucose levels carefully upon start of diuretic therapy, periodically thereafter; monitor for glucose intolerance; incidence greatest with thiazides
Elevated blood urea nitrogen, creatinine, hematocrit levels	Oliguria, poor renal function	May be due to excessive salt, water depletion, progressive renal dysfunction; notify physician at once if urine output falls markedly; question orders calling for increased diuretic dose, especially of thiazides
Increased serum triglyceride, LDL, and total cholesterol levels; decreased HDL levels		Limits or requires cautious use, monitoring, in patients with preexisting hyperlipidemias, history of atherosclerosis; risk greatest with thiazides

(continued)

Table 32–S | **Major Side Effects of and Contraindications for Diuretics (*Continued*)**

BODY SYSTEM/ Side Effect	CONTRAINDICATION/ PRECAUTION	COMMENTS AND NURSING IMPLICATIONS
CARDIOVASCULAR Hypotension, arrhythmias	Hypotension, arrhythmias	Hypotension most likely to occur due to excessive fluid, sodium depletion, or use of other antihypertensive drugs; cardiac irregularities often indicate hypokalemia, are more ominous in digitalized patient; measure electrolytes, BP, monitor ECG frequently
GASTROINTESTINAL Anorexia, nausea, vomiting		May indicate electrolyte imbalances (check lab data); mild GI upset may be alleviated by taking drug with meals
Acute abdominal pain		Rare, may indicate pancreatitis, jaundice (observe color of skin, eyes, urine); report severe pain to physician at once
Thiazides, High-Ceiling Diuretics, Acetazolamide		
BLOOD Hypokalemia	Hypokalemia	Incidence as high as 50% with chronic thiazide therapy, may occur with any potassium-wasting diuretic; particularly dangerous for patients with poor respiratory status, uncontrolled diabetes, severe diarrhea, those taking digitalis; check pulse, ECG periodically; report irregular pulse, muscle weakness, malaise, GI disturbances at once; see Table 32-3 for major signs, symptoms
Thiazides		
BLOOD Hypercalcemia	Hypocalcemia	Innocuous for most patients; may increase risk of arrhythmias in digitalized patients; clinically useful for reducing systemic, bone calcium loss
Potassium-Sparing Diuretics		
BLOOD Hyperkalemia	Relative contraindication: concurrent use of oral potassium supplements	Question orders for both potassium-sparing diuretics and oral potassium supplements
Endocrine (spironolactone) Gynecomastia, abnormal menses, deepening of the voice, oily skin		Incidence, severity usually increase with increased dose, duration of therapy; side effects wane when dosage is reduced, drug is discontinued
Acetazolamide		
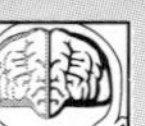 **NEUROLOGIC** Paresthesias, vertigo		May be due to either hyponatremia or systemic acidosis; check serum electrolytes, blood gases, and pH

(continued)

Table 32–S | **Major Side Effects of and Contraindications for Diuretics (*Continued*)**

BODY SYSTEM/ Side Effect	CONTRAINDICATION/ PRECAUTION	COMMENTS AND NURSING IMPLICATIONS
Ostmotic Diuretics		
CARDIOVASCULAR Hypertension, stroke, acute heart failure, pulmonary edema	Hypertension, stroke, heart failure, pulmonary edema, intracranial bleeding, aneurysms	Monitor BP, urine output; check for signs, symptoms of heart failure; notify physician and be prepared to discontinue mannitol administration if they develop; dilute concentrated mannitol as indicated for specific use; administer appropriate fluids to compensate for fluid, electrolyte loss due to diuresis

Table 32–I | **Major Interactions between Diuretics and Other Agents**

AGENT	RESULT OF INTERACTION	COMMENTS AND NURSING IMPLICATIONS
Interactions Involving Most Orally Effective Diuretics		
Alcohol (Chapter 22)	Potentially excessive fluid, electrolyte loss or imbalance, BP fall	Assess for alcohol use as part of medication history; advise patient to restrict alcohol use, preferably under physician's supervision
Antihypertensive drugs, other classes (Chapter 33)	Additive or greater BP lowering	Interaction advantageous when therapy planned, monitored properly
Laxatives, cathartics (Chapter 41)	As for alcohol, above	As for alcohol, above; laxative use, abuse, more prevalent in elderly
Lithium (Chapter 24)	Increased risk of lithium toxicity, potentially severe	Diuretic-induced sodium loss reduces lithium excretion; avoid interaction if possible; otherwise, monitor responses, blood sodium and lithium levels more closely; stress need for consistent, proper dietary sodium intake to reduce risk of hyponatremia
Methylxanthines (eg, caffeine, theophylline; Chapter 38)	Potentially excessive fluid loss, BP fall, owing to additive diuretic effect	Encourage patient to restrict intake of caffeine-containing beverages (colas, coffee, tea), preferably under physician's supervision; theophylline use need not be avoided if combined therapy is supervised closely
Interactions Involving All Potassium-Wasting Diuretics		
Amphotericin B (Chapter 57)	Increased risk of hypokalemia	Risk greatest with parenteral amphotericin; avoid combined use if possible, monitor if unavoidable
Corticosteroids (oral or parenteral; Chapter 45)	Antagonism of diuretic's sodium-depleting, BP-lowering effects; excessive potassium wasting	Risks greater with steroids having appreciable mineralocorticoid activity (eg, cortisone, prednisone); monitor accordingly if prolonged systemic steroid therapy unavoidable
Digoxin, other digitalis glycosides (Chapter 31)	Increased risk of digitalis toxicity	Combined use of interactants is common; problems arise from potassium and magnesium loss; anticipate need for potassium supplements or potassium-sparing diuretics based on lab test results, other assessment tools

(continued)

Table 32–I **Major Interactions Between Diuretics and Other Agents**

AGENT	RESULT OF INTERACTION	COMMENTS AND NURSING IMPLICATIONS
Interactions Involving Mainly the Thiazides and Thiazide-Like Agents		
Diazoxide (Chapter 33)	Additive increases of blood glucose levels; potential signs, symptoms of diabetes mellitus	Avoid interaction if possible, anticipate need to reduce dose of one or both agents; most important when diazoxide is given orally, chronically, for hypoglycemia
Probenecid (Chapter 53)	Reduced uric acid excretion, increased serum urate levels, poor control of hyperuricemia, gout	Thiazides and probenecid have opposing effects on urate excretion; avoid thiazide use in gout patients, if possible; allopurinol can reduce the diuretic's hyperuricemic effects, is usually preferred alternative for gout patients who require diuretics
Tolbutamide, other oral hypoglycemic drugs (Chapter 46)	Increased blood glucose levels, reduced ability of interactant to control diabetes	Signs of interaction may take months to appear; may require increased hypoglycemic drug dosages if interaction unavoidable; interaction may be less common, severe, with newer hypoglycemics (glipizide, glyburide); insulin therapy may require adjustments also
Interactions Involving High-Ceiling Diuretics		
Aminoglycoside antibiotics (Chapter 56)	Ototoxicity	Risk greater with (1) parenteral therapy; (2) high dosages; (3) preexisting hearing or renal impairment. Hearing impairment usually occurs suddenly, may be mild or severe, temporary or permanent; use alternative drugs if possible
Cisplatin (Chapter 59)	Ototoxicity	See aminoglycosides, above
Nonsteroidal antiinflammatory drugs (Chapter 52)	Decreased diuretic efficacy	Arises from inhibited prostaglandin synthesis; mainly applies to ibuprofen, indomethacin, sulindac; alternative antiinflammatory drugs preferred if interaction occurs
Interaction Involving Potassium-Sparing Diuretics		
Indomethacin (Chapter 52)	Renal failure	Avoid combination
Potassium-containing drugs (including oral potassium supplements) (p 611 and Chapter 61)	Hyperkalemia, potentially symptomatic; severe	Avoid interaction unless it is impossible to control potassium levels with either agent alone; stress importance of following dietary guidelines regarding potassium intake; monitor serum electrolyte levels frequently
Interaction Involving Acetazolamide		
Aspirin, other salicylates (Chapter 52)	Increased acetazolamide blood levels, effects	Aspirin displaces acetazolamide from plasma proteins
	Increased risk of CNS toxicity of salicylate	Metabolic acidosis caused by acetazolamide increases salicylate penetration into CNS. Avoid interaction if possible; probably applies to dichlorophenamide also

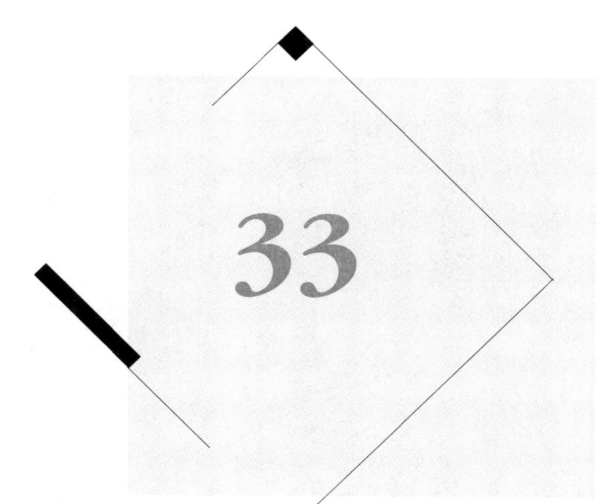

PROTOTYPES

33 Antihypertensive Drugs

Thousands of people are killed or incapacitated each year by the consequences of **hypertension** (high blood pressure). Certain drugs, and certain medical conditions can cause hypertension (Table 33–1). However, the most common type of hypertension is *essential hypertension,* meaning that the cause is unknown. Its treatment is the focus of this chapter.

Part I of the chapter is a brief review of how blood pressure is normally controlled; some characteristics of hypertension and its effects on the body; factors affecting the decision to treat it; and general treatment goals. Part II discusses the drugs that are used for long-term management of hypertension. Part III focuses on the treatment of hypertensive emergencies. Part IV discusses some general nursing implications for successful therapy of hypertension. Part V is an overview of how to optimize therapy and make it safer for patients with unique needs and characteristics.

Major reference tables appear beginning on p. 665.

Table 33–1 Some Identifiable Causes of or Contributors to Hypertension

Alcohol: acute or chronic ingestion, acute alcohol withdrawal

Aortic coarctation

Atherosclerosis

Brain lesions, including increased intracranial pressure

Diabetes

Drugs
- Sympathomimetics
- Mineralocorticoids, glucocorticoids
- Estrogens
- Thyroid hormones

Hyperaldosteronism
- Primary: adrenal cortical tumors
- Secondary: impaired hepatic function (eg, cirrhosis, which may be related to alcohol ingestion)

Pheochromocytoma

Pregnancy (preeclampsia/eclampsia)

Renal disease, including atherosclerosis and other causes of renal artery stenosis

Smoking

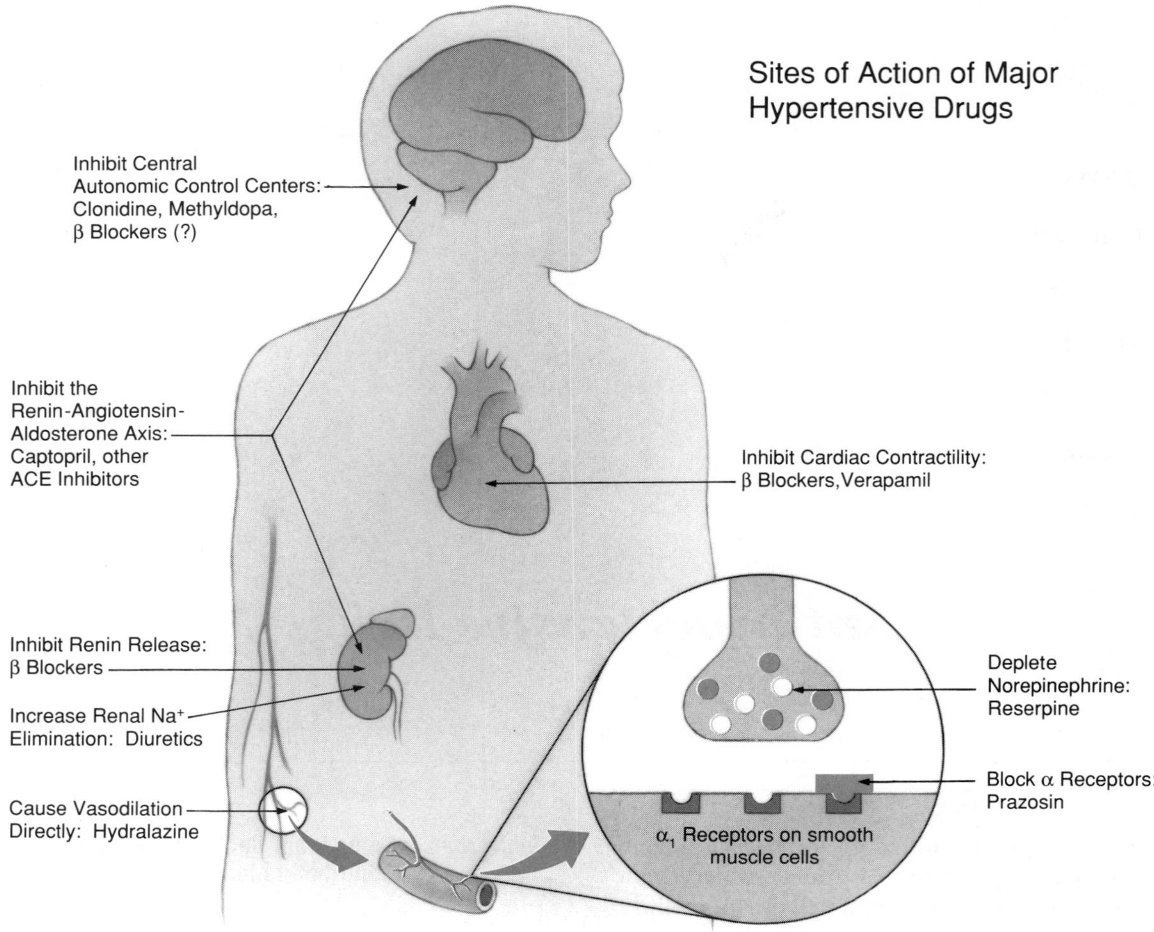

Figure 33–1

Drugs used to treat chronic hypertension act at various sites that play a role in the etiology of essential hypertension. Some drugs, such as *β* blockers, exert beneficial effects in several ways. For simplicity, the figure shows only drug classes or prototype agents in each class.

I. Background

Control of Blood Pressure

Blood pressure rises when blood vessels constrict, when cardiac contractility is too intense, or when blood volume rises too high. The *sympathetic nervous system*, the *kidneys*, and the *renin-angiotensin-aldosterone system* are among the key blood pressure regulators. They evolved to restore blood pressure when it falls, as with hemorrhage; when they operate abnormally, however, they contribute to the pathophysiology of hypertension—and congestive heart failure (CHF). Antihypertensive drugs act on one or more of these control mechanisms (Figure 33–1; Table 33–2).

Classification of High Blood Pressure

Defining high blood pressure is not as straightforward as it might seem. "High" blood pressure is obviously some value above "normal," but the norm varies, mainly according to age. For example, 120/80 mm Hg is the typical norm for younger adults, but pressures significantly higher than this are common in the elderly. For the elderly, such increased values may be *statistically* normal but not necessarily harmless. Conversely, a pressure of 120/80 in an infant is considered dangerously high.

In 1978, a committee organized by the National Institutes of Health concluded that an adult (>18 years old) is hypertensive if blood pressure at rest, in the sit-

Table 33–2 **Oral Antihypertensive Drugs for Essential Hypertension: Classes, Prototypes, and Mechanisms of Action***

Class	Prototype	Mechanism(s)
Diuretics	Hydrochlorothiazide	Increase renal sodium loss; reduce blood volume; reduce vasoconstriction in response to vasoconstrictors (eg, epinephrine, norepinephrine)
β blockers	Propranolol	Reduce cardiac contractility; inhibit renin release; act in CNS by ill-defined mechanism
Calcium channel blockers	Verapamil	Reduce cardiac contractility and vasoconstriction and directly dilate blood vessels by blocking cell calcium influx
ACE inhibitors	Captopril	Inhibit synthesis of angiotensin II, a vasoconstrictor; inhibit renin release, aldosterone levels
Centrally acting α agonists	Clonidine	Stimulate α receptors in cardiovascular control center of brain, reducing sympathetic constriction of blood vessels, stimulation of heart
Peripheral, selective α blockers	Prazosin	Block ability of epinephrine, norepinephrine to cause vasoconstriction via normal α receptor stimulation
Peripheral catecholamine depleters	Reserpine, guanethidine	Partially reduce (reserpine) or completely eliminate (guanethidine) norepinephrine stores in sympathetic nerves, thereby reducing vasoconstrictor effects of sympathetic stimulation
Direct-acting vasodilators	Hydralazine	Directly relaxes arteriolar smooth muscle

*Listed in general order of use in stepped-care approach, except for guanethidine, which is usually a last-choice drug.

ting and standing positions, is greater than 120/80 mm Hg during two or more blood pressure measurements made under the same conditions at different times. Elevated *diastolic* blood pressure was of most concern. In 1988, a new committee report placed more emphasis on the assessment and follow-up of hypertension and its treatment, issues related to special patient populations, the need to communicate disease- and therapy-related information to patients, and economic factors (National Institutes of Health, 1988). The committee also provided more specific criteria to define hypertension and addressed both systolic and diastolic pressures. (The latter is still of more concern over the long run.) Key points of the classification of hypertension are summarized in Table 33–3.

Consequences of Hypertension

Prolonged or severe hypertension can damage the vasculature and, eventually, the major organs. Important consequences include heart and kidney failure and stroke. *The higher the pressure and the longer it is elevated, the greater the risk of serious organ damage and death.* In short, *hypertensive patients have a greater morbidity and mortality rate than individuals with normal (or lower) blood pressure.*

Factors Influencing the Decision to Treat Hypertension

The benefits of treating moderate or severe hypertension are generally accepted. Clinicians disagree more about whether and how to treat mild hypertension. (Some data suggest that mildly hypertensive patients have twice the risk of serious cardiovascular problems than normotensive persons.) A small number of clinicians believe that nondrug measures alone may be effective and appropriate and that avoiding medication spares patients from unpleasant or potentially serious drug side effects. Nevertheless, the consensus is that, over the long run, decreasing any persistently elevated pressure is desirable.

In addition to the actual blood pressure, other factors must be considered in the assessment:

Table 33–3 Classifications of Hypertension in Adults

Pressure (mm Hg)	Category	
	Diastolic	
< 85	Normal	Recheck within 2 years
85–89	High-normal	Recheck within 1 year
90–104	Mild hypertension	Confirm within 2 months
105–114	Moderate hypertension	Confirm within 2 weeks or refer promptly to source of care
≥ 115	Severe hypertension	Evaluate/refer for care at once
	Systolic (if diastolic pressure is < 90)	
< 140	Normal	Recheck within 2 years
140–159	Borderline isolated systolic hypertension	Confirm within 2 months
160–199	Isolated systolic hypertension	Confirm within 2 months
≥ 200	Isolated systolic hypertension	Evaluate/refer for care at once

Source: Adapted from *The 1988 Report of the Joint National Committee on Detection, Evaluation, and Treatment of High Blood Pressure.* NIH Publication 88-1088. U.S. Government Printing Office, 1988.

- *Age.* The longer the blood pressure remains elevated, the greater the risk of complications or death. Therefore, for a given blood pressure increase, younger patients are more likely to obtain greater long-term benefit from therapy. Also, younger patients generally tolerate antihypertensive drugs better than the elderly and are less likely to be taking other medications with which antihypertensive drugs might interact.
- *Sex and race.* For a given age and blood pressure, blacks and females have a greater cardiovascular risk. They are more likely to be treated than Caucasians or males. There are also race-related differences in the efficacies of certain antihypertensive drugs.
- *Other risk factors.* Treatment is particularly important for patients with other cardiovascular risk factors, including preexisting vascular or organ damage, hyperlipidemias, diabetes, and so on. The pretreatment work-up includes an assessment of these factors by means of appropriate tests. Test outcomes can help determine which antihypertensive drug is more suited for a particular patient.
- *Family history of cardiovascular disease.* A positive history argues in favor of treating even mild hypertension.
- *How fast pressure rises.* A rapid or constant pressure rise is of more concern than a slow increase. Continued pressure rises despite normally effective drug therapy may be difficult to halt. They may also indicate *malignant hypertension,* which is associated with arteriolar damage. It may be rapidly fatal.
- *Whether the measured high blood pressure persists or is an isolated incident, perhaps due to identifiable factors.* Everyone experiences short periods of elevated blood pressure. However, even though those occasional increases may be detected during a physical exam, usually they do not need to be treated. In contrast, a prolonged blood pressure increase is more worrisome. Ideally, to help make the diagnosis of hypertension, the clinician establishes the presence of increased blood pressure on several occasions, with the patient at rest. Table 33–3 gives some guidelines about how often follow-up exams should be provided.
- *Whether high blood pressure can be reduced by surgical or other nondrug means.* Hypertension from such causes as pheochromocytoma or adrenal cortical tumor may be treated surgically. Reducing body weight and sodium intake and stopping smoking help many more patients. Even if such measures are implemented, antihypertensive drug therapy still plays an important role.
- *Whether hypertension is caused by drugs that elevate blood pressure.* If pressure-elevating drugs are not absolutely necessary for the patient's health,

Table 33–4 | A Typical Plan for the Stepped-Care Approach to Essential Hypertension Therapy*

STEP I

1. Start with low doses of one of the following:
   - a diuretic (eg, hydrochlorothiazide) *or*
   - a β-adrenergic blocker (eg, propranolol) *or*
   - a calcium channel blocker (eg, verapamil) *or*
   - an ACE inhibitor (eg, captopril)

STEP II

1. Cautiously increase dose of initial drug, *or*
2. Add a sympathetic inhibitor *or*
3. Substitute a sympathetic inhibitor for the starting agent:
   - a centrally acting α agonists (eg, clonidine) *or*
   - a selective peripheral α antagonist (eg, prazosin) *or*
   - a peripheral catecholamine depleter (eg, reserpine)

STEP III

1. Add a vasodilator (eg, hydralazine) *or*
2. Use a vasodilator instead of the drug added in Step II

STEP IV

1. Add a third drug if only two were used in Step III *or*
2. Add a fourth drug (usually guanethidine)

*Prototypes are shown in parentheses. If a diuretic was not used in Step I, it will probably be needed in later steps. Using hydralazine (Step III) usually requires both a diuretic and a β blocker.

discontinuing them or at least reducing their dosage is preferred to using still other drugs to counteract their effects.

Therapeutic Goals

A goal of drug therapy is to lower blood pressure safely toward, but not necessarily to, the age-related norm for the healthy population. For some patients it may be possible to reach normal values. For others, especially those with severe acute or longstanding hypertension, this may be impossible, and aiming for the norm could actually be dangerous. For these patients, any appreciable pressure decrease is a therapeutic gain.

The "Stepped-Care" Approach to Drug Therapy of Essential Hypertension

Antihypertensive drugs are often used in a sequence called the "stepped-care" approach (Table 33–4). The idea is to begin treatment with a single drug, if possible. That drug is used as a foundation for any necessary further treatment. This is Step I. If greater blood pressure control is needed, Step II, the use of small doses of several agents, is implemented. A different drug might be substituted for the first, or small doses of another drug can be added to the foundation. This approach capitalizes on the fact that *antihypertensive drugs in different classes have additive blood pressure-lowering effects.* (The alternative approach, ie, increasing the dose of a single drug as much as possible, usually does little more than increase the risk and severity of dose-dependent side effects and adverse responses.)

If the response is still inadequate, other (Step III) drugs can be added to or substituted for current agents. For *refractory hypertension*—high blood pressure that does not respond to usually effective treatments—still other drugs can be tried (Step IV).

The chosen drug(s) should provide some evidence of a desired effect on blood pressure by 1 month of use (assuming proper dosages and compliance), and certainly after a 3-month trial. If the response has not occurred within this therapeutic window, therapy should

TRENDS AND CONTROVERSIES IN PHARMACOLOGY

Why Do We Need Another Antihypertensive Drug?

Given the many drugs available to treat hypertension, the appearance of new drugs on the market often seems unwarranted. Certainly resources spent on drug development contribute significantly to the rising costs of prescription drugs. These costs are of increasing concern to both consumers and health professionals; they raise questions about the reasons behind the development of new therapeutic agents. Within the pharmaceutical industry, the role of the "profit motive" in drug development cannot be disregarded. However, efforts aimed at developing therapeutic alternatives are based on many considerations.

The major classes of antihypertensive drugs—angiotensin converting enzyme (ACE) inhibitors, β blockers, calcium channel antagonists, and diuretics—are each effective in lowering blood pressure but are characterized by different profiles of limitations. These limitations include specific side effects, contraindications, and relative lack of effectiveness in some patient groups. The focus of new development in the major drug categories often addresses the limitations of existing drugs.

Beta-blockers provide a good example. Although propranolol is still widely prescribed, the development of cardioselective ß blockers has allowed this class of drugs to be used in situations where it was previously contraindicated. Changes have also been important for patient adherence, since the newer drugs require less frequent administration. There is a caveat; the list of approved ß blockers keeps growing, but with relatively few therapeutic gains characterizing the most recently added drugs.

Hypertension is associated with increased risks of atherosclerosis, stroke, and myocardial infarction. Therefore, when antihypertensive drugs are compared, equal blood pressure lowering ability does not *necessarily* translate into equal efficacy as antihypertensive treatments. For example, ß blockers may offer cardioprotective effects not observed with calcium channel antagonists or diuretics. However, selected advantages are often accompanied by other disadvantages. Beta blockers have been shown to increase plasma lipid levels, although the clinical significance of these changes has not been determined.

A large number of antihypertensive medications are available, but heterogeneity in blood pressure responses to specific antihypertensive treatments supports the need for a variety of drugs. Furthermore, existing drugs do not fully address the therapeutic needs of reducing associated complications without adverse sequelae. With an estimated 60 million Americans affected by hypertension, the development of new drugs can be justified by the importance of meeting unmet goals for therapy in a form that is safe, easy to use, and acceptable to patient populations. This is not to say that all new development is appropriate. But by communicating with manufacturers and holding them accountable, both health care professionals and health care consumers can express their opinions when new drug development appears to add unnecessarily to rising health care costs.

American Heart Association. *Heart Facts.* Dallas, TX: American Heart Association 1988.

Gorlin, R: Do we need another antihypertensive agent? *Am Heart J* 1991; 121: 670-676.

be modified by using another drug in another pharmacologic class.

The sequence of drug use in the traditional stepped-care approach was formerly quite rigid—it almost always began with a diuretic or a β blocker. The consensus now is that any one of several drug classes can be a reasonable choice for initial therapy. The choice of a specific drug is based mainly on its side effects, adverse responses, or drug interactions that would be particularly unsuitable for a given patient. With experience gained from using newer agents, it is now common and acceptable to start treatment with some drugs that only a few years ago were rarely used early on.

NURSING IMPLICATIONS

Although the stepped-care approach is more flexible than it was, the underlying principle behind it remains basically the same: The drug should be chosen according to the severity of hypertension, and the patient's individual traits. For example, an antihypertensive drug suited for severe hypertension but administered to a mildly hypertensive individual will certainly reduce blood pressure but needlessly cause significantly more or more distressing side effects not caused by another equally effective alternative.

II. Drug Therapy

Step I Drugs: Starting Therapy

Treatment of mild hypertension usually starts with a drug in one of the following classes:

- diuretics, almost always a thiazide or thiazide-like agent;
- β-adrenergic blockers;
- calcium channel blockers; or
- angiotensin converting enzyme (ACE) inhibitors.

Diuretics

Diuretics (Chapter 32) probably help lower blood pressure by lowering total body sodium levels and sodium levels of blood vessel smooth muscle cells. This sodium loss reduces the sensitivity of the arterioles to the constrictor effects of epinephrine and norepinephrine.

For many years, thiazide diuretics were preferred starting agents for managing mild hypertension in most patients. However, they have lost some popularity in that role, mainly because they raise serum triglyceride and cholesterol levels, both of which are recognized risk factors for cardiovascular disease. Other common side effects—hypokalemia, hypomagnesemia, hypercalcemia, and increases of serum glucose and lipid levels—are also of concern for many patients with related contraindicating conditions. Indapamide (LOZOL; p 607), which has thiazide-like antihypertensive actions but is thought to cause fewer metabolic side effects, is another reasonable alternative.

Diuretics still play an important role in hypertension therapy, in conjunction with other drugs. They exert additive pressure-lowering effects when used with other medications. Moreover, some other antihypertensive drugs trigger renal sodium and water retention, which tends to maintain blood pressure; diuretics counteract this unwanted effect. The use of diuretics with other antihypertensive medications is so common that many fixed-dose combination products are available (Table 33–5).

NURSING IMPLICATIONS

Several treatment options are available if the pressure-lowering effects of a thiazide are not adequate. Some are likely to work, others are not. Increasing the dosage of the current drug, switching to another thiazide, or even switching to another class of diuretics usually does little to lower pressure. The best approach usually is to add, or switch to, an antihypertensive drug in a completely different class. Many fixed-dose antihypertensive drug combinations are available. However, none of them is used to start therapy. Each drug is assessed first to determine its effectiveness and proper dosage; then, a suitable combination can be used for convenience.

Beta-Adrenergic Blockers

Drugs that block β-adrenergic receptors (discussed as a group in Chapter 15), lower pressure in two major ways: They reduce cardiac contractility somewhat, thereby reducing the arterial pressure pulses that occur each time the heart contracts; and they inhibit renin release, thereby interrupting the renin-angiotensin-aldosterone system. As a result, β blockers are particularly useful for some patients with tachycardia, high plasma renin levels, or both.

All the orally effective β blockers are approved as antihypertensives (see pp 231–240, for an overview). Like the thiazides, however, β blockers are now less frequently chosen as starting drugs because of side effects. Of most concern, perhaps, are the abilities of β blockers to increase serum lipid levels, cause hypoglycemia, and aggravate such conditions as heart failure, asthma, or emphysema.

In terms of adverse effects on serum lipids, there are some differences among the β blockers. Nonselective agents (eg, propranolol, the overall prototype) increase triglycerides more than any other antihypertensive drugs and cause significantly greater reductions of high density lipoprotein (HDL) levels. Beta blockers with the property of cardioselectivity (eg, atenolol, metoprolol), intrinsic sympathomimetic activity (eg, pindolol), or combined α- and β-blocking actions (labetalol) have less adverse lipid effects. These drugs also tend to cause somewhat fewer problems for patients with cardiac or pulmonary disease (eg, heart failure, asthma, emphysema) that can be aggravated by β

Table 33–5 Selected Fixed-Dose Combination Antihypertensive Products

Proprietary Name	Ingredients
Products Containing an ACE Inhibitor	
CAPOZIDE	25 or 50 mg captopril, 15 or 25 mg HCTZ*
PRINZIDE, ZESTORETIC	20mg lisinopril, 12.5 or 25 mg HCTZ
VASERETIC	10 mg enalapril, 25 mg HCTZ
Products Containing a β Blocker	
CORZIDE	40 or 80 mg nadolol, 5 mg bendroflumethiazide
INDERIDE	40 or 80 mg propranolol, 25 mg HCTZ
INDERIDE LA	80, 120, or 160 mg propranolol, 50 mg HCTZ
LOPRESSOR-HCT	50 or 100 mg metoprolol, 25 or 50 mg HCTZ
NORMOZIDE	100, 200, or 300 mg labetalol, 25 mg HCTZ
TENORETIC	50 or 100 mg atenolol, 25 mg chlorthalidone
TIMOLIDE	10 mg timolol, 25 mg HCTZ
Product Containing Clonidine	
COMBIPRES	0.1 or 0.2 mg clonidine, 15 mg chlorthalidone
Products Containing Diuretics Only	
DYAZIDE	50 mg triamterene, 25 mg HCTZ
MAXZIDE	75 mg triamterene, 50 mg HCTZ
Products Containing Methyldopa	
ALDOCLOR	250 mg methyldopa, 150 or 250 mg chlorothiazide
ALDORIL	250 mg methyldopa, 15 or 25 mg HCTZ; 500 mg methyldopa, 30 or 50 mg HCTZ
Product Containing Prazosin	
MINIZIDE	1, 2, or 5 mg prazosin, 0.5 mg polythiazide
Products Containing Reserpine or Related Rauwolfia Alkaloids	
DEMI-REGROTON	0.125 mg reserpine, 25 mg chlorthalidone
DIUPRES	0.125 mg reserpine, 250 or 500 mg chlorothiazide
ENDURONYL FORTE	0.5 mg deserpidine, 5 mg methyclothiazide
HYDROPRES	0.125 mg reserpine, 25 or 50 mg HCTZ
RAUZIDE	50 mg Rauwolfia serpentina alkaloids, 4 mg bendroflumethiazide
REGROTON	0.25 mg reserpine, 50 mg chlorthalidone
RENESE-R	0.25 mg reserpine, 2 mg polythiazide
SERP-AP-ES	0.1 mg reserpine, 25 mg hydralazine, 15 mg HCTZ
Products Containing Hydralazine	
APRESAZIDE	25, 50, or 100 mg hydralazine, 25 or 50 mg HCTZ
APRESOLINE-ESIDRIX	25 mg hydralazine, 15 mg HCTZ
SERPASIL-APRESOLINE	see above

*HCTZ = hydrochlorothiazide.

blockers in general. Thus, for certain patients, the alternatives may have some advantages over a drug such as propranolol. However, if one *β* blocker does not work well to lower the patient's blood pressure, switching to another is not likely to work better.

Even though a *β* blocker alone may not be fully effective for some hypertensive patients, *β* blockers still can be useful adjuncts to other antihypertensive drugs because of their additive antihypertensive effects and because they can minimize reflex tachycardia, which is a side effect of several other antihypertensive medications. Chapter 30 discusses the use of *β* blockers as antiarrhythmics; Chapter 34 covers their use in managing angina pectoris.

NURSING IMPLICATIONS

All the contraindications and drug–drug interactions that apply to using *β* blockers for other indications apply to their use for hypertension (see Table 15–S, p 248). Beta blocker therapy should never be dis-

TRENDS AND CONTROVERSIES IN PHARMACOLOGY

Sublingual Nifedipine—An Appropriate Route?

Despite the fact that nifedipine is not manufactured in a sublingual form for patient use, there are numerous reports describing the efficacy of sublingual nifedipine in the treatment of angina pectoris, congestive heart failure, and hypertension. As a recent review by Schumann (1991) points out, these studies are difficult to interpret. Because of variations in the techniques used to deliver nifedipine, it can't be determined whether the effects of the drug are caused by absorption of the drug across buccal membranes or are actually due to swallowing and gastric absorption. The potential for gastric absorption is evident in some of the methods used by nurses to administer sublingual nifedipine, described in a study by Kedas et al.

The basis for decisions to prescribe nifedipine by the sublingual route is not well established. There are claims that this route increases absorption and peak activity of the drug. However, existing evidence demonstrates that the absorption of nifedipine occurs mainly in the stomach. Studies examining sublingual or buccal administration of nifedipine in anesthetized patients that were unable to swallow indicate that little, if any, sublingual or transbuccal absorption occurs (Nussmeier et al., 1983; Weaver, 1989).

Nifedipine is used to treat hypertensive emergencies and is particularly useful in this setting because hypotension rarely occurs. However, if the sublingual route is chosen in order to achieve a more rapid and greater effect than can be obtained using oral routes, it appears that patients could be placed at risk since absorption is unlikely to occur until the drug reaches the stomach. Furthermore, differences in administration techniques lead to variations in the nifedipine dosage received by the patient. One strategy suggested for the effective administration of "sublingual" nifedipine to conscious patients is the "bite and swallow" method in which the capsule is broken before swallowing to aid gastric absorption (Schumann, 1991).

Nurses can and do have an impact on the prescription and administration of medications. Because prescribers don't usually administer drugs, they may be unaware of some of the difficulties encountered. Questions are likely to occur when medications are prescribed by routes other than those formally approved by the FDA, since information about the route may be hard to obtain. Even when a drug is prescribed by an approved route, problems can arise when there is a need to give the drug by an alternate method, such as through a feeding tube. Nurses should discuss these problems as well as concerns about the route selected with physicians and pharmacists. In hospitals and other health care facilities, nursing practice committees as well as pharmacy and therapeutics committees provide excellent forums for dealing with issues concerning medication and their administration.

Kedas A, Shively M, Burris J: Nursing delivery of sublingual nifedipine. *J Cardiovasc Nurs* 1989; 3(4): 31-37.

Lange MP, Dahn MS, Jacobs LA: Patient-controlled analgesia versus intermittent analgesia dosing. *Heart Lung* 1988; 17: 495-498.

Nussmeier NA, Curling PE, Murphy DA, et al: Nifedipine: Cardiovascular effects after sublingual administration during fentanyl-pancuronium anesthesia in man. *Anesthesiology* 1983; 59(suppl3A): A34.

Schumann D: Sublingual nifedipine controversy in drug delivery. *Dim Crit Care Nurs* 1991; 6: 314-320.

Weaver WF. Administration of nifedipine. *Cathet Cardiovasc Diagn* 1989 16: 80.

Simpson R et al.: The effects of epidural versus parenteral opioid analgesia on postoperative pain and pulmonary function in adults who have undergone thoracic and abdominal surgery: A critique of research. *Heart Lung* 1992;21: 125-138.

continued abruptly unless there is a life-threatening emergency and other antihypertensive drugs can be substituted. Abrupt discontinuation may cause **rebound hypertension**—acute increases of blood pressure to levels that may exceed predrug levels—and may also be accompanied by severe tachycardia. Overall, there is a risk of stroke, arrhythmias, angina, or myocardial infarction.

Calcium Channel Blockers

Calcium channel blockers are also called calcium antagonists. The prototype is verapamil (ISOPTIN, CALAN). It and related agents are covered in more detail in Chapter 34, which deals with their use as antianginal drugs. The calcium channel blockers inhibit the influx of calcium ion muscle cells. In the blood vessels, this reduces vasoconstriction in response to a variety of stimuli, including sympathetic stimulation. Total peripheral resistance and blood pressure fall. Decreased cardiac contractility also tends to reduce blood pressure.

Calcium channel blockers are now viewed favorably as starting drugs in antihypertensive therapy. They not only are effective but also lack the ability to elevate serum lipids or interfere much with autonomic reflexes—problems associated with diuretics or β blockers. Blacks seem to respond particularly well to calcium channel blockers, especially in comparison with their relatively poor response to β blockers.

The individual calcium channel blockers (see below) differ in terms of how intensely and selectively they affect the heart and the blood vessels. This, in turn, affects their clinical uses somewhat. About half of the approved calcium antagonists are used for hypertension. They are given orally. The drugs are sustained-release dosage forms of diltiazem (CARDIZEM SR) and nifedipine (PROCARDIA XL); and immediate-acting dosage forms of felodipine (PLENDIL), isradipine (DYNACIRC), and nicardipine (CARDENE). Both immediate- and sustained-acting verapamil formulations are indicated for treating high blood pressure. Dosages are given in Table 34–C.

There are also drug- and dose-dependent differences in the incidence and severity of side effects. The most common side effect for all is *constipation*. Verapamil, in particular, can cause excessive cardiac depression, especially if used with other drugs that depress contractility (eg, β blockers) or electrical activity (β blockers, quinidine, digitalis); or if given to patients with preexisting heart failure, bradycardia, or heart block.

Angiotensin Converting Enzyme (ACE) Inhibitors

Captopril (CAPOTEN) is the prototype and oldest approved member of a group of drugs called angiotensin converting enzyme (ACE) inhibitors. When captopril was first approved, it was used mainly for severe hypertension that did not respond to most other medications. However, the ACE inhibitors now are widely used for initial therapy of hypertension *in persons with normal renal function*.

There are about half a dozen ACE inhibitors in addition to the prototype, and more are likely to be approved soon. Some of these agents, including the prototype, are also indicated for managing CHF.

PROTOTYPE

Captopril

Absorption, Distribution, Metabolism, and Excretion

Captopril and all other ACE inhibitors are available in oral dosage forms. About 75% of the administered captopril dose is absorbed; significantly less is absorbed when the drug is taken with food. About half the absorbed dose is metabolically inactivated by the liver; the rest is excreted unchanged by the kidneys. The need to reduce dosage is due more often to renal dysfunction than to hepatic impairment.

NURSING IMPLICATIONS

Administer captopril 1 hour before meals to maximize the drug's absorption. Timing of administration with respect to meals seems to be less a problem with related ACE inhibitors (eg, enalapril, lisinopril). Nevertheless, stress to patients the need to take these drugs at a consistent time each day.

Pharmacologic Effects

Angiotensin converting enzyme plays a critical role in the renin-angiotensin-aldosterone system's involvement in blood pressure control. The ACE inhibitors interrupt parts of this system, causing three important effects that help lower blood pressure. They

- inhibit formation of angiotensin II, a vasoconstrictor; this reduces vasoconstriction mediated by angiotensin II.
- reduce aldosterone secretion. This increases renal sodium and water excretion, which in turn lowers blood volume and blood pressure. Another outcome is reduced potassium excretion. (Potassium excretion is normally another renal effect of aldosterone.)
- reduce metabolic inactivation of bradykinin, a local hormone with vasodilator activity. This occurs because bradykininase, the enzyme that breaks down bradykinin, is inhibited by drugs such as captopril. (Bradykininase and ACE are probably the same enzymes, despite their different names.)

These same effects are desirable for patients with CHF because the renin-angiotensin-aldosterone system contributes to the pathophysiology of that common cardiovascular disease also (see Fig. 31–1, p 579). They account for the use of ACE inhibitors as treatments for chronic heart failure. As noted in Chapter 31, ACE inhibitors also seem to cause some other effects, the mechanisms of which are not fully known, that appear to decrease mortality in some heart failure patients.

Clinical Indications and Administration

Hypertension

ACE inhibitors can be used as initial treatments of essential hypertension. Ideally, they are chosen as starting drugs only if the patient has normal renal function. The ACE inhibitors can be used alone or with a potassium-wasting diuretic, usually a thiazide or thiazide-like agent. These diuretics provide additive antihypertensive effects and help counteract the potassium retention that occurs when ACE inhibitors lower aldosterone levels. Usual starting dosages are listed in Table 33–C1. Half the typical starting dose is used if the patient is already being treated with a diuretic. This is done to reduce the risk of hypotension.

If possible, other antihypertensive drugs that the patient may be taking already, including diuretics, are discontinued gradually a week or so before ACE inhibitor therapy is started. These drugs are discontinued to help avoid hypotension from drug interactions. However, discontinuing other medications may not be safe and feasible for some patients, particularly those who have severe or rapidly progressing hypertension. Such patients often cannot tolerate even brief antihypertensive drug withdrawal and are hospitalized when ACE inhibitor therapy is started.

There is some evidence that parenteral captopril is useful for the management of hypertensive emergencies. However, other drugs that are discussed later are almost always used instead.

Heart Failure

The values and uses of ACE inhibitors for patients with chronic CHF are discussed in Chapter 31. Currently, only captopril and enalapril are approved for this use. See Table 31–C for dosages of these drugs for heart failure.

Side Effects, Adverse Reactions, and Contraindications

The types and severity of side effects of ACE inhibitors (Table 33–S1) vary among the individual drugs, but some generalizations can be made about the drug class. These unwanted responses can also occur when the ACE inhibitor is used for managing heart failure.

Renal side effects and adverse responses include hyperkalemia, and renal tubular damage. Increased serum potassium levels seem to be dose related. They can be managed by adjunctive use of potassium-wasting diuretics (eg, thiazides or, for patients with poor renal function, a high-ceiling agent such as furosemide).

Usually the first indication of drug-induced renal tubule damage is proteinuria. Blood urea nitrogen (BUN) and serum creatinine levels may also rise. These signs and symptoms do not necessarily require immediate discontinuation of the drug, and they may not be dose related. However, they do require increased monitoring; if they become worse, the ACE inhibitor may need to be discontinued. The incidence appears to be greater in patients who have renal dysfunction at the time ACE inhibitor therapy is started. As a general rule, if the patient has evidence of poor renal function when ACE inhibitor therapy is to be started, other classes of antihypertensive drugs are tried first.

Another important side effect is excessive hypotension, which can be one cause of dizziness or headache. Hypotension is more common and more intense in patients who are being treated with other antihypertensive drugs; who are sodium-depleted (eg, because of diuretic therapy or other causes, such as inadequate dietary sodium intake); or who receive ACE inhibitor doses that may be too high. Hypotension tends to occur within an hour or two after ACE inhibitor administration, and especially after the first one or two doses are given. However, hypotension may occur later after a dose or continue as treatment continues.

Gastrointestinal (GI) side effects include nausea and vomiting, diarrhea or constipation, and gut pain. **Dysguesia,** an altered sense of taste, can occur (especially with captopril). This may contribute to anorexia in some patients.

Other side effects to anticipate include skin rashes and cough. Rashes tend to be mild, but may be accompanied by pruritus, fever, and joint pain. They usually occur during the first month of therapy and tend to resolve when the ACE inhibitor dose is reduced. Antihistamine treatment may be indicated. The cough is usually nonproductive. It affects as many as one-third of all patients taking ACE inhibitors, and can be so disturbing that the patient will wish to discontinue the drug. More serious potential adverse responses include blood dyscrasias and angioedema.

NURSING IMPLICATIONS

Instruct patients to report signs of blood dyscrasias (eg, sore throat, fever, abnormal bruising), renal damage (eg, weight gain; edema; and urine protein, which can be detected easily at home with a chemical test strip), excessive hypotension (eg, dizziness), and rashes. Some of the more important side effects of ACE inhibitors, such as altered blood counts and hyperkalemia, cannot be detected easily by the patient; therefore, stress the need for frequent follow-up examinations for blood and urine testing.

There is no firm guideline about what to do for rashes, other than to have the physician evaluate them promptly. They may disappear after the drug dose is reduced, be managed by giving antihistamines and maintaining or reducing the ACE inhibitor dose, or they may become worse.

◆ Use During Pregnancy and Lactation

No ACE inhibitor should be given to pregnant women, either for hypertension or heart failure, owing to the risk of serious or fatal renal problems in the newborn (see the section on antihypertensive therapy during pregnancy, p 659). Breast-feeding is not encouraged during ACE inhibitor therapy.

◆ Use in Children

There is little information about the safety and effectiveness of using captopril or other ACE inhibitors in children. If these drugs are used, dosages are adjusted for the child's body weight and other considerations, such as kidney or renal function.

◆ Use in the Elderly

Impaired renal or hepatic function, the potential for excessive hypotension, or sudden drops in blood pressure are the major concerns with the use of captopril or other ACE inhibitors in the elderly. Smaller or less frequent doses are generally indicated, especially if the patient is already taking a diuretic. As noted earlier, diuretics are often preferred starting antihypertensive drugs for the elderly, and when they are used with ACE inhibitors, the risk of excessive hypotension increases.

Interactions with Other Drugs

If therapy is not carried out properly, the desired antihypertensive effects of using diuretics with ACE inhibitors can be overshadowed by an increased risk of hypotension. Vasodilators, β blockers, or other adrenergic inhibitors are used with extreme care, if at all, for the same reason. Potassium-sparing diuretics, potassium supplements, and other drugs that increase serum potassium increase the risk of hyperkalemia and are used with great caution. Indomethacin, one of the most powerful nonsteroidal antiinflammatory (NSAI) drugs, can antagonize the therapeutic effects of captopril. This is thought to occur because indomethacin inhibits synthesis of prostaglandins, which seem to play a role in captopril's antihypertensive actions. This interaction may apply to many other NSAI drugs, including aspirin and ibuprofen, and to the related ACE inhibitors.

Food is also an important interactant, especially with captopril. Taking this ACE inhibitor with a meal can reduce drug absorption by about one-third. Thus, it is important to administer oral captopril 1 hour before meals and time the administration consistently.

Related Drugs

The related ACE inhibitors are benazepril (LOTENSIN), enalapril (VASOTEC), fosinopril (MONOPRIL), lisinopril (PRINIVIL, ZESTRIL), quinapril (ACCUPRIL), and ramipril (ALTACE). Enalapril is partly metabolized; lisinopril is excreted unchanged; benazepril, fosinopril, and ramipril are *prodrugs* that produce an active metabolite.

In general, these drugs differ in the degree to which dosages must be reduced for persons with liver or kidney dysfunction. Each of these drugs has a longer duration of action than captopril and are therefore administered just once a day. This facilitates compliance, but it is a potential disadvantage if adverse responses related to the diuretic (eg, hypotension) occur. A fixed-dose enalapril-hydrochlorothiazide product (VASERETIC) is available. Enalaprilat (VASOTEC IV injection) is available for parenteral therapy.

Most adverse responses and drug interactions noted for captopril apply to the alternatives. The risk of proteinuria and renal damage is presumably less than that associated with the prototype, but patients must nevertheless be monitored for these problems. Of all the ACE inhibitors, enalapril seems to present the greatest risk of angioedema, which usually develops within weeks after therapy is started. It is a life-threatening emergency.

Step II Drugs: Other Agents That Alter the Sympathetic Nervous System

The agents used to start therapy (discussed above) can be tried, at higher doses, if initial treatment does not work adequately. Alternatively, the patient may be started on one of the drugs discussed next. One of these Step II drugs can be added to or substituted for the Step I agent. Often, a diuretic, if it was not used in Step I, becomes a part of the overall treatment plan in Step II and later steps.

All the drugs discussed in this section inhibit actions of the sympathetic nervous system (ie, cause a **sympatholytic** effect) in one way or another, but none of the mechanisms involves β blockade. There is no overall prototype sympathetic inhibitor, but a most representative drug in each subclass can be identified:

1. Centrally acting α-adrenergic agonists: clonidine. Related drugs are methyldopa, guanabenz, and guanfacine.
2. Peripherally acting, selective α_1-adrenergic blockers: prazosin. Similar agents are doxazosin and terazosin.
3. Peripherally acting catecholamine depleters: reserpine. A related drug is guanadrel.

Unwanted Responses Common to All the Sympathetic Inhibitors

Drugs in all three subclasses share several other properties, including some side effects (Table 33–S1) and drug interactions. The prevalence and intensity of these responses vary according to the drug, the dose, and the individual patient.

- Any of these drugs may cause resting orthostatic hypotension. Centrally acting adrenergic agonists (eg, clonidine) are least likely to do so; the selective α blockers (eg, prazosin) have a moderate ability to do so. Catecholamine depleters (eg, reserpine), however, cause significant orthostatic hypotension. It is important to instruct the patient about proper measures (eg, standing slowly, consuming adequate but permissible amounts of salt) that help minimize the severity and risks of a sudden or excessive blood pressure fall.
- Adjunctive use of other antihypertensive drugs can enhance the antihypertensive effects of a sympatholytic and in some cases is necessary. However, such combinations also increase the risk of excessive drops in blood pressure.
- All the sympathetic inhibitors can, to varying degrees, reduce renal blood flow. This can activate the renin-angiotensin system, increasing sodium and water retention and favoring weight gain. These are compensatory responses to overcome the very effect for which the antihypertensive drug is given—a reduction of blood pressure. Unless other measures are taken or diuretics are prescribed adjunctively, such responses can counteract desired antihypertensive actions. Thus, close monitoring of blood pressure, body weight, and other clinical signs is important.
- Most sympathetic inhibitors cause some degree of sedation and psychic disturbances (eg, altered sleep patterns, nightmares). Any other drug with CNS-depressant activity (alcohol, barbiturates, benzodiazepines, narcotics, and others), can cause excessive CNS depression if they are administered also. Sedation usually becomes less of a problem with continued use. Nevertheless, it is best to administer these drugs at bedtime and to discourage alcohol consumption, especially in excess.
- The sympatholytic antihypertensive drugs may impair sexual performance. In general, these agents cause greater sexual dysfunction, especially ejaculatory dysfunction, than do other antihypertensive medications. Living with this side effect may be a necessary trade-off if the patient is to control a dangerous medical condition.

The drug class (and drug) chosen depends mainly on patient-related characteristics, including relative or absolute contraindications to a particular agent. Dosing schedules, which may affect compliance, are also important. The drug selected may have to be changed (either to another drug in the same class or, preferably, to one in a different class) because of side effects or interactions.

NURSING IMPLICATIONS

Once Step II is reached, the nurse and patient must anticipate the need to try several drugs to identify one or more that will control blood pressure with the fewest side effects. To simplify patient education, first teach the side effects shared by most sympathetic inhibitors (noted earlier). Then focus on the important side effects and precautions that are unique to the selected agent, particularly those requiring immediate notification of the physician. Suggest nondrug measures that can deal with common side effects: sucking hard candies to alleviate dry mouth; taking initial doses at bedtime to alleviate daytime sedation; avoiding motor vehicle operation or other tasks made dangerous by sedation or drowsiness; sitting up and standing slowly and avoiding strenuous exercise, alcohol consumption, dehydration, and hot baths or showers to minimize hypotension. These interventions apply to therapy with virtually any antihypertensive drug.

Reaching Step II also often means that the patient must be responsible for taking several medications. Although all-in-one fixed-dose antihypertensive drug combinations are available, which can simplify self-medication, some patients will need to take two or three separate drugs. If patients have other medical problems that require drug treatment, their medication list may be long. Some drugs interact and should not be taken simultaneously; others may or may not be taken with meals. Make a special effort to discuss all aspects of therapy, and devise a suitable treatment plan that helps the patient take each drug properly.

Centrally Acting Alpha-Adrenergic Agonists

Clonidine, methyldopa, guanabenz, and guanfacine work gradually in the central nervous system (CNS) to lower pressure. They do not significantly interfere with the cardiovascular reflexes (eg, those involving the baroreceptors) that are needed for fine control of the circulatory system, such as those which prevent a sudden blood pressure fall when the patient stands quickly. The oldest and most representative group member is clonidine.

PROTOTYPE

Clonidine

Absorption, Distribution, Metabolism, and Excretion

Clonidine (CATAPRES), given orally, is absorbed well from the GI tract. Transdermal delivery systems ("patches"; CATAPRES-TTS), which release a constant daily dose over a week, are also available. Clonidine crosses the blood–brain barrier easily, reaching its major site of action. About half the absorbed dose is metabolized by the liver. The kidneys excrete the metabolites, plus the unmetabolized drug. Patients with renal or hepatic dysfunction usually require reduced doses.

Pharmacologic Effects

Clonidine and the related centrally acting antihypertensives can lower blood pressure or elevate it. Both effects occur because these drugs stimulate α_2-adrenergic receptors. First, these drugs stimulate α_2 receptors in the cardiovascular control centers of the brain. This decreases sympathetic outflow to the periphery, causing vasodilation and slight decreases of heart rate, cardiac contractility, and renin release—all of which help lower blood pressure. Decreased sympathetic outflow also reduces the severity of reflex tachycardia that might otherwise occur when blood pressure falls.

Clonidine can also stimulate α_2-adrenergic receptors on arterioles, thereby increasing blood pressure. This effect, however, occurs mainly when the blood level of the drug is very high, either from excessive oral dosages or from injecting it. (The drug is rarely administered by injection.) With usual doses, given orally or transdermally, the central pressure-lowering effect predominates. However, other drugs can interact to provoke the hypertensive effects of clonidine (see Drug Interactions, below).

Clinical Indications and Administration

Clonidine is used mainly for moderate hypertension as a Step II agent. The usual initial oral dose is 0.1 mg twice a day (Table 33–C1). When a thiazide diuretic is part of the medication plan, oral clonidine can be given as a separate agent or as a fixed-dose combination (COMBIPRES) with the long-acting thiazide-like diuretic chlorthalidone. (The dose is based on the amount of clonidine in the product.) Transdermal clonidine is indicated only for maintenance therapy; treatment starts with the oral dosage form.

Side Effects, Adverse Reactions, and Contraindications

In addition to the side effects common to all the sympathetic inhibitor antihypertensive drugs (noted above), clonidine frequently causes drowsiness and dry mouth; these occur in about 50% of patients taking this drug.

These side effects may be severe enough to cause a few patients to discontinue therapy, but they usually can be managed by giving the drug at bedtime and by nondrug measures. Other important but less frequent side effects include constipation, headache, and impaired ejaculation. Most side effects diminish in intensity with time or with reduced doses.

Clonidine's most dangerous side effect occurs when the drug is suddenly discontinued (or the dose is lowered dramatically) after long-term therapy. Clonidine was the first antihypertensive drug linked to a rebound hypertension phenomenon: an episode of intense and potentially dangerous hypertension that occurs shortly after administration is stopped quickly (see Nursing Implications for β blockers, p 237). With clonidine, this is thought to occur because the α receptors in blood vessels become supersensitive when they are chronically deprived of normal sympathetic stimuli. When the clonidine is no longer present, epinephrine and norepinephrine cause vasoconstriction that is much more intense than usual. Should such an episode occur, it is managed either by restarting clonidine therapy or by administering another antihypertensive drug.

NURSING IMPLICATIONS

Oral clonidine is best administered in the evening to minimize daytime sedation. If the dose must be increased, give the first higher dose in the evening. If clonidine must be discontinued, reduce the dose gradually over a period of about four days, and monitor the patient carefully. Assess for nervousness, agitation, and headache, followed by a rapid rise of blood pressure, which may indicate discontinuation of treatment without supervision or approval. Stress the dangers of abrupt withdrawal. Assess for signs of heart failure, including weight gain and edema, during therapy.

◆ Use During Pregnancy and Lactation

Based on current information, clonidine should not be administered to pregnant women. Discourage breast-feeding while the drug is used.

◆ Use in Children

Clonidine is not indicated for use in children.

◆ Use in the Elderly

Clonidine's adverse effects are, in general, more disturbing for the elderly than for younger adults. The drug is best used when alternative Step I or Step II agents have proved inadequate. Anticipate the need for reduced doses to compensate for decreased renal or hepatic function, and for careful assessment and precautions for problems owing to sedation.

Interactions with Other Drugs

Two specific interactions are very important for clonidine and the related centrally acting sympathetic inhibitors (Table 33–1). *Beta-adrenergic blockers* (eg, propranolol) can counteract the pressure-lowering effects of these medications; severe hypertension may result if the two types of drugs are given to the same patient. In the absence of a β blocker, clonidine's vasoconstrictor effects (caused by α-receptor stimulation) are slight; moreover, circulating epinephrine stimulates β-adrenergic receptors, thereby dilating some blood vessels and lowering pressure. However, in the presence of β blockade, clonidine's peripheral vasoconstrictor (α-stimulating) effects are unopposed. This tends to reduce the drug's antihypertensive effects. Moreover, if the sympathetic nervous system is activated (as by stress or exercise), the vasoconstrictor effects of epinephrine and norepinephrine will become more intense: An actual hypertensive episode can occur.

Tricyclic antidepressants (eg, imipramine) are likely to counteract clonidine's antihypertensive effects, possibly because the tricyclics block the central α receptors that clonidine must stimulate in order to lower blood pressure.

NURSING IMPLICATIONS

If possible, avoid these interactions; if this is not possible, check blood pressure more often than usual. Blood pressure increases owing to these interactions usually require discontinuing one or both of the interactants, or at least reducing the dose. If the clonidine dose is to be reduced or discontinued altogether, be sure that this is done as slowly but as safely as possible to avoid further rebound pressure increases. Monitor accordingly, and anticipate the need to control blood pressure with other medications that do not interact.

Overdose and Toxicity

Clonidine overdoses can cause CNS depression and bradycardia. Blood pressure changes are expected, but they vary with the patient and the amount of drug taken.

Most patients experience *hypotension,* which is an extension of clonidine's major and expected effect. However, because of the drug's ability to cause vasoconstriction via stimulating α-adrenergic receptors in the periphery, very severe overdoses can cause *hypertension.*

The hypotensive patient may require intravenous fluids, dopamine (to raise blood pressure and heart rate carefully), or both. Alpha-adrenergic blockers (eg, phentolamine), diuretics, or nitroprusside have been used to manage hypertension. Atropine can be used for severe bradycardia.

Seizures, cardiac arrhythmias, and *respiratory depression* can occur. Parenteral anticonvulsants (eg, diazepam) or antiarrhythmics (eg, lidocaine) are used as needed. Respiratory depression is managed with oxygen, artificial airways, and ventilatory support, as needed. Some physicians are tempted to give analeptic (CNS-stimulating) drugs to overcome CNS or respiratory depression. However, the dosages needed are more likely to cause seizures than the desired effects.

NURSING IMPLICATIONS

Given the variable changes of blood pressure and other vital signs, proper management of a clonidine overdose depends on thorough and frequent assessment and anticipation of what might occur next. Question medication orders calling for administration of CNS stimulants to patients experiencing a clonidine overdose. Be aware that although respiration or overall CNS function appears depressed (eg, if the patient is comatose), seizures can occur. Be prepared.

Related Drugs

Methyldopa, guanabenz, and guanfacine are the related drugs. Methyldopa has been in use longer than the others, and more is known about its actions and uses.

Methyldopa

Methyldopa (ALDOMET) is available in oral dosage forms, including fixed-dose combination products containing chlorothiazide or hydrochlorothiazide (ALDOCLOR, ALDORIL, respectively). These are used for essential hypertension. A parenteral dosage form, methyldopate hydrochloride (ALDOMET Ester HCl), is used mainly for treating hypertensive emergencies that are not life-threatening (see p 654). Methyldopa crosses the placental barrier and enters the fetal circulation. However, it is one of the few antihypertensive agents recommended for use during pregnancy on an acute or long-term basis.

Methyldopa, like clonidine, works mainly as a central α-adrenergic agonist. Methyldopa is also metabolized, inside adrenergic nerves, to a substance called methylnorepinephrine. This substance is a much weaker vasoconstrictor than norepinephrine itself and has been referred to as a "false neurotransmitter."

Methyldopa's side effects profile is much like clonidine's. However, methyldopa does have some unique side effects. About 20% of patients treated long term with this drug develop antibodies to the drug, giving a positive Coombs test and indicating the potential for developing hemolytic anemia. Fewer than 1% of Coombs-positive patients taking methyldopa actually develop hemolysis, but this condition is potentially fatal. Therefore, a predrug blood count and periodic tests after therapy is started are essential. A positive Coombs test does not necessarily require stopping methyldopa, but evidence of hemolysis does—and at once. Other antihypertensive drugs must be substituted in its place. Thrombocytopenia, leukopenia, or other blood dyscrasias may also occur.

Methyldopa seems to be the only major antihypertensive drug that causes hepatotoxicity and hepatitis. Although these side effects are uncommon, periodic liver function studies are indicated, and the drug is generally contraindicated in patients with poor hepatic function. Methylnorepinephrine, the methyldopa metabolite, can cause falsely elevated urinary catecholamine levels, and a false-positive diagnosis of pheochromocytoma.

Patients taking methyldopa seem to be overly sensitive to the actions of traditional sympathomimetic drugs. The interactants include prescription agents such as epinephrine and norepinephrine; and sympathomimetics found mainly in over-the-counter (OTC) cold remedies, such as phenylpropanolamine. These drugs do not merely counteract the antihypertensive effects of methyldopa; they may cause further pressure increases. The best approach is to avoid this interaction, if possible; otherwise, reduced doses of the sympathomimetic are indicated. If severe hypertension occurs, prompt antihypertensive drug intervention (eg, with nitroprusside or an α-blocker) may be needed.

Signs, symptoms, and treatment of methyldopa overdoses are generally similar to those of clonidine. Be aware that if sympathomimetics must be used to raise an excessively low blood pressure, lower than usual dosages are needed to avoid causing hypertension.

NURSING IMPLICATIONS

Discourage all hypertensive patients from taking excessive doses of OTC products that contain sympathomimetics. For patients being treated with methyldopa, this advice may be even more important. Caution patients with respiratory or ocular conditions that might benefit from OTC sympathomimetics to use these interactants under the guidance of a physician.

Explain the need for baseline and in-treatment blood and liver function tests. Advise patients to report promptly signs of hemolysis, anemia (hematuria, unusual or excessive fatigability), or liver dysfunction (discolored urine, jaundice, upper abdominal pain). Urine of methyldopa-treated patients may darken when left standing and exposed to air; this does not indicate liver dysfunction.

◆ Use During Pregnancy and Lactation

Although methyldopa crosses the placental barrier and enters the fetal circulation, it is one of the few antihypertensive drugs indicated for hypertension that requires drug therapy during pregnancy. Nevertheless, assess newborns' vital signs with extra care for the first two to three postpartum days. Discourage breast-feeding during methyldopa therapy.

◆ Use in Children

Reduced doses of methyldopa have been used to treat hypertension in children.

◆ Use in the Elderly

Precautions for the elderly are the same as those noted for clonidine.

Guanabenz, Guanfacine

Guanabenz (WYTENSIN) and guanfacine (TENEX) are newer central α_2 agonists that also are quite similar to clonidine. An alleged advantage of these drugs is that they appear to cause less rebound hypertension if treatment is stopped too fast. Nevertheless, abrupt discontinuation is not recommended.

Peripherally Acting Selective Alpha$_1$-Adrenergic Blockers

Blocking the peripheral adrenergic receptors on blood vessels offers another approach to lowering blood pressure. The prototype agent is prazosin.

PROTOTYPE

Prazosin

Prazosin (MINIPRESS) is very effective, and causes no unwanted effects on serum lipids. However, because of a common and disturbing side effect—orthostatic hypotension—prazosin is used as a starting drug much less frequently than the drugs mentioned so far.

Absorption, Distribution, Metabolism, and Excretion

Prazosin is absorbed well from the GI tract. It is extensively bound to plasma proteins. Although the drug is almost completely metabolized in the liver, either impaired hepatic or renal function generally calls for reduced doses.

Pharmacologic Effects

Prazosin lowers blood pressure by selectively blocking α_1-adrenergic (postsynaptic) receptors in the peripheral vasculature, leading to vasodilation. Because these receptors are blocked, blood vessels cannot constrict well when the patient stands suddenly. This causes orthostatic hypotension, a key side effect. Reflex tachycardia is usually slight because norepinephrine, released by sympathetic cardiac nerves, is still able to act on the unblocked presynaptic α_2 receptors, thereby turning off further transmitter release and blunting cardiac stimulation (see p 198 for further explanation).

Clinical Indications and Administration

Prazosin is mainly used when other antihypertensive drugs are not suited to the patient or have failed to work well. Prazosin desirably lowers total cholesterol and triglyceride levels and increases HDL levels. This drug may therefore be particularly suited for patients who also have hyperlipidemias. Prazosin is also useful for hypertension caused by a pheochromocytoma. Beta-adrenergic blockers are used adjunctively for these patients.

Regardless of the indication, prazosin therapy should *always* be started with the lowest available dose, 1 mg (see Table 33–C1). A combination product, MINI-

ZIDE, contains prazosin and polythiazide (a hydrochlorothiazide-like diuretic). The diuretic helps lower blood pressure and counteracts renal sodium and water retention that can occur when blood pressure falls.

Side Effects, Adverse Reactions, and Contraindications

The most notable side effect of prazosin is called the "first-dose faint" effect—pronounced hypotension, especially orthostatic hypotension, that occurs suddenly within about 2 hours after the first dose. It is often severe enough to cause syncope and a fall if the patient happens to be standing at the time. (For this reason, treatment is started with the smallest dose, and the patient is kept under observation for several hours.) Postdose hypotension becomes more gradual with the first few doses. However, it may recur after the first increased dose during dosage elevations; when therapy is resumed after a few missed doses; or when another antihypertensive drug is added.

Sodium depletion, which can be caused by diet, exercise, or diuretic drug therapy, increases the incidence and severity of resting and orthostatic hypotension. Concomitant therapy with β-adrenergic blockers does the same.

With continued prazosin treatment, some lightheadedness, headache, generalized fatigue, and nasal stuffiness remain as more common side effects. Reflex tachycardia or palpitations may persist, but they are seldom severe with therapeutic doses. Peripheral edema may develop; diuretics usually alleviate this.

NURSING IMPLICATIONS

Ideally, the first prazosin dose should be administered under medical supervision; check vital signs frequently until it is safe to leave the patient. Record baseline blood pressures (both arms; sitting and standing) immediately before giving the first dose, and, when possible, every 15 to 30 minutes for the first 2 hours afterward. Instruct all patients to take the first few prazosin doses lying on a bed, to remain there for a couple of hours, and to stand gradually and with support in case of dizziness. The same precautions should be taken at other times when the first-dose effect is likely to occur, as identified earlier. Caution patients about the expected duration of hypotension and sedation as therapy continues, and teach appropriate ways to deal with or avoid their consequences.

◆ Use During Pregnancy and Lactation

The safety of prazosin during pregnancy has not been established. The drug may be used when preferred alternative drug or nondrug therapies are not satisfactory, and the possible benefits of prazosin outweigh potential risks. Prazosin is excreted in maternal milk, so breast-feeding must be avoided.

◆ Use in Children

The safety and effectiveness of prazosin in children have not been established.

◆ Use in the Elderly

The major concern associated with prazosin therapy in elderly persons is acute or severe hypotension, which can exacerbate peripheral vascular disease or organ ischemia, especially if the heart or brain is involved.

Interactions with Other Drugs

All antihypertensive drugs can increase the hypotensive effects of prazosin. However, β blockers (see above) seem to cause the greatest risk of excessive hypotension. Signs and symptoms of the interaction are likely to be most intense when prazosin therapy is started in a patient who is already taking a β blocker.

Overdose and Toxicity

Prazosin overdoses cause severe hypotension, tachycardia, and potential cerebral or cardiac ischemia or generalized cardiovascular collapse. Parenteral fluids and vasoconstrictors ("pure" α-agonists, eg, phenylephrine) may be needed to restore blood pressure. These interventions simultaneously slow the heart rate via the baroreceptor reflex. Higher doses of α-agonists may be needed to overcome prazosin's α-blockade and restore blood pressure. Avoid epinephrine or norepinephrine; their β agonist actions can cause severe cardiac stimulation before they elevate blood pressure sufficiently.

Related Drugs

Terazosin and Doxazosin

Terazosin (HYTRIN) and doxazosin (CARDURA) are similar to prazosin in many ways. However, they have a longer duration of action, which allows once-daily administration (preferably at bedtime). Doxazosin is claimed to cause less first-dose hypotension than the other two, so physicians may be more willing to prescribe it. Nevertheless, all precautions noted for prazosin apply.

Peripherally Acting Catecholamine Depleters

Depletion of norepinephrine in peripheral sympathetic nerves offers a third approach to lowering blood pressure through actions on the sympathetic nervous system. Reserpine is the most representative catecholamine depleter.

PROTOTYPE

Reserpine

Reserpine (SERPASIL, others) is a rauwolfia alkaloid, derived from the plant *Rauwolfia serpentina*.

Absorption, Distribution, Metabolism, and Excretion

Reserpine is absorbed well from the GI tract and is extensively metabolized by the liver. Its plasma half-life is much shorter than its antihypertensive action, which suggests that small but effective amounts of drug remain for prolonged periods at important sites of action.

Pharmacologic Effects

Reserpine, like the drugs just discussed, is a sympatholytic agent; however, its mechanism of action is different. Reserpine acts in sympathetic nerve endings, where it prevents norepinephrine uptake into neurotransmitter storage granules. This exposes the norepinephrine to the enzyme monoamine oxidase (MAO). The enzyme destroys and partially depletes the norepinephrine within the nerve. The eventual outcome is decreased stimulation of all structures innervated by the sympathetic nervous system, including arterioles. The antihypertensive effect develops gradually: it may take 4 to 6 weeks of daily use to lower blood pressure desirably.

Other cardiovascular effects owing to peripheral catecholamine depletion include decreased heart rate and contractility. There is little or no reflex tachycardia, even if blood pressure falls significantly. Cardiac output falls slightly in persons with normal cardiac function. The effect is greater, and potentially dangerous, in patients with heart failure. Renin release falls because of decreased sympathetic stimulation, but reduced renal perfusion counteracts this effect and triggers sodium and water retention.

Reserpine also depletes catecholamines in the brain. This contributes to certain side effects and adverse responses (discussed below).

Clinical Indications and Administration

Oral reserpine is used mainly when alternative antihypertensive drugs are unsuitable or ineffective. Reserpine use usually requires adjunctive diuretics to counteract sodium and water retention. Reserpine is also used as an adjunct to reduce reflex tachycardia caused by direct vasodilator antihypertensives (see the discussion of hydralazine, p 652). The availability of many fixed-dose products (Table 33–5) containing reserpine or a reserpine-like drug with thiazide diuretics, vasodilators, or both attests to the drug's formerly widespread adjunctive use.

Side Effects, Adverse Reactions, and Contraindications

Reserpine causes many side effects (Table 33–S1) that are common and sometimes quite severe. They affect many key body systems, including the CNS, and some preexisting diseases can contraindicate reserpine use altogether because side effects can make them worse. Overall, these side effects are a major reason why reserpine is no longer a preferred agent for hypertension.

Most of the side effects of reserpine occur because the drug depletes catecholamines (norepinephrine, epinephrine, and dopamine). Many body systems are controlled by opposing effects of the parasympathetic nervous system and its neurotransmitter, acetylcholine. Thus, reserpine's ability to "turn off" sympathetic activity lets the opposing effects predominate, causing unusually excessive influences on a body system. The overall clinical picture is sometimes referred to as *parasympathetic predominance*.

Effects on Peripheral Body Systems

- *Cardiovascular side effects.* Postural hypotension is the most common cardiovascular side effect, and it is often severe. Reserpine decreases heart rate and contractility, leading to decreased cardiac output. The overall effect can be dangerous for patients with CHF. Reduced blood pressure and renal blood flow trigger sodium and water retention. These add to the problems of patients with CHF and further increase the need for adjunctive use of diuretics. No rebound hypertension or tachycardia results when reserpine therapy is stopped abruptly.

- *Ocular problems.* These include excessive lacrimation and *miosis,* a condition in which the pupils are constricted and do not open adequately in dim light.
- *Respiratory tract alterations.* Increased mucus secretions and nasal or respiratory tract congestion may occur.
- *GI side effects.* These include salivation, diarrhea and increases in gastric acid secretion. The drug is contraindicated for persons with peptic ulcer disease, and long-term therapy can actually cause ulcers. Colitis, gallbladder disease, or other disorders aggravated by increased gut motility or acid secretion also contraindicate reserpine use.
- *Impaired ejaculation and gynecomastia in males or females.* Both are reversible when reserpine is stopped or the dose is reduced. There may be a link between reserpine use and breast cancer in women. This has not been proved, however, and reserpine is not contraindicated for women. Nevertheless, as a precaution it is not given to women with a personal or family history of breast carcinoma or recurrent mastitis.

Effects on the Central Nervous System

Some key activities in parts of the brain also depend on a balance between the effects of catecholamines and the opposing effects of other neurotransmitters, including acetylcholine. Catecholamine depletion caused by reserpine can, therefore, cause chemical imbalances and related side effects.

- *Sedation and drowsiness.* These common side effects probably reflect depletion of norepinephrine, which normally acts as an excitatory transmitter. These side effects are intensified by the use of other CNS depressants, including alcohol. These substances must be avoided if possible.
- *Suicidal depression.* This, the most serious CNS side effect, also appears to be caused by decreased norepinephrine (or dopamine) activity in the brain. The risk is greatest with prolonged administration of reserpine doses over 0.5 mg per day. These dosages are quite high, and they are rarely justified for treating hypertension. Regardless of the dose, reserpine is not to be used for patients with a history of depression or suicidal tendencies. All patients receiving the drug are evaluated periodically for signs of depression, and the drug is discontinued immediately at the first sign of it. Depression may last several months after stopping reserpine therapy, so the patient should be under observation during that time.
- *Parkinsonism.* Involuntary movement of skeletal muscles is regulated by a balance between dopamine and acetylcholine (see Chapter 25 for more information) in the brain's extrapyramidal system. Reserpine depletes dopamine there, upsets the balance, and causes all the signs and symptoms of true Parkinson's disease. Reserpine should not be used for patients with a history of parkinsonism.

NURSING IMPLICATIONS

Specifically ask about a history of mental illness; ask female patients about a history of breast disorders or cancer. Notify the physician if either history is positive. Even in the absence of prior mental illness, always assess predrug emotional status for comparison with in-treatment evaluations to help detect depression.

Assess all patients carefully for signs of significant parasympathetic predominance, which may be simply annoying (nasal congestion) or dangerous (abdominal pain owing to ulcers; edema owing to heart failure).

Assess for muscle tremor, rigidity, or other potential signs of parkinsonism. Notify the physician at once if any potentially dangerous untoward response occurs. The risk of rebound hypertension on abrupt discontinuation is low because of reserpine's long duration of action.

◆ Use During Pregnancy and Lactation

Reserpine enters the fetal circulation and is not used during pregnancy unless absolutely necessary. If it is used, assess newborns for hypotension, bradycardia, and evidence of parasympathetic predominance. Increased respiratory tract secretions and pulmonary congestion may cause impaired gas exchange and hypoxia or cyanosis after birth. Reserpine is excreted in breast milk, so discourage breast-feeding. If the mother chooses to breastfeed, assess the infant for the signs and symptoms noted above and for poor feeding habits that might be caused by sedation.

◆ Use in Children

Reserpine is not recommended for children.

◆ Use in the Elderly

Reserpine is not a preferred antihypertensive drug for the elderly because of its greater risk of causing depression, parkinsonism, and decreased cardiac output, all of which are more prevalent in older persons.

Interactions with Other Drugs

Reserpine, given long enough to lower blood pressure, significantly increases all the key actions of direct-acting sympathomimetics, such as epinephrine and norepinephrine. This occurs because the receptors become supersensitive to the effects of these sympathomimetics after having been deprived of their stimulating effects for so long. If usual dosages of the interactants are given to a reserpine-treated patient—for example, to treat hypotension caused by an overdose or another drug interaction—an excessive and possibly dangerous sympathomimetic response can result.

By contrast, reserpine significantly reduces the actions of mixed- or indirect-acting sympathomimetics (eg, phenylpropanolamine, ephedrine, amphetamines). Normally, the actions of these drugs depend (partly or completely) on their ability to release norepinephrine from adrenergic nerves. However, because reserpine depletes norepinephrine stores in the neurons, the actions of these drugs are diminished significantly or lost altogether.

Overdose and Toxicity

Nearly all the peripheral side effects noted above also occur with reserpine overdoses, but they are more intense. CNS depression also occurs, and coma is possible. Reserpine's adverse effects—and the need for close monitoring—may last several days after an acute overdose.

The first goal is to normalize the cardiovascular system. Sympathomimetic drugs such as norepinephrine or dopamine are the only agents likely to restore heart rate, contractility, and blood pressure. However, lower doses must be given to compensate for receptor supersensitivity and to avoid causing hypertension or excessive cardiac stimulation. Respiratory support and pulmonary suctioning to remove increased secretions are often needed. Signs of parasympathetic predominance in the gut usually are intense, but they are seldom life-threatening. As noted for clonidine overdoses (p 645), CNS stimulants are not administered.

Related Drug

Guanadrel

Guanadrel (HYLOREL) acts faster than reserpine. It also causes an initial norepinephrine release at the start of treatment, which can lead to a potentially important increase of blood pressure and cardiac stimulation. Guanadrel has little or no CNS activity. Overall, its side effects (ie, intense and prolonged orthostatic hypotension), contraindications, and drug–drug interactions are more like those of guanethidine (a powerful and seldom used antihypertensive; see p 654) than for reserpine. Adjunctive diuretic therapy is usually necessary when guanadrel is used.

Step III Drugs: Direct-Acting Vasodilators

When the Step I and Step II drugs fail to reduce blood pressure well, whether tried alone or in combination, the usual next step is to use hydralazine. It is the prototype of a group of direct-acting vasodilators. In practical terms, it is the only drug of its group that is used for long-term antihypertensive therapy.

PROTOTYPE

Hydralazine

Absorption, Distribution, Metabolism, and Excretion

Hydralazine (APRESOLINE) is absorbed well from the GI tract. The drug is metabolized in the liver by a process called *acetylation.* The metabolites are less active and less toxic than the parent drug. The activities of hepatic acetylation enzymes vary greatly among certain ethnic groups because of genetic factors. This difference affects the doses of hydralazine needed to cause therapeutic or adverse effects.

Pharmacologic Effects

Hydralazine directly dilates arterioles without affecting sympathetic nerves or adrenergic receptors on smooth muscle cells. Arteriolar dilation decreases peripheral resistance, lowering blood pressure. This also triggers reflex tachycardia. Overall, cardiac output rises unless blood pressure falls too much.

Clinical Indications and Administration

Hypertension

Hydralazine has some very desirable properties. It is a powerful drug that often can lower blood pressure when other agents cannot. Its ability to dilate renal arterioles makes it particularly useful for patients with poor renal function. Overall, hydralazine is very effective, and it is fairly easy to titrate its dose. The dose can be increased or decreased quickly, and blood pressure will soon follow. Nevertheless, hydralazine is not preferred for earlier stages of hypertension because two other drugs are often required to counteract its side effects. Parenteral hydralazine can be used for hypertensive emergencies.

Heart Failure

Hydralazine is gaining more attention as a valuable treatment for CHF. Its benefits probably arise from its antihypertensive (afterload-reducing) effects, which ease the failing heart's workload. See Chapter 31 for more information.

Side Effects, Adverse Reactions, and Contraindications

Intense reflex tachycardia and palpitations are common side effects. Tachycardia necessitates cautious use of hydralazine in patients with coronary artery disease, aortic aneurysms, mitral valve disease, or a history of stroke. Beta blockers (or, less often, reserpine) are important adjuncts to reduce this unwanted reflex cardiac stimulation. These adjunctive drugs may also prevent the headache that is often caused by hydralazine—a consequence of cerebral vasodilation and increased cardiac output.

Hydralazine's ability to lower blood pressure triggers renal sodium and water retention. Therefore diuretics are often used adjunctively also. Hydralazine seldom causes severe orthostatic hypotension because it does not interfere with cardiovascular reflexes that result in vasoconstriction.

Hydralazine causes two relatively unique adverse effects. An arthritis-like syndrome resembling systemic lupus erythematosus (SLE) occurs in about 10% to 20% of patients taking high daily doses (400 mg or more) but can occur with more typical therapeutic doses. The syndrome is more common in "slow acetylators"—persons who metabolize hydralazine much slower than others. Signs and symptoms of SLE require prompt evaluation, including appropriate blood tests, to determine whether to continue hydralazine therapy. Signs and symptoms disappear when therapy is stopped.

Also, chronic therapy may cause *peripheral neuritis*. It often presents as numbness or paresthesias in the extremities. This is thought to occur because hydralazine interferes with pyridoxine (vitamin B_6) metabolism in nerve tissue. Vitamin B_6 supplements may be indicated for prophylaxis or treatment.

Hydralazine (or other vasodilators) ordinarily should not be given to patients with pheochromocytomas. Reduction of blood pressure causes reflex activation of the sympathetic nervous system. In the pheochromocytoma patient, the massive outpouring of catecholamines can cause severe hypertension, cardiac stimulation, and arrhythmias. Likewise, using hydralazine alone is also dangerous for persons with aortic aneurysms. These special patient populations are considered at the end of the chapter.

NURSING IMPLICATIONS

Hydralazine is seldom given without β blockers, diuretics, or both. Whether it is used alone or with other agents, always assess for signs of heart failure in addition to checking blood pressure and heart rate. Advise patients to report possible indicators of an SLE-like state or peripheral neuritis. Unless there is a specific contraindication, such as concurrent treatment of parkinsonism with levodopa/carbidopa (see Chapter 25), advise patients that nonprescription vitamin supplements containing B_6 may be useful for prophylaxis of neuritis. Patient-related differences in drug acetylation rates are rarely known before therapy is begun. Because metabolic rates affect the likelihood of side effects and the doses at which they appear, monitor all patients closely during hydralazine therapy.

◆ Use During Pregnancy and Lactation

The safety of hydralazine during pregnancy has not been established. Petechial bleeding, hematomas, and thrombocytopenia in newborns have been reported.

◆ Use in Children

Hydralazine has been used in children, but the drug's safety and efficacy have not been established.

◆ Use in the Elderly

The lack of a sedative effect makes hydralazine more desirable than many other antihypertensive drugs for the elderly. However, the greater prevalence of other cardiovascular diseases that might be worsened by the drug's side effects requires more careful assessment during therapy.

Interactions with Other Drugs

Hydralazine can increase the absorption and blood levels of oral propranolol (and perhaps the related β blocker, metoprolol), leading to an excessive hypotensive effect. The interaction is thought to be caused by reduced metabolism of the β blocker.

Overdose and Toxicity

Hydralazine overdoses cause hypotension and, if β blockers are not present, tachycardia. The greater the overdose, the greater the changes. If an excessive dose is taken all at once, blood pressure can fall very quickly. Fluid retention and edema may also occur. These cardiovascular changes can lead to myocardial ischemia or infarction, stroke, or acute renal failure. Intravenous fluids are preferred for restoring blood pressure, but these should be given carefully if there is evidence of fluid retention. If it is necessary to raise blood pressure pharmacologically, a pure α agonist/vasoconstrictor (eg, phenylephrine) is preferred. Sympathomimetics that have cardiac-stimulating (β_1) activity (dopamine, norepinephrine, epinephrine) should be avoided because they can make cardiac problems worse. The overdose picture and its management are more complex if hydralazine was ingested in a combination product that also contains a β blocker, reserpine, and/or a diuretic (Table 33–5).

Related Drug

Minoxidil

Minoxidil (LONITEN) is an orally effective antihypertensive drug that works, much like hydralazine, as a vasodilator. Minoxidil is recommended only for severe, refractory hypertension because of its more serious adverse effects: cardiac lesions that may lead to pericardial effusion and tamponade; and pulmonary damage. As with hydralazine, minoxidil therapy may require adjunctive use of a diuretic and a β blocker. Signs and symptoms of acute minoxidil toxicity are very similar to those of hydralazine toxicity.

A unique side effect of minoxidil is *hirsutism,* excessive growth of body hair. It occurs in about 80% of patients taking this drug orally for high blood pressure. This discovery led to the eventual marketing of topical minoxidil (ROGAINE) for baldness. (It is unlikely that applying this baldness remedy to the skin, even for prolonged periods of time, will cause the potentially serious reactions caused by long-term oral minoxidil therapy. However, ingesting topical minoxidil is likely to cause a serious overdose: just 1 teaspoon of the product contains a full day's maximum antihypertensive dose.)

NURSING IMPLICATIONS

Advise patients to expect cosmetically unpleasant hair growth and not to stop taking the drug because of it. Unfortunately, it is often the price to be paid for controlling refractory, severe hypertension. Frequent examinations to assess cardiac and pulmonary status are essential for detecting minoxidil toxicity. Any abnormality requires immediate notification of the physician, reevaluation of the treatment plan, immediate cessation of minoxidil administration, and administration of alternative drugs.

Other Oral Antihypertensive Agents

Three other drugs or drug groups were formerly reserved for treating later stages of severe or refractory hypertension: ACE inhibitors, MAO inhibitors, and guanethidine. As noted earlier, ACE inhibitors are now widely accepted as starting drugs, probably because initial fears over the seriousness of the side effects have been found to be overestimated. The same cannot be said for the other drugs.

MAO Inhibitors

Only one MAO inhibitor, pargyline (EUTONYL), had been approved in recent years for hypertension. (Others are used for treating refractory depression; Chapter 24). The MAO inhibitors are very effective for treating hypertension (and depression), but they gained a reputation for being among the most dangerous of all drugs. The danger arises from interactions with some very common foods and drugs that contain mixed- or indirect-acting sympathomimetic (mono)amines—for example, foods containing tyramine, and such drugs as phenylpropanolamine or pseudoephedrine in prescription and OTC cold/allergy remedies. The interaction results in a severe and sometimes fatal hypertensive crisis. Pargyline's use has all but stopped.

Guanethidine

Guanethidine (ISMELIN) is another very powerful oral antihypertensive drug. However, it usually causes such intolerable side effects that it is rarely used except as a last choice.

One way to describe guanethidine is to compare and contrast it with reserpine (p 649). Both drugs deplete norepinephrine from adrenergic nerve endings. This accounts for several common properties: antihypertensive actions, the lack of reflex tachycardia, and nearly all the side effects and related contraindications. Reserpine depletes catecholamines gradually, and only partially. It acts in both the peripheral and central nervous systems. Guanethidine works much faster and causes almost complete loss of norepinephrine from nerves, but it works mainly in the periphery. Thus, nearly all of guanethidine's desired and unwanted peripheral autonomic effects are just like those of reserpine, but they occur faster and are much more intense. All the drug interactions noted for reserpine apply to guanethidine also.

Guanethidine is likely to cause significant renal fluid and salt retention, so diuretics are often needed as adjuncts. Beta-adrenergic blocking drugs and, probably, calcium channel blockers are likely to cause excessive cardiac depression if used with guanethidine. They should be used with extreme caution, if at all. Because guanethidine virtually eliminates all activity of the sympathetic nervous system, other sympathetic inhibitors are not needed. Indeed, they are likely to make the already severe side effects caused by guanethidine seem even worse.

III. Drugs for Acute Hypertension

Regardless of the cause, severe and abrupt increases of blood pressure require prompt treatment. The clinical goal is same as for treatment of essential hypertension: *safely lower blood pressure to an acceptable level.* Reaching the so-called norm of 120/80 mm Hg is an acceptable goal for previously normotensive adults, but those values may be dangerously low for patients with longstanding severe hypertension, or for those whose vital organs (eg, the kidneys, heart, or brain) have been damaged because of elevated blood pressure. For those patients, "normalizing" pressure could cause underperfusion of vital organs that have adapted to higher pressures.

Hypertensive Crises

Different terms have been used to describe conditions in which blood pressure is elevated acutely. A *hypertensive crisis* can be defined as a "severe" elevation of blood pressure, usually when diastolic pressures are above 120 to 130 mm Hg. Patients in this category should be evaluated in a hospital emergency department; a physician's office does not have the facilities necessary for a complete work-up or the means to intervene properly if the situation proves to be an emergency. If there is no evidence that vital organs have been damaged—for example, no brain dysfunction or stroke, no cardiac ischemia, and no renal insufficiency—the situation can be called an *urgent hypertensive crisis.* In many cases, the patient can be monitored for several hours after antihypertensive therapy is started and then discharged for follow-up examinations and possible changes of drug therapy soon thereafter.

Treatment might start with oral medications, often with clonidine or verapamil. If the patient is already on an antihypertensive medication, the dose of the same medication might be adjusted. Alternatively, and depending on the patient, a parenteral form of an orally effective agent might be used: methyldopa, reserpine, hydralazine, or labetalol (NORMODYNE; the only injectable β blocker approved for hypertension).

Sometimes specific antihypertensive drugs might be indicated. For example, hypertension caused by a sympathomimetic vasoconstrictor (α agonist) might be treated first with an α blocker. Most of the side effects, contraindications, and drug interactions noted for oral administration of these drugs apply to their parenteral use.

NURSING IMPLICATIONS

Obtain a thorough medical and medication history for evaluation and treatment planning, but do not allow history taking to take excessive time away from the physical examination and intervention. Evidence of organ involvement, such as headache, slurred speech, or altered reflexes, can give important clues about the patient's condition and are relatively easy and quick to assess for. It is not enough to determine whether the pressure is high by means of a single blood pressure measurement. More important is to determine whether the pressure is high and still going up and, if so, how much and how fast. Frequent measurements are the only way to detect a clear-cut signal of an impending emergency. They are not simply a part of routine nursing care; they help guide proper pharmacologic intervention.

There are other important considerations. For example, if parenteral methyldopa is to be given, be aware that this drug can act initially like a high dose of clonidine: Stimulation of α-receptors can occur first, elevating blood pressure somewhat for a while. Also, question medication orders that call for parenteral administration of methyldopa or reserpine if there is any hint of brain dysfunction or head injury. These drugs cause CNS depression that can mask or mimic underlying brain dysfunction or trauma, and they can thus impair neurologic evaluation.

Hypertensive Emergencies

If the hypertension is accompanied by acute or ongoing end-organ damage, the situation can be called a *hypertensive emergency*. Patients in this category should be admitted to the hospital, preferably to an intensive care setting. Parenteral antihypertensive therapy should be used. The usual drug of choice is sodium nitroprusside, which has now become the prototype of all emergency antihypertensive agents.

PROTOTYPE

Nitroprusside

Absorption, Distribution, Metabolism, and Excretion

Nitroprusside, formerly marketed under the familiar trade name, NIPRIDE, is given only intravenously. Aside from other pharmacologic factors, the drug has such a powerful antihypertensive action, such an extremely fast onset of action, and such an exceedingly short duration of action because of rapid metabolism that intravenous administration is the only feasible way to control its actions. One metabolite is cyanide. Normally, cyanide is quickly metabolized to thiocyanate, which is then excreted by the kidneys.

Pharmacologic Effects

Nitroprusside, like hydralazine, is a "pure" vasodilator. It has no direct autonomic effects. Nitroprusside's major effects include direct arteriolar and venous dilation. These direct effects trigger reflex tachycardia and increased cardiac contractility. Antihypertensive effects occur almost instantaneously on administration and disappear just as fast when administration is stopped or slowed. The close dose–effect relationship allows precise and prompt regulation of blood pressure through control of the infusion rate and provides a quick way of restoring pressure should it fall too much.

Clinical Indications and Administration

Nitroprusside is the major drug for nearly all hypertensive emergencies. It is also used during certain surgical procedures to cause controlled hypotension, which reduces bleeding from surgical sites. Another use is afterload reduction for management of severe heart failure. Typical dosages are shown in Table 33–C2.

Because nitroprusside works so fast and well, and because patients receiving it are usually critically ill, this drug should be administered by a calibrated infusion pump. Never inject nitroprusside directly from a syringe. Invasive monitoring of cardiovascular status (arterial and central venous pressures, for example) is essential during nitroprusside administration.

NURSING IMPLICATIONS

Nitroprusside is supplied in vials containing 50 mg of the drug. It must be diluted before use in sterile water containing 5% dextrose to concentrations of 200, 100, or 50 μg/mL. Do not use other diluents or add other drugs to a nitroprusside solution. Discard diluted solutions within 24 hours.

Fresh nitroprusside solutions that are prepared properly have a faint brownish tint. However, the drug is light-sensitive; the solution darkens, and becomes less active, when exposed to light. Therefore, wrap nitroprusside containers and IV tubing with aluminum foil or some other opaque material to protect it from light.

Side Effects, Adverse Reactions, and Contraindications

Reflex tachycardia is the most common side effect (Table 33–S2) and it is usually managed with a β blocker. Tachycardia is usually accompanied by increased cardiac contractility. The combination of tachycardia, increased contractility, and reduced blood pressure is particularly dangerous for patients with ischemic heart disease; these side effects increase the risk of angina pectoris and myocardial infarction. The cardiovascular changes are also dangerous for persons with aortic aneurysms: More intense pulsations of blood pressure, owing to increased cardiac contractility, can hasten or cause aneurysm rupture. Overall, β blockers are very important adjuncts for patients with ischemic heart disease or aneurysms, but they must be used cautiously.

If nitroprusside doses are too high or the drug is infused too fast, blood pressure can also fall too much or too quickly. This is particularly dangerous for patients with a history of renal or cerebral vascular disease or stroke. Organ ischemia can occur. The patient need not become "hypotensive" for ischemia to occur; any marked and abrupt pressure reduction in a previously hypertensive patient may cause serious problems. Therefore, when nitroprusside is given *blood pressure is usually stabilized initially at only 30% or 40% below predrug levels.*

Hypovolemia, hypotension, or anemia contraindicate nitroprusside use.

NURSING IMPLICATIONS

Notify the physician immediately if usual doses of nitroprusside do not reduce blood pressure adequately within 10 minutes of administration, or if pressure falls to less than 30% or 40% of predrug levels.

◆ Use During Pregnancy and Lactation

Nitroprusside can be used during pregnancy, but only in emergencies in which the anticipated benefits clearly outweigh risks of cyanide poisoning (see below) to both the mother and fetus. It is not used for routine management of hypertension associated with preeclampsia or eclampsia. These conditions generally require long-term antihypertensive drug administration—and long-term use of nitroprusside is known to increase the risk of cyanide toxicity. Mothers must not breast-feed their infants during drug administration.

◆ Use in Children and the Elderly

Dosage adjustments are based on the actual response to nitroprusside.

Interactions with Other Drugs

There are no specific drug interactions that involve nitroprusside. The drug will, however, cause additive pressure-lowering effects when administered to patients who are already taking antihypertensive medications. Therefore, anticipate the need for reduced doses (based on the individual patient's responses) when nitroprusside is given to such patients.

Overdose and Toxicity

Nitroprusside overdoses cause profound hypotension and reflex tachycardia. These are usually handled initially, and adequately, simply by slowing or stopping administration. Vasoconstrictors may be given cautiously if blood pressure fails to recover sufficiently.

Cyanide poisoning is a manifestation of nitroprusside toxicity. The risks are very real when the maximum recommended dose (10 μg/kg/min) is exceeded or the drug has been infused too long. Indeed, revised (1991) labeling now warns that fatal cyanide poisoning can occur when the maximum dose is infused for longer than only 10 minutes. Signs and symptoms of cyanide poisoning include metabolic acidosis; dizziness, headache, ataxia, or coma; thready pulse; impaired reflexes; and cherry-red coloration of the blood and skin.

Another indication of poisoning is what appears to be a loss of nitroprusside's vasodilator activity (tolerance)—a steady or even rising blood pressure despite the administration of large doses. The "logical" response might be to increase the infusion rate. This will only make the problem worse by further increasing cyanide levels. That, in turn, further reduces the vasodilator response and causes blood pressure to rise more. The underlying cause of tolerance—cyanide poisoning—must be treated.

If there is *any* evidence of cyanide poisoning, notify the physician at once and start administering oxygen. The nitroprusside administration should be stopped and other drugs given to control blood pressure if needed. Treatment of the poisoning itself usually involves a commercially available cyanide poisoning kit, which should be stocked in any facility that uses nitroprusside. The first step is having the patient inhale amyl nitrite; then, an IV infusion of sodium nitrite is started. These drugs cause the formation of methemoglobin, which binds excess cyanide in the bloodstream (forming cyanmethemoglobin). Sodium thiosulfate is then injected intravenously; it reacts with cyanmethemoglobin to form sodium thiocyanate, which is excreted by the kidneys. (See nitroprusside package inserts for details.) Be aware that the antidotes for cyanide poisoning can lower blood pressure further.

Other Injectable Antihypertensive Drugs

Nitroprusside usually is the ideal antihypertensive drug for use when proper administration and monitoring facilities are available. However, other injectable drugs can be used for managing acute hypertension (see the Annotated Bibliography), for producing controlled levels of hypotension (eg, during some surgeries), or both.

Nitroglycerin (Chapter 34), the most widely used antianginal drug, comes closest to nitroprusside in terms of uses and actions, and it does not lead to cyanide poisoning. However, the drug requires special IV tubing sets (it binds to some types of plastics, so only a part of the dose reaches the patient), and its dose–response relationship is not quite as good as that of nitroprusside.

Another alternative is the ganglionic blocker trimethaphan (ARFONAD; p 251). Its efficacy and dose–response relationship are good. However, the drug works by blocking all autonomic reflexes, which, normally, help the cardiovascular system adapt to sudden or excessive pressure falls. These reflexes are also important in diagnosing underlying medical problems, such as brain dysfunction owing to a stroke or trauma. Trimethaphan eliminates these diagnostic clues.

Alpha-adrenergic blockers, such as phentolamine (REGITINE; p 225), can also be used. They are best used to counteract pressure increases caused by catecholamines—hypertension caused by pheochromocytomas or by excessive effects of α-adrenergic agonist drugs given for vasoconstrictor effects.

Another injectable drug that may be particularly useful in special situations is diazoxide.

Diazoxide

Diazoxide (HYPERSTAT), another vasodilator, is indicated for emergency treatment of malignant hypertension in hospitalized patients. It is a second-choice drug for other hypertensive episodes when suitable administration devices or the intensive monitoring facilities needed for giving nitroprusside are not available.

Diazoxide has several advantages. The drug can (and should) be given simply as a bolus injection of the total dose (1 to 3 mg/kg) directly into a peripheral vein. The total dose is given in 30 seconds or less (slower infusions do not seem to work as well). The first dose often works, and blood pressure usually begins falling within 5 minutes. Pressure may rise again over the next 10 to 30 minutes. However, repeated doses may be given, and they usually cause a more longlasting pressure reduction.

Diazoxide also has limitations. It is nearly impossible to titrate the dose to achieve a relatively constant blood pressure or to target a particular pressure. Although diazoxide seldom causes hypotension, it may drop pressure too fast, and there is no satisfactory way to elevate it quickly if this should happen. Either hypotension or too fast a pressure fall can cause organ ischemia.

Diazoxide stimulates heart rate and contractility reflexly and through direct cardiac-stimulating effects. Beta blockers are commonly used adjunctively to control the cardiac responses and are essential pretreatments if diazoxide is given to a patient with a known dissecting aortic aneurysm. Diazoxide usually causes sodium and water retention, so diuretics are also indicated.

Diazoxide can also increase blood glucose levels. Diazoxide's hyperglycemic effect counteracts the hypoglycemic actions of oral antidiabetic drugs (eg, tolbutamide) and adds to the hyperglycemic effects of thiazide diuretics. The drug may also stimulate the metabolic inactivation of phenytoin, leading to reduced seizure control. However, the outcomes of these interactions develop slowly and are not likely to cause problems when only one or even several doses of diazoxide are used to treat hypertensive episodes. The interactions may become important when oral diazoxide (marketed as PROGLYCEM) is used on a long-term basis to manage hypoglycemia.

NURSING IMPLICATIONS

Keep the patient supine before and for at least half an hour after diazoxide injection, and closely monitor all vital signs, particularly heart rate, blood pressure, neurologic status, and blood glucose levels.

IV. General Nursing Implications for Antihypertensive Drug Therapy

Knowledge of the pathophysiology of hypertension and its treatment, the use of nondrug interventions, and the avoidance of pressure-elevating drugs are all important in controlling the disease. Nurses must teach this information to patients and their families in a way they can understand. There are also many misconceptions about these issues and other problems that can interfere with therapy. Here too, educating patients about what is myth and what is fact can facilitate a satisfactory clinical outcome. What follows is a brief overview of some of these topics.

Emotional Stress

Day-to-day stress is a recognized contributor to hypertension. (Surprisingly, many lay persons think that hypertension means *only* excessive nervous tension—

"hyper-tension"—and that it has nothing to do with increased blood pressure. Nondrug strategies to avoid or deal with stress, including relaxation techniques and exercise within the patient's limits, may help. However, they are not substitutes for proper drug therapy, especially for moderate or severe hypertension. The same applies to the use of sedative or anxiety-relieving drugs, prescription or OTC. They not only are unreliable pressure-reducing drugs, but also pose an added risk of variable and often unpredictable interactions.

Sodium Intake, Obesity, and Smoking

There is no doubt that reducing salt intake, losing excess weight, and quitting smoking are beneficial. An appropriate low-sodium diet helps the actions of all antihypertensive drugs, and sodium restriction alone can normalize blood pressures in some individuals. Additionally, lowering salt intake reduces potassium loss and may help reduce the risk of diuretic-induced hypokalemia. An acceptable daily sodium intake for most hypertensive patients is about 4 to 6 g of sodium chloride (about 2 g or 100 mEq of sodium). A "no salt added" diet may accomplish this goal and be acceptable to most patients. It includes avoiding highly processed foods, including most canned foods; milk and milk products; and baked goods (most contain large amounts of sodium in the form of baking soda or baking powder). For obese patients, also consider other dietary measures to limit caloric intake and to attain a more acceptable weight.

Nicotine activates the sympathetic nervous system, increasing blood pressure and counteracting the effects of most antihypertensive drugs. Quitting smoking altogether is preferred. If this is impossible, any reduction in smoking is considered a therapeutic gain. Nicotine-containing transdermal delivery systems (skin patches; p 257) may help many patients stop smoking. Nevertheless, they do deliver nicotine to the circulation, and so can cause unwanted and potentially dangerous effects for hypertensive patients.

Other Pressure-Elevating Drugs

Drugs that raise blood pressure or counteract antihypertensive drug actions must be avoided as much as possible. These include most OTC cold or allergy decongestant remedies, which usually contain sympathomimetics. Many antacids contain much sodium. Recommend products that are labeled sodium-free, and advise the patient to avoid sodium bicarbonate (baking soda). *Systemic corticosteroids,* which are used for arthritis or pulmonary disease, increase sodium and water retention and potassium loss. These effects may cause added problems for patients taking a potassium-wasting diuretic.

Compliance and Noncompliance

Antihypertensive therapy is usually lifelong. Even if treatment can be discontinued eventually, which is sometimes the case, compliance is essential during therapy. Unfortunately, compliance is not always achieved. There are several reasons; many may apply to the same patient, and many can be minimized or prevented with proper advice and good communication between patient and nurse:

- Hypertension is often symptomless. This fact can delay the detection of hypertension, because people who feel well tend not to have medical examinations. Once treatment starts, the patient may still feel well, or better. This can be interpreted as being "cured," and can lead the patient to stop taking medications. Alternatively,
- Antihypertensive drugs can cause side effects that the patient perceives to be worse than a disease that is often symptomless. Advise the patient ahead of time what to expect; indicate which side effects are likely to become less bothersome with continued drug use, and suggest simple nondrug ways to deal with some of them. All these important measures may facilitate compliance and reassure the patient that the health-care team is both aware of and concerned about them.
- Hypertension treatment can be expensive in terms of time and money. Follow-up examinations to track the progress of treatment, detect adverse effects, and change medications can be frustrating, inconvenient, and annoying. The examinations and the medications used to treat high blood pressure can be costly, as well. Stress the importance of repeated examinations, and make sure the patient understands why they and various tests should be done. If cost is a concern, notify the physician. Generic antihypertensive medications usually are as effective as brand-name products. Indeed, when treatment can be provided with one of two (or more) drugs, each with the same potential benefits and risks for a given patient, the less expensive choice might prove to be more acceptable. Skipping doses or stopping treatment altogether may save money in the short run. In the long run, how-

ever, such practices may increase cost if hypertension becomes more severe or if complications occur. Moreover, they can be dangerous.

- Pharmacotherapy may seem haphazard. Switching from one antihypertensive drug to another or adding other medications is often necessary and unavoidable. When this must be done, explain the reasons so that the patient is not left feeling that the physician is uncertain of what he or she is doing.

V. Hypertension in Special Patient Populations

The discussions of antihypertensive drug therapy in this chapter generally assume the patient is an "otherwise healthy young adult male." Some comments have been made about the use of specific drugs used for certain patient populations, such as pregnant women, children, and the elderly. What follows is a brief overview of hypertension and its therapy in these and other common patient groups.

Pregnancy

Slight and gradual blood pressure increases during pregnancy usually require no drug intervention. Bedrest is often the safest and most effective treatment. If hypertension existed before pregnancy and was being treated with antihypertensive drugs, and if the drug(s) used are not contraindicated during pregnancy, the important steps are to

- monitor the mother and fetus closely, and
- make no major changes of therapy unless pressure rises excessively or quickly or unless there are other causes for concern. For example, the combined appearance of maternal hypertension, edema, and proteinuria usually indicates preeclampsia, a condition characterized by profound and rapidly progressing hypertension, organ damage, and seizures. It can be fatal to both the mother and child, and it requires prompt evaluation. Delivery of the fetus puts an end to eclampsia, but sometimes that cannot be done safely.

If drug therapy is necessary for the remainder of pregnancy, there are three major guidelines to follow:

- control maternal pressure to avoid harm to the mother, child, or both;
- avoid maternal *hypo*tension and resulting fetal ischemia from treatment that is too aggressive, and
- avoid drugs that are contraindicated, including those that are contraindicated by pregnancy.

Many physicians consider methyldopa a treatment of choice for chronic hypertension; β blockers or hydralazine are alternatives for oral therapy if methyldopa does not work or cannot be used. For preeclampsia, when delivery of the fetus is not possible, hydralazine or a calcium channel blocker is often chosen.

The use of diuretics is controversial. Any diuretic may deplete maternal blood volume and cause underperfusion of the placenta; thiazides may directly lower placental blood flow; and diuretics do not prevent preeclampsia or eclampsia. A conservative approach is to avoid diuretics or use them only in low doses to manage fluid retention caused by other drugs.

ACE inhibitors are to be avoided, especially during early pregnancy or for long-term use during the gestational period. A growing number of reports show that children born to mothers taking these drugs during pregnancy have nonfunctioning or poorly functioning kidneys. Many of these children are either stillborn or die soon after delivery.

Relatively new evidence indicates that *low* doses of aspirin (80–160 mg/day, or one-quarter to one-half a regular aspirin tablet) administered during the second and third trimester can significantly and safely reduce morbidity and mortality associated with pregnancy-induced hypertension or preeclampsia. Aspirin may inhibit the overproduction of prostaglandins that make blood vessels hypersensitive to factors that cause vasoconstriction. This use for aspirin is not approved, and such therapy must be carried out only under a physician's supervision. Moreover, as noted in Chapter 52 there are risks associated with aspirin use even during normal pregnancy. Therefore, it is still important to advise all pregnant women to avoid use of this drug indiscriminately, even for the drug's usual indications (eg, mild pain, inflammation, and fever).

Hypertensive emergencies during pregnancy may involve use of hydralazine, diazoxide, or the parenteral α and β blocker, labetalol. If these more conventional therapies do not work in an emergency, nitroprusside is used. Magnesium sulfate has been given as an antihypertensive drug for eclampsia because eclampsia is accompanied by excessively low serum magnesium levels. This drug will *not* lower blood pressure; it is effective only as an anticonvulsant. The definitive treatment for eclampsia is delivery of the fetus. Obviously, this cannot be done if the fetus is not developed enough to survive or if other contraindications to delivery are present at the time. In these situations, drug therapy is the only choice.

Children

Kidney disease accounts for about 80% of pediatric hypertension cases. Other common causes are obesity and adrenal gland disorders. If specific therapies such as surgery or diet cannot be used, drugs may be the only way to prolong life. Most of the same antihypertensive drugs used for adults can be used for children. Keep in mind that the "normal" 120/80 mm Hg pressure is not reached until puberty. Pressures near or even slightly above that value in a young child may indicate a major disorder.

The Elderly

High blood pressure, especially systolic hypertension from atherosclerosis, is common in the elderly. No antihypertensive drug can dilate hardened vessels, but many can lower blood pressure in other ways. If the patient is otherwise symptom-free, is relatively healthy, or has mild hypertension of recent onset or slowly progressing, there may be little reason to cause undue distress with excessive drug treatment. Nondrug approaches are often useful if the patient can comply with them, and if they seem to work.

If therapy is indicated, the drug and its dose are chosen in such a way that they do not worsen other common age-related disorders. Also, the drug must not cause sudden changes of blood volume, postural hypotension, or excessive sedation—side effects that are not tolerated well by the elderly. For this reason, α blockers (eg, prazosin and related agents) and catecholamine depleters (eg, reserpine) are less than ideal. Calcium channel blockers seem to be ideally suited, for many reasons, in the absence of heart failure. Methyldopa or β blockers (particularly cardioselective ones, eg, metoprolol or atenolol) are suitable if the patient does not have other cardiac or pulmonary diseases. ACE inhibitors are acceptable if renal function is good, and they also exert favorable effects on heart failure that might also be present. Thiazides, at low starting doses, seem to work very well, but metabolic side effects and other side effects related to fluid and electrolyte imbalances can cause problems. High-ceiling diuretics are likely to make these problems even greater. Be aware of the need for age-related dosage adjustments, and be responsive to complaints of side effects that cause more discomfort than therapeutic benefits.

Racial and Ethnic Differences

The genetic characteristics of some ethnic groups can alter the response to drugs, including antihypertensive agents such as hydralazine. Racial differences are also important. For example, hypertension and the related illnesses and deaths are more common and serious in blacks. The response of blacks to some antihypertensive drug classes seems quite different from that of whites. (This may reflect differences in the underlying pathology, a topic that is too complex to discuss here.) In initial therapy, blacks tend to respond very well to calcium channel blockers and to thiazides. They seem to respond less to usually effective doses of ACE inhibitors (high doses work better), and much less to β blockers (on the average, blacks have lower plasma renin levels, a fact which may explain why β blockers, which lower renin secretion, may not work so well). There is less information about racial differences in the response to other classes of antihypertensives.

Diabetes, Hyperlipidemia, Atherosclerosis

Diabetes, hyperlipidemia, atherosclerosis, and hypertension often occur together. They significantly increase the risk of organ damage and early death. Drug-induced side effects related to metabolic abnormalities such as serum lipid profiles can complicate treatment (Table 33–6).

Calcium channel blockers or ACE inhibitors (in the absence of renal disease) are considered good choices for initial treatment because they do not adversely affect these other disorders. In contrast, thaizides tend to cause hyperglycemia and hyperlipidemias; β blockers tend to cause hypoglycemia and inhibit the recovery from hypoglycemia. Beta blockers also block the tachycardia that signals hypoglycemia in some diabetic patients. If a β blocker must be used, low doses of a cardioselective agent are preferred because their effect on blood glucose levels is less than that of nonselective ones. In addition, both thiazides and β blockers tend to interact with other antidiabetic therapies. Potassium-sparing diuretics or oral potassium supplements are used cautiously to counteract diuretic-induced hypokalemia; hyperglycemia, a hallmark of diabetes, increases the risks and consequences of hyperkalemia.

Asthma or Obstructive Pulmonary Disease

For patients with asthma or obstructive pulmonary disease, the obvious goal is to control blood pressure without causing bronchoconstriction or counteracting the

Table 33–6 | Effects of Selected Antihypertensive Drug Groups on Serum Lipid Profiles

Agent	Total Cholesterol	TG	LDL	HDL	HDL/Total Cholesterol
Thiazides	↑	↑↑	↑	↓	↓
β blockers, nonselective (eg, propranolol)	0	↑↑↑	0	↓↓	↓
β Blocker + ISA (eg, pindolol)	0	0	0	0	0
α & β blocker (labetalol)	0	0	0	0	0
Selective α_1 blocker (eg, prazosin)	↓	↓↓	↓	↑	↑
ACE inhibitors	0	0	0	0	0
Calcium channel blockers	0	0	0	0	0

Key: TG, triglycerides; LDL, low density lipoproteins; HDL, high density lipoproteins; ISA, intrinsic sympathomimetic activity; ACE, angiotensin converting enzyme.

Source: Modified from Grimm RH Jr: *Am Heart J* 1990; 119(3,Pt 2): 729-732.

desired effects of bronchodilator drugs. A good choice is a calcium channel blocker (they also seem to cause bronchodilation); selective α antagonists (eg, prazosin) or ACE inhibitors are other choices. Antihypertensive drugs that deplete catecholamines (reserpine) or work as centrally acting α agonists (clonidine) may worsen pulmonary problems. Beta blockers, even those with cardioselectivity or intrinsic sympathomimetic activity, are most likely to make the pulmonary problems worse.

Pheochromocytoma

Antihypertensive drugs are usually indicated for pheochromocytoma patients, even if the tumor can be removed surgically. Drug treatment is absolutely necessary during surgery, because manipulating the tumor causes massive catecholamine release. The major cardiovascular problems caused by a pheochromocytoma are due to excessive levels of epinephrine and norepinephrine, through stimulation of α- and β-adrenergic receptors. Therefore, α and β blockers are a logical choice. They can be prescribed separately, or a combined α and β blocker, labetalol (NORMODYNE), might be just as effective. Phentolamine, the short-acting injectable α blocker, has been used to help diagnose pheochromocytoma (a positive response is a large and sudden blood pressure fall), but this test is potentially dangerous. The drug can also be used in emergencies to lower pressure acutely. Phenoxybenzamine (DIBENZYLINE), the long-acting orally effective α blocker, is the historical agent for chronic use, but the newer prazosin alternatives are gaining much popularity.

If α and β blockers are given separately for severe, acute hypertension in a pheochromocytoma patient, it is important to give the α blocker first. Giving the β blocker first will cause pressure to rise even more, because it leaves the α-mediated vasoconstrictor effects of epinephrine unopposed. If the two are given simultaneously, the β blocker will depress contractility of the heart. The combination of increased pressure and a weakened heart can lead to acute heart failure.

Avoid vasodilators (eg, hydralazine) and rapidly acting catecholamine depleters (guanethidine, guanadrel); they usually do more harm than good because they abruptly release catecholamines, either reflexly or directly.

Dissecting Aortic Aneurysms

Blood pressure is the major force that causes ballooning and eventual rupture and death from aneurysms, so antihypertensive therapy is clearly beneficial. However, drugs that lower blood pressure but also increase cardiac contractility (directly or reflexly) can make the aneurysm dissect (tear) or rupture by causing intense pressure pulsations each time the heart beats. The preferred drugs are ones that inhibit, or at least do not increase, contractility: sympathetic inhibitors, including oral β blockers, for chronic therapy; or trimethaphan (an autonomic ganglionic blocker discussed on p 251) for emergencies. Vasodilators, whether given orally (hydralazine) or parenterally (nitroprusside, hydralazine, diazoxide, nitroglycerin), are given only after the patient is pretreated with a β blocker to prevent reflex cardiac stimulation.

SUMMARY OF NURSING IMPLICATIONS

◆ Assessment

Review past or present use of antihypertensive medications: name of drug, length of time on drug, any side effects; determine use of OTC drugs that may interact with antihypertensives or are contributing to an elevated blood pressure.

Establish baseline physical and emotional status: complete physical assessment, determine vital signs, review laboratory tests.

Review patient history for risk factors associated with hypertension (stress, family history); level of high blood pressure; duration of hypertension (if known); smoking habits; history of physical or emotional factors that may contraindicate use of specific antihypertensive drugs or drug groups.

Obtain both sitting and standing pressure on at least two different occasions at least one to two weeks apart, and when the patient is under no stress, as baseline data.

During follow-up visits, assess for worsening of other preexisting conditions caused by antihypertensive drug therapy (eg, gout or diabetes with thiazides; diabetes, breathing disorders, or heart failure with beta blockers).

◆ Nursing Diagnoses

Decreased cardiac output related to adverse drug effects (hypotension) or disease process (hypertension).

Knowledge deficit related to antihypertensive drug therapy and lifestyle changes (exercise, weight reduction, sodium restriction).

Noncompliance related to disturbing drug side effects.

Sexual dysfunction related to adverse drug effects.

High risk for injury related to untoward side effects.

◆ Planning Implementation

Observe for pertinent signs of excessive drug effects indicating inadequate cerebral blood flow (dizziness, confusion, mental clouding) or imminent stroke (slurred speech, localized muscle weakness).

Measure blood pressure 5 to 10 minutes after initial dose of antihypertensive medication.

Observe for signs of side effects or adverse reactions pertinent to the drug or drug class.

Recognize pertinent signs indicating drug-induced cardiac or pulmonary damage (edema, weight gain, dyspnea) or electrolyte imbalances.

Administer nitroprusside with an infusion pump. Protect the drug from light.

◆ Patient and Family Education

Teach the patient/family:

The basis of the stepped-care approach that probably will be used.

The possibility that in the future more than one drug may be used.

That therapy must be reevaluated periodically and perhaps changed several times.

The potential dangers of hypertension.

The major potential drug-induced side effects that are common to the overall drug class or unique to the agent that is prescribed.

Which side effects or adverse responses that necessitate immediate attention by the nurse or physician.

The potential need to accept some side effects to achieve prolonged health and reduced blood pressure.

The kinds of nondrug therapy (diet, behavior modification) that are likely to help reduce blood pressure.

Which medications, including OTC drugs, to avoid.

The need for female patients of childbearing age to discuss with the physician the potential fetal risks associated with some antihypertensive drugs, the possibility that breast-feeding may be contraindicated, the possibility that conception should be avoided, and the need to inform the physician immediately if pregnancy occurs.

The need to be compliant with therapy, including the need for periodic follow-up evaluations.

About the possible benefits of active participation in self-evaluation of therapy, including daily monitoring of blood pressure and body weight, as examples.

The fact that lowering of blood pressure or an overall sense of well-being is not a signal that drug therapy can be stopped.

The fact that antihypertensive therapy will probably be lifelong.

Nondrug measures to help reduce dry mouth (sucking hard candies); and daytime sedation (taking the drug at bedtime if possible; avoiding other sedative drugs or alcohol); to avoid operating a car or hazardous machinery; to stand slowly to prevent postural hypotension.

Doses and schedules for multiple-drug therapy.

About the potential dangers of abrupt discontinuation of therapy.

About "first-dose faint" with prazosin, doxazosin, terazosin and how to prevent it; to take drug in bed; that lightheadedness may persist during therapy.

About the almost certain abnormal growth of body hair with minoxidil.

To report swelling of face, lips, or eyelids, or breathing difficulties at once if taking ACE inhibitors; may indicate angioedema leading to closure of glottis or airway.

◆ Evaluation

The patient/family will:

Achieve blood pressure control: blood pressure within acceptable limits.

Tolerate undesirable drug effects; verbalize frustration and acceptance.

Comply with drug therapy as directed; continue therapy uninterrupted; verbalize principles of drug safety, storage, and expected side effects.

Monitor drug effects; measure weight weekly; measure and record blood pressure daily.

Discuss sexual problems openly with health professional and partner; request needed information and assistance from available resources.

Avoid OTC medications, alcohol, and smoking while receiving antihypertensive medication.

Report serious side effects; avoid physical injury associated with adverse effects.

Annotated Bibliography

Amadio P Jr, Amadio PB, Cummings DM: ACE inhibitors: A safe option for hypertension and congestive heart failure. *Postgrad Med* 1990;87(1):223–226, 231–232, 235–243. *An excellent review of the benefits of ACE inhibitor therapy and what to look for when monitoring patients taking these and other drugs.*

Black HR: Choosing initial therapy for hypertension: A personal view. *Hypertension* 1990;13(Suppl I):I-149–I-153. *Reviews patient- and drug-related factors that can help you evaluate whether the drugs your patient is taking are the right ones. Also discusses why thiazides or β blockers are no longer automatically used as starting drugs.*

Calhoun DA, Oparil S: Treatment of hypertensive crisis. *N Engl J Med* 1990;323:1177–1183. *An excellent review of drug therapy of hypertensive emergencies and urgent hypertensive crises.*

Cerrato PL: Hypertension: The role of diet and lifestyle. RN 1990;53:46–51. *Identifies the values and limitations of some important nondrug adjuncts to blood pressure control.*

Christleib AR: Treatment selection considerations for the hypertensive diabetic patient. *Arch Intern Med* 1990;150:1167–1174. *The author makes a case for using ACE inhibitors or calcium channel blockers to start therapy in patients with hypertension and diabetes. The article includes a treatment flow-sheet that may prove useful.*

Cooper K, Albrezzi B: Emergency! It's cyanide! *Am J Nurs* 1990;90(11):42–44. *Practical tips for recognizing and managing cyanide poisoning, a consequence of nitroprusside overdoses.*

Croog SH, Kong W, Levine S, Weir MR, Baume RM, Saunders E: Hypertensive black men and women: Quality of life and effects of antihypertensive medications. *Arch Intern Med* 1990;150:1733–1741. *Summarizes a comprehensive study on the incidence of hypertension, the response to specific antihypertensive drugs, and quality of life in black men and women.*

Gifford RW Jr: Management of hypertensive crises. *JAMA* 1991; 266:829–835. *A noteworthy review because of the author's caution that even when oral therapy might be indicated for acute treatment, parenteral therapy (nitroprusside) has some distinct advantages.*

Gifford RW Jr, Borazanian RA: Traditional first-line therapy: Overview of medical benefits and side effects. *Hypertension* 1989;13(Suppl I):I-119–I-124. *Succinctly compares the pros and cons of using thiazides or β blockers for Step I therapy.* The tables alone are worth a look.

Gorlin R: Do we need another antihypertensive agent? *Am Heart J* 1991;121(2, Pt 2):670–676. *Why so many antihypertensive drugs? This short article summarizes the limitations of current agents and what is (and is not) known about underlying pathophysiology. The article also makes a case for why newer agents may be needed.*

Grimm RH Jr,: Alpha-1 antagonists in the treatment of hypertension. *Hypertension* 1989;13(Suppl I):I-131–I-136. *Concisely reviews the pharmacologic profiles of prazosin and related drugs and compares them with other classes of antihypertensive drugs.*

Grimm RH Jr, Mlack JM: Management of hypertension: Potential tradeoffs on coronary risk. *Am J Med* 1989;87(Suppl 2A):62S–65S. *Has useful tables comparing lipid effects of a variety of antihypertensive agents, discusses their clinical implications, and helps explain why thiazides and β blockers have lost some popularity as starting drugs.*

Hockenberry B: Multiple drug therapy in the treatment of essential hypertension. *Nurs Clin North Am* 1991;26(2):417–436. *Clearly identifies nursing roles and responsibilities in all aspects of hypertension therapy.*

Kaplan NM: The appropriate goals of antihypertensive therapy: Neither too much nor too little. *Ann Intern Med* 1992;116:686–690. *Explores two important and often overlooked aspects of hypertension therapy: undertreatment and overtreatment, and their consequences for patients.*

Lamy PP: Potential adverse effects of antihypertensive drugs in the elderly. *J Hypertens* Suppl 1988;6(1):S81–S85. *This excellent article identifies issues that still apply to drug therapy of elderly hypertensive patients.*

Lopez LM: Hypertension in the elderly: Conventional wisdom revisited. *Pharmacotherapy* 1991;11(3):225–236. *Tread carefully with your elderly hypertensive patient. Implementing nondrug measures and making sure they are followed can be just as important as (and potentially less dangerous than) careful use of antihypertensive drugs.*

Materson BJ, et al: Treatment of hypertension in the elderly: I. Blood pressure and clinical changes. *Hypertension* 1990;15:348–360. *A multicenter Veterans Administration study that focuses on the efficacy and other clinical considerations of hydrochlorothiazide, still viewed as a preferred starting drug for treating hypertension in the elderly.*

National Institutes of Health. *The 1988 Report of the Joint National Committee on Detection, Evaluation, and Treatment of High Blood Pressure.* NIH Publication 88-1088. U.S. Government Printing Office, 1988. *A consensus viewpoint on all key aspects of hypertension and its treatment.*

Palevsky HI, Fishman AP: The management of primary pulmonary hypertension. *JAMA* 1991;265(8):1014–1020. *Excellent coverage of drug therapy for a disorder that may lead to heart–lung transplantations or death.*

Remuzzi G, Ruggenenti P: Prevention and treatment of pregnancy-associated hypertension: What have we learned in the last 10 years? *Am J Kidney Dis* 1991;18(3):285–305. *An excellent review of the classification, pathophysiologic mechanisms, and treatment of pregnancy-associated hypertension.*

Rodman MJ: Hypertension: First-line drug therapy. *RN* 1991;54(1):32–40. Step-care management. *RN* 1991;54(2):24–31. *Although lacking information on some of the latest drugs, these well-written papers explain the key actions and uses of antihypertensive medications.*

Roe DA: Drug and nutrient interactions in elderly cardiac patients. *Drug Nutr Interact* 1988;5(4):205–212. *Although it covers cardiovascular medications in general, this article has useful comments focusing on hypertension and its therapy and the role nutritional factors can play in the outcome.*

Saunders E: Tailoring treatment to minority patients. *Am J Med* 1990;88(3B):21S–23S. *Three pages pack a wealth of practical, thought-provoking information about hypertension and its treatment in minorities, especially blacks, who are at very great risk.*

Schmieder RE, Rockstroh JK, Messerli FH: Antihypertensive therapy. To stop or not to stop? *JAMA* 1991;265(12):1566–1571. *Treat forever? Stopping antihypertensive therapy, at least temporarily, may be acceptable for some patients. This paper identifies what is involved in making this decision.*

Schulze C: Aortic dissection—an ICU crisis. *RN* 1990;53(8):42–47. *Good nursing insight into the complications and therapy of this life-threatening, hypertension-related medical emergency.*

Schwartz GL: Initial therapy for hypertension—individualizing care. *Mayo Clin Proc* 1990;65(1):73–87. *Helps explain why there isn't one "right" antihypertensive therapy for the nearly 60 million Americans who have high blood pressure.*

Sibai BM: Diagnosis and management of chronic hypertension in pregnancy. *Obstet Gynecol* 1991;78(3, Pt 1):451–461. *This easy to read article hits the key points about the epidemiology, complications, treatment strategies, and monitoring for this common population.*

Stein PP, Black HR: Drug treatment of hypertension in patients with diabetes mellitus. *Diabetes Care* 1991;14(6):425–448. *Reviews the combined adverse effects of diabetes and hypertension, discusses pertinent side effects of antihypertensive drugs, and suggests a stepped-care approach to therapy for patients with both diseases.*

Systolic Hypertension in the Elderly Program (SHEP) Cooperative Research Group. Prevention of stroke by antihypertensive drug treatment in older persons with isolated systolic hypertension: Final results of the Systolic Hypertension in the Elderly Program. *JAMA* 1991;265(24):3255–3264. *Demonstrates that isolated systolic hypertension can be effectively, safely, and economically treated, and serious consequences reduced, with a stepped-care regimen that includes low doses of a diuretic (chlorthalidone) and a β blocker (atenolol).*

Taylor RB: Patient profiling: Individualization of hypertension therapy. *Am Fam Physician* 1990;42(5 Suppl):29S–31S, 34S–36S. *Identifies key factors to consider beyond the high blood pressure and the drugs used to treat it.*

Weber MA: Antihypertensive treatment: Considerations beyond blood pressure control. *Circulation* 1989;80(Suppl IV):IV-120–IV-127. *A clearly written summary of the many factors that should be considered before and after what seems to be the "right" antihypertensive drug is prescribed.*

Weiss RJ: Effects of antihypertensive agents on sexual function. *Am Fam Physician* 1991;44(6):2075–2082. *Discusses an important and often overlooked side effect that can limit successful antihypertensive therapy.*

Table 33–C1 Drugs Indicated for Oral Therapy of Hypertension*

AGENT	DOSAGE AND ROUTE OF ADMINISTRATION
	Step I Agents
Diuretics	See Chapter 32, p 624
β-adrenergic blockers	See Chapter 15, p 244
Calcium channel blockers	See Chapter 34, p 697
	ACE Inhibitors
PROTOTYPE	
Captopril (CAPOTEN)	Initially 25 mg bid or tid; average maintenance dose 50 mg, bid or tid, up to 450 mg/day maximum in divided doses; start with half the usual starting dose if patient is already taking diuretics
RELATED DRUGS	
Benazepril (LOTENSIN)	Initially, 10 mg/day (5 mg if taking diuretic), increase to 20–40 mg/day as single dose or in 2 equal divided doses
Enalapril (VASOTEC)	Initially, 5 mg once daily (2.5 mg if taking diuretic); average maintenance dose 10–40 mg/day as single dose or in 2 equal divided doses
Fosinopril (MONOPRIL)	Initially, 10 mg/day (5 mg if taking diuretic); maintain with up to 40 mg/day
Ramipril (ALTACE)	Initially, 2.5 mg/day (1.25 mg if taking diuretic), increase to 20 mg/day as single dose or in 2 equal divided doses
	Step II Agents
PROTOTYPES	
Clonidine (CATAPRES)	Initially, 0.1 mg bid; average maintenance dose 0.1–0.4 mg bid; maximum 2.4 mg/day
(CATAPRES-TTS)	Topical: Apply patch (delivers 0.1, 0.2, or 0.3 mg/day for 1 week) every 7 days to hairless area of intact skin on upper arm or torso
Prazosin (MINIPRESS)	Initially, 1 mg bid or tid; average maintenance dose 2–5 mg, 3 tid
Reserpine (SERPASIL, others)	Initially, single dose of 0.5 mg/day; average maintenance dose 0.1–0.25 mg/day

(continued)

Table 33–C1 **Drugs Indicated for Oral Therapy of Hypertension*(*Continued*)**

AGENT	CLINICAL USES	DOSAGE AND ROUTE OF ADMINISTRATION
RELATED DRUGS		
Doxazosin (CARDURA)		Initially, 1 mg once daily; usual maintenance dose 4 mg once daily
Guanabenz (WYTENSIN)		Initially, 4 mg bid; average maintenance dose about 8 mg bid; maximum 32 mg bid
Guanadrel (HYLOREL)		Initially, 5 mg bid; average maintenance dose is 20–75 mg/day in 2 doses
Guanfacine (TENEX)		Initially, 1 mg at bedtime; increase, at 3- or 4-week intervals, to 2 mg/day, then 3 mg/day, if needed; daily doses above 3 mg increase the risk and severity of side effects and adverse reactions
Methyldopa (ALDOMET)		Initially, 250 mg bid or tid; average maintenance dose 500 mg–3 g in 2–4 doses
Terazosin (HYTRIN)		Initially, 1 mg qhs; increase gradually to maintenance dose, usually 1–5 mg taken once daily; daily doses greater than 20 mg are not likely to be effective
Step III Agents		
PROTOTYPE		
Hydralazine (APRESOLINE)		Initially, 10 mg qid; average maintenance dose 50 mg, qid; fast acetylators, most blacks require higher daily doses
RELATED DRUG		
Minoxidil (LONITEN)		Initially, 5 mg/day; average maintenance dose 10–40 mg in 1 or 2 divided doses
Step IV Agent		
PROTOTYPE		
Guanethidine (ISMELIN)		Initially, 10 mg/day for ambulatory patients, 25 or 50 mg/day or every other day for hospitalized patients; average maintenance dose 25–50 mg/day

*Drugs are listed first according to the usual stepped-care sequence and then alphabetically. Prototypes appear at the beginning of each step sequence. Consult the index for uses of drugs having indications in addition to treatment of hypertension. Dosages of drugs used for hypertensive emergencies are found in Table 33–C2.

Table 33–S1 **Side Effects of and Precautions or Contraindications for Orally Effective Drugs Used for Essential Hypertension***

BODY SYSTEM/ Side Effect	CONTRAINDICATION/ PRECAUTION	COMMENTS AND NURSING IMPLICATIONS
Thiazide Diuretics		
See Table 32–S, p 627		
Beta Blockers		
See Table 15–S, p 248		
Calcium Channel Blockers		
See Table 34–S, p 699		
Captopril, Other ACE Inhibitors		
BLOOD Neutropenia, agranulocytosis (mainly captopril)	Serious autoimmune disease (eg, SLE)	Periodic blood analysis is necessary; look for onset of fever, flu-like symptoms, or other signs of blood dyscrasias
CARDIOVASCULAR Excessive hypotension	Preexisting hypotension, ongoing therapy with other antihypertensive drugs	Usually occurs with combined drug therapy, discontinue other antihypertensives first, if possible
RENAL Proteinuria (mainly captopril)	Renal damage, especially collagen vascular disease	Due to renal tubular damage; frequent urinalysis is essential; use low doses in presence of renal dysfunction, including that accompanied by heart failure
OTHER Angioedema (mainly enalapril, lisinopril)	History of this reaction with prior ACE inhibitor therapy	Advise patients to report immediately any swelling of face, mouth, lips, eyelids, or difficulty breathing or swallowing; may progress quickly to medical emergency
Cough		Common, usually nonproductive, often disturbing and relentless; notify physician if it becomes bothersome to patient
Clonidine, Guanabenz, Guanfacine		
CENTRAL NERVOUS SYSTEM Sedation, drowsiness; nightmares, altered sleep patterns		If severe during early therapy, have patient avoid tasks requiring mental acuity; tolerance usually develops with continued therapy; may be drug-related or a response to reduced BP
CARDIOVASCULAR Decreased cardiac output; Severe CHF orthostatic hypotension (mild, infrequent); weight gain due to edema; poor blood pressure control	Severe CHF	Although not common, clonidine may reduce renal blood flow, causing increased salt and water retention; manage with diuretics
Rebound hypertension with abrupt discontinuation		Never discontinue abruptly; taper dose over 4 days or more

(continued)

*Listed in general sequence of use in the stepped-care approach.

Table 33–S1 **Side Effects of and Precautions or Contraindications for Orally Effective Drugs Used for Essential Hypertension* (*Continued*)**

BODY SYSTEM/ Side Effect	CONTRAINDICATION/ PRECAUTION	COMMENTS AND NURSING IMPLICATIONS
GASTROINTESTINAL Dry mouth		Common: reported in about 40% of patients taking the drug; manage with nondrug measures (sipping water, sucking hard candies)
GENITOURINARY Impotence; urinary retention	Use cautiously in patients with prostatic hypertrophy	Impotence cited as cause of poor compliance; explain potential risks of discontinuing therapy because of it
Methyldopa		
CENTRAL NERVOUS SYSTEM See clonidine		
BLOOD Hemolysis, hemolytic anemia		Recommend periodic Coombs' test and tests for anemia, blood dyscrasias
RESPIRATORY See clonidine		
CARDIOVASCULAR See clonidine		
GASTROINTESTINAL See clonidine		
LIVER Hepatotoxicity	Use cautiously in patients with history of hepatic dysfunction	Recommend periodic hepatic function tests
GENITOURINARY See clonidine		
Guanabenz		
See clonidine		
Prazosin, Doxazosin, Terazosin		
CARDIOVASCULAR Initial, acute postural hypotension, syncope		Hypotension, syncope common with first few doses or after increasing dose; may be marked in sodium-depleted patients; give initial doses to patient in bed; take precautions against syncope, injury from falls; tolerance develops with continued use

(continued)

Table 33–S1 Side Effects of and Precautions or Contraindications for Orally Effective Drugs Used for Essential Hypertension* (*Continued*)

BODY SYSTEM/ Side Effect	CONTRAINDICATION/ PRECAUTION	COMMENTS AND NURSING IMPLICATIONS
CENTRAL NERVOUS SYSTEM		
See clonidine		
RESPIRATORY		
See clonidine		
GASTROINTESTINAL		
See clonidine		
GENITOURINARY		
See clonidine		
Reserpine		
CENTRAL NERVOUS SYSTEM		
Sedation, drowsiness		See clonidine
Parkinsonism	Parkinson's disease	Observe patient for parkinsonian signs (increased involuntary movements) and report to physician if they occur
Depression, possibly suicidal	Personal or familial history of depression, suicide attempts	Depression may develop during reserpine therapy or 2 or 3 months after termination, most likely to occur with daily doses greater than 0.5 mg; assess, evaluate patient for personality, mood changes
EYE		
Mydriasis; increased lacrimation	Potential aggravation of glaucoma	Administer cautiously to glaucoma patients; encourage periodic measurement of intraocular pressure
RESPIRATORY		
Increased respiratory tract secretions	Severe bronchial asthma, COPD	Monitor for dyspnea, excessive secretions in respiratory tract
CARDIOVASCULAR		
Postural hypotension; decreased cardiac output due to decreased contractility, heart rate; renal salt, water retention	CHF	Postural hypotension apt to be more prominent than with clonidine and related drugs
GASTROINTESTINAL		
Diarrhea	Active peptic ulcer disease	May be severe
Acid hypersecretion		Prophylactic antacid therapy may be recommended for some patients
GENITOURINARY		
Impotence		See clonidine

(continued)

Table 33–S1 Side Effects of and Precautions or Contraindications for Orally Effective Drugs Used for Essential Hypertension* (*Continued*)

BODY SYSTEM/ Side Effect	CONTRAINDICATION/ PRECAUTION	COMMENTS AND NURSING IMPLICATIONS
Guanadrel		
See guanethidine		
Hydralazine		
CARDIOVASCULAR Reflex tachycardia, renal salt, water retention	Coronary atherosclerosis, severe angina pectoris; dissecting aortic aneurysm unless pretreated with β blocker	β blockers and diuretics are almost always given adjunctively
Headache		Due to cerebral vasodilation
OTHER SLE-like syndrome: arthralgia, fever, etc		Monitor for characteristic signs of SLE-like state; discontinue and reevaluate therapy if they occur
Peripheral neuritis; paresthesias, numbness		Vitamin B_6 supplements may be used to prevent or treat neuritis
Minoxidil		
CARDIOVASCULAR Reflex tachycardia; renal salt, water retention		See hydralazine
Myocardial lesions; pericardial effusions; tamponade		Periodic noninvasive cardiac monitoring is essential; have patient report dyspnea, which might indicate problems
OTHER Hirsutism		Cosmetically displeasing; may cause poor compliance; because patients receiving minoxidil have severe and refractory hypertension stress the importance of continued therapy
Guanethidine		
RESPIRATORY Possible dyspnea in COPD patients; severe nasal congestion, lacrimation	Severe COPD	May be due to either decreased circulating catecholamines or increased secretions
CARDIOVASCULAR Orthostatic hypotension, bradycardia; decreased cardiac output	Severe CHF; cerebral or coronary ischemia	Orthostatic hypotension likely to be severe; take appropriate precautions
Transient hypertension, tachycardia with initial administration	Aneurysm; stroke; pheochromocytoma	Monitor BP closely
GASTROINTESTINAL Diarrhea		Explosive diarrhea may occur with initial dose; chronic severe diarrhea requires reduced doses

Table 33–I | **Major Interactions Between Orally Effective Antihypertensives and Other Agents**

AGENT	RESULT OF INTERACTION	COMMENTS AND NURSING IMPLICATIONS
Interactions Involving All Antihypertensive Drugs		
All other antihypertensive drugs, any drugs that can lower BP (eg, narcotics, sedatives, antidepressants, antipsychotics, alcohol, others)	Additive and desired BP reduction; excessive and unwanted effects (hypotension)	Interaction provides basis for combination therapy in stepped-care approach; obtain complete medication history, including OTC drug use; discourage unsupervised use of OTC drugs that can lower blood pressure; assess for potential cause(s) of unexpected, excessive BP falls
STEP I AGENTS		
Interactions Involving Diuretics		
See Chapter 32, Table 32–I, p 629 and specific interactions below		
Interactions Involving β-Adrenergic Blockers		
See Chapter 15, Table 15–12, p 249, and other drugs below		
Interactions Involving Calcium Channel Blockers		
See Chapter 34, Table 34–I, p 701, and other drugs below		
Interactions Involving ACE Inhibitors		
Diuretics, potassium-sparing (eg, triamterene; see Chapter 32)	Increased risk of hyperkalemia	ACE inhibitors cause potassium retention; normally avoid use of interactant; monitor BP and serum potassium levels if use is required
Indomethacin (Chapter 52)	Reduces effects of ACE inhibitor	Interactant interferes with prostaglandin synthesis, a component of ACE inhibitor's mechanism of action; monitor for reduced BP (or CHF) control; discontinue interactant or use other nonsteroidal antiinflammatory drug if interaction poses problems
Potassium-containing drugs (eg, potassium penicillins)	Increased risk of hyperkalemia	Monitor serum potassium levels frequently if combined use is necessary
STEP II AGENTS		
Interactions Involving Centrally Acting α-Adrenergic Agonists: Clonidine, Guanabenz, Guanfacine, Methyldopa		
Antidepressants, tricyclics (Chapter 24)	Poor BP control, potential hypertension	Avoid interaction by using alternative drug(s) if possible
β Blockers (Chapter 15)	Significantly reduced antihypertensive effect of clonidine, potential for severe hypertension	Monitor BP closely and often, if combined use necessary, if necessary to discontinue one or both drugs, discontinue slowly to avoid rebound BP increase; probably, discontinue α agonist first
Additional Interaction Involving Methyldopa		
Sympathomimetics, mixed- and indirect-acting (Chapter 14)	Increased sympathomimetic effects, potential hypertension	Obtain history of OTC medication use (eg, cold, allergy products) and discourage unsupervised use; assess for use of interactant as potential cause of antihypertensive failure

(continued)

Table 33–1 Major Interactions Between Orally Effective Antihypertensives and Other Agents (*Continued*)

AGENT	RESULT OF INTERACTION	COMMENTS AND NURSING IMPLICATIONS
Interactions Involving Selective α-Adrenergic Blockers: Prazosin, Doxazosin, Terazosin		
β Blockers (Chapter 15)	Significantly increased risk of hypotension, esp. orthostatic	Interactant prevents heart from speeding up as BP falls, esp. on standing; forewarn patient, instruct about measures to reduce symptoms; avoid interaction if possible
Calcium channel blockers (eg, verapamil; Chapter 34)	As for β blockers	Precautions basically same as for β blockers
Interactions Involving Peripheral Catecholamine Depleters: Reserpine, Guanadrel		
Sympathomimetics, direct-acting (eg, epinephrine, norepinephrine; Chapter 14, pp 191–206)	Increased, potentially severe sympathomimetic response	Occurs because catecholamine depleters cause adrenergic receptors to become supersensitive to agonists; avoid indiscriminant use of interactants; use low doses if needed to treat hypotension or cardiac depression owing to reserpine overdose
Sympathomimetics, mixed-acting (eg, ephedrine), indirect-acting (eg, amphetamines, phenylpropanolamine; Chapter 14)	Reduced sympathomimetic drug effects	Effects of interactants depend partially or completely on ability to release catecholamines; if sympathomimetics needed to treat reserpine overdoses or to cause other desired effects, use low doses of direct-acting agents (see above)
STEP III AGENTS		
Interactions Involving Vasodilators: Hydralazine, Minoxidil		
β Blockers (Chapter 15)	Increased serum levels, effects, of both drugs	β blockers often used adjunctively with hydralazine, but lower doses often needed; monitor accordingly, anticipate need to adjust dosages of one or both drugs
STEP IV AGENT		
Interactions Involving Guanethidine		
Antidepressants, tricyclics (Chapter 24)	Reduced or abolished effects of guanethidine	Avoid interaction, monitor BP otherwise, or use antihypertensive drugs other than guanethidine
Phenothiazines (eg, chlorpromazine; Chapter 23)	Reduced antihypertensive effect of guanethidine	Avoid interaction; use other antihypertensives if combined therapy with antipsychotic is needed
Sympathomimetics, direct-acting (see reserpine, above)	Increased, potentially excessive sympathomimetic effects	See reserpine, above
Sympathomimetics, indirect-acting (see reserpine, above)	Reduced antihypertensive effect of guanethidine; greatly reduced or absent response to these sympathomimetics	Avoid combined use; if unavoidable, anticipate need for increased guanethidine doses during use, need to lower antihypertensive dose when interactant is discontinued

Table 33–C2 **Clinical Uses and Administration of Major Antihypertensive Drugs Indicated for Hypertensive Crises**

AGENT	CLINICAL USES	DOSAGE AND ROUTE OF ADMINISTRATION
PROTOTYPE		
Nitroprusside sodium	Most hypertensive emergencies; afterload reduction; to produce controlled hypotension	IV infusion: Usually 3 μg/kg/min, adjusted as needed based on invasive measurements of systemic and pulmonary arterial, venous pressures
OTHER DRUGS		
Diazoxide (HYPERSTAT)	Emergency treatment of malignant hypertension; alternative therapy of hypertensive emergencies	IV bolus: Usually 1-3 mg/kg, up to maximum total of 150 mg, repeated as necessary; administer entire dose in < 30 sec
Hydralazine (APRESOLINE)	Subacute hypertensive emergencies	IM or IV: 20 or 40 mg
Labetalol (NORMODYNE, TRANDATE)	Hypertensive emergency, especially if caused by sympathomimetic drug overdoses or accompanied by excessive cardiac stimulation	IV: Start with 20 mg or 0.25 mg/kg, whichever is less, injected over 2 min; if needed, give additional 40 or 80 mg at 10-min intervals, up to cumulative dose of 300 mg; alternatively, dilute drug to 1 mg/mL or 2 mg/3mL IV solution and infuse at 2 mg/min
Methyldopa (ALDOMET Ester Hydrochloride)	Subacute hypertensive emergencies	IV: Usually 250 or 500 mg every 6 hr as needed
Nitroglycerin	Adjunctive treatment of acute hypertension; induced (eg, intraoperative) hypotension	See Chapter 31
Trimethaphan, mecamylamine	Hypertensive emergencies, especially with pheochromocytoma or MAO inhibitor interactions; intraoperative blood pressure control	See Chapter 16

Table 33–S2 Major Side Effects of and Precautions or Contraindications for Nitroprusside and Diazoxide Crises

BODY SYSTEM/ Side Effect	CONTRAINDICATION/ PRECAUTION	COMMENTS AND NURSING IMPLICATIONS
	Diazoxide	
METABOLIC Hyperglycemia	Use cautiously in diabetics	May be intensified by concurrent use of diuretic; monitor diabetic patient's blood glucose, vital signs, closely; give insulin as needed
CARDIOVASCULAR Reflex tachycardia	Severe angina; dissecting aortic aneurysm	Pretreat with β blocker if diazoxide use is unavoidable in presence of contraindication, give β blocker if excessive tachycardia occurs in any patient receiving diazoxide
Salt, water retention	Severe CHF	Use diuretic (thiazide or furosemide) adjunctively
	Nitroprusside	
CARDIOVASCULAR Reflex tachycardia; renal salt, water retention	Coronary atherosclerosis, severe angina pectoris; dissecting aortic aneurysm unless pretreated with β blocker	β blockers and diuretics may be required adjuncts; assess all vital signs constantly, preferably invasively; also applies to parenteral use of nitroglycerin, hydralazine
OTHER Cyanide poisoning; acidosis; tolerance to vasodilator effect; altered sensorium; obtunded reflexes		Discontinue drug; give amyl nitrite inhalation followed by IV sodium thiosulfate, give oxygen; use vasopressors as needed to restore blood pressure; avoid use, especially if prolonged and in high doses, in pregnant women

PROTOTYPES

Nitroglycerin 677

Verapamil 686

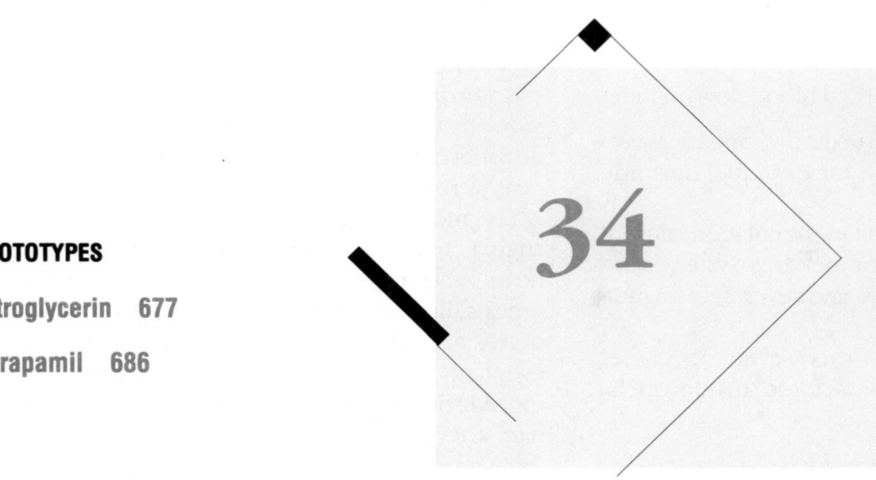

Antianginal Drugs

Angina pectoris—a Latin term meaning "chest pain"—is a symptom of myocardial ischemia. **Ischemia** can be defined as an inadequate flow of oxygenated blood to a tissue or organ—in this case, the heart muscle. The underlying pathophysiology can quickly cause a loss of cardiac contractility, rate, or rhythm. When myocardial ischemia is too widespread, severe, or prolonged, heart muscle begins to die quickly, or become infarcted (dead). Thus, angina is also a potential indicator of heart attack—a myocardial infarction (MI)—which can be fatal in minutes.

Ischemia is, in essence, an imbalance between oxygen supply and demand. This chapter discusses the drugs used to treat or prevent anginal attacks through one or more actions on this imbalance.

Myocardial Oxygen Supply and Demand

The major metabolic energy fuel for the heart muscle (as for most other organs) is adenosine triphosphate (ATP). Large amounts of oxygen and other nutrients delivered by the coronary arteries are needed to replenish the large amounts of ATP that the heart uses constantly. Any factor that increases myocardial oxygen demands or decreases coronary blood flow and the related oxygen delivery can trigger myocardial ischemia and angina if the resulting imbalance is too great.

Factors that increase myocardial oxygen demands include those that increase

- the force with which the heart contracts during systole (afterload, which is related to blood pressure),
- diastolic heart volume and size (preload, or ventricular wall tension during diastole), or
- heart rate.

These changes can be caused by disease (pathophysiology), hormonal influences, environmental stresses, and by many drugs. Exercise, and the release of cardiac-stimulating catecholamines (epinephrine, norepinephrine) that occurs with it, is one of the best examples of a physiologic factor that increases myocardial oxygen demands in several ways at once: through increases of heart rate, force of contraction, and blood pressure. Hypertension itself is another important cause of increased myocardial oxygen demands, because it forces the heart to develop greater pressures to expel blood into the arterial system; that is, hypertension increases afterload.

Major reference tables appear beginning on p. 696.

Factors that decrease myocardial blood flow include

- physical narrowing or obstruction of one or more coronary arteries caused by, for example, thrombi or atherosclerotic plaques;
- vasoconstriction in the coronary circulation caused by, for example, sympathetic nervous system activation, vasoconstrictor drugs, and several other mediators; and
- hypotension, especially if it is severe, because blood pressure is the major force that propels blood through the vessels.

Like the abnormalities that can increase oxygen demand, those that decrease blood and oxygen delivery can be caused by disease, drugs, and other stressors.

Whether any of these changes lead to ischemia and angina depends on how severe the supply–demand imbalance becomes. For persons with "healthy" hearts, the imbalance may need to be very great before ischemia occurs. In contrast, for persons with significant cardiac disease, such as severe coronary artery occlusion, even slight increases in oxygen demand can trigger severe ischemia and pain.

The drugs used to treat angina work in one way or another on this supply–demand can trigger severe ischemia and pain.

The drugs used to treat angina work in one way or another on this supply–demand imbalance. Most work by reducing oxygen demand. The choice of drug depends, to a great degree, on the type of angina that the patient has. In some cases, there are multiple causes, and the patient may need two or more drugs.

Types of Angina

There are basically two major types of angina (Table 34–1): chronic-stable and vasospastic angina. *Chronic-stable* (also called *exercise-induced*) angina is caused mainly by obstruction or narrowing of one or more coronary arteries by thrombi, atherosclerotic plaques, or both. These obstructions do not reduce blood flow enough to trigger signs and symptoms when the patient is at rest and oxygen demand is normal. However, when oxygen demands increase, as during exercise, blood flow cannot increase enough; it becomes inadequate for the heart, and angina occurs. The attack is accompanied by electrocardiogram (ECG) abnormalities, but usually there is no permanent heart muscle damage. Autopsies of patients with chronic-stable angina usually show some evidence of coronary occlusion by thrombi or plaques.

Chronic-stable angina can progress to *unstable angina*. In this case, the obstructions to coronary blood flow become so great that signs and symptoms can appear at rest, and they are more severe. Unstable angina is the most worrisome and potentially lethal form of angina. It can lead to permanent heart damage or a heart attack (one reason why unstable angina is sometimes called *preinfarction angina*). Unstable angina requires drug therapy but may not respond to it well; the eventual treatment is thrombolytic drug therapy or more invasive procedures, such as angioplasty or coronary artery bypass surgery, for example.

Vasospastic angina (also called *Prinzmetal's angina* or *variant angina*) is the second major type. It is caused by episodes of intense coronary artery vasoconstriction (spasm), not by artery obstruction or narrowing due to plaques of thrombi. (Indeed, autopsies on persons with vasospastic angina show coronary arteries that look quite normal and free of blockage or narrowing.) The causes of spasm usually are unknown, and exercise is not a consistent trigger. Symptoms usually occur at the same time each day, often in the early morning hours or shortly after awakening.

Treatment of Angina

Angina is treated first with drugs. When drugs fail to give adequate relief or when the risk of cardiac damage, dysfunction, or death is great or immediate, other approaches may be needed. These include thrombolytic drug administration (Chapter 35), angioplasty, or surgery.

The antianginal drugs fall in one of three major classes:

organic nitrate vasodilators (nitroglycerin, others),

calcium channel blockers, and

β-adrenergic blockers (eg, propranolol).

Depending on the type or severity of the angina and on other characteristics of the patient, a drug in any one of these three groups might be used first. Some patients require treatment with two antianginal drug classes; a few might require all three.

Objectives and Limitations of Antianginal Drug Therapy

The initial treatment goal during an acute angina attack is to relieve the pain and discomfort as quickly as possible. This involves bringing the supply–demand imbal-

Table 34–1 | Comparison of Chronic-Stable Angina and Variant Angina

Characteristic	Chronic-Stable Angina	Vasospastic Angina
Basic underlying cause	Myocardial oxygen demand > oxygen supply (ischemia)	Same as for chronic-stable angina
Cause of ischemia	Coronary artery obstruction with thrombi, atherosclerotic plaques	Coronary artery vasospasm
Appearance of coronary arteries at autopsy	Partially or completely obstructed (one or more) vessels	Usually "clean" unless patient also had history of chronic-stable angina
Intensity of attack	Very variable	Often severe
Common trigger(s) for attack, onset	Physical stress (eg, exercise), emotional stress	Unknown; often occurs in AM shortly before or after awakening
Usual effects of exercise ("stress") testing	Pain, ST segment depression on ECG (indicator of ischemia)	Pain, ST segment changes not common
Effects of antianginal drugs	All reduce myocardial oxygen demands; nitrates reduce only afterload (systemic BP); β blockers, some calcium channel blockers also lower HR	Nitrates, calcium channel blockers reduce oxygen demand as in chronic-stable angina; calcium channel blockers also reduce vasospasm; β blockers generally contraindicated (see p 692)
Occurrence of arrhythmias during attack	Variable	In about 50% of attacks

ance (the cause of ischemia and pain) back into balance. The long-term treatment goals are to maintain the balance, thereby reducing the frequency and severity of anginal pain and discomfort; to prevent or at least delay ischemic cardiac damage that can be potentially fatal; and to enable the patient to maintain a lifestyle that is as enjoyable, productive, and active as possible.

For most patients with angina, antianginal drug therapy only reduces or prevents a symptom; it does not cure or treat the underlying pathology. For example, if the angina is caused by atherosclerotic coronary artery disease, antianginal drugs may prevent ischemia and pain but will do nothing to reduce the artery blockage.

Organic Nitrate Vasodilators

PROTOTYPE

Nitroglycerin

Nitroglycerin is the prototype of several organic nitrate compounds that exert antianginal activity. Of all the available antianginal drugs, nitroglycerin is the drug of choice for treating ongoing attacks, and it has important prophylactic use as well. Plain nitroglycerin is not only effective but also the cheapest antianginal medication.

Table 34–2 Time-Course of Action of Nitroglycerin and Other Nitrates When Taken by Various Routes

Route of Administration	Onset of Action	Duration of Action
Nitroglycerin		
Sublingual tablet	1–3 min	30–60 min
Lingual spray	1–2 min	30–60 min
Buccal	1–2 min	3–5 hr*
Oral, sustained release	20–45 min	3–8 hr
Topical ointment	30–60 min	2–12 hr
Transdermal disc	30–60 min	18–24 hr
Amyl nitrite		
Inhalation	30 sec	3–5 min
Erythrityl tetranitrate		
Sublingual or chewable tablets	5 min	3 hr
Oral	30 min	6 hr
Isosoribide dinitrate		
Sublingual or chewable tablets	2–5 min	1–3 hr
Oral tablets	20–40 min	4–6 hr
Oral, sustained release	>1 h	6–8 hr
Isosorbide mononitrate		
Oral	30 min	—
Pentaerythritol tetranitrate		
Oral	20–60 min	3–6 hr
Oral, sustained release	30 min	about 12 hr

*The effects of nitroglycerin tablets administered buccally will last up to five hours if the tablet remains intact. Eating, drinking, or excessive salivation and swallowing will hasten tablet dissolution and shortens its duration of action.

Source: Adapted from *Drug Facts and Comparisons*, Facts and Comparisons, Inc., St. Louis, 1992.

Absorption, Distribution, Metabolism, and Excretion

Nitroglycerin is absorbed rapidly from the gastrointestinal (GI) tract. However, it is not very effective when taken orally because it is extensively metabolized in the liver before reaching the systemic circulation (via first-pass metabolism; see p 60). Nitroglycerin is absorbed well through the oral mucous membranes, the major site of nitroglycerin administration, and adequately through the skin. The liver and several other tissues metabolize nitroglycerin and related nitrate vasodilators to water-soluble compounds that are readily excreted by the kidneys. The effects of various routes of administration on nitroglycerin's duration of action are shown in Table 34–2.

Pharmacologic Effects

Nitroglycerin and related nitrates are given to patients with angina for their beneficial effects on the heart. However, their major cardiac actions are indirect and due to primary effects outside the heart. The major hemodynamic effects of nitroglycerin and other nitrates are summarized and compared with the actions of the other two major classes of antianginals, the calcium channel blockers and the β blockers, in Table 34–3. Although nitroglycerin and related drugs manage the symptom of ischemia—angina—they seldom affect the underlying causes.

Peripheral Vasodilation

Nitroglycerin and the other nitrates dilate peripheral arterioles and veins by relaxing vascular smooth muscle. (This effect does not involve inhibition of the sympathetic nervous system or blockade of the α-adrenergic receptors that mediate vasoconstriction.) Arteriolar dilation reduces peripheral resistance so that arterial pressure (afterload) decreases. Dilation of veins reduces venous return, which lowers diastolic ventricular filling pressure (preload) and the resting tension of the ventricular walls. Both effects decrease myocardial oxygen demand and prevent or alleviate anginal pain.

TRENDS AND CONTROVERSIES IN PHARMACOLOGY

Transdermal Drug Therapy

Some transdermal drug formulations have been available since the 1950s, but their use became widespread in the 1980s and can be expected to increase over the next decade. Ideal candidates for this formulation are drugs for which transdermal application should improve therapeutic control with fewer side effects and greater patient adherence, as compared to conventional formulations given by other routes. Cardiovascular drugs, hormones, narcotic analgesics, antineoplastic drugs, insulin, and drugs to combat motion sickness (eg, scopolamine) are some of the drugs now or soon to be available in this form.

Transdermal therapy has potential advantages over oral drugs. Transdermal drug formulations are significantly longer-acting and therefore allow for less frequent dosing. In the case of nitrates vasodilator/antianginal drugs for example, the duration of action of some common oral products is two to four hours, while nitroglycerin ointment lasts six to eight hours and nitroglycerin patches work for 24 hours (even though much shorter times for wearing the patch are recommended to reduce the risk of tolerance). Increased duration of action may translate into better patient acceptance and increased compliance. CATAPRES TTS-2, the transdermal formulation of the antihypertensive clonidine, is applied only once a week, resulting in greater convenience than oral drugs which are taken every 6 to 12 hours.

A drug that is absorbed through the skin avoids the problems inherent in GI absorption. Drugs entering the body through the GI tract have to compete with food and other drugs for absorption, and are subject to biorhythmic variation in GI motility that can increase or decrease the drug's effects. In addition, many drugs—nitroglycerin is one—undergo substantial first pass inactivation by the liver that eliminates much of an oral dose before it has a chance to enter the general circulation. Transdermal drugs also provide more consistent blood levels than oral formulations. In theory at least, once transdermal absorption is underway, a continuous feed of the drug from the product reservoir eliminates the peaks and valleys in serum levels that are inevitable with oral dosing. This should result in a more consistent therapeutic effect. And, because transdermal drugs don't have to hit high serum peaks to maintain a minimum effective concentration for a reasonable length of time, they should result in fewer side effects during the course of therapy.

The biggest disadvantage of transdermal drug products is probably their cost. For example, many consumers who change from an oral, short-acting nitrate to a transdermal form are taken aback when they learn that the new product costs two to six times as much as the oral medication. When the patient can afford this, and when transdermal therapy results in better control than oral drugs, the increased cost may be perfectly acceptable. For some people though, the actual benefit of transdermal drug therapy is not significant enough to offset the cost problem.

Remember, too, that while transdermal drugs offer convenience and potentially improved therapeutics they are hard for some people to manipulate. With arthritic or tremulous hands, it is virtually impossible to handle the ointment tube and paper or to separate the backing from a transdermal patch. A theoretically ideal drug product is not necessarily practical for everyone.

Berba J, Banakar U: Clinical efficacy of current transdermal drug delivery systems: A retrospective evaluation. *Am Pharm* 1990; NS30(11): 33-41.

When taking a medication history, determine not only whether the patient is taking nitroglycerin and the dosage, but also the dosage form. Different dosage forms have different proper uses; knowing which form the patient is taking provides more insight into the frequency or severity of the patient's coronary artery disease. Check further.

Allow sublingual or transmucosal nitroglycerin tablets to dissolve slowly under the tongue; advise the patient not to eat, drink, or smoke while some undissolved tablet remains.

Instruct the patient to swallow sustained-release nitroglycerin capsules or tablets whole; not to chew them or administer them sublingually; and not to open the capsules.

Use transdermal delivery systems as directed, usually on a cycle of 10 to 12 hours on and 10 to 12 hours off. Apply the patches to hairless areas of healthy, undamaged skin that are not subject to excessive motion or abrasion, preferably areas on the trunk or upper arms. Advise the patient not to bathe with patches on; to avoid excessively hot or humid environments (which could speed up drug absorption); and not to reuse patches. Rotate application sites to minimize the risk of local irritation.

Measure nitroglycerin ointment doses carefully, preferably with a ruler; use a disposable applicator stick, rubber gloves, or both to spread the drug evenly over 2 to 3 square inches of skin area; cover the application site with plastic wrap, if instructed to do so; and rotate application sites.

Be sure that patients who are treated with long-acting nitrates have a sublingual dosage form on hand at all times. If a long-acting preparation is the only one prescribed, double-check the medication order and the overall medication plan with the prescribing physician.

Institutional policies differ about nitroglycerin administration for hospitalized patients. If the patient has not been hospitalized for angina or cardiac disease, is able to self-medicate, has no other contraindicating conditions, and has a supply of immediate-acting nitroglycerin, the person might be allowed to keep the drug at the bedside. Advise these patients to notify the nurse each time they take their nitroglycerin; the nurse should chart each dose. For patients who are admitted for angina, many facilities require that medication be administered only by the nurse—often via nitroglycerin IV drip (see below). Always check with the physician first.

Help all patients learn to identify the lowest effective dosage of their immediate-acting dosage form. This requires some trial and error, but it can help maximize therapeutic effectiveness and minimize problems from side effects. If previously effective doses seem to lose their effectiveness with time, have the patient notify the physician at once.

◆ Medication Storage and Effectiveness

Review storage recommendations (see the package insert or label, or consult *The Physician's Desk Reference* or pharmacist) for each drug or product. Because heat, moisture, and light inactivate the drug, nitroglycerin sublingual tablets are dispensed in small amber glass bottles with metal screw caps. Advise patients not to transfer the drug to other containers.

Recommend that patients discard unused nitroglycerin tablets six months after the container is opened, but to be sure they have a fresh supply first. Some nitroglycerin tablets cause a tingling or slight burning sensation when placed under the tongue. For many years this has been used as an indicator of the drug's "freshness" or effectiveness. Do not rely on this; older patients may not experience this sensation, even with new nitroglycerin tablets, and some of the newer tablet formulations may not cause these responses in any patient. Advise patients that if they doubt the potency of their medication, they should have their prescription refilled and discard the old medication. Nitroglycerin sprays have about a three-year storage life at room temperature; nevertheless, they should not be exposed to excessive heat, such as in the glove box or on the dashboard of an automobile.

◆ Identification and Prevention of Angina Triggers

Help patients identify stressors that trigger anginal attacks so that they can avoid or minimize these factors. When drug pretreatment is needed in anticipation of stress, have patients administer the proper sublingual drug 5 to 10 minutes before stress onset. Encourage them to keep a written log of symptom onset, dosages used, and the responses (desired and otherwise) to drug administration.

◆ Recognizing Signs of a Possible Heart Attack

Stress the importance of calling 911 (or a suitable emergency number) if three sublingual doses, taken over 15 minutes, fail to relieve all distress. Other responses to this potential emergency—calling the doctor or hospital (unless personnel can dispatch an ambulance or fire department crew) or driving the patient to the doctor or hospital, for example—are unsuitable and outright dangerous.

Indications for Intravenous Nitroglycerin

Nitroglycerin solutions formulated for slow IV infusion, or "drips" (NITRO-BID-IV, TRIDIL) have several indications. Typical dosages, which must be individualized for each patient based on their clinical response, are given in Table 34–S. For each of these uses, the prototype emergency antihypertensive drug nitroprusside (Chapter 33) can be used instead. Nitroglycerin has one major advantage over the alternative: It will not cause potentially fatal cyanide poisoning, which can occur with prolonged or high-dosage nitroprusside administration.

Severe or Refractory Angina

Nitroglycerin can be administered intravenously to control angina when maximum doses of other nitrates and adjuncts (calcium channel blockers, β blockers), given by more common administration routes, do not give adequate relief. (Even for patients whose only antianginal medication is nitroglycerin, the IV dosage form may be used instead of others in the hospital setting.) Nitroglycerin therapy for these indications is usually followed by more invasive procedures, such as thrombolysis, angioplasty, or bypass.

Heart Failure Following Myocardial Infarction

Nitroglycerin can be used to reduce afterload (blood pressure) in the post-MI patient with acute heart failure. In this instance, the goal is to reduce the failing heart's workload and improve cardiac output, not to relieve chest pain.

Perioperative Blood Pressure Control

Intravenous nitroglycerin can be used for short-term control of hypertension that might occur before, during, or after various surgical or diagnostic procedures (eg, anesthesia induction, intubation, skin incision). The drug can also be used to induce slight hypotension intraoperatively, as might be done to reduce bleeding from surgical wounds (eg, in neurosurgery).

NURSING IMPLICATIONS

Several general guidelines apply to all infused nitroglycerin preparations:

- Nitroglycerin must be diluted before administration and then used within 24 hours. Consult the manufacturer's instructions or the hospital pharmacy before diluting the drug, because different products come in different strengths. Normal saline containing 5% dextrose is the recommended diluent.
- Nitroglycerin binds to the polyvinylchloride (PVC) plastic that is used to make most IV solution bags and infusion sets. So much drug can bind to the plastic that very little—often an unpredictable amount—reaches the patient's circulation. Therefore, store the diluted solution in a glass bottle, and use the infusion sets, which are made of special plastic, supplied by the nitroglycerin manufacturer or distributor. Use PVC sets only when proper sets are not available, and anticipate the need for dosage increases when they are used. Continuously monitor key vital signs (eg, ECG, arterial pressures, and central venous pressure if possible); the clinical responses provide essential information needed to adjust the dose.

Side Effects, Adverse Reactions, and Contraindications

Table 34–S summarizes the side effects for nitroglycerin. Most of them involve effects on the cardiovascular system.

Cardiovascular Side Effects

The most common side effects of nitroglycerin (Table 34–S) result from the drug's ability to cause peripheral vasodilation and, potentially, to lower blood pressure. They can arise regardless of the dosage form that is used. However, the cardiovascular side effects are most likely to appear suddenly with the formulations meant for self-administration, and are more intense with the immediate-acting dosage forms.

Headache is relatively common and potentially distressing, especially during the first few weeks of sublingual nitroglycerin therapy. It is thought to occur because of nitrate-induced dilation of the cerebral blood vessels (and so has been called "vascular headache"). Fortunately, tolerance usually develops after one to two weeks of therapy. Until then, analgesic drugs (aspirin or acetaminophen, depending on other relevant medical conditions or drug use) can be used to relieve the pain. Headache may persist in some patients, however.

For many patients, cerebral vasodilation and the headache it causes are mainly annoying. However, cerebral vasodilation also can increase intracranial pressure, which can be very dangerous for patients with a history of stroke, brain neoplasms, or closed-head injury. Nitroglycerin is therefore relatively contraindicated for these patients.

Hypotension is another side effect that may pose risks or dangers to some patients, including those with strokes or a history of cerebral ischemia. Hypotension is dose-dependent. When nitroglycerin or other nitrates are used to manage angina, the dose is adjusted so that systolic blood pressure does not fall by more than 10 mm Hg. (See Chapter 33 for general goals for reducing blood pressure during a hypertensive episode.) Blood pressure falls that are too fast or too great can cause dizziness or fainting and feelings of generalized weakness or uneasiness. Excessive blood pressure falls can also deprive organs (eg, the brain and heart) of blood flow, thereby worsening myocardial or cerebral edema.

Hypotension can trigger another side effect that can be particularly dangerous, especially for persons with cardiac disease—**reflex tachycardia**. Tachycardia occurs when the baroreceptors (located in the carotid sinus and aortic arch) sense a blood pressure fall that is too great or too fast. The outcome is an increase of sympathetic nervous system activity that leads to increased heart rate. Palpitations or arrhythmias may also occur. In addition, generalized sympathetic activation increases cardiac contractility and can cause vasoconstriction.

These reflex responses are the body's attempts to counteract drug-induced blood pressure changes. However, all these effects increase the heart's workload, thereby reducing the antianginal drug's effectiveness in normalizing the oxygen supply–demand imbalance. In short, reflex sympathetic activation counteracts some of the desired direct effects of the drug. The outcome can be poorer control of angina and the underlying ischemia, an increased frequency of severity of anginal attacks, or a worsening or appearance of other cardiac problems, particularly arrhythmias.

These risks underscore the need to adjust nitrate dosages to prevent excessive falls in blood pressure. For those patients in whom reflex tachycardia and other related responses pose a real risk or problem, adjunctive drugs, such as β-adrenergic blockers (see below), may be needed to control them.

Other Side Effects

A small number of patients experience GI upset or fecal or urinary incontinence. Sublingual or buccal nitroglycerin administration can cause burning or tingling in the mouth (see Nursing Implications for medication storage and effectiveness, above). Nitroglycerin ointment or transdermal systems can cause dermatitis.

NURSING IMPLICATIONS

Review the expected side effects with patients when they are started on nitrate therapy. Advise them of side effects to which they are likely to develop tolerance, and instruct them to report side effects that seem intolerable or unusual or that persist after several weeks of treatment. It is particularly important to assess for headache, dizziness, increases of heart rate, and palpitations. Teach standard precautions to minimize lightheadedness caused by hypotension on standing. For patients receiving IV nitroglycerin, continuously monitor blood pressure and the ECG.

◆ Use During Pregnancy and Lactation

Therapeutic doses of nitroglycerin are probably not harmful to the pregnant woman or fetus. However, as with other drugs, the potential risks and benefits of drug therapy, or withholding it, must be evaluated before and during treatment. A major concern is excessive maternal hypotension, which can reduce placental blood flow. Ensuring that the dose does not lower maternal blood pressure excessively can minimize this problem.

◆ Use in Children

Nitroglycerin is used mainly as an IV afterload-reducing drug for severe heart failure or for intraoperative blood pressure control. Dosages are based on body weight, the indication, and the response.

◆ Use in the Elderly

Elderly persons are generally less tolerant of sudden or dramatic changes of blood pressure. The risks of postural hypotension and fainting are greater. Likewise, the prevalence of cardiac and vascular disease in this population increases other risks associated with hypotension and tachycardia. Physical, mental, or sensory impairments may cause elderly outpatients great difficulty in using nitroglycerin properly. (For example, there have been reports of nitroglycerin overdoses caused by mistaking nitroglycerin ointment for toothpaste.) Devise strategies to improve proper use (eg, large labels, screw caps), recruit the help of another responsible person, and provide written lists of proper drug use for whoever will supervise therapy.

Interactions with Other Drugs

As a general rule, *all* antianginal drugs can interact with

- virtually all antihypertensive agents, which can cause excessive hypotension and worsening of myocardial or cerebral ischemia;
- nearly all sympathomimetics (α- or β-adrenergic agonists, including those available over the counter [OTC]), which can cause excessive cardiac stimulation, vasoconstriction, or both (depending on the specific sympathomimetic), thereby counteracting desired antianginal drugs;
- thyroid hormones, which also stimulate the heart;
- nicotine (ie, from smoking), which causes vasoconstriction and stimulates the heart;
- alcohol, which can cause significant vasodilation; and
- ergot alkaloids, such as dihydroergotamine. These drugs have been cited as particularly important interactants because they can simultaneously increase

systemic blood pressure and directly constrict the coronary arteries (Table 34–I).

NURSING IMPLICATIONS

Prescription drugs that can interact with antianginal drugs are often administered with the latter agents. Monitor the patient's responses and vital signs accordingly, and closely. Discourage the patient from using OTC interactants (eg, cold, decongestant, or weight-loss medications that contain sympathomimetics) unless such use is approved by a physician. For most patients, moderate alcohol consumption causes no problems; nevertheless, each patient should discuss this with the physician. Smoking should be stopped altogether. The use of nicotine-containing smoking deterrents (eg, HABITROL, NICODERM, PROSTEP; see Chapter 16) by angina patients must be evaluated on a case-by-case basis by the physician; they should not be administered to any recent post-MI patient.

Overdose and Toxicity

Nitrate overdoses cause dose-dependent hypotension and reflex tachycardia. Simultaneous increases of oxygen demand and decreases of oxygen supply may cause acute myocardial ischemia and possibly myocardial infarction. Hypotension may also cause cerebral ischemia and stroke. Clinically significant hypotension may occur even when "recommended" doses are administered to patients who are hypovolemic or who are receiving other antihypertensive medications. Proper management includes temporary discontinuation of nitroglycerin administration, because the drug's short duration of action usually allows blood pressure to rise in a relatively short time. If an intentional overdose is taken orally, induced emesis (as permitted by the patient's condition) and other measures to reduce drug absorption may be indicated. Vasopressors may be given to correct excessive hypotension. However, they must be used cautiously to avoid coronary artery vasoconstriction, which may further aggravate angina. Epinephrine should *not* be used: it may lower myocardial blood flow and oxygen supply by reducing diastolic pressure and almost always increases oxygen demands by causing tachycardia. Oxygen therapy is indicated. It helps overcome inadequate tissue oxygenation owing to hypotension and methemoglobinemia, another potential accompaniment of nitrate overdoses. If the patient becomes cyanotic or other indicators of tissue hypoxia are present, oxygen is administered.

Nitroglycerin allergy is relatively uncommon. If it does occur, alternative nitrates may be substituted to maintain therapy. Most individuals who experience an allergic reaction can tolerate another nitrate.

Related Drugs

Amyl Nitrite, Erythrityl Tetranitrate, Isosorbide Mononitrate and Dinitrate, and Pentaerythritol Tetranitrate

Amylnitrite, erythrityl tetranitrate, isosorbide mononitrate and dinitrate, and pentaerythritol tetranitrate are alternatives to nitroglycerin. In general, they act in the same way as the prototype, share similar uses (depending on the dosage form) and drug interactions, and cause similar side effects. Table 34–2 summarizes typical onsets and durations of action of these alternatives. These pharmacokinetic factors determine whether the drug is suitable for prophylaxis or treatment of angina (like sublingual nitroglycerins) or for long-term prevention of recurrences. Specific indications and usual dosages are listed in Table 34–C.

Amyl nitrate is supplied as a capsule that is administered by crushing it, waving it under the nose, and inhaling the vapors. It is indicated for immediate relief of angina. Erythrityl tetranitrate (CARDILATE) tablets can be administered sublingually for prophylaxis of acute angina or taken orally. Isosorbide mononitrate (ISMO), isosorbide dinitrate (ISORDIL, SORBITRATE, many others), and pentaerythritol tetranitrate (eg, PERITRATE), are available in standard and sustained-release tablets for oral administration. These drugs and dosage forms should be used only for long-term prophylaxis. (Pentaerythritol tetranitrate is listed as "possibly effective" for angina relief and prophylaxis.) Isosorbide dinitrate is also available in sublingual and chewable tablets; these are indicated for immediate relief of angina.

NURSING IMPLICATIONS

Overall, all nursing implications noted for nitroglycerin apply to these drugs. It is important to reemphasize two points:

- Patients who are being treated with any long-acting oral nitrate must have a supply of an immediate-acting dosage form on hand in case it is needed.

- When taking a medication history, identify the name, the dose, and the dosage form of the antianginal drug(s) that has been prescribed.

Dipyridamole

Dipyridamole (PERSANTINE) has been used for many years for the long-term prophylaxis of angina. Supposedly, the drug acts as a "selective" coronary vasodilator. Nevertheless, dipyridamole's effectiveness for angina has been questioned, and in the near future the drug will no longer be approved for that use.

Dipyridamole also seems to reduce the ability of blood platelets to attach to the surfaces of artificial heart valves. Such attachment eventually destroys the platelets. Because of this effect, dipyridamole is approved as an adjunct to anticoagulant drugs for preventing thromboembolism in patients who have received a heart valve prostheses. This use is discussed further in Chapter 35.

Calcium Channel Blockers

Most cell membranes have special ion channels that allow calcium to flow into the cell. Calcium influx through the channels, which is normally controlled by neurotransmitters or hormones such as norepinephrine and epinephrine, plays an essential role in several aspects of cardiovascular function. For example, calcium influx is necessary for initiating contraction of all muscles in the body, including cardiac and vascular smooth muscle. It regulates the intensity of force during cardiac contraction and regulates blood pressure by controlling the intensity of vasoconstriction. Calcium entry into the cells is also important in the generation and conduction of electrical impulses through the heart. This is especially important in nodal tissues and the specialized conduction pathways linking various heart regions, which regulate cardiac rate and rhythm.

Drugs that inhibit the entry of calcium ions through cell membrane channels are called *calcium channel blockers,* or *calcium antagonists.* Through their major pharmacologic actions, and because of the importance of calcium influx in cardiovascular control, calcium channel blockers can affect many aspects of cardiovascular function. Verapamil (ISOPTIN, CALAN) was the first calcium channel blocker approved for use in the United States. Several related agents are now approved and widely used. They fall in different chemical classes, but verapamil still serves as the prototype of the entire group.

PROTOTYPE

Verapamil

Absorption, Distribution, Metabolism, and Excretion

Verapamil is absorbed well from the GI tract. It undergoes extensive first-pass metabolism in the liver. With continued administration, the plasma half-life is about 12 hours.

Pharmacologic Effects

The ability of verapamil to block calcium entry affects the function of all muscle cells in the body. From a therapeutic viewpoint, however, the effects on cardiac and vascular smooth muscle and on the specialized nodal and impulse-conducting tissues of the heart are most important. These actions and their related therapeutic uses include the following:

- Verapamil decreases myocardial contractile force, thereby reducing cardiac workload and oxygen demands. The use of verapamil and some other calcium channel blockers as antianginal agents is attributable to this action.
- Verapamil decreases heart rate, automaticity, and electrical impulse conduction. The decrease in heart rate contributes to the drug's antianginal effects. Actions on automaticity and other electrophysiologic properties of the heart account for the antiarrhythmic activity of some of these agents.
- Verapamil decreases vasoconstriction (ie, allows vasodilation) in the coronary and systemic circulations. This can lower blood pressure, and accounts for the use of verapamil and some of the alternatives as antihypertensive agents. Because calcium influx into smooth muscle cells occurs during coronary artery spasm, the ability of verapamil and related drugs to inhibit that process also explains their effectiveness in treating vasospastic angina.

For a given dose or blood level of verapamil, each of these effects occurs to roughly equal degrees. Thus, verapamil has the most uses (indications) of all the calcium channel blockers. The uses of the related calcium channel blockers are more limited. Some are much more effective as vasodilators but have a much lower cardiac-depressant effect, for example.

	Bepridil	Diltiazem	Diltiazem SR,CD	Diltiazem IV	Felodipine SR	Isradipine	Nicardipine	Nicardipine SR	Nicardipine IV	Nifedipine	Nifedipine SR	Nimodipine	**Verapamil**	**Verapamil SR**	**Verapamil IV**
Angina															
Chronic-stable	X	X					X			X	X		X		
Unstable													X		
Vasospastic		X								X	X		X		
Essential hypertension			X		X	X	X	X			X		X	X	
Acute hypertension									X						
Arrhythmias				X											X
Subarachnoid hemorrhage												X			

Figure 34–1

Calcium channel blockers: drugs, dosage forms, and approved uses. X = approved use; SR = sustained-release oral dosage form (manufacturers may use other designations for these formulations); IV = intravenous dosage form; all others are oral dosage forms.

Clinical Indications and Administration

Typical dosages of verapamil for its various indications and dosage forms are summarized in Table 34–C and Figure 34–1.

Angina Pectoris

Immediate-acting oral dosage forms of verapamil are indicated for treating chronic-stable, unstable, and vasospastic, angina. Currently, verapamil is the only calcium channel blocker approved for all these types. Regardless of the type of angina that is being treated, however, verapamil's onset of action is too slow to prevent or stop an angina attack quickly. (For that use, a rapidly acting nitrate is indicated and must therefore be kept on hand.) Thus, the approved calcium channel blockers are used only for long-term prophylaxis of angina.

Arrhythmias

Verapamil is an important antiarrhythmic drug. Immediate-acting oral dosage forms and a parenteral formulation given as a slow IV injection are used to control supraventricular arrhythmias. The antiarrhythmic actions and uses of verapamil and other antiarrhythmic agents are discussed further in Chapter 30.

NURSING IMPLICATIONS

Do not add the IV verapamil solution to any IV fluid that has a neutral or alkaline pH (eg, those containing sodium bicarbonate); the drug will precipitate. Albumin and several other injectable drugs also cause precipitation or inactivation. Check the package insert first if you must dilute the verapamil before administration. Always have resuscitation facilities readily available when giving this drug by the IV route.

Essential Hypertension

Oral verapamil is indicated for treating essential hypertension. Indeed, verapamil or another calcium antagonist (see below) is often the first drug to be prescribed for many hypertensive patients. The patient can be started with immediate-acting oral dosage forms and then switched to maintenance therapy with a sustained-acting formulation. (Treatment of essential hypertension is currently the only approved use for sustained-acting preparations.) The use of calcium channel blockers and other medications for treating essential hypertension is covered in more detail in Chapter 33.

Unapproved Uses

Oral verapamil, and some of the related calcium channel blockers, appear to be effective for managing several conditions for which these drugs are not currently approved. Cardiovascular uses include management of paroxysmal supraventricular tachycardia and nocturnal leg cramping. In neurology, these drugs are being studied for prophylaxis of migraine and cluster headache. Verapamil and some of the related drugs may reduce bronchoconstriction in persons with exercise-induced asthma. Blocking calcium influx into muscle cells seems to account for the effectiveness of these drugs. Calcium channel blockers are also being evaluated for their ability to help alleviate signs and symptoms of manic-depressive illness. The mechanism of action has not been fully determined. With further clinical testing and the development of new dosage forms and drugs, many of these uses will no doubt become approved, and many other uses will be found.

Side Effects, Adverse Reactions, and Contraindications

Side Effects During Administration

Table 34–S summarizes the key side effects associated with verapamil therapy. In practice, they are seldom serious enough to cause discontinuation of the drug or major dosage changes. They are more likely to occur with long-term administration of oral verapamil (ie, during outpatient therapy) than with short-term use of the injectable dosage form. Persons with impaired liver function tend to be at a greater risk of side effects, owing to decreased verapamil metabolism; therefore, they require dosages lower than those recommended for patients with normal liver function.

Constipation is the most common side effect of oral verapamil. Somewhat fewer than 10% of patients experience this side effect, but for some of these individuals it may be severe enough to require a dosage reduction or discontinuation of the drug altogether. The incidence is probably higher in the elderly. Other noteworthy side effects, listed in decreasing order of frequency, include dizziness or lightheadedness, hypotension and peripheral edema, nausea, and headache. Collectively, these unwanted responses affect fewer than 1% to 2% of all patients taking this prototype agent.

Hypersensitivity reactions to verapamil are uncommon, but they contraindicate further use. These reactions include hives, skin rashes, and the like. These are unrelated to any of the main pharmacologic effects of the drug. Other contraindications involve, in one way or another, verapamil's cardiovascular actions. Because of its potential hypotensive and cardiac-depressant actions, the drug should not be administered to persons with preexisting hypotension (including hypotension associated with shock or severe heart failure); heart block greater than first degree; and sick sinus syndrome. For *all* patients with heart failure, verapamil must be used with more care, and closer assessment is required. One paradoxical effect of the drug is a rapid increase in ventricular rate in some patients with atrial fibrillation or flutter. See Chapter 30 for more information about this side effect.

Verapamil is being used as a treatment for some patients with idiopathic hypertrophic subaortic stenosis (IHSS), a serious cardiomyopathy that involves severe narrowing of the left ventricle's blood outflow pathway. However, several patients with advanced or refractory IHSS have died during verapamil therapy.

Potential Adverse Effects on Sudden Discontinuation of Therapy

There is some evidence that abruptly stopping long-term administration of calcium channel blockers can cause more frequent or more severe angina attacks. Whether this finding is common or clinically important is controversial. (There is no doubt that this type of "withdrawal syndrome" occurs on abrupt discontinuation of β blockers [see below] and can be fatal.) Nevertheless, the best advice is not to stop antianginal therapy with drugs such as verapamil quickly but to taper the dose, if possible.

NURSING IMPLICATIONS

Recommend adequate daily intake of water and bulk-forming foods as the preferred method for dealing with constipation. Laxatives should be used under a physician's supervision.

◆ Use During Pregnancy and Lactation

There are no reports of fetal harm caused to humans by usual dosages of verapamil. The drug can be used during pregnancy as long as maternal vital signs (eg, blood pressure, cardiac function) are within normal limits. Verapamil is excreted in maternal milk, where the drug's concentrations may come close to those found in the mother's serum. However, it is unclear whether the drug causes adverse effects in the newborn. If the drug is used and the mother wishes to breast-feed, monitor the child for side effects.

◆ Use in Children

The IV dosage form of verapamil is generally used as an antiarrhythmic in children. Dosages are adjusted to body weight. Children less than six months old may, for one reason or another, be unresponsive to verapamil.

◆ Use in the Elderly

Because of reduced hepatic and cardiac function, the elderly usually require reduced dosages of verapamil. Anticipate a greater incidence of side effects, even when the dosage is adjusted.

Interactions with Other Drugs

Table 34–I summarizes the major drugs that can interact with verapamil. Many of these interactants are cardiovascular drugs that are often administered with verapamil or a related agent. They include β-adrenergic blockers, digitalis (especially digoxin), quinidine, and the α-blocking antihypertensive drug prazosin. The combined use of one of these interactants with verapamil is fairly common, because one drug can increase the desired actions of the other. If the dosages are not adjusted (in most cases, reduced) properly, however, the effects of one or both interactants can be excessive and potentially toxic.

Other important interactants are carbamazepine, an anticonvulsant, and cyclosporine, which is widely used to suppress rejection of transplanted organs. Verapamil inhibits their metabolic inactivation and thus can increase their effects or the risk of toxicity. In contrast, rifampin (an antitubercular drug) can stimulate verapamil's metabolic inactivation, lower its blood levels, and reduce its effectiveness.

Verapamil weakly blocks calcium influx that is necessary for skeletal muscle contraction. When the drug is administered alone and at usual dosages, side effects on skeletal muscle rarely occur. However, this action can significantly increase skeletal muscle paralysis caused by tubocurarine and related neuromuscular blockers. The outcome of the interaction is greater and more prolonged muscle dysfunction.

Overdose and Toxicity

Nausea is a common symptom of verapamil overdoses. Other common signs and symptoms include generalized weakness, drowsiness, dizziness, confusion, and slurred speech. These are usually caused by inadequate cerebral blood flow that results from decreased cardiac function and blood pressure. The major cardiovascular changes include depressed cardiac contractility, rate, and electrical impulse conduction and an inability of the blood vessels to constrict adequately. Therefore, assessment shows bradycardia, hypotension, and rhythm disturbances such as atrioventricular (AV) block. At the extreme, cardiac failure, edema, and cardiogenic shock can develop.

For recent overdoses that involve oral dosage forms, induced emesis and gastric lavage are indicated (see Appendix C). If needed, further treatment of any overdose, by any administration route, involves supportive care of symptoms.

Initially, place the patient in Trendelenburg's position to help increase cerebral blood flow. The goal is then to normalize cardiovascular function, and the approach usually involves drugs used to treat acute heart failure of any other cause (see Chapter 31, pp 591–592). These include inotropic catecholamines (eg, isoproterenol, dopamine, or dobutamine), which stimulate cardiac output and normalize abnormal impulse conduction. Improving cardiac function usually helps restore blood pressure. Diuretics are used as needed to combat edema. Calcium chloride is often given intravenously to "drive" calcium through blocked calcium channels, thereby helping to restore normal cardiac and vascular function.

NURSING IMPLICATIONS

With calcium channel blocker overdoses, anticipate that the patient will be critically ill. Invasive, constant monitoring is indicated until vital signs become and remain stable and within acceptable limits.

Remember that decreased cardiac output or true shock caused by calcium channel blocker overdoses is cardiogenic; it is *not* due to hypovolemia. Therefore, do not administer large volumes of IV fluids to raise blood pressure. Excessive volume will "fill up" the dilated vasculature, and the heart will be too weak to circulate it effectively. Overall, administering IV fluids worsens edema and heart failure, doing more harm than good. Maintain venous access, and infuse fluids slowly and carefully. Adjust the infusion rate according to the patient's condition and the response to drugs given to support the cardiovascular system.

Related Drugs

More than a half dozen calcium channel blockers, in addition to verapamil, are approved for use in the United States. More are on the way. All the related calcium channel blockers are extensively metabolized, but some form active metabolites that must be eliminated by renal excretion. Thus, for any of these drugs impaired liver function requires a reduced dose, and impaired renal function may affect the dosage as well.

All the related calcium channel blockers share verapamil's basic mechanism of action on cardiac and vascular smooth muscle. However, they differ in the intensity of vasodilation that a typical therapeutic dose or blood level causes, as compared to the degree that they depress cardiac contractility or electrical activity. To some extent, these differences affect the clinical uses of these drugs, especially with oral administration routes.

Some of the related agents are indicated for treating only angina or only essential hypertension; some are indicated for both. Moreover, for some of these drugs the oral dosage form (immediate-acting or sustained-release) affects the use. (See Figure 34–1 for a quick overview of the indications for each dosage formulation, and Table 34–C for dosages.) These differences also affect the side effects profiles to some extent (Table 34–S).

Most of the drug–drug interactions noted for verapamil apply to the related drugs. However, a few interactions apply more to one related agent than to the others (Table 34–I). Overall, the safety of using one of these alternatives with nitrates, a β blocker, or other antihypertensive agents depends on which drugs will be used, their dosages, the patient's overall needs and condition, and the ability of care providers to monitor the desired and potentially unwanted responses adequately.

NURSING IMPLICATIONS

Although many of the other calcium channel blockers are indicated for angina, none should be relied on to manage acute angina. Only rapidly acting nitrates (eg, sublingual or IV nitroglycerin) should be used for that purpose.

Bepridil

Bepridil (VASCOR) is very different from verapamil and the other related drugs. It is available only in immediate-acting oral dosage forms and is approved only for preventing attacks of chronic-stable angina. However, bepridil is not a first-line antianginal drug. Alternatives should be tried first because bepridil therapy has been associated with two potentially serious adverse effects that are not as common when other agents are used:

- *Agranulocytosis.* This depression of the white blood cell count can make the body susceptible to potentially fatal infections.
- *Arrhythmias.* Bepridil has pharmacologic properties that are similar to those of several Class IC antiarrhythmics (see encainide and flecainide, Chapter 30, for more details). Paradoxically, these arrhythmia-treating drugs can cause serious or fatal cardiac arrhythmias (a proarrhythmic effect) in some patients, particularly those who have recently suffered a heart attack and have or are prone to developing arrhythmias. The risk may apply to bepridil. This potential danger is important, because myocardial ischemia causes not only angina but also arrhythmias.

Bepridil also tends to cause dizziness and lightheadedness, headache, or nausea much more often than most of the other calcium channel blockers.

NURSING IMPLICATIONS

Before bepridil therapy is started, check the medication history to determine whether other antianginal drugs have been tried. During treatment, monitor as you would for verapamil, but also assess closely for evidence of infection and the appearance of new or worsening arrhythmias. Teach patients how to assess their pulse for irregularities, and encourage them to report changes. Teach patients to anticipate bepridil's more common side effects and to report them if they become prolonged or intolerable.

Diltiazem

Diltiazem (CARDIZEM), used for angina or hypertension, is more similar to verapamil than any other currently approved calcium channel blocker. Diltiazem is available in immediate- and long-acting oral and parenteral (IV) dosage forms. Like verapamil, diltiazem causes peripheral vasodilation, decreases myocardial contractility, and inhibits automaticity and impulse conduction rates to roughly equal degrees for a given dose.

The side effects caused by diltiazem and verapamil are similar in most respects. However, diltiazem appears to cause depression of AV conduction or heart rate, peripheral edema, dizziness, and headache more often than the prototype.

Felodipine, Isradipine, Nicardipine, and Nifedipine

Felodipine (PLENDIL), isradipine (DYNACIRC), nicardipine (CARDENE), and nifedipine (ADALAT, PROCARDIA) belong to the largest chemical class of calcium channel blockers, called *dihydropyridines.* Each of these drugs comes in at least one oral dosage form. They are used for essential hypertension, angina prophylaxis, or both, depending on the drug and dosage form (Figure 34–1 and Table 34–C). An injectable formulation of nicardipine is indicated for treating acute hypertensive episodes. It is given by slow IV injection.

Compared with the other calcium channel blockers that are used for angina or hypertension, these agents are much more active as vasodilators than as depressants of cardiac contractility, rate, or electrical activity. The decreased peripheral resistance contributes to the antianginal and antihypertensive actions. Bradycardia is very uncommon with these drugs, because they cause reflex increases of cardiac stimulation. Indeed, reflex tachycardia may occur. All these drugs tend to increase cardiac output significantly.

Overall, the most common side effects caused by felodipine, isradipine, nicardipine, and nifedipine are peripheral edema, flushing, lightheadedness or dizziness, and headache. (These side effects have been noted for diltiazem, but they occur much more often with the dihydropyridines.)

NURSING IMPLICATIONS

Of the four drugs mentioned in this section, only nifedipine is available in immediate- and long-acting oral dosage forms. Both dosage forms are indicated for angina, but only the former is used to start treatment.

Tablets and capsules of these and other calcium channel blocking drugs should be swallowed whole—not crushed, broken, or chewed. However, with immediate-acting nifedipine, in particular, this guideline is sometimes broken. Immediate-acting nifedipine is supplied in soft capsules that contain the drug in the form of a thick liquid. When the clinical goal is a faster antihypertensive or antianginal effect than can be achieved by swallowing the capsule whole, some care providers pierce the capsules many times and then give them to the patient to chew; sometimes they are inserted as a rectal suppository or the drug squeezed into the sublingual area.

These approaches do give high blood levels rather quickly (with sublingual or rectal administration, the drug is absorbed by a route that avoids significant first-pass metabolic inactivation by the liver). However, the use of these administration routes is controversial. They may work in an emergency, when other drugs are not available. But when there is an urgent need to alleviate acute angina, the preferred treatment is a rapidly acting nitrate (eg, sublingual nitroglycerin). When the goal is to reduce blood pressure quickly, a suitable injectable antihypertensive, such as nitroprusside (Chapter 33), is used.

Nimodipine

Nimodipine (NIMOTOP), like nifedipine and the other dihydropyridines, exerts little cardiac-depressant activity but is a very effective vasodilator. However, it differs from the other calcium channel blockers because, in clinical practice, its vasodilator and antivasospasm actions appear to be particularly strong on cerebral arteries. Nimodipine exerts a much less pronounced effect on the peripheral vasculature. Its major effect on the brain's vascular supply is probably due to nimodipine's high lipid solubility, which allows it to cross the blood–brain barrier easily.

Because of these unique properties and site of action, nimodipine has a unique indication. It is currently used only in the therapy of subarachnoid hemorrhage. Presumably, nimodipine alleviates cerebral vasospasm that occurs in this condition. Effectiveness is assessed, in part, by an increased level of consciousness and greater mental and motor function.

The most common side effect caused by nimodipine is facial flushing. The drug rarely causes the other systemic side effects noted for other calcium channel blockers.

Beta-Adrenergic Blockers

Beta blockers block the β subtypes of the adrenergic receptors, which are normally stimulated by drugs such as epinephrine. The β blockers are discussed in detail in Chapter 15; only major points that relate to their use as antianginal drugs are summarized here.

Only four of the 12 β blockers marketed in the United States are approved for treating angina: two of the cardioselective (β_1) drugs, atenolol (TENORMIN) and metoprolol (LOPRESSOR); and two nonselective (β_1 and β_2) blockers, nadolol (CORGARD) and propranolol (INDERAL, the group prototype). Although the number of β blockers approved for angina is much smaller than the number approved for treating essential hypertension—another major indication for the overall group (see Chapter 33)—these drugs are important for many patients with angina nonetheless. Usual dosages are given in Table 34–C.

Antianginal Actions and Uses

The β blockers are useful in their own right for the prophylaxis of chronic-stable angina. For some patients these may be the only drugs used for preventing attacks. The major beneficial actions affect the heart: they all lead to decreased myocardial oxygen demands, and they all are due to the ability of these drugs to block the cardiac-stimulating effects of norepinephrine and epinephrine.

Proper doses of a β blocker decrease heart rate and contractility, thereby reducing myocardial oxygen demands. Through these effects, β blockers also reduce blood pressure slightly, particularly in hypertensive patients. This afterload-reducing effect also reduces the heart's workload.

The β blockers are also important adjuncts to therapy of chronic-stable or unstable angina involving other drugs (eg, nitroglycerin or other nitrates, and some of the calcium antagonists) that trigger reflex cardiac stimulation. As noted before, this reflex effect is counterproductive to angina treatment because it increases oxygen demands. Beta blockade prevents this unwanted response.

General Precautions

When β blockers are used for any indication, side effects and related contraindications may prevent their safe use, or at least increase the risk of problems. These include

- cardiac failure, bradycardia, or AV conduction blocks, especially if severe (β blockers can weaken an already failing heart, slow heart rate more, or worsen the conduction problem);
- asthma or severe chronic obstructive pulmonary disease (β blockers prevent the bronchodilator activity of epinephrine in the bloodstream, favoring bronchoconstriction or bronchospasm that has, occasionally, been fatal); and
- diabetes mellitus (β blockers lower blood glucose levels and can prolong hypoglycemic episodes that may occur).

The β blockers can also interact, in desired or unwanted ways, with many drugs. Interactions with other classes of antianginal drugs have been noted above. See Table 15–I (pp 249–250) for a more complete listing.

Special Precautions for Use in Angina

Even when the indication is angina, the nurse must be aware of several aspects of β blocker therapy:

- *Beta blockers are for prophylaxis only.* No β blocker acts quickly enough to alleviate an ongoing attack. Do not administer them with the assumption that they will, and be sure the patient understands that also. Only such drugs as sublingual or intravenous nitroglycerin are acutely effective.
- *Beta blockers can worsen vasospastic angina.* These drugs should be used with care, if at all, when the patient's major or only form of angina is vasospastic. The coronary arteries contain both α-adrenergic receptors, which cause vasoconstriction, and β receptors, which cause vasodilation. Normally, the circulating epinephrine that is constantly bathing these blood vessels causes some β-mediated vasodilation that simultaneously cancels out some of the opposing α-mediated vasoconstriction. Blocking just the β receptors favors vasoconstriction and vasospasm, and the frequency or severity of vasospastic anginal attacks can increase. (When the cause of angina is *not* vasospasm, the desired cardiac-depressant [oxygen-sparing] effects of β blockers predominate, and anginal attacks are lessened.)
- *Beta blockers must not be discontinued abruptly.* Never stop β blocker therapy abruptly unless the situation is an emergency (eg, an overdose or an extreme untoward reaction) and other antianginal drugs can be administered during withdrawal. In brief, during long-term therapy the β receptors on the heart muscle and blood vessels compensate for the presence of the drug by becoming supersensitive. When the β blocker is taken away abruptly, these overresponsive receptors are excessively stimulated by the always available epinephrine and norepinephrine. Acute and severe increases of heart rate and contractility (and blood pressure) often occur. The outcome can be severe myocardial ischemia (or hypertension) leading to fatal arrhythmias or infarction (or stroke). The problem also applies to the use of β blockers as antihypertensive drugs (see p 638).

NURSING IMPLICATIONS

General precautions for the use of any β blocker for any indication apply to their use for angina. In addition, for the angina patient,

make sure that outpatients have a supply of an immediate-acting nitrate on hand at all times and that they know when and how to use it;

- reemphasize the need for patients to keep a log of pertinent information and to call their physician immediately if angina worsens after β blocker therapy is started (this could indicate underlying vasospasm or an incorrect diagnosis);
- emphasize the need to continue taking β blockers as directed. Withdrawing these drugs or reducing the dose should be done under a physician's care and supervision;
- encourage patients to carry identification that indicates their history and drug therapy; other health care providers need to be aware of it in cases of emergency.

Adjuncts to Antianginal Therapy

Prescription sedatives or anxiety-relieving drugs may be used adjunctively to alleviate emotional stress, a common trigger for chronic stable angina. However, they are not appropriate substitutes for antianginal drugs, and they have little if any ability to normalize the oxygen supply–demand imbalance. More importantly, barbiturate sedatives may reduce the effectiveness of antianginal drugs by stimulating their hepatic metabolism. Moderate alcohol consumption may interact similarly, and acute alcohol consumption may inhibit hepatic metabolism of antianginal drugs, leading to profound hypotension and other manifestations of toxicity. Stress-avoidance and stress-management techniques may be good alternatives to sedative drugs for some patients and should be recommended for all patients with angina.

SUMMARY OF NURSING IMPLICATIONS

◆ Assessment

Gather baseline data—frequency, severity, onset of angina; vital signs; ECG; and peripheral perfusion status—as basis for determining drug effects.

Assess patient's current knowledge of cardiac condition and drug therapy.

Identify with patient situations that bring on anginal attacks.

Review patient history for known contraindications to drugs or conditions requiring cautious use of drugs (eg, diabetes, hyperthyroidism).

Identify current drug therapies that involve potential drug–drug interactants with specific antianginal drugs (eg, verapamil with digoxin, blockers, disopyramide, or quinidine).

Review history for patterns, times of onset of angina (eg, exercise-induced, occurs at rest or in early morning) to ensure that improper drugs are not prescribed (eg, β blockers not suitable for vasospastic angina).

◆ Nursing Diagnoses

Decreased cardiac output related to disease process (angina and coronary artery disease).

Chest pain related to inadequate blood flow to myocardium.

Constipation related to drug (particularly verapamil) side effects.

Knowledge deficit related to limited understanding of prescribed antianginal drugs.

Ineffective individual coping related to job and/or family pressures (stress).

Noncompliance related to dietary and lifestyle changes.

Activity intolerance related to chest pain.

Fear related to chest pain and possible myocardial infarction.

◆ Planning/Implementation

Have nitroglycerin sublingual tablets or translingual spray available to patient at all times to terminate an anginal attack; keep at bedside unless otherwise ordered.

Observe vital signs continuously during IV nitroglycerin administration.

Observe during therapy for edema or weight gain (indicating heart failure), slow or irregular pulses (bradycardia or arrhythmias), or difficulty breathing (bronchoconstriction or heart failure) indicating adverse response.

Question any medication order that calls for abrupt discontinuation of a β blocker or calcium channel blocker in patients who have been taking the drug chronically.

Observe for signs of hepatotoxicity with verapamil (jaundice, abdominal pain).

Check blood pressure and pulse regularly when a calcium channel blocker and a nitrate are taken together; additive hypotension and reflex tachycardia may occur.

◆ Patient and Family Education

Teach the patient/family:

That immediate-release nitroglycerin tablets may be crushed between the teeth first for quicker relief; side effects may be more intense.

That sublingual or buccal tablets must not be swallowed; long-acting oral preparations must be swallowed.

To seek medical attention if anginal pain is unrelieved by three successive doses (administered five minutes apart) of a previously effectively sublingual nitroglycerin preparation.

To store nitroglycerin sublingual tablets in a tightly capped glass container protected from excessive heat or moisture.

The proper administration technique for topical nitroglycerin ointment: apply with applicator stick or spatula to chest, upper arm, upper thigh, or back on area free of body hair; rotate sites to avoid dermatitis.

The major side effects related to hypotensive changes: headache (tolerance will develop); flushing of face or upper extremities, tachycardia or palpitations; and dizziness or fainting (sit in head-low position until feelings subside).

Always to carry nitroglycerin sublingual tablets or spray to treat acute attacks; to sit and rest when the drug is used.

About the danger of abruptly discontinuing a β blocker or calcium channel blocker.

Appropriate stress-managing techniques.

Not to use sedatives as substitutes for antianginal drugs.

Methods to assist in quitting smoking.

◆ Evaluation

The patient/family will:

Report rapid relief from chest pain.

Experience minimal side effects; verbalize ability to manage headache, dizziness, constipation if present.

Discuss correct administration technique of antianginal drug.

Identify precipitating causes of chest pain and take steps to reduce their incidence.

Alter diet according to recommendations; avoid alcohol and cigarettes.

Use stress-reduction techniques to manage effects of stressful life events and feelings of fear.

Establish a regular exercise program, prescribed by the physician, to improve cardiac function.

Annotated Bibliography

Alpert JS: Nitrate therapy in the elderly. *Am J Cardiol* 1990; 65:23J–27J. *A valuable review of the aging cardiovascular system and basic changes in drug responsiveness, plus an overview of nitrate pharmacology and how these changes can affect safe, effective antianginal therapy in the elderly.*

Anderson KA: A practical guide to nitrate use. *Postgrad Med* 1991; 89(1):67–70, 75–76, 78. *Covers such issues as antianginal drug choice, tolerance associated with continuous therapy, and specific aspects of nitrate treatment of elders.*

Campbell RW: The deficiencies of current medical therapy for the management of angina pectoris. *Postgrad Med J* 1991;67 (Suppl 3):S37–S40. *Is the drug plan for your angina patient rational? Is it doing little to modify the underlying disease? Read this short paper to get more insight into these important questions.*

Fletcher A: Transdermal nitroglycerin: Does it really work in the treatment of angina? *Drugs Aging* 1991;1(1):6–16. *Assesses the efficacy of a commonly used and unquestionably convenient nitrate dosage form for the elderly.*

Fung HL: *Nitrate therapy: Is there an optimal substance and formulation? Eur Heart J* 1991;12 (Suppl A):9–12. *Discusses the important differences of the various nitrate preparations and considers these properties in practical terms of how they affect use, efficacy, and patient acceptability.*

Gleeson B: Loosening the grip of anginal pain. *Nursing* 1991;21(1): 33–40. *A good synopsis of major points about pathophysiology and therapy, along with a self-test you can use to evaluate your knowledge and understanding.*

Gleeson B: Teaching your patient about his antianginal drugs. *Nursing* 1991;21(2):65–72. *A collection of forms you can copy and give to patients who will be self-medicating with various antianginal drugs and dosage forms. Those for sublingual nitroglycerin tablets or sprays should be modified to convey a greater sense of urgency and suitable action when three doses fail to alleviate acute pain.*

Gold ME: Pharmacology of the nitrovasodilators: Antianginal, antihypertensive, and antiplatelet actions. *Nurs Clin North Am* 1991; 26(2):437–450. *An excellent overview of pertinent pathophysiology, insight into current thoughts about the biochemical mechanisms of antianginal drugs and nitroprusside, and specific guidance about nursing interventions.*

Horowitz, BZ, Rhee KJ: Massive verapamil ingestion: A report of two cases and a review of the literature. *Am J Emerg Med* 1989;7(6): 624–631. *Successfully treating severe calcium channel blocker overdoses is more complicated than administering the logical "antidote," calcium. Read this article for more insight into what to expect and do should an overdose victim be in your care.*

Lambert CR: Combination therapy with nicardipine and beta-adrenergic blockade for angina pectoris. *Clin Cardiol* 1992; 15(4):231–234. *A review of one of the newest calcium antagonists, and circumstances in which combined therapy with a β blocker might be of particular value to some angina patients.*

Lazar EJ, Frishman WH, Grover N: Medical therapy of the hypertensive patient with concomitant angina pectoris. *Cardiol Clin* 1991; 9(1):167–176. *You will encounter many patients with both high blood pressure and ischemic heart disease. Learn why and how to "tailor" therapy for them.*

Maseri A: Aspects of the medical therapy of angina pectoris. *Drugs* 1991;42 (Suppl 1):28–30. *A wealth of information in three pages: well worth reading, especially with regard to pathophysiology, regardless of the type of angina your patient has.*

Munger TM, Oh JK: Unstable angina. *Mayo Clin Proc* 1990;65(3): 384–406. *A good review of relevant pathophysiology, the variable symptomatology, and both pharmacologic and invasive interventions used for this serious form of angina and ischemia.*

Ridker PM, Manson JE, Gaziano JM, Buring JE, Hennekens CH: Low-dose aspirin therapy for chronic stable angina: A randomized, placebo-controlled clinical trial. *Ann Intern Med* 1991;114:

835–839. *This study showed that alternate-day treatment with 325 mg aspirin significantly reduced the risk of a first MI. Further testing may find a new clinical role for this already versatile, inexpensive OTC drug with significant antiplatelet actions.*

Shively M, Riegel B: Effect of nitroglycerin ointment placement on headache and flushing in healthy subjects. *Int J Nurs Stud* 1991; 28(2):153–161. *The outcome of this study suggests that in terms of side effects it makes little difference where nitroglycerin ointment is applied or whether the application site is rotated.*

Shub C: Stable angina pectoris: 3. Medical treatment. *Mayo Clin Proc* 1990;65(2):256–273. *Reviews treatment goals, drug selection, individualization of therapy based on the presence of other diseases, and a host of other important issues.*

Thadani U: Medical therapy of stable angina pectoris. *Cardiol Clin* 1991;9(1):73–87. *A comprehensive review and comparison of the actions and uses of nitrates, calcium channel blockers, and β blockers for angina.*

Todd PA, Goa KL, Langtry HD: Transdermal nitroglycerin (glyceryl trinitrate): A review of its pharmacology and therapeutic use. *Drugs* 1990;40(6):880–902. *Focuses on nitrate tolerance, especially from the use of transdermal administration; contains valuable, practical information about therapy planning and monitoring.*

Weintraub M, Horn J, Krakoff L, Vetrovec G: P&T Committee review of nifedipine GITS: New modality for angina and hypertension. *Hosp Formul* 1990;25 (Suppl A):10–14. *Nifedipine GITS—a GI therapeutic system for this antianginal and antihypertensive drug—will soon come into widespread use. This article provides more information about a novel, convenient, and effective drug delivery system.*

Table 34–C **Clinical Uses and Administration of Major Antianginal Drugs**

AGENT	CLINICAL USES	DOSAGE AND ROUTE OF ADMINISTRATION
	Nitrates (Representative Products)	
PROTOTYPE		
Nitroglycerin (generic and various proprietary forms)	Treatment of acute angina attacks; prophylaxis of angina	Sublingual or buccal: 0.15 to 0.3 mg at onset or in anticipation of attack (eg, 5–10 min before engaging in exercise); for faster relief in acute attack, crush tablet between teeth; some physicians advise use every 2–3 hr and at bedtime for prophylaxis (see text); limit 3 doses over 15 min for acute attack
(NITROLINGUAL)	Treatment, prophylaxis of angina	Sublingual spray: 1 or 2 sprays on/under tongue at onset of attack, limit to 3 sprays within 15-min period; for prophylaxis, 1 (or 2) sprays 5–10 min before engaging in activity
(NITROGARD)	Prophylaxis of angina	Buccal: Usually start with 1 mg tid (every 5 hr during waking hours); usual maintenance dose is 2 mg
(NITROCINE TIMECAPS; NITROGLYN; NITRO-BID PLATEAU CAPS)	Prophylaxis of angina	Oral: Sustained-action tablets or capsules: 2.5–9 mg, bid or tid
(NITROL; NITRO-BID)	Prophylaxis of angina	Topical ointment: 2–3 in. to upper chest or upper arm q8h; spread evenly, cover with plastic wrap
(DEPONIT; NITRODISC; NITRO-DUR; TRANSDERM-NITRO)	Prophylaxis of angina	Transdermal infusion system: Apply one patch qd as directed (see text)
(NITRO-BID IV, TRIDIL)	Adjunctive treatment of severe heart failure, myocardial infarction; controlled perioperative hypotension or management of hypertension	IV: Average effective dose 10–20 μg/min when manufacturer's IV tubing is used; higher rates needed when standard PVC tubing used (adsorbs drug); adjust response by adjusting infusion rate
RELATED DRUGS		
Amyl nitrite	Treatment of acute angina	Inhalation: Crush ampul (contains 0.3 mL liquid), wave under nose for 1–6 inhalations; repeat in 3–5 min if needed
Erythrityl tetranitrate		
(CARDILATE)	Prophylaxis of angina	Sublingual: Usually 5 or 10 mg before each anticipated angina trigger, and at bedtime if needed to prevent nocturnal angina Oral: 10 mg ac; additional midmorning, midafternoon, bedtime doses as needed *Note:* Identical tablet formulation is used for either route of administration

(continued)

Table 34–C | Clinical Uses and Administration of Major Antianginal Drugs (*Continued*)

AGENT	CLINICAL USES	DOSAGE AND ROUTE OF ADMINISTRATION
Isosorbide dinitrate		
(ISORDIL; SORBITRATE)	Acute angina	Sublingual: 2.5 or 5 mg Oral: 5 mg (chewable tablet)
	Initial angina prophylaxis	Sublingual or oral (chewable tablet): Initially 5 or 10 mg, taken every 2 or 3 hr
	Maintenance prophylaxis of angina	Oral: Initially 5–20 mg of immediate-release tablet or 40-mg sustained-release tablet; maintain with 10–40 mg immediate-release tablet q6h, or a 40- or 80-mg sustained-release tablet every 8 to 12 hr
Pentaerythritol tetranitrate		
(DUOTRATE; PENTYLAN; PERITRATE; PERITRATE-SA)	Angina prophylaxis	Oral: Usually 10 or 20 mg chewed or swallowed whole, qid; 80-mg sustained-acting tablet or 30–60 mg timed-release capsule in AM and 12 hr later
Isosorbide mononitrate		
(ISMO)	Angina prophylaxis	Oral: 20 mg bid; give first dose on awakening, second 7 hr later
Calcium Channel Blockers (All Approved Drugs, Indications)		
PROTOTYPE		
*Verapamil**		
(CALAN, ISOPTIN)	Angina prophylaxis (chronic-stable, unstable, vasospastic)	Oral: Usually 80–120 mg tid to start, increase weekly as needed to 480 mg/day (maximum) in divided doses
	Essential hypertension	Oral: Usually 80 mg tid, increase to maximum of 360 mg/day in divided doses if needed; may switch to same total daily dose (mg) of sustained-acting preparation when patient is stabilized
	Atrial fibrillation or flutter (as adjunct to digitalis)	Oral: 240–320 mg/day in 3 or 4 doses
	Prophylaxis of supraventricular tachycardia (nondigitalized patients)	Oral: 240–480 mg/day in 3 or 4 doses
	Treatment of supraventricular tachyarrhythmias	IV: Initially 75-150 μg/kg bolus over 2 min, repeat 150 μg/kg 30 min after first dose if needed Elderly: infuse over 3 min (may need to reduce dosage); children ≤ 1 yr: 100–200 μg/kg over 2 min; 1–15 yr: 100–300 μg/kg over 2 min; monitor ECG continuously
(CALAN SR, ISOPTIN SR, VERELAN)	Essential hypertension	Oral (sustained-release): Usually 240 mg in AM (with food); 240 mg in AM, 120 mg in evening, if needed; start therapy with immediate-acting dosage form (see above)

(continued)

*Note: Oral dosages of verapamil are for immediate-acting preparations unless noted otherwise.

Table 34–C Clinical Uses and Administration of Major Antianginal Drugs (*Continued*)

AGENT	CLINICAL USES	DOSAGE AND ROUTE OF ADMINISTRATION
Calcium Channel Blockers (All Approved Drugs, Indications)		
RELATED DRUGS		
Bepridil		
(VASCOR)	Angina prophylaxis (chronic-stable)	Oral: Usually 200 mg once daily; average maintenance dose 300 mg/day
Diltiazem		
(CARDIZEM)	Angina prophylaxis (chronic-stable or vasospastic)	Oral: Initially 30 mg qid (before meals and at bedtime; increase gradually to 180–360 mg/day in 3 or 4 doses)
	Atrial fibrillation, flutter, paroxysmal	IV: Single bolus injection of 0.25 mg/kg over 2 min initially; 0.35 mg/kg over 2 min 15 min after first dose if needed; adjust subsequent doses as needed
		IV infusion: After initial bolus, infuse 5–15 mg/hr (as 0.45–1 mg/mL diluted solution) for up to 24 hr
(CARDIZEM CD, CARDIZEM SR)	Essential hypertension	Oral (sustained-release): Initially 60–120 mg bid; adjust (usually after 14 days of treatment) to 120–180 mg bid as needed
Felodipine		
(PLENDIL)	Essential hypertension	Oral (sustained-release): Initially 5 mg qd; adjust at 2-week intervals if needed to usual maintenance dose of 5–10 mg/day (20 mg/day maximum)
Isradipine		
(DYNACIRC)	Essential hypertension	Oral: Initially 2.5 mg bid; increase at 2–4-week intervals by 5 mg/day if needed
Nicardipine		
(CARDENE)	Angina prophylaxis (chronic-stable)	Oral: 20–40 mg tid
	Essential hypertension	Oral: 20–40 mg tid
(CARDENE SR)	Essential hypertension	Oral (sustained-release): 30–60 mg once daily
(CARDENE IV)	Acute hypertension	IV: Dilute to 0.1 mg/mL, infuse 5 mg/hr initially (15 mg/hr for faster effects); titrate maintenance dose to desired effect; if switching to oral nifedipine, give first oral dose 1 hr before stopping infusion; if switching to other oral calcium antagonists, start when IV therapy is stopped
Nifedipine		
(ADALAT, PROCARDIA, others)	Angina prophylaxis (chronic-stable or vasospastic)	Oral: Initially 10 mg tid; usual maintenance dose 10 or 20 mg tid; may switch to equivalent mg of sustained-release form when patient stabilized
(PROCARDIA XL)	Essential hypertension	Oral (sustained-release): 30 or 60 mg once daily
	Angina	See above
Nimodipine		
(NIMOTOP)	Improvement of neurologic status after subarachnoid hemorrhage	Oral: 60 mg q4h for 21 consecutive days

(continued)

Table 34–C | **Clinical Uses and Administration of Major Antianginal Drugs (*Continued*)**

AGENT	CLINICAL USES	DOSAGE AND ROUTE OF ADMINISTRATION
	Beta Adrenergic Blockers*†	
Atenolol (TENORMIN)	Prophylaxis of angina	Oral: 50 mg once daily; some patients may require up to 200 mg/day
Metoprolol (LOPRESSOR)	Prophylaxis of angina	Oral: 50 mg bid or 100 mg once daily
Nadolol (CORGARD)	Prophylaxis of angina	Oral: 40 or 80 mg once daily
Propranolol (INDERAL; INDERAL-LA)	Prophylaxis of angina	Oral: (immediate-acting) 10–20 mg ac and qhs; long-acting preparation 80 mg once daily up to 320 mg/day if needed; optimal daily dose is 160 mg/day (immediate- or long-acting)

†See Chapter 30 for the use of β blockers as antiarrhythmics and Chapter 33 for their use in hypertension. Chapter 15 contains general information about β blockers.

Table 34–S | **Major Side Effects of and Contraindications for Antianginal Drugs**

BODY SYSTEM/ Side Effect	CONTRAINDICATION/ PRECAUTION	COMMENTS AND NURSING IMPLICATIONS
	Nitroglycerin and Related Nitrates	
CARDIOVASCULAR Hypotension	Shock; hypovolemia; preexisting hypotension; severe coronary artery or cerebrovascular disease; pericardial tamponade	Transient hypotension common, especially with rapid-acting (eg, sublingual) administration; avoid marked hypotension in patients with severe coronary artery disease (may cause MI or stroke)
Flushing of extremities		Related to vasodilation; usually occurs with rapid-acting preparations
Headache	Increased intracranial pressure; head trauma; stroke	May be intense; due to cerebral vasodilation; manage with common analgesics until tolerance develops (1 or 2 weeks)
Reflex tachycardia	Severe preexisting tachyarrhythmias	Usually managed by adding beta blockers to drug plan; severe tachycardia plus hypotension predisposes to MI: longstanding tachycardia can aggravate CHF
	Calcium Channel Blockers	
CENTRAL NERVOUS SYSTEM Dizziness, lightheadedness		Most common with bepridil, nifedipine; least with diltiazem, verapamil; teach patient to stand slowly to avoid orthostatic hypotension that can trigger these CNS responses
Headache	Caution in patients with increased intracranial pressure, head trauma	Most common with felodipine, nifedipine, bepridil, isradipine; incidence lowest with verapamil; cerebral vasodilation can increase intracranial pressure; have patient report severe or persistent headache; recommend consultation with physician before use of medications for headache relief

(continued)

Table 34–S Major Side Effects of and Contraindications for Antianginal Drugs (*Continued*)

BODY SYSTEM/ Side Effect	CONTRAINDICATION/ PRECAUTION	COMMENTS AND NURSING IMPLICATIONS
CARDIOVASCULAR Hypotension	Hypotension, shock	Usually mild, dose-dependent; possible with all calcium channel blockers; monitor accordingly
Bradycardia, decreased cardiac output, AV block	Systolic BP < 90 mm Hg, decreased cardiac output (severe heart failure, shock); sick sinus syndrome, AV block > 1st degree	Most common with diltiazem, is dose-dependent; monitor accordingly; teach, encourage patient to monitor pulse rate, rhythm, quality
Tachycardia (reflex); potential worsening of angina if excessive	Tachycardia	Dose-dependent, most common with nicardipine, but overall incidence about 1%; may require adjunctive β blocker to control HR (if not contraindicated)
Peripheral edema		Monitor; triggered by hypotension, decreased cardiac output; 20% to 30% incidence with felodipine and nifedipine, much less with others; may require therapy with diuretics
Extremity flushing		Most common with nifedipine, nicardipine; seldom problematic
Arrhythmias (new or worsened, possibly acute or fatal, eg, VTACH, VFIB)		Risk greatest with bepridil, which should be last choice of calcium channel blockers; monitor pulse; see discussion of encainide, other related antiarrhythmics on p 562
Calcium Channel Blockers		
GASTROINTESTINAL Constipation		Most common with verapamil (about 10% incidence), especially in elderly; best managed with diet (fluid, bulk-forming foods); discourage laxative use without physician's approval
Nausea		Most common with bepridil, nifedipine
SKIN Hypersensitivity reactions (hives rash, etc)	Prior reaction to same drug	Monitor, report
BLOOD Agranulocytosis	Suppressed immune system	Risk apparently greatest with bepridil; recommend periodic blood tests; teach patient to recognize and report signs, symptoms of potential immunosuppression (eg, fever, sore throat, flulike illness)
Beta Blockers		
See Table 15–S2		

Table 34–1 **Major Interactions Between Antianginals and Other Agents**

AGENT	RESULT OF INTERACTION	COMMENTS AND NURSING IMPLICATIONS
General Interactions Involving Most Antianginal Drugs		
Alcohol	Risk of hypotension, worsening of angina and underlying ischemia	Alcohol, especially at high blood levels, causes vasodilation; encourage patients to moderate alcohol intake, especially at one sitting
Antihypertensive drugs (all; Chapter 33)	As for alcohol	Combined use is common; requires close monitoring, especially of BP and HR, to help adjust dosages properly; antihypertensive drugs other than β blockers, calcium channel blockers, and catecholamine depleters (eg, reserpine) also increase risk, severity of reflex tachycardia
Sympathomimetics, other drugs that increase heart rate and/or contractility, blood pressure (Chapter 33); thyroid hormones (Chapter 47)	Poor control, or worsening, of angina and underlying cardiac ischemia	Avoid combined use of these agents if possible; if combined use is necessary, use lowest effective doses, monitor accordingly; identify OTC drugs that can cause unwanted interactions (eg, cold, allergy, decongestant, and weight-loss medications), and encourage patient to consult with physician before using them
Interactions Involving Nitroglycerin, Other Nitrates		
Ergot alkaloids (eg, dihydroergotamine; Chapter 15)	Increased blood pressure and increased incidence and severity of angina	Nitroglycerin decreases ergot metabolism, thereby increasing systemic hypertensive, coronary vasoconstrictor (proanginal) effects of interactant; monitor for BP increases and anginal/ischemic signs and symptoms if interaction unavoidable
Interactions Involving Most Calcium Channel Blockers		
Calcium salts	Reduced therapeutic and toxic effects of calcium channel blocker	Advise patients stabilized on calcium channel blockers to minimize intake of calcium-containing drugs (eg, as mineral supplements, some antacids [Chapter 40]) especially without physician's supervision; IV calcium is used to reverse calcium channel blocker toxicity

(continued)

Table 34–I Major Interactions Between Antianginals and Other Agents (*Continued*)

AGENT	RESULT OF INTERACTION	COMMENTS AND NURSING IMPLICATIONS
Major Interactions Involving Verapamil		
β–Adrenergic blockers (Chapter 15)	Increased antianginal and antihypertensive effects of both drugs (desired); potentially excessive depression of BP, ventricular contractility, AV conduction (unwanted)	Combined use common; interaction likely to occur soon after starting combined therapy; monitor accordingly
Carbamazepine (Chapter 26)	Increased risk of carbamazepine side effects, toxicity	Verapamil may reduce carbamazepine metabolism; monitor carbamazepine levels closely, and anticipate dosage reduction when adding verapamil
Cyclosporine (Chapter 54)	Increased risk of cyclosporine toxicity (especially renal)	Decreased cyclosporine metabolism: Interaction well documented: appears and may disappear spontaneously within 1 week of adding verapamil; monitor cyclosporine blood levels at start of combined therapy; anticipate need to reduce dosage
Digitoxin, digoxin (Chapter 31)	Increased digitalis blood levels and effects; additive, potentially serious depression of AV conduction	Monitor digitalis blood levels; assess for clinical evidence of excessive effects (eg, AV block) or worsening of heart failure; anticipate reducing dosage of one or both drugs; interaction best established, and more likely to be significant, for digoxin
Quinidine (Chapter 30)	Increased effects, usually excessive/toxic: cardiac depression (hypotension, bradycardia, edema), AV block, VTACH	Avoid combined use unless absolutely necessary; monitor quinidine blood levels and clinical status closely; anticipate need to discontinue one or both drugs
Rifampin (Chapter 57)	Increased verapamil metabolism, decreased effects	Applies mainly to oral verapamil; monitor accordingly; use IV verapamil or substitute noninteracting alternatives for either or both interactants
Tubocurarine, other nondepolarizing neuromuscular blockers (Chapter 17)	Increased, more prolonged, muscle (eg, ventilatory) impairment or paralysis	Additive skeletal muscle depression; avoid interaction if possible; otherwise, anticipate result of interaction and need for longer ventilatory support
Prazosin (Chapter 33)	Worsening of prazosin-induced postural/orthostatic hypotension	Remind patients to anticipate and how to avoid or minimize hypotension (eg, avoid standing suddenly); monitor supine, sitting, standing BP
Interaction Involving Bepridil		
Digoxin	See verapamil-digoxin interaction above	
Interactions Involving Diltiazem, Nicardipine		
Cyclosporine	See verapamil-cyclosporine interaction above	

(continued)

Table 34–1 **Major Interactions Between Antianginals and Other Agents (*Continued*)**

AGENT	RESULT OF INTERACTION	COMMENTS AND NURSING IMPLICATIONS
Interactions Involving Felodipine		
Barbiturates (Chapter 22)	Decreased felodipine blood levels and effects	Interactants (especially phenobarbital) stimulate felodipine metabolism: monitor for decreased antianginal or antihypertensive effects; higher felodipine dosages may be needed
Carbamazepine (Chapter 26)	Decreased felodipine blood levels and effects	See felodipine-barbiturate interaction above
Cimetidine (Chapter 40)	Increased felodipine effects, potentially excessive	Inhibition of felodipine metabolism; monitor clinical responses during combined use; interaction probably less likely with cimetidine alternatives
Phenytoin, other hydantoins (Chapter 26)	Decreased felodipine blood levels, effects	See felodipine-barbiturate interaction above
Interaction Involving Nifedipine		
Cimetidine	See felodipine-cimetidine interaction above	
Interaction Involving Beta Blockers		
See Table 15–12		

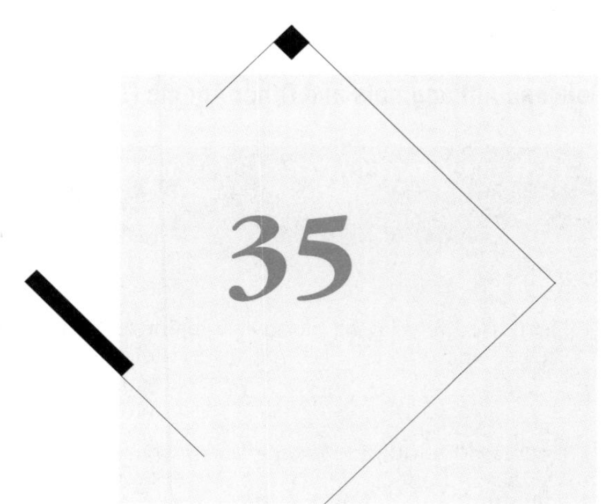

PROTOTYPES

35 Anticoagulant, Antiplatelet, and Thrombolytic Drugs

To deliver oxygen and nutrients throughout the body, the blood must remain in a fluid state. But when injury occurs and blood vessels are severed, the blood must coagulate locally to prevent excessive bleeding and to initiate tissue repair. Once repair is complete, blood clots must be dissolved. These processes describe *hemostasis,* which normally provides an important protective mechanism for the host. However, in several clinical situations clotting processes must be inhibited intentionally and in a controlled way; in others, the consequences of clotting must be reversed. Four major components are involved in clot formation. One occurs mainly in the blood vessel (vascular) endothelium; the others occur in the cellular or fluid phases of the blood.

The vascular component of hemostasis involves reactions within the blood vessel wall that usually prevent coagulation but can trigger it when vascular damage occurs. Endothelial cells normally synthesize prostacyclin (also called prostaglandin I_2, or PGI_2), a lipid-like derivative of arachidonic acid that causes vasodilation and prevents platelets from adhering to the vessel wall. Inhibiting prostacyclin synthesis in the endothelium favors vasoconstriction and platelet aggregation ("stickiness"), which is the second major component of hemostasis.

Damage to the vascular endothelium exposes underlying collagen-rich connective tissue that stimulates platelets to aggregate. Endothelial damage also releases adenosine diphosphate (ADP) and produces another arachidonic acid derivative called thromboxane A_2 (TXA_2), both of which stimulate platelet aggregation. Thromboxane A_2 also causes local vasoconstriction, which reduces blood flow and restricts coagulation to the site of damage. Activated platelets release many substances that attract other platelets to the injured area, and they eventually aggregate to form a plug, or **thrombus,** that helps limit further blood loss. Thrombi may become dislodged, forming **emboli** that can circulate throughout the body, lodge in small blood vessels, and thereby dramatically reduce organ blood flow and cause ischemia. Emboli may also form directly within the bloodstream without prior thrombus formation.

Two other major components of blood clotting are the *intrinsic* and *extrinsic coagulation pathways* (Fig. 35–1). The intrinsic pathway (also called the *cascade pathway*) involves a series of sequential reactions that, in general, convert inactive coagulation factors into

Major reference tables appear beginning on p. 721.

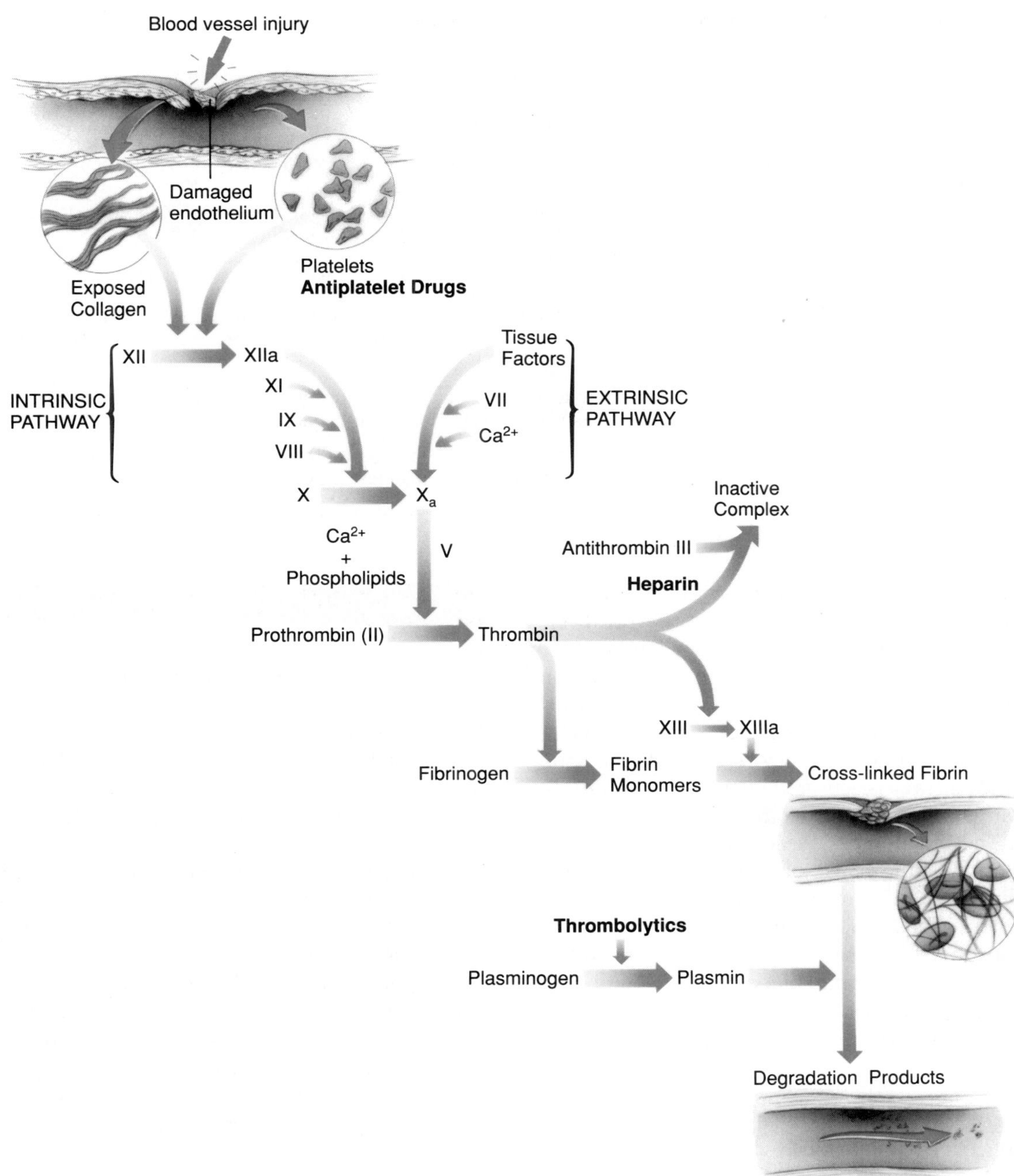

Figure 35–1

Overview of the intrinsic and extrinsic coagulation pathways leading to the formation of a fibrin clot and clot breakdown (thrombolysis). Aspirin and other antiplatelet drugs inhibit platelet aggregation. Warfarin and other oral anticoagulants inhibit hepatic synthesis of vitamin K-dependent clotting factors (VII, IX, X), and inhibit the actions of some activated clotting factors (eg, II, VIIa, Xa). Heparin stimulates formation of an inactive complex between thrombin and antithrombin III. Streptokinase and other thrombolytics convert plasminogen to plasmin, which helps break down clots.

Table 35–1 **Overview of Drugs Used to Inhibit Blood Clotting or Increase Clot Breakdown**

Class	Prototype	Site, Mechanism(s) of Action	Specific Antidote
Injectable anticoagulant	Heparin sodium	Acts in blood; increases activity of antithrombin III, eventually inhibiting conversion of prothrombin to thrombin; high doses also inactivate thrombin and prevent conversion of fibrinogen to fibrin; response measured as activated partial thromboplastin time (APTT)	Protamine sulfate
Oral anticoagulant	Warfarin sodium	Acts in liver; inhibits synthesis of vitamin K–dependent clotting factors; response measured as prothrombin time (PT)	Vitamin K_1 (phytonadione)
Thrombolytic drug	Streptokinase	Acts in clot; converts plasminogen to plasmin, which dissolves fibrin and fibrinogen in clots	Aminocaproic acid
Antiplatelet drug	Aspirin	Acts on platelet; inhibits synthesis of thromboxane A_2, which normally triggers platelet aggregation	None

active ones. Most of the coagulation factors are synthesized in the liver, which explains why severe liver disease may be accompanied by impaired blood coagulation. The intrinsic pathway is triggered by contact of clotting factor XII (Hageman factor) with collagen or foreign substances. Some reactions of the intrinsic pathway require platelet-derived factors and calcium ion. The extrinsic pathway is activated by thromboplastin released from damaged tissue. Both pathways act simultaneously. The reactions of the extrinsic and intrinsic pathways join with the activation of factor X (Stuart factor), leading to the conversion of prothrombin to thrombin. Thrombin catalyzes the transformation of fibrinogen, a soluble plasma protein, to insoluble fibrin, which serves as the backbone of a clot.

Four major groups of drugs (Table 35–1) are used to inhibit one or more of these processes, and each has a prototype:

- injectable anticoagulants (heparin sodium);
- oral anticoagulants (warfarin sodium)
- thrombolytic (clot-dissolving) drugs (streptokinase); and
- antiplatelet drugs (aspirin)

Injectable Anticoagulants

Anticoagulant drugs interfere with one or more steps in the coagulation pathways. They prevent clotting but do not dissolve existing blood clots.

PROTOTYPE

Heparin Sodium

Heparin is an extremely effective and fast-acting anticoagulant. It is an endogenous substance that is found in mast cells and basophils throughout the body. Controversy exists about whether endogenous heparin has important physiologic roles. However, during anaphylaxis blood heparin levels rise as the result of widespread mast cell activation, and in this setting heparin may serve as a natural anticoagulant, yet at the same time contribute to excessive bleeding.

Heparin that is used clinically is isolated and purified from organs of slaughterhouse animals. The sodium salt is used most commonly. Heparin is an acidic mucopolysaccharide that carries a high negative electrostatic charge, which seems to account for many of its actions and provides a way to inactivate it should its effects be too great.

Absorption, Distribution, Metabolism, and Excretion

Heparin is not absorbed well from the gastrointestinal (GI) tract, so it is given only parenterally. Intravenous (IV) administration produces an almost immediate anticoagulant action. When more gradual, longer-lasting actions are desired, heparin can be given subcutaneously (SC). Heparin should not be given intramuscularly (IM) because it is absorbed erratically and can cause bleeding, irritation, and pain at the injection site. Heparin is distributed throughout the body, although its actions are limited primarily to the blood.

Some heparin is metabolized by the liver enzyme heparinase; the rest is excreted unchanged by the kidneys. In normal individuals the anticoagulant effects of a single heparin dose disappear in four to six hours. For most heparin doses, impaired renal function prolongs heparin's half-life more than does impaired liver function.

Pharmacologic Effects

Low doses of heparin enhance the activity of antithrombin III (sometimes called AT-III or heparin cofactor) to neutralize activated factor X, which is the common link between the intrinsic and extrinsic coagulation pathways. The conversion of prothrombin to thrombin is inhibited. Larger heparin doses inactivate thrombin and prevent conversion of fibrinogen to fibrin.

The major clinical indicator of heparin action is the activated partial thromboplastin time (APTT). The APTT test is a general (but quick, sensitive, and reproducible) test of the entire coagulation process and is preferred to other assays such as the whole blood clotting time. Heparin prolongs the APTT in a dose-dependent manner. The usual goal of heparin therapy is an APTT that is 1.5 to 2 times the normal value of 30 to 40 seconds. Greater effects on the APTT, from greater heparin doses, may be required in special situations.

NURSING IMPLICATIONS

Obtain baseline measurements of the APTT, platelet count, and other relevant hematologic indicators before administering any anticoagulant. In most instances these data are also obtained at regular intervals during anticoagulant therapy. Blood samples must be drawn immediately before the next scheduled heparin administration, at least five to six hours after the last IV injection or 24 hours after the last SC injection.

Clinical Indications and Administration

Heparin has several clinical uses (Table 35–C), and the recommended doses vary considerably depending on the indication. Heparin doses are expressed in Units (U), which are standardized by all manufacturers using a bioassay to ensure consistent potency. Approved preparations of heparin contain a minimum of 120 U/mg of dry powder. It is available as sterile solutions with concentrations ranging from 1000 to 40,000 U/mL.

Prophylactic Anticoagulation with Low-Dose Subcutaneous Heparin

Low doses of heparin may be given preoperatively for prophylaxis of postoperative venous thrombosis, particularly for high-risk patients who will undergo orthopedic, abdominal, or thoracic surgery. Thrombosis frequently occurs in the deep veins of the legs, causing ischemia. Venous thrombosis may lead to the development of pulmonary, cerebral, or myocardial embolism, which generally is a medical emergency. These surgical patients are likely to be confined to bed and have limited physical activity after surgery. Stasis of blood caused by severely restricted physical activity increases the chance of thrombosis. The low doses of heparin that are used for this indication usually have negligible effects on normal hemostasis and do not increase the patient's risk of intraoperative or postoperative hemorrhage. Most coagulation parameters are unchanged, and there is usually little need to monitor the effects of low-dose heparin if the patient's coagulation processes were previously normal.

Other risk factors that increase the likelihood of needing prophylactic low-dose heparin therapy for surgical or nonsurgical patients include a history of phlebitis or thromboembolism; oral contraceptive or estrogen use; peripheral vascular disease; obesity; and atrial fibrillation accompanied by thrombi in the atrial wall (mural thrombi). Surgical patients over the age of 40, and most debilitated patients, also are at high risk.

Low-dose prophylaxis usually involves giving 5000 U, SC, about two hours before surgery. This dose is repeated every 8 to 12 hours after surgery until the patient is ambulatory. Patients who are over 40 years old or have other factors that increase their risk of thrombosis may require prophylactic heparin therapy for up to a week after surgery.

Full-Dose Anticoagulation

When more complete anticoagulation is needed, larger doses of heparin are given either by intermittent IV injection or by continuous IV infusion (see Table 35–C). Some indications for high-dose heparin include treatment of disseminated intravascular coagulation (DIC), treatment of embolism or thrombosis, and management of myocardial infarction. Heparin has been advocated for use in patients with evolving stroke, but some authorities believe that the increased risk of intracranial

SPOTLIGHT ON NURSING RESEARCH

Subcutaneous heparin is used for prophylactic anticoagulation in hospitalized patients. The therapy is often associated with bruising and induration at the site of injection, producing patient discomfort and limiting future injection sites. A variety of administration techniques have been advocated to reduce these problems, but their effectiveness has not been established, and a specific procedure for subcutaneous heparin injection has not been generally accepted.

To address this issue, these nurses compared two techniques for heparin injection in 50 hospitalized, adult volunteers receiving heparin, 5000 units SC every 12 hours. Basic elements of the two techniques were held constant, but selected factors thought to contribute to bruising and induration at injection sites were varied. In both techniques, 1 mL of heparin (5000 units/mL) was administered over a period of 10 seconds, and injections were made using a 25 gauge, 5/8 inch needle inserted at a 90° angle through a gently raised fold of skin. All sites were cleansed with alcohol and allowed to dry before injection.

Variables studied included syringe size, use of a 0.2 mL air bubble, needle change after drawing heparin into the syringe, and the use of alcohol swabs following injection. The investigators postulated that increased syringe diameter would reduce the force of injection and that an air bubble and needle change would reduce leaking and superficial tracking of injected heparin—thereby decreasing bruising and induration. They also speculated that alcohol swabs might disrupt clot formation and continue to contribute to bleeding.

Based on these ideas, they hypothesized that injection technique A—which involved a 3 mL syringe in combination with an air bubble, needle change, and sterile dry sponge—would result in fewer and smaller areas of bruising and induration as compared to technique B—which incorporated a tuberculin syringe without an air bubble or needle change and did use an alcohol swab after injection.

Subjects in this study served as their own controls, with each receiving injections using both techniques. Two injections were given in random order, at 24 hour intervals, by a single investigator. Areas of bruising and induration were measured 52 hours after injection by an investigator who was not aware of the technique used.

Bruising occurred with most injections, but the number of bruises did not differ significantly between techniques A (82%) and B (94%). In contrast, areas of induration occurred infrequently, and their occurrence was significantly less with technique A (4%) than with technique B (16%). Although the number of bruises in the sample was not affected by injection technique, the size of both bruises and of indurated areas was significantly less with technique A versus B in men and women. In women over age 60, technique appeared to be particularly important; the mean size of bruises was 13 mm^2 with technique A as compared to 72 mm^2 with technique B.

The authors conclude that the administration of subcutaneous heparin using Technique A results in less tissue trauma than technique B. As they point out, however, costs associated with this alternative—an extra needle and a dry sterile sponge—must be considered. Additional work is needed to determine if these factors are essential to the reduction in local trauma seen with this injection technique.

Wooldridge JB, Jackson JG: Evaluation of bruises and areas of induration after two techniques of subcutaneous heparin injection. *Heart Lung* 1988;17:476–482.

hemorrhage contraindicates routine use of high doses of heparin. Patients who receive high doses of heparin require periodic measurements (every six hours is common) of coagulation parameters to assess the response. Draw blood samples before giving the next dose.

The initial dose for slow intermittent IV injection is 10,000 U. Thereafter, 5000 to 10,000 U are injected every four to six hours. Intermittent injections cause marked anticoagulant effects shortly after the drug is given, but negligible anticoagulation just before the next dose is given. When continuous or more stable effects are needed, a slow IV infusion of heparin can be used. The patient gets an initial IV injection of 5000 U, followed by an infusion of around 1000 U per hour.

Anticoagulation for Cardiac or Vascular Surgery

Patients who undergo open-heart or vascular surgery may receive heparin doses ranging from 150 to 400 U/kg of body weight. Such high doses, which almost completely prevent coagulation, are used to prevent widespread thrombosis that would otherwise occur in response to cutting and suturing of blood vessels or blood passing through extracorporeal pumps and oxygenators. When surgery is completed, protamine (discussed later) is administered to counteract most of the actions of heparin and prevent postoperative hemorrhage. Low doses of heparin may then be given to prevent postoperative thrombosis or embolism.

Anticoagulation of Indwelling Arterial Catheters

Small amounts of a dilute heparin-saline solution (10 to 100 U/mL) can be injected into catheters that are used for invasive hemodynamic monitoring, or for indwelling catheters used for intermittent drug or fluid administration. The doses used in this ***heparin lock*** technique prevent clotting in the catheters but usually are too low to cause systemic anticoagulation if the volume of drug used is sufficient to fill only the catheter.

Anticoagulation of Blood for Transfusion or During Hemodialysis

When it is necessary to anticoagulate transfused whole blood, heparin can be added to give a concentration of approximately 500 U/100 mL of blood.

In Vitro Anticoagulation of Blood Samples for Laboratory Analysis

Many laboratory tests require unclotted blood. Heparin (75–150 U per 10–20 mL of collected blood) is the preferred anticoagulant when it is essential to prevent hemolysis and preserve red blood cell size. Prepared collection tubes containing heparin are commercially available. Other anticoagulants used for laboratory assays are EDTA (ethylenediamine tetraacetic acid; versene), oxalate, or citrate. Consult other texts for information about preferred anticoagulants for specific blood assays.

NURSING IMPLICATIONS

Because several concentrations of heparin solution are available, always double-check the package and container labels before giving the drug. Hospital policy may require that two professionals check the dose and concentration. The proper technique for SC heparin administration is controversial. Applying ice to the site 10 to 15 minutes before injection may reduce hematoma formation and pain. Relatively concentrated heparin solutions are preferred, to minimize tissue damage and bleeding that might occur if larger volumes of more dilute solutions were injected. The objective is to achieve a deep subcutaneous or ***intrafat*** injection. A preferred injection site is the lower abdominal wall between the iliac crests. If this is inaccessible, sites on the lateral plane of the upper thigh, the posterior arm, or fat pads above the scapulae can be used. Systematically rotate injection sites when repeated administration is anticipated; mark each site to avoid multiple injections into the same place. Do not aspirate the syringe when giving heparin SC. Apply gentle pressure to the site for about one minute after injection.

Nondrug interventions such as early ambulation, moderate exercise, and intermittent use of elastic leg stockings help prevent postoperative thrombosis and embolism, and they should be used when possible since they may allow reduced heparin doses or a shorter duration of anticoagulant therapy.

Calibrated infusion pumps are preferred for IV heparin infusion; they are essential when concentrated heparin solutions (40,000 U/mL) are being administered, to avoid infusing large volumes of fluid. It is best not to mix heparin with other drugs. The drug should not be mixed with aminoglycoside antibiotics and related drugs (amikacin, gentamicin, tobramycin, vancomycin), barbiturates, diazepam, furosemide, meprobamate, morphine, nitroprusside, or phenytoin. If you have doubts about compatibility, check with the hospital pharmacy.

Side Effects, Adverse Reactions, and Contraindications

The major adverse effects of heparin are bleeding or hemorrhage (Table 35–S). Uncontrolled bleeding may occur from any site, but common locations are the GI tract, the urinary tract, and such mucosal surfaces as the gums and nasal passages. Intracranial bleeding may occur, and the consequences can be severe, because it may be difficult to detect early enough to avoid significant brain damage. Prolonged administration of high doses of heparin can also cause excessive bleeding owing to thrombocytopenia.

Other recognized adverse reactions include osteoporosis, alopecia, and suppression of aldosterone release. They usually occur when high doses of heparin are given frequently, and they seem to be more common in patients over 40 years old, particularly women. Alopecia may not occur until several months after heparin therapy is discontinued. It is generally reversible, and the patient should be reassured about this. Since heparin is a large molecule that is isolated from animal sources, it has antigenic properties and may cause mild to severe allergic reactions. Modern recombinant DNA techniques are being used to produce human heparin, which should eliminate allergic responses.

The major contraindications for heparin administration are those that place the patient at high risk of bleeding. Patients with active or occult bleeding or an increased danger of hemorrhage should not receive any anticoagulant. These may include some women during menstruation, who may experience greater or prolonged menstrual flow. Patients with hemophilia, thrombocytopenia (which may be heparin-induced), or other blood dyscrasias also should not receive the drug. Other high-risk groups are patients with GI ulcers, patients who have had recent brain, spinal cord, or ocular trauma or surgery (including diagnostic lumbar punctures), or women who may shortly abort or deliver a fetus. Heparin is used cautiously in patients with a history of bleeding disorders, or postoperative patients who have surgical drains in place. Pregnancy-related aspects of heparin therapy are noted later.

Anticoagulants should be used cautiously in patients who are receiving ulcerogenic drugs. These include nonsteroidal antiinflammatory drugs (which, as noted elsewhere, also have antiplatelet actions), systemically administered corticosteroids, and catecholamine-depleting drugs, such as guanethidine or reserpine.

NURSING IMPLICATIONS

In addition to measuring the APTT and other hematologic indicators of anticoagulation, assess the patient frequently for signs of excessive heparin action. The more obvious ones include bleeding from the gums, nosebleeds (epistaxis), petechiae, hematoma at the site of injection, tarry or bloody stools that might indicate GI bleeding, and hematuria. If heparin is given for prevention of limb thrombosis, assess the limb for signs of possible bleeding into the tissues, such as changes in limb size or color.

If frequent venous or arterial punctures are required during heparin therapy, apply sufficient pressure to the puncture site to reduce bleeding, and check frequently all sites of skin penetration, whether by incisions or catheters. Be sure that typed and cross-matched blood is readily available for any patient at risk of excessive bleeding.

◆ Use During Pregnancy and Lactation

Heparin does not cross the placenta, and there is no information that it causes birth defects. Nevertheless, the drug should be used with extreme care, and only if absolutely necessary, during the last trimester and during and immediately after labor or abortion. Unlike other anticoagulants, heparin is not excreted in maternal milk. Therefore, breast-feeding need not be avoided as long as there is no other contraindication to using the drug.

◆ Use in Children

Heparin doses in children are based on the child's weight—usually 50 U/kg—for systemic anticoagulation.

◆ Use in the Elderly

Elderly patients are prone to developing thromboembolism, particularly if they are immobilized. However, bleeding complications and mortality associated with anticoagulant use also appear to increase with age. The incidence is higher in women over 60 years old, but the reasons are not known.

Interactions with Other Drugs

As a general rule, all drugs that affect some aspect of the coagulation pathway can interact with one another. These include heparin and the other drugs discussed later in the chapter: oral anticoagulants (eg, warfarin), antiplatelet drugs (aspirin), and thrombolytic agents (eg, streptokinase). The result of all these interactions is an increased bleeding risk due to simultaneous inhibition of several parts of the coagulation process. In clinical practice, it is common to administer two or more of these interactants. However, this necessitates extra vigilance: frequent monitoring of coagulation profiles and assessing for key signs and symptoms of excessive effects—petechiae, mucosal bleeding, bruising, and so on.

Aspirin (see Chapter 52 and Table 35–11) is basically the only drug for which there is good evidence of a relatively common and clinically significant interaction with heparin. An increased bleeding risk can develop quickly after combined administration, even with very low aspirin doses (eg, one standard 300 mg tablet) and regardless of the reason for which the aspirin was given. The heparin–aspirin interaction is avoided if possible.

The risks and precautions apply to generic and brand-name aspirin products alike, and also to all aspirin formulations (eg, buffered or enteric-coated preparations). The interaction is less likely to occur with other salicylates that have a less pronounced antiplatelet effect—choline and magnesium salicylates, for example. Similarly, other nonsteroidal antiinflammatory drugs (NSAIDs) are less likely than aspirin to interact with heparin. See Chapter 52 for more information on these medications.

Parenterally administered cephalosporin and penicillin antibiotics and nitroglycerin (when given IV) are potential interactants with heparin; the risks are not as clear-cut as they are for the heparin-aspirin interaction. The antibiotics may increase bleeding tendencies by inhibiting platelet aggregation; evidence of an interaction necessitates a reduction of the heparin dose. In contrast, IV nitroglycerin may antagonize heparin's effects and require an increase in the anticoagulant dose. These interactants can be administered to patients receiving heparin, provided that they can also receive proper monitoring to detect problems and make correct dosage changes.

Overdose and Toxicity

Heparin overdoses are managed by discontinuing heparin administration and by giving the specific heparin antidote protamine sulfate. This antidote must be readily available whenever heparin is administered.

Protamine Sulfate as a Heparin Antidote

Protamine molecules carry positive electrostatic charges that combine with and inactivate the negatively charged heparin molecules. The drug does not counteract the effects of any other drug that affects blood function. Besides its important role in treating heparin overdoses, protamine is routinely administered postoperatively to reverse the actions of high-dose heparin given during surgery. Protamine is available as a 1% solution (10 mg/mL) or as a powder that should be reconstituted to 1%. One milligram of protamine sulfate neutralizes approximately 100 U of heparin; the actual dose is based on the amount of heparin the patient has received and on laboratory measurements of coagulation, such as the APTT.

NURSING IMPLICATIONS

Give protamine by slow IV injection or infusion, and give no more than 50 mg in any 10-minute period. Rapid administration may cause excessive coagulation, hypotension, bradycardia, or dyspnea. Monitor vital signs continuously during protamine administration.

Related Drugs

Heparin Calcium

Heparin calcium (CALCIPARINE) is pharmacologically equivalent to heparin sodium, but the sodium salt is used more often.

Oral Anticoagulants

PROTOTYPE

Warfarin

Heparin is not convenient for long-term anticoagulation because it must be injected or infused frequently. An orally effective anticoagulant is used instead (see Table 35–C). Warfarin sodium (COUMADIN, PANWARFIN) is the sole agent and therefore the prototype. Chemically, it is a coumarin derivative.

Absorption, Distribution, Metabolism, and Excretion

Warfarin is absorbed rapidly and completely from the GI tract, so it is almost always given orally. Warfarin can be injected (IM or IV), but injection does little to hasten its onset of activity, and so parenteral administration is seldom justified. Warfarin is extensively bound to plasma protein and metabolized by hepatic enzymes. These enzymes can be stimulated or inhibited by many interacting drugs that cause a host of problems, as discussed later. Some warfarin metabolites are excreted in the urine. Others are excreted in the bile and may be reabsorbed (enterohepatic recirculation) before fecal excretion. Warfarin normally has a half-life of about 36 hours.

Pharmacologic Effects

Unlike heparin, warfarin's site of action is not the blood. Warfarin acts in the liver to inhibit the synthesis of active vitamin K-dependent clotting factors (factors X, IX, VII, and prothrombin). (This hepatic site of action explains why adding warfarin to a tube of fresh blood will not prevent coagulation.) Prolonged coagulation associated with inhibited factor synthesis does not become apparent for several days after warfarin therapy is begun. During this time, preformed (active) clotting factors can provide relatively normal hemostasis until they are depleted and replaced by inactive factors formed by warfarin.

Clinical Indications and Administration

Warfarin is used for long-term prophylaxis and treatment of venous thrombosis or pulmonary embolism, as adjunctive treatment of acute myocardial infarction, and to manage atrial fibrillation when atrial-wall thrombi are apt to be present (see Table 35–C). The usual starting dose is 10 to 15 mg. Maintenance doses are individualized for each patient, based on measurements of prothrombin time, and are usually between 2 and 10 mg per day. The therapeutic goal is a prothrombin time of 18 to 30 seconds, which is between 1.5 to 2.5 times the normal value of 12 seconds.

Heparin and warfarin can be given together for rapid anticoagulation in patients who will require long-term anticoagulation. Heparin is given for its immediate effects; it is continued for two or three days, until the actions of warfarin have developed, at which time the heparin is discontinued.

NURSING IMPLICATIONS

Giving heparin and warfarin together will affect many laboratory measurements of coagulation and will complicate evaluation of the individual effects of each drug. When treatment is changed from heparin to warfarin (or a related oral anticoagulant), blood samples obtained sooner than six hours after the switch will not give useful information about the effects of the oral agent, owing to residual effects of the heparin.

Alterations in diet or general health, and addition or discontinuation of other medications, can alter warfarin action. Once the patient has been stabilized in the hospital, frequent follow-up evaluations will be needed after discharge to ensure that coagulation parameters are acceptable and to determine whether the anticoagulant dose needs to be changed. Instruct the patient to take warfarin at approximately the same time each day.

Side Effects, Adverse Reactions, and Contraindications

Several side effects of and adverse reactions to warfarin are similar to those caused by heparin (see Table 35–S). Excessive bleeding is the major problem. The contraindications for warfarin are also similar to those for heparin. Dietary vitamin K deficiency intensifies the actions of warfarin, as does excessive loss of vitamin K in the feces, which may be caused by steatorrhea. High dietary vitamin K intake may significantly antagonize warfarin's actions.

NURSING IMPLICATIONS

Advise outpatients taking warfarin to avoid vigorous activity that could cause bruising or damage to sensitive structures such as the kidneys, joints, and GI tract. Monitor patients for tarry stool or vomitus, hematuria, and joint pain or deformity.

◆ Use During Pregnancy and Lactation

Warfarin enters the fetal circulation and may cause fetal birth defects or excessive bleeding in the newborn. It should not be taken by pregnant women before the third trimester. If pregnancy occurs during warfarin therapy, the pros and cons of terminating either the pregnancy or the anticoagulant treatment should be considered. Warfarin is excreted in maternal milk and may alter coagulation in the nursing infant. Breast-feeding should be avoided.

◆ Use in Children

Warfarin doses for children have not been established.

◆ Use in the Elderly

The presence of complicating disease or malnutrition in elderly patients may increase their sensitivity to even small warfarin dosages. Anticipate that elderly patients will be taking one or more of the many drugs that can interact with warfarin, and monitor accordingly.

Interactions with Other Drugs

Clinically significant interactions between warfarin and other medications (Table 35–12) are far more common and potentially more dangerous than those described for heparin. One reason is that the list of interactants is very long. It includes drugs in many different pharmacologic classes that are used for treating a variety of disorders, and it includes both prescription and nonprescription medications. Another reason is that most patients who receive warfarin are outpatients: they are self-medicating, possibly with little supervision, and may not have ready access to proper monitoring facilities that can help prevent or detect unwanted effects.

There are about twice as many drugs or drug groups that increase the actions of warfarin—and the related risks of excessive bleeding—as there are medications that reduce anticoagulant effects. Some interactions must be avoided; all require careful monitoring of coagulation profiles to determine any need to reduce the anticoagulant dose.

Agents that increase the actions of warfarin include

- the antiarrhythmic drugs amiodarone and quinidine, the latter of which is often used, particularly with oral anticoagulants, to prevent thromboembolism in patients with atrial fibrillation or flutter;
- several antibiotics and other antimicrobial agents, including cephalosporins, chloramphenicol, erythromycin, metronidazole, nalidixic acid, and the sulfonamides;
- certain androgenic steroids, including danazol and some testosterones;
- most NSAIDs, of which aspirin poses one of the greatest risks;
- clofibrate, a commonly used lipid-lowering drug;
- histamine H_2 receptor blockers such as cimetidine, which are widely used to treat peptic ulcer disease and other GI disorders; and
- thyroid hormones.

These drugs can interact in different ways. Some exert their own anticoagulant or antiplatelet effects (eg, the antibiotics, quinidine, and aspirin); others inhibit the anticoagulant's metabolic inactivation in the liver (amiodarone, cimetidine); and others (eg, aspirin and other antiinflammatory drugs) displace the anticoagulant from plasma protein binding sites, increasing blood levels of free (active) warfarin.

As noted above, aspirin and related antiinflammatory drugs pose risks in more than one way: they inhibit platelet aggregation, thereby altering another component of the coagulation process, and they displace warfarin from binding sites. In addition, these drugs irritate and potentially damage the gastric mucosa. That effect favors local bleeding. When such local bleeding occurs and clotting processes are simultaneously inhibited, the risk of serious local blood loss or true hemorrhage rises considerably. It is important to note that usual analgesic/antipyretic doses of acetaminophen (TYLENOL, others) do not interact with warfarin; they are preferred for relief of minor pain and fever.

Drugs that antagonize the effects of warfarin—and may require increased anticoagulant doses to maintain the desired prothrombin time—include

- aminoglutethimide, a drug occasionally used to inhibit adrenal steroid synthesis; and
- barbiturates and phenytoin, both of which are widely used, and ethchlorvynol and glutethimide, which are seldom used nonbarbiturate hypnotics/sedatives.

These drugs stimulate the metabolic inactivation of warfarin. Importantly, benzodiazepines (eg, diazepam; Chapter 22, pp 355–359) do not interact similarly. They are almost always preferred to barbiturates or other CNS depressants, regardless of whether the patient is or is not taking anticoagulant also.

NURSING IMPLICATIONS

Ideally, obtain baseline prothrombin time measurements just before starting therapy with an interactant and frequently after combined administration starts. This will help determine how the dosage must be adjusted and when prothrombin times have stabilized again. This frequent monitoring of coagulation profiles and the clinical response, along with dosage readjustments, will be needed once again when therapy with the interactant is stopped.

Advise all outpatients who are treated with warfarin to carry identification (eg, a MedicAlert bracelet and ID card) indicating the medication(s) they are taking. Educate them to avoid interacting drugs (especially nonprescription agents), to recognize and report key signs and symptoms that could indicate unwanted effects, and to have periodically scheduled blood tests to assess the progress of therapy.

Overdose and Toxicity

Mild bleeding episodes caused by warfarin may be managed by omitting one or two doses. Complete discontinuation of warfarin administration is not appropriate, because it may induce a hypercoagulable state. Administration of vitamin K_1, the antidote for warfarin, as well as transfusions with whole blood or plasma concentrates rich in clotting factors, may be needed to control bleeding.

Vitamin K_1 as an Oral Anticoagulant Antidote

Vitamin K_1 (phytonadione; AQUAMEPHYTON, KONAKION) counteracts the inhibitory effects of warfarin on hepatic synthesis of vitamin K–dependent clotting factors, including prothrombin. Vitamin K_1 has no effect on excessive anticoagulation caused by heparin.

The usual dose of vitamin K_1 for managing slight warfarin overdoses is 2.5 to 10 mg, given orally or injected IM or SC. Higher doses, or IV administration, should be used only for severe bleeding. Vitamin K_1 administration can be repeated 8 to 10 hours after the initial dose if the prothrombin time has not decreased satisfactorily. Patients who fail to respond to the second dose are not likely to respond at all.

Vitamin K_1 can be used to treat hemorrhagic disorders in newborns of mothers who have been taking oral anticoagulants. It is also indicated for hypoprothrombinemia owing to inadequate vitamin K absorption from the GI tract, as may occur in some individuals with jaundice, sprue, or ulcerative colitis. Oral therapy with some antibiotic drugs may also reduce vitamin K absorption. Dosages are noted in Table 35–C.

Adverse responses to vitamin K_1 include flushing or hypotension; a few severe allergic reactions have been reported. Repeated injection may cause local erythema and pain. High doses of vitamin K_1 may cause reappearance of the clotting problems for which an oral anticoagulant was originally prescribed.

Related Drug

Dicumarol

Dicumarol (no proprietary names) has the same mechanism of anticoagulant action as warfarin. Unlike warfarin, however, dicumarol is incompletely and erratically absorbed from the GI tract, and its duration of action varies greatly with the dose. These unpredictable pharmacokinetic properties explain, in part, why dicumarol was recently withdrawn from the American market.

Thrombolytic Drugs

Thrombosis and embolism occur as the result of trauma or disease. Such interruptions of blood flow require prompt, definitive therapy to dissolve the obstruction before ischemic tissue damage occurs, especially when organs such as the brain, lungs, or heart are involved. The anticoagulants discussed above can prevent thrombosis and embolism but cannot dissolve thrombi or emboli. When such effects are necessary, **thrombolytic** drugs are used. Streptokinase is the prototype.

PROTOTYPE

Streptokinase

Streptokinase is an enzyme synthesized by β-hemolytic streptococci. The drug form (STREPTASE; KABIKINASE) contains purified, sterilized bacterial product.

Absorption, Distribution, Metabolism, and Excretion

Streptokinase is a protein and therefore cannot be given orally because it is destroyed by gastric acid. The drug is given parenterally. Little is known about its biologic fate.

Pharmacologic Effects

Streptokinase reacts with plasminogen, which is normally found in clots and in plasma, and converts it to plasmin, another proteolytic enzyme. Plasmin dissolves fibrin clots, fibrinogen, and several other proteins found in the clot and free in the plasma.

Clinical Indications and Administration

Lysis of Pulmonary or Systemic Emboli or Thrombi

Streptokinase can be infused IV to dissolve pulmonary emboli or thrombi in systemic arteries or veins. A loading dose of 250,000 International Units (IU) is first infused into a peripheral vein over 30 minutes. This is followed by a maintenance dosage of 100,000 IU per hour. If streptokinase is administered to dissolve pulmonary emboli, the maintenance dose infusion generally is continued for 24 hours; dissolution of arterial emboli or thrombi usually requires infusions lasting 24 to 72 hours, and deep venous thrombi usually require a full 72-hour infusion period.

Management of Acute Myocardial Infarction

Intracoronary infusion of streptokinase is sometimes used to manage acute myocardial ischemia and the resulting symptoms of acute myocardial infarction associated with coronary artery thrombosis. The overall goal of restoring coronary blood flow is to limit the extent of ischemic tissue death and dysfunction, which contribute to arrhythmias and heart failure. The likelihood of restoring myocardial blood flow seems best when ischemia is due to obstruction of only one major vessel. A common dose is 20,000 IU, given as a bolus, followed by a maintenance infusion of 2000 IU given over one hour. This is usually sufficient to restore blood flow, but it is not known whether the treatment salvages ischemic myocardium or reduces mortality. If streptokinase therapy fails or is contraindicated, other treatments, such as balloon angioplasty (mechanical distention of the vessel to disrupt and dislodge the thrombus) or coronary artery bypass surgery, are generally required.

Clearing Clogged Arterial or Venous Catheters

Streptokinase may be used to clear arterial or venous catheters that have become occluded by clots. Mechanical techniques and heparinized saline should be tried first to restore catheter patency.

NURSING IMPLICATIONS

Thrombolytic drugs are most effective when used immediately to manage acute thrombosis. Reconstitute the drug in 5% dextrose-normal-saline. Do not shake the contents; gently roll and tilt the bottle to mix. Aspirate the reconstituted drug into a syringe through a 0.22- or 0.45-μm filter. Streptokinase contains no preservatives, so the reconstituted solution should be refrigerated if not used immediately, and remaining unused solution should be discarded within 24 hours. Discard any solutions that contain appreciable flocculation. If possible, use an infusion pump to regulate the dose when thrombolytic drugs are used to dissolve thrombi or emboli.

Once streptokinase administration is completed, and coagulation profiles have returned toward normal, anticipate that the patient will be placed on anticoagulant therapy to prevent the formation of new thrombi. Anticoagulation therapy is usually started with an IV infusion of heparin; oral anticoagulant administration should be started at the same time, as discussed earlier.

Side Effects, Adverse Reactions, and Contraindications

Streptokinase prolongs normal coagulation processes; the thrombin time, APTT, and PT are all increased. Collectively, these effects may increase the risk of minor bleeding, especially at injection sites. Major contraindications include active internal bleeding; recent (within the last two months) intracranial bleeding or intracranial or intraspinal surgery; and brain neoplasms or vascular defects, including aneurysms. Otherwise, the general precautions and contraindications noted for anticoagulant drugs apply to thrombolytic drugs. Streptokinase may cause *reperfusion-induced arrhythmias* (mainly ventricular tachycardia or fibrillation) when used to dissolve coronary artery thrombi or emboli. Arrhythmias are not unique to streptokinase; they may be caused by any drug or surgical intervention that restores coronary blood flow abruptly.

Streptokinase can cause allergic reactions. Most are mild and can be managed by administration of antihistamines or corticosteroids. Streptokinase may also cause mild fever. If antipyretic therapy is needed, acetaminophen should be used because the antiplatelet actions of alternatives such as aspirin may increase bleeding tendencies.

NURSING IMPLICATIONS

Monitor for signs of excessive bleeding, particularly at injection sites. Avoid IM injections and nonessential handling of the patient during thrombolytic therapy. If venipuncture is absolutely essential, perform the technique carefully. Arterial puncture wounds will require firm pressure for at least 30 minutes to control bleeding. Minor bleeding usually can be controlled by applying pressure dressings, and streptokinase administration can be continued. Major bleeding must be managed by immediate discontinuation of streptokinase, and transfusion of whole blood, packed red cells, or plasma. Aminocaproic acid (p 716) may also be administered to help control excessive bleeding. Be prepared to administer appropriate antiarrhythmic drugs and to defibrillate the heart when streptokinase or other thrombolytic drugs are given for acute myocardial infarction.

◆ Use During Pregnancy and Lactation

The safety of administering streptokinase during pregnancy has not been established.

◆ Use in Children

The safety and efficacy of streptokinase for children have not been established.

Interactions with Other Drugs

Unless streptokinase is being used with heparin for coronary artery thrombosis, avoid using other drugs with effects on coagulation. It is best not to administer heparin or other anticoagulants before or during thrombolytic therapy, but heparin may be indicated when streptokinase is used for coronary thrombosis. To reduce risks from puncture wounds further, discontinue parenteral medications if possible, and substitute appropriate oral dosage forms. Platelet-active drugs such as aspirin and dipyridamole should be avoided. Specific actions with heparin are noted in Table 35–I1; those involving warfarin are listed in Table 35–I2.

Overdose and Toxicity

The major concern with streptokinase overdoses is excessive bleeding or hemorrhage. Transfusions, preferably with whole blood, are the most effective way to deal with these problems. When bleeding is not life-threatening, aminocaproic acid can be given.

Aminocaproic Acid as a Thrombolytic Drug Antidote

Aminocaproic acid (AMICAR) inhibits plasminogen activation and antagonizes plasmin. The drug can be given orally or IV (see Table 35–C for dosages). If aminocaproic acid is given IV, it should be injected slowly to reduce the risk of hypotension, bradycardia, and cardiac arrhythmias. The drug should not be administered to patients with active disseminated intravascular coagulation (DIC) unless heparin is given also.

Related Drugs

Alteplase, Recombinant

Alteplase (ACTIVASE) is also called tissue plasminogen activator, or t-PA. It is a thrombolytic agent indicated for dissolving obstructive coronary artery thrombi, as occurs with acute myocardial infarction (MI), and for improving ventricular function and lowering the incidence of heart failure associated with acute infarction.

Alteplase activates plasminogen to help dissolve thrombi. These effects depend on the presence of thrombin, which is found only in clots and is not free in the circulation. This dependency on thrombin tends to localize alteplase's effects to clots and dramatically reduces—but does not eliminate—the risk of widespread effects on coagulation throughout the rest of the bloodstream. Therefore, the risk of hemorrhage is much less than that associated with any other approved thrombolytic drug. In addition, alteplase has a very short half-life, which makes it easier to titrate the dose precisely.

Another potential advantage of alteplase is the way it is made. It is synthesized with modern recombinant DNA technology. This gene-cloning method makes alteplase, the drug, identical to human t-PA. This virtually eliminates the risk of the serious allergic reactions that are more commonly caused by the other thrombolytics, all of which are "foreign" and therefore antigenic materials.

Antistreplase

Antistreplase (EMINASE), the newest thrombolytic drug, is indicated for managing acute coronary artery thrombosis. Antistreplase is a complex of streptokinase and a derivative of human plasminogen. Once in the bloodstream, the drug is metabolized to a compound that converts plasminogen to plasmin, which causes fibrin (clot) breakdown. The usual dose is 30 units, injected into a peripheral vein over three to five minutes, starting as soon as possible after symptoms of coronary occlusion begin.

Antistreplase is very similar to the prototype, streptokinase, in several ways. Both drugs break down fibrin in clots and also attack circulating fibrinogen. Thus, the risks of internal (eg, intracranial) bleeding or hemorrhage are comparable. The risks of an allergic reaction or hypotension also seem to be equal. And, when treatment is started shortly after vessel occlusion (or symptoms appear), the two drugs seem to be equally effective in dissolving clots or preventing rethrombosis and reocclusion. Overall, all the major precautions and contraindications that apply to the prototype apply to antistreplase.

One advantage of antistreplase—at least in some settings—relates to its simple administration method: a brief injection into a peripheral vein. This can make antistreplase a good choice to use "in the field" (eg, on medical helicopter transports) or in any facility where staffing or equipment is limited.

Urokinase

Urokinase (ABBOKINASE; BREOKINASE) is used mainly for systemic thrombolysis. The drug is given IV (see Table 35–C) and is not indicated for intracoronary administration. Compared with streptokinase, urokinase may be associated with a lesser risk of plasminogen inactivation, bleeding, and fibrinolysis, and because the drug is derived from human tissue sources, fewer allergic reactions may occur.

Drugs Used to Inhibit Platelet Function

Drugs that inhibit platelet aggregation prevent thrombosis and are useful for managing some circulatory disorders in which thrombosis or thromboembolism seem to play an important role.

Aspirin

Aspirin (acetylsalicylic acid), which is discussed more fully in Chapter 52, has been mentioned throughout this chapter as a key interactant with anticoagulant and thrombolytic drugs. Aspirin also inhibits platelet aggregation. This effect occurs because the drug inhibits an enzyme called thromboxane synthase. The enzyme is crucial for the synthesis of thromboxane A_2, a potent stimulus for platelet–platelet aggregation, or "stickiness." Just one aspirin tablet (300–325 mg) doubles bleeding time for about seven days. That is the time needed for the body to synthesize new platelets, with intact biochemical processes, that can replace the platelets that were permanently altered by the aspirin. If aspirin doses are repeated, the antiplatelet effects will continue. Aspirin doses as low as 100 mg can cause the same effects; higher doses also cause the desired effects on platelets, plus other unwanted effects on blood vessels (and elsewhere; Table 52–S1). The antiplatelet effects of plain aspirin, generic or brand names, and special aspirin formulations (eg, buffered or enteric-coated) are the same.

These antiplatelet effects are clinically useful. One use is the prophylaxis of myocardial infarction (MI). Aspirin can reduce the risk of fatal or nonfatal heart attacks in patients who have suffered a heart attack already or who have unstable angina pectoris. The usual dose is 300 or 325 mg per day. Some physicians continue this therapy for the rest of the patient's life (unless contraindications develop). There is also a growing trend toward administering an aspirin tablet in the emergency department or clinic or physician's office to patients as soon as an MI is suspected. This may quickly prevent further thrombosis and vessel occlusion and can help the actions of other drugs—such as the thrombolytics—that may be administered later.

Another approved use of aspirin is the prophylaxis of recurrent transient ischemic attacks (TIAs, sometimes called "ministrokes"), or strokes, in men. The approved dose for this indication is 1300 mg per day, but there is good evidence that 300 mg is just as effective. Aspirin does not appear to prevent strokes in women (the reasons are unclear) and has no benefits once a stroke has developed fully in any patient.

See Tables 52–S1 and 52–I1 for summaries of aspirin's side effects, contraindications, and drug-drug interactions.

Dipyridamole

Dipyridamole (PERSANTINE) inhibits the ability of platelets to adhere to themselves or to other biologic or artificial structures. The drug is indicated for preventing thromboembolism, a potential complication after surgery to replace heart valves with prostheses. Artificial valves tend to attract and activate platelets, which may aggregate into thrombi and dislodge to cause embolism elsewhere. Dipyridamole is used as an adjunct to warfarin. Some of the mechanisms by which the drug inhibits platelet adhesion, including inhibited synthesis of thromboxane A_2, also block constriction of blood vessels. Hypotension may occur and may cause dizziness, the most common side effect of dipyridamole therapy. Dipyridamole must be used cautiously in hypotensive patients. Otherwise, there are no known contraindications. Dipyridamole allegedly causes few adverse fetal effects, but the drug should be administered during pregnancy only when absolutely necessary. The drug's safety in children under 12 years has not been established. Dipyridamole overdoses may cause brief episodes of hypotension.

The use of dipyridamole as an antianginal drug is mentioned briefly in Chapter 34 (p 686).

Sulfinpyrazone

Sulfinpyrazone (ANTURANE); approved for management of hyperuricemia (see Chapter 53), inhibits platelet aggregation. The drug appears to be an effective adjunct for reducing the risk of thrombosis, and permitting reduced heparin doses, in hemodialysis patients. This is an unapproved use of which the nurse should be aware. It is more important to be aware that sulfinpyrazone may cause excessive effects on coagulation when given for its approved use, and especially when used with other anticoagulant or antiplatelet drugs, including aspirin or other salicylates. See Table 53–S for a list of side effects and contraindications, and Table 53–I for more drug interactions.

Ticlopidine

Ticlopidine (TICLID) is an orally effective antiplatelet drug. It is approved for reducing the incidence of thrombotic stroke in patients who are at high-risk of that event, and for administration to patients who have had a completed stroke caused by thrombi. Dosages are listed in Table 35–C. There are several other uses related to ticlopidine's ability to inhibit platelet aggregation, but they are not approved and are not discussed further here.

Aspirin shares ticlopidine's indication for reducing the risk of stroke. Aspirin should be tried first because ticlopidine use is associated with a risk of neutropenia and agranulocytosis. Although the overall incidence is less than about 2% for all ticlopidine-treated patients, neutropenia can allow otherwise minor infections to become serious, and agranulocytosis can be fatal. When neutropenia and agranulocytosis occur, ticlopidine therapy should be stopped. To detect these problems early, complete blood counts should be performed frequently through the third month of therapy. After that, the risk of blood dyscrasias seems to decrease dramatically. Nevertheless, periodic blood tests are still important.

Ticlopidine therapy also includes an increased risk of prolonged or excessive bleeding, especially if used with other drugs that affect blood coagulation. The related precautions and assessment tools are the same as those used during therapy with aspirin or other antiplatelet agents. Aspirin and ticlopidine should not be used together owing to an even greater risk of bleeding.

The most common side effects of ticlopidine therapy are nausea, diarrhea, and gastric upset or pain. Taking ticlopidine with meals to reduce GI discomfort is preferred to administering antacids, which can reduce ticlopidine absorption.

The information about drug interactions involving ticlopidine is relatively scant, aside from the previously mentioned interactions with antacids and aspirin. It is known that the drug can significantly interfere with theophylline metabolism, leading to an increased risk of theophylline toxicity. Monitor accordingly, and anticipate the need to reduce the bronchodilator dose. Cimetidine can reduce ticlopidine's metabolic inactivation, and ticlopidine may lower digoxin blood levels. At this time, however, it is not known whether the cimetidine or digoxin interactions are clinically significant. Proper monitoring is recommended, however.

NURSING IMPLICATIONS

Explain to patients the need for and importance of blood tests. Advise them not to self-medicate with aspirin, acetaminophen, or ibuprofen if they develop a fever, chills, or nonspecific aches and pains. These could be signs and symptoms of infection caused by a blood dyscrasia, and masking them with an analgesic or antipyretic drug could delay prompt evaluation and proper treatment. Instead, urge patients to consult their physician at once. He or she should perform the necessary blood tests to rule out serious problems before prescribing a drug to manage the patient's complaints.

Miscellaneous Drug

Pentoxifylline

Pentoxifylline (TRENTAL) reduces the adhesiveness of red blood cells and reduces overall blood viscosity. It is an orally effective drug indicated for treatment of intermittent claudication, as occurs in chronic occlusive arterial disease of the extremities. Pentoxifylline merely reduces symptoms of the disorder; it is not a replacement for other pharmacologic or surgical therapies for vascular disease.

Pentoxifylline may be used with other drugs that affect coagulation, but more frequent monitoring of coagulation parameters is necessary to detect bleeding tendencies. The drug may cause hypotension, which requires periodic blood pressure monitoring. Pentoxifylline should be used cautiously in pregnant women, and breast-feeding should be discouraged. Little is known about its use in children under 18 years old. Pentoxifylline is structurally related to the methylxanthines (caffeine, theophylline, aminophylline), and should not be administered to patients with prior intolerance to any of these agents.

SUMMARY OF NURSING IMPLICATIONS 

◆ Assessment

Determine the presence of conditions that may place the patient at added risk for hemorrhage (eg, liver or renal disease).

Complete a nursing history to include allergies, and use of OTC drugs.

Complete baseline blood tests (eg, PT, PTT); results must be reviewed by physician before beginning therapy.

Review past and present medication history for contraindications to anticoagulant, thrombolytic, or antiplatelet therapy.

Assess for signs of excessive or abnormal bleeding or bruising throughout therapy.

Table 35–C **Clinical Uses and Administration of Major Anticoagulant, Thrombolytic, and Antiplatelet Drugs (*Continued*)**

AGENT	CLINICAL USES	DOSAGE AND ROUTE OF ADMINISTRATION
	Drugs Affecting Platelet Function	
Aspirin	Reducing risk of stroke in male patients with recurrent TIA	Oral: Usually 1300 mg/day in 2 or 4 divided doses
	Reducing risk of myocardial infarction in patients with prior infarction or unstable angina pectoris	Oral: Usually 300-1500 mg/day in divided doses
	Other uses	See Chapter 52
Dipyridamole (PERSANTINE)	Adjunct to oral coagulants for preventing postoperative thromboembolic complications of cardiac valve replacement	Oral: Usually 75–100 mg qid
Ticlopidine (TICLID)	Reducing the risk of thrombotic stroke in high-risk patients; adjunctive management of evolved thrombotic stroke	Oral: 250 mg bid with meals
	Miscellaneous	
Pentoxifylline (TRENTAL)	Treatment of intermittent claudication from chronic occlusive arterial disease of the limbs	Oral: Usually 400 mg tid with meals

Table 35–S | **Major Side Effects of and Contraindications for Anticoagulant, Thrombolytic, and Antiplatelet Drugs***

BODY SYSTEM/ Side Effect	CONTRAINDICATION/ PRECAUTION	COMMENTS AND NURSING IMPLICATIONS
Side Effects and Contraindications for All Anticoagulants		
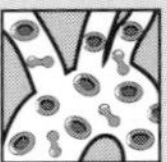 **BLOOD** Increased risk of excessive bleeding, hemorrhage	Active bleeding; history of bleeding disorders; recent head or eye trauma; imminent parturition or abortion; lumbar puncture; CNS or ophthalmic surgery; peptic ulcer disease; severe hypertension or risk of stroke, aneurysm	Problems likely to be greatest with excessive doses of any drug affecting hemostasis, failure to reduce doses when indicated, use of interacting drugs; aim anticoagulant therapy to achieve APTT that is 1.5 to 2 times normal value (30–40 sec) with heparin; PT 1.5 to 2.5 times normal (12 sec) with oral anticoagulants
Side Effects and Contraindications Mainly for Heparin		
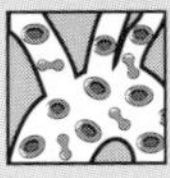 **BLOOD** Excessive bleeding	See above	Monitor APTT closely; discontinue heparin if evidence of bleeding occurs; be prepared to administer antidote, protamine sulfate, then observe for excessive coagulation caused by antidote
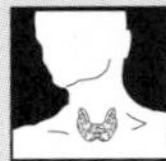 **ENDOCRINE** Hypoaldosteronism and resulting hyperkalemia		Most likely with chronic high-dose treatment
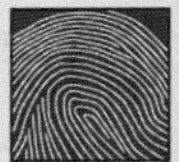 **SKIN** Alopecia		Advise patient that hair loss may occur, even up to several months after heparin therapy; alopecia is usually reversible
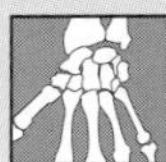 **BONE** Osteoporosis, susceptibility to fractures		Most common in postmenopausal women
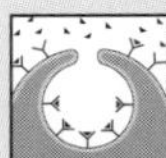 **IMMUNE SYSTEM** Allergic reactions, mild to severe: rhinitis, urticaria, hypotension, bronchospasm, etc.	Known hypersensitivity; use with care in patients with high incidence of hypersensitivity reactions, asthma	May depend on brand of heparin, animal source of drug; patients may tolerate other brands/sources better
Side Effects and Contraindications Mainly for Warfarin		
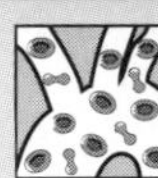 **BLOOD**	Severe debilitating disease (eg, heart, hepatic, or renal dysfunction)	Probably due to impaired synthesis of hepatic clotting factors; use reduced dosages, monitor PT closely, skip one or two anticoagulant doses if PT excessively prolonged or evidence of bleeding occurs

(continued)

Table 35–S **Major Side Effects of and Contraindications for Anticoagulant, Thrombolytic, and Antiplatelet Drugs* (*Continued*)**

BODY SYSTEM/ Side Effect	CONTRAINDICATION/ PRECAUTION	COMMENTS AND NURSING IMPLICATIONS
Side Effects and Contraindications for Thrombolytic Drugs		
BLOOD Excessive bleeding	See heparin, oral anticoagulants, above	Control minor bleeding at injection site or other sites of body penetration (eg, surgical wounds, catheter insertion sites) with direct pressure; if major bleeding occurs, discontinue thrombolytic drug, infuse whole blood or packed red cells or plasma; administer aminocaproic acid as needed
IMMUNE SYSTEM Minor to severe allergic reactions	History of allergic reaction to thrombolytic agent(s)	Check history of reaction to thrombolytic drugs; discontinue administration at once if signs of anaphylaxis occur; be prepared to administer epinephrine, steroids, antihistamines as needed; lowest risk with alteplase, which is derived from human genetic material.
Side Effects and Contraindications for Antiplatelet Drugs		
BLOOD Excessive bleeding	Recent bleeding disorder, including recent history of bleeding gastric ulcers, stroke; surgery anticipated within next 2 weeks	Monitor accordingly; teach proper self-assessment
Additional Side Effects and Contraindications Involving Aspirin		
	See Table 52-S1	
Additional Side Effects and Contraindications Involving Sulfinpyrazone		
	See Table 53-S	
Additional Side Effects and Contraindications Involving Ticlopidine		
GASTROINTESTINAL Nausea, GI pain or discomfort		Administer ticlopidine with meals
BLOOD Neutropenia, agranulocytosis, and related blood dyscrasias; potentially serious or fatal	Neutropenia, infection, compromised immune system	Blood tests should be performed frequently, especially during first 3 months of ticlodipine treatment; advise patient to report immediately any sign, symptom, of potential underlying infection, to withhold OTC analgesic/antipyretic drug self-administration until evaluated by physician

*For side effects and contraindications for aspirin, see Chapter 52.

Table 35–I1 Major Interactions Between Heparin and Other Drugs

AGENT	RESULT OF INTERACTION	COMMENTS AND NURSING IMPLICATIONS
Cephalosporin antibiotics, parenteral (Chapter 56)	Potential for increased bleeding risk	Combined therapy acceptable but necessitates closer monitoring of coagulation profiles
Nitroglycerin, intravenous (Chapter 34)	Potential reduction of heparin's effects	Combined use acceptable, but monitor coagulation profiles often for potential interaction
Penicillins, parenteral (Chapter 56)	Potential for increased bleeding risk	As for parenteral cephalosporins
Salicylates (eg, aspirin; Chapter 52)	Increased bleeding risk likely	Evidence of interaction may occur quickly; applies to all formulations of aspirin (eg, buffered, enteric-coated); avoid interaction if possible; otherwise, monitor coagulation profiles closely, and treat bleeding symptomatically

Table 35–I2 Major Interactions Between Warfarin and Other Drugs

AGENT	RESULT OF INTERACTION	COMMENTS AND NURSING IMPLICATIONS
Aminoglutethimide (Chapter 59)	Increased anticoagulant metabolism, decreased effects	Monitor prothrombin time (PT) to help determine when and how to increase anticoagulant dose
Amiodarone (Chapter 30)	Increased, potentially serious anticoagulant effects (bleeding, hemorrhage) from inhibited anticoagulant metabolism	Interaction almost certain; decrease anticoagulant dose by 30% to 50% of usual; monitor closely to make further dosage adjustments, especially during first month of combined therapy: interaction longlasting owing to amiodarone's prolonged effects
Androgens, 17-alkyl (eg, danazol, methandrostenolone, oxymetholone, stanozolol; Chapter 48)	Potentially serious increase of anticoagulant effects, bleeding tendencies	Avoid interaction if possible; otherwise, monitor PT closely; interaction not likely to involve "nonalkyl" derivatives, eg, testosterone
Antiinflammatory drugs, nonsteroidal (NSAIDS; Chapter 52)	Increased anticoagulant effects, potential risk of bleeding (especially in GI tract) or hemorrhage	Risks vary with individual NSAIDs (see phenylbutazone and salicylates, below); mechanisms involve one or more of the following: displacement of anticoagulant from plasma protein binding sites and direct antiplatelet and gastric-irritating effects of NSAID; monitor PT closely if combined therapy unavoidable
Aspirin	See salicylates	
Barbiturates (Chapter 22)	Increased anticoagulant metabolism, decreased effects	Avoid interaction if possible, eg, by using benzodiazepine alternative; monitor closely; anticipate need to increase anticoagulant dosage after start of barbiturate use and reduce anticoagulant dosage when interactant therapy is stopped

(continued)

Table 35–12 **Major Interactions Between Warfarin and Other Drugs (*Continued*)**

AGENT	RESULT OF INTERACTION	COMMENTS AND NURSING IMPLICATIONS
Carbamazepine (Chapter 26)	As for barbiturates	Avoid if possible; otherwise, monitor as noted for barbiturates
Cephalosporin antibiotics (Chapter 56)	Additive, potentially serious increase of bleeding risk	Monitor PT if interaction is unavoidable; anticipate potential need for reduced anticoagulant dosage
Chloramphenicol (Chapter 56)	As for cephalosporins	As for cephalosporins
Cholestyramine (Chapter 36)	Reduced anticoagulant effects	Ideally, separate administration of interactants by at least 3 hr, but stress need for daily consistency with whatever schedule is used; monitor PT
Clofibrate (Chapter 36)	Serious, potentially fatal increase of anticoagulant effects	Avoid combination if possible; otherwise monitor PT often
Disulfiram (Chapter 22)	Increased anticoagulant effects	Monitor PT often as guide for potential dosage adjustments
Erythromycin (Chapter 56)	Increased anticoagulant effects, potentially serious	Monitor PT closely; anticoagulant dose may need to be reduced significantly or discontinued altogether during combined therapy
Ethchlorvynol (Chapter 22)	Decreased anticoagulant effects	See barbiturates, above
Glutethimide (Chapter 22)	Decreased anticoagulant effects	See barbiturates, above
Griseofulvin (Chapter 57)	Decreased anticoagulant effects	Monitor PT often when starting or stopping griseofulvin therapy
Cimetidine (Chapter 40)	Increased anticoagulant effects; potential hemorrhage	Cimetidine significantly reduces anticoagulant metabolism; avoid combination; interaction reported with ranitidine, presumably less likely with famotidine or nizatidine (preferred alternatives)
Metronidazole (Chapter 57)	Significantly increased anticoagulant action, risk of hemorrhage	Monitor PT if interaction unavoidable; anticipate need for reduced anticoagulant dosage
Nalidixic acid (Chapter 57)	Significantly increased anticoagulant action, potential hemorrhage	Monitor PT; anticipate reduced anticoagulant dosage during combined therapy
Phenylbutazone, oxyphenbutazone (Chapter 52)	Significantly increased risk of bleeding or hemorrhage	Avoid by using alternative NSAIDs; interactions involving these drugs pose greater risks than with any other NSAIDs owing to three factors: decreased anticoagulant metabolism, displacement from plasma proteins, gastric mucosal irritation
Phenytoin (Chapter 26)	Increased blood levels and potential toxicity of phenytoin; increased risk of excessive anticoagulation	Closely monitor phenytoin levels, evidence of seizure control and PT during combined therapy
Quinidine, quinine (Chapter 30)	Potential increased risk of bleeding	Combined quinidine-anticoagulant therapy is common; monitor PT closely as guide for possible anticoagulant dosage reduction
Rifampin (Chapter 57)	Increased anticoagulant metabolism, decreased effects	Monitor PT; anticipate need to increase anticoagulant dose during combined therapy and to decrease when rifampin therapy is stopped

(continued)

Table 35–I2 Major Interactions Between Warfarin and Other Drugs (*Continued*)

AGENT	RESULT OF INTERACTION	COMMENTS AND NURSING IMPLICATIONS
Salicylates, acetylated (eg, aspirin; Chapter 52)	Increased risk of bleeding, hemorrhage	Aspirin displaces oral anticoagulant from plasma proteins, irritates gut mucosa, and exerts antiplatelet actions; monitor PT closely during combined use; discourage self-prescribed aspirin use (all dosages, forms, products); recommend acetaminophen for relief of minor fever, pain; nonacetylated salicylates (eg, choline or magnesium salicylate) are less likely to interact
Sulfinpyrazone (Chapter 53)	Increased risk of bleeding, hemorrhage	Monitor PT; anticipate need to reduce anticoagulant dosage; when goal is to increase uric acid excretion, probenecid seems to be preferred noninteracting alternative
Sulfonamides, especially sulfamethoxazole-trimethoprim combination (Chapter 56)	Increased risk of bleeding, hemorrhage	Monitor PT closely; anticipate need for reduced anticoagulant dose during combined therapy
Thyroid hormones (eg, dextrothyroxine, levothyroxine, liothyronine; Chapter 47)	Potentially serious increase of anticoagulant effects	Anticipate need for reduced anticoagulant dosages based on PT monitoring

Table 35–I3 Interactions Between Antiplatelet Drugs and Other Agents

AGENT	RESULT OF INTERACTION	COMMENTS AND NURSING IMPLICATIONS
General Interactions Involving All Antiplatelet Drugs		
Anticoagulants, thrombolytics	Risk of excessive bleeding	Monitor all relevant coagulation parameters if combined use is necessary; discourage self-medication with aspirin for other uses (eg, fever, pain) without physician's approval
Additional Interactions Involving Aspirin		
	See Table 52–I1	
Additional Interactions Involving Sulfinpyrazone		
	See Table 53–I	
Additional Interactions Involving Ticlopidine		
Theophylline (Chapter 37)	Increased theophylline blood levels, effects, potential toxicity	Ticlopidine inhibits theophylline metabolism; assess accordingly, monitor theophylline blood levels, anticipate reducing dose, especially when starting ticlopidine therapy; reassess when ticlopidine therapy is stopped

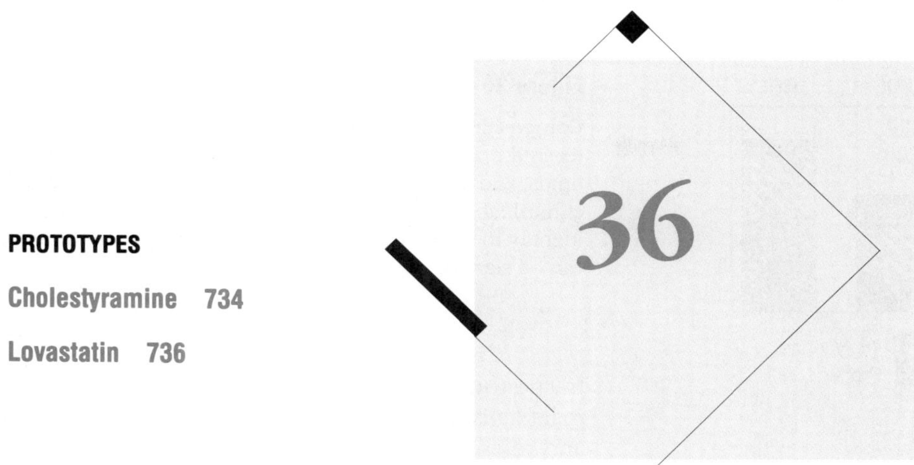

PROTOTYPES

36 Drugs for Regulating Blood Lipid Levels

Atherosclerosis ("hardening of the arteries") contributes to over 500,000 deaths in the United States each year. Most of the deaths are caused by atherosclerotic coronary artery disease, leading to cardiac ischemia and infarction. The brain and kidneys are also common sites of atherosclerotic damage. Atherosclerosis is usually caused by an abnormal increase of blood lipid levels, particularly those of cholesterol and triglycerides (hypercholesterolemia and hypertriglyceridemia, respectively). This chapter identifies the major serum lipids and how they are regulated; cardiovascular risk factors caused by hyperlipidemias; the importance of diet to control hyperlipidemias; and the use of lipid-lowering (antihyperlipidemic) drugs.

Plasma Lipids, Lipoproteins, and Their Regulation

The major plasma lipids are composed of cholesterol, cholesteryl esters, triglycerides, phospholipids, and free fatty acids. These substances serve as essential structural components of cell membranes. Plasma lipids are not water-soluble. They are carried by protein-containing particles, called *lipoproteins,* from their sites of synthesis in the liver and intestines to their sites of utilization, mainly muscle and adipose tissue.

The three major classes of lipoproteins differ in terms of the types of lipids and proteins they contain (Fig. 36–1) and their size, shape, and density. Their unique properties provide a way for the clinical laboratory to separate, identify, and measure them. That information, in turn, helps make the diagnosis and plan treatment.

- *Very-low-density lipoproteins* (VLDL; sometimes called pre-β-lipoproteins) are triglyceride-rich but also contain cholesterol and phospholipids; they are synthesized in the liver and intestines, and mainly transport triglycerides and cholesterol.
- *Low-density lipoproteins* (LDL, or β-lipoproteins), also produced in liver and intestine, are rich in cholesterol. They account for about two thirds of the circulating cholesterol in humans.
- *High-density lipoproteins* (HDL) contain relatively small amounts of cholesterol and triglyceride. Unlike the other major lipoproteins, HDL seems to provide an important way to transport cholesterol from the peripheral tissues to the liver for eventual excretion in the bile.

Major reference tables appear beginning on page 744.

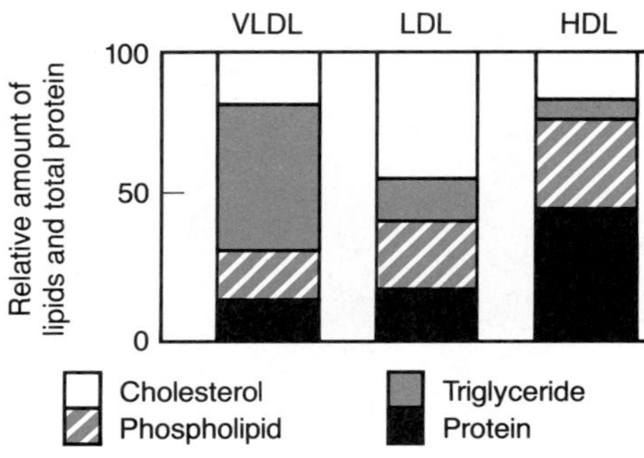

Figure 36–1

Composition of plasma lipoproteins. VLDL, LDL, and HDL differ in the amounts of cholesterol, triglycerides, phospholipids, and protein they contain. These differences help the clinical laboratory separate and measure each, and help identify the type of hyperlipidemia so that proper treatment can be started.

Some cholesterol is absorbed from the diet, but dietary cholesterol is not essential, because most tissues in the body, and the liver and intestines in particular, can synthesize it in sufficient amounts. Some cholesterol is converted to bile acids, which are then excreted in the feces. Bile acids also increase fecal elimination of unconverted cholesterol.

Hyperlipidemias

Increased blood levels of cholesterol, triglycerides, or both—and of the lipoprotein fractions in which they are mainly found (LDL and VLDL, respectively)—are associated with an increased risk of organ disease. The heart, brain, and kidneys are common and important sites of damage. There is a very strong link between elevated LDL cholesterol levels and coronary heart disease (CHD). In contrast, higher levels of the cholesterol-poor HDL seem to be associated with a reduced risk. (For this reason, HDL is often casually referred to as the "good cholesterol.")

Lipid Changes, and Detecting Them

Hyperlipidemias often do not involve increased levels of all the lipoprotein fractions or the lipids in them. As shown in Table 36–1, one or more values may be increased, whereas others may stay normal. The pattern of the changes provides the basis for classifying, diagnosing, and treating the abnormality. Measurements of the individual lipoprotein fractions—such as VLDL, LDL, and HDL—and the cholesterol and triglyceride levels associated with them are far more useful than measurements of total cholesterol or triglyceride levels.

These tests, which should be done on a fasting blood sample, are routine. The test results are analyzed to help classify the hyperlipidemia and determine its severity. Values for each measured lipid and lipoprotein fraction in the patient's blood are compared with normal (statistical) values that are tabulated in various texts and references to assess the extent of change. The normal values are reported as averages and a range of upper and lower limits. Normal values differ according to age and sex.

Classifications

The lipid abnormalities are classified in several ways. The basic system (Table 36–1) uses Roman numerals, and each numeric class has one or more names that usually describe the alteration. For example, Type IIb hyperlipidemia is characterized by increased cholesterol levels (in various lipoprotein fractions) but normal triglyceride levels. It is often called *hypercholesterolemia,* or *familial hypercholesterolemia.*

Primary and Secondary Hyperlipidemias

Hyperlipidemias can also be described in terms of their underlying cause. A small number of hyperlipidemias are idiopathic: the cause is unknown. Nearly 95% of all hyperlipidemias are *primary hyperlipidemias.* They are usually caused by genetic (hereditary or familial) factors, and the traits are passed on to the offspring. (This is one reason why obtaining a thorough family history from the patient is a crucial part of the assessment.) In simplest terms, these genetic characteristics affect one or more metabolic steps that are important in lipid or lipoprotein metabolism and regulation.

Secondary hyperlipidemias have other identifiable causes. The common ones are diet (eating too much altogether, or simply eating too much of the wrong foods), smoking, and excessive alcohol consumption. Other causes include diabetes mellitus, hypothyroidism, and renal or hepatic disease. As noted below, some drugs can also increase lipid levels.

Only about 5% of hyperlipidemic patients have "pure" secondary hyperlipidemia—ie, lipid levels that would be normal if it were not for an "outside" cause.

Table 36–1 | A Simplified Classification of the Major Hyperlipidemias

		Lipoprotein Abnormality			Plasma Lipid Changes		Relationship to Increased Coronary Disease
Type	**Synonym**	**VLDL**	**LDL**	**HDL**	**Cholesterol**	**Triglyceride**	
I	Familial hyperchylomicronemia (exogenous hypertriglyceridemia)	NC	↓	↓	↑	↑	None
IIa	Familial hypercholesterolemia	NC	↑	↓	↑	NC	Positive
IIb	Combined hyperlipoproteinemia (familial multiple-type hyperlipoproteinemia)	↑	↑	NC	↑	↑	Positive
III	Broad-β disease (familial dysbetalipoproteinemia)	↑	↑	NC	↑	↑	Positive
IV	Familial hypertriglyceridemia (exogenous hypertriglyceridemia)	↑	NC	NC or ↓	NC	↑	Unclear
V	Familial mixed hyperlipemia (mixed hypertriglyceridemia)	↑	NC	NC or ↓	↑	↑	Unclear

Key: ↑ = increased; ↓ = decreased; NC = no change (compared to normal values for age and sex).

Nevertheless, secondary factors must also be assessed for because they can, and often do, aggravate an underlying primary lipid abnormality. Correcting or eliminating secondary causes may reduce the need for drugs given to treat the primary disorder.

Nondrug Aspects of Therapy

There are three nonpharmacologic aspects to the management of essentially all hyperlipidemias, primary or secondary: modifying the diet and alcohol intake, stopping smoking, and exercising. Each is clearly important, and each should be implemented at the outset of treatment, based on the patient's individual health, needs, and abilities. For patients with mild lipid abnormalities and no apparent organ damage, these nondrug measures alone may reduce or delay risks. However, even when drugs are prescribed, the nondrug measures remain as integral and essential parts of a holistic treatment plan. They may allow adequate lipid control with lower drug dosages than would be needed otherwise.

Diet

Dietary modifications should be tried, and the effects evaluated, *before* drug therapy is started. This general guideline applies to all patients except those who are at imminent risk (ie, patients with severe hyperlipidemias or one or more coronary heart risk factors). If the desired outcomes of a change in diet alone are not attained and maintained, then drug therapy can be implemented, but as an ongoing adjunct to diet.

Dietary changes are usually implemented in steps to achieve goals gradually, and in a way that makes lifestyle changes more tolerable for the patient; and to determine whether and how well the patient will follow recommendations. Periodic follow-up to assess compliance and progress are therefore essential. The exact dietary changes that might be prescribed are based on medical and other characteristics of each patient. However, several aspects of diet and general dietary goals apply to all patients. They include reducing daily intake of total fat, saturated fat, cholesterol, and calories; reducing cholesterol, triglyceride, and lipoprotein levels to the age-dependent norms; and reducing body weight to norms for age and stature. All diets must strive to maintain an overall adequate nutritional status.

Alcohol intake must be considered part of an overall dietary plan. Modest alcohol consumption may have some protective effects on cardiovascular risk. In contrast, high-dose, long-term alcohol intake exerts many adverse effects on many organs and metabolic processes, including those that regulate serum lipid levels. The patient should therefore limit alcohol intake.

Relatively few nurses (and physicians) have adequate training in nutrition or the ability or time to provide proper, individualized counseling. Registered nutritionists are usually the best source of information about diet and related aspects (eg, what to eat and shop for, how to prepare palatable yet nutritious meals, and the like). Ideally, these professionals are part of the overall treatment team, engaging in one-to-one contact with the patient.

Smoking

Stopping smoking, or at least cutting down on smoking drastically, is another critical nondrug aspect of therapy for many patients. Just as it is important to start dietary therapy early on, the patient should also take measures to curb smoking immediately. Smoking causes or worsens the key lipid abnormalities, favors atherosclerosis, and causes increases of heart rate and blood pressure (and other changes) that can put further stress on a diseased heart.

Drugs marketed to help a person quit smoking are available by prescription (see Chapter 16, p 256). However, the agents that are most likely to be effective contain nicotine. Their safety for persons with hyperlipidemias and other cardiovascular risk factors remains to be established. Their use has to be determined on a case-by-case basis by the physician.

Exercise

Adequate aerobic exercise helps bring about desired changes in lipid profiles, aids in weight reduction, and improves overall fitness. Exercise also seems to facilitate an overall change in a person's attitudes toward wellness, which can carry over into diet and smoking habits. Because persons differ in their overall health and exercise tolerance, exercise plans should be tailored for each patient by a professional who has experience in the field and familiarity with the patient's medical and lifestyle history.

NURSING IMPLICATIONS

It may be easy to prescribe any or all of these nondrug approaches. Unfortunately, implementing them adequately—perhaps for the rest of the patient's life—requires major lifestyle changes that may not be easy to accept for long. It also requires much effort in patient teaching and counseling, time and money for consultation with experts (eg, registered nutritionists), and frequent follow-up assessments. Furthermore, most patients are well aware that drugs can treat their medical condition and that taking a pill or two each day can provide desirable effects with much less personal effort. Therefore, over the long run it may be difficult or impossible to rely on nondrug measures. Nevertheless, each of these nondrug factors must be considered and encouraged for every patient. Optimal therapy also requires engaging the patient as an active partner with all members of the health-care team.

Lipid-Elevating Drugs

A variety of drugs can cause unwanted effects on serum lipid levels. Avoiding these drugs or using alternatives, if possible, should be considered. Perhaps the worst offenders are estrogens (and oral contraceptives; Chapter 49), thiazide diuretics (Chapter 32), and some β-adrenergic blockers (Chapter 15).

Thiazides and β blockers deserve special mention because of their widespread use in treating cardiovascular diseases, such as heart failure, hypertension, and angina pectoris—disorders that often accompany (or may be caused or worsened by) hyperlipidemias. As mentioned elsewhere (eg, see pp 660 and 661 and Table 36–2), alternative drugs that cause the same desired effects but fewer of the unwanted lipid changes are available. Thus, it is important to assess whether one of these more suitable agents can be used for patients with hyperlipidemias plus other medical conditions.

Antihyperlipidemic Drugs

There is good evidence that all of the antihyperlipidemic drugs are effective when the proper drug is selected, correct dosages are prescribed and taken, and the patient follows dietary and other nondrug advice. The drugs can reduce the progression of atherosclerosis; some can reduce morbidity and mortality; and some drugs—current and future—may be able to reverse atherosclerotic damage to blood vessels and organs. Overall, most of the antihyperlipidemic drugs provide long-term benefits to the patient that outweigh the potential risks caused by the drugs themselves—and long-term therapy is exactly what is needed.

No one drug can correct all hyperlipidemias in all patients. The medication plan therefore involves selecting a drug that is best suited for the individual's lipid abnormalities and treatment goals. Quite often, two drugs are administered, usually for one of three reasons:

Table 36–2 Some Factors That Increase or Decrease LDL or HDL Cholesterol

Factor	Effect on HDL or LDL Level	Comments
Sex	↓ HDL ↑ LDL	HDL levels are generally higher in women; LDL levels are usually higher in males than in premenopausal women, and higher in postmenopausal women than in men of identical age
Age	↑ HDL ↓ LDL	HDL levels rise slightly with age, mainly in females; LDL levels generally rise up to age 60
Diet		
Alcohol	↑ or ↓ HDL	HDL levels rise with moderate alcohol consumption, fall with excessive intake
Carbohydrates	↓ HDL	
Cholesterol	↑ LDL	
Fat, polyunsaturated	↓ LDL	
Fat, saturated	↑ LDL	Cereals, fruits, and vegetables generally have favorable effect on HDL and LDL
Fiber	↓ LDL	
Fish	↑ HDL	
Vegetarian diet	↓ HDL	
Exercise	↑ HDL	Exercise also helps overall weight control, improves cardiovascular status
Smoking	↓ HDL	Encourage reduction or complete cessation of smoking
Diseases, disorders		
Obesity	↓ HDL ↑ LDL	Weight loss tends to beneficially reverse effects on HDL and LDL
Hypothyroidism	↑ HDL ↑ LDL	Treatment of hypothyroidism may lower LDL levels
Renal disease	↓ HDL ↑ LDL	
Diabetes mellitus	↓ HDL	Control of diabetes tends to lower overall cardiovascular risk
Drugs		
Oral contraceptives	↑ or ↓ HDL ↑ LDL	Change of HDL depends on composition of contraceptive: decreased by progestins, increased by estrogens, especially in postmenopausal women; LDL may rise with pregnancy; oral contraceptives may decrease actions of drugs used to lower serum lipid levels
β-blockers	↓ HDL ↑ LDL	
Thiazide diuretics	↓ HDL ↑ LDL	

Key: ↑ = increased, ↓ = decreased (from baseline)

- Some drugs have additive effects on one or more lipids, so greater effects can be achieved with combined therapy.
- Some drugs cause desired effects on a particular lipid, but unwanted effects on another; the second drug may counteract the unwanted actions.
- Some patients have multiple lipid abnormalities, each of which is best treated with a different drug.

Although the various drugs may be effective, individually or when used in combination, they differ in their adverse effects. These effects range from common, relatively minor ones to those that can be considered adverse or plainly dangerous. This consideration is important in therapy planning and monitoring. Moreover, some drug combinations should be avoided altogether, and some must be chosen with care; when less than ideal combinations must be prescribed, especially close monitoring for adverse effects is needed.

There are two major groups of antihyperlipidemic drugs—the *bile acid sequestrants* and the *cholesterol synthesis inhibitors*—plus several other miscellaneous agents. For many patients, drug treatment starts with one of the bile sequestrants. However, there is a growing trend toward starting patients on one of the cholesterol synthesis inhibitors early on, particularly patients who have severe hyperlipidemias, who have suffered a heart attack, or who have hyperlipidemia accompanied by diabetes mellitus or other risk factors.

I. Bile Acid Sequestrants

Cholestyramine and a related drug, colestipol, are classified as bile acid sequestrants based on their major mechanism of action. These drugs have a long track record of safe use and have been shown to be effective in the primary prevention of CHD. One of these drugs is often chosen first when drug therapy is started.

PROTOTYPE

Cholestyramine

Absorption, Distribution, Metabolism, and Excretion

Cholestyramine (CHOLYBAR, QUESTRAN) acts solely in the gastrointestinal (GI) tract. It is not absorbed. The drug is excreted in the feces.

Pharmacologic Effects

Cholesterol is the metabolic building block for the bile acids, which are crucial for the digestion and absorption of dietary fats. During digestion, bile acids are secreted into the intestine by way of the gallbladder. However, cholesterol is reabsorbed into the hepatic portal circulation, eventually reaching the systemic circulation once again. This process is called **enterohepatic recirculation**.

Cholestyramine sequesters (binds) bile salts in the gut, forming an insoluble complex that cannot be reabsorbed. Thus, bile salts and cholesterol are excreted in the stool. Gradually, serum cholesterol and LDL levels fall. Indirect effects include an increase of cholesterol synthesis and bile secretion. Although increased cholesterol synthesis can raise serum cholesterol levels, the drug's cholesterol-lowering effects are greater, so serum cholesterol levels fall to below pretreatment levels. (This mechanism is basically the same one by which dietary fiber, eg, that in oat bran and legumes, can reduce serum cholesterol levels.)

Clinical Indications and Administration

Treatment of Hyperlipoproteinemias

Cholestyramine or the related drug colestipol is often a preferred agent for adjunctive therapy (along with diet) of primary hypercholesterolemias. In this disorder, the major lipid abnormality is an elevation of LDL levels. Blood tests taken after only about a week of cholestyramine treatment will show falls of LDL levels, and after a month or so cholesterol levels also decrease. Dosages are listed in Table 36–C. Cholestyramine or colestipol are often used along with nicotinic acid (see below).

Patients with elevated LDL cholesterol and triglycerides usually should not be treated first with cholestyramine inhibits digitalis absorption and interrupts its return to the bloodstream via enterohepatic recirculation. (See Chapter 31, p 589, for more details.)

Biliary Tract Obstruction

Cholestyramine is approved for managing puritus that can accompany partial obstruction of the bile ducts.

Other Uses

Cholestyramine has several unapproved uses that depend on the drug's ability to bind, and enhance the fecal excretion of, various bacterial toxins and ingested poisons. Its most common unapproved use is adjunctive therapy of overdoses of digoxin or digitoxin. Cholestyramine inhibits digitalis absorption and interrupts its return to the bloodstream via enterohepatic recirculation. (See Chapter 31, p 589, for more details.)

NURSING IMPLICATIONS

Cholestyramine comes in two major oral dosage forms. One is a granular powder (QUESTRAN). The cheapest form of this is dispensed in bulk (in cans), along with a scoop to measure the dose. Premeasured packets of drug may be more convenient, but they are much more expensive and obviously no more effective. In either case, for each dose the drug should be added to at least 2 ounces (60 mL) of water, fruit juice (preferred, because it masks the unpleasant taste), some other noncarbonated beverage, or a fluidy soup. Stir the mixture well before it is swallowed. The dose can also be mixed in applesauce or similar semisolid fruit products. Inform the patient not to take the dry powder; it is nearly impossible to swallow safely and very unpleasant in addition.

The other cholestyramine dosage form is a chewable bar (CHOLYBAR) flavored with caramel or raspberry. These should be chewed thoroughly and taken with plenty of fluids.

Side Effects, Adverse Reactions, and Contraindications

Cholestyramine, taken alone, is a relatively harmless drug because it is not absorbed. Its major side effects involve the GI tract (Table 36–S). Constipation is common; its incidence and severity are greater when high doses are used and in elderly patients. Cholestyramine may also cause fecal impactions. The drug should be used cautiously in patients with preexisting constipation. Other, less common, GI side effects include flatulence, nausea, vomiting, and abdominal pain.

Cholestyramine's ability to bind lipid in the GI tract may cause steatorrhea and impaired absorption of the fat-soluble vitamins A, D, E, and K.

Impaired vitamin A absorption can interfere with night vision. Decreased vitamin D absorption may cause osteoporosis in susceptible patients. Impaired vitamin K absorption can cause hypoprothrombinemia and increased bleeding tendencies, because vitamin K has an essential role in the hepatic synthesis of several clotting factors. Since cholestyramine indirectly increases bile formation, it should not be administered to patients with complete obstruction of the biliary ducts. Cholestyramine should not be given to patients with a history of allergic reactions to the drug.

NURSING IMPLICATIONS

To minimize problems caused by constipation, encourage patients to drink large amounts of water and to include appropriate amounts of fiber (bran, raw vegetables) in the diet. A high-fiber diet not only helps prevent constipation, but also helps reduce the daily fat intake, which may further lower serum lipid levels. If these nondrug interventions fail to prevent or alleviate constipation, the physician may recommend occasional use of a stool softener. Discourage the use of laxatives or cathartics without a physician's approval.

Monitor patients receiving high-dose, long-term cholestyramine therapy for signs of inadequate absorption of fat-soluble vitamins. Oral multivitamin supplements may be indicated.

◆ Use During Pregnancy and Lactation

Cholestyramine apparently causes no fetal harm, but no well-controlled study has proven this. One concern is impaired vitamin absorption, which may adversely affect the mother and child, whether before conception or during breast-feeding.

◆ Use in Children

The effects of long-term cholestyramine therapy in pediatric patients are unknown. There are no recommended pediatric doses.

◆ Use in the Elderly

The presence of diabetes or other disorders requiring therapy with interacting drugs, common in elderly patients, requires extra care when cholestyramine is used. Anticipate more problems related to constipation.

Interactions with Other Drugs

Cholestyramine binds not only bile acids and fat-soluble vitamins, but also many drugs the patient may be taking orally (Table 36–I). The interaction can markedly reduce the systemic absorption of these agents and enhance their fecal elimination, thereby causing subtherapeutic blood levels of the interactant. Significant interactions have been reported with orally administered digitalis, thiazide diuretics, anticoagulants, thyroid hormone preparations, and corticosteroids.

NURSING IMPLICATIONS

If patients are taking interacting drugs, keep the administration interval as great as possible. A general guideline is to administer the interactant no less than three hours before cholestyramine, or no sooner than four to six hours after. Increased doses of the interactant may be needed if systemic absorption is still reduced. If the patient is stabilized on an interactant during cholestyramine therapy, and cholestyramine is discontinued, assess closely and anticipate the need to reduce the dose of the interactant.

Overdose and Toxicity

The physical form and bulk of cholestyramine are such that it is not likely to be a common cause of overdose. If acute overdose occurs, the major concern is obstruction of the GI tract. Treatment is based on assessment of the location and severity of the obstruction.

Related Drugs

Colestipol

The only approved use for colestipol (COLESTID) is management of hyperlipidemias, as an alternative to cholestyramine. Administration instructions for the drug, which is dispensed in bulk or premeasured packets, are identical to those for cholestyramine. Dosages are listed in Table 36–C.

II. Cholesterol Synthesis Inhibitors

Drugs that inhibit cholesterol synthesis through a specific biochemical action provide the newest pharmacologic approach to treating some common hyperlipidemias. The prototype of the class, also known as HMG-CoA reductase inhibitors, is lovastatin. Lovastatin is also called mevinolin; the drug is marketed as MEVACOR. Related drugs are pravastatin and simvastatin.

Compared with cholestyramine or colestipol, lovastatin and the related drugs cause greater reductions of serum cholesterol levels. All are formulated as tablets, so they are easier and more pleasant to take, facilitating compliance. Lovastatin has become the most widely prescribed cholesterol-lowering drug because of these properties. However, the trade-off is a greater incidence of side effects or adverse responses that are potentially more serious than those seen with cholestyramine or colestipol.

PROTOTYPE

Lovastatin

Absorption, Distribution, Metabolism, and Excretion

Lovastatin is poorly absorbed from the GI tract, and that portion of the dose which is absorbed is extensively metabolized by first-pass hepatic metabolism. Thus, very little of a given dose reaches the bloodstream and causes pharmacologic effects. Lovastatin absorption is reduced further in the fasting state.

NURSING IMPLICATIONS

Administer lovastatin with meals. If a once-daily administration schedule is used, advise the patient to take the drug with the evening meal.

Pharmacologic Effects

Lovastatin inhibits an enzyme, HMG-CoA reductase, that controls a critical step in cholesterol synthesis. The outcome of HMG-CoA reductase inhibition is a decrease in total cholesterol levels, as well as cholesterol associated with low-density and very-low-density lipoproteins. In addition, triglyceride levels fall and HDL cholesterol levels rise. Although lovastatin and the related drugs inhibit cholesterol synthesis, and although cholesterol is the chemical backbone of steroid hormones, these antihyperlipidemic drugs do not seem to have a significant effect on steroid hormone levels or biologic activities in otherwise normal adults.

Clinical Indications and Administration

Similar to cholestyramine and colestipol, lovastatin is approved as an adjunct to the therapy of primary hypercholesterolemias that have not responded to diet alone. Usual dosages are listed in Table 36–C. Lovastatin is being tested for effects on other types and causes of hyperlipidemias, but these uses are not approved.

Side Effects, Adverse Reactions, and Contraindications

Lovastatin seldom causes significant or bothersome side effects (see Table 36–S). The most common side effect is headache. The GI tract can be affected in many ways; patients may develop flatulence, nausea or vomiting, and gastric or other abdominal pains. Some patients develop diarrhea, whereas others experience constipation. Other side effects include muscle aches (myalgia) and skin rashes that are often pruritic.

Lovastatin should be prescribed with extra care for any patient with liver dysfunction or a history of high, long-term alcohol intake (which can cause liver dysfunction). Before lovastatin is administered, the patient's liver function should be tested to establish a baseline and rule out significant dysfunction. These tests should be repeated once a month or every other month for the first year, and about twice yearly thereafter. Increased blood transaminase (eg, AST, ALT) levels are the most common indicator of drug-induced liver dysfunction; if the increases become significant, lovastatin therapy may need to be stopped.

Myalgia, a side effect reported in a small number of patients taking lovastatin, may progress to true skeletal muscle damage (*myopathy*) and eventual cell disintegration (*rhabdomyolysis*). The outpouring of myoglobin from muscle cells into the bloodstream, which can eventually be detected in the urine, may cause serious damage to the renal tubules. Skeletal muscle cell integrity is usually tracked by measurements of other serum enzymes, including creatine phosphokinase (CPK). (These tests can be done on blood samples withdrawn to monitor liver function.) Slight increases of CPK levels are common when lovastatin therapy is started, but levels usually fall toward normal. If they do not, further testing is required to determine whether lovastatin therapy should be continued. The combined use of lovastatin with other drugs (especially immunosuppressants; see below) seems to increase the risk of myopathy and secondary renal damage.

NURSING IMPLICATIONS

Stress the importance of periodic blood tests. Advise patients to report any severe or prolonged muscle aches or tenderness, which could indicate early development of myopathy that might progress to more serious complications.

◆ Use During Pregnancy and Lactation

Lovastatin and the related HMG-CoA reductase inhibitors are absolutely contraindicated during pregnancy because of their potential ability to cause birth defects in utero. Do not give these drugs to any woman of childbearing age unless it is determined that she is not pregnant and she is taking precautions to prevent conception. If the woman conceives during drug therapy, drug treatment should be stopped at once and the progress of fetal development should be monitored closely. Discourage breast-feeding during drug therapy.

◆ Use in Children

Lovastatin and the related drugs should not be used in children under the age of 18 years.

◆ Use in the Elderly

Age-related declines in liver function may increase the risk of drug-induced liver dysfunction. Monitor elderly patients closely with recommended blood tests.

Interactions with Other Drugs

Several drugs listed in Table 36–I can increase the risk of severe myopathy or rhabdomyolysis. The greatest risk seems to be associated with concurrent use of cyclosporine, but other immunosuppressant drugs may interact similarly. This interaction should be avoided, mainly by the use of antihyperlipidemics other than lovastatin (and perhaps the other HMG-CoA reductase inhibitors). If the interaction cannot be avoided, the maximum daily lovastatin dose is 20 mg—roughly one-fourth the maximum daily dose for most other patients.

The interaction between lovastatin and cyclosporine can be very serious. However, cyclosporine is not used as often as some other interactants that can cause the same serious outcome when given with lovastatin. Gemfibrozil, another antihyperlipidemic drug (see below), is the best example of such an interactant. Erythromycin, a widely used antibiotic, and another antihyperlipidemic drug, nicotinic acid, can also interact with lovastatin to cause myopathy, rhabdomyolysis, and potential renal complications. However, there is not much data to indicate that the interaction with erythromycin or nicotinic acid is as common or severe as with cyclosporine or gemfibrozil. Nevertheless, all these interactions should be avoided if possible and noninteracting alternative drugs should be used instead.

NURSING IMPLICATIONS

Advise patients receiving any drug that is a potential interactant with lovastatin, or the other HMG-CoA reductase inhibitors, to report muscle aches, pain, or tenderness at once. These patients should receive appropriate testing as soon as possible and HMG-CoA reductase therapy discontinued, at least temporarily, until the evaluation and diagnosis can be done. Help patients understand the importance of undergoing periodic blood tests during therapy.

Overdose and Toxicity

There is very little information about overdoses with lovastatin or the related HMG-CoA reductase inhibitors. Available reports indicate no serious signs or symptoms. Acute overdoses are treated with standard first-aid measures to reduce further drug absorption (Appendix C). Further treatment is supportive, addressing the patient's symptoms.

Related Drugs

Pravastatin and Simvastatin

Pravastatin (PRAVACHOL) and simvastatin (ZOCOR) are the newer HMG-CoA reductase inhibitors. Either can be used instead of lovastatin. A major difference is that with these alternatives once-daily dosing is adequate, and food does not affect their absorption or action. Thus, these drugs can be taken before, with, or after meals. Bedtime administration is generally recommended for convenience and compliance.

Side effects noted for lovastatin apply to the alternatives. For the most part, however, the incidence of side effects is lower with the newer drugs than with the prototype. Similar drug–drug interactions can be assumed. In addition, cholestyramine and colestipol seem to reduce pravastatin absorption significantly when these drugs are given together. Pravastatin is given one hour before or four hours after giving a bile acid sequestrant.

III. Miscellaneous Antihyperlipidemics

The drugs discussed next are placed in the miscellaneous category mainly because they are neither bile acid sequestrants nor HMG-CoA reductase inhibitors. Many of these drugs are second-choice agents, used when the usually preferred agents are not effective or should be avoided for other reasons. A noteworthy exception is nicotinic acid, which is clearly a first-line agent for many patients. These drugs are described, briefly, in alphabetical order.

Clofibrate and Gemfibrozil

Clofibrate (ATROMID-S) and gemfibrozil (LOPID) are derivatives of a substance called fibric acid. These drugs mainly lower serum triglyceride levels. They are indicated for treating Type III hyperlipoproteinemia (see Table 36–C), as adjuncts to diet, when diet alone has failed to control the disorder. Clofibrate and gemfibrozil probably work by inhibiting the hepatic synthesis or release of VLDL, the plasma fraction that is responsible for carrying most of the triglyceride in the blood. Cholesterol levels also tend to fall.

Clofibrate and gemfibrozil share similar mechanisms of action, some key clinical indications, and relatively equal lipid-lowering efficacies. However, they differ in terms of the types and frequencies of side effects, drug interactions, and other adverse responses. The differences affect the choice of one of these agents over another. Of these two drugs, clofibrate is usually the poorer choice of the two.

Owing to side effects and true adverse responses, clofibrate is generally used only if gemfibrozil therapy has been unsuccessful—ie, the patient still has severe hypertriglyceridemia and a risk of pancreatitis. Clofibrate is also indicated for managing very high triglyceride levels (750 mg/100 mL or more) that may accompany Types IV or V hyperlipoproteinemias. These disorders are associated with a high risk of pancreatitis.

Clofibrate's minor side effects include nausea (the most common side effect) and loose or fatty stools. The drug may also cause hypoglycemia, but this seems to be more of a problem in diabetes patients who are taking antidiabetic medications.

In terms of more serious side effects, clofibrate (much more so than gemfibrozil) can increase the amount of cholesterol in the bile, leading to an increased risk of forming cholesterol-rich gallstones in the biliary tract. This often necessitates surgery (cholecystectomy). Young, healthy patients may tolerate this surgery well, but it poses greater risks for patients who are older, debilitated, or have other diseases. Overall, compared with placebo, long-term clofibrate therapy increases the mortality rate by about 40%. Most of the deaths are caused by complications of either pancreatitis or cholecystectomy. Long-term clofibrate therapy is also associated with a higher incidence of malignancies in various organs.

Finally, clofibrate can cause a significant and potentially dangerous interaction with oral anticoagulants; fatal bleeding episodes have occurred. Clofibrate can also increase the hypoglycemic effects of insulin or oral antidiabetic (hypoglycemic) drugs.

Gemfibrozil is generally well tolerated. It is often selected for patients with mixed hyperlipidemias and low levels of HDL cholesterol. Gemfibrozil's main side effects involve upper GI distress, but the overall incidence is low. There is also an increased risk of cholesterol stone formation in the gallbladder; the frequency is lower than that associated with clofibrate.

The only drug–drug interaction that has been shown to be clinically important involves gemfibrozil and the HMG-CoA reductase inhibitors (lovastatin and others; see above and Table 36–I).

Dextrothyroxine

Dextrothyroxine (CHOLOXIN) is closely related, chemically and pharmacologically, to the thyroid hormone supplement levothyroxine (see Chapter 47 for more information). Of the two, only dextrothyroxine is indicated for lowering increased cholesterol and LDL levels. It presumably works by increasing the metabolic breakdown and excretion of cholesterol.

Not all patients with increased LDL or cholesterol levels should receive dextrothyroxine, owing to its thyroid hormone–like actions. Patients who are candidates for treatment with dextrothyroxine must be euthyroid (ie, have normal thyroid gland status and thyroid hormone levels) and free of any other disorders that contraindicate thyroid hormone use. Cardiovascular and cardiac disorders (eg, tachycardia, arrhythmias, ischemic heart disease, and advanced heart failure), a history of cerebrovascular disease, and severe liver or kidney disease are among the most important contraindications for the overall population. Pregnancy and breastfeeding contraindicate dextrothyroxine use in women.

Dextrothyroxine interacts with the same drugs as do the other thyroid hormone supplements. One interactant is cholestyramine, which can reduce dextrothyroxine's absorption if the two are taken together (see Table 47–I for more details).

Neomycin

Neomycin is an antibiotic that belongs to a large class of drugs known as aminoglycosides. Neomycin differs from the rest of the aminoglycoside antibiotics mainly because it is not absorbed well from the GI tract. Unlike all the other antihyperlipidemics, neomycin is sometimes used for hypercholesterolemia, but it is not officially approved for that use. Thus, dosages are not listed in Table 36–C.

Neomycin causes modest reductions of LDL cholesterol. It may also undesirably lower HDL cholesterol levels. Neomycin's exact mechanism of action is not known, but it probably works locally in the gut either to decrease cholesterol absorption (or enterohepatic recirculation) or to increase cholesterol excretion in the feces.

Neomycin's most common side effects are nausea and vomiting. Its most serious side effects include nephrotoxicity and potentially severe and permanent hearing loss (ototoxicity). These are well-known adverse responses that can be caused by any of the aminoglycosides. Thus, although neomycin is poorly absorbed, it appears that sufficient amounts can reach the bloodstream to cause these unwanted actions. Drug interactions that apply to the aminoglycosides, in general, apply to neomycin. See the complete description for aminoglycosides in Chapter 56 for more information.

Nicotinic Acid

Nicotinic acid (niacin; vitamin B_3; marketed as NICOLAR and under several other brand and generic names) has many desired properties that make it a first-line antihyperlipidemic drug for many patients. Nicotinic acid is effective, and generic products are also the cheapest antihyperlipidemic drugs prescribed (brand-name products cost much more).

Nicotinic acid causes virtually all the desired effects on lipids: triglyceride, VLDL, total cholesterol and LDL levels fall, and HDL levels rise. The drug is indicated for treating hypertriglyceridemia, hypercholesterolemia, or combined elevations of both lipids. For combined hypertriglyceridemia and elevated LDL cholesterol, nicotinic acid is preferred over cholestyramine or colestipol. Long-term use of nicotinic appears to reduce mortality or morbidity from coronary heart disease.

Despite all the positive properties of nicotinic acid, the drug's use for hyperlipidemias is limited by some common and annoying side effects. They are caused, in part, by the relatively high dosages that are used for these indications (Table 36–C)—dosages much higher than those used when nicotinic acid is given as a vitamin supplement (Chapter 61). Many of nicotinic acid's side effects are caused by, or are related to, the drug's vasodilator actions. Facial flushing, skin rashes or tingling, and a sense of overall warmth are common. They are most disturbing during the first few weeks of therapy. These side effects often appear within an hour or two after taking a dose. Other related side effects are headache and hypotension. Nicotinic acid may cause GI upset. Administering the drug with meals tends to reduce the severity of side effects, particularly flushing.

Nicotinic acid is contraindicated in persons with peptic ulcer or liver disease, severe hypotension, or ongoing hemorrhage. Severe ischemic heart or cerebrovascular disease also weigh against nicotinic acid therapy. Persons with diabetes mellitus may experience glucose intolerance and may need readjustment of their antidiabetic drug therapy or diet.

As noted earlier, the combination of nicotinic acid and lovastatin (or other HMG-CoA reductase inhibitors) can cause myopathy, rhabdomyolysis, and renal complications. Combined therapy should therefore be avoided.

NURSING IMPLICATIONS

If nicotinic acid's side effects become troublesome during early therapy, as they often do, check with the physician. Most side effects can be minimized if treatment starts with very low doses (eg, 100 mg three times daily). Increase the dosage gradually to the usual maintenance dose, 2 to 6 g per day in two or three divided doses.

Advise patients who experience significant flushing in response to nicotinic acid to take 325 to 650 mg of aspirin about 30 minutes before, provided that there are no contraindications to aspirin use. Hypotension associated with nicotinic acid is usually orthostatic: advise patients to stand slowly, with support, if they become dizzy.

Omega-3 Polyunsaturated Fatty Acids (Fish Oil Concentrate)

Years ago it was recognized that Eskimos have an unusually low incidence of fatal coronary artery disease. This was attributed to their high dietary intake of cold-water fish, which contains large amounts of omega-3 polyunsaturated fatty acids. These fatty acids, when ingested in large amounts each day as part of the diet, seem to lower total cholesterol and triglyceride levels and have desired effects on LDL and HDL levels. The fatty acids also inhibit platelet aggregation, which otherwise can lead to thrombus formation and coronary artery occlusion.

Capsules containing these fatty acids are marketed over-the-counter (OTC) under such trade names as PROMEGA. These products are used as nondrug dietary supplements to lower an early risk of coronary artery disease.

Owing to the antiplatelet effects of the omega-3 fatty acids, long-term use may increase the risk of bleeding tendencies, especially when the patient is taking anticoagulants or other antiplatelet drugs (eg, warfarin or aspirin, respectively). These agents may also increase blood glucose levels and impair insulin release. Thus, they should be used cautiously in patients with diabetes who are not being treated with insulin.

NURSING IMPLICATIONS

Since these products are available OTC, patients with diabetes or other conditions that may relatively contraindicate their use may self-prescribe them. Advise these patients to consult with their physician first.

There is conflicting information about these supplements: the recommended dosages may be too low to cause desired lipid effects consistently; they may be high enough to cause unwanted effects on platelets or to interact with other drugs; and some products contain ingredients that may cause unwanted serum lipid changes. Also, be aware that none of these products are replacements for proper, nutritious lipid-lowering diets or for any of the antihyperlipidemic drugs discussed in this chapter.

Probucol

Probucol (LORELCO) is indicated for treating primary hypercholesterolemia. However, it is seldom used as a first-line drug for several reasons: its effects on total and LDL cholesterol are modest; it may also lower HDL levels; and it can cause potentially serious adverse effects.

The most common side effects associated with probucol therapy are generally mild and limited to the GI tract (eg, flatulence, diarrhea, and discomfort). The most worrisome adverse effect is a potential ability to prolong the Q–T interval on the electrocardiogram (ECG). This part of the ECG reflects the time needed for the ventricles to depolarize and then repolarize. When the Q–T interval is excessively prolonged (the normal value depends on heart rate), the risk of serious ventricular arrhythmias increases. Thus, probucol is contraindicated for patients with ventricular arrhythmias, QT prolongation, or progressive cardiac disease or damage.

No specific drugs interact with probucol. However, other drugs can prolong the Q–T interval and cause excessive cardiac effects when given with probucol. They include antiarrhythmic drugs such as quinidine and procainamide; and phenothiazine antipsychotics and tricyclic antidepressants. Hypocalcemia can cause the same outcome.

NURSING IMPLICATIONS

It is important to obtain a baseline ECG before starting probucol therapy. The ECG should be followed periodically thereafter. Report evidence of Q–T prolongation or other ventricular abnormalities. Check the medication history or plan for simultaneous use of other drugs that may prolong the Q–T interval.

Administer probucol with meals to reduce the incidence and severity of GI disturbances. Advise patients to report severe or prolonged GI side effects.

Drugs Used to Dissolve Cholesterol-Containing Gallstones

Stones that block the flow of bile cause excruciating pain and potentially serious organ damage until and unless they are removed. Cholecystectomy is the most common and effective treatment, and for patients who are young and otherwise healthy, this surgical procedure is quite safe, even for elective (nonemergency) surgery. Newer, less traumatic surgical techniques and nonsurgical techniques, such as shock wave lithotripsy, are being used more and more.

For some patients, however, elective cholecystectomy is not indicated or acceptable, either because of poor physical status (and the associated risks of surgery) or because the patient refuses the operation. For such individuals, drugs can be used in an attempt to dissolve the stones, provided that the gallstones are composed mainly of cholesterol and are not calcified. (Such stones are called *radiolucent,* because they do not appear well on radiographs.)

Two drugs are approved for oral therapy of cholesterol-containing gallstones: chenodiol (chenodeoxycholic acid; CHENIX) and ursodiol (ursodeoxycholic acid; ACTIGALL). A third drug, monooctanoin (MOCTANIN), is administered by direct perfusion of the common bile duct. Monooctanoin is indicated for dissolving gallstones that remain after cholecystectomy and cannot be removed by other means. None of these drugs dissolve stones that are composed of mineral salts (eg, calcium).

Overall, these drugs are rarely used; indeed, chenodiol and monoctanoin are classified as orphan drugs, mainly because of their infrequent use. For this reason, only a brief overview of these agents follows; data on dosages, side effects, and drug interactions are not included in the tables. See package inserts for more information.

Chenodiol and Ursodiol

Chenodiol and ursodiol are naturally occurring bile acids. When given in pharmacologic doses, they decrease the hepatic synthesis of cholesterol and cholic acid, which are poorly soluble ingredients in some bile stones. With prolonged administration, these drugs help bile stones to dissolve slowly. Stones that become sufficiently small may then pass out of the bile ducts spontaneously.

Treatment with chenodiol or ursodiol may last anywhere from six months to two years. Even with such long-term therapy there is no guarantee that all stones will dissolve completely or become small enough to pass spontaneously. The response is, therefore, very variable and sometimes unpredictable for a given patient. It depends on many factors, such as the size, number, and chemical makeup of the stones. Treatment with these drugs, which are used to avoid surgery, may actually necessitate surgical intervention in some patients. Even if treatment with chenodiol or ursodiol is successful, about 30% to 50% of patients develop new stones within two to five years after therapy is stopped.

Chenodiol is noteworthy because it is hepatotoxic. It is absolutely contraindicated during pregnancy; indeed, it should not be given to women who might become pregnant during treatment. Ursodiol appears to be somewhat safer in this regard, but liver damage is still a potential complication. GI upset, pain, nausea and vomiting, and diarrhea are relatively common side effects with either drug.

Cholesterol-lowering drugs may be prescribed during chenodiol or ursodiol therapy to reduce further stone formation. However, they should be chosen and administered carefully. Clofibrate and gemfibrozil (see above) should be avoided, owing to their ability to increase the risk of stone formation. Estrogens and oral contraceptives, which increase cholesterol synthesis, may do the same. Cholestyramine or colestipol may be used as systemic lipid-lowering drugs, but their administration should be timed properly so that they do not interfere with the absorption of the oral gallstone-dissolving agent.

NURSING IMPLICATIONS

Advise patients who receive chenodiol or ursodiol that therapy may be longlasting and that there is no guarantee of successful treatment. Inform them of the risks, and stress the need for frequent tests to evaluate liver function and the progress of treatment. Advise patients to report at once severe upper abdominal pain or the onset of severe nausea or vomiting.

Monooctanoin

Monooctanoin is administered via a tube placed directly in the bile duct either at the time of surgery (a T-tube) or later, guided by an endoscope. The drug is then infused slowly, usually be gravity. Drug that directly bathes the stones helps the stones dissolve. Two to ten days of infusion are usually necessary to cause the desired effect. The most common side effect is abdominal pain or discomfort; it is usually alleviated by slowing or temporarily stopping the drug infusion and aspirating the duct. Nausea, diarrhea, and vomiting are the other most common side effects.

SUMMARY OF NURSING IMPLICATIONS

◆ Assessment

Establish baseline laboratory values (cholesterol, triglycerides, total plasma phospholipids) and ECG (particularly with probucol).

Review patient history for the four major risk factors for hyperlipidemia: family history, diseases such as diabetes, diet, and smoking.

Complete a nutritional history to determine dietary needs before therapy is initiated.

Complete nursing history to include past and present bowel pattern (constipation or poor bowel function).

◆ Nursing Diagnoses

Constipation related to drug side effects (particularly with cholestyramine).

Altered nutrition: less than body requirement related to impaired fat-soluble vitamin absorption.

Knowledge deficit related to antihyperlipidemic drug therapy.

Noncompliance related to dietary restriction (low fat) and drug side effects.

Pain (headache) related to drug side effects (lovastatin).

◆ Planning/Implementation

Monitor for signs of deficiency in fat-soluble vitamins (eg, night blindness with low vitamin A, abnormal bleeding with low vitamin K, bone fragility with low vitamin D).

If patient is taking other drugs concurrently with cholestyramine or colestipol, separate administration of interactants as much as possible: give interactant no less than three hours before or four to six hours after antilipidemic; monitor for inadequate medication responses.

◆ Patient and Family Education

Teach the patient/family:

The role of dietary modification: provide list of foods to avoid and those to be eaten; refer to nutritionist for counseling.

To mix powdered cholestyramine or colestipol in a liquid or fluidy food (eg, applesauce, soup, noncarbonated beverages) to reduce unpleasant taste.

To report significant constipation during therapy; encourage liberal intake of fluids and bulk-forming foods (cereals, raw vegetables); consult physician before taking laxatives.

To report at once muscle aches, pain, or tenderness with lovastatin.

To take lovastatin or probucol with evening meal to enhance absorption; food reduces GI distress.

The need for periodic testing of prothrombin time, and to note signs of excessive or abnormal bleeding.

To expect flushing, pruritus, and possible dizziness with nicotinic acid.

◆ Evaluation

The patient/family will:

Show signs of effective drug therapy: decreased serum lipids.

Follow low cholesterol diet as planned; lose weight.

Verbalize presence of optimal bowel pattern and consistency.

Modify lifestyle to reduce controllable risk factors contributing to hyperlipidemia.

Annotated Bibliography

Blankenhorn DH, Hodis HN: Treating serum lipid abnormalities in high-priority patients. *Postgrad Med* 1991;89(1):81–82, 87–90, 93–96. *Identifies and discusses treatment for high-risk hyperlipidemic patients; includes comments on specific drugs, drug groups, and diet.*

Burke LE: Dietary management of hyperlipidemia. *J Cardiovasc Nurs* 1991;5(2):23–33. *Discusses principles and applications of dietary treatment, ideas for counseling and instruction, and strategies to improve compliance.*

Dart AM: Managing elevated blood lipid concentrations: Who, when and how? *Drugs* 1990;39(3):374–387. *Valuable discussion of the main components in decision making for the treatment of hyperlipidemias.*

DiPalma JR, Thayer WS: Use of niacin as a drug. *Annu Rev Nutr* 1991;11:169–187. *In-depth coverage of this interesting and important lipid-lowering nutrient.*

Gotto AM Jr: Rationale for treatment. *Am J Med* 1991;91(1B):31S–36S. *Summarizes several large clinical studies dealing with hyperlipidemia and its consequences and identifies treatment benefits that can be anticipated or hoped for.*

Hoeg JM: Pharmacologic and surgical treatment of dyslipidemic children and adolescents. *Ann N Y Acad Sci* 1991;623:275–284. *Reviews diet, drug, and surgical therapies for youngsters with hyperlipidemias.*

Illingworth DR: Management of hyperlipidemia: Goals for the prevention of atherosclerosis. *Clin Invest Med* 1990;13(4):211–218. *A practical guide to assessing patients, identifying treatment goals, and implementing therapy with diet and drugs.*

LaRosa JC: At what levels of total low- or high-density lipoprotein cholesterol should diet/drug therapy be initiated? United States guidelines. *Am J Cardiol* 1990;65(12):7F–10F. *Gives the generally accepted guidelines for the detection, evaluation, and treatment of hypercholesterolemia in adults. These data are also used as part of a public health education program.*

Maryniuk MD: Hyperlipidemia and diabetes: The role of dietary fats. *Diabetes Educ* 1989;15(3):258–265. *A self-study format that focuses on the meaning and implementation of national guidelines for dietary therapy of hyperlipedemia, with emphasis on diabetes patients and nonphysician health care providers.*

McCann BS, Retzlaff BM, Dowdy AA, Walden CE, Knopp RH: Promoting adherence to low-fat, low-cholesterol diets: Review and recommendations. *J Am Diet Assoc* 1990;90(10):1408–1414. *Valuable for its many explicit recommendations about how to increase acceptance of and compliance with the most important element of hyperlipidemia therapy—diet.*

Milander MM, Kuhn M: Lipid-lowering drugs. *AACN Clin Issues Crit Care Nurs* 1992;3(2):494–506. *A good review of general and current information about hyperlipidemias, therapeutic strategies, and related nursing measures.*

National Cholesterol Education Program (NCEP) Panel: Report of the National Cholesterol Education Program Panel on detection, evaluation and treatment of high blood cholesterol in adults. *Arch Intern Med* 1988;148:36–69. *A comprehensive, authoritative, and widely cited summary of experts on all aspects of the topic.*

Scott D, Kurenitz M: Using lipid-lowering agents effectively: When diet is not enough. *Postgrad Med* 1990;87(8):171–176, 179–181, 186. *Emphasizes that long-term planning for and implementation of therapy is much more important than setting short-term goals.*

Steinberg D, Olefsky JM, eds: *Hypercholesterolemia and Atherosclerosis: Pathogenesis and Prevention.* Churchill Livingstone, New York, 1987. *This remains a valuable yet easy-to-read (and even enjoy) compilation of chapters dealing with all aspects of the subject. Nurses working in the area of atheroscelerosis are guaranteed to find worthwhile material here.*

Steiner A, Weisser B, Vetter W: A comparative review of the adverse effects of treatments for hyperlipidaemia. *Drug Saf* 1991;6(2):118–130. *Because antihyperlipidemic drugs are effective, it is wise to focus on their unwanted and potentially dangerous effects. That is the theme of this review.*

Waters D, Lesperance J: Regression of coronary atherosclerosis: An achievable goal? Review of results from recent clinical trials. *Am J Med* 1991;91(1B):10S–17S. *Drugs and diet may reduce the development or worsening of atherosclerotic lesions; this article discusses what can be done to reverse the lesions.*

Watson JE: Nutritional intervention in hyperlipidemia. *Prog Cardiovasc Nurs* 1989;4(4):131–137. *Provides guidelines for nurses in screening and educating patients promoting wellness via behavioral change, monitoring patient outcomes, and integrating nutritional intervention with other therapies.*

Table 36–C **Clinical Uses and Administration of Major Lipid-Lowering Drugs***

AGENT	CLINICAL USES	ORAL DOSAGE
	Bile Acid Sequestrants	
PROTOTYPE		
Cholestyramine (CHOLYBAR, QUESTRAN)	Primary (Type IIa or IIb) hypercholesterolemia (elevated LDL)	4 g 1–6 times daily
	Short-term management of pruritus due to partial biliary tract obstruction	See above
RELATED DRUG		
Colestipol (COLESTID)	Primary hypercholesterolemia	15–30 g/day (total) in 2–4 divided doses
	Cholesterol Synthesis (HMG-CoA Reductase) Inhibitors	
PROTOTYPE		
Lovastatin (MEVACOR)	Primary hypercholesterolemia	Initially 20 mg with evening meal; maintenance 20–80 mg/day in single or divided doses
RELATED DRUGS		
Pravastatin (PRAVACHOL)	Primary hypercholesterolemia	Initially 10–20 mg qhs (10 mg for elderly); maintenance 10–40 mg qhs
Simvastatin (ZOCOR)	Primary hypercholesterolemia	Initially 5–10 mg qhs (5 mg for elderly); maintenance 5–40 mg qhs
	Miscellaneous Antihyperlipidemics	
Clofibrate (ATROMID-S)	Refractory Type III hyperlipidemia	2 g/day in divided doses (starting and maintenance)
Dextrothyroxine (CHOLOXIN)	Primary hypercholesterolemia in euthyroid patients	Adults: Initially 1–2 mg/day; maintenance 4–8 mg/day Children: Initially 50 μg/kg/day, maintenance 100 μg/kg/day or 4 mg/day (whichever is less)
Gemfibrozil (LOPID)	Hypertriglyceridemia (Type IV or V hyperlipidemia)	1.2 g/day in 2 divided doses 30 min before morning and evening meals
Nicotinic acid (niacin; NICOLAR)	Hypercholesterolemia and/or hypertriglyceridemia	1–2 g tid with or following meals; 8 g/day maximum

(continued)

Table 36–C | Clinical Uses and Administration of Major Lipid-Lowering Drugs* (*Continued*)

AGENT	CLINICAL USES	ORAL DOSAGE
Omega-3 polyunsaturated fatty acids (PROMEGA, others)	Nutritional supplement for regulating serum lipids	1 or 2 capsules tid with meals
Probucol (LORELCO)	Primary hypercholesterolemia with or without secondary hypertriglyceridemia	500 mg with morning and evening meals (or once daily)

*Unless noted otherwise, all drugs are used as adjuncts to dietary modifications and other nondrug measures for hyperlipidemias, and dosages are for adults

Table 36–S | Major Side Effects of and Contraindications for Lipid-Lowering Drugs

BODY SYSTEM/ Side Effect	CONTRAINDICATION/ PRECAUTION	COMMENTS AND NURSING IMPLICATIONS
Bile Acid Sequestrants: Cholestyramine, Colestipol		
GASTROINTESTINAL Constipation, bloating, flatulence	Partial or complete bowel obstruction, hypomotility	Most common side effects; administer with recommended amounts of fluid; use laxatives only on physician's approval
OTHER Deficiencies in fat-soluble vitamins (A,D,E,K)	Caution: pregnancy, breast-feeding	Assess for signs and symptoms of deficiencies, especially of D (bone fragility), K (impaired coagulation profiles, abnormal bruising or bleeding); vitamin supplements may be required
HMG-CoA Reductase Inhibitors: Lovastatin, Pravastatin, Simvastatin		
CENTRAL NERVOUS SYSTEM Headache		Most common side effect; tolerance usually develops; consult physician about use of OTC analgesics
GASTROINTESTINAL Flatulence, nausea/ vomiting, miscellaneous GI discomforts		May be dose-dependent, usually self-limiting; have patient report severe or longlasting reactions
HEPATIC Hepatotoxicity	Liver dysfunction; excessive alcohol intake or alcohol-induced liver dysfunction	Obtain baseline blood tests for liver status (eg, AST, ALT) and monitor monthly or bimonthly for first 12–15 months of therapy, semiannually thereafter; advise patient to report upper abdominal pain, tenderness, or jaundice at once

(continued)

Table 36–S **Major Side Effects of and Contraindications for Lipid-Lowering Drugs (*Continued*)**

BODY SYSTEM/ Side Effect	CONTRAINDICATION/ PRECAUTION	COMMENTS AND NURSING IMPLICATIONS
SKELETAL MUSCLE Myalgia, myopathy, rhabdomyolysis	Impaired renal function	May lead to serious renal damage due to myoglobin loss from muscle; obtain baseline blood work-ups (eg, CPK), monitor periodically thereafter; urge patients to report muscle pain or tenderness at once, especially if accompanied by fever or malaise
REPRODUCTIVE	Pregnancy	Avoid use in women of childbearing age; discourage breast-feeding during use
Miscellaneous Drugs **Clofibrate, Gemfibrozil**		
GASTROINTESTINAL Nausea, loose or fatty stools		Nausea is most common side effect; monitor stool frequency and consistency; report severe diarrhea or prolonged fatty stools
Increased risk of gallstones, pancreatitis, deaths secondary to cholecystectomy complications		Relatively common, more so with clofibrate; advise patient to report upper abdominal pain or tenderness; may require cholecystectomy or drug discontinuation
ENDOCRINE Hypoglycemia	Caution: non-insulin-dependent diabetes	Mainly with clofibrate; monitor blood glucose levels periodically; assess for signs and symptoms of hypoglycemia; antidiabetic drug regimen and diet may need changes
Dextrothyroxine **(See levothyroxine, Table 47–S for more information.)**		
CARDIOVASCULAR Tachycardia, tachyarrhythmias, palpitations, angina, infarction	Ischemic heart disease, heart failure, hypertension (other than mild)	Monitor for onset of side effects in patients with previously good cardiovascular status; side effects are dose-dependent
HEPATIC	Advanced liver disease	Monitor liver function (blood tests) periodically
RENAL	Advanced renal disease	Perform urinalysis periodically
ENDOCRINE	Hyperthyroidism	Confirm euthyroid status of patient before starting therapy
REPRODUCTIVE	Pregnancy, breast-feeding	

(continued)

Table 36–S | **Major Side Effects of and Contraindications for Lipid-Lowering Drugs (*Continued*)**

BODY SYSTEM/ Side Effect	CONTRAINDICATION/ PRECAUTION	COMMENTS AND NURSING IMPLICATIONS
	Neomycin (Unappoved for hyperlipidemias: See streptomycin and other aminoglycosides, Chapter 55)	
	Nicotinic Acid (Niaqcin)	
CENTRAL NERVOUS SYSTEM Headache		Probably secondary to cardiovascular effects; see below
CARDIOVASCULAR Facial flushing, rashes, feeling of warmth or tingling	Hypotension, ischemic heart disease; cerebrovascular disease, stroke; hemorrhage	Most problematic during first few weeks of therapy and within hours after dosing; incidence and severity reduced by administering with meals, starting with lower doses (eg, 100 mg tid), and increasing gradually to maintenance levels; aspirin (325–650 mg, 30 min before nicotinic acid dose, if not contraindicated) may alleviate flushing and headache
GASTROINTESTINAL Peptic ulcer disease	Active or history of peptic ulcer disease	Monitor for gut pain and black, tarry stools
ENDOCRINE Hypoglycemia	Caution: diabetes	Monitor accordingly; antidiabetic drug therapy or diet may need change
	Omega-3 Polyunsaturated Fatty Acids	
BLOOD Impaired platelet function	Thrombocytopenia, anticoagulant drug therapy (caution)	Monitor accordingly; have patient report abnormal bruising or bleeding and follow up with suitable blood tests
ENDOCRINE Hyperglycemia	Diabetes mellitus	Monitor accordingly; caution diabetics to use these OTC drugs only under physician's supervision
	Probucol	
CARDIOVASCULAR Ventricular arrhythmias, Q–T interval prolongation	Arrhythmias (current, recurrent, or recent history of), ischemic heart disease, serum (eg, K, Mg) electrolyte abnormalities	Obtain baseline ECG and serum electrolyte levels; correct electrolytes as needed; monitor regularly during probucol therapy
GASTROINTESTINAL Flatus, diarrhea, pain or discomfort		Common; administer with meals; advise patient to report severe or prolonged side effects at once

Table 36–I Major Interactions Between Antihyperlipidemics and Other Drugs

AGENT	RESULT OF INTERACTION	COMMENTS AND NURSING IMPLICATIONS
Interactions Involving Cholestyramine, Colestipol		
Anticoagulants, oral (eg, warfarin; Chapter 35	Decreased absorption and effects of interactant	Separate administration of interactants by 3 or more hr; monitor prothrombin time; assess for need to increase anticoagulant dose
Corticosteroids, oral (eg, hydrocortisone; Chapter 45)	See anticoagulants, above	True incidence of interaction unknown; space administration by several hours if possible; monitor for reduced steroid effects
Digitalis (digitoxin, digoxin; Chapter 31)	See anticoagulants, above	Clinical importance of interaction probably least with digoxin capsules (nearly 100% absorbed normally), most with digitoxin (only partially absorbed; undergoes significant enterohepatic recirculation); separate administration of interactants by several hours; monitor digitalis blood levels, clinical response (eg, weight gain, edema, dyspnea); interaction used intentionally to manage digitalis overdoses (see p 589)
Pravastatin	Reduced pravastatin absorption and effects	Give pravastatin 1 hr before or 4 hr after giving cholestyramine or colestipol
Thiazide diuretics, oral (eg, hydrochlorothiazide; Chapter 31)	See anticoagulants, above	Separate administration of interactants by 2 hr if possible; monitor response to diuretic, the dosage of which may need to be increased
Thyroid hormones, oral (eg, dextrothyroxine, levothyroxine; Chapter 47)	Decreased hormone absorption, effects	Separate administration of interactants (6 hr is recommended); monitor for return of hypothyroid state or lessening of dextrothyroxine's antihyperlipidemic effects
Interactions Involving Clofibrate		
Anticoagulants, oral (Chapter 35)	Significantly increased anticoagulant effects, risk of bleeding, hemorrhage	Bleeding-related deaths have occurred; avoid interaction if possible; otherwise, monitor prothrombin time closely, and assess for abnormal bleeding or bruising; anticipate need to reduce anticoagulant dose
Antidiabetic drugs (insulin, oral hypoglycemics; Chapter 46)	Risk of excessive hypoglycemia	Additive or synergistic effects of these drugs; monitor blood glucose levels closely if these drugs must be used together
Interactions Involving Dextrothyroxine		
See cholestyramine, above, and Table 47–I		
Interactions Involving Gemfibrozil		
Lovastatin	Increased risk of myopathy and rhabdomyolysis	Risk appears to be significant; avoid interaction if possible by using noninteracting alternatives; otherwise, advise patient to report muscle aches, pain, or tenderness at once for follow-up; discontinue lovastatin on evidence of untoward effects; interaction may apply to lovastatin alternatives (pravastatin, simvastatin)

(continued)

Table 36–I Major Interactions Between Antihyperlipidemics and Other Drugs (*Continued*)

AGENT	RESULT OF INTERACTION	COMMENTS AND NURSING IMPLICATIONS
Interactions Involving Lovastatin (and Pravastatin, Simvastatin)		
Cholestyramine, colestipol	Reduced pravastatin absorption, effects	See cholestyramine-pravastatin, above
Cyclosporine (Chapter 54)	Increased risk of myopathy and rhabdomyolysis	Avoid interaction if possible by using alternative(s) to one of the interactants; otherwise, limit lovastatin dose to 20 mg/day maximum, and advise patient to report muscle pain or tenderness at once; assess renal function if interaction is suspected, and discontinue lovastatin; risks may apply to related HMG-CoA reductase inhibitors
Erythromycin	See cyclosporine, above	Little data regarding potential interaction; use alternatives when possible, and monitor accordingly
Gemfibrozil	See gemfibrozil-lovastatin, above	
Nicotinic acid	Myopathy and rhabdomyolysis, as noted above for cyclosporine-lovastatin interaction	Scant data to document interaction; nevertheless, use noninteracting alternatives to HMG-CoA reductase inhibitors or to niacin if possible; monitor
Interactions Involving Neomycin		
	See Table 56–I	
Interactions Involving Nicotinic Acid		
Lovastatin	See lovastatin-nicotinic acid, above	
Sulfinpyrazone (Chapter 53)	Reduced ability of interactant to lower serum uric acid levels	Potential interaction; use of alternatives to either drug advised; interaction of nicotinic acid with major sulfinpyrazone alternative, probenecid, not reported

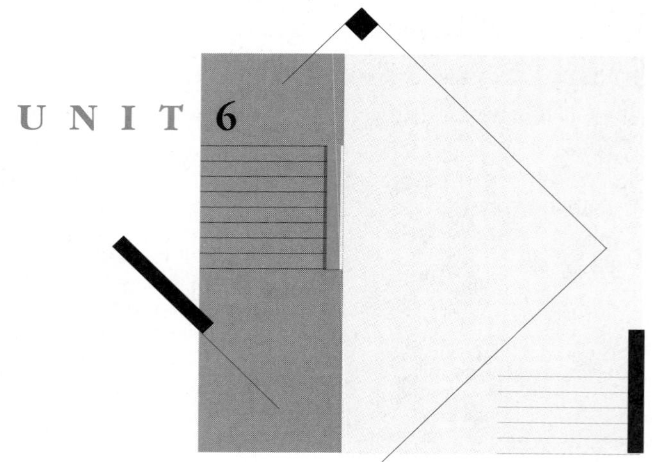

Drugs That Affect the Respiratory System

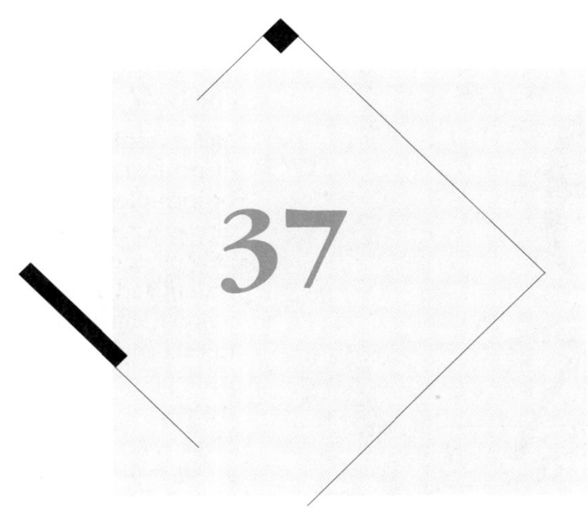

Structure and Function of the Respiratory System

The respiratory system, in conjunction with the circulatory system, is responsible for supplying the body cells with oxygen and for eliminating the carbon dioxide that cells produce as metabolic waste. The respiratory system also has a major role in maintaining the blood's acid–base balance. The following sections review the anatomy and physiology of the respiratory system, to provide an introduction to the drugs that affect it in desired or unwanted ways. Most of the drugs are discussed in Chapter 38.

Respiratory System Structures

Figure 37–1 illustrates the respiratory system organs, and briefly describes their functions. The upper respiratory tract comprises the nasal cavities, the bronchi, and all components in between. These structures bring expired air to the lungs' alveoli, where oxygen and carbon dioxide exchange occurs. In addition to serving as passageways, these structures also warm, humidify, and purify incoming air so that air reaching the alveoli contains far fewer irritants than it does when first inspired. Cells lining the tracheobronchial tree secrete and help eliminate mucus. The smooth muscles of the bronchi and bronchioles have a crucial role in regulating the flow of air, as discussed in more detail later.

Pulmonary Structure and Function

Gas Exchange

The gases of most importance to pulmonary function and overall well-being are oxygen and carbon dioxide. The body's oxygen source is inspired air, while the most important sources of carbon dioxide are the body cells. In the alveolar capillaries, oxygen from inspired air diffuses into the oxygen-poor pulmonary arterial blood, and carbon dioxide diffuses from the carbon dioxide–rich blood to the alveolar air. Both processes occur simultaneously. Most of the oxygen in the blood binds to hemoglobin molecules inside erythrocytes, forming oxyhemoglobin, which carries oxygen to the systemic tissues. Only a small amount of oxygen is dissolved in the plasma.

Carbon dioxide is carried in the blood mainly in the form of bicarbonate ions. Carbon dioxide that enters the blood flowing through systemic capillaries diffuses into erythrocytes, which have an abundant supply

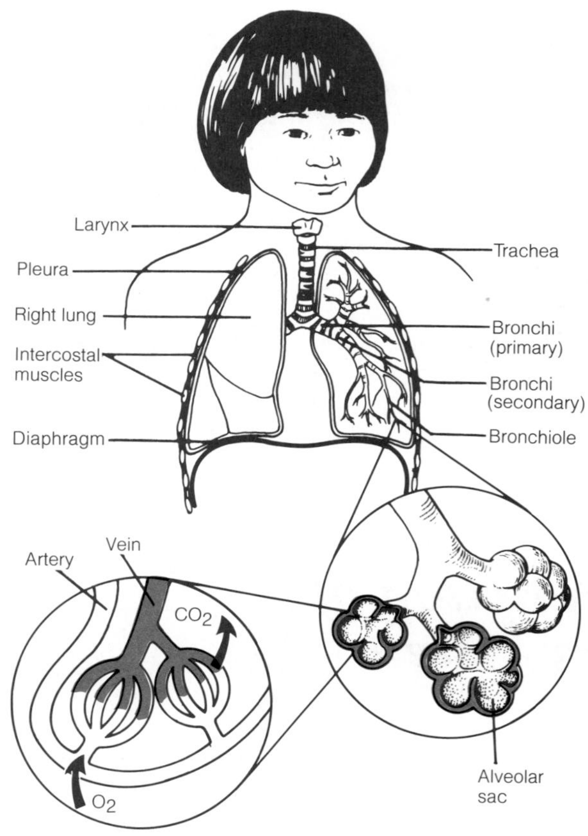

Figure 37-1

Major respiratory system structures and their functions. Structures that extend from the pharynx and larynx to the bronchioles contain smooth muscles and glands that regulate airway tone and secretions. Their activities depend considerably on endogenous regulation by the autonomic nervous system and mediators released by cells such as mast cells. Smooth muscle tone, gland secretory activity, and the ability to exchange gases adequately, play important roles in the pathophysiology of asthma and chronic obstructive lung diseases.

(*Source:* Reprinted from S James and S Mott, *Child Health Nursing,* p. 660. Addison–Wesley, 1988.)

of the enzyme *carbonic anhydrase.* The enzyme quickly forms carbonic acid through the reaction between carbon dioxide and water. Carbonic acid, in turn, quickly dissociates into hydrogen and bicarbonate ions, which promptly leave the red cells and enter the blood. In the alveolar capillaries, the reactions are reversed. Since the carbon dioxide concentration in alveolar capillary blood (at least on the arterial side) is higher than in inspired air, carbon dioxide is unloaded from the blood and eliminated in the expired air.

Three properties of the alveoli allow efficient gas exchange:

1. The huge exchange (alveolar) surface.
2. The extremely thin alveolar wall and adjacent capillary membranes.
3. The action of surfactant molecules on the alveolar surfaces, which lower the surface tension, oppose the tendency of the alveoli to collapse, and significantly reduce the energy needed to expand the lungs.

Deficiencies in the formation of surfactants play a crucial role in the respiratory distress syndrome seen in some premature infants. Dilation and collapse of the alveoli (atelectasis) play an important role in such common pulmonary disorders as emphysema, which is mainly a disorder of older adults.

Respiratory Tract Secretions

Cells lining the tracheobronchial tree secrete mucus, which forms a protective fluid blanket that entraps irritant particles and microorganisms entering the respiratory passages. Other cells lining these passageways have cilia that propel the mucus, and its entrapped particles, out of the respiratory passages; the process is called *mucociliary clearance.*

The volume of mucus formation, the viscosity (thickness) of the mucus, and the process of mucociliary clearance are all under physiologic control. They can be affected adversely by pulmonary diseases or local irritants (including tobacco smoke and air pollutants), and can be affected adversely or desirably by various chemicals. For example, parasympathetic nervous system influences, through released acetylcholine (ACh), cause the formation of thin, watery mucus. In contrast, sympathetic influences, sympathomimetic drugs, and antimuscarinic (atropine-like) agents decrease the volume of mucus but increase its viscosity. Excessive mucus secretion often is considered undesirable. However, administration of drugs that form a thick and dry mucus that is difficult to expel (inspissation) is also undesirable, particularly if a condition is present that might reduce the free flow of air through the airways, such as asthma and some forms of obstructive pulmonary disease.

Roles and Regulation of Bronchial Smooth Muscle Tone

The smooth muscle cells of the bronchi and bronchioles are important participants in the overall process of respiration. Like the mucus-secreting cells, they are under opposing control of both divisions of the autonomic nervous system. They also are affected by other endogenous chemical mediators. Bronchoconstriction is one of the key contributors to the pathophysiology and symptoms of asthma, and is also an important factor in chronic obstructive pulmonary disease (COPD). These diseases, and others, are discussed later.

Acetylcholine

The primary neural control of bronchial smooth muscle tone is conferred by ACh released from parasympathetic nerves. Acetylcholine, acting on muscarinic receptors on smooth muscle cells, and through formation of a second messenger (cyclic GMP), stimulates smooth muscle cell contraction, decreases the diameter of bronchioles (that is, causes bronchoconstriction), and increases airway resistance. (This same process accounts for the ability of ACh or parasympathetic drugs to increase mucus production by other cells in the airways.)

Individuals with asthma appear to be extremely sensitive to the effects of ACh or parasympathomimetic drugs.

Epinephrine

There appears to be little or no sympathetic *neural* control of smooth muscle function and airway diameter. Instead, circulating epinephrine is the major stimulus for bronchial smooth muscle dilation (relaxation). Epinephrine's bronchodilator actions are the result of its ability to interact with β_2-adrenergic receptors on the smooth muscle cells, leading to the formation of cyclic AMP as a second messenger. The involvement of β_2 receptors in bronchodilation provides the rationale for using beta agonists (or epinephrine) when bronchodilation must be induced therapeutically. It also explains why norepinephrine, which cannot stimulate β_2 receptors, is useless as a physiologic regulator or therapeutic agent.

Other substances affect airway smooth muscle tone, mucus secretion, or both. The two most important ones are histamine and some of the prostaglandins.

Histamine

Histamine clearly has pathologic relevance in terms of pulmonary function. It is found in mast cells that are abundant in the respiratory tree, and is released in response to allergens and several common drugs (morphine, for example). Histamine exerts powerful bronchoconstrictor effects on smooth muscles. Histamine is but one of several mast cell mediators (see Chapter 50 and Table 50–3) that are particularly important in the pathophysiology of asthma. Fortunately, and as discussed in the next chapter, the drug cromolyn is available to prevent mast cell mediator release.

Prostaglandins

Prostaglandin E_2 (PGE_2) is a bronchodilator. It probably serves a physiologic role in all persons, but it appears to be less important than epinephrine in normal individuals. In persons with asthma, the true importance of PGE_2 becomes much greater, particularly when its synthesis is inhibited by aspirin and many other nonsteroidal antiinflammatory agents. The manifestation of its inhibited synthesis is bronchoconstriction, which can be life-threatening.

Mechanics of Ventilation

The process of ventilation and its two components, inspiration and expiration, depend on the activities of skeletal muscles in the diaphragm and the thoracic cage, and on the elastic or recoil properties of the lung tissues. Impaired lung elasticity is important in the etiology of some restrictive lung disorders; skeletal muscle dysfunction causes the breathing difficulty associated with such diseases as myasthenia gravis.

Ventilatory Volumes and Rates

The processes of inspiration and expiration, and the volume and speed with which air is moved with each normal or forced breath, are important and relatively easy to measure clinically with a technique called spirometry. A full discussion of such tests—what they measure and how they are interpreted—is beyond the scope of this book. However, such parameters as inspiratory and tidal volumes, expiratory volumes, and inspiratory and expiratory air flow rates, are crucial for the proper diagnosis of many pulmonary disorders.

That information in turn often determines the drugs to be selected to treat them. Moreover, pulmonary function tests provide quantitative measurements of the success of therapeutic interventions.

For the most part, and unlike the situation with asthma or COPD, pulmonary problems involving skeletal muscle dysfunction or loss of lung elasticity are not very responsive to pharmacotherapy.

Respiratory Rhythm and Depth

The neural centers that control respiratory rhythm and rate are located in both the medullary and pons regions of the brainstem. The basic ventilatory rate, 14 to 18 respirations per minute, seems to be set by the medullary inspiratory center. However, reflexes (coughing, sneezing, and so on), peripheral sensory input, and voluntary controls all can influence respiratory rate and force.

Changes of blood carbon dioxide tensions and pH are sensed by chemoreceptors in the brain. Peripheral chemoreceptors, mainly in the carotid bodies and aortic arch, respond to changes of blood oxygen tensions and convey neural stimuli to the brain's respiratory control centers. Unless a patient suffers marked hypoxia, it appears that blood carbon dioxide and pH levels provide the most important and sensitive ventilatory "drives."

Carbon dioxide retention (hypercapnia), caused by decreased respiratory rate or depth, or both, tends to cause respiratory acidosis. Conversely, excessive falls of blood carbon dioxide levels, such as those caused by hyperventilation, cause respiratory alkalosis. The body corrects such changes in several ways. For example, rising levels of blood carbon dioxide lower blood pH, and the increased levels of protons stimulate medullary chemoreceptors. Ventilation increases, primarily via increased ventilatory rate. (It is clinically important to note that morphine and most other narcotics, which depress ventilation, also block this critical carbon dioxide–related mechanism for correcting hypoventilation.) Rising blood carbon dioxide levels also act on airway smooth muscles to cause bronchodilation. Renal mechanisms to adjust and compensate for blood acid–base imbalances are also important.

Most central nervous system (CNS) depressant drugs are capable of depressing respiration. The narcotic analgesics (morphine and others) exert the most obvious and clinically important respiratory depression, even with therapeutic doses. Because such depressants are widely used and abused, their effects on ventilation are commonly encountered by health-care providers. Drugs that stimulate respiration (analeptics and cerebral stimulants; Chapter 27) are also available. Their adverse respiratory effects are encountered much less frequently because they are seldom used.

Pulmonary Dysfunction

Chronic pulmonary dysfunction usually is classified as being restrictive or obstructive. In some cases both types of dysfunction occur simultaneously. Pulmonary function tests are clearly important components of diagnosis and selection of proper treatment. However, astute assessment of the presenting signs and symptoms—including their nature, intensity, and clinical course (fluctuating or steady)—and a thorough history are also important. The nurse has an essential role in these aspects of diagnosis, in the evaluation of therapeutic responses, and in providing information to patients that will help ensure safe and effective treatment.

Restrictive Pulmonary Diseases

Most restrictive pulmonary diseases involve reduced elastic properties of the lungs or chest wall. Examples include pulmonary edema; pulmonary fibrosis (whether disease-induced or caused by such drugs as the antiarrhythmic agent amiodarone; the antihypertensive agent minoxidil; or the anticancer drug bleomycin); pneumonitis; bronchiolar smooth-muscle hypertrophy; granuloma formation; and lung neoplasms. Disorders of the pleura or the chest wall musculature (as might be caused by quadriplegia or myasthenia gravis), and thoracic deformities (scoliosis, for example), also may cause or contribute to diminished lung capacity. They are also causes of restrictive pulmonary disease.

Obstructive Pulmonary Diseases

Obstructive disorders are the largest and most frequently encountered group of pulmonary diseases. Increased airway resistance (bronchoconstriction) is the common finding, but the mechanisms by which it occurs vary. It is common to refer to all the major obstructive pulmonary diseases using the generic term chronic obstructive pulmonary disease (COPD), but contemporary pulmonologists are encouraging use of more precise terms. Each of the major obstructive pulmonary diseases is identified and described briefly here to set the stage for later discussions of drug treatment. Asthma and COPD are treated with many of the same drugs.

Asthma

Asthma is characterized by *reversible* narrowing of the airways caused by bronchoconstriction. Other pathologic components include bronchial mucosal edema, excessive mucus secretions, and inflammation.

The major signs and symptoms of asthma are shortness of breath, cough, chest tightness, wheezing, tachycardia, and tachypnea (rapid breathing). Mucus production usually increases. The symptoms may be brief or prolonged, and mild, severe, or even life threatening (as in *status asthmaticus*). Usually there are intervening periods during which the patient is symptom-free.

The treatment of asthma, discussed in the next chapter, involves a variety of drugs that can be used alone or in combination. The major drug interventions include bronchodilators, (theophylline), mast cell stabilizers (cromolyn), and corticosteroids.

Chronic Obstructive Pulmonary Disease (COPD)

Chronic obstructive pulmonary disease (also called chronic obstructive lung disease [COLD]) encompasses chronic bronchitis and emphysema. Chronic bronchitis and emphysema often occur together. Cigarette smoking is, without doubt, the number one cause of COPD; *all* smokers have bronchitis. Some evidence suggests that air pollution is an important contributing factor for both smokers and nonsmokers. Morbidity and mortality from COPD are high; the overall death rate has doubled every five years over the past 30 years. About half of long-term smokers may have advanced COPD by middle age. Unfortunately, COPD often is not diagnosed early, and so the implementation of treatment and preventive measures is delayed.

The typical findings in chronic bronchitis are mucus plugging, inflammation, fibrosis, narrowing, and overall destruction of the small terminal bronchioles. Patients with this condition tend to develop severe episodes of wheezing, coughing, hypoxemia, and hypercapnia; experience weight gain from systemic edema; and eventually have most of the findings associated with congestive heart failure. Right heart failure (*cor pulmonale*) and cyanosis usually occur before generalized cardiac failure. Because of cyanosis and edema, patients with severe bronchitis often are called "blue bloaters." Bronchiolar damage and poor air flow tend to make breathing difficult and fatiguing. Patients with chronic bronchitis tend to be younger than those with emphysema.

Emphysema mainly affects the terminal alveoli, and is characterized by alveolar dilation and eventual collapse. The term "pink puffer" often is applied to persons with emphysema. Such individuals typically appear thin or wasted, and breathe with rapid, shallow breaths. Blood gas studies show reduced blood oxygen tensions, but not elevated blood carbon dioxide levels.

The pharmacologic treatment for COPD involves the bronchodilators that are used for asthma. Antibiotics and corticosteroids may be indicated for some patients. The success of the pharmacologic approach depends greatly on getting the patient to quit smoking altogether.

Bronchiectasis

Bronchiectasis is pathologic dilation of the bronchi caused by bronchial wall destruction. The damage provides an ideal location for the growth of infectious organisms, which cause a vicious cycle of pulmonary damage and resulting symptoms. A common cause of bronchiectasis used to be repeated or prolonged episodes of pneumonitis, especially during early childhood. However, the use of antibiotics has reduced this cause dramatically, at least in some parts of our society and culture. Cystic fibrosis and hypogammaglobulinemia (deficiencies of IgA, IgG, and IgM) are other causes of bronchiectasis.

Drug therapy usually involves administration of one or more antibiotics to suppress infection, and mucolytic (mucus-thinning) drugs to help expel mucus. Although bronchodilator drugs typically used for asthma may be indicated for some patients with bronchiectasis, they are not primary therapies.

NURSING IMPLICATIONS

As with all areas of therapeutics, be aware not only of drugs that cause desired pulmonary effects, but also of those that may cause unwanted effects, whether in patients with preexisting pulmonary disorders or in persons with previously good pulmonary status. Pulmonary or ventilatory dysfunction is a direct or indirect consequence of overdoses of many drugs that are discussed in this book; it is an untoward response to many more drugs, even when therapeutic doses are given. Many

Table 37–1 Selected Examples of Ways in Which Drugs Can Cause Adverse Pulmonary Effects*

Effect	Examples	Chapter
Bronchoconstriction	Acetylcholinesterase inhibitors	12
	Alpha-adrenergic agonists	14
	Beta-adrenergic blockers	15
	Histamine releasers: any allergen or allergenic drug; curare and related neuromuscular blockers; morphine	17, 21
	Nonsteroidal antiinflammatory drugs	52
	Parasympathomimetics	11
Central nervous system (respiratory) depression or other types of decreased respiratory drive	Most CNS depressants, including high doses of alcohol, barbiturates, benzodiazepines; therapeutic doses of morphine, other narcotics	21, 22
Mucus hypersecretion or accumulation	Acetylcholinesterase inhibitors	12
	Antitussives	—
	Histamine releasers (see above)	—
	Parasympathomimetics	11
Mucus plugging (inspissation; decreased, thickened secretions)	Anticholinergics, including atropine and derivatives; antipsychotics; antidepressants; and antihistamines (H_1 blockers)	13, 23, 24 25, 51
	Diuretics (in doses sufficient to cause dehydration)	32
Pulmonary fibrosis, other manifestations of lung pathology	Amiodarone	30
	Bleomycin	59
	Minoxidil	33

*The drugs or drug groups listed are selected only to encourage awareness of their potential adverse effects. The conditions under which they may cause unwanted effects, and the extent of the problems caused, may vary. Consult the chapters noted for more details, especially regarding how they cause adverse effects and how to assess for and avoid them.

of these drugs, summarized by group in Table 37–1, are given for desired effects that have nothing to do with treating pulmonary problems. But if their pulmonary effects are overlooked, the consequences can be serious.

The potential adverse effects of nonprescription drugs are just as important as those of drugs prescribed by a physician or other authorized health-care provider. For example, drugs such as aspirin, antihistamines, decongestants, and cough suppressants may be safe and effective when used properly, especially by persons with normal lung function. When used inappropriately, however, they may be very dangerous.

In short, it is important not only to assess pulmonary function before administering drugs, but also to assess for and avoid, when possible, the potential adverse effects of drugs on the respiratory system.

PROTOTYPE

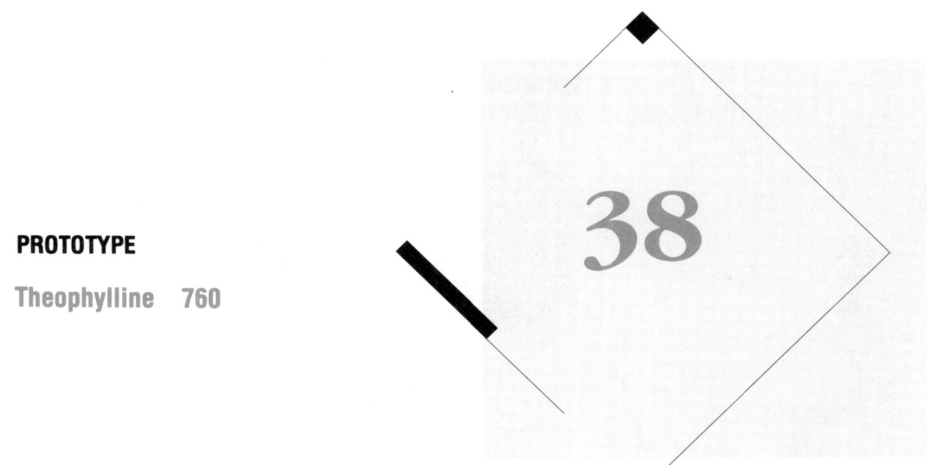

Drugs for Managing Asthma

Asthma is the most common pulmonary disorder in children, adolescents, and nonsmoking young adults. About one in 10 children have the disease, and asthma affects about 4% of the adult population. Each year asthma directly causes approximately 2000 deaths, and it is an important contributor to about 5000 others. Chronic obstructive pulmonary diseases (COPD)—chronic bronchitis and emphysema—disable another 35,000 or so Americans each year.

This chapter discusses the drugs used to treat these disorders. The emphasis is on asthma, but several of the drugs used to treat asthma are useful for COPD also.

In the mid-1800s, prescriptions for asthma included such recommendations as "two breakfast cups of strong coffee" or "violent emotions." There was some scientific wisdom to these remedies, although it was not well understood until years later. Coffee contains caffeine. Violent emotions release epinephrine.

Nowadays these chemicals, or ones related to them, have been purified, standardized, and put into widespread use for treating asthma and COPD. Unfortunately, data collected between 1970 and 1990 show that asthma therapy has not been as successful as we might hope or expect. Even in the United States, with its high quality health-care system, the overall *prevalence* of asthma increased by slightly more than 20%; the *hospitalization rate* nearly doubled for adults, and rose about five times for children; and the *death rate* from asthma nearly *doubled* overall. Affected most were the elderly and blacks. (Among children aged 10 to 14 years, the death rate for blacks was three to nine times higher than for whites.)

One explanation is that health-care providers and patients alike need more knowledge about the available drugs and how to use them properly. However, probably the most important explanation is that for years scientists and clinicians focused on bronchoconstriction as if it were the only important pathophysiologic contributor to asthma. That idea was probably wrong.

Overall, asthma may be underdiagnosed, undertreated, or simply treated improperly.

Asthma Symptoms: Causes and Rationales for Antiasthma Drug Use

Asthma symptoms include wheezing, cough, dyspnea, and tightness of the chest. Symptom severity and duration can be mild and brief, even without drug treatment;

Major reference tables appear beginning on page 779.

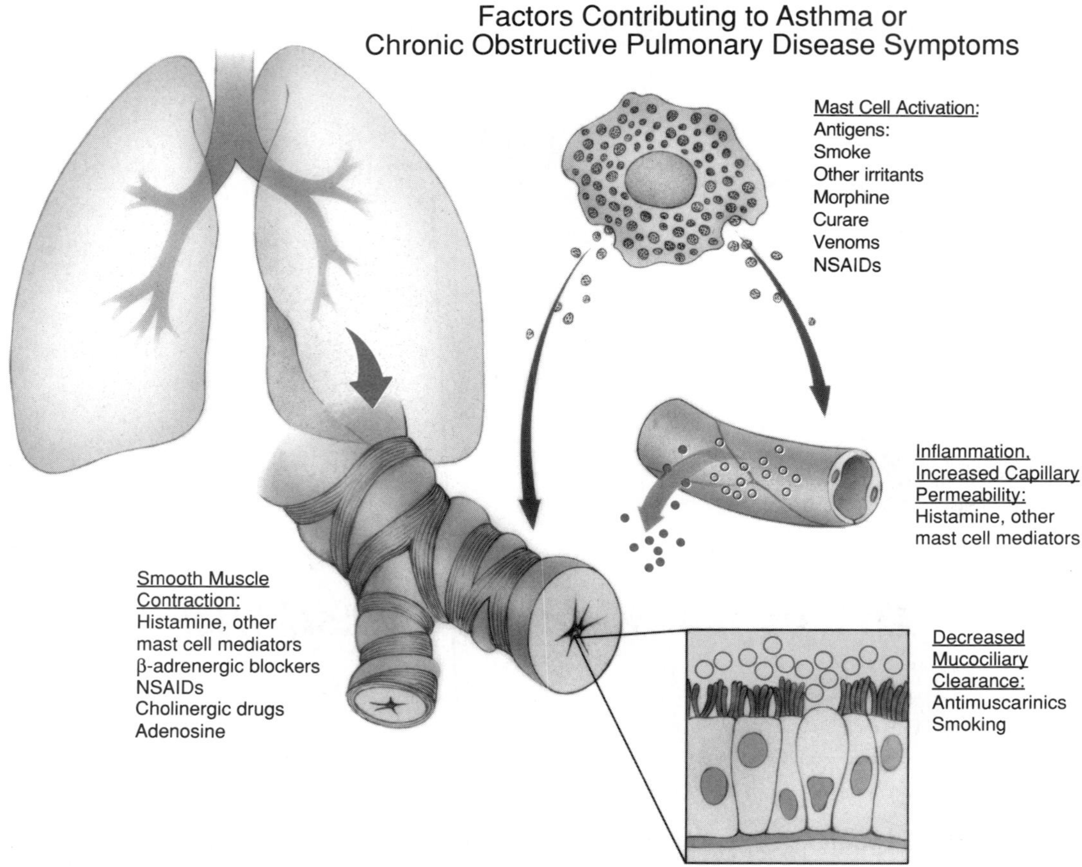

Figure 38–1

Factors contributing to asthma or chronic obstructive pulmonary disease symptoms. Many drugs, antigens, and other environmental factors trigger one or more of these underlying symptom causes. NSAID-nonsteroidal antiinflammatory drugs such as aspirin.

or severe and unrelenting, leading to potentially fatal *status asthmaticus.* The impaired ability of the lungs to exchange oxygen and carbon dioxide can affect the body as a whole, and the consequences may be very serious.

There are three major components to asthma (Figure 38–1): bronchoconstriction; inflammation, including changes of capillary permeability; and increased mucus production and reduced mucus removal. For years bronchoconstriction was considered the key problem to attack therapeutically. Bronchoconstriction *is* important, and it is probably the most important target of intervention in managing *acute* symptoms.

However, it is now apparent that we underestimated the role of respiratory tract inflammation. Suppressing airway inflammation is very important, whether the asthma symptoms are acute or chronic. The key substances that cause inflammation come from mast cells that are abundant in the airways. These chemical mediators include histamine, kinins, and eosinophil-attracting factors.

Another pathophysiologic factor is a reduced ability of cilia on epithelial cells in the respiratory passages to remove airway secretions that can be profuse and thick. This diminished ciliary function is called *decreased mucociliary clearance.*

Asthma Types and Triggers

Extrinsic asthma is the term used to describe asthma that is caused by external factors. Some of these factors (see Figure 38–1) can trigger an acute attack or sustain the disease long-term. They include airborne pollutants; exercise, cold air, and other physical stresses; emotional

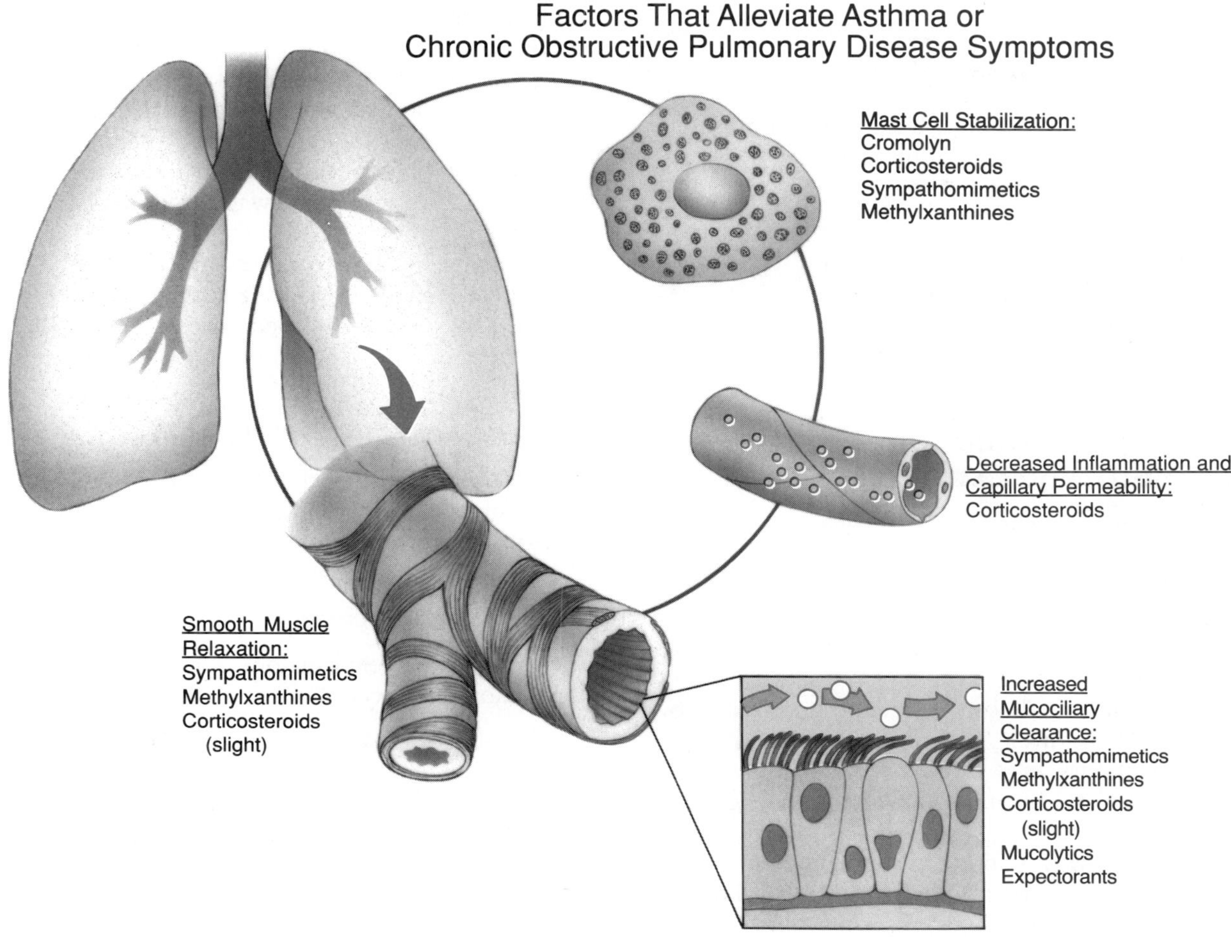

Figure 38–2

The drugs used to treat asthma and chronic obstructive lung disease tend to act on one or more of the underlying causes of symptoms. Some drugs, such as the methylxanthine and sympathomimetic "bronchodilators," actually have more than one beneficial action.

stress; infection; and certain drugs such as aspirin and morphine.

Antigen-antibody reactions trigger symptoms in patients with *atopic* (meaning allergy-mediated) asthma, which is a form of extrinsic asthma. In *intrinsic* asthma, the trigger is unknown.

Treatment

There are a variety of nondrug measures that can reduce the frequency or severity of asthma attacks. These are discussed briefly at the end of the chapter. For the majority of patients, drug treatment will be required at some time. The main drugs are classified as bronchodilators, corticosteroids, and mast cell stabilizers.

Figure 38–2 summarizes how these drugs affect one or more of the pathophysiologic changes that contribute to asthma or COPD. It also shows the actions of some miscellaneous drugs that may be indicated for some patients. These drugs are discussed briefly on pages 759 to 774.

I. Bronchodilators

There are two major chemical classes of bronchodilators that are used widely for asthma: *methylxanthines* and *sympathomimetics.* A third class of bronchodilators, the inhaled antimuscarinics, have special and somewhat limited use. They are discussed in a separate section beginning on page 773.

Methylxanthines

Methylxanthines are related chemically to caffeine. The prototype methylxanthine is *anhydrous theophylline.* It is still a common and usually effective drug for asthma and COPD, but its use is declining as the use of sympathomimetic bronchodilators rises.

PROTOTYPE

Theophylline (Anhydrous)

Absorption, Distribution, Metabolism, and Excretion

Anhydrous theophylline usually is given orally. The drug is poorly soluble and is absorbed irregularly from the gut. Theophylline distributes throughout the body and enters the central nervous system (CNS) well. About half the drug molecules in the bloodstream are bound to plasma proteins.

Theophylline is almost completely inactivated by metabolism in the liver. The plasma half-life is about three to six hours in a healthy adult, and three to four hours (or less) for most individuals younger than 16 years.

There are many important and common factors such as diseases and interacting drugs that can alter significantly theophylline's metabolism, its blood levels, and its biologic actions.

Pharmacologic Effects

Theophylline's main therapeutic effects are in the airways. Other potentially important targets of action are the cardiovascular and central nervous systems. Some of these effects should be familiar to persons who drink large amounts of caffeine-containing beverages, such as coffee or colas (see Chapter 26).

Pulmonary Effects

Theophylline's most obvious pulmonary effect is bronchodilation. However, it also stabilizes mast cells and increases mucociliary clearance. Theophylline has no true antiinflammatory effect, however.

Cardiovascular and Renal Effects

Theophylline's cardiovascular effects are seldom intense or important with therapeutic doses given to healthy persons. Nevertheless, they can become important, and unwanted, for some patients. They are clearly important with overdoses.

Theophylline increases heart rate, the force of contraction, and automaticity, and also dilates most peripheral blood vessels. Overall, cardiac output increases. These effects, plus the drug's ability to dilate renal arterioles and increase blood flow to the kidneys, can cause diuresis.

Theophylline also constricts arterioles in the brain. (Caffeine is found in some headache remedies; presumably, the cerebral vasoconstrictor effects alleviate headache.)

Central Nervous System Effects

Methylxanthines cause dose-dependent CNS stimulation, mainly in the cerebral cortex and the respiratory control centers (medulla).

Mechanisms of Action

There are many explanations for how theophylline might exert its effects

1. It inhibits an enzyme called *phosphodiesterase* (Figure 38–3). Inhibiting phosphodiesterase leads to a buildup of cyclic AMP in cells, because normally phosphodiesterase breaks down cyclic AMP. Cyclic-AMP buildup causes bronchial smooth muscle relaxation, inhibits mucus secretion, and decreases mediator release from mast cells. In the heart, cyclic-AMP buildup owing to phosphodiesterase inhibition contributes to cardiac stimulation.
2. Theophylline blocks receptors for adenosine, a naturally occurring bronchoconstrictor substance.
3. Theophylline, through its actions in respiratory control centers, may stimulate "ventilatory drive."

However, despite much experimental evidence, the theophylline concentrations needed to cause these effects are much higher than those reached with therapeutic doses. In reality, we don't know how methylxanthines work.

Clinical Indications and Administration

Theophylline is an important drug for pediatric asthma patients. Its use for adults has declined as the use of sympathomimetics has increased. Some physicians think the most important role for theophylline in adult asthma is to control symptoms that affect about one in three asthma patients on a nightly basis. Sustained-acting dosage forms are best used for this purpose.

Figure 38–3

Role of cyclic AMP (c-AMP) in regulation of smooth muscle tone and mast cell activity. Interventions that elevate cyclic AMP levels dilate the bronchi and stabilize mast cells, probably by stimulating a pump that lowers cell calcium (Ca) levels. Sympathomimetics ① act mainly by increasing formation of cyclic AMP. Methylxanthines ② inhibit breakdown of cyclic AMP, and also block smooth muscle cell receptors for adenosine, a bronchoconstrictor.

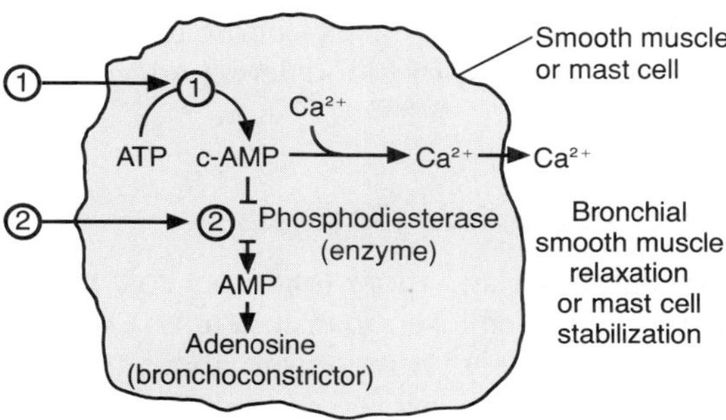

The Therapeutic Goal

The therapeutic goal with theophylline—as with all the other antiasthma drugs—is to reduce the frequency and severity of asthma symptoms without causing side effects. With theophylline, that goal usually is reached when serum levels are maintained consistently between 10 and 20 μg/mL, which is the generally accepted therapeutic range. Blood levels less than 10 μg/mL usually are subtherapeutic; levels above 20 μg/mL usually are associated with significant side effects or toxicity.

Dosage Forms

Oral dosage forms of theophylline include "immediate-acting" tablets and elixirs, and sustained-release preparations. Both oral and rectal formulations are for prophylaxis only. No oral or rectal formulation acts fast enough to cause immediate bronchodilation and acute relief of an asthma attack. Only immediate-acting tablets or elixirs should be used to start therapy. Sustained-acting preparations should be used only after blood levels have stabilized, and symptoms have been controlled after starting treatment with another oral dosage form.

A related theophylline salt, aminophylline, usually is used when parenteral therapy is needed for faster effects. It is discussed below.

Standard theophylline tablets and elixirs are relatively inexpensive. The elixirs have a very poor taste, and the need for frequent administration of elixirs or standard tablets may be a nuisance. Overall, compliance may be a problem. The sustained-release preparations, although more expensive, have several advantages: they tend to cause less gastrointestinal upset, and they only need to be administered every six or 12 hours. These factors may improve compliance, and the longer duration of action may reduce bronchospasm near the end of the dosing interval. That can be particularly important when the main therapeutic goal is to prevent symptoms throughout the night. However, many sustained-release theophylline preparations are large and difficult for some patients, especially children and elders, to swallow.

Doses and Dosage Adjustments

Typical methylxanthine doses (Table 38–C) are for the "average, otherwise healthy" patient. Actual doses must be individualized because many factors—especially those that affect the drug's metabolism—can make an otherwise right dose the wrong dose. Metabolic changes affect theophylline's duration of action, blood levels, and the proper dosages. These considerations are very important, because theophylline and related drugs have a *narrow margin of safety:* therapeutic blood levels are not far below toxic blood levels.

The starting dose usually is based on the patient's body weight; age; smoking habits; the presence of other diseases (especially liver dysfunction); and the use of interacting drugs. Once the best estimates are made and treatment is started, the dose is adjusted again, if necessary, based on measurements of serum theophylline levels, assessments of the adequacy of the response, and assessment for side effects.

Typical Adult Dosages and Dosage Adjustments

For the average nonsmoking adult with good liver function, the starting dose of anhydrous theophylline per day is 16 mg/kg or 400 mg, whichever is less. Give it in three or four divided doses per day. After about three days there should be a change to the typical maintenance dose, 13 mg/kg per day or 900 mg per day (whichever is less), also in divided doses.

Patients who smoke may require 50% to 100% higher doses, expressed as milligrams of theophylline per kilogram of body weight, than otherwise identical nonsmokers. Patients with severe hepatic, cardiac, or respiratory dysfunction require doses (mg per kg) lower than those for a generally healthy adult. The physician should determine the exact dose for each patient, and adjust according to blood levels and the clinical response.

Typical Pediatric Dosages

Methylxanthines play a more important role in treating asthma in young children than in adults. Children between approximately six months to about 16 years old require higher doses, expressed as milligrams of drug per kilogram of body weight, than adults. This relationship occurs because the younger the patient, the faster he or she will metabolize the drug. (This age-related effect with theophylline is quite different from what is found with most other drugs.) However, infants younger than six months old usually require lower milligram-per-kilogram doses than older children do.

NURSING IMPLICATIONS

◆ Methylxanthine Administration and Use

Question medication orders that initiate therapy with sustained-release theophylline preparations. Be sure patients understand that there is no self-administered theophylline preparation that can stop an ongoing asthma attack quickly.

When a sustained-release theophylline product is prescribed, and the patient has trouble swallowing it, advise him or her to open the capsule and sprinkle the contents onto a cold semisolid food such as applesauce, pudding, or ice cream. Alternatively, notify the physician of the problem; theophylline products made specifically to sprinkle on foods are available.

Advise patients not to crush or chew a sustained-release theophylline capsule. This can lead to the rapid absorption of large amounts of the drug, and may cause toxicity.

◆ Blood Level Monitoring

Blood tests to measure theophylline levels should be done when starting therapy, during maintenance therapy, and when changing the dose. Check serum theophylline levels often during the start of treatment, and in severely ill patients. Once the patient is stabilized on theophylline, drug levels may need to be checked only once or twice a year if no adverse or side effects occur. Recheck levels at once, and change doses if needed, if there are side effects or signs of toxicity, or if the response is inadequate.

Dosage adjustments based on blood level measurements are reliable only when peak serum theophylline levels can be measured. Draw samples one to two hours after oral administration of standard theophylline, or six to seven hours after giving a sustained-release product.

Be aware that measuring theophylline blood levels is useful, but it does not eliminate the need for careful assessment and common sense to ensure effective and safe therapy.

Side Effects, Adverse Responses, and Contraindications

Side effects and other unwanted actions (Table 38–S) account for the decreased use of theophylline as a preferred treatment for asthma or COPD. Gastrointestinal (GI) intolerance and dose-dependent CNS stimulation—problems less likely to be caused by sympathomimetics—contribute to the decline in the use of theophylline and related drugs.

Gastrointestinal Side Effects

Therapeutic doses of methylxanthines irritate the gastric mucosa and increase mucosal blood flow. Gastrointestinal upset or pain, and nausea are common, especially with standard theophylline tablets or elixirs. Taking the medication with a full glass of water or milk, or with meals, tends to reduce the frequency and severity of GI distress. However, regardless of what precautionary measures are taken, methylxanthines are relatively contraindicated for patients with peptic ulcer disease.

Central Nervous System Side Effects

Nervousness, anxiety, or agitation are the major side effects related to CNS stimulation. The severity of these responses is dose-dependent. They may occur with therapeutic blood levels, but are more likely to occur and be bothersome when blood levels are 20 μg/mL or more—about the therapeutic range. If therapy is continued but blood levels are kept in the therapeutic range, most patients develop tolerance to CNS stimulation. Insomnia can be a problem if the patient takes methylxanthine too close to bedtime.

Do not administer prescription or OTC sedative drugs, or alcohol, to counteract CNS stimulation caused by methylxanthines. They can cause drug interactions and mask signs and symptoms of potential toxicity.

Cardiovascular Side Effects

Cardiovascular side effects usually are not serious or common when blood theophylline levels are normal and the patient has no cardiovascular disease. Serum concentrations at the high end of normal, or more, may cause tachycardia, palpitations, or anginal pain (indicating potential myocardial ischemia).

NURSING IMPLICATIONS

◆ Use During Pregnancy and Lactation

Theophylline may be used cautiously during pregnancy and breast-feeding. Close monitoring of the mother and fetus or child is important. Women who wish to breast-feed should do so just before the next dose, when blood levels are lowest. This helps reduce the infant's ingestion of the drug. Bottle-feeding may be needed if the child shows signs of drug effects (eg, irritability, poor eating or sleep habits). Assess the child for these effects.

◆ Use in Children

Many children who receive proper therapeutic doses of methylxanthines initially develop such disturbing CNS stimulation that their parents would rather tolerate wheezing than have the child disrupt the house. Advise the parents or guardians that this behavior is common; that tolerance to CNS stimulation should develop in a week or two; and that both wheezing and excess "energy" should subside. Nevertheless, if CNS stimulation is severe or prolonged, recheck the prescribed dosage and compliance with it, and assess the child in other ways; toxicity may be occurring. Advise parents not to medicate their children with OTC sedatives, such as pediatric antihistamine preparations, without consulting the physician first.

◆ Use in the Elderly

Elderly patients require reduced doses of methylxanthines, per kilogram of body weight, because of age-associated decreases in liver function. Other common age-related diseases (and the use of interacting drugs to treat them), as well as changes in body weight, usually require further dosage adjustments. Close monitoring of blood levels and the overall response is essential.

Interactions with Other Drugs

Several often-used drugs can cause clinically significant interactions (Table 38–1) with theophylline. The frequency and severity of these interactions also account for the decreased use of methylxanthines, and the increased use of alternative noninteracting drugs.

Many interactants alter theophylline metabolism.

1. *Barbiturates, phenytoin, rifampin, thyroid hormone supplements, and components in tobacco smoke* are among the key interactants that stimulate theophylline metabolism. Use of these drugs, or smoking, may reduce theophylline blood levels and the control of symptoms, unless the theophylline dose is increased carefully.
2. *Beta-adrenergic blockers, cimetidine, and several antibiotics* are common inhibitors of theophylline metabolism. Using them may increase theophylline blood levels and the risk of toxicity if theophylline dosages are not reduced properly.
3. Theophylline is often used as an adjunct to *sympathomimetic (adrenergic) bronchodilators.* The combination increases the degree of asthma symptom control. However, it also can increase the risk of excessive and potentially dangerous degrees of cardiovascular and CNS stimulation. Many physicians are wary of prescribing a methylxanthine and a sympathomimetic for outpatients who cannot be trusted to use their medications properly; sudden death has occurred.
4. *Halothane,* the prototype inhaled general anesthetic, may cause serious or fatal arrhythmias in patients who are taking theophylline. Avoid this interaction by making sure anesthesia staff are aware of theophylline use.

NURSING IMPLICATIONS

If theophylline must be used with an interacting drug, anticipate the need to remeasure theophylline blood levels often, and to adjust doses accordingly, until theophylline levels restabilize in the therapeutic range. This is most important when starting and stopping administration of the interactant.

◆ Food as a Theophylline Interactant

Food usually causes no clinically significant problems when theophylline is given in an immediate-acting dosage form. Taking such products with meals helps reduce GI side effects. However, taking sustained-release theophylline products with a full meal can increase or decrease drug absorption. The outcome depends on the theophylline product. Consult package inserts for information about the product your patient is taking.

There is also some evidence that the composition of the meal can affect theophylline absorption or metabolism, thereby changing blood levels and drug effects. Diets that include very large amounts of charcoal-broiled foods contain substances (much like those in tobacco smoke) that stimulate theophylline metabolism, thereby reducing theophylline blood levels and effectiveness. High-protein diets can do the same. In contrast, diets that are rich in carbohydrates and low in protein can reduce theophylline metabolism and cause blood levels of the drug to rise.

NURSING IMPLICATIONS

Stress proper theophylline administration with respect to meals. If otherwise correct doses of theophylline cause inadequate or excessive effects, consider rechecking the diet history for possible clues. Despite the usefulness of laboratory measurements of theophylline levels, careful patient assessment is still the best indicator of adequate and safe therapy.

Other Uses of Methylxanthines

The methylxanthine caffeine, which is rarely used as a bronchodilator, is used as a diuretic (Chapter 32), a CNS and respiratory stimulant (Chapter 27), and as an ingredient in headache remedies.

Overdose and Toxicity

Signs and Symptoms

Indicators of toxicity are extensions of the side effects noted above. Some appear when serum levels are only slightly above 20 μg/mL. Earliest indicators are CNS stimulation, headache or confusion, and GI upset (nausea, vomiting, anorexia). Palpitations, tachycardia, and rapid, shallow breathing (tachypnea), may occur.

If theophylline blood levels continue to rise, severe toxicity may develop soon after milder signs and symptoms appear. Serious toxicity includes seizures (status epilepticus is the usual cause of death), inadequate ventilation, and ventricular fibrillation. Such serious complications usually occur when theophylline levels reach 40 μg/mL.

Treatment

If toxicity cannot be prevented, the next best thing is to recognize it early so treatment can be started quickly.

There is no antidote for theophylline. If toxicity is from recent ingestion of an orally administered preparation, use standard first-aid measures to reduce further drug absorption (administration of active charcoal, inducing emesis, gastric lavage; see Appendix C). These measures have better chance of success when the overdose is detected quickly, and when sustained-acting preparations are swallowed whole. Mechanical ventilatory support may be needed.

Question medication orders to give CNS depressants to counteract respiratory stimulation; it is difficult to pick the right depressant dose and avoid causing another problem that is just as bad—respiratory depression. If seizures do occur, give proper drugs (eg, IV diazepam) at once.

Manage hypotension with IV fluids, but do *not* use sympathomimetic vasopressors (eg, norepinephrine, phenylephrine) routinely: they can potentiate adverse cardiovascular effects of methylxanthines. Antiarrhythmic drugs should be given as needed.

NURSING IMPLICATIONS

Even "therapeutic" blood levels of a methylxanthine may cause signs and symptoms that could signal toxicity in patients who are seriously ill or are taking interacting drugs. Therefore, adjust dosages, monitor blood levels, and assess each patient carefully.

Any signs or symptoms noted above should be considered as a warning of potential toxicity that might become serious. Sudden or severe CNS or cardiovascular stimulation are most worrisome. They may necessitate immediate (but perhaps temporary) discontinuation of the drug, and measurement of blood levels to guide subsequent intervention.

If serum theophylline levels are between 25 and 30 μg/mL, skip the next scheduled dose and reduce subsequent doses if needed. If levels are 30 μg/mL or more, anticipate skipping one or two doses, and reducing the maintenance dose by as much as 50%. Any indicator of toxicity, or a resulting dosage alteration, requires frequent monitoring of blood levels until they have stabilized at a lower, safe level.

Related Drugs

Anhydrous theophylline, the prototype or "gold standard," is poorly soluble. There are about six other generic drugs (and many formulations and brand names

Table 38–1 Approximate Equivalent Doses of Theophylline and Theophylline-Like Drugs*

Drug	% Theophylline	Dose Equivalent to 900 mg Anhydrous Theophylline
Theophylline, anhydrous	100	900 mg
Theophylline monohydrate (BRONKOTABS, QUIBRON, THEOLAIR)	91	990 mg
Aminophylline (SOMOPHYLLIN)	79	1260 mg
Dyphylline (DILOR, LUFYLLIN)	70	1290 mg
Oxtriphylline (choline theophyllinate; CHOLEDYL)	64	1400 mg
Theophylline sodium glycinate (SYNOPHYLATE)	49	1800 mg
Theophylline calcium salicylate (QUADRINAL)	48	1880 mg

*Table shows that all substitutes for anhydrous theophylline are less potent on a milligram-for-milligram basis, and therefore dosage adjustments are required when switching between theophylline and a substitute. For example, a patient stabilized on 900 mg of anhydrous theophylline would require approximately 1800 mg of SYNOPHYLATE. All of the above, except diphylline (not a theophylline salt), are converted to and measured as theophylline in the blood.

of each) in which theophylline is combined with another simple molecule or ion that increases solubility and absorption. These are theophylline *salts* (Table 38–1). They can be used instead of anhydrous theophylline. One of the more important theophylline salts is aminophylline. Another theophylline-like drug, dyphylline, is a theophylline derivative, not a salt. Because of their unique characteristics, aminophylline and dyphylline are discussed separately below.

There are some therapeutically important properties to remember about all of the related drugs.

1. They are less potent, on a milligram-for-milligram basis, than anhydrous theophylline (see Table 38–1). For example, 900 mg per day of a related theophylline preparation is not therapeutically equivalent to 900 mg per day (the average adult maintenance dose) of anhydrous theophylline. Therefore, dosage adjustments are necessary when substituting one drug for another.
2. Side effects, adverse reactions, and signs and symptoms of toxicity are the same for all of these drugs.

There are other important properties of theophylline salts; that is, of all the related drugs except dyphylline.

1. They are converted in the bloodstream to free theophylline. The free theophylline is responsible for therapeutic, side, and toxic effects. It is also what is measured in blood samples to determine drug levels.
2. Owing to the formation of free theophylline, subtherapeutic, therapeutic, and toxic serum levels noted for anhydrous theophylline are the same as those used to monitor therapy with a theophylline salt.
3. All precautions and dosage adjustments noted for anhydrous theophylline (for age, health, multidrug therapy, smoking, etc) apply to all the theophylline salts.
4. All drug interactions noted for anhydrous theophylline apply to all the theophylline salts.

Aminophylline

Aminophylline (eg, SOMOPHYLLIN) is the ethylenediamine tetraacetic acid (EDTA) salt of theophylline. It is the most important alternative to anhydrous theophylline because it is very soluble, and so is better suited for parenteral use. Aminophylline also can be given orally or per rectum; rectal suppositories or solutions are absorbed erratically.

Aminophylline is used mainly for severe, acute bronchoconstriction in hospitalized patients. (Here, too, its popularity is falling as sympathomimetic bronchodilator use increases.) A loading dose usually is given by slow IV injection, and maintenance doses then are given by IV infusion. Doses are based on the patient's age and weight; see Table 38–C for guidelines.

NURSING IMPLICATIONS

Aminophylline IV solutions must be diluted to concentrations no stronger than 25 mg/mL. They are best made in 5% dextrose injection or 0.9% sodium chloride. Inject the loading dose at 25 mg per minute or less if the patient is taking no other methylxanthines. Reduce the dose and injection rate if the patient already is taking methylxanthines.

Aminophylline is physically or chemically incompatible with many IV drugs, so do not mix them in the same container or syringe. If aminophylline will be "piggy-backed" on an IV set with another drug-containing IV solution, turn off the other drug before starting the aminophylline. Better yet, use a separate line altogether.

Each 0.6 mg/kg of aminophylline causes about a 1 μg/mL increase of serum theophylline levels. Typical maintenance infusion rates for a nonsmoking adult patient are about 0.6 mg/kg per hour. Periodically draw blood samples for measurements of serum levels during the infusion. Monitor blood pressure frequently, especially soon after starting therapy.

Dyphylline

Dyphylline (DILOR) differs from anhydrous theophylline and its salts in that dyphylline *cannot* be measured with standard theophylline assays. It also is excreted almost completely unchanged by the kidneys; it does not depend on metabolism. Therefore, dyphylline may be preferred for some patients with liver disease, or those taking other (interacting) drugs that alter hepatic metabolism. Conversely, dyphylline is a poor choice for persons with renal dysfunction.

Fixed-Dose Combinations of Theophylline and Other Drugs

There are dozens of medications such as ephedrine, phenobarbital, expectorants, or several of them together, that contain drugs in addition to theophylline or one of its salts. Consult *Physicians' Desk Reference* or *Drug Facts and Comparisons* for more information about their composition and use.

These multiple-drug medications may be no more effective than a medication that contains nothing more than a methylxanthine, and they are more expensive. In addition, some combinations are illogical or can increase the risk of drug interactions. For example, ephedrine (see Chapter 14 and below) increases the risk of cardiovascular and CNS side effects. Barbiturates (Chapter 22) can cause respiratory depression and stimulate methylxanthine metabolism. And, as with all fixed-dose combinations of drugs, it is impossible to change the dosage of one ingredient without altering the dosage of others.

Sympathomimetic Bronchodilators

Sympathomimetic bronchodilators belong to a large class of drugs that are also known as adrenergic receptor agonists. This section reviews general aspects of sympathomimetic drugs and their actions, and focuses on their use in asthma and COPD therapy. See Chapter 14 for more details about these drugs, their actions and uses, unwanted effects, and drug interactions.

Review of Adrenergic Receptors and Effects

Sympathomimetics stimulate one or more of the three major subtypes of adrenergic receptors—α, β_1 and β_2. These receptors control the activities of smooth and cardiac muscles, glands, and metabolic processes throughout the body. (Table 14–2 summarizes the receptor subtypes and the key responses that occur when they are stimulated.)

For asthma and COPD therapy, desired sympathomimetic effects require stimulation of β_2 receptors only. The effects are bronchodilation (bronchial smooth-muscle relaxation), decreased mucus secretion, increased mucociliary clearance, and mast-cell stabilization.

All these effects are the same as noted above for theophylline, and they all involve the same cyclic-AMP pathway in target cells (see Figure 38–3). However, whereas theophylline works by inhibiting cyclic-AMP breakdown, the sympathomimetics work by increasing cyclic-AMP synthesis. The ability of sympathomimetics and theophyllines to build up cyclic-AMP levels in the same target cells (admittedly in different ways) accounts for their combined use in some patients.

Beta$_2$ stimulation can cause other (extrapulmonary) effects that usually are not wanted in asthma or COPD therapy. These effects include dilation of the large blood vessels (which can decrease blood pressure) and metabolic effects such as increased blood glucose levels.

For years, the only major sympathomimetics that were available, and could be used for treating bronchoconstriction, were epinephrine, isoproterenol, and ephedrine. Their use for pulmonary dysfunction is limited because they cause more than the desired β_2-stimulating effects by also stimulating α receptors, β_1 receptors, or both. The resulting effects may be unneeded, unwanted, or even dangerous for pulmonary patients. For example, they could alleviate asthma or COPD symptoms, but aggravate the patient's cardiovascular disorder.

Drugs that are *relatively* β_2-selective have been developed, and they are used widely. *Albuterol* is the prototype.

"Selective" Beta₂ Agonists

There are six drugs in this class. Some have only one administration route and others have several. The administration route is important not only in terms of how the drug is given, but also in terms of uses and side effects that are due to drug actions outside the lungs.

1. *Albuterol* (PROVENTIL; VENTOLIN) and *metaproterenol* (ALUPENT; METAPREL) are formulated for administration orally or by inhalation.
2. *Terbutaline* (BRETHINE; BRETHAIRE; BRICANYL) can be given orally, by injection, or by inhalation.
3. *Isoetharine* (BRONKOMETER; BRONKOSOL), *bitolterol* (TORNALATE), and *pirbuterol* (MAXAIR) are given by inhalation only.

Formulations, Routes, Dosages, and Uses

Parenteral sympathomimetics are used to treat severe, acute bronchoconstriction. Inhaled agents can be used as initial treatments for adolescent or adult patients with mild and relatively infrequent episodes of wheezing. They can be used prophylactically or for terminating ongoing (but not severe or life-threatening) attacks. Their onsets of action are five minutes or less, and the effects last for about six hours, depending on the drug. All of the inhaled products are available in *metered-dose inhalers* (MDIs). These are pressurized canisters that deliver a fixed dose of drug each time the canister is activated. They are designed so that two activations (inhalations, or "puffs") give the usually prescribed dose. The drugs are inhaled *orally,* not nasally.

Oral formulations of sympathomimetics—those meant to be swallowed—may be used instead of, or in addition to, a methylxanthine for round-the-clock prophylaxis. Oral formulations act too slowly to terminate ongoing attacks; do not rely on them for that purpose.

All β agonists have durations of action that are too short to be of much use for relieving symptoms in patients who experience nocturnal asthma. For those patients, sustained-acting oral theophylline preparations appear to offer the best effectiveness. However, longer-acting β agonists are being tested, and they may become available for clinical use in the next few years.

NURSING IMPLICATIONS

All MDIs of sympathomimetics or other drugs to be mentioned later work on the same principle. Proper use of any inhaler requires good coordination of exhalation, inspiration, and activation of the canister; plus strength and dexterity. However, there are important differences in how each of the various inhalers is designed. These differences affect how the product should be used for best results. For example, the mouthpieces on some inhalers are meant to be placed between the lips. For others, the mouthpiece should be held slightly away from pursed lips.

Some MDIs are used with devices, called spacers, that are designed to give the proper distance between the mouth and the site where the drug is released from the canister. Spacers increase the amount of drug that reaches the airways, and decrease the amount that is deposited in the oral cavity. Each type of spacer has its own directions for proper use. Some of these devices have a very intimidating look.

Other accessories that greatly simplify and improve the administration of drugs packaged in MDIs are available from pharmacies. One example is the AERO CHAMBER, which is available with a soft face mask. Consult the physician or a pharmacist for more information.

Familiarize yourself with the instructions for each inhaler design or device so you can instruct patients to use them properly to ensure optimal results. Regardless of the products available, inhalers are usually inappropriate for patients who cannot be trusted to use them properly and safely, or who have physical impairments that affect proper use of the inhaler.

Instruct patients using any MDI bronchodilator to wait one to two minutes between the first and second puffs. The first inhaled dose opens the airways so the second can get further down. For the same reason, if the patient is using another type of inhaled drug, have him or her use the sympathomimetic first, followed in one to two minutes by the other.

Actions and Side Effects of "Selective" Bronchodilators

The term "selective β_2 agonist" is widely used and recognized, but it is misleading. These drugs are so-called because of the way they appear to act in the test tube or in other experimental settings. At usual doses they stimulate β_2 receptors much more effectively than the β_1 (cardiac) receptors. In practical terms, compared with nonselective beta agonists (β_1 and β_2 agonists such as isoproterenol), albuterol and the related agents have a greater ability to dilate the bronchi than to stimulate the heart directly. Thus, β_2 selectivity is partial or relative, not absolute.

In addition, none of these drugs is a "pure" (totally selective) bronchodilator. They can, and usually do, cause stimulation of β receptors outside the pulmonary system. The drug, the dose, and the administration route determine what other effects will occur, and how widespread and intense they will be.

These drugs come closest to being selective bronchodilators when they are administered by inhalation at low doses (ie, the usually recommended two puffs). Even then, β_2-mediated effects outside the lungs can occur.

These drugs are *much less* selective when they are given orally or by injection, at any dose; or when excessive doses are inhaled. They can cause all the cardiovascular and metabolic side effects or adverse responses that can be caused by isoproterenol (see Table 14–S). Thus, many contraindications that apply to the use of isoproterenol can apply to albuterol and related agents. The noteworthy ones are:

1. *Direct stimulation of heart rate, contractility, and automaticity.* Give these drugs with extra caution if the patient has tachycardia, arrhythmias, ischemic heart disease, or poorly controlled hyperthyroidism.
2. *Reflex cardiac stimulation.* This is triggered by β_2-mediated vasodilation and a slight fall of blood pressure, which activates the sympathetic nervous system via the baroreceptors.
3. *Hyperglycemia.* Give these drugs cautiously to patients with diabetes mellitus.
4. *Uterine relaxation.* Give these drugs cautiously to pregnant women, especially in the third trimester as labor and delivery approach, because they may delay or prolong labor. (To emphasize the concept that these agents are not totally selective as β_2 agonists or bronchodilators, consider another related drug, ritodrine (YUTOPAR). It too is classified as a selective β_2 agonist. However, ritodrine's sole use is as a parenteral or oral uterine relaxant to manage preterm labor.)
5. Two other side effects that can occur regardless of the administration route are *CNS stimulation* (anxiety, irritability, etc) and *skeletal muscle tremor.* CNS stimulation might indicate overdose. However, even mild CNS stimulation associated with proper doses can be annoying. It also can contribute to insomnia, a problem that is avoided best by not administering sympathomimetics too close to bedtime, unless immediate symptom relief is needed.

   Tremor is common, especially with high doses of inhaled sympathomimetics. It is more of an annoying side effect than a warning sign, and it can be severe. Some physicians use the appearance of skeletal muscle tremor as one indicator of proper dosages. They will advise the patient to increase the dose of the drug gradually, until tremor appears, then reduce the dose gradually. For many patients, tremor may persist.

NURSING IMPLICATIONS

To be safe, assume that *all* precautions (and contraindications, drug interactions, etc) for isoproterenol apply to these special agents. Assess for possible complications before giving the sympathomimetic, and periodically during treatment.

Tolerance to Sympathomimetic Bronchodilators

Chronic Tolerance

If used alone, inhaled adrenergic bronchodilators often are unsatisfactory for patients with frequent, severe asthma symptoms. Controlling such symptoms would require frequent use of high doses, with an added risk of side effects or toxicity. In addition, over the long run, frequent sympathomimetic use may lead to tolerance to the desired bronchodilator actions. One common way to handle drug tolerance is to increase the drug dosage to overcome the diminished response. With sympathomimetics, however, such dosage increases often increase side effects or may cause toxicity more than they will help alleviate bronchoconstriction, and this plan can actually make tolerance develop more quickly and become more severe. The medication plan must be reevaluated and changed.

Acute Tolerance

One of the most important limitations of *all* sympathomimetic bronchodilators, including the selective β_2 agonists, is a significant loss of bronchodilator activity in the presence of hypoxia and acidosis (hypoxemia). Hypoxemia, and the resulting tolerance, often occur in patients with chronically poor respiratory function due to inadequate bronchodilator therapy or severe illness. It also can occur acutely, as in anaphylaxis or status asthmaticus.

In these situations, even very large doses of sympathomimetics given by injection may not produce satisfactory bronchodilation. More likely, they will cause excessive and potentially dangerous cardiovascular stimulation.

If sympathomimetics are given to these patients, correct blood oxygenation by effectively administering oxygen; treat acidosis with suitable IV fluids (eg, sodium bicarbonate), if needed; and administer corticosteroids. Corticosteroids are discussed in a separate section below.

NURSING IMPLICATIONS

An inhaler may need to be used more often than prescribed for symptom relief, because of improper use or true lack of drug effectiveness (eg, because of advancing disease). Encourage patients to keep a written log of how often they use the product so outcome of therapy, possible development of tolerance, and overall compliance can be assessed. All this information is necessary for deciding what to do next if treatment must be reevaluated or changed.

Patients using inhalers often increase the dose on their own to get desired relief. That is potentially dangerous. Medication changes may be needed, but they should be made by the physician.

Use of Beta Blockers for Overdoses

Excessive cardiac stimulation is the greatest concern with overdoses of sympathomimetic bronchodilators. Ordinarily, a β blocker (eg, propranolol, INDERAL) is the most logical pharmacologic antidote for β-agonist overdoses. However, when the patient has asthma or COPD, a β blocker may correct cardiovascular adverse effects, but simultaneously may trigger acute or severe bronchoconstriction. Administer β blockers very cautiously, and monitor respiratory status very closely.

As noted below, β blockers can be deadly for any asthma or COPD patient, regardless of how or why the β blocker is being used.

Nonselective Sympathomimetic Agonists: Epinephrine, Isoproterenol, and Ephedrine

Nonselective sympathomimetic agonists have very limited uses for long-term management of asthma or COPD. However, it is important to know what their limitations are, when they should be used, and how to use them best. Refer to Table 14–C1 for dosages.

Epinephrine

Epinephrine stimulates all adrenergic receptors—α, β_1, and β_2. In doing so, it causes far more effects than are wanted when the main goal is bronchodilation. Epinephrine solution, given by subcutaneous injection, is the drug of choice for treating *anaphylaxis,* for which the drug's bronchodilating, cardiac-stimulating, and blood pressure–raising effects are all required.

Epinephrine seldom is used for acute bronchoconstriction of status asthmaticus. Its bronchodilator effects are useful, but the cardiovascular effects that always go along with them are unwanted; other drugs are preferred.

Epinephrine inhalers (eg, ASMANEFRIN, BRONKAID MIST, PRIMATENE MIST) are sold over-the-counter (OTC) as remedies for infrequent, mild asthma attacks. Here, too, cardiovascular side effects can occur.

NURSING IMPLICATIONS

The actions of subcutaneous injections of epinephrine solution may be too short-lived for some situations. If more prolonged effects are needed, repeated injections can be given. Usually, however, the longer-acting epinephrine suspension (eg, SUS-PHRINE) is used. It is given by SC injection; *never* give it IV.

Advise all patients, whether they have asthma or not, to avoid using OTC epinephrine inhalers except under a physician's supervision. In all likelihood, the physician will not recommend use of the OTC product; if a sympathomimetic is indicated, one of the β_2 agonists will be prescribed instead.

Isoproterenol

Isoproterenol's lack of α-stimulating (vasopressor) activity makes it unsuitable for anaphylaxis. Like epinephrine, isoproterenol can be injected or inhaled (inhalers are available by prescription only) for acute asthma symptoms. Given the availability of the more selective β agonists discussed above, there is little reason to use isoproterenol routinely as a bronchodilator.

Ephedrine

Ephedrine (see Chapter 14) has been used for years as a bronchodilator to treat asthma and some other pulmonary disorders. Ephedrine has one advantage over epinephrine and isoproterenol: it is orally effective. That means it is better suited for long-term outpatient therapy. Nevertheless, ever since newer drugs (even theophylline) have been approved, the use of ephedrine has fallen sharply. There are good reasons for this.

- Ephedrine is a weak bronchodilator, at best.
- Tolerance develops rapidly with continued administration—probably much faster than with other oral sympathomimetics. Thus, higher doses that increase the risk of side effects may be needed to overcome tolerance.
- Therapeutic doses often cause significant CNS stimulation; higher doses needed to overcome tolerance usually do so.
  Ephedrine, like epinephrine, stimulates *all* adrenergic receptors. Thus, it can cause all the unwanted cardiac and metabolic effects noted for epinephrine.
- Ephedrine participates in more drug-drug interactions than other sympathomimetics. Many interactants are very common drugs, and the outcomes of some interactions can be serious.

II. Corticosteroids

Glucocorticosteroids (corticosteroids, or steroids, for short) are very important drugs in asthma therapy. This section focuses on how these drugs are used in the overall treatment plan for asthma. In general, corticosteroids are used much less, and are less effective, for treating COPD. Refer to Chapter 45 for general information about corticosteroids.

Background

Before the late 1980s, corticosteroids were used mainly for acute and severe symptoms (eg, status asthmaticus), or for chronic symptoms that could not be controlled with full doses of theophylline or sympathomimetics, or both. The use of corticosteroids was limited because of fears of systemic side effects and a belief that treating bronchoconstriction was the best therapeutic approach.

Corticosteroids are used now much more often, and they are prescribed much earlier in the treatment plan, because physicians have learned how to prescribe steroids in a better way, and to monitor for unwanted effects. Also, there are newer inhaled corticosteroids that pose a lower risk of systemic side effects than the older oral drugs. Finally, we now realize that inflammation of the airways is a key component in the pathophysiology of asthma, and that suppressing inflammation is a major way to achieve asthma relief.

Actions of Corticosteroids in Asthma

Corticosteroids reduce inflammation and edema in the respiratory tract. They also stabilize mast cells, thereby reducing the release of mediators that cause inflammation and edema. In acute bronchoconstriction accompanied by hypoxemia, steroids also restore the bronchodilator response to sympathomimetics. Corticosteroids are not bronchodilators.

Use and Therapeutic Options

How and when to start steroid therapy, and the drugs to use, depend on symptom onset and severity. It is important not only to start therapy correctly, but also to stop it as quickly and safely as possible. There are three administration routes to choose from: parenteral or oral (systemic); and inhaled (local).

Systemic Administration

Parenteral steroids (eg, hydrocortisone) generally are given to patients with severe and acute bronchoconstriction to overcome a poor response to sympathomimetics. Long-term effects are maintained, if needed, by switching to oral therapy (eg, prednisone). Oral therapy can be started directly in some patients, without using injectable steroids first.

Systemic therapy usually is effective, but it may cause side or adverse effects during administration and after discontinuation. The severity and duration of these problems depend on the dose, the duration of use, and the actual steroid drug that is given.

Problems During Systemic Therapy

During therapy, high circulating steroid levels cause renal sodium and water retention. This retention can lead to electrolyte imbalances (hypernatremia, hypokalemia), edema, weight gain, and hypertension. These effects can cause or worsen heart failure or hypertension, both of which are contraindications to systemic steroids. Other side effects include muscle weakness or wasting, redistribution of body fat, osteoporosis, and psychic changes. Systemic steroids also can cause or worsen peptic ulcer disease, which is another contraindication. In children, chronic systemic steroid administration can inhibit growth.

Problems on Stopping Systemic Therapy

Systemic steroid therapy suppresses the adrenal-pituitary axis. It inhibits the natural synthesis of cortisol—often called the "stress hormone"—and its release into the bloodstream. These effects can occur after only a couple of weeks of full-dose systemic steroid therapy; and they can be great and last many months after steroid therapy is stopped.

Because of significant, long-term inhibition of normal steroid production and release, abrupt discontinuation of corticosteroid drugs can cause a severe withdrawal syndrome owing to adrenal insufficiency. Acute withdrawal is associated with distressing physiologic and psychologic (emotional) changes. For up to a year after steroid discontinuation, patients can be greatly susceptible to the consequences of trauma or infection. The outcome can be fatal. These problems can be minimized by keeping systemic steroid therapy as short as possible; using the lowest possible doses; using alternate-day therapy; and by weaning the dose gradually over a period of several weeks.

Inhaled Steroids

If it weren't for the adverse effects caused by systemic steroids, they would be ideal antiasthma drugs. To maintain the effectiveness of these drugs for asthma, but to limit their common side effects and the risks of withdrawal, several orally inhaled corticosteroids were developed. These drugs exert their effects mainly in the lungs. Their chemical structures, and their administration route, do not cause blood levels that are anywhere near those associated with oral or parenteral therapy. They are sold in metered-dose dispensers for ease and consistency of self-administration.

The orally inhaled steroids are *beclomethasone dipropionate* (BECLOVENT; VANCERIL), which can be considered the prototype of the inhaled steroids; *dexamethasone phosphate* (DECADRON PHOSPHATE RESPIHALER); *flunisolide* (AEROBID); and *triamcinolone acetonide* (AZMACORT).

The inhaled steroids are used as adjuncts to bronchodilators. The expected treatment outcome is a reduced frequency and severity of asthma attacks, and decreased dosages of other drugs. Inhaled steroids are *not* effective treatments for ongoing attacks or for anaphylaxis, since their effects do not develop until several weeks of use.

The usual adult dose of an inhaled steroid is two puffs taken four times a day. Children between six and 12 years old should receive lower doses. However, some adult and pediatric patients require higher doses. Inhaled steroids should not be used for children five years old or younger. Table 38–C lists dosages for each of the inhaled steroids.

Some asthma patients who need steroids may be started directly on an inhaled product; this rarely causes problems, but it may take several weeks for obvious signs of symptom improvement. Many patients start with parenteral or oral steroids, then are switched to an inhaled one.

A serious and common error is to stop systemic steroids abruptly at the same time inhaled steroid therapy starts. Very little of an inhaled steroid dose reaches the bloodstream. Inhaled steroids will not, therefore, prevent the sudden decrease of blood steroid levels, and effects, that occur when systemic therapy is stopped. Thus, patients who will be switched from a systemic steroid to an inhaled preparation should be started on it one to two weeks before the lowest dose of the oral steroid is expected to be reached, and the dose of oral steroid should be reduced gradually during this time. Have the patient keep a small supply of oral steroids on hand for flare-ups of asthma symptoms, since the inhaled steroid won't be of much help initially.

Side Effects of Inhaled Steroids

Hoarseness is common. Inhaled steroids also may alter the normal flora in the oral cavity, leading to an overgrowth of fungi—especially *Candida albicans.* These fungi can be detected by throat culture in more than two-thirds of patients who use inhaled steroids. If this fungus is allowed to proliferate, it can cause an infection of the oropharynx known as thrush. White patches in the mouth are good indicators of fungal infestation. If left unchecked, the oral infection can progress to serious systemic fungal infections that can be very difficult to treat. Oral *Candida* infestations are nearly 100 percent preventable if the patient swishes his or her mouth with water, then expectorates, after each use of the steroid inhaler.

Although inhaled steroids are much less likely than systemic steroids to suppress the adrenal-pituitary axis, they have the potential to do so. The risk increases if high doses are used for a long time (months).

Steroid Nasal Sprays

Nasal sprays containing beclomethasone (BECONASE, VANCENASE), dexamethasone phosphate (DECADRON PHOSPHATE TURBINAIRE), flunisolide (NASALIDE), and triamcinolone (NASACORT) are used to manage seasonal or perennial rhinitis (hay fever) symptoms that do not respond to other treatments. Some also are indicated for management of nasal polyps. Therapy with these products should be limited to a few weeks, despite the fact that it may take two weeks for symptomatic relief to occur.

III. Mast Cell Stabilizer

Cromolyn Sodium

Cromolyn (INTAL), a drug that is inhaled or applied topically, has one major pharmacologic action: it "stabilizes" mast cells. The drug reduces release of the many mast cell chemicals that cause bronchoconstriction, edema, and inflammation. Cromolyn does not dilate the bronchi, and has no steroid-like antiinflammatory action. It causes minimal side effects and poses virtually no risk of serious chronic or acute toxicity owing to overdoses. Cromolyn has little use in managing COPD.

Cromolyn is indicated for the prophylaxis of asthma attacks. It often is used adjunctively with a bronchodilator, steroids, or both. Like inhaled steroids, cromolyn's effects may not develop fully until several weeks of daily use. The drug will not relieve an attack once it has begun, and so it should not be relied on for an immediate effect.

Cromolyn has been considered most effective for atopic asthma, mainly because it can prevent mediator release from mast cells that are acted on by allergens. However, it also appears to work for extrinsic asthma, and even for exercise-induced bronchoconstriction in persons (eg, joggers) who otherwise experience no typical asthma symptoms. Cromolyn works best in pediatric patients, but many adults respond well too. In general, the drug should be used 10 to 15 minutes before the patient is exposed to factors that are known to trigger an asthma attack.

There are three cromolyn formulations for asthma:

1. Capsules containing the powdered drug, which must be administered using a special device (SPINHALER) provided by the manufacturer;
2. MDIs; and
3. A solution for nebulizer administration by health-care professional.

Dosages are summarized in Table 38–C.

A positive response to cromolyn is similar to that of inhaled steroids: fewer and milder asthma attacks and a decreased need for (or dosages of) other antiasthma drugs. Sometimes, when cromolyn is fully effective, it is possible to discontinue other medications completely.

If the patient already is taking other asthma drugs, cromolyn should be added to the treatment plan. The other medications should be continued for several weeks, at their current dosages, until asthma symptoms appear better controlled. If symptom control appears to have been achieved, then doses of other drugs can start to be reduced gradually and cautiously with close monitoring. This gradual reduction of doses of other drugs is particularly important if the patient is taking systemic steroids.

Cromolyn does not cause serious side effects. It may cause wheezing, sneezing, or coughing. Occasionally, it can cause bronchoconstriction. Rare reactions to cromolyn include signs and symptoms of a drug allergy, such as urticaria, angioedema, or joint pain and swelling. Patients who experience what might be allergic reactions to cromolyn should not receive the drug again.

There are no known, clinically important, drug interactions involving cromolyn. The consequences of administering cromolyn during pregnancy are unknown.

NURSING IMPLICATIONS

Make sure patients understand that cromolyn will not stop an ongoing asthma attack. They should carry an inhaled sympathomimetic with them to use if an attack occurs.

Other Cromolyn Formulations and Uses

Cromolyn nasal drops, marked as NASALCROM, are indicated for prophylaxis or treatment of allergic rhinitis symptoms. Use of this formulation may cause an unpleasant taste, or a burning sensation in the nose. A topical ophthalmic solution of cromolyn (OPTICROM) is used to alleviate ocular allergy symptoms, such as watery or irritated eyes. The ocular formulation occasionally causes eye discomfort or irritation. See Table 38–C for dosages.

Related Drug

Nedocromil Sodium

Nedocromil sodium (TILADE) should be available soon. It is a "second-generation" antiasthma drug that probably will serve as just another drug to use instead of cromolyn.

IV. Other Respiratory Drugs with Special Uses or Actions

Drugs Affecting the Actions of Acetylcholine

Acetylcholine (ACh) is the parasympathetic nervous system's neurotransmitter. It is a powerful bronchoconstrictor, mast cell activator, and stimulant of mucus secretion, particularly in asthmatic persons.

Methacholine

Persons with asthma are so sensitive to bronchoconstriction caused by ACh and drugs that act like it that the inhaled parasympathomimetic drug methacholine (PROVOCHOLINE) is used, along with pulmonary function tests, to help confirm an otherwise uncertain diagnosis of asthma. Very low doses of methacholine will reduce various measures of ventilatory function in persons with asthma. The same low doses have little or no effect on persons without the disease. (Because of the obvious risks of administering methacholine to a person with asthma, methacholine should never be given when the diagnosis of asthma is known.)

Antimuscarinic Drugs

The effects of ACh and other parasympathomimetic drugs are mediated by muscarinic receptors, so it would appear that atropine (the prototype antimuscarinic drug; Chapter 13), or another drug that blocks the ability of ACh to stimulate muscarinic receptors, would be useful for treating asthma. In practice, the benefits or possible risks of these drugs depend on the drug itself, and on how it is administered.

Systemic Antimuscarinics

Systemically administered antimuscarinics (or any drug with atropine-like activity) usually are contraindicated in asthmatic patients. Reasons for this include the risks of systemic side effects and the worsening of other common medical conditions, and mucus thickening and plugging in the airways. See the section on Drugs to Be Avoided, below, for more information.

Inhaled ("Topical") Antimuscarinics

Although orally or parenterally administered anticholinergics could do more harm than good for persons with asthma, inhaled formulations have some use for persons with pulmonary disease. Inhaled antimuscarinics tend to act locally in the respiratory passages. The main effect is bronchodilation. For reasons that are not fully known, inhaled antimuscarinics appear to be less effective than inhaled β agonists for persons with asthma. In contrast, they appear to be more effective for patients with emphysema and chronic bronchitis.

Ipratropium

Ipratropium (ATROVENT), an inhaled antimuscarinic bronchodilator that is indicated for adjunctive maintenance therapy of chronic bronchitis or emphysema, will not cause prompt bronchodilation. It is not approved for asthma. The drug is supplied in an MDI. The dosage is shown in Table 38–C.

Atropine

Inhaled atropine, given by nebulizer, is used for *status asthmaticus* because of its desired bronchodilating activity. However, it can cause other unwanted pulmonary effects, including mucus plugging. Therefore, inhaled atropine should be used as an adjunct to other drug and nondrug treatments, including mucolytics, oxygen and airway suctioning, and postural drainage.

NURSING IMPLICATIONS

Inhaled antimuscarinics tend to cause fewer side effects on body structures outside the airways. Nevertheless, such extrapulmonary effects can occur, and for patients with other medical conditions that may be worsened by an antimuscarinic drug, the unwanted effects can be serious. Thus, contraindications noted for systemic atropine (see Table 13–S) apply.

Other Therapies

Other pharmacologic and nondrug interventions play important roles in the management of patients with asthma, COPD, or other common respiratory disorders. What follows is an overview. Typical dosages for most of these agents are listed in Table 38–C.

Mucolytic Drugs

Mucolytic drugs reduce the viscosity (thickness or stickiness) of mucus. Reducing mucus viscosity helps remove secretions and reduces inspissation. The main mucolytic drug is acetylcysteine (MUCOMYST). It is used for some patients with asthma or other acute or chronic lung disorders (eg, emphysema, bronchitis, pneumonia, cystic fibrosis, or postoperative respiratory complications). It is inhaled, and is an adjunct to other respiratory drugs. Nebulized acetylcysteine has a foul odor, similar to rotten eggs.

Acetylcysteine is also an oral antidote for poisoning with acetaminophen (eg, TYLENOL). This special use is discussed in Chapter 52.

Expectorants

Expectorants such as *guaifenesin* (formerly called glyceryl guaiacolate) sometimes are prescribed to decrease mucus viscosity and help convert a nonproductive cough into a productive one. Guaifenesin is found in many prescription and OTC medications. Other expectorants include *potassium iodide* (use cautiously in patients with thyroid disease); *ammonium chloride* (also acidifies the urine, may enhance the excretion of drugs such as aspirin); and low doses of *ipecac* (the prototype emetic drug; see Chapter 42).

The true effectiveness of expectorants in asthma therapy is controversial. Expectorants will not cause bronchodilation or suppress inflammation.

Antibiotics

Pulmonary disease caused or accompanied by infection should be treated with the appropriate antibiotics, plus adjunctive drugs that cause faster symptomatic relief. See Chapter 56 for specific information about the antibiotics.

Desensitizing Injections

When allergy-related asthma triggers can be identified (eg, pollen, dust), desensitizing injections can be given by repeatedly administering small, then gradually increasing doses, of the allergen(s); these injections usually are given intradermally. This treatment is expensive, time-consuming, and not always completely effective. Therapy with bronchodilators, steroids, and cromolyn may be needed until desensitization develops.

Sedatives

Sedatives occasionally are prescribed for some patients, mainly to counteract CNS stimulation caused by drugs such as theophylline or ephedrine, or to reduce emotional stress that may trigger asthmatic attacks. Sedatives may be effective in some cases, but there is much controversy over whether they are suitable, safe, or necessary. Barbiturates, in particular, stimulate theophylline metabolism and could cause drug interactions. Sedatives should never be used instead of a bronchodilator, steroid, or cromolyn when those drugs would be indicated.

Nondrug Adjuncts

Many nondrug measures are important adjuncts to drug therapy of asthma or COPD. These measures include maintaining an adequate but safe degree of hydration to reduce mucus viscosity and the risk of physical airway narrowing or plugging; suctioning; postural drainage; and chest percussion.

Drugs to Be Avoided

Several drugs or drug classes can worsen signs and symptoms of pulmonary disorders such as asthma. Avoiding them or reducing their use (or dosage) increases the potential success of antiasthma therapy, and may reduce the number or dosages of antiasthma drugs needed for symptom control. It is important to know what these drugs are and how they may cause problems. They are listed in Table 38–2 and discussed briefly here.

Cholinergic Drugs

The ability of methacholine to cause unusually intense bronchoconstriction in persons with asthma was noted earlier. Other cholinergic drugs (eg, bethanechol, URECHOLINE; used for bladder dysfunction), including the acetylcholinesterase inhibitors (eg, neostigmine; PROSTIGMIN; a major drug for myasthenia gravis), can cause the same serious effects. Therefore, they are contraindicated in asthma or COPD. This warning applies to topical cholinergic drugs and cholinesterase inhibitors that are used for managing glaucoma: fatal bronchoconstriction can occur.

Systemic Antimuscarinic (Anticholinergic) Drugs

In contrast to the desirable effects of inhaled antimuscarinics, systemic administration of antimuscarinics poses some potentially great problems. Usual doses cause significant extrapulmonary side effects. As noted in more detail in Chapter 13 (and Table 13-S), dry mouth, blurred vision, and other disturbing side effects are common. These drugs also can cause great harm to persons with narrow-angle glaucoma, prostatic hypertrophy, and other contraindicating conditions.

More importantly for asthma patients, systemic antimuscarinics dry the often profuse airway mucus secretions. This can cause mucus plugging of the airways

Table 38–2 Major Drugs Asthmatic Patients Should Avoid or Use Cautiously

Drug	Possible Adverse Effect
Alpha-adrenergic agonists: phenylephrine, others	May cause bronchoconstriction
Antimuscarinics, drugs with antimuscarinic activity: atropine (unless given by inhalation); antidepressants; antihistamines (H_1 blockers); antiparkinson drugs with central anticholinergic activity (benztropine, trihexyphenidyl); antipsychotics; belladonna alkaloids; scopolamine	Dry mucus, may cause inspissation
Beta-adrenergic blockers: propranolol and others	Reduced effectiveness of antiasthma drugs, possible serious or fatal bronchoconstriction; avoid; applies to both systemic and topical (ophthalmic) β blockers
Cholinergic agonists: acetylcholinesterase inhibitors parasympathomimetic drugs	Are potent bronchoconstrictors in asthmatic patients
Histamine releasers: tubocurarine and most related nondepolarizing neuromuscular blockers morphine dextran	Cause bronchoconstriction
Nonsteroidal antiinflammatory drugs: all "rapidly-acting" agents, including aspirin and ibuprofen at doses found in OTC products	Cause bronchoconstriction by inhibiting prostaglandin synthesis

(inspissation), leading to partial or sometimes complete (and potentially fatal) airway blockage.

Atropine itself seldom is used on an outpatient basis, but there are many more oral drugs and drug classes that can cause atropine-like actions or side effects. They include scopolamine (a widely used drug for motion sickness); most antipsychotics (Chapter 23); most *antidepressants* (Chapter 24); and most *antihistamines* (see below).

See Table 38–S for a longer listing of other drugs that cause significant atropine-like effects and should be avoided if possible.

Antihistamines

Antihistamines (H_1 blockers) such as diphenhydramine (BENADRYL; Chapter 51) might appear to be logical treatments for asthma because of histamine's action as a powerful bronchodilator that is released from mast cells. However, mast cells release many more mediators besides histamine, and antihistamines have *no* ability to block the adverse responses mediated by those other substances. More important, most antihistamines cause significant antimuscarinic side effects, and favor mucus plugging. Thus, systemic use of these drugs usually is contraindicated.

Beta-Adrenergic Blockers

Beta blockers, which have many clinical uses (see Chapter 15), can cause severe bronchoconstriction in patients with asthma. Systemically administered nonselective (β_1 and β_2) β blockers (eg, propranolol, nadolol) pose the greatest risk. The β blockers that are called "cardioselective" (β_1-selective; eg, atenolol, metoprolol), and those with intrinsic sympathomimetic activity (eg, pindolol), may be somewhat safer for asthma patients. However, they are not completely without risk, especially when high doses must be used. Even β blockers that are administered topically on the eye, as used for treating glaucoma, have caused *fatal* bronchoconstriction in asthmatics.

All β blockers, regardless of how they are classified or used, must be used with extreme caution, and only when potential benefits outweigh their potentially greater risks, if the patient has asthma or COPD.

Histamine-Releasing Drugs

Drugs that cause histamine release from mast cells can cause serious adverse effects also. Common examples are morphine, curare and some related neuromuscular blockers, and dextran (a parenteral plasma expander). When possible, avoid these drugs or use alternatives.

Nonsteroidal Antiinflammatory Drugs

Inflammation is clearly an important contributor to asthma, and nonsteroidal antiinflammatory drugs (NSAIDs)—aspirin and related NSAIDs, including indomethacin and ibuprofen—clearly suppress inflammation. However, they also inhibit the synthesis of a prostaglandin (PGE_2) that is a physiologically important bronchodilator and mast cell stabilizer. When its synthesis is inhibited, bronchoconstriction can occur. In addition, aspirin, and some other NSAIDs simultaneously unmask the bronchoconstrictor and mast cell–activating effects of another prostaglandin ($PGF_{2\alpha}$). Severe or fatal bronchoconstriction has been reported in asthma patients who have taken only one or two aspirin tablets. Asthmatics with nasal polyps appear to be at greater risk than those without polyps.

A history of wheezing or hives in an asthma patient who has received aspirin or a related NSAI drug may contraindicate future use of any NSAID. If NSAIDs are essential for treating inflammatory states (eg, arthritis), careful patient monitoring and adequate "coverage" with proper antiasthma drugs are necessary.

There is some evidence that gradually desensitizing asthma patients with aspirin offers some eventual reduction of asthmatic responses to the drug. However, patients who might benefit from such treatment must be identified carefully; the treatment itself should be given only by physicians who are experienced in this area and who can provide immediate emergency care when it is needed.

Table 38–3 Diseases That Might Increase a Patient's Risk of Adverse Responses to Antiasthmatic Drugs

Disease	Drugs*
Hypertension or ischemic heart disease; coronary or cerebral vascular disease; aneurysm; hyperthyroidism	Sympathomimetics; methylxanthines; systemic corticosteroids
Cardiac arrhythmias (especially tachyarrhythmias); angina	Any inhaled preparation using halogenated hydrocarbons as a propellant; sympathomimetics; methylxanthines; atropine, ipratropium
Narrow-angle glaucoma; prostatic hypertrophy; paralytic ileus or obstructive bowel disease	Atropine, ipratropium; ephedrine Sympathomimetics; methylxanthines; atropine, ipratropium
Hepatic failure, hyperuricemia, gout	Methylxanthines
Diabetes mellitus	Sympathomimetics; systemic corticosteroids
Peptic ulcer disease	Systemic corticosteroids; methylxanthines
Seizure disorders	Methylxanthines

*In some cases the drugs noted are absolutely contraindicated. In others, appropriate therapeutic modifications may be needed to increase the safety of administering the drugs.

NURSING IMPLICATIONS

Give asthma patients a written list of drugs to avoid, especially those available OTC. Make special note of aspirin and ibuprofen (ADVIL, NUPRIN, etc); and nonprescription cough, cold, or allergy remedies that contain antihistamines, scopolamine, or belladonna alkaloids—all are anticholinergics. Recommend acetaminophen for minor pain or fever; it is much less likely to cause bronchoconstriction than aspirin.

Disorders That Can Be Worsened by Drugs Used for Asthma or COPD

In children and younger adults, asthma may be the only medical problem for the patient. However, in older adults, and especially in the elderly, other diseases may be present also. Long-term, heavy smokers also represent a special category, since pulmonary and various cardiovascular disorders (eg, hypertension, heart failure) may go hand-in-hand.

Just as some drugs used to treat those disorders may cause unwanted pulmonary side effects, so can pulmonary drugs aggravate other conditions. Thus, assessment must address the potential unwanted consequences of pulmonary drugs on other body systems. Table 38–3 summarizes problems that may be caused, the drugs that may be responsible, and explanations of why these unwanted effects may occur.

SUMMARY OF NURSING IMPLICATIONS

◆ Assessment

Determine the patient's ability to move air (absence or presence of wheezing, dyspnea) and the amount of distress experienced (eg, diaphoresis, use of accessory muscles, presence of orthopnea).

Assess characteristics of cough (moist, harsh, etc) and sputum (color, amount, viscosity).

Establish baseline vital signs, pulmonary function, hydration status, activity tolerance, and, for very ill patients, blood gases.

Obtain a complete nursing history to include contraindications to drug therapy, potential drug interactions, and smoking habits.

◆ Nursing Diagnoses

Knowledge deficit related to drug therapy: dose, administration techniques.

Pain related to gastric irritation from methylxanthines.

Decreased cardiac output related to tachycardia or arrhythmias.

Sensory/perceptual alterations related to CNS effects (nervousness, tremors, delirium, hyperactivity).

Sleep pattern disturbance related to insomnia, restlessness.

Ineffective breathing pattern related to bronchospasm from inadequate drug therapy, contraindicated or interacting drugs.

Anxiety related to difficulty breathing.

Ineffective airway clearance related to tenacious secretions and bronchospasm.

High risk for fluid volume deficit related to diuresis from methylxanthines.

◆ Planning/Implementation

Administer theophylline and related drugs as ordered to promote optimum absorption: on an empty stomach with a full glass of water; with or after meals only if gastric distress occurs.

Give methylxanthines three hours before sympathomimetics, to avoid interactions.

Monitor theophylline levels frequently while stabilizing patient.

Do not exceed aminophylline infusion rates of 25 mg/min.

Monitor pulse and blood pressure before, during, and after all drug treatments in hospitalized patients.

Observe for signs of drug toxicity: methylxanthines and sympathomimetics—irregular heart beat, signs of CNS stimulation; steroids—weight gain, hypertension, and altered psyche.

Use therapeutic nursing measures to relieve anxiety, decrease oxygen demands, and increase respiratory efficiency: reassurance, positioning, quiet environment, breathing techniques.

Maintain minimum daily fluid intake (eight glasses of water) as permitted by patient's condition.

Encourage smokers to quit, and support smokers in their effort to stop.

◆ Patient and Family Teaching

Teach the patient/family:

The proper use of hand-held nebulizers and metered-dose drug delivery systems, and the proper sequence of administration of inhaled drugs. Reinforce the importance of oral hygiene following treatment, especially with inhaled steroids.

To avoid self-medicating with nonprescription drugs for colds, coughs, and allergies, provide a list of drugs to avoid.

If taking systemic corticosteroids, to continue drug unless gradually withdrawn by physician, and to follow weaning process as directed. Teach patients key signs of adrenal insufficiency, triggers of insufficiency, and the need to carry a medication alert.

Effective deep breathing and coughing techniques.

About signs, symptoms, and changes that should be reported: increasing shortness of breath, fever, purulent sputum, etc.

◆ Evaluation

The patient/family will:

Obtain relief from bronchospasm: no wheezing or dyspnea.

Experience minimal adverse drug effects: gastric distress minimized; able to sleep at night; regular heart rhythm.

Quit smoking.

Maintain theophylline levels within therapeutic range (10–20 μg/mL).

Wear medical alert tag or carry card.

Return for follow-up assessment.

Be able to complete self-care responsibilities; tolerate activity.

Annotated Bibliography

Anderson B: An overview of drug therapy for chronic adult asthma. *Nurse Pract* 1991;16(12):39–47. *Reviews all contemporary asthma drugs and presents a stepped-care approach with excellent orientation to nursing.*

Chapman KR: The role of anticholinergic bronchodilators in adult asthma and chronic obstructive pulmonary disease. *Lung* 1990; 168 Suppl: 295–303. *Explains why drugs such as ipratropium seem to work better for COPD than for asthma, and what should you look for when your patient is taking this drug.*

DiMarco AF: Asthma in the pregnant patient: A review. *Ann Allergy* 1989;62(6):527–533. *Topics include physiologic respiratory alterations during pregnancy, maternal-fetal gas exchange, and safe use of virtually all the antiasthma drug classes available today.*

George RB, Owens MW: Bronchial asthma. Dis Mon 1991;37(3): 137–196. *A good article to consult for comprehensive information.*

Hannaway PJ: *The Asthma Self-help Book. A Comprehensive Guide to Management of Asthma in Children and Adults.* Lighthouse Press, 1989. *An award-winning book for nurses, adult patients, and parents of pediatric patients.*

Hendeles L, Weinberger M, Szefler S, Ellis E: Safety and efficacy of theophylline in children with asthma. *J Pediatr* 1992;120(2 Pt 1):177–183. *A well-written, contemporary review that is essential reading for nurses whose asthma patients are children taking any methylxanthine.*

Hofford JM: Metered dose inhaler therapy for asthma, bronchitis, and emphysema. *J Fam Pract* 1992;34(4):485–492. *Learn how physicians' inconsistent and suboptimal prescribing habits for inhalers may explain why some useful drugs don't work as well as they should, and why inadequate instruction of the patient may be a limitation, too.*

Kelly, HW, Lindley C: Asthma products. In: *Handbook of Nonprescription Drugs.* Ninth ed. American Pharmaceutical Association, 207–224. *Essential reading if your patient is, or asks about, taking OTC asthma medications; covers pathophysiology, assessment, OTC medication ingredients, and their use.*

Kelly HW, Murphy S: Corticosteroids for acute, severe asthma. *DICP* 1991;25(1):72–79. *Essential, practical information if your asthma patient is taking any corticosteroid, no matter the route or the expected duration of use.*

Kerrebijn KF: Long-term drug treatment of asthma in children. *Lung* 1990;168 Suppl: 142–153. *Includes valuable information on treatment plans for maintenance therapy.*

Levin RH: Advances in pediatric drug therapy of asthma. *Nurs Clin North Am* 1991;26(2):263–272. *A practical guide to the stepwise use of bronchodilators, steroids, and cromolyn in children with asthma and* status asthmaticus.

Lindell KO, Mazzocco MC: Breaking bronchospasm's grip with MDIs. *Am J Nurs* 1990;90(3):34–39. *Clearly shows proper use of "typical" metered-dose inhalers, gives good general patient teaching information.*

Lipworth BJ: Risks versus benefits of inhaled beta 2-agonists in the management of asthma. *Drug Safety* 1992;7(1):54–70. *As you read about newer and unapproved β agonists, you will appreciate the limitations of the drugs your patients are taking now, and learn about how to use them better.*

Nathan RA: Beta 2 agonist therapy: Oral versus inhaled delivery. *J Asthma* 1992;29(1):49–54. *Discusses the pros and cons of oral and inhaled sympathomimetic treatment, supports the better use of inhaled drugs, and emphasizes how to optimize their effectiveness.*

O'Connell EJ, Rojas AR, Sachs MI: Cough-type asthma: A review. *Ann Allergy* 1991;66(4):278–282, 285. *Learn more about a common but often undiagnosed (and untreated) type of asthma, in children or adults, for which cough is the major sign.*

Plaut T: *Children with Asthma: A Manual for Parents.* Second ed. Pedipress, Amherst, MA, 1989. *Practical and accurate information, at an easily understood level, for parents of children with asthma. Must reading for parents and nurses alike.*

Poe RH, Utell MJ: Theophylline in asthma and COPD: Changing perspectives and controversies. *Geriatrics* 1991;46(4):55–56, 61–65. *Discusses when and why inhaled β agonists might be preferred to theophylline, and tells when and why theophylline might be given to the elderly patient.*

Rachelefsky GS: The inflammatory response in asthma. *Am Fam Physician* 1992;45(1):153–160. *A contemporary perspective that focuses on the primary importance of corticosteroids.*

Reisman JJ, Canny GJ, Levison H: Management of asthma in early life. *Pediatrician* 1991;18(4):280–286. *Describes the challenges of treating asthma, and ways to accomplish successful treatment of it in infants and preschoolers.*

Rumbak MJ: New concepts in treatment of chronic persistent asthma. Using a stepwise protocol to control inflammation. *Postgrad Med* 1991;90(3):81–84, 89–90. *Discusses not only treatment of asthma, but also the need for patients to learn what asthma is, what its symptoms are, and how they can help in the treatment plan.*

Salinger L, Low MB: Asthma in pregnancy. *NAACOGS Clin Issu Perinat Womens Health Nurs* 1990;1(2):165–176. *Addresses "the interplay between asthma and pregnancy, as well as current treatment modalities." This information is vital for nurses caring for obstetric patients and their families.*

Silverman M: The role of anticholinergic antimuscarinic bronchodilator therapy in children. *Lung* 1990;168 Suppl: 304–309. *Focuses on the safe use of ipratropium and other medications for pediatric asthma and other pulmonary disorders.*

Skinner MH: Adverse reactions and interactions with theophylline. *Drug Saf* 1990;5(4):275–285. *Describes how to prevent, recognize, and manage theophylline toxicity.*

Sly PD, Le Souef PN: Inhaled therapy in paediatrics. *J Paediatr Child Health* 1991;27(1):7–10. *Focuses on the use of aerosolized drugs by pediatric asthma and cystic fibrosis patients, and gives practical insight into dosage schedules and adjustments.*

Spector SL: Asthma and chronic obstructive lung disease: A pharmacologic approach. *Dis Mon* 1991;37(1):1–58. *Discusses what's done now for asthma; identifies limitations and controversies of current therapies; and gives a glimpse of what to expect in terms of using old drugs for new uses in asthma and COPD treatment.*

Truwit JD: Toxic effects of drugs used in the ICU. Toxic effects of bronchodilators. *Crit Care Clin* 1991;7(3):639–657. *An excellent review of what to expect, and do, if any of the bronchodilators often used in the intensive care unit cause toxicity.*

Zahr LK, Connolly M, Page DR: Assessment and management of the child with asthma. *Pediatr Nurs* 1989;15(2):109–114. *Not "just another" article on pediatric asthma; this one takes a valuable holistic approach that addresses interventions beyond drugs.*

Table 38–C | Clinical Uses and Administration of Major Drugs for Asthma and Other Common Respiratory Disorders

AGENT	CLINICAL USES	DOSAGE AND ROUTE OF ADMINISTRATION	
	Methylxanthines		
PROTOTYPE			
Theophylline (many proprietary and generic products)	Treatment, prevention of reversible bronchoconstriction in asthma, chronic bronchitis, emphysema	Oral: Adults, children >16 years: Initially, the lesser of 16 mg/kg or 400 mg per day, in 3 or 4 divided doses. Maximum maintenance doses: Adults: the lesser of 13 mg/kg or 900 mg per day in 3 or 4 divided doses. Children aged 12–16 years: 18 mg/kg day; 9–12 years: 20 mg/kg/day; 6 months–9 years: 24 mg/kg/day. In addition to adjustments for age, doses should be reduced, or dose intervals prolonged, for older patients, patients with heart failure, cor pulmonale; doses often need to be increased for smokers. Timed-release products, total daily dose in 2 or 3 divided doses separated by 8 or 12 h Infants (<6 months old): Loading dose for all ages is 1 mg/kg for each 2 μg/mL increase of serum theophylline level; thereafter, maintenance doses are: 8 weeks–6 months: 1–3 mg/kg every 6 h; 4–8 weeks: 1–2 mg/kg every 8 h; term–4 weeks: 1–2 mg/kg every 12 h; preterm: 1 mg/kg every 12 h	
RELATED DRUGS			
Aminophylline (many proprietary and generic products)	Treatment of acute asthma attacks	Oral: Adults: 500 mg immediately, followed by 250–300 mg every 6–8 h. Children: 7.5 mg/kg immediately, followed by 5–6 mg/kg every 6–8 h IV: Dilute to ≤25 mg/mL; give all patients loading dose of 6 mg/kg at ≤25 mg/min. Maintenance infusion doses (reduce if patient already taking methylxanthines):	
		mg/kg/h	
		First 12 h	After 12 h
	Otherwise normal adults (non-smokers)	0.7	0.5
	Children 9–16 years, young adult smokers	1.0	0.8
	Older patients, patients with cor pulmonale	0.6	0.3
	Patients with heart failure, liver disease	0.5	0.1–0.2
	Children 6 months–9 years	1.2	1.0
	Prevention of bronchoconstriction in asthma, other forms of COPD	Oral: See above Rectal suppositories: Adults: 500 mg 1 or 2 ×/day. Children: 7 mg/kg every 6 h: daily dose should not exceed 1 g for any patient	
Other theophylline salts, dyphylline		Calculate daily theophylline dose, use equivalent dose of substitute as shown in Table 38–1	

(continued)

Table 38–C **Clinical Uses and Administration of Major Drugs for Asthma and Other Common Respiratory Disorders (*Continued*)**

AGENT	CLINICAL USES	DOSAGE AND ROUTE OF ADMINISTRATION
Sympathomimetics		
Albuterol sulfate (PROVENTIL, VENTOLIN) *Bitolterol mesylate* (TORNALATE) *Epinephrine* (many products) *Ethylnorepinephrine* (BRONKEPHRINE) *Isoetharine* (BRONKOMETER, BRONKOSOL) *Isoproterenol* (ISUPREL) *Metaproterenol* (ALUPENT, METAPREL) *Pirbuterol* (MAXAIR) *Terbutaline sulfate* (BRETHINE, BRICANYL, BRETHAIRE)		See Table 14–C1 for details concerning specific uses, routes of administration, and dosages
Corticosteroids		
Systemic Steroids		
See Chapter 45		
Orally Inhaled Steroids for Asthma		
Beclomethasone dipropionate (BECLOVENT, VANCERIL)	Adjunctive treatment of asthma in steroid-dependent patients	Oral inhaler: Adults, children >12 years: Usually 2 inhalations tid or qid; patients with severe asthma may require inhalations 6–8 ×/day. Children 6–12 years: 1–2 inhalations tid or qid, not to exceed 10 inhalations (total) daily
Dexamethasone sodium phosphate (DECADRON PHOSPHATE RESPIHALER)	See beclomethasone	Oral inhaler: Adults, children >12 years: Usually 3 inhalations tid or qid; do not exceed 12 inhalations/day or 3/dose. Children 6–12 years: 2 inhalations tid or qid, not to exceed 8/day or 2/dose
Flunisolide (AEROBID)	See beclomethasone	Oral inhaler: Adults, children >6 years: Initially, 2 inhalations bid (morning and evening); adults may increase as needed to 4 inhalations bid

(continued)

Table 38–C Clinical Uses and Administration of Major Drugs for Asthma and Other Common Respiratory Disorders (*Continued*)

AGENT	CLINICAL USES	DOSAGE AND ROUTE OF ADMINISTRATION
Triamcinolone acetonide		
(AZMACORT)	See beclomethasone	Oral inhaler: Adults: Usually 2 inhalations tid or qid, not to exceed 16 inhalations per day. Children 6 to 12 years: 1 or 2 inhalations tid or qid, not to exceed 12 inhalations per day
Nasally Inhaled Steroids for Seasonal, Perennial Allergies		
Beclomethasone dipropionate		
(BECONASE, VANCENASE)	Symptomatic relief of seasonal or perennial allergic rhinitis in patients who fail to respond well to other therapies (decongestants, antihistamines); *not* indicated for asthma Prevention of nasal polyps after surgical removal	Nasal inhaler: Adults or children >12 years: 1 inhalation into each nostril bid–qid. Children 6–12 years: 1 inhalation into each nostril tid
Dexamethasone sodium phosphate		
(DECADRON PHOSPHATE TURBINAIRE)	Rhinitis, nasal polyps, (see beclomethasone)	Nasal spray: Adults: 2 sprays per nostril bid–qid,; Children 6–12 years: 1–2 sprays per nostril bid; reduce or discontinue when symptoms improve/disappear
Flunisolide		
(NASALIDE)	Rhinitis: See beclomethasone	Nasal spray: Adults, children >14 years: Usually 2 sprays in each nostril bid, increased to tid as needed, but not to exceed 8 sprays per nostril per day. Children 6–14 years:1 spray per nostril tid or 2 sprays per nostril bid, not to exceed 4 sprays per nostril per day
Triamcinolone acetonide		
(NASACORT)	Rhinitis: See beclomethasone	Nasal spray: Adults, children >12 years: Initially 2 sprays per nostril qid
Mast Cell Stabilizer		
Cromolyn		
(INTAL)	Chronic management, prophylaxis of asthma	Oral inhaler or nebulizer: 20 mg (1 capsule or ampul) inhaled tid or qid
(NASALCROM)	Prevention, treatment of allergic rhinitis	Nasal spray: Adults, children ≥6 years: 1 spray in each nostril tid or qid
(OPTICROM)	Treatment of allergic ocular disorders	Topical: 1 or 2 drops of 4% solution in each eye 4–6 times daily at regular intervals

(continued)

Table 38–C Clinical Uses and Administration of Major Drugs for Asthma and Other Common Respiratory Disorders (*Continued*)

AGENT	CLINICAL USES	DOSAGE AND ROUTE OF ADMINISTRATION
	Antimuscarinic Bronchodilators	
Atropine	Short-term treatment or prevention of bronchospasm in asthma, COPD	Nebulizer inhalation: Adults: 25 μg/kg tid–qid up to 2.5 mg total. Children: 50 μg/kg 3–4 times daily
Ipratropium bromide (ATROVENT)	Maintenance treatment of bronchospasm in COPD	Oral inhaler: 2 inhalations qid
	Other Adjuncts	
Acetylcysteine (MUCOMYST)	Reduction of mucus viscosity in patients with acute or chronic bronchopulmonary disease (asthma, emphysema, bronchitis, pneumonia, cystic fibrosis, etc); usually adjunctive with bronchodilators	Inhalation with nebulizer: Usually 3–5 mL of 20% solution or 6–10 mL of 10% solution nebulized into face mask, mouthpiece, or tracheostomy tid or qid
Guaifenesin (ingredient in numerous prescription, OTC products)	Expectorant/mucolytic	Oral: Adults, children >12 years: Usually 100–400 mg every 4–6 h, not to exceed 2.4 g/day. Children 6–12 years: 100–200 mg every 4–6 h (1200 mg/day maximum); 2–6 years; 50–100 mg every 4 h (600 mg/day maximum)
Potassium iodide (found in several prescription and OTC medications)	See guaifenesin	Oral: Adults, children >12 years: Usually 500 mg every 4–6 h. Children 2–12 years: 175–350 mg every 4–6 h

Table 38–S **Major Side Effects of and Contraindications for Antiasthma Drugs**

BODY SYSTEM/ Side Effect	CONTRAINDICATION/ PRECAUTION	COMMENTS AND NURSING IMPLICATIONS
Methylxanthines		
CENTRAL NERVOUS SYSTEM Various signs of CNS stimulation (restlessness, anxiety, etc)	History of seizure disorders (cautious use)	May indicate imminent toxicity; tolerance may develop to CNS stimulation associated with therapeutic blood levels; do not take before bedtime (see text); seizures develop at toxic blood levels
RESPIRATORY Increased respiratory rate		Most likely with rapid IV injection of aminophylline; monitor respiratory status; respiratory arrest may occur
CARDIOVASCULAR Increased heart rate, force; palpitations, arrhythmias	History of cardiovascular disorders, hyperthyroidism	Monitor heart rate, BP; advise patient to report irregularities, chest pain, at once for further evaluation
GASTROINTESTINAL Nausea, vomiting, epigastric distress	Peptic ulcer disease	Take drug with milk or meals if GI distress is great; may produce gastroesophageal reflux if patient is recumbent or sleeping after medication is taken
Rectal irritation, bleeding	Hemorrhoids, anorectal	Occurs with aminophylline suppositories; use other route of administration
RENAL Increased urine output	Dehydration	Report unusual increases of urine output; monitor ill patients for signs of dehydration; urinary retention may occur in presence of prostatic hypertrophy
Sympathomimetics		
See Chapter 14		
Corticosteroids, Systemic		
See Chapter 45		
Corticosteroids, Inhaled		
OROPHARYNX Hoarseness; drying of mucous membranes; *Candida* infection (thrush)		Rinse mouth or gargle with warm water after use of inhaler; inspect mouth periodically for sores or eruptions that may indicate *Candida* infection
ENDOCRINE Adrenal suppression: psychologic changes, myalgia, arthralgia, malaise	Adrenal cortical tumors	Risk is low, but present, with inhaled steroids, especially if recommended doses are exceeded chronically, wean inhaled steroid, as for systemic steroids, if high doses are used for prolonged periods, monitor for potential withdrawal (eg, intolerance of stress)

(continued)

Table 38–S **Major Side Effects of and Contraindications for Antiasthma Drugs (*Continued*)**

BODY SYSTEM/ Side Effect	CONTRAINDICATION/ PRECAUTION	COMMENTS AND NURSING IMPLICATIONS
Corticosteroids, Inhaled		
RESPIRATORY Coughing, wheezing, bronchoconstriction		May need to discontinue if side effects are severe
CARDIOVASCULAR Sodium, water retention; hypokalemia; edema; hypertension	Poorly controlled heart failure or hypertension	Monitor body weight, skin turgor, lung sounds, and cardiovascular status in presence of history of cardiovascular disease; risk low with inhaled steroids unless recommended doses are chronically exceeded
Cromolyn, Orally Inhaled		
RESPIRATORY Cough, nasal congestion, bronchoconstriction		A warm water rinse or gargle after cromolyn use may reduce minor irritation of upper respiratory passages and mouth
Acetylcysteine		
RESPIRATORY Bronchospasm		May occur in asthmatic patients; discontinue acetylcysteine, administer inhaled adrenergic bronchodilator
OTHER Nausea, vomiting		Drug's offensive odor, plus large volume of loose mucus, may cause nausea, gagging, vomiting; have suction device handy; encourage patient to cough
Antimuscarinics, Inhaled (eg, Ipratropium)		
See Chapter 13		

Table 38–I Major Interactions Between Methylxanthines and Other Agents

AGENT	RESULT OF INTERACTION	COMMENTS AND NURSING IMPLICATIONS
Antithyroid drugs, oral	See thioamides, below	
Barbiturates (eg, phenobarbital; Chapter 22)	Increased theophylline metabolism, decreased blood levels and effects	Remeasure theophylline blood during start and discontinuation of interactant; monitor clinical responses to theophylline
Benzodiazepines (eg, diazepam; Chapter 22)	Decreased sedative effect of interactant	Monitor response to drug(s)
β-Adrenergic blockers (eg, propranolol; Chapter 15)	Decreased theophylline metabolism; increased blood levels, effects; risk of toxicity	These drugs pharmacologically antagonize each other's actions; avoid combination if possible; if β blocker treatment is essential, cardioselective β blockers usually preferred; monitor theophylline levels, clinical responses; do not reduce theophylline dose to overcome interaction: that can worsen symptom control
Cimetidine (Chapter 40)	Decreased theophylline metabolism; increased blood levels, effects; risk of toxicity	Combined use may require 20% to 40% reduction in theophylline dose (monitor blood levels); cimetidine alternatives (famotidine, nizatidine, ranitidine) less likely to interact, usually are preferred
Ciprofloxacin, other quinolone antibiotics (Chapter 56)	Decreased theophylline metabolism, increased blood levels, effects, toxicity risk	Monitor theophylline levels, clinical response; anticipate need to reduce theophylline dose
Contraceptives, oral (Chapter 49)	Decreased theophylline metabolism, increased blood levels, effects, risk of toxicity	Lower-than-usual daily theophylline doses may be required; monitor theophylline levels to guide dosage adjustment
Disulfiram (Chapter 22)	Decreased theophylline metabolism, increased blood levels, effects, risk of toxicity	Anticipate need for lower theophylline maintenance doses; monitor theophylline levels
Erythromycin, troleandomycin (Chapter 56)	Reduced antibiotic effects, reduced theophylline metabolism, increased blood levels, toxicity	Monitor theophylline levels and responses to both drugs; noninteracting antibiotics may be preferred
Food	Variable effects; see text	
Halothane (Chapter 20)	Serious risk of fatal cardiac arrhythmias	Must avoid combined use; make sure use of any theophylline is plainly noted as warning on charts of all patients scheduled for surgery or anesthesia
Mexiletine (Chapter 30)	Increased blood levels, toxicity risk of theophylline	Mechanism unknown; monitor theophylline levels closely
Phenytoin, other hydantoins (Chapter 26)	Increased theophylline blood levels, toxicity; increased metabolism; decreased blood levels and effects of phenytoin	Monitor levels of both drugs to guide dosage adjustments; assess clinical responses
Quinolone antibiotics	See ciprofloxacin, above	
Rifampin (Chapter 57)	Increased theophylline metabolism; decreased blood levels and effects	Monitor theophylline levels, clinical response; anticipate cautious increase of theophylline maintenance doses
Thiabendazole (Chapter 57)	Increased theophylline blood levels, toxicity	Mechanism unknown; anticipate need to reduce theophylline dose based on blood level measurements

(continued)

Table 38–I Major Interactions Between Methylxanthines and Other Agents (*Continued*)

AGENT	RESULT OF INTERACTION	COMMENTS AND NURSING IMPLICATIONS
Thioamides (eg, propylthiouracil; Chapter 47)	Reduced theophylline metabolism; increased blood levels, toxicity	Hyperthyroid patients metabolize theophyllines faster; controlling hyperthyroidism with thioamides reduces theophylline metabolism, may require reduced theophylline dose based on frequent blood level measurements
Thyroid hormones (Chapter 47)	Increased theophylline metabolism; decreased blood levels, effects	Hypothyroid patients metabolize theophyllines slower; normalizing thyroid hormone levels with supplements increases metabolism, may require increased theophylline dose based on frequent blood level measurements
Ticlodipine (Chapter 35)	Decreased theophylline metabolism; increased blood levels, toxicity risk	Mechanism unknown; anticipate need to reduce theophylline dose based on blood level measurements
Tubocurarine, pancuronium (Chapter 17)	Decreased neuromuscular blockade	Record theophylline use on preoperative or preanesthesia charts; use of higher-than-usual neuromuscular blocker doses generally needed

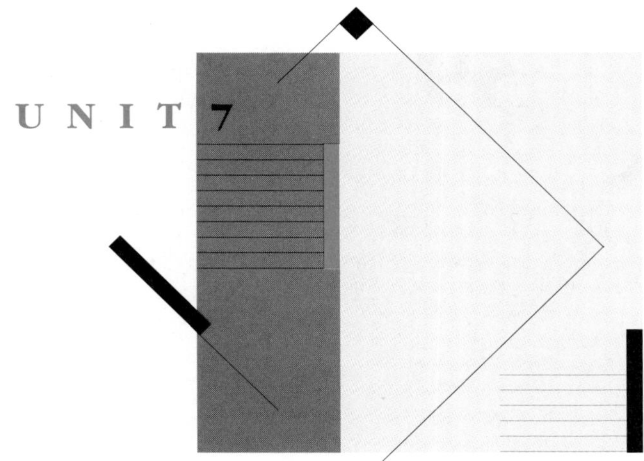

Drugs That Affect the Gastrointestinal Tract

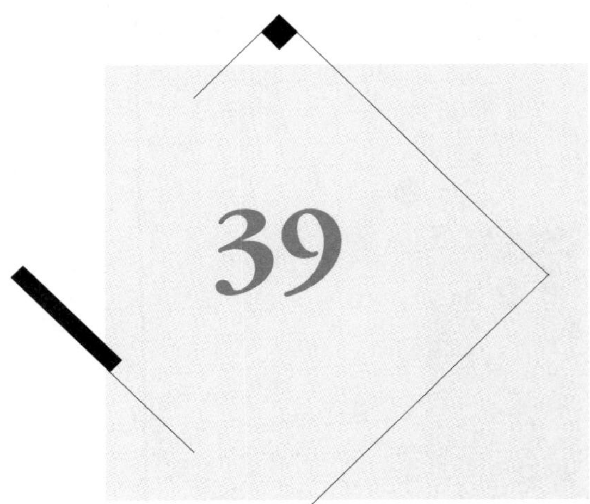

Structure and Function of the Gastrointestinal Tract

Disorders of the gastrointestinal (GI) tract are varied and common. Whether acute or longstanding, they account for some of the most common problems faced by health-care professionals. This chapter highlights general aspects of GI tract structure and the physiologic control mechanisms that enable the GI tract to carry out its intended functions.

General Features of the Gastrointestinal Tract

The GI tract is essentially a tube, starting at the mouth and ending at the anorectum, which conveys food as it undergoes digestion. In addition to the structures of the alimentary tube itself, the GI tract uses several accessory organs, including the salivary glands, gallbladder, liver, and pancreas, that are essential to digestion and elimination. The structure of the alimentary tube wall, with the exception of the oral cavity and a portion of the esophagus, is basically the same along its entire length. It is composed of four distinct tissue layers: the mucosa, the submucosa, the muscularis externa, and the serosa, or adventitia.

The major functions of the alimentary tube are

- movement of food;
- secretion of enzymes, ions, and other substances;
- absorption of food metabolites (from protein, fat, and carbohydrates) and vitamins, water, and salts; and
- excretion of wastes.

In terms of therapeutics, the GI tract's major role is absorption of orally administered drugs. Some drugs are also metabolized by or excreted via the gut. The two intrinsic properties of the GI tract, motility and secretory activity, are under neural and hormonal control, and are key targets of drug action.

Although some regions of the gut are structurally and functionally similar, each region is specialized to perform a more or less specific task. Many parts of the GI tract are sites of exocrine and endocrine gland activity. The primary functional roles of the major GI tract structures, plus those of some of the accessory organs, are summarized in Table 39–1.

The alimentary tube undergoes both tonic and rhythmic contractions of its circular and longitudinal smooth muscles. Tonic contractions, though changing

Table 39–1 General Functions and Activities of Major Gastrointestinal Tract Structures and Accessory Organs

Structure	Function	Exocrine Activity	Endocrine or Other Activity
Mouth and pharynx	Chew, mix food Initiate chewing reflex		
Salivary glands		Release salts, water, mucus to moisten food; release amylases to begin carbohydrate digestion	
Esophagus	Propels food toward stomach	Produces mucus to lubricate food	
Stomach	Temporarily stores, mixes food for digestion	Produces hydrochloric acid (HCl) to kill bacteria, disintegrate food; produces pepsinogen, activated to the proteolytic enzyme pepsin by HCl; produces mucus to lubricate food, protect gastric mucosa	Releases gastrin, which stimulates HCl secretion and gastric motility; stimulates ileum and mass movements in large intestine Releases histamine, which stimulates HCl secretion; probably mediates acid secretion caused by other stimuli (gastrin, parasympathetic stimulation); histamine acts as autacoid, not true hormone
Pancreas		Produces bicarbonate to neutralize HCl delivered from stomach, enzymes to digest proteins (eg, trypsin, chymotrypsin), fats (lipases), carbohydrates (amylases)	Releases insulin and glucagon
Liver	Initial site of drug metabolism before orally administered drug reaches systemic circulation; metabolizes other body wastes	Produces bile salts to help dissolve fats; produces bicarbonate	
Gallbladder	Stores, concentrates, releases bile and some drugs or their metabolites		
Small intestine	Continues, terminates most digestive processes; adjusts osmolality of chyme; secretes sodium, potassium, chloride, etc; absorbs water		Releases cholecystokinin, which stimulates gallbladder contraction, relaxes sphincter of Oddi, increases pancreatic enzyme and bicarbonate secretion; potentiates effects of secretin on bicarbonate production by liver Releases secretin, which inhibits gastric acid secretion and motility; stimulates pancreatic and hepatic bicarbonate production; potentiates effects of cholecystokinin on pancreatic enzyme secretion

(continued)

Table 39–1 General Functions and Activities of Major Gastrointestinal Tract Structures and Accessory Organs (*Continued*)

Structure	Function	Exocrine Activity	Endocrine or Other Activity
Large intestine	Stores undigested matter; concentrates wastes by absorption of salts, water; mixes and lubricates wastes with mucus; propels feces toward rectum		
Rectum	Initiates defecation reflex when distended by feces		

in intensity, are continuous. They regulate the amount of pressure in various segments of the GI tract and the tone of the various sphincters. In the stomach, for example, rhythmic contractions mix food with the acid and enzymes needed for digestion. In the small and large intestines, rhythmic segmental movements mix food and digestive juices, while peristaltic movements provide propulsive force to move chyme or feces toward the anus.

The intensity and frequency of contractions vary in the different parts of the GI tract, ranging from the almost continuous but relatively mild contractions that occur in the stomach when food is present to the strong contractions that occur only a few times a day in the large intestine.

Many substances are secreted in various parts of the GI tract. Cells lining the stomach wall secrete, among other chemicals, gastric acid (hydrochloric acid); pepsinogen, which is converted by acid to the protein-digesting enzyme pepsin; and mucus, which lubricates and protects the GI tract lining. In contrast, most of the substances added to the small intestine, such as bicarbonate, bile salts, and digestive enzymes, come from accessory organs such as the pancreas and liver. The continual destruction of mucosal cells in the intestines also adds essential cell-derived regulatory chemicals to the gut lumen.

The products released into the GI tract are essential not only for processes such as digestion but also for the absorption and metabolism of drugs that are taken orally. For example, although the liver is considered an accessory organ, substances absorbed from the GI tract enter the hepatic portal circulation, and are presented to the hepatocytes, before entering the systemic circulation. This process has a dramatic influence on the fate of orally administered drugs, many of which undergo extensive first-pass metabolism before reaching distant parts of the body.

Also important is the process of **enterohepatic recirculation**, by which drugs in the bloodstream are processed by the liver, concentrated in bile, secreted into the GI tract, and eventually reabsorbed. The cardiac glycoside digitoxin is a prime example of a drug that has a long half-life partly because of this process. Enterohepatic recirculation affects the fate of many orally administered drugs, as well as those given by other routes. These aspects of GI function were described in Chapter 4.

Control of Motility and Secretions

The central nervous system (CNS) is one of the systems controlling motility and secretion. The ability of sensory stimuli, such as the smell or sight of enjoyable—or offensive—food to trigger a variety of events (for example, salivation in anticipation of a good meal; retching, vomiting, and perhaps diarrhea from a meal that is not good) is but one example of this central, or *cephalic,* neural phase of GI regulation.

Autonomic Control

The major link between the brain and the gut is the autonomic nervous system. Both parasympathetic and sympathetic nerve fibers innervate the smooth muscle and glands of the gut, although there are regional anatomic differences. These two autonomic branches serve basically antagonistic roles in most parts of the GI tract. Of the two, the parasympathetic nervous system, through release of acetylcholine, exerts the major control, tending to stimulate secretions and motility. The sympathetic nervous system has a lesser role, inhibiting secretions and motility.

The roles of each autonomic branch can be modified by sympathomimetic and parasympathomimetic drugs, and in particular by their antagonists. The effects can be either unwanted or therapeutically useful. For example, blockade of parasympathomimetic influences by a drug such as atropine may cause unwanted constipation by inhibiting motility, or it may have clinically useful effects when the goal is to treat diarrhea or suppress gastric acid secretion.

Local Neural Control

The GI tract is endowed with its own nervous system network—the myenteric and submucosal nerve plexuses—that help control motility and secretion. These plexuses interact with one another, and are found the full length of the GI tract, starting with the esophagus. This arrangement allows changes in the motile or secretory activity of one part of the GI tract to affect other regions through reflexes, so that the entire alimentary tube, or specific parts of it, can coordinate activity as needed. Local nerve influences can be modified by input from the autonomic nervous system.

In general, only a few types of local stimuli affect the gut wall and trigger or modulate reflexes to regulate motility and secretions. They include mechanical factors such as distention of the gut wall by the presence of food, chyme, or feces; osmotic factors, such as caused by the ingestion of large amounts of salt; metabolic stimuli, arising largely from products of protein, fat, and carbohydrate digestion; and pH (local acidity or alkalinity). Most of these factors can be categorized as belonging to the *gastric* or *intestinal phases* of GI tract control.

Local Hormones

Local hormones—gastrin, cholecystokinin (CCK), and secretin—provide the major nonneural control and integration of gut motility and secretion. Like neural processes, they participate in feedback mechanisms that regulate motility and the composition of the lumen in various parts of the GI tract, particularly the stomach and small intestine. Since they reach their targets only after being delivered to them by the bloodstream, each hormone has the opportunity to affect more than one structure. Thus, a given aspect of motility or secretion in a particular part of the GI tract is controlled by more than one hormone.

Some local hormones exert opposing effects on a particular process. For example, gastrin stimulates gastric acid secretion, while secretin inhibits it. In other instances, hormones act synergistically, as exemplified by the effects of secretin and CCK on pancreatic bicarbonate secretion. Currently, there are no approved drugs that specifically mimic or antagonize the effects of any of these hormones.

Other substances, such as gastric inhibitory peptide (GIP) and vasoactive intestinal peptide (VIP), are produced locally and affect the GI tract (as well as other distant structures). However, not enough is known about them to call them true hormones. As with gastrin, CCK, and secretin, there are no therapeutic agents that specifically alter the activity of these mediators.

A list of mediators of secretion, particularly of gastric acid, cannot be complete without mention of histamine. This substance, which has important roles in the pathophysiology of allergy and inflammation, probably serves as the single most important physiologic stimulus for gastric acid secretion. It is an autacoid, released at or near its site of action on the parietal cells (see Chapter 51 for more information). Although histamine itself does not exert typical neural or hormonal control of secretion, it is clearly a part of the neural and hormonal control systems. For example, increased acid secretion, whether caused by parasympathetic stimulation, gastrin, or other stimuli, appears to be mediated ultimately by the effects of histamine on a specific subclass of histamine receptors, the H_2 receptors.

Common Gastrointestinal Tract Disorders

The etiology of many GI disorders is obscure. Their pharmacologic management is, in many cases, directed at controlling symptoms or preventing progression of the problems rather than eliminating the underlying and often unknown cause. Since the two major aspects of GI tract activity—secretion and motility—are intimately linked, most GI disorders involve alterations of both processes. The common GI disorders are ulcers, constipation, diarrhea, and vomiting.

Ulcers

Ulcers of the mucosa and underlying structures develop mainly when there is a failure of physiologic processes to maintain the normal acidic environment in the stomach, the normal alkaline environment in the duodenum, or the normal protective functions of mucus. In some cases the underlying cause is a mechanical failure in the small intestine to separate adequately the acidic gastric juice and the alkaline chyme. In other cases, excessive secretion of gastric acid, perhaps through deficits in the normal feedback control of that process, is the cause. Also, as discussed in Chapter 40, bacteria may cause ulcers or gastritis.

Drugs such as alcohol, aspirin and its related anti-inflammatory drugs, and corticosteroids alter the mucosal barrier and often cause ulcer development. Gastric tumors that cause excessive production of gastrin, or pancreatic tumors that release large amounts of gut mediators, are less common but nevertheless important causes. Pharmacologic approaches to treating ulcer disease include the use of antacids, to neutralize acid that is already secreted; histamine antagonists, to suppress acid production; and drugs that coat the ulcer crater, to facilitate healing. They are discussed in Chapter 40.

Constipation

A decrease in the motility of the large intestine, or failure to heed the defecation reflex stimulus, results in retention of fecal waste in the colon and rectum for prolonged periods of time. Physical damage to the intestine, excessive dilation of the intestinal wall, and gut infections may damage the nerve plexuses and cause serious and potentially permanent loss of spontaneous intestinal motility. The diminished gut motility that is characteristic of constipation also allows more time for some orally administered drugs to be absorbed, which could lead to increased and potentially adverse effects of those agents.

A variety of drugs classified as laxatives or cathartics (see Chapter 41) can affect either the feces, the smooth muscle in the gut wall, or the underlying nerve plexuses, to facilitate defecation and alleviate constipation. As noted in Chapter 41, excessive or prolonged use of laxatives or cathartics can damage the gut wall and its underlying nerve plexuses, and cause serious, permanent damage.

Diarrhea

When motility of the large bowel is enhanced abnormally, excessively hydrated fecal residue is excreted frequently and rapidly, leading to what is typically considered diarrhea. Common causes of diarrhea include drugs (especially antibiotics that alter normal gut flora), foods, and toxins that are byproducts of infectious organisms. Diarrhea typically is considered a disorder only of gut motility. However, other common causes—and consequences—of diarrhea include impaired absorption of water or fatty acids from the intestinal lumen into the bloodstream, and excessive secretion of fluid (as with cholera) or mucus (as in some inflammatory bowel diseases) into the lumen. Prolonged diarrhea leads to systemic dehydration and depletion of essential nutrients and electrolytes. Diarrhea also reduces the time during which orally administered drugs can be absorbed, resulting in decreased therapeutic effects.

Antidiarrheal drugs may act locally to **adsorb** noxious stimuli, or more directly on GI tract musculature or secretory cells. These medications also are discussed in Chapter 41.

Vomiting

Vomiting is a complex reflex involving a series of effects on smooth muscle in the upper alimentary tract, such as relaxation of the lower esophageal sphincter, and skeletal muscles of the abdomen and thorax. The reflex activates a variety of autonomic responses, including increased salivation and sweating. Although vomiting may be triggered by local irritation of the GI tract, more often it is caused by noxious stimuli (motion; unpleasant odors or sights; intense pain; intracranial pressure; drugs) affecting the vomiting center in the brainstem's medulla. Severe or prolonged vomiting can lead to severe acid–base and electrolyte imbalances.

In terms of therapy, vomiting usually is controlled with antiemetic drugs that act in the brain's vomiting center. When it is desirable to cause vomiting, as in the management of ingested poisons, emetic drugs can be administered. Like the antiemetics, most of these drugs also work in the brain. They are discussed in Chapter 42.

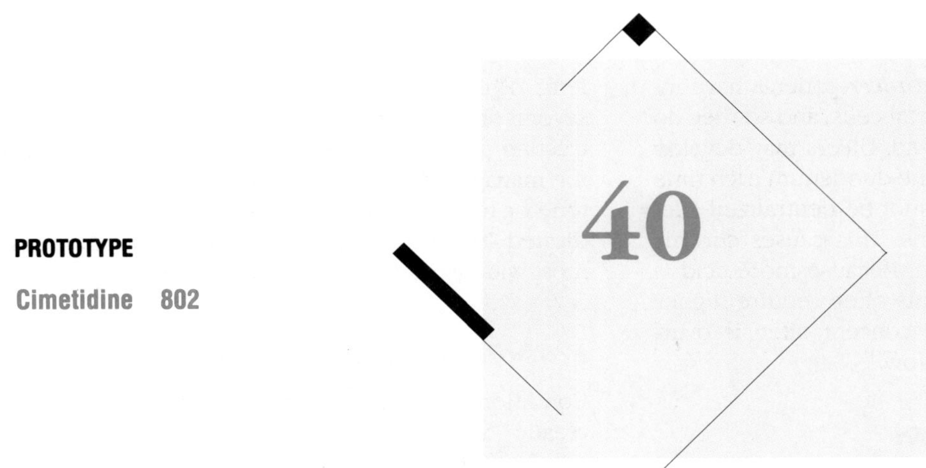

PROTOTYPE

Cimetidine 802

Pharmacologic Management of Peptic Ulcer Disease

Peptic ulcer disease (PUD) generally involves digestion and erosion of the gastric or duodenal mucosa through the combined actions of acid and proteolytic enzymes (pepsins). PUD affects three to four million persons each year. Over the lifetime, about 5% of the general population will develop PUD. The incidence rises to about 20% for some high-risk groups. These include patients with chronic respiratory, coronary, or renal disease; those suffering acute, severe trauma; or those taking ulcerogenic (ulcer-causing) drugs. Many patients die, either of PUD directly or of associated complications. The disease carries an annual estimated cost of more than $3 billion for medical care, drugs, and lost work. Millions of dollars more are wasted on improper self-medication with over-the-counter (OTC) drugs.

Benign Peptic Ulcer Disease

Benign PUD is that which is not caused by malignancies. It is the most common form of the disorder.

Major reference tables appear beginning on page 810.

The Roles of Acid and Pepsins

Hydrochloric acid (HCl) is secreted by the parietal cells in response to histamine, acetylcholine, and local hormones (eg, gastrin). Acid is the cause of ulcer pain, but acid per se is not terribly damaging to the gut wall. It is important because it activates the proteolytic activity of the pepsins. Normally, pepsins digest proteins such as those found in foods. However, when the protective mucus layer that lines the gut breaks down, or is not secreted in adequate amounts, the pepsins literally can digest the mucosal, muscular, and vascular tissues of the gut. Pepsins are most active in the normally acidic environment of the stomach, with a pH value of around two. When there is insufficient acid, proteolytic activity is inhibited.

Contrary to popular belief, not all ulcers are caused by excessive acid secretion. Most patients with benign *gastric ulcers* secrete normal amounts of acid. They may develop gastric ulcers because the pyloric sphincter that separates the stomach and duodenum is weak; this allows reflux of the alkaline duodenal contents, leading to chronic inflammation (gastritis) and, eventually, gastric ulcers. There is also a likely bacterial cause of gastric ulcers, which is mentioned below.

In contrast, most *duodenal ulcer* patients have increased numbers of active parietal cells, and so they do secrete excessive amounts of acid. Ulcers may develop because so much acid reaches the duodenum each time the stomach empties that it cannot be neutralized adequately by pancreatic secretions. This causes chronic duodenal irritation and erosion. Because more acid is secreted, duodenal ulcer patients often require higher doses of antiulcer drugs. This concept often is overlooked. It is discussed more below.

The Role of Gut Bacteria

Heliobacter pylori is an acid-stable bacterium (gram-negative rod) that releases toxins that can irritate the gastric mucosa. Several recent studies found *H. pylori* in the gut mucosa of nearly *all* patients with benign gastric or duodenal ulcers that were not caused by ulcerogenic drugs. *H. pylori* also may play an important role in the persistence of ulcers that do not respond well to pharmacotherapy, and in the pathophysiology of antral gastritis.

Drug-Induced Ulcers

A variety of drugs, listed near the end of this chapter, are ulcerogenic. Some, such as ethanol, probably are nonspecific mucosal irritants. Others may have a more discrete ulcerogenic action. Aspirin is one example. The drug appears to accumulate in the gut mucosal cells as it is being absorbed, and may reach local levels that cause cell damage. In addition, aspirin and all other nonsteroidal antiinflammatory drugs (NSAIDs; the drug class to which aspirin belongs) inhibit the synthesis of prostaglandins that normally protect the gut mucosa, perhaps by stimulating mucus formation. Corticosteroids may be ulcerogenic through the prostaglandin mechanism also. As noted later, avoidance of ulcerogenic drugs is a crucial part of ulcer therapy.

Other Ulcer Diseases or Related Gastrointestinal Conditions

Gastroesophageal Reflux Disease

All of us suffer reflux of the acidic gastric contents into the esophagus from time to time. However, when these episodes become too frequent, there is an increased risk of erosive damage to the esophageal tissues. The chronic disorder, gastroesophageal reflux disease (GERD), usually is caused by anatomic or functional (motility) problems of the lower esophageal sphincter. Antacids and several drugs that inhibit gastric acid secretion, used for treating gastric or duodenal ulcers, also are indicated for management of GERD. Other agents that alter the tone or motility of the gut musculature also may be indicated. These agents, of which metoclopramide is the most widely used, are discussed in Chapter 42.

Pathologic Acid-Hypersecretory States

Conditions such as Zollinger-Ellison syndrome, pancreatic tumors, systemic mastocytosis, or multiple tumors of the adrenal cortex are called *pathologic acid-hypersecretory states.* These somewhat uncommon conditions, which are not considered benign ulcer disease, are accompanied by the secretion of massive amounts of gastric acid. Ulcers may be large and numerous, and may be found in both the stomach and duodenum. Patients with pathologic acid-hypersecretory states require intensive antiulcer therapy, plus other treatments appropriate for the many systemic effects that arise from an endocrine tumor.

Acute Stress Ulcers

The term *acute stress ulcer* specifically refers to ulcers that develop quickly—in as little as a few days—in response to severe physical insults that initially do not involve the gut. These stressors include major burns, accidental or surgical trauma, renal or hepatic failure, serious respiratory disease, and sepsis.

Before the seriousness and frequency of stress ulcers were realized, morbidity and mortality in high-risk patients were very high. Patients who were treated "successfully" for their major presenting illness or condition died suddenly from gut hemorrhage, often failing to survive emergency attempts to intervene. The cause of stress ulcers may involve significantly reduced gut mucosal blood flow (ischemia), leading to cell damage that eventually exposes underlying structures to acid and pepsins. Acute stress ulcers may be rapidly fatal due to hemorrhage if the lesion affects a large blood vessel. If the ulcers perforate, peritonitis and sepsis can occur. The last section of this chapter summarizes some of the medication plans used to prevent acute stress ulcers.

Drug Therapy

Drug therapy for PUD and the other conditions mentioned above is usually effective, and it is always tried before subjecting the patient to the risks of the other main treatment alternative—surgery. Surgery, to denervate or remove part of the gut, usually is reserved for patients with ulcers that fail to respond to intensive drug therapy; ulcers that recur despite drug treatment; perforated or excessively bleeding ulcers; or intestinal obstruction.

Treatment Goals

Several classes of drugs are used, alone or in combination. Drugs are given to achieve three main therapeutic goals:

1. Relieve and then *totally* prevent pain. In terms of general ulcer and esophageal reflux therapy, relieving pain is the easiest goal to achieve. However, this is relief of a symptom, not a cure of the underlying disease.
2. Hasten the rate of ulcer healing.
3. Prevent recurrences and complications.

Concern over acute stress ulcers adds a fourth goal for critical care medicine:

4. Recognize at-risk patients and prevent acute stress ulcers from forming.

Therapeutically, these goals can be met by giving drugs that

- Neutralize acid that already has been secreted. This is how *antacids* work.
- Reduce further acid secretion. This is how drugs classified as *histamine H_2–receptor blockers* (eg, cimetidine), **antimuscarinic** drugs, and agents called "*proton pump inhibitors*" (eg, omeprazole) work. To some extent, *prostaglandins* work in this way also.
- Form a protective coating over the ulcer crater. This is how the drug *sucralfate* works. Prostaglandins cause a similar effect by stimulating mucus secretion.

The next three sections of the chapter discuss the three drug groups according to the mechanisms of action outlined above. These parts are followed by a brief discussion of newer drug therapies; an overview of nondrug aspects of treatment that can benefit all patients; and short comments on acute stress ulcers.

Acid-Neutralizing Drugs: Antacids

Antacids are simple chemicals that neutralize gastric acid that already has been secreted. There are four major drugs: aluminum hydroxide (or other Al salts); magnesium hydroxide (or other salts); calcium carbonate; and sodium bicarbonate. They share a few properties, but their differences are more important. No one agent can be considered a prototype. Most ulcers are treated with a commercially formulated combination of an aluminum antacid and a magnesium antacid.

Absorption, Distribution, Metabolism, and Excretion

Antacids are given orally. However, the traditional parameters of absorption, distribution, metabolism, and excretion that apply to most other orally administered drugs do not really apply to antacids. Antacids are given for their local effects in the gut. They are not supposed to be absorbed. As noted below, however, some antacids are absorbed, which usually leads to unwanted systemic effects.

Pharmacologic Effects and Therapeutic Uses Common to Antacids

Antacids work locally in the gut to neutralize gastric acid. The goal is to neutralize enough gastric acid to raise gastric pH to around 3.5 sufficient to reduce pepsin activity. Increasing pH much more is unnecessary, and can trigger an unwanted reflex increase of acid secretion called *acid rebound.* Acid is the substance that causes pain. By neutralizing only modest amounts of acid, antacids easily achieve the first therapeutic goal, relief and prevention of pain. This is the "*no acid, no pain*" concept. It assumes, of course, that the antacids are prescribed properly and taken as directed.

Antacids are used to treat active ulcers, to prevent ulcer recurrence or the development of new ones, and to manage gastroesophageal reflux disease. Antacids can be used as the only antiulcer medication, or they can be used as adjuncts to other classes of antiulcer drugs. They are often referred to as the cornerstones, or foundations, of ulcer therapy; because of their ability to stop pain quickly and effectively, antacids have an essential role in the treatment plan for most ulcer or esophageal reflux patients, even when other medications are or will be used.

The effective dose of an antacid drug or combination product depends on the amount of acid that needs to be neutralized (Table 40–C). That amount is based roughly on how much acid is secreted in a given time. The dose also depends on the *acid-neutralizing capacity* (ANC) of the antacid drug or product. The ANC is a way of expressing antacid potency. It is determined by the volume of liquid antacid, or number of antacid tab-

Table 40–1 Acid-Neutralizing Capacity and Sodium Content of Selected Liquid Antacids*

Product	Acid-Neutralizing Capacity (mEq/mL)	Approximate mL Needed to Neutralize 70 mEq HCl	mg Na per 5 mL	Active Ingredients
CAMALOX	18.5	4	1.2	AH, MH, CC
GAVISCON	4	18	13	AH, MC
GELUSIL	12	6	0.7	AH, MH, S
GELUSIL M	15	4.5	1.2	AH, MH, S
GELUSIL II	24	3	1.3	AH, MH, S
MAALOX PLUS, EXTRA-STRENGTH	29	2.5	1.2	AH, MH, S
MAALOX	13.3	5	1.4	AH, MH
MAALOX THERAPEUTIC CONCENTRATE (TC)	27	2.5	0.8	AH, MH
MYLANTA	12.7	4.5	0.7	AH, MH, S
MYLANTA II	25.4	3	1.1	AH, MH, S
RIOPAN PLUS	15	4.5	<0.1	AH, MH, S, Magaldrate
RIOPAN PLUS 2	30	2.5	<0.3	AH, MH, S, Magaldrate

Key: AH-aluminum hydroxide; AP-aluminum phosphate; CC-calcium carbonate; MC-magnesium carbonate; MH-magnesium hydroxide; S-simethicone (not an antacid).

Sources: Modified from manufacturer's data, *Drug Facts and Comparisons*, 1992, © Facts & Comparisons. Reprinted with permission.

lets, needed to neutralize a certain amount (expressed in milliequivalents, mEq) of HCl.

The ANC and, therefore, the proper dosage, varies from drug to drug and product to product (Tables 40–1 and 40–2). The average gastric ulcer patient needs to take enough antacid to neutralize about 70 mEq HCl per dose. The average duodenal ulcer patient, who typically secretes more acid, may need twice the dose. More information on this is given below.

Antacids may stop ulcer pain after only a day or two of use, but complete ulcer healing takes about eight to 10 weeks of continued, proper therapy. Antacids do not *cause* healing; they create a local environment that favors it. There isn't a "no pain, no ulcer" relationship. During the pain-free time, effective doses still must be taken until the ulcer heals fully. Eight weeks is considered the usual duration of this "intensive" therapy for active ulcers.

Quick pain relief actually can be a therapeutic limitation of antacids. It often is perceived incorrectly and prematurely as a signal that the ulcer is gone, so the patient (or careless prescriber) stops therapy too soon. Avoid this noncompliance by giving explicit instructions to the patient to keep taking the medication, and ensure that the advice is heeded.

Another therapeutic limitation is how often the stomach empties, or the rate of gastric emptying. When antacid passes to distal parts of the gut, it is removed from its sites of action. Food in the stomach delays gastric emptying somewhat. This is one reason why some clinicians advise ulcer patients to eat small meals frequently during the day. Antimuscarinic drugs, which are discussed below, also delay gastric emptying. However, their side effects limit their usefulness.

The best way to deal with the problem of gastric emptying is to administer effective doses of an antacid frequently, usually one and three hours after meals, and at bedtime.

NURSING IMPLICATIONS

Be sure patients understand that ulcer pain or discomfort may stop soon after treatment starts, and they should continue taking their medication for as long as directed. The goal in ulcer pain management is not to

Table 40–2 In Vitro Acid Neutralizing Capacity and Sodium Content of Selected Antacid Tablets*

Product	Neutralizing Capacity (mEq) per Tablet	Tablets to Neutralize 70 mEq Hcl	mg Na per Tablet	Active Ingredients
CAMALOX	18	4	1.0	AH, MH, CC
GELUSIL	11	6	0.8	AH, MH, S
GELUSIL M	12.5	6	1.3	AH, MH, S
GELUSIL II	21	3	2.1	AH, MH, S
MAALOX PLUS	11.4	6	0.8	AH, MH, S
MAALOX	9.7	7	0.7	AH, MH
MAALOX TC	28	5	0.5	AH, MH
MYLANTA	11.5	6	0.77	AH, MH, S
MYLANTA II	23	3	1.3	AH, MH, S
RIOPAN PLUS	13.5	5	<0.1	Magaldrate, S
ROLAIDS	7.5	9	53	ASC
TUMS	10	7	<2	CC

Key: AC-aluminum carbonate; AH-aluminum hydroxide; AP-aluminum phosphate; ASC-dihydroxyaluminum sodium carbonate; CC-calcium carbonate; MH-magnesium hydroxide; S-simethicone (not an antacid).

Sources: Modified from manufacturer's data, *Drug Facts and Comparisons,* 1992, © Facts & Comparisons. Reprinted with permission.

reduce the discomfort partially, or make painful attacks less frequent, but to make the patient pain-free and discomfort-free, and to prevent recurrences of the distress. This requires proper dosages and compliance.

Important Properties of Antacids

Dozens of antacid products are available, but they are not all alike. It is often hard to choose one that is "best." The properties to consider include

1. How much acid it neutralizes per dose (ANC; potency);
2. How fast it neutralizes acid (onset of action);
3. How long it neutralizes acid (duration of action);
4. Whether it alters gut motility;
5. The risks of causing electrolyte imbalances, including changes of blood pH;
6. Its physical form (liquid or tablet) and how convenient it is to take as directed;
7. Taste; and
8. Cost.

Each factor will be examined more closely later.

Individual Antacid Chemicals

Aluminum Salts

Aluminum salts are used widely as antacids. The most common one is aluminum hydroxide. The aluminum salts are not absorbed well into the systemic circulation, so aluminum-containing antacids are classified as ***nonsystemic.*** (Increased blood aluminum levels ***may*** occur in patients with very poor renal function who take very large doses of these drugs chronically. However, this is seldom a problem.)

Compared with other antacids, the ANC of aluminum compounds is relatively low. This low potency is one reason aluminum salts rarely are used alone to treat PUD. Instead of neutralizing acid, aluminum salts work by forming a gelatinous mass in the GI tract, which effectively ***adsorbs*** acid and pepsins. Through the same action, they also can adsorb other oral drugs the patient might be taking, interfering with their ***absorption.*** This can cause drug-drug interactions, which are discussed below.

The most common side effect of any aluminum salt, given alone, is constipation. Therefore, aluminum antacids usually are administered with magnesium salts, which tend to cause diarrhea.

All aluminum salts except aluminum phosphate, given long-term in high doses, significantly reduce phosphate absorption from the gut. Over the long run, they increase phosphate loss from the body. Hypophosphatemia can occur. Decreased phosphate absorption also can cause loss of bone calcium, making the bones more brittle and the patient susceptible to fractures. Bone calcium loss can cause hypercalcemia indirectly and increase the risk of urinary tract calcium stones. The phosphate-depleting effect of aluminum-containing antacids can be used therapeutically (intentionally) for patients with hyperphosphatemia, which is seen commonly in patients with such severe renal failure that they require hemodialysis.

Aluminum phosphate gel (PHOSPHALJEL) differs from other aluminum salts because it contains phosphate, and so does not cause phosphate depletion. It is used mainly to treat hypophosphatemia. Its acid-neutralizing potency is so low that it is unsuitable for treating ulcers.

Magnesium Salts

Magnesium oxide and hydroxide (milk of magnesia) are potent and rapidly acting. Magnesium ion is absorbed quickly into the bloodstream, but it is excreted rapidly by patients with normal renal function. However, magnesium intoxication (hypermagnesemia) is a risk if the patient has impaired renal function. Signs include nausea, vomiting, hypotension, and depressed peripheral and central neurologic status.

Magnesium salts cause a dose-dependent laxative effect that can be clinically useful (see Chapter 41, which discusses laxatives and cathartics) or unwanted (as in PUD therapy). Diarrhea is the most common side effect when magnesium salts are used alone. Excessive or long-term use can cause significant fluid and electrolyte loss from profuse diarrhea, and may impair spontaneous bowel activity over the long run.

Like aluminum salts, magnesium salts can interact with other orally administered drugs by adsorbing them in the gut, and reducing their absorption into the bloodstream. In addition, increased gut motility allows less time for orally administered drugs to be absorbed.

NURSING IMPLICATIONS

Closely monitor patients who are taking magnesium salts, and who have poor renal function, for evidence of hypermagnesemia. Advise them to avoid self-prescribing magnesium-containing antacids or laxatives, and to avoid excessive use of those that are prescribed. This general advice should be given to all elderly patients, in whom the risk of decreased renal function is relatively high.

Calcium Carbonate

Calcium carbonate (which is similar to ordinary blackboard chalk) is an effective and cheap antacid. However, it has several properties that make it unsuitable for routine use, especially by itself, for PUD or esophageal reflux.

Calcium carbonate neutralizes gastric acid quickly and effectively. However, it can stimulate acid secretion, and too much of the drug can alkalinize the gut contents. This is a dose and pH-dependent excessive effect that triggers "acid rebound," which is a reflex increase of acid secretion. In addition, calcium ion directly stimulates acid secretion by the parietal cells.

Calcium carbonate is not very water soluble, so it generally is considered a nonsystemic antacid. However, in the presence of acid it is converted to calcium chloride. Both the calcium and chloride ions are absorbed. With high doses or prolonged use, hypercalcemia can occur and lead to formation of renal calcium stones. The risk is high in patients who are dehydrated, have poor renal function, or who are taking thiazide diuretics (which reduce renal calcium excretion). Hypercalcemia also increases the risk of digitalis intoxication.

The most common side effect of calcium carbonate is constipation. At the extreme, it can cause fecal impactions.

Overuse of calcium carbonate, especially when combined with bland diets rich in calcium-containing dairy products (once popular ulcer treatments), can cause the *milk-alkali syndrome.* It is characterized by systemic alkalosis and hypercalcemia. These electrolyte and blood pH abnormalities can be severe.

Because of these problems, products that contain calcium carbonate alone (eg, TUMS), rarely are used alone for ulcer therapy.

NURSING IMPLICATIONS

Discourage patients from using products that contain only calcium as an antacid, unless their physician directs them to do so. As the use of OTC calcium-containing antacids decreased because of their therapeutic limitations, they were advertised more heavily as calcium supplements, particularly for women. The same problems that could occur when these drugs are used as antacids apply to their use as a mineral supplement.

Sodium Bicarbonate

Sodium bicarbonate (baking soda) is one of the most common home remedies for simple GI upset, but it seldom is prescribed for PUD. It is an extremely effective and quick-acting acid neutralizer. In fact, its efficacy is so great that unless the dose is adjusted carefully it will not elevate gastric pH slightly and desirably, but actually will alkalinize the stomach contents. Thus, it can cause acid rebound. Sodium bicarbonate does this much easier than calcium carbonate can.

Both sodium and bicarbonate ions are absorbed readily into the bloodstream, so sodium bicarbonate is clearly a systemic antacid. Absorbed bicarbonate can cause systemic metabolic alkalosis. The usual dose (one-half teaspoon every two hours as needed, up to four teaspoons per day) contains about 21 mEq (0.5g) of sodium. With long-term therapy, that extra sodium intake can be enough to cause significant problems for patients with hypertension, heart failure, or edema. Prolonged use of sodium bicarbonate can cause the milk-alkali syndrome, as noted for calcium carbonate.

Sodium bicarbonate reacts with acid to form carbon dioxide. Expelling the gas may provide some subjective relief (belching, properly called "eructation") for an ulcer-free patient who ate or drank too much. However, stretching of the stomach wall by gas may cause bleeding or hemorrhage if there is a gastric ulcer. There are also reports of stomach rupture after sodium bicarbonate ingestion. Sodium bicarbonate rarely causes constipation or diarrhea.

NURSING IMPLICATIONS

At best, recommended doses of sodium bicarbonate might be safe and effective if used infrequently for minor GI upset by persons who have no other contraindications, including PUD. Patients with suspected or diagnosed ulcers should avoid the drug. The best advice to give patients is to have them consult with a physician before ingesting sodium bicarbonate for any reason.

Antacid Combinations

The typical therapeutic approach to treating ulcers or esophageal reflux with antacids is to use a commercially available combination product. Usually, these include a magnesium salt mixed with an aluminum salt. Less often, calcium carbonate will be used instead of or in addition to the aluminum compound. Most antacid products contain two or more separate chemicals, mixed together. Some contain a substance called *magaldrate,* which is a true chemical complex of magnesium and aluminum, not a simple mixture. RIOPAN is an example of an antacid that contains magaldrate.

The theoretical advantage of aluminum and magnesium combinations is a balance between diarrhea-producing actions of one drug and constipating actions of the other. In practice, altered gut motility still may occur, depending on the patient and the antacid product.

NURSING IMPLICATIONS

It is usually wrong to start pharmacotherapy for any disorder with a medication that contains two or more drugs formulated together as a fixed-dose combination. However, the use of fixed-dose antacid combinations is a major (and uncommon) example of an instance in which such treatment is rational, clinically acceptable, and almost always done.

General Comparison of Antacid Combinations

Tables 40–1 and 40–2 compare and contrast several popular antacid combinations in terms of acid-neutralizing capacity, which determines the dose; the sodium content; and active ingredients.

Differences of Acid-Neutralizing Capacity

Products differ widely in terms of this potency indicator. Consider that a typical gastric ulcer patient requires 70 mEq of acid neutralization one hour after meals and at bedtime. Then consider only liquid antacids. As shown in Table 40–1, 5 mL of some products provides the desired effect, but the same volume of some others does not. Therefore, the simple recommendation to "take a teaspoonful (or two) of whatever antacid you like" is not always adequate. The same applies to antacid tablets, because of their different potencies.

Differences Between Tablets and Liquids

Antacid tablets are not preferred for intensive, long-term antacid therapy because of their lower ANC per unit (compare data in Tables 40–1 and 40–2). Three or four tablets of a typical antacid (what you might expect a reasonable person to tolerate chewing) neutralize much less acid than one or two teaspoons of a typical liquid. A duodenal ulcer patient may need to chew 15 or more tablets at a time to get an effective dose. Few patients are willing to do this for long. This is important, because tablets must be chewed thoroughly to be maximally effective. (In addition, antacid tablets are far too large to swallow whole safely.)

In contrast, liquid antacids are suspensions of tiny drug particles with a large surface area, which helps neutralize acid quickly and effectively. The best use of tablets is when the need is infrequent, the required dosages are low, and it is not convenient for the patient to carry a bottle of liquid.

Sodium Content

Many antacid combination products that do not include sodium bicarbonate as an active ingredient contain sodium that is left over from the manufacturing process. With high-dose, long-term therapy, the added sodium load can be important if the patient has a condition that is aggravated by it and the water retained by the kidneys. Antacid tablets usually contain more sodium than equivalent doses of liquids.

Manufacturers have recognized the importance of sodium content, and sell low-sodium or no-sodium antacids. At-risk patients should be instructed explicitly to use them. Even if low-sodium antacids are used, the patient's cardiovascular status should be assessed before starting intensive therapy and followed thereafter. Diuretic, antihypertensive, or heart failure therapies may need to be modified if excessive salt intake causes problems.

Taste

This important factor often is overlooked by the prescriber. However, it is worthless to recommend a potent antacid that the patient refuses to take because it tastes bad. Once acid-neutralizing requirements are assessed, give the patient a list of several products, and their equivalent doses, from which to select one that tastes acceptable. Some antacid products contain sugar or artificial sweeteners to improve taste. If the patient must control sugar intake (eg, for diabetes), consult product summaries in current drug references (see Nursing Implications, below) for details about ingredients. The sweetener type or amount generally is not listed on the package label.

Cost

Cost is another often overlooked factor that can add 40 or more dollars per month to the patient's expenses. Expense is another potential contributor to patient noncompliance and the failure to achieve successful treatment. Antacid liquid dosage forms are generally cheaper than tablets.

NURSING IMPLICATIONS

Ensuring the proper therapeutic dosage of an antacid is essential. It depends mainly on the indication for which the drug is given, and in general it should not be varied. However, so long as the proper dosage can be provided, factors such as taste and cost permit some flexibility in selecting an antacid that is not only effective, but also acceptable to the patient. This is most important, of course, for outpatient therapy.

Be sure to double-check the prescribed antacid dosage (which depends on the amount of acid that needs to be neutralized per dose) and dosage schedule. Also be sure to follow-up on what antacid, other than the specific product that was recommended, the patient actually may be using. This follow-up should identify not only the specific brand, but also the formulation—liquid, tablet, or both—and what other ingredients are in the chosen medication.

Antacid products often are reformulated; active ingredients, other additives, and potency are among the things that may change. However, the antacid product's name may not change also. Thus, dosages may have to be adjusted, or a change of composition may make a product that was more (or less) suitable for the patient less (or more) appropriate.

Labels on antacid bottles or tablet packets generally are not of much help in terms of gaining all the information that may be needed for proper patient education and advice. Sources such as textbooks and the *Handbook of Nonprescription Drugs,* which contain helpful information that is timeless and helpful in other respects, are not updated often enough to reflect changes in composition. Check with a pharmacist, or consult the latest issue of a frequently updated drug information source (eg, *Physicians' Desk Reference* supplements, the *Physicians' Desk Reference for Nonprescription Drugs,* or perhaps the best source, *Drug Facts and Comparisons* and its monthly supplements), for the most up-to-date information.

Side Effects, Adverse Reactions, and Contraindications

Changes of gut motility are the most common side effects of the common antacid combination products (Table 40–S). For a given antacid product, and a given dose, some patients will develop diarrhea; others may become constipated. Thus, monitor for both possibilities, and have the patient report significant changes in bowel function or stool consistency.

The best initial measure to deal with diarrhea or

Side Effects, Adverse Responses, and Contraindications

The most common side effects caused by cimetidine (Table 40–S) involve the central nervous system (CNS). They include headache (sometimes severe), drowsiness, and occasional delusional states (eg, delirium, disorientation, hallucinations). These are more likely to occur when high doses are given, or when usual dosages are given to patients who cannot eliminate the drug normally. The overall incidence of CNS side effects caused by cimetidine is somewhat greater than that associated with the other H_2 blockers. This may be because cimetidine's chemical structure enables it to cross the blood–brain barrier better than the other drugs. Cimetidine also can cause antiandrogenic effects such as gynecomastia and reduced sperm count. All these effects are dose-related and are generally reversible. None of the H_2 blockers cause atropine-like (antimuscarinic) side effects; this is a tremendous advantage over the atropine-like drugs that, before the availability of cimetidine, were used widely to treat PUD.

NURSING IMPLICATIONS

Anticipate side effects, particularly those affecting the CNS, in any patient who receives parenteral cimetidine. In most cases, excessive side effects can be eliminated or reduced, while maintaining the desired therapeutic responses, by switching to another H_2 blocker. Switching drugs is also the best way to handle drug interactions, which are discussed below.

◆ Use During Pregnancy and Lactation

Cimetidine should be given to pregnant women only when absolutely necessary. Cimetidine is excreted in maternal milk, and drug levels in the milk can be much greater than those in the maternal blood. If the mother must take cimetidine, the infant should be bottle-fed.

◆ Use in Children

Cimetidine is not recommended for children younger than 16 years old unless the anticipated benefits outweigh possible risks.

◆ Use in the Elderly

Assess for renal dysfunction, and anticipate the need for dosage reductions, or a less frequent dosage schedule. Central nervous system side effects are likely to occur, especially if needed dosage adjustments are not made.

Interactions with Other Drugs

Cimetidine, more so than the alternative H_2 blockers that are discussed below, inhibits the hepatic metabolism of many other drugs. In doing so, cimetidine can increase blood levels, and effects, of the interactants. Cimetidine does this by reducing hepatic blood flow, which delivers drugs to the liver for metabolism. Interactions may necessitate reducing dosages of one or both drugs, or switching to another H_2 blocker.

In theory, virtually any drug that depends on the liver for metabolism can be an interactant with cimetidine. However, even when one considers only those drugs for which there is good evidence of a clinically significant interaction (see Table 40–I), the list is still long. The interactants include several important cardiovascular drugs (eg, some antiarrhythmics, β blockers, and oral anticoagulants); CNS drugs (most antidepressants and benzodiazepines, and several anticonvulsants); quinolone antibiotics (eg, ciprofloxacin); theophylline; and even alcohol.

NURSING IMPLICATIONS

Cimetidine is capable of interacting with many other medications, and the outcome can be an increased risk of side effects, adverse responses, or toxicity of the interactant. Therefore, double-check the patient's overall medication plan to verify the potential interaction; refresh your memory about potential effects of the interactant (ie, its pharmacologic actions and toxicity); assess for evidence of an interaction accordingly; and anticipate the need to adjust dosages, discontinue cimetidine or the interactant, or switch to another noninteracting drug.

There are two main reasons to advise patients who are taking cimetidine to avoid alcohol consumption: the interaction, which risks greater-than-usual CNS depression caused by decreased alcohol metabolism; and the ability of alcohol to directly worsen the conditions for which cimetidine is given (see below).

Overdoses and Toxicity

The major signs of acute toxicity include tachycardia and delirium or other acute changes of mental status, which are best managed only by closely observing the patient and protecting the patient from self-injury. Respiratory difficulty may occur. Symptomatic, supportive treatment, and temporarily stopping cimetidine administration, are usually all that is required. Severe tachycardia may require treatment with a β-adrenergic blocker. However, as noted above, these drugs can interact and lead to excessive β blocker effects (eg, bradycardia or heart failure).

Related H_2 Blockers

Famotidine, Nizatidine, and Ranitidine

Famotidine (PEPCID), nizatidine (AXID), and ranitidine (ZANTAC) are the other H_2 blockers. They inhibit acid secretion in exactly the same way as cimetidine, and they share many of the prototype's indications. However, their potencies (and, therefore, their dosages) differ (see Table 40–C). The alternatives tend to cause fewer side effects (especially in the CNS) and drug interactions than cimetidine. One exception appears to be a greater incidence of headache with famotidine.

Some patients with PUD or pathologic hypersecretory states appear to be unresponsive or poorly responsive to even high doses of cimetidine; many of them seem to respond better, with fewer side effects, to an alternative.

NURSING IMPLICATIONS

Check laboratory test results to assess the patient's renal status (eg, serum creatinine levels) before administering any of these H_2 blockers. Renal dysfunction usually requires a dosage reduction.

Antimuscarinics

Antimuscarinics provide another way to inhibit gastric acid secretion. The antimuscarinic drugs include atropine and several related natural or synthetic agents that block muscarinic receptors for ACh (see Chapter 13 for more information). Through this effect, antimuscarinics block that portion of gastric acid secretion that is triggered by the parasympathetic nervous system.

The drugs, and their dosages, are listed in Table 13–C2. These drugs have been used for years to manage PUD. However, ever since the H_2 blockers became available, the use of antimuscarinics has fallen significantly.

There are several reasons for the dramatic decline in antimuscarinic drug use for PUD. Usual doses of these drugs inhibit acid secretion only about half as well as a typical H_2 blocker. Moreover, antimuscarinics routinely cause systemic side effects, including dry mouth, blurred vision, urinary retention, and constipation. These are not only potentially disturbing for most patients, but also potentially dangerous for many patients with prostatic hypertrophy, narrow-angle glaucoma, or tachycardia—all of which are contraindications for antimuscarinic agents (Table 12–S). The main indication for using an antimuscarinic instead of an H_2 blocker is when gut hypermotility or spasm (which are suppressed by antimuscarinics) accompanies ulcer disease.

Pirenzipine

Pirenzipine is a new antimuscarinic drug that preferentially blocks the subtype of ACh receptors (designated M_1 receptors) that mediate gastric acid secretion. Because of this selectivity, pirenzipine causes few of the bothersome or potentially dangerous side effects associated with typical antimuscarinics. Pirenzipine is being studied extensively for managing PUD, but it is not yet approved for use in the United States. The future for this drug as an antiulcer agent appears promising. However, the drug probably will be no more effective than an H_2 blocker, and H_2 blockers cause *no* antimuscarinic side effects.

Misoprostol

Misoprostol (CYTOTEC) is a new orally effective semisynthetic analog of the prostaglandin PGE_2. Like H_2 blockers and antimuscarinics, misoprostol inhibits gastric acid secretion. However, misoprostol does not block the receptors for histamine or ACh. Its actions are not known for sure. Unlike histamine or ACh blockers, misoprostol also stimulates the secretion of mucus, which protects the gut mucosa. The latter action is called a *mucotropic* effect.

Misoprostol is not used for routine management of PUD. Its only approved use is for preventing gastric ulcers in high-risk patients who are taking large doses of nonsteroidal antiinflammatory drugs (NSAIDs; Chapter 52), including aspirin, as for arthritis. These drugs cause ulcers by inhibiting prostaglandin synthesis; misoprostol overcomes that effect through its own prostaglandin-like activity. Misoprostol should be administered for as long as the patient is taking NSAIDs. It is absorbed best when taken with meals.

Misoprostol's prostaglandin activity accounts for its key side effects and contraindications. It stimulates gut motility, so diarrhea (dose-dependent) is common, especially during early therapy. Its uterine-stimulating activity (an *oxytocic* effect) may cause spotting or menstrual irregularities in nonpregnant women. *Pregnancy absolutely contraindicates misoprostol use:* the drug may cause uterine bleeding, partial or complete abortion, or premature labor.

Based on current information, there are no common, clinically significant drug interactions that involve misoprostol. The drug's efficacy and safety for children younger than 18 years old have not been established.

NURSING IMPLICATIONS

Advise patients to expect diarrhea, especially during the first two weeks of misoprostol therapy. Encourage them to take the drug with meals and at bedtime to minimize the severity of this side effect.

Abortion-related concerns are critically important. If misoprostol must be given to any woman who has the potential to become pregnant during treatment, she must be advised in writing and verbally of the risks; she should have a serum pregnancy test performed no more than two weeks before misoprostol therapy is to start, and the test must be negative; she must be given explicit instructions about effective contraceptive methods, and she must be capable of following them. Once these can be assured, misoprostol therapy should start only on the second or third day of the next menstrual period. Question medication orders, and do not give misoprostol, if these precautions have not been taken.

Omeprazole

Omeprazole (PRILOSEC) offers another way to inhibit gastric acid secretion. Omeprazole is a **prodrug**—a drug that is inactive in its administered form, but becomes pharmacologically active once it is metabolized. Omeprazole's metabolite binds to and inhibits an enzyme on the parietal cell membrane. This enzyme, an adenosine triphosphatase (ATPase), secretes acid (protons) in response to a variety of mediators, including histamine and acetylcholine. The enzyme often is called the "proton pump," and it is inhibited by omeprazole.

Omeprazole's ability to inhibit the proton pump and acid secretion is longlasting. For acid secretion to return, omeprazole therapy must be stopped and the parietal cells must have sufficient time to synthesize new enzyme. That usually takes about three weeks once treatment is discontinued.

Omeprazole is not indicated for routine use as an antiulcer drug. Its approved uses are: short-term treatment of severe or refractory gastroesophageal reflux; and long-term treatment of pathologic acid-hypersecretory states. Dosages are listed in Table 40–C. Clinical data suggest that omeprazole is more effective for these conditions than other standard therapies (eg, an H_2 blocker). However, owing to potentially greater long-term safety, an H_2 blocker should be tried before trying omeprazole.

Omeprazole's short-term side effects are nausea, diarrhea, and headache. They affect about one in 10 patients, or less, and the severity is usually mild. The major concern with this drug involves the unknown consequences of long-term, intense suppression of acid secretion from prolonged administration. This triggers a compensatory increase in secretion of gastrin, which exerts a trophic (growth-stimulating) effect on the gastric mucosa. Animal studies show that long-term omeprazole administration causes gastric carcinoid tumors, and these lesions have been reported in a few patients receiving high omeprazole doses for Zollinger-Ellison syndrome.

Another concern related to long-term and intense suppression of acid secretion is an overgrowth of certain bacteria in the gut. This may increase the risk of superinfection and the microbial production of carcinogenic chemicals (eg, nitrosamines) from substances in the diet.

Omeprazole can inhibit the liver's drug-metabolizing enzymes, leading to potential drug interactions similar to those noted for cimetidine. However, the most important interaction involves benzodiazepines, especially diazepam. Omeprazole inhibits benzodiazepine metabolism, and can cause excessive CNS depressant effects of the interactant. A similar interaction may apply to phenytoin and related hydantoin anticonvulsants.

Pregnancy contraindicates omeprazole use, and women who take the drug should not breast-feed their infants.

NURSING IMPLICATIONS

Since the long-term safety of omeprazole is not established, question medication orders if omeprazole is given for a reason other than an approved indication, or if approved dosages are not prescribed. Also question the order if effective doses of H_2 blockers have not been tried first.

As omeprazole use increases, the list of interacting drugs may grow. In general, monitor for altered (usually excessive) effects of other medications that are being administered, particularly if they depend on hepatic metabolism for their inactivation.

Omeprazole is formulated in capsules; they should be swallowed whole.

Drugs That Coat Ulcer Craters

Sucralfate

Sucralfate (CARAFATE), another oral medication, differs from all of the drugs discussed so far. It is structurally similar to aluminum hydroxide, the antacid, but sucralfate itself has very little antacid activity. Sucralfate works by chemically combining with chemicals that are released from damaged cells in exposed ulcer craters, forming a coating over the ulcer. This coating protects the cells from the damaging effects of acid, pepsins, and other noxious stimuli. Sucralfate is the only approved drug that works only through this action.

Sucralfate is indicated for short-term (up to eight weeks) adjunctive treatment of duodenal ulcers. Dosages are listed in Table 40–C. The drug should be administered on an empty stomach one hour before meals, and at bedtime. If antacids are used also, space the administration of the two drugs by at least 30 minutes.

Sucralfate seems to be quite harmless. Constipation is the most common side effect, but the overall incidence is low. Sucralfate causes far fewer side effects than cimetidine, but there appears to be little difference between the two in terms of efficacy or cost. Since some H_2 blockers can be taken with meals, with little concern that food will interfere with absorption, but sucralfate should not, patients may prefer the convenience of an H_2 blocker. Another consideration related to the use of sucralfate is whether the patient is taking other oral drugs: the properties that enable sucralfate to bind to ulcer craters enable it to bind to, and reduce the absorption of, other orally administered drugs (Table 40–I). Key interactants are hydantoins (eg, phenytoin), penicillamine, and quinolone antibiotics (eg, ciprofloxacin).

Antibiotic Therapy

Antibiotics that can kill or inhibit the growth of *H. pylori,* the acid-stable bacterium implicated in gastritis and ulcer disease, may help heal ulcers and prevent recurrences. However, suitable antibiotic treatment plans have not been approved.

H. pylori is sensitive to several subsalts (basic salts) of bismuth. Thus, there is growing interest in these compounds as therapeutic agents for ulcer disease. One familiar OTC product that contains bismuth is PEPTO-BISMOL, which is widely used as a remedy for such maladies as "upset stomach," "heartburn," and "traveller's diarrhea." Although its manufacturer describes its action as "coating the stomach" (it does), its antibiotic action may be important. Although PEPTO-BISMOL is not approved for treating PUD—and should not be used for that purpose—the future may hold new indications for it or others like it.

PEPTO-BISMOL contains bismuth subsalicylate, a chemical form of bismuth that shares many of the unwanted actions of the prototype salicylate, aspirin. Salicylates cause many adverse effects, they have contraindications, and participate in many drug-drug interactions (see Chapter 52). There is much interest in bismuth subcitrate, another bismuth salt, as a treatment for ulcer disease, GERD, and other disorders that may involve *H. pylori.*

Other Aspects of Therapy

Several other pharmacologic and nondrug factors have been said to be important in the etiology and treatment of PUD. Some are more myth than fact. Be aware of these in order to provide optimal ulcer therapy and teaching information for patients.

Common Emotional Stress

Patients with chronic physical or emotional complaints *may* have a greater risk of developing ulcers. Stress avoidance or reduction may help. And, antianxiety or sedative drugs (eg, benzodiazepines) may be useful adjuncts for selected patients in whom excessive stress is thought to contribute to the cause, persistence, or recurrence of PUD. However, these drugs should not be used instead of the proper antiulcer drugs discussed above. When they are prescribed, be aware of potential interactions with antiulcer drugs.

Diet

Many patients think their ulcers are caused by what they eat, but there is little proof that typical balanced diets play a role. Also, many patients expect that ulcer treatment will involve poor-tasting and hard-to-follow "bland" diets that once were commonly prescribed.

Dietary recommendations have changed dramatically. For example, bland diets, which are rich in calcium-containing dairy products, may do more harm than good. Dairy products neutralize acid for a short time, but their high calcium and protein content stimulates acid secretion. The milk-alkali syndrome, caused by consuming high doses of antacids with large amounts of dairy products, was described above.

Many physicians think that what is in the diet is not important, as long as irritating substances such as caffeine and alcohol (and *perhaps* some very spicy foods) are not part of a patient's "normal" diet. Food does stimulate acid secretion, but it also acts as a natural antacid and inhibitor of gastric emptying. Thus, some clinicians recommend frequent small meals throughout the day for patients with *benign gastric ulcers.* Things may be different for *duodenal ulcer patients,* who usually secrete excessive amounts of acid after eating even small amounts of food. For these persons, many physicians recommend three normal meals a day, and avoiding snacking, so episodes of food-induced acid secretion occur less often.

Virtually all patients with ulcers or GERD should be advised not to eat or snack before bedtime, even if they are taking a bedtime dose of an antiulcer medication.

Smoking

Smoking should be reduced or stopped. Chemicals in tobacco smoke, including nicotine, increase gastric acid secretion, motility, and mucosal blood flow. They also stimulate hepatic metabolism of other drugs, including cimetidine, and so may counteract effective therapy in yet another way.

Avoidance of Ulcerogenic Drugs

Several drugs may cause ulcers or aggravate existing lesions. They include:

- *alcohol,*
- *caffeine,*
- *corticosteroids* (with the exception of "nonsystemic" inhaled steroids, such as beclomethasone, that are used for asthma),
- *NSAIDS,* including aspirin and ibuprofen (both are common OTC remedies), and
- *antihypertensive drugs such as reserpine,* which tend to cause "parasympathetic predominance," an accompaniment of which is increased gastric acid secretion.

Avoiding these drugs, when possible, can help prevent or alleviate ulcers, and facilitate antiulcer therapy. If these drugs must be administered to persons who already have (or have had) PUD, antiulcer drug dosages may need to be increased or restarted. Prophylactic antiulcer therapy may be needed for previously ulcer-free patients who must take an ulcerogenic drug. (The use of misoprostol for patients taking NSAIDs is an example of the latter instance.)

NURSING IMPLICATIONS

Check the patient's medication history to assess whether poor antiulcer therapy might be due to ulcerogenic drugs. Advise patients to take acetaminophen, rather than aspirin or ibuprofen, for minor headache, fever, or musculoskeletal discomfort. All forms of aspirin, including enteric coated preparations, which are broken down in the alkaline environments produced by antacids, should be avoided. Patients taking salicylates or other nonsteroidal antiinflammatory/analgesic drugs for conditions such as arthritis often need medication changes or dosage adjustments.

Management of Acute Stress Ulcers

Because of the high morbidity and mortality of stress ulcers and the GI hemorrhage that may be associated with them, the therapeutic goal is prophylaxis. Antacids, H_2 blockers (cimetidine has been studied most), sucralfate, and combinations of these drugs are being used successfully as prophylactics. Many physicians have individual preferences about how best to prevent stress ulcers, and there are conflicting data about the superiority of intensive antacid therapy versus histamine antagonists.

When antacids are used, treatment often involves frequent (every hour or two) nasogastric suctioning and subsequent administration of between 10 and 120 mL of a potent aluminum-magnesium combination. Once the antacid is given, suction is withheld for about 45 minutes, the stomach contents are aspirated and assayed (the goal is to keep gastric pH between 5 and 6), and the sequence is repeated until the patient's overall condition has improved such that stress ulcer development is no longer likely.

A typical cimetidine protocol might involve IV administration of the drug in doses of up to 3.2 g per day in divided doses.

Each approach has advantages and disadvantages. For example, antacids are inexpensive compared with H_2 blockers, but the need for frequent suctioning and drug administration is costly in terms of personnel time. Administering a more costly drug such as cimetidine is less labor intensive. However, there may be an increased risk of more serious adverse effects, particularly in critically ill patients with an impaired ability to excrete the drug, and who also must receive interacting medications. Although there is disagreement about which treatment is best, there is no argument about the need for some form of intervention. Withholding prophylactic therapy could be a fatal error.

NURSING IMPLICATIONS

Assume that all critically ill patients are at risk of developing stress ulcers, and anticipate the possibility of serious GI bleeding and a sudden decline in the patient's condition if stress ulcers develop. Anticipate the use of prophylactic antacids or H_2 blockers for these patients so that adjustments in the doses or timing of interacting drugs can be made easily and with forethought.

Check the stool of all patients who are likely to develop stress ulcers, assessing for a black, tarry appearance that might indicate upper GI bleeding. (Teach this precaution to all ulcer patients, so that they may detect GI bleeding before it becomes serious.) Assess laboratory tests of peripheral blood or gastric aspirate for other indicators of blood loss. Monitor blood pressure and the pulse rate and quality as an indicator of serious and possibly life-threatening GI bleeding.

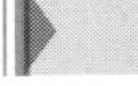

SUMMARY OF NURSING IMPLICATIONS

◆ Assessment

Obtain a complete nursing history that includes the pattern of GI pain or discomfort, factors that may possibly cause or worsen gastrointestinal discomfort, and factors that may aggravate ulcer disease or limit the effectiveness of antiulcer drugs. This should include assessment of current medications; diet, particularly sources of caffeine and alcohol; smoking habits; and work habits, recreational outlets, and sources of relaxation and stress.

Review current use of antacids to determine adequacy and need for modifications of treatment plan.

Obtain baseline data that includes information about renal, hepatic, cardiovascular, and mental status.

◆ Nursing Diagnoses

Altered comfort: pain related to hyperacidity and gastric irritation.

Altered bowel elimination: constipation related to use of calcium or aluminum salts.

Altered bowel elimination: diarrhea related to use of magnesium salts.

Knowledge deficit related to drug therapy.

Ineffective individual coping: stress and anxiety related to disease process.

Fluid volume deficit related to GI tract bleeding, altered gut motility, electrolyte imbalances.

Altered thought processes related to absorption of drug (magnesium salts; cimetidine).

◆ Planning/Implementation

Monitor patients taking high doses of aluminum-containing antacids for signs of hypercalcemia.

Note evidence of increased bone demineralization in elderly patients, postmenopausal women, or others with prior phosphate depletion states.

Observe for changes in mental status, reflexes, or muscular activity in patients taking magnesium-containing products.

Learn the ingredients and properties of several popular antacids.

Monitor patients on multidrug therapy for inadequate responses to other medications, which might indicate impaired absorption.

Monitor patients with hypertension or congestive heart failure for a worsening of condition with chronic high-dose intake of sodium bicarbonate or antacid combinations that are not low in sodium.

Monitor patients taking antimuscarinics for eye pain indicating possible undiagnosed glaucoma; changes of bowel function such as constipation; difficulty urinating; and discomfort or other problems due to dry mouth, blurred vision.

Monitor patients taking cimetidine for CNS side effects (eg, dizziness, confusion) that might warrant reduced doses.

Monitor patients taking cimetidine for gynecomastia and impotence; reassure patient that these responses are usually reversible.

Observe for signs of upper GI bleeding (eg, black tarry stools, possible hypotension) and stress ulcers in critically ill patients.

Anticipate the need for therapy to prevent stress ulcers in critically ill patients, and the possible need to alter other drug regimens when prophylaxis is begun.

Encourage and support ulcer patients in efforts to quit smoking and decrease intake of alcohol and caffeine, all of which stimulate acid secretion.

◆ Patient and Family Education

Teach the patient/family:

That the recommended antacid dose must be taken frequently and long after pain relief occurs; to continue to take antacids even with other antiulcer drugs, but generally one hour before or one to two hours after ingesting the other medication(s).

To report severe or prolonged diarrhea with magnesium compounds, which could lead to dehydration and electrolyte imbalances.

To avoid self-prescribing antacids that contain calcium carbonate or magnesium salts as the sole ingredient.

To chew antacid tablets thoroughly before swallowing, and drink approximately four ounces of water afterward.

To measure liquid antacids accurately.

To take antacids after meals, cimetidine with meals, and sucralfate on an empty stomach.

To avoid concurrent drug ingestion, particularly with antacids and sucralfate.

About differences in antacid preparations: liquids are generally more effective; tablets may be best for infrequent use or when carrying a bottle of liquid is inconvenient.

Relaxation techniques to reduce stress.

To take frequent sips of water or suck hard sugarless candies to manage dry mouth (if patient is taking anticholinergics); advise to expect difficulty focusing eyes; wear sunglasses to reduce discomfort from photophobia; report changes in bowel or bladder function.

◆ Evaluation

The patient/family will:

Obtain relief of ulcer pain.

Show signs of ulcer healing (based on endoscopy, X-ray films).

Comply with drug regimen to prevent progression of disease.

Quit or reduce smoking and ingestion of alcohol and caffeine.

Modify lifestyle to reduce stress.

Experience no adverse drug effects (eg, electrolyte imbalance, headache, disorientation, altered bowel function).

Annotated Bibliography

Brooks WS: Short- and long-term management of peptic ulcer disease: Current role of H_2-antagonists. *Hepatogastroenterol* 1992;39 Suppl 1:47–52. *Topics include pathophysiology, efficacy, compliance, relapse rates, side effects, and drug interactions.*

Clearfield HR: Management of NSAID-induced ulcer disease. *Am Fam Physician* 1992;45(1):255–258. *Identifies factors that increase the risk of antiinflammatory drug-induced ulcers, and gives practical advice about what to do about the disorder pharmacologically.*

Garnett WR: Antacid products. In Handbook of Nonprescription Drugs. Ninth ed. American Pharmaceutical Association, 1990: 243–281. *An excellent overview of the actions, uses, and misuses of antacids, and disorders for which they are given; includes timeless information on assessing patients, implementing therapy, and evaluating therapeutic outcomes.*

Gilbert G, Chan CH, Thomas E: Peptic ulcer disease. How to treat it now. Postgrad Med 1991;89(4):91–93, 96, 98. *Focuses on traditional therapies and newer options, and addresses the necessity of nondrug measures in successful therapy.*

Hixson LJ, Kelley CL, Jones WN, Tuohy CD: Current trends in the pharmacotherapy for gastroesophageal reflux disease. *Arch Intern Med* 1992;152(4):717–723. *Considers a holistic approach—including nondrug therapies—that are important for treating GERD and preventing recurrences.*

Hixson LJ, Kelley CL, Jones WN. Tuohy CD: Current trends in the pharmacotherapy for peptic ulcer disease. *Arch Intern Med* 1992; 152(4):726–732. *Reviews current therapy with single and combined drugs, and gives good insight into the likelihood of therapeutic "successes." This article also addresses the importance of the bacterium H. pylori.*

Holland EG, Taylor AT: Practical management of stress-related gastric ulcers. *J Fam Pract* 1991;33(6):625–632. *There is no one "ideal" way to manage acute stress ulcers, and many factors, including nursing availability, often help determine the choice for a given patient.*

Hopkins S: Drugs update. Undermining ulcers. *Nurs Times* 1992; 88(16):62–64. *Worth a look for its focused, nurse-oriented summary information.*

Isenberg JI: Should safety concerns with available ulcer treatment influence drug selection? *J Clin Gastroenterol* 1990;12 Suppl 2:S48–53. *For the most part, all the major antiulcer drugs have comparable effectiveness. Thus, safety becomes a major issue when choosing and monitoring therapy.*

Johnson DA: Medical therapy for gastroesophageal reflux disease. *Am J Med* 1992;92(5A):88S–97S. *Reviews treatment options for GERD; gives a good background on pathophysiology as a frame of reference.*

Katz KD, Hollander D: Practical pharmacology and cost-effective management of peptic ulcer disease. *Am J Surg* 1992;163(3): 349–359. *An excellent overview of therapeutic options, with coverage of an often overlooked topic—cost.*

Keithley JK: Histamine H_2-receptor antagonists. *Nurs Clin North Am* 1991 Jun;26(2):361–373. *Solid pharmacology and good clinical connections presented in a way the nurse-practitioner will appreciate.*

McCarthy DM: Acid peptic disease in the elderly. *Clin Geriatr Med* 1991;7(2):231–254. *Identifies three major risk factors for peptic ulcer disease in the elderly; discusses likely complications; and addresses therapeutic approaches that may, or may not, lead to a successful treatment outcome. Close monitoring is one of the keys to success.*

McCarthy DM: Sucralfate. N Engl J Med 1991;325(14):1017–1025. *Complete coverage of this interesting drug.*

McQuaid KR, Isenberg JI: Medical therapy of peptic ulcer disease. *Surg Clin North Am* 1992;72(2):285–316. *A comprehensive, worth-reading review of ulcer disease etiologies, and how pathophysiology and drug actions may relate to one another when treatment is being planned and evaluated.*

Richter JE: Gastroesophageal reflux: Diagnosis and management. *Hosp Pract* (Off Ed) 1992;27(1):59–66. *An excellent article that focuses on the potential consequences and current treatments of a common gut disorder.*

Table 40–C | **Clinical Uses and Administration of Major Drugs for Peptic Ulcer Disease**

AGENT	CLINICAL USES	DOSAGE AND ROUTE OF ADMINISTRATION
Antacids	Treatment, prophylaxis of gastric, duodenal ulcers; gastroesophageal reflux disease (GERD)	Oral: For benign gastric ulcer: 70 mEq acid-neutralizing capacity 1 and 3 hr after meals and at bedtime (the antacid volume or number of tablets depends on potency of individual product). For duodenal ulcers: up to 140 mEq of acid-neutralizing capacity, at same dosage schedule. (See Tables 40–1 and 40–2 for potencies of various antacids)
	Prophylaxis of acute stress ulcers	Oral (or via nasogastric tube): Usually suction stomach contents, give 30–60 mL of aluminum-magnesium antacid, repeat every 1 or 2 hr as needed
Histamine (H_2) Antagonists		
PROTOTYPE		
Cimetidine (TAGAMET)	Treatment of active duodenal ulcers	Oral: Usually 800 mg daily (at bedtime); patients with large ulcers or heavy smokers (>1 pack cigarettes/day) may require 1600 mg daily; reduce dose with severe renal impairment; may substitute divided doses for single dose, but generally is not recommended
	Maintenance therapy for duodenal ulcers	Oral: 400 mg at bedtime
	Treatment of active benign gastric ulcers	Oral: 300 mg qid or 800 mg at bedtime
	GERD	Oral: 800 mg bid or 400 mg qid
	Pathologic acid-hypersecretory states (eg, Zollinger-Ellison syndrome)	Oral: 300 mg qid (with meals, at bedtime); maximum of 2400 mg/day (600 mg 4 times daily) may be needed
	Pathologic hypersecretory conditions; short-term alternative to oral therapy; other indications	IM: 300 mg every 6–8 hr (use supplied solution undiluted) IV injection: Dilute 300 mg in 20 mL 0.9% sodium chloride injection, inject over 2 min every 6–8 hr Intermittent IV infusion: Dilute 300 mg in ≥50 mL 5% dextrose-water, infuse over 20–30 min every 6–8 hr (or use prediluted drug supplied by manufacturer)
RELATED DRUGS		
Famotidine (PEPCID)	Active duodenal ulcers	Oral: 40 mg at bedtime, or 20 mg bid, for minimum of 4 wks
	Maintenance therapy of duodenal ulcers	Oral: 20 mg at bedtime
	Benign gastric ulcers	Oral: 40 mg at bedtime
	GERD	Oral: 20 mg bid for up to 6 wks (20–40 mg bid for up to 12 wks for erosive GERD)
	Pathologic acid-hypersecretory states	Oral: 20–160 mg every 6 hr IV 20 mg, injected over 2 min or infused over 15–30 min every 12 hr

(continued)

Table 40–C **Clinical Uses and Administration of Major Drugs for Peptic Ulcer Disease**

AGENT	CLINICAL USES	DOSAGE AND ROUTE OF ADMINISTRATION
Nizatidine		
(AXID)	Treatment of active duodenal ulcers	Oral: 300 mg once daily at bedtime (preferred) or 150 mg bid
	Maintenance therapy of healed duodenal ulcers	Oral: 150 mg once daily at bedtime
Ranitidine		
(ZANTAC)	Active duodenal ulcers	Oral: 150 mg in morning and at bedtime, or 300 mg once daily at bedtime
	Maintenance therapy of duodenal ulcers	Oral: 150 mg at bedtime
	Benign gastric ulcers or gastroesophageal reflux disease (GERD)	Oral: 150 mg bid; parenteral administration not recommended
	Pathologic acid-hypersecretory states	Oral: 150 mg bid
	Intractable duodenal ulcers, pathologic hypersecretory conditions; short-term alternative to oral therapy for above conditions in patients who cannot take oral medication	IM, IV injection, or intermittent IV infusion: 50 mg every 6–8 hr; give IV doses over at least 5 min
	Antimuscarinics	
	See Tables 13–C1 and 13–C2	
	Prostaglandin Analog: Misoprostol	
Misoprostol		
(CYTOTEC)	Prevention of nonsteroidal anti-inflammatory drug (NSAID)–induced gastric ulcers in high-risk patients	Oral: 200 μg qid with meals while NSAID therapy lasts
	Proton Pump Inhibitor: Omeprazole	
Omeprazole		
(PRILOSEC)	Active duodenal ulcer; refractory GERD or erosive gastritis	Oral: 20 mg/day for 4–8 weeks, before meals
	Pathologic acid-hypersecretory conditions	Oral: 60 mg/day to start, adjust maintenance dose as needed; give doses >80 mg in divided doses
	Ulcer Protectant	
Sucralfate		
(CARAFATE)	Short-term treatment of duodenal ulcer	Oral: 1 g qid, taken on empty stomach 1 hr before meals and at bedtime; maintenance therapy; 1 g bid

Table 40–S **Major Side Effects of and Contraindications for Antiulcer Drugs**

BODY SYSTEM/ Side Effect	CONTRAINDICATION/ PRECAUTION	COMMENTS AND NURSING IMPLICATIONS
	All Antacids	
GASTROINTESTINAL Altered gut motility: diarrhea or constipation	Current diarrhea or constipation; obstructive bowel disease	Assess bowel function before and periodically during antacid therapy
	Aluminum Salts	
GASTROINTESTINAL Constipation	Gut hypomotility or obstruction	Monitor frequency, consistency of stool; risk, severity of constipation reduced by administering with magnesium salt
OTHER Loss of bone calcium; hypercalcemia; hypophosphatemia (except aluminum phosphate)	Osteomalacia; tendency for bone fractures	Encourage patient to take precautions against falls if they are in high-risk group; monitor for signs of hypercalcemia (eg, muscle weakness, bone pain or fractures, flank pain due to renal calcium stone formation)
	Magnesium Salts	
GASTROINTESTINAL Diarrhea	Diarrhea, malabsorption syndrome	Monitor frequency, consistency of stool; risk severity of diarrhea reduced by administering with aluminum or calcium salt
OTHER Hypermagnesemia	Poor renal function	Restrict use, dose, in patients with poor renal function; observe for signs of hypermagnesemia (nausea, vomiting, hypotension, hyporeflexia, lethargy, muscle hypoactivity)
	Calcium Carbonate	
GASTROINTESTINAL Constipation, fecal impaction (when used alone)	See aluminum salts	See aluminum salts
OTHER Hypercalcemia (when used alone or in combination products) Systemic (metabolic) alkalosis (milk-alkali syndrome)	Use cautiously in patients receiving digitalis	Monitor response to digitalis; check serum calcium levels; limit use of calcium carbonate, especially with diets rich in dairy products; check for increased muscle rigidity, tetany; observe for signs of hypercalcemia (see aluminum salts, above)
	Sodium Bicarbonate	
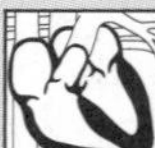 **CARDIOVASCULAR** Salt, fluid accumulation; edema, hypertension, heart failure; milk-alkali syndrome	Edema, congestive heart failure, hypertension	Encourage all patients to avoid taking sodium bicarbonate unless prescribed by a physician; see also milk-alkali syndrome above (calcium carbonate)

(continued)

Table 40–S **Major Side Effects of and Contraindications for Antiulcer Drugs (*Continued*)**

BODY SYSTEM/ Side Effect	CONTRAINDICATION/ PRECAUTION	COMMENTS AND NURSING IMPLICATIONS
	Histamine (H_2) Blockers (especially Cimetidine)	
CENTRAL NERVOUS SYSTEM Dementia, confusion, combativeness, other mental changes		Side effects occur mainly when high doses are used or in patients with liver dysfunction; reassure, orient patient, take precautions to guard against self-inflicted injury
REPRODUCTIVE Transiently reduced sperm count		Advise patient that effect is dose-dependent and reversible
OTHER Gynecomastia		Is dose-dependent and reversible; affects males and females
	Sucralfate	
GASTROINTESTINAL Constipation (uncommon)		Advise patient to increase intake of fluids and dietary fiber
	Antimuscarinics	
	See Table 13–S	
	Misoprostol	
CENTRAL NERVOUS SYSTEM Headache		
GASTROINTESTINAL Diarrhea, abdominal pain		Diarrhea affects up to 4 in 10 patients, is most common side effect; GI side effects often dose-dependent, most common, severe in first few weeks of therapy; take with meals
REPRODUCTIVE Uterine spotting, cramping; hyper- or amenorrhea; premature labor; abortion	Pregnancy (absolute contraindication); any woman of child-bearing age (relative contraindication)	Rule out pregnancy before starting drug; instruct patient about risks, need for effective contraception; see text for other guidelines
	Omeprazole	
CENTRAL NERVOUS SYSTEM Headache, dizziness		Headache most common side effect, but is usually mild
GASTROINTESTINAL Diarrhea, abdominal pain, nausea, vomiting		
Potential gastric carcinogenesis		Consequences of long-term, intense acid suppression unknown; question orders for unapproved uses, dosages, or treatment durations

Table 40–I **Major Interactions Between Antiulcer Drugs and Other Agents**

AGENT	RESULT OF INTERACTION	COMMENTS AND NURSING IMPLICATIONS
General Interactions Involving Antacids and Common Antacid Combination Products		
Antibiotics, quinolones and tetracyclines (Chapter 56) Iron salts (Chapter 61) Nitrofurantoin (Chapter 57) Penicillamine (Chapter 52) Quinidine (Chapter 30) Salicylates, including aspirin (Chapter 52)	Reduced oral absorption, effects, of interactant	Avoid combined use, or separate administration of interactant and antacid as much as possible; monitor accordingly for evidence of reduced effectiveness of interactant; interactions with unlisted oral medications are possible, apparently less clinically significant, but require appropriate monitoring anyway
Interactions Involving H_2 Blockers (Mainly Cimetidine)		
Aminophylline	See theophylline, below	
Antidepressants, tricyclics and related agents (Chapter 24)	Reduced antidepressant metabolism; increased risk of side effects, toxicity	Monitor accordingly, especially for excessive central nervous system (CNS) depression, hypotension, antimuscarinic effects; monitoring serum antidepressant levels may be needed to guide dosage adjustments; interaction involves cimetidine, possibly ranitidine; less likely with cimetidine alternatives
Benzodiazepines (eg, diazepam; Chapter 22)	Reduced benzodiazepine metabolism; increased blood levels, effects	Monitor accordingly, especially for excessive CNS depression, which requires decreased dose or increased dosage interval of interactant; affects most, not all, benzodiazepines, less likely with cimetidine alternatives
Carbamazepine (Chapter 26)	Reduced carbamazepine metabolism; increased risk of toxicity	Monitor accordingly, especially when adding cimetidine; measure carbamazepine blood levels to guide possible dosage reductions
Ethanol (Chapter 22)	Reduced ethanol metabolism, excessive CNS depression, ataxia	Discourage use of alcohol during cimetidine therapy
Lidocaine (Chapters 19, 30)	Reduced lidocaine metabolism, risk of excessive cardiac depression and/or hypotension	Cimetidine alternatives less likely to interact, are preferred; if cimetidine must be used, monitor lidocaine levels, ECG, CNS status, other vital signs closely; lidocaine dose may need to be reduced
Nifedipine (Chapter 34)	Reduced nifedipine metabolism; increased blood levels, effects (especially hypotension)	Monitor accordingly if interaction cannot be avoided, alternatives cannot be used

(continued)

Table 40–I **Major Interactions Between Antiulcer Drugs and Other Agents**

AGENT	RESULT OF INTERACTION	COMMENTS AND NURSING IMPLICATIONS
Phenytoin (Chapter 26)	Reduced phenytoin metabolism; excessive side effects, toxicity	Use cimetidine alternatives if possible; otherwise monitor serum phenytoin levels to guide dosage changes
Procainamide (Chapter 30)	See lidocaine	See lidocaine
Quinidine (Chapter 30)	As for lidocaine; increased risk of cinchonism or true quinidine toxicity	See lidocaine
Theophylline (Chapter 38)	Reduced theophylline metabolism; increased risk of toxicity	Monitor for theophylline toxicity (eg, excessive CNS stimulation, potential seizures); theophylline blood levels should be rechecked to guide dosage when adding, discontinuing cimetidine; anticipate need for significantly reduced theophylline dosages; interaction applies to all theophyllines except diphylline; cimetidine alternatives almost always preferred
Warfarin (Chapter 35)	Reduced warfarin metabolism; increased risk of excessive effects, bleeding	Highly clinically significant interaction; avoid; H_2 blockers other than cimetidine less likely to interact, nevertheless require close monitoring (eg, prothrombin times)
Interactions Involving Antimuscarinics		
	See Table 13–I	
Interactions Involving Misoprostol		
	None; see text	
Interactions Involving Omeprazole		
Benzodiazepines (eg, diazepam, Chapter 22)	Reduced benzodiazepine metabolism; increased blood levels, effects	Monitor for excessive CNS effects (eg, ataxia, drowsiness); may need to reduce benzodiazepine dose or prolong dose interval during combined therapy
Interactions Involving Sucralfate		
Penicillamine (Chapter 52)	Reduced penicillamine absorption, effects	Separate administration times as much as possible; increased penicillamine dosages may be needed
Phenytoin (Chapter 26)	Reduced absorption, effects	See penicillamine, above; monitoring phenytoin blood levels may be needed to adjust dose, monitor response
Quinolone antibiotics (eg, ciprofloxacin; Chapter 56)	Reduced absorption, effects	Avoid combined use if possible; otherwise, use precautions noted for penicillamine, above

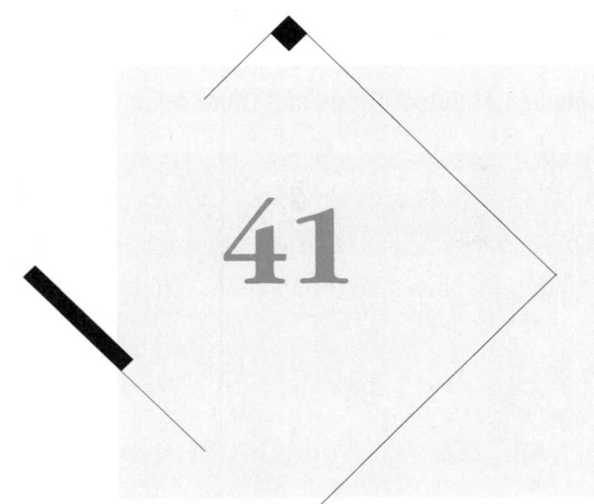

Laxatives, Cathartics, and Antidiarrheal Medications

Many of us are preoccupied with our bowel habits, and we think that regular bowel movements are an indication of overall health. This perception is perhaps most common in the elderly. Drugs that relieve what is perceived either as constipation or diarrhea have a few valid therapeutic uses, but they are widely abused by the lay public. The mass media do not help. Many advertisements in magazines and on television stress the importance of "regularity."

Drugs that affect bowel function fall into two major categories, laxatives and cathartics, to relieve constipation; and antidiarrheals. There are subclasses of each, based on their mechanisms of action. Unfortunately, no single class of laxative, cathartic, or antidiarrheal agent can be considered a prototype. Therefore, the general characteristics of the drug categories are presented first, followed by a brief discussion of each subclass. Dozens of proprietary products are available, and there are considerable differences in their ingredients and actions.

Major reference tables appear beginning on p. 828.

Laxatives and Cathartics

Drugs that increase the frequency or volume of the stool are classified as laxatives or cathartics. A popular belief is that they are panaceas capable of relieving the common cold and virtually every other common illness. In reality, these drugs have only a handful of valid medical uses. More important is the widespread and potentially dangerous misuse of self-prescribed laxatives, for which the public wastes hundreds of millions of dollars each year.

Drug Therapy of Constipation

Normal Gut Function and Constipation

Most individuals who have reached adolescence have developed some regularity of bowel movements. For some, regularity means defecating once or twice a day, while for others regularity means defecating only a few times a week. The frequency of defecation is affected by diet, exercise, emotional stress, and travel. Nevertheless, many individuals who deviate even slightly from what they consider normal bowel habits, even for a day or so, will turn to one of the many readily available over-the-counter (OTC) laxative or cathartic drugs, trying to force regularity in the face of natural and innocuous stimuli that cause brief changes of normal bowel function.

In view of the wide individual variability in bowel habits, general definitions of constipation can be:

- a decreased number of bowel movements from what is normal for the individual in question;
- the development of stools that are painful or otherwise difficult to expel; or
- fewer than two bowel movements during any consecutive seven-day period.

General Characteristics of Laxatives and Cathartics

A laxative can be defined as a drug that gradually softens or facilitates passage of a formed stool. Cathartics can be defined as drugs that produce a more prompt, complete, and watery evacuation of the gastrointestinal (GI) tract. In many instances the nature of the stool produced by a given drug is dose-related, with a low dose causing laxation and higher doses causing catharsis.

Laxatives and cathartics can be grouped into six general categories (some texts classify some of the individual agents differently):

- bulk-forming agents such as psyllium and bran;
- saline laxative-cathartics such as milk of magnesia;
- hyperosmotic agents such as glycerin;
- stimulant-irritants such as bisacodyl, phenolphthalein, senna, and castor oil;
- stool-softeners such as docusate sodium; and
- lubricants, for which mineral oil is the main example.

Absorption, Distribution, Metabolism, and Excretion of Laxatives and Cathartics

Laxatives and cathartics usually are given orally. Some also can be given per rectum as instilled liquids (enemas) or suppositories. Laxatives and cathartics are given for their local actions in the gut, not for systemic action, but some drugs may be absorbed. Most of the drugs are excreted in the feces unchanged; others may be metabolized in the gut or, following absorption, in the liver.

Major Effects of Laxatives and Cathartics

Laxatives and cathartics affect fluid and electrolyte movement, and muscle tone, in the gut. Some stimulate muscle tone indirectly by increasing the size and water content of the feces; others stimulate muscular activity directly. The drugs are classified based on their major mechanism of action, as noted later. Some proprietary products contain drugs belonging to two or more classes.

Misuse of, Valid Indications for, and General Dangers of Laxatives and Cathartics

Uses for laxatives can be considered best by identifying the more common causes for which they should *not* be used. Ordinarily, these drugs should not be self-prescribed to manage constipation that can be traced to relatively simple causes, which usually can be determined from the patient's history. A simple initial nondrug approach to the problem usually can be instituted effectively. Common causes of constipation are:

- Inadequate water intake. Often, increasing the daily intake of water, pulpy juices, or other nonalcoholic beverages may alleviate constipation.
- Inadequate intake of fiber-rich food (raw vegetables, fresh or dried fruit, cereals or breads made with whole grains such as bran). Increasing the daily intake of these foods may help.
- Excessive intake of low-fiber or constipating foods (meat products, sweets, highly processed baked goods, processed cheeses). Reducing consumption of these foods may normalize bowel function.
- Inadequate exercise. Increasing physical activity, as permitted by the patient's overall status, may be beneficial.
- Use of constipating drugs. Stopping or limiting the use of such drugs, if they are not essential for the patient's well-being, may resolve the problem. Habitual use of laxatives/cathartics, often as part of a cycle with antidiarrheal drugs, is a common cause of constipation. Other drugs that commonly cause constipation include:
  - antacids that are rich in calcium or aluminum salts;
  - any drug with antimuscarinic (anticholinergic) activity (for example, atropine, scopolamine, most antidepressants, antihistamines, and antipsychotics);

- calcium salts, which are becoming popular as mineral supplements;
- iron salts (as supplements, hematinics); and
- opiates (narcotic analgesics).

Laxatives

Laxative administration, under the direction of a physician, is indicated when constipation that lasts for more than one week is not managed effectively by the above regimens. Other patients who should not strain to defecate may appropriately receive laxatives or cathartics. These include persons

- with hemorrhoids or other anorectal disease;
- many pre- and postoperative patients;
- patients with recent myocardial infarction;
- patients who are immediately pre- or postpartum;
- patients with hernias;
- hypertensive patients (straining to defecate may elevate blood pressure in some patients);
- hypotensive patients ("pushing" to defecate involves marked increases of intrathoracic pressure—the Valsalva maneuver—that dramatically reduces venous return to the heart, and then abruptly increases venous return when straining stops); and
- some bedridden patients who develop constipation because of physical inactivity.

In most of these cases *bulk-forming laxatives* (see below) should be tried first, followed by stool softeners.

Cathartics

Cathartics, which cause more complete fluid evacuation, generally are indicated to evacuate the gut before and sometimes after diagnostic procedures, such as radiologic studies of the GI tract, or before surgery. They also may be used adjunctively in the treatment of helminth (worm) or parasitic infestations of the gut, for which they help eliminate invading organisms from the bowel.

Cathartics often are administered as enemas, which generally provide more prompt and complete effects than orally administered agents, and with a lower risk of systemic side effects. In general, far fewer valid indications exist for self-administration of cathartics than for laxatives.

General Laxative/Cathartic Contraindications

No laxative or cathartic, regardless of its mechanism of action or route of administration, should be given to patients with nausea, vomiting, or diarrhea, mainly because of the great risk of serious fluid and electrolyte loss and resulting imbalances. These agents should be avoided in any individual with abdominal pain or tenderness unless obstruction or weakness of the GI tract can be absolutely ruled out as the cause. Administration of these drugs in the presence of gut obstruction can cause serious mechanical damage, or even bowel perforation. Likewise, additional doses of a laxative or cathartic should not be given if severe abdominal pain, nausea, or vomiting occur after administration. Since cathartic drugs almost always produce defecation after one recommended dose is given, further doses should be withheld if the expected effect does not occur, and the patient should be evaluated further.

NURSING IMPLICATIONS

When assessing patients with a constipation problem, inquire about their previously "normal" bowel habits and possible expected and innocuous causes for temporary irregularity (listed above). The history also should consider other potential causes of constipation, such as recent surgery and drug (prescription and OTC) use. Inquire about medical conditions that are likely to cause constipation, such as most disorders associated with neurologic or muscular dysfunction (diabetes, multiple sclerosis, parkinsonism, and so on); hypothyroidism; hypercalcemia (such as from hyperparathyroidism); and pregnancy. Ask about general or abdominal discomfort, weight loss, nausea, vomiting, and the appearance of the stool.

Discourage self-medication unless under a physician's direction, and stress the dangers of frequent laxative or cathartic use. Recommend the nondrug interventions, including dietary modification, for occasional constipation.

Enemas

Enemas provide a convenient and effective means of cleansing the lower GI tract. They are best used in controlled settings such as a hospital, where the patient's status is known, the means to assess and treat untoward consequences are available, and the results of administration can be monitored.

In outpatient settings, enemas, which are available without prescription, should mainly be used with the advice of a physician or other health-care professional. When administered according to label directions, approved OTC enemas are generally safe. However, the lay public frequently misuses enemas, and the results are potentially dangerous. Many problems arise because self-prescribers do not consider these agents, especially "home-recipe" enemas composed of tap water or "cleansing" soapsuds, as drugs. Like any laxative or cathartic, and any route of administration, even tap water or soapsuds can cause adverse effects on the rectum and large bowel, excessive fluid and electrolyte loss or imbalance, systemic effects if the ingredients are absorbed, and loss of spontaneous bowel tone and rhythm if used too frequently.

NURSING IMPLICATIONS

As a general rule, all the precautions noted for oral cathartics apply to enemas. Enemas that are premixed by the manufacturer and supplied in single-dose packages are preferred for self-administration. If a premixed preparation is not being used, the product should be diluted as directed to prevent irritation of the colon. Enema use for more than one week absolutely should be discouraged unless a physician orders otherwise. Enemas should not be administered to children younger than two years without a physician's order, and infants should be in a hospital setting if an enema must be given.

Major Classes of Laxatives and Cathartics

Bulk-Forming Laxatives

The most common ingredient in bulk-forming laxatives is the plant gum psyllium (as in METAMUCIL products), which is obtained from plantago seeds. Other products contain as the active ingredient bran, calcium polycarbophil, chondrus, guar gum, malt soup extract, or methylcellulose (or carboxymethylcellulose). They often are supplied in powder form, which must be mixed thoroughly with water or other suitable beverage before ingestion. Some brand name products are expensive, and probably no more effective than less costly generic brands.

Actions

The bulk-forming agents produce a laxative effect in the same way as a diet that is naturally rich in whole grains, fresh vegetables, dried fruits, and adequate amounts of water. They act in the small and large intestines by absorbing water and forming a soft bulky mass that stimulates the normal intestinal reflexes, and leads to passage of the fecal mass through the intestine and out of the body.

Effects usually occur in 12 hours, but may not occur for one to three days for some patients and products. Their effects are enhanced by the ingestion of large amounts of liquid, which prevents the drug from becoming dry in, and eventually blocking, the intestines.

Uses

Bulk-forming laxatives are probably the safest type of laxative to recommend to outpatients who are bothered by simple constipation that is not responsive to diet, fluid intake, and exercise, mainly because little or none of the active ingredient is absorbed systemically, and because the risk of diarrhea is lowest if too high a dose is taken. Recommended dosages for common bulk-forming laxative drugs or products are listed in Table 41–C.

Precautions

Bulk-forming laxatives should not be taken without the recommendation of a physician if the patient has dysphagia, obstruction of the gut, or ulcers, or by individuals who seem constipated because of long-term abuse of other laxative drugs. Calcium polycarbophil (MITROLAN) contains calcium in amounts that can cause side effects and drug interactions noted for calcium-containing antacids (Chapter 40). Bran, a popular health food, should be used as part of an otherwise balanced diet to reduce bloating and interference with the absorption of important dietary nutrients.

NURSING IMPLICATIONS

When bulk-forming laxatives are prescribed, instruct the patient to stir the powder well into a full glass of cool liquid, and to drink six to eight glasses of water or other nonalcoholic liquid per day until normally soft stools are formed or until directed otherwise. Suitable liquids for administering these agents include water, milk, or fruit juice. Advise patients to avoid all alcohol- or caffeine-containing beverages. Advise them to avoid taking bulk-forming laxatives before bedtime, to reduce the risk of intestinal obstruction. A high dietary intake of bran increases the risk of impaction when bulk-forming laxative products also are used. Bulk-forming laxatives generally should not be administered to children younger than six years without a physician's recommendation.

Saline Laxatives and Cathartics

Magnesium salts used orally as laxatives or cathartics include hydroxide (milk of magnesia; also used as an antacid), sulfate (epsom salts), and citrate (citrate of magnesia). They are the best examples of saline laxatives or cathartics. Whether laxation or catharsis occurs depends on the dose taken, but it appears easiest to titrate the dose and achieve only a laxative effect with milk of magnesia. Sodium phosphates are used as enemas for catharsis (FLEET PHOSPHO-SODA).

Actions

The saline products, when given orally, act in the small and large intestines to osmotically withdraw water from the capillaries into the gut lumen. They also may cause the release of enteric hormones that stimulate secretion of fluid into the intestine and enhances gut motility. The cathartic effects of magnesium citrate or sulfate, or the sodium phosphate salts, usually appear within 30 minutes to three hours after ingestion. They usually cause a watery evacuation. Milk of magnesia may take twice as long for effects to appear, especially if a low dose is given, and a semisolid stool may occur under these conditions. Sodium phosphate salt enemas work mainly in the colon and rectum, producing a watery evacuation within two to 15 minutes. Typical dosages are given in Table 41–C.

Uses

The saline laxatives are used to cause rapid or complete bowel evacuation.

Precautions

There are potential problems associated with the use of any saline laxative or cathartic (Table 41–S). Their GI actions may be too prompt and complete at times when these effects are not wanted. This could lead to excessive fluid and electrolyte loss when used chronically or even when taken acutely by individuals with dehydration or electrolyte imbalances. Used long-term, they will interfere with adequate absorption of dietary nutrients or other orally administered drugs that the patient may be taking (Table 41–I). Chronic use also inhibits rhythmic bowel reflexes that are responsible for regular defecation. This can lead to cyclic dependency on laxatives and antidiarrheal drugs. The salts in virtually all the saline laxatives or cathartics are absorbed well. This is more of a problem with oral administration, since prompt evacuation of the bowel when an enema is given reduces the time during which absorption can occur.

The magnesium salts pose the risk of hypermagnesemia and its associated neuromuscular changes (see Chapter 40), particularly in patients with poor renal function, for whom these products are contraindicated.

Products containing sodium phosphates require additional precautions owing to their composition. In particular, both sodium and phosphate can be absorbed, leading to hypernatremia and dehydration, hyperphosphatemia, increased blood volume, and secondary effects such as worsening of heart failure or hypertension, hypocalcemia, and acidosis. Do not administer them to patients with congestive heart failure or megacolon because of the increased risk of systemic absorption.

NURSING IMPLICATIONS

Monitor patients taking saline laxatives or cathartics for signs of excessive fluid and electrolyte loss or imbalance. If they are taking magnesium salts (such as milk of magnesia), look for pertinent neuromuscular signs of magnesium intoxication. Recommend geriatric or debilitated patients not to take these drugs without a recommendation by their health-care provider. Generally, magnesium salts should be taken early in the day to reduce sleep interruption. The oral products should be taken with a full glass of alcohol- and caffeine-free fluid before eating to ensure that the drug reaches the bowel easily. If magnesium sulfate is recommended, suggest mixing it in chilled fruit juice or pouring the liquid over ice chips to increase palatability.

In general, magnesium-containing saline laxatives or cathartics should not be administered to children younger than two years. Pediatric doses are listed in Table 41–C.

Hyperosmotic Laxatives

Glycerin (glycerol), the major nonelectrolyte (nonsalt) hyperosmotic laxative, usually is given as a suppository. Liquid glycerin can be given as an enema. Glycerin evacuates the colon within 15 minutes to one hour after administration. It is a common home remedy for constipation.

Glycerin's actions are, like the saline laxatives and cathartics, due to local osmotic (water-withdrawing) actions, which also stimulate defecation by stretching the rectum. Since glycerin (like other osmotic agents) withdraws water from surrounding tissues, anticipate the possibility of anorectal irritation.

Stimulant (or Irritant-Stimulant) Laxatives and Cathartics

Drugs in this category include bisacodyl (as in DULCOLAX), phenolphthalein (as in AGORAL; CORRECTOL; EX-LAX; FEEN-A-MINT; PHENOLAX), and senna (SENOKOT). Castor oil, placed in its own category in some texts, may act through one of its metabolites as a stimulant laxative or cathartic.

Most of these agents stimulate gut motility and fluid movement into the intestines through actions on muscle and secretory cells. These drugs may cause a toxic effect on the intestinal mucosal cells.

Laxative or cathartic effects are dose-dependent, but for most patients initial administration of recommended doses usually produces a watery evacuation, with an onset from a few to six or eight hours, usually associated with gripping or cramping.

Virtually all the drugs are indicated for oral administration, but some are available as suppositories.

Most of the stimulants are excreted in maternal milk and should not be administered to nursing mothers without a physician's order. Castor oil, often used as a home remedy, should be used only for purging the gut before surgery or diagnostic procedures.

As a group, the effects of stimulant laxatives/cathartics on the GI tract are the least "natural." They should not be used as initial treatment of constipation, and they should not be administered for more than one week. All these drugs can produce excessive fluid loss, and their strong gut-stimulating actions can cause intestinal rupture if obstruction or weakening of the intestinal wall is present.

Chronic use can, like the magnesium salts, suppress normal bowel reflexes. They also pose the risk of causing "cathartic colon," in which the organ is paralyzed, dilated, and suffers increased mucosal permeability leading to possibly severe fluid and electrolyte alterations (similar in many ways to ulcerative colitis). This often can be detected as a decrease in bowel sounds on auscultation, and by altered tone of the abdomen on palpation.

Some stimulant-laxatives, such as CORRECTOL, PERI-COLACE, and SENOKOT S, are available as proprietary mixtures with docusate, a stool softener. However, as noted in the section on stool softeners, below, mixing these classes of drugs may be dangerous.

NURSING IMPLICATIONS

Discourage use of stimulants for initial treatment of constipation, and stress the need for acute administration only. Time the dose so that the relatively prompt effects do not disturb sleep. Advise patients that most liquid dosage forms of these drugs are poor tasting, and that administration with fruit juice, carbonated beverages, or ice chips may help increase palatability.

Be aware of the unique properties or side effects of the individual agents:

- Enteric-coated bisacodyl tablets should be swallowed whole, and should not be administered with alkaline substances (milk, milk of magnesia, other antacids), since doing so will cause premature tablet dissolution in the stomach, leading to severe GI distress.
- Advise lactating women that senna may cause a brown discoloration of the breast milk, and that drug excreted in the milk may cause diarrhea in nursing infants (and so should be avoided).
- Advise all patients taking phenolphthalein that if the urine is alkaline the drug may cause a pink or red discoloration. Also assess for respiratory distress, hypotension, or skin rashes, which may indicate a potentially (although uncommon) allergic response.
- Administer castor oil only on an empty stomach, since the drug inhibits gastric emptying, and discourage self-prescribing.

Stool Softeners

Stool softeners reduce surface tension of the stool and help form an emulsion between fats and water in the intestines, which can penetrate hard, dry stools. Because of this action they are sometimes classified as *emollient* laxatives. The most common stool softener is docusate sodium (dioctyl sodium sulfosuccinate), which is marketed under several brand names (eg, COLACE; MODANE SOFT). Related drugs are docusate calcium (SURFAK) and potassium (KASOF). They are supplied as capsules, tablets, or liquids for oral administration, and are one of the most common ingredients in single- and multiple-drug laxative products.

Stool softeners are best used to ease painful passage of hard stools, or to help the patient avoid straining during defecation. Effects occur between 12 and 72 hours after the first dose is taken.

These products are generally considered to be nonabsorbable and free from systemic toxicity. Nevertheless, their use should be limited to one week in the absence of a physician's prescription. Docusate apparently does not interfere with the absorption of nutrients from the GI tract. However, the stool softeners may increase the absorption of other drugs that the patient may take orally, including mineral oil. As a result, docusate products are labeled with a warning against concomitant use with other prescription drugs or mineral oil.

The sodium in docusate sodium may cause problems for patients with hypertension, edema, or heart failure. Docusate potassium or calcium contain less sodium, but the potassium and calcium may be absorbed and cause problems for patients at risk of hyperkalemia or hypercalcemia, respectively.

NURSING IMPLICATIONS

Monitor patients taking stool softeners for signs of increased effects or toxicity from other oral medications. Instruct them not to take other drugs, particularly mineral oil, concurrently, since the risk of adverse effects may be increased. Advise the patient that effects may not be seen for several days after initial drug administration.

Lubricants

Mineral oil (liquid petrolatum) is the only lubricant laxative available. The drug coats the fecal mass with an oily film that lubricates it and facilitates the passage of feces through the gut. The oily coat also serves as a barrier against absorption of water from the feces into the intestinal mucosa—an effect that otherwise tends to dry or harden the stool.

Mineral oil can be taken orally or given per rectum as an enema (FLEET MINERAL OIL ENEMA). The rectal route generally is preferred, for reasons to be noted shortly. Only pure mineral oil should be given as an enema; the pure product also is preferred for oral use over combination products containing other classes of laxatives.

Oral use of mineral oil can cause significant problems, including

- reduced absorption of dietary fat-soluble vitamins (A, D, E, and K), which may cause vitamin deficiency;
- leakage past the anal sphincter, causing anorectal irritation (pruritis ani) and aggravation of hemorrhoids or other anorectal lesions;
- possible damage to the spleen or liver owing to systemic absorption and eventual entry into the reticuloendothelial-lymphatic system; and
- possibly serious or fatal pneumonitis or pneumonia if fine droplets of the oil are aspirated owing to careless ingestion.

Risks associated with systemic absorption are increased by concomitant administration of stool softeners. The risk of lung problems is particularly great in geriatric patients.

NURSING IMPLICATIONS

Advise patients to avoid regular or frequent use of orally administered mineral oil, especially if the patient is elderly or debilitated. Concomitant use of mineral oil and stool softeners absolutely should be avoided.

Since food delays gastric emptying and delivery of mineral oil to its site of action, the drug should not be taken with meals. Bedtime administration is acceptable for most patients, but children, the elderly, and debilitated individuals may aspirate the drug during sleep.

Advise patients taking oral mineral oil to suck on a lemon or orange slice afterward to reduce the unpleasant oily aftertaste.

Monitor patients taking anticoagulants concurrently for increased bleeding tendencies associated with impaired absorption of vitamin K.

As for any patient who might require a laxative on an outpatient basis, be aware of the pertinent history of the pediatric, geriatric, or pregnant individual, the specific needs and limitations for each, and the relative safety of dietary modifications as a starting point. The following discussion assumes that potentially serious underlying problems have been ruled out.

◆ Use During Pregnancy and Lactation

Constipation in pregnancy is relatively common. Prime contributors include uterine pressure on the colon and the ingestion of constipating iron and calcium supplements. Here, too, if diet, fluid intake, and exercise are not satisfactory, careful use of a laxative may be appropriate; stool softeners or bulk-forming laxatives may be best.

Castor oil should be avoided because of its uterine-stimulating effect; mineral oil, used excessively, may interfere with maternal vitamin absorption, causing adverse fetal effects; and saline products may further increase maternal blood pressure if significant amounts are absorbed, or cause significant hypotension if excessive fluid and electrolyte loss occur.

Stimulants should be avoided, except on the advice of a physician, during both pregnancy and lactation.

◆ Use in Infants and Children

Increasing fluid or sugar intake may work best with infants, whereas older children are more apt to benefit from increased dietary intake of cereals, fruits, and vegetables. If laxatives are needed for neonates, consult a physician. For older children requiring drug intervention, palatability and ease of administration are almost as important as safety and efficacy. This largely limits the initial selection to glycerin suppositories or, for older children, a stool softener administered in three or four divided doses throughout the day. Discourage parents from giving stimulants, mineral oil, or enemas, or any product or route of administration for more than a week, without the supervision of a physician.

Use in the Elderly

Laxative therapy for the elderly person must consider age-related factors that increase the incidence of slow passage of the gut contents. They include inadequate diet or anorexia, the inability to chew food properly (as due to poor-fitting dentures or tooth loss), disease, decreased physical activity, and the likelihood of ingestion of many drugs that may cause constipation. The widespread advertising of drugs to help achieve regularity in the elderly patient also increases the risk of constipation as part of a laxative-antidiarrheal cycle.

Stool softeners or bulk-forming agents generally are preferred for mild constipation when alteration of lifestyle factors contributing to constipation cannot be corrected, or cannot be remedied quickly. Large amounts of water should be consumed with these products, not only to increase their efficacy, but also to reduce the risk of obstruction by powders and to facilitate swallowing.

Cathartics and enemas should be avoided because of the elderly patient's intolerance of marked fluid and electrolyte shifts. Saline laxatives and cathartics, in particular, are not suitable because of the increased systemic load of salts such as magnesium or sodium, which often are not excreted with sufficient speed to prevent systemic effects. Mineral oil should be avoided unless prescribed by a physician.

Antidiarrheal Drugs

Diarrhea can be defined as a significant increase in the frequency of defecation compared with what is normal for the individual. Because frequent defecation often does not allow for adequate absorption of water from the fecal mass into the circulation, diarrhea usually involves excreta that are very watery and poorly formed, although blood or fats may predominate in diarrhea of more serious functional or metabolic causes. Significant amounts of electrolytes and nutrients are also lost.

Like constipation, the causes and consequences of diarrhea can be trivial or serious, and in some cases no drug treatment is required. Diarrhea may be caused by diet, emotional factors, and numerous drugs. Bacteria or protozoa often contribute to "travelers' diarrhea," and viruses are perhaps the most common cause of diarrhea in infants and young children. Diarrhea is often a common accompaniment of systemic disorders that may be common and relatively innocuous (such as flu), or it may be due to more serious problems such as cancer, neuropathy, sepsis, or gut disorders such as ulcerative colitis. The changes of gut motility that occur in diarrhea are often secondary to either decreased absorption of water from the GI tract or increased secretion of ions and fluid into it.

General Characteristics of Antidiarrheal Drugs

Pharmacologic Effects

The four general groups of antidiarrheal agents are the adsorbents, opiates, antimuscarinics (atropine-like drugs), and antibiotics. The adsorbents act locally in the GI tract to bind noxious substances that are stimulating gut motility or secretions. Antimuscarinics and opiates act systemically to suppress gut motility, either through a direct action on intestinal smooth muscle or via the nerves that stimulate the muscle.

Agents in any of these classes may be suitable for treating diarrhea due to a variety of "nonspecific" causes. Antibiotics are used specifically for diarrhea caused by infection.

Some brand name products contain more than one class of antidiarrheal drug. Many OTC antidiarrheal products are available; those containing opiates are usually available only by prescription.

Misuse of, and Valid Indications for, Antidiarrheal Drugs

Acute diarrhea lasts three days or less. It usually has a sudden onset and may be accompanied by a generalized feeling of weakness, flatulence, periodic mild intestinal cramping, a slight fever, and perhaps vomiting. In most instances, and when the patient is otherwise healthy, diarrhea caused by travel, emotional changes, diet, the first meal after a fast, or acute intolerance of recently started drug therapy, will subside spontaneously. For these individuals, who suffer acute nonspecific diarrhea, antidiarrheal drug therapy need not (and usually should not) be instituted.

Acute diarrhea is not likely to cause dehydration unless the patient is very young, very old, or debilitated.

Recommend professional evaluation for these patients. In infants, for example, only a couple of days of severe diarrhea can deplete body water and electrolyte stores sufficiently to cause circulatory collapse.

Advise adults complaining of acute nonspecific diarrhea that is not accompanied by fever or more worrisome symptoms to assess the possible causes and eliminate them if possible. They should begin a bland diet that excludes spicy foods, alcohol, and other substances that, based on their personal experience, cause GI distress. Recommend clear broths, gelatin desserts, and caffeine-free soft drinks that have been allowed to go flat (stir well in an open glass). Milk should be avoided since most patients with diarrhea are intolerant of the lactose (sugar) that it contains. (This is one reason why breast-feeding infants who experience chronic or recurrent diarrhea may be switched to a lactose-free formula.) If diarrhea can be traced to a prescribed drug that the patient has begun taking, a health-care professional should be consulted.

Misuse of laxative and cathartic drugs also may lead to inappropriate use of antidiarrheal agents. Patients who take excessive doses of laxatives or cathartics for perceived constipation then may perceive that they have developed diarrhea, and may take one of the readily available OTC antidiarrheal medications, often excessively, to combat the problem. Doing so may harden the stool or decrease the frequency of movements, so that they have again become "constipated." A laxative-antidiarrheal cycle starts, and it may be difficult to break.

Physicians may prescribe one of the drugs noted in the following section for acute nonspecific diarrhea. Other accepted indications for drug therapy of acute diarrhea are for persons who travel to areas where water or food supplies are likely to be unsanitary, and for young children who develop diarrhea caused by enteric infections.

Chronic diarrhea lasts more than three days, is not responsive to the nondrug measures noted above, or is recurrent. It requires immediate evaluation by a health-care professional so that serious underlying causes such as infection or disease can be identified or eliminated.

The medication history should give particular attention to drugs that are well known for their ability to cause diarrhea. These include antacids (particularly magnesium salts); many antibiotics (especially broad-spectrum agents likely to alter gut flora: ampicillin, erythromycin and related agents, tetracyclines, cephalosporins, and trimethoprim/sulfamethoxazole); most cancer chemotherapeutic agents; radiation therapy; and virtually all laxatives/cathartics (especially if used excessively). The antihypertensive drug reserpine, which causes a syndrome of "parasympathetic predominance," also usually causes diarrhea. If diarrhea is drug-induced, discontinuation of the drug, or substitution of another drug, may be all that is indicated.

Failure to treat chronic diarrhea can lead to severe fluid and electrolyte imbalances in any patient. Other situations requiring immediate medical evaluation and care include diarrhea accompanied by high fever (greater than 101°F; this implies that the temperature of all patients with diarrhea should be checked), severe abdominal pain, severe vomiting, evidence of blood loss from the GI tract (coffee-ground stools; bloody stool or vomitus), or fatty stool (steatorrhea). Physicians usually will start antidiarrheal therapy after initial attempts to make the diagnosis.

NURSING IMPLICATIONS

Few antidiarrheal agents are better than a placebo, or the nondrug treatment plan noted earlier, for managing *acute nonspecific diarrhea*. In general, they should not be recommended for self-medication without prior evaluation by a health-care professional. Evaluation always should attempt to identify underlying causes, including the use of diarrhea-causing drugs and serious disease.

All antidiarrheal drugs should be used with extreme care in any patient in whom constipation must be avoided.

Depending on the type of antidiarrheal agent, the actions of other orally administered drugs may be increased or decreased by altered systemic absorption, and patients must be monitored for signs of drug overdose. If concomitant drug administration is necessary for hospitalized patients, inquire about alternative routes of administration of potential interactants. Patients should take at least 3000 mL of fluid per day until diarrhea resolves, to compensate for fluid loss. Parenteral fluid and electrolyte administration may be required for patients with severe or prolonged diarrhea, or for patients who are debilitated.

Major Classes of Antidiarrheals

Adsorbents

Adsorbents act locally to bind noxious substances that can stimulate the gut and produce diarrhea, including irritating foods, drugs, and bacterial products. Activated charcoal, which is used routinely in the emergency management of oral drug overdoses, acts as an adsorbent, but it is not used often for routine diarrhea. Adsorbents are generally safe drugs, but few of them have demonstrated efficacy for managing acute diarrhea. Their beneficial adsorbent action, which accounts for their efficacy in managing diarrhea, also accounts for their significant and often unwanted ability to reduce the absorption of other drugs that the patient may be taking orally. Unlike the opiate and antimuscarinic antidiarrheal agents, adsorbents may be used safely for diarrhea caused by enteral bacteria or some cases of drug ingestion.

The most widely used antidiarrheal adsorbent is kaolin (hydrated aluminum silicate). It is combined with another adsorbent compound, pectin, in proprietary medications such as KAOPECTATE. They are common ingredients in OTC antidiarrheal drugs. The recommended dose (see Table 41–C) should be taken after every loose stool.

Calcium polycarbophil (MITROLAN), identified earlier as a bulk-forming *laxative,* can be used to treat diarrhea. When polycarbophil is taken as a laxative it is taken with large amounts of water. The bulky mass that forms facilitates normal defecation. When used for diarrhea, polycarbophil is taken with only the small amount of water needed to enable swallowing after the tablets are chewed thoroughly. Limited ingestion of water allows the drug to adsorb the extra fluid in the gut; this tends to help form the stool and suppress diarrhea.

Bismuth subsalicylate, the active ingredient in PEPTO-BISMOL and some other proprietary products, is one of the few nonprescription medications with some demonstrated efficacy for preventing and managing traveler's diarrhea, in which the major problem is impure food or water supplies. Bismuth "subsalts" act not only as adsorbents but also as GI protectants. Bismuth salts also have some local antimicrobial action. The recommended dose should be taken with the onset of diarrhea and following each unformed stool.

Although the amount of salicylate in bismuth subsalicylate that is absorbed is relatively low, the drug nevertheless should be used with care in any patient who should not take the prototype salicylate, aspirin (Chapter 52).

Other adsorbents include attapulgite (KAOPECTATE ADVANCED FORMULA; CHILDREN'S KAOPECTATE, others), which generally is used for nonspecific diarrhea; and cholestyramine resin (QUESTRAN), which is used mainly for diarrhea resulting from excess secretion of bile salts.

NURSING IMPLICATIONS

Administer adsorbents after every loose stool unless instructed otherwise by a physician. Advise patients that bismuth-containing products will cause a harmless darkening of the tongue or stool. The stool should be examined closely, since discoloration may be confused with bleeding or melena. Frequent administration of adsorbents usually interferes significantly with the absorption of most other orally administered drugs. Monitor for signs of apparent underdosing of interactants, and be prepared to use alternative dosage schedules or routes of administration if needed actions are diminished.

Opiates

The constipating effects of morphine, codeine, and other narcotic analgesics have been known for years. However, because of their central nervous system (CNS) depressant actions and their potential for abuse, they are not used commonly to treat diarrhea. Paregoric (camphorated tincture of opium) has similar constipating effects, and less abuse potential than the narcotic analgesics. However, sale of this Schedule V drug without prescription may be restricted in some states.

Two narcotic derivatives, diphenoxylate (in LOMOTIL, combined with atropine) and loperamide (IMODIUM, IMODIUM A-D, which is available without prescription), are used more frequently because they are relatively free of analgesic, euphoric, or abuse-promoting effects. Their main effects are on the gut; they cause few effects elsewhere. Diphenoxylate and loperamide decrease the propulsive movements of the ileum and colon, allowing more time for water to be absorbed from the fecal contents. They also increase the tone of the external anal sphincter and blunt the subjective response to sensations caused by a full rectum. They generally are used for managing acute diarrhea of nonspecific origin, or for chronic diarrhea from causes such as inflammatory bowel disease. Dosages are noted in Table 41–C.

The dose of atropine in LOMOTIL is subtherapeutic in terms of antidiarrheal activity. Atropine is included to increase the likelihood of unpleasant side effects so that potential drug abusers would be less likely to take high doses for the opiate-like effects of diphenoxylate. Nevertheless, the amount of atropine in this product is sufficient to cause serious adverse effects in persons for whom atropine or other antimuscarinics are contraindicated (see Chapter 13).

Prescribe opiates cautiously for patients with a history of drug abuse. Although they can potentiate the actions of any other oral medication, the greatest problems are likely to occur when taken with other CNS-depressant drugs (see Table 41–I). Opiates and antimuscarinics, both of which have antispasmodic action but no ability to adsorb substances in the gut, generally are contraindicated when diarrhea is due to enteric bacteria or toxic drugs.

NURSING IMPLICATIONS

Monitor patients taking diphenoxylate or loperamide for CNS depression that may indicate excessive doses, systemic absorption, or interactions with other CNS-depressant drugs. Observe patients taking LOMOTIL for signs of adverse atropine-like side effects as well (see the next section). Caution patients about potential risks from occasional drug-induced dizziness or drowsiness, which might interfere with safe performance of tasks requiring alertness and good reflexes. Be aware of laws that govern the availability of opiate antidiarrheal agents. These drugs, and products that contain them, are abused by the lay public and health-care professionals alike.

Antimuscarinics

Atropine and many related agents block both the spasmogenic and acid secretory effects of acetylcholine. They are used mainly to manage diarrhea that is secondary to peptic ulcer disease or irritable bowel syndromes. The major disadvantage of these drugs, compared with drugs such as diphenoxylate, is that they lack GI specificity. Systemic atropine-like side effects are common (see Chapter 13). Some proprietary products (eg, DONNAGEL; DONNAGEL-PG; DONNATAL) combine atropine with two other atropine-like alkaloids, hyoscyamine and scopolamine. Some of these formulations also contain powdered opium, phenobarbital, or kaolin and pectin. They have questionable efficacy, and clearly are contraindicated in patients who should not take atropine.

NURSING IMPLICATIONS

Rule out glaucoma, prostatic hypertrophy, and obstruction of the GI or urinary tracts before administering drugs with atropine-like actions, including LOMOTIL. Observe patients for signs of adverse atropine-like effects such as eye pain, impaired micturition, or constipation. Nursing measures to relieve atropine-like side effects are discussed in Chapter 13.

Antibiotics

Some cases of diarrhea are caused by bacteria, usually *Escherichia coli* or shigella. Bacterial-induced diarrhea is most common in children and travelers. Colistin sulfate (COLY-MYCIN S) oral suspension is used commonly in pediatric patients. Colistin acts mainly in the GI tract, but small amounts of the drug can be absorbed systemically; signs of renal toxicity, such as azotemia, should be looked for. Doxycycline, taken at a dose of 100 mg per day, may also significantly reduce the incidence of traveler's diarrhea.

The probable antibiotic/antidiarrheal effects of bismuth salts were noted above. See Chapter 56 for more information.

SUMMARY OF NURSING IMPLICATIONS

◆ Assessment

Determine previously normal bowel habits and possible expected and innocuous causes for temporary irregularity (travel, diet changes, stress).

Establish self-medicating history with laxatives, cathartics, or antidiarrheal agents, or any other drug that may cause constipation or diarrhea.

Obtain a complete nursing history that includes indications for immediate medical care; prolonged gut irregularity of any sort; severe abdominal or rectal pain; GI bleeding; fatty stool; high fever; excessive drug use; underlying disease; recent changes in drug therapy or disease symptoms; extremes of age.

Check for normal bowel sounds, evidence of fecal impaction, gut bleeding, abdominal pain, tenderness, or distention before administering laxatives or cathartics.

Review history for glaucoma, prostatic hypertrophy, or obstruction of the GI or urinary tract before administering drugs with atropine-like actions.

◆ Nursing Diagnoses

Constipation or diarrhea related to inactivity, dietary changes, disease process, or medication:

Altered nutrition: less than body requirements related to impaired bowel absorption.

High risk for fluid volume deficit related to diarrhea.

Knowledge deficit related to newly prescribed medication (specify laxative, cathartic, antidiarrheal, or other).

◆ Planning/Implementation

Monitor all patients taking laxatives, cathartics, or antidiarrheals for inadequate therapeutic response, decreased or increased (toxic) effects of other orally administered medications.

Administer potential interactants at least one or two hours before or after giving laxatives, cathartics, or antidiarrheals. Be prepared for alternate routes of administration if interactions occur because of altered absorption of drug.

Monitor all patients taking laxative/cathartics, especially saline agents, for signs of excessive fluid or electrolyte loss.

Observe for signs of neuromuscular changes owing to magnesium intoxication when magnesium salts (eg, milk of magnesia) are given (see Chapter 40).

Administer milk of magnesia at bedtime or earlier; give other magnesium salts, which act faster, early in the day to avoid interrupted sleep.

Give adsorbent-type antidiarrheals after every loose stool unless instructed otherwise.

Monitor patients taking diphenoxylate or loperamide for CNS depression that may indicate overdose, systemic absorption, or interactions with other CNS depressants.

Observe for signs of adverse atropine-like effects with anticholinergic drugs or medications containing them (eg, LOMOTIL): eye pain, impaired micturition, constipation, tachycardia.

◆ Patient and Family Education

Teach the patient/family:

Nondrug measures to prevent irregularity (eg, bulk in diet, exercise for constipation, bland diet for diarrhea, fluids to soften stool).

That laxatives, cathartics, or antidiarrheal drugs are indicated for specific problems and for short-term use only.

To stir bulk-forming laxatives well in a full glass of cool liquid before taking.

To drink six to eight glasses of nonalcoholic liquid per day until the stool softens or until otherwise directed.

To avoid taking oral bisacodyl with alkaline laxatives, antacids, beverages, or stool softeners.

To record the frequency and characteristics of bowel movements.

◆ Evaluation

The patient/family will:

Establish a normal pattern of bowel elimination.

Comply with medication regimen; report side effects or lack of drug effectiveness.

Recognize the importance of dietary factors, hydration, and activity in maintaining or restoring normal bowel function.

Avoid or resolve untoward side effects.

Annotated Bibliography

Ashkenazi S, Cleary TG: Antibiotic treatment of bacterial gastroenteritis. *Pediatr Infect Dis J* 1991; 10(2):140–148. *Good coverage of assessment, diagnosis, and treatment, when the cause of diarrhea is thought to be bacterial.*

Castle SC, Cantrell M, Israel DS, Samuelson MJ: Constipation prevention: Empiric use of stool softeners questioned. *Geriatrics* 1991; 46(11):84–86. *This short article addresses important issues related to the almost routine use of "mild" laxatives.*

Ericsson CD, Johnson PC: Safety and efficacy of loperamide. *Am J Med* 1990; 88(6A):10S–14S. *Compares and contrasts ioperamide with another OTC antidiarrheal, bismuth subsalicylate (in PEPTO-BISMOL), and diphenoxylate atropine.*

Gorbach SL: Bismuth therapy in gastrointestinal diseases. *Gastroenterol* 1990; 99(3):863–875. *Covers diarrhea therapy, a current use for bismuth, and a potential new role in peptic ulcer disease. Important reading, given the frequent use and potential misuse of OTC bismuth (as in PEPTO-BISMOL).*

Longe RL: Antidiarrheal and other gastrointestinal products. In: *Handbook of Nonprescription Drugs,* E.G. Feldmann, ed. Washington, D.C., American Pharmaceutical Association 1990:313–332. *Perhaps the best all-in-one-place source for information about the uses, actions, and formulations of OTC antidiarrheals; indispensable patient teaching information.*

Spees DN: Health risks of foreign travel. Preparing adults for jaunts abroad. *Postgrad Med* 1991; 89(8):147–150, 153, 156. *Good advice for preparing travelers to areas where diarrhea can do much more than spoil an otherwise enjoyable trip.*

Yakabowich M: Prescribe with care. The role of laxatives in the treatment of constipation. *J Gerontol Nurs* 1990; 16(7):4–11. *Learn more about alternatives to laxatives and cathartics, plus what to do when these drugs must be used; an excellent review of the topic.*

Table 41–C **Clinical Uses and Administration of Laxatives, Cathartics, and Antidiarrheal Drugs***

AGENT	CLINICAL USES	DOSAGE AND ROUTE OF ADMINISTRATION
	Laxatives and Cathartics	
	Bulk-Forming Agents	
Calcium polycarbophil (FIBERCON, MITROLAN)	Management of constipation when drug therapy is indicated	Oral: Adults: Chew and swallow, with at least 8 oz. of water per dose, 2 tablets qid or as needed (not to exceed 12 tablets/24 hr). Children 6–12 years: 1 tablet tid (do not exceed 6 tablets/24 hr); 3–6 years: 1 tablet bid (not to exceed 3 tablets/24 hr); take with water as for adults
Psyllium (eg, METAMUCIL)	Management of constipation as for calcium polycarbophil; constipation associated with anorectal disorders	Oral: Adults: Usually 1 unit dose (about 3.4 g) mixed with cool water or fruit juice 1–3 times daily until return of regularity (usually 2 or 3 days). Children ≥6 years: Usually half the adult dose
	Hyperosmotic Laxative	
Glycerin	Evacuation of colon	Suppository: Adults: 1 suppository (3 g). Children ≥6 years: Pediatric suppository or one third–one half adult suppository
	Lubricant	
Mineral oil (liquid petrolatum)	See docusate sodium	Oral: Adults: 15–45 mL. Children ≥6 years: 5–15 mL Retention enema: Adults 90 to 120 mL, once daily. Children 2–11 years: 30–60 mL
	Saline Laxatives/Cathartics	
Magnesium citrate	Bowel evacuation prior to surgery, diagnostic procedures; gut cleansing in parasitic or worm infestations, etc	Oral: Usually 1 dose of 200–240 mL/day as bottled (11–18 g/day). Children: 2–6 years: Usually one fourth the adult dose; 6–12 years: Usually one half the adult dose
Magnesium hydroxide (milk of magnesia)	Short-term management of functional constipation not remedied by diet, etc	Oral: Adults: 30–60 mL. Children: <6 years: 5–15 mL; 6–12 years: 15–30 mL.
Magnesium sulfate (epsom salts)	See magnesium citrate, hydroxide	Oral: Adults: 10 to 30 g in glass of water or juice; Children: 5–10 g in glass of water or juice Rectal: Adults 135 mL. Children: 2–12 years: 34–68 mL.
Sodium phosphate plus biphosphate (FLEET PHOSPHO-SODA)	See magnesium citrate, hydroxide	Oral: Adults: Usually 20–30 mL of solution containing 18 g sodium phosphate and 48 g sodium biphosphate per 100 mL, mixed in cool water. Children: Usually 5–15 mL of above solution
Bisacodyl (DULCOLAX)	Short-term management of functional constipation; gut evacuation as for magnesium citrate	Oral: As laxative, 10–15 mg; as cathartic, up to 30 mg. Children ≥6 years: 5–10 mg Rectal suppository: Adults: 1 10-mg suppository. Children ≥6 years: one half adult suppository For preoperative or prediagnostic gut evacuation, may give tablets night before, suppository on morning of procedure

(continued)

Table 41–C | Clinical Uses and Administration of Laxatives, Cathartics, and Antidiarrheal Drugs* (*Continued*)

AGENT	CLINICAL USES	DOSAGE AND ROUTE OF ADMINISTRATION
	Stimulant Laxatives/Cathartics	
Castor oil	Evacuation of lower bowel	Oral: Adults, children ≥12 years: 15–30 mL. Children 2–12 years: 5–15 mL
Phenolphthalein (EX-LAX, FEEN-A-MINT, MODANE)	See danthron	Oral: 60–200 mg; not recommended for children
Senna (SENOKOT; X-PREP)	See bisacodyl	Oral: Powder: Adults: 0.5–2 g. Children >2 years: One third to one half adult dose. Fluid extract: Adults 2 mL. Syrup: Adults: 8 mL. Children 6–12 years: 2 mL Rectal suppository: Adults: 625 mg–1 g. Children >60 lbs: 0.5 g
	Stool Softeners	
Docusate sodium (COLACE, MODANE SOFT)	Softening of hard, dry stool, especially in patients who should not strain to defecate	Oral: Adults, children ≥12 years: 50–500 mg daily; initial doses usually in high range, reduced with onset of action. Children 2–12 years: 25–150 mg daily Rectal: 5 to 10 mL of 10 mg/mL solution added to retention enema
	Antidiarrheal Drugs	
	Adsorbents	
Bismuth salts (PEPTO-BISMOL)	Short-term management of diarrhea, including traveler's diarrhea (prophylaxis and treatment)	Oral: Adults: 300–600 mg at onset of diarrhea and after every loose stool. Children: 100–300 mg at onset of diarrhea and after every loose stool.
Calcium polycarbophil (MITROLAN)	Diarrhea, especially due to irritable bowel syndrome, related disorders	Oral: Doses are same as for polycarbophil as laxative (see above), but should *not* be taken with water; dose may be repeated every 30 min, but total daily dose should not be exceeded
Kaolin plus pectin (eg, KAOPECTATE)	Short-term management of diarrhea	Oral: Adults: Dosage varies with product; usually 60 to 120 mL after each loose stool; each 30 mL of regular-strength product contains about 6 g kaolin plus 130 mg pectin; see product information for concentrates. Children: One fourth to one half the adult dose.

(continued)

Table 41–C **Clinical Uses and Administration of Laxatives, Cathartics, and Antidiarrheal Drugs* (*Continued*)**

AGENT	CLINICAL USES	DOSAGE AND ROUTE OF ADMINISTRATION
	Opiates	
Diphenoxylate		
(in LOMOTIL)	See kaolin	Oral: Adults: Usually 2 tablets or tsp 3 or 4 times daily. Children >2 years: Usually 0.3–0.4 mg/kg daily in 4 equal divided doses
Loperamide		
(IMODIUM)	See kaolin	Oral: Adults: Initially, 4 mg, followed by 2 mg after each unformed stool; do not exceed total of 8 mg/day for more than 2 days. Children 2–12 years: One fourth to one half the adult dose.
	Antibiotic	
Colistin		
(COLY-MYCIN)	Treatment of diarrhea due to *E coli,* shigella, in children	Oral: 5–15 mg/kg daily in 3 divided doses

*Dosages and proprietary names are for single-ingredient products only. Most laxatives and cathartics are available OTC; review dosage information on the label of each product with the patient or person responsible for administration. Many products are packaged as unit doses; one "unit" (packet, measuring spoon, etc) provides the usual dose.

Table 41–S Major Side Effects of and Contraindications for Laxatives, Cathartics, and Antidiarrheal Drugs

BODY SYSTEM/ Side Effect	CONTRAINDICATION/ PRECAUTION	COMMENTS AND NURSING IMPLICATIONS
Major Side Effects Involving Laxatives aad Cathartics		
For All Classes		
GASTROINTESTINAL Mechanical damage to gut (eg, rupture)	Gut weakness or obstruction	Do not administer in presence of gut pain, swelling, tenderness, or fever (might indicate appendicitis, other GI infection or inflammation); avoid additional doses if first does not produce anticipated effect by expected onset of activity
Excessive fluid/electrolyte loss, systemic imbalances	Vomiting, diarrhea	Most likely with saline laxatives/cathartics, stimulant-irritants; withhold drug if vomiting or diarrhea (other than expected drug effect) are present or develop
	Simple acute constipation	Discourage laxative or cathartic use for simple acute constipation that can be corrected with nondrug measures
Bulk-Forming Agents and Stool Softeners (eg, psyllium)		
GASTROINTESTINAL Gastrointestinal pain, obstruction; fecal impactions	Dysphagia; preexisting obstruction or perforation of gut	Mix powder well in full glass of water or other cool liquid before swallowing; recommend drinking additional liquid after taking drug; immediately report esophageal or other GI pain, or constipation lasting more than 2 days.
Saline Laxatives/Cathartics (eg, magnesium salts)		
NEUROMUSCULAR AND CARDIOVASCULAR Weakness, depressed reflexes, lethargy, hypotension, bradycardia	Renal failure	Are major signs of hypermagnesemia; risk increased in geriatric patients, those with poor renal function
Edema, weight gain, increased blood pressure, worsening of CHF	Edema, hypertension, CHF	Applies mainly to products containing sodium phosphates
GASTROINTESTINAL Cramping, retching, vomiting, diarrhea	Renal failure; preexisting gut obstruction or perforation; fluid and electrolyte imbalances	Because of prompt effect and to prevent interruption of sleep, administer in morning; counsel patient against frequent or prolonged use.
Stimulant Laxatives/Cathartics (eg, bisacodyl)		
GASTROINTESTINAL See saline laxatives/cathartics		Side effects, precautions, interventions similar to those of saline agents; will not cause hypermagnesemia; rectal irritation may occur with suppositories

(continued)

Table 41–S | **Major Side Effects of and Contraindications for Laxatives, Cathartics, and Antidiarrheal Drugs (*Continued*)**

BODY SYSTEM/ Side Effect	CONTRAINDICATION/ PRECAUTION	COMMENTS AND NURSING IMPLICATIONS
	Lubricant (mineral oil)	
RESPIRATORY Pneumonitis, pneumonia		Pulmonary damage can occur due to aspiration or absorption of ingested drug; discourage use in geriatric, pediatric, debilitated patients
GASTROINTESTINAL Diarrhea; pruritis ani; impaired healing of rectal wounds, hemorrhoids	See saline laxative/cathartics for major contraindications	Discourage use in geriatric, pediatric, debilitated patients; discourage any frequent use
NUTRITIONAL Deficiencies of fat-soluble vitamins (A, D, E, K)		Occurs with repeated oral use; discourage this practice
	Major Side Effects Involving Antidiarrheal Drugs	
	For All Classes	
GASTROINTESTINAL Constipation, risk of impaction, gut damage	Simple acute constipation; intestinal obstruction	Discourage use for mild, acute diarrhea, especially due to minor causes that can be dealt with using nondrug measures
	Adsorbents	
GASTROINTESTINAL Constipation, fecal impaction; darkening of the stool	Constipation; gut obstruction	Discourage frequent use or use after normalization of stool; monitor for signs of bloating, abdominal pain, hard stools; stool darkening may mask blood in stool; do not use in patients with suspected GI bleeding or ulcer disease
	Antimuscarinics/Anticholinergics	
EYE Ocular pain; mydriasis; blurred vision	Glaucoma	Assess for eye pain that may indicate undiagnosed glaucoma; occurs with LOMOTIL due to atropine content
GASTROINTESTINAL, GENITOURINARY Constipation; paralytic ileus; urinary hesitancy or retention	Obstruction of gut or urinary tract; prostatic hypertrophy	May be due to both opiate and (in LOMOTIL) atropine; monitor, have patient report, difficulty or pain associated with defecating, urinating
Dry mouth		Due to atropine in LOMOTIL
Persistent diarrhea	Diarrhea due to ingested drugs, poisons	Antispasmodic drugs cause retention of toxins, drugs, in GI tract: remove poisons or toxins from GI tract first, either by suction, emesis, or cathartics, before beginning antidiarrheal therapy
	Antibiotics	
	See Individual Agents in Chapter 56	

Table 41–I **Major Interactions Between Laxatives, Cathartics, and Antidiarrheal Agents and Other Agents**

AGENT	RESULT OF INTERACTION	COMMENTS AND NURSING IMPLICATIONS
Interactions Involving Most Laxatives/Cathartics		
Most other drugs given orally	Decreased therapeutic response to interactant	Increased gut motility may decrease time for other drugs to be absorbed; take other oral medications no sooner than 1 or 2 h before or after a saline agent (or use alternate administration routes); monitor responses to interactant
Interactions Involving Calcium Polycarbophil (Bulk-Forming Laxative)		
Tetracycline antibiotics (Chapter 56)	Reduced tetracycline absorption, antibiotic effect	Due to release of free calcium from laxative, which binds, reduces absorption of tetracyclines; avoid interaction, use alternative bulk-forming laxatives; also applies to polycarbophil use as antidiarrheal
Interactions with All or Selected Stimulant Laxatives/Cathartics		
Antacids	Gastric irritation due to bisacodyl	Antacids (and milk) increase gastric pH and cause premature dissolution of enteric-coated bisacodyl tablets; take interactants no sooner than 1 h before or after bisacodyl
Interactions with Stool Softeners		
Mineral oil	Increased risk of systemic toxicity of mineral oil	Docusate reduces surface tension, increases absorption of mineral oil, increasing deposition in lymph nodes, spleen, liver; avoid interaction
Stimulant laxatives	Increased risk of hepatotoxicity, other systemic effects, elimination into breast milk	Docusate increases system absorption of stimulant laxatives (eg, bisacodyl); avoid interaction
Interactions with Lubricant (Mineral Oil)		
Oral anticoagulants (Chapter 35)	Increased or decreased anticoagulant action	Impaired vitamin K absorption due to mineral oil may potentiate anticoagulant action; decreased anticoagulant absorption may antagonize anticoagulant effect; assess for signs of excessive bleeding or thrombosis; monitor prothrombin time more closely if necessary; discourage use during pregnancy
Stool softeners	See above	
Interactions Involving Antidiarrheal Drugs		
Interactions with Adsorbents		
Most other oral drugs	Decreased therapeutic response to interactant	Adsorbents bind, reduce absorption of most other oral medications; due to frequent need to administer adsorbents, monitor response to interactions with particular care
Interactions with Opiates		
Alcohol, anticonvulsants, antidepressants, antipsychotics, barbiturates, benzodiazepines, narcotic analgesics (Chapters 21–26)	Increased risk of excessive CNS depression	Decreased GI transit of other drugs may increase their absorption; potentiation of CNS depression possible
Interactions with Antidiarrheal Drugs Containing Antimuscarinics		
Other drugs with atropine-like actions (antidepressants, antihistamines, antipsychotics; disopyramide) (Chapter 13, Table 13-2)	Increased risk of atropine poisoning	Interaction due to possible increased absorption of interactant that produces cholinergic blockade

PROTOTYPE

Syrup of Ipecac 835

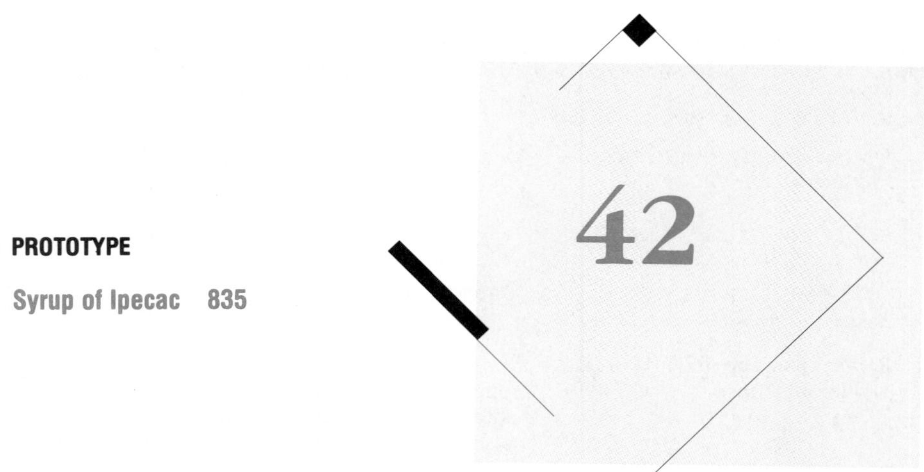

42

Emetic and Antiemetic Drugs

The drugs discussed in this chapter are used either to produce **emesis** (emetics) or to prevent or treat nausea and vomiting (antiemetics). Although the unpleasant sensations of nausea and vomiting are commonly attributed to the gastrointestinal (GI) tract, their triggers originate in the brain, which is the major site of action of emetic and antiemetic drugs.

Vomiting

The vomiting center, located near the medulla oblongata, integrates sensory nerve impulses caused by noxious stimuli from peripheral sites such as the gastric mucosa and the labyrinth of the ear. Some incoming impulses are processed by the chemoreceptor trigger zone (CTZ), a structure that lies near the medulla. The CTZ itself can be a source of noxious sensory stimuli. It lies outside the blood–brain barrier and is bathed by the systemic circulation, which exposes it to many drugs that cause nausea or vomiting as side effects.

Stimulation of the vomiting center sends neural impulses centrally to autonomic control centers located near the CTZ, and to peripheral structures such as the GI tract. Dopamine appears to have an important role in this process, and drugs with dopamine-like activity (for example, dopamine itself, levodopa, and morphine) often cause nausea and vomiting.

Stimulation of the CTZ first causes generalized activation of the autonomic nervous system, producing salivation, sweating, peripheral vasoconstriction, and rapid or irregular heart rates. Respiration accelerates or becomes labored. Shortly thereafter, respiration deepens and intraabdominal and thoracic pressures rise. These effects, combined with cyclic stimulation and relaxation of the gastric and esophageal musculature, propel the gastric contents back and forth between the stomach and esophagus. Eventually there is a deep inspiration, the glottis closes, and vomitus is propelled up the esophagus.

Drugs that stimulate the CTZ cause nausea and vomiting, whereas drugs that suppress its activity suppress these symptoms.

I. Emetic Drugs

Only two drugs, syrup of ipecac and apomorphine, are used clinically to induce vomiting. Ipecac is used much more, and is considered the prototype.

Major reference tables appear beginning on p. 843.

PROTOTYPE

Syrup of Ipecac

Syrup of ipecac is prepared from the dried roots of a South and Central American plant. The drug is available over-the-counter (OTC) as a first-aid measure for drug poisoning, and is found in virtually every hospital emergency room and poison center.

Absorption, Distribution, Metabolism, and Excretion

Ipecac is given orally. It can be absorbed from the GI tract, but the expected emetic effect expels drug from the GI tract and normally limits absorption and resulting systemic effects.

Pharmacologic Effects

The actions of ipecac are not fully known. They probably involve stimulation of the CTZ and local irritation of the GI tract. Since the CTZ is located close to respiratory and autonomic control centers, emetics may cause many of the peripheral autonomic and respiratory signs and symptoms that usually occur before vomiting, as described earlier.

Clinical Indications and Administration

Inducing Emesis

Ipecac is used to induce vomiting in patients who have ingested toxic doses of drugs, poisons, or other dangerous chemicals. Emetics act according to a very simple principle: by evacuating the contents of the stomach they reduce the time available for absorption of substances that have been taken orally. As noted in the following section, there are several general but very important situations in which induced vomiting is contraindicated.

Neither ipecac nor the related drug apomorphine is a specific antidote for any other drug or poison, but they are valuable first-aid measures, when used properly, for treating oral poisoning from a variety of agents. A more complete discussion of the treatment of poison emergencies is presented in Appendix C.

The usual emetic dose of syrup of ipecac for adults or children 10 years or older is 30 mL. Emetics do not work well when given on an empty stomach, so give at least three to four glasses of water (reduce the volume, based on body weight, for children) immediately after giving the ipecac. Vomiting usually occurs in less than 30 minutes. A second dose may be given if vomiting does not occur in this time. Adults should receive no more than 60 mL of ipecac. Dosages and dose limits for younger patients are noted in Table 42–C.

If the patient has ingested a toxin that can be absorbed systemically, activated charcoal may be (and often is) administered orally after emetic drug administration. This is another way to limit toxin absorption. The charcoal then is removed by direct gastric suction. If there will be an unavoidable delay in administering an emetic, the charcoal can be given first, followed by parenteral administration of apomorphine. Ipecac should not be used after administration of charcoal, which antagonizes its effects.

NURSING IMPLICATIONS

Determine the name and amount of substance ingested, if possible, before administering an emetic. Do not give more than two doses of an emetic to an individual to induce vomiting; if the patient is younger than one year old, give only one dose. Excessive doses of any emetic may cause violent and relentless vomiting, resulting in fluid and electrolyte loss, and possibly circulatory collapse. Many poison centers recommend administering an emetic drug in the hospital to induce vomiting, even if the poisoning has caused spontaneous vomiting earlier.

Expectorant

One of ipecac's expected actions is to stimulate respiratory tract secretions, and so the drug sometimes is used as an expectorant. It is found in a few proprietary antitussive products. The usual dose of ipecac in these products is less than 2 mg, about a thousand times less than the average emetic dose. Nevertheless, some GI upset or nausea and vomiting may occur when recommended or excessive doses are taken. Expectorants using guaifenesin or terpin hydrate generally are preferred. If an ipecac-containing product is used, limit administration to one week.

Side Effects, Adverse Reactions, and Contraindications

Emetics cause most of the unpleasant symptoms associated with vomiting. They initially produce central nervous system (CNS), respiratory, and cardiovascular stimulation (Table 42–S). After vomiting occurs, these systems may be depressed enough to require intervention. Aspiration of vomitus, another adverse effect, can cause pneumonitis or pneumonia.

Emetic drug administration is contraindicated for semiconscious or unconscious patients; patients with seizures; or any person with impaired gag reflexes, whether due to head trauma or to drugs (such as excessive doses of alcohol, sedative-hypnotic drugs, or opiates).

Administration of an emetic to a person who is not fully conscious and does not have intact reflexes greatly increases the risk of aspiration and lung damage, for which there is already a high risk in a severely poisoned, critically ill patient.

Emetic drug administration also is contraindicated if the ingested substance is highly corrosive (strong acids or alkali); is a volatile petroleum-based product (gasoline, kerosene, paint thinners, and so on); or is a rapidly acting convulsant (eg, strychnine) or depressant (eg, cyanide). Inducing emesis after ingestion of a corrosive agent worsens damage to the esophageal and pharyngeal mucosa by the vomitus. Induced vomiting after ingestion of a petroleum product increases the risk of inhaling the offending substance, and the risk of lung damage or infection. The toxic effects of agents such as strychnine or cyanide progress too quickly to be managed well with an emetic, and they are likely to impair consciousness or reflexes, or cause seizures, all of which contraindicate safe emetic use.

NURSING IMPLICATIONS

Recommend having syrup of ipecac available in the home to manage oral poisonings. However, it is just as essential to teach the proper use of this drug (indications, contraindications, dose limits, and so on). Poisoning for which ipecac might be indicated or actually is used requires subsequent and immediate professional evaluation by a physician, preferably in an emergency room or poison control center. This is especially important if ipecac administration fails to induce vomiting and there is the risk of excessive ipecac use.

Position the patient on his or her side to reduce further the risk of aspiration once ipecac is given.

Many patients will sleep deeply after induced emesis, and respiration and cardiovascular status may be depressed. Additionally, emetic drug administration may not have completely prevented absorption of the ingested poison or drug. Therefore, monitor vital signs not only before giving an emetic but also for at least two hours thereafter. Have equipment for gastric lavage, airway suctioning, and respiratory support available for subsequent management of the poisoning. Atropine should be available to manage severe bradycardia, which may develop in response to any emetic.

Save the vomitus for inspection and possible chemical analysis, which may help diagnose poisoning by an unknown substance.

◆ Use During Pregnancy and Lactation

Neither pregnancy nor lactation absolutely contraindicates the use of an emetic for management of poisoning emergencies. However, fetal vital signs must be monitored closely to assess both the effects of a poison and the potential adverse effects of the emetic drug.

Breast-feeding should be discontinued until the mother has recovered completely from the cause for which an emetic was given, and has recovered from residual effects of the emetic.

◆ Use in Children

Give only a single ipecac dose to children younger than 10 years old. If this dose fails to induce emesis, institute alternative or adjunctive treatments for poisoning (activated charcoal, gastric lavage, cathartic administration) immediately. The risk of aspiration of vomitus is greater in children than in adults.

Milk has been recommended as a substitute for water or other fluids to facilitate vomiting in a child. However, milk delays the onset of emetic activity, and so it should be avoided. Gently bouncing the child may speed the onset of emesis.

◆ Use in the Elderly

Emetics can be used for the elderly, but these individuals are less tolerant than younger persons of the expected autonomic effects and the risks of fluid and electrolyte loss. Preexisting cardiac or vascular impairment increases the risk of untoward responses.

Interactions with Other Drugs

Vomiting interferes with the absorption of all orally administered drugs. However, emetics, when used properly, are not contraindicated for fear of potential interactions with any other class of therapeutic agent, except for drugs with central *antiemetic* actions.

Antiemetics markedly reduce the efficacy of emetics, and attempts to overcome this antagonism by giving high emetic doses are likely to cause serious adverse cardiovascular and respiratory effects. This is one reason why only two doses of an emetic should be given to adults, and only one dose to small children.

If recommended doses of an emetic fail to act, or when antiemetics are known to be the cause of overdose, start alternative treatments at once. Activated charcoal, one of the key pharmacologic interventions in the treatment of poisoning by the oral route, adsorbs and inhibits the activity of ipecac. It should not be administered first.

Overdose and Toxicity

Overdoses of ipecac are relatively common because it often is administered by persons who are not familiar with proper use.

Overdoses are treated symptomatically and supportively, with major emphasis on the cardiovascular and respiratory systems. Gastric lavage and administration of activated charcoal are important adjunctive treatments for ipecac overdose, since the route of poisoning is almost always oral. Never give more emetic, nor an antiemetic drug.

Ipecac Abuse

Ipecac is abused by individuals with anorexia nervosa and bulimia. After eating even small amounts of food, patients self-administer ipecac to prevent the food from being digested and contributing to their caloric intake. Over the long run, this practice potentially leads to cardiotoxicity and seizures due to absorbed ipecac; malnutrition, emaciation, fluid and electrolyte imbalances because of frequent vomiting after eating; and oral mucosal and dental problems due to frequent exposure of the soft tissues and teeth to acidic vomitus. This is a potentially fatal OTC drug abuse problem.

Related Drug

Apomorphine

Apomorphine is a morphine-like drug with little analgesic activity or other actions commonly associated with the opiates (see Chapter 21). The drug is not absorbed well from the GI tract, and its emetic actions are not reliable when the drug is ingested. Therefore, it is given by injection (usually subcutaneously). Apomorphine is metabolized in the liver and excreted in the urine.

Apomorphine structurally resembles dopamine, which accounts for its ability to stimulate the CTZ. However, apomorphine's actions are more selective. Recommended doses seldom cause the significant cardiovascular effects seen with dopamine. When given to adults, apomorphine produces vomiting in 15 minutes or less. The onset is usually less than five minutes for children. Do not give repeat doses.

Anticipate the abrupt development of myoclonic jerking, head-bobbing, and dyskinesia when apomorphine is given to patients with parkinsonism. It is due to the drug's central dopamine-like actions.

Neither gastric lavage nor administration of activated charcoal alters the effects of apomorphine, since it is given parenterally. The narcotic antagonist, naloxone, may counteract some excessive effects of apomorphine overdoses, but the most effective treatment is merely symptomatic and supportive.

II. Antiemetic Drugs

Most of the antiemetic drugs work in the CNS, at the CTZ. They block receptors for one or more of the neurochemicals that appear to trigger the signs and symptoms of nausea and vomiting: acetylcholine, dopamine, serotonin, and perhaps histamine. The drugs belong to major drug classes that have other members, and other clinical uses, that are discussed elsewhere in this book. Therefore, the following highlights the antiemetics and their uses. Refer to cross-referenced material for more information about these drug groups.

Antimuscarinics

Scopolamine is the major antiemetic drug that is most closely related to atropine, the prototype antimuscarinic (anticholinergic) drug (see Chapter 13). Scopolamine is probably most familiar to the lay public for its dosage form and administration route—a self-adhesive transdermal delivery system ("skin patch")—and perhaps its trade name, TRANSDERM-SCOP (or, simply, "scop"). This drug and administration route are used widely and are quite effective for preventing motion sickness. Owing to slow absorption, this preparation has very little immediate value when motion sickness symptoms already have begun.

Although scopolamine is administered topically, sufficient amounts of drug can enter the circulation. Thus, the potential and common side effects include dry mouth and blurred vision; contraindications to atropine apply (eg, glaucoma, prostatic hypertrophy; Table 13–S); and drug–drug interactions that apply to atropine (Table 13–I) also can apply. In addition, scopolamine tends to cause more CNS depression than atropine, but whether a person using the drug becomes drowsy is variable.

The elderly are more likely to have contraindicating conditions, or be taking other drugs, that require extra caution before scopolamine is used. CNS depression and atropine-like side effects—and the precautions and risks associated with them—apply to drugs in two other major classes of antiemetics, the antihistamines and the phenothiazines, which are discussed next.

Antihistamines

Diphenhydramine (BENADRYL) is the prototype of many drugs that block the H_1 subtype of histamine receptor (Chapter 51). It has clinically useful antiemetic activity, but other effects of this drug limit its usefulness, especially for outpatients. These effects include significant CNS depression and atropine-like side effects, just as noted above for scopolamine. In terms of antiemetic activity, the actions of antihistamines probably depend more on their ability to block acetylcholine (or other) receptors than on their histamine receptor-blocking effects. Histamine H_2 receptor blockers such as cimetidine (TAGAMET) have no antiemetic activity at all.

Related antihistamine antiemetics are listed in Table 42–C, along with usual dosages. Some of these drugs are available for administration by several routes, including parenteral routes that can be used for controlling active nausea or vomiting; some are available OTC. Several of the OTC agents have brand names that are familiar to the lay public: DRAMAMINE (dimenhydrinate); MAREZINE (cyclizine); and BONINE (meclizine). The prescription and nonprescription agents differ in terms of onsets and durations of action. Those properties affect both the dosing interval and the suitability of a particular drug for fast or prolonged effects, depending on the need.

Compared with diphenhydramine, most of the related antihistamine antiemetics have better (or more selective) antiemetic activity, and cause less CNS depressant and atropine-like side effects. This somewhat lessens the risks of side effects, the number of contraindicating conditions (Table 13–S), and problems owing to drug interactions (Table 13–I). Nevertheless, assume that all the precautions that should be taken for diphenhydramine apply to these other agents.

Phenothiazines

Phenothiazines such as the prototype, chlorpromazine (THORAZINE), are regarded mainly as antipsychotic agents, but several drugs in this class have prominent antiemetic actions. The effect is due mainly to blockade of central dopamine receptors. (See Chapter 23 for more details.) Chlorpromazine can be used as an antiemetic, but other phenothiazines are used more commonly for this purpose. They include perphenazine (TRILAFON), prochlorperazine (COMPAZINE), promethazine (PHENERGAN), and thiethylperazine (TORECAN).

The phenothiazines are indicated for treatment of severe nausea and vomiting, particularly in pre- and postoperative patients. Some of these drugs are available for administration orally, per rectum, or by injection. The major side effects of the phenothiazines include atropine-like actions, orthostatic hypotension and cardiac stimulation, and parkinsonian movement disorders (extrapyramidal side effects).

Other Antiemetics

Several other antiemetic drugs do not fit easily into one of the pharmacologic or chemical classes noted above.

Bismuth Salts

A familiar brand name drug that contains a bismuth salt is PEPTO-BISMOL. This OTC product contains bismuth subsalicylate, which causes a variety of useful GI effects including control of nausea, indigestion, and diarrhea. The bismuth salts probably work through local antibiotic and antisecretory actions; this distinguishes them from most other antiemetics, which act in the CNS.

Bismuth subsalicylate is relatively safe and free from side effects for most persons. However, it can cause adverse effects, some of which can be serious, if taken by persons who should not take other salicylates, such as aspirin. Avoid combined use of bismuth subsalicylate and other salicylates to reduce the risk of salicylate side effects or toxicity. See Chapter 40 for more information about the actions and uses of bismuth subsalicylate.

Dronabinol

Dronabinol is the main psychoactive substance in *Cannabis sativa,* better known as marijuana. It is marketed as MARINOL, a prescription drug that is given orally. Dronabinol is indicated only for treating nausea and vomiting that is associated with cancer chemotherapy, and that cannot be controlled with other, more traditional antiemetic drugs.

Because of its marijuana-like actions, dronabinol can cause all the adverse psychiatric effects of marijuana smoking. Those effects, plus the drug's abuse potential, have led to its classification as a Schedule II agent—the same narcotics schedule for morphine.

Metoclopramide

Metoclopramide (REGLAN) stimulates GI tract motility, presumably by increasing sensitivity of the gut muscles to acetylcholine. This property is used to treat gastric stasis that often occurs in diabetic patients, and to stimulate the gut when needed to facilitate some diagnostic procedures. However, metoclopramide also has phenothiazine-like actions in the CTZ, and so it is indicated for antiemetic actions.

Metoclopramide is used mainly as a pretreatment to reduce nausea and vomiting during and shortly after parenteral cancer chemotherapy.

Metoclopramide can cause restlessness, drowsiness, or fatigue. Headache, insomnia, and, paradoxically, nausea may occur. It also may produce the extrapyramidal side effects noted for the phenothiazines. Extrapyramidal effects may be reduced by pretreating with diphenhydramine. The side effects disappear when metoclopramide administration is discontinued.

Ondansetron Hydrochloride

Ondansetron (ZOFRAN) appears to work by blocking a subclass of serotonin (5-hydroxytryptamine) receptors that trigger nausea and vomiting. It is indicated for the prophylaxis of nausea and vomiting caused by cancer chemotherapeutic agents. Treatment for each course of chemotherapy involves three ondansetron doses (see Table 42–C) infused intravenously: one starting 30 minutes before chemotherapy and the other two at four and eight hours after chemotherapy. Constipation is ondansetron's most common side effect.

NURSING IMPLICATIONS

Several general principles apply to the use of virtually all antiemetic drugs.

◆ Prevent Anticipated Nausea and Vomiting

When nausea or vomiting can be anticipated because of travel, drug administration, or a certain medical or surgical procedure, pretreatment is preferred. Compared with treating nausea and vomiting, prophylactic therapy helps make the patient more comfortable; allows the use of lower drug dosages; and may prevent potentially serious complications that could arise if vomiting occurs.

◆ Identify the Underlying Cause of Idiopathic Nausea and Vomiting

Nausea and vomiting can be symptoms and signs of serious underlying disorders, or drug toxicities. Antiemetic drugs can mask important diagnostic clues. If time permits, and it is safe to do so, withhold antiemetic drug administration until at least a partial diagnosis of a cause of nausea and vomiting can be made. Assess as thoroughly as possible (history, vital signs, etc) before giving the medication.

Advise patients who self-prescribe OTC antiemetics (except for controlling motion sickness) to consult a physician if the drug fails to work after a day of treatment.

◆ Review the Drug and Administration Route

Choose the drug and administration route to meet the needs of each patient. Oral administration generally is preferred (except for scopolamine) for adults. Rectal administration is best for small children, or for adults who cannot swallow or keep an oral medication in the gut long enough for it to be absorbed effectively. Parenteral administration works fastest and is indicated for severe or intractable vomiting. Question medication orders calling for oral or rectal therapy when the situation is acute. Adverse effects of the drug given parenterally are likely to be more intense, and appear faster, than when oral or rectal routes are used.

◆ Rule Out Contraindications, Prevent Further Harm

Since most antiemetics fall in a major drug class, become familiar with the overall contraindications for the class. The majority of antiemetics, in the various classes, share atropine's side effects and contraindications. It is usually unsafe to administer a contraindicated antiemetic, even if only one dose may be needed.

Most antiemetics, including those available OTC, can cause drowsiness, or impair mental or motor skills. Caution patients against participating in activities that can become hazardous because of these effects. If both alertness and the use of an antiemetic are necessary, it may be helpful for the user to try the drug ahead of the time of actual need to assess its effects. Discourage alcohol use.

◆ Recognize the Importance of Fluid and Electrolyte Administration

Antiemetic drugs do not replace fluid and electrolytes that have been lost because of prolonged or severe vomiting. Also, they may not work quickly enough to prevent worsening of imbalances that initially are only mild or asymptomatic. Anticipate the need for replacing lost fluids, electrolytes, and nutrients. Intravenous administration almost always is preferred to oral therapy, even when only relatively small amounts of fluid and electrolytes might be needed. It works the fastest, it is the most reliable route, and it offers a ready way to administer other drugs that may be needed if the patient's condition worsens.

◆ Use of Antiemetic Drugs During Pregnancy and Lactation

Nausea and vomiting ("morning sickness") are common during pregnancy. It once was relatively common to administer antiemetics formulated specifically for use during pregnancy, for morning sickness. However, these drugs were linked to fetal malformations; some products were withdrawn from the market, and the use of others has declined dramatically. The consensus is that non-drug measures (for example, chewing crackers or eating a small meal in the morning) should be stressed. Even in the absence of proven fetal problems, antiemetic drugs should be reserved only for severe, intractable nausea and vomiting associated with pregnancy, and they should be used in low doses and only as long as needed. Additionally, women receiving antiemetic drugs, often at their insistence, should be asked to give written informed consent after the potential fetal effects have been explained to them.

Buclizine, cyclizine, meclizine, perphenazine, prochlorperazine, and thiethylperazine are absolutely contraindicated for pregnant women, even for occasional low-dose use. These drugs belong to a chemical class of antihistamines or phenothiazines—the *piperazine derivatives*—that is widely known for teratogenic effects. Pregnancy should be ruled out before beginning therapy with centrally acting antiemetic drugs in any woman of child-bearing age.

◆ Use in Children

Children younger than 12 years are particularly susceptible to the extrapyramidal side effects of the phenothiazines, and to the peripheral autonomic effects of any drug with atropine-like activity. Phenothiazines also may contribute to the development of Reye's syndrome in viral illness.

◆ Use in the Elderly

The extrapyramidal side effects of phenothiazines are exaggerated. Parkinsonism, which is more prevalent in the elderly population, also increases the risk of these side effects. More careful monitoring is essential. Glaucoma is also more prevalent; attempt to rule out this ocular disorder before giving any antimuscarinic, antihistamine, or phenothiazine antiemetic.

Drug Interactions Common to All Centrally Acting Antiemetic Drugs

All these drugs cause generalized CNS-depressant actions and peripheral atropine-like activity, which may be intensified significantly by concomitant administration of any other drug that produces similar effects (Table 42–I). They are likely to mask nausea and vomiting that often are used as indicators of adverse responses to, or overdoses of, other drugs. Concomitant administration of antacids or adsorbent-type antidiarrheal agents may reduce antiemetic drug activity.

Antiemetic Drug Overdoses

Excessive doses of most centrally acting antiemetics cause signs and symptoms typical of atropine poisoning. Central effects include possibly severe CNS depression, followed by stimulation and possibly seizures. The phenothiazines also may produce severe hypotension that may require administration of parenteral fluids and vasopressor drugs; and profound extrapyramidal side effects. Antiparkinson drugs should be used cautiously, however, since most of them are likely to increase CNS depression and atropine-like peripheral problems.

In general, treatment of antiemetic drug overdoses involves symptomatic management of vital signs. Activated charcoal and gastric lavage are generally useful adjunctive treatments for oral overdoses. Emetic drugs should not be used, since they are not likely to be effective. If signs and symptoms of severe atropine poisoning are apparent, the antidote, physostigmine (ANTILIRIUM; see Chapter 12) may be indicated.

SUMMARY OF NURSING IMPLICATIONS

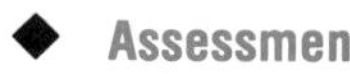

◆ Assessment

Determine the nature of the substance swallowed before giving an emetic drug; vomiting should not be induced when caustic substances, petroleum products, or agents such as cyanide or strychnine have been ingested.

Assess for level of consciousness and intact reflexes before administering an emetic, to reduce the chance of aspiration.

Determine underlying causes of nausea and vomiting before giving antiemetics, which may mask important diagnostic signs or symptoms.

Obtain a complete nursing history to rule out contraindications for antimuscarinic drugs (antiemetics).

◆ Nursing Diagnoses

Fluid volume deficit related to uncontrolled vomiting.

Altered nutrition: less than body requirements (electrolyte imbalance) related to excessive vomiting or nausea.

Impaired gas exchange related to aspiration of vomitus.

High risk for injury related to improper/unsafe use of emetics for weight control.

Altered oral mucous membranes related to ingestion of caustic agent or irritation from vomiting.

High risk for aspiration related to vomiting.

◆ Planning/Implementation

Administer 8 to 32 ounces of water to adults (proportionally less for children) shortly after administering an emetic.

Give no more than two doses of an emetic (one dose for children younger than one year old).

Observe for significant fatigue, excessive sleep, and cardiovascular or respiratory depression after induced emesis.

Monitor vital signs before and for several hours after giving an emetic.

Have appropriate suctioning and cardiovascular/respiratory support equipment, and drugs to manage seizures or cardiovascular collapse, available before giving an emetic.

Know the most effective route of administration for antiemetics: oral for most adults; rectal suppositories for small children or patients with difficulty swallowing or frequent vomiting; parenteral for prompt effects in adults with severe nausea or vomiting.

Give intramuscular antiemetic injections deep into the upper outer quadrant of the buttocks; anticipate that side effects will appear sooner and be more severe than when other administration routes are used.

Give oral antiemetics on an empty stomach, about one hour before anticipated need (eg, travel).

Monitor all patients for atropine-like adverse responses.

Observe for muscle tremor, rigidity, or involuntary movements with patients receiving phenothiazine antiemetics or metoclopramide. Report side effects to a physician at once.

Observe for signs of excessive CNS depression.

Administer replacement fluids and electrolytes as ordered for severe vomiting.

Monitor vital signs, fluid intake and output, and body weight if vomiting persists.

◆ Patient and Family Teaching

Teach the patient/family:

To avoid driving or operating hazardous machinery; centrally acting antiemetics may cause drowsiness or sedation.

To abstain from ingesting alcohol or other drugs that cause sedation unless recommended by a physician.

To avoid use of antiemetic drugs, including OTC medications, during pregnancy; teach nondrug measures to control pregnancy-related nausea and vomiting.

◆ Evaluation

The patient/family will:

Vomit with less frequency; cease vomiting.
Remain free of aspiration; breath sounds clear.
Eat and retain food and fluids.
Maintain body weight.
Seek psychologic counseling if indicated.

Annotated Bibliography

DiPalma JR: Metoclopramide: A dopamine receptor antagonist. *Am Fam Physician* 1990;41(3):919–924. *An excellent review of an important drug that has antiemetic properties.*

Egan AP, Taggart JR, Bender CM: Management of chemotherapy-related nausea and vomiting using a serotonin antagonist. *Oncol Nurs Forum* 1992;19(5):791–795. *Discusses the pharmacodynamics and pharmacokinetics of ondansetron, gives suggestions for adverse events, identifies implications for nursing practice and future research.*

Hockenberry-Eaton M, Benner A: Patterns of nausea and vomiting in children: Nursing assessment and intervention. *Oncol Nurs Forum* 1990;17(4):575–584. *Focuses on assessment, incidence, etiology, and patterns of nausea and vomiting, developmental influences on nursing intervention (including behavioral), innovative nursing strategies, therapy, and home care.*

Krenzelok EP, Dunmire SM: Acute poisoning emergencies. Resolving the gastric decontamination controversy. *Postgrad Med* 1992; 91(2):179–182, 185–186. *Covers the pros and cons of inducing emesis with ipecac, versus other and perhaps better measures once the poisoned patient reaches the emergency department.*

Mataruski MR, Keis NA, Smouse DJ, Workman ML: Effects of steroids on postoperative nausea and vomiting. *Nurs Anesth* 1990;1(4): 183–188. *This interesting clinical study suggests that prelaminectomy treatment with corticosteroids reduces postoperative nausea, vomiting, and requirements for pain medications.*

Peters CA: Myths of antiemetic administration. *Cancer Nurs* 1989; 12(2):102–106. *Distinguishing between fact and fiction, and intervening accordingly, can help you provide more comfort for patients with chemotherapy-induced nausea and vomiting.*

Storey P, Hill HH, Jr., St. Louis RH, Tarver EE: Subcutaneous infusions for control of cancer symptoms. *J Pain Symptom Manage* 1990; 5(1):33–41. *An interesting approach to controlling pain, vomiting, seizures, and other common adverse responses to chemotherapy. Gives useful tips for safe and effective procedures for hospitalized and home-care patients.*

Tortorice PV, O'Connell MB: Management of chemotherapy-induced nausea and vomiting. *Pharmacotherapy* 1990;10(2):129–145. *Useful information on assessment, treatment, and the pharmacology of several antiemetic drug classes; presents guidelines for managing chemotherapy-induced emesis.*

Watcha MF, White PF: Postoperative nausea and vomiting. Its etiology, treatment, and prevention. *Anesthesiology* 1992;77(1):162–184. *Essential reading for any nurse caring for postoperative or immediate preoperative patients—inpatient or ambulatory. Covers risk factors, prevention, assessment, and treatment.*

Wilder-Smith CH, Schuler L, Osterwalder B, Naji P, Senn HJ: Patient-controlled antiemesis for cancer chemotherapy-induced nausea and vomiting. *J Pain Symptom Manage* 1990;5(6):375–378. *Patient-controlled antiemetic therapy, like patient-controlled analgesia, may offer a more effective and more acceptable approach to intermittent dosing.*

Table 42–C | **Clinical Uses and Administration of Major Emetic and Antiemetic Drugs**

AGENT	CLINICAL USES	DOSAGE AND ROUTE OF ADMINISTRATION
	Emetic Drugs	
PROTOTYPE		
Syrup of ipecac	Induction of vomiting	Oral: Adults, children ≥10 years: Usually 30 mL, followed by 2–4 glasses of cool water; no more than 1 additional dose if first dose fails to induce vomiting. Children 1–10 years: 15 mL, followed by water (volumes proportionally reduced based on body weight). Children 6 mos–1 year: 10 mL, followed by water; limit to 1 dose for children <10 years
RELATED DRUG		
Apomorphine	Induction of vomiting	SC: Adults: 5 mg. Children: Usually 0.1 mg/kg; do not repeat dose for adults or children
	Antiemetic Drugs	
	Antimuscarinic	
Scopolamine (TRANSDERM-SCOP)	Prophylaxis, treatment of motion sickness, drug- or disease-induced nausea, vomiting	Oral: Adults: 0.25–0.5 mg taken 30–60 min before anticipated onset of symptoms, higher doses may be needed whan used to treat symptoms
	Prophylaxis of motion sickness	Percutaneous: Apply one 1.5-mg drug delivery system on neck behind ear lobe before travel; replace in 3 days if needed
	Antihistamines	
Buclizine (BUCLADIN-S)	Prophylaxis of motion sickness	Oral: Adults 50-mg tablet chewed or swallowed whole, 30 min before travel; take second dose 4–6 h later if needed
Cyclizine (MAREZINE)	Prophylaxis of motion sickness	Oral: Adults: 50 mg every 4–6 hr as needed (up to 200 mg/day); best taken 30 min before travel. Children 6–12 years: 25 mg every 4–6 hr (up to 75 mg/day)
		IM (lactate salt): 50 mg every 4–6 hr (adults only)
Dimenhydrinate (DRAMAMINE)	See cyclizine	Oral: Adults: 50–100 mg every 4 hr. Children: 2–6 years: 12.5–25 mg every 6–8 hr; 6–12 years 25–50 mg every 6–8 hr
		IM, IV: 50 mg (inject IV dose slowly). Children: 1.25 mg/ kg qid
Diphenhydramine (BENADRYL)	Treatment of nausea, vomiting due to surgery, drugs, radiation, some inner ear disorders	Oral, IM, IV: Adults: 25–50 mg every 4–6 hr; do not exceed 400 mg per day. Children: 1–2 mg/kg qid (not to exceed 300 mg/day)

(continued)

Table 42–C Clinical Uses and Administration of Major Emetic and Antiemetic Drugs (*Continued*)

AGENT	CLINICAL USES	DOSAGE AND ROUTE OF ADMINISTRATION
	Antihistamines	
Meclizine (ANTIVERT; BONINE)	See buclizine	Oral: Adults: 25–50 mg per day as single dose; best taken 1 hr before travel
Trimethobenzamide (TIGAN)	See diphenhydramine	Oral: Adults: 250 mg tid or qid. Children 30–90 lbs: 100–200 mg tid or qid IM: Adults: 200 mg tid or qid Rectal: Adults: 200 mg tid or qid. Children 30–90 lbs: 100–200 mg tid or qid. Children <30 lbs: 100 mg tid or qid
	Phenothiazines	
Chlorpromazine (THORAZINE)	Management of severe nausea, vomiting due to surgery, drugs, radiation	Oral: Adults: 10–25 mg every 4–6 hr IM: Adults: 25 mg; if patient stays normotensive give 25–50 mg every 3 hr until vomiting stops Rectal: Adults: 50–100 mg every 6-8 hr
Perphenazine (TRILAFON)	See chlorpromazine	Oral: Adults: 4 or 8 mg bid or one 16-mg repeat-action tablet daily IM: 5 mg (10 mg if necessary) then 5 mg every 6 hr if needed; pediatric use not recommended
Prochlorperazine (COMPAZINE)	See chlorpromazine	Oral: Adults: 5–10 mg tid or qid; sustained-release capsules; 15 mg in AM or 10 mg every 12 hr Rectal: 25 mg bid IM or slow IV injection: 5–10 mg IV: 20 mg; dilute in at least 1 L isotonic saline, infuse over at least 1 hr
Promethazine (PHENERGAN)	See chlorpromazine	Oral or rectal: Adults or children: 25 mg every 4–6 hr as needed IM: 12.5 to 25 mg every 4–6 hr as needed
Thiethylperazine (TORECAN)	See chlorpromazine	Oral, IM, or rectal: Adults: 10 mg 1–3 times daily; pediatric use not recommended
	Others	
Dronabinol (MARINOL)	Nausea and vomiting due to chemotherapy	IM: 5 mg/m^2 body surface area 1–3 hr before chemotherapy; limit to 4–6 doses per day. Not recommended for children

(continued)

Table 42–C | **Clinical Uses and Administration of Major Emetic and Antiemetic Drugs (*Continued*)**

AGENT	CLINICAL USES	DOSAGE AND ROUTE OF ADMINISTRATION
	Others	
Metoclopramide (REGLAN)	See dronabinol	IV: Adults or children: Infuse 1 mg/kg (or 2 mg/kg for highly emetogenic drugs) 30 min before starting chemotherapy; repeat every 2 hr for 2 doses, then every 3 hr for the final 3 doses
Ondansetron HCl (ZOFRAN)	See dronabinol	IV: 3 doses of 0.15 mg/kg: 30 min before chemotherapy, 4 and 8 hr post-chemotherapy

Table 42–S | **Major Side Effects of and Contraindications for Emetic and Antiemetic Drugs**

BODY SYSTEM/ Side Effect	CONTRAINDICATION/ PRECAUTION	COMMENTS AND NURSING IMPLICATIONS
	Ipecac	
CENTRAL NERVOUS SYSTEM Stimulation, then depression with high doses	Epilepsy or other seizure disorders; semiconscious, unconscious patients	Gastric suctioning, activated charcoal administration preferred when contraindications present
RESPIRATORY Profuse secretions; aspiration of vomitus	See CNS	Always be prepared for suctioning of upper respiratory tract
CARDIOVASCULAR Hypotension, syncope; tachycardia	Severe hypotension; poor cardiac status	Monitor vital signs; administer emetic with water, no more than 2 doses, to reduce chance of overdose; plan on gastric suctioning if emetic fails; high or frequent doses of ipecac may be directly cardiotoxic
GASTROINTESTINAL Severe retching, persistent vomiting; fluid and electrolyte imbalances	Fluid and electrolyte imbalances	Usually caused by overdoses; may be managed with antiemetic drugs if severe, prolonged

(continued)

Table 42–S Major Side Effects of and Contraindications for Emetic and Antiemetic Drugs (*Continued*)

BODY SYSTEM/ Side Effect	CONTRAINDICATION/ PRECAUTION	COMMENTS AND NURSING IMPLICATIONS
Centrally Acting Antiemetics		
CENTRAL NERVOUS SYSTEM Sedation or stimulation; drowsiness, coma, restlessness; agitation; seizures	Seizure disorders; drug-induced CNS depression or stimulation	Use cautiously; assess to determine whether CNS changes due to prolonged vomiting (eg, fluid and electrolyte imbalances), drug overdose, or interaction with other CNS-active drugs
High fever		Determine whether fever is due to infection from vomitus aspiration or due to poisoning; flushed dry skin usually indicates problem due to antimuscarinic drug effects
Abnormal involuntary extrapyramidal movements (tremor, rigidity, other dyskinesias); see Chapter 25	Use cautiously in patients with Parkinson's disease or drug-induced parkinsonism	Produced by phenothiazines (especially chlorpromazine) and metoclopramide, especially in children or young adults; signs may be reduced by decreasing dose or cautiously administering antimuscarinic (eg, diphenhydramine)
EYE Mydriasis; cycloplegia; ocular pain	Glaucoma	Due to antimuscarinic actions of most centrally acting antiemetics (except dronabinol); monitor, report eye pain to physician at once
CARDIOVASCULAR Tachycardia; hypotension (including orthostatic)	Tachycardia; hypotension; myocardial infarction; angina pectoris; cerebrovascular disease	Tachycardia due to antimuscarinic activity; orthostatic hypotension frequently caused by α-blocking activity of phenothiazines, may be caused by fluid and electrolyte losses
GASTROINTESTINAL, GENITOURINARY Constipation; paralytic ileus; impaired urination; urinary retention; dry mouth	Obstructive bowel, bladder disease including prostatic hypertrophy	Due to anticholinergic activity of scopolamine, antihistamines, phenothiazines; bothersome dry mouth may be relieved by sipping water, sucking hard candies
	Pregnancy	Discourage antiemetic drug use during pregnancy, recommend nondrug interventions; reserve antiemetic drug therapy for severe, intractable nausea, vomiting, under care of physician; piperazine antiemetics (see text) absolutely contraindicated

Table 42–I Major Interactions Between Emetics and Antiemetics and Other Agents

AGENT	RESULT OF INTERACTION	COMMENTS AND NURSING IMPLICATIONS
Interactions Involving Emetic Drugs		
Adsorbents, antacids, antidiarrheals (activated charcoal; antacids, bismuth salts; kaolin and kaolin-pectin combinations) (Chapters 40, 41)	Antagonism of ipecac action	Adsorbents bind to ipecac and render it ineffective; continued ipecac action may fail to produce vomiting while increasing risk of systemic absorption, toxicity; interaction does not affect apomorphine
Antiemetic drugs (antimuscarinics, antihistamines, phenothiazines)	Antagonism of emetic drug action (ipecac or apomorphine)	If emetic drug is being used to help manage drug overdose, try to determine whether offending drug has antiemetic action; if so, use activated charcoal, gastric lavage instead; repeated emetic drug administration can lead to systemic toxic effects, especially if emesis does not occur
Interactions Involving Antiemetic Drugs		
Antidiarrheal drugs (activated charcoal; bismuth salts; kaolin and kaolin-pectin combinations; antacids) (Chapter 41)	Antagonism of antiemetic action; persistent vomiting	Adsorbents bind to and render orally administered drugs inactive by inhibiting systemic absorption; space administration of interactant by at least 1 h
Antimuscarinics, others with atropine-like actions (antidepressants; antihistaminics, including most cough and cold remedies; antipsychotics; centrally acting anticholinergic/antiparkinsonism drugs; diazepam; MAO inhibitors)	Increased risk of antimuscarinic side effects, toxicity	Avoid interaction when possible; monitor for pertinent signs of atropine side effects or poisoning (see Chapter 13, Table 13-2)
CNS depressants (alcohol; antidepressants; antihistaminics; antipsychotics; anxiolytics, hypnotic/sedatives; narcotic analgesics) (Chapters 21–26)	Increased risk of excessive CNS and/or respiratory depression	Avoid interaction when possible; determine whether drowsiness or marked sedation is due to excessive vomiting or drug–drug interaction; counsel patient against alcohol consumption
Dopamine agonists (bromocriptine; carbidopa; levodopa; morphine and other opiate analgesics; dopamine) (Chapters 21, 25)	Persistent vomiting or reduced antiemetic drug effect	These drugs stimulate the CTZ and may directly provoke vomiting
Laxatives/cathartics (Chapter 41)	Decreased antiemetic drug action; increased risk of fluid and electrolyte loss	Avoid interaction; monitor fluid and electrolyte status
Other orally administered drugs	Increased or decreased absorption, action of interactant	See text

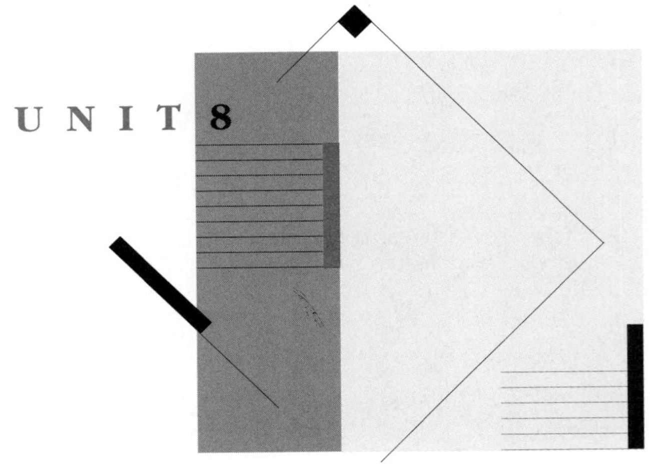

Hormones, Hormone Antagonists, and Drugs That Affect Endocrine Disorders

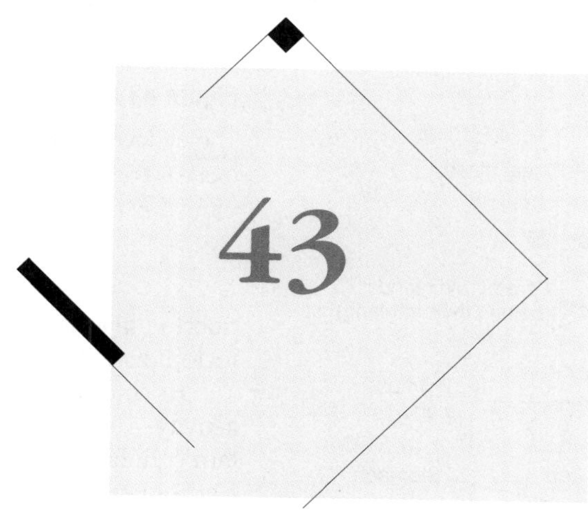

Structure and Function of the Endocrine System

The endocrine system, in conjunction with the nervous system, controls homeostasis by coordinating and integrating the activity of the cells of the other body systems. Endocrine control is exerted via hormones. **Hormones** are chemical substances that are released into the blood by the various endocrine organs and that act as messengers to other body systems. Drugs that block or stimulate endocrine activity thus have widespread effects on the body.

This chapter considers the endocrine system as a functional unit. Endocrine organ anatomy and the functions of specific hormones are discussed in Chapters 44 through 49.

Anatomic Features of the Endocrine System

The *endocrine glands* are ductless structures that secrete hormones directly into extracellular spaces. Hormones excreted by endocrine glands enter the bloodstream and are transported throughout the body. The major components of the endocrine system (Fig. 43–1) are the pituitary, adrenal, thyroid, and parathyroid glands; and the pancreas and gonads (which have both endocrine and exocrine functions). The endocrine glands produce the majority of the body's hormones, but other organs, such as the stomach, small intestine, and kidneys, also have hormone-producing cells.

Physiologic Roles of the Endocrine System

Whereas the nervous system bears primary responsibility for promoting rapid adjustments to changes occurring both within and outside the body, the endocrine system has a prominent role in regulating processes for relatively long periods of time. Examples of hormonally controlled processes include reproduction, growth and development, response to stress and injury, maintenance of fluid balance, regulation of cellular metabolism, and control of certain digestive system activities (Table 43–1).

Hormones

Chemical Nature and Mechanism of Action

Most hormones are synthesized either from amino acids (the protein, peptide, and catecholamine hormones) or from cholesterol (the steroid hormones). The various hormones synthesized by the different en-

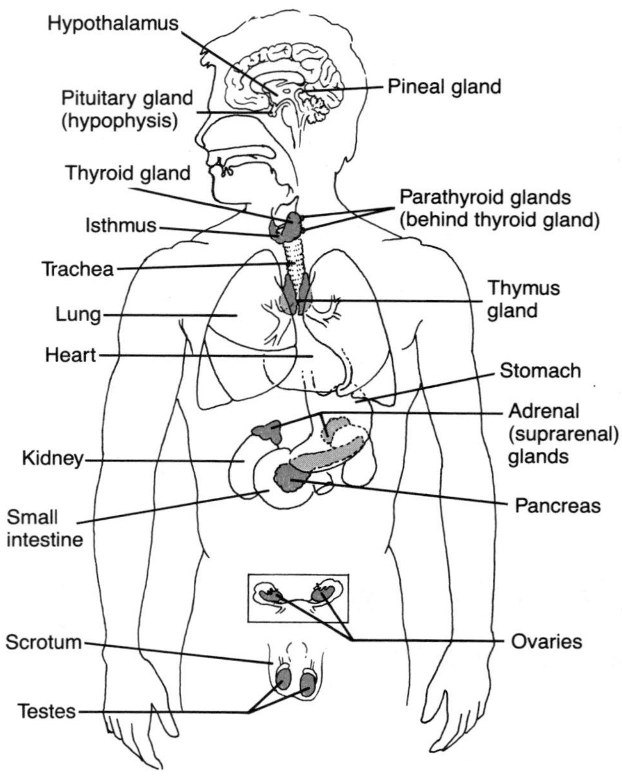

Figure 43–1

The endocrine glands and related structures.

(*Source:* From Ames SW, Kneisl CR: *Essentials of Adult Health Nursing,* p. 753. Addison-Wesley, 1988.)

docrine glands, and their representative effects and selected disorders, are summarized in Table 43–2.

Hormones produce their effects by altering cellular activity—either increasing or decreasing the rate of certain cellular biochemical processes. However, they cannot initiate previously nonexistent functions. Although hormones circulate throughout the body, most hormones affect only specific organs or body tissues (their target organs or cells). The ability of a target cell to respond to a given hormone depends on the hormone's ability to bind to specific receptors.

In general, peptide hormones interact with membrane receptors coupled to the adenyl cyclase system. Hormone binding activates the system, converting adenosine triphosphate (ATP) into cyclic 3′,5′-adenosine monophosphate (cyclic AMP), which acts as an intracellular mediator, or second messenger. Cyclic AMP regulates such processes as cell membrane perme-

Table 43–1 | Activities Regulated by the Endocrine System

Activity	Endocrine Function
Reproduction	Fertility is maintained through a delicately timed interaction among several different hormones produced by the hypothalamus (gonadotropin-releasing hormone), anterior pituitary gland (gonadotropins), and gonadal axis (estrogen, progesterone, and testosterone)
Growth and development	The endocrine system, in cooperation with the hypothalamus, controls normal growth and development. Growth hormone (somatotropin), produced by the anterior pituitary gland, influences overall body growth. Gonadotropins, also produced by anterior pituitary, promote maturation of reproductive organs at puberty. Thyroid hormones are necessary for normal growth of the skeleton
Response to stress and injury	Epinephrine and norepinephrine, catecholamines produced by the adrenal medulla, enhance the "flight or fight" response of the sympathetic nervous system. Adrenal hormones are mobilized in the presence of longer term stressors such as infection, physical trauma, and psychosocial problems
Maintenance of ionic/water balance of the blood	Aldosterone and antidiuretic hormone, produced by the adrenal cortex and hypothalamus respectively, help maintain homeostasis by promoting alterations in the water and sodium ion levels of the blood. As a result of sodium ion adjustment, potassium levels are adjusted simultaneously as well
Regulation of cellular energy metabolism	The thyroid hormones determine the basal metabolic rate. Normal energy metabolism also is influenced by pancreatic, adrenal, and pituitary hormones
Control of digestive system secretory activity and motility	Local hormones produced by the stomach and small intestine influence GI motility and secretions of digestive enzymes

Table 43–2 Major Endocrine Glands and Their Hormones

Gland	Hormones	Representative Effects	Selected Disorders
PITUITARY (Including hypothalamic-releasing factors) (Chapter 44)	Antidiuretic hormone (ADH [vasopressin])	Promotes reabsorption of water from the kidney's collecting ducts	Undersecretion leads to diabetes insipidus
	Oxytocin	Stimulates contraction of uterine smooth muscle and myoepithelial cells around alveoli of mammary glands. Is involved in birth processes and milk "letdown" during nursing	
	Follicle-stimulating hormone (FSH) and luteinizing hormone (LH)	Stimulate gonads to produce gametes and sex hormones	Undersecretion causes gonadal inactivity in males and impairment or cessation of menstruation in females
	Thyroid-stimulating hormone (TSH)	Stimulates thyroid gland to secrete thyroid hormones	Undersecretion leads to symptoms of hypothyroidism
	Adrenocorticotropin (ACTH)	Stimulates adrenal cortex to secrete glucocorticoids (such as cortisol)	Undersecretion leads to symptoms of adrenal cortical insufficiency. Oversecretion leads to symptoms of adrenal cortical hyperfunction.
	Growth hormone (GH)	Stimulates growth in general, growth of skeletal system in particular. Also affects metabolic functions	Undersecretion produces pituitary dwarfs. Oversecretion causes gigantism or, in adults, acromegaly
	Prolactin	Involved in milk production in females	Undersecretion may cause failure to lactate after giving birth. Oversecretion may lead to lactation without recently having given birth
ADRENAL CORTEX (Chapter 45)	Mineralocorticoids (such as aldosterone)	Promote reabsorption of sodium and excretion of potassium from kidney tubules	Undersecretion may lead to decreased fluid volume and circulatory difficulties, and contribute to Addison's disease. Oversecretion may cause increased fluid volume, edema, hypertension
	Glucocorticoids (such as cortisol)	Affect many aspects of carbohydrate metabolism; tend to increase blood glucose levels	Undersecretion contributes to Addison's disease. Oversecretion leads to Cushing's syndrome
PANCREAS (Chapter 46)	Insulin	Affects many aspects of carbohydrate metabolism; tends to lower blood glucose levels	Relative deficiency of insulin leads to hyperglycemia, diabetes mellitus
	Glucagon	Affects metabolism in fashion generally opposite of insulin; raises blood glucose levels	
THYROID (Chapter 47)	Thyroxine (T_4 or tetraiodothyronine) and triiodothyronine (T_3)	Increase oxygen consumption, heat production (calorigenic effect). Important for normal growth and development. Affect many metabolic processes	Undersecretion leads to symptoms of hypothyroidism, possibly causing cretinism in children or myxedema in adults. Oversecretion leads to symptoms of hyperthyroidism
	Calcitonin	Lowers blood calcium and phosphate levels	
PARA-THYROIDS (Chapter 47)	Parathyroid hormone	Affects calcium and phosphate metabolism to raise plasma calcium levels and decrease plasma phosphate levels	Undersecretion leads to nervous excitability, tetanus. Oversecretion leads to bone decalcification, calcification of soft tissues such as kidneys

(continued)

Table 43–2 Major Endocrine Glands and Their Hormones (*Continued*)

Gland	Hormones	Representative Effects	Selected Disorders
GONADS			
Testes (Chapter 48)	Androgens (such as testosterone)		
Ovaries (Chapter 49)	Estrogens Progesterone	Involved in the processes of reproduction. Their functions are discussed in Chapters 48 and 49	Deficiencies cause such problems as delayed sexual maturation, infertility

Source: Adapted from Spence AP, Mason EB: *Human Anatomy and Physiology*, 3rd ed. pp. 499–500. Benjamin/Cummings, 1987.

ability, synthesis or destruction of intracellular regulatory molecules, and the activity of key cellular enzymes (Fig. 43–2). However, there are exceptions. For example, insulin appears to act through cyclic guanosine monophosphate (GMP), and thyroxine appears to bind to intracellular (nuclear and cytoplasmic) receptors as well as receptors located on the plasma membrane. The final site of action of steroid hormones appears to be the cell nucleus, where they stimulate DNA transcription, thus promoting synthesis of a particular enzyme or enzymes (Fig. 43–3).

Prostaglandins also act as chemical messengers, mediating or modifying the effects of hormones on target cells. These fatty acid-based molecules are made by nearly all body tissues. Although some investigators claim that prostaglandins travel through the bloodstream and act as hormones, most believe that they act primarily as local messengers, exerting their effects in the tissues in which they are synthesized.

Regulation of Hormone Release and Activity

Hormones are exceptionally potent agents that are rapidly degraded within target cells and blood and by the kidney and liver. Their half-lives usually range from 10 to 30 minutes, but the value is much shorter for some. There is also a wide range in the onset and duration of activity of the various hormones. For this reason it is essential that their blood concentrations be controlled precisely. For most hormones, this is accomplished by some type of negative-feedback system. Hormone synthesis and release are promoted by internal or external stimuli—neural, hormonal, or humoral—and, as blood levels rise, physiologic changes provide signals that inhibit further hormone synthesis. A stylized feedback control loop is illustrated in Figure 43–4.

Neural Stimuli

In a few cases, nerve fibers stimulate hormone-producing cells. A classic example is the stimulation of the adrenal medulla by preganglionic sympathetic nervous system fibers during periods of stress.

Hormonal Stimuli

Hormone-releasing hormones produced by the hypothalamus regulate most anterior pituitary hormones. They, in turn, stimulate other endocrine organs to release their hormones into the bloodstream. These hormonally controlled feedback systems tend to be rhythmic; the hormone blood concentrations rise and fall in a specific pattern. The female menstrual cycle depends on this type of control. In this case the terminal endocrine gland is the ovary, and the rhythm produces a monthly cyclic rise and fall of ovarian hormone levels.

Humoral Stimuli

Chemicals other than hormones also can trigger hormone release. For example, when blood calcium levels fall below the physiologic range, parathormone is released, stimulating metabolic changes in bone, the small intestine, and kidney tubule cells. These changes increase serum calcium levels, which, in turn, inhibit parathormone secretion until blood calcium levels rise and once again begin to fall.

Another example of humoral control is pancreatic release of insulin, which is triggered by increasing blood glucose levels and inhibited by hypoglycemia.

Although these mechanisms explain most regulatory systems of hormone release, they are by no means inclusive. For example, release of aldosterone by the adrenal cortex is stimulated both by humoral factors

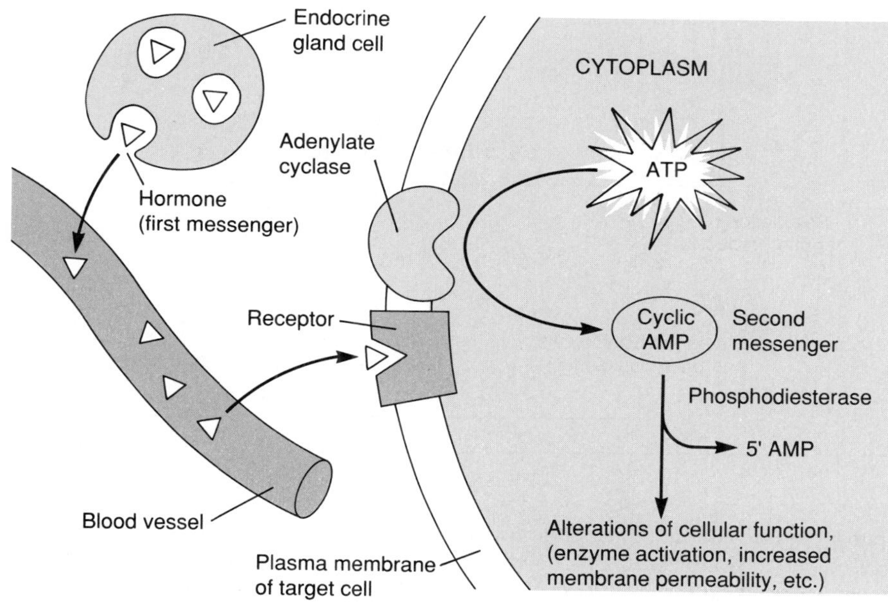

Figure 43–2

Second messenger model of hormone action. A hormone (first messenger) binds to its receptor on the plasma membrane, activating a membrane-bound enzyme called adenylate cyclase. This enzyme catalyzes the conversion of ATP to cyclic AMP, which then serves as an intracellular mediator (second messenger). Cyclic AMP eventually is broken down to an inactive form by the cytoplasmic enzyme phosphodiesterase, which terminates the response to the hormone.

(*Source:* From Campbell NA, *Biology,* p. 886. Benjamin/ Cummings, 1988.)

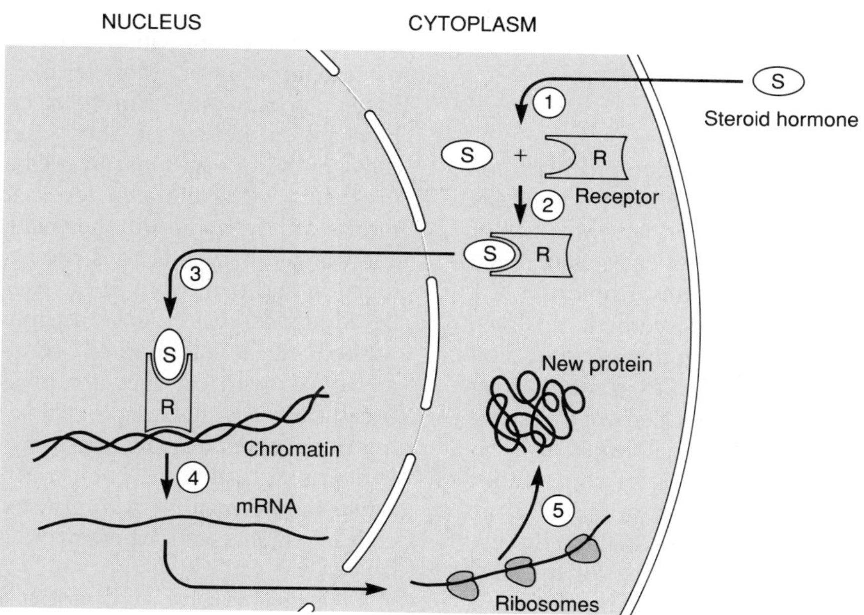

Figure 43–3

Steroid hormone action. The lipid-soluble steroid passes through plasma membrane and binds (**1**) to a receptor protein present in target cells. Hormone-receptor complex (**2**) enters the nucleus and binds (**3**) to specific receptor sites, activating the expression of certain genes (**4**). In turn, ribosomal protein synthesis is stimulated (**5**) in the cytosol.

(*Source:* Adapted from Campbell NA, *Biology,* p. 885. Benjamin/Cummings, 1988.)

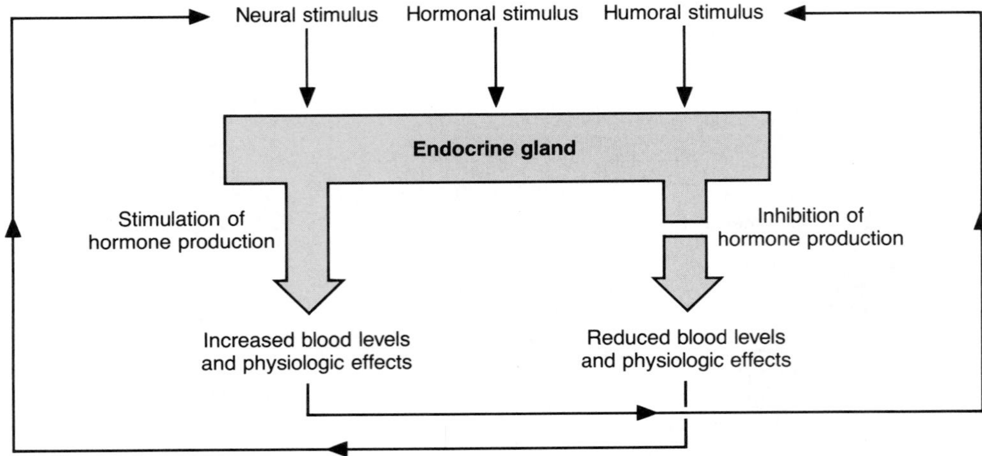

Figure 43–4

Feedback control loop that regulates hormone secretion. The endocrine gland is stimulated to synthesize and release hormone. As the hormone is released into the bloodstream, blood concentrations rise and it produces its effects. When sufficient hormone has been released, the endocrine gland is signaled to reduce synthesis of the hormone (right-hand loop) until the stimulus for increased hormone production is triggered again (left-hand loop).

(declining sodium or increasing potassium ion concentrations in the blood) and by a drop in renal blood pressure (mediated by the sympathetic nervous system). Additionally, hormones produced by the stomach and small intestine are liberated in response to increased acidity or other chemical fluctuations occurring in those organs.

Clinical Uses for Hormones

Most endocrine abnormalities are related to hypo- or hyperactivity of an endocrine organ. Problems also may result when there are deficiencies or abnormalities of specific hormone receptors on target cells, as in some forms of diabetes mellitus and diabetes insipidus.

Clinically, hormones (or their synthetic analogs) are used commonly for replacement therapy, to inhibit the action of other hormones, and to treat certain nonendocrine disorders. In general, replacement therapy is aimed at restoring normal hormonal levels and responses in the body; low hormone doses (which mimic or reproduce normal hormonal levels) are used. Common examples of replacement therapy include the use of insulin for diabetes mellitus; thyroxine for hypothyroidism; and adrenocorticosteroids for acute or chronic adrenocortical insufficiency.

Hormones also may be used as diagnostic agents to assess the function of a specific target organ. For example, adrenocorticotropic hormone (ACTH) may be administered to assess the capability of the adrenal cortex to produce glucocorticoids, and thyroid-stimulating hormone (TSH) is used to evaluate the thyroid gland's ability to produce thyroxine.

Some cases of undesirable hormone production may be handled by administering hormones or other drugs that interfere with the action or regulation of the natural hormone, or destroy the hormone-producing tissue. Perhaps one of the best examples of hormone blockade is the use of birth control pills (containing estrogen and progestins) to create a state of "pseudopregnancy." The elevated levels of the externally administered ovarian hormones inhibit the hypothalamic-anterior pituitary axis, thus preventing normal ovarian function and ovulation. In other cases, a hormone can be administered to antagonize physiologically the unwanted effects of another. Androgen administration to women with estrogen- or progesterone-dependent breast cancer is an example of this type of therapy. Nonhormonal agents usually are used when destruction of endocrine gland tissue is desired. For example, radioactive iodine may be administered to destroy thyroid cells in patients with hyperthyroidism caused by thyroid cancer.

Pharmacologic ("hyperphysiologic") hormone doses may be given to produce effects that are *not* seen at only physiologic concentrations. Such doses usually are used to manage nonendocrine disorders. An example is the use of adrenocorticosteroids for severe arthritis. Regulating the response to pharmacologic doses of a hormone is much more difficult, and care must be exercised to avoid toxic responses during treatment and on its discontinuation.

Many nonhormonal drugs also are used to inhibit hormone synthesis or release. Common examples are the use of high concentrations of iodide to inhibit the release of thyroid hormones, as in the treatment of thyrotoxicosis; the administration of danazol to treat endometriosis or fibrocystic breast disease (it inhibits gonadotropin release from the pituitary); and the administration of bromocriptine, which inhibits prolactin release, to treat hyperprolactinemia. Bromocriptine also reduces serum growth hormone levels; hence its approved use for treating some cases of acromegaly. There are also drugs that are not given to inhibit release of a hormone, but do so as a side effect. Alcohol's ability to inhibit antidiuretic hormone release is an example.

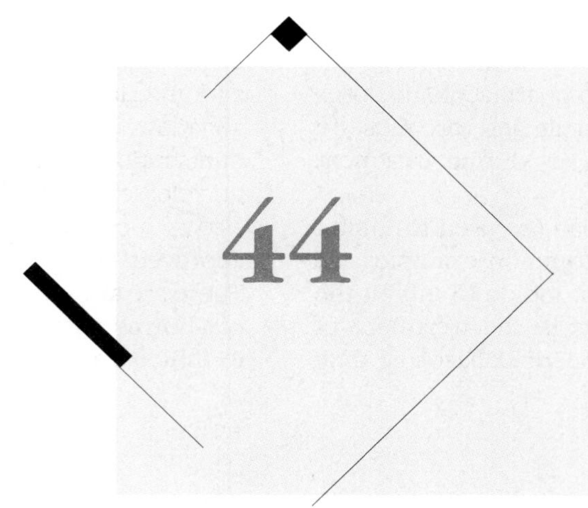

Pituitary-Hypothalamic Relationships

The hypothalamus is an important autonomic center that controls thirst, body temperature, and water balance, as well as biologic rhythms, drives, and emotions. Hypothalamic neurons involved in pituitary regulation make widespread synapses with other brain areas, and the hypothalamic peptides are broadly distributed in the brain, thus allowing central nervous system (CNS) input to anterior pituitary function.

In addition, the lack of a blood–brain barrier in the hypothalamic-pituitary area renders it accessible to circulating plasma factors, including hormones, ions, sugars, and drugs. Thus, a single external stimulus, such as acute blood volume loss or a severe wound, can be followed by widespread neuroendocrine adjustments. The hypothalamic-pituitary linkage also accounts for the pulsatile nature of pituitary hormone secretion, which is dependent on biologic rhythms, and the hormonal deficits seen in patients with hypothalamic tumors.

Major reference tables appear beginning on p. 880.

The Normal Pituitary Gland

The pituitary gland, or hypophysis, is located at the base of the brain in the sella turcica. It is composed of two histologically distinct areas—the posterior pituitary, or neurohypophysis, primarily composed of nerve fibers; and the anterior pituitary, or adenohypophysis, composed of glandular tissue.

The posterior pituitary derives from a downgrowth of hypothalamic tissue and maintains its connection with the brain via the hypothalamic-hypophyseal tract—neural pathways that run through the connecting infundibular stalk. Neurosecretory cells in the hypothalamus produce two neurohormones, vasopressin and oxytocin, which are transported down the length of their axons to the posterior pituitary. They are stored temporarily and released into the bloodstream in response to appropriate stimuli (Fig. 44–1).

The anterior pituitary is formed from a superior outpocketing (Rathke's pouch) of the pharyngeal mucosa. In contrast to the posterior pituitary, the anterior pituitary has no direct neural connection with the brain. Instead, a vascular connection (Fig. 44–2), the hypophyseal portal system, allows blood to flow from the hypothalamus to the anterior pituitary.

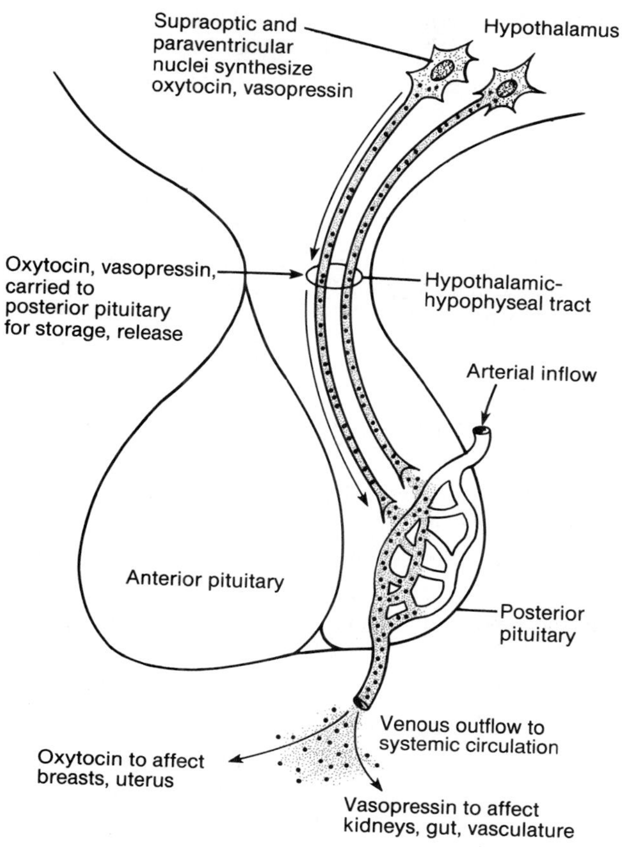

Figure 44–1

The posterior pituitary gland, its vascular supply, and secretory activity. Neurons in hypothalamus synthesize oxytocin and vasopressin (●), which are carried to the termini of the axons where they await release by hypothalamic stimuli. Stimulated axons release these hormones into bloodstream via venous outflow from the posterior pituitary. Hormones then are delivered to target tissues, where they exert their major effects.

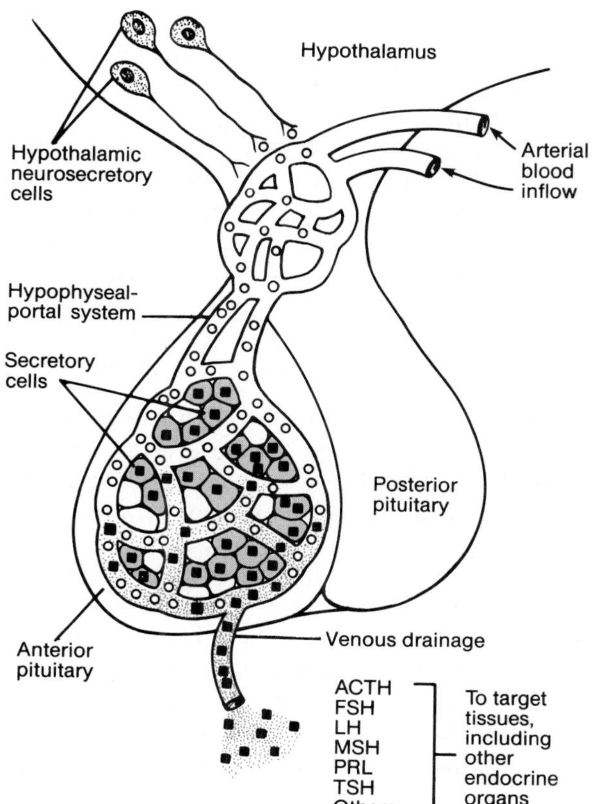

Figure 44–2

The anterior pituitary gland. Neural stimuli (or other stimuli delivered by the arterial inflow to the hypothalamus) trigger release of local releasing or inhibiting hormones (○) into the hypophyseal portal system from neurosecretory cells. They are carried to the anterior pituitary gland, where they regulate the release of other hormones (■) from secretory cells into the systemic circulation. Released hormones and factors affect other targets, some of which (eg, the adrenal cortex and the thyroid) release still other hormones.

Table 44–1 Hypothalamic Releasing and Inhibiting Hormones

Factor	Effects
Corticotropin-releasing hormone (CRH)	Stimulates anterior pituitary release of adrenocorticotropin (ACTH)
Gonadotropin- or luteinizing hormone–releasing hormone (GnRH or LHRH)	Stimulates anterior pituitary release of follicle-stimulating hormone (FSH) and luteinizing hormone (LH)
Growth hormone–inhibiting hormone (GHIH; somatostatin)	Inhibits anterior pituitary release of growth hormone (GH)
Growth hormone–releasing hormone (GHRH)	Stimulates anterior pituitary release of GH
Prolactin-inhibiting hormone (PIH)	Inhibits anterior pituitary release of prolactin
Prolactin-releasing hormone (PRH)	Stimulates anterior pituitary release of prolactin
Thyrotropin-releasing hormone (TRH)	Stimulates anterior pituitary release of thyroid-stimulating hormone (TSH) and probably prolactin

Neurons in the hypothalamus produce small polypeptides, releasing and inhibiting hormones that are released into the portal capillary blood (Table 44–1). This anatomic adaptation prevents dilution of the hypothalamic factors in the general circulation, and guarantees a high concentration of the releasing and inhibiting hormones in the anterior pituitary, where they regulate the secretory activity of hormone-producing target cells.

I. Anterior Pituitary Hormones

Traditionally, the anterior pituitary has been called the "master endocrine gland" because of the many hormones it produces. However, recent findings suggest a more important role for hypothalamic control of endocrine function.

Over a half-dozen distinct anterior pituitary peptide hormones with specific physiologic actions have been identified. Several of these hormones—thyroid-stimulating hormone, gonadotropins (follicle-stimulating hormone and luteinizing hormone), and adrenocorticotropic hormone—control the secretory activity of target organs that are also endocrine glands. Prolactin, growth hormone, and melanocyte-stimulating hormone, the other anterior pituitary hormones, exert their primary effects on nonendocrine targets. The effects and regulation of anterior pituitary hormones are summarized in Table 44–2.

Anterior Pituitary-Hypothalamic Interactions

The anterior pituitary hormones are secreted in response to hypothalamic-releasing hormones. Hormonal release is inhibited by direct-feedback inhibition of target organ hormones (in the case of tropic hormones), by hypothalamic-inhibiting hormones, and by CNS-mediated neurotransmitters. As noted earlier, various blood-borne substances may alter pituitary secretory activity by acting on the brain itself or via the hypophyseal portal system.

Pituitary hormones are extremely important physiologically, but few of them are used therapeutically because endocrine organ dysfunction caused by pituitary failure usually can be treated by administering target organ hormones.

Growth Hormone

Physiologic Effects

Growth hormone (GH), also known as somatotropin (STH), is a polypeptide composed of 191 amino acids. It is the only anterior pituitary hormone that targets nearly all body tissues. Growth hormone promotes generalized somatic growth. Its major growth-stimulating or anabolic effects are on long bones and skeletal muscle. Growth hormone initiates changes in cellular protein, carbohydrate, and fat metabolism. Growth hormone exerts some of its effects directly on target tissues, and exerts others indirectly through *somatomedins,* intermediate growth-promoting proteins produced by the liver. The important effects of GH on metabolism, muscle, bone, cartilage, and most other body cells, are summarized in Table 44–2.

Growth hormone's direct effects are limited by its short half-life (approximately 20 minutes); however, indirect effects mediated through somatomedins are much more prolonged.

Regulation

Secretion of GH is regulated primarily by two hypothalamic factors (see Table 44–1) with effects antagonistic to one another: *growth hormone–releasing hormone*

Table 44–2 | Anterior Pituitary Hormone Regulation and Effects

Hormone	Regulation of, Drug Effects on, Release	Target(s) and Effect(s)	Effects of Hyposecretion	Effects of Hypersecretion
Adrenocorticotropic hormone (ACTH)	↑ by CRH, fever, hypoglycemia, stress; *Drugs:* corticotropin, cosyntropin ↓ by feedback inhibition from circulating cortisol; *Drugs:* corticosteroids	1. Promotes release of glucocorticoids, androgens, and, to a lesser extent, mineralocorticoids, which affect many target tissues	Addison's disease	Cushing's disease
Follicle-stimulating hormone (FSH)	↑ by GnRH (LHRH), tumors; *Drug:* clomiphene ↓ by feedback inhibition of estrogen in females, and of testosterone in males; *Drug:* danazol	1. Females: stimulates ovarian follicle maturation and estrogen production 2. Males: stimulates sperm production by seminiferous tubules	Failure of sexual maturation	Unknown
Growth hormone (GH)	↑ by growth hormone–releasing hormone (GHRH), hypoglycemia, increased blood amino acid levels (especially arginine), estrogen, vasopressin, hypoglycemia; ↓ by growth hormone–inhibiting hormone (GHIH), hyperglycemia, increased blood free fatty acid levels, progestins; *Drugs:* β-adrenergic agonists, α adrenergic, serotonin, or dopamine receptor blockers; effects antagonized by corticosteroids	1. Stimulates cell uptake of amino acids, protein synthesis, causing increased muscle cell size and number 2. Stimulates uptake of sulfur into cartilage matrix, synthesis of collagen, condroitin sulfate 3. Stimulates glucagon release from pancreatic alpha cells, increasing blood glucose levels that stimulate insulin release 4. Mobilizes fats, increases serum triglyceride levels 5. In children may antagonize insulin's effects on carbohydrate and fat metabolism (ie, diabetogenic effect) 6. May induce insulin resistance in normal adults 7. Influences internal organ size, increases red cell mass	Pituitary dwarfism in children	Gigantism in children; acromegaly in adults
Luteinizing hormone (LH)	↑ by GnRH (LHRH) ↓ by feedback inhibition by progesterone in females, by testosterone in males	1. Females: triggers ovulation, converts ruptured follicle to corpus luteum 2. Males: stimulates Leydig cells to secrete androgens	As for FSH	As for FSH
Melanocyte-stimulating hormone (MSH)	Unknown	Causes melanocytes to form melanin deposits	Unknown	Unknown

(continued)

Table 44–2 **Anterior Pituitary Hormone Regulation and Effects (*Continued*)**

Hormone	Regulation of, Drug Effects on, Release	Target(s) and Effect(s)	Effects of Hyposecretion	Effects of Hypersecretion
Prolactin	↑ by prolactin-releasing hormone (PRH), which is increased by serotonin, estrogens; ↓ PIH by dopamine receptor blockers (most antipsychotic drugs), reserpine ↓ by prolactin-inhibiting hormone (PIH), which is increased by dopaminergic agonists (eg, bromocriptine, levodopa)	1. Females: promotes lactation through actions on breast secretory tissues 2. Males: probably potentiates testosterone's effects on various target cells	Poor milk production postpartum	Galactorrhea; anovulation; impotence in males
Thyroid-stimulating hormone (TSH)	↑ by thyrotropin-releasing hormone; protirelin ↓ by circulating thyroid hormones via feedback mechanism *Drugs:* corticosteroids	1. Stimulates thyroid hormone synthesis in, release from, follicular cells of thyroid gland	Eventual thyroid atrophy, depressed secretory activity, signs and symptoms of hypothyroidism, myxedema, cretinism	Overproduction of thyroid hormones, hyperthyroidism, Graves' disease

Key: = ↑ increased; = ↓ decreased.

(GHRH) and *growth hormone–inhibiting hormone* (GHIH) (or *somatostatin*).

Typically, GH secretion has a diurnal cycle, with the highest levels occurring during sleep. However, its release can be extremely variable, and responds to several secondary triggers such as α-adrenergic, dopaminergic, or serotoninergic stimuli; β-adrenergic blockade; estrogen; vasopressin; glucagon and hypoglycemia; decreased free fatty acid levels; increased arginine levels; and vigorous exercise or stress.

Growth hormone release can be inhibited by somatostatin; β-adrenergic stimuli; α-adrenergic, serotoninergic, or dopaminergic receptor blockade; glucocorticoids and increased blood glucose and free fatty acid levels; and progestins.

Effects of Growth Hormone Hyper- and Hyposecretion

Hypersecretion of GH in children results in *gigantism,* a syndrome in which growth rate is accelerated. Gigantism results in abnormally tall stature (seven to eight feet), but fairly normal body proportions. The term *acromegaly* is the term used to describe the onset of excessive GH secretion occurring after puberty and epiphyseal plate closure. Acromegaly is characterized by enlargement and thickening of bony areas still responsive to GH effects (or those of somatomedins), particularly the bones of the fingers, feet, and face. Enlargement of facial bones and cartilages, and thickening of some of the soft tissues, results in coarse and often malformed facial features. Excessive GH levels are determined routinely by sensitive radioimmunoassay techniques.

Almost all conditions of GH hypersecretion are caused by pituitary tumors, and are treated surgically or by radiation therapy of the pituitary. One drug, bromocriptine, is indicated for pharmacotherapy of acromegaly.

Hyposecretion of GH in children results in *pituitary dwarfism,* characterized by small stature (heights of four feet or less) but normal body proportions. The lack of malproportion is a reason pediatric patients with GH deficits may go undiagnosed initially. True pediatric GH hyposecretion is diagnosed by objective tests. Children should be screened for GH deficiency if their height is less than two to three standard deviations below the mean for children of the same age.

Other tests include radiographic examinations to assess bone age, measurement of plasma somatomedin-C levels, and functional tests (such as insulin to induce hypoglycemia or intravenous arginine infusions) that normally stimulate GH release. If such challenges fail to increase GH levels above 5 to 7 ng/mL, GH deficiency may be suspected.

Growth hormone deficits are seldom problematic in otherwise normal adults after somatic growth is complete. However, diabetic patients with an onset of GH deficiency may require lower doses of insulin or other hypoglycemic drugs, since the normal antagonism between GH and insulin is decreased.

Therapeutic Products

The use of human cadaver–derived GH was stopped because it often caused Creutzfeldt-Jakob disease (a severe and fatal neuromuscular discorder caused by degeneration of the brain's pyramidal and extrapyramidal tracts), and because sufficient quantities of GH were difficult to obtain. Recombinant DNA technology is now used to produce GH from bacteria. That has increased the supply of GH, but the drug is still expensive, with costs up to about $20,000 per year.

Bromocriptine

Bromocriptine mesylate (PARLODEL) is indicated for treating acromegaly and other endocrine disorders. The drug often is used for treating parkinsonism. Chapter 25 discusses this use, and provides a more complete discussion of the pharmacokinetics, side effects, and drug interactions.

Absorption, Distribution, Metabolism, and Excretion

Bromocriptine is administered orally, but gastrointestinal (GI) tract absorption is irregular. The drug is metabolized completely before excretion.

Pharmacologic Effects, Clinical Indications, and Administration

All of bromocriptine's therapeutic effects result from its ability to act as a dopamine-like agonist. Some are based on its ability to inhibit prolactin release, which reduces serum GH levels.

Treatment of Pituitary Tumors and Acromegaly

Bromocriptine can be used alone or as an adjunct to radiation therapy directed at destroying a pituitary tumor. Typical doses are noted in Table 44–C1. Bromocriptine's desired effects in acromegaly appear much sooner than those caused by radiation therapy, which may not be seen for months or a year or more. In persons with acromegaly, bromocriptine lowers GH levels by 50% or more in about half of treated patients, but it seldom normalizes GH levels. Prolactin levels usually are decreased, but the levels of other anterior pituitary hormones seldom are changed.

Uses Based on Reduced Serum Prolactin Levels

There are two major indications for bromocriptine based on its ability to lower prolactin levels: treatment of hyperprolactinemia, and suppression of physiologic lactation after stillbirth, abortion, or after normal delivery for women who will not be breast-feeding. In both cases, the drug acts through a dopamine-like agonist action, which stimulates hypothalamic PIH release. Typical dosages are summarized in Table 44–C1.

Hyperprolactinemia

Amenorrhea, with or without galactorrhea or hypogonadism (infertility), is a symptom of a hyperprolactinemic condition in which bromocriptine is indicated to lower serum prolactin levels. One of the related therapeutic goals is pregnancy.

Another indication is the presence of a prolactin-secreting adenoma, which often is the underlying cause of amenorrhea. Bromocriptine can be used alone, or in conjunction with surgical or radiation therapy of prolactin-secreting adenomas. Bromocriptine may shrink the tumor.

About two thirds of all patients receiving bromocriptine for suppression of hyperprolactinemia experience mild side effects. Nausea is the most common side effect, followed by headache and dizziness. Hypotension, a common side effect when bromocriptine is used for any purpose, also may occur. These side effects may appear with therapeutic doses, usually 5 to 7.5 mg per day, which are much lower than typical doses used for acromegaly or parkinsonism. Rhinorrhea caused by cerebrospinal fluid leakage in persons with large adenomas has been reported, but usually this has occurred after pituitary surgical or radiation therapy.

Suppression of Physiologic Lactation

Bromocriptine indirectly inhibits milk secretion and breast engorgement (the latter of which often can be managed with nondrug measures), thus inhibiting milk production. Three conditions should be met before bromocriptine is administered for this purpose: the need to suppress lactation; the mother's desire not to breast-feed; and a stable and normal maternal blood pressure. Bromocriptine therapy to suppress lactation usually lasts 14 days.

Of the side effects noted earlier, hypotension is common and significant. Other relatively frequent side effects include headache, dizziness, vomiting, fatigue, and nausea. Pregnancy-related precautions previously noted for the use of bromocriptine for acromegaly also apply to its use for suppressing prolactin levels.

Even though postpartum therapy with bromocriptine is brief, it is not without danger. There have been reports of stroke, myocardial infarction, and seizures during such use, mainly in women with uncomplicated pregnancies. In many cases, strokes or seizures were preceded by a progressively worsening headache, or visual disturbances. Rebound breast engorgement and pain may occur after bromocriptine therapy is stopped.

NURSING IMPLICATIONS

Since bromocriptine often increases the risk of pregnancy before the return of menses, but the drug should not be administered during pregnancy, advise patients of the need for frequent and periodic pregnancy tests. Such tests are recommended every four weeks during the amenorrheic phase of bromocriptine therapy, and after every missed menstrual period once menstruation returns.

Bromocriptine therapy should be stopped as soon as pregnancy is detected. Advise pregnant women of the need for continued follow-up, since prolactin-secreting tumors may grow quickly once bromocriptine therapy is stopped. If pregnancy is not a desired outcome of therapy, stress the importance of contraception by means other than birth-control pills.

Notify the physician immediately if a patient receiving bromocriptine develops any side effects. Of most concern are blood pressure changes, headaches, increased CNS irritability or frank seizures, visual disturbances, or a watery nasal discharge.

Before administering bromocriptine postpartum, confirm the mother's desire not to breast-feed; the drug's effects on lactation are essentially irreversible until the next pregnancy. Assess for breast engorgement and mild pain after stopping bromocriptine therapy for suppressing lactation. Provide nondrug comfort measures, and mild analgesics as ordered, to reduce discomfort.

Side Effects, Adverse Reactions, and Contraindications

Bromocriptine usually causes side effects (Table 44–S1), but they are rarely severe. Nausea, constipation, and dizziness are common when bromocriptine is used for acromegaly. Dizziness probably is caused by the drug's hypotensive action, particularly with postural changes. This postural or orthostatic hypotension, caused by peripheral vasodilation, is often sufficient to cause fainting, and rarely may be sufficient to trigger significant reflex cardiac stimulation or to aggravate preexisting arrhythmias.

Hypotension is the most common cardiovascular side effect caused by bromocriptine, although hypertension caused by vasoconstriction has been reported. Blood pressure changes may occur early during therapy, or after one or two weeks of treatment. Some persons with acromegaly experience cold-induced vasospasm in the extremities, and bromocriptine may increase the severity or frequency of this response. Dosage reductions and keeping the extremities warm alleviate the problem.

Therapeutic doses of bromocriptine often cause drowsiness or sedation, which usually diminish with continued administration of the drug or with reduced doses. High doses of bromocriptine may cause confusion and mental disturbances, but these are more likely to occur in persons with parkinsonism. Bleeding ulcers and pituitary tumor growth during bromocriptine therapy of acromegaly have been reported. Whether these were caused by the drug is not known, but appropriate monitoring nevertheless is indicated. Long-term, high-dose bromocriptine therapy (ie, six to 36 months at daily doses between 20 and 100 mg) may cause pulmonary infiltrates and pleural effusions or thickening. Confusion, hallucinations, and other mental disturbances also may occur. These doses and therapy durations are relatively common when bromocriptine is used to treat acromegaly or parkinsonism, and the side effects should be looked for during assessment. Both the pulmonary and mental changes appear to be reversible when bromocriptine doses are reduced or stopped.

Bromocriptine is contraindicated in patients with uncontrolled hypertension, eclampsia or preeclampsia, or sensitivity to ergot alkaloids. The drug should be used cautiously and with appropriate monitoring in any patient with excessively high or low blood pressure, unstable blood pressure, or ischemic heart or brain disease.

NURSING IMPLICATIONS

Advise all patients taking bromocriptine that nausea, constipation, dizziness or lightheadedness, or sedation may occur during early therapy. The drug should be taken with meals to lessen GI upset. Monitor to assess the frequency and severity of these problems, and implement nondrug interventions to alleviate them when possible (eg, increasing intake of fluids and bulk-forming foods for constipation; standing slowly with support to guard against syncope; avoiding motor vehicle operation).

Advise patients to report these side effects if they are excessive or prolonged, and to report other potential side effects such as palpitations; abdominal pain or discolored stools (may indicate underlying peptic ulcer disease); headache (could indicate stroke); and paresthesias, pain, or discoloration of the extremities. Explain to patients and their families that bromocriptine only halts the progression of acromegaly; it will not reverse prior changes. Advise that periodic blood tests of GH levels are necessary to help evaluate and guide therapy.

Other nursing implications, particularly those associated with the use of bromocriptine for parkinsonism, are discussed in Chapter 25.

◆ Use During Pregnancy and Lactation

Pregnancy and lactation are two of the most interesting contraindications for bromocriptine. The drug should be used during pregnancy only if anticipated benefits outweigh possible risks to the mother or fetus. However, because of its endocrine effects, particularly suppression of prolactin levels, bromocriptine increases the likelihood of conception. Extra precautions to prevent pregnancy are essential.

Oral contraceptives contain estrogens, which antagonize bromocriptine's desired endocrine effects. Therefore, recommend other contraceptive methods.

Hypertension associated with preeclampsia or eclampsia, and hypotension caused by postpartum maternal bleeding, are common pregnancy-related symptoms that absolutely contraindicate bromocriptine use. Even if maternal blood pressure is normal and stable, very close monitoring of the maternal and fetal responses to bromocriptine is always essential.

Bromocriptine inhibits breast milk production, so women who wish to breast-feed should not receive this drug.

◆ Use in Children

There is no information about the efficacy or safety of bromocriptine in children younger than 15 years.

◆ Use in the Elderly

Bromocriptine seldom is administered to elderly persons for endocrinologic effects. The drug's major use in the elderly is for parkinsonism. Special precautions for this use are discussed in Chapter 25.

Interactions with Other Drugs

Bromocriptine increases the risk of hypotension when administered with other drugs that lower blood pressure, and combined use should be avoided or at least supervised closely. Drugs that block dopamine receptors in the brain, primarily antipsychotic drugs and metoclopramide, and drugs that deplete catecholamines (reserpine, guanadrel, and related agents) may antagonize bromocriptine's therapeutic effects and may increase the risk of hypotension.

Related Drugs

Somatrem and Somatropin

Somatrem (PROTROPIN) and somatropin (HUMATROPE) are biosynthetic forms of human GH. Both drugs are pharmacologically identical to human GH and are used in identical ways.

Absorption, Distribution, Metabolism, and Excretion

Somatrem and somatropin have half-lives equivalent to endogenous GH, about 10 to 50 minutes. Their effects last for several days because of the intermediary action of somatomedin.

Pharmacologic Effects

The bioengineered growth hormones are used to stimulate somatic growth, but they also cause all the other effects ascribed to endogenous GH.

Clinical Indications and Administration

Somatrem and somatropin are used exclusively for replacement therapy in children shown to have growth retardation caused by a lack of GH. These drugs are not indicated for treating dwarfism of other causes, or for use after epiphyseal plate closure. The dosages of somatrem and somatropin are slightly different (see Table 44–C1).

Regardless of which drug is chosen, it is administered by intramuscular (IM) injection three times a week, with a minimum of 48 hours between successive injections. The therapeutic response is assessed by measurement of body growth and development, which should be apparent within six to 12 months after treatment starts.

Side Effects, Adverse Reactions, and Contraindications

Somatrem and somatropin cause few side effects (see Table 44–S1). Some patients develop neutralizing antibodies to these products, but they generally do not interfere with drug efficacy. There have been a few reports of therapeutic failure, however. If the response during treatment declines, tests to detect anti-GH antibodies should be performed. Somatrem or somatropin may cause hypothyroidism during treatment. Insulin resistance, an expected consequence of GH itself, may cause added problems if the patient has diabetes.

Somatrem and somatropin are contraindicated in persons with closed epiphyses, and in all persons with evidence of an active intracranial lesion. The drugs may be used after completion of antitumor therapy or inactivation, but should be stopped if there is any evidence of tumor growth or renewed activity. Somatrem contains benzyl alcohol as a preservative, and somatropin includes glycerin and the preservative, *m*-cresol. Prior adverse responses to these agents contraindicate use of the respective drugs.

Interactions with Other Drugs

Somatrem and somatropin, like GH itself, may antagonize the effects of insulin. Therefore, insulin doses in diabetic patients may need to be increased as GH levels rise. Corticosteroids antagonize the growth-promoting effects of somatrem or somatropin. Patients with adrenal cortical dysfunction who are receiving corticosteroid replacement therapy may require reduced steroid doses to compensate for the interaction.

NURSING IMPLICATIONS

Somatrem and somatropin are supplied as powders that should be reconstituted with the diluent provided by the manufacturer. The diluents for each drug differ, and cannot be interchanged. The volume of diluent to be used depends on the desired concentration of the final solution. This, in turn, depends on the dose to be administered, which is based on the patient's weight. Both products must be stored in the refrigerator before use. Inject the diluent into the vial using aseptic technique, taking care to direct the stream of diluent down the sides of the vial, rather than directly into the drug. Rotate the vial gently; never shake it. The product should be clear; discard it if there is evidence of cloudiness or solid matter; once reconstituted, store in a refrigerator. Reconstituted somatrem can be stored and used within seven days; somatropin is stable up to 14 days.

Be familiar with child growth and development norms to help assess potential candidates for GH replacement therapy, and to help assess the response of treated children. In general, candidates for GH therapy are children who are below the third percentile for growth.

Encourage parents or guardians to monitor and record the child's height and weight weekly, to report significant deviations from anticipated changes (based on estimates provided by the physician), and to obtain an identification bracelet for the child indicating GH replacement therapy. The wait for a positive drug response can be frustrating to the patient, parents, and health-care providers. Assist the patient and family to achieve a positive outlook as normal maturation occurs, and reinforce positive progress.

If the GH-treated patient also has diabetes, use proper assessment to monitor the course of antidiabetic therapy; anticipate the potential need for altered dietary or drug therapy if insulin resistance develops. Also assess for signs and symptoms of hypothyroidism during therapy, since hypothyroidism could contribute to inadequate growth and development during GH therapy.

If the patient also is receiving corticosteroids, anticipate the need to reduce steroid doses to avoid an inhibitory effect on growth. Slipped capital femoral epiphyses may occur more frequently in patients with endocrine disorders. Be alert to complaints of hip or knee pain, or the development of a limp, in patients treated with somatrem or somatropin.

Prolactin

Prolactin is a protein that arises from the same precursor as GH. Its major function in women is to stimulate the enzymes necessary for milk production. In men, prolactin appears to potentiate the effects of testosterone on that hormone's target cells.

Regulation

Prolactin levels are controlled by two hypothalamic factors, *prolactin-releasing hormone (PRH)* and *prolactin-inhibiting hormone (PIH)* (see Table 44–1). In men and nonpregnant women, the hypothalamus inhibits prolactin release, indicating that PIH is the major influence. This basal control differs from the control of other anterior pituitary hormones. Damage to the hypothalamus in a man or nonpregnant woman usually inhibits secretion of other pituitary hormones, but increases prolactin levels.

Other factors that control prolactin secretion are dopamine and dopaminergic drugs (levodopa, bromocriptine, and ergot alkaloids, for example), which enhance PIH release and reduce eventual prolactin secretion. In contrast, dopamine-receptor blockers (eg, phenothiazines, haloperidol) and catecholamine-depleting drugs (such as reserpine) inhibit PIH release and may cause inappropriate lactation (galactorrhea).

Galactorrhea is a relatively common side effect of phenothiazine therapy. Serotonin, morphine, estrogens, and thyrotropin releasing hormone may promote PRH release, thereby increasing prolactin secretion.

During pregnancy, the usual inhibition of prolactin release is overcome by rising estrogen levels. Lactation occurs as a result of high prolactin and low estrogen levels near the end of pregnancy. Suckling stimulates further prolactin secretion, and stimulates oxytocin release from the posterior pituitary. The prolactin stimulates milk production. Oxytocin stimulates milk ejection (the "let-down" reflex). As nursing continues, levels of prolactin fall gradually, ultimately reaching nonpregnant levels.

Effects of Prolactin Hypersecretion

Hyperprolactinemia is more common than prolactin deficiency. Prolactin overproduction is the most common abnormality associated with pituitary tumors. Other causes of hyperprolactinemia include primary hyperthyroidism, chronic renal failure, and the use of drugs that stimulate prolactin release.

Important symptoms of hyperprolactinemia include galactorrhea, amenorrhea, and infertility in women and impotence in men. Hyperprolactinemia is diagnosed by measuring prolactin blood levels. Many cases of hyperprolactinemia are controlled by administration of bromocriptine, which was described earlier.

Effects of Prolactin Hyposecretion

Prolactin hyposecretion occurs in conditions of panhypopituitarism resulting from pituitary tumors or other causes. It is diagnosed by baseline prolactin measurements and the lack of serum prolactin increases after stimulation by administering thyrotropin-releasing hormone or chlorpromazine. In rare cases, a condition of postpartum hypoprolactinemia (Sheehan's syndrome) occurs in new mothers who have developed pituitary necrosis secondary to severe hemorrhage or shock. Characteristics of the syndrome include poor milk production, fatigability, and loss of axillary and pubic hair.

Purified sources of prolactin are presently unavailable for replacement therapy, and pharmacologic treatment of hypoprolactinemia is not recommended.

Thyroid-Stimulating Hormone

Physiologic Effects and Regulation

Thyroid-stimulating hormone (TSH) is a glycoprotein tropic hormone required for normal development and function of the thyroid gland. When TSH attaches to thyroid gland cell membranes, it activates the enzyme adenyl cyclase, which triggers thyroid hormone synthesis and release. Thyroid-stimulating hormone release occurs when thyrotropin-releasing hormone (TRH) is released from the hypothalamus into the hypophyseal portal system; thyroid hormones in the systemic circulation cause feedback-inhibition of TSH release (see Tables 44–1 and 44–2). Animal-derived TSH and synthetic TRH are available for diagnosing thyroid gland dysfunction.

Effects of Thyroid-Stimulating Hormone Hyper- and Hyposecretion

Overproduction of TSH may cause hyperthyroidism, but this is not common. Most cases of hyperthyroidism are caused by pituitary macroadenomas, pituitary resistance to circulating thyroid hormone levels, or Graves' disease, all of which involve failure of the normal feedback regulatory system. The clinical manifestations of hyperthyroidism, and its treatment with surgery, irradiation, or antithyroid drugs, are discussed in Chapter 47.

Hyposecretion of TSH results in atrophy and depressed secretory activity of the thyroid gland, leading to such syndromes as myxedema in adults and cretinism in children. Thyroid hormone replacement therapy is also discussed in Chapter 47. In addition to agents used commonly to treat thyroid dysfunction, two other agents have important diagnostic uses.

Thyrotropin

Thyrotropin (THYTROPAR) is a purified extract of TSH isolated from bovine anterior pituitary glands. The drug is administered by intramuscular (IM) or subcutaneous (SC) injection. Once absorbed, it is eliminated rapidly by the kidneys. Thyrotropin's half-life is about 30 minutes in euthyroid (normal) individuals; it is longer in persons with hypothyroidism, and shorter in persons with hyperthyroidism.

Thyrotropin is used diagnostically to help differentiate between primary and secondary hypothyroidism, and to assess for decreased thyroid reserve. When the drug is injected in a normal individual, it acts like endogenous TSH to increase thyroid hormone release and, in turn, to stimulate the basal metabolic rate.

For diagnostic testing, a 10 International Unit (IU) dose of the agent is injected, and a radioiodine (^{131}I) uptake study is performed 24 hours later. In euthyroid individuals a predictable increase of ^{131}I uptake occurs. If the patient has primary hypothyroidism (failure of the thyroid gland to synthesize and release thyroid hormones), there will be little or no radioisotope incorporation. In patients with hypothyroidism caused by pituitary failure (secondary hyperthyroidism), the sudden availability of TSH will increase ^{131}I uptake to levels much greater than those seen in euthyroid patients.

Common side effects of thyrotropin injection (see Chapter 47 for more details) include facial flushing, nausea, vomiting, and headache. Transient hypotension and tachycardia, nervousness, diaphoresis, and diarrhea may occur. In some patients these reflect expected effects of normal or excessive thyroid hormone release, including signs and symptoms of acute hyperthyroidism (thyroid storm), which may include arrhythmias, angina, or acute heart failure. In others, they may reflect hypersensitivity to the drug. Anaphylactic reactions have been reported.

Thyrotropin is contraindicated for patients with prior hypersensitivity or allergy to it, patients with untreated Addison's disease, and patients with most cardiac disorders.

NURSING IMPLICATIONS

Thyrotropin must be dissolved with the diluent provided by the manufacturer immediately before use. Once reconstituted, however, the solution can be stored in a refrigerator for up to two weeks.

Before administration, assess patients for prior allergic reactions or cardiovascular disorders, either of which contraindicate thyrotropin use. Obtain baseline vital signs for comparison with changes caused by drug administration, and report any adverse effects caused by thyrotropin administration (eg, symptoms of acute drug-induced hyperthyroidism) immediately. Likewise, notify the physician if evidence of severe hypothyroidism (myxedema) exists, which may delay testing until thyroid hormone replacement therapy has been started.

Have epinephrine and the means for assisted ventilation available in case of anaphylaxis.

Advise all patients receiving this agent to keep appointments for scheduled follow-up testing the next day. Explain the various parts of the test procedure, and that subsequent therapy depends on the test's outcome.

Little is known about the safety of administering thyrotropin during pregnancy or to children. In pregnancy, the drug's ability to provide useful diagnostic information must be weighed against potential risks to the mother and fetus. Anticipate that worsening of cardiovascular disease by thyrotropin is more likely to be important for elderly patients; monitor accordingly.

Protirelin

Protirelin is the generic name for synthetic thyrotropin-releasing hormone (TRH). The product's trade names are RELEFACT TRH and THYPINONE. Protirelin is used diagnostically to provide additional evidence of thyroid disease or pituitary or hypothalamic dysfunction (secondary and tertiary hypothyroidism, respectively) as causes of thyroid hypofunction. The test involves measuring the baseline levels of TSH in a blood sample immediately before an intravenous (IV) protirelin injection (see Table 44–C1 for adult and pediatric doses).

In persons with normal pituitary, hypothalamic, and thyroid function, protirelin will increase serum TSH levels significantly because the complete hypothalamic-to-thyroid system is functioning as expected. If the diagnostic agent increases TSH levels, it is likely that the pituitary gland is responding normally, but the hypothalamus is not making enough TRH to release TSH. Alternatively, the thyroid gland may be unable to release thyroid hormone in response to TSH. If protirelin does not increase TSH levels, the pituitary gland may not be functioning normally because it does not release TSH in response to the normal stimulus. These test results, combined with the results from other tests and from patient assessments, help identify the source and cause of hypothyroidism.

The diagnostic use of synthetic TRH is relatively safe, and adverse reactions usually are mild and last only a few minutes. Perhaps the most common and unwanted side effect is a change of blood pressure—usually increases of about 20 to 30 mm Hg systolic, diastolic, or both; hypotension is less common. Signs and symptoms of hyperthyroidism may occur if protirelin increases thyroid hormone levels. Other reactions include severe headaches and temporary blindness (mainly in persons with large pituitary tumors), and, uncommonly, seizures in persons with a history of seizure disorders. Women who are lactating may experience breast enlargement or milk leakage that lasts for two or three days. There is little information about adverse effects of protirelin during pregnancy, but it is best to avoid it.

Thyroid hormone supplement therapy interferes with the use of protirelin for diagnosing the cause of underlying thyroid dysfunction. If the patient is taking liothyronine (triiodothyronine; T_3) alone, it should be discontinued one week before testing. Any other thyroid supplement should be discontinued two weeks before the protirelin test. Thyroid supplements should not be discontinued if protirelin is being used to assess the adequacy of hormone therapy.

Other agents that might suppress the expected response to protirelin include levodopa, high doses of corticosteroids, and aspirin. Although it may be easy to discontinue aspirin before testing, stopping levodopa or corticosteroid therapy may not be feasible or safe.

Protirelin itself interferes with subsequent testing if done within one week of a prior test. High serum lipid levels also interfere with thyroid testing.

NURSING IMPLICATIONS

Protirelin is supplied in 1 mL ampuls containing 500 μg (the usual adult dose). The dose should be administered as an IV bolus over about 15 to 30 seconds. Instruct most patients to fast overnight before the test; if this is not feasible or safe (as in persons with hypopituitarism), recommend a low-fat meal. Ensure that patients have discontinued other medications that might alter test results. Explain that the test may need to be repeated to confirm results of earlier testing, but that at least one week must pass to help ensure accurate results.

To minimize hypotension, make sure the patient is recumbent before and during the test, and until the last blood sample is collected (30 minutes later).

Following administration, monitor vital signs (especially blood pressure and heart rate) until the last blood sample is collected. If significant blood pressure changes occur, continue monitoring closely until pressure and other vital signs have normalized and stabilized.

Gonadotropic Hormones

Physiologic Effects

Gonadotropic hormones (or gonadotropins) regulate the activity of the gonads (ovaries and testes; see Table 44–2). The two gonadotropins, *follicle-stimulating hormone* (FSH) and *luteinizing hormone* (LH), are glycoproteins secreted by the anterior pituitary, and are similar in structure to TSH. Like nearly all peptide-based hormones, their cellular effects are mediated by receptor-binding activation of adenyl cyclase.

Secreted in increasing levels at puberty, FSH stimulates the production of gametes, or sex cells. In males, FSH promotes the maturation of the seminiferous tubules of the testes, and initiates sperm production (spermatogenesis).

In females, FSH promotes the maturation of ovarian follicles (each containing an immature egg). It causes the follicular stage of the ovarian cycle. As the follicles enlarge they secrete estrogen, and the immature ovum that each follicle contains undergoes the first maturation division in preparation for ovulation. This ovarian response represents the major action of FSH.

Luteinizing hormone stimulates the gonads to produce their hormones. In females, LH works synergistically with FSH to cause follicle maturation, and triggers ovulation approximately 14 days after follicle maturation has started. Following ovulation, LH initiates the luteal phase of the ovarian cycle, promoting the conversion of the ruptured follicle to a glandular corpus luteum and stimulating luteal production of the second ovarian hormone, progesterone.

In males, LH targets the Leydig (interstitial) cells of the testes, causing them to secrete androgens, or male sex hormones. (For this reason, LH has also been called interstitial cell-stimulating hormone, or ICSH.) The androgens (primarily testosterone), in turn, act locally in the testes to stimulate spermatogenesis.

The onset of estrogen and testosterone production in prepubertal girls and boys promotes maturation of the reproductive system and the appearance of secondary sex characteristics. A detailed consideration of the functional roles of the gonadal hormones appears in Chapters 48 and 49.

Regulation

The control of gonadotropin secretion of the progressive stages of the life (and reproductive) cycle is more complex than that of other anterior pituitary hormones. In both sexes, gonadotropin-releasing cells of the anterior pituitary are stimulated to release FSH and LH by the same hypothalamic factor, *gonadotropin-releasing hormone* (GnRH). (The term luteinizing hormone–releasing hormone [LHRH] is used to describe the factor that specifically increases luteinizing hormone secretion, but the same chemical appears to cause FSH release also, so the general term GnRH can be used. The abbreviation LHRH will be reserved for agents used therapeutically to test LH release.)

Gonadal hormones, produced in response to the gonadotropins, inhibit FSH and LH release via a feedback mechanism. Feedback of testosterone in males maintains fairly constant levels of gonadotropin release and testosterone production. In addition, gonadotropin release is inhibited by *inhibin,* a protein product of both male and female gonads.

In contrast, feedback inhibition of the two ovarian hormones results in cyclic peaks and troughs of FSH and LH release. These recur at approximately 28-day intervals and result in the sequential follicular, ovulatory, and luteal stages of the ovary. The follicular stage, initiated by rising FSH levels in the plasma, results in follicular estrogen production; estrogen feedback to the anterior pituitary inhibits FSH release (and thus its own release), and stimulates release of LH.

Rising LH blood levels, in turn, trigger luteal secretion of progesterone. Increasing progesterone levels inhibit LH release; as LH levels decline, luteal stimulation ends. By the 28th day of the ovarian cycle, both the gonadotropins and the ovarian hormones are at their lowest levels in the blood, which results in menses, and the resumption of FSH release.

Thus it appears that modification of gonadotropin release in females—that is, a choice for FSH or LH—is exerted at the level of the pituitary gland via differences in blood levels of the different ovarian hormones. Prolactin, cortisol, and androgens, when present in high levels, suppress the effects of gonadotropins.

Effects of Gonadotropic Hormone Hyper- and Hyposecretion

Ectopic, excessive gonadotropin secretion can occur with testicular or ovarian cancers (germinomas), lung carcinomas, hepatomas, and other tumors. Pituitary gonadotropin-secreting tumors are relatively common. Excessive secretion causes precocious puberty in children and gynecomastia in men; no distinct clinical syndrome occurs in women with gonadotropin hypersecretion.

Gonadotropin deficiency seriously interferes with the reproductive capabilities of both sexes. The cause may involve either hypothalamic or pituitary dysfunction. Permanent genetic deficits of hypothalamic GnRH, such as Kallman's syndrome, result in congenital gonadotropin deficiency and a failure of sexual maturation.

Therapeutic Products

Several products are useful for treating or diagnosing hypogonadotropic states. Many of them are intimately involved with regulating gonadal activity and reproductive processes. Therefore, they will be mentioned only briefly here and discussed in more detail in Chapter 49.

Gonadotropins

Purified gonadotropin products are human chorionic gonadotropin (hCG; marketed as A.P.L., PREGNYL, PROFASI, and many more; obtained from the urine of pregnant women), urofollitropin, and menotropins (METRODIN and PERGONAL; both obtained from postmenopausal urine). One indication for hCG is inducing ovulation and pregnancy in women who are infertile because of causes other than ovarian failure. The hCG is administered after pretreatment with urofollitropin or menotropins, which stimulate follicular development. Other uses for hCG, given by IM injection, are treatment of prepubertal cryptorchidism (failure of the testicles to descend) and some cases of male hypogonadism caused by pituitary failure.

Menotropins, as commercially prepared for clinical use, contain equal amounts of FSH and LH. Menotropins, also injected IM, can be used adjunctively with hCG to stimulate spermatogenesis in males with hypogonadism caused by gonadotropin deficiencies.

Nonhormonal Agents

Nonhormonal products stimulate or inhibit pituitary gonadotropin release. Clomiphene citrate (CLOMID; SEROPHENE), similar to hCG, promotes pituitary release of FSH and LH. It is used to treat infertility in women who have normal ovarian and pituitary function, but lack the normal hypothalamic stimulus (GnRH) for FSH and LH release. Danazol (DANOCRINE) is a synthetic androgen that depresses FSH and LH release. It is used frequently to treat endometriosis, a common cause of female infertility. These agents are discussed in Chapter 49.

Gonadotropin Releasing Hormone Analogs

Gonadorelin

Gonadorelin (FACTREL) is a synthetic LHRH used to evaluate pituitary gonadotropic function, either in patients with suspected dysfunction or after pituitary surgery or irradiation for a tumor (see Table 44–C1 for dosages). The drug should be administered in the early follicular stage of the menstrual cycle (days 1 through 7). Given as an IV or SC injection, gonadorelin normally increases release of LH from the anterior pituitary, and causes a measurable rise of blood LH levels. Two predrug blood samples are collected and analyzed for baseline LH levels; after the drug is given, five more samples are collected and analyzed at 15, 30, 45, 60, and 120 minutes postinjection. The patient's data can be compared with normal responses noted in the package insert.

When used diagnostically, an abnormally low response to a single injection of gonadorelin will not distinguish between pituitary or hypothalamic dysfunction, so other tests and evaluations are necessary. When used to assess the effectiveness of treatments to remove or destroy the pituitary, the rise (or lack thereof) of LH levels provides insight into the residual pituitary function.

Gonadorelin causes only mild headache, nausea or abdominal discomfort, lightheadedness, and flushing (see Table 44–S1). Subcutaneous injections may cause localized pain or localized or generalized pruritic rashes. Allergic reactions after administration of several doses have been reported.

If possible, patients should not be taking drugs that interfere with pituitary function, including steroids and drugs with steroid-like structures (androgens, estrogens, progestins, glucocorticoids, and digoxin); steroid antagonists (spironolactone); and drugs that mimic or block the effects of dopamine and related agonists (levodopa and phenothiazines, for example).

NURSING IMPLICATIONS

Remind women to record their menstrual cycle so gonadorelin testing can be timed properly. Before administering gonadorelin, rule out the use of interfering drugs, or a prior allergic response to the agent. Explain the nature of the test to the patient, including the need for seven blood samples over slightly more than two hours. The use of a single indwelling catheter, rather than seven venipunctures, is preferred. Discuss this with the patient to allay apprehension.

Gonadorelin is supplied as a freeze-dried powder (100 and 500 μg) that should be stored at room temperature and reconstituted with the manufacturer's diluent immediately before use. Reconstituted but unused product can be stored at room temperature for up to a day.

Handle blood samples according to institutional laboratory protocol, since this is critical to the accuracy of the test. Assess for signs of allergic reactions (bronchospasm, hypotension, etc) and for injection site irritation or pain especially if injected SC.

Leuprolide

Leuprolide (LUPRON) is a synthetic analog of LHRH that possesses greater potency than the natural hormone. This drug occupies and desensitizes LHRH receptors, which eventually inhibits gonadotropin secretion. Chronic leuprolide administration suppresses ovarian and testicular steroidogenesis. It is indicated for palliation of advanced prostatic cancer. Prostatic cancer growth is stimulated by androgens (which can be eliminated by surgically removing the testes) and inhibited by estrogens, which can be administered therapeutically. Leuprolide can be used as an alternative when neither surgery nor estrogen administration is feasible for or acceptable to the patient.

Goserelin

Goserelin (Gonadorelin; LHRH) is a synthetic GnRH analog that stimulates short-term gonadotropin and sex hormone release, then causes suppression of release with continued administration. Goserelin is therapeutically useful as an alternative to surgery or estrogen therapy in prostatic cancer, possibly palliation of breast cancer in premenopausal women, and for managing the signs and symptoms of endometriosis. Goserelin is administered as an SC biodegradable depot that constantly releases the drug over four weeks.

Adrenocorticotropic Hormone

Adrenocorticotropic hormone (corticotropin; ACTH) is the major anterior pituitary hormonal stimulus for adrenal cortical release of androgens, glucocorticoids, and (to a lesser extent) mineralocorticoids. When ACTH binds to adrenal cortical cells it activates adenyl cyclase, leading to the formation of cyclic AMP. Cyclic AMP, in turn, acts as a second messenger to trigger enzymatic reactions that synthesize adrenal cortical hormones. The normal actions of these hormones, and characteristics of insufficiencies and excesses, are discussed in Chapter 45. This section focuses on the factors that affect their ultimate release.

Regulation

Synthesis and release of ACTH are stimulated by *corticotropin-releasing hormone* (CRH), which is secreted by the hypothalamus (see Table 44–2). There is a circadian rhythm to ACTH secretion, with highest levels occurring early in the morning and lowest levels in the late evening. Adrenal cortical cells respond to ACTH by increasing their output of glucocorticoids (primarily cortisol, also called hydrocortisone). Cortisol exerts feedback inhibition on ACTH and CRH release. Thus, there is an important hypothalamic-pituitary-adrenal interaction that normally regulates CRH, ACTH, and cortisol levels.

Release of ACTH also is triggered, via hypothalamic pathways, by fever, hypoglycemia, physiologic or mental trauma, pain, infection, intense heat or cold, falling glucocorticoid levels, and other factors that help the body adapt to stress. All these situations are accompanied by catecholamine release, which overcomes the normal inhibitory effects of cortisol on ACTH and CRH release. This provides a way for the entire organism to respond to and compensate for stress. Inhibition of this natural hypothalamic-pituitary-adrenal axis by long-term administration of glucocorticoid drugs is a major reason for iatrogenic adrenal gland atrophy and failure.

Effects of Adrenocorticotropic Hormone Hyper- and Hyposecretion

Causes of ACTH hypersecretion include excessive CRH release by the hypothalamus, pituitary-dependent bilateral adrenal hyperplasia, and excessive ACTH release by nonendocrine or pituitary tumors. Overall, the signs and symptoms reflect excessive cortisol levels and effects (see Chapter 45). Cushingoid signs and symptoms also may be caused by long-term administration of large corticosteroid doses.

Cushingoid symptoms are diagnosed by several laboratory tests. Some tests detect a loss of the diurnal patterns for ACTH and cortisol levels. Others involve administration of a potent glucocorticoid such as dexamethasone, which normally should suppress ACTH release.

If the cause of cushingoid symptoms is drug-induced, discontinuation of the causative agent (carefully and slowly, as described in Chapter 45) is indicated. The treatment of choice for pituitary-initiated cushingoid symptoms, when permissible, is surgical excision or irradiation of the tumor. The anticancer drug mitotane (LYSODREN), which selectively destroys the adrenal cortex, can be used for hypersecretion caused by an adrenal cortical tumor.

Hyposecretion of ACTH is rare. Usually it is the result of panhypopituitarism. Its pharmacologic management involves replacement therapy with corticosteroid drugs (see Chapter 45.)

Corticotropin

Corticotropin is purified ACTH derived from porcine anterior pituitary glands. It is used mainly as a diagnostic agent for adrenal insufficiency. Corticotropin is available as a stable aqueous solution for IV, IM, or SC injection (ACTHAR and others), and in two long-acting parenteral dosage forms, corticotropin injection repository (ACTH GEL, others) and corticotropin zinc hydroxide (CORTROPHIN-ZINC), which cannot be injected IV. A synthetic corticotropin, cosyntropin (CORTROSYN), which has biologic activity equivalent to that of corticotropin, is also available. See Table 44–C1 for dosages.

Absorption, Distribution, Metabolism, and Excretion

Corticotropin solution is absorbed readily from injection sites. Once absorbed, the drug binds to plasma proteins and concentrates in several body tissues. Corticotropin's plasma half-life after IV administration is about 15 minutes, and the effects of a single injection rarely last more than two hours.

When prolonged effects are needed, the alternatives are to give frequent IM injections, use a slow IV drip, or administer the slowly absorbed repository form. The actions of repository injections of corticotropin last up to three days.

Physiologic and Pharmacologic Effects

The pharmacologic effect of corticotropin is identical to the physiologic effect of endogenous ACTH. Within about five minutes of injection, corticotropin directly stimulates corticosteroid release from the adrenal cortex, and does so only when the adrenal cortex is functional. This corticosteroid-releasing effect is unique, and it provides a rationale for corticotropin's diagnostic use. However, when corticotropin is used on a long-term basis for treatment, the indirect effects of the released steroids are the ones that are clinically important.

Many steroids are available for clinical use, most of which can be administered by routes that do not require injections. Direct steroid administration always is preferred for treatment. The actions of released steroids also account for the majority of corticotropin's side effects, contraindications, and drug interactions. (see Chapter 45).

Clinical Indications and Administration

Corticotropin aqueous solution is used mainly for diagnostic testing of adrenal cortical function. Blood and urinary levels of adrenal corticosteroids and their metabolites are measured before corticotropin administration, and then measured again after the diagnostic agent is given. Failure of the agent to increase circulating cortisol levels generally indicates primary adrenal cortical failure.

The long-acting repository formulations of corticotropin can be used to treat most of the same disorders for which corticosteroid administration is indicated. These include arthritic, collagen, endocrine, nervous system, ocular, and dermatologic disorders, and manifestations of allergic reactions. Dosages are summarized in Table 44–C1.

Side Effects, Adverse Reactions, and Contraindications

The major side effects and contraindications that apply to corticotropin are the same as those for most corticosteroids (see Chapter 45) and are most likely to be problematic with long-term administration. The major side effects caused by corticotropin include all the manifestations of drug-induced Cushing's syndrome:

- The glucocorticoid effects of released cortisol, including alterations of fat, protein, and carbohydrate metabolism;
- Muscle-wasting and fat redistribution;
- Suppression of wound healing and the immune response;
- An increased risk of GI tract ulceration; and
- Cataracts or other visual disturbances.

Corticotropin's side effects also reflect the mineralocorticoid effects of released aldosterone, particularly renal potassium-wasting, and sodium and water retention that contributes to hypertension, edema, and heart failure. Wound healing may be delayed, the susceptibility to infection may be increased (since glucocorticoids suppress the immune response), and symptoms of infection may be masked.

Unlike the corticosteroids themselves, which are steroids, corticotropin is a protein that can trigger an allergic reaction. The manifestations can range from mild to life-threatening (anaphylaxis).

Prolonged administration of high doses of corticotropin may cause adrenal cortical hyperplasia, hypertrophy, and hypersecretion. In addition, prolonged and high circulating levels of corticosteroids released by corticotropin can suppress the hypothalamic-pituitary-adrenal axis, leading to a potentially severe or fatal steroid-withdrawal syndrome once corticotropin administration is stopped. As discussed in Chapter 45, the withdrawal syndrome greatly reduces the body's ability to respond to stress, and supplemental doses of corticosteroid drugs usually will be needed to support the individual during times of stress. Corticotropin therapy that has lasted for more than about a week should never be stopped abruptly.

All the contraindications for corticosteroid administration, plus a few significant others, apply also to corticotropin. Those shared by both agents include heart failure and hypertension; recent surgery; peptic ulcer disease; fungal infections or ocular herpes simplex; scleroderma; osteoporosis; and chronic diseases in which corticosteroids might suppress signs and symptoms without desirably affecting the underlying condition.

Hyperglycemia caused indirectly by cortisol release requires extra care, and often necessitates alterations in the therapy of diabetes mellitus.

Corticotropin, like glucocorticoids, can reactivate latent tuberculosis. Administration of live or attenuated vaccines should be avoided during corticotropin therapy because of potential failure to form an immune response, and the risk of inducing a severe infection, due to immunosuppression.

Corticotropin is contraindicated for treating conditions accompanied by primary adrenocortical insufficiency (a situation for which corticosteroid administration is indicated) or hyperfunction. Corticotropin aqueous solution or cosyntropin may be injected IV; this route is best reserved for diagnostic purposes. Corticotropin products are contraindicated for patients with prior allergic reactions to these products or to porcine proteins.

NURSING IMPLICATIONS

Before initial administration of any corticotropin product for any reason, check the history to rule out prior allergic responses. Do not administer any corticotropin preparation for treatment purposes unless laboratory data prove increased steroid release by the adrenal gland using the route of administration chosen for treatment.

Reconstitute corticotropin aqueous injection with sterile water for injection or sodium chloride injection. When the drug is used IM for treatment purposes the total desired dose should be contained in 1 to 2 mL of final solution. When infused IV for diagnostic purposes, the solution can be diluted further in 500 mL of 5% dextrose in water and administered over eight hours. Cosyntropin also may be diluted in dextrose or saline solution for IV infusion.

Repository corticotropin preparations are supplied ready to use, and must be given only by IM or SC injection. Store these products in a refrigerator before use and after dilution. Use reconstituted corticotropin or cosyntropin within 24 hours.

Warm repository forms to room temperature immediately before injection, and advise patients that injection of a repository form may be painful. If the IM route is used, administer the drug slowly via deep injection with a large bore (22 gauge) needle.

Monitor patients receiving their first injection of these drugs for signs of hypersensitivity or allergy. Thereafter, focus assessment on evidence of excessive glucocorticoid and mineralocorticoid effects (Cushing's syndrome) and infection, as would be done for corticosteroid therapy (see Chapter 45).

Since steroid release suppresses such signs of infection as fever, redness, and swelling, use pain, diminished function, and other indicators for assessment. Also assess for evidence of adverse effects or interactions in special patient populations: poor control of diabetes symptoms; hypokalemia in persons taking potassium-wasting diuretics; abdominal pain or bleeding in ulcer patients or patients taking other ulcerogenic drugs. Report adverse responses at once so proper corrective therapy can be started, and corticotropin administration stopped, as needed. Teach patients the key signs and symptoms of adverse effects so they will be able to recognize and report them.

Advise patients receiving steroid-releasing drugs that supplemental steroid doses may be needed during times of severe stress (illness, surgery, trauma). Caution patients against discontinuing therapy except under the supervision of a physician.

◆ Use During Pregnancy and Lactation

Animal studies have demonstrated an embryocidal effect of corticotropin. Corticotropin and related products should not be administered during pregnancy unless anticipated benefits outweigh possible risks. The same recommendation applies to breast-feeding. If corticotropin is used during pregnancy, check the newborn for evidence of decreased adrenal function.

◆ Use in Children

Prolonged corticotropin administration to children may inhibit skeletal growth and should not be used unless clearly necessary. Use the drug intermittently. Advise parents or guardians to keep written monthly records of the child's height and weight; review this information at each clinical visit.

◆ Use in the Elderly

The major concerns associated with corticotropin use in elderly patients relate to the prevalence of cataracts, diabetes, immune system dysfunction, and cardiovascular diseases, all of which can be aggravated by corticosteroids released after corticotropin administration.

Interactions with Other Drugs

Interactions that would apply to corticosteroid administration are potential concerns with corticotropin, especially with long-term use; aspirin and other nonsteroidal antiinflammatory drugs (increased risk of GI tract ulcers); amphotericin B, thiazides, and high-ceiling diuretics (increased risk of hypokalemia); and insulin or oral hypoglycemic drugs (poor control of blood glucose levels).

Melanocyte-Stimulating Hormone

The remaining known anterior pituitary hormone is melanocyte-stimulating hormone (MSH). Both MSH and ACTH are derived from the same precursor molecule. Melanocyte-stimulating hormone stimulates melanocytes to form melanin, a pigment that disperses in epidermal cells. An excess of MSH has a role in the hypermelanosis of Addison's disease.

There are no therapeutic products available to stimulate or inhibit MSH release or activity.

Table 44–3 | **Posterior Pituitary Hormone Regulation and Effects**

Hormone	Regulation of, Drug Effects on, Release	Target(s) and Effect(s)	Effects of Hyposecretion	Effects of Hypersecretion
Oxytocin	↑ by impulses from hypothalamic neurons in response to cervical and uterine stretching and by suckling of the breast by newborn ↓ by lack of appropriate neural or tactile stimuli	1. Stimulates rhythmic uterine contractions, mainly near and at term (see Chapter 49) 2. Stimulates milk ejection (letdown reflex)	Unknown	Unknown
Vasopressin (ADH)	↑ by hypothalamic impulses in response to increased plasma osmolality, decreased blood volume or pressure *Drugs* (either increase release or sensitize kidneys to effects of ADH): β-adrenergic agonists, carbamazepine, chlorpropamide, cholinergic agonists (including nicotine), clofibrate, cyclophosphamide, morphine, some tricyclic antidepressants, vinca alkaloids (vinblastine, vincristine) ↓ by adequate body hydration, blood volume, or BP *Drug:* alcohol	1. Increases permeability of renal collecting ducts to water, thereby reducing urine volume and increasing urine concentration, osmolality, specific gravity	Diabetes insipidus	Dilutional hyponatremia (SIADH)

Key: ↑ = increased; ↓ = decreased.

II. Posterior Pituitary Hormones

The posterior pituitary gland is composed of the termini of specific hypothalamic neurons. These neurons synthesize two peptide neurohormones, *oxytocin* and *vasopressin,* which then are transported within neurosecretory granules down the axonal fibers to the posterior pituitary, where they are stored. The hormones are released into the bloodstream in response to neural stimuli from the same hypothalamic neurons. Damage to the hypothalamic-hypophyseal tract interferes with oxytocin and vasopressin release.

Both oxytocin and vasopressin are composed of only nine amino acids. Seven of the nine in each are identical, and so the two substances share similar actions (Table 44–3). A mixture of the compounds stimulates uterine smooth muscle tone, vascular smooth muscle (which increases blood pressure), and water reabsorption by the kidney tubules (an antidiuretic effect, resulting in reduced urine volume).

When the compounds are separated in pure form, the slight structural differences dramatically affect the intensities of their effects. Oxytocin stimulates the uterus but has little effect on the kidneys; vasopressin has a marked effect on the kidneys, but little effect on the uterus. The effects of each on vascular smooth muscle are intermediate.

Oxytocin

Oxytocin release and its resulting effects are significant only during childbirth and in lactating women. See Chapter 49 for more information.

Vasopressin

Vasopressin derived one of its names from its ability to increase blood pressure, a (vaso)pressor response. Even though the hormone's renal antidiuretic effect is more important physiologically, and antidiuretic hormone (ADH) is a more descriptive name, the term vasopressin is used because some of the therapeutic products are so named.

As an antidiuretic hormone, the principle role of vasopressin is to conserve body water and plasma osmolality. Acting through the second messenger, cyclic AMP, vasopressin enhances the water permeability of the kidney's collecting ducts (and, to a lesser extent, that of the distal tubules). In the presence of vasopressin, water is reabsorbed from the urine and returned to the blood as the urine passes through the increasing osmotic gradient from the renal cortex to the medulla. Through removal of water, the resulting urine is more concentrated but reduced in volume.

Vasopressin does cause a vasopressor effect, but whether and how much blood pressure changes depends on the dose and how fast it is given. The vasoconstrictor effect is greatest in hepatic portal and splanchnic vessels.

Purified, synthetic antidiuretic hormones exert little or no effects on the uterus, and only modest effects on GI motility and tone.

Regulation

Antidiuretic hormone is released more or less continuously in response to changes of blood osmolality. The major control is exerted by osmoreceptor neurons in the hypothalamus that respond to increased plasma solute concentrations. When activated, these neurons stimulate other hypothalamic neurons to release vasopressin into the blood from the posterior pituitary. Increased hormone levels cause the kidneys to return more water to the blood, so that plasma osmolality falls.

Mild shifts in blood volume and pressure do not significantly affect vasopressin release, but larger shifts stimulate baroreceptors (pressure sensors) in the left atrium and carotid sinus. This triggers vasopressin release from the hypothalamus.

Neurotransmitters and neuromodulators, including dopamine and other catecholamines, angiotensin II, and endorphins, affect regulatory pathways to the hypothalamus, thereby affecting vasopressin release. Autonomic effects on vasopressin release may be important contributors to the antidiuresis that often accompanies congestive heart failure, hepatic cirrhosis, and the nephrotic syndrome. Head trauma, tumors, meningitis, and encephalitis are common causes of a syndrome of inappropriate antidiuretic hormone (vasopressin) secretion (SIADH), with hormone output failing to respond to normal control mechanisms.

Drugs also affect vasopressin release. For example, α-adrenergic agonists, carbamazepine, chlorpropamide, cholinergic agonists (including nicotine), clofibrate, cyclophosphamide, some tricyclic antidepressants, and the vinca alkaloids (vinblastine and vincristine) stimulate vasopressin release or sensitize the kidney to vasopressin. The diuresis that often accompanies alcohol ingestion reflects ethanol's ability to inhibit vasopressin release.

Effects of Vasopressin Hyper- and Hyposecretion

Hypersecretion of vasopressin, except that caused by drugs or associated with conditions noted earlier, is rare. When it occurs, however, as in SIADH, excessive water retention can lead to serious dilutional hyponatremia. The disorder is equivalent to an "overdose" of vasopressin, which is discussed later.

Hyposecretion of vasopressin (independent of drug effects) is more common, and it causes neurogenic (hypothalamic) diabetes insipidus, a syndrome characterized by the excretion of large amounts of dilute urine (polyuria). Polyuria causes secondary effects, mainly intense thirst and polydipsia (increased water intake).

Neurogenic diabetes insipidus can be caused by brain neoplasms, head trauma, or hypothalamic or pituitary surgery. Usually the cause is unknown (idiopathic). The polydipsia and polyuria of diabetes insipidus is annoying, but not dangerous if the thirst center is functional and the individual can drink enough water to prevent dehydration. However, it can lead to life-threatening electrolyte imbalances and dehydration in unconscious, comatose, or ill individuals. The usual treatment is replacement therapy by administration of vasopressin or its analog. (Nephrogenic diabetes insipidus is a less common form of the disorder in which vasopressin levels are adequate but the collecting ducts cannot respond to it. Thiazide diuretics, which exert a paradoxical antidiuretic effect in this condition, have an important therapeutic role. See Chapter 32.)

Therapeutic Products

Vasopressin and its analogs are used mainly to treat neurogenic diabetes insipidus. Several preparations are available. They are all synthetic products that exhibit mainly vasopressin activity, with virtually no oxytocic activity. The prototype agent is vasopressin aqueous injection (PITRESSIN), which can be injected IM or SC. Related agents are the vasopressin-like drugs lypressin and desmopressin, which also lack oxytocic activity.

Absorption, Distribution, Metabolism, and Excretion

Aqueous synthetic vasopressin (PITRESSIN), injected IM or SC, causes an antidiuretic effect that lasts about two to eight hours. Vasopressin does not bind extensively to plasma proteins. The kidneys play an important part in eliminating vasopressin and its metabolites. Tissue peptidases also degrade vasopressin rapidly.

Pharmacologic Effects

Synthetic vasopressins and their analogs act on the kidneys' collecting ducts in a manner identical to that of endogenous vasopressin (ADH). They cause vasoconstriction and increased GI smooth muscle tone. Therapeutic doses used to control polyuria seldom cause significant blood pressure increases.

Clinical Indications and Administration

Vasopressin injection has several clinical uses (Table 44–C2) in addition to the treatment of neurogenic diabetes insipidus.

Treatment of Neurogenic Diabetes Insipidus

This is the major indication for all vasopressin formulations and analogs. The primary therapeutic goal is to lower urine output. Secondary effects include a reduced risk of electrolyte imbalances and dehydration, reduced polydipsia, less disruption of daytime activities, and improved sleep as nocturia is relieved. None of the vasopressins cure the disorder. Fluid intake and output and periodic measurements of urinary and plasma osmolality and electrolytes are used to monitor therapy.

Injectable vasopressin, because of its short duration of action, is best suited for short-term effects in the management of diabetes insipidus. It is also useful for unconscious patients.

Aqueous vasopressin for injection also can be administered intranasally, either in drops, sprays, or applied to cotton pledgets inserted into the nostrils. This is seldom done because products made specifically for intranasal administration are available.

Gastrointestinal Tract Uses

The ability of vasopressin to increase the tone of GI tract smooth muscles or vascular smooth muscle has therapeutic use. The drug can be used to treat postoperative abdominal distention, to control bleeding esophageal varices, and to eliminate intestinal gas that might interfere with X-ray diagnostic tests of the GI tract. Dosages and administration routes are summarized in Table 44–C2.

Side Effects, Adverse Reactions, and Contraindications

The most serious concern with any vasopressin product is an allergic reaction, including anaphylaxis. The risk appears to be greatest with pituitary extract, the animal-derived product, which is another reason why it is not used widely. Use of the offending drug is contraindicated for any person who has experienced a prior hypersensitivity or allergic reaction to it.

Therapeutic doses of any pure vasopressin or analog seldom cause side effects (Table 44–S2). Excessive doses, regardless of the administration route, may cause excessive antidiuretic effects, leading to fluid retention (water intoxication) and hyponatremia (called dilutional hyponatremia to indicate that blood sodium concentrations are low because normal amounts of sodium are diluted by the large amount of retained water). Early signs and symptoms include drowsiness, listlessness, and headache, which may be followed by seizures, coma, and death. Treatment usually includes discontinuation of vasopressin administration and temporary restriction of fluid intake.

Large doses, through their effects on smooth muscles in the gut, respiratory tract, and blood vessels, may cause cramping and diarrhea, bronchoconstriction and dyspnea, varying degrees of hypertension (usually slight), plus headache, heartburn, substernal pain, and pallor. Cardiac arrest has been reported.

Intranasal administration may also cause nasal congestion, irritation, inflammation, ulceration, or rhinorrhea. The incidence of nasal irritation is probably greatest with pituitary extract powder, but any of the intranasal vasopressins may cause this problem.

Because of the potential for peripheral and coronary artery vasoconstriction and a potentially sudden rise in circulating fluid volume, vasopressins should be used with extreme care in persons with cardiac disease, especially ischemic heart disease and angina; peripheral vascular diseases; asthma; a history of seizures; and hypertension, including that associated with preeclampsia/eclampsia. Other important pregnancy-related contraindications are noted later.

Vasopressin and desmopressin injections occasionally cause local reactions including pain, swelling, and erythema. The untoward responses noted earlier are more likely to be severe and appear faster with parenteral administration, and especially with IV injection. Extravasation of an IV injection may cause intense vasoconstriction, leading to severe pain, tissue necrosis, and possibly gangrene.

Desmopressin is contraindicated in patients with Type II von Willebrand's disease, hemophilia B, persons with factor VIII antibodies, and most patients with factor VIII levels below 5% of normal. Platelet aggregation and thromboembolism, or allergic reactions, may occur.

NURSING IMPLICATIONS

Obtain a thorough history before administering any vasopressin product to rule out prior allergic reactions and contraindications, including pregnancy. Obtain baseline body weight, blood pressure, and fluid intake and output for comparison with measurements made during treatment.

Parenteral dosage forms of the vasopressin products are supplied ready for use. With the exception of desmopressin, for which IV administration may be indicated, all other parenteral products should be injected IM or SC. Use a large-bore needle, avoid injecting into the deltoid, and rotate sites if repeated injections will be needed. Advise patients that the injection may be painful. Observe for and report redness or swelling at the injection site.

Teach patients the proper administration technique for the specific intranasal product to be used. Desmopressin, a liquid, is drawn up into a calibrated plastic tube and blown by mouth into the nasal passages. (If desmopressin is administered to a child or obtunded patient, an air-filled syringe may be used instead.) Lypressin is supplied in plastic bottles as a nasal spray (solution) that should be administered with the patient sitting or standing with the head upright. Consult the package insert accompanying the product to be used.

Assess for the reappearance of polyuria before the next scheduled dose. If this occurs, the best management is usually to increase the frequency of administration, rather than the amount administered for each dose. If large volumes are administered at one time (for example, more than three sprays of lypressin), the drug can drain down the nasopharynx and eventually into the GI tract. As a result, a portion of the dose is wasted.

Also assess for nasal congestion, which may interfere with drug absorption.

Patients who have had hypothalamic surgery or head trauma require careful monitoring of intake and output, serum osmolality, and urine osmolality and specific gravity. This is necessary to detect and document excessive diuresis, especially at the onset of ADH replacement therapy.

Teach outpatients who will be self-medicating with vasopressins how to measure fluid intake and output. Encourage them to keep a daily log of intake and urine output to help document the effectiveness of treatment. Teach and encourage them to avoid fluids, foods, or drugs that might alter water and electrolyte balance. Inquire about and report nocturia, which may be managed with an added bedtime dose prescribed by the physician.

Patients receiving vasopressin injection may experience abdominal cramping or nausea. Often this can be minimized by drinking one or two glasses of water with each dose. This strategy also might be useful for related drugs and other routes of administration.

Assess for, and have the patient report, sudden changes in urine output, or the need for altered fluid intake, that are not expected with drug therapy. Other responses that require immediate physician notification include anginal pain, dyspnea, sudden or large increases of blood pressure, and sudden changes in body weight. Headache, drowsiness, listlessness, or confusion might indicate underlying water intoxication, and also should be reported at once.

With the exception of desmopressin, most preparations of vasopressins can be stored at room temperature. Desmopressin should be refrigerated. If the patient using desmopressin nasal solution cannot keep the product refrigerated between use, as during travel, protecting the drug from excessive heat should maintain drug activity for up to three weeks.

◆ Use During Pregnancy and Lactation

No controlled studies have shown adverse effects of the vasopressin products on the fetus. Posterior pituitary (inhaled or injected), which contains both vasopressin and oxytocin, clearly should not be used during pregnancy. There is a high risk of inducing fetal distress, asphyxia, premature labor, and uterine rupture when given before labor is complete. Breast-feeding is discouraged when these drugs are used.

◆ Use in Children

Vasopressin and its analogs can be used to manage diabetes insipidus in children. Extra precautions to monitor and regulate fluid intake and output are necessary, since children are extremely intolerant of sudden blood volume and osmolality changes. The greatest concern in children is the risk of dilutional hyponatremia and resulting seizures when excessive doses are administered. The safety and effectiveness of desmopressin as a treatment for diabetes insipidus in children younger than 12 years are not known. Desmopressin injection is not indicated for treating hemophilia or von Willebrand's disease in children younger than three months.

◆ Use in the Elderly

The prevalence of coronary artery disease in the elderly increases the risk of anginal attacks, even when small doses of vasopressins are administered. Instruct patients to report anginal pain at once. Elderly patients also are less tolerant of sudden or significant changes of blood pressure, volume, and composition. Monitor and regulate fluid intake and output closely during therapy.

Interactions with Other Drugs

Vasopressin and its analogs should be used cautiously, and with close monitoring, in patients receiving other drugs that increase vasopressin levels or activity: carbamazepine, chlorpropamide, and clofibrate. Even though the vasoconstrictor activity of vasopressin is relatively low, it should be administered cautiously in persons receiving other drugs with vasoconstrictor activity.

Related Drugs

Desmopressin

Desmopressin acetate (DDAVP) is a synthetic analog of endogenous vasopressin. The drug can be administered intranasally as a spray, or by injection. Desmopressin acetate is the preferred agent for long-term treatment of diabetes insipidus both because of its long duration of action (around 20 hours when administered intranasally) and because of the ease and effectiveness of intranasal administration. The drug is administered into the nares through a flexible nasal tube marked for measuring doses of the solution from the drug vial. Once the dose has been individualized for the patient (see Table 44–C2), twice-daily administration for adults or once-daily administration for children usually suffices.

Desmopression acetate nasal spray is indicated for the management of primary nocturnal enuresis. It may be used alone or in combination with nondrug interventions such as behavioral conditioning.

Another indication for desmopressin, but not for the other vasopressins, is the management of hemophilia A and some cases of von Willebrand's disease (Type I). Hemophilia A is a congenital bleeding disorder in which the procoagulant activity of factor VIII (antihemophilic factor) is deficient. Factor VIII is a complex of two proteins, with von Willebrand protein constituting the largest part. Desmopressin acetate injection raises levels of factor VIII. The drug is indicated for short-term prevention or treatment of bleeding episodes, as might arise because of trauma or surgery, in persons with mild to moderate factor VIII deficiencies. The desired response is assessed with hematologic studies (factor VIII and factor VIII antigen levels, and activated partial thromboplastin times).

Lypressin

Lypressin (DIAPID) is a synthetic compound that is very similar to natural human vasopressin. Lypressin is absorbed well across the mucous membranes in the nasal passages, causing peak effects in about 30 to 60 minutes. Generally one to two sprays per nostril will control polyuria and secondary symptoms for about three to eight hours. Lypressin is used mainly for controlling mild polyuria in patients who have experienced allergic reactions or are unresponsive to animal-derived products, or for adjunctive therapy between injections of other agents.

Posterior Pituitary

Posterior pituitary is available in a parenteral formulation (PITUITRIN S) for all the indications noted above except hemophilia and von Willebrand's disease. The powder, administered intranasally, is indicated only for treating diabetes insipidus.

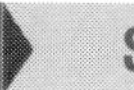

SUMMARY OF NURSING IMPLICATIONS

◆ Assessment

Growth hormone: Assess for growth and development delays in children.

Accurately weigh patient and record height.

Bromocriptine: Obtain a complete patient history to determine contraindications for therapy or concurrent medications that may interact with bromocriptine.

Gonadorelin: Establish baseline LH levels with blood drawn 15 minutes and immediately before initiation of test.

Obtain a complete patient history to identify any medications that could interfere with gonadotropin levels, such as spironolactone, digoxin, phenothiazines and dopamine, androgens, estrogens, progestins or glucocorticosteroids.

In females, administer the test in days 1 through 7 of the menstrual cycle.

Corticotropin (ACTH): Obtain a complete patient history to determine if any contraindications apply.

Accurately weigh patient and establish vital signs.

Vasopressin: Obtain a complete patient history to rule out contraindications to therapy and to identify drugs known to potentiate ADH.

Accurately weigh patient to establish hydration status during treatment for diabetes insipidus.

◆ Nursing Diagnoses

Growth hormone: Body image disturbance related to short stature.

Altered growth and development related to hormone deficiency.

Ineffective individual coping related to chronic illness (hypothyroidism).

Bromocriptine: High risk for injury related to dizziness, headache, lightheadedness, hypotension or hypertension.

High risk for activity intolerance related to fatigue.

Decreased cardiac output related to cardiac arrhythmias.

Gonadorelin: Pain related to headache, abdominal discomfort.

High risk for injury-related lightheadedness.

Ineffective breathing pattern related to bronchospasm (hypersensitivity reaction).

Corticotropin (ACTH): Body image disturbance related to drug side effects (weight gain, acne, hyperpigmentation).

Fluid volume excess related to sodium and water retention.

High risk for injury related to osteoporosis (fractures), impaired wound healing, intolerance to stress.

Vasopressin: Alteration in fluid volume: excess or deficit related to drug dosage or disease effects.

Ineffective individual coping related to chronic illness (diabetes insipidus).

◆ Planning/Implementation

Growth hormone: Reconstitute medication correctly; avoid shaking GH after dissolution. Note stability durations and refrigerate.

Provide for the physical and emotional needs of patients requiring hormonal replacement—mood and personality changes, sensitivity to cold, and physical sluggishness with hypothyroidism.

Instruct parents on proper maintenance of height and weight charts, and the need to report significant deviations.

Be alert for complaints of hip or knee pain or new limp in patients treated with GH, and alert parents to watch for these symptoms.

Bromocriptine: Teach patients to recognize possible adverse effects and particularly to report unremitting and progressively severe headache, which may precede seizure or stroke.

Teach female patients to use mechanical contraceptives during bromocriptine administration.

Have patients take bromocriptine with meals.

Caution patients not to engage in activities requiring rapid and precise responses, such as operating a motor vehicle.

Carefully record blood pressure.

Gonadorelin: Explain blood draws necessary for test and purpose of the test to the patient. Be sure manufacturer's insert with the gonadorelin package is available to compare patient values with known normal values, depending on the route of administration. Watch patient for flushing, headache, nausea, lightheadedness, or abdominal discomfort. Be alert for uncommon but possible hypersensitivity reactions, such as bronchospasm or skin rash.

Reconstitute the vial immediately before use.

Ensure appropriate laboratory handling of blood samples at appropriate times.

Corticotropin (ACTH): Reconstitute carefully, and be certain the product is administered by the correct route.

Teach home monitoring of blood glucose if hyperglycemia occurs.

Prepare patient if ACTH is being used as a diagnostic agent.

Carefully observe patient for cushingoid signs and symptoms associated with prolonged corticotropin therapy: edema (sodium and water retention) with weight gain, acne, symptoms of peptic ulcer, impaired wound healing, hyperpigmentation, menstrual irregularities, loss of muscle mass, mood changes, aseptic necrosis of bones, fractures, osteoporosis, or signs or symptoms of infections.

Never administer smallpox immunization to patients taking corticotropin therapy; administer other vaccinations with great caution.

Be aware of possible interacting drugs, and caution patient about them.

Teach patients about possible adverse effects and which symptoms require immediate attention by their physician: thirst, muscle weakness or cramping, gastric pains, mood swings, cloudy vision.

Be aware of intolerance to stress, signs and symptoms of fatigue, nausea, sluggishness.

Vasopressin: Teach patient how to use the intranasal product and provide manufacturer's insert explaining administration technique.

Carefully follow appropriate reconstitution and administration procedures for each product; do not filter vials of vasopressin tannate in oil.

Teach patient how to control polyuria by appropriate dosing schedule.

Observe patient for weight gain or loss, indicating fluid status.

Be alert for rare but possible hypersensitivity reactions. If giving larger doses, be alert for smooth muscle constriction, bronchiolar constriction, nausea, abdominal cramping and diarrhea, and extreme fluid retention leading to water intoxication.

Observe IV infusion site closely for extravasation.

◆ Evaluation

The patient/family will:

Growth hormone: Achieve normal stature.

Bromocriptine: Achieve end point of bromocriptine therapy (depending on the indication being treated).

Gonadorelin: Monitor pretreatment menstrual cycle closely to ensure proper timing of drug administration.

Corticotropin (ACTH): When used therapeutically observe for signs of disease remission and report adverse effects; see Chapter 45 for details.

Vasopressins: Maintain normal weight: hydrated, no polyuria, polydipsia, or nocturia following vasopressin therapy.

Understand correlation between symptoms and appropriate dosing; manage schedule and dose well.

Annotated Bibliography

Blackman MR: Pituitary hormones and aging. *Endocrin Metab Clin North Am* 1987;16(4):981–994. *This extensively referenced article addresses the misconception that aging merely reflects age-related hormone deficiency states. The author brings attention to the possibility that hormonal changes may instead reflect other common age-related factors: disease (including nonendocrine illness), diet, drugs, sleep, and physical and nervous system activity.*

Bradley CA, Sodeman TM: Human growth hormone. Its use and abuse. *Clin Lab Med* 1990;10(3):473–477. *Focuses on the potential appeal of human growth hormone to athletic competitors, and the possible overuse of growth hormone in children and adolescents.*

Cunnah D, and Besser M: Management of prolactinomas. *Clin Endocrinol* 1991;34:231–235. *Describes the types of interventions useful in treating prolactinomas, and how these treatments correct the presenting symptoms of gonadal dysfunction and infertility.*

Molitch ME, ed: Pituitary tumors. *Endocrin Metab Clin North Am* 1987;16(3):475–828. *Many well-written articles that are valuable for nurses dealing with patients who have pituitary tumors, including articles on neurologic and ophthalmologic features of the tumors; an extensively illustrated discussion of common pituitary surgical approaches that is invaluable for pre- and postoperative teaching and care; acromegaly; and adenomas involving hypersecretion of prolactin, gonadotropins, and thyrotropin.*

Reisine T: Neurohormonal aspects of ACTH release. *Hosp Pract* 1988; 23(3):77–96. *As with so many well-written reviews appearing in this journal, this article discusses key aspects in the physiologic roles of ACTH, providing a basis for understanding its involvement in important endocrine disorders and therapeutic approaches to managing them.*

Robertson GL, Harris A: Clinical use of vasopressin and analogues. *Hosp Pract* 1989;24:114–118, 126–128. *Reviews the actions and uses of vasopressin analogs.*

Williams DM, Barnes ND: Recombinant growth hormone in pediatrics. *Br J Hosp Med* 1991;45:224–225. *Describes indications and rationales for the use of growth hormone in deficiency states and other conditions in children.*

Table 44–C1 Clinical Uses and Administration of Anterior Pituitary Hormones and Releasing Factors or Their Antagonists

AGENT	CLINICAL USES	DOSAGE AND ROUTE OF ADMINISTRATION
	Adrenocorticotopic Hormones	
Corticotropin		
("ACTH"; ACTHAR; others)	Diagnosis of adrenal cortical function	IV: 10–25 U in 500 mL of 5% dextrose-water, infused over 8 h
	Rarely, to treat conditions usually managed by corticosteroids	IM or SC: 20 U injected qid
	Acute treatment of multiple sclerosis	IM or SC: 80–120 U/day for 2–3 weeks
Corticotropin repository injection		
(CORTROPHIN GEL; HP ACTHAR GEL; others)	Steroid-responsive conditions noted above	IM or SC: 40–80 U every 24–72 h
Corticotropin zinc hydroxide		
(CORTROPHIN ZINC)	Steroid-responsive conditions noted above	IM: 40–80 U every 24–72 h into gluteus
Cosyntropin		
(CORTROSYN)	Diagnosis of adrenal cortical function	IM: Adults: 250 μg to 750 μg in sterile saline. Children <2 years: Usually 125 μg
		IV: 250 μg as IV infusion, 40 μg/h over 6 h
	Gonadotropin-Releasing Hormone	
Gonadorelin HCl		
("LHRH"; "GnRH"; FACTREL)	Diagnosis of anterior pituitary ability to produce LH	IV or SC: 100 μg during first 7 days of menstrual period
	Growth Hormone, Analogs, and Related Diagnostic Agent	
Somatrem		
(PROTROPIN)	Growth failure caused by GH deficit	IM: 100 μg/kg (0.2 IU/kg) 3x weekly
Somatropin		
(HUMATROPE)	As for somatrem	IM: 60 μg/kg (0.16 IU/kg) 3x weekly
Arginine HCl		
(R-GENE 10)	Diagnosis of pituitary function/reserve by stimulating HGH release	IV: Adults: 300 mL infused over 30 min. Children: 5 mL/kg; administer after overnight fast

(continued)

Table 44–C1 **Clinical Uses and Administration of Anterior Pituitary Hormones and Releasing Factors or Their Antagonists (*Continued*)**

AGENT	CLINICAL USES	DOSAGE AND ROUTE OF ADMINISTRATION
	Prolactin-Release Inhibitor	
Bromocriptine mesylate (PARLODEL)	Acromegaly	Oral: Initial dose 1.25 mg–2.5 mg for 3 days, with food at bedtime; if tolerated, add 1.25–2.5 mg every 3 to 7 days; usual maintenance dose, 20–30 mg/day
	Prevention of physiologic lactation	Oral: Initially, 2.5 mg bid; usual maintenance dose 2.5–7.5 mg/day; treatment usually 14 days
	Parkinsonism	See Chapter 25
	Thyroid-Releasing and -Stimulating Hormones	
Protirelin ("TRH"; RELEFACT TRH; THYPINONE)	Differential diagnosis of pituitary vs hypothalamic hypothyroidism	IV: Adults: 200–500 μg bolus; Children 6–16 years: 7 μg/kg, up to 500 μg; infants and children up to 6 years: up to 7 μg/kg
Thyrotropin ("TSH"; THYTROPAR)	Differential diagnosis of pituitary vs thyroid hypothyroidism in conjunction with radioiodine uptake studies	IM or SC: 10 U for 1–3 days, followed by radioiodine study 24 h after last injection

Table 44–S1 Major Side Effects of and Contraindications for Anterior Pituitary Hormones and Releasing Factors or Their Antagonists

BODY SYSTEM/ Side Effect	CONTRAINDICATION/ PRECAUTION	COMMENTS AND NURSING IMPLICATIONS
Bromocriptine		
CENTRAL NERVOUS SYSTEM Confusion, hallucinations, other emotional or psychic alterations		May occur with high doses and prolonged treatment, as for acromegaly or parkinsonism; risk appears to be greater in elderly or debilitated patients treated for parkinsonism; assess for and report behavioral or psychologic abnormalities not apparent before or during early treatment
ENDOCRINE/ METABOLIC Inhibited lactation	Desire to breast-feed	When administering after childbirth, ensure that woman does not wish to breast-feed
Rebound breast pain, engorgement on drug discontinuation		May occur on discontinuation of bromocriptine for suppression of physiologic lactation; provide necessary comfort measures
RESPIRATORY Pulmonary infiltrates, pleural effusions	Poor pulmonary function (use cautiously)	May occur with prolonged, high-dose therapy (as indicated for treatment of acromegaly, parkinsonism); assess for dyspnea, altered lung sounds
CARDIOVASCULAR Orthostatic hypotension with reflex tachycardia; hypertension may occur	Severe ischemic heart disease, uncontrolled hypertension, eclampsia/preeclampsia; caution in patient with unstable BP	Assess BP before and after administration; report BP changes, excessive cardiac stimulation (eg, dizziness, syncope, headache, palpitations, arrhythmias, angina)
GASTROINTESTINAL Nausea, GI upset		Administer with meals; report intense nausea or abdominal pain at once
Gonadotropin-Releasing Hormone and Analogs		
GENERAL Mild headache, nausea, abdominal discomfort, lightheadedness		Explain expected side effects to patient before testing; report excessive side effects at once; indwelling IV catheter usually used for repetitive blood sampling provides quick access for drugs, fluids for managing severe allergic reactions (uncommon)
Growth Hormone, Analogs, and Related Diagnostic Agents		
ENDOCRINE/ METABOLIC Renewed or accelerated growth of intracranial tumor	Active brain tumors	Periodic CAT scans, X-rays, other diagnostic tests may be useful for assessing presence, growth of cranial neoplasms; assess for headache, visual changes, paresis, or paralysis that might indicate underlying problems caused by tumor
Hypothyroidism	Hypothyroidism	Assess for and report lethargy, weight gain, other indicators of hypothyroidism
Hyperglycemia (insulin resistance)		For diabetic patients assess blood glucose levels periodically, anticipate potential need for increased insulin or oral hypoglycemic drug doses

(continued)

Table 44–S1 **Major Side Effects of and Contraindications for Anterior Pituitary Hormones and Releasing Factors or Their Antagonists (*Continued*)**

BODY SYSTEM/ Side Effect	CONTRAINDICATION/ PRECAUTION	COMMENTS AND NURSING IMPLICATIONS
OTHER	Closed epiphyses	Growth hormone analogs are ineffective once epiphyses have closed; drug administration may increase the risk of other side effects
	Prolactin Release Inhibitor: Bromocriptine	
OTHER Allergic reactions ranging from mild urticaria to anaphylaxis	Prior allergic reactions to these or other drugs	Complete history should include prior allergic reactions (name of substance; date of reaction; manifestations/severity of response) before administering in full doses; have emergency drugs, devices ready for immediate use when administering first dose

Table 44–C2 **Clinical Uses and Administration of Vasopressins***

AGENT	CLINICAL USES	DOSAGE AND ROUTE OF ADMINISTRATION
Desmopressin acetate		
(DDAVP)	Chronic therapy of neurogenic diabetes insipidus	Nasal spray: Adults: 0.1–0.4 mL as a single dose, or 2 to 3 doses/day, using manufacturer's dispensing tube; usual adult dose 0.2 mL/day in two divided doses. Children 3 months–12 years: usually 0.05 to 0.3 mL/day, as single or 2 divided doses
	Prevention, treatment of bleeding in persons with hemophilia A or von Willebrand's disease, Type 1	IV: 0.3 μg/kg diluted in sterile physiologic saline, infused over 15–30 min; use 50 mL diluent for adults, children >10 kg, and 10 mL diluent for children 10 kg or less; if used to control intraoperative bleeding, administer 30 min before scheduled procedure
(*DDAVP injection*)	Primary nocturnal enuresis	IV or SC: Usually 0.5–1.0 mL (2–4 μg) per day in 2 divided doses
Lypressin		
(DIAPID)	Chronic therapy of neurogenic diabetes insipidus	Nasal spray: 1 or 2 sprays in one or both nostrils qid or on increased urination or thirst; additional bedtime doses may be needed; if patient requires more than 2 sprays per dose, shorten dosage interval instead of increasing amount per dose
Vasopressin aqueous injection		
(PITRESSIN)	Acute or chronic therapy of neurogenic diabetes insipidus	SC, IM, or intranasal: 5–10 IU (0.25–0.5 mL) bid or tid; parenteral solution intranasally as spray, drops, or on cotton pads
	Prevention or treatment of postoperative abdominal distention	IM: Usually 5 U (0.25 mL) initially, repeated in 3–4 h; increases to 0.5 mL may be needed. Children: reduce dose based on body weight
	Elimination of abdominal gas before radiography	IM: Usually 2 injections of 0.5 mL to start; give first injection 2 h before, second injection 30 min before, anticipated time for radiographic study

*See Chapter 49 for information related to oxytocin use.

Table 44–S2 **Major Side Effects of and Contraindications for Vasopressin and Related Agents***

BODY SYSTEM/ Side Effect	CONTRAINDICATION/ PRECAUTION	COMMENTS AND NURSING IMPLICATIONS
FLUID/ELECTROLYTE Dilutional hyponatremia: drowsiness, lethargy, headache, and potential seizures, coma if severe	History of seizures, preeclampsia/eclampsia, require cautious use	Assess for and report side effects and sudden appearance of oliguria, weight gain that may indicate "water intoxication;" encourage patient to keep written log of fluid intake and output (especially important for pediatric patients); teach how to measure fluid intake and urine output; temporarily stopping drug administration, restricting fluid intake, may be adequate for mild symptoms; severe symptoms may require forced diuresis, anticonvulsant drugs
CARDIOVASCULAR Vasoconstriction leading to systemic hypertension or coronary artery vasoconstriction	Hypertension, angina pectoris, coronary atherosclerosis, preeclampsia/eclampsia, require cautious use	Risk of coronary vasoconstriction, myocardial ischemia, and its consequences (angina, arrhythmias, infarction) may occur with any vasopressin product or analog or route of administration; most likely with parenteral administration in persons with ischemic heart disease, especially elderly; obtain baseline data; report anginal pain, pulse irregularities at once, be prepared to administer nitroglycerin for relief of angina; precautions apply to vasopressin use for any indication
GASTROINTESTINAL Cramping, diarrhea		Side effects usually occur with parenteral administration, often can be alleviated by having patient drink one or two glasses of water when drug is administered; assess for diminished bowel sounds, abdominal distention, or pain when vasopressin injection is used for abdominal distention or expulsion of intestinal gas
REPRODUCTIVE Increased uterine tone, premature labor, fetal distress or death (with posterior pituitary extract)	Pregnancy	Rule out pregnancy; controlled administration of synthetic vasopressins may be acceptable
OTHER Allergic reactions		See Table 44-S1, GH

*Unless noted otherwise, side effects, contraindications, and comments apply to synthetic vasopressin and analog. See Chapter 49 for information related to oxytocin and related agents.

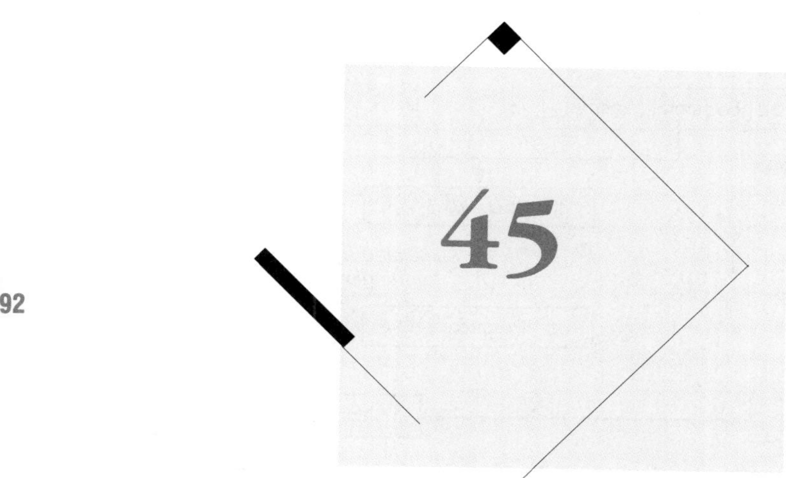

PROTOTYPE

Adrenocorticosteroids

The adrenal glands are each composed of two distinct parts, the medulla and the cortex. Hormones from the adrenal medulla (epinephrine and norepinephrine) are important in counteracting short-term stress. They are discussed in Chapters 10 and 14.

The adrenocorticosteroids discussed in this chapter (aldosterone, desoxycorticosterone, cortisone, and cortisol) are produced in the adrenal cortex, and have more long-lasting effects. They influence cardiovascular and cerebral function, the immune system, maintenance of healthy bone and muscle, and nearly all aspects of carbohydrate, fat, and protein metabolism.

In addition to the adrenocorticosteroids, the adrenal cortex also produces small amounts of androgenic hormones. These are discussed more completely in Chapter 48.

A clear understanding of the therapeutic principles of steroid drug use is essential to good nursing care of patients receiving these drugs. To help achieve that understanding, this chapter considers the normal physiology of adrenocortical hormones, the effects of hypo- and hypersecretion, and the advantages and adverse effects of their pharmacologic use.

Major reference tables appear beginning on p. 907.

The Normal Adrenal Cortex

The cells of the adrenal cortex are arranged in three histologically distinct zones. The outermost zone (zona glomerulosa) produces hormones known as the *mineralocorticoids,* which include *aldosterone, desoxycorticosterone* (DOC), and *corticosterone.* The predominant and most potent of these hormones is aldosterone. The mineralocorticoids influence salt and water balance in the body by promoting renal tubular reabsorption of sodium ions and secretion of potassium ions.

The zona fasciculata and zona reticularis regions produce two other categories of hormones, *glucocorticoids* and *gonadocorticoids* (adrenal androgens), respectively.

The glucocorticoids include *cortisol* (also called *hydrocortisone*) and *cortisone.* Cortisone is slightly less active than cortisol, but the two hormones are interconverted readily in the liver and are considered identical. Glucocorticoids exert their primary effects on carbohydrate, fat, and protein metabolism, but they have many other important effects that are discussed more fully later in the chapter.

The gonadocorticoids, chemically identified by the term "17-keto" steroids, are weak anabolic androgens (*dehydroepiandrosterone* [DEA] and *androstenedione*), but some testosterone and estrogens are produced also.

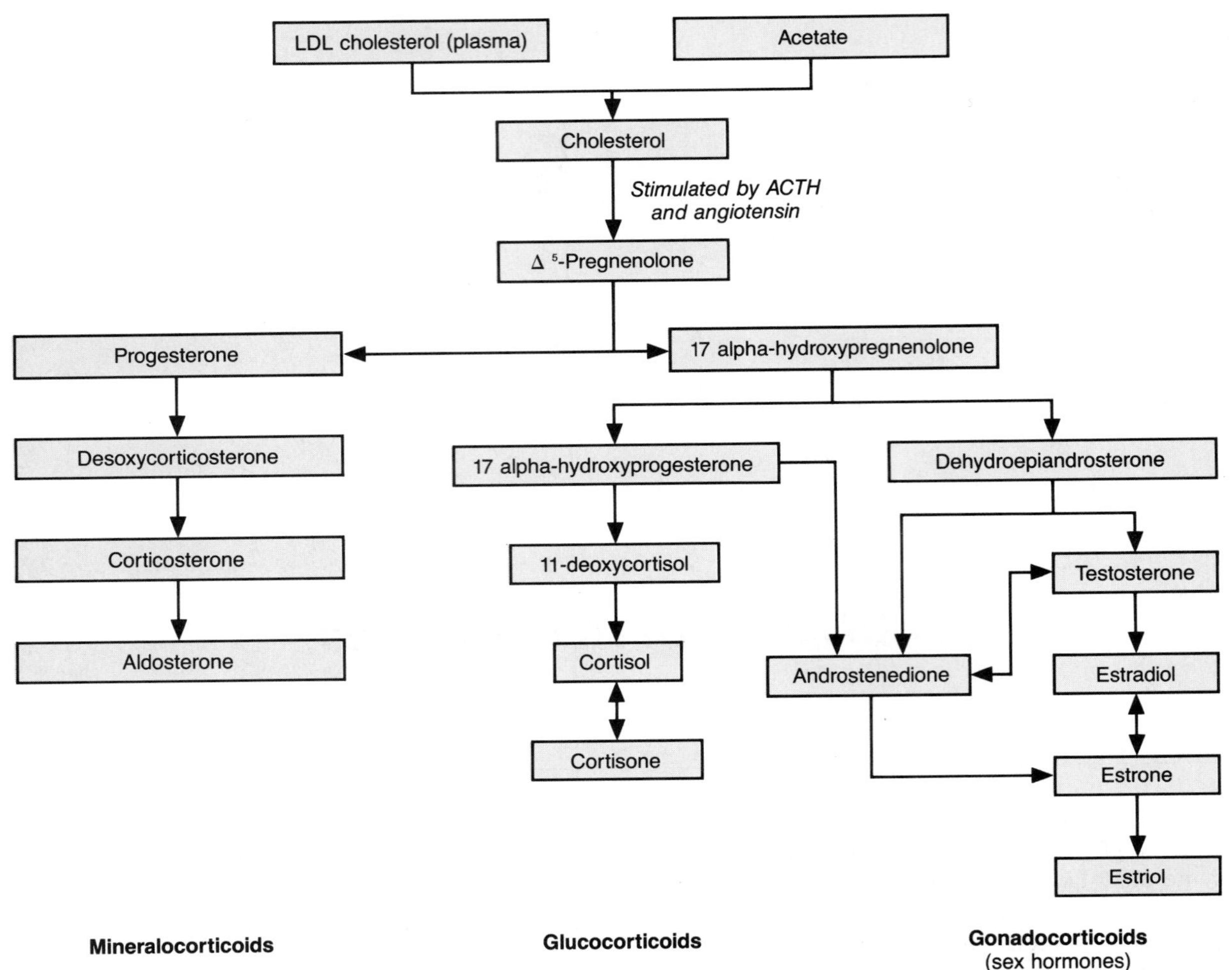

Figure 45–1

Biosynthesis of adrenocorticosteroids.

Biosynthesis, Transport, and Metabolism

Biosynthesis of the adrenal corticosteroids begins with cholesterol. Cholesterol is converted into pregnenolone. Thereafter the synthetic pathways separate to form the various active adrenal corticosteroids. Figure 45–1 summarizes corticosteroid biosynthesis. Pregnenolone appears to be the pivotal intermediate. It is susceptible to control by such regulatory substances as adrenocorticotropic hormone (ACTH) and angiotensin. This control is discussed in more detail later.

I. Glucocorticoids

In the absence of stress, about 15 to 20 mg of cortisol is secreted daily. Immediately on release it binds to cortisol-binding globulin (CBG). Cortisol-binding globulin serves as a carrier for cortisol. The normal range of CBG-bound cortisol is 10 to 20 μg/100 mL of plasma, representing 85% to 90% of the total amount of cortisol in the blood. Thus, only about 10% to 15% of total blood cortisol is free and biologically active.

Cortisol is inactivated by hepatic metabolism through a series of steps that eventually lead to conjugation with glucuronic acid or sulfate. The glucuronate or sulfate conjugates are water-soluble and readily excreted in the urine as 17-hydroxycortisol products. Both cortisol inactivation and CBG synthesis are impaired significantly in persons with hepatic dysfunction. That explains the prevalence of signs and symptoms of hypercortism in such persons. Cortisol elimination is reduced in the nephrotic syndrome and other disorders involving diminished renal function.

The normal plasma half-life of cortisol is about 90 minutes. Disorders of either the liver or kidneys, decreased metabolic states (such as hypothyroidism), or drugs that inhibit hepatic metabolism, including high and acute alcohol intake, may prolong the half-life significantly. Conversely, hyperthyroidism or hepatic enzyme-inducing drugs (phenobarbital and phenytoin) shorten the half-life. The plasma half-life of cortisol is much less important physiologically and pharmacologically than its duration of action, which is approximately 12 hours.

Physiologic Effects

The glucocorticoids influence the metabolic activity of most body cells. Physiologic amounts promote homeostasis in the body through adaption to changes in the external environment; they are absolutely essential to life. In general, their effects are concentration-dependent: they are increased when blood levels are high, and decreased when blood levels are too low.

The basic mechanism of glucocorticoid activity is unclear, but it is known that steroid hormones pass through the cell membrane and bind to cytoplasmic receptors. The receptor-hormone complex enters the nucleus and regulates gene expression, the ultimate effect being increased protein synthesis.

Perhaps the most important physiologic effects of the burst-like release of cortisol during the stress response are increases in blood glucose levels and systemic blood pressure. Hyperglycemia is mediated by cortisol's effects on cellular catabolism of tissue proteins and fats, and the conversion of their breakdown products to glucose—a process called gluconeogenesis. Increased arterial blood pressure, a desirable condition during emergency situations, results from cortisol's ability to increase epinephrine's vasoconstrictor effect, and its maintenance of adequate extracellular fluid volumes. However, these protective responses are only part of the total spectrum of body responses to glucocorticoids.

Glucocorticoids depress bone metabolism, the immune system, and the inflammatory response, and promote changes in cardiovascular, neural, and gastrointestinal (GI) function. In the absence of glucocorticoids with mineralocorticoid activity (such as cortisone and hydrocortisone), renal function (and thus fluid and electrolyte balance) is impaired.

Under conditions of prolonged cortisol excesses, such as might arise from adrenocortical hyperactivity (Cushing's syndrome) or therapeutic dosages, the enhanced responses may be serious and potentially life-threatening. Physiologic effects of cortisol, as well as effects of its excess or deficit, are presented in Table 45–1. This table summarizes nearly all side effects that can be anticipated during glucocorticoid therapy, and provides the indications for nursing actions.

Regulation

Glucocorticoid blood levels exhibit a well-established diurnal rhythm that reflects the oscillations of anterior pituitary release of ACTH and hypothalamic release of corticotropin-releasing hormone (CRH). There is a burst of ACTH release at approximately 3 AM; levels peak at 6 AM, which induces a brisk rise in cortisol levels between 6 AM and 9 AM. Increased serum cortisol levels feed back to inhibit the hypothalamic-pituitary-adrenal axis, which inhibits ACTH release temporarily.

As cortisol is metabolized progressively throughout the day, its level declines and reaches a low around midnight. At this point, lack of feedback inhibition causes ACTH release once again. Although often referred to as a "sleep-wake cycle," adrenal activity is independent of sleep; the normal rhythm of cortisol release is abolished by unconsciousness and (typically) by Cushing's syndrome.

The diurnal rhythm of cortisol release is interrupted by many stressors acting on the body. Under stressful conditions, the inhibitory effect of elevated cortisol levels is counteracted by sympathetic nervous system activity, which triggers hypothalamic release of CRH. This is followed shortly by rising plasma levels of ACTH and an outpouring of glucocorticoids by the adrenal cortex. This regulatory scheme is shown in Figure 45–2.

Effects of Glucocorticoid Hyper- and Hyposecretion

Cushing's Syndrome

With the exception of iatrogenic Cushing's syndrome, caused by pharmacologic doses of cortisol and its analogs, the syndrome of chronic glucocorticoid excess is exceptionally uncommon. Of the nondrug-induced cases, nearly two-thirds arise from excess ACTH pro-

Table 45–1 Major Effects of Glucocorticoids

Process/System	Physiologic Effects	Effects of Hypersecretion	Effects of Hyposecretion
Metabolism of proteins, fats, and carbohydrates	Hyperglycemic effect: 1. Stimulates glyconeogenesis; ↑ protein catabolism in muscle and peripheral tissues via conversion to glucose, leading to ↑ blood glucose and deposit of glycogen in muscle tissue 2. Enhances liver uptake of amino acids, stimulates liver enzymes, promoting gluconeogenesis, ↑ glucose released to blood, ↑ glycogen deposited in the liver 3. Exerts a permissive action: cortisol must be present for epinephrine and glucagon to cause glucose release from the liver	Steroid diabetes; may aggravate existing diabetes mellitus or initiate the appearance of latent diabetes	Hypoglycemia
	4. Stimulates the release of insulin, which stimulates cellular uptake of amino acids and glucose	When prolonged, amino acids and glucose are converted to fat because cortisol inhibits glucose oxidation; fat accumulates in face, neck, trunk—at expense of body protein (protein wasting)	
	Catabolic effect: Antagonizes use of amino acids for anabolism, in addition to breaking down protein (muscle)	Muscle wasting, negative nitrogen balance; osteoporosis; poor wound healing	
	Hyperlipidemic effect: Enhances fat absorption from the gut; acting in conjunction with epinephrine, growth hormone, and insulin (permissive effect) promotes mobilization of fatty acids from adipose tissue and their use for energy metabolism	Hyperlipidemias: accelerates atherosclerotic processes	
Hematopoietic tissue	↓ number of lymphocytes eosinophils, monocytes, basophils; ↑ number of neutrophils, platelets, and red blood cells	Involution of thymus and lymph nodes—↓ B lymphocytes and greater ↓ of T cells for cellular immunity; ↓ allergic response; polycythemia; enhanced clotting with tendencies to form thromboemboli	Anemia

Table 45–1 Major Effects of Glucocorticoids (*Continued*)

Process/System	Physiologic Effects	Effects of Hypersecretion	Effects of Hyposecretion
Inflammatory response	Antiinflammatory effects: ↓ connective tissue response to injury; ↓ redness and swelling at injured site; ↓ white blood cell migration into area of injury; ↓ reactions to antigen-antibody complexes; stabilizes lysosomal membranes, ↓ cellular damage; stabilizes mast cell membranes, ↓ mediator release caused by antigen-antibody reaction	Masks or prevents protective inflammatory response to tissue trauma and infection	
Fluid/electrolyte balance	↑ diuresis; prevents shift of water into cells, maintaining blood volume and assuring adequate glomerular filtration	Mineralocorticoid effect: sodium and water retention; hypertension; edema; increased renal potassium excretion, hypokalemia	Hypovolemia; hyperkalemia; hyponatremia; hypotension
Central nervous system	↓ threshold for brain electrical activity; analgesic properties	Seizures; psychologic abnormalities: irritability, insomnia, mood elevation	Psychologic abnormalities: apathy, depression
Cardiovascular system	Potentiates vasoconstrictor effect of epinephrine; enhances angiotensinogen and aldosterone production; lipolytic effect (see metabolism) leads to hyperlipidemia	Hypertension; edema; heart failure; atherosclerosis	Hypotension; decreased vasoconstrictor effect of catecholamines; cardiovascular collapse
Gastrointestinal system	↓ gastric acidity and pepsin production; thinning of gastric mucosa	Peptic ulcers	
Skeletal system	Antagonizes bone formation; prevents bone remodeling; ↓ cartilage and bone matrix formation and calcium salt deposit; antagonizes stimulating effect of vitamin D on calcium absorption by gut (may interfere with growth hormone effects)	Severe osteoporosis; fractures (most severe limiting factor in long-term use of glucocorticoids); growth retardation in children	
Skeletal muscle	Maintains muscle strength	Muscle wasting owing to catabolism of muscle proteins	Muscle weakness

Key: ↑ = increased, ↓ = decreased.

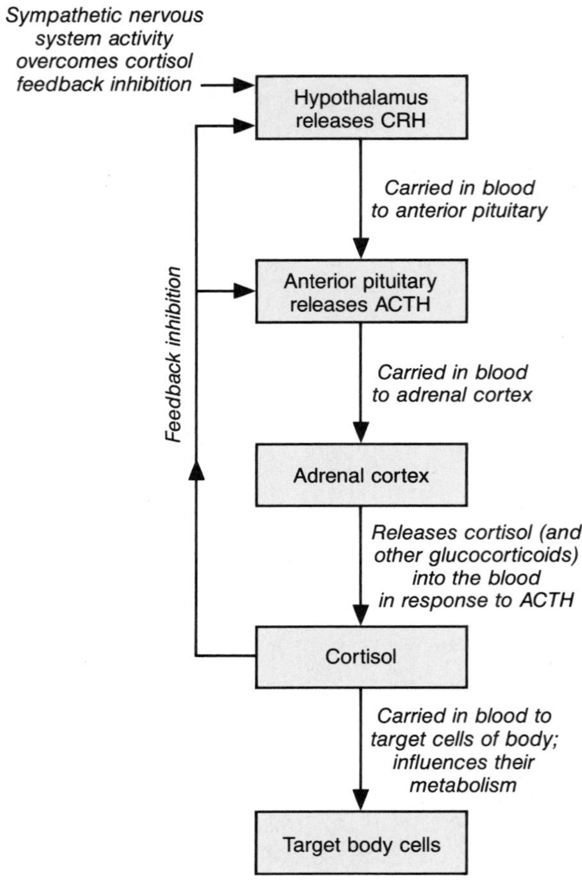

Figure 45–2

Regulation of glucocorticoid release. The diurnal rhythm of cortisol release reflects the hormonal interactions of the hypothalamic-pituitary-adrenocortical axis. Stressors act through sympathetic nervous system pathways to overcome cortisol feedback inhibition and to induce CRH, ACTH, and cortisol release.

duction by pituitary adenomas or in response to excessive hypothalamic CRH release. Other causes include ectopic ACTH synthesis and release by malignant neoplasms (most commonly of the lungs, kidneys, pancreas, or thymus), and adrenal hyperplasia or neoplasms.

Common presenting signs of Cushing's syndrome are those typical of excess cortisol (see Table 45–1). The so-called cushingoid signs include a swollen plethoric face (moonface and rosy cheeks); characteristic fat deposits on the posterior neck (buffalo hump), abdomen, and trunk; cutaneous striae; bruising; thin extremities; and thin fragile skin. However, the syndrome has many clinical variants that reflect hypersecretion of mineralocorticoids or androgens as well as cortisol.

When excessive mineralocorticoids are produced, the clinical picture includes hypertension, hypernatremia, and hypokalemic alkalosis accompanied by muscle weakness. Androgen excess leads to hirsutism and masculinization in women. When Cushing's syndrome results from a pituitary adenoma, typical signs of cortisol excess are likely to be coupled with menstrual irregularity in women and impotence in men (owing to alterations in secretion of pituitary gonadotropins).

Table 45–2 lists various tests used to determine the level of adrenocortical function. The most appropriate diagnostic test for Cushing's syndrome is the dexamethasone suppression test. Plasma cortisol levels are measured the morning after a midnight dose of dexamethasone (a potent synthetic glucocorticoid). If plasma cortisol is less than 5 μg/100 mL, ACTH suppression by glucocorticoids is verified and Cushing's disease is ruled out. If plasma cortisol levels are greater than 5 μg/100 mL, more complete testing is indicated.

Surgery is the preferred treatment for Cushing's disease initiated by pituitary, ectopic, or adrenal neoplasms. Preoperative treatment with metyrapone (Chapter 45) or other adrenal suppressant drugs modulates the effects of hypercortisolism, making surgery relatively safe. Bilateral removal of the adrenal glands requires lifelong corticosteroid replacement therapy. When surgery is contraindicated, various adrenal suppressant drugs (discussed later) may be prescribed. In iatrogenic Cushing's syndrome, a decision must be made about the advisability (in terms of patient benefit) of corticoid drug withdrawal (discussed later).

Adrenogenital Syndrome

An extreme clinical variant of adrenocortical hyperfunction is *adrenogenital syndrome,* which most often results from congenital lack of an enzyme needed for cortisol synthesis. A deficit of plasma cortisol induces high ACTH blood levels that, in turn, enhance production of the nonglucocorticoid adrenocorticoids. The exceptionally large amounts of androgens secreted lead to virilization. This disorder is treated by the administration of cortisol or related analogs, which inhibit ACTH secretion and replace the deficient corticosteroids.

Adrenocortical Insufficiency

Adrenal Crisis

Adrenocortical insufficiency is a disorder in which both glucocorticoids and mineralocorticoids are lacking. Spontaneous or acute adrenal insufficiency (*adrenal crisis*) is extremely rare, but it is always life-threatening.

Table 45–2 Tests to Evaluate Adrenocortical Function

Test	Goal of Measurement	Method	Normal Values	Comments
ACTH screening test	Adrenal responsiveness to ACTH stimulation when adrenal insufficiency is suspected; rule out adrenal insufficiency	Baseline cortisol levels measured, 25 U of ACTH administered IM; cortisol levels measured one hour later	Cortisol levels increase by 25%	Lack of cortisol increase indicates adrenal insufficiency; does not differentiate between primary and secondary adrenal insufficiency
Cosyntropin test	As for ACTH screening test	Baseline plasma cortisol levels measured, 0.25 mg cosyntropin administered IV one hour later; plasma cortisol levels measured again	Baseline cortisol levels double with normal adrenal function	As for ACTH screening test
ACTH infusion test	Differentiate between primary and secondary adrenal insufficiency	Urinary levels of 17-hydroxycortisol measured at 1, 2, and 24 hours. 10–25 U of ACTH administered daily for 3 days and urinary 17-OHCS levels measured	17-hydroxycortisol levels are 2–4 times base levels in normal individuals; increased by half that amount with secondary insufficiency; levels not increased in primary disease	Observed results elevated by obesity and decreased by hepatic and renal disease
Dexamethasone suppression test	Susceptibility of hypothalamic-pituitary-adrenal axis to feedback inhibition	One mg dexamethasone administered between 11 PM and midnight; plasma cortisol measured at 8 AM the following morning	Plasma cortisol levels less than 5 μg/100 mL are normal	Levels over 5 μg/100 mL indicate nonsuppressibility of the axis, which is characteristic of Cushing's disease
Metyrapone test	Assess for pituitary-adrenal insufficiency (metyrapone inhibits synthesis of cortisol by blocking 11 β-hydroxylation)	3 g metyrapone administered orally at midnight and plasma 11-deoxycortisol and cortisol levels obtained at 8 AM the following morning	Plasma cortisol levels remain below 10 μg/100 mL, and 11-deoxycortisol levels rise to over 7 μg/100 mL, in normal individuals	Subnormal response establishes diagnosis of adrenal insufficiency; if patient has a normal ACTH test, but an abnormal metyrapone test, the patient has a secondary adrenal insufficiency
Plasma cortisol levels	Diagnose adrenal hyperfunction	Plasma cortisol levels measured in the morning and evening	10–25 μg/100 mL in AM; 2–10 μg/100 mL in PM	Values increased by increased estrogen and decreased hepatic disease
24-Hour urinary free cortisol	Diagnose adrenal hyperfunction	24-Hour urinary free cortisol measured		Less useful for diagnosis of hypofunction; levels increased in obese individuals

It can result from massive adrenal cortex hemorrhage, and is seen most often in patients taking anticoagulants. It occurs infrequently in patients with overwhelming sepsis. The important clinical signs of acute adrenal insufficiency are hypotension, confusion, nausea and vomiting, and back pain. Unless treated promptly by intravenous (IV) adrenocorticoid administration, the patient's condition deteriorates rapidly to circulatory collapse, shock, and death.

Addison's Disease

Addison's disease is primary adrenal insufficiency characterized by reduced output of glucocorticoids and mineralocorticoids. (An infrequent clinical variant involves mineralocorticoid deficits only.) Usual causes include chronic granulomatous infections (such as tuberculosis) or, more commonly, an autoimmune disorder in which the adrenal gland is invaded by lymphocytes and antiadrenal antibodies.

Patients with Addison's disease characteristically have anorexia, weight loss, hypotension caused by hypovolemia, hypoglycemia, hyperkalemia, and muscle weakness. (See Table 45–1 for other signs.) A useful diagnostic sign is hyperpigmentation of the skin, particularly over palmar creases and pressure points. Although the actual cause of the hyperpigmentation is not known, it is believed to result from the stimulatory effect of chronic ACTH (and possibly melanocyte-stimulating hormone [MSH]) excess on skin melanocytes.

Secondary adrenal insufficiency, resulting from a deficiency of ACTH, can be distinguished from the primary disease by the absence of hyperpigmentation and the finding that mineralocorticoid functions are less impaired.

Addison's disease may be diagnosed by intramuscular (IM) injection of ACTH gel (H.P. ACTHAR GEL) or an IV challenge with synthetic ACTH (ACTHAR), followed by measurement of cortisol levels. In healthy individuals, plasma cortisol levels increase after ACTH stimulus. When adrenocortical insufficiency is strongly suspected, more involved testing must be done and is always accompanied by administration of adrenocorticoid drugs to prevent adrenal collapse during testing. Addison's disease is treated by replacement therapy with drugs that have both glucocorticoid and mineralocorticoid activity.

Glucocorticoid Replacement Drugs

A number of natural and synthetic glucocorticoid products are available for therapeutic use. Unlike most other hormone drugs, which are used primarily for replacement therapy in cases of endocrine organ hypofunction, the glucocorticoids also are employed for conditions unrelated to disturbances of adrenal gland function. The prototype drug is cortisol (also called hydrocortisone).

PROTOTYPE

Cortisol

Absorption, Distribution, Metabolism, and Excretion

Cortisol and its analogs are well absorbed after oral administration or deep IM injection. The effects of oral administration are more rapid, but less prolonged, than those obtained by IM injection. Topical forms provide maximal antiinflammatory activity at the site of application; used in excess, they produce systemic effects as well.

Glucocorticoids are transported bound to CBG, metabolized by the liver, and excreted in urine as previously described for endogenous cortisol. Synthetic glucocorticoids (prednisone, prednisolone, and others) are absorbed rapidly, transported, and metabolized in a manner similar to cortisol. However, structural differences influence the degree of protein binding, rate of reduction and activation, and end products excreted. The duration of activity and dose equivalents of representative corticosteroid products are noted in Table 45–3.

Pharmacologic Effects

The many pharmacologic effects of cortisol are described in Table 45–1. The most important ones include widespread metabolic and antiinflammatory effects. Pharmacologic doses of cortisol depress the activity of both adrenal cortical cells and ACTH-secreting anterior pituitary cells; if prolonged, irreversible adrenal gland atrophy occurs.

In pharmacologic (supraphysiologic) doses, all natural glucocorticoids and some of the chemically modified synthetic forms have significant water- and sodium-retaining (mineralocorticoid) activity. Chemical modification of the basic steroid ring structure forms several synthetic glucocorticoids (eg, dexamethasone, methyprednisolone, betamethasone, paramethasone, triamcinolone) that almost completely lack mineralocorticoid activity. However, they have significantly great-

Table 45–3 | **Comparison of Activities of Selected Natural and Synthetic Corticoids***

Drug	Equivalent Oral Dose (mg)	Duration of Action (hr)	Relative Gluco-corticoid Activity	Relative Mineralo-corticoid Activity
Natural glucocorticoids				
Cortisol (hydrocortisone)	20	8–12	1	1
Cortisone	25	8–12	0.8	2
Synthetic glucocorticoids				
Prednisone	5	18–36	4	1
Methylprednisone	4	18–36	5	0
Prednisolone	5	18–36	4	1
Triamcinolone	4	18–36	5	0
Dexamethasone	0.75	36–54	20–30	0
Betamethasone	0.6	36–54	20–30	0
Natural mineralocorticoid				
Aldosterone	†	1	0.2	3000
Synthetic mineralocorticoid				
Fludrocortisone	0.1–0.2	18–36	10	125

**Source:* Modified from *Drug Facts and Comparisons,* 1992, and *Goodman and Gilman's Pharmacological Basis of Therapeutics,* 8th ed., 1991. Reprinted with the permission of the copyright owners.
†Not used clinically.

er antiinflammatory activity than cortisol. Since these products have less potential for producing the troubling side effects of sodium and water retention, they provide a more satisfactory alternative for long-term therapy of nonadrenal disorders that benefit from glucocorticoid therapy. The relative glucocorticoid (antiinflammatory) and mineralocorticoid activities of some of the glucocorticoid products are given in Table 45–3.

Clinical Indications and Administration

The various therapeutic uses, and rationales for use, of glucocorticoid drugs are summarized in Table 45–4. Dosages for representative drugs administered for systemic actions are summarized in Table 45–C1. Selected steroid preparations indicated for topical application to the skin are summarized in Table 45–5, and Table 45–6 identifies steroid preparations indicated for ophthalmic or otic disorders accompanied by inflammation.

Management of Adrenal Insufficiency

The most obvious use for cortisol is for replacement therapy in cases of adrenocortical insufficiency. In addition, the glucocorticoid analogs that lack mineralocorticoid effects are used in clinical practice in supraphysiologic doses for their antiinflammatory, antiallergic, and antiimmune effects. These properties suggest a usefulness for glucocorticoids to relieve characteristic symptoms of many acute and chronic diseases.

The goal of replacement therapy is to restore normal hormonal concentrations. Thus, physiologic, or minimally supraphysiologic, doses are used; for cortisol the replacement dose would be 15 to 25 mg/day. (See Table 45–C1 for equivalent doses of the other glucocorticoids.)

Replacement therapy must provide not only glucocorticoids but also drugs with mineralocorticoid activity. For many patients, administration of the natural corticoids (cortisol and cortisone) serves both functions well. In others, however, additional supplementation with a separate mineralocorticoid drug may be necessary.

Generally, replacement drugs are administered in a schedule that attempts to mimic the normal diurnal rhythm. For short-acting drugs, two-thirds of the daily dose is taken in the morning, the balance at night. Longer-acting glucocorticoids are taken once daily, in the morning. Dosages are adjusted to individual patient needs and monitored by laboratory testing to provide the desired results.

Table 45–4 Clinical Uses of Glucocorticoids

Use	Basis for Use
Replacement therapy in acute or chronic adrenal insufficiency and congenital adrenal hyperplasia (genetic deficiency preventing cortisol synthesis)	Replacement of deficient hormones to restore physiologic effects; systemic administration; requires glucocorticoid with mineralocorticoid activity or separate administration of both glucocorticoid and mineralocorticoid supplements
Joint disorders; osteoarthritis, gout, rheumatoid arthritis; ankylosing spondylitis; acute bursitis/tendinitis	Used for progressive disease accompanied by joint swelling, disability, pain; antiinflammatory and antiautoimmune effects; systemic administration; intraarticular administration for rheumatoid arthritis
Collagen diseases: systemic lupus erythematosus, rheumatic carditis and rheumatoid arthritis; polyarteritis nodosa and others; multiple sclerosis	Antiinflammatory, and antiautoimmune effects; decreased connective tissue reactivity and damage; systemic administration
Allergic or hypersensitivity reactions: drug reactions; anaphylaxis, urticaria, asthma, contact dermatitis, and status asthmaticus	Antiinflammatory, antiallergy activity; decreases number of eosinophils and histamine production; enhances response of cardiovascular system, bronchial smooth muscle to sympathomimetics
Head trauma; cerebral edema and increased intracranial pressure	Antiinflammatory effect; systemic administration; reduces cerebral swelling
Gastrointestinal: celiac sprue, chronic ulcerative colitis, regional enteritis	Antiinflammatory and antiautoimmune effects; systemic administration
Liver disease: hepatic necrosis; chronic/alcoholic hepatitis	Antiinflammatory effects; systemic administration
Renal disease: nephrotic syndrome, glomerulonephritis	Decreases edema and proteinuria; antiinflammatory and antiautoimmune effects; if ineffective, therapy discontinued
Shock	May enhance cardiovascular response to epinephrine; increases vasoconstriction and restores blood volume; IV administration required for immediate effect
Ocular inflammation not due to infection: conjunctivitis, keratitis, iritis, corneal ulcers, others	Antiinflammatory effect; prevents damage to eye
Malignancies: leukemia, lymphoma (lymphatic tissue cancers), other cancer types	Antilymphocytic activity; increases response to other chemotherapeutic agents; systemic administration
Prevention of organ transplant rejection	Lympholytic and antiinflammatory actions; often prophylactic; systemic administration

Management of Inflammation: Arthritis and Asthma

Glucocorticoids are used for their antiinflammatory actions in such disorders as arthritis and asthma, for which pharmacologic doses of cortisol analogs are administered to produce high glucocorticoid levels at the desired sites of activity. The preferred drugs are those with minimal mineralocorticoid activity. Whether used for arthritis or asthma, steroids are not first-line agents. Generally they should be used only if the disorder fails to respond to other drugs that cause fewer or less severe side effects.

Dosages vary widely, depending on the nature and severity of the disorder being treated. A cardinal rule of long-term glucocorticoid therapy is to use the smallest dose that will provide the desired therapeutic effects. Usually any systemic dose larger than the equivalent of 20 mg per day of cortisol is considered a large dose. For management of severe symptoms, an equivalent of as much as 300 mg of cortisol may be given initially, with the dose gradually tapered to a lower maintenance

Table 45–5 Selected Topical Steroids Used for Cutaneous Inflammation and Pruritis

Product	Formulation and Composition
Betamethasone benzoate (BENISONE)	C, G, L: 0.025%
Betamethasone dipropionate (DIPROLENE; DIPROSONE; others)	A: 0.1% C, L, O: 0.05%
Betamethasone valerate (VALISONE; others)	C, L, O: 0.1%
Dexamethasone (DECADERM; DECASPRAY)	G: 0.1% A: 0.04%, 0.01%
Dexamethasone sodium phosphate (DECADRON PHOSPHATE)	C: 0.1%
Fluandrenolide (CORDRAN; others)	C: 0.025%, 0.05% L: 0.05% O: 0.025%, 0.05% Tape: 4 μg/cm^2
Hydrocortisone (CORT-DOME; others)	A: 0.5% C, L: 0.25%–2.5% S: 1% O: 0.5%, 1%, 2.5%
Hydrocortisone acetate (CORTAID; others)	C: 0.5%, 1% G, L, O: 0.5%
Methylprednisolone acetate (MEDROL ACETATE TOPICAL)	O: 0.25%, 1%
Triamcinolone acetonide (ARISTOCORT; KENALOG; others)	A: 0.2 mg per 2 sec spray C, O: 0.025%–0.5% L: 0.025%–0.1%

Key to abbreviations: **A:** aerosol spray; **C:** cream; **G:** gel; **L:** lotion; **O:** ointment; **S:** solution.

Table 45–6 Selected Topical Corticosteroids for Management of Ocular or External Ear Inflammation

Ocular*	
Dexamethasone (MAXIDEX)	Suspension: 0.1%
Dexamethasone sodium phosphate (DECADRON PHOSPHATE)	Suspension: 0.1% Ointment: 0.05%
Fluoromethalone (FML)	Suspension: 0.1%, 0.25% Ointment: 0.1%
Prednisolone acetate (PRED-MILD, PRED-FORTE)	Suspension: 0.12%, 0.125%, 1.0%
Prednisolone sodium phosphate (AK-PRED)	Solution: 0.125%–1.0%
Otic†	
Hydrocortisone (CORTISPORIN)	Solution or suspension: 0.5%, 1.0% (combined with polymyxin G and/or neomycin sulfate)
Hydrocortisone acetate (COLY-MYCIN S OTIC)	Suspension: 1% (usually combined with colistin, neomycin)

*The usual dose of an ophthalmic steroid preparation varies greatly, from one to two drops of suspension hourly to one drop tid or qid. Ointments provide more long-lasting effects, initial application may be tid or qid, decreasing to qd when desired response develops.

†Usual dose of an otic preparation is four drops, instilled tid or qid

dose. The average maximum daily cortisol-equivalent dose is 30 to 80 mg, administered in divided doses. The overall goal is to provide relief as quickly as possible, and to use systemic steroids for as short a time as possible to reduce the risk of adrenal suppression.

Arthritis

The use of glucocorticoids for arthritis is discussed in Chapter 55. Preferred use involves periodic intraarticular injections of a steroid into one or two inflamed joints during arthritis flare-ups. Systemic (oral) steroids should be used only for selected arthritis patients with severe symptoms that are potentially life-threatening, or patients who cannot tolerate traditional nonsteroidal antiinflammatory drugs.

Asthma

Glucocorticoids are used for asthma that has failed to respond to sympathomimetic bronchodilators, methylxanthines such as theophylline, or both. Oral steroids may be needed for severe asthma symptoms, but inhaled steroids such as beclomethasone are preferred if long-term use is anticipated. The inhaled steroids suppress inflammation in the respiratory tract, and when used properly there is a very low risk of causing systemic effects and adrenal suppression. The growing use of steroids for asthma is discussed in Chapter 38.

Adjunctive Therapy of Anaphylaxis

Glucocorticoids are also important emergency drugs for managing life-threatening situations such as anaphylaxis, status asthmaticus, septic shock, myxedema coma, and acute adrenal crisis. In anaphylaxis and status asthmaticus in particular, steroids are valuable for their ability to restore airway responsiveness to sympathomimetic bronchodilators. A single large IV dose is used, and more can be given if the desired effects do not occur. Since a rapid response is essential, water-soluble drug forms, such as hydrocortisone sodium succinate or dexamethasone phosphate, are selected. In these potentially fatal situations, the precaution of making a definitive diagnosis before treatment becomes less important than usual since the risks of acute steroid administration are low compared with the risks of not administering them. If the patient's symptoms are thought to be caused by an adrenal crisis, blood samples for cortisol measurements should be drawn before IV glucocorticoid administration, to help make the diagnosis.

Other Indications

Systemic administration of corticosteroids with predominant glucocorticoid activity also is indicated for management of

- severe erythema multiforme and exfoliative dermatitis;
- ocular inflammation;
- management of hematologic disorders such as thrombocytopenia in adults;
- palliation of leukemias and lymphomas;
- adjunctive management of acute phases of ulcerative colitis or regional enteritis;
- reduction of intracranial pressure in persons with brain neoplasms;
- management of such collagen disorders as systemic lupus erythematosus and acute rheumatic carditis; and
- suppression of organ graft rejection in transplant patients.

Steroids may be applied topically for some forms of ocular, cutaneous, or otic inflammation. Oral inhalation is used often for asthma therapy.

NURSING IMPLICATIONS

Glucocorticoid use, except for replacement therapy, relieves signs and symptoms, but does not cure the underlying disorder. Regardless of the disease (or patient) being treated, the dosage that will provide the best therapeutic effect must be determined by trial and error. The patient's condition must be reevaluated continually to determine the necessity of dosage changes.

Only succinate and phosphate steroid drug forms should be administered IV. Never inject the suspensions or poorly absorbed acetate forms IV; they are intended for IM, intraarticular, and intralesional injection. To prevent muscle atrophy, use deep IM injections.

Warn patients receiving intraarticular or intrabursal injections that temporary discomfort will follow drug injection. Instruct patients using ointments or creams for dermatologic and ocular problems on how the preparation is to be applied. If occlusive dressings are indicated, teach the patient the technique of dressing application.

Advise patients to carry a medical alert card indicating their diagnosis and medication. Advise them to anticipate and report stressful situations, since dosage increases may be necessary during such times. Encourage patients to return for biannual follow-up visits to monitor the success of drug therapy.

Glucocorticoid products must be stored in tightly capped, light-proof containers.

Side Effects, Adverse Reactions, and Contraindications

Adverse responses and side effects caused by corticosteroids fall into two categories: those that appear during therapy and are caused by the administered drug; and those that occur on discontinuation of steroid therapy and are caused by suppression of the adrenal gland and its release of endogenous hormones once free of drug influences and negative feedback.

Untoward Responses During Glucocorticoid Therapy

Undesirable complications of glucocorticoid use seldom are true toxic effects. More often they are exaggerations of normal hormonal actions (see Table 45–1) that lead to the clinical picture of iatrogenic Cushing's disease. The rate of appearance of cushingoid symptoms depends on the glucocorticoid dose and the individual drug's relative glucocorticoid and mineralocorticoid potencies. When such symptoms appear, the dose should be reduced, if the severity of the condition being treated and such other patient-related factors as overall health allow it.

The speed with which corticosteroid doses can be reduced or discontinued also depends on the degree of adrenal suppression that has occurred, as discussed later. In some cases it may be difficult to convince patients to reduce the dose of a drug that has provided them with appreciable symptomatic relief.

Metabolic Side Effects

These include the appearance of hyperglycemia, fat mobilization and redistribution, and muscle wasting. The hyperglycemic effects of the drugs normally can be counteracted by increased insulin secretion in normal individuals. However, individuals with diabetes and pre- or subclinical diabetes (a condition found in many elderly individuals) are unable to compensate and may develop clinical signs of diabetes mellitus. As a result, persons with diabetes may need larger doses of insulin or oral hypoglycemic agents. Some normoglycemic individuals also may require supplementary hypoglycemic medications during steroid therapy.

Relocalization of fat deposits often leads to changes in physical appearance (round face and thick trunk) and cutaneous striae. The catabolic effects of the drugs result in muscle wasting, depression of bone metabolism, and poor wound healing. Severe myopathy and accelerated osteoporosis are serious adverse effects and are often sufficient indications for drug withdrawal.

Glucocorticoid therapy should be used with extreme caution for persons with preexisting osteoporosis. Postmenopausal women are at particular risk. Vertebral compression and spontaneous fractures may occur, particularly in immobilized and elderly patients, and in those with rheumatoid arthritis. Impaired growth may occur in children.

Central Nervous System Side Effects

Prolonged use of glucocorticoids occasionally produces central nervous system (CNS) effects including elevated mood (often alternating with depression), irritability, insomnia and, infrequently, overt psychotic reactions. In patients developing corticosteroid-induced behavioral changes, the dosage should be reduced if possible.

The enhanced sense of well-being and diminished pain perception experienced by some patients may encourage them to become more active physically. When the underlying problem is a joint or rheumatoid disorder, worsening of joint deterioration may follow such increases in activity.

Ocular Side Effects

Increased intraorbital pressures can occur during prolonged use of topical steroids on the eye. Cataract formation, another consequence, appears to be dose-related.

Cardiovascular Side Effects

Glucocorticoids, administered for prolonged times (as with replacement therapy), can elevate serum lipid and cholesterol levels and may cause or accelerate atherosclerosis. If the drug being administered has even slight mineralocorticoid activity, renal sodium and water retention can cause or worsen hypertension or congestive heart failure.

Gastrointestinal Side Effects

Glucocorticoids tend to thin mucus secretions that line and normally protect the GI tract. They also depress regeneration of gastric mucosal cells. Both actions contribute to the ulcerogenic effect of systemic steroids. Antacids or histamine-receptor antagonists (cimetidine, for example) may be required adjunctive therapies during prolonged glucocorticoid treatment. Patients at high risk of peptic ulcer disease are extremely susceptible to this adverse response, and long-term glucocorticoid use generally is contraindicated for them.

Fluid and Electrolyte Balance

Natural glucocorticoids and some synthetic analogs have substantial renal water- and sodium-retaining activity and potassium-wasting effects (mineralocorticoid activity; see Table 45–3). Fluid and electrolyte disturbances may occur. In severe hypokalemia, reduced steroid doses or potassium supplementation may be necessary. Hypokalemic alkalosis is uncommon with triamcinolone, dexamethasone, paramethasone, and betamethasone, all of which have minimal mineralocorticoid activity.

Immune and Inflammatory Responses

Glucocorticoids depress the immune response and increase susceptibility to infection. Since the usual inflammatory signs (heat, redness, pain, swelling) are absent during steroid use, symptoms of preexisting or new infections may be masked. Infections may become broadly disseminated before they are recognized.

No effective therapy exists for most viral infections. Therefore, corticosteroid therapy generally is contraindicated when viral infections are present, except in specific cases in which the benefits outweigh the disadvantages. Glucocorticoids are contraindicated when systemic fungal infections are present. Topical glucocorticoids are contraindicated in fungal or herpes simplex eye inflammations.

NURSING IMPLICATIONS

Corticosteroid therapy is not without risk, but careful nursing care can help maximize the therapeutic benefits while helping to minimize the dangers. For all patients, obtain a complete history to identify persons at high risk of steroid-induced untoward responses.

Careful monitoring for side and adverse effects of glucocorticoids will help keep serious complications to a minimum. Monitor all patients for signs and symptoms of hyperglycemia and glucosuria, to identify those at risk for steroid-induced diabetes and exacerbation of diabetes mellitus symptoms. Report persistent hyperglycemia, since supplemental or increased doses of hypoglycemic drugs may be needed to restore normal carbohydrate metabolism during glucocorticoid therapy in diabetic patients.

Advise patients that physical appearance changes may occur with prolonged therapy. Reassure them that the changes are reversible when therapy is discontinued.

Monitor patients for antianabolic effects, and instruct them to report muscle weakness. Instruct patients to report slow wound healing and make them aware that routine skeletal X-rays should be taken during prolonged therapy to assess for osteoporosis. Inform postmenopausal women (and others at risk for skeletal wasting) of their risk status during the course of glucocorticoid therapy. Advise patients to report symptomatic back or chest pain, and to sleep on a firm mattress. Instruct patients to eat a high-protein diet and to take calcium and vitamin D supplements to antagonize bone-wasting effects of the steroid drugs.

Take baseline and routine measurements of blood pressure for patients with cardiovascular disease, clotting problems, and for all elderly patients. Report marked increases in blood pressure promptly. Instruct patients to report any incidences of fainting, lightheadedness, or nosebleed.

Careful monitoring for thrombophlebitis or thromboembolytic disease is mandatory. Instruct patients to report any episodes of throbbing leg pain, which may require prophylaxis with anticoagulant drugs. Prothrombin time must be monitored in patients receiving concurrent anticoagulant therapy, to assess for diminished effects of anticoagulant therapy.

Assess for signs of infection, particularly after drug withdrawal. Examine the oral mucosa for signs of fungal infection, especially in patients using oral preparations. Carefully instruct patients to report any signs of malaise or any unusual symptoms of any type that may indicate an underlying infectious process. Advise patients to avoid vaccinations and immunizations (which depress the immune response) during glucocorticoid therapy. Teach patients who are using corticoid ointments or creams, and applying occlusive dressings, to inspect for and report any signs of secondary infection.

Monitor patients taking corticosteroids with mineralocorticoid activity (prednisone, prednisolone, cortisone, and hydrocortisone) for edema, and instruct them to report any muscle weakness or tetany (hypokalemic effects). Patients using diuretics or digitalis must be monitored very closely and carefully instructed to report signs of hypokalemia. Monitor fluid intake and output daily in hospitalized patients. Advise outpatients to keep weekly weight charts. Instruct them to follow a low-sodium diet to minimize salt and fluid retention, and to report severe edema to the physician for consideration of drug changes or initiation of diuretic measures.

Monitor stools of hospitalized patients for an increase of occult blood loss as one indication of steroid-induced ulcers. Be particularly alert for these signs in patients with rheumatoid arthritis, since they are exceptionally susceptible to the GI effects of these drugs. Advise outpatients to report any vomitus with a "coffee grounds" appearance or black tarry stools, since these are signs of GI bleeding.

Be meticulous in history-taking to identify patients at risk for severe mood changes—those with a previous history of psychotic or neurotic tendencies and individuals with chronic seizure disorders. Patients who exhibit mood swings, progressing abruptly from a happy talkative state to severe depression, should be watched closely since suicidal tendencies are common in depressed persons. Additionally, depressed individuals do not cope well with disease. Report prolonged bouts of depression to the physician for consideration of drug withdrawal.

Advise patients with underlying joint disorders who report diminished pain that lack of previous symptoms does not indicate cure; instruct patients to follow a safe regimen of physical activities.

Patients accustomed to symptom reduction and the often exhilarating effects of glucocorticoids are difficult to deal with when drug withdrawal is indicated. Patience and a calm reassuring manner are always required when working with these patients.

Instruct patients administering topical steroids to their eyes to obtain ophthalmoscopic and tonometer examinations at maximum intervals of three months.

Since individual patient susceptibility to pancreatitis is unknown, and symptoms are likely to be masked, urge all patients to report any episodes of GI distress that persist for more than a day.

Advise patients on replacement therapy to take the hormones for the rest of their lives. Instruct them to take the prescribed doses to try to replicate normal hormonal levels.

Provide patients with the rationale for their oral dosage scheduling so that they will understand the importance of taking their medication at the scheduled times. Advise patients taking the hormone drug once daily to take it in the morning for best therapeutic results.

Urge patients to appear for scheduled visits for monitoring their conditions throughout therapy. Instruct patients to notify the doctor immediately when they are faced with sudden and unavoidable stressors, since steroid supplementation will be necessary.

◆ Use During Pregnancy and Lactation

Adequate studies of the use of glucocorticoids during pregnancy have not been done. Therefore, their use in pregnant women, nursing mothers, or women of childbearing age requires weighing risks and benefits. Observe infants born of mothers receiving corticosteroids for signs of hypoadrenalism.

◆ Use in Children

Monitor the growth of children receiving glucocorticoids carefully, since glucocorticoids can increase bone demineralization. Instruct parents to maintain weekly height and weight charts, and reassure them that permanent growth stunting with glucocorticoid therapy is rare. If stunting occurs, most children experience a growth spurt when therapy is stopped.

◆ Use in the Elderly

Monitor immobilized, elderly, and arthritis patients for progression of osteoporosis. Use extra care in turning immobilized patients to avoid causing fractures. Report changes in cardiovascular status and monitor immobilized patients for thrombophlebitis. Elderly patients generally have an increased risk of infection due to immune suppression, which can be worsened by glucocorticoids.

Corticosteroid Withdrawal

Glucocorticoid therapy with any agent that is given more than a few times for *systemic* effects poses the risk of adrenal suppression when drug treatment is stopped. For this reason, discontinue steroid therapy gradually, with slow daily dosage reductions.

The risk of withdrawal symptoms is low with inhaled steroids (as for asthma) or steroids applied topically to the skin, eye, or ear. However, when systemic steroids are administered for prolonged times, as for arthritis, or when replacement therapy is stopped abruptly, the risk of withdrawal is significant. It may be life-threatening.

Signs and Symptoms

Typical withdrawal signs and symptoms include hypotension, hypoglycemia, nausea, anorexia, such emotional changes as depression and lability of mood, and extreme intolerance of physical stress, as might be caused by illness, trauma, or surgery.

A state of adrenal insufficiency can last from several days to a year or more after therapy is stopped. Paradoxically, patients may have withdrawal symptoms despite having normal cortisol levels and pituitary responses to an ACTH challenge. If systemic therapy must be stopped, it may be necessary to taper the dose over several weeks or months before stopping administration altogether.

Minimizing Withdrawal Signs and Symptoms

The major ways to avoid adrenal suppression include limiting treatment to only a couple of days, or using steroid preparations (ie, topical or inhaled steroids) that are not likely to cause appreciable rises of blood steroid levels. Obviously, neither approach is feasible for replacement therapy or for other indications in which systemic effects are wanted. If long-term treatment is necessary, the risk of adrenal suppression can be reduced (but not eliminated) with alternate-day dosing. This involves stabilizing the patient on the lowest possible multiple or once-daily steroid dose, then switching to a schedule in which the total 48-hour dose is administered in a single dose every other day. There are variations on this theme.

NURSING IMPLICATIONS

The degree of adrenal suppression is a function of the length of time the patient has been on therapy. The steroid dose is unimportant once the threshold for suppression has been exceeded. Thus, anticipate adrenocortical depression with prolonged administration of both physiologic and pharmacologic doses. Provide supportive therapy during times of severe stress to all patients receiving extended glucocorticoid therapy.

The minimum duration of systemic corticosteroid therapy that will cause adrenal suppression is not known. It may be as short as a couple of weeks of continued administration. To help minimize adrenal suppression, reinforce the need to follow the recommended dosing schedule. Monitor for signs and symptoms of adrenal insufficiency (hypotension, hypoglycemia, nausea, anorexia, and mood changes such as depression) during dosage changes and during planned drug withdrawal. Use the same assessment skills to help determine whether the patient has been noncompliant or has discontinued therapy on his or her own.

Advise patients whose systemic steroid therapy is to be stopped that the process may take several weeks of gradual dosage reductions to maximize withdrawal safety. Also indicate that because of long-lasting adrenal suppression, their response to illness, trauma, or surgery may be compromised. For this reason, instruct patients during withdrawal to notify all health-care providers of prior steroid treatment so that proper care can be rendered to compensate for adrenal hypofunction.

Interactions with Other Drugs

Corticosteroids interact with many drugs. The greatest risk of a clinically significant interaction arises with long-term oral steroid therapy. The risks are much less with brief systemic steroid therapy (whether by oral or parenteral routes); usually there is no risk with orally inhaled steroids, as often used for treating asthma, provided recommended doses are not exceeded.

The key interactants plus several other drugs that may cause potential problems, are summarized in Table 45–1. The major interactions also are discussed briefly below.

Cholestyramine, the cholesterol-binding resin (also classified as a bile acid sequestrant), can bind orally administered steroids in the gut if the two medications are taken together. The outcome is a decreased corticosteroid effect. The interaction can be prevented by separating administration of the two drugs as much as possible. Colestipol, a drug with cholestyramine-like actions and uses, and antacids may interact with orally administered steroids similarly.

Drugs that induce (stimulate) the liver's drug metabolizing enzyme systems can speed the metabolic breakdown of systemically administered steroids, and lead to a decreased steroid effect. The main drugs that interact in this way are the *barbiturates, phenytoin* (and other hydantoins), *rifampin,* and perhaps even *low doses of alcohol* consumed often.

In contrast, *estrogens,* administered alone or in the form of *oral contraceptives,* may reduce corticosteroid metabolism and increase corticosteroid effects, possibly to the point of toxicity unless steroid dosages are reduced if needed.

Aspirin, and probably other nonsteroidal antiinflammatory drugs, can interact with steroids in two major ways. Both types of drugs are ulcerogenic, and so the risk of gastric lesions increases when the two drugs are administered together. Moreover, the corticosteroids appear to increase the metabolic inactivation or renal elimination of salicylates. The outcome is reduced symptom control by the salicylate. This interaction can be common, since both steroids and salicylates are indicated for managing some cases of arthritis. It probably is also the most clinically significant interaction; there do not appear to be significant problems with infrequent aspirin use for minor pain, headache, or fever.

Another potentially serious interaction affects persons with myasthenia gravis. The main drugs for maintenance therapy of that disorder are the *acetylcholinesterase inhibitors,* such as neostigmine. When the disease progresses, and when the primary drugs do not exert as much symptom control as desired, corticosteroid therapy may be started. However, and for reasons that are unclear, such patients may experience profound muscle weakening. What amounts to a myasthenic crisis (see Chapter 12) can develop. It usually occurs within a few days of when the patient started systemic steroids, and the muscle weakness can be so severe that some patients may require mechanical support or assistance with ventilation. Because the interaction can become a medical emergency, steroid treatment should be started while the patient is hospitalized.

The sodium- and water-retaining effects of systemic steroids also can elevate blood pressure and aggravate heart failure. Thus, the desired effects of antihypertensive drugs or digitalis might be counteracted, and their dosages might need to be increased. These are not specific drug-drug interactions, however.

Related Drugs

With the exception of cortisone, synthetic steroids have greater glucocorticoid than mineralocorticoid potency (see Table 45–3). Although glucocorticoids share essentially similar indications, some of the drugs are available as different salts (Table 45–7), each of which is suitable for a particular route of administration and spe-

Table 45–7 Key Properties of Selected Corticosteroids and Their Salts

Glucocorticoid Prototype	
Hydrocortisone (Cortisol)	Water-insoluble preparation with both glucocorticoid and mineralocorticoid actions for replacement therapy, given orally or IM only; various dosage forms for topical or rectal administration; suitable for long-term use
Acetate	Prolonged actions at injection sites when given IM, intraarticular, or intralesionally; not for IV use; topical dosage forms, intrarectal foam, available
Cypionate	Oral administration only
Sodium succinate	Highly soluble, allows IV administration of large doses in small volumes; recommended for short-term management of emergency conditions (anaphylaxis, status asthmaticus, shock, etc.)
Related Glucocorticoids	
Beclomethasone	Dipropionate salt: available as oral inhaler for asthma, nasal spray for seasonal allergies, nasal polyps (see Chapter 38)
Betamethasone	Intense glucocorticoid activity with no mineralocorticoid actions; administered orally
Sodium phosphate	Very soluble, suitable for IV, IM, or local injection; prompt onset of action; intraarticular injection provides both local and systemic effects
Sodium phosphate plus acetate	Sodium phosphate salt provides prompt action, acetate salt provides long duration; for IV use; used mainly for arthritic conditions, has been used 2 to 3 days before premature birth to help fetal lung maturation
Cortisone	Supplied as water-insoluble acetate salt; for IM or oral administration only; has about 80% of activity of cortisol; slow onset, prolonged actions; suitable for replacement therapy
Dexamethasone	Extremely potent antiinflammatory (glucocorticoid) activity, lacks mineralocorticoid activity, therefore not suitable for replacement therapy; administered orally, often after initial parenteral treatment with dexamethasone sodium phosphate, for acute and self-limited allergic disorders, or flare-ups of chronic disorders (eg, arthritis); used for Cushing's syndrome diagnosis
Acetate	Prompt-acting repository preparation with long duration of action; suitable for IM, intralesional, intraarticular injection, but not IV
Sodium phosphate	More soluble than dexamethasone; injectable by IM, IV, intraarticular, or intralesional routes; rapid onset and short duration, as might be needed for shock, acute adrenal crisis, cerebral edema, or emergency management of systemic lupus erythematosus; has been used to induce fetal lung maturation; oral inhaler, nasal spray, available for asthma, seasonal rhinitis, respectively (see Chapter 38)
Flunisolide	Available as oral inhaler for asthma, nasal spray for rhinitis from seasonal allergies (see Chapter 38)
Methylprednisolone	More potent antiinflammatory activity than prednisone; almost lacks mineralocorticoid actions; oral therapy only
Acetate	Low solubility provides long-lasting effects; suitable for IM, intraarticular, intralesional, soft-tissue injection, not for IV use; retention enema available
Sodium succinate	Most soluble form of methylprednisolone; rapid effects when given IM or IV
Paramethasone	Acetate salt only: twice the glucocorticoid potency of triamcinolone; oral administration only
Prednisolone	Partially metabolized to, potency equivalent to, more expensive than, prednisone; tablets or syrup for oral administration, mainly indicated for multiple sclerosis; ointments, creams, ophthalmic formulations available

(continued)

Table 45–7 Key Properties of Selected Corticosteroids and Their Salts (*Continued*)

Prednisolone (cont.)	
Acetate	Poorly soluble form that provides long-lasting effects, slow systemic absorption; suitable for most common parenteral routes except IV
Sodium phosphate	Very soluble, rapid-acting preparation for common parenteral routes, including IV; short duration; available as liquid for oral administration
Sodium phosphate plus acetate	Suspension providing fast onset of sodium phosphate, long action of acetate
Tebulate	Slightly soluble, providing slow onset and prolonged action similar to acetate; for local injection in arthritic states, not for IV use
Prednisone	Greater glucocorticoid activity, less but still significant mineralocorticoid activity, therefore suitable for replacement therapy; commonly used for arthritic conditions; available only in oral dosage forms
Triamcinolone	Five times the antiinflammatory potency of cortisol; virtually lacks mineralocorticoid activity; for oral or topical administration
Acetonide	Insoluble, poorly absorbed; very long-lasting effects (weeks to months) when given by most parenteral routes (except IV); creams, ointments, aerosol for topical use; oral inhaler for asthma
Diacetate	Slight solubility provides prompt onset but prolonged action; suspension for injection except IV; oral syrup
Hexacetonide	Similar to acetonide when injected (intraarticular, intralesional), but not for IM or IV use
Mineralocorticoid	
Fludrocortisone	Acetate only: Used for mineralocorticoid effects, but has some glucocorticoid activity; is preferred for acute adrenal insufficiency; oral dosage forms only

cific use. Usual dosages for systemic and local effects are summarized in Tables 45–C1, 45–5, and 45–6.

Betamethasone, Dexamethasone

These drugs are approximately 10 to 30 times as potent as cortisol in terms of doses and glucocorticoid activity. Usual therapeutic doses cause virtually no mineralocorticoid effects. Betamethasone and dexamethasone have biologic half-lives of two to two and one half days. As with many other steroids, several salts of these drugs are available for different uses and routes of administration.

Methylprednisolone, Prednisolone, Prednisone, and Triamcinolone

These drugs are about four to five times as potent as cortisol in terms of antiinflammatory activity and actual doses. Prednisone and prednisolone have about half the mineralocorticoid activity of cortisol, whereas methylprednisolone and triamcinolone have virtually no mineralocorticoid activity. The biologic half-lives of each of these drugs are approximately 18 to 30 hours, compared with about eight to 12 hours for cortisol.

These drugs are available in different salts, each of which is indicated for a particular route of administration and clinical use. Insoluble salts of some of these drugs, administered as repository IM injections, have longer biologic half-lives than those noted above.

Inhaled Steroids for Asthma

Beclomethasone dipropionate, dexamethasone sodium phosphate, flunisolide, and triamcinolone acetonide are available in dosage forms for oral inhalation, nasal sprays, or both, for managing asthma or rhinitis. They are discussed in Chapter 38.

II. Mineralocorticoids

Biosynthesis, Metabolism, and Transport

Aldosterone is the major mineralocorticoid hormone. With moderate salt intake, it is secreted at the rate of 75 to 175 μg/day. Plasma protein binding of aldosterone is minimal. Aldosterone is metabolized in the liver and is excreted in urine. The metabolic clearance rate of aldosterone is very dependent on hepatic blood flow; when hepatic blood flow is reduced (as in hepatic disease), hyperaldosteronism may result.

Physiologic Effects

Aldosterone stimulates reabsorption of sodium ions and excretion of potassium and hydrogen ions by the renal tubules. Mineralocorticoids also enhance sodium ion reabsorption at other body sites, including sweat and salivary glands and GI mucosa. These effects are mediated by the actions of aldosterone on specific aldosterone receptors. They can be antagonized pharmacologically by spironolactone (ALDACTONE), which was identified in Chapter 32 as a potassium-sparing diuretic.

Aldosterone is far more potent in initiating sodium retention than is cortisol. In contrast, cortisol causes many widespread antiinflammatory and metabolic effects, but aldosterone causes very few.

Regulation

A fall of blood volume, blood pressure, or serum sodium levels, or rises of serum potassium levels, triggers the kidney's juxtaglomerular cells to release renin. Renin initiates a series of chemical pathways that result in the formation of angiotensin II, a powerful stimulant of aldosterone production. The impact of the renin-angiotensin cascade extends far beyond simply triggering aldosterone release. It provides a crucial response to decreased blood volume or alterations in serum electrolyte profiles, as might arise from hemorrhage, excessive diuresis, vomiting, or diarrhea. More importantly, the renin-angiotensin-aldosterone system plays a key role in the pathophysiology of congestive heart failure and hypertension, as discussed in Chapters 31 and 33, respectively.

Conditions that normally trigger aldosterone release, or excessive sodium or fluid intake, will depress the renin-angiotensin-aldosterone system. They also will reduce the effects of endogenous mineralocorticoids.

Unlike the glucocorticoids, mineralocorticoid secretion is increased only minimally in response to increased plasma ACTH levels. The minute amounts of mineralocorticoids that actually are released have insignificant feedback-inhibitory effects on ACTH release.

Effects of Mineralocorticoid Hyper- and Hyposecretion

Hyperaldosteronism

Primary hyperaldosteronism results from overproduction of mineralocorticoids. The usual etiology is adrenocortical neoplasm in adults and bilateral adrenocortical hyperplasia in children. The patient presents with two major clinical problems: hypertension and edema caused by excessive renal sodium and water retention; and hypokalemia caused by enhanced renal potassium elimination. The preferred therapy is surgical removal of the tumor. As discussed in Chapter 32, the potassium-sparing diuretic spironolactone can be used preoperatively to suppress symptoms, or it can be used as primary treatment in patients in whom surgery is contraindicated.

The signs and symptoms of secondary hyperaldosteronism are similar to those noted for primary hyperaldosteronism. The underlying cause often is impaired hepatic metabolism of aldosterone, whether caused directly by hepatic dysfunction (as occurs in alcoholics) or indirectly by such disorders as advanced heart failure. Spironolactone is used frequently to suppress symptoms of secondary hyperaldosteronism.

Although aldosterone is the prototypic mineralocorticoid, it seldom is used clinically because of its limited availability, its high cost, and the fact that it must be injected.

Fludrocortisone

Fludrocortisone acetate (FLORINEF) is the only drug with considerable mineralocorticoid activity available for oral administration and is the preferred mineralocorticoid for acute adrenal insufficiency. It also has glucocorticoid activity. Fludrocortisone is absorbed readily from the GI tract, and peak serum concentrations occur in about 90 minutes. Its plasma half-life is about three and one half hours, but its duration of action is 18 to 36 hours. Fludrocortisone is indicated for therapy of chronic adrenal insufficiency or adrenogenital syndrome, and it is used adjunctively with cortisone or hydrocortisone. Dosages are summarized in Table 45–C2.

Fludrocortisone may induce negative nitrogen balance, so encourage patients to eat a protein-rich diet during therapy. If fludrocortisone therapy is prolonged, the patient must be assessed for all the untoward responses noted for glucocorticoids.

Other Drugs That Affect Adrenal Cortical Function

Metyrapone

Metyrapone (METOPIRONE) is used for evaluating hypothalamic-pituitary ACTH function. The drug inhibits a key step in the biosynthetic pathway that forms cortisone and corticosterone in the adrenal cortex. It leads to the formation of steroid precursors that normally are present in very low amounts, and that exert very weak effects on pituitary ACTH release. When the crucial enzyme is inhibited by metyrapone, the strong inhibitory feedback normally exerted on the pituitary by circulating steroids is lost, and the pituitary will release more ACTH. ACTH then acts on the adrenal cortex, leading to increased formation of cortisol precursors. These precursors and their metabolites can be measured in the urine. Although careful physical examinations and other tests are essential for diagnosing altered pituitary or adrenal cortical function, metyrapone may help confirm the diagnosis.

Testing with metyrapone requires six days. On the first day, a 24-hour urine sample is collected, in which corticosteroid precursor levels are measured. On the second day, an ACTH test is administered (infusing 50 U ACTH over eight hours, and measuring steroid levels in the 24-hour urine sample). If the ACTH test is normal, the usual interpretation is normal adrenal cortical function but impaired pituitary ACTH release. The metyrapone test continues with a rest period on days three and four. On the fifth day, six doses of metyrapone (approximately 15 mg/kg) are administered at four-hour intervals, and another 24-hour urine sample is collected through day six. Steroid levels in this sample are measured. In persons with normal pituitary and adrenal cortical function, metyrapone causes an obvious rise in blood and urinary steroid precursor levels. Little or no rise in response to metyrapone suggests some pituitary hypofunction. If metyrapone causes an excessive rise in blood or urinary steroid precursor levels, adrenal hyperplasia may be present.

Common side effects caused by metyrapone include GI upset; headache, dizziness, or sedation; and occasional skin rashes suggesting allergy to the drug. Blood dyscrasias are rare. The major acute toxicity of metyrapone involves signs and symptoms of acute adrenocortical insufficiency. The drug should not be administered to pregnant or breast-feeding women.

NURSING IMPLICATIONS

Advise all patients who will be tested with metyrapone that the full test may require six days, during which all instructions provided by the physician must be followed closely. Stress the need to collect and properly store all urine excreted during the crucial test periods. Administer each dose of metyrapone with milk or a snack to reduce GI distress.

Mitotane

Mitotane (LYSODREN) is an anticancer drug used exclusively to treat inoperable adrenal cortical carcinoma. The precise mechanism by which the drug works is unknown, but it appears to concentrate in adrenal cortical cells, inhibiting corticosteroid synthesis without actually destroying the cells. Dosages are noted in Table 45–C2. The drug can be given intermittently to treat acute flare-ups of symptoms caused by elevated blood steroid levels, but it works best when therapy is continuous. Most patients show obvious symptomatic relief, and reduced circulating steroid levels after about three months of daily treatment. Between the onset of mitotane treatment and the development of its optimum effects, spironolactone may be administered to counteract excessive effects of mineralocorticoids on their receptors.

Gastrointestinal distress, including nausea, vomiting, anorexia, and diarrhea, occurs in about 80% of patients taking mitotane. Less frequent untoward responses include CNS depression or dizziness, and occasional skin rashes. The drug should not be administered during pregnancy; breast-feeding should be discouraged.

SUMMARY OF NURSING IMPLICATIONS

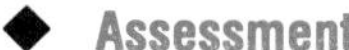

Assessment

Obtain a complete nursing history to identify special risks associated with corticosteroid therapy—history of diabetes; peptic ulcer disease; use of diuretics, digitalis, antibiotic agents; or previous corticosteroid use.

Recognize signs of adrenal insufficiency: hypotension, hypoglycemia, depression.

Assess for signs and symptoms of hyperadrenalism: hyperglycemia, glycosuria, hypertension, poor wound healing, buffalo hump, "moon" face.

Check blood pressure, urine sugar, and weight regularly.

◆ Nursing Diagnoses

Body image disturbance related to cushingoid appearance.

Altered nutrition: less than body requirements related to potassium loss and protein wasting with replacement therapy; more than body requirements related to sodium retention and hyperglycemia with replacement therapy.

High risk for injury related to osteoporosis, poor wound healing, infection, stress ulcers.

Altered tissue perfusion (cardiopulmonary or peripheral) related to hypertension, atherosclerosis, clotting tendency.

Fluid volume excess related to water retention.

Ineffective individual coping related to mood changes, irritability, insomnia with drug changes and chronic illness.

Knowledge deficit related to adrenocorticosteroid therapy.

◆ Planning/Implementation

Administer oral medication with food to minimize gastric upset.

Provide emotional support during drug therapy, particularly with the development of a cushingoid appearance.

Assist patient in obtaining a MedicAlert card or bracelet.

Prepare for stressful events: medication adjustments, life support.

◆ Patient and Family Teaching

Teach the patient/family:

About the need for lifelong therapy and adherence to medication schedule and exact dosage.

Signs and symptoms indicating excesses or deficiencies in drug therapy that must be reported—edema, weight gain, nausea with excesses.

To limit dietary intake of high-sodium foods and increase potassium-rich sources; to avoid alcohol and coffee, which increase gastric irritation.

◆ Evaluation

The patient/family will:

Experience minimal to no adverse effects (increased sodium, low potassium, muscle wasting, peptic ulcers).

Appear for follow-up visits with physician for monitoring of drug therapy and physical condition.

Comply with medication regimen.

Maintain sodium-restricted diet.

Maintain blood pressure and blood glucose within normal limits.

Cope with physical appearance and emotional impact of chronic illness.

Annotated Bibliography

Ansell BM: Overview of the side effects of corticosteroid therapy. *Clin Exp Rheumatol* 1991;9 Suppl 6:19–20. *A succinct review of common side effects during corticosteroid therapy of rheumatoid arthritis. The emphasis is on children.*

Barnetson RS, White AD: The use of corticosteroids in dermatological practice. *Med J Aust* 1992;156(6):428–431. *This literature review identifies the values and risks associated with corticosteroid therapy of skin diseases and cutaneous reactions to allergies.*

Crowley P: Corticosteroids after preterm premature rupture of membranes. *Obstet Gynecol Clin North Am* 1992;19(2):317–326. *Discusses benefits and risks of corticosteroids in premature birth and premature membrane rupture.*

Davenport J, Kellerman C, Reiss D, Harrison L: Addison's disease. *Am Fam Physician* 1991;43(4):1338–1342. *Discusses the link between tuberculosis, automimmune disease, and Addison's disease; addresses diagnosis and management very well.*

Fink CW: Overview of corticosteroid therapy in the different rheumatic diseases of childhood. *Clin Exp Rheumatol* 1991;9 Suppl 6:9–13. *Sets the stage for other important papers covering corticosteroid therapy of arthritis and lupus erythematosus in children; includes illustrative cases.*

Greenberger PA: Corticosteroids in asthma. Rationale, use, and problems. *Chest* 1992;101(6 Suppl):418S–421S. *Short but good coverage of oral, inhaled, and parenteral steroids in this common pulmonary disorder.*

Gumowski J, Proch M, Kessler CA: Endocrinopathies of hyperfunction: Cushing's syndrome and aldosteronism. *AACN Clin Issues Crit Care Nurs* 1992;3(2):331–349. *An excellent review of these disorders, their management, and nursing roles.*

Jones KL: The Cushing syndromes. *Pediatr Clin North Am* 1990; 37(6):1313–1332. *A comprehensive review of all key aspects of the topic.*

Loriaux DL: The treatment of Cushing's syndrome and adrenal cancer. *Endocrinol Metab Clin North Am* 1991;20(4):767–771. *Describes why an accurate diagnosis is one of the keys to proper treatment.*

Millikan LE, Shrum JP: An update on common skin diseases. Acne, psoriasis, contact dermatitis, and warts. *Postgrad Med* 1992; 91(6):96–98, 101–104, 107–110. *Excellent insight into pharmacologic and nondrug measures, and patient education for these disorders.*

Moeser PJ: Corticosteroid therapy for rheumatoid arthritis. Benefits and limitations. *Postgrad Med* 1991;90(8):175–176, 178–182. *Covers indications, treatment goals and strategies, benefits and risks, and monitoring when steroids are used.*

Prihoda JS, Davis LE: Metabolic emergencies in obstetrics. *Obstet Gynecol Clin North Am* 1991;18(2):301–318. *Covers many endocrine emergencies, including Cushing's syndrome and addisonian crisis.*

Putterman C: Modern approaches to the therapy of septic shock. *Am J Emerg Med* 1990;8(2):152–161. *Reviews the role of corticosteroids, plus other drugs, in treating septicemia.*

Woster PS, LeBlanc KL: Management of elevated intracranial pressure. *Clin Pharm* 1990;9(10):762–772. *Discusses the use of steroids, barbiturates, other drugs, and overall management of patients with head trauma, stroke, and brain neoplasms.*

Zuckerman JD, Meislin RJ, Rothberg M: Injections for joint and soft tissue disorders: When and how to use them. *Geriatrics* 1990; 45(4):45–52, 55. *Reviews principles of diagnostic and therapeutic use of joint, soft-tissue injections; recommends injection sites; techniques for aspirating and injecting joints, bursae, and soft tissue. Focuses on judicious use of corticosteroids.*

Table 45–C1 Typical Dosages and Uses of Corticosteroids

DRUG	TYPICAL DOSAGES, USES
PROTOTYPE	
Hydrocortisone	
(cortisol; CORTEF)	Oral: Initially, 20–240 mg/day, depending on symptom severity
(CORTENEMA)	Rectal (for adjunctive therapy of ulcerative colitis, proctitis, and related intestinal disorders as retention enema): One enema (contains 100 mg/60 mL unit) for 21 consecutive nights, or until direct proctoscopic evidence shows positive response
Hydrocortisone acetate	
(HYDROCORTONE ACETATE)	Intralesional, intraarticular, or soft-tissue injection: Dose depends on administration site, symptom severity; usually 5–12.5 mg for tendon sheaths; 25 mg for large joints (knee, hip, etc); 25–50 mg for soft tissues, bursae; 10–25 mg for small joints, ganglia
(CORTIFOAM)	Rectal foam (for adjunctive treatment of ulcerative proctitis): Fill applicator with foam, use 1 applicator amount (90 mg) once or twice daily for 2–3 weeks, every other day thereafter or until proctoscopic evidence of response (usually occurs within a week)
Hydrocortisone cypionate	
(CORTEF)	Oral: 20–240 mg/day; each 5 mL of oral suspension contains 10 mg hydrocortisone equivalent
Hydrocortisone sodium phosphate	
(HYDROCORTONE PHOSPHATE)	IM, IV, SC: Initially, 15–240 mg/day, or one third to one half usual oral dose, administered every 12 h
Hydrocortisone sodium succinate	
(SOLU-CORTEF)	IM or IV: 100–500 mg/day
RELATED DRUGS	
Betamethasone	
(CELESTONE)	Oral: 0.6–7.2 mg/day
Betamethasone sodium phosphate plus betamethasone acetate	
(CELESTONE SOLUSPAN)	IM: 0.5–9 mg/day, or roughly one third to one half oral dose, given every 12 h Intraarticular, intralesional, intradermal: 0.25–2 mL, depending on size of area affected. *Note:* Each mL of the proprietary product contains 3 mg of the sodium phosphate salt and 3 mg of the acetate
Betamethasone sodium phosphate	
(CELESTONE PHOSPHATE, others)	IV, IM: Usually 3–9 mg/day
Dexamethasone	
(DECADRON, HEXADROL, others)	Oral: 0.75–9 mg/day for most indications; see text for dexamethasone suppression test IV (for acute but self-limiting allergic symptoms): Start with 4–8 mg of dexamethasone sodium phosphate, IV; switch to 3 mg/day of dexamethasone, orally, in two divided doses, then taper to no drug over one week

(continued)

Table 45–C1 Typical Dosages and Uses of Corticosteroids (*Continued*)

DRUG	TYPICAL DOSAGES, USES
Dexamethasone acetate	
(DECADRON LA, others)	IM: Usually 8–16 mg when systemic effects desired, repeat in 1–3 weeks Intralesional: 0.8–1.6 mg per site Intraarticular, soft-tissue injections: 4–16 mg, repeat in 1–3 weeks
Dexamethasone sodium phosphate	
(DECADRON PHOSPHATE, others)	IM: For most indications: Initially 0.5–9 mg/day, or one third to one half oral dose, when systemic effects desired IV: For cerebral edema: Initially 10 mg, then 4 mg IM, every 6 h; switch to oral administration as soon as possible. Refractory hypotension (shock): Doses vary from 1–6 mg/kg as single IV injection, to 40 mg every 6 h Intraarticular, intralesional, or soft-tissue injections: 0.4–6 mg per site, depending on size of area. *Note:* Dexamethasone sodium phosphate is available with lidocaine for injection into soft tissue; dose ranges from 0.1–0.75 mL, depending on injection site
Fludrocortisone acetate	
(FLORINEF ACETATE)	Oral: Usually 0.1 mg per day for Addison's disease, administered along with glucocorticoid (cortisone, hydrocortisone); 0.1–0.2 mg per day for androgenital syndrome
Methylprednisolone	
(MEDROL)	Oral: Usually 4–48 mg/day, or twice that amount administered every other day
Methylprednisolone acetate	
(DEPO-MEDROL; others)	IM: Daily dose varies with indication: Androgenital syndrome: 40 mg every other week; asthma, allergic rhinitis: 80–120 mg; rheumatoid arthritis: 40–120 mg, administered weekly; skin lesions: 40–120 mg, single dose or weekly for chronic conditions Intraarticular or soft-tissue injections: 4–80 mg depending on size of affected area
Methylprednisolone sodium succinate	
(SOLU-MEDROL; others)	IV, IM: Adults: Slowly inject 10–40 mg IV initially, subsequent doses (same, less, more, depend on condition, initial response) IM or IV. Dosages of $\leq$ 30 mg/kg over 20 minutes IV for severe symptoms requiring immediate control. Children: Usually 0.5 mg/kg/day
Prednisolone	
(DELTA-CORTEF; PRELONE)	Oral: 5–60 mg/day for most uses; treatment of acute flare-ups of multiple sclerosis may require 200 mg/day for 1 week then 80 mg every other day for 1 month
Prednisolone acetate	
(PREDALONE; others)	IM: Initially 4–60 mg/day for systemic effects; flare-ups of multiple sclerosis may require doses noted for prednisone Intralesional, intraarticular, or soft-tissue injection: 5–100 mg per injection, depending on size of area to be injected (see hydrocortisone acetate for typical dose relationships)
Prednisolone sodium phosphate	
(HYDELTRASOL; others)	IM or IV: Usually 4–60 mg/day to start Intralesional, intraarticular, or soft-tissue injection: Usually 2–30 mg per injection, depending on size of area to be injected (see hydrocortisone acetate for typical dose relationships)

(continued)

Table 45–C1 Typical Dosages and Uses of Corticosteroids (*Continued*)

DRUG	TYPICAL DOSAGES, USES
Prednisolone tebutate (PREDALONE TBA; others)	Intralesional, intraarticular, or soft-tissue injection: Usually 4–20 mg per injection, depending on size of area to be injected (see hydrocortisone acetate for typical dose relationships)
Prednisone (DELTASONE; ORASONE; others)	Oral: Adults: Usually 5–60 mg/day. Children: Usually 0.1–0.15 mg/kg/day, or 4–5 mg/m^2 body surface area/day, in divided doses every 12 h (for replacement therapy); oral solutions or syrups contain 1 mg/mL
Triamcinolone (ARISTOCORT; KENACORT; others)	Oral (daily doses are for all indications unless noted otherwise): Adrenal cortical insufficiency: 4–12 mg, plus supplementation with mineralocorticoid; asthma, most rheumatic and dermatologic disorders: 8–16 mg; other respiratory disorders: 16–48 mg; systemic lupus erythematosus: 20–32 mg; hematologic disorders: 16–60 mg; acute leukemias, lymphomas in adults: 16–40 mg or more; acute leukemias in children: 1–2 mg/kg; acute rheumatoid carditis: 20–60 mg; ocular inflammation, other indicated eye disorders: 12–40 mg
Triamcinolone acetonide (KENALOG -10, -40; KENALONE; others)	IM: 2.5–60 mg/day Intradermal: 1 mg per injection site Intraarticular, intrabursal: Usually 2.5–40 mg, depending on size of area to be treated
Triamcinolone diacetate (ARISTOCORT FORTE; others)	IM: Initially 40 mg, once weekly Intrarticular, intrasynovial: 5–40 mg Intralesional: Usually 25 mg per lesion, no more than 12.5 mg per injection site
Triamcinolone hexacetonide (ARISTOSPAN preparations)	Intraarticular: 2–20 mg depending on size of area to be treated Intralesional: 0.5 mg or less per square inch of affected area

Table 45–C2 Clinical Uses and Administration of Other Drugs Affecting Adrenal Cortical Function

AGENT	CLINICAL USES	DOSAGE AND ROUTE OF ADMINISTRATION
Metyrapone		
(METOPIRONE)	Diagnosis of pituitary adreno-corticotropic function	Oral: Adults: Usually 750 mg every 4 h (or 15 mg/kg), with milk or a snack, for 6 doses. Children: 15 mg/kg at times noted for adults; see text for details about test protocol
Mitotane		
(LYSODREN)	Treatment of inoperable adrenal cortical carcinoma	Oral: Initially 2–6 g/day in 3 or 4 divided doses; increase gradually to 9–10 g/day in divided doses; start therapy in hospital; positive response should occur after about 3 months of continuous treatment

Table 45–1 **Interactions Between Systematically Administered Corticosteroids* and Other Agents**

AGENT	RESULT OF INTERACTION	COMMENTS AND NURSING IMPLICATIONS
Acetylcholinesterase inhibitors (eg, neostigmine) (Chapter 12)	Reduced effectiveness of cholinesterase inhibitor in supporting muscle strength of myasthenia gravis patients	Be prepared for potentially serious decline of muscle strength, possibly necessitating ventilatory support, 2–3 days after starting corticosteroid therapy in patients receiving cholinesterase inhibitors; such combined use common in advanced myasthenia gravis, patient should be hospitalized when it is begun
Alcohol (Chapter 22)	Increased risk, worsening, of peptic ulcers	Discourage alcohol use during systemic corticosteroid therapy; both steroids and alcohol are ulcerogenic, see phenobarbital, below, for possible effects of alcohol on steroid metabolism
Antacids (Chapter 40)	Reduced steroid absorption, effect	Applies only to orally administered corticosteroids; separate administration of interactants by as much time as possible
Anticoagulants, oral (Chapter 35)	Potentially reduced anticoagulant effects	Monitor prothrombin times, assess for evidence of reduced anticoagulant effect, particularly when starting, stopping steroid
Aspirin, all other nonsteroidal antiinflammatory drugs (Chapter 52)	Increased risk of, or worsening of, gastric ulcers	Glucocorticoids, aspirin, all other nonsteroidal antiinflammatory drugs are ulcerogenic; if combined use is unavoidable, assess carefully for pain or evidence of GI bleeding; antiulcer drugs (H_2 blockers, antacids, sucralfate) may be used, as long as combined use is done properly to avoid other interactions with oral steroids
	Reduced aspirin blood levels, effects	Corticosteroids may increase salicylate clearance, potentially necessitating increased aspirin dose when used concomitantly (with probable increased ulcer risk); reduced aspirin doses may be indicated if steroid administration is stopped after combined therapy
Cholestyramine, colestipol (Chapter 36)	Reduced steroid absorption, effect	See antacids
Contraceptives, oral (Chapter 49)	Enhanced steroid effects, possibly excessive	May inhibit corticosteroid metabolism, increase blood glucose levels; monitor, especially in persons with frank or borderline diabetes; corticosteroid doses may need to be reduced or alternative contraceptive methods used
Estrogens	See contraceptives, above	
Phenobarbital, other barbiturates, phenytoin, rifampin, chronic low-dose alcohol consumption (Chapters 22, 26, 57)	Increased metabolism, decreased actions, of corticosteroids	Interactants induce hepatic drug-metabolizing enzymes; if interaction unavoidable, assess for indicators of inadequate steroid effects
Vaccines, attenuated virus (Chapter 54)	Potential increased risk of infection	Immunosuppression caused by high-dose glucocorticoids increases risk; avoid vaccination with attenuated virus vaccines during steroid therapy and until complete recovery once steroid therapy is stopped; assess for infection if interaction cannot be avoided

*None of these interactions are likely to apply to orally inhaled corticosteroids such as beclomethasone that are used for asthma and other respiratory tract disorders, if administered properly to minimize systemic absorption. See Chapter 38 for more details.

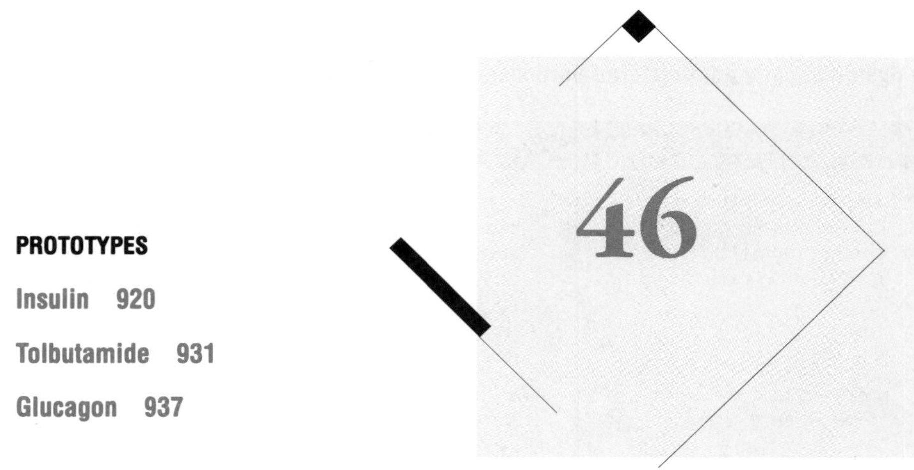

PROTOTYPES

Drugs for Managing Diabetes Mellitus and Hypoglycemia

The pancreas is a mixed gland that has important exocrine and endocrine functions. Acinar cells, forming the bulk of the gland, produce enzyme-rich pancreatic juice that is excreted into the small intestine during food digestion. Scattered amid the acinar tissue are the islets of Langerhans, clusters of cells involved in the production of pancreatic hormones. The islets contain four major populations of hormone-producing cells: glucagon-producing alpha cells, insulin-producing beta cells, somatostatin in the D cells, and pancreatic polypeptide in the F cells.

The most important endocrine disorders of the pancreas are associated with excessive or inadequate secretion of insulin. Thus the following discussion concentrates on the physiologic role of insulin, as well as the effects of its excess or deficiency.

Diabetes mellitus is the most common endocrine pancreatic disorder. It usually is the result of hypoinsulinism, and is perplexing and difficult to treat. Its manifestations, etiology, and pharmacologic management are the major focus of this chapter. The chapter ends with a discussion of glucagon, the major physiologic antagonist of insulin. It is also a drug with a few important clinical uses.

Major reference tables appear beginning on p. 942.

I. Physiology of Insulin

Insulin is a 51-amino acid protein consisting of two linked amino acid chains. It is synthesized from a single longer chain called *proinsulin.* Insulin is stored in membrane-bound secretion granules (beta granules) for later release in response to appropriate stimuli. In normal individuals, approximately 2 mg (50 units) of insulin is released daily.

After secretion, small amounts of insulin are bound to serum globulins, but most of the hormone is transported in the free and active form. Insulin released by the pancreas initially enters the hepatic portal circulation, but very little is metabolized by a first-pass effect. Therefore, much remains to enter the systemic circulation and to produce widespread effects.

Circulating insulin is distributed throughout the extracellular fluid volume and is taken up rapidly by the liver and most other body tissues except the brain and red blood cells. Its plasma half-life is approximately 10 minutes, but its duration of activity is five to seven hours. Less than 10% of circulating insulin is excreted unchanged in urine.

Insulin metabolism occurs mainly in the liver. It involves proteolysis of the peptide chains. Insulin degradation also occurs in the kidneys, and, to a lesser extent, in muscle and plasma.

Regulation of Insulin Secretion

The single most important factor controlling the rate of insulin synthesis and release is the plasma glucose level. An increase in circulating glucose elicits an initial burst of insulin release. It reaches a peak in minutes and then rapidly declines. This is followed by a second, longer-lasting period of insulin release, peaking in about one hour. Falling glucose levels inhibit insulin release.

Aside from rising blood glucose levels, other plasma factors that stimulate insulin release directly or indirectly include:

- Other sugars such as fructose;
- Increasing levels of free fatty acids and certain amino acids;
- Adrenocorticotropic hormone (ACTH), growth hormone, and glucagon;
- Vagal nerve (parasympathetic) stimulation;
- β-Adrenergic stimuli; and
- Oral hypoglycemic drugs.

There is also evidence that specific enteric signals such as gastric inhibitory peptide (GIP), pancreozymin, and secretin, released into the blood as a meal is ingested, enhance β-cell secretory activity that has been triggered by other stimuli. Insulin release is inhibited by somatostatin.

Sympathetic nervous system effects on insulin release are complex but important. The β cells of the pancreas are endowed with both α- and β-adrenergic receptors. Alpha receptors, when stimulated, inhibit insulin release, Beta$_2$ receptors mediate increased insulin release. Therefore, epinephrine, which stimulates both α and β receptors, causes variable effects on insulin release. Overall, it increases insulin release through both its β-adrenergic effects on the pancreatic cells and its ability to increase blood glucose levels. Norepinephrine, which has α-stimulating activity but no effects on β_2 receptors, inhibits insulin release.

The actions of insulin on its target cells throughout the body are *antagonized* by epinephrine and cortisol. During stress, both epinephrine and cortisol counteract insulin's effects and promote mobilization of energy sources from stored fat and tissue proteins. Usually the result is a further rise in blood glucose levels, even when hyperglycemia is present. All these interactions attest to the fact that the regulation of insulin release is very complex.

Metabolic Effects of Insulin

Insulin is a pivotal mediator of carbohydrate metabolism, and it exerts important effects on protein and fat metabolism as well. The most important metabolic effects of insulin are summarized in Table 46–1.

Insulin is a hypoglycemic hormone, and it is the *only* hypoglycemic hormone. (All other hormones directly influencing blood sugar levels promote hyperglycemia and antagonize insulin's effects.) In the presence of insulin, glucose is transported out of the blood into most body cells, reducing blood sugar levels. The exact mechanism by which insulin facilitates cellular entry of glucose is not known.

Tissue-Specific Effects

Insulin's effects are tissue-specific. It enhances membrane transport of glucose (as well as other monosaccharides, amino acids, and various ions) into muscle, adipose, and connective tissue cells, and into leukocytes. It does not facilitate glucose entry into liver, kidney, or brain cells, or into red blood cells, which apparently have glucose transport systems independent of insulin's effects. Thus, in cases of insulin deficiency, glucose uptake is not impaired in the brain, liver, or kidneys.

In all body cells that respond to insulin, the hormone activates enzymes that catalyze

1. the oxidative breakdown of glucose for cellular energy (adenosine triphosphate [ATP]) production,
2. the polymerization of glucose into glycogen, and
3. the conversion of glucose to fat (lipogenesis).

In general, energy needs are met first, followed by glycogen synthesis and deposition. If excess glucose is still present, lipogenesis and fat deposition occur.

Insulin promotes protein synthesis in muscle, and the conversion of glucose to amino acids or glycogen. Glucose conversion to fatty acids is the predominant effect in adipose tissue. All these conversions occur in the liver.

Responses to a Meal

Insulin inhibits glycogenolysis and lipolysis (breakdown of glycogen and fat, respectively), and the conversion of amino acids and fatty acids to glucose (gluconeogenesis). Thus, insulin antagonizes any process that increases serum levels of glucose or fatty acids.

Table 46–1 Metabolic Effects of Normal, Excessive, and Deficient Insulin Levels

Metabolic Effect	Normal Insulin Activity	Hyposecretion/ Diabetes Mellitus	Hypersecretion/ Hypoglycemia
Cellular uptake of glucose	↑ glucose transport into body cells (except liver, brain, kidney, and red blood cells)	Glucose unable to enter cells, leading to hyperglycemia and glycosuria	Glucose uptake ↑ over normal levels leads to hypoglycemia; less glucose available to the brain leads to lethargy, confusion, impaired mental function, seizures, coma; early signs include hunger, weakness, sweating, tachycardia, anxiety, tingling and tremor
Carbohydrate metabolism	↑ glucose oxidation for energy and glucose storage as glycogen; ↓ gluconeogenesis and glycogenolysis	↓ glucose use; ↑ glycogenolysis in liver and muscle leads to ↑ glucose in blood	Glycogenolysis in the liver increases blood sugar levels (secondary effect of release of epinephrine, glucagon, and cortisol)
Lipid metabolism	↑ conversion of glucose to fat for deposit; prevents lipolysis in adipose tissue and liver	↑ lipolysis in fat tissue and liver; ↑ fatty acid and ketone levels in blood lead to ketosis and ketonuria	↑ lipolysis leads to ↑ plasma levels of fatty acids via secondary effect of hyperglycemia-inducing hormones (growth hormone, epinephrine, cortisone, others)
Protein metabolism	↑ uptake of amino acids and conversion of glucose to amino acids; protein anabolism	↓ amino acid uptake; protein depletion; ↑ gluconeogenesis to provide intracellular glucose for metabolism; muscle wasting, fatigue, weight loss	↑ gluconeogenesis (secondary effect of epinephrine and corticosteroid release)

Key: ↑ = increased, ↓ = decreased.

Since insulin release is stimulated primarily by increased blood glucose levels, its effects are most obvious in individuals who have just eaten. Shortly after a meal, plasma levels of glucose and free fatty acids are lowered markedly and amino acid uptake and tissue protein synthesis are accelerated. Glucose uptake is so rapid that blood sugar levels rarely change more than 20% to 40% over the normal range of 80 to 120 mg/dL, even after eating a high-carbohydrate meal. In young healthy individuals, venous glucose levels may not increase at all, resulting in a flat glucose tolerance test.

As dietary stimuli decline, insulin release is depressed. As cellular glucose uptake continues and blood glucose drops, the hyperglycemic hormones come into play to maintain blood sugar at physiologic levels. Liver glycogen stores typically are exhausted within six hours after a meal. If additional food is not ingested by this time, muscles begin to release amino acids, which are converted to glucose. Lipolysis occurs in adipose tissue, and free fatty acid levels rise in the blood. Free fatty acids are used for energy metabolism by muscle and liver cells, thus conserving glucose for use by the brain. Metabolic effects of the hyperglycemic hormones are summarized in Table 46–2.

Responses to Fasting and Starvation

With prolonged fasting, by-products of hepatic lipolysis (acetoacetic acid, acetone, and β-hydroxybutyric acid), commonly called *keto acids* or *ketone bodies,* enter the blood in increasing amounts. The resulting ketoacidosis depresses muscle protein catabolism and hepatic gluconeogenesis. At this point, blood sugar levels are very low and the brain begins to use fatty acids for fuel.

Insulin release is influenced markedly by diet. For example, a mixed carbohydrate, fat, and protein meal

Table 46–2 **Action of Selected Hormones and Other Mediators on Metabolic Regulation**

Hormone	Decreased Glucose Uptake	Increased Amino Acid Release	Increased Gluconeo-genesis	Increased Lipolysis	Decreased Insulin Secretion	Decreased Insulin Effects
ACTH	N	N	Y	Y	N	N
Cortisol	Y	Y	Y	Y	N	Y
Epinephrine	Y	N	Y	Y	Y/N*	Y
Glucagon	N	N	N	Y	N	N
Growth hormone	Y	N	N	Y	N	N

Key: Y = hormone exerts effect; N = hormone does not exert effect.

*Epinephrine, through its actions as an α-adrenergic agonist, inhibits insulin release. However, it stimulates insulin release through actions as a β_2-adrenergic agonist. Epinephrine also increases insulin release indirectly through its ability to elevate blood glucose levels. See text for further discussion of adrenergic effects on insulin release.

provokes insulin levels of approximately 150 μU/mL, whereas a protein-only meal results in insulin levels of only 50μU/mL. During short-term fasting (such as occurs overnight), insulin levels are approximately 12 μU/mL; after several weeks of starvation, insulin levels may reach 6μU/mL. Thus, the patterns of fuel metabolism form a continuum that reflects insulin levels, timing of food intake, and the interacting effects of hyperglycemic hormones.

II. Diabetes Mellitus

Diabetes mellitus is characterized by a broad range of physiologic and anatomic abnormalities, but its most notable feature is disturbed glucose metabolism and inappropriate hyperglycemia.

Metabolic Changes

Two major pathophysiologic phenomena—*hyperglycemia* and *ketosis*—account for essentially all metabolic abnormalities of diabetes mellitus. When insulin activity is absent, blood sugar levels remain high after a meal because glucose cannot enter tissue cells. The affected individual begins to feel nauseated when blood sugar levels are elevated abnormally. A stress reaction is triggered. It results in all the reactions that normally occur in the hypoglycemic or fasting state—glycogenolysis, lipolysis, and gluconeogenesis. However, in diabetes mellitus, the already hyperglycemic patient becomes even more hyperglycemic.

When blood sugar levels reach 180 to 200 mg/dL, the renal tubules become unable to reabsorb excess amounts of glucose and glucose begins to spill into the urine (glycosuria). The literal translation of diabetes mellitus—that is, "something sweet passing or siphoning through"—refers specifically to this manifestation of the disease.

The presence of glucose in urine promotes osmotic diuresis, causing **polyuria.** It is one of the cardinal signs of diabetes mellitus. Excessive fluid loss results in hyperosmolarity of blood which, in turn, causes the osmotic transfer of water from cells to the bloodstream and stimulates hypothalamic thirst centers. Consequently, the individual with diabetes tends to drink large volumes of water to satisfy thirst, which causes the second cardinal sign, *polydipsia.* In ambulatory individuals with normal thirst centers, dehydration usually is prevented. However, in unconscious, bedridden, or nonambulatory patients, dehydration can occur and be fatal.

Increased blood levels of fatty acids and ketone bodies result from the breakdown of fat stores in the absence of insulin. The nervous system attempts to compensate for the metabolic acidosis by increasing respiratory rate and depth to "blow off" carbon dioxide. Excess ketone bodies spilling into the urine carry sodium and potassium ions with them, thus causing electrolyte imbalances.

Because most cellular activities (especially those of neurons and muscle) are critically dependent on electrolyte and acid–base balance, ketoacidosis is the most serious acute complication of diabetes mellitus. When blood pH drops to around 7.25, symptoms of cardiac irritability occur. As the pH drops still further, to the 7.1

Table 46–3 Comparison of Signs of Severe Diabetic Ketoacidosis, Hyperglycemic Hyperosmolar Coma, and Hypoglycemia

	Diabetic Ketoacidosis	Hyperosmolar Coma	Hypoglycemia
Duration of onset	Hours to days	Days	Minutes to hours; may be prolonged in elderly patients taking long-acting oral hypoglycemic agents
Patient's appearance	Very sick	Sick	Healthy but confused
Appearance of skin	Flushed, dry	Dry	Pallor; moist
Respiration	Hyperventilation; rapid deep breathing; acetone breath	Normal	Shallow, rapid
Cardiovascular	Possible heart irregularity	Tachycardia, hypotension	Tachycardia, hypotension
Nervous system; mental status changes	Headache, abdominal pain, numbness of fingers and toes; progresses to unconsciousness and coma	No early symptoms; progresses to unconsciousness and coma	Apprehension, hunger, anxiety, fatigue, weakness, lethargy, confusion; progresses to coma; personality changes include emotional lability and hostility
Glycosuria/polyuria	Present	Present	Absent
Glucose levels	High	Very high	Low
Ketoacidosis	Present	Absent	Absent
Treatment	Insulin and fluids	Insulin and fluids	Oral and IV glucose

to 6.9 range, higher brain centers are depressed and coma occurs. Untreated ketoacidotic coma is associated with high mortality rates.

Ketoacidotic coma is most frequent in persons with Type I (insulin-dependent) diabetes. It also may occur suddenly in old people with previously undiagnosed diabetes mellitus as a result of severe stress. More commonly, elderly patients slip into the comatose state as a result of hyperosmolarity (often due to dehydration) without ever developing ketoacidosis; that is, they develop a *nonketotic coma*. Because unconsciousness and coma occur in diabetic ketoacidosis, in hyperosmolarity without ketosis, and in hypoglycemia, it is important to know the distinguishing characteristics of each condition. These are summarized in Table 46–3.

The most common early symptoms of diabetes mellitus—fatigue, polyuria, and polydipsia—can be correlated easily with the metabolic changes described. A state of constant fatigue occurs as body cells continually are deprived of adequate energy sources, even in the face of excessive food intake. Figure 46–1 and Table 46–1 summarize these metabolic consequences.

Anatomic Changes in Diabetes

The major anatomic complications of chronic diabetes mellitus are vascular and neural changes.

Vascular Problems

The most significant diabetic vascular problems are atherosclerosis and microangiopathic lesions. Atherosclerosis is the greatest risk for all patients with diabetes. It appears early in the disease and progresses rapidly, causing hypertension and significantly increasing the incidence of stroke, myocardial infarctions, and peripheral vascular problems. Peripheral vascular changes lead to impaired circulation in the limbs, predisposing the patient to tissue breakdown (ulcers) and necrosis. Abnormal platelet aggregation and clotting, and depressed high-density lipoprotein (HDL) serum levels, also occur in uncontrolled diabetes mellitus.

Microangiopathic lesions—abnormal thickenings in capillary basement membranes—result in leaky capillary walls throughout the body (particularly in the

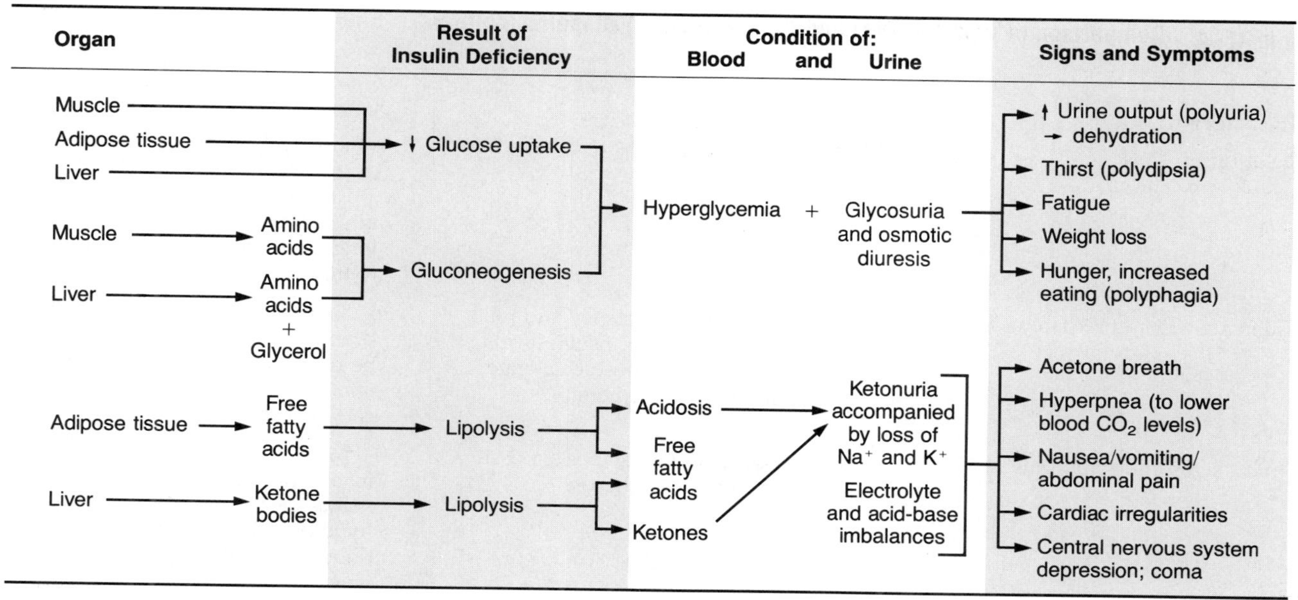

Figure 46–1

Hyperglycemia is caused by increased glucose production and, because of the insulin lack, an inability of body cells to take up glucose from blood. In diabetes, blood glucose levels are high enough to overcome the kidney's ability to reclaim glucose from the urine, causing glycosuria, osmotic diuresis, and other secondary signs and symptoms. The lack of intracellular glucose for use as a metabolic fuel increases lipolysis, generates acidic ketone bodies, eventually causing ketosis, and more secondary signs and symptoms. Diet and exercise help correct these imbalances, and provide the foundation for all forms of diabetes treatment. Pharmaco-therapy supplies either exogenous insulin or drugs that increase the release and activity of endogenous insulin.

eyes and kidneys). Within three to five years after the onset of disease, most persons with diabetes have developed some form of retinopathy. These persons are 25 times more prone to partial loss of vision or blindness than are people without diabetes, and two and six times more at risk for developing glaucoma and cataracts, respectively.

Renal changes involve thickening of the glomerular wall, which alters glomerular filtration. In five to 10 years, gross alterations are likely to occur and lead to deteriorating renal function (nephrotic syndrome), signaled by proteinuria, rising serum creatinine levels, and other clinical markers.

Neuropathies

A depression in the rate of neural conduction velocity occurs as clinical signs develop. Essentially every person with diabetes has demonstrable neuropathy within several years of disease onset. Ultimately, approximately half of all persons with diabetes have significant disabling symptoms. Commonly reported neuropathies include paresthesias or loss of sensation (particularly in the limbs), pain, and various symptoms of autonomic nervous system dysfunction, including impaired bladder function, diarrhea or fecal incontinence, postural hypotension, and impotence in men.

Other neural abnormalities, such as demyelination and deterioration of peripheral nerves resulting from inadequate blood supply, occur. Age appears to be an important factor in the degree of neuropathy observed. The neural changes are most frequent in middle-aged adults and appear unrelated to the degree of insulin deficiency. Local trauma and toxic substances such as alcohol aggravate the neural changes.

Other Complications

Two other important complications of the diabetic state are increased susceptibility to infection and delayed wound healing. Contributing factors include depressed protein synthesis, inadequate cellular energy sources, impaired phagocytosis, and the immunosuppressive effects of elevated blood cortisol levels.

Table 46–4 **Comparison of Type I (IDDM) and Type II (NIDDM) Diabetes Mellitus***

Characteristic	Type I	Type II
Age at onset	Often before age of 15; sudden onset	In individuals 40 years or older; occurrence increases with advanced age and obesity; gradual onset; may be asymptomatic for a long time; often detected during routine physical examination
Insulin activity and requirements	Absolute insulin deficiency and total insulin requirement; insulin levels fail to rise after glucose challenge, resulting in hyperglycemia	Insulin is made but released slowly or in subnormal amounts, or may be released in normal amounts but effects reduced by inadequate tissue (receptor) response
Clinical signs and symptoms	Hyperglycemia; ketoacidosis; possible weakness, weight loss	Hyperglycemia, but sufficient insulin produced to protect from ketoacidosis; may present with hyperosmolar (nonketotic) syndrome; patients are often overweight
Etiology	Not fully known; may result from β-cell destruction by viral infection or autoimmune process; some genetic component	Not fully known; strong genetic predisposition
Management	Insulin injections; may be difficult to control; diet controls and exercise regimen also required; oral hypoglycemic drugs ineffective because of lack of endogenous insulin	Diet, exercise; possible use of sulfonylurea oral hypoglycemic agents (or insulin) in cases that cannot be controlled by diet and weight reduction alone

*IDDM, insulin-dependent diabetes mellitus; NIDDM, noninsulin-dependent diabetes mellitus.

Classification of Diabetes Mellitus

The severity of diabetic manifestations is related to disease etiology, age of onset, and other factors. Two major diabetic categories are recognized, *Type I,* or *insulin-dependent diabetes mellitus (IDDM),* and *Type II,* or *noninsulin-dependent diabetes mellitus (NIDDM).* Types I and II diabetes mellitus are compared in Table 46–4.

Type I

Type I diabetes mellitus most often develops early in life, so this form of the disease previously was called juvenile-onset diabetes. Other terms used formerly include ketosis- and acidosis-prone diabetes.

Examination of Table 46–4 reveals that these terms, taken together, provide a characteristic clinical picture of persons with Type I diabetes. They totally lack insulin, tend to exhibit ketoacidosis, require insulin to prevent ketotic symptoms, and their disease is difficult to control (ie, "brittle").

This lack of insulin renders oral hypoglycemic drugs ineffective, since their therapeutic effects depend on the presence of endogenous insulin stores. Because of the ketotic tendency and the early onset of Type I diabetes, serious vascular and neural complications are more prevalent in this group. Children developing diabetes tend to perform poorly at school, and to be restless and irritable. Weakness and weight loss may be dramatic, and the craving for sweets, particularly sweet, cold fluids, becomes intense.

Type II

Type II diabetes occurs mainly in individuals older than 40, with the incidence increasing with age. Type II or NIDDM diabetes has been referred to variously as adult-

or maturity-onset diabetes, and ketosis- or acidosis-resistant diabetes mellitus.

Most persons with Type II diabetes do not have an absolute insulin deficiency. A gradual decline in β-cell function is more typical. Some patients exhibit diminished peripheral tissue responses to insulin, although insulin may be present in normal amounts. This is thought to reflect a decrease in the number or activity of the insulin receptors, and is correlated closely with obesity and inactivity. (More than 90% of the people with Type II diabetes are overweight.) Most cases of Type II diabetes can be handled by weight reduction, appropriate physical activity, dietary measures, and the administration of oral hypoglycemic drugs.

Heredity appears to have an important role in all cases of diabetes mellitus, but the genetic component is particularly strong in Type II diabetes. If an identical twin has Type II diabetes, the probability that both twins will have the disease is very high. In Type I identical twins, the genetic correlation is more in the range of 20% to 50%, and other causative factors appear to be more important.

The two categories of diabetes are not totally exclusive; there is some overlap of symptoms and treatment. For example, some Type II patients deteriorate to the point where insulin is required to control hyperglycemia.

Prevalence of Diabetes Mellitus

Diabetes mellitus incidence figures are imprecise, largely because there is no general agreement as to exactly what glucose blood levels should be considered excessive. Of the more than 200 million people in the United States, there are approximately 6 million diagnosed cases of diabetes. It is assumed that an additional 2 million cases are undiagnosed. Since Type I diabetes is overt, whereas symptoms of Type II may be masked temporarily, most undiagnosed cases are believed to be in older persons.

Diagnosis of Diabetes Mellitus

Procedures used to diagnose or monitor diabetes mellitus include the fasting blood sugar (FBS) test, the glucose tolerance test (GTT), the two-hour postprandial blood sugar test, and various other blood and urine tests.

The GTT is considered by many physicians to be the most reliable diagnostic test; it identifies both overt and borderline cases. Seventy-five grams (1.75 g/kg for a child) of glucose are administered orally; blood samples are obtained before glucose administration, and at one- and two-hour intervals thereafter. In healthy individuals, plasma glucose levels rise in response to the glucose load, and trigger insulin release. As a result, glucose levels begin to fall and are below 160 mg/dL within one hour and return to normal (below 120 mg/dL) by two hours after glucose loading. (Glucose tolerance declines with age, but age-related normal values are not discussed here.) In contrast, plasma glucose levels fall more slowly in persons with diabetes because insulin release is impaired or absent, and plasma glucose levels remain high (over 200 mg/dL) two hours after the glucose load.

The two-hour postprandial blood glucose test and "dipstick" tests for the presence of glucose in blood or urine are primarily screening procedures. Dipsticks make urine testing fast and inexpensive. However, a positive test indicates only relatively high blood sugar levels, since the renal threshold is not exceeded until blood sugar levels are in the range of 180 to 200 mg/dL. In addition, renal thresholds vary from person to person and with health and activity conditions; certain drugs (aspirin, for example) may cause inaccurate results; the differences between the "+" readings of the various urine test strips are not uniform (percent values must be used to prevent erroneous readings); and any condition leading to concentrated or diluted urine will distort the readings.

Blood tests are clearly the best both for screening procedures and for self-monitoring. They are more accurate and avoid many of the ambiguities of the urine dipsticks. Urine testing generally is a poor indicator of diabetes and its management.

Management of Diabetes Mellitus

The major goal of diabetes treatment is to reduce symptoms so that the patient can be as healthy and active as possible. This goal is attainable by the use of insulin or oral hypoglycemic agents, and by careful attention to diet, weight, and activity levels.

Diet, Weight Control, and Exercise

The importance of these nondrug interventions to successful diabetes management cannot be overstated. Dietary intake that is properly timed and matched to the pattern of insulin absorption is particularly important for patients requiring insulin therapy. The diabetic diet is similar to a nutritious diet eaten by normal individuals, with the exclusion of sweets. In general, the diet is calculated carefully to provide adequate nutrients and divides caloric intake into three meals and—especially for persons with Type I diabetes—several snacks taken at fixed times.

Obesity accentuates the disease process and introduces special problems. Overweight individuals need more insulin than otherwise identical nonobese persons, as it appears as if they have "lost" a fraction of functional insulin receptors. When obese patients reach their ideal weight, their body cells regain normal numbers of insulin receptors. In a successful weight-reduction program, hyperglycemia, glycosuria, and the requirement for drug therapy will diminish together. Thus, weight reduction is an extremely important part of diabetes control for obese persons.

Exercise, as permitted by the patient's condition, helps control weight and causes beneficial metabolic effects.

III. Drug Therapy of Diabetes Mellitus

The use of insulin and orally effective antidiabetic drugs is discussed next. They should be considered as adjuncts—and very important ones—to nondrug measures.

Insulins

PROTOTYPE

Insulin

Therapeutic Products

A number of highly purified forms of insulin derived from pork and beef pancreas are available for therapeutic use. Chemical modification of pork insulin has provided a semisynthetic human insulin product (NOVOLIN). In addition, human insulin derived from recombinant DNA techniques (HUMULIN, NOVOLIN) has been available since 1982.

The various insulin products can be divided into three general categories (rapid-, intermediate-, and long-acting types) depending on the speed and duration of action following their subcutaneous (SC) administration.

A rapid-acting insulin solution, *insulin injection,* is considered the prototype insulin drug. Since all insulins are injected, insulin injection will be referred to as *regular insulin* in the discussion that follows, to avoid semantic confusion.

Absorption, Distribution, Metabolism, and Excretion

Because insulin is a protein, it is destroyed by gastric acid and enzymes and so must be injected. (Insulin nasal sprays are being developed, but they are not yet approved for use.) The most common injection method is SC, but intramuscular (IM) or intravenous (IV) injections can be used with some insulin products and under some circumstances that are identified below.

The site of SC insulin injection affects the speed with which the drug will be absorbed, and therefore the time course of action. In resting individuals, insulin uptake is fastest and most consistent when the drug is injected in the abdominal SC tissues. Absorption is slower from injection sites on the extremities. Exercising a limb will speed insulin absorption, but the effects can be unpredictable and so abdominal administration sites generally are preferred.

Hypotension, hypovolemia, and other conditions associated with poor tissue perfusion, will reduce insulin absorption from SC or IM injection sites significantly. Patients with these conditions should be hospitalized for IV administration and proper monitoring.

As noted in the clinical indications and administration section, there are many different insulin preparations available for use. The way in which the insulin is prepared is another major factor in the speed of insulin absorption and effect, and the insulin formulation also affects many other aspects of drug use.

Once insulin is absorbed into the bloodstream, it is distributed and is eliminated by the kidneys and the liver just like endogenous insulin.

Pharmacologic Effects

Insulin that is injected exerts the same effects as natural insulin. By restoring the ability to metabolize carbohydrates, it acts as a hypoglycemic agent and antagonizes ketotic tendencies. As peripheral tissue carbohydrate use is enhanced, glucose tolerance (the rate of glucose removal from the circulation) increases and the use of fats and body protein for energy sources is depressed.

Therapeutic Products and Their General Use

There are many types of insulin (Table 46–5). Once they reach the bloodstream, all of them work identically to insulin that is released from the human pancreas. However, there are important differences among the various products, and those differences affect such things as administration routes and onsets and dura-

Table 46–5 Selected Examples of Insulins Available in the United States*

Action	Source
Short-acting (regular and semilente)	Human (HUMULIN REGULAR; HUMULIN BR; NOVOLIN R; VELOSULIN HUMAN R) Pork (ILETIN II regular†; purified pork regular; VELOSULIN) Beef (ILETIN II regular; semilente) Beef and pork (ILETIN I regular; ILETIN I semilente)
Intermediate-acting (lente and NPH)	Human (HUMULIN L, NOVOLIN L (both lente); HUMULIN N, NOVOLIN N (both NPH); INSULATARD NPH human) Pork (ILETIN II lente; ILETIN II NPH; purified pork lente; purified pork NPH) Beef (ILETIN II lente; ILETIN II NPH; lente insulin; NPH insulin) Beef and Pork (ILETIN I NPH; ILETIN I lente)
Long-acting (ultralente)	Human (HUMULIN U) Beef (ultralente) Beef and Pork (ILETIN I ultralente)
Fixed combination (premixed)‡	Human (HUMULIN 70/30; NOVOLIN 70/30; MIXTARD HUMAN 70/30) Pork (MIXTARD)

*All are U-100 insulins. Other concentrations available in some countries other than the United States. Names in full capital letters are brand names, except NPH, which is the abbreviation of the protein (neutral protein Hagedorn) used to prepare some insulins.

†Also available as U-500.

‡Contain 70% NPH and 30% regular insulins. Mixtures in addition to 70/30 available in some countries other than the United States.

Source: Modified from Campbell RK: The changing insulin market. *Diabetes Educator* 1991; 17(6):496–500. Reprinted with permission of the copyright owner.

tions of action. The differences also mean that many insulins cannot be substituted for or mixed with one another.

Insulin Potencies

The strength or concentration of all insulins is expressed in terms of units (U). A unit of insulin represents a standardized activity (or potency) for lowering blood glucose levels. The main insulin concentration used in the United States is U-100, or 100 units of insulin per mL of product.

Standardizing insulins to U-100 makes it easy to measure and administer equivalent dosages of different insulins, with reduced risks of dosage errors due to incorrect calculations or dilutions, or accidental substitution of the wrong "strength" of insulin for the proper one. Syringes designed specifically for insulin administration also are marked in units. Since U-100 insulin is now the standard, U-100 syringes—syringes with marks up to 100 U on the barrel—are also standard; this also simplifies measurement.

A U-500 insulin is also available, but this very concentrated drug is used only for patients who have very high daily insulin requirements, mainly more than 200 units per day. The U-500 insulin is administered with a tuberculin syringe. U-40 insulin (ILETIN) is also available for patients with very low insulin requirements. It requires a special U-40 syringe for administering the correct dose. Insulin concentrations in addition to U-40, U-100 and U-500 are available outside the United States.

Insulin Sources

Insulin preparations come from two main sources: animal pancreata and human insulin genes.

Some insulins are obtained from beef or pork pancreas, and some are combinations of beef and pork insulins. These *animal-derived insulins* are treated to remove impurities, including most of the proinsulin that also is isolated when the gland is processed. Animal insulins are very similar to human insulin, but even after purification they are not identical to human insulin. One or two amino acids in the polypeptide chains of the animal insulins are different from those in the human hormone. These differences slightly affect onsets and durations of action. Because they are not quite

Table 46–6 Pharmacokinetic Properties of Insulins*

Name	Onset of Action (hr)	Time to Peak Effect (hr)	Duration (hr)
Rapid-Acting Insulins			
Regular insulin (IV)	0.2–0.5	0.25–0.5	0.5–1
Regular insulin	0.5–1	2.5–5	6–8
Semilente insulin	1–1.5	5–10	12–16
Intermediate-Acting Insulins			
NPH insulin	1–1.5	4–12	24
Lente insulin	1–2.5	7–15	24
Long-Acting Insulins			
Ultralente insulin	4–8	10–30	>36
Premixed Insulin Combination Products			
(70% NPH, 30% regular)	0.25–1	2–8	24

*Times are for SC injection unless noted otherwise.

Source: Adapted from *Drug Facts and Comparisons*. St. Louis: Facts & Comparisons, Inc., 1992. Reprinted with permission of the copyright owner.

identical to the insulin made by the patient's own pancreas, they also can trigger an immune response in some patients.

Other insulins are more similar to, or identical with, human insulin. Because of the technology involved in preparing them, they are generally more expensive than pork or beef insulins. *Semisynthetic insulins* are obtained initially from pork insulin, which then is purified and chemically modified to convert one of the amino acids that is characteristic of pork insulin to the amino acid found naturally in human insulin. *Biosynthetic insulin* is obtained by inserting the gene for human insulin into bacteria using modern recombinant DNA technology ("genetic engineering"). The bacteria then synthesize insulin that is identical to insulin secreted by human beings, and the hormone is processed further. However, even these so-called human insulins have a low but real potential to cause allergic reactions in some patients.

Insulin Onsets and Durations of Activity

The animal and human insulins can be divided further into three general categories according to whether their actions appear rapidly (eg, regular insulin) or whether they have intermediate or long durations of action (Table 46–6).

In general, the faster the onset of action, the shorter the duration of effects. A preparation with a fast onset of action would be used when prompt effects are needed, and a longer-acting preparation would be chosen when more prolonged blood glucose control is the goal. Often two insulins with different onsets are used together—either injected separately or mixed together before injection—when both prompt and longlasting effects are needed. (As noted below, however, some insulin mixtures are not compatible.)

The onsets and durations of action depend on how the insulin is manufactured. All insulins are prepared with zinc ions. However, the manufacturer can alter the drug's absorption rate and time-dependent profiles of action by varying the amount of zinc and diluents (buffers), or by adding other substances.

Rapid-Acting Insulins

The rapid-acting insulins include *regular insulin* and *semilente insulins*.

Regular Insulin

Regular insulin is comprised of insulin crystals that are so small that they dissolve completely in the product. Because the insulin is fully dissolved, regular insulin can be injected IV. (Regular U-100 insulin also can be given SC or IM, and SC and IM are the only accepted routes for U-500 insulin).

Regular insulin is also the only insulin formulation that looks clear if it is suitable for injection. If it looks cloudy, it must never be used. All other insulins are suspensions—particles of undissolved insulin suspended in liquid—and they should look cloudy. Moreover, none of the insulins except regular insulin can be injected IV because of the serious risks of injecting drug particles directly into a vein. They are usually given by SC injection, but IM injections sometimes are used.

Semilente Insulins

Semilente insulins are prepared so that the insulin stays in small crystals that do not dissolve completely in their bathing medium. Nevertheless, crystals in semilente insulins are small enough that when they are injected into SC tissues they dissolve quickly, and the insulin is absorbed quickly into the bloodstream. The onset of action after SC injection of a semilente insulin is called "rapid," but it is not quite as rapid as when regular insulin is injected by the same route (Table 46–6).

Intermediate-Acting Insulins

There are two types of intermediate-acting insulins: *NPH insulins* and *lente insulins.*

NPH Insulins

These insulins are prepared with a protein called neutral protein Hagedorn. This protein additive binds the insulin and slows insulin absorption after SC injection. It also prolongs the duration of action, compared with rapid-acting insulins.

Lente Insulins

Lente insulins are identical, chemically, to semilente insulins. The only difference between the two is that insulin crystals in lente insulins are larger than those in semilente insulins. Because of the larger crystal size, lente insulins are absorbed more slowly than the smaller semilente insulin crystals. This slows the onset of action and prolongs the duration of action.

Long-Acting Insulins

The long-acting (or extended-acting) insulins also are known as *ultralente insulins.* Ultralente insulins are suspensions of insulin crystals that are even larger than those found in lente insulins. Ultralente insulins therefore have the slowest onset of action and the longest duration of action.

An insulin known as protamine-zinc insulin is prepared in the presence of another protein, protamine. It is no longer available for use in the United States.

Mixing Insulins

The natural pattern of insulin release and blood glucose levels involves rises and falls during the day in response to meals or exercise. Since the clinical goal is to mimic these patterns as much as possible, and to compensate for sudden changes of blood glucose levels, insulin therapy poses a problem because no one insulin can provide both rapid and sustained effects. Thus, for many patients, two insulins may be required: one for fast effects, another for more longlasting actions.

This can be achieved in two ways once the patient's insulin requirements have been determined. One way is to inject the two insulins separately, each at the proper dose. This is an added burden, and added pain, for some patients. However, for some patients it may be necessary.

The other way to tailor the drug effects is to mix insulins, each in the proper dose. The patient may buy and use commercially prepared insulin mixtures. In the United States, these mixtures contain 70% NPH insulin for more prolonged effects, and 30% regular insulin for fast action. These formulations are convenient, because they make measuring the dose and injecting it relatively easy, and the commercial preparations have a long shelf life if stored properly. However, for some patients, the 70–30 mix is not the right proportion for optimal diabetes control. Thus, the patient either should inject the right doses of the right insulins separately, or mix the insulins (or have someone else do it). (Many NPH-regular insulin mixtures in addition to 70–30 are available outside the United States, and a 50–50 mix may be available in the United States soon.)

Not all insulins are compatible with one another (see Table 46–7). Semilente, lente, and ultralente insulins can be mixed together in any ratio, and they are stable for a long time because they differ from one another only in terms of crystal size (and onsets and durations of action). Thus, they can be prepared well ahead of the time when they will be injected. Some patients prefill several syringes with the proper mixture, and store them before use. Regular and NPH insulins also can be mixed in any ratio by the patient or care provider (if the premixed NPH-regular insulins are not suitable).

Table 46–7 General Insulin Mixing Guidelines

Insulin Type	Guidelines
Semilente, lente, and ultralente insulins	These insulins are chemically identical, differ only in terms of particle size in suspension; may mix two or more of these insulins in any ratio; mixtures stable for 18 months (with proper storage)
Regular and NPH insulins	May mix in any ratio; mixtures stable; mixtures of regular and NPH insulins are preferred mixtures for combining a rapidly acting insulin with an intermediate-acting one
Regular and lente insulins	These insulins start to bind to one another immediately; binding slows onset of activity of regular insulin, lowers peak effect, prolongs overall action; binding and altered activity continue for about 24 h; if using *nonhuman* regular and lente insulins, inject immediately after mixing; binding of human regular and human lente insulins more problematic: inject immediately after mixing or inject in separate sites, do not mix; for all regular-lente mixtures, always maintain constant time between mixing and injection; do not mix VELOSULIN regular or HUMULIN BR
Lente and phosphate-buffered insulins (all NPH insulins, all insulins marketed by Novo Nordisk and HUMULIN BR are phosphate-buffered)	Never mix. Phosphate buffer "converts" the intermediate-acting insulin to a rapidly acting form

Source: Modified from Anderson JH, Campbell RK: Mixing insulins in 1990. *Diabetes Educator* 1991; 16(5):380–385. Reprinted with permission of the copyright owner.

Special guidelines apply to the mixing of other insulins, and some insulins should not be mixed together at all. Regular and lente insulins react for about 24 hours after they are mixed. Ingredients in the lente insulin convert some of the regular insulin to what is more like lente insulin, and the onset of action of the regular insulin is delayed. There is one way to get around this problem: when regular and lente insulins are mixed, inject them within five minutes. If that cannot be done, use a *constant* time interval between mixing and injecting. *Never* change the mix-inject interval with regular and lente insulins.

Lente and NPH insulins (and other insulins prepared in phosphate buffer; see Table 46–7) must *never* be mixed together.

Storing Insulins

Insulin should not be frozen or exposed to extreme heat or direct sunlight. Most insulins keep their activity well when stored at room temperature, but storage in a refrigerator is preferred for syringes that have been filled with insulin in advance of intended use (consult manufacturers' recommendations for commercially prefilled syringes, and see comments above on incompatible mixtures); and for opened or unopened multiple-dose containers. Opened multidose containers should be discarded if they have not been used for several weeks.

Injecting Insulins

Proper, consistent insulin administration is essential, regardless of whether it is done by the patient or a caregiver. With SC administration, the most common route, teach proper technique to the patient and be sure he or she is capable of following instructions. Instructions go far beyond knowing how to mix insulins (if necessary), or the mechanics of withdrawing drug from its container and injecting it consistently and safely. (See Appendix A and general medical-surgical nursing texts for more information.)

The SC injection sites must be rotated to avoid local tissue damage (see side effects section) and erratic drug absorption and effects that can occur when the same site is used too often over months and years. In general, avoid injections into the same site (or within one inch of a given site) more often than every four to six weeks. Anatomic diagrams, such as the one shown in Figure 46–2, should be used to devise a methodical site rotation plan. Patients should be given a supply of such charts, and then educated about why and how to use

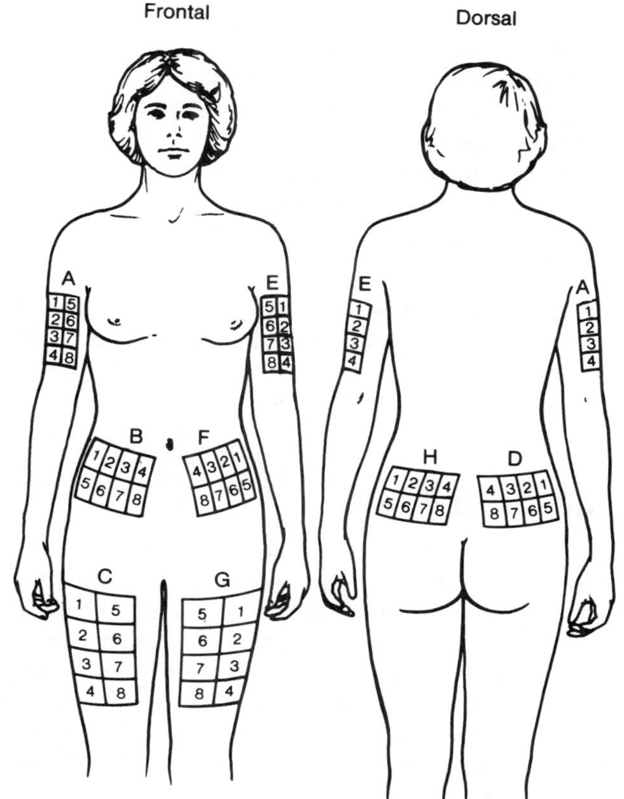

Figure 46–2

Insulin injection sites. Use diagrams such as this to teach patients to develop a consistent rotation plan. Tailor the plan to the patient's needs; avoid sites that are scarred, poorly accessible, or with compromised tissue integrity; use abdominal sites if possible, rather than those on limbs subjected to intermittent or excessive exercise, which can alter insulin absorption rates. Avoid injecting into the same site (or within one inch of it) more often than once every four to six weeks.

them. Some patients have trouble reaching specific sites, or find that injections into certain spots are unusually painful. Help them find and stay with an acceptable plan.

Special considerations for IM or IV insulin injections are discussed in the context of their clinical uses below.

NURSING IMPLICATIONS

Information that is important for the nurse eventually becomes important for the patient who will be self-medicating with insulin, or for other caregivers.

Become familiar with the various insulin groups—sources, onsets, and so on. Learn which insulins can or cannot be mixed, and the proper timing needed when mixes that are not commercially supplied will be used. Before drawing insulin into a syringe, check the medication container(s) for expiration date and other pertinent label information. Never use regular insulin that has any cloudiness; it should be crystal clear.

When preparing mixtures that include regular insulin, always draw up the regular insulin first; this will avoid contaminating the unused regular insulin that is left in the bottle with other insulins that can react with it and change its activity profile. When drawing up or mixing any insulin suspension, roll the bottle between the palms several times, or shake it gently. Otherwise, because insulin crystals may have settled in the bottom of the container, the amount of active drug that will be removed and injected will vary.

Consistency of insulin therapy is one of the most important keys to smooth, successful insulin treatment. It is important when adjusting the insulin dosages for persons with newly diagnosed diabetes, and it is equally important once the patient's blood glucose levels have been brought under control, and therapy continues.

Besides following mixing and administration guidelines, the patient and caregiver should not change the types of insulin (animal or human; fast-, intermediate-, or slow-acting), the brand or product, or even the type and manufacturer of the insulin syringe. Although some of these changes may appear to be insignificant, they all can contribute to poor or less than ideal treatment outcomes. Changes should be made only by a physician who has evaluated the patient.

If your patient will be traveling out of the United States, where other insulins and syringes are available, make sure he or she has an adequate supply of material, and a way to store it properly. If the trip is so long that new insulins or syringes may have to be purchased, provide the patient with explicit instructions about what to use. Plan ahead.

There are too many other aspects of outpatient insulin therapy, and nursing implications related to them, to cover adequately in this general pharmacology text. The important areas include not only the proper use of drugs (eg, mixing, storing, and injecting insulin), which have been mentioned above, but also such things as

- Adapting syringes and purchasing special syringes, needle guides and guards, or other accessories for safe and effective self-use by persons with manual or visual impairments;
- The care and use of implantable insulin infusion pumps;

- Selecting and properly using devices to obtain blood samples and measure blood glucose levels;
- Planning diets and exercise activities;
- Identifying and dealing with psychosocial and economic concerns; and
- Preventing and recognizing adverse consequences of diabetes (eg, infections, tissue ischemia, foot problems) and diabetes therapy (eg, adverse drug effects).

For more detailed information, refer to specialty texts and journals, publications by the American Diabetes Association, and local care providers and support groups specializing in diabetes.

Therapeutic Uses

Insulin has several uses. When long-term therapy is indicated, virtually any of the insulin formulations available can be used, and they usually are given by the standard SC injection route. Some patients with unstable ("brittle") diabetes may require IV infusions of regular insulin; implantable insulin pumps are available for use by carefully selected outpatients. In emergencies, or when the patient is acutely unstable, start with regular insulin by IV injection or infusion.

Uses of Therapeutic Products

Type I Diabetes

Insulin is the only hypoglycemic agent that is effective for Type I diabetes. There is no "average" dose. Twenty-four-hour insulin requirements are determined for each patient by injecting regular insulin 15 minutes before each meal, and the daily maintenance dose is estimated.

In a daily maintenance program, many persons with Type I diabetes require a prebreakfast injection of a mixed dose of *rapid-acting* regular or semilente insulin (one quarter to one third the total daily dose) and NPH or lente insulin (three quarters to two thirds the total daily dose). A premixed 70%–30% NPH–regular insulin product often is used. This is followed by an additional injection of intermediate-acting insulin before the evening meal or at bedtime to maintain blood sugar levels as close to the normal range as possible and to prevent evening glycosuria. Routinely, two thirds of the total daily insulin dose is administered in the morning and the balance is administered in the evening. Table 46–C1 summarizes the usual range of daily insulin doses.

In some particularly difficult cases, regular insulin also is added to the presupper injection of an intermediate-acting (NPH or lente) insulin. The rapid-acting insulin prevents glycosuria and hyperglycemia in the later evening; the intermediate-acting form maintains the same control between midnight and the following morning. The additional dose of rapid-acting insulin in the evening provides greater control of hyperglycemia after the evening meal in refractory diabetes.

A frequently used plan for patient preparation of a mixed insulin dose is a combination of regular insulin and NPH insulin. An alternative plan involves injection of small doses of regular insulin before each meal and the administration of a long-acting (ultralente) preparation before breakfast and dinner. However, the use of long-acting preparations has declined markedly, largely because of the difficulty in controlling both glycosuria and hypoglycemia with these products. Some patients with Type II diabetes receiving insulin may require only a single early-morning dose of NPH or lente insulin.

The main goal of diabetes care is optimal use of glucose throughout each 24-hour interval. The insulin-mixing and split administration plans just outlined permit a fairly close approximation of the normal physiologic pattern of insulin release, particularly the rapid insulin rise precipitated by each meal. However, average glucose blood levels achieved with these protocols tend to be substantially higher than those seen in nondiabetic individuals (200 to 300 mg/dL vs 100 mg/dL).

Moreover, with this type of regimen, there may be an excess of insulin in the midafternoon and around bedtime; snacks are indicated at these times, particularly if a second insulin dose is given later in the day. An insulin deficiency may occur at midday and can be compensated for by moderate exercise after the noon meal.

Patients on a mixed- and split-dose regimen need to test their blood (preferred) or urine (or both) several times daily. Insulin dosages then can be modified on the basis of the degree and frequency of hyperglycemia.

One way to modify insulin dosages to supplement maintenance therapy is based on a "sliding scale" approach. It is used most often when the patient is hospitalized, but can be adapted to self-care settings. Blood glucose levels that are above a specified level are managed by administering a small, supplemental dose (eg, 10 U) of regular insulin. The greater the blood glucose level, the greater the supplemental dose.

However, the sliding scale system has been criticized because blood glucose levels are allowed to rise above desired levels before supplemental insulin is administered. The trend is toward closer assessment of the patient, and better planning of insulin needs, so that blood glucose levels are kept within normal limits as much as possible. This amounts to preventing hyperglycemia, rather than reacting to it. See the Annotated Bibliography for more information.

Emergency Management of Acute Diabetic Ketoacidosis or Hyperosmolar Conditions

Insulin is the only effective hypoglycemic agent for acute diabetic manifestations and ketosis, where therapy must be initiated as rapidly as possible. Insulin therapy is accompanied by infusions of isotonic saline to correct hypovolemia and to prevent circulatory collapse. Blood is withdrawn for determination of blood glucose, ketone, and potassium levels.

Laboratory findings of hyperglycemia and ketoacidosis usually require initial IV infusion of regular insulin (20 to 50 U), followed by single SC injections or IV injections or infusions. A typical goal is to deliver 5 to 10 U per hour, depending on the patient's response to the initial dose. Higher insulin doses are administered when the patient's usual daily requirements are 100 U or more, or for insulin-resistant patients. Concentrated insulin solutions (U–500) may be used in this setting, but extra care must be taken to ensure that the product is not mistaken for a 100 U/mL product. The U–500 product should never be given IV, because of the great risk of causing acute hypoglycemia.

As blood glucose levels fall and glycosuria and polyuria subside, a mixture of isotonic saline, 5% dextrose, and potassium salts (often potassium phosphate, to correct simultaneous hypophosphatemia) is infused to prevent hypoglycemia, counteract dehydration, and normalize and maintain electrolyte balance.

For patients with hyperosmolar coma, rehydration with saline (first isotonic, then hypotonic to prevent edema) should be started immediately. Generally, such patients respond well to much lower doses of insulin (10 U), which can be administered IV or SC. Serum potassium levels also may need correction. As therapy continues, a dextrose-saline solution is infused to prevent hypoglycemia.

Management of Type II Diabetes

Insulin is a preferred and often necessary therapy for persons with Type II diabetes who do not respond adequately to oral hypoglycemic drugs (the usual pharmacologic approach for Type II diabetes), diet, and exercise.

Insulin is also the safest and most effective way to temporarily manage persons who have changing drug requirements owing to surgery or other physical stressors, even if they have been managed well previously with diet, exercise, and orally effective antidiabetic drugs.

Major stress of any sort releases catecholamines, corticosteroids, and glucagon, all of which increase blood glucose levels. Caloric demands also are affected by the body's attempts to heal tissues and fend off infections. These processes already may be compromised in persons with diabetes. Stress, and recovery from it, also change fluid and electrolyte balances and demands, which are more difficult to meet in a person with diabetes.

If the patient's blood glucose levels are well controlled (regardless of how the control is achieved), and surgery is minor, little more than added vigilance during and after the procedure may be necessary. However, if diabetes is poorly controlled, if the patient is debilitated, or if major surgery is anticipated, insulin therapy becomes essential.

It is common and wise to admit all preoperative diabetes patients a day or two before surgery to perform proper tests and achieve good control of blood glucose. The actual approach depends on the patient, the institution, the physician's preferences, and the procedure to be performed. If the patient was being treated with oral hypoglycemic drugs, they may be discontinued and replaced with insulin doses calculated to maintain normoglycemia. Another approach calls for insulin-treated patients to be switched from intermediate-acting insulins to regular insulin, given in single doses or as additives to an IV infusion of dextrose. Still another plan may continue use of an intermediate-acting preparation, but in split doses.

Insulin needs will be very different in the immediate postoperative period, and they are likely to change dramatically once the patient stabilizes and begins eating a regular diet. Often the nurse will obtain ordered blood tests, perform urinalyses, assess their results, and administer supplemental insulin doses based on test results and patient status. Regardless of what is done, assessment and treatment procedures must be planned and organized carefully, all members of the health-care team must be made aware of what is to be done, and the nurse must be ready to adapt to the patient's changing needs.

Diabetes in Pregnancy

Whether maternal diabetes exists before conception, or develops during pregnancy (gestational diabetes mellitus), tight control of blood glucose levels during pregnancy is usually more difficult to achieve, yet it is absolutely essential to do so. Poorly controlled diabetes is associated with a higher incidence of fetal malformations and mortality than in the normal population. Fetal mortality rates can be reduced significantly by proper management.

As with all other situations, dietary modification can help prevent hyperglycemia. If diet alone fails, multiple daily insulin injections would be indicated also. Insulin is the preferred pharmacologic agent during pregnancy, even for patients with Type II diabetes that has been treated with oral hypoglycemic drugs. (As noted later, the risk of adverse fetal effects is greater with the oral hypoglycemic drugs than with insulin.)

In addition to routine prenatal care, monitor blood glucose levels more closely, and anticipate changes in insulin requirements. It is essential to assess weight, blood pressure, and fetal status frequently. Signs of fetal distress must be reported at once. If they occur, delivery usually is initiated as soon as possible, if it is safe to do so.

Infants born to women receiving insulin should be monitored closely for hypoglycemia. Maternal insulin requirements often drop in the first one to three days after delivery, rising to prepregnancy levels thereafter. Careful monitoring is, once again, crucial.

Management of Hyperkalemia

Regular insulin, administered parenterally with glucose, will drive glucose into the body cells, carrying with it large amounts of potassium. Thus, insulin may be used to treat severe hyperkalemia in persons either with or without diabetes.

NURSING IMPLICATIONS

When the diabetes patient is hospitalized and will not be self-administering insulin, and you must administer insulin SC or IM to a patient who has been self-medicating with the drug, try to learn the patient's administration pattern. Then select suitable injection sites that are normally inaccessible to the patient. All nurses who are caring for a given patient should agree on an injection site rotation plan, and should chart the use of sites with an anatomic diagram.

Be aware of the risks of administering insulin SC or IM to patients with hypovolemia, hypotension, or other conditions in which blood flow through the tissues is reduced. Insulin will be absorbed more slowly than usual, and often in an unpredictable way, in these conditions; blood glucose levels may not respond adequately. This low or slow response might be interpreted incorrectly as insulin resistance, and so it might be managed by giving another (perhaps larger) insulin dose. However, when the patient's hemodynamic status improves, blood flow to the injection site rises, the insulin will be absorbed more quickly, and an acute hypoglycemic reaction can occur. Giving insulin intravenously in these situations usually is safer.

When giving insulin IV, be aware that the drug tends to bind to plastic IV fluid bags and infusion tubing. Some of the drug may not reach the patient's circulatory system. Insulin loss in this way is greater when more dilute insulin solutions are being used. The results may be unpredictable, and so follow blood glucose measurements to guide therapy.

If the patient's bladder is catheterized, whether for collecting urine samples or for other purposes, use meticulous technique in insertion and catheter care. It is easy to introduce infectious organisms through the urethra, the sugar-rich urine in patients with glycosuria provides an excellent medium for rapid microorganism growth, and infections that may occur can be serious and difficult to treat.

Side Effects, Adverse Reactions, and Contraindications

Important adverse effects of insulin administration include hyperinsulinism (resulting in hypoglycemia and hypokalemia), allergy, and lipodystrophy. Insulin resistance is a significant problem in some patients.

Hyperinsulinism

Hyperinsulinism resulting from unanticipated changes in the patient's insulin requirements is the single most common adverse reaction to insulin administration. Type I diabetes patients may have unpredictable spontaneous reductions in their insulin requirements, particularly in the early course of the disease. In other patients, excessive insulin activity (hypoglycemia) more likely reflects failure to eat at the proper time, unusual exercise, or inadvertent administration of too much insulin.

The particular hypoglycemic signs and symptoms vary with the type of insulin preparation used, and depend on the speed at which blood glucose levels fall. For example, injection of rapid-acting regular insulin produces early symptoms of hunger and weakness, followed by symptoms of sympathetic nervous system activation such as lightheadedness, sweating, tachycardia, anxiety, and tremor.

The symptoms usually caused first by long-acting

preparations occur more gradually and typically involve headache, and mental, emotional, and visual disturbances. Intermediate-acting preparations produce symptoms between the two extremes.

Expect serum potassium levels to fall as insulin drives glucose into cells and the blood glucose level falls. Symptomatic hypokalemia (eg, cardiac arrhythmias and neuromuscular disturbances) may occur. Regardless of initial symptoms, all cases of severe hypoglycemia will progress to coma if left untreated. In acute conditions, treatment consists of IV administration of 50% glucose solution to restore consciousness. Blood glucose levels also may be enhanced by the administration of glucagon.

Allergic Reactions

Before the highly purified insulins came into use, approximately 25% of insulin-dependent persons with diabetes demonstrated an allergic reaction to insulin at some time. Most of these reactions involve transient and localized itching, swelling, and erythema at the injection site. A few individuals (primarily those using insulin on an intermittent basis) develop a generalized urticaria and have detectable antiinsulin antibodies in their serum. The antibodies interact with and neutralize the administered insulin. In such cases, a change to a human insulin product is advisable in spite of its comparatively high cost.

Local Tissue Damage

Lipodystrophies (lipoatrophy and lipohypertrophy) are local tissue responses to frequent (or cold) insulin injections at the same site. Lipoatrophy is atrophy of the fatty tissue and irregular cavity formation, whereas lipohypertrophy is localized tissue thickening, which may delay insulin absorption. Both conditions may be prevented or reversed by not using a particular injection site more often than once every four weeks. If a patient has been injecting insulin into a dystrophic site (because it is usually painless), insulin dosage reductions are usually necessary when moving to another site. Observe closely for hypoglycemia.

Insulin Resistance

Insulin resistance requires that large doses of insulin (200 U per day or more) be administered to produce the desired hypoglycemic effects. In some cases, the poor response to insulin may be caused by the development of antibodies to insulin. As discussed earlier, the insulin resistance of obese individuals is believed to be a consequence of diminished insulin receptor activity. Losing weight usually helps lower insulin requirements.

NURSING IMPLICATIONS

Help patients learn the onset, peak, and duration of action of the insulin product(s) they are using. This helps anticipate the onset of hyperglycemia or hypoglycemia, allows for proper treatment, and helps prevent overdoses. Patients should understand clearly the signs and symptoms of hypoglycemia. Advise them to have some simple sugar source available at all times to manage it promptly: hard candies or sugar cubes, or one of the commercially available nonprescription products such as B-D GLUCOSE, GLUCTOSE, INSTA-GLUCOSE, or MONOJEL.

Alert patients to the symptoms of an allergic response to insulin, including local irritation, swelling, and erythema. Advise them to report such responses at once.

Stress again the need for patients to administer insulin at room temperature, and to rotate injection sites, to prevent lipodystrophies.

Encourage all patients with diabetes to carry or wear (preferred) some form of identification indicating that they have diabetes, and other pertinent information. This becomes particularly important in cases of profound hypoglycemia, in which the patient will be unable to communicate information vital for proper and prompt treatment.

◆ Use During Pregnancy and Lactation

The issue of pregnancy and diabetes was discussed earlier. Insulin is not excreted in breast milk, and so breast-feeding is not contraindicated. Many women who breast-feed appear to require lower insulin doses than women who do not breast-feed; their insulin requirements may rise again when they stop nursing.

◆ Use in Children and the Elderly

Age is an important factor in determining the need for insulin, insulin requirements, the understanding of therapy, activity levels, and the ability for self-care. Each factor must be assessed to optimize care. Elderly patients may have poor vision or motor skills that may affect their ability to perform required tasks. They are also more likely to have other disorders that may complicate diabetes and its management, and may be taking other medications that may interact with insulin or alter blood glucose levels. Recognize the needs associated with age, and involve family members or other caregivers as needed.

Interactions with Other Drugs

Table 46–I1 summarizes the drugs that cause clinically significant interactions with insulin. The list includes not only prescription drugs, but also aspirin and alcohol. Most of the drugs interact indirectly, either by increasing or decreasing blood glucose levels. Thus, they can either potentiate insulin's glucose-lowering effects, increasing the risk of hypoglycemia, or they can counteract insulin's desired actions and lead to persistent hyperglycemia. In either case, the interaction makes provision of predictable control of blood glucose levels much less consistent. (As noted later, many of these same drugs also interact with oral antidiabetic drugs.)

Beta-adrenergic blockers deserve special attention. Diabetes mellitus in adults often is accompanied by cardiovascular disorders such as hypertension or angina pectoris, for which β blockers are indicated. The β blockers pose problems for diabetes patients in several ways. They inhibit insulin release (which is most important for Type II diabetes but potentially important for insulin-dependent diabetes as well), and in this and other ways β blockers lower blood glucose levels on their own. By blocking the cardiac β receptors (β_1 receptors) they also block the tachycardia that many persons with diabetes use as one of the signals that their blood glucose levels are falling too low, whether because of excessive insulin dosages, inadequate diet, or too much exercise or stress. The β blockers also prolong recovery from a hypoglycemic episode, even when glucose or other interventions are used to help normalize glucose levels that have become too low.

Interactions tend to be greater and more clinically important with nonselective (β_1 and β_2) blockers such as propranolol than with the cardioselective (β_1) blockers, atenolol and metoprolol (Table 15–C2). The nonselective agents will affect both heart rate and blood glucose levels; the cardioselective agents will have less of an effect on blood glucose, but they certainly can inhibit heart rate increases.

Finally, interactions involving β blockers and insulin (or oral hypoglycemic drugs) can occur not only when systemic administration routes (eg, oral) are used, but also with topical administration of β blockers for glaucoma and ocular hypertension.

None of the interactions mentioned above or in Table 46–I1 need to be avoided absolutely, but the use of interacting drugs should be known to and regulated by the physician so that expected outcomes can be anticipated and perhaps prevented by adjusting the dosage of the insulin or the interacting drug(s). In some cases, noninteracting alternatives can be used. For example, many drugs other than β blockers can be used for managing hypertension (Chapter 33) or angina pectoris (Chapter 34), and so they may be preferred for the patient who also has diabetes. Regardless of what is done, frequent monitoring of therapy and of blood glucose levels is essential for achieving stable and safe therapy. Monitoring is especially important when starting or stopping therapy with a drug that interacts with an antidiabetic medication.

Overdose and Toxicity

Profound hypoglycemia and its many consequences are the major problems of insulin overdoses. The time course of symptom onset depends on the insulin formulation used.

Administration of an insulin dose greater than the patient's usual dose is not the only cause of overdoses. Even usual doses can cause profound hypoglycemia if the patient has failed to eat, has exercised excessively, or has received other drugs that lower blood glucose levels. Patients with "brittle" diabetes are also at greater risk, since their insulin needs often fluctuate dramatically.

Whereas some persons can adapt to blood glucose levels as low as 40 mg/dL, some persons with insulin-dependent diabetes may experience intense signs and symptoms with reasonably normal blood glucose levels (100 mg/dL) if the blood glucose level falls rapidly from much higher levels (300 to 400 mg/dL). This suggests that the severity and speed of the fall may be more important than the actual blood glucose level.

The most serious concerns with insulin toxicity are blood glucose levels that are inadequate to support brain metabolism. Seizures and coma are eventual consequences, leading to death if blood glucose and electrolyte levels are not corrected promptly.

Prompt intervention is essential. Unfortunately, the disorientation and confusion associated with some hypoglycemic episodes, or the occurrence of hypoglycemia during sleep, may prevent patients from obtaining proper care or intervening with self-treatment. In addition, some cases of profound hypoglycemia have been misdiagnosed as diabetic ketoacidosis, and have been treated with more insulin.

Ingestion of simple sugars (juice, candy, or commercial glucose preparations) is the treatment for persons who are conscious and can ingest these foods. In the hospital, IV glucose administration is preferred to begin treatment. For outpatients, an injection of the hyperglycemic hormone glucagon, discussed later, is a reasonable emergency intervention if simple sugars are ineffective or cannot be administered.

Normalizing blood glucose levels usually restores consciousness and more or less full function almost immediately unless hypoglycemia has lasted sufficiently long to cause some brain damage. Beta blockers, noted earlier as sometimes unavoidable interactants, will prolong the recovery from hypoglycemia, even when glucose, glucagon, or both, are administered.

NURSING IMPLICATIONS

Virtually all the nursing interventions noted earlier for preventing mild hypoglycemia apply to preventing overdose-related hypoglycemia. Teach patients and their families to react properly and promptly (and call for help) at the first signs of potential overdose. Advise all patients to carry some form of simple sugar at all times, but discuss with the physician the feasibility of prescribing a glucagon emergency kit (a vial of glucagon and a syringe prefilled with the proper diluent) for patients at great risk of profound hypoglycemia. If they are prescribed, explain their proper use to the patient and family.

Health-care providers should be familiar with the signs and symptoms of insulin-induced hypoglycemia and of diabetic ketoacidosis to facilitate proper diagnosis and the prompt administration of proper care.

Oral Hypoglycemic Drugs

Several orally effective drugs that lower blood glucose levels have essential rôles in the treatment of diabetes. All share a common mechanism of action that depends on the presence of reasonable amounts of endogenous insulin. Because of this, they are not suitable for treating the majority of patients with Type I (IDDM) diabetes mellitus, in whom insulin levels are very low or lacking altogether.

Sulfonylureas

The therapeutically useful oral hypoglycemic drugs are classified chemically as sulfonylureas. The historical prototype is tolbutamide. Related agents are acetohexamide, chlorpropamide, and tolazamide, which have been in use for many years. Two newer ("second-generation") sulfonylureas, usually preferred because of a lesser risk of drug interactions, are glipizide and glyburide. The dosages of these agents are summarized in Table 46–C2.

PROTOTYPE

Tolbutamide

Absorption, Distribution, Metabolism, and Excretion

Tolbutamide is quickly and almost completely absorbed after oral administration. More than 90% of tolbutamide molecules in the bloodstream are bound to plasma proteins. Tolbutamide is metabolized completely to inactive substances that are excreted by the kidneys. Tolbutamide is the shortest acting of the sulfonylureas, having a serum half-life of four to six hours in persons with normal hepatic function. Its average duration of action is six to 12 hours. Tolbutamide often is considered a preferred drug for patients with impaired renal function because of its short half-life and complete dependence on hepatic function for elimination. The related sulfonylureas, discussed later, differ in terms of their durations of action (Table 46–8), but they all depend on hepatic metabolism.

Pharmacologic Effects

All the oral hypoglycemic drugs lower blood glucose levels, but in a manner that is very different from that of insulin. On initial administration they increase pancreatic insulin release, although with continued administration insulin levels do not rise much above pretreatment values. More likely explanations of their actions are that they inhibit hepatic release of glucose; increase peripheral tissue sensitivity to insulin, probably by increasing the number of cell insulin receptors; and increase sensitivity of the β cells to the insulin-releasing effects of glucose. Although these drugs can lower blood glucose levels, there is no proof that they prevent the long-term cardiovascular or neurologic complications of diabetes.

Clinical Indications and Administration

Tolbutamide and related agents are indicated only for patients with Type II diabetes mellitus that cannot be controlled by diet or exercise alone, and such patients

Table 46–8 Pharmacokinetic Properties of Oral Hypoglycemic Drugs

Drug	Serum Half-life (hr)	Duration of Action (hr)	Fate, Usual Administration Times
Tolbutamide	4–5	6–12	Rapid hepatic metabolism; metabolites inactive, excreted in urine; short-acting; given in two (sometimes three) equal divided doses
			Related Drugs
Acetohexamide	6–8	12–24	Hepatic metabolism; major metabolite more active than parent drug; depends on renal excretion for termination of activity; intermediate-acting; once- or twice-daily administration
Chlorpropamide	36	≥60	Hepatic metabolism to less active substances excreted mainly in urine; long-acting; once-daily administration
Glipizide	2–4	10–24	Hepatic metabolism; metabolites inactive, excreted in urine; intermediate-acting; administered once or twice daily, depending on dose
Glyburide	~10	24	Hepatic metabolism; metabolites inactive, excreted in equal extent in urine, bile; intermediate-acting; usually given once daily
Tolazamide	7	12–24	Hepatic metabolism; major metabolites have some hypoglycemic activity, depend on renal excretion for elimination; usually administered once daily

who are not overweight or are overweight but refuse to diet. A daily insulin requirement of 40 U or less is usually another prerequisite, although some patients with insulin needs above this may be candidates for oral hypoglycemic drug therapy.

The oral hypoglycemics are not a substitute for insulin, and so are not used in drug therapy of Type I diabetes mellitus. More importantly, oral hypoglycemics should be used as adjuncts to diet and exercise, not as replacements for them.

Any oral hypoglycemic agent can be used as the first pharmacologic agent used to treat diabetes, but usually the patient's daily insulin needs should be determined first to be sure maintenance therapy with insulin is not required. When initial diabetes therapy is begun with tolbutamide, the usual daily starting dose is 1 to 2 g. Thereafter, based on the patient's response, the maintenance dose (Table 46–C2) can be established with gradual dosage adjustments. Weight reduction, which appears to increase the number of cell insulin receptors or increase their sensitivity to insulin, is a valuable therapeutic aid to keep dosages of any antidiabetic drug as low as possible.

If the patient is started on insulin, and the daily insulin requirement is less than 20 U, insulin administration can be stopped abruptly on the day oral hypoglycemic therapy begins. If daily insulin requirements are between 20 and 40 U, a 30% to 50% reduction in the previous insulin dose is given along with the first day's tolbutamide dose. Insulin doses then are tapered gradually until the effects of the oral agent appear, at which time insulin administration is stopped. For those patients requiring more than 40 U of insulin per day, the insulin dose is reduced by 20% on the first day, followed by gradual discontinuation over several days.

Patients also may be switched to tolbutamide after starting therapy with another oral hypoglycemic drug. It is acceptable to stop administration of most other agents abruptly, and directly begin therapy with another drug such as tolbutamide. The related sulfonylurea, chlorpropamide, is an exception. It is discussed separately on page 935. Starting doses of the new agent should be low, and blood glucose should be checked several times a day for the first week or two after the switch.

The effectiveness of tolbutamide and related drugs can vary with time. For example, enhanced effects are likely during the first four to six weeks of treatment. An apparent loss of efficacy may occur, often after about a year of treatment. One explanation for this is accelerated metabolic inactivation of the drug. If this occurs, two options are to increase the dose and assess its effects, or switch to another oral hypoglycemic.

Many patients who do not respond adequately to

tolbutamide may respond to one of the related oral hypoglycemic drugs. At any time during oral hypoglycemic therapy, factors such as infections, trauma, or other illnesses may necessitate the use of supplemental insulin, at least temporarily.

NURSING IMPLICATIONS

The daily dose of tolbutamide can be administered all at once or in divided doses. Splitting the dose, and administering doses shortly after meals, help reduce GI upset, a relatively common side effect. Impaired hepatic function, and to a lesser extent renal dysfunction, may cause accumulation of hypoglycemic drugs or their metabolites. This will require extra monitoring for adverse reactions, including excessive hypoglycemic effects, and possibly a dosage reduction.

If the patient is switched from insulin to an oral hypoglycemic drug, or from one oral agent to another, blood testing should be performed three times daily during the transition period. If ketonuria or hyperglycemia persist, the oral hypoglycemic drug should be discontinued and insulin therapy restarted, at least until the cause of the failure can be determined and corrected.

Advise patients of the continued need for prescribed diet and exercise, and the probable need for insulin during stressful times or illness. To assess the initial response to oral hypoglycemic drug therapy, instruct the patient to contact the physician or nurse daily with the results of blood and urine tests during the first month of therapy. Advise patients to keep scheduled appointments for physical examinations; usually these are done weekly for the first month, and monthly thereafter for the duration of therapy.

Side Effects, Adverse Reactions, and Contraindications

Most unwanted responses to sulfonylurea therapy are transient and dose-related (Table 46–S2). The overall incidence of side effects is about 5% to 10%, and is greatest with long-acting drugs such as chlorpropamide.

Signs and symptoms often reflect GI upset, and include nausea; vomiting or diarrhea; heartburn or abdominal pain; and, occasionally, GI bleeding. Some of these problems may arise from the drug's ability to increase gastric secretory activity.

Common central nervous system (CNS) manifestations include confusion, vertigo, and ataxia (most common with large doses of chlorpropamide).

More severe responses include hepatic dysfunction, manifested as altered liver function tests and cholestatic jaundice. Cardiomyopathy may occur, largely as a consequence of prolonged drug use.

Severe hypoglycemia, an exaggeration of expected drug action, is uncommon except with overdoses. Common causes other than true overdose include inadequate food intake, excessive exercise, or the use of other drugs that lower blood glucose levels—the same as noted for insulin. With tolbutamide, which depends on hepatic inactivation, age, excessive alcohol intake, and hepatotoxicity caused by other drugs will increase the risk of hypoglycemia.

Tolbutamide and the related drug chlorpropamide appear to stimulate release of antidiuretic hormone (ADH; vasopressin). The hormone acts on the kidney's collecting ducts, causing water retention. The consequences include increased blood volume and pressure, hyponatremia (blood sodium concentration is reduced because of the extra retained water), reduced serum osmolality, and a concentrated urine. This untoward response is of most concern to patients with heart failure, hypertension, or hepatic cirrhosis.

Miscellaneous but uncommon adverse responses to tolbutamide include goiter or blood dyscrasias, including thrombocytopenia, leukopenia, and anemia. These are usually reversible on discontinuation of the drug.

Allergic reactions can occur. They usually involve urticaria or other rashes. Fever, eosinophilia, jaundice, and perhaps blood dyscrasias also may reflect allergic reactions. They require immediate evaluation; if allergy is documented, further use of the offending drug is contraindicated.

There is some evidence that patients with diabetes receiving long-term (five to eight years) tolbutamide plus dietary therapy have a significantly higher risk of sudden cardiac death than an otherwise similar group treated with diet alone. The data are controversial, and there is little explanation for the phenomenon. It is not known whether the risk applies to all oral hypoglycemic drugs. Nevertheless, one important implication is that the cardiovascular risks of oral hypoglycemic drug therapy should be weighed against the potential benefits, and against the risks and benefits of using diet alone.

Overall, oral hypoglycemics should not be used for persons with Type II diabetes that can be controlled with diet and exercise alone. Oral hypoglycemic drugs are ineffective, and contraindicated, in most patients with Type I diabetes and in all patients with diabetic ketoacidosis (with or without coma).

NURSING IMPLICATIONS

Assess for signs and symptoms of the adverse responses noted earlier, and teach patients to assess for and report them. Extra assessment is required for patients with heart failure, hypertension, or cirrhosis, to detect an antidiuretic effect. Manifestations may include weight gain, dyspnea, and increased blood pressure. Assess for lethargy, listlessness, or drowsiness, which may indicate hyponatremia. Notify the physician if any of these responses occur. Inquire about the development of GI distress, and recommend taking the drug shortly after meals. If this does not alleviate the problem, consult with the physician about the suitability of administering divided doses (where appropriate for the drug). All precautions noted for detecting and managing hypoglycemia during insulin apply also to the use of oral hypoglycemic agents.

◆ Use During Pregnancy and Lactation

Oral hypoglycemic agents should not be used during pregnancy. If diet alone will control diabetes during pregnancy, that is the preferred approach. Of the available oral drugs, the related agent glyburide appears to carry the lowest risk of pregnancy-related adverse effects. Overall, however, insulin is the safest choice when antidiabetic drug therapy is required during pregnancy.

If oral hypoglycemic therapy is continued during pregnancy, attempts should be made to discontinue their administration, and switch to insulin if needed, during the last two weeks before the due date. The long-acting drugs chlorpropamide and glipizide generally should be discontinued one month before parturition.

If oral hypoglycemic drugs are administered through labor, anticipate and assess for prolonged hypoglycemia in the newborn. Breast-feeding should be discouraged if oral hypoglycemic drug therapy is necessary. This is another instance in which insulin has an advantage.

◆ Use in Children

There is little solid information about the safety and effectiveness of oral hypoglycemic drugs in children. Since diabetes in children is usually Type I, oral hypoglycemic agents would not be indicated.

◆ Use in the Elderly

Additional concerns regarding the use of oral hypoglycemic drugs in the elderly patient are the potential difficulty in maintaining adequate diet and exercise, age-related declines in drug metabolism or excretion; the prevalance of heart failure or other disorders that may be worsened by an antidiuretic effect; and the prevalence of other disorders that might require therapy with interacting drugs.

Interactions with Other Drugs

Many of the drugs cited in Table 46–11 as interactants with insulin also interact with the oral hypoglycemics (Table 46–12). They include alcohol, aspirin and other salicylates, β-adrenergic blockers, clofibrate, thiazide diuretics, and monoamine oxidase inhibitors. The causes and outcomes of the interactions are similar to those noted for insulin: the interactants increase or decrease blood glucose levels; potentiate or counteract effects of the oral hypoglycemic; and lead to inconsistent control of diabetes.

Several other drugs that do not interact with insulin, or interact in ways that probably are not clinically significant, can cause problems with oral hypoglycemic therapy. These include the antimicrobial agents chloramphenicol, some of the sulfonamides, and rifampin. They alter the hypoglycemic drug's hepatic metabolism, or the ability of the hypoglycemic agent to bind to plasma proteins. The usual outcome of administering one of these interactants is an increased or excessive hypoglycemic response unless dosages of one or both drugs are adjusted properly. Oral hypoglycemics also interact with oral anticoagulants, leading to a potentially excessive effect of the anticoagulant.

Alcohol intolerance is an interesting and important interaction that involves tolbutamide and other "first-generation" sulfonylureas. These drugs have a disulfiram-like action (see Chapter 22) to inhibit a crucial step of alcohol metabolism, leading to accumulation of acetaldehyde, a toxic intermediate. Headache and facial flushing are some of the milder consequences of this interaction. More dangerous responses include severe dyspnea, hypotension, and shock. Since alcohol not only interacts in this way, but also can interfere with hypoglycemic drug metabolism and can lower blood glucose levels, discourage alcohol use, especially in excess.

Overdose and Toxicity

The major concern with an overdose of any oral hypoglycemic drug, as with insulin, is hypoglycemia and its many consequences. Induced emesis (as permitted by the patient's level of consciousness and gag reflexes) and gastric lavage are important adjuncts for managing recent overdoses. Otherwise, treatment is the same as noted for insulin: temporary discontinuation of the drug, dietary modifications, and, if hypoglycemia is severe, administration of parenteral glucose. Intensive-care monitoring and treatment will be required for a few days.

Related Drugs

There are five sulfonylureas in addition to tolbutamide. Three of them are older, or "first-generation" agents. They are very similar to the prototype in terms of uses, desired and side effects, and drug-drug interactions. Dosages for these drugs are summarized in Table 46–C2, and their pharmacokinetic properties are compared in Table 46–8.

Other First-Generation Sulfonylureas

Acetohexamide

Acetohexamide (DYMELOR) has an intermediate duration of action (12 to 24 hours) in persons with normal renal and hepatic function. As with tolbutamide, the drug is metabolized extensively. However, acetohexamide is converted to an active metabolite that depends on renal excretion for its elimination. Thus, either hepatic or renal dysfunction will require dosage adjustments to optimize blood glucose control. Otherwise, acetohexamide is unremarkable.

Chlorpropamide

Chlorpropamide (DIABINESE) has the longest duration of action of all the oral hypoglycemic drugs. The biologic half-life is about 36 hours, and hypoglycemic effects may last up to 60 hours after a dose. The vast majority of the drug in the bloodstream is bound to plasma proteins. Chlorpropamide is eliminated in the urine after prior metabolism.

Chlorpropamide's long duration of action, and the resulting steady effect once the proper dose and dosage schedule have been established, makes the drug advantageous for patients who have extremely stable blood glucose levels. However, it becomes a disadvantage for patients who have unstable or frequently changing blood glucose levels.

The long half-life accounts for other drawbacks. Chlorpropamide blood levels, and the related effects on blood glucose levels, will require more than a week to stabilize once treatment starts. That is much longer than with any other oral hypoglycemic agent. Thus, there is an appreciable lag time between dosage increases and corresponding falls of blood glucose levels. Conversely, chlorpropamide's long duration of action can be more problematic if the patient experiences hypoglycemia in response to an excessive dose or overdose, or because of drug interactions. With this drug it will take much longer for blood glucose levels to rise toward normal than it would if another oral hypoglycemic drug had been the cause of the problem. Obviously, glucose will be administered in such situations to correct blood glucose levels, but this treatment (and other supportive measures) will have to continue for a longer time until chlorpropamide is cleared from the patient's circulatory system. Patients with severe chlorpropamide overdoses may require a week or more of intensive care.

Chlorpropamide's slow onset of action and long duration also necessitate extra care, monitoring, and patience, when switching the patient to or from insulin, or to or from another oral hypoglycemic agent. For example, if the patient were to be switched from tolbutamide to another agent with a comparably short duration of action (eg, glipizide; see below and Table 46–8), the tolbutamide dose could be stopped abruptly, or at least tapered quickly, as glipizide treatment is begun simultaneously. A similar situation would apply when starting tolbutamide therapy after an initial trial of insulin.

However, if the switch were to chlorpropamide, there would have to be much more overlap in the administration of both drugs, and slower tapering of the shorter-acting tolbutamide's dosage. This more gradual switch is needed to maintain good blood glucose control with the original agent as effective blood levels of the chlorpropamide are reached slowly.

Despite these limitations, chlorpropamide is an effective drug, and with proper management is as safe as any other sulfonylurea. Indeed, it is a preferred agent by some physicians.

All drug interactions noted for tolbutamide apply to chlorpropamide. Alcohol intolerance may be more pronounced with chlorpropamide. Chlorpropamide also has a marked ability to stimulate release of antidiuretic hormone; direct additional monitoring toward assessing for weight gain, hypertension, worsening of heart failure, and hyponatremia.

Tolazamide

Tolazamide (TOLINASE) has a short to intermediate duration of action, up to about 14 hours. It is metabolized extensively in the liver to several compounds, all of which are less active as hypoglycemic agents that tolazamide itself. Otherwise, there is little that is remarkable about tolazamide.

Second-Generation Sulfonylureas

Glipizide and Glyburide

Glipizide (GLUCOTROL) and glyburide (DIABETA, MICRONASE) are the newer oral hypoglycemic drugs. They are, on the average, about 100 times more potent than the first-generation agents. That does not mean they are 100 times more effective, but rather that 2.5 mg of one of the newer agents tends to cause effects that are roughly equal to 250 mg of an agent such as tolbutamide. Overall, this potency difference is not important as long as the proper dosage (see Table 46–C2) is used.

The more important differences relate to their durations of action, side effects, and drug interactions. Glipizide and glyburide have durations of action on the order of 24 hours. Thus, whereas some of the older agents may need to be given twice daily, once daily dosing is clearly adequate with the newer drugs. This may help compliance.

The side effects profile for the second-generation sulfonylureas is generally the same as for the older drugs. However, glipizide and glyburide tend to cause these unwanted responses less often, and they tend to be milder. Likewise, drug interactions noted for the prototype apply, but they also tend to be less common and less intense. This includes less severe alcohol intolerance, which can be of significant value to patients who wish to consume small and otherwise safe amounts of alcohol occasionally. It can be critically important for patients who wish not or are unable to abstain from alcohol altogether. Nevertheless, all the precautions and nursing implications noted for tolbutamide apply to these newer drugs.

Glipizide may help prevent a potentially serious interaction in a patient trying to maintain what they consider to be a normal lifestyle. Glipizide does not eliminate either the dangers of alcohol-induced hepatic damage or alcohol's ability to cause hypoglycemia, especially in the presence of another hypoglycemic drug.

Glipizide is bound extensively to plasma protein, and is almost completely dependent on hepatic metabolism to inactive products for termination of its activity.

Food delays glipizide absorption, so the drug should be taken about 30 minutes before eating. Encourage patients to be consistent in their timing of meals and drug administration.

Glyburide is absorbed well, and a major portion of the drug is eliminated in the bile and urine. Like other sulfonylureas, glyburide binds extensively to plasma proteins. However, the type of binding is different from that of the others. Glyburide is not displaced easily by aspirin and other nonsteroidal antiinflammatory drugs, nor by oral anticoagulants. Theoretically, this suggests that interactions with these drugs are less likely to occur. Nevertheless, all the precautions noted above for similar drug interactions should be taken when glyburide is used.

Biguanides

Two oral hypoglycemic drugs, phenformin and metformin, are chemically classified as biguanides. They were once available in the United States, but are no longer available routinely because they were implicated in the development of fatal lactic acidosis. Because they may be effective in a highly specialized group of patients with Type II diabetes, mainly those who fail to respond to the sulfonylureas, they are available only on written request to the manufacturer.

IV. Hypoglycemia and Its Treatment

Hypoglycemia is characterized by blood sugar levels of 40 mg/dL or less, but symptoms begin to occur at levels below 80 mg/dL. Clinically documented cases of hypoglycemia usually occur in persons with diabetes who have taken overdoses of insulin or oral hypoglycemic drugs, or have taken usual doses at times when blood glucose levels have fallen dramatically for such reasons as exercise, inadequate food intake, drugs, and other factors noted earlier. The metabolic consequences of hypoglycemia, and its various signs and symptoms, also have been discussed.

Diagnosis and Management

In diagnosing hypoglycemia consider whether it occurs in the fasting state (solely or in conjunction with the administration of hypoglycemic agents or drugs that antagonize the effects of a hypoglycemic agent), or after a meal.

A failure of insulin levels to decrease as glucose levels fall indicates inappropriate insulin secretion. Fasting blood glucose levels of 40 to 60 mg/dL, accompanied by episodes of confusion, often indicate islet-cell dysfunction. Symptomatic relief within minutes of oral or IV glucose administration almost always confirms this diagnosis. Tumors such as fibrosarcomas and mesotheliomas are responsible for some cases of hypoglycemia in middle-aged or elderly patients. If possible, surgery is indicated for the removal of such insulin-secreting tumors.

Alcohol ingestion in fasting individuals induces hypoglycemia because hepatic alcohol metabolism interferes with the liver's ability to perform gluconeogenesis. The obvious solution is abstinence, but this is often difficult to achieve. Secondary hypoglycemia occurs in acute liver failure, congestive heart failure, and uncontrolled leukemia, but in these cases the primary disease usually is apparent.

Postprandial hypoglycemia routinely occurs in patients who have had total gastrectomy surgery. As noted earlier, it also is displayed in certain individuals who produce excessive insulin after food ingestion (reactive hypoglycemics). Such cases are managed by dietary measures—several small meals with low concentrations of rapidly absorbed carbohydrates.

Hypoglycemia also may result from the production of antiinsulin antibodies. Periodic dissociation of insulin from its antibodies can cause periods of insulin "excess" and hypoglycemia. This situation is fairly common in patients receiving animal insulins, but may occur in patients who have never received exogenous insulin.

Three major clinical approaches are used to increase blood glucose levels in hypoglycemic episodes. The most common method is oral or IV administration of concentrated glucose solutions. Drugs that effectively increase blood sugar include glucagon and diazoxide.

PROTOTYPE

Glucagon

Glucagon is a polypeptide hormone produced by the α cells of the pancreatic islets. As with insulin, glucagon released from the pancreas enters the hepatic portal system first. Unlike insulin, however, virtually all the released glucagon acts in the liver to stimulate glycogenolysis, and is metabolized in the liver so that little or none reaches the systemic circulation. The gastric and duodenal mucosae also produce a glucagon-like hormone in response to ingestion of glucose or sugary foods. Glucagon isolated from animal sources, used as a therapeutic product, exerts effects identical to those of endogenous glucagon.

It appears that glucagon release is affected by circulating insulin levels and is connected intimately to disorders of insulin hypo- or hypersecretion. Hypoglycemia is caused primarily by excessive insulin, and glucagon may be used to treat it.

Absorption, Distribution, Metabolism, and Excretion

Glucagon is inactivated in the GI tract, and so is ineffective when given orally. Administered parenterally, glucagon has a plasma half-life of three to six minutes. It is metabolized and excreted in the same manner as endogenous glucagon.

Pharmacologic Effects

In addition to the effects of endogenous glucagon, discussed above, exogenously administered glucagon also increases the force of cardiac contraction (a positive inotropic effect), but does not appear to increase the tendency toward arrhythmias. These effects are not prevented by β-blocking agents. Parenteral glucagon also relaxes smooth muscle in the GI tract.

Clinical Indications and Administration

Treatment of Hypoglycemia

Glucagon is used in conjunction with glucose to manage acute hypoglycemic reactions (Table 46–C3). It may be the sole hyperglycemic agent administered when glucose administration is not possible, such as in the management of a hypoglycemic episode in a person with Type I diabetes who becomes unconscious or comatose at home. Since glucagon's hyperglycemic action depends on adequate hepatic glycogen stores, it is of little value in persons with chronic hypoglycemia, adrenal insufficiency, or prolonged starvation.

Glucagon dosages are listed in Table 46–C3. The response to glucagon, indicated by a rise in blood glucose levels, generally occurs within five to 20 minutes. Unresponsive individuals may need a second (or third) dose. If there is still no response after a third dose, glucose must be administered, if possible, to prevent brain damage. Since blood glucose levels eventually again fall to normal or hypoglycemic levels within one to two hours, the initial glucagon or glucagon-dextrose therapy must be followed by administration of glucose to prevent later unconsciousness or coma.

Other Uses

Glucagon is indicated for relaxing portions of the GI tract to facilitate certain radiologic examinations, for which the drug is injected intramuscularly (IM) or IV (see Table 46–C3). The onset of action after IM injection is usually between five and 10 minutes; effects appear almost immediately after IV injection. Ordinarily, effects last about 15 minutes with either administration route.

Side Effects, Adverse Reactions, and Contraindications

With the exception of occasional nausea and vomiting, which appear to be dose-related, there are few reported adverse responses to glucagon. Hypotensive reactions are uncommon. The most serious adverse response is an allergic reaction, which contraindicates further use of the drug. Allergic reactions to the parenteral use of other animal-derived proteins may predict an allergic response to glucagon.

Pheochromocytomas or insulin-secreting tumors are relative contraindications to glucagon use. In persons with pheochromocytoma, glucagon can cause sudden catecholamine release and severe hypertension or cardiac stimulation. In persons with insulinomas, glucagon will increase blood glucose levels. This may indirectly cause further insulin release and trigger profound hypoglycemia.

NURSING IMPLICATIONS

Glucagon is supplied as a freeze-dried powder that can be kept at room temperature prior to reconstitution. One mg of glucagon is equivalent to 1 U. Use the manufacturer's diluent when the total glucagon dose is likely to be 2 U or less. Use sterile water for injection when higher doses are needed. Never prepare glucagon in, or add to, solutions containing chloride, since the drug will precipitate. Do not prepare glucagon solutions that are stronger than 1 U per mL. Reconstituted glucagon solutions should be clear and colorless. They may be stored in a refrigerator for up to 48 hours.

Patients with Type I diabetes and their families should be taught the signs and symptoms of hypoglycemia, and how to reconstitute and administer glucagon. Emergency kits that contain a vial of glucagon (1 U) and a syringe prefilled with suitable diluent are available by prescription.

Whenever glucagon is administered, assess for signs and symptoms of allergic reactions; give patients and their families similar assessment information. Whenever glucagon must be administered in an outpatient setting, the patient should receive professional follow-up care. Expect that any use of glucagon for treating hypoglycemia will require subsequent testing of blood glucose levels, and may require administration of oral or parenteral glucose once glucagon's effects have waned, about one to two hours later.

◆ Use During Pregnancy and Lactation

No information is available about the safety of glucagon when administered to pregnant women. Glucagon administration should not be withheld during pregnancy to treat acute hypoglycemia. Glucagon should be administered cautiously during breast-feeding, since it is not known whether the drug is excreted in breast milk. Since glucagon is inactivated rapidly in the GI tract, effects are not likely to be great or prolonged even if the infant were to ingest the drug.

◆ Use in Children and the Elderly

There are no special age-related implications for glucagon.

Overdose and Toxicity

The major consequences of glucagon overdoses are hyperglycemia, hypokalemia, nausea, and vomiting. The drug's plasma half-life is about five minutes, so none of the effects should be long lasting. The major intervention is to monitor serum potassium levels (and correct them as needed), and to make the patient comfortable until nausea and vomiting subside.

Other Hyperglycemic Drugs

Diazoxide

Diazoxide is related chemically to thiazide diuretics, and is unrelated chemically to glucagon. Its oral dosage form, PROGLYCEM, is used to treat chronic hypoglycemia. The parenteral dosage form of diazoxide, HYPERSTAT, is used to treat malignant hypertension, as discussed in Chapter 33.

Absorption, Distribution, Metabolism, and Excretion

Orally administered diazoxide is absorbed rapidly. It is bound extensively to plasma proteins, and is eliminated mainly by renal excretion without prior metabolism.

Diazoxide's plasma half-life is about one day in persons with normal renal function.

Pharmacologic Effects

Diazoxide causes dose-dependent increases in blood glucose levels by stimulating epinephrine release from the adrenal medulla, inhibiting insulin release, increasing hepatic release of glucose, inhibiting glucose by peripheral tissues, and enhancing fat mobilization.

Other important pharmacologic effects include cardiac stimulation and relaxation of vascular smooth muscle. This latter effect accounts for the parenteral use of diazoxide to treat malignant hypertension (see Chapter 33). However, hypotension is not likely to occur with oral diazoxide. Diazoxide exerts important effects on the kidneys. Like the thiazide diuretics, it reduces renal excretion of uric acid. But unlike the thiazides, diazoxide reduces renal sodium excretion, which indirectly causes renal water retention.

Clinical Indications and Administration

Oral diazoxide is used to manage hypoglycemia of organic cause, such as that arising from insulin-producing tumors (pancreatic islet-cell tumors and extrapancreatic malignancies) that have failed to respond to surgery or irradiation (see Table 46–C3 for dosages). The hyperglycemic effect begins in about one hour and lasts for about eight hours in persons with normal renal function.

Side Effects, Adverse Reactions, and Contraindications

The most common adverse effect caused by oral diazoxide is sodium and water retention, which may cause or worsen heart failure or hypertension (Table 46–S3). This may be alleviated with diuretics, but as noted later, other problems arising from a drug interaction may occur. Use extreme care when diazoxide is given to patients with hypertension or cardiac failure.

A less common but equally serious adverse response is hyperglycemia complicated by ketoacidosis. Coma may occur, and must be managed as for treatment of regular diabetic ketoacidosis (insulin, fluids, electrolytes). Since diazoxide has a long half-life, prolonged monitoring is necessary. More often, diazoxide causes hyperglycemia that is moderate but still sufficient to cause glycosuria. If persistent, the diazoxide dose should be reduced. Impaired renal function also requires reduced doses of diazoxide and close monitoring.

Nausea, vomiting, and other manifestations of GI upset may occur, particularly with high-dose therapy. Cardiovascular effects such as hypotension, tachycardia, and palpitations may occur, but they are far more common when diazoxide is administered parenterally. Hirsutism, thrombocytopenia (with or without purpura), and neutropenia may occur. Hyperuricemia is another potential consequence, and it requires cautious use of diazoxide in persons with a history of hyperuricemia or gout. There have been reports of ocular changes such as transient cataracts or diplopia, skin rashes, and occasional neurologic abnormalities such as paresthesias, extrapyramidal tract disorders, and neuritis.

The major contraindications for oral diazoxide are functional hypoglycemia and a history of allergic reactions to thiazide diuretics.

NURSING IMPLICATIONS

Always carefully obtain an initial history to rule out contraindications and to identify interacting drugs or medical conditions that may increase the risk of untoward responses. Supervise patients closely during initial diazoxide treatment, with emphasis placed on monitoring blood glucose and electrolyte levels and blood pressure.

Alert patients to the signs and symptoms of hyperglycemia, and teach them simple ways to test urinary glucose and ketone levels. Advise them of potential adverse responses to this drug, and encourage them to report such responses at once. Instruct patients using the oral suspension to shake the bottle well before dispensing the drug.

◆ Use During Pregnancy and Lactation

Diazoxide should not be used during pregnancy unless absolutely necessary. The drug crosses the placenta and can exert adverse effects on the fetus. There have been reports of fetal or neonatal hyperbilirubinemia, thrombocytopenia, altered carbohydrate metabolism, and other adverse responses like those occurring in adults. Alopecia and unusually heavy growth of the lanugo (*hypertrichosis lanuginosa*) have been reported when diazoxide was administered to women during the last two months of pregnancy. Intravenous administration of diazoxide during labor may inhibit uterine contractions. It is not known whether oral diazoxide will do the same, but if the drug must be given at this time, monitor uterine motility; oxytocic drugs may be necessary.

◆ Use in Children

Infants are more prone to sodium and water retention and their consequences than older children. In addition to regular monitoring for untoward and expected responses, assess closely and frequently for evidence of fluid retention, including excessive or rapid weight gain.

◆ Use in the Elderly

The prevalence of cardiovascular disease, renal disease, and hyperuricemia requires added caution when diazoxide is administered to elderly persons. More frequent physical assessments and laboratory tests are recommended.

Interactions with Other Drugs

Diuretics appear to be reasonable drugs to manage diazoxide-induced sodium and water retention, but they interact to increase the risk of hyperglycemia and hyperuricemia. This is particularly true for the thiazides. Overall, if this drug combination must be used, close monitoring of blood glucose and uric acid levels is imperative.

Diazoxide may stimulate the metabolism or excretion of phenytoin, leading to loss of seizure control. In general, diazoxide potentiates the effects of other drugs that elevate blood glucose levels, and antagonizes the effects of those that lower blood glucose levels (mainly insulin). Diazoxide also antagonizes the effects of oral hypoglycemic drugs, and the effects of each may be reduced if they are administered together. With this interaction, it appears that hyperglycemia is the most likely outcome. The important interactions involving diazoxide are summarized in Table 46–13.

Overdose and Toxicity

The most serious concerns with oral diazoxide overdoses are hyperglycemia and ketoacidosis. Cautious administration of insulin, and correction of serum electrolytes, are indicated. Diazoxide's long half-life necessitates intensive monitoring and treatment of overdoses for as long as a week.

SUMMARY OF NURSING IMPLICATIONS

◆ Assessment

Obtain a complete nursing history to include: patient preferences for dietary changes (cultural and religious); daily routine; current medical management of disease; patient responses to hypo- or hyperglycemic episodes; contraindicated drugs; allergies to pork- or beef-derived drugs.

Identify areas that could limit the patient's self-care abilities: stress level, learning ability, physical dexterity, visual deficits, sensory impairment.

Assess financial/insurance resources: ability to cover cost of medication, equipment for testing, supplies; ability to afford prescribed diet.

Recognize signs and symptoms of hyperglycemia (including diabetic ketoacidosis) or hypoglycemia (including insulin shock).

◆ Nursing Diagnoses

Ineffective individual coping related to chronic disease and therapy.

High risk for injury related to glucose intolerance, vascular impairment, infection.

Knowledge deficit related to diabetes, drug therapy, dietary restrictions.

Sensory/perceptual alterations related to blindness, neuropathies.

Altered tissue perfusion related to atherosclerosis: occlusive disease leading to gangrene, myocardial infarction, stroke.

High risk for infection related to diabetes mellitus.

Altered nutrition: more than or less than body requirements related to metabolic imbalance or lack of dietary control.

◆ Planning/Implementation

Instruct patient and family in the pathophysiology of diabetes, safe administration of insulin, blood and urine testing, dietary management, skin and foot care, signs and symptoms of insulin reaction or hyperglycemia.

Administer insulin at the same time daily, 15 to 30 minutes before a meal.

Rotate injection sites; use upper outer aspect of upper arms, back, abdomen (avoid area 1½ in. around umbilicus), upper thighs, and buttocks. Allow at least four to six weeks before reusing the same area if possible. When hospitalization is necessary, use sites not easily reached by patient.

Provide source of simple sugar in the event of hypoglycemia (sugar cubes, hard candy, commercial preparations.)

Establish guidelines for patient to follow if illness occurs: do not omit insulin; ingest liquid carbohydrates if unable to eat; increase frequency of blood and urine testing to at least four times daily; notify physician if vomiting or diarrhea occur or illness lasts more than two days.

◆ Evaluation

The patient/family will:

Comply with medical regimen; blood glucose and urine sugar and acetone indicate diabetic control.

Demonstrate ability to self-administer insulin, test blood and/or urine, plan a balanced diet, and care for skin (particularly feet).

Experience few episodes of metabolic imbalance; recognize and report signs and symptoms of hyperglycemia or hypoglycemia.

Experience minimal or no long-term complications.

Accept need for lifelong adjustments and therapy.

Annotated Bibliography

Anderson JH, Campbell RK: Mixing insulins in 1990. *Diabetes Educ* 1990;16(5):380–387. *Excellent text and tables on how to mix and store insulins the right, easy way; important advice for nurses and patients alike.*

Bubb JA, Pontious SL: Weight loss from inappropriate insulin manipulation: An eating disorder variant in an adolescent with insulin-dependent diabetes mellitus. *Diabetes Educ* 1991;17(1):29–32. *An interesting case of substance use; the paper describes the assessment, diagnosis, and treatment of a young woman with IDDM who manipulated her insulin inappropriately to lose weight.*

Campbell RK: The changing insulin market. *Diabetes Educ* 1991; 17(6):496–498, 500. *Discusses reasons for discontinuing U-40 and protamine zinc insulins, and how this can influence health-care providers and insulin users; notes new insulins that are likely to be approved; reviews overall therapy goals, regardless of which insulin is used.*

Diabetes Educator and *Diabetes Care. Consult these journals for the latest information about drug therapy and other aspects of diabetes care, especially patient teaching information. Some recent articles are cited in this bibliography, but there are too many more to mention individually.*

Francisco GE: Antidiabetic agents. *Prim Care* 1990;17(3):499–519. *Careful attention to initial assessment of patients with diabetes and establishment of drug requirements and maintenance therapy to tailor drug administration to the patient's needs. Includes valuable guidelines for adequate glucose control, and identifies problems when the goal for control is too tight.*

Guthrie DW, Guthrie RA: Approach to management. *Diabetes Educ* 1990;16(5):401–406. *Plan for your patient's changing insulin needs—don't just react to what's happened. This paper considers the physiology of glucose control and stresses the importance of intensive patient education, intelligent self-management, and frequent blood glucose monitoring.*

Hollander P: Premixed insulins. How do they compare with other insulin preparations? *Postgrad Med* 1991;89(4):52–54, 57–58, 61. *Practical information about how premixed NFH and regular insulin can be an asset to diabetes caregivers and recipients alike.*

Katz CM: How efficient is sliding-scale insulin therapy? Problems with a "cookbook" approach in hospitalized patients. *Postgrad Med* 1991;89(5):46–48, 51–54, 57. *Sliding-scale insulin therapy often is used but is seldom the best way to treat hospitalized patients with diabetes. Describes when it is appropriate, how to manage it optimally, and how to organize alternative approaches that might be more effective and efficient.*

McAvoy KH: Oral hypoglycemic agents in the management of non-insulin–dependent diabetes mellitus among the elderly. *Diabetes Educ* 1991;17(5):411–413. *A useful review of pitfalls of diabetes therapy in elders, and how good assessment skills can help prevent complications.*

Sann L: Neonatal hypoglycemia. *Biol Neonate* 1990;58 Suppl 1:16–21. *Discusses unique features of neonatal hypoglycemia and glucose metabolism, recommends lipid and triglyceride supplementation to prevent it.*

Stein PP, Black HR: Drug treatment of hypertension in patients with diabetes mellitus. *Diabetes Care* 1991;14(6):425–448. *Diabetes and hypertension often go hand in hand, and treating one can affect the other. This paper discusses the efficacy and side effects of various antihypertensive drug classes and suggests a stepped-care approach to drug treatment of patients with both disorders.*

Ulchaker MM, Sheehan JP: Iatrogenic brittle diabetes: The hold-the-insulin decision. *Diabetes Educ* 1991;17(2):111–113. *Discusses the potential catastrophic consequences of withholding insulins in patients dependent on multiple daily insulin injections.*

Zehrer, C, Hansen R, Bantle J: Reducing blood glucose variability by use of abdominal insulin injection sites. *Diabetes Educ* 1990; 16(6):474–477. *Varying rates of insulin absorption from SC injection sites may be the most important contributor to significant variability in blood glucose control. The authors advise patients with Type I diabetes not to use rotating injection sites on the extremities, but to confine sites to a single anatomic region (eg, the abdomen).*

Table 46–C1 Insulin Dosage Ranges

INDICATION	DOSE AND ROUTE OF ADMINISTRATION
Maintenance therapy of Type I diabetes mellitus Intermittent or temporary therapy for hospitalized patients, pregnant women, with Type II diabetes	SC (preferred) or IM: Adults, children: 0.5–1.0 U/kg/day; individualize dose, dosage schedule, usually to achieve preprandial and bedtime blood glucose levels of 100–140 mg/dL; see text for more information; Adolescents in growth spurt: 0.8–1.2 U/kg/day; individualize as above; adjust doses to maintain desired blood glucose levels
Diabetic ketoacidosis	(Regular insulin only): Adults: 25–150 U IV immediately, repeat hourly as needed; switch to SC q6h; or, 50–100 U IV plus 50–100 U SC, then additional SC doses q 2–6 hr as needed; or 5–10 U or 0.33 U/kg as IV bolus, then infuse 7–10 U/hr as needed; Children: 0.25–0.5 U/kg IV plus 0.25–0.5 U/kg SC, then 0.5–1 U/kg IV every 1–2 hr as needed; or: 0.1 U/kg IV bolus, then infuse 0.1 U/kg/hr until blood glucose reaches 250 mg/dL, then begin SC therapy as needed

Table 46–S1 Side Effects and Adverse Responses to Insulin

BODY SYSTEM/ Side Effect	CONTRAINDICATION/ PRECAUTION	COMMENTS AND NURSING IMPLICATIONS
METABOLIC Hypoglycemia		See Table 46–3 for signs, symptoms; usually caused by true overdose, missed meals, excessive exercise; other causes include SC administration in patients with low cardiac output, normalization of tissue perfusion leading to abrupt insulin absorption (give IM or IV instead); measure blood glucose, then administer fast-acting carbohydrate by route permitted by patient's condition; give carbohydrate first if glucose testing cannot be done immediately; assess further for cause(s)
Hyperglycemia		See Table 46–3 for signs, symptoms; usually caused by inadequate insulin dose or mix, may be caused by excessive carbohydrate intake, insulin resistance, repeated injection into dystrophic or hypoperfused tissue. Monitor blood glucose levels; anticipate need to give supplemental insulin, hydrate patient with oral or IV fluids/electrolytes depending on severity of response; assess further for cause(s)
IMMUNE Allergic reactions	Prior allergic reaction to same or similar insulin product	More likely with pork or beef insulins; do not readminister; switch to human insulin, but change and dosage adjustments must be supervised by physician
SKIN Lipodystrophy, lipoatrophy		Usually caused by failure to rotate SC injection sites properly and/or use of cold insulins; also may contribute to poor or erratic insulin response; reteach proper techniques

Table 46–I1 **Major Interactions Between Insulin and Other Agents**

AGENT	RESULT OF INTERACTION	COMMENTS AND NURSING IMPLICATIONS
Alcohol (Chapter 22)	Hypoglycemia, ketosis	Alcohol lowers blood glucose levels, particularly when large amounts are ingested acutely; calories provided by alcohol, and potential for inadequate diets with chronic alcoholism, further complicate diabetes management; discourage all alcohol use, or strive for the lowest acceptable alcohol intake
Aspirin, other salicylates (Chapter 52)	Possible potentiation of insulin-induced hypoglycemia	Salicylates increase baseline insulin levels, hypoglycemic response; supervised long-term salicylate therapy may allow reduced insulin dosages; haphazard (self-) administration can complicate insulin therapy, should be avoided; recommend acetaminophen or ibuprofen when OTC pain, fever relief is needed
Beta-adrenergic blockers (propranolol, most others; Chapter 15)	Increased risk of hypoglycemia, prolonged recovery from a hypoglycemic episode	Nonselective β blockers (all except atenolol and metoprolol) inhibit insulin release, have other effects that lower blood glucose levels; effects of nonselective blockers likely to be greatest in IDDM patients with some residual endogenous insulin release, and in patients with NIDDM; nonselective β blockers usually contraindicated in persons with diabetes; if β blocker therapy is essential, cardioselective agents (atenolol, metoprolol) may be preferred, but close, frequent monitoring of blood glucose levels is essential
Clofibrate (Chapter 36)	Increased sensitivity to insulin, risk of hypoglycemia	Clofibrate may lower blood glucose levels, requiring decreased insulin doses
Epinephrine, other β-adrenergic agonists (Chapter 14)	Increased blood glucose levels, poor control of diabetes	Interactants increase blood glucose levels; monitor if long-term therapy with interactant required (eg, sympathomimetic bronchodilators for pulmonary disease); increased insulin doses may be required
Fenfluramine, related anorexigenic drugs (Chapter 27)	Decreased blood glucose levels, increased risk of hypoglycemia	Anorexigenic drugs that may be prescribed as weight-reducing agents may lower blood glucose levels; interaction may be beneficial, allowing reduced insulin (or oral hypoglycemic drug) doses, or unwanted, if response is excessive; diet may require adjustments; monitor blood glucose levels frequently during combined therapy
Monoamine oxidase inhibitors (Chapter 24)	Decreased blood glucose levels, possible risk of hypoglycemia	Anticipate additive effect to lower blood glucose levels, need to reduce doses of hypoglycemic drugs (based on measurements of blood glucose levels), or increased dietary carbohydrate intake

Table 46–C2 Dose and Administration of Oral Hypoglycemic Drugs*

AGENT	DOSAGE AND ROUTE OF ADMINISTRATION
PROTOTYPE	
Tolbutamide (ORINASE)	Usually start with 1–2 g once daily (or in 2 equal divided doses if GI upset is a problem); maintenance doses 250 mg–3 g per day)
RELATED DRUGS	
Acetohexamide (DYMELOR)	Initially 250 mg once daily before breakfast; adjust as needed in 250–500 mg increments at 5–7 day intervals to maintenance dose, 250 mg–1.5 g per day; daily doses of 1 g or less can be taken once daily, higher doses may be split in two equal parts, administered before morning and evening meals
Chlorpropamide (DIABINESE)	Initially 250 mg once daily (100–125 mg per day for high-risk patients*); if needed, increase by no more than 50–125 mg at 3–5 day intervals; maintenance dose usually 250 mg once daily, may range from 100–500 mg once daily; should not exceed 750 mg per day
Glipizide (GLUCOTROL)	Initially 5 mg 30 min before breakfast (2.5 mg for high-risk patients*); as needed, increase dose in 2.5–5 mg increments at several day intervals to maintenance doses between 5 and 40 mg/day; daily doses >15 mg should be administered as 2 divided doses, one 30 min before breakfast, the other 30 min before the evening meal
Glyburide (DIABETA; MICRONASE)	Initially 2.5 or 5 mg once daily with breakfast or first main meal of day (1.25 mg for high-risk patients*); if needed, increase by no more than 2.5 mg per week to maintenance dose, 2.5–20 mg once daily
Tolazamide (TOLINASE)	Initially 100–250 mg with breakfast or first main meal of day (100 mg for elderly or high-risk patients); if needed, increase in 100–250 mg increments at weekly intervals; average maintenance dose 250–500 mg/day

*All doses are adult doses; not recommended for children. Use reduced doses for persons prone to hypoglycemia, including elderly or debilitated patients and those who are malnourished or eating poorly. See text for general strategies for switching from insulin to an oral hypoglycemic drug, or switching between oral hypoglycemics.

Table 46–S2 | Major Side Effects of and Contraindications for Oral Hypoglycemic Drugs

BODY SYSTEM/ Side Effect	CONTRAINDICATION/ PRECAUTION	COMMENTS AND NURSING IMPLICATIONS
CENTRAL NERVOUS SYSTEM Confusion, vertigo, ataxia		Risk may be greatest with large doses of chlorpropamide; patients with significant CNS symptoms should be assessed promptly for hypoglycemia, hyperglycemia, electrolyte imbalances
METABOLIC Hypoglycemia		In addition to overdoses and drug interactions, risk increased by excessive exercise, skipping meals, or poor nutrition; stress adherence with prescribed drug, diet, and exercise therapy; discourage alcohol use; teach patient/family ways to detect hypoglycemia; encourage patient to carry source of simple sugars (candy, commercial glucose supplements) at all times; emergency kits containing glucagon may be prescribed; if so, teach proper storage and use; encourage wearing of some identification tag indicating that the patient has diabetes
Hyperglycemia		Patients with widely fluctuating blood glucose levels periodically may require supplemental insulin, particularly during times of excessive physical or emotional stress; advise patients of this potential need, and the need to keep a supply of insulin if prescribed
CARDIOVASCULAR/ RENAL Renal sodium, water retention; dilutional hyponatremia (syndrome of inappropriate ADH secretion)	Heart failure, hypertension, and hepatic dysfunction necessitate care	Tolbutamide, chlorpropamide, possibly other sulfonylureas may stimulate ADH release; monitor body weight, blood pressure, serum electrolytes, and blood and urine osmolality periodically, assess for signs of heart failure; consider CNS, GI, or neuromuscular problems as potential reflections of hyponatremia caused by excessive water retention
Risk of sudden death		Some oral hypoglycemic drugs increase risk of sudden cardiac death compared with control group with similar blood glucose levels managed with only diet and exercise/weight reduction; it is not known whether problem applies to all sulfonylureas; patients should be advised of potential risks and benefits of therapy; oral hypoglycemics should be used only when necessary
GASTROINTESTINAL Nausea, vomiting, diarrhea; heartburn or epigastric distress	Peptic ulcer disease necessitates care	Timing of drug administration with respect to meals, dividing dose may alleviate problem; actual approach depends on offending drug; severe or persistent side effects require notification of physician; prophylactic antiulcer drug therapy (antacids, others) may be indicated in persons with ulcer disease, should be administered so that they do not interfere with absorption of oral hypoglycemic drug
OTHER Allergic reactions manifest as skin rashes, hepatotoxicity with or without jaundice, blood dyscrasias	Prior allergic reaction	Notify, advise patient to notify, physician at any sign of potential allergic reaction; other sulfonylureas may or may not exhibit cross-sensitivity with offending agent

Table 46–I2 **Major Interactions Between Oral Hypoglycemics and Other Agents**

AGENT	RESULT OF INTERACTION	COMMENTS AND NURSING IMPLICATIONS
Alcohol (Chapter 22)	Moderate to profound hypoglycemia (including hypoglycemic coma); applies to any hypoglycemic drug	Alcohol lowers blood glucose levels; actual response depends on amount of alcohol ingested, whether acute or long-term, overall dietary/nutritional status, actual hypoglycemic drug being administered; advise patients to limit or avoid alcohol use, strive for lowest possible and acceptable alcohol intake
	Disulfiram-like reaction: facial flushing, headache, hypotension, and possibly cardiovascular collapse	Tolbutamide, other "first-generation" sulfonylureas stop alcohol metabolism at acetaldehyde, a toxic intermediate; severity of response depends on hypoglycemic drug, amount of alcohol consumed; as many as one third of patients experience facial flushing; more serious responses may occur; if alcohol consumption cannot be stopped, glipizide, glyburide interact less
Anticoagulants, oral (Chapter 35)	Increased risk of acute prolonged hypoglycemia; possible prolongation of dicumarol's anticoagulant effects, increased risk of bleeding	Interaction presumably most important, most serious, for dicumarol; may displace sulfonylurea from plasma proteins, inhibit sulfonylurea metabolism; monitor blood glucose levels and prothrombin times in patients receiving interactants; interaction thought to be less with warfarin, glipizide, glyburide
Aspirin, other salicylates (Chapter 52)	Increased hypoglycemic effect	Mechanism complex; monitor accordingly; may reduce hypoglycemic drug dose during stable, long-term salicylate therapy; discourage haphazard salicylate self-medication
Beta-adrenergic blockers (propranolol, most others; Chapter 15)	Increased risk of hypoglycemia, prolonged recovery from hypoglycemic episode	See Table 46–I1. Use β blockers, especially nonselective agents, with extreme caution in persons with NIDDM; they inhibit release of remaining insulin stores, also may inhibit metabolism of oral hypoglycemic drugs, thereby prolonging duration of action; if β blocker therapy essential, may need to adjust overall treatment plan; frequent monitoring of blood glucose levels essential; cardioselective β blockers usually preferred, but close monitoring of blood glucose levels still important
Chloramphenicol (Chapter 56)	Excessive falls of blood glucose levels, or prolonged hypoglycemia	Chloramphenicol may reduce renal excretion of oral hypoglycemic; monitor blood glucose levels during combined therapy to aid dosage adjustments
Clofibrate (Chapter 36)	Increased risk of hypoglycemia	Clofibrate lowers blood glucose levels, may interfere with chlorpropamide excretion, may displace any sulfonylurea from plasma proteins; monitor accordingly if combined therapy necessary, anticipate need for reduced oral hypoglycemic drug dose; interaction not likely to affect glipizide and glyburide, which may be preferred
Diuretics (mainly thiazides; Chapter 32)	Increased blood glucose levels, poor control of diabetes symptoms	Diuretics, particularly thiazides, increase blood glucose levels, reduce responsiveness of peripheral tissues to insulin; dosage requirements for oral hypoglycemics, and possibly for insulin (in IDDM) may be increased if interaction unavoidable; monitor blood glucose levels as guide to dosage adjustments

(continued)

Table 46–I2 Major Interactions Between Oral Hypoglycemics and Other Agents (*Continued*)

AGENT	RESULT OF INTERACTION	COMMENTS AND NURSING IMPLICATIONS
Monoamine oxidase inhibitors (Chapter 24)	Increased hypoglycemic effects	Monitor accordingly; may need to reduce hypoglycemic drug dose
Phenylbutazone (Chapter 52)	Increased risk of acute, severe, and potentially fatal hypoglycemia	Interaction more serious than with aspirin (see above), but phenylbutazone rarely used
Rifampin (Chapter 57)	Reduced hypoglycemic drug duration, effect	Monitor accordingly; anticipate possible need to increase hypoglycemic drug dose during combined therapy
Sulfamethizole (other sulfonamide antibiotics?) (Chapter 56)	Increased risk of severe or acute hypoglycemia	Severity of interaction depends on hypoglycemic drug, sulfonamide antibiotic used; may involve reduced hepatic metabolism or plasma protein displacement of hypoglycemic drug; monitor blood glucose levels closely, frequently, especially during onset of combined therapy; be prepared to reduce hypoglycemic drug dose or intervene to increase blood glucose levels

Table 46–C3 Clinical Uses and Administration of Glucagon and Diazoxide

AGENT	INDICATION	DOSAGE AND ROUTE OF ADMINISTRATION
Glucagon		*Note:* Glucagon should be reconstituted with solution supplied by manufacturer if total dose to be administered is less than 2 U; use sterile water for injection for higher doses. 1 mg glucagon = 1 U glucagon; reconstituted solution should be no more concentrated than 1 mg (or 1 U) per mL
	Treatment of acute hypoglycemia	IV (preferred), IM, or SC: 0.5–1 U; if first dose fails to restore consciousness or raise blood glucose levels, may inject second, third doses; inject glucose IV if third glucagon dose ineffective
	Adjunct to radiologic examinations of the GI tract	IV or IM: 0.25–2 U usually injected 10 min before diagnostic test
Diazoxide		
(PROGLYCEM)	Treatment of chronic hypoglycemia, as from insulinomas	Oral: Adults, children: 3–8 mg/kg/day in divided doses every 8–12 hr. Infants: usually 8–15 mg/kg/day at intervals noted above
(HYPERSTAT)	Treatment of hypertensive emergencies, malignant hypertension	See Chapter 33

Table 46–S3 Major Side Effects of and Contraindications for Oral Diazoxide*

BODY SYSTEM/ Side Effect	CONTRAINDICATION/ PRECAUTION	COMMENTS AND NURSING IMPLICATIONS
EYE		
Diplopia, transient cataracts, other eye or visual disturbances		Usually dose-related and reversible; frequent assessment advised
METABOLIC		
Hyperglycemia, with or without ketoacidosis		Dose-related, often induced by other drugs that elevate blood glucose levels (eg, thiazide diuretics); monitor dose and response closely; check blood glucose levels immediately at suggestion of hyperglycemia (eg, altered sensorium); insulin, fluid and electrolyte replacement preferred treatment; anticipate need for prolonged monitoring, care, as diazoxide's half-life is very long
Hyperuricemia	Hyperuricemia of any cause, impaired renal function, necessitate extra care	High risk patients require close monitoring of serum uric acid levels, assessment for gout if diazoxide must be used; hyperuricemia risk increased by alcohol consumption, high-protein diets, most diuretics
CARDIOVASCULAR/ RENAL		
Tachycardia, palpitations	Cardiac disease necessitates care	Diazoxide stimulates heart directly, indirectly (reflexively) if BP falls; risk relatively low with oral diazoxide, but requires close monitoring in patients with cardiac disease
Edema, hypertension sodium and water retention, weight gain	Cardiac disease, hypertension, renal disease necessitate extra care	Common and serious, particularly in young infants or the elderly; assess; use reduced doses in patients with impaired renal function; diuretics may alleviate sodium and water retention, but may increase risk of hyperglycemia and hyperuricemia
SKIN		
Hirsutism; alopecia; hypertrichosis lanuginosa in newborns of women receiving diazoxide during last two months of pregnancy	Pregnancy is relative contraindication to diazoxide use	Usually reversible

*See Chapter 33 for information about parenteral use of diazoxide.

Table 46–I3 Major Interactions Between Oral Diazoxide and Other Agents

AGENT	RESULT OF INTERACTION	COMMENTS AND NURSING IMPLICATIONS
Diuretics (thiazides, thiazide-like, and indapamide) (Chapter 32)	Increased risk of hyperglycemia	These diuretics increase blood glucose levels; monitor accordingly if combined therapy used, anticipate need to reduce dose of one or both interactants
Phenytoin (Chapter 26)	Poor control of seizure disorder	Diazoxide may stimulate phenytoin metabolism or excretion; assess for seizures if combined therapy essential; more frequent monitoring of serum phenytoin levels advised

PROTOTYPES

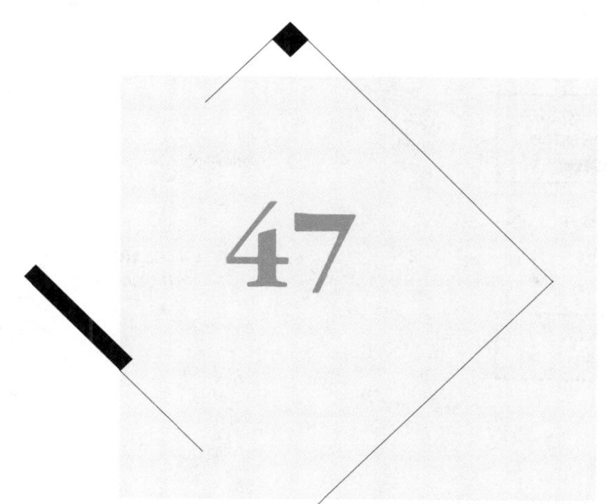

Thyroid and Parathyroid Hormones and Antithyroid Drugs

The major topics of this chapter are the hormones of the thyroid and parathyroid glands, and the hormonal and nonhormonal drugs used to manage dysfunction of these two endocrine organs. Both glands have close anatomic relationships, but in most other respects they are very different.

I. The Thyroid Gland and Its Hormones

Thyroid hormone, often called the body's "metabolic hormone," is actually two hormonal products: *thyroxine* (also called levothyroxine, tetraiodothyronine, or T_4) and *liothyronine* (also called triiodothyronine, or T_3). These hormones usually will be referred to as T_4 and T_3 in the following discussion. The main function of thyroid hormone is to control the rate of body metabolism and cellular oxidation. It affects every cell in the body. In addition, it is an important regulator of tissue growth and development, especially in the reproductive and nervous systems.

The thyroid's parafollicular cells produce calcitonin, which antagonizes the effects of parathyroid hormone on calcium metabolism. Calcitonin and parathyroid function in general are discussed later in this chapter.

Since nearly all thyroid disorders result from defects in hormonal synthesis or release, it is important to review these processes.

Thyroid Hormone

Biosynthesis, Transport, and Metabolism

The biosynthesis of thyroid hormone in the follicular cells essentially involves three interrelated processes:

1. formation of thyroglobulin, a storage colloid;
2. iodine attachment to thyroglobulin; and
3. coupling of iodine-containing thyroglobulin amino acids to form T_3 and T_4 (Fig. 47–1).

The thyroid's ability to store and to slowly release its hormones makes it unique among the endocrine glands. In the normal thyroid gland, the thyroglobulin colloid contains sufficient reserves of T_3 and T_4 to provide normal levels of hormone release (a *euthyroid* state) for more than three months.

Major reference tables appear beginning on p. 970.

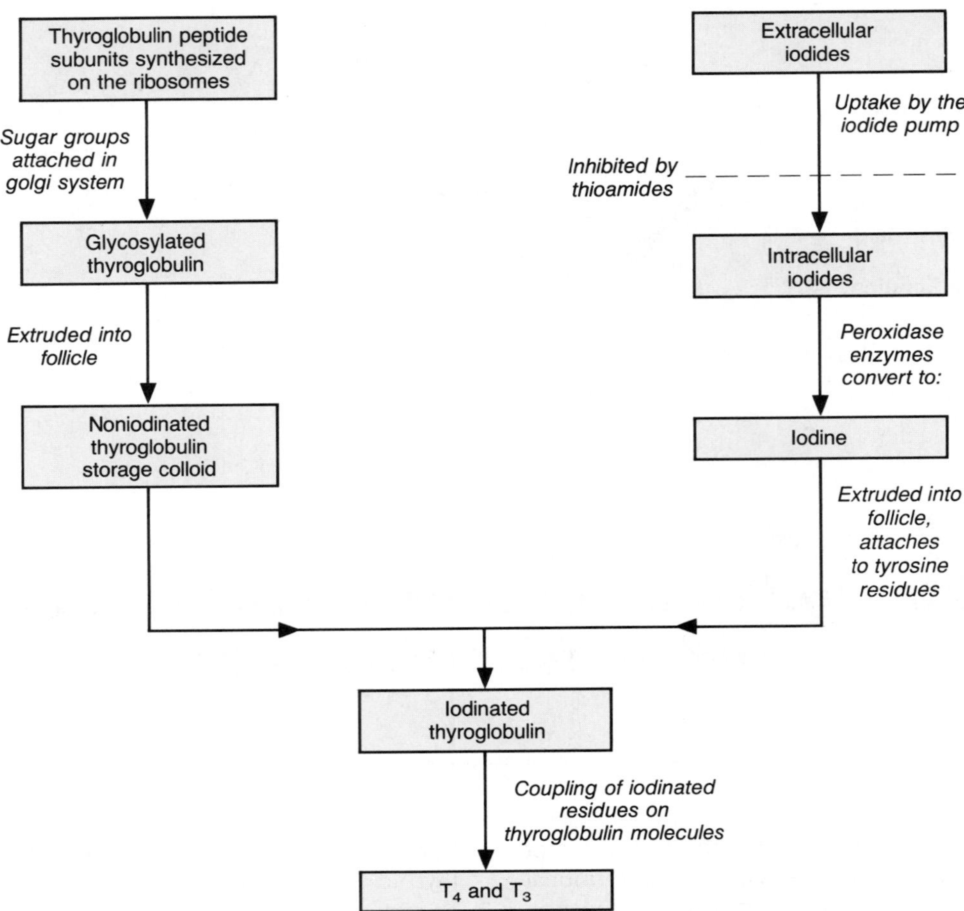

Figure 47–1

Synthesis of the thyroid hormones, T_4 and T_3.

Thyroid hormone release involves the reentry of iodinated thyroglobulin into the follicle cells and its subsequent splitting to release T_3 and T_4. The colloid is taken up by endocytosis to form a colloid-filled vacuole or phagosome, and the phagosome is combined with a lysosome, within which proteolysis occurs. The released T_3 and T_4 then diffuse from the cell into the bloodstream. Precursor fragments are retained and their iodine is recycled for new hormonal synthesis. Large amounts of iodine inhibit thyroglobulin proteolysis.

Released thyroid hormones almost immediately bind to several plasma proteins, but most importantly to thyroxine-binding globulin (TBG). Normal levels of thyroid hormone binding to transport proteins is 4 to 8 μg/100 mL of plasma. This measurement is referred to as the *protein-bound iodine,* or *PBI,* value. Thyroxine-binding globulin is capable of binding two to three times more hormone than it ordinarily transports. When its limit is reached, the excess thyroid hormones bind primarily to albumin and prealbumin in the bloodstream. Only very low levels of T_4 (0.03%) and T_3 (0.3%) exist in the free, active state in the circulation.

Although circulating blood contains both T_4 and T_3, 95% of the total circulating hormone is T_4. Approximately 80% (equivalent to 30 μg per day) of serum T_3 arises peripherally from the action of extrathyroidal enzymes found in many tissues (liver, kidneys, and others) that deiodinate T_4 to form T_3.

Because T_3 is less tightly bound to the transport proteins than T_4 and is generated rapidly from T_4 in the peripheral tissues, T_3 is the most abundant form of thyroid hormone found in the target tissues. Additionally, the serum half-life of T_4 is approximately 7 days, which is considerably longer than that of T_3 (approximately 12 hours). For these reasons, T_3 is considered to be the more important hormone physiologically.

Regulation and Release

The major regulatory influences on thyroid gland activity are thyroid-stimulating hormone (TSH), released by the anterior pituitary gland, and intrathyroidal iodine concentrations. Binding of TSH to thyroid gland membrane receptors stimulates hormone synthesis and release via effects mediated by cyclic AMP.

Thyroid-stimulating hormone release, in turn, is responsive to blood levels of thyroid hormones; increased levels effectively inhibit TSH release. (The regulatory effect of thyroid-releasing hormone [TRH] on pituitary release of TSH is discussed in Chapter 44.) As T_4 levels fall, TSH release is initiated once again.

High intrafollicular concentrations of iodine suppress hormone synthesis and release, thus modulating the stimulatory effect of TSH. Failure of any of the control mechanisms in the hypothalamic-pituitary-thyroid axis results in hypo- or hypersecretory thyroid gland disease.

Several pharmacologic agents influence thyroid hormone release; for example, glucocorticoids and dopamine are inhibitory via hypothalamic pathways. Others inhibit the uptake or use of iodide. These include the antithyroid drugs, which are discussed later in this chapter.

Physiologic Effects of Thyroid Hormones

Both T_3 and T_4 bind to target tissue receptors. However, T_3 is bound 10 to 20 times more readily than T_4 and bears the major responsibility for initiating thyroid hormonal effects.

Presently, three theories exist concerning the mechanism of action of thyroid hormones on target cells. All are supported by experimental evidence. The first theory presumes that the cAMP mechanism typical of most protein hormones is at work. The remaining theories state that T_3 enters the cell and first binds to a cytoplasmic binding protein (CBP). It then detaches and moves to bind to receptors located either within the mitochondria (which stimulates enzymatic activity and oxygen uptake) or within the nucleus, where it initiates protein synthesis. The mechanism of thyroid hormone action on its target cells may vary depending on the specific receptor types available.

Just how these multiple mechanisms actually relate to the biologic effects of thyroid hormones is still unclear. However, the major end result is stimulation of cellular metabolism, reflected in increased oxygen consumption and calorigenesis. The long half-life, slow onset, and prolonged action of T_4 predict effects that are important in promoting long-term functions such as growth and development, and maturation of various organ systems. Thyroid hormones are particularly critical for skeletal development, reproductive capability, and brain development and maturation.

These and other physiologic effects of the thyroid hormones on the body organ systems and functional processes are outlined in detail in Table 47–1.

Hypothyroidism

Hypothyroidism is a general term indicating that body tissues are exposed to subnormal amounts of thyroid hormones. The clinical picture of hypothyroidism depends on the etiology, age, and sex of the patient, and the speed of onset of thyroid hormone deficiency.

Causes of hypothyroidism may be secondary (resulting from failure of TRH or TSH release by the anterior pituitary) or primary (arising in the thyroid gland itself). Primary hypothyroidism is expected when the thyroid gland is removed surgically or destroyed by radioiodine or irradiation; these are treatments for hyperthyroidism. Other factors rendering the thyroid hypofunctional include lack of dietary iodine, acute or chronic inflammation (eg, viral infections or Hashimoto's disease, an autoimmune disorder), and certain drugs (eg, lithium, sulfonamides, thioamides, and occasionally β-adrenergic blockers).

Myxedema and Myxedema Coma

In adults, a full-blown hypothyroid syndrome (see Table 47–1) is called *myxedema*. Manifestations include cold intolerance, constipation, loss of initiative, thick dry skin, a notably puffy appearance of the skin around the eyes, slowed intellectual function including retarded speech and apathy, and low metabolic rate.

A complication of myxedema is *myxedema coma*. It occurs primarily in elderly patients with long standing hypothyroidism. The precise cause is unknown, but triggers include cold exposure, hypoventilation accompanied by carbon dioxide retention (as may be caused by sedative or anesthetic drugs), illness or infection, and trauma. Signs include lethargy or coma accompanied by hypothermia. Although relatively rare, myxedema coma is a possibly fatal medical emergency.

Table 47–1 Major Effects of Thyroid Hormones

Process/System	Physiologic Effects	Effects of Hyposecretion	Effects of Hypersecretion
Basal metabolic rate (BMR), temperature regulation	Promotes normal oxygen consumption/calorigenesis	BMR subnormal; decreased body temperature; cold intolerance; decreased appetite; tendency toward weight gain	BMR supranormal; increased body temperature; heat intolerance; increased appetite; weight loss
	Potentiates effects of catecholamines involved in increasing body temperature and decreasing heat loss during cold exposure	Decreased sensitivity to catecholamines and adrenergic drugs	Increased sensitivity to catecholamines and adrenergic drugs
Carbohydrate, lipid, and protein metabolism	Promotes glucose catabolism; increases cholesterol synthesis and enhances liver cholesterol secretion; mobilizes fats; essential for development of protein tissues; promotes normal nitrogen balance	Decreased glucose catabolism; elevated serum cholesterol/triglyceride levels; decreased protein synthesis; deposit of mucoproteins in subcutaneous tissues that attract water, leading to edema	Hypercatabolism of glucose and fats; weight loss; increased protein catabolism; loss of muscle mass; increased nitrogen secretion
Central nervous system	Promotes normal development of nervous system in fetus/infant; necessary for normal adult nervous system function	Infants: Slowed/deficient brain development and retardation, plus effects noted for adults. Adults: Mental dulling, decreased sensation, paresthesias; memory impairment; listlessness; sleepiness; hypoactive reflexes; retarded speech; emotional dullness/affect; depression	Irritability; excitability; restlessness; insomnia; emotional lability; extreme responsiveness to environmental stimuli; tremors; exophthalamos; personality changes ranging from mild to frank psychosis
Cardiovascular system	Promotes normal cardiac growth, function	Decreased cardiac metabolism and output and pulse pressure; bradycardia; hypotension	Increased metabolism of cardiac muscle; tachycardia; increased cardiac output and pulse pressure; palpitations; hypertension; if prolonged, leads to cardiac hypertrophy/failure
Gastrointestinal system	Promotes normal GI motility and tone; secretion of digestive juices	Depressed GI motility and tone; depressed secretion of digestive juices; constipation	Frequent stools; diarrhea; anorexia common in elderly; hepatic congestion
Skin	Promotes normal hydration, secretory activity	Skin pale, thickened, dry; facial/periorbital edema; hair coarse and thin; nails hard and thick	Skin flushed, thin, moist; hair fine; nails soft
Reproductive system	Synergistic effect with other hormones in development and maintenance of female reproductive cycle; necessary for normal lactation	Depressed ovarian function; amenorrhea; possible habitual abortion; sterility (anovulation); depressed lactation	Women: Depressed ovarian function; oligomenorrhea. Men: Impotence/gynecomastia; increased serum estrogen and testosterone levels
Muscular system	Promotes normal development, tone, and function	Sluggish or decreased vigor of muscle action; muscle cramps; myalgia	Muscular protein catabolism; muscle atrophy and weakness (may be exaggerated in older men); fine muscle tremor
Skeletal system	Promotes normal growth and maturation	Children: Growth retardation and skeletal stunting/malproportion. Adults: Arthralgia	Children: Excessive skeletal growth initially, then early epiphyseal closure and possible short stature: Adults: Demineralization of skeleton

Cretinism

Severe congenital hypothyroidism, presenting at birth, is called *cretinism.* It results in developmental abnormalities, such as short, disproportionate body stature, mental retardation, and a thickened tongue and neck. Cretinism may arise from inborn genetic defects of the fetal thyroid, or as a result of thyroid-interfering maternal factors, such as a lack of dietary iodine or treatment with antithyroid drugs.

Persons afflicted with cretinism or myxedema typically express many, if not most, of the signs and symptoms of thyroid hormone deficiency.

Typical Acquired Hypothyroidism

Expression of mild or borderline symptoms of hypothyroidism is a more common situation. The symptoms tend to be vague and the disease progresses slowly and subtly over several years. Signs and symptoms of apparent hypothyroidism are particularly common in the elderly, but often they are manifestations of other disorders common in old age, such as congestive heart failure, constipation, lethargy, and cold intolerance.

Thyroid enlargement may be a presenting sign in some hypothyroid patients, particularly if dietary iodine intake is deficient or the patient is receiving an antithyroid drug. In such situations the thyroid gland produces colloid, but is unable to iodinate the hormones; therefore, no functional hormone is produced. As a result, TSH levels are elevated continuously and thyroid gland hyperplasia occurs. This type of hyperplasia is called *simple* or *colloidal goiter.*

Diffuse hyperplasia also occurs in some types of thyroiditis; nodular enlargement of the thyroid gland is more likely to be cancerous. Benign nodular adenomas ("hot nodules") often mimic the hormonal function of normal thyroid gland cells—they concentrate iodine and produce the functional hormones. In many cases this leads to persistent TSH suppression and a resultant hypofunction of the remaining thyroid gland tissue. Most individuals with nodular adenomas are euthyroid. (In contrast, cancerous nodules do not show hormonal differentiation and are referred to as "cold nodules.")

Diagnosis of Hypothyroidism

Diagnosis of hypothyroidism is often difficult and complicated. The various tests used to determine the etiology of hypothyroidism are summarized in Table 47–2. Most individuals with signs and symptoms of primary hypothyroidism exhibit elevated serum TSH levels and depressed serum T_3 and T_4 levels. The most frequently used tests to diagnose hypothyroidism measure serum TSH levels and total T_4 levels. Once diagnosed, treatment of hypothyroidism involves replacement therapy with one of the natural or synthetic thyroid hormones.

II. Treatment of Hypothyroidism: Thyroid Preparations

Several products containing natural or synthetic thyroid hormones are available to treat hypothyroid syndromes. These include preparations containing both T_4 and T_3 activity, such as thyroid extract, thyroglobulin, and the synthetic liotrix. Other synthetic products exert only T_4 or T_3 activity.

Although thyroid extract can be considered the prototype drug, levothyroxine is prescribed more frequently because of its predictable bioavailability. The characteristics of these products are compared in Table 47–3.

Absorption, Distribution, Metabolism, and Excretion

Thyroid preparations are well absorbed from the gastrointestinal (GI) tract; most forms are supplied (in tablet form only) in a wide range of dosages. They are distributed, metabolized, and excreted like endogenous hormones.

Preparations containing both T_3 and T_4 activity (liotrix, for example) provide both the slow onset and prolonged activity of T_4 and the more rapid but shorter-lasting activity of T_3. Such preparations produce serum blood levels of T_3 and T_4 that can be used to assess the patient's clinical progression toward the euthyroid state.

Preparations containing only levothyroxine provide only the more prolonged activity of T_4, producing inappropriately high PBI, total T_4, and free T_4 levels.

Liothyronine (T_3) preparations produce inappropriately low results for the same tests.

When patients are switched from one thyroid medication to another, modifications must be made to account for the difference in time course of the different drugs. Levothyroxine therapy is preferred by many (if not most) physicians, but desiccated (dried) thyroid, thyroglobulin, and liothyronine all can normalize TSH levels.

Pharmacologic Effects

Expected effects of thyroid product administration are equivalent to those of endogenous hormones—maintenance of normal metabolic capabilities of body cells

Table 47–2 Tests Used to Evaluate Thyroid Function

Test	Goal of Determination	Method	Normal Values	Comments
Percent free T_4 (% FT_4)	To assess free T_4 levels; diagnostic use as for total T_4	Equilibrium dialysis	1.0–2.5 ng/100 mL serum	Independent of TBG levels; elevated in hyperthyroidism; depressed in hypothyroidism
Protein-bound iodine (PBI)	To distinguish euthyroid from hypothyroid and hyperthyroid states	Measurement of total protein-bound iodine	6–13 μg/100 mL serum	Measures all protein-bound iodine in blood; assumes that 80%–90% is T_4; test less accurate than other tests listed for determination of T_4/T_3 values, thus use declining
Radioactive iodine uptake (RAIU)	To distinguish hypothyroid, euthyroid, and hyperthyroid conditions; to determine extent of thyroid function	Measurement of percent uptake of iodine tracer dose after 4, 6, and 24 hr	Normal gland incorporates 10%–35% of the radioisotope in 24 hr	Test may be affected by dietary iodine or antithyroid drug therapy; less frequently used than other tests for determining thyroid functional status; hyperthyroidism does *not* always result in high ^{131}I uptake
Resin T_3 uptake (RT_3U)	To assess free T_3; diagnostic use as for total T_4	Binding of T_3 to resin compared with T_3 binding to TBG in patient's serum	25%–45%	Ratio increased in hyperthyroidism, decreases in hypothyroidism; clarifies whether alterations in T_4 are due to thyroid pathology or alterations in T_4 binding proteins
Serum antibody	To assess status of thyroid hypertrophy and nodular goiters	Complement fixation test, antimicrosomal antibodies, and others		High titer suggests Hashimoto's thyroiditis
Serum T_3	To assess free T_3; used to determine hyperthyroidism	RIA*	0.08–0.20 μg/100 mL	Misleadingly low when patient has cirrhosis, uremia, malnutrition; low values do *not* necessarily indicate hypothyroidism
Serum TSH	Diagnostic use; serum TSH levels are an index of thyroid status	RIA	0.5–5 μU/mL	Elevated TSH with primary hypothyroidism, little or no TSH with secondary hypothyroidism; most sensitive test for primary hypothyroidism because TSH levels are high before T_4 levels decrease; less reliable for diagnosis of secondary hypothyroidism

(continued)

Table 47–2 **Tests Used to Evaluate Thyroid Function (*Continued*)**

Test	Goal of Determination	Method	Normal Values	Comments
Thyroid scan	To assess functional status of thyroid nodules; to diagnose thyroid cancer	Radionucleotide scanning of thyroid gland after administration of isotope tracer	Outlines functionally active hormone-producing thyroid tissue; areas not taking up isotope appear blank on scan	Most often used for examination of nodular or asymmetric thyroid masses; benign hyperplasias generally take up radioactive iodine ("hot" nodules); malignant tissue does not ("cold" nodules); Technetium or ^{123}I preferred to ^{131}I, which gives excessive radio-exposure
Thyrotropin-releasing hormone (TRH) test	To determine if hypothyroidism is a result of pituitary failure (ie, secondary hypothyroidism)	Synthetic TRH (500 μg) given IV; causes peak release of TSH 30 min later	Peak concentration of TSH 5–35 μU/mL serum if pituitary function is normal	No rise in TSH levels seen with hyperthyroidism; normal elderly males show blunted or absent response to TRH; no rise in TSH levels if pituitary nonfunctional in TSH release
Total serum T_4	To assess T_4 levels; to differentiate euthyroid, hyperthyroid, and hypothyroid conditions	Competitive protein binding or radioimmunoassay (RIA)	5–12 μg/100 mL serum	Misses fewer than 10% of hyperthyroid patients; affected by changing levels of TBG—ie, misleadingly elevated in conditions that elevate TBG levels (eg, estrogen therapy and pregnancy), low in hepatic cirrhosis and nephrosis; values low in primary and secondary hypothyroidism

*RIA, radioimmunoassay.

and promotion of the maturation and proper function of the various organ systems, as previously described.

Clinical Indications and Administration

The clinical aim of thyroid hormone replacement therapy is to alleviate symptoms and to produce a euthyroid state. Thyroid hormone replacement therapy is the most successful of the hormonal replacement therapies. Thyroid hormone replacement is reliable, easily regulated, nontoxic in doses that are generally used, rarely allergenic, and inexpensive. In addition, it provides effects indistinguishable from those of endogenous hormones.

Thyroid drug administration is indicated for replacement therapy in cretinism, myxedema, and subacute or chronic thyroiditis (including Hashimoto's disease), and to promote regression of simple goiter (via feedback inhibition of TSH).

Oral administration is the norm. Only levothyroxine is readily available in parenteral dosage forms, for use in emergencies or in patients unable to take oral medications. If parenteral liothyronine treatment is necessary, it must be obtained by special request to the manufacturer.

Adult patients with newly diagnosed hypothyroidism are started on very low levels of the selected thyroid medication. Myxedema patients, in particular, are extremely sensitive to replacement therapy. The dose is increased at varying intervals (routinely, mixed-product preparation doses are doubled biweekly and the single

Table 47–3 Comparison of Various Thyroid Hormone Replacement Products

Agent	Description	Advantages	Disadvantages	Dosage Equivalent
Levothyroxine (LEVOTHROID; SYNTHROID; others)	Pure synthetic sodium salt of T_4	Exhibits all effects of endogenous T_4; provides long-lasting effects; preferred by many physicians; available in both oral and parenteral dosage forms	Causes inappropriately high protein-bound iodine (PBI), total T_4, free T_4 levels; variable absorption from GI tract	0.1 mg = 65 mg thyroid
Liothyronine (CYTOMEL; others)	Pure synthetic sodium salt of T_3	Less binding to TBG than T_4 or mixed preparations; rapid onset; also used for T_3 suppression test	Higher incidence of cardiac side effects than T_4 or mixed preparations; brief duration of action; causes inappropriately low PBI, total T_4, and free T_4 levels; parenteral dosage form for treating myxedema coma available only on special request from manufacturer	15–37.5 μg = 65 mg thyroid
Liotrix (EUTHROID; THYROLAR)	Pure synthetic preparation containing T_4 and T_3 in 4:1 ratio	Lab tests show normal range for T_4:T_3; stable on storage	Commercial preparations contain different amounts of each hormone (although hormone ratio is similar)	50–60 μg T_4 and 12.5–15 μg T_3 = 65 mg thyroid
Thyroglobulin (PROLOID)	Purified extract of hog thyroid; contains T_4 and T_3 in 2.5:1 ratio	Standardized according to hormone activity, providing more accurate dosages	Degrades on prolonged storage	65 mg = 65 mg thyroid
Thyroid desiccated (Thyroid USP)	Desiccated (dried) preparation of animal thyroid glands; contains T_4 and T_3 in anticipated ratio of 2.5:1	Relatively inexpensive	T_4:T_3 ratio unpredictable, may range from 2:1 to 5:1 (most products are standardized by iodine content, not hormone activity); degrades on storage when damp	65 mg = 65 mg thyroid

T_3 or T_4 preparation doses are increased weekly), until the euthyroid state is achieved as indicated by laboratory tests.

Regression of hypothyroid symptoms normally occurs within two weeks, regardless of the thyroid medication used. Dosages for the various products can differ considerably and must be adjusted to the patient's response. Dosage equivalents of the various thyroid products are listed in Table 47–3. Table 47–C1 summarizes the usual dosages of these agents. Once a patient has been brought to the desired hormone levels and rendered euthyroid, daily maintenance doses are prescribed to retain that condition.

During continued therapy, it may be desirable to switch patients from mixed hormone preparations to a single hormone preparation, or from one type of single drug preparation to another. Since there are differences in onsets and durations of activity, such changes must be planned carefully and explained well to the patient.

When switching from prolonged-acting levothyroxine to liothyronine, levothyroxine therapy is stopped and liothyronine therapy is begun with low doses; the dose is increased in small increments after residual effects of levothyroxine have disappeared. When changing from liothyronine to levothyroxine, levothyroxine therapy is begun several days before liothyronine withdrawal, to avoid relapse.

Cretinism is rarely obvious at birth and may be an unanticpated outcome, particularly if the maternal history is incomplete. Once diagnosed, replacement therapy is started immediately, since anatomic changes caused by thyroid hormone deficiency are not reversible. In most cases, the infant is given an adult dose of hormone. During childhood, however, larger doses are required to maintain normal growth.

Side Effects, Adverse Reactions, and Contraindications

When administered in the smallest doses necessary to obtain the desired therapeutic effects, thyroid medications cause few undesirable side effects. If doses are excessive or are increased too rapidly, or side effects occur for any other reason, any of the replacement products will cause effects that resemble those described for hyperthyroidism (see Table 47–1). These symptoms include nervousness, instability, sweating, increased bowel motility, tachycardia, angina, and induced or aggravated congestive heart failure (and possible shock). Massive doses may cause *thyroid storm,* which is discussed later.

Thyroid medications are contraindicated for patients with uncontrolled adrenal insufficiency. If thyroid replacement therapy is necessary, it should be preceded by cortisone or related steroid drug therapy to prevent adrenal crisis. Cardiac disease is another relative contraindication. If thyroid hormone therapy is necessary, very small initital doses are given and therapy is monitored by routine blood pressure and pulse measurements. *Thyrotoxicosis,* an extreme acute hyperthyroid state, contraindicates thyroid hormone therapy except in conjunction with antithyroid drug therapy.

NURSING IMPLICATIONS

Before starting therapy, obtain a careful drug and medical history to screen for patients who are taking interacting drugs or patients in whom hormone therapy is contraindicated. Obtain baseline blood pressure, temperature, pulse, and weight measurements.

When caring for patients with myxedema coma, assess for infection and electrolyte disturbances that are also likely to be present. Anticipate the need for parenteral electrolyte supplementation (guided by laboratory tests), administration of antibiotics, the almost routine need for corticosteroids, as well as very cautious administration of thyroid hormone products.

Outpatient hormonal therapy is the norm with hypothyroidism. Whether initiating therapy or caring for someone with longstanding disease, emphasize that the patient will most likely require lifelong drug treatment, and that regular drug administration is needed to prevent relapse. All patients should be advised to carry a MedicAlert card or tag indicating diagnosis, hormone replacement drug, and their physician's name.

Constipation is a common problem with hypothyroidism that may need attention by nurses, at least during the start of therapy. Monitor for bowel movements. When appropriate, teach bowel training measures, and recommend adding bulk-forming foods to the diet. The physician may prescribe stool softeners or laxatives to prevent impaction.

Generally, patient instruction at the start of therapy includes directions to take the medication regularly at the same time each day (preferably before the morning meal to help prevent insomnia) to maintain constant hormone blood levels.

The apathetic nature characteristic of many patients with myxedema may result in medication lapses, so provide a follow-up system. In addition, inability to concentrate may necessitate repetition of teaching instructions. Involve a responsible family member when necessary.

Advise patients to keep their thyroid medications in tight, light-proof containers. What appears to be therapy failure may, in fact, reflect a loss of product potency, particularly in the case of thyroid extract and thyroglobulin.

Understand the differences in action of the mixed- and single-ingredient products. Products with different trade names are not necessarily equivalent (eg, the composition of liotrix produced by different manufacturers varies), and during medication changes from one replacement drug to another patients need careful instruction to avoid overdose or relapse. Advise patients not to switch to another brand or to a generic medication without consulting their health-care provider.

Alert patients to the signs and symptoms of hyperthyroidism and the need to report palpitations, diaphoresis, chest pain, dyspnea, and other signs of overdose.

Instruct patients to avoid excessive intake of foods that inhibit thyroid secretion, including turnips, cabbage, carrots, peaches, peas, strawberries, spinach, and radishes.

Advise patients to take thyroid hormones on an empty stomach to minimize irregular absorption caused by food.

◆ Use During Pregnancy and Lactation

Thyroid hormones do not readily cross the placental barrier. No adverse fetal effects have been reported. Consequently, replacement therapy during pregnancy can and should continue, but with close monitoring of the mother and fetus. Minimal amounts of the hormones are excreted in human breast milk. Use caution when administering thyroid hormones to a nursing woman.

Use in Children

Obtain weight and height records routinely for infants and children receiving replacement therapy, to ensure normal growth. Report deviations from anticipated results. Children need to be carefully monitored for signs of toxicity. Typical pediatric dosages are summarized in Table 47–C1.

Use in the Elderly

If thyroid hormones must be given to elderly patients, especially those with cardiovascular disease, careful blood pressure and pulse monitoring is mandatory since these individuals are particularly susceptible to toxic effects. Do not administer the medication if the pulse rate is more than 100 beats per minute. Cardiac effects may be enhanced if the patient is also receiving sympathomimetics, such as bronchodilators.

Liothyronine (T_3) has been associated with acute myocardial infarction in the elderly. Elderly patients require lower initial doses, and smaller dosage increases, than younger adults. The presence of myxadema or cardiac disease necessitates use of even lower doses.

Interactions with Other Drugs

There is an important relationship between a person's thyroid hormone status and the actions of several drugs (Table 47–I1). Thus, changing thyroid status (eg, when thyroid supplements are given to treat hypothyroidism) can lead to drug interactions. These interactions may affect the ability of cells to respond to certain dosages of an interacting drug, or can affect the absorption, distribution, metabolism, or excretion of the interactant. Overall, administering thyroid hormones can make a previously "right" dose of some drugs too little or too much. (Similar problems can occur when antithyroid drugs are given to treat hyperthyroidism.)

The main interactions that occur because of changing thyroid hormone status involve:

- *Beta blockers:* If their dosages are not changed, their therapeutic effects may decrease as euthyroidism is reached during thyroid hormone treatment of hypothyroidism;
- *Digitalis:* The effects of digoxin or digitoxin also may decrease if their dosage is not increased;
- *Oral anticoagulants such as warfarin:* An increased effect during the transition to euthyroidism often requires a decreased anticoagulant dose;
- *Theophylline, aminophylline, and related bronchodilators:* Their effectiveness decreases with hypothyroidism treatment, because of increased drug metabolism rates, so dosages may need to be increased as the patient becomes euthyroid;
- *Cholestyramine,* the orally administered cholesterol-lowering resin, is also an important interactant. If it is taken along with a thyroid hormone it will prevent hormone absorption.

NURSING IMPLICATIONS

Interactions that involve β blockers, digitalis, oral anticoagulants, or theophyllines, are most important when the patient already is stabilized on one (or more) of these drugs, hypothyroidism is diagnosed, and thyroid hormone supplement therapy is started. Monitor for changed effects of these drugs, and anticipate a need to adjust their dosages. Once the hypothyroid patient is stabilized at a euthyroid level, the new, proper maintenance dose of the interactant can be identified. If thyroid hormone supplementation is stopped, anticipate the need to readjust the dosage of interactants once again.

If the patient requires both cholestyramine and a thyroid preparation, instruct him or her to separate the administration of the interactants by at least six hours.

Hyperthyroidism

In hyperthyroid states (except those caused by excessive doses of thyroid hormone supplements) supraphysiologic amounts of thyroid hormones are produced and enter the circulation. The term *thyrotoxicosis* is used as a synonym for severe hyperthyroidism.

Like hypothyroidism, hyperthyroidism tends to develop slowly. Depending on the degree of hormone excess, the patient may exhibit a broad range of signs and symptoms (see Table 47–1). Hyperthyroidism may result from hyperfunction of the entire thyroid gland (Graves' disease), excessive output of hormones by toxic nodular goiters or toxic adenomas of the thyroid, and, rarely, excessive TSH output by the anterior pituitary gland.

Graves' Disease

The most common hyperthyroid syndrome is *Graves' disease*, also called diffuse toxic goiter or exophthalmic goiter. Women are afflicted more frequently than men.

Common precipitating factors include puberty, pregnancy, and menopause, all periods characterized by substantial hormonal changes. Typically, the patient reports excessive perspiration, heat intolerance, nervousness, and irritability, palpitations, and weight loss despite adequate food intake. Exophthalmos (ocular bulging) may or may not be present, but it is common in this syndrome.

Graves' disease is a unique hyperthyroid condition in several ways. The thyroid gland appears to act in an unregulated, autonomous manner: T_4 production is excessive, T_3 feedback does not result in thyroid suppression, and TSH does not stimulate the thyroid gland.

A breakthrough finding revealed that the serum of many patients with Graves' disease contained the same factor—long-acting thyroid stimulator (LATS)—that stimulates thyroid function, and which is not inhibited by high T_3 levels. Long-acting thyroid stimulator has been found to be equivalent to two types of thyroid-stimulating antibodies—one stimulating adenyl cyclase (and thus thyroid tissue) and the other an active TSH competitor for thyroid cell receptor binding sites. Graves' disease is thought to be an autoimmune disorder reflecting defects in suppressor T cells such that there is an overproduction of the abnormal or undesirable antibodies.

Thyroid Storm

Thyroid storm is an acute and serious episode of hyperthyroidism that sometimes occurs in hyperthyroid individuals. Precipitating factors include acute infection, surgical or other physical trauma, severe diabetic ketosis, and other stressors that are metabolically challenging. Unless rapidly controlled, this condition may result in fatal congestive heart failure, cardiac arrhythmias, and myocardial ischemia.

Antithyroid drugs (described later) are used adjunctively to manage this condition, but they do not control symptoms quickly because of their relatively slow onset of action. Immediate control of serious cardiovascular symptoms is achieved by administering β-adrenergic blockers (eg, propranolol).

Subacute Hyperthyroidism

Subacute or mild cases of hyperthyroidism are often extremely hard to recognize. For example, in a fairly common condition called monosymptomatic hyperthyroidism, only one symptom (more often associated with other diseases) is seen, or symptoms of hyperthyroidism may be manifested as those of a preexisting pathology. Indeed, the presence of cardiac disease is the single most important factor modifying the clinical manifestations of mild hyperthyroidism in elderly patients.

In such patients, hypersecretion of thyroid hormones is manifested commonly as the appearance or worsening of angina, unexpected congestive heart failure, or atrial arrhythmias. Because the tendency is to focus on cardiac findings in elderly patients (rather than the possibility of hyperthyroid disease), these changes are often attributed to a progression of the underlying cardiac disease. As a result, the hyperthyroid condition goes undiagnosed and untreated. This may account for the relatively high risk of thyroid storm in this patient population.

Treatment

Three principle therapies are used, alone or in combination, to treat hyperthyroidism:

- subtotal thyroidectomy,
- antithyroid drugs, and
- radioiodine therapy.

The therapy selected depends on the etiology of the hyperthyroid state and the patient's age and choice. Of the three therapies, antithyroid drug therapy has the lowest success rate in producing total remissions of hyperthyroidism. Radioiodine therapy is usually the most successful. All three can produce hypothyroidism. However, antithyroid drugs do not irreversibly destroy thyroid tissue, so there is less potential for producing permanent hypothyroid disorders.

Subtotal thyroidectomy is the preferred treatment for persons who, for various reasons, are not candidates for drug therapy. This procedure induces remission of hyperthyroidism in most patients with Graves' disease. Although surgery may be the primary approach for treating hyperthyroidism, antithyroid drug therapy plays an essential preoperative role in rendering the patient euthyroid before operation. This is essential to reduce the risk of intraoperative thyroid storm and other complications such as excessive bleeding from a highly vascular gland.

III. Antithyroid Drugs

Drugs that interfere with the synthesis, release, or activity of thyroid hormones are called antithyroid drugs. This term generally is used to designate drugs that are chemically classified as thioamides, of which propylthiouracil (sometimes abbreviated PTU) is the prototype. Thioamides are discussed first. Iodides represent the other major class of drugs with antithyroid activity.

Before discussing the traditional antithyroid drugs, it is important to note the role of β-adrenergic blockers such as propranolol (INDERAL). When used judiciously in conjunction with thioamides, β blockers help manage many signs and symptoms of hyperthyroidism, such as tachycardia, palpitations, nervousness, and tremor. The β blockers exert rapid symptom control that is valuable while the patient is awaiting the gradual onset of symptomatic relief afforded by a thioamide. Propranolol and related drugs are discussed extensively in Chapter 15.

A. Thioamides

PROTOTYPE

Propylthiouracil

Thioamides have the broadest clinical use as antithyroid drugs because of their predictability, efficacy, and relative safety. Either propylthiouracil ("PTU"; formerly marketed as PROPACIL) or the related drug, methimazole, can be used. The choice between the two depends largely on the personal experience and preference of the prescribing physician, and on patient-related factors that are identified later.

Absorption, Distribution, Metabolism, and Excretion

The thioamides are available only for oral adminstration. They are absorbed readily from the GI tract, and concentrate in the thyroid gland within minutes of ingestion. Peak serum levels occur one to two hours after drug administration. The half-life of PTU is about one hour. The thioamides are metabolized rapidly and excreted in the urine. They cross the placental barrier and are excreted in breast milk.

Pharmacologic Effects

Propylthiouracil inhibits thyroid hormone synthesis by blocking reactions responsible for iodide conversion to iodine and its coupling to the thyroglobulin colloid (see Fig. 47–1). It does not interfere with iodide trapping or with the release of colloid-stored hormones. The major effects outside the thyroid gland include inhibition of T_4 conversion to T_3 in peripheral tissues, possible inhibition of anti-TSH receptor antibody formation, and enhancement of T-suppressor cell activity.

Clinical Indications and Administration

Thioamides are used to treat hyperthyroid conditions. The aim is to return the patient to the euthyroid state. However, these drugs are not curative. In cases of severe thyrotoxicity that can be treated with surgery or radioiodine therapy, the thioamides are used to induce the euthyroid state prior to those procedures.

Antithyroid effects, indicated by the decreased thyroid hormone output, are seen almost immediately after drug therapy has begun. However, clinical improvement is not apparent until the stored thyroid hormones have been depleted—approximately two weeks. This is the period during which adjunctive use of propranolol is most important. Usual PTU dosages (Table 47–C2) will render nearly all hyperthyroid patients euthyroid in eight to 12 weeks, or at most within six months. Occasionally, doses have to be increased considerably to achieve these effects.

Once patients have been rendered euthyroid, the thioamide dosage is reduced to maintenance levels (generally 25% to 50% of the initial dose). It is extremely important that the drug dosage be reduced as soon as the patient's TSH levels begin to rise. When this precaution is not observed, symptoms of hypothyroidism, particularly thyroid gland enlargement (goiter), paresthesias, and arthralgias, may occur. To lessen this possibility, many physicians prescribe a thyroid product together with the antithyroid drug.

In most clinical settings, treatment is continued for 12 to 24 months; the drugs then are withdrawn to determine if the patient will remain in remission. This approach is being challenged by reports of equivalent remission rates when drug withdrawal is initiated as soon as the euthyroid state is achieved.

Thirty to forty percent of patients remain euthyroid after discontinuance of thioamides, and require no further therapy. Factors that appear to favor permanent remission are a short history of hyperthyroidism, mild or borderline disease, and an initially small toxic goiter. However, the factor that seems most predictive of positive drug therapy outcome is observation of low thyroid-stimulating antibody levels; when levels remain elevated, relapse is highly probable. In patients experiencing relapse within a few months after antithyroid drug withdrawal, a second course of drug therapy may be initiated and may be successful in inducing permanent remission.

Side Effects, Adverse Reactions, and Contraindications

Adverse reactions to the thioamides occur in only 1% to 5% of patients, but these drugs are not risk-free. Manifestations of hypothyroidism are potential expected unwanted consequences of these drugs if excessive doses are administered. However, other problems may occur (Table 47–S). The most frequent complications of thioamide therapy are a transient drug-induced leukopenia, and hypersensitivity reactions indicated primarily by skin rash, urticaria, sore throat, fever, and nausea.

Agranulocytosis (occurring in 0.5% of cases) and toxic hepatitis are serious but rare occurrences that usually result from unnecessarily large doses. Drug-related hepatotoxicity is associated almost exclusively with PTU administration. The appearance of either blood dyscrasias or hepatotoxicity requires immediate drug withdrawal. In case of bone marrow depression, broad-spectrum antibiotics and whole-blood transfusions should be considered. Hepatitis complications require the usual regimen of rest and adequate diet.

NURSING IMPLICATIONS

Hyperthyroid patients tend to be irritable and have difficulty concentrating. For this reason, carefully explain and reinforce instructions for taking antithyroid drugs. Noncompliance in drug administration may result in the recurrence of hyperthyroidism signs and symptoms.

Patients experiencing remission should be encouraged to report for reevaluation of their condition every six to 12 months. Explain to patients who experience a relapse after discontinuation of antithyroid drug therapy that remission is still possible with subsequent treatment.

Instruct patients to take their medication with food to lessen gastric distress. Emphasize that to prevent relapse, they need to take the drug at regularly spaced intervals, as ordered, and must avoid iodide-containing foods and drugs. Advise patients to store the drugs in light-resistant containers.

Complete blood counts and prothrombin times need to be monitored routinely and periodically, particularly with surgical candidates.

Be alert for signs of hypothyroidism (periorbital edema and reports of lethargy or cold intolerance) or other signs and symptoms of adverse effects (fever, sore throat, skin eruptions, jaundice). Remind patients that if these symptoms appear they should stop taking their medication and report the symptoms immediately.

Advise patients that exophthalmos is not reversible, and that drug therapy alone may not produce permanent remission. Other therapy may be necessary. Early detection of the problem obviously is preferred.

◆ Use During Pregnancy and Lactation

Thioamides cross the placenta and may depress fetal thyroid function enough to cause congenital hypothyroidism. Alert pregnant women to these potential effects.

Although about four times more methimazole crosses the placenta than propythiouracil, any thioamide should be used cautiously during pregnancy, and only if the anticipated benefits to the mother outweigh potential fetal risks.

Previously, thioamide therapy was accompanied by thyroid hormone therapy to counteract untoward fetal effects of the antithyroid drug. This is no longer recommended because thyroid hormones enter the fetal circulation less well than the antagonists; they do not prevent fetal effects, as predicted; and they may mask signs and symptoms of maternal antithyroid drug-induced hypothyroidism, which could cause needless and dangerous administration of high antithyroid doses to the mother. In addition, hyperthyroid conditions tend to lessen or completely resolve temporarily during the last trimester. This may allow reduced doses, or complete cessation, of antithyroid drug therapy. Thus, if antithyroid drug therapy is needed during pregnancy, frequent monitoring is needed to guide treatment.

Oral antithyroid drugs are excreted in maternal milk, and may exert goitrogenic effects in the nursing infant. In general, breast-feeding should be discouraged. Otherwise, PTU is the preferred drug because its concentrations in maternal milk are roughly 75% lower than those of the alternative, methimazole.

◆ Use in Children

Thioamide therapy is used to treat hyperthyroidism in children. Dosage levels begin at 5 to 15 mg daily for children six to 10 years old.

◆ Use in the Elderly

Cardiovascular disease and arthritic conditions are more prevalent in the elderly, and some drugs commonly used to treat these disorders (see Table 47–I2) interact with the thioamides. Use caution and assess carefully.

Interactions with Other Drugs

The drug interactions section dealing with thyroid hormone supplements stated that bringing a hypothyroid patient to a euthyroid state can cause several important drug-drug interactions. The same principle applies, but basically in reverse, when hyperthyroid patients receiving several other drugs (Table 47–I2) are treated with thioamides. The main and potentially the most serious interactants are:

- Oral anticoagulants;
- Beta blockers;
- Digitalis;
- Oral anticoagulants such as warfarin; and
- Theophyllines

NURSING IMPLICATIONS

Monitor for changed effects of these drugs, and anticipate a need to adjust their dosages. Once the hyperthyroid patient is stabilized at a euthyroid level with thioamide therapy, the new and proper maintenance dose of the interactant can be identified. If antithyroid drug supplementation is stopped for some reason, anticipate the need to readjust the dosage of interactants once again.

NURSING IMPLICATIONS

If antithyroid drugs must be administered with interactants, monitor carefully and frequently for expected outcomes of the interaction, notify the physician if they occur, and be prepared for dosage adjustments. If the patient is receiving a thioamide, caution him or her to avoid iodine-rich foods (seafoods, iodized salt) and drugs such as cough and cold remedies that may contain iodine as an agent for reducing mucus viscosity.

Related Drug

Methimazole

Methimazole (TAPAZOLE) and PTU share similar mechanisms of action, uses, and drug interactions. However, methimazole has about 10 times the antithyroid potency of the prototype, based on typical doses (see Table 47–C2). Thus, 10 mg of methimazole is roughly equivalent to 100 mg of PTU.

Methimazole has a plasma half-life of about five hours, much longer than that of PTU. Methimazole usually is administered every eight to 12 hours. However, because of its relatively long duration of action, once-daily dosing has been suggested. This approach is controversial, but might be advantageous for patients who are poorly compliant. The risk of hepatotoxicity with methimazole therapy is much less than with PTU therapy.

B. Iodides

Iodides, supplied as inorganic sodium or potassium salts, or administered as the precursor, iodine, exert dose-dependent effects on thyroid function. Low amounts of iodide are essential for thyroid hormone synthesis; high doses inhibit thyroid function. Strong iodine solution (LUGOL'S SOLUTION), which consists of 5% iodine and 10% potassium iodide, is considered the prototype.

PROTOTYPE

Strong Iodine Solution

Absorption, Distribution, Metabolism, and Excretion

Iodide, whether administered as a drug product or as part of the diet, is absorbed readily. Iodine is reduced to iodide in the intestine before absorption. Iodide accumulates in the thyroid gland and is excreted slowly from the body in the urine.

Pharmacologic Effects

The essential role of physiologic amounts of iodide to facilitate thyroid hormone synthesis was discussed earlier. In pharmacologic doses, iodides inhibit thyroid hormone secretion, inhibit thyroid hormone synthesis, and reduce the size and vascularity of the thyroid gland.

Clinical Indications and Administration

Strong iodine solution generally is administered three times daily. Usual dosages are summarized in Table 47–C2.

The iodides act rapidly; the basal metabolic rate (BMR) begins to fall within 24 hours of administration. Maximal effects are observed after 10 to 15 days of continued therapy. However, the effects of iodine and iodides are short-lived, unreliable, and temporary. Incomplete thyroid suppression may occur, or the thyroid gland may become refractory to iodide and unresponsive to its effects. In addition, failure to continue with iodide therapy may result in recurrence of hyperthyroidism in an even more severe form.

For these reasons, and because the more satisfactory thioamides are available, the use of iodides is restricted to

- emergency treatment of thyroid storm;
- control of hyperthyroid symptoms *after* radioiodine therapy, until the desired response has been achieved; and
- presurgical preparation of hyperthyroid patients to reduce the size and vascularity of the gland, thus decreasing the chance of excessive intraoperative bleeding as the gland and its vessels are dissected.

Although iodides may be used as the sole agent to prepare surgical patients, the preferred approach is to start drug therapy with a thioamide several weeks before anticipated surgery. Iodides then are administered, in addition, during the final 10 to 14 days of the preparatory period. The administration of iodides first, followed by thioamides, is contraindicated because it may worsen the hyperthyroid condition.

Side Effects, Adverse Reactions, and Contraindications

The major side effect of iodides is mild GI distress. Skin rashes and salivary gland swelling also may occur. Some adverse responses that develop quickly may reflect hypersensitivity to iodides. Others that develop later during treatment may indicate toxicity, which is discussed later.

Iodides may cause hypersensitivity reactions ranging from fever, arthralgia, and swelling of the face or body; to more serious cases involving edema of the respiratory mucosae and larynx, angioedema, multiple cutaneous hemorrhages, eosinophilia, or full-blown anaphylaxis. Individuals with allergic reactions to iodides may require emergency medical care. Further iodide administration is contraindicated.

Iodide administration also is contraindicated for persons scheduled for radioiodine therapy. If the thyroid gland is saturated with iodine stores, radioiodine therapy will be ineffective. Moreover, if iodide therapy is started and then discontinued before radiotherapy, the hyperthyroid state may be worsened when previously synthesized thyroid hormones are released rapidly into the bloodstream from damaged and dying cells.

NURSING IMPLICATIONS

Obtain a complete history before administering iodine or iodides to identify patients with contraindicating conditions or interacting drugs (see below). Inquire about prior problems with or reactions to this group of antithyroid drugs.

Most patients find the taste of liquid iodine or iodide preparations unpleasant. Instruct them to administer the preparation after meals, and to dilute it in juice, milk, or another beverage of their choice to mask the taste. They should sip the solution through a straw to hide the taste and help prevent staining of the teeth. Store the medication in an air-tight dark container. Instruct patients to avoid iodine-containing foods and OTC medications, which might increase the risk of toxicity. Stress the importance of adhering to drug protocols, especially when the patient is being prepared for thyroid surgery.

Monitor carefully for signs of allergic or hypersensitivity reactions, especially after the first iodide dose. Thereafter, assess for signs of toxicity. Teach patients to report warning signs and symptoms, including GI distress or responses resembling a head cold, at once. Always be prepared to deal with reactions such as anaphylaxis or overdoses, and to discontinue drug administration at once.

◆ Use During Pregnancy and Lactation

The use of therapeutic doses of iodine or iodides is contraindicated during pregnancy because of potential adverse effects on the fetal thyroid gland.

◆ Use in Children

Iodine or iodides may be indicated for treating hyperthyroidism in children or adolescents. The drugs may trigger or worsen acne in adolescents.

Interactions with Other Drugs

Iodides and lithium (used for treatment of manic-depressive disease) both inhibit the thyroid gland. Used together, they act synergistically and may induce a hypothyroid state. This interaction should be avoided; monitor the patient's thyroid status closely if it cannot.

Overdose and Toxicity

Chronic iodide toxicity is called *iodism*. It is a syndrome characterized by a metallic aftertaste, burning mouth and throat, sore gums, increased salivation, productive cough, headache, rashes, and mucous membrane inflammation. Iodide therapy should be stopped at the first sign of iodism.

Acute iodine overdoses irritate the GI tract and cause intense pain. Vomiting and diarrhea, possibly bloody, may occur. Death may be caused by GI hemorrhage, generalized shock, or airway edema and asphyxiation. Symptomatic and supportive care to normalize vital signs is necessary. Gastric lavage with cornstarch or flour in water may be indicated to bind iodine and remove it from the stomach. Oral sodium thiosulfate is an antidote. It converts iodine to iodide.

C. Radioactive Iodine

The radioactive isotope of iodine, ^{131}I, has an important role in the diagnosis of thyroid function. It is the agent most commonly used for therapy of hyperthyroidism in adults. ^{131}I is supplied in a colorless, tasteless form of sodium iodide. One commercial product is IODOTOPE.

Chemically, the radioisotope behaves in a manner identical to nonradioactive iodine, concentrating in the thyroid gland. However, this isotope is unstable, and as it disintegrates it liberates β particles and gamma rays. The radioactive half-life is 8.06 days, so radioactivity leaves the body quickly.

Small oral doses of ^{131}I are used diagnostically to assess the ability of the thyroid gland to concentrate iodine (see Tables 47–2 and 47–C2). The drug is administered on the morning of testing, on an empty stomach. The thyroid's ability to accumulate iodide is determined by measuring urinary excretion of the isotope.

In persons with hypothyroidism or thyroid carcinoma, very little isotope is taken up by the gland; most is excreted rapidly in the urine. In contrast, the thyroid glands of persons with hyperthyroidism incorporate and retain a large fraction of the isotope, and very little is detected in the urine.

Thyroid scans also are done using low doses of ^{131}I given intravenously (IV). The radiologic scan will show "hot" areas that pick up and concentrate the iodine rapidly (such as nodular goiters) and "cold" areas (such as nonfunctioning cancerous nodules) that do not function in the same way as other thyroid tissue and do not accumulate and concentrate the ion.

When used therapeutically in substantially larger doses, ^{131}I is administered orally to destroy thyroid tissue deliberately. The actual dose, which can be administered in a single large dose or a series of smaller ones, is determined according to laboratory test results and the severity of the condition being treated. Treatment of Graves' disease is the major indication, but radioiodine may be used to treat selected cases of thyroid carcinoma, since functioning cancerous neoplasms frequently concentrate iodide.

Usual indications for radioiodine therapy include age over 40 years; disease recurrence after thyroidectomy; or refractoriness to thioamide drug therapy. It is used most frequently in persons who are not surgical candidates, such as poor surgical risks, the elderly, or patients with preexisting or hyperthyroidism-related cardiac conditions.

Once accumulated in the thyroid, the isotope destroys the tissue primarily through emission of its β particles. Although β particles have relatively low penetrating power, and mainly affect the thyroid, they do pose the risk of irradiating and destroying adjacent tissue.

Clinical results are obvious within 12 weeks. By that time sufficient thyroid tissue destruction has occurred to render the patient euthyroid. During the time between radiotherapy and full clinical effects, antithyroid drugs (thioamides or iodides) are administered to suppress hyperthyroid symptoms.

Side Effects, Adverse Reactions, and Contraindications

Hypothyroidism, caused by excessive destruction of thyroid tissue by ^{131}I, is the main unwanted outcome of therapy. Its symptoms may not appear until as long as 10 years after treatment. Since thyroid damage is permanent, such patients will require replacement thyroid hormone therapy. A minor adverse effect of ^{131}I is transient thyroiditis shortly after therapy.

Radioiodine, like most other radioactive substances, is mutagenic, teratogenic, and carcinogenic. These properties contraindicate use of the agent for most patients except adult males, or females who cannot become pregnant.

As noted earlier, nonradioactive iodine or iodides should not be administered before radioiodine use. They will compete with the isotope for uptake into the thyroid gland, and they may either precipitate an episode of hyperthyroidism or alter the diagnostic or therapeutic effects of the isotope.

NURSING IMPLICATIONS

When administering any radioactive substance, pay scrupulous attention to the precautions listed in the product literature. Follow all applicable protocols for administration; disposing of patient excreta, and reporting and decontaminating spillage.

When radioiodine is being administered for diagnosis, be sure that the patient is maintained NPO on the morning of the test. Carefully check the history to identify the use of iodides or other contraindicated drugs or conditions. Be sure the patient understands the risks of thyroiditis and hypothyroidism. Be prepared to provide appropriate comfort measures if thyroiditis occurs. Stress the need for periodic and long-term follow-up after ^{131}I is used to treat hyperthyroidism.

◆ Use During Pregnancy and Lactation

Radioiodine is contraindicated during pregnancy and breast-feeding, and for virtually all women of child-bearing age. The only major exception is life-threatening hyperthyroidism that is impossible to treat surgically or with other drugs.

◆ Use in Children

To reduce the risk of cancer and chromosome damage, radioiodine should be administered to children only for hyperthyroidism that cannot be controlled with surgery or other drugs.

◆ Use in the Elderly

Radioiodine therapy is a preferred treatment for elderly persons with hyperthyroidism. The morbidity and mortality of this treatment are much less than those associated with thyroidectomy (and even with oral antithyroid drug therapy). Signs and symptoms of thyroid disorders may mimic those of such age-related illnesses as dementia and heart failure. A thorough work-up, including thyroid function tests, is essential before starting treatment of any kind.

IV. Parathyroid Glands and Hormone

The tiny parathyroid glands are located on the posterior aspect of the thyroid gland. There are usually four such glands. The hormonal product, called parathormone (PTH) or parathyroid hormone, is an 84-amino acid protein that is split off from a larger prohormone molecule.

Parathormone

Regulation and Physiologic Effects

Parathormone is the single most important hormone regulating ionic serum calcium levels. Its release is triggered by decreasing blood levels of ionic calcium (Ca^{2+}) and inhibited by hypercalcemia. The major effect of PTH is to increase blood calcium levels by actions exerted primarily on three target organs—bone, the kidneys, and the intestine. Parathormone release

- activates the osteoclasts which, in turn, solubilize some of the bony matrix releasing calcium to the blood;
- increases absorption of calcium by intestinal mucosal cells; and
- increases calcium reabsorption (and decreases phosphate reabsorption, allowing for enhanced mobilization of calcium) by the kidney tubule epithelial cells.

In the kidneys, parathormone also stimulates hydroxylation reactions that lead to the production of calcitriol, the active form of vitamin D. Calcitriol stimulates the production of a protein that transports calcium through the intestines and into the blood. Homeostasis of blood calcium levels is essential for many cellular functions, including membrane transport processes and integrity, conduction of nerve impulses, muscle contraction, and blood clotting. Normal serum calcium levels are between 9 and 11 mg/dL (4.5 and 5.5 mEq/L).

Effects of Hyper- and Hyposecretion

Hyperparathyroidism, accompanied by excessive output of PTH, may arise from an adenoma. The results are hypercalcemia accompanied by decalcification of the skeleton, and deposition of calcium salts in body tissues. The most dangerous place where this "heterotopic ossification" can occur is in the kidneys. It can lead to permanent renal damage.

At present, no PTH-inhibiting drug is available. Routine treatment of hyperparathyroidism is surgical removal of hyperactive parathyroid tissue. On rare occasions, calcitonin is used briefly to control the symptoms. Its use is discussed later.

Hypoparathyroid disorders are rare. They may arise from autoimmune mechanisms, genetic disorders, or pharmacologic treatment of other conditions (eg, phenobarbital and phenytoin treatment of epilepsy). However, presenting hypoparathyroidism is most often the result of parathyroid tissue removal during thyroidectomy. The classic symptoms of hypoparathyroidism are the result of hypocalcemia. They include tetany, paresthesias, muscle spasm, and convulsions. Untreated, the symptoms progress to respiratory paralysis, GI hemorrhage, and death.

Therapeutic Products

Pharmacologic products used routinely for PTH excess or deficit act primarily to decrease or increase blood calcium levels, rather than to replace or inhibit PTH activity. The major products include calcitonin, biphosphonates (eg, etidronate), and gallium, which depress blood calcium concentrations; and vitamin D products, which increase blood calcium levels. Parathyroid hormone is used occasionally for short-term treatment of acute hypoparathyroidism accompanied by tetany. The drug is administered parenterally (see Table 47–C3).

Therapy of Hypercalcemia

Calcitonin

Calcitonin-salmon (CALCIMAR), a synthetic polypeptide with hypocalcemic properties, has the same amino acid sequence as salmon-derived calcitonin hormone. Human calcitonin (CIBACALCIN) is available to treat Paget's disease. It is relatively free of the possible allergic reactions that can occur with the salmon-derived product. Therefore, it is preferred for any patient with a history of allergies or sensitivity to animal products.

Absorption, Distribution, Metabolism, and Excretion

Calcitonin is metabolized rapidly by the kidneys (and to a lesser extent in the blood and peripheral tissues) to inactive fragments. Its plasma half-life is approximately 10 minutes. It is excreted in the urine. Calcitonin does not cross the placental barrier.

Pharmacologic Effects

Calcitonin's major action is antagonistic to that of PTH. It directly inhibits bone resorption and enhances bone formation by altering osteoclast and osteoblast activity. Calcitonin produces a marked, but transient, reduction in the rate of bone reabsorption and blood calcium levels, and increases renal excretion of phosphorus, calcium, and sodium. Overall, calcitonin lowers blood calcium levels.

Clinical Indications and Administration

Calcitonin is indicated for early, short-term management of hypercalcemic emergencies. Therapy is initiated by intramuscular (IM) or subcutaneous (SC) injections every 12 hours (Table 47–C3). (An inhaled dosage form is being developed.)

Calcitonin also is used therapeutically for management of symptomatic Paget's disease, a disease recognized by increased urinary levels of hydroxyproline and increased serum alkaline phosphatase levels. Initially, calcitonin administration causes a fall in both values in approximately 66% of the patients treated. However, with continued therapy, its effectiveness often diminishes and relapse occurs.

Dosages are listed in Table 47–C3. Drug effects are monitored by periodic measurements of serum alkaline phosphatase and calcium levels, and of 24-hour urinary hydroxyproline excretion.

Side Effects, Adverse Reactions, and Contraindications

Calcitonin may cause tachycardia secondary to hypocalcemia. Calcitonin-salmon is a foreign protein that may cause allergic reactions, including anaphylaxis. For this reason, initial skin testing should be done prior to therapeutic use.

Less serious side effects occur in approximately 10% of patients. These include nausea with or without vomiting (which decreases in severity with subsequent therapy), and local inflammatory reactions at the injection site.

Since the effectiveness of calcitonin is transitory at best, it is contraindicated for therapy of osteoporosis, a chronic and progressive disorder.

NURSING IMPLICATIONS

Have epinephrine and resuscitation equipment available when giving calcitonin-salmon, and be prepared to use them if signs of anaphylaxis appear. During administration of the first full dose of any calcitonin product, assess for signs of hypocalcemia (tachycardia, paresthesias, muscle cramps) and have parenteral calcium available for reversal. Continue to be alert for systemic hypersensitivity reactions or anaphylaxis.

Use IM injections for volumes over 2 mL, and rotate injection sites. Teach outpatients who will be self-administering calcitonin proper technique and the need to rotate sites; SC administration generally is preferred for outpatient use. If the injection site becomes inflamed, teach and provide comfort measures.

Advise patients that nausea and vomiting may occur. Antiemetic drugs may be helpful. Teach and provide additional comfort measures for the management of these side effects. Encourage adequate fluid intake to decrease the possibility of renal calculi, and advise patients that the effectiveness of calcitonin injections may diminish with time. Some OTC medications, such as multivitamins and antacids, may contain calcium. Advise patients to consult their health-care provider before using one of these products.

Use During Pregnancy and Lactation

Calcitonin should not be used during pregnancy unless the benefits justify the potential risks to the fetus. Calcitonin's effects on lactation by human beings are not known, but it should not be used by nursing mothers.

Use in Children

There are no conclusive data to recommend the use of calcitonin in children.

Use in the Elderly

Calcitonin is contraindicated in osteoporosis, a condition that is prevalent in elderly females.

Etidronate and Pamidronate

Etidronate disodium (DIDRONEL) and disodium pamidronate (AREDIA) are classified chemically as biphosphonates. Biphosphonates prevent bone resorption by binding to bone mineral and by being absorbed into newly formed bone matrix. They also may inhibit the activity of the bone-wasting osteoclasts. Dosages are listed in Table 47–C3.

Etidronate and pamidronate are available in parenteral dosage forms for IV infusion, which are indicated for treating hypercalcemia associated with malignancies. Cancer-related hypercalcemia is relatively common, especially in advanced stages of cancer, when bone breakdown starts accelerating.

Etidronate is also available in an oral dosage form. Its uses include hypercalcemia associated with Paget's disease of the bones, hyperparathyroidism, osteoporosis after menopause, and heterotopic ossification. The latter disorder involves the formation of bone-like calcium deposits in the soft tissues, and it is fairly common after hip replacement surgery or spinal cord injury. An oral dosage form of pamidronate is likely to be approved soon.

Both drugs are relatively safe. Mild diarrhea or nausea, and transient fever and leukopenia, are the most common side effects. These effects appear to be dose-dependent. Maintaining adequate hydration, and monitoring urine output for decreases that might indicate renal dysfunction, are essential parts of therapy when these drugs are used. Severe nausea, vomiting, and potentially serious renal dysfunction are the main concerns with overdoses.

There is little information about the safety of administering these drugs to pregnant women or to women who wish to breast-feed their infants. The best advice is to avoid giving it to pregnant women, if possible, and to stop breast-feeding during drug use.

Gallium Nitrate

Gallium nitrate (GANITE) is another drug that inhibits bone resorption and thereby can reduce elevated serum calcium levels associated with bone breakdown. Gallium nitrate is approved for malignancy-related hypercalcemia. It should not be used unless the patient clearly has symptomatic hypercalcemia that cannot be controlled with other measures, including hydration.

The drug is given by IV infusion continually (around the clock) for five days straight, unless normal serum calcium levels are reached before then. Dosages are listed in Table 47–C3.

The most common side effects with gallium administration are hypocalcemia, hypophosphatemia, and systemic alkalosis. Serum calcium and phosphate levels should be checked during administration. Some patients may require oral calcium or phosphorus supplementation. The alkalosis is usually mild and requires no intervention.

The most serious potential adverse effect of gallium administration is renal damage. Apparently, the excreted drug can plug the renal tubules, especially if the patient is not hydrated adequately. Therefore, ensure that the patient is well hydrated before and during gallium therapy, monitor serum creatinine levels and urine output, and perform urinalyses (as indicators of renal status) frequently during the infusion.

Gallium therapy should be avoided in persons with severe renal dysfunction. It should not be used at all with other nephrotoxic drugs (eg, aminoglycoside antibiotics).

Treatment of Hypocalcemia

Just as with hypercalcemia, the severity of hypocalcemia can range from mild and asymptomatic to severe or even life-threatening. The key players in regulating serum calcium levels are diet—through the intake of adequate amounts of calcium and D vitamins—and parathyroid hormone. The hormone is important because it stimulates the final metabolic step that forms active vitamin D (1,25–dihydroxyvitamin D_3) from precursors that are less active or inactive.

Dietary deficiencies of vitamin D and calcium are, in general, more important and common causes of hypocalcemia than deficiencies of parathyroid hormone. The dietary deficiencies are the main causes for rickets, a disorder mainly affecting children. Rickets is far more common in economically deprived countries in other regions of the world than in the United States. Dietary deficiencies also play an important role in osteoporosis, another important osteodystrophy that affects far more adults than children.

Calcium and Vitamin D

The administration of calcium salts is clearly the most effective—if not the only safe—way to manage acute, severe hypocalcemia. Nevertheless, the combined use of supplemental calcium and vitamin D can be important for many patients who require long-term control of hypocalcemia, whether or not the electrolyte imbalance is caused by parathyroid hormone deficiencies. Refer to Chapter 61, which discusses the actions and uses of these and other important minerals and vitamins in more detail.

SUMMARY OF NURSING IMPLICATIONS

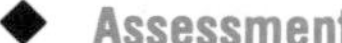

◆ Assessment

Recognize and report signs and symptoms of hyperthyroidism: palpitations, diaphoresis, chest pain, dyspnea; hypothyroidism: weight gain, weakness, cold intolerance; hypercalcemia: polyuria, confusion, lethargy, bradycardia; hypocalcemia: tetany.

Obtain a complete nursing history to establish necessary baseline data and identify underlying medical conditions or contraindications to therapy.

Note vital signs, laboratory values, fluid intake and output, and body weight and height to chart progress of underlying condition.

◆ Nursing Diagnoses

Constipation related to hypothyroidism; diarrhea related to thyroid drug therapy or hyperthyroidism.

Decreased cardiac output related to drug effects (thyroid imbalance).

Knowledge deficit related to disease condition and drug therapy.

Body image disturbance related to unresolved exophthalmos with hyperthyroidism.

Altered nutrition: more than body requirements (hypothyroidism, hypercalcemia) or less than body requirements (hyperthyroidism, hypocalcemia).

Anxiety related to need for long-term drug therapy.

Altered tissue perfusion (renal) related to gallium therapy.

◆ Planning/Implementation

Establish a system with the patient and with a responsible family member to ensure regular medication schedule and follow-up care.

Develop a medication schedule that prevents complications from thyroid and concurrent therapy with: anticoagulants (take thyroid one hour before or six hours after); antihyperlipidemics (four to five hours between drugs).

Support patient and family in dealing with long-term therapy; provide encouragement and opportunity to express fears and concerns.

Notify physician if side effects occur (see Evaluation); withhold thyroid medication if pulse >100 beats per minute.

Stress the importance of taking medications continually unless advised otherwise by physician.

Ensure adequate hydration during gallium therapy; monitor urine output and serum creatinine.

◆ Patient and Family Teaching

Teach the patient/family:

The proper and safe administration of prescribed drugs: thyroid—before breakfast, empty stomach; antithyroid—as scheduled with food; antihypercalcemics—oral, two hours before meals, on empty stomach with full glass of water; injectables—rotate sites, SC in ½ mL volumes; antihypocalcemics—oral, 1 to 1½ hours before meals, with milk.

About drug interactions and contraindications: thyroid—avoid aspirin, anticoagulants; antithyroid—avoid OTC preparations and foods high in iodides; antihypocalcemics—avoid mineral oil, which increases vitamin D absorption; spinach, bran, and whole grains interfere with calcium absorption; antihypercalcemics—may need to reduce consumption of leafy green vegetables and dairy products.

◆ Evaluation

The patient/family will:

Maintain blood chemistry values within normal limits.

Wear MedicAlert bracelet indicating disease condition and drug therapy.

Demonstrate correct administration of medication.

Avoid foods, prescription drugs, and OTC preparations that interfere with drug effects.

Cope in a positive manner with condition and treatment regimen.

Keep appointments for follow-up care.

Experience minimal to no adverse drug effects: thyroid—tachycardia, sweating; antithyroid—pruritus, urticaria, sore throat; calcium—nausea, vomiting, constipation; anticalcium—nausea, vomiting, tetany.

Annotated Bibliography

Adami, S, Rossini M: Hypercalcemia of malignancy: Pathophysiology and treatment. *Bone* 1992;13 Suppl 1:S51–55. *An excellent, short review that will be particularly useful for oncology nurses.*

Drinka PJ, Nolten WE: Subclinical hypothyroidism in the elderly: To treat or not to treat? *Am J Med Sci* 1988;295(2):125–128. *Several years old, but still valuable for its to-the-point approach to common problems in diagnosing and treating elders with few or mild symptoms that may or may not be caused by hypothyroidism.*

Geffner DL, Hershman JM: Beta-adrenergic blockade for the treatment of hyperthyroidism. *Am J Med* 1992;93(1):61–68. *Describes how and when, in general, β blockers can be useful for hyperthyroidism.*

Gruters A: Congenital hypothyroidism. *Pediatr Ann* 1992;21(1):15, 18–21, 24–28. *Discusses the importance of a newborn screening program for early diagnosis, potential treatment, of these disorders.*

Horowitz E, Miller JL, Rose LI: Etidronate for hypercalcemia of malignancy and osteoporosis. *Am Fam Physician* 1991;43(6):2155–2159. *This well-written article discusses pamidronate and other biphosphonates that will be approved.*

Lowe TW, Cunningham FG: Pregnancy and thyroid disease. *Clin Obstet Gynecol* 1991;34(1):72–81. *Important reading if your patient has thyroid disease and is, or is likely to be, pregnant.*

Sawin CT: Thyroid dysfunction in older persons. *Adv Intern Med* 1992;37:223–248. *Comprehensive insight into both hypo- and hyperthyroidism in the elderly.*

Sibai BM: Medical disorders in pregnancy, including hypertensive diseases. *Curr Opin Obstet Gynecol* 1991;3(1):28–40. *A discussion of thyroid disorders is only a part of this good article, which gives the "big picture" of medical and metabolic disorders—and their treatment—during pregnancy.*

Singer FR, Ritch PS, Lad TE, Ringenberg QS, Schiller JH, Recker RR, Ryzen E: Treatment of hypercalcemia of malignancy with intravenous etidronate. A controlled, multicenter study. The Hypercalcemia Study Group. *Arch Intern Med* 1991;151(3):471–476. *The results of this study are detailed, but they give much valuable information about what to expect when your patient will be receiving etidronate.*

Todd PA, Fitton A: Gallium nitrate. A review of its pharmacological properties and therapeutic potential in cancer related hypercalcemia. *Drugs* 1991;42(2):261–273. *How gallium's actions and uses compare with those of other hypocalcemic drugs, including calcitonin and the biphosphonates.*

Wolf PG, Meek JC: Practical approach to the treatment of hypothyroidism. *Am Fam Physician* 1992;45(2):722–731. *Useful, to-the-point insight into pathophysiology and etiology, diagnosis, decisions about whether and how to treat, and how to monitor therapy.*

Yeomans AC: Assessment and management of hypothyroidism. *Nurse Pract* 1990;15(11):8, 11–16. *Worth reading for nursing-related information on assessment, treatment, and monitoring.*

Table 47–C1 Clinical Uses and Administration of Major Thyroid Hormone Replacement Products

AGENT	CLINICAL USES	DOSAGE AND ROUTE OF ADMINISTRATION
Levothyroxine		
(LEVOTHROID; SYNTHROID; others)	Hypothyroidism	Oral: Adults: Initially, 50–100 μg/day, or as little as 25 μg/day for elderly patients, patients with myxedema, cardiovascular disorders; increase over 2–3 weeks (healthy adults; 3–4 weeks for elderly, etc) to average daily maintenance dose of 100–200 μg
		IV or IM: For patients previously taking oral thyroid preparations: Half previous oral dose once daily, switch to oral therapy as soon as possible
	Myxedema coma	IV: Adults: Initially 200–500 μg, plus 100–200 μg on next day if needed; avoid IV administration or use extremely low doses if myxedema coma accompanied by severe heart disease
	Congenital hypothyroidism	Oral: Doses vary by age: 0–6 months; 25–50 μg or 8–10 μg/kg; 6 months–1 year: 50–75 μg or 6–8 μg/kg; 1–5 years: 75–100 μg or 5–6 μg/kg; 6–12 years: 100–150 μg or 4–5 μg/kg; >12 years: 150 μg or 2–3 μg/kg; dosage modifications may be needed to provide maximal growth
Liothyronine		
(CYRONINE; CYTOMEL)	Mild hypothyroidism in adults	Oral: Adults: Initially 25 μg/day; increase by 12.5–25 μg weekly or biweekly to average daily maintenance dose of 25–75 μg. Elderly: start with 5 μg/day, increase by 5 μg at intervals
	Myxedema	Oral: Adults: Initially 5 μg/day; increase by 5–10 μg/day weekly or bi-weekly; once 25 μg/day is reached, may increase dosage by 12.5–25 μg weekly or biweekly to average daily maintenance dose of 50–100 μg
	Congenital/hypothyroidism	Oral: Initially, 5 μg/day, increased by 5 μg every 3–4 days as needed; daily maintenance doses 20 μg for children <6 months, 50 μg for children 1 year, full adult doses for children >3 years
	Simple (nontoxic) goiter	Oral: Adults: Initially, 5 μg/day; increase by 5–10 μg weekly or biweekly to average daily maintenance dose of 75 μg
	T_3 suppression test	Oral: Usually 75–100 μg/day for 7 days, followed by radioiodine uptake test
Liotrix		
(EUTHROID; THYROLAR)	Hypothyroidism	Oral: Usually start with 1 tablet (contains 25–30 μg T_4 and 6.25–7.5 μg T_3); increase every 1–2 weeks for adults, every 2 weeks for children, to average daily maintenance doses equivalent to 50–180 μg T_4, 15–45 μg T_3 (each μg of T_4 activity equivalent to 1 mg thyroid).

(continued)

Table 47–C1 Clinical Uses and Administration of Major Thyroid Hormone Replacement Products (*Continued*)

AGENT	CLINICAL USES	DOSAGE AND ROUTE OF ADMINISTRATION
Thyroglobulin		
(PROLOID)	Hypothyroidism	Oral: Adults: Initially, 30 mg per day, with dosage increases at 2–3-week intervals as needed; usual daily maintenance dose 60–180 mg
Thyroid desiccated		
(Thyroid USP)	Replacement therapy for hypothyroid adults with myxedema	Oral: Initially, 15 mg per day for 2 weeks; increase to 30 mg/day for 2 more weeks; assess and adjust dose as needed; usual daily maintenance dose is 60 mg, may be as high as 180 mg
	Adults without myxedema	Oral: Initially, 60 mg/day, increased by 60 mg/day every month as needed; maintenance doses as noted above
	Cretinism or severe pediatric hypothyroidism	Oral: Generally as for adults with myxedema, dosage increases usually at 2-week intervals as needed

Table 47–I1 Major Interactions BetweenThyroid Hormone Supplements and Other Agents

AGENT	RESULT OF INTERACTION	COMMENTS AND NURSING IMPLICATIONS
Anticoagulants, oral (eg, warfarin; Chapter 35)	Increased anticoagulant effects, bleeding risk	Interaction potentially serious; anticipate need to reduce anticoagulant dosage when thyroid supplementation started in anticoagulated patient; monitor accordingly, including more frequent prothrombin time measurements; teach patients signs, symptoms of excessive effects, to notify physician
Cholestyramine (Chapter 36)	Reduced thyroid hormone absorption, effects	Space administration of these agents by as much as possible (at least 6 hr)
Digitalis (digoxin, digitoxin; Chapter 31)	Reduced digitalis effects	Digitalis' cardiac effects increased in hypothyroidism, decreased when bringing hypothyroid patient to euthyroidism; monitor responses to, blood levels of, digitalis; anticipate need to increase digitalis dose as patient brought to euthyroidism
Theophyllines (Chapter 38)	Decreased theophylline effects	Bringing theophylline-stabilized patient from hypothyroidism to euthyroidism increases theophylline metabolism, reduces effects; anticipate need to increase theophylline dosage to new (higher) maintenance levels; monitor theophylline levels and clinical response (eg, wheezing, dyspnea) often

Table 47–C2 **Clinical Uses and Administration of Antithyroid Drugs**

AGENT	CLINICAL USES	DOSAGE AND ROUTE OF ADMINISTRATION
	Thioamides	
PROTOTYPE		
Propylthiouracil ("PTU"; PROPACIL)	Management of hyperthyroidism	Oral: Adults: Initially, 300–400 mg/day in 3 divided doses; average maintenance dose 100–150 mg/day. Children: 6–10 years: Initially, 50–150 mg/day; >10 yrs: Initially, 150–300 mg/day; maintenance doses depend on response
RELATED DRUG		
Methimazole (TAPAZOLE)	As for propylthiouracil	Oral: Adults: Initially, 15–60 mg/day in 3 divided doses; average maintenance dose 5–15 mg/day. Children: Initially about 0.4 mg/kg/day; maintenance doses usually one-half initial dose
	Iodides	
PROTOTYPE		
Strong iodine solution (LUGOL'S SOLUTION)	To reduce size, vascularity of thyroid before thyroid surgery	Oral: Usually 2–6 drops (0.1–0.3 mL) of liquid (contins 8 mg iodide per drop) tid, after meals, for 10 days before surgery
RELATED DRUGS		
Potassium iodide, saturated ("SSKI")	Prethyroidectomy management as for strong iodine solution	Oral: Adults: Usually 50–250 mg 3 or 4 times daily for 10–12 days preoperatively
	Expectorant	Oral: Adults: Usually 300–1000 mg (0.3–1.0 mL) 2–3 times daily after meals; optimal dose may be as high as 1–1.5 g tid. Children: Usually one-half adult dose
Sodium iodide I-131 (IODOTOPE)	Diagnosis of thyroid function	See Table 47–2
	Treatment of hyperthyroidism	Oral (or IV): Usually 4–10 millicuries (mCi)
	Treatment of thyroid carcinoma	Oral (or IV): Usually 50–100 mCi

Table 47–12 **Major Interactions Between Thioamides and Other Antithyroid Agents**

AGENT	RESULT OF INTERACTION	COMMENTS AND NURSING IMPLICATIONS
Propylthiouracil, Methimazole		
Anticoagulants, oral (Chapter 35)	Decreased or increased (excessive, toxic) anticoagulant effects	Response unpredictable but potentially serious; monitor accordingly, including frequent prothrombin time measurements, when combined therapy is started (to reach euthyroid state) or stopped; anticipate need to change anticoagulant dosages until PT stabilizes; teach self-assessment to patients
β blockers (eg, propranolol; Chapter 15)	Reduced β blocker clearance, increased or potentially toxic effects	Anticipate need to reduce β blocker dosage as hyperthyroidism is controlled; assess accordingly
Digitalis (digitoxin, digoxin; Chapter 31)	Increased digitalis effects, potential	Digitalis' cardiac effects decreased in hyperthyroidism, increased when bringing hyperthyroid patient to euthyroidism; monitor responses to, blood levels of, digitalis; anticipate need to decrease digitalis dose until euthyroid state reached, maintained
Theophyllines (Chapter 38)	Increased theophylline effects	Bringing theophylline-stabilized patient from hyperthyroidism to euthyroidism decreases theophylline metabolism, increases effects; anticipate need to decrease theophylline dosage to new (lower) maintenance levels; monitor theophylline levels and clinical response (eg, for CNS stimulation) often
Iodine/Iodides		
Lithium (Chapter 24)	Added risk of hypothyroidism	Avoid combined use; otherwise, monitor accordingly; anticipate need to administer thyroid hormone supplements to reverse hypothyroidism, manage goiter, or to reduce dosage of one of the interactants

Table 47–S | **Major Side Effects of and Contraindications for Antithyroid Drugs***

BODY SYSTEM/ Side Effect	CONTRAINDICATIONS/ PRECAUTION	COMMENTS AND NURSING IMPLICATIONS
Thioamides		
METABOLIC Hypothyroidism	Pregnancy	Thioamides enter fetal circulation and breast milk, may cause fetal or neonatal hypothyroidism; discourage breast-feeding; if necessary propylthiouracil may be preferred to methimazole
BLOOD Blood dyscrasias	Blood dyscrasias	May involve white cells, red cells, or platelets; assess for infection, abnormal bleeding, or bruising, notify physician for immediate follow-up, discontinuation of drug administration
HEPATIC Hepatotoxicity	Liver dysfunction (relative or absolute contraindication, depending on severity)	Almost exclusively with propylthiouracil; assess for jaundice, abdominal pain; periodic liver function tests may be indicated for patients with prior liver dysfunction; hepatotoxicity requires immediate discontinuation of drug; liver dysfunction may continue for a couple of months after discontinuation of drug, but usually is reversible
Iodine/Iodides		
TEETH Staining		Caused by iodine-containing solutions (eg, LUGOL'S); medication through a straw, which also helps mask poor taste
RESPIRATORY Increased secretions	Prior hypersensitivity or allergic response to iodine/iodides in which dyspnea or more serious respiratory difficulty has occurred; pulmonary edema, tuberculosis	Increased secretions not surprising, since low iodide doses used as expectorants; swelling of mucosae, larynx, glottis could suggest allergic reaction (usually rapid onset), more likely reflects chronic toxicity (iodism); either requires prompt treatment
GASTROINTESTINAL GI distress		Mild GI distress common; intense pain, especially if accompanied by vomiting, diarrhea, pain in throat, mouth, gums, are potential indicators of iodism, should be assessed immediately; bloody diarrhea or vomitus may indicate acute iodine poisoning
SKIN Rashes, acne		Worsening of acne more likely in adolescents; other rashes, especially macropapular, bullous, or vesicular, may indicate iodism; report at once for further assessment, discontinuation of drug administration

*Does not include expected signs, symptoms of hypothyroidism that might occur with excessive doses of antithyroid drugs.

Table 47–C3 Clinical Uses and Administration of Drugs Used to Manage Hypercalcemia*

AGENT	CLINICAL USES	DOSAGE AND ROUTE OF ADMINISTRATION
Calcitonin-human		
(CIBACALCIN)	Paget's disease	SC: Initially, 0.5 mg/day; maintenance doses range from 0.5 mg 2 or 3 times a week to 0.25 mg daily
Calcitonin-salmon		
(CALCIMAR)	Skin testing prior to any other use	Intracutaneous: 1.0 U in 0.1 mL sodium chloride injection
	Short-term management of hypercalcemic crisis	IM or SC: Usually 4 IU/kg every 12 hr; increase to 8 IU/kg every 12 hr if needed based on response assessed 1 or 2 days after initial dose. *Note:* Skin test first (see below)
	Long-term management of Paget's disease	SC or IM: Initially, 100 IU/day (SC preferred for outpatient self-administration); maintenance doses 50 IU/day or every other day may be sufficient
	Adjunct to vitamin D and calcium supplement therapy of postmenopausal osteoporosis	SC or IM: Usually 100 IU/day
Disodium pamidronate		
(AREDIA)	Hypercalcemia associated with malignancies	IV: 60–90 mg infused over 24 h
Etidronate disodium		
(DIDRONEL)	Paget's disease	Oral: Initially, 5 or 10 mg/kg/day for 6 months; 11–20 mg/kg/day (maximum) may be tried for ≤ 3 mos if necessary; 90-day treatment-free period should precede attempt to restart etidronate therapy
	Heterotopic ossification	Oral: Total hip replacement patients: 20 mg/kg/day starting 1 mo before and lasting 3 mo after surgery. Spinal cord injury: 20 mg/kg/day for 2 weeks, followed by 10 mg/kg/day for 10 weeks, started as soon as feasible after injury
	Hypercalcemia associated with malignancies	IV: 7.5 mg/kg, infused over 2 h for 3 consecutive days
Gallium nitrate		
(GANITE)	Refractory symptomatic hypercalcemia	IV: 200 mg/m^2 body surface area daily for 5 consecutive days; infuse over 24 h; discontinue if serum calcium level normal in <5 days
Parathyroid hormone	Short-term treatment of acute hypoparathyroidism (hypocalcemia) accompanied by tetany	IV, IM, or SC: Adults: Usually 50–100 U every 12 h. Children: 25–50 U every 12 h; therapy typically lasts 1–3 days

*See Chapter 61 for dosages of vitamin D supplements as therapies for hypocalcemia.

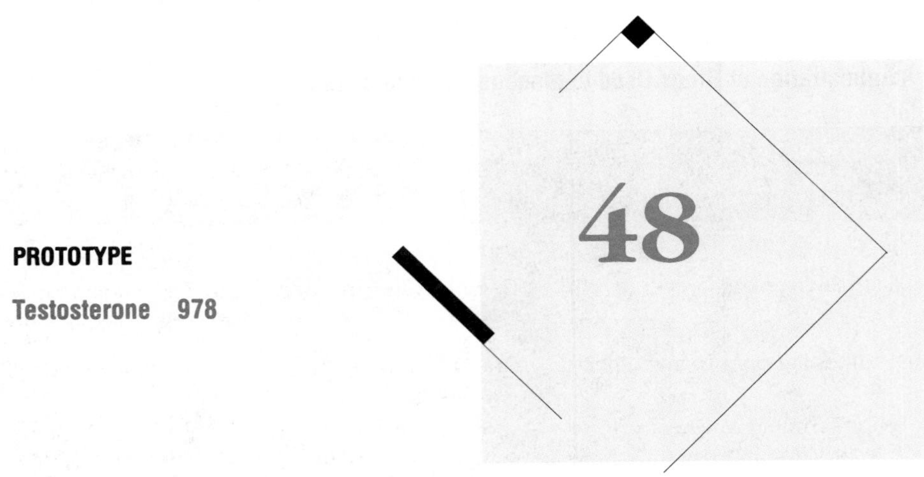

PROTOTYPE

Androgens and Anabolic Steroids

The primary sex organs of males, the testes, produce both sperm and male hormones (androgens). While the testes do not produce sperm until puberty, testicular androgens (primarily testosterone) play various roles during all the life stages of the male.

This chapter describes the normal role of the testes in sperm and androgen production, the physiologic role of endogenous androgens, and clinical uses of both natural and synthetic androgen products. The role of the ovaries, female sex hormones, and hormones of pregnancy are discussed in the next chapter.

Testicular Hormonal Function: Regulation and General Effects

The testis has both gametogenic (sperm production) and endocrinologic (testosterone production) functions. All other male reproductive structures are either conduits (epididymis, vas deferens, and urethra) or sources of secretions (prostate, seminal vesicles, and Cowper's glands) that aid in the safe delivery of sperm to the body exterior or the female reproductive tract.

Sperm production in the seminiferous tubules is promoted by anterior pituitary release of follicle-stimulating hormone (FSH) and is stimulated by testicular androgens. Anterior pituitary function is regulated by gonadotropin-releasing hormone (GnRH), a hypothalamic-releasing hormone. Gonadotropin-releasing hormone also stimulates the anterior pituitary to release luteinizing hormone (LH), also called interstitial cell-stimulating hormone (ICSH). As ICSH plasma levels rise, the interstitial (or Leydig) cells (found outside and interspersed between the seminiferous tubules) begin to produce and secrete increasing amounts of testosterone, the major androgen product. The rising testosterone plasma levels effectively decrease subsequent ICSH and androgen release by exerting feedback inhibition on the hypothalamus.

The Sertoli cells of the testes also produce some estrogen, as well as a peptide hormone called ***inhibin***. Inhibin and testicular estrogen are believed to suppress the release of FSH by the anterior pituitary. Thus, testosterone feeds back to depress its own release by blocking ICSH release, whereas nonandrogenic testicular hormone feedback results in inhibition of FSH and a subsequent decrease in sperm production. Inhibin currently is being investigated as a possible male birth control preparation.

Major reference tables appear beginning on p. 987.

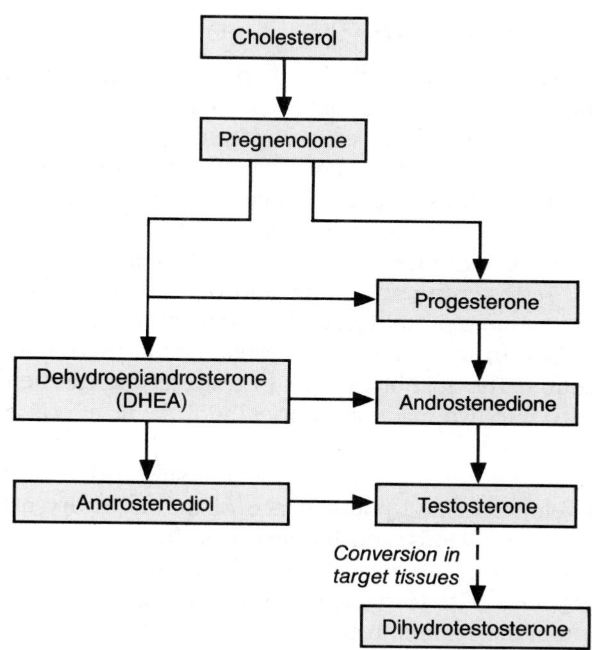

Figure 48–1
An overview of testosterone synthesis.

During male fetal development, the immature testes secrete testosterone in response to chorionic gonadotropin, a placental hormone. Testosterone causes the indifferent structures of the reproductive duct system to differentiate to form the male duct system. (When testosterone is absent, the female duct system forms, regardless of the sex of the fetus.) In newborn males, testosterone levels reach levels close to those of a midpubertal boy. After the first few months of life, pituitary-testicular function subsides and FSH and testosterone levels decrease; they remain low throughout childhood. It is presumed that this depression of the axis is a result of an extreme sensitivity of the hypothalamus to very low testosterone levels.

In the prepubertal male, hypothalamic sensitivity to testosterone progressively declines. This decline results in marked increases in FSH and ICSH release and increasingly higher levels of testosterone secretion until the adult anterior pituitary-testicular hormonal balance is achieved. Initially, gonadotropin bursts occur only during sleep, but as puberty advances gonadotropin secretion begins to occur during waking hours as well. The complete maturation of the pituitary-testicular interaction requires about three years.

As testosterone levels rise, the young man experiences the adolescent growth spurt. The external genitalia and internal reproductive ducts and glands enlarge, and sperm formation is gradually initiated. The male secondary sex characteristics appear: increased muscularity and skeletal mass, loss of subcutaneous fat, deepening of the voice, the appearance of axillary and pubic hair followed by growth of the beard, and the emergence of the male sex drive (libido) and potency.

Other testosterone-induced changes include enhanced vascularization and circulation, which cause darkening of the skin; increased activity of the sebaceous glands, often indicated by acne; and the first indications of genetically programmed patterned baldness (frontal balding).

Testosterone not only initiates accelerated growth in height, but also limits growth via hypothalamic inhibition of growth hormone release. When the growth spurt ends and epiphyseal bone closure occurs, the young man is several inches taller and possesses the body mass and proportions of an adult.

Testosterone

Biosynthesis, Transport, and Metabolism

Testosterone is a 19-carbon steroid. Like adrenocorticoids and female sex hormones, it is synthesized from cholesterol by two synthetic pathways. Pregnenolone is the intermediate common to both pathways, which are depicted in abbreviated form in Figure 48–1.

Testosterone is secreted at a slow, steady rate. The testes secrete approximately 8 mg of testosterone each day. Adult testosterone plasma levels are approximately 0.6 μg per 100 mL and show little variation with age. Testosterone is also present in the plasma of females in concentrations of 0.02 μg per 100 mL. The testosterone sources in females are the ovaries and the adrenal cortex.

Approximately 65% of circulating testosterone is bound to plasma proteins. Testosterone is reduced to relatively inactive metabolites (androsterone and others) in the liver. These metabolites are then conjugated to sulfates or glucuronides and excreted in the urine. Testosterone metabolism also yields low amounts of estrogens (estriol and estrone), which are detectable in urine. The amount of testosterone that is metabolically broken down daily appears to equal that released by the testes.

Physiologic Effects

Little is known about the mechanism of testosterone action in the target cells, but it appears to enter the cells, where it is transformed to dihydrotestosterone. A dihydrotestosterone-androgen receptor complex then enters the nucleus, where it induces protein synthesis. The metabolic effects of testosterone are antagonized by female sex hormones and their synthetic analogs.

Testosterone and other androgens are hormones that promote protein anabolism and antagonize protein catabolism, thus leading to greater systemic nitrogen retention. The anabolic effects of testosterone can be divided into two major categories: androgenic effects and myogenic effects.

The androgenic effects include stimulation of the development and maintenance of the accessory male ducts and glands, and induction of the secondary sex characteristics, as described earlier. The local (testicular) effect of testosterone is to stimulate sperm production in the seminiferous tubules.

Testosterone's myogenic effects are exerted primarily on skeletal muscles. Muscle growth is stimulated, and muscle bulk increases. Since testosterone also causes salt retention (potassium, sodium, chloride, and phosphorus), it is believed that a part of the increased muscle bulk and body weight is due to increased water retention by the muscle cells.

In adult women, excessive androgen production may occur with certain adrenal disorders, such as Cushing's syndrome, and with rare uterine tumors. Such androgen production in females precipitates changes in the female similar to those seen in the prepubertal boy—growth of facial and body hair, frontal baldness, voice deepening, and enlargement of the musculature and the clitoris may occur.

Effects of Hyper- and Hyposecretion

Androgen hypersecretion rarely is of testicular origin. More often it is secondary to massive secretion of adrenal cortical androgens (adrenogenital syndrome). The management of adrenogenital syndrome with adrenocortical suppressant drugs is discussed in Chapter 45.

Androgen deficiency may be primary (for example, as a result of testicular failure to respond to gonadotropin stimulation) or secondary (arising from deficits in hypothalamic or anterior pituitary function, for example). Whatever the cause, when testosterone is lacking in a prepubertal boy, puberty fails to occur and eunuchoidism occurs. In the eunuchoid condition, the boy continues to grow, often becoming unusually tall; the vocal folds fail to thicken, so voice changes do not occur; the skin remains thin and pale; subcutaneous fat is retained (producing a feminine appearance); skeletal muscles remain underdeveloped; the beard doesn't develop; external genitalia and accessory reproductive structures remain infantile; and a sex drive is absent.

After pubertal changes have occurred, testosterone deficiency has little or no effects on the body proportions already established. However, the prostate and seminal vesicles begin to atrophy, semen volume is diminished, and the male sex drive is greatly reduced or absent. Replacement therapy with testosterone or one of the synthetic androgens is routine for managing testosterone deficiencies in both prepubertal and adult males.

Androgens and Anabolic Steroids

Testosterone is considered the prototype testicular androgenic drug. Most of the various natural and synthetic androgens used clinically mimic the effects of endogenous testosterone.

PROTOTYPE

Testosterone

Absorption, Distribution, Metabolism, and Excretion

Testosterone is readily absorbed when injected intramuscularly (IM) as an aqueous or oily solution. However, its metabolism and excretion are so rapid that its resulting therapeutic effects are short-lived. Chemically modified testosterone—testosterone esters—are absorbed more slowly when injected IM and therefore have a more prolonged duration of action and are preferred for long-term therapy.

Testosterone propionate is given in an oily solution that is absorbed at a moderately slow rate and produces steady hormonal effects when injected at two- or three-day intervals. The large esters, testosterone cypionate and enanthate, are also given in oil and provide even more prolonged effects. These esters can be given in large doses at one- to six-week intervals.

Oral testosterone is adequately absorbed. However, virtually all the hormone is degraded by hepatic first-pass metabolism before it reaches the general circula-

Table 48–1 **Characteristics of Testosterone, Related Androgens, and Anabolic Steroids**

Generic Name	Anabolic:Androgenic Ratio	Half-Life or Relative Duration of Action
Testosterone and Its Esters		
Testosterone Aqueous suspension	1:1	Short (10–100-min half-life)
Testosterone cypionate in oil	1:1	3–4-week duration of action, 8-day half-life (approximate)
Testosterone enanthate in oil	1:1	3–4-week duration of action
Testosterone propionate in oil	1:1	Slightly longer than testosterone
Chemically Modified Testosterones		
Fluoxymesterone	1:1	Slightly longer than testosterone; 9- to 10-hr
Methyltestosterone	1:1 (oral) 2:1 (buccal)	Slightly longer than testosterone; 3-hr half-life (approximate)
Anabolic Steroids		
Nandrolone decanoate in oil	2.5:1	Intermediate-acting (suitable for once-weekly injection)
Nandrolone phenpropionate in oil	2.5:1	Suitable for once-weekly injection
Oxymetholole	2.5:1	Short-acting
Stanozolol in oil	3:1	Short-acting

tion. Testosterone and its derivative, methyltestosterone, can also be administered buccally, but absorption is often unpredictable. This administration problem has been largely overcome by the chemically modified synthetic androgen fluoxymesterone, which is fully effective when taken in tablet form.

The testosterone esters are transported, metabolized, and excreted in the same manner as testosterone. However, other chemical changes in the testosterone molecule (as in methyltestosterone and fluoxymesterone) have produced products that are metabolized and excreted in a different (and largely unknown) manner.

Pharmacologic Effects

The pharmacologic effects of aqueous testosterone injection, testosterone esters (cypionate, enanthate, and propionate), and the chemically modified agents fluoxymesterone and methyltestosterone are equivalent to those of endogenous testosterone. Each drug causes androgenic effects equal in intensity to their anabolic effects (that is, an anabolic:androgenic ratio of 1:1; Table 48–1). These agents promote the development and maintenance of the male sex organs and secondary sex characteristics. In high concentrations they depress the anterior pituitary-hypothalamic axis, thereby inhibiting spermatogenesis.

Many of the synthetic androgens have enhanced anabolic activity (anabolic:androgenic ratios of 2.5:1 or 3:1; see Table 48–1). The anabolic steroids were developed from a systematic search for chemically modified testosterone agents that were essentially free of masculinizing (androgenic) effects but that would promote positive nitrogen balance and stimulate muscle and bone growth in debilitated patients. Given in low doses, the anabolic steroids are nearly devoid of masculinizing effects. However, when used in high doses, androgenic effects are seen and manifested as priapism (constant erection) in men and virilization in women. As a result, the uses of many of these agents have been similar to that of testosterone.

Clinical Indications and Administration

Testosterone and Its Analogs

Testosterone and its analogs have several important therapeutic uses, which include replacement therapy and treatment of male infertility. In women they are used to treat a variety of gynecologic disorders and to provide symptomatic relief in metastatic breast cancer. Specific indications and typical dosages are summarized in Table 48–C.

Replacement Therapy

Testosterone is used for replacement therapy for primary or secondary hypogonadism arising in males during the prepuberty period or later in life. Testosterone replacement therapy can provide all the systemic effects of the endogenous hormone.

Hypogonadism is rarely recognized in children. The first indication of a problem is delayed puberty. Because the onset of puberty is highly individualized, the possibility of hypotestosteronism is generally not considered until the boy is 15 to 17 years of age.

When testosterone or its analogs are given to the prepubertal or young eunuchoid man, the results are dramatic. Within hours, the skin darkens (owing to increased circulation). By the second day of therapy, erections begin and occur with a frequency that is likely to be disturbing. As therapy continues, the excessive penile response ceases, muscle strength and mass increase, pubic and axillary hair appear, and the external genitalia increase in size. Linear growth during the first year of therapy may add as much as four to five inches to the young man's height, and growth may continue at the same pace for two to three years more or until epiphyseal closure. During therapy, oily skin and acne often occur and are distressing side effects to many teenagers.

Because puberty is a gradual process, replacement therapy begins with low doses that are gradually increased to adult levels. The goal of therapy is to mimic the natural hormonal progression in boys undergoing normal puberty changes. The changes that are induced are permanent for the most part. However, testosterone replacement therapy must be continued indefinitely to maintain the man's physical vigor and sex drive and to prevent a partial regression of secondary sex characteristics. It is important to recognize that testosterone replacement therapy does not ensure spermatogenesis in cases of primary testicular deficits involving the seminiferous tubules.

If hypotestosteronism is caused by hypothalamic or anterior pituitary problems, treatment of the prepubertal male may be started with products possessing gonadotropin activity. One such approach is to use human chorionic gonadotropin (which possesses ICSH-like activity) in conjunction with menotropins (which provide FSH activity). These agents are discussed in Chapter 49. Regardless of the initial therapy, the teenager is switched eventually to an androgen replacement regimen that is less expensive and more convenient.

Adult men displaying valid signs of testosterone deficit, such as loss of sex drive and potency, partial regression of the accessory sex organs, and very low levels of circulating testosterone, may regain their former sexual state by receiving relatively low doses of methyltestosterone or oral androgens. For permanent replacement or testosterone substitution in adults, one or two IM injections of 50 mg of testosterone propionate weekly usually provide the desired response. If longer-acting preparations are desired, testosterone cypionate or enanthate is the preferred treatment.

Testosterone replacement therapy is not used to treat complaints of impotence not accompanied by low testosterone levels. In most such cases, failure to achieve and maintain an erection represents functional rather than organic deficits. However, since other hormonal deficits (of thyroxine or insulin, for example) and certain drugs, as well as specific genitourinary, cardiovascular, or nervous system pathologies, lead to impotence, the cause should be sought carefully.

Androgen replacement therapy is sometimes used to manage distressing symptoms arising from surgical or traumatic castration or interstitial cell failure in later life (male climacteric). The symptoms are similar to those experienced by women undergoing menopause (hot flashes, palpitations, and other vasomotor effects, irritability, anxiety, inability to concentrate, emotional lability, and insomnia). Because many of the same symptoms may reflect a psychogenic disorder (for example, depressive neurosis or psychosis), differential diagnosis is extremely important.

Treatment of Male Infertility

Testosterone has limited usefulness for treating men who fail to produce sperm. Most often, azoospermia (the absence of sperm in semen) stems from duct system blockages that are correctable by surgery, or from a genetic deficiency. However, selected types of sperm deficiencies (oligospermia) may respond to testosterone therapy via a "rebound effect." High doses of testosterone suppress spermatogenesis by inhibiting the pituitary-hypothalamic axis. However, when testosterone hormone is withdrawn, the testicular tissue may be more sensitive to FSH stimulation than before. This treatment is extremely unpredictable and is useful only in the presence of essentially normal testicular tissues. Most often, male infertility is treated by human chorionic gonadotropin and menotropin administration.

Since several medications (sulfasalazine, antimalarial agents, cimetidine, propranolol, lidocaine, chlorpromazine, vincristine, and others) are known to depress sperm formation or to interfere with sperm motility, a thorough investigation of the patient's drug history must precede any orders for testosterone therapy.

Management of Gynecologic Disorders

Androgens inhibit gonadotropin release and antagonize the physiologic effects of estrogen. Recognition of these effects has led to their use in a variety of female gynecologic disorders and to provide symptomatic relief in cases of metastatic breast carcinoma.

Testosterone and its analogs have been used to relieve dysmenorrhea and, in combination with estrogens, to minimize menopausal symptoms. They are also indicated to suppress postpartum breast engorgement and lactation. However, because of the undesirable masculinizing effects of androgens, their use for these disorders has been largely replaced by oral estrogen-progesterone therapy or other drugs.

Palliation of Breast Cancer in Women

Commonly, testosterones are administered in large doses to provide palliative relief to premenopausal patients with metastatic breast cancer that is not responsive to surgery or radiation therapy. Usually, it takes about three months for improvement from androgen therapy to become evident. The masculinizing effects that inevitably occur are considered by most patients to be an acceptable exchange for the pain relief and sense of well-being that androgen therapy provides. Unfortunately, symptomatic relief is temporary and rarely exceeds one year. Androgen therapy of cancer is discussed in detail in Chapter 59.

Because large-dose testosterone therapy may cause hypercalcemia, the short-acting testosterone propionate or fluoxymesterone (which are less likely to cause hypercalcemia) are the drugs of choice for therapy of cancers.

Anabolic Steroids

Drugs that produce a relatively greater anabolic effect than an androgenic effect have clinical uses that differ from those noted for testosterone and its analogs. The important uses include management of refractory anemias and treatment of catabolic states such as osteoporosis or those caused by long-term corticosteroid administration. The specific indications for the anabolic steroids, and related dosages, are summarized in Table 48–C.

Management of Refractory Anemias

The observation that large doses of androgens promote excessive erythropoiesis and polycythemia has provided a useful approach to manage aplastic and hemolytic anemias, as well as various anemias associated with metastatic conditions (myeloid metaplasia, leukemia, lymphoma, and others). It is thought that testosterone and its analogs stimulate the kidneys to produce erythropoietin and directly stimulate heme production in the bone marrow. Because large androgen doses are required for this particular therapy, the anabolic androgens are preferred to testosterone, to minimize virilization.

Although the bone marrow response is variable in the different conditions treated, desirable results are usually seen within three months of drug therapy initiation. Red blood cell formation is stimulated first (as indicated by a substantial rise in hematocrit) and is followed by significant rises in platelets and leukocytes.

Management of Catabolic States

The therapeutic use of the anabolic androgens to promote anabolism and reverse a catabolic state is controversial. The goal of this use is to reverse negative nitrogen balance, stimulate protein synthesis, and promote appetite and weight gain.

The two most common applications of anabolic steroids include the treatment of debilitated patients, including those with wasting diseases such as tuberculosis and cancer and those suffering from extensive burns, major physical trauma, severe viral or bacterial infections, or disuse osteoporosis; and as adjunctive drug therapy to counteract the catabolic effects in patients receiving long-term corticosteroids for the treatment of rheumatic, allergic, or other chronic conditions. Anabolic steroid therapy is accompanied by a diet high in quality protein foods, vitamins, and minerals.

The anabolic steroids have been used to accelerate growth in childhood, usually as a last resort in children exhibiting signs and symptoms of deprivation dwarfism (growth retardation, anemia, and poor appetite and sleeping habits). The most important shortcoming is that an initial stimulation of longitudinal growth and weight may be followed by premature epiphyseal closure. The net result is that the child's ability to achieve full adult height has been permanently compromised. For these reasons, the use of androgens in children remains controversial.

NURSING IMPLICATIONS

Intramuscular preparations must be administered deep into heavy muscles, preferably gluteal muscle. Use a dry needle and rotate injection sites. Warm oil-based preparations between the hands, and shake thoroughly to resuspend the drug crystals before administration. Carefully assess IM injection sites for signs of inflammation.

Instruct patients who have received a prescription for androgens administered by the buccal route to place the tablet between the gum and cheek and allow it to dissolve; to refrain from swallowing the tablet; and to avoid eating, drinking, and smoking while the tablet is in place. The oral site chosen for tablet dissolution should be continually changed. Advise patients taking oral androgen preparations (those to be swallowed) to administer the tablets shortly before or with meals to avoid gastrointestinal upset.

Advise patients receiving anabolic steroids for their metabolic effects to eat a diet high in protein, vitamins, and minerals to support the drug therapy. Referral to a dietician may be beneficial.

Side Effects, Adverse Reactions, and Contraindications

Testosterone, its analogs, and the anabolic steroids cause several important side effects and untoward responses. Many are expected actions on normal tissue targets of androgen action. Table 48–S summarizes these unwanted actions.

The risks of serious adverse effects are real, but comparatively low, when these drugs are used for valid therapeutic uses under a physician's supervision. The risks increase greatly when the anabolic steroids are self-prescribed, and abused, by persons wishing to increase their muscle mass and strength. (Anabolic steroid abuse is discussed in Chapter 28, and several references are cited in the annotated bibliography.) Because of the abuse risks, the anabolic steroids are classified by the Food and Drug Administration as Schedule III agents. Some states are more restrictive, classifying these drugs as Schedule II agents—the same schedule that includes morphine and many other drugs with a high abuse potential.

When androgens are used in women, their normal physiologic effects are considered adverse effects. Amenorrhea and other menstrual disorders are common results of inhibited gonadotropin secretion. All the androgen preparations cause virilization in women. The first indications of virilization are acne, growth of facial hair, and deepening of the voice. If therapy is discontinued when these adverse effects are first noted, a slow reversal occurs. With prolonged therapy (as in treatment of mammary carcinoma), pattern baldness, hirsutism, enlargement of the clitoris, and increasing bulkiness of the voluntary muscles ensue. With the exception of clitoral enlargement, all these effects are reversible.

Edema

A common response to androgen administration is renal retention of sodium and water. With doses used to treat testosterone deficiency syndromes, noticeable edema is uncommon but can be troublesome when large doses are used. As a general rule, the edematous effects may be managed by reducing dietary sodium intake or by using diuretics. The use of androgens is contraindicated in patients with cardiovascular deficits or those who are edema-prone owing to other causes (cirrhosis, renal disease, or hypoproteinemia), to avoid precipitation of congestive heart failure.

Psychologic Changes and Hyperandrogenism

In large doses, testosterone and its analogs cause increased libido and priapism in men. Prolonged high-dose administration may result in testicular atrophy, impotence, and oligospermia. Personality changes, aggressiveness, and emotional lability may also occur. In some cases, suicidal or homicidal behaviors have resulted.

Liver Damage

Long-term high-dose administration of any androgen may cause serious and potentially irreversible hepatic damage, including hepatic cancer or a hemorrhagic liver disorder known as pelosis hepatis. Jaundice, reflecting cholestatic hepatitis, may be the first clue that something is wrong. Even relatively low doses of fluoxymesterone, methandrostenolone, or methyltestosterone may cause cholestatic hepatitis. Therefore, periodic liver function tests should be performed routinely when one of these three drugs is administered, or whenever prolonged and high-dose therapy with any androgen is used. Abnormal test results, or any other evidence of hepatic dysfunction, require prompt discontinuation of androgen therapy and further evaluation. Jaundice usually is reversible when detected early and androgen administration is stopped. The overall risk is generally low when low doses of testosterone or its esters are administered.

Enhanced Growth and Metastasis of Testosterone-Dependent Tissues

Men receiving androgen therapy must be continually monitored for prostate gland hypertrophy. Prostatic cancer and breast carcinomas in males should be ruled out before therapy, since they contraindicate androgen use.

Osteolysis and Hypercalcemia

Patients with breast cancer and immobile patients require frequent serum calcium determinations. Drug therapy must be discontinued when excessive calcium loss is detected or symptomatic hypercalcemia (indicated by vomiting, constipation, loss of muscle tone, polyuria, and lethargy) occurs. Advise these patients to drink large amounts of fluid to help prevent the formation of renal calculi.

Gynecomastia

Patients being treated for hypogonadism frequently develop gynecomastia. In young patients, this adverse effect usually subsides. However, it should be recognized that gynecomastia may be a result of therapy with such other drugs as cimetidine, spironolactone, and some chemotherapeutic agents.

Increased Risk of Atherosclerosis

Androgen or anabolic steroid administration may cause sudden or dramatic decreases in circulating levels of high-density lipoproteins (HDL), and may also increase low-density lipoprotein (LDL) levels. Both changes are risk factors in the development of atherosclerosis; they may be detrimental for patients with atherosclerosis and, in particular, for patients with a risk of coronary vascular disease.

Allergic Reactions

The androgens and anabolic steroids themselves are not likely to cause allergic reactions. However, preservatives or other additives, such as dyes or benzyl alcohol, in some of the products may cause allergic reactions in susceptible individuals. Some oral fluoxymesterone or methyltestosterone tablets contain tartrazine dye (FD&C Yellow #5), which may cause allergic reactions, mainly affecting the respiratory tract, in some individuals. The risk appears to be greatest in patients with asthma or an allergy to aspirin. Some formulations of testosterone cypionate and propionate, and of nandrolone decanoate and phenpropionate, contain benzyl alcohol.

Effects on Laboratory Tests

Androgens inhibit hepatic clotting factor synthesis and can result in excessive prolongation of prothrombin time (also see drug interactions section). Androgens also raise plasma LDL cholesterol and lower HDL cholesterol concentrations. Liver function tests are often altered (for example, increases in bilirubin concentration and the activities of liver enzymes AST and ALT). Androgens have also been shown to affect thyroid function tests.

NURSING IMPLICATIONS

Urge all patients to wear a MedicAlert or similar tag indicating their diagnosis and androgen medication.

Monitor women receiving androgen therapy for vaginal bleeding and for signs of virilization. Outpatients must be instructed to report immediately any vaginal bleeding, the appearance of facial hair, or hoarseness. When such adverse effects are noted, notify the physician for consideration of drug withdrawal. Advise women receiving palliative androgen therapy for breast carcinoma that improvement is likely to be slow and that virilizing effects will occur. Reassure women receiving temporary androgen therapy that early signs of virilization are reversible and will disappear after therapy is discontinued.

Use particular caution when androgens are administered to patients with medical conditions that might be aggravated by fluid retention, particularly cardiovascular or renal disease. Monitor all patients for edema, weight gain, and changes in liver function tests. Obtain pretreatment measurements of blood pressure, weight, and plasma calcium levels for all patients scheduled for androgen therapy, and monitor these parameters periodically during therapy. Other tests that must be done for selected patients include

- monitoring hemoglobin and hematocrit results in patients receiving high doses of androgens; report high levels if this is not the desired therapeutic effect;
- monitoring males for prostatic hypertrophy and gynecomastia;
- monitoring blood calcium levels and for signs of hypercalcemia (nausea, vomiting, lethargy) in bedridden or immobilized patients and in those receiving androgens for palliative relief of breast carcinoma symptoms.

Advise patients of the possible adverse effects of androgen therapy, and instruct them to notify the physician if nausea, vomiting, edema, jaundice, or priapism occurs.

Encourage patients receiving high-dose androgen therapy to drink large volumes of fluids to reduce the risk of renal calcium stone formation and intractable constipation caused by hypercalcemia.

Carefully check the medication history for prior allergies. The major goal is to identify a history of asthma, allergic or other untoward responses to aspirin, and adverse responses to drugs containing benzyl alcohol or tartrazine dye. Notify the physician if there is a positive history, or a suspicion of one. Alternatives to most products containing these triggers of allergic responses are available, and are preferred when the history is positive or suspect.

Use During Pregnancy and Lactation

Androgen therapy during pregnancy, and especially during the first trimester, causes virilization of the external genitalia of the female fetus. Androgen use is therefore absolutely contraindicated during pregnancy and is strongly discouraged for any woman of childbearing age. It is not known whether androgens are excreted in human milk. Because of potential adverse effects on the nursing infant, androgens are usually contraindicated during breastfeeding.

Use in Children

Instruct parents of children receiving androgen or anabolic drug therapy to make and keep appointments for medical evaluation at six-month intervals. At this time, bone growth should be monitored by X-rays of the hand and wrist to detect and then prevent premature ossification and growth retardation.

Scrupulous hygiene and application of an appropriate drying acne lotion are recommended if drug therapy aggravates oiliness of the skin and acne.

Assess children for signs of premature puberty (enlarged phallus, precocious sexuality), which requires withdrawal of the drug.

Use in the Elderly

Careful monitoring of older patients for signs of edema and possible aggravation of cardiac or hypertensive disease is important. Prostatic enlargement is common in older men, and androgen therapy may increase the gland size, interfering with voiding. The risk of prostatic carcinoma also increases. Elderly males frequently experience excessive sexual stimulation and priapism.

Interactions with Other Drugs

Several testosterone analogs, including methyltestosterone and stanozolol, can cause serious interactions in patients receiving an oral anticoagulant. The mechanism is not known. However, the likely outcome is a potentiation of the anticoagulant's effects and a significant increase in the risk of bleeding or hemorrhage unless prothrombin times are monitored closely and the anticoagulant dosage is adjusted accordingly. Indeed, you should anticipate the need to reduce anticoagulant dosages when testosterone analog therapy is started in a patient who is stabilized on warfarin and to increase the dosage when hormone therapy is stopped.

The interaction is much less likely to occur with testosterone itself. Nevertheless, close monitoring is still important.

NURSING IMPLICATIONS

Always obtain a complete drug history to identify and thereby minimize or avoid drug interactions. Because of the potential interaction between androgens and antacids that are available over-the-counter (OTC), be sure to ask about nonprescription drug use. Advise the physician of any interacting drugs the patient is taking.

Assess patients for conditions noted earlier that might be aggravated or precipitated by androgens, particularly if therapy with interacting drugs is unavoidable. Baseline data obtained before starting androgen therapy is important for assessing changes once treatment has begun and for helping determine whether drug dosages should be changed or combined therapy should be stopped. For persons taking oral anticoagulants, check prothrombin times and assess for unusual bleeding, bruising, or petechiae, and report abnormalities at once. Blood glucose levels should be checked carefully in persons with diabetes. Encourage diabetic patients to report signs and symptoms of hypoglycemia at once and to follow dietary recommendations with extra care. Measure body weight, blood pressure, and other indicators of related adverse effects of interactions between androgens and other drugs that cause sodium and water retention.

SUMMARY OF NURSING IMPLICATIONS

Assessment

Review the patient's history for contraindications to testosterone or anabolic steroids: prostatic hypertrophy; cancer of breast or prostate; preexisting cardiac, renal, or liver disease; allergy to preparations containing tartrazine (yellow dye #5) or aspirin; asthma.

Obtain a complete nursing history to identify medications the patient may be taking that interact with androgens: anticoagulants (increase bleeding tendency); insulin and oral hypoglycemics (hypoglycemia); adrenal corticosteroids, antihypertensives, antacids, phenylbutazone (edema).

Establish baseline height, weight, nutritional status, laboratory values, and blood pressure.

Nursing Diagnoses

Knowledge deficit related to androgen therapy.

Sexual dysfunction related to impotence, menstrual irregularities, changes in libido.

Body image disturbance related to virilism in women, puberty in hypogonadal boys, acne.

Noncompliance with drug therapy related to body image changes.

Fluid volume excess related to sodium and water retention.

Altered nutrition: high risk for more than body requirements related to hypercalcemia.

Planning Implementation

Administer drug safely: IM—upper outer quadrant gluteal muscle; buccal—dissolve between gum and cheek (ensure that patient avoids eating, drinking, and smoking until tablet fully absorbed, about 60 minutes); oral—administer shortly before or with meals.

Monitor for local effects from method of administration: soreness in mouth with buccal form.

Select foods high in protein, vitamins, and minerals (except calcium) when using anabolic steroids; refer to dietician as needed.

Report drug side effects to physician: weight gain, edema, nausea, jaundice, vaginal bleeding, facial hair, hoarseness, priapism, difficulty voiding.

Increase fluid intake to 2000 to 3000 mL per 24 hours if hypercalcemia is present.

Monitor laboratory values and vital signs: hemoglobin and hematocrit with high doses; Ca^{2+} in bedridden, immobilized, or breast cancer patients; liver function tests; glucose in persons with diabetes; sodium, phosphorus, and creatinine; blood pressure.

Weigh patient daily.

Provide emotional support and an opportunity for patient to talk about changes in body image and sexual drive.

Patient and Family Teaching

Teach the patient/family:

The name of the drug, the reason for the drug's administration, and that the drug should be taken only as directed and not given to other people.

That the oral drug can be taken with food to decrease stomach upset.

That many side effects can be expected as a result of the drug's actions in the body—increase in facial hair, balding tendencies, acne, weight gain, increased muscle development, changes in sexual drive, growth (children), menstrual irregularities (women).

That this drug should be kept out of the reach of children.

That MedicAlert tag should be worn to alert health care providers that the patient is taking this drug.

Caution patients about the need for regular medical follow-up and evaluation; provide a calendar or other means to remind the patient of return visits and need for further drug.

Evaluation

The patient/family will:

Know action, use, dosage, and side effects of prescribed medication.

Maintain weight within normal limits; increases with anabolic androgens.

Maintain blood pressure within normal limits.

Comply with medication regimen; state need for long-term therapy.

Keep appointments for follow-up care.

Wear MedicAlert bracelet or tag.

Take measures to minimize or resolve adverse effects.

Annotated Bibliography

Bhasin S: Clinical review 34: Androgen treatment of hypogonadal men. *J Clin Endocrinol Metab* 1992;74(6):1221–1225. *A succinct review of the topic.*

Kaiser FE: Sexuality and impotence in the aging man. *Clin Geriatr Med* 1991;7:63–72. *Discusses normal physiologic changes and the pathologic events that can lead to erectile difficulties in elderly men.*

Lee PA, O'Dea LS: Primary and secondary testicular insufficiency. *Pediatr Clin North Am* 1990;37(6):1359–1387. *Focuses on etiology and treatment, with an emphasis on children, from the general practice perspective.*

Parker LN: Control of adrenal androgen production. *Endocrinol Metab Clin North Am* 1991;20:401–421. *Takes a detailed look at the mechanisms of adrenal androgen release and factors that regulate such a release.*

Ray OS, Ksir C: *Drugs, Society, and Human Behavior.* Fifth ed. St. Louis, Times Mirror/Mosby, 1990. *An excellent source for easy-to-read information about historical, cultural, and social foundations of substance abuse—anabolic steroids and more—plus insight into actions of the drugs themselves.*

Rogol AD: Anabolic steroid therapies for growth disorders. *Hosp Pract* 1989;24:89–92. *Discusses the use of metabolic steroids to promote growth and development. Also addresses growth hormone dynamics and its impact on therapy.*

Rogol AD, Yesalis CE 3d: Anabolic-androgenic steroids and the adolescent. *Pediatr Ann* 1992;21(3):175, 183, 186–188. *Reviews hormonal and behavioral maturation during adolescence and risks associated with anabolic steroid misuse.*

Strauss RH, Yesalis CE: Anabolic steroids in the athlete. *Annu Rev Med* 1991;42:449–457. *Describes reasons why anabolic steroids are banned by most sports organizations and reviews the deleterious side effects of these agents.*

Williams G: Erectile dysfunction-advances. *Practitioner* 1991;235:114, 117–18. *Describes recent developments, both mechanical and pharmacologic, in the treatment of impotence.*

Winters SJ: Androgens: Endocrine physiology and pharmacology. *NIDA Res Monogr* 1990;102:113–130. *A comprehensive review of both physiologic and therapeutic aspects of androgens and anabolic steroids.*

Yesalis CE, Anderson WA, Buckley WE, Wright JE: Incidence of the nonmedical use of anabolic-androgenic steroids. *NIDA Res Monogr* 1990;102:97–112. *Chronicles a long history of misuse of these drugs, plus current abuse patterns and statistics.*

Zachmann M: Therapeutic indications for delayed puberty and hypogonadism in adolescent boys. *Horm Res* 1991;36(3–4):141–146. *Discusses current trends and recommendations for androgen use in these disorders.*

Table 48–C **Clinical Uses and Administration of Testosterone, Related Androgens, and Anabolic Steroids**

AGENT	CLINICAL USES	DOSAGE AND ROUTE OF ADMINISTRATION
Testosterone and Esters		
Testosterone aqueous suspension		
(ANDRO 100; HISTERONE-50, -100; others)	Replacement therapy for androgen deficiency (eunuchism, eunuchoidism, male climacteric, some forms of impotence)	IM: Usually 25–50 mg 2 or 3 times per week
	Palliation of breast cancer	IM: Usually 50–100 mg 3 times a week
	Prevention of postpartum breast pain and engorgement	IM: Usually 25–50 mg daily, starting at time of delivery and lasting 3 or 4 days
Testosterone propionate in oil		
(TESTEX; various generic products)	Indications and dosages as for testosterone aqueous suspension	
Testosterone cypionate in oil		
(ANDRO-CYP; ANDRONATE; DEPO-TESTOSTERONE; other brands and generic products)	Replacement therapy in eunuchism (male hypogonadism)	IM: Usually 50–400 mg every 2–4 weeks (not to exceed 400 mg/month)
	Treatment of delayed puberty in males	IM: Usually 50–200 mg every 2–4 weeks as needed for a limited duration
	Palliation of breast cancer	IM: Usually 200–400 mg every 2–4 weeks
Testosterone enanthate in oil		
(ANDRO LA 200; DELATEST; DELATESTRYL; other brands and generic products)	Indications and dosages as for testosterone cypionate	
Chemically Modified Testosterones		
Fluoxymesterone		
(ANDROID-F; HALOTESTIN; others)	Replacement therapy in male hypogonadism	Oral: Usually 5–20 mg/day
	Delayed puberty	Oral: Usually 2.5–10 mg/day for 4–6 months
	Palliation of breast cancer	Oral: Usually 10–40 mg/day in divided doses for 1–3 months or more, depending on response
	Postpartum breast pain and engorgement	Oral: Usually 2.5 mg shortly after childbirth, then 5–10 mg daily in divided doses for 4 or 5 days
Methyltestosterone		
(ANDROID-5, -10, -25; METANDREN; ORETON METHYL; others)	Male hypogonadism, climacteric, impotence	Oral: Usually 10–40 mg/day Buccal: 5–20 mg/day
	Replacement therapy for male androgen deficiency	Oral: 10–50 mg/day Buccal: 5–25 mg/day
	Postpubertal cryptorchidism	Oral: 30 mg/day Buccal: 15 mg/day
	Postpartum breast pain and engorgement	Oral: 80 mg/day, usually for 3–5 days Buccal: 40 mg/day, as for oral
	Breast cancer	Oral: 50–200 mg/day Buccal: 25–100 mg/day

(continued)

Table 48–C **Clinical Uses and Administration of Testosterone, Related Androgens, and Anabolic Steroids (*Continued*)**

AGENT	CLINICAL USES	DOSAGE AND ROUTE OF ADMINISTRATION
Anabolic Steroids		
Nandrolone decanoate (ANDROLONE-D 100; DECA-DURABOLIN; other brands and generic products)	Adjunctive treatment of anemias, mainly those caused by renal insufficiency	IM: Adults: Males: Usually 100–200 mg once weekly. Females: 50–100 mg once weekly. Children 2–13 years old: Usually 25–50 mg every 3–4 weeks
Nandrolone phenpropionate (DURABOLIN; other brands, generic products)	Metastatic breast carcinoma	IM: Usually 50–100 mg administered once weekly
Oxymetholone (ANADROL-50)	Anemias	Oral: Usually 1 to 2 mg/kg once daily; administration usually lasts 3–6 months to assess adequacy of effect; therapy often may be discontinued, but congenital aplastic anemia may require continuous administration
Stanozolol (WINSTROL)	Hereditary angioedema	Oral: Initially, 2 mg tid; if permissible and edema subsides decrease dosage at 1- to 3-month intervals to 2 mg once daily or every other day; long-term therapy in children not recommended; should be based on frequency and severity of edema and semiannual radiographic assessment for premature epiphyseal maturation

Table 48–S | **Major Side Effects of and Contraindications for Testosterone, Related Androgens, and Anabolic Steroids**

BODY SYSTEM/ Side Effect	CONTRAINDICATION/ PRECAUTION	COMMENTS AND NURSING IMPLICATIONS
ENDOCRINE, METABOLIC, REPRODUCTIVE Hypercalcemia (and related signs and symptoms, including constipation, vomiting, lethargy, muscle dystonias, etc), renal calcium stone formation	Severe renal disease	Risk and need for frequent assessment of serum calcium levels greatest in women with metastatic breast cancer, immobile patients; usually necessary to discontinue androgen administration when laboratory tests indicate hypocalcemia or when symptomatic hypocalcemia occurs
Accelerated bone maturation without proportional increase in linear skeletal growth		Use with great care in children, and only in selected cases for delayed puberty; stress need for semiannual X-rays of hand and wrist to assess bone maturation; accelerated bone maturation usually requires discontinuation of androgentherapy
Gynecomastia	Preexisting gynecomastia (use with great care)	Monitor males and females during androgen therapy; breast enlargement may persist after treatment stopped
Male pattern baldness, acne, seborrhea in men or women		Monitor accordingly; skin-drying acne remedies may provide relief; good skin hygiene essential
Women: amenorrhea, other menstrual irregularities; virilization caused by inhibited gonadotropin secretion, including characteristic deepening of the voice, clitoral enlargement, changes of facial, body hair noted above		Very common during androgen therapy; monitor closely during treatment; most of these side effects, with possible exception of clitoral enlargement, may be reversible with prompt recognition, discontinuation of androgen therapy
Permanent virilization of female fetus	Pregnancy (absolute contraindication); woman of childbearing age	Report pregnancy, discontinue androgen therapy at once
Men: oligospermia, azoospermia, reduced ejaculate volume, priapism		Monitor postpubertal males accordingly during prolonged high-dose androgen administration
Prostatic hypertrophy or carcinoma	Prostatic hypertrophy or carcinoma	Careful pretreatment assessment essential; assess adult males for inguinal pain and changes in urinary comfort or pattern periodically during therapy

(continued)

Table 48–S Major Side Effects of and Contraindications for Testosterone, Related Androgens, and Anabolic Steroids (*Continued*)

BODY SYSTEM/ Side Effect	CONTRAINDICATION/ PRECAUTION	COMMENTS AND NURSING IMPLICATIONS
BLOOD Prolonged prothrombin times, polycythemia, porphyria	History of porphyria (requires cautious use)	Monitor accordingly; notify physician if bleeding, bruising, etc, appear; periodic blood tests (hemoglobin, hematocrit) recommended during use of high doses of androgens; avoidance of OTC drugs with antiplatelet activity (aspirin, ibuprofen) may be helpful if PTT times are slightly prolonged; attempt to rule out history of porphyria, monitor for acute attacks (neuritis, etc) if androgen therapy must be used in persons with positive history
CARDIOVASCULAR/ RENAL Renal sodium, water retention leading to or worsening of hypertension, edema, heart failure, etc	Severe cardiovascular or renal disease	Assess all patients, particularly those receiving high-dose or prolonged androgen therapy, for expected consequences of renal or cardiovascular dysfunction, including increased blood pressure, body weight; edema; venous distention; dyspnea; fatigability; use androgens cautiously in the elderly
Onset or acceleration of hyperlipidemias, hypercholesterolemia, atherosclerotic vascular disease	Severe or refractory hyperlipidemias, hypercholesterolemias, etc	Recommend periodic hematologic studies to detect possible hypercholesterolemia, decreased LDL, increased HDL levels, especially in patients with a history of hyperlipidemia or cerebral, coronary, or peripheral atherosclerotic vascular disorders
LIVER Cholestatic hepatitis with jaundice; hemorrhagic liver damage (pelosis hepatis); hepatic cancer	Severe liver dysfunction	Risk present with long-term high-dose administration of any androgen, may occur with low doses of fluoxymesterone, methandrostenolone, methyltestosterone; assess for jaundice, recommend periodic liver function tests whenever above drugs or dosages are used; evidence of hepatic changes requires prompt notification of physician, discontinuation of androgen therapy; jaundice, hepatitis usually reversible

Table 48–I Major Interactions Between Androgens and Other Agents

AGENT	RESULT OF INTERACTION	COMMENTS AND NURSING IMPLICATIONS
Anticoagulants, oral (Chapter 35)	Significantly increased risk of excessive bleeding, hemorrhage	Interaction likely with testosterone analogs (eg, methyltestosterone, stanozolol), much less with testosterone itself; monitor prothrombin time; assess for bruising, bleeding; anticipate need to reduce anticoagulant dosage when adding hormone and to recheck PT and readjust anticoagulant dosage when hormone stopped

PROTOTYPES

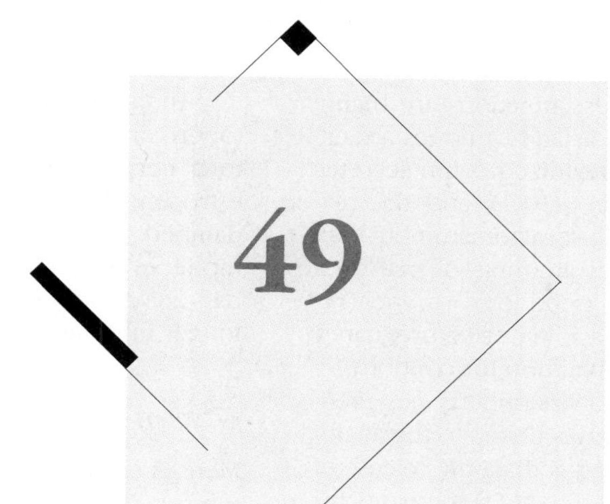

Ovarian Hormones and Hormones Related to Pregnancy

The ultimate biologic function of the reproductive system is to perpetuate the species. Thus, the reproductive system is unique, because the other organ systems of the body function primarily to sustain the individual. The essential female reproductive role is to produce ova; the male's role is to manufacture sperm. If fertilization occurs, the uterus provides a nurturing environment in which the fetus develops until birth. The reproductive process is complex and involves many interlocking neural and hormonal controls. Both gametogenic and hormonal dyscrasias can diminish or abolish reproductive capability.

This chapter begins with an overview of the endogenous ovarian hormones. The first main drug-oriented section of the chapter is divided into two main parts: one focuses on estrogen; the second focuses on progesterone. Estrogen and progesterone are the two main ovarian hormones, and so they may be considered prototype agents. Discussions of these hormones are divided into the usual parts that have been used elsewhere in the book for prototypes. As you will see, however, synthetic and semisynthetic estrogen-like and progesterone-like agents are used much more in clinical practice. Their actions are so similar to the naturally occurring hormones that discussions of the therapeutic agents are integrated into the discussions of the natural hormones.

Section two of the chapter discusses oral contraceptives—another large group of agents that will be considered, collectively, as a prototype. Section three covers miscellaneous drugs used as ovulatory and fertility stimulants. Section four discusses drugs used to alter uterine muscle motility. The emphasis is on uterine stimulants and the prototype drug, oxytocin. Uterine relaxants are discussed briefly at the end of the chapter.

Major reference tables appear beginning on p. 1027.

Ovarian Hormonal Function: Regulation and General Effects

The female reproductive system can be viewed as a four-tiered system involving the hypothalamus; the anterior pituitary gland; the gonads; and a duct system (fallopian tubes, uterus, and vagina). The duct system provides passageways for sperm entry, menstrual outflow, and the birth of a baby. The female reproductive system is unique, compared to the male's, in its ability to house and nurture a developing fetus until birth.

The ovaries begin to assume their adult functions—gametogenesis (ova production) and secretion of ovarian hormones—at puberty. These functions are highly integrated. The predominant ovarian hormones are estrogen and progesterone. The fertilized ovum secretes human chorionic gonadotropin (HCG), and the placenta secretes human chorionic somatomammotropin. The ovaries also produce small amounts of male sex hormones (androgens) and a peptide hormone (relaxin), which is thought to play a role during pregnancy to relax pelvic ligaments in preparation for childbirth.

Initiation of ovarian function at puberty is genetically and centrally controlled and is linked to the attainment of a critical body weight. Hypothalamic release of gonadotropin releasing hormone (GnRH) increases for three to four years after puberty, eventually resulting in a cyclic release of gonadotropins (follicle stimulating hormone [FSH] and luteinizing hormone [LH]) by the anterior pituitary gland. Increasing levels of FSH stimulate follicle maturation in the ovary and follicular production of estrogen.

Estrogen production in females, like that of testosterone in males, is largely responsible for the changes that take place at puberty. Estrogen causes feminization and prepares the young woman's body for childbearing. Estrogen directly stimulates the growth of the female reproductive duct system and causes enlargement of the breasts by promoting fat deposit and growth of the milk duct system. Estrogen also promotes the pubertal growth spurt and its cessation (via epiphyseal closure), skeletal changes leading to widening of the female pelvis, a feminine pattern of fat distribution, and growth of axillary and pubic hair.

Generally, by the second year of puberty, sufficient estrogen is produced to induce irregular sloughing of the endometrium and the initial manifestations of menses (menarche). After the first several bleeding episodes and ovarian cycles (which are, most likely, anovulatory), normal ovarian cyclic function is established with a rhythmic uterine (or menstrual) cycle.

Normal reproductive function depends on the proper sequential balance of anterior pituitary and ovarian hormones and is exquisitely susceptible to neural and hormonal interference. The major events of the female ovarian and uterine cycles are depicted in Figure 49–1.

Ovarian Cycle

Oscillations between pituitary and ovarian hormones result in the sequential follicular and luteal ovarian stages. Rising FSH levels promote the follicular stage and estrogen secretion. Estrogen stimulates pituitary release of LH.

The peak LH levels trigger ovulation at midcycle (approximately day 14). The ruptured follicle converts to a corpus luteum, and releases progesterone and estrogen. As progesterone levels rise, LH release is damped. The corpus luteum atrophies and ovarian hormone levels fall to their lowest levels at approximately day 28. A new cycle is initiated as FSH release (no longer inhibited) begins once again.

Uterine (Menstrual) Cycle

Menses occurs during the first two to seven days of the uterine cycle, when ovarian hormone levels are low. Then, under the influence of rising estrogen levels, the uterine mucosa proliferates rapidly to form a thick velvety lining. Vascularization increases and secretory glands form in preparation for the next phase.

Beginning approximately at ovulation, rising progesterone levels antagonize endometrial proliferation but enhance its vascularization and secretory activity. Progesterone modifies the endometrium in the direction of pregnancy.

In the absence of fertilization, the sudden drop in ovarian hormone levels by day 28 causes the uterine blood vessels to become spastic. Deprived of nutrients and oxygen, the endometrium becomes necrotic, and menses begins. Although both estrogen and progesterone levels have diminished, the drop in progesterone levels is the more important determinant of menses onset. Control of the ovarian cycle is a result of hormonal feedback between the anterior pituitary and the ovary, but the menstrual cycle is a direct uterine response to ovarian hormones only.

If fertilization occurs, the developing embryo produces HCG, which has LH-like activity. In its presence, the corpus luteum continues to produce estrogen and progesterone, which act to maintain the pregnancy until the placenta can assume the hormonal functions of pregnancy.

In adult women, estrogen primes the uterus for menstrual cycling and maintains the mature state of the reproductive organs. In nonpregnant women, progesterone is important for promoting the secretory phase of the menstrual cycle and feedback inhibition of LH and FSH secretion. During pregnancy, both estrogen and progesterone blood levels increase, but the source of these hormones is the placenta, not the ovaries.

In middle age, a natural decline in ovarian estrogen production occurs, marking the onset of menopause, or the female climacteric. Ovulation and menstruation become less regular and more infrequent, reflecting the variations in estrogen levels. Just as estrogen is the first

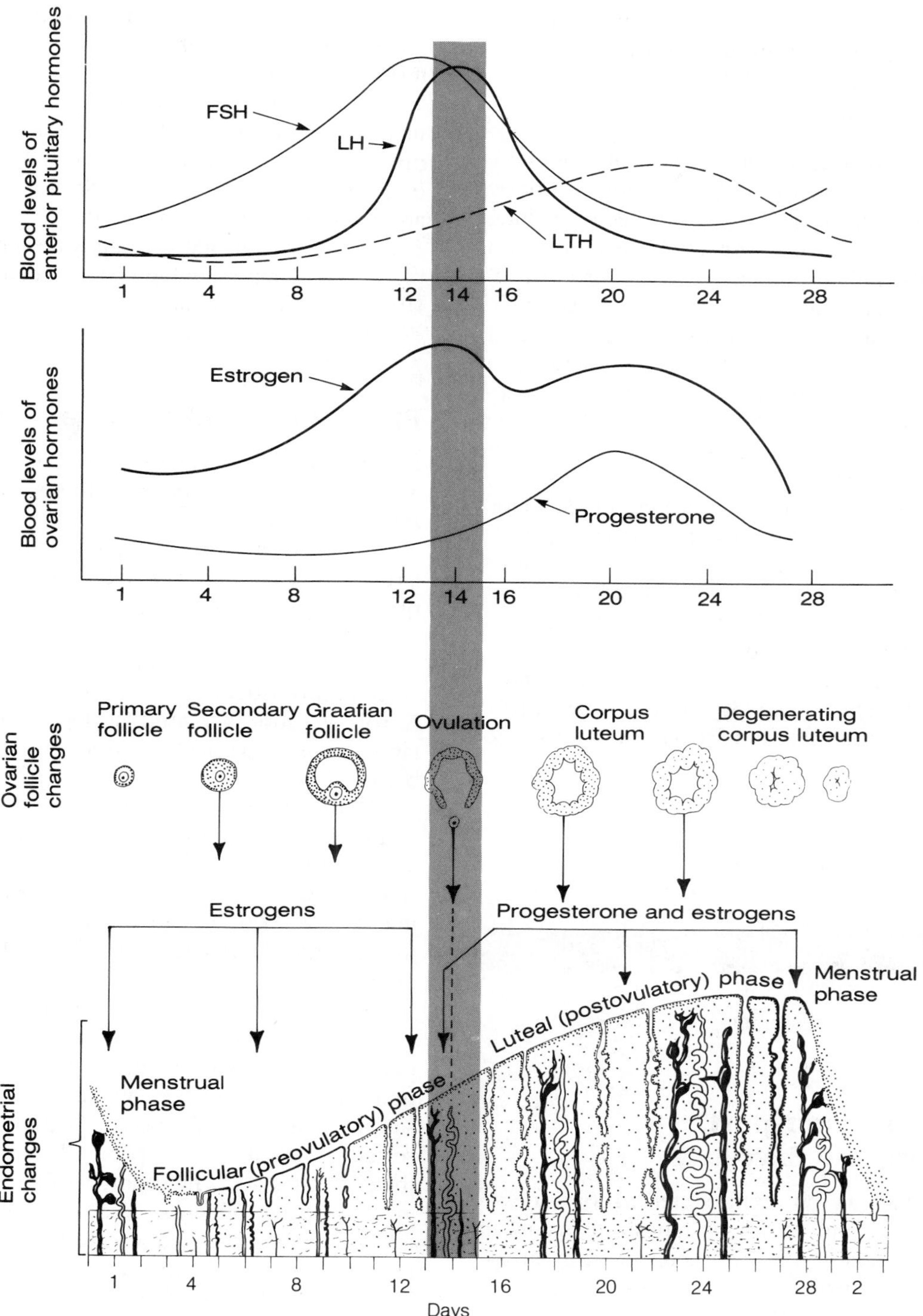

Figure 49–1

Hormonal interactions of the female cycles. Anterior pituitary hormone levels are correlated with the follicular and luteal stages of the ovary and with ovarian hormone release. The menstrual cycle is also depicted.

Source: Marieb EN, *Human Anatomy and Physiology Laboratory Manual, Cat Version,* 2nd ed., 1985 Benjamin/Cummings, p 393.

ovarian hormone to appear during puberty, it is the last hormone to disappear as reproductive capacity wanes.

Irregular Cycles

Disturbances of cyclic function are relatively common. The etiology of most menstrual irregularities is poorly understood, but many of the minor problems resulting in anovulatory cycles or amenorrhea are functional and tend to be self-limiting. Certain emotional or environmental changes, such as severe anxiety or excessive physical exercise, can inhibit hypothalamic release of GnRH and inhibit menses. Other causes of amenorrhea include excessive prolactin secretion, leading to inappropriate lactation, and excessive androgen production (usually a result of an androgen-secreting adrenal cortical or ovarian tumor).

When ovarian hormones are lacking or deficient, reproduction is not possible. Without estrogen, prepubescent girls fail to mature and secondary sex characteristics never appear. The variety of possible causes of ovarian hormone deficits and reproductive dyscrasias is beyond the scope of this text. Ovarian hormones (or their synthetic analogs) are used clinically for replacement therapy, to treat some types of gynecologic problems, in birth control pills, and for other indications to be discussed later.

I. Ovarian Hormones

PROTOTYPE

Estrogen

Biosynthesis, Transport, Metabolism, and Excretion

Estrogen is actually a group of three steroid hormones—estradiol, estrone, and estriol—synthesized mainly in the liver from cholesterol. Many intermediates in the estrogen synthesis pathway are identical to those involved in testosterone synthesis (Chapter 48).

Estradiol is secreted at a rate ranging from 50 to 350 μg per day, depending on the time of the female cycle. Estrogen plasma levels peak at ovulation and remain high during the life of the corpus luteum. Estrogens are transported in the circulation both in free and conjugated forms (50% or more is bound to plasma proteins). The plasma half-life of estrogens is approximately one hour; but their duration of action is two to three days.

Estrogen is metabolized and conjugated to glucuronides or sulfates by the liver. The bulk of estrogen metabolites are eliminated in urine. A small amount is excreted into the bile, reabsorbed by intestinal cells, and recirculated back to the liver.

During pregnancy, estrogens are produced by the placenta and appear in high concentration in the urine. Urine from pregnant mares is a major source of natural estrogens for commercial use.

Physiologic and Pharmacologic Effects

Estrogen enters target cells and binds to receptors, where it influences protein synthesis and promotes enzyme activation.

Estrogen is weakly anabolic; its primary anabolic targets are the secondary sex organs. However, it also promotes protein synthesis in other body tissues, and some tissue wasting (particularly of skeletal tissue) occurs in its absence, as demonstrated by the rapid acceleration of osteoporosis in postmenopausal women. Estrogens cause increased fat deposition in the subcutaneous tissue, particularly in the thighs, buttocks, and breasts.

Estrogen directly stimulates endometrial growth and thickening. Prolonged or excessive estrogen exposure causes abnormal endometrial hyperplasia, which is associated with abnormal (functional) uterine bleeding. Its action on the uterine myometrium and smooth muscle in the fallopian tube walls is to increase motility or contractile activity.

Peaking estrogen levels at ovulation cause the cervical mucus to become thinner and more watery, thus easing sperm passage into the uterus. Estrogen also promotes thickening of the vaginal mucosa and glycogen storage by the vaginal mucosa. Glycogen metabolism by resident vaginal bacteria produces lactic acid, creating the protective acid environment of the vagina.

Under the influence of estrogen, the skin thickens and becomes more hydrated. Estrogen also decreases platelet adhesiveness, increases serum levels of vitamin K–dependent clotting factors, depresses the release of gonadotropins by the anterior pituitary, and suppresses lactation in postpartum women.

Important metabolic effects of estrogen include

- depression of bone resorption, conservation of calcium and phosphorus, epiphyseal closure, and enhancement of bone formation;

- modification of carbohydrate absorption and metabolism by reducing intestinal motility (and thus the rate of sugar absorption) and by antagonizing the hypoglycemic activity of insulin;
- alteration of liver metabolism, which results in higher plasma levels of thyroxin and cortisol binding proteins; and
- enhancement of α-lipoprotein and triglyceride plasma levels and depression of β-lipoprotein and cholesterol plasma levels. This overall action, in conjunction with the capillary dilatation and vascular maintenance activities of estrogen, is believed to be the basis for estrogen's cardiovascular protective effect.

Therapeutic Products

Ethinyl estradiol and mestranol are the two synthetic estrogens most commonly used in oral contraceptives. Estradiol is the most potent estrogen secreted by the ovary. It is rapidly oxidized to produce estrone, which is half as potent. Estrone is then hydrated to produce estriol. Estradiol or its metabolites are commonly used in drug preparations of nonsynthetic estrogens.

Preparations used clinically are broadly classified into natural estrogens, their esters, and semisynthetic derivatives; and synthetic nonsteroidal compounds with estrogenic activity. Preparations are available in oral, parenteral, and topical forms.

Estradiol and estrone are poorly absorbed when administered orally and are almost immediately inactivated by the liver. However, conjugated estrogens, esterified estrogen derivatives, and chemically modified synthetic forms are effective after oral and parenteral administration. Topical forms are readily absorbed and may cause systemic effects.

Conjugated estrogens are mixtures of estrogens isolated from the urine of pregnant mares. They are relatively inexpensive, well absorbed orally, and effective for many clinical purposes. As a result, they are widely used.

When injected in oil or suspensions, the estradiol esters (dibenzoate, cypionate, dipropionate, and others) provide prolonged activity (one month or more) because of their slow absorption from intramuscular (IM) injection sites.

Ethinyl estradiol is a synthetic steroid ester. Because of specific chemical alterations, it persists in the body much longer than the natural estrogens.

The synthetic steroid esters are presumed to be distributed, metabolized, and excreted in the same manner as endogenous estrogens. Metabolism of ethinyl estradiol and its congeners is different; inactivation by the liver and other tissues is considerably slower, but the actual degradative process is not known.

Diethylstilbesterol (DES) was the first ***nonsteroidal estrogen*** discovered, and it is the most potent. Compared to natural estrogens, it is highly active when administered orally, and its duration of activity is much longer. Little is known about its metabolic fate.

Both the steroidal and nonsteroidal estrogens effectively reproduce the whole spectrum of physiologic effects caused by endogenous estrogens. Supraphysiologic doses

- predispose patients to edema and effects on other systems, which may complicate the therapy of elderly, bedridden, or malnourished patients;
- increase the incidence of gallbladder disease, thromboembolic disease, benign hepatic adenoma, hypertension and glucose intolerance; and
- alter the composition of circulating lipids. This includes increases in high-density lipoproteins (HDLs) and plasma triglycerides and decreases in plasma cholesterol and low-density lipoproteins (LDLs).

Clinical Indications and Administration

Equivalent doses of all clinically useful estrogenic compounds cause virtually the same therapeutic responses and side effects. The choice of preparation depends on cost, duration of action, convenience, route of administration, approved indication, and physician's choice. Oral preparations are often preferred because of their ease of administration, prompt effects, and easy termination of treatment. Intramuscular administration has few advantages since onset of activity is slow. Table 49–C1 provides a partial summary of the treatment forms and usual dosages of estrogen products currently in clinical use.

Estrogens are used for a wide variety of clinical conditions. Important indications for estrogen-only products relate to three major use categories:

- replacement therapy in girls with primary hypogonadism, and relief of vasomotor symptoms in menopausal women;
- palliative treatment of advanced breast or prostate cancer; and
- treatment of estrogen deficiency–induced osteoporosis.

Estrogen is used infrequently to suppress lactation and breast engorgement in postpartum women.

Estrogens used in combination with progesterone have their broadest use as oral contraceptive agents. Combination products are also used to treat various gynecologic conditions, including endometriosis and hypermenorrhea, and to produce cyclic withdrawal bleeding. Estrogen-progesterone combinations are discussed as a separate topic. This discussion considers clinical indications and rationales for the use of estrogen-only products.

Menopausal/Postmenopausal Use

As a woman ages, the functional life of the ovaries declines. The average age at onset of menopause is 48 years, but many women retain full reproductive capability well into their fifties.

During menopause, estrogen secretion declines slowly, continuing for several years after menses has ended. This decline causes symptoms such as hot flashes and inappropriate sweating (vasomotor symptoms), palpitations, and atrophic vaginitis. Headache, dizziness, fainting, paresthesias, and muscle and joint aches, as well as feelings of anxiety or emotional lability, may occur. Obese females may show fewer of these symptoms, presumably because their greater body fat is an important source of extraovarian estrogen synthesis.

Estrogen replacement therapy is specific and effective in relieving vasomotor symptoms after menopause, and continued therapy will prevent vaginal atrophy. Estrogens also prevent vulvovaginal atrophy, a condition that makes women susceptible to vaginitis and dyspareunia. However, there is no evidence that estrogens relieve emotional lability or alter the natural aging or arteriosclerotic processes.

Estrogen replacement therapy for vasomotor symptoms of menopause is treated with the lowest dose that will control symptoms. The use of local estrogenic medications in the form of creams or vaginal suppositories is effective in managing atrophic vaginitis or kraurosis vulvae, a distressing itchy condition of the vulva.

Estrogen therapy for relief of "nervous symptoms" or depression is controversial for several reasons. A universally safe therapeutic dose does not exist—there is an increased incidence of endometrial cancer in postmenopausal women given unopposed estrogens. More important, no controlled randomized trials have shown estrogen therapy to be effective at relieving nervous symptoms. As a result, the risks of this therapy outweigh its benefits.

Nevertheless, fixed-dose proprietary products containing estrogens and other agents are available. For example, conjugated estrogens are combined with meprobamate, a barbiturate-like sedative, or chlordiazepoxide. Such products are claimed to be beneficial for menopausal vasomotor symptoms accompanied by anxiety or tension not responsive to estrogens alone. Products containing estrogen and androgens (eg, PREMARIN with methyltestosterone) are also marketed for use when estrogens alone fail to control menopausal vasomotor and other symptoms.

Prevention of Osteoporosis

Osteoporosis commonly occurs in postmenopausal women and is associated with estrogen deficiency. Reduced bone mass will also occur in women with bilateral oophorectomy before natural menopause. Factors thought to be associated with a higher incidence of osteoporosis are cigarette smoking, immobility, low dietary calcium, high caffeine consumption, high alcohol consumption, and thin stature. Clinical signs of osteoporosis are not evident until the later stages, when preventive estrogen therapy is no longer helpful. The difficulty in diagnosing and treating osteoporosis is the lack of clear diagnostic criteria in the early, symptomless, stage of the disease.

The NIH Consensus Development Conference on Osteoporosis concluded that estrogen replacement therapy is the most effective single modality in prevention of osteoporosis. Estrogen replacement therapy at doses of at least 0.625 mg conjugated estrogens per day prevents or retards bone loss as long as therapy continues. Doses less than this have not been shown to be effective, and doses greater than this were equally effective as 0.625 mg. Conjugated estrogens, mestranol, or estradiol are generally used. One product, ESTRADERM, is available as a topical patch that releases estradiol over a period of less than one week. Estrogen replacement therapy is more effective at preventing osteoporosis than reversing it, and so should be started early after menopause. Variables other than declining estrogen levels have been suggested to be associated with osteoporosis, but evidence is inconclusive.

Progestin is used to supplement estrogen therapy to reduce the risk of endometrial hyperstimulation. This is why cyclic estrogen with added progestin may reduce the risk of endometrial cancer.

Most randomized trials show calcium supplementation results in a small protective effect against loss of some bone mass. However, the effect is much less than that provided by estrogen and will not replace previously lost bone mass, which can be achieved with appropriate estrogen use.

TRENDS AND CONTROVERSIES IN PHARMACOLOGY

Myths About Calcium, Estrogen, and Osteoporosis

The media's oversimplification of the relationships among calcium and estrogen and bone health has fostered misconceptions about what women can and cannot do to avoid osteoporosis. Strong bones are not solely the result of high calcium intake or premenopausal estrogen levels.

Many factors predispose people to osteoporosis. Medical conditions such as hypopituitarism, thyrotoxicosis, and Cushing's syndrome contribute to the condition. Prolonged therapy with many drugs—including aluminum-based antacids, corticosteroids, cytotoxic agents, furosemide, heparin, phenobarbital, phenytoin, and thyroid hormones—can weaken bones. Three "social" drugs are also detrimental to bone health: caffeine, nicotine, and alcohol.

For women, the rate of bone loss increases after menopause. When menopause takes place abruptly following oophorectomy ("surgical menopause"), a woman's chances of developing osteoporosis increase dramatically. This iatrogenic contribution to osteoporosis is significant; more than half a million oophorectomies are performed every year in the United States. The average age at hysterectomy—a procedure frequently accompanied by oophorectomy—is 35.6 years. For women who lose their ovaries so young, there are many more years of accelerated bone loss, and their risk of developing osteoporosis is high.

The role of estrogen loss in bone health remains far from clear. Estrogen replacement has been found to reduce postmenopausal bone loss. However, long-term therapy of five to ten years is probably needed to reduce fracture risk, making it difficult to evaluate the effectiveness of treatment (Stork and Hosking, 1991). Even after a natural menopause, all women don't have an equal probability of developing osteoporosis. White women are at greater risk than black women; the rates of osteoporosis for black women and black men are similar.

The fact that osteoporosis occurs late in life may be due not simply to hormonal changes, but in part to the sedentary lifestyle of most Americans. Even a short period of bedrest causes a loss of calcium from bones. Studies of the effects of regular, moderate, weight-bearing exercise on bones in older people are encouraging (Chow, Harrison, and Notarius, 1987), and point to exercise as a significant, easily initiated method of slowing bone loss later in life.

Many dietary factors influence bone health. Inadequate vitamin D intake decreases calcium absorption, although this occurs only rarely. Excess protein, fat, salt, sugar, or phosphorus—substances found in red meats, soft drinks, and processed foods that are consumed in abundance by many people—all increase the body's calcium needs by decreasing calcium absorption or increasing its excretion.

For many years, osteoporosis was considered to reflect normal aging, and so it received little attention. But growing interest in the prevention and treatment of osteoporosis over the past decade marks an encouraging trend in the recognition of issues concerning women's health. Without ever purchasing a calcium supplement or undergoing estrogen replacement therapy, women can do several things to maintain or improve bone health: exercise regularly; spend at least a few minutes in the sun every day; avoid caffeine, nicotine, and alcohol; and limit dietary fat, protein, salt, sugar, and phosphorus.

Chow R, Harrison JE, Notarius C: Effect of two randomized exercise programmes on bone mass of healthy postmenopausal women. *Br Med J* 1987; 295:1441–1444.

MacPherson KI. Osteoporosis and menopause: A feminist analysis of the social construction of the syndrome. *ANS* 1985; 7(4):11–22.

Stork, MD, Hosking DJ. Treatment of osteoporosis: current and future. *Ann Rheum Dis* 1991; 50:663–665.

Treatment of Female Hypogonadism

A variety of conditions may cause failure of ovarian function at puberty. These include chromosomal abnormalities, such as Turner's syndrome; hypofunction of the pituitary or hypothalamus; and others. In such cases, estrogen replacement therapy reproduces pubertal events (except for the growth spurt) and, of course, normal ovarian changes. Estrogen therapy is initiated with larger estrogen doses and then slowly decreased when menstrual periods are initiated.

Treatment of Cancer

Estrogens are used as palliative agents for advanced prostatic cancer in men and for the treatment of inoperable radiation-resistant metastatic breast carcinoma in both women (five years or more postmenopausal) and men for whom bilateral orchidectomy is contraindicated. The final outcome of the disease is not changed by estrogen therapy, but it may reduce the patient's symptoms. Lower estrogen doses are used for palliation of prostatic cancer. Feminizing effects such as gynecomastia and loss of libido routinely occur with estrogen therapy in men. DES is the estrogen most commonly used for prostatic cancer (see Chapter 59).

NURSING IMPLICATIONS

Roll all containers of estrogen suspensions and solutions between the palms to resuspend the drug before aspirating into a syringe. Refrigerate parenteral conjugated estrogen preparations before reconstitution, and shake gently after reconstitution. Inject dosage forms for IM injection deeply, and rotate injection sites if repeated administration is necessary.

Instruct patients using vaginal suppositories to store the product in the refrigerator. Instruct them how to insert the suppository, and to wash their hands before and after drug administration. Teach patients using estrogen creams for external or vaginal (mucosal) use proper administration techniques. When vaginal creams or suppositories are used, advise the patient that lying down for 30 minutes after insertion, and wearing a perianal pad, will help prevent soiling clothes. Instruct patients using transdermal estrogen delivery systems (eg, ESTRADERM) to apply the patch to a clean, dry area of skin on the trunk.

Side Effects, Adverse Reactions, and Contraindications

Estrogens may cause many side effects. Effects on the reproductive system are discussed first, since that is the primary site of estrogen action. Table 49–S1 summarizes the side effects associated with estrogen use.

Effects on Reproductive Organs and Secondary Sexual Characteristics

Estrogen-induced side effects on the female reproductive tract include

- breast tenderness, enlargement, or secretion; breakthrough bleeding, changes in menstrual flow, dysmenorrhea, or amenorrhea during and after treatment;
- a syndrome resembling premenstrual syndrome;
- vaginal candidiasis;
- changes in cervical eversion and cervical secretions;
- a cystitis-like syndrome;
- endometrial cystic hyperplasia; and
- uterine fibromyomata.

As discussed later, pregnancy absolutely contraindicates estrogen use. Males may experience feminization and impotence; these effects are reversible after estrogen therapy is stopped.

Endometrial, Breast Cancers

Estrogens increase the risk of endometrial carcinoma, compared with the incidence in otherwise matched nonusers. The risk appears to parallel the dose and duration of treatment, especially in postmenopausal women receiving estrogens uninterrupted for a year or more. The risk with cyclic administration of estrogens may be lower. Women with a personal or family history of cancer may be at a higher risk than those without such a history. Persistent or recurrent abnormal vaginal bleeding must be evaluated at once, with the specific aim of diagnosing the cause and identifying a possible malignancy. Such episodes may contraindicate further use of estrogens or products containing them, especially until an underlying cause can be diagnosed.

Studies of thousands of women taking oral contraceptives (with cyclic estrogen administration) indicated no increased risk of breast cancer. There is no evidence that a given estrogen preparation is more or less hazardous than others. However, estrogens should be used with great caution in women who have a strong family history of breast cancer or who have breast nodules, fibrocystic disease, or abnormal mammograms. Estrogens are absolutely contraindicated for patients with known or suspected breast cancers, unless the patient has been specifically selected for estrogen therapy of a metastatic disease.

Other Cancers

Long-term, continuous estrogen administration to some animals has increased the frequency not only of breast, cervix, and vaginal carcinomas, but also carcinomas of the liver and kidney. Although benign and rare, estrogen-related hepatic carcinomas may occur in human beings, causing rupture and death from intraabdominal hemorrhage. Hepatic lesions must be considered in any estrogen user with abdominal pain and tenderness, an abdominal mass, or hypovolemic shock. Hepatocellular carcinoma has been reported during estrogen therapy, but whether the drug caused the cancer is uncertain. A known or suspected estrogen-dependent neoplasm in any site absolutely contraindicates the use of this hormone.

Central Nervous System Side Effects

Estrogen therapy may cause changes in libido. Headache (including migraine), dizziness, chorea, and seizures have been reported. There is also evidence of an increased risk of depression during estrogen therapy, and patients with a history of depression should be assessed closely.

Cardiovascular Side Effects

Elevated blood pressure is common during estrogen therapy. Usually the pressure rise is small, but this vital sign should be monitored closely and periodically in all patients receiving any estrogen. Significant hypertension has been reported. Increased weight and edema, probably related to fluid retention, also may occur. Some patients may lose weight. It is likely that fluid retention may worsen not only prior renal or cardiovascular dysfunction, but also noncardiac disorders such as asthma, migraine, and seizures.

Estrogen use, including oral contraceptive use, is associated with an increased risk of thromboembolism (including thrombophlebitis, pulmonary embolism, stroke, and myocardial infarction). Cases of retinal and mesenteric thrombosis, of optic neuritis, and of postsurgical thromboembolic complications have been reported. These thromboembolic effects have not occurred as often in women taking estrogens after menopause.

Males taking large doses of conjugated estrogens (5 mg per day or more) are at increased risk of nonfatal myocardial infarction, pulmonary embolism, and thrombophlebitis, and men receiving estrogens for prostatic cancer are at increased risk of thrombosis.

For any patient, cigarette smoking increases the risk of serious cardiovascular side effects from estrogens. The risk increases with age and the number of cigarettes smoked. The risk is dramatically increased in women smokers over the age of 35 years.

Overall, any person with active thrombophlebitis or a thromboembolic disorder should be treated with estrogens cautiously. A history of such disorders precipitated or worsened by previous estrogen therapy contraindicates further use of these agents. Exceptions are patients for whom estrogens are considered essential, such as those with refractory and advanced breast or prostate malignancy. Estrogens should be used with great caution in patients with cerebrovascular or coronary artery disease, and only when such drugs are clearly needed.

Gastrointestinal Tract and Accessory Organ Side Effects

Estrogens commonly cause nausea. Taking the drug with the evening meal usually is effective in reducing the incidence and severity of this problem. Some patients develop vomiting, abdominal cramps, bloating, colitis, and acute pancreatitis. Patients with a history of jaundice during pregnancy have an increased risk of recurrence while receiving estrogen-containing oral contraceptives. Studies suggest a doubled risk of gallbladder disease in postmenopausal women taking estrogens. If jaundice occurs, the estrogen should be discontinued while the cause is being evaluated. Estrogens are metabolized poorly in patients with impaired liver function, and so should be administered to such patients with caution. Cholestatic jaundice may occur.

Dermatologic Side Effects

Estrogens can cause chloasma (hyperpigmentation of the skin), which may persist when the drug is discontinued. Erythema nodosum or multiforme, hemorrhagic eruptions, urticaria, dermatitis, loss of scalp hair, and hirsutism have all been reported. Some estrogen-induced skin rashes are photosensitive.

Metabolic Side Effects

Decreased glucose tolerance has occurred in patients taking estrogens, which requires monitoring in prediabetic or diabetic individuals. These drugs may cause severe hypercalcemia in patients with breast cancer, bone metastases, or renal insufficiency.

Other Side Effects

Estrogens have been reported to precipitate acute intermittent porphyria. A positive history, whether induced by estrogens or other common causes of this response (barbiturates, for example), requires cautious use of estrogens, if they are administered at all. Estrogens may steepen the cornea's curvature, and may cause intolerance to contact lenses.

NURSING IMPLICATIONS

Manufacturers of estrogen preparations provide information written especially for the patient. That information must be supplied to and reviewed with the patient.

All patients should have pretreatment physical examinations that include assessment of the breasts, abdomen, pelvic organs, and the menstrual pattern. For women of appropriate ages, a pretreatment Papanicolaou (Pap) test should be performed. All patients should have pretreatment blood pressure and body weight measurements, measurements of serum lipid profiles, and other tests related to the individual's history. Obtain a personal and family history to assess prior cancers and breast disease, cardiovascular diseases and risk factors (including smoking habits), and to rule out interacting drugs. Complete physical examinations, including a Pap smear, should be repeated every six months (preferred) to one year. No patient should receive estrogens for longer than one year without an intervening physical examination. The risks of endometrial cancer in women make this critically important.

Teach women breast self-examination techniques, and encourage them to perform them regularly. Advise patients of potential estrogen side effects. It is important for them to report at once evidence of possible

- thromboembolism (thigh or calf pain, swelling, warmth or redness; chest pain or dyspnea; headache, dizziness, faintness; numbness or weakness of a body part; any visual disturbances);
- cardiovascular problems (edema or weight gain);
- hepatic dysfunction or gallbladder disease (jaundice or severe abdominal pain);
- untoward endocrine or precancerous changes (breast lumps or abnormal vaginal bleeding); and
- mental depression.

Strongly encourage smokers to quit or drastically reduce smoking. Recommend taking oral estrogen preparations with meals to reduce the incidence of gastrointestinal (GI) side effects and the risk of missing a dose.

Anticipate the need to discontinue estrogens or estrogen-containing drugs about four weeks before elective surgery, especially surgery that carries a high risk of thromboembolism (eg, orthopedic surgery or procedures likely to require prolonged periods of bed rest and immobility). If your patient is scheduled for such a procedure, ask the physician whether estrogens are to be discontinued, and, if so, advise the patient. Careful assessment is indicated not only for these patients, but also for those receiving estrogen therapy who encounter major trauma, unscheduled surgery, or other insults that increase the risk of thrombosis and embolism.

Educate women receiving estrogen and progesterone replacement therapy of the importance of cyclic timing of drug administration. Teach them to report any breakthrough bleeding at once, and make them aware that such bleeding does not indicate that fertility has been restored. Any suspicion of pregnancy should be reported to the physician at once.

Advise male patients to anticipate feminization, and offer support when such changes or impotence occurs. Reassure the patient that these effects are reversible when estrogen therapy is discontinued.

Stress to diabetic patients the need for careful adherence to diet, exercise, and drug therapy; to monitor closely their blood or urine glucose or ketone levels (as prescribed by the physician); and to report any sudden changes in symptoms or overall feeling of well being.

◆ Use During Pregnancy and Lactation

Use of estrogen early in pregnancy may result in serious damage to the fetus. Female offspring exposed to DES in utero are at increased risk to develop a rare form of vaginal cancer or cervical cancer in their teens or twenties. These is no evidence that estrogen is effective in treating threatened or habitual abortion. In utero exposure to estrogen has been associated with congenital anomalies, including congenital heart defects and limb reduction defects. Therefore, estrogen therapy is contraindicated in pregnancy. Women desiring to breast-feed should not use estrogen for suppression of lactation.

◆ Use in Children

Estrogen therapy is not indicated for use in children owing to insufficient data on the effects of estrogens in children. These drugs should be used with caution prior to completion of bone growth (epiphyseal closure).

Interactions with Other Drugs

Estrogens interact with several common drugs (Table 49–11). They enhance hepatic inactivation of oral anticoagulants and increase formation of active clotting factors by the liver. Both effects may require increased anticoagulant doses to maintain the desired anticoagulant effect. Insulin or oral hypoglycemic drug requirements of diabetic patients may be increased; tricyclic antidepressant doses may need to be lowered or discontinued to reduce the risk of toxic reactions. Estrogens, through their ability to increase biliary cholesterol secretion and gallstone formation, counteract the effects of chenodiol, which is used to dissolve gallstones.

Drugs that induce hepatic drug-metabolizing enzymes (barbiturates, meprobamate, phenytoin, rifampin, and others) may increase the metabolism of estrogens, thereby counteracting their effects. The greatest related concern is failure of estrogens to act as oral contraceptives. Alterations of normal gut flora caused by broad-spectrum antibiotics can reduce the reabsorption of orally administered estrogens, which undergo enterohepatic recirculation. Here, too, the major concern is pregnancy during combined treatment.

NURSING IMPLICATIONS

Assess for the anticipated responses to interactions between estrogens and other drugs. Some interactions, whether short-term (broad-spectrum antibiotics, rifampin) or long-term (phenobarbital and phenytoin, used for treating chronic seizures), may be unavoidable. They are particularly important when estrogens are administered as contraceptives. Advise women to assess for vaginal spotting or breakthrough bleeding, which may be early indicators of contraceptive failure. If these responses occur, the patient should report them at once, and either abstain from intercourse or use supplemental contraceptive methods.

PROTOTYPE

Progesterone

Progesterone is the prototype *progestin* (progesterone-like) drug. Progestins available for clinical use include both the natural steroid hormones and synthetic derivatives.

Biosynthesis, Transport, Metabolism, and Excretion

Progesterone is produced by the corpus luteum, testes, and adrenal glands, and by the placenta during pregnancy.

In the luteal phase, the corpus luteum secretes approximately 20 to 30 mg of progesterone daily. During the follicular phase, progesterone secretion is suppressed and amounts secreted are only slightly higher than those secreted in males (1 to 5 mg per day).

The plasma half-life of progesterone is about five minutes, but its activity persists for approximately 24 hours. Small amounts of progesterone are stored in body fat. Most of the circulating hormone is metabolized in the liver. The major portion of its metabolites is excreted in urine as pregnanediol glucuronide. Urinary content of pregnanediol provides an indirect but clinically useful index of progesterone secretion and metabolism. Small amounts are excreted in breast milk.

Physiologic and Pharmacologic Effects

Like estrogen, progesterone enters the target cell to influence protein synthesis. Its major physiologic effect in nonpregnant women is to promote changes in the estrogen-primed endometrium to convert it to a secretory mucosa. Both estrogen and progesterone are necessary to produce the normal endometrial cycle. Progesterone also influences the cervical glands, causing the abundant watery secretion promoted by estrogen to be changed to a scant, viscous secretion shortly after ovulation. Progesterone is responsible for alveolobular development of the secretory breast.

Rising progesterone levels influence the spontaneous contractile activity of the uterus: contraction amplitude increases, but frequency decreases. Then, as progesterone levels decline toward the end of the menstrual cycle, uterine contractions increase in force, sometimes becoming tetanic. This may be the basis of idiopathic dysmenorrhea, since it is clear that progesterone sensitizes the uterus to oxytocin, which causes premenstrual cramping. Progesterone also plays a part in labor induction, which occurs when levels drop near term.

Progesterone's metabolic effects are fewer than those of estrogen. It decreases plasma amino acid levels and causes a slight catabolic effect, leading to enhanced nitrogen excretion. By competing with aldosterone, progesterone inhibits sodium ion reabsorption by the kidney tubules, which, in turn, promotes enhanced aldosterone release.

Progesterone increases body temperature, perhaps through an action on hypothalamic heat regulating centers.

Therapeutic Products

Progestins that are given as drugs exert the same physiologic effects as endogenous progesterone—they convert a proliferative endometrium into a secretory endometrium, induce changes in cervical mucus consistency, inhibit spontaneous uterine contractions, and at high doses can damp release of hypothalamic GnRHs. High doses of progestins suppress endometrial bleeding; progestin withdrawal induces endometrial sloughing and has antineoplastic activity against some cancers.

Progesterone itself is poorly absorbed when given by mouth; thus, the natural progestins are administered parenterally, by IM injection. Synthetic progestins are available for oral and parenteral administration. Absorption by all routes is rapid, and inactivation by hepatic enzymes is prompt. All progestins are eliminated in the urine.

Clinical Indications and Administration

Progestin-only preparations are used for the treatment of functional uterine bleeding and some types of amenorrhea; as adjunctive and palliative therapy for metastatic endometrial or renal carcinoma and endometriosis; and investigationally as a long-acting contraceptive in females and for management of paraphilia—deviant sexual practices—in males (Table 49–C2). Progestins are used in combination with estrogen in oral contraceptives.

Progestins are also used investigationally as diagnostic agents to determine if the ovary is functional in estrogen production. There is growing interest in their use to manage premenstrual syndrome. The various progestins provide useful therapeutic effects for treating specific conditions, and they cannot be interchanged. Because progesterone injections tend to be painful and may cause local inflammation, the oral preparations are almost always preferred for daily dosing schedules.

Treatment of Functional Uterine Bleeding

Functional uterine bleeding occurs when the hypothalamic-pituitary-ovarian axis is altered, causing irregular ovulation. It is much more common at the extremes of reproductive life—that is, at menarche and menopause. It usually results from continuous estrogenic stimulation of the endometrium without cyclic opposition by progesterone. In the absence of a dramatic drop in ovarian hormones, complete desquamation of the endometrium does not occur, so bleeding is not self-limiting. Alternatively, estrogen levels may be slightly low, resulting in a poorly developed proliferative endometrium. The endocrine basis of both conditions is similar: steady, poorly cycling estrogen activity unopposed by progesterone action.

The immediate goal of therapy is to stop the bleeding; the long-range goal is to regulate the cycle. Acute bleeding can be controlled by both estrogen and androgens, but progesterone has more specific activity and is preferred. Therapy may be initiated by daily administration of IM injections of progesterone, or an oral synthetic progestin such as norethindrone for one to two weeks; or by administration of a long-acting progestin such as medroxyprogesterone acetate, or hydroxyprogesterone caproate. Withdrawal of progesterone results in endometrial shedding within three to seven days, which approximates a normal menstrual flow. This approach, sometimes referred to as a medical dilatation and curettage (D&C), is highly reliable for controlling bleeding caused by anovulation.

Occasionally, more than one course of treatment may be needed to restore normal cycles. In women at the end of the usual reproductive life, normal cycling may not be possible. Such women may benefit from cyclic administration and withdrawal of progestins to stimulate periodic endometrial sloughing.

Treatment of Amenorrhea

Amenorrhea may reflect emotional problems, pregnancy, completion of menopause, reproductive organ defects, endocrine dysfunction, or systemic disease. Primary amenorrhea occurs in hypogonadal females who have never menstruated. Secondary amenorrhea occurs in women who have previously demonstrated menstrual cycling. Both types are treated with cyclic administration of estrogen and progesterone (or more commonly, estrogen-progestin combinations).

Diagnostic Testing for Endogenous Estrogen Production

Progestins may be used as diagnostic agents to determine if the ovaries are capable of producing estrogen. One procedure involves IM injection of 250 mg of hydroxyprogesterone caproate. Because administration of a progestin will produce a secretory endometrium and withdrawal bleeding only if the endometrium has been estrogen-primed, failure to bleed indicates a deficit of endogenous estrogen. Normal ovarian function is indicated by the initiation of menses seven to 14 days after the progestin challenge.

Treatment of Endometriosis

In its most severe form, endometriosis involves the implantation and enlargement of extrauterine masses of endometrial tissue that have been carried to host organ sites in the pelvic cavity by retrograde menstrual flow. These ectopic masses bleed and slough in response to cyclic changes in ovarian hormones, in the same manner as the uterine endometrium. As the masses bleed, surface swelling of the host organs occurs, causing pain and possible sterility if the ovaries are damaged or the fallopian tubes become blocked.

Danazol and nafarelin are the drugs for initial endometriosis therapy.

Management of Premenstrual Syndrome

Premenstrual syndrome (PMS) encompasses a broad range of physical and emotional symptoms, including irritability, mood swings, depression, breast swelling and tenderness, abdominal bloating, and fatigue. Both the timing and degree of the symptoms vary widely among women. Some are troubled only the day before menses onset, whereas others are affected for up to 14 days before onset. The symptoms may be mild enough to be disregarded, or they may severely disrupt the woman's life. It is estimated that approximately 30% of women of reproductive age suffer from PMS. The etiology of PMS is still unknown, but ovarian dysfunction has been implicated; both high and low progesterone levels have been demonstrated during the period of PMS symptomatology.

High-dose progesterone therapy (25 to 100 mg per day, IM or SC, or 200 to 400 mg up to 4 times daily administered via rectal or vaginal suppositories) has been shown to ameliorate PMS symptoms in a few cases. The results have been variable and controversial; in many cases, placebos had equivalent effects. Therapy with GnRH agonists is also being evaluated.

Other Uses

Some of the synthetic progestins, such as megestrol acetate and medroxyprogesterone acetate, are used to treat advanced endometrial cancer and other hormone-dependent cancers. They can be used in conjunction with traditional anticancer drugs, surgery, or radiation therapy. Medroxyprogesterone acetate is also being used investigationally to treat menopausal symptoms, paraphilia, hirsutism, and a variety of other disorders.

Progestins have been used to manage threatened abortion and to treat infertility, but these uses are not recommended.

Side Effects, Adverse Reactions, and Contraindications

Usual complaints associated with progestin therapy are gastrointestinal (GI) upset, headache, and dizziness. Prolonged administration of high doses enhances GI disturbances, and promotes edema, weight gain, breast congestion, and menstrual abnormalities. Progestins may decrease glucose tolerance. Other effects include thromboembolism, cholestatic jaundice, depression, breakthrough bleeding, amenorrhea, insomnia, alopecia, acne, and hirsutism. These and other adverse effects of the progestins are listed in Table 49–S1.

Progestins are contraindicated in patients with any of the following:

- demonstrated hypersensitivity to these drugs;
- current or past history of thromboembolic disease;
- missed abortion or undiagnosed vaginal bleeding;
- known or suspected cancer of the breast or genital organs;
- markedly impaired liver function or liver disease;
- thrombophlebitis;
- cerebral hemorrhage (current or past).

The use of progestins as therapeutic or diagnostic test agents during pregnancy is also contraindicated.

NURSING IMPLICATIONS

Administer parenteral progestin preparations as deep IM injections, and rotate injection sites for repeated injections. Inspect the injection site for inflammation.

Provide instructions about proper use of orally administered progestins. Instruct patients complaining of GI distress to take the drugs with food.

The pretreatment physical examination should include breast and pelvic exams and a Pap smear. Observe patients for depression, particularly those with a history of depression. Acute intermittent porphyria may be precipitated. Caution patients about possible skin photosensitization. Assess patients for medical conditions in which edema may aggravate the underlying disease (migraines, asthma, seizures, cardiac or renal dysfunction). Observe diabetic patients for a decrease in glucose tolerance. Instruct patients to report any symptoms of possible thromboembolic disease, such as headache; thigh or calf pain, particularly if accompanied by swelling, warmth, and redness; acute chest pain or sudden shortness of breath; visual changes; dizziness or fainting; and numbness in an arm or leg. Instruct the patient how to monitor basal body temperature to determine ovulation, and advise her that conception can occur during treatment for hormonal imbalance.

◆ Use During Pregnancy and Lactation

The use of progestins during the first four months of pregnancy is not recommended, owing to possible harm to the fetus. Several reports have suggested an association between intrauterine exposure to female sex hormones and congenital anomalies. If the patient is exposed to progestins during the first four months of pregnancy, or if she becomes pregnant while taking this drug, she should be apprised of the potential risks to the fetus.

Other Drugs Used for Endometriosis

Danazol

Danazol (DANOCRINE) is used for managing endometriosis. It is a synthetic *androgen* that suppresses the pituitary-ovarian axis by inhibiting pituitary gonadotropin output. Danazol alters normal and ectopic endometrial tissue so that it becomes inactive and atrophic. Complete resolution of endometrial lesions occurs in the majority of cases. As a result, many women with this disorder have been able to retain or reachieve their ability to bear children. See Table 49–C2 for dosages.

The side effects of danazol and the high cost of therapy are the major drawbacks to its use. Androgenic reactions (see Chapter 48 for details) include acne, oily skin or hair, and hirsutism; edema and weight gain; voice deepening; and decreased breast size.

Nafarelin

Nafarelin (SYNAREL) is a synthetic agonist of GnRH that desensitizes pituitary GnRH receptors. This desensitization leads to decreased gonadotropin release. Nafarelin is comparable to danazol in the management of endometriosis, but there are potentially fewer side effects. Common adverse effects include hot flashes and other signs of hypoestrogenemia, such as vaginal dryness.

Nafarelin is rapidly absorbed following intranasal administration. Other therapeutic uses are the management of uterine leiomyoma, precocious puberty (for which nafarelin is classified as an orphan drug), and palliation of prostate and breast cancers.

II. Oral Contraceptives

In the 1950s, progestins were used experimentally to induce ovulation in women who appeared normal but failed to conceive. Instead researchers found that ovulation could be abolished pharmacologically, and for as long as desired, by combination estrogen and progesterone therapy. The original preparation used, ENOVID, was a combination of norethynodrel (a progestin) and mestranol (an estrogenic compound). Subsequent studies helped optimize the drug combinations and discovered lower effective doses. The earlier high-dose sequential pills were taken off the market because their use was associated with a greatly increased risk of endometrial cancer. Today, the combination oral contraceptives are among the most widely used drugs in the world, with well over 50 million women taking them to prevent pregnancy. However, data on their long-term effects are just now becoming available, and the drugs are becoming better understood.

There are three classes of oral contraceptive (OC) drugs marketed today: estrogen-progestin combinations; progestin-only preparations; and estrogen-only (for emergency postcoital use only) preparations. All three share several common properties, but their differences are important.

Estrogen-Progestin Combination Contraceptives

The estrogen-progestin combinations are associated with the lowest pregnancy rate—0.005% to 0.01% per user per year. In spite of side effects arising mainly from their estrogenic activity, they are effective contraceptives. These are the agents commonly called birth control pills or, simply, "the pill." Table 49–1 lists some of these products and their compositions.

Absorption, Distribution, Metabolism, and Excretion

All the combination OC products are well absorbed following administration. Their individual components are metabolized and excreted as described earlier. Small amounts are excreted in breast milk.

Pharmacologic Effects

The most important action of the OC combinations is suppression of ovulation by suppression of FSH and LH release. There may also be a direct action on reproductive tract organs: depressed fallopian tube motility and thickening of the cervical mucus, which prods the early secretory endometrium into a stage of secretory exhaustion that is inhospitable to an implanting embryo. These effects interfere with sperm motility and prevent implantation. (Progestin-only contraceptives also alter the cervical mucus, interfere with implantation, and

Table 49–1 Oral Contraceptives

Trade Name	Estrogen Content	Progestin Content
	Monophasic*	
GENORA 1/50	50 μg mestranol	1 mg norethindrone
NORINYL 1 + 50-21	50 μg mestranol	1 mg norethindrone
ORTHO-NOVUM 1/50-21	50 μg mestranol	1 mg norethindrone
OVCON-50	50 μg ethinyl estradiol	1 mg norethindrone
NORLESTRIN 1/50-21	50 μg ethinyl estradiol	1 mg norethindrone acetate
NORLESTRIN Fe 1/50	50 μg ethinyl estradiol	1 mg norethindrone acetate
DEMULEN 1/50-21	50 μg ethinyl estradiol	1 mg ethynodiol diacetate
NORLESTRIN 21-2.5/50	50 μg ethinyl estradiol	2.5 mg norethindrone acetate
OVRAL	50 μg ethinyl estradiol	0.5 mg norgestrel
GENORA 1/35	35 μg ethinyl estradiol	1 mg norethindrone
NORINYL 1 + 35-21	35 μg ethinyl estradiol	1 mg norethindrone
ORTHO-NOVUM 1/35-21	35 μg ethinyl estradiol	1 mg norethindrone
BREVICON-21	35 μg ethinyl estradiol	0.5 mg norethindrone
MODICON	35 μg ethinyl estradiol	0.5 mg norethindrone
OVCON-35	35 μg ethinyl estradiol	0.4 mg norethindrone
DEMULEN 1/35-21	35 μg ethinyl estradiol	1 mg ethynodiol diacetate
LOESTRIN-21 1.5/30	30 μg ethinyl estradiol	1.5 mg norethindrone acetate
LOESTRIN Fe 1.5/30	30 μg ethinyl estradiol	1.5 mg norethindrone acetate
LO/OVRAL-21	30 μg ethinyl estradiol	0.3 mg norgestrel
NORDETTE-21	30 μg ethinyl estradiol	0.15 mg levonorgestrel
LEVLEN-21	30 μg ethinyl estradiol	0.15 mg levonorgestrel
LOESTRIN-21 1/20	20 μg ethinyl estradiol	1 mg norethindrone acetate
LOESTRIN Fe 1/20	20 μg ethinyl estradiol	1 mg norethindrone acetate
	Biphasic	
ORTHO-NOVUM 10/11-21	Phase I: 10 days 35 μg ethinyl estradiol	0.5 mg norethindrone
	Phase II: 11 days 35 μg ethinyl estradiol	1 mg norethindrone
	Triphasic	
ORTHO-NOVUM 7/7/7	Phase I: 7 days 35 μg ethinyl estradiol	0.5 mg norethindrone
	Phase II: 7 days 35 μg ethinyl estradiol	0.75 mg norethindrone
	Phase III: 7 days 35 μg ethinyl estradiol	1 mg norethindrone

(continued)

Table 49–1 **Oral Contraceptives (*Continued*)**

Trade Name	Estrogen Content	Progestin Content
TRI-NORINYL	Phase I: 7 days 35 μg ethinyl estradiol	0.5 mg norethindrone
	Phase II: 9 days 35 μg ethinyl estradiol	1 mg norethindrone
	Phase III: 5 days 35 μg ethinyl estradiol	0.5 mg norethindrone
TRI-LEVULEN-21		
TRIPHASIL-21	Phase I: 6 days 30 μg ethinyl estradiol	0.05 mg levonorgestrel
	Phase II: 5 days 40 μg ethinyl estradiol	0.075 mg levonorgestrel
	Phase III: 10 days 30 μg ethinyl estradiol	0.125 mg levonorgestrel
	Progestin-Only	
MICRONOR		0.35 mg norethindrone
NOR-QD		0.35 mg norethindrone
OVRETTE		0.075 mg norgestrel
	Estrogen-Only (postcoital emergency use only)	
Diethylstilbesterol	25 mg twice daily for 5 days	

*Monophasic oral conceptives are listed in order of decreasing estrogen content. Many brand-name oral contraceptives are marketed with the suffix "28" instead of "21" (not listed by brand name). The medication dispenser contains 28 tablets for 28 sequential days of use. Tablets used for the first 21 days contain estrogen and progestin in amounts identical to those of products listed above. The remaining 7 tablets contain inert ingredients to increase compliance by having the patient take one tablet every day and may differ in appearance for those used for the prior 21 days. Some oral contraceptive products (not listed) may also include the designation "Fe," indicating the presence of an iron supplement.

may suppress ovulation.) Other effects, usually considered beneficial, include more regularity of menstrual cycles, and a lower incidence of dysmenorrhea.

Most patients resume normal menstrual patterns within three months after terminating OC therapy. However, women with a history of amenorrhea are prone to relapse after ceasing use of any OC.

Clinical Indications and Administration

The most important use of combination OC products is, of course, prevention of pregnancy. Other investigational uses include management of some types of menstrual irregularities, including amenorrhea, functional bleeding, and endometriosis. These uses were discussed earlier.

Many combination OC products are *monophasic*—that is, they consist of fixed and unchanging doses of a potent estrogen (ethinyl estradiol or its methyl ester derivative, mestranol), and one of several synthetic progestins (ethynodiol diacetate, levonorgestrel, norethindrone, norethynodrel, or norgestrel). Each ingredient causes different effects, providing a selection for the best preparation for each individual. For example, and as summarized in Table 49–2, the progestin component can exert estrogenic or antiestrogenic activity, or androgenic actions. The relative amounts and activities of both the estrogen and progestin ingredients (Table 49–3), considered together, are also important in terms of product selection and potential side effects (discussed later).

Table 49–2 **Relative Hormonal Activities of Progestins Used in Oral Contraceptives**

Drug	Activity			
	Progestin	**Estrogen**	**Antiestrogen**	**Androgen**
Ethynodiol diacetate	2+	1+	1+	1+
Levonorgestrel, norgestrel	3+	0	2+	3+
Norethindrone	1+	1+	1+	1+
Norethindrone acetate	1+	1+	3+	1+
Norethynodrel	1+	3+	0	0

Listed alphabetically. The relative activities are useful when selecting a drug or drug combination for achieving specific effects, and for helping predict likely side effects.

Key to pharmacologic effect 3+, pronounced; 2+, moderate; 1+, slight; 0, no effect.

Source: Adapted from *Drug Facts and Comparisons*, 1992:108b. Copyright Facts and Comparisons, St. Louis, 1992.

Table 49–3 **Relative Estrogen/Progestin Potencies of Selected Oral Contraceptive Combination Products**

Progestin Activity	Estrogen Activity: **Low**	Estrogen Activity: **Intermediate**
Low	BREVICON LOESTRIN 1/20 MODICON NORINYL 1+35, 1+50 ORTHO-NOVUM 1/35, 1/50, 10/11, 7/7/7 OVCON-35 TRI-NORINYL TRIPHASIL	NORLESTRIN 1/50 OVCON 50
Intermediate	DEMULIN 1/35 LO/OVRAL NORDETTE	NORLESTRIN 2.5/50 DEMULIN 1/50
High		OVRAL

Listed alphabetically within groups.

Source: Adapted from *Drug Facts and Comparisons*, 1992:108b. Copyright Facts and Comparisons, 1992.

Biphasic oral contraceptives contain one estrogen-progestin dose ratio during the first 10 days of the treatment cycle and a larger progestin dose during the last 11 days of therapy.

The newest combination products marketed in the United States are ***triphasic*** oral contraceptives—the tablets, taken in a specific sequence during treatment, have three estrogen-progestin concentrations and ratios. These products were developed to achieve two major goals: to reduce the total hormone content (dose); and to provide hormone delivery that mimics more closely that associated with normal physiologic processes. Current evidence suggests that the triphasic products are equal in efficacy to the monophasic products described earlier, and it is hoped that long-term studies will prove a lower incidence of side effects.

Regardless of the product selected, menstrual flow normally occurs two to three days after the last hormone-containing tablet is taken. This response occurs more reliably with the triphasic agents. The prescribed schedule should be adhered to regardless of the presence or absence of breakthrough bleeding (a side effect) or the anticipation of menstrual flow.

Missed doses increase the chance of ovulation or breakthrough bleeding. The chance is least with a single missed dose, and increases dramatically when consecutive doses are missed. The overall risk of intramenstrual bleeding is lower with the triphasic products, even with a dose omission.

NURSING IMPLICATIONS

Nurses have close contact with women practicing birth control, whether through the use of oral contraceptives or other means. Nurses are in an excellent position to provide trusted advice about proper OC use and their advantages and potential risks. The nurse should be knowledgeable about these drugs and convey that information to the patient regardless of personal views about birth control and birth control methods.

Taking any OC as directed is important to achieve successful therapy. Compliance is particularly critical with the triphasic products, which have low total hormone doses. Oral contraceptive products are packaged for easy use. Some require administration of one tablet daily for 20 or 21 days, starting on day five of the menstrual cycle. Others are supplied in packets of 28 tablets to be taken every day. The last seven tablets of the combination 28-tablet regimen are hormone-free and contain inert substances or, in some products, ferrous fumarate. Discuss with the patient the proper use of the product selected for her. Encourage her to take the medication at the same time each day to establish a routine and reduce further the chance of missing a dose.

Pretreatment teaching should include advice about what to do if a dose is missed:

- One dose: take the drug as soon as the omission is realized, then resume the regular administration schedule.
- Two consecutive doses: either take two tablets per day for the next two days, or take both of the two missed doses as soon as the omission is realized, then resume the normal schedule.
- Three consecutive doses: usually stop therapy, begin a new sequence with a fresh pack of tablets, and discard the supply that had been used up to the time of the missed doses. Instruct patients to use an alternative or additional nonhormonal method of birth control for seven days after two missed doses and for 14 days (or until the next menses) after three missed doses.

Table 49–4 Adverse Effects Related to Estrogen/Progestin Concentrations in Oral Contraceptive Pills

Concentration	Adverse Effect
Estrogen excess	Nausea, bloating, cervical mucorrhea, edema, breast fullness and tenderness, hypertension, headache, hypermenorrhea, fibroid growth
Estrogen deficit	Early/midcycle breakthrough bleeding, spotting, hypomenorrhea, hot flashes
Progestin excess	Weight gain, fatigue, depression, monilial vaginal infections, reduction in breast size, increased appetite, acne, oily skin, hirsutism, hypomenorrhea
Progestin deficit	Late-cycle breakthrough bleeding, hypermenorrhea, amenorrhea

Two other times during which an additional birth control method should be used are during the first monthly drug therapy cycle at the onset of OC use; and for at least the first three months after the woman discontinues OC use to become pregnant.

Side Effects, Adverse Reactions, and Contraindications

Combination OC products may cause any of the side effects or complications noted for estrogens and progestins (see Table 49–S1). Overall, the most common side effects include nausea and vomiting, headache, fluid retention and weight gain, and breast tenderness.

The types and incidences of common side effects reflect the total hormone dose in the particular product, as well as the relative amounts of estrogen or progestin components. Table 49–4 provides information that should help determine whether side effects reflect excesses or deficits of estrogen or progestin in the product being used. Combination OC products containing more estrogen than others (see Table 49–3) produce a heavier menstrual flow and more nausea. Preparations containing more progestins than others cause more weight gain, acne, and fatigue. They also exert more anabolic and androgenic effects. Breakthrough bleeding is common during the first few cycles of monophasic OC administration. If it persists, a product with a different estrogen-progestin balance should be tried. Menstrual flow usually declines after several months of any OC use.

Adverse cardiovascular responses and cancer are the greatest concerns with OC therapy. There is a positive association between the dose of estrogen in OC products and the risk of thromboembolism. The risk of cerebrovascular disorders (idiopathic thromboembolic disease, postoperative thromboembolic complications, thrombotic or hemorrhagic stroke, and myocardial infarction) also increases. Women who smoke and are over the age of 30 have a greater risk of myocardial infarction. Compared with age-matched nonsmokers taking OC drugs, there is a fivefold increase in the risk of a fatal heart attack; compared with women who neither smoke nor take OC drugs, the risk is 10 to 12 times greater. The cardiovascular conditions noted as contraindications for estrogen use apply to the combination OC drugs.

The increased risk of estrogen-linked endometrial cancer was noted earlier, and it applies to estrogen-containing OC drugs as well. Recent studies suggest no increased risk of breast cancer. However, a personal or family history of breast abnormalities (fibrosis, cysts, recurrent cystic mastitis, other lesions, abnormal mammograms) requires very careful use of OC drugs, including frequent monitoring. Cervical dysplasia also requires cautious use because of the risks of cancer.

Oral contraceptives are contraindicated in women with known or a history of thrombophlebitis, thromboembolic disorders, deep vein thrombophlebitis, cerebral vascular disease, myocardial infarction, or coronary artery disease. Women with carcinoma of the breast, estrogen-dependent neoplasia, undiagnosed abnormal genital bleeding, or known or suspected pregnancy should not receive OCs. Women who developed benign or malignant liver tumors during prior use of OCs or other estrogen-containing products should not be given OCs.

NURSING IMPLICATIONS

Consider the possibility of pregnancy when a patient has missed doses and reports a missed menstrual period. Consider the same possibility in persons who have failed to menstruate for two consecutive cycles, even though they have adhered to the medication schedule. In either case, pregnancy must be ruled out before continuing with OC administration. Advise the patient to see her physician at once. Also advise patients to seek prompt reexamination if persistent bleeding occurs, to rule out nonfunctional causes of bleeding.

The nursing implications noted for the side effects caused by estrogens and progestins also apply to combination OC drugs. There is an increased risk of congenital anomalies, such as heart and limb defects, when OC drugs are administered during pregnancy. They will decrease the quantity and composition of breast milk, and are also excreted in milk. Therefore, OC drugs are contraindicated during pregnancy and should not be administered postpartum before weaning to women who wish to breast-feed their infants.

Interactions with Other Drugs

Oral contraceptives, including the combination agents, participate in important interactions with many other drugs. Most of the interactions noted for estrogens alone apply (see Table 49–11). Because oral contraceptives are usually taken for long times, and interruption of therapy and the potential risks of pregnancy generally are undesirable, it may not be possible to avoid interactions with other drugs required by the patient. As a result, knowing the potential interactants and consequences of the interactions may be the best way to anticipate and recognize clinically important problems, and to help modify therapy properly.

Progestin-Only Contraceptives

Progestin-only oral contraceptives, which contain low doses of norethindrone or norgestrel, are sometimes called “minipills.” Their mechanism of action is not fully known, but probably involves alterations of the endometrium that decrease the probability of successful ovum implantation. In some patients these preparations may also suppress ovulation. The pregnancy rate associated with minipills is about 3 pregnancies per 100 women per year, versus less than 1 per 100 women per year for the combination products. Thus, minipills are less effective as contraceptives.

Minipill therapy is started on the first day of menses and continues without interruption thereafter. Patients should be instructed to use other means of contraception during the first 14 days of therapy when the norgestrel-containing product is used.

Special measures must be taken when minipill doses are missed. A single missed dose should be taken as soon as the omission is realized. If two doses are missed, one tablet should be taken at the usual time. In addition, the woman should use an alternative method of birth control until the next 14 tablets have been taken. If more than two consecutive doses are missed, drug therapy should be discontinued, and alternative contraceptive methods used, until menses occurs. Then the usual treatment plan is started again.

Minipills were introduced to eliminate estrogen, the hormone component responsible for most of the adverse effects of the combination OC products. However, the potential adverse effects of the minipills still are not fully known. Therefore, adverse effects, warnings, contraindications, and drug interactions for the minipill should be considered equivalent to those noted for the combination products. In addition, because the minipill is taken continuously, withdrawal bleeding does not occur. Often the user's menstrual pattern becomes irregular and unpredictable. These problems are thought to account for the high dropout rate among patients taking the minipill.

NURSING IMPLICATIONS

All nursing implications noted for combination OC drugs apply. Instruct patients to discontinue minipill administration if they have been amenorrheic for more than 45 days, regardless of the cause, and to request immediate pregnancy testing. All minipill products are contraindicated during pregnancy and lactation.

Progestin-Only Contraception by Other Administration Routes

Progestin-Containing Intrauterine Device

An intrauterine device (IUD) that releases progesterone in small daily doses (65 μg/day) over a year (PROGESTASERT) is available for contraception. Because the progesterone effects are exerted locally, natural hormonal rhythms are not disrupted and systemic effects are largely avoided. The presence of progesterone in the uterine cavity is thought to prevent endometrial proliferation and inhibit sperm capacitation and survival. The pregnancy rate with this product approximates that with the minipill.

A complete pelvic examination is conducted before the device is inserted. The device is inserted during or shortly after menses, checked within three months after insertion, and replaced yearly. The major disadvantages of this product are those of IUDs in general. Their effectiveness results from the mild inflammation induced in the endometrium. Adverse effects include the possibility of severe pelvic infection and uterine perforation. If the patient conceives while wearing the device, ectopic pregnancy, pelvic inflammatory disease (PID), and septic abortion are much more likely than in nonusers. Long-term effects on the fetus are not known. The manufacturer provides an extensive patient education packet with the IUD. It requires the patient's signature, indicating patient education and awareness of the risks associated with the progesterone IUD.

The progesterone-containing IUD is contraindicated in the following conditions:

- pregnancy;
- a history of ectopic pregnancy;
- current or past pelvic infection or PID;
- multiple sex partners;
- endometriosis;
- a history of pelvic surgery;
- current or past venereal disease;
- a history of postpartum endometritis or infected abortion;
- incomplete involution of the uterus after childbirth or abortion;
- a history of pelvic surgery that might be associated with an increased risk of ectopic pregnancy;
- uterine abnormalities resulting in distortion of the uterine cavity;
- known or suspected uterine or cervical malignancy;
- genital bleeding of unknown cause;
- genital actinomycosis;
- acute cervicitis; and
- conditions or treatments associated with increased susceptibility to infections that might be introduced into the uterus during IUD insertion.

In addition, progesterone-containing IUDs are contraindicated in patients with another inserted IUD in place.

NURSING IMPLICATIONS

Advise patients that some bleeding and cramping are likely during the first few weeks after insertion of the device, but to report these adverse effects if they continue or are severe. Immediate reporting of abnormal symptoms, such as abdominal cramping or pain, vaginal discharge, or flu-like symptoms that may indicate septicemia, is mandatory. The increased risk of spontaneous abortion, should pregnancy occur during use, should be made clear.

Give patients the following instructions:

- Check to see if the threads are still in place after each menstrual period. Wash hands before checking.
- Do not tug or pull on the threads.
- If the threads are not detected or pain during sex occurs, notify the physician; use an alternate (nonhormonal) contraceptive method in the interim.
- Return every 12 months for replacement or removal.

Long-Acting Injectable Progestins

There has been a demand for a longer-acting injectable or implantable contraceptive. The need for such a product is especially important for use in underdeveloped countries, where the typical user is not likely to be compliant with daily oral therapy.

Intramuscular injections of medroxyprogesterone acetate have proved to be exceptionally effective contraceptives when administered in high dosages (150 to 300 mg) every three to six months. However, this administration route causes both short-term problems (prolonged or irregular vaginal bleeding and a high risk of amenorrhea and infertility) and an increased risk of birth defects in children of mothers who took medroxyprogesterone acetate in the first four months of pregnancy. The only current approved indication for parenteral medroxyprogesterone acetate (DEPO-PROVERA) is as adjunctive treatment and palliation of inoperable, recurrent metastatic endometrial or renal cancer.

NORPLANT SYSTEM

The NORPLANT SYSTEM (levonorgestrel implants) represents a novel birth control product. NORPLANT consists of six thin capsules, made of soft, flexible material, that are placed in a fan-like pattern under the skin via a small incision on the upper arm. Norplant should be inserted within five to seven days after the onset of menstrual bleeding. The contraceptive effect begins within 24 hours and continues for five years. The average annual pregnancy rate over a five-year period is less than 1%, a rate comparable to surgical sterilization. The capsules can be removed at any time, and fertility will resume.

Adverse effects of NORPLANT consist mainly of menstrual bleeding irregularities. Other risks and adverse effects associated with combination progestin-estrogen oral contraceptives may also occur (see Table 49–S1).

Estrogen-Only Contraceptives

Diethylstilbestrol, a potent synthetic estrogen, has been used as an emergency postcoital contraceptive. The precise mechanism of action of DES is not clear, but it is believed to prevent implantation.

Doses of DES required for postcoital contraception cause unpleasant and potentially dangerous side effects. Therefore, its use is limited to a single five-day course for postcoital contraception in emergency treatment. To increase the drug's effectiveness, treatment should start within 24 hours (and certainly not later than 72 hours) after intercourse (see Table 49–C1). Severe nausea and vomiting are common. In the occasional case in which pregnancy occurs despite DES therapy, an abortion generally is advised because of the risk of inducing vaginal or cervical cancer later in the offspring's life.

III. Ovulatory Stimulants and Fertility Drugs

Anovulation is a normal physiologic state in women who are pregnant, lactating, or postmenopausal. It is a pathologic finding in women with abnormal bleeding patterns and infertility.

The etiology of infertility is often difficult to ascertain. It may result from failure of the adrenal, thyroid, or anterior pituitary glands or from ovarian or testicular failure. Thyroid hormone or corticosteroid replacement therapy is appropriate and may induce ovulation when deficits of those hormones promote infertility. However, the emphasis here is on agents that stimulate the release or mimic the action of endogenous pituitary gonadotropins.

Products used to stimulate the ovaries and induce fertility include the synthetic agent clomiphene citrate and the human-derived hormonal drugs menotropin and urofollitropin. The latter two are used in conjunction with HCG for inducing fertility and selected other indications.

NURSING IMPLICATIONS

A complete endocrinologic work-up is essential before starting any fertility-inducing therapy. Pretreatment assessment should include a thorough history to identify potential medical or drug-induced causes, and assessment of the sperm.

Once the decision to start treatment is made, the patient (and her partner) must be informed of the potential for, and hazards of, multiple births. Drug related potential adverse effects should always be explained.

Teach the importance of the need for daily intercourse as directed by the physician. Provide instructions on how to use a thermometer correctly to determine the time of ovulation. Monitor vaginal secretions to help assess whether ovulation has occurred: mucus becomes clear and can be stretched into a fine thread at the peak of ovulation. Since it will be necessary to measure hormone levels in the woman's urine samples to assess ovulation and the response to therapy, teach proper collection and storage methods. Stress the need to avoid missing scheduled appointments.

Provide the patient with the emotional support needed to cope with the disappointment in being unable to conceive, the lengthy treatment cycles, painful injections (some drugs), possible loss of spontaneity during sexual intercourse, and other subjective responses.

Clomiphene Citrate

Clomiphene citrate (CLOMID; SEROPHENE) is a nonsteroidal drug that is commonly used as a fertility agent. Its structure is similar to that of synthetic estrogens.

Clomiphene is readily absorbed after oral administration. About half the absorbed dose is excreted in the feces within five days of administration, but fecal metabolites can be detected for up to six weeks after a single dose.

Clomiphene stimulates gonadotropin secretion by binding competitively to estrogen receptors in the hypothalamus and anterior pituitary gland. This diminishes the number of receptors available to endogenous estrogen, signalling the hypothalamus and pituitary to increase output of gonadotropin releasing factor and, subsequently, of pituitary gonadotropins. The gonadotropins (FSH and LH), in turn, stimulate ovarian function and induce ovulation.

Clomiphene, given orally, is used to induce ovulation in selected anovulatory patients. The prospective patient must have normal levels of endogenous estrogen and normal liver function.

Therapy usually is started on the fifth day of the menstrual cycle in women who ovulate, or at any time in anovulatory women. The usual initial oral dose is 50 mg, taken for five consecutive days. About 80% of patients become pregnant after the first course of treatment (Table 49–C3). If the woman ovulates but fails to conceive, a second (and third, if needed) treatment cycle (up to 100 mg per day) can be tried at 30-day intervals. With each trial, the likelihood of inducing pregnancy diminishes. No more than three treatment courses are recommended. About 90% of clomiphene-facilitated pregnancies result in single live births. Thus, the incidence of multiple births, most of which involve twins, is much higher than that found in the general population.

Clomiphene is being used investigationally to treat male infertility.

Clomiphene's side effects are usually mild (Table 49–S2). They are unlikely to interfere with therapy, and more likely to occur with high doses. About 11% of women receiving this drug experience mild vasomotor symptoms that disappear after the treatment course is over. About 2% of patients report breast tenderness, nausea and vomiting, or visual changes such as blurring, flashes, or prolonged afterimages. Less than 1% experience central nervous system responses such as insomnia, headache, depression, or fatigue; reversible hair loss; urticaria or other allergic manifestations; urinary frequency; weight gain; or dizziness.

Ovarian enlargement, which usually regresses spontaneously, may occur. However, there have been reports of massive ovarian enlargement in patients with polycystic ovaries, who appear to be unusually sensitive to the drug. Signs and symptoms include massive ovarian enlargement, abdominal distention, pain, and possibly severe hemorrhage (hemoperitoneum) if the cyst(s) ruptures. Thus, the complications are potentially serious. Ovarian hyperstimulation may occur with other fertility-inducing drug regimens, discussed later.

The major contraindications for clomiphene use include current or prior hepatic dysfunction, abnormal bleeding of undetermined origin, evidence of ovarian cysts, and pregnancy. The incidence of congenital birth defects in children of women treated with clomiphene before conception is, overall, no different from that of the general population. The risks rise when the drug is given during pregnancy, which stresses the need for frequent monitoring for pregnancy and the need to discontinue clomiphene therapy at once.

NURSING IMPLICATIONS

Ensure that the contraindications to clomiphene therapy have been ruled out, and advise the woman of the greater incidence of multiple births, before treatment is started. Advise patients to report promptly signs of pregnancy and any of the side effects noted earlier. Encourage patients to avoid operating a motor vehicle or performing other tasks that require alertness or that may be made dangerous by dizziness and visual impairments. Patients who experience visual changes should discontinue treatment at once and seek a complete ophthalmic examination.

Teach the woman to assess for the various signs and symptoms of excessive ovarian stimulation and to report them and other untoward effects (vaginal bleeding, weight gain, etc) at once. Intercourse should be discontinued if there is a suspicion of the hyperstimulation syndrome, and the physician should be consulted immediately.

When caring for women hospitalized for ovarian hyperstimulation, anticipate the need for frequent monitoring of fluid and electrolyte balance (including intake, output, blood and urine tests, assessment for evidence of internal bleeding, and monitoring of weight gain). Advise patients of the need for bedrest, and administer analgesics as ordered. Caution women with significant ovarian enlargement to avoid sexual intercourse, which could rupture ovarian cysts and cause hemoperitoneum. Be aware that pelvic examinations may also cause cysts to rupture.

Menotropins

Menotropins are a preparation of human gonadotropins extracted from the urine of postmenopausal women. The drug product (PERGONAL) is supplied as a biologically standardized powder containing FSH and LH in an activity ratio of 1:1. Little is known about the product's exact metabolic fate, other than that it is probably identical to that of endogenous FSH and LH.

Menotropins are used to promote follicular growth and maturation in anovulatory women with otherwise functional ovaries. Then, HCG is given in the hope of promoting pregnancy. Therapy for anovulation can be started only after assessment to rule out pregnancy, ovarian failure, endometrial cancer, and other uterine and tubal pathologies. The pretreatment work-up and teaching sessions should include the general guidelines noted in the introduction to this section.

Once treatment is deemed appropriate, one ampule of 75 IU FSH/75 IU LH is reconstituted and injected IM daily for nine to 12 days during the seventh to fourteenth day of the menstrual cycle. Urinary estrogen levels are measured, and if the results indicate sufficient follicular maturation a dose of 10,000 USP units of HCG is administered on the day after the last menotropin dose.

The couple should have sexual intercourse daily, beginning on the last day of menotropin administration (the day before HCG administration) and continuing until ovulation is demonstrated by clinical evidence of progesterone production (increased basal temperature, urinary pregnanediol excretion, and so on). If ovulation occurs but pregnancy does not, the dosage regimen may be repeated for two more courses before doubling the daily menotropin dose (150 IU each of FSH/LH), and repeating the courses again. Additional dosage information is given in Table 49–C3.

Pregnancy generally occurs in 20% to 45% of women within four to six treatment cycles. Eighty percent of such pregnancies produce single births. Therefore, 20% are multiple births, a rate that is much higher than that found in the general population. Most of these (15%) are twins, with a relatively high live birth rate (about 93%).

Menotropins and HCG are also used to stimulate spermatogenesis in men with primary or secondary hypogonadotropism but functional testes. See Table 49–C3 for dosages.

Minor side effects associated with menotropins include nausea, vomiting, diarrhea, and fever (see Table 49–S2). The risks of multiple births were noted earlier. The incidence of birth defects is about 1.4%. About one in five treated women will develop mild, uncomplicated ovarian enlargement. As with clomiphene, there is a risk of ovarian enlargement and, possibly, the more severe ovarian hyperstimulation syndrome. Ovarian enlargement usually develops within two weeks following menotropin-HCG treatment. In the hyperstimulation syndrome, which has an overall incidence of about 1.5% with menotropin-HCG therapy, symptoms tend to develop rapidly over three to four days. A small subset of patients may develop sudden ovarian enlargement with ascites, and possible pleural effusion. These symptoms also tend to regress without treatment in two to three weeks. Other potential adverse effects caused by menotropins include arterial thromboembolism and hypersensitivity or febrile reactions. Thromboembolism is a relatively infrequent but serious adverse effect of menotropin use.

The major contraindications to starting or continuing menotropin administration include pregnancy; abnormal vaginal or uterine bleeding, which includes evidence of ovarian hyperstimulation syndrome; ovarian cysts other than polycystic ovarian syndrome; high gonadotropin levels indicating primary ovarian failure; overt thyroid or adrenal dysfunction; and any cause of infertility other than anovulation or organic intracranial lesion.

Gynecomastia is the most common side effect in men. Erythrocytosis occurs rarely. Contraindications for males include elevated gonadotropin levels (primary testicular failure), and infertility arising from causes other than hypogonadotropic hypogonadism.

NURSING IMPLICATIONS

Menotropin preparations may be stored at room temperature or refrigerated. Inject them only by the IM route, immediately after reconstituting the product with sterile saline.

Before they consent to menotropin therapy, advise women of the greater risk of multiple births and of increased infant mortality rates. If they accept these and other risks, advise them to keep scheduled appointments, which usually will be daily or every other day during treatment and for two weeks after HCG administration. Stress the importance of intercourse at the scheduled time and assessing for the common indicators of pregnancy. Precautions noted for clomiphene-induced ovarian hyperstimulation apply also to menotropin-HCG therapy. Advise men receiving menotropins of the risk of gynecomastia.

Related Drugs

Urofollitropin

Urofollitropin (METRODIN), also extracted from human postmenopausal urine, exerts biologic effects equivalent to those of FSH. Urofollitropin stimulates ovarian follicular growth but does not induce ovulation. Therefore, HCG administration is part of the treatment plan for inducing ovulation in patients with polycystic ovarian disease who have elevated LH/FSH ratios and have failed to respond to adequate clomiphene citrate therapy. The usual starting treatment involves once daily IM injections of one ampule of the product (contains 75 IU of FSH activity) for seven to 12 days, followed by 5000 or 10,000 units of HCG on the day after the last urofollitropin dose. Daily intercourse should be started on the day before scheduled HCG injection. Other dosage information is given in Table 49–C3.

Virtually all the side effects and contraindications noted for menotropins apply to urofollitropin. In addition, a few women will experience such dermatologic reactions as dry skin, hair loss, and rashes or urticaria. Precautions concerning proper pretreatment diagnosis, and surveillance for desired responses (including pregnancy) and side effects during and after treatment, are basically the same for urofollitropin as for menotropins. Anticipate a similar incidence and time-course of mild ovarian enlargement and of ovarian hyperstimulation and the need to implement the same nursing implications as noted earlier.

Human Chorionic Gonadotropin

The placenta produces large amounts of HCG during a normal pregnancy. The therapeutic products (A.P.L.; PREGNYL; PROFASI HP; and several other brand and generic names) are derived from the urine of pregnant women.

Human chorionic gonadotropin activity is virtually identical to that of endogenous LH. It has only slight FSH activity. In females, HCG triggers ovulation and maintains corpus luteum production of progesterone. In males, HCG stimulates testosterone production.

The use of HCG with menotropins or urofollitropin for promoting pregnancy was noted earlier. In males, HCG is used to treat cryptorchidism in young boys, usually between the ages of four and nine years, and to manage hypogonadism resulting from pituitary deficiency. However, if hypogonadism caused by pituitary dysfunction has existed for several years before therapy is begun, irreparable testicular damage may have occurred and HCG will have no effect.

Human chorionic gonadotropin may cause headache, irritability, fatigue, gynecomastia, restlessness, edema, and depression. Ovarian hyperactivity, noted in the discussion of menotropins, may occur, as well as multiple births and arterial embolism. Precocious puberty may occur in boys, and it contraindicates further HCG administration. Males are liable to experience gynecomastia. This possibility requires cautious use in persons with conditions aggravated by fluid retention and related electrolyte imbalances, including those with cardiac, renal, or obstructive pulmonary disease, seizures, or migraine headache. Other contraindications to HCG therapy include prostatic cancers or other androgen-dependent neoplasms and allergy to HCG.

NURSING IMPLICATIONS

Reconstituted HCG preparations are stable for 90 days after reconstitution if kept refrigerated. Advise patients that HCG injections are likely to be painful. Inject the drug slowly into a relaxed muscle to minimize tissue trauma and pain. Instruct patients about suitable measures to reduce discomfort (limb exercise, application of heat).

Because the onset of precocious puberty contraindicates further HCG use and parents are in the best position to detect it, teach them the pertinent signs and symptoms. Advise all patients of the side effects noted earlier, and have them report severe or intolerable responses at once.

IV. Drugs Influencing Uterine Motility

A variety of drugs are used before, during, and after labor and delivery to control pain and anxiety, and for other purposes. They have been discussed in other chapters of this text. This section focuses on important drugs that stimulate or inhibit uterine contractile activity.

A. Oxytocics

Oxytocic drugs stimulate contractile activity of uterine smooth muscle. There are three major groups: oxytocin, certain ergot alkaloids, and certain prostaglandins. Although these drugs exert their primary and desired effects on the uterus, they have the potential to cause unwanted effects elsewhere. Oxytocin, one of the two major endogenous stimulants of uterine activity, is discussed first.

PROTOTYPE

Oxytocin

Oxytocin (PITOCIN; SYNTOCINON) and the related hypothalamic hormone vasopressin (antidiuretic hormone; ADH) were discussed in Chapter 44. Oxytocin clearly is the most important endogenous regulator of uterine motility during parturition.

As childbirth becomes imminent during a normal pregnancy, large amounts of oxytocin are released from the hypothalamus. This, in turn, initiates normal stages of labor and delivery. When the effects of endogenous oxytocin are inadequate, or labor and delivery must be induced for medical reasons, oxytocin (PITOCIN; SYNTOCINON) is administered as a therapeutic product.

Absorption, Distribution, Metabolism, and Excretion

Oxytocin is given IV, IM, or as a nasal spray. Oxytocin cannot be given orally because it is a protein that is rapidly degraded in the stomach. The route of administration differs for the different indications. The usual plasma half-life is about five minutes. The short duration of action allows prompt termination of effects when the infusion is stopped.

Oxytocin is metabolized primarily in the liver and kidneys. During pregnancy, and especially at term, high levels of a plasma enzyme that degrades oxytocin and ADH (called oxytocinase or vasopressinase) appear.

Physiologic and Pharmacologic Effects

The effects of therapeutic oxytocin products are identical to those of the endogenous hormone. The major effect is stimulation of uterine contractile force and the frequency of contractions. Increases in tone and frequency in response to oxytocin rise dramatically as parturition draws near. Oxytocin does not stimulate the nongravid uterus nor act well during the first two trimesters of pregnancy.

Oxytocin stimulates mammary myoepithelial cells, ejecting milk into the large sinusoids. Compared with vasopressin, oxytocin has much less activity as a vasopressor and as an antidiuretic. Nevertheless, these slight activities are clinically important, as discussed in the section on side effects.

Clinical Indications and Administration

Oxytocin has both prepartum and postpartum uses. It is the drug of choice for inducing labor. The various oxytocin products, their uses, and their dosages are summarized in Table 49–C4.

Induction of Labor

Oxytocin may be used to stimulate uterine contractility when the normal progression of labor and vaginal delivery is too slow or too distant for the well-being of the mother or fetus. Such conditions include maternofetal Rh factor incompatibilities; maternal diabetes mellitus or preeclampsia syndrome at or near term; premature maternal membrane rupture that necessitates delivery; or the need to reinforce labor slowed by uterine inertia. In any case, the fetus must be in a position compatible with safe vaginal delivery. Intravenous infusion is the only acceptable route of oxytocin administration for this indication.

Abortion

Oxytocin IV infusion may be used, alone or with other drugs, to induce an inevitable abortion or to expel uterine contents after an incomplete abortion during the second trimester. Oxytocin is not indicated for managing abortions during the first trimester, when the uterine response to the drug is very low.

Control of Postpartum Bleeding

Oxytocin, given by IV infusion or IM injection after delivery of the placenta, is indicated for controlling postpartum bleeding or hemorrhage. The drugs ergonovine or methylergonovine maleate are preferred for this use, as discussed later.

Facilitation of Breast Milk Ejection

Oxytocin, administered as a nasal spray, can be used to trigger milk ejection postpartum when physiologic mechanisms usually responsible for this process are inadequate.

Side Effects, Adverse Reactions, and Contraindications

Oxytocin must be used with careful regard for its warnings and contraindications to prevent potential harm or death to the mother or infant (Table 49–S3). Uterine stimulants should only be used by trained personnel who are familiar with their use and management of possible complications. Even when carefully administered, some patients may be especially sensitive to oxytocic drug action. Thus, the physician must weigh potential benefits against the risks in every patient. Oxytocin should be used only with an indication for medical necessity.

Cardiovascular adverse reactions to oxytocin that may occur in the mother include premature ventricular contractions or other cardiac arrhythmias. Hematologic effects include pelvic hematoma, postpartum hemorrhage, and fatal afibrinogenemia. Excessive dosage or high sensitivity to the drug may result in uterine hypertonicity, spasm, tetanic contraction, or rupture.

Fetal effects that could result from induced uterine motility include bradycardia or other arrhythmias; permanent central nervous system (CNS) or brain damage; low Apgar scores; jaundice; retinal hemorrhage; and death.

There are reports of maternal seizures and deaths caused by excessive fluid retention ("water intoxication") as a result of the antidiuretic effects of oxytocin. Consequently, fluid intake should be closely monitored during prolonged oxytocin infusions.

Prolonged or high dose oxytocin use during delivery may cause uterine tetany. Prolonged contractions without intervening relaxation may result in uterine rupture, cervical and vaginal lacerations, postpartum hemorrhage, uteroplacental hypoperfusion, and fetal hypoxia, hypercapnia, bradycardia or death.

Contraindications to the use of oxytocin include cases of significant cephalopelvic disproportion; unfavorable fetal positions or presentations; fetal distress where delivery is not imminent; obstetric emergencies where surgical intervention is favored; uterine hyperactivity; other cases in which vaginal delivery is contraindicated; or in patients who are hypersensitive to the drug. Except in unusual circumstances, it is preferable not to use oxytocin for mothers with previous major surgery of the cervix or uterus, cesarean section, overdistension of the uterus, grand multiparity, or invasive cervical carcinoma. Fetal prematurity also rules out the use of oxytocin.

Interactions with Other Drugs

The most important interaction involving oxytocin is with other drugs that elevate blood pressure (Table 49–I2). The greatest risk is with parenteral oxytocin administration. In the typical obstetric settings in which oxytocin is used, the most common pressure-elevating interactants are the vasoconstrictors (mainly epinephrine) often included in local anesthetic preparations used for alleviating pain during parturition. The most serious risk is an acute hypertensive episode that could cause maternal and possibly fetal death.

Aspirin and other nonsteroidal antiinflammatory drugs are not routinely cited as interactants with oxytocin or other oxytocic agents; however, there are reasons to recommend avoidance or at least very cautious use of these drugs during pregnancy (see Chapter 52), especially near term. They may interfere with the synthesis of endogenous prostaglandins, which have oxytocic activity, and so could prolong labor. More important, perhaps, their ability to inhibit platelet aggregation could prolong uterine bleeding or increase postpartum blood loss.

NURSING IMPLICATIONS

Oxytocin for parenteral administration is supplied in ampules or prefilled syringes; the concentration of all such preparations is 10 U/mL. When used for IV administration, the drug should be added to a suitable diluent to give a final concentration of 10 mU/mL (ie, 10 U of oxytocin in 1 L of solution).

When used prepartum, whether to facilitate live childbirth or as an abortifacient, oxytocin must be administered only by IV infusion, and an infusion pump is always preferred. During administration, it is essential to monitor maternal blood pressure, heart rate, and fluid intake and output; and to assess for potential allergic reactions and other adverse effects that could reflect fluid overload or hypertension (headache, confusion, drowsiness; dyspnea, appearance of edema). When oxytocin is used prior to what is expected to be a live birth, appropriate devices must be used to monitor uterine contractile activity and fetal heart rate. Such information is essential for adjusting oxytocin doses and for determining whether alternative therapies, including surgery, might be indicated. As a rule, oxytocin administration should be stopped if there is evidence of fetal distress; if uterine contractions are frequent (for example, less than two minutes apart) or prolonged (longer than about 90 seconds); or if intrauterine pressure exceeds 50 mm Hg. Evidence of maternal distress, particularly that reflecting hypertension and edema and their potential consequences, also require reducing the dose or discontinuing oxytocin administration altogether, at least temporarily. If there is any evidence of maternal or fetal distress, notify the physician immediately, place the woman on her left side, and administer oxygen.

Adequate hydration and electrolyte balance must be ensured, but it must be done carefully. The goal is to replace fluids and electrolytes lost during the normal stresses of labor, but to avoid causing fluid overload that might add to oxytocin's hypertensive and fluid-retaining effects. Intravenous fluid and electrolyte therapy is the rule, because oral fluid intake might cause serious problems if surgery becomes necessary. Conservative use of ice chips to alleviate oral dryness and discomfort is acceptable. Usually, any physiologic IV fluid that is deemed appropriate for the mother will be compatible with oxytocin, except those containing bisulfite. (There are no good data on compatibility between oxytocin and bicarbonate.) Nevertheless, sodium chloride (0.9%) or lactated Ringer's solution is preferred. The oxytocin-containing solution should be piggy-backed onto an existing IV fluid line. This makes it possible to discontinue drug administration yet maintain IV access to administer fluids or other drugs.

When oxytocin nasal spray is used to cause milk ejection, the mother should be sitting in a chair or in bed. Advise her to keep her head and the squeeze-bottle upright and to deliver one spray per nostril. If the patient prefers, it is acceptable to allow her to tilt her head back, invert the bottle, and gently squeeze out the drop. Advise the patient to administer the drug two or three minutes before planned breast-feeding or breast pumping.

Other Oxytocic or Uterine-Stimulating Drugs

Ergot Alkaloids

Drugs classified as ergot alkaloids include a number of compounds that possess the ability to cause α-adrenergic receptor blockade, vasoconstriction, and oxytocic effects. As discussed in Chapter 15, there are three major subclasses of ergot alkaloids, distinguished mainly in terms of the predominance of one of these three pharmacologic activities (Table 15–2). Methylergonovine and ergonovine cause relatively intense oxytocic effects, modest vasoconstriction, and little or no α-blocking actions. The two drugs are so similar that they will be discussed together.

Ergonovine and Methylergonovine

Ergonovine (ERGOTRATE) and methylergonovine (METHERGINE) are used as postpartum oxytocic agents. Their primary effect is on uterine smooth muscle tone.

Absorption, Distribution, Metabolism, and Excretion

Both drugs are absorbed well when given orally or by IM injection. They may be injected IV, but this route is not recommended for routine use. The onset of action of methylergonovine is two to five minutes when injected IM, compared to about eight minutes for ergonovine. Oxytocic effects occur almost instantaneously with IV injections. Uterine stimulant effects persist for about three hours, regardless of the drug or parenteral route used. Overall, the differences between the two drugs are so slight that they do not affect the choice of a particular agent. When given orally, the effects of either drug appear in five to ten minutes.

Ergonovine is eliminated mainly by hepatic metabolism and biliary excretion of the metabolites. Methylergonovine appears to depend on both hepatic metabolism and renal excretion. Such differences may affect drug choice when, for example, a patient has hepatic dysfunction.

Pharmacologic Effects

Oxytocic Effects

Ergonovine and methylergonovine are roughly equipotent in exerting oxytocic effects. Typical doses of these agents almost always cause prolonged and intense uterine contractions (tetany), unlike those that occur when usual doses of oxytocin are given prepartum. The indirect consequence of the uterine tetany is mechanical hemostasis—occlusion of bleeding vessels by the contracted uterine muscle. This pattern of oxytocic effect has great importance to the proper use of ergonovine and methylergonovine.

As with oxytocin, nongravid uterine smooth muscle is not very sensitive to the ergot compounds, nor is the gravid uterus before the third trimester. Thus, the ergot drugs are not effective for inducing therapeutic abortion. Used improperly in the first or second trimester, however, they may cause serious adverse effects, including abortion.

Vasoconstrictor and Alpha-Adrenergic Blocking Effects

Ergonovine and methylergonovine have vasoconstrictor activity, mainly in the large arteries. However, significant increases of blood pressure seldom occur in otherwise normal individuals given therapeutic doses orally or IM. Hypertension is more likely to occur with ergonovine, or with either drug given IV. Regardless of the administration route, however, the vasoconstriction produced may be sufficient to cause unwanted and potentially serious adverse responses in patients with peripheral, cerebral, or coronary vascular diseases. Therapeutic doses of ergonovine or methylergonovine do not cause such manifestations of α-blockade as hypotension.

Endocrine Effects

Ergonovine lowers serum prolactin levels and inhibits postpartum lactation. Methylergonovine may do the same.

Clinical Indications and Administration

Oxytocic Activity

Ergonovine and methylergonovine, by virtue of their oxytocic effects, are used to prevent and treat postpartum bleeding or hemorrhage after delivery of the fetus and placenta, and to hasten uterine involution. Uterine atony, a common cause of postpartum bleeding, usually lasts about 48 hours, the typical duration of oral ergonovine or methylergonovine therapy. Dosages are summarized in Table 49–C4. Overall, the drugs shorten Stage 3 of labor and reduce blood loss.

Methylergonovine (0.2 mg) can be given routinely (but certainly not to every patient) as a prophylactic measure. For this indication, IM injection is preferred. The same dose of either drug can be given IV for true emergencies. However, IV administration carries a greater risk of side effects. If needed to control bleeding, the dose can be repeated at two- to four-hour intervals.

Methylergonovine (IM) can also be administered in the second stage of labor, after delivery of the child's anterior shoulder, to complete labor. This use is associated with a higher risk to both mother and child and should be reserved for those situations in which full obstetric facilities and supervision are present.

Side Effects, Adverse Reactions, and Contraindications

Methylergonovine appears to cause fewer and less severe side effects than ergonovine. Thus, methylergonovine usually is preferred. Either drug, at usual doses, may cause uterine cramping, an expected result of the drug's intended actions. When used improperly, particularly during the early stages of labor, most of the adverse effects noted for excessive doses of oxytocin (see Table 49–S3) may occur. The ergot drugs may also cause nausea, vomiting, and diarrhea, but the overall incidence of these side effects is relatively low.

Adverse cardiovascular responses caused by vasoconstriction are possible, particularly with ergonovine or parenteral (especially IV) administration of either ergonovine or methylergonovine. For any patient, the major potential cardiovascular risk is hypertension with or without related headache, dizziness, and transient chest pain. Blood pressure rises may be dangerous in hypertensive patients, including those with hypertension associated with eclampsia, for whom these drugs are generally contraindicated. Cerebrovascular accidents resulting in brain damage, paralysis, seizures, or death may occur, especially with IV use. Persons with peripheral vascular diseases such as Raynaud's disease are at greater risk of experiencing paresthesias, or even total limb ischemia caused by reduced blood flow to the extremities that might lead to gangrene. Persons with Prinzmetal's angina are at greater risk of experiencing myocardial ischemia and its consequences.

Another potential complication, most important for women who must be confined to bed during the puerperium, is thromboembolism. It is caused by the combined effects of physical inactivity and the drug's vasoconstrictor actions. Both effects tend to promote blood stasis, setting the stage for thrombosis.

The drugs are contraindicated for the induction of labor, for any stages of pregnancy other than those noted earlier, in the presence of threatened abortion, in patients with hypertension, preeclampsia/eclampsia, or in patients hypersensitive to these drugs. Because ergonovine can lower serum prolactin levels and suppress lactation, it should be administered to women who wish to nurse their infants only if potential for inhibited lactation is less important than the need to control uterine bleeding. Methylergonovine is less likely to suppress lactation, but may do so.

Allergic reactions, including shock, have been reported rarely.

Interactions with Other Drugs

The greatest concern for drug interactions with ergonovine and methylergonovine involve vasoconstrictors, including those found in local anesthetic products. See Table 49–12 and refer to the discussion of oxytocin's drug interactions. Hypocalcemia counteracts the desired oxytocic effects of ergonovine and methylergonovine. Measurements and possible correction of serum calcium levels with parenteral calcium administration (usually the gluconate salt) may be indicated if the drugs fail to cause their anticipated effects.

Overdose and Toxicity

There have been reports of accidental overdoses of ergonovine or methylergonovine when administered therapeutically. The major consequence is a syndrome called *ergotism*. It is characterized by nausea, vomiting, GI upset, and intensification of all the potential systemic and organ-related consequences of vasoconstriction and hypertension noted earlier. Seizures and hypercoagulability of the blood may also occur.

Treatment is symptomatic and supportive, and guided by the intensity and nature of major problems and the overdose route. For example, if severe hypertension occurs, IV administration of nitroprusside may be indicated. If chest pain occurs, indicating potential coronary vasospasm, sublingual or IV administration of nitroglycerin is recommended. If vasoconstriction causes paresthesias or other signs of reduced peripheral blood flow, nitroprusside or an α-adrenergic blocker (phentolamine, chlorpromazine) might be tried. The goal is to prevent tissue necrosis and potential gangrene, which may require surgical amputation. Anticonvulsant drugs are indicated for seizures.

NURSING IMPLICATIONS

Parenteral and oral dosage forms of ergonovine and methylergonovine are supplied in ready-to-use forms. Room-temperature storage is adequate, but protect all preparations from exposure to light. Do not use parenteral solutions that have become discolored.

Be sure to check the history to rule out contraindications to these drugs. Assess baseline maternal blood pressure, pulse rate and quality, and abdominal (uterine) tone, and assess for evidence of uterine bleeding, before and periodically after administering the ergot products. Such monitoring is particularly important when these drugs are injected.

If methylergonovine is given during Stage 2 of labor, assess fetal vital signs, maternal vital signs and uterine activity, and the overall progression of labor, as noted for oxytocin. Never give the drug at this time unless you are sure that complete maternal and fetal monitoring, emergency drugs and devices, and skilled medical obstetric care are available.

If the ergot preparations must be given IV, infuse the total dose (which should be no more than the usual IM dose) slowly, over at least 60 seconds. Monitor closely for untoward uterine or systemic responses.

Assess for hypocalcemia as a possible cause of failure of usual doses of the ergot products to produce their expected effects. Be prepared to administer calcium salts parenterally, with caution and constant monitoring of maternal vital signs, including the ECG. Do not administer calcium salts to persons taking digitalis; the risk of accidentally inducing hypercalcemia may trigger digitalis-induced arrhythmias.

Always assess for signs and symptoms of ergotism, and be prepared to intervene, as discussed earlier.

Advise women who wish to breast-feed their infants that methylergonovine may interfere with this process (even though it is less likely to do so than ergonovine).

Prostaglandin Abortifacients

There are several therapeutic ways in which pregnancy can be terminated intentionally, or incomplete spontaneous abortion can be completed quickly and safely. Prostaglandins offer one way to produce such an *abortifacient* effect. Intraamnionic injection of hypertonic (20%) sodium chloride generally is a preferred pharmacologic approach for inducing abortion. The major advantage of this approach is fewer untoward and intolerable maternal side effects than are caused by prostaglandins for patients with no cardiovascular diseases that might be worsened by added salt load. The major disadvantage of saline for most patients is the relatively slow onset of action.

Prostaglandins (PGs) are derivatives of arachidonic acid, a component of virtually all cell membranes. They are among the most ubiquitous regulatory chemicals in the body, affecting such processes as vascular, intestinal, and airway smooth muscle tone, coagulation, and hypothalamic temperature regulation.

Prostaglandins have important effects on the reproductive system. Indeed, they derived their name because they were first identified as arising from the prostate gland, being released in large amounts into the semen. They regulate sperm motility, stimulate anterior pituitary release of LH, inhibit activity of the corpus luteum, and control uterine smooth muscle tone. There are several chemical families of prostaglandins, distinguished by their biologic activities, chemical structures, and the metabolic pathways by which they are synthesized (see Chapter 50 for an overview). Concentrations of PGE_2 and $PGF_{2\alpha}$ increase exponentially in peripheral blood and amnionic fluid during the natural course of labor. Prostaglandins have essential roles in the birth process.

Prostaglandin products are available as abortifacients, and one product is indicated for treatment of postpartum hemorrhage. The drugs are carboprost and dinoprostone. The discussion that follows focuses on the actions and uses of these drugs in obstetrics.

Carboprost Tromethamine

Carboprost (PROSTIN/15M) is administered by IM injection. One indication is in second trimester abortion (between weeks 13 and 20 measured from the first day of the last normal menstrual period) characterized by failure of expulsion of the fetus, premature rupture of membranes and absent uterine activity, or membrane rupture in the presence of a previable fetus, and absence of uterine expulsion. Several doses, spaced by 1.5 to 3.5 hours, may be needed. Carboprost is also indicated for control of postpartum uterine hemorrhage, caused by uterine atony, that has failed to respond to conventional management.

Dinoprostone

Dinoprostone (prostaglandin E_2; PROSTIN E2) is used as an abortifacient during weeks 12 to 20. It is supplied as a suppository that is inserted high into the vagina, with repeated administration at three- to five-hour intervals as needed. Dinoprostone is indicated for uterine evacuation in the case of missed abortion or intrauterine fetal death up to 28 weeks gestational age.

Clinical Indications and Administration

Carboprost and dinoprostone are effective uterine stimulants. Like oxytocin, they stimulate the gravid uterus well near term. Unlike oxytocin, they also stimulate the nonpregnant uterus, as well as the uterus during early stages of pregnancy. This activity accounts for one common use for the drugs: to induce abortion during the second trimester. Dosages are summarized in Table 49–C4. Nondrug procedures such as suction curettage usually are used for abortions performed during the first trimester. Prostaglandins have the potential to induce incomplete abortions, in which case other therapies such as intraamnionic injection of hypertonic sodium chloride may be necessary.

Side Effects, Adverse Reactions, and Contraindications

The prostaglandin abortifacients may cause untoward effects on all major body systems (see Table 49–S3). It is rare for some side effects not to occur during administration of these drugs. The severity of the side effects ranges from mild, to intensely distressing, to life-threatening episodes which, fortunately, are uncommon.

Gastrointestinal side effects occur more often than those involving other body systems. Vomiting occurs in one half to two thirds of patients receiving recommended doses of these drugs. Diarrhea and nausea occur in roughly one third of patients. Diarrhea may last for several days.

The most serious adverse responses are uterine rupture, or uterine or cervical perforation. Any hemorrhage requires immediate surgical intervention. Other genitourinary side effects include uterine pain, cramping, inflammation, urinary tract infection, and endometritis. Acute pelvic inflammation contraindicates the use of any prostaglandin abortifacient.

Central nervous system side effects include drowsiness, dizziness, feelings of anxiety or tension that may be accompanied by hyperventilation, headache, paresthesias, and fever. A recent history of epilepsy requires great caution when prostaglandins are used. Cardiovascular effects include arrhythmias, hypertension, hypotension sufficient to cause syncope or more serious problems, and chest discomfort that could reflect myocardial ischemia. Active cardiovascular disease contraindicates the use of prostaglandin abortifacients. Constriction of airway smooth muscles may occur, causing cough, dyspnea, wheezing, or bronchospasm. Active pulmonary disorders, hepatic or renal disease, and acute PID contraindicate prostaglandin use. Allergic reactions, including anaphylaxis and cardiac arrest, have occurred. Dinoprostone may cause chills in about 10% of treated patients.

The prostaglandin abortifacients are not indicated if the fetus has reached the stage of viability and are not feticidal agents. Thus, transient life signs could be present in a fetus aborted by these agents. Dinoprostone and carboprost should be used cautiously in patients with a history of asthma, hypotension or hypertension, cardiovascular, adrenal, renal, or hepatic disease, anemia, jaundice, diabetes, epilepsy or compromised uteri. Dinoprostone suppositories should be used cautiously in the presence of cervicitis, infected endocervical lesions or acute vaginitis.

Prostaglandin abortifacients are potential teratogens. Therefore, if they are administered to induce abortion and fail to do so, other methods will be required to complete the abortion.

Interactions with Other Drugs

The major obstetric-related interactions between prostaglandins and other drugs involve other oxytocic agents, including oxytocin, ergot alkaloids, and hypertonic sodium chloride. The potential consequences of such interactions include excessive uterine stimulation (and the potential consequences of such an effect), plus a greater risk of such cardiovascular problems as hypertension and heart failure.

Aspirin, ibuprofen, and most other nonsteroidal antiinflammatory drugs (see Chapter 52) have been cited as interactants because they antagonize the effects of prostaglandins. They do inhibit some pathways of prostaglandin synthesis in the body, but they do not significantly antagonize the effects of exogenous prostaglandins administered therapeutically. However, as discussed in Chapter 52 and summarized in the section on oxytocin, prolonged antiplatelet effects of nonsteroidal antiinflammatory drugs may favor excessive uterine bleeding. Avoid administering them within two weeks of scheduled abortion, and advise patients to avoid them also. Acetaminophen may be preferred if an antipyretic drug is indicated shortly before or after an abortion.

NURSING IMPLICATIONS

Store carboprost in a refrigerator. Keep dinoprostone suppositories in a freezer, and remove before use to allow warming to room temperature.

Help allay anxiety and other emotional patient responses in anticipation of abortion. Be supportive and nonjudgmental.

Before prostaglandin administration, check the patient's history to rule out contraindications; gather baseline vital signs, including blood pressure, pulse rate and quality, respiratory status; and assess the patient's mental state. Assess pretreatment uterine tone, and check for uterine bleeding before and after drug administration. Inquire specifically about the recent use of aspirin or ibuprofen during the pretreatment interview.

Always administer carboprost via deep IM injection. Do not exceed a total dose of 2 mg or administer carboprost for more than two days.

Advise the patient of likely side effects, particularly GI upset and uterine discomfort. The medication order should include antiemetics and antidiarrheal drugs. Since prostaglandins do not directly cause fetal death, anticipate the possibility that the abortus may show signs of transient viability. Ensure that intensive care monitoring and treatment facilities are readily available in case untoward responses occur.

Patients who receive dinoprostone suppositories should remain supine for at least 10 minutes after drug insertion to reduce the risk of drug loss. Administer subsequent suppositories at three- to five-hour intervals until abortion occurs.

Always monitor during the immediate postadministration period for evidence of potential anaphylaxis (dyspnea, hypotension, rashes, etc). Monitor for bleeding, hypotension, or other vasomotor symptoms; for GI upset or nausea; and for evidence of abortion and uterine bleeding. Report sudden changes to the physician at once. Regardless of whether the abortus shows signs of viability or not, provide it with humane care until the arrival of a physician. Make no comments that may cause the mother undue alarm.

One important nursing role in the posttreatment period is to help assess the cause of fever, which can be drug-induced or due to endometrial inflammation or infection. Drug-induced fever typically occurs within one to 16 hours after carboprost administration or within 15 to 45 minutes of dinoprostone administration. Body temperature usually falls spontaneously after discontinuation of therapy. Moderate or slight abdominal or uterine tenderness occurs, and the vaginal discharge appears and smells normal. Infection-related fever tends to occur on the third day after abortion and may continue to rise. The uterus will remain boggy and tender; pelvic examination or simple movement may provoke significant pain, and the discharge is discolored and foul smelling. Assessing for these signs (and encouraging the patient to do the same) helps guide proper treatment and prevent the development or spread of a severe pelvic infection.

B. Uterine Relaxants

Just as there are instances in which it is desirable to stimulate uterine motility, there are others in which the opposite effect is wanted. A variety of drugs have been used to suppress uterine motility to manage premature labor. They include progesterone, prostaglandin synthesis inhibitors (aspirin, indomethacin, others), ethanol, and β-adrenergic agonists. None of these agents exerts selective uterine effects, and the attendant systemic maternal and fetal effects may be deleterious. Nevertheless, drug intervention may be necessary. Only one drug is indicated for this use—ritodrine.

PROTOTYPE

Ritodrine

Ritodrine (YUTOPAR and others) is classified as a sympathomimetic drug that stimulates *mainly* the β_2 subclass of adrenergic receptors, which causes inhibition of uterine smooth muscle contractility. Ritodrine belongs to the same pharmacologic family as albuterol and related agents, which are widely used to cause bronchodilation and manage asthma. Despite the pharmacologic similarities of ritodrine and the other β_2 agents, ritodrine is indicated only for management of preterm labor. None of the other β_2 agonists share this approved use. This section focuses on ritodrine's use in obstetrics. Other aspects of β agonists are discussed in detail in Chapter 14.

Clinical Indications and Administration

Ritodrine is indicated for managing preterm labor in selected patients who have been pregnant 20 weeks or more and in whom ritodrine therapy is not contraindicated. The drug's relatively selective ability to stimulate the β_2 receptors in the uterus causes decreased uterine activity, thus prolonging gestation in the majority of patients. However, because it stimulates β_2 receptors that mediate other responses in the body, and also stimulates β_1 receptors that mediate still other responses, particularly those in the cardiovascular system, ritodrine causes many other sympathomimetic effects that are often unwanted and potentially dangerous.

Once preterm labor has been diagnosed and the decision to treat it is made, ritodrine therapy is started with an IV infusion. The initial dosage, 0.1 mg/min, is increased gradually up to a maximum of 0.35 mg/min (if needed; see Table 49–C4). Actual dosages are titrated, based on assessment of uterine contractions and maternal and fetal vital signs. The IV infusion is continued for at least 12 hours after uterine contractions have stopped. Before discontinuing the IV infusion the patient is started on oral ritodrine, which is continued for as long as it is deemed desirable to prolong pregnancy. If there are periods of premature labor during oral maintenance therapy, repeated courses of parenteral ritodrine therapy are indicated.

Side Effects, Adverse Reactions, and Contraindications

Probably the most important side effects and adverse reactions caused by ritodrine, as caused by most other beta agonists, involve the cardiovascular system. They are more common or intense during IV administration of maximal doses (see Chapter 14, Table 14–S). Under these conditions ritodrine exerts its vasodilator activity and lowers diastolic blood pressure by an average of 20 to 25 mm Hg. The heart is stimulated by both the drug's direct actions and via the baroreceptor reflex, in response to lowered blood pressure. As a result, maternal and fetal heart rates almost always increase. For example, expect maternal heart rates of about 130 beats per minute, and fetal rates of 160 to 170 (assuming normal pretreatment rates), with IV infusions. Cardiac stimulation, seen mainly with IV administration, also increases maternal systolic blood pressure by 10 to 15 mm Hg. Palpitations occur in about one third of patients receiving ritodrine intravenously. Cardiac stimulation may also cause arrhythmias, or chest discomfort that might indicate underlying myocardial ischemia. Dosage decreases reduce the severity of these side effects. Cardiovascular changes of the magnitude described above seldom occur when ritodrine is given orally.

Maternal heart rates persistently over 140 beats per minute require immediate discontinuation of ritodrine administration. Such tachycardia, if allowed to continue, may lead to pulmonary edema. Heart rate usually declines toward predrug levels when the ritodrine dose is reduced or discontinued altogether. Maternal and fetal bradycardia may occur if the infusion is discontinued abruptly. If tachycardia persists, even after discontinuing the drug, it should be considered as a warning sign of potential pulmonary edema. Prepare for emergency treatment, as deaths have occurred. Fluid overload, as caused by administration of large volumes of IV fluids during ritodrine administration, also increases the risk of pulmonary edema. When it is deemed medically necessary, the use of a more concentrated ritodrine infusion (see Nursing Implications) may help reduce this risk, but does not prevent it altogether. Prior or current cardiovascular disorders may contraindicate ritodrine use. They include arrhythmias, ischemic heart disease, uncontrolled hypertension (including pulmonary hypertension), pheochromocytoma, and hyperthyroidism.

Other side effects associated with β-adrenergic agonist administration (see Chapter 14) should be anticipated when ritodrine is given, especially IV. Nausea, vomiting, headache, erythema, or skeletal muscle tremor occur in up to 50% of patients. Central nervous system responses including nervousness, anxiety, and restlessness are less likely to occur (about a 5% incidence).

Ritodrine, especially when given IV, can increase blood glucose and insulin levels and lower serum potassium levels. These are expected responses to systemic administration of sympathomimetics with β-agonist activity. In otherwise healthy persons, blood glucose levels tend to fall spontaneously toward normal in two to three days, even during continued IV ritodrine administration. However, ritodrine is contraindicated in persons with uncontrolled diabetes mellitus, for whom the drug's effects on insulin, glucose, and serum electrolytes may cause serious complications. Since ritodrine is a bronchodilator, dyspnea should be uncommon. If it occurs, it should be assessed immediately, in conjunction with other signs and symptoms, as possible evidence of pulmonary edema or myocardial ischemia.

Ritodrine is contraindicated before the twentieth week of pregnancy because fetal blood concentrations of the drug approach or equal those in the mother, and the potential exists for adverse developmental effects. The drug is also contraindicated whenever continuing pregnancy or ritodrine administration is dangerous for either the mother or fetus. Such situations include pulmonary edema, severe cardiovascular disease, diabetes, antepartum hemorrhage, intrauterine fetal death, eclampsia or severe preeclampsia syndrome, and bacterial infection and inflammation of the fetal membranes (chorioamnionitis).

Ritodrine solutions for parenteral use contain the preservative sodium metabisulfite, which may trigger mild or severe allergic reactions in persons with sulfite allergies. The greatest risk is in persons with both allergies to sulfites themselves and asthma or a history of allergic responses to other substances.

NURSING IMPLICATIONS

Ritodrine for IV administration is supplied in vials or prefilled syringes that contain the drug at a concentration of 1.5 mg/mL. This must be diluted before administration, usually to 0.3 mg/mL (that is, 150 mg of drug in a final volume of 500 mL). More concentrated solutions may be prepared, as when there is a risk of pulmonary edema from volume overload. The preferred diluent is 5% dextrose in water, because this further reduces the risk of salt overload that might favor pulmonary edema. A salt solution (sodium chloride or Ringer's) might be preferred if the patient has diabetes; check the patient's history and consult with the physician first, and be prepared to monitor blood glucose levels before and during ritodrine administration. Ritodrine solutions should be clear and colorless; discard the solution if it is discolored or contains particulate matter, or if it has not been used within 48 hours of dilution. It is always best to administer the diluted solution as soon as possible after preparation.

Always infuse ritodrine with a system that permits accurate drug delivery and the ability to alter the infusion rate without compromising continual IV access or the ability to administer another drug. Thus, use an IV microdrip chamber or (preferably) an infusion pump; piggyback the ritodrine or use a separate IV infusion site altogether.

Before giving ritodrine, rule out disorders or drugs that would absolutely contraindicate its use. Monitor all pertinent maternal and fetal vital signs including the mother's electrocardiogram, before ritodrine administration and before each dosage increase. Advise the patient that it will be necessary for her to avoid oral fluid or food intake (NPO except for ice chip administration; the major concern here is to avoid complications if anesthesia and surgery become necessary). If evidence of any significant adverse response occurs, notify the physician at once, and be prepared to reduce or discontinue ritodrine administration and implement necessary treatments.

Continue ritodrine infusion for at least 12 hours after uterine contractions cease, then give the first oral dose of ritodrine approximately 30 minutes before IV therapy is to be stopped.

When the patient is discharged on oral maintenance therapy, advise her to report at once any untoward effects, including signs of possible premature delivery. Food interferes with the absorption of oral ritodrine, so advise the patient to take the drug one or two hours before or after meals. Make patients aware of the need to take ritodrine four to six times a day, unless prescribed otherwise. Provide a written list of interacting over-the-counter drugs to avoid during ritodrine therapy. Encourage following prescribed bedrest and avoiding intercourse.

Interactions with Other Drugs

The drugs that interact with most sympathomimetics (see Chapter 14 and Table 14–I) are potential interactants with ritodrine. In the setting of typical ritodrine use, the interactants can be placed in three major groups.

1. Drugs that intensify or cause cardiac stimulation or blood pressure changes. This includes sympathomimetics, antimuscarinics, magnesium sulfate, diazoxide, meperidine, and potent general anesthetic agents.
2. Drugs that increase the risk of pulmonary edema. This mainly applies to systemic corticosteroids, which may also increase the incidence or severity of hypertension and hypokalemia in patients taking ritodrine.
3. Beta-adrenergic blockers, which antagonize ritodrine's effects.

Overdose and Toxicity

Ritodrine overdoses cause the adverse reactions of other β-adrenergic agonists. These include maternal and fetal tachycardia, arrhythmia, hypotension, dyspnea, nervousness, tremor, nausea and vomiting. Overdoses are treated symptomatically, supportively, and with administration of a β-adrenergic blocker such as propranolol. See Chapter 14 for details and nursing implications.

Other Uterine Relaxants

Terbutaline

Terbutaline, belonging to the same pharmacologic class as ritodrine, is used sometimes to suppress premature labor. This is not an approved use. In general, however, therapy parallels that noted for ritodrine: initial IV infusion, followed by oral maintenance therapy. If terbutaline is used, anticipate the same side effects, contraindications, and drug interactions as noted for ritodrine.

Ethanol

Ethyl alcohol (ethanol), infused IV as a 5% or 10% solution in 5% dextrose, is also used to suppress premature labor. In this setting alcohol inhibits uterine contractions through a direct effect on the muscle and through inhibition of oxytocin release from the pituitary gland. This is not an approved use. If the drug is used, side effects and contraindications noted in Chapter 22 apply.

SUMMARY OF NURSING IMPLICATIONS

Assessment

Obtain a complete nursing history to identify present and past medical conditions that contraindicate therapy with the prescribed drug (for example, breast or genital cancer, thromboembolic disorders, unexplained vaginal bleeding, pregnancy, cerebral or coronary vascular disease with estrogens or progestins; complications of pregnancy, cardiovascular disease or instability with oxytocics, ritodrine).

Establish baseline vital signs (maternal and fetal when indicated), weight, menstrual pattern, and specified laboratory tests (eg, serum lipids, glucose) to evaluate drug responses.

Review current medications for potential drug–drug interactions.

Nursing Diagnoses

Knowledge deficit related to drug therapy.

Body image disturbance related to drug effects (feminization in males with estrogen).

Altered role performance related to infertility.

Fluid volume excess related to edema and water intoxication.

Sexual dysfunction related to estrogen therapy in men (impotence).

Ineffective individual coping related to long-term drug therapy, infertility problems, threatened abortion, etc.

Pain related to contractions or drug side effects.

Altered tissue perfusion: maternal and fetal.

◆ Planning/Implementation

Weigh the patient weekly; check blood pressure at regular intervals (to check for possible fluid retention); limit sodium intake.

Encourage the patient to stop smoking to prevent aggravation of thromboembolic problems with estrogens or progestins.

Inform the patient fully about anticipated or important side effects associated with the prescribed drug. Stress the need to report immediately any side effects that require prompt assessment or intervention.

Administer preparation safely: for example, warm oil-based parenteral formulations to room temperature; ensure that solutions are clear; wash the hands before inserting suppositories, and have patient lie down for 30 minutes after insertion if possible. Administer oral form in proper relation to meals, adhere to drug cycle.

Provide emotional support to patients receiving any of the drugs discussed in this chapter for any indication; reassure them that most drug-induced effects are reversible.

Instruct patient on the correct technique for: breast self-examination with estrogen and progesterone; basal temperature monitoring with fertility drugs.

◆ Evaluation

The patient/family will:

Experience minimal or no adverse drug effects (edema, thromboembolism, breakthrough bleeding); vital signs within normal limits.

Comply with medication schedule (eg, cyclic pattern with oral contraceptives).

Maintain laboratory values within normal limits.

Cope with condition in a positive manner; verbalize concerns and anxieties; seek counseling when needed; return for medical follow-up.

Achieve pregnancy and carry to term when pregnancy-inducing drugs are used.

Demonstrate correct administration techniques.

Annotated Bibliography

Ansbacher R: Interchangeability of low-dose oral contraceptives: Are current bioequivalent testing measures adequate to ensure therapeutic equivalency? *Contraception* 1991;43(2):139–147. *Essential reading. Even with oral contraceptives that seem to be similar, changing product formulations, brand names, packaging, and generic substitutions can have a dramatic effect on preventing pregnancy.*

Barrett-Connor E: Risks and benefits of replacement estrogen. *Annu Rev Med* 1992;43:239–251. *Focuses on risks of cardiovascular disease and cancers during estrogen replacement therapy.*

Beard MK: Atrophic vaginitis: Can it be prevented as well as treated? *Postgrad Med* 1992;91(6):257–260. *Concise coverage of how to prevent this common accompaniment of menopause using both estrogens and other drug and nondrug measures.*

Bracero LA, Leikin E, Kirshenbaum N, Tejani N: Comparison of nifedipine and ritodrine for the treatment of preterm labor. *Am J Perinatol* 1991;8(6):365–369. *Learn more about potential complications of β-agonist therapy for premature labor and why the calcium channel blocker nifedipine might become a preferred treatment.*

Burckhardt P: Treatment of osteoporosis. *Curr Opin Rheumatol* 1992;4(3):402–409. *Good integration of content about hormone replacement therapy and the use of calcitonin, biphosphonates, calcium, and vitamin D (see Chapter 47).*

Burry KA: Nafarelin in the management of endometriosis: Quality of life assessment. *Am J Obstet Gynecol* 1992; 166(2):735–739. *Compares and contrasts efficacies and side effects of nafarelin and danazol as they relate to patient satisfaction and compliance with therapy.*

Canadian Preterm Labor Investigators Group: Treatment of preterm labor with the beta-adrenergic agonist ritodrine. *N Engl J Med* 1992;327(5):308–312. *The conclusions of this multicenter study of the most widely used drug for slowing preterm labor may be shocking: ". . . ritodrine . . . had no significant beneficial effect on perinatal mortality, the frequency of prolongation of pregnancy to term, or birth weight." Read the article, and an accompanying editorial, to appreciate the implications better.*

Coleman FH: Safety and efficacy of combined ritodrine and magnesium sulfate for preterm labor: A method for reduction of complications. *Am J Perinatol* 1990;7(4):366–369. *Discusses complications of combined therapy, and how proper assessment might allow restarting treatment that was initially stopped because of adverse effects. A useful article for perinatology nurses.*

Flattum-Riemers J: Norplant: A new contraceptive. *Am Fam Physician* 1991;44:103–108. *A comprehensive discussion of NORPLANT, including side effects and other patient responses to the drug.*

Garner CH, Webster BW: Endometriosis. *J Obstet Gynecol Neonatal Nurs* 1985;14(6 Suppl):10S–20S. *Still valuable for its emphasis on education, the disease, and physical and psychologic implications of treatment.*

Harlap S: The benefits and risks of hormone replacement therapy: An epidemiologic overview. *Am J Obstet Gynecol* 1992;166(6 Pt 2): 1986–1992. *Concludes that hormone replacement therapy with estrogen and a progestin of minimal androgenicity is a rational alternative to unopposed estrogen therapy, and that benefits of hormone replacement therapy with or without progestins strongly outweigh the risks.*

Leonardi MR, Hankins GD: What's new in tocolytics. *Clin Perinatol* 1992;19(2):367–384. *Comprehensive, but certainly important reading if you want to keep up to date on latest trends in managing premature labor with drug therapy.*

Lobo RA: The role of progestins in hormone replacement therapy. *Am J Obstet Gynecol* 1992;166(6 Pt 2):1997–2004. *Discusses roles and potential benefits and risks of adjunctive progestin use in postmenopausal osteoporosis prevention.*

MacPherson KI: Cardiovascular disease in women and noncontraceptive use of hormones: A feminist analysis. *ANS* 1992;14(4): 34–49. *A provocative yet interesting discussion of potential links between menopause, hormone replacement therapy, and risks of cardiovascular disease.*

Rubin CD: Age-related osteoporosis. *Am J Med Sci* 1991;301:281–298. *Reviews age-related changes in bone physiology as they relate to osteoporosis; considers the use of estrogen and calcium supplements in the elderly patient.*

Walling M, Andersen BL, Johnson SR: Hormonal replacement therapy for postmenopausal women: A review of sexual outcomes and related gynecologic effects. *Arch Sex Behav* 1990;19(2):119–137. *Discusses both physiologic and behavioral consequences of hormone replacement therapy after menopause.*

Weinstein L: Hormonal therapy in the patient with surgical menopause. *Obstet Gynecol* 1990;75(4 Suppl):47S–50S. *Succinct coverage of the benefits of estrogen replacement and the controversial use of adjunctive androgens; good advice on assessment and planning.*

Table 49–C1 **Clinical Uses and Administration of Natural and Synthetic Estrogen-Only Products**

AGENT	CLINICAL USES	DOSAGE AND ROUTE OF ADMINISTRATION
	Natural Estrogenic Steroids and Derivatives	
Estradiol		
(ESTRACE)	Replacement therapy for menopause	Oral: Usually 1–2 mg/day (usually cyclic: 3 weeks on drug, 1 week off)
	Breast carcinoma	Oral: 10 mg tid for at least 3 months
	Prostatic carcinoma	Oral: Usually 1–2 mg tid
	Atrophic vaginitis, kraurosis vulvae (dry, brittle vulva)	Vaginal cream: Initially, 2–4 g/day for 1–2 weeks, reducing to 1–2 g/day for another 2 weeks; maintenance dose 1 g 1–3 times weekly if needed (contains 0.1 mg drug per gram of cream)
	Female hypogonadism	Oral: Usually 1–2 mg/day, adjust as necessary
(ESTRADERM)	Menopausal replacement therapy, female hypogonadism, atrophic vaginitis, kraurosis vulvae	Transdermal patch: Apply new patch twice weekly initially, then once weekly for 3 weeks, one week off
	Estradiol Esters	
Estradiol cypionate in oil (various)	Menopausal replacement therapy	Deep IM: 1–5 mg every 3–4 weeks
	Replacement therapy in female hypogonadism	Deep IM: 1.5–2 mg once monthly
Estradiol valerate in oil (various)	Menopausal replacement therapy, female hypogonadism, atrophic vaginitis, kraurosis vulvae	Deep IM: 10–20 mg every 4 weeks
	Prevention of postpartum breast engorgement	Deep IM: 10–25 mg, single dose, given at end of first stage of labor
	Prostatic carcinoma	Deep IM: 30 mg or more every 1–2 weeks
Quinestrol		
(ESTROVIS)	Menopausal replacement therapy, atrophic vaginitis, female hypogonadism, primary ovarian failure	Oral: Initially 100 μg for 7 days; continue with 100–200 μg once weekly, starting 2 weeks after original start of treatment
	Estrone Products	
Estrone aqueous suspension (various)	Menopausal replacement therapy, atrophic vaginitis or kraurosis vulvae	IM: 0.1–0.5 mg, 2 or 3 times weekly
	Female hypogonadism, castration, or primary ovarian failure	IM: 0.1–1 mg/week in single or divided doses; weekly maintenance doses up to 2 mg
	Prostatic carcinoma	IM: 2–4 mg, given 2 or 3 times weekly until disease resumes progression
Estrogenic substance (various)	Contains mainly estrone; uses, dosages, as for estrone	

(continued)

Table 49–C1 **Clinical Uses and Administration of Natural and Synthetic Estrogen-Only Products (*Continued*)**

AGENT	CLINICAL USES	DOSAGE AND ROUTE OF ADMINISTRATION
Esterified estrogens (various)	Menopausal replacement therapy	Oral: 0.3–1.25 mg/day
	Primary ovarian failure	Oral: 1.25 mg/day
	Female hypogonadism	Oral: 2.5–7.5 mg daily in divided doses for 20 days; cycle with progestins for ovarian failure
	Prostatic carcinoma	Oral: 1.25–2.5 mg tid
	Breast carcinoma	Oral: 10 mg tid for 3 months
Estropipate		
(piperazine estrone sulfate; OGEN)	Menopausal replacement therapy, atrophic vaginitis, kraurosis vulvae	Oral: Usually 0.625–5 mg daily, given cyclically (see estradiol)
	Atrophic vaginitis, kraurosis vulvae	Vaginal cream: 2–4 g of cream daily (contains 1.5 mg drug/g cream); for 1–2 weeks, then reduce maintenance dose 1 g 1–3 times weekly
	Female hypogonadism, primary ovarian failure	Oral: 1.25–7.5 mg daily, given cyclically
Conjugated estrogens		
(PREMARIN; others)	Menopausal replacement therapy	Oral: 1.25 mg per day, given cyclically
	Atrophic vaginitis, kraurosis vulvae	Vaginal cream: 2–4 g of cream daily (contains 0.625 g drug/g cream)
		Oral: 0.3–1.25 mg or more daily
	Female hypogonadism	Oral: 2.5–7.5 mg/day in divided doses; use cyclic 20-day-on/10-day-off schedule; if bleeding occurs during 10-day-off period, resume 20-day estrogen course, adding oral progestin to last 5 days of estrogen treatment
	Treatment of abnormal uterine bleeding from hormone imbalance	IV (preferred) or IM: Usually one 25-mg dose, repeated in 6-12 hr if needed
	Prevention of postpartum breast engorgement	Oral: 3.75 mg q4h for 5 doses, or 1.25 mg q4h for 5 days
	Osteoporosis	Oral: 0.625 mg/day, cyclically
	Primary ovarian failure	Oral: 1.25 mg/day
	Breast carcinoma	Oral: 10 mg tid for 3 months
	Prostatic carcinoma	Oral: 1.25–2.5 mg tid
Semisynthetic Estrogen Derivatives		
Ethinyl estradiol (various)	Menopausal replacement therapy	Oral: 0.02–1.5 mg daily, cyclically (21 days on, 7 days off adding a progestin, in some, every other day)
	Female hypogonadism	Oral: 0.05 mg, 1–3 times daily during first 2 weeks of theoretical menstrual cycle, followed by oral progestin for last 2 weeks; continue for 3–6 months
	Oral contraception	See Table 49–1
	Breast carcinoma	Oral: 1 mg tid
	Prostatic carcinoma	Oral: 0.15–2 mg/day
Mestranol	Oral contraception	See Table 49–1

(continued)

Table 49–C1 Clinical Uses and Administration of Natural and Synthetic Estrogen-Only Products (*Continued*)

AGENT	CLINICAL USES	DOSAGE AND ROUTE OF ADMINISTRATION
	Nonsteroidal Estrogens	
Chlorotrianisene		
(TACE)	Menopausal replacement therapy	Oral: 12–25 mg/day, cyclically in 30-day courses
	Female hypogonadism	Oral: 12–25 mg once daily for 21 days, followed by 100 mg IM progesterone or oral progestin during last 5 days
	Atrophic vaginitis, kraurosis vulvae	Oral: 12–25 mg/day, cyclically, for 30–60 days
	Postpartum breast engorgement	Oral: Usually 12 mg qid for 7 days, or 50 mg q6h for 6 doses, or 72 mg bid for 2 days; treatment should start within 8 hr of delivery
	Prostatic carcinoma	Oral: 12–25 mg daily
Diethylstilbestrol		
("DES")	Emergency postcoital contraception	Oral: 25 mg bid for 5 consecutive days; begin treatment within 24 hr of coitus, no later than 72 hr after
	Breast carcinoma	Oral: 15 mg/day
	Prostatic carcinoma	Oral: Initially, 1–3 mg/day
	Atrophic vaginitis, kraurosis vulvae	Oral: 0.2 mg–2 mg daily, may administer with suppository for 10–14 days
		Suppository: 1–2 full applicators daily for 1–2 weeks, then reduce to half this dose

Table 49–C2 Clinical Uses and Administration of Progestins Commonly Used in Progestin-Only Therapy, and of Danazol and of Nafarelin

AGENT	CLINICAL USES	DOSAGE AND ROUTE OF ADMINISTRATION
Progesterone (aqueous or in oil, various products)	Amenorrhea, abnormal uterine bleeding	IM: Usually 5–10 mg once daily for 6–8 consecutive days; anticipate withdrawal bleeding in 2–3 days after last dose if ovarian activity restored and endometrium proliferates
	Functional uterine bleeding	IM: Usually 5–10 mg daily for 6 doses; discontinue when bleeding stops (usually occurs in 6 days); if estrogen therapy is used adjunctively, begin progesterone administration after 2 weeks of estrogen therapy
	Progesterone Derivatives	
Hydroxyprogesterone caproate in oil (various)	Primary or secondary amenorrhea; abnormal uterine bleeding caused by hormonal imbalances	IM: Usually 375 mg; after 4 days of desquamation, or if bleeding does not start within 21 days, start 28-day (4-week) cyclic therapy: 20 mg estradiol valerate on day 1; 250 mg hydroxyprogesterone caproate + 5 mg estradiol valerate 2 weeks later; repeat cycle 4 times
	Production of secretory endometrium and desquamation	IM: For patients not currently on estrogen therapy, start cycle as for amenorrhea; for patients on estrogen therapy, begin with 375 mg then continue described cycle after 4 days
	Advanced uterine corpus adenocarcinoma	IM: Initially 1 g or more; give repeated doses 1–7 times per week, stop when relapse occurs or after 12 weeks if it does not occur
	Diagnosis of endogenous estrogen production	IM: 125–250 mg, repeated in 4 weeks if confirmation needed; bleeding 1–2 weeks after injection indicates responsive endometrium in nonpregnant woman
Medroxyprogesterone acetate (PROVERA; others)	Secondary amenorrhea	Oral: 5–10 mg daily for 5–10 days; should be preceded by estrogen therapy
	Abnormal uterine bleeding caused by hormonal imbalances	Oral: Usually 5–10 mg daily for 5–10 days, starting on 16th or 21st day of menstrual cycle. Should be preceded by estrogen therapy
	Endometrial or renal carcinoma	IM: 400–1000 mg/week; see also Chapter 59
Megestrol acetate (MEGACE)	Palliation of advanced breast carcinoma	Oral: 40 mg qid
	Palliation of advanced endometrial carcinoma	Oral: 40–320 mg daily in divided doses
	19-Nortestosterone Derivatives	
Norethindrone (NORLUTIN)	Amenorrhea	Oral: 5–20 mg daily, starting on 5th day of menstrual cycle, ending on 25th day

(continued)

Table 49–C2 **Clinical Uses and Administration of Progestins Commonly Used in Progestin-Only Therapy, and of Danazol and of Nafarelin (*Continued*)**

AGENT	CLINICAL USES	DOSAGE AND ROUTE OF ADMINISTRATION
	Endometriosis	Oral: Usually 10 mg daily for 2 weeks; increase in 5 mg/day increments every 2 weeks, up to maximum of 30 mg daily; continue for 6–9 months or until breakthrough bleeding occurs
Levonorgestrel implants (NORPLANT SYSTEM)	Contraceptive agent	Subdermal: 6 capsules implanted during first 7 days of onset of menses; contraceptive efficacy up to 5 yr if capsules not removed
Norethindrone acetate (NORLUTATE, AYGESTIN)	Amenorrhea, abnormal uterine bleeding	Oral: 2.5–10 mg; timing as for norethindrone
	Endometriosis	Oral: 5 mg daily for 2 weeks, increase in 2.5 mg/day increments every 2 weeks, up to maximum of 15 mg/day; continue as noted for norethindrone
Synthetic Androgen		
Danazol (DANOCRINE)	Endometriosis	Oral: Initially, 800 mg/day in 2 doses starting during menstruation or with other assurance patient is not pregnant; may reduce maintenance dose, based on response; continue uninterrupted for 3–9 months; reinstitute therapy if symptoms recur; discontinue if pregnancy suspected or documented; may initiate mild cases with 100–200 mg bid
	Fibrocystic breast disease	Oral: 100–400 mg/day in 2 doses. Pain usually relieved by first month, nodularity decreased by 4–6 months of uninterrupted therapy
	Hereditary angioedema	Oral: Start at 200 mg bid or tid; titrate dose to response
Synthetic GnRH Analog		
Nafarelin (SYNAREL)	Endometriosis	Intranasal: One spray (200 μg) in one nostril in AM, one spray into other nostril in PM; start treatment between days 2 and 4 of menstrual cycle

Table 49–S1 | Major Side Effects of Estrogens and Progestins

BODY SYSTEM	ESTROGENS	PROGESTINS
CENTRAL NERVOUS SYSTEM	Headache (migraine); nervousness; cerebral thrombosis, paresthesias; chorea; dizziness; mental depression	Depression; migraine; cerebral thrombosis; headache; nervousness; dizziness
EYE	Retinal thrombosis; optic neuritis; steepening of corneal curvature; intolerance to contact lenses	Sudden partial or complete loss of vision; proptosis; diplopia; papilledema; retinal vascular lesions; retinal thrombosis; optic neuritis
METABOLISM	Slight impairment of glucose tolerance; alterations in levels of plasma triglycerides, cholesterol, and lipoproteins; hypercalcemia, reduced carbohydrate tolerance	Moderate catabolic effect; increased nitrogen excretion; glucose intolerance
BREASTS	Tenderness; enlargement; secretion; carcinoma; gynecomastia in men	Tenderness; secretion
CARDIOVASCULAR	Hypertension; increased risk of MI; enhanced clotting tendencies; thrombophlebitis pulmonary embolism; stroke and myocardial infarction	As for estrogens
GASTROINTESTINAL	Nausea; bloating, vomiting; anorexia; diarrhea; abdominal cramping; increased incidence of gallbladder disease; cholestatic jaundice and increased risk of recurrence in those with history of jaundice during pregnancy; hepatic carcinoma; benign hepatic adenoma; mesenteric thrombus	Changes in appetite; nausea, cholestatic jaundice
WATER BALANCE	Edema; weight gain	Edema; weight gain
SKIN	Local dermatitis, chloasma, or melasma that may persist when the drug is withdrawn; hemorrhagic eruption; hirsutism; loss of scalp hair, photosensitivity; erythema multiforme; erythema nodosum	Hair loss; hirsutism; acne; melasma or chloasma; rash; erythema multiforme; erythema nodosum
GENITOURINARY	Breakthrough bleeding; changes in menstrual flow (amenorrhea, dysmenorrhea, hypomenorrhea); cystitis-like syndrome, premenstrual-like syndrome; cervical erosion; vaginal candidiasis; growth of uterine fibromas; cervical and vaginal carcinoma; excessive endometrial proliferation; increased risk of endometrial cancer when used alone (ie, not with progestins); testicular atrophy, feminization and reversible impotence in men	Breakthrough bleeding; changes in menstrual flow; changes in cervical secretions; amenorrhea; cystitis-like syndrome
FETUS	Increased risk of congenital abnormalities (heart, limb); possible increased vaginal cancer or vaginal adenosis in adult life	Masculinization of the female fetus; increased risk of congenital anomalies
OTHER	Aggravation of porphyria; changes in libido	Precipitation of acute intermittent porphyria; insomnia; somnolence, pyrexia; premenstrual-like syndrome; changes in libido; fatigue

Table 49–I1 **Interactions Between Estrogens and Other Agents***

AGENT	RESULT OF INTERACTION	COMMENTS AND NURSING IMPLICATIONS
Antibiotics, broad spectrum (Chapter 56)	Decreased actions of estrogen or estrogen-containing product (eg, oral contraceptive)	Effective blood levels of estrogens, estrogen-containing products are maintained in part by enterohepatic recirculation; destruction of gut flora by antibiotics may reduce this process, lowering estrogen blood levels and increasing risk of pregnancy; monitor women taking oral contraceptives for spotting, breakthrough bleeding; if they occur, recommend use of supplemental contraceptive measures during combined therapy
Anticoagulants, oral (Chapter 35)	Decreased actions of anticoagulant; increased risk of thromboembolism	Interaction important because oral anticoagulants are often given for thromboembolic disorders, the risk of which is increased by estrogens or estrogen-containing products; occurs because estrogens may increase hepatic inactivation of anticoagulant, may increase hepatic formation of active clotting factors; monitor prothrombin times, other objective and subjective indicators anticoagulant effect; anticipate need to increase anticoagulant dose and continue monitoring
Anticonvulsants (carbamazepine, phenytoin, primidone) (Chapter 26)	Decreased plasma levels of estrogens	Caused by increased estrogen metabolism. See barbiturates
Antidepressants, tricyclics (Chapter 24)	Increased risk of antidepressant side effects or toxicity	Through unknown mechanisms, estrogens may increase risk of antidepressant side effects (see Chapter 24); estrogen use may cause depression symptoms, which might be interpreted as need to increase antidepressant dose; assess closely for antidepressant side effects, small doses of ethinyl estradiol enhance therapeutic response to imipramine, but larger doses increase toxicity
Antidiabetic drugs (oral; insulin) (Chapter 46)	Reduced effectiveness of antidiabetic drug	Estrogens may increase blood glucose levels; if patient is diabetic and is prescribed estrogen-containing products (eg, oral contraceptives), reinforce need for strict monitoring for hyperglycemia
Ascorbic acid (vitamin C) (Chapter 61)	Increased effects of ethinyl estradiol	
Barbiturates (Chapter 22)	Reduced plasma levels of estrogen	Caused by ability to stimulate hepatic metabolism; one concern is oral contraceptive failure (pregnancy); if interaction cannot be avoided (as when barbiturates used for long-term seizure control in persons with epilepsy), have patients assess for and report breakthrough bleeding, spotting; such responses generally require either discontinuing barbiturate or increasing estrogen dose; regardless of plan, recommend use of alternative (and effective) nondrug contraceptive methods until interaction can be eliminated or resolved
Chenodiol (Chapter 36)	Increased risk of cholesterol gallstone, gallbladder pain, inflammation	Estrogens increase biliary cholesterol secretion, risk of gallstones; assess for abdominal pain, especially after meals; alternative therapies may be required
Dantrolene (Chapter 20)	Hepatotoxicity	Causative relationship unclear, but use special caution in women over 35 receiving both dantrolene and estrogen therapy
Rifampin (Chapter 57)	See barbiturates	Temporary use of additional contraceptive measures may be needed during combined therapy; assess for breakthrough bleeding, spotting, as evidence of interaction

*Interactions apply not only to estrogen-only products but also to products containing estrogens, including most oral contraceptives.

Table 49–C3 Clinical Uses and Administration of Ovulatory Stimulants and Fertility Drugs

AGENT	CLINICAL USES	DOSAGE AND ROUTE OF ADMINISTRATION
Chorionic gonadotropin, human		
("HCG"; A.P.L.; FOLLUTEIN; PREGNYL; PROFASI; others)	Treatment of prepubertal cryptorchidism in the absence of anatomic obstruction	IM: 4000 USP units 3 times weekly for 3 weeks; or 5000 units every other day for 4 injections; or 15 injections of 500–1000 units over a 6-week period; or 500 units 3 times weekly for 4–6 weeks, raising to 1000 units per injection for repeated course if needed; dosage, treatment duration, vary according to patient, physician's experiences
	Treatment of selected cases of male hypogonadotropic hypogonadism	IM: 500–4000 units 3 times weekly; dosage, treatment duration, vary depending on patient, physician
	Adjunct to menotropins for male hypogonadism; adjunct to menotropins, urofollitropin, in anovulatory women	See menotropins, urofollitropin
Clomiphene citrate		
(CLOMID; SEROPHENE)	Treatment of ovulatory failure, in selected women with normal liver function and endogenous estrogen levels	Oral: Initially, 50 mg/day for 5 days; if first course fails, 100 mg/day for 5 days, usually started 30 days after first; some patients may need third (final) course
Menotropins		
(PERGONAL)	Induction of ovulation, pregnancy in women with functional anovulation	IM: Reconstitute 1 ampul (contains 75 IU of FSH and LH activity in 1–2 mL sterile saline); inject once daily for 9–12 consecutive days (maximum), then 5000–10,000 IU HCG 1 day after last menotropin dose; in absence of side effects, pregnancy, and in presence of ovulation, repeat above course at least twice; may repeat course twice more with 150 IU FSH/150 IU LH
	Stimulation of spermatogenesis in males with primary or secondary hypogonadotropic hypogonadism	IM: Pretreat initially with HCG (usually 5000 IU 3 times weekly for 4–6 months) to increase testosterone levels, induce secondary sexual characteristics (may require 4–6 months); then give 75 IU FSH/LH menotropins 3 times weekly plus 2000 IU HCG twice weekly, continue for at least 4 months; if therapy fails, maintain or double menotropin weekly dosage, maintain HCG dose
Urofollitropin		
(METRODIN)	Induction of ovulation, pregnancy, in selected anovulatory women failing to respond to clomiphene citrate	IM: Reconstitute 1 ampul (contains 75 IU FSH activity) in 1–2 mL sterile saline, inject once daily for 7–12 days, followed by 5000–10,000 U of HCG 1 day after last urofollitropin dose; in absence of side effects, pregnancy, but in presence of ovulation, repeat course at least twice, before then increasing dose to 150 IU/day for 7–12 days, followed by 5000–10,000 U HCG

Table 49–S2 Side Effects of and Contraindications for Ovulatory Stimulants and Fertility Drugs

BODY SYSTEM/ Side Effect	CONTRAINDICATION/ PRECAUTION	COMMENTS AND NURSING IMPLICATIONS
Urofollitropin and Menotropins		
CENTRAL NERVOUS SYSTEM Dizziness, drowsiness, fatigue, lethargy, etc	Organic intracranial lesion	Advise of potential for these diverse reactions, and to notify physician immediately if severe or persistent
ENDOCRINE Ovarian hyperstimulation syndrome	High gonadotropin levels indicating primary ovarian failure	Ensure thorough pretreatment work-up to rule out primary endocrine failure; assess for ovarian hyperstimulation syndrome as noted above; women in later years of reproductive life should have surgical D&C performed before menotropin therapy starts
Gynecomastia in males		Advise of possible side effect (usually reversible), monitor accordingly
	Males: normal or elevated gonadotropin levels, indicating normal pituitary function or primary testicular failure, infertility disorders other than hypogonadotropic hypogonadism	Advise males of need for thorough pretreatment work-up to ensure proper drug use Rule intracranial lesions out as causes or accompaniments of disorder for which menotropins or urofollitropin are administered
CARDIOVASCULAR Thromboembolism	Thromboembolism	Check history, assess for evidence of thrombosis or embolism, report at once
GASTROINTESTINAL Nausea, vomiting, diarrhea		Advise patient to expect these side effects; provide usual comfort measures, administer prescribed drugs to alleviate symptoms if ordered
REPRODUCTIVE Birth defects	Pregnancy	Notify physician at once if any evidence of pregnancy during therapy
Multiple births	Any cause of infertility other than anovulation; ovarian cysts or enlargement not due to polycystic ovary syndrome	Fertility-inducing drugs increase overall incidence of multiple births; when triplets or more are conceived, live birth-rate falls; advise women of the potential risks before treatment starts
Uncomplicated ovarian enlargement or symptomatic ovarian hyperstimulation syndrome; ovarian cyst rupture, bleeding or hemorrhage	Ovarian cysts or enlargement not due to polycystic ovary syndrome	Assess, and have patients assess, for abdominal pain, tenderness, or distention; weight gain; dyspnea, that might indicate ascites or pleural effusions; assess for vaginal/uterine bleeding; symptom onset usually develops within 2 weeks after treatment, intensity then progresses rapidly; advise patients to report such symptoms at once and to discontinue intercourse immediately; advise of the need for hospitalization for proper observation, treatment
	Abnormal uterine bleeding of undetermined etiology	Rule out abnormal bleeding, possible endometrial cancer, before starting treatment; notify physician at once if abnormal bleeding develops during therapy

(continued)

Table 49–S2 Major Side Effects of and Contraindications for Ovulatory Stimulants and Fertility Drugs (*Continued*)

BODY SYSTEM/ Side Effect	CONTRAINDICATION/ PRECAUTION	COMMENTS AND NURSING IMPLICATIONS
Chorionic Gonadotropin		
ENDOCRINE Precocious puberty in males	Precocious puberty	Assess for evidence of early or rapidly developing secondary sexual characteristics; teach assessments to parents, who are in best position to observe child during treatment; discontinue HCG administration if signs appear
Stimulation of androgen-dependent cancers	Androgen-dependent cancers or prostatic carcinoma	Assess before administration and during therapy for development or enlargement of any responsive lesions (eg, of prostate)
CARDIOVASCULAR Fluid retention and its potential consequences		Use with care, frequent assessment, in patients at risk from androgen-induced fluid overload: hypertension, edema, heart failure, seizures, migraine headache, renal disease
Clomiphene Citrate		
EYE Visual spots, flashes, persistent afterimages; possible reduced visual acuity	Abnormal uterine bleeding, pregnancy or liver disease	Generally reversible; often intensified in bright light; may be severe enough to interfere with vision, requiring cautious motor vehicle operation, performance of other potentially dangerous tasks, especially if accompanied by drowsiness, dizziness; severe or persistent symptoms require prompt ophthalmologic examination

Table 49–C4 **Clinical Uses and Administration of Oxytocics, Abortifacients, and Uterine Relaxant (Ritodrine)**

AGENT	CLINICAL USES	DOSAGE AND ROUTE OF ADMINISTRATION
	Oxytocics	
PROTOTYPE		
Oxytocin		
(PITOCIN; SYNTOCINON)	Induction, stimulation of labor	IV infusion: Dilute 10 U (1 ampul) in 0.9% sodium chloride or lactated Ringer's to 10 mU/mL (0.01 U/mL); start with infusion of 1 mU/min, increase to dose giving desired uterine contractions at rate of 1 mU/min every 15 minutes; dosage increases should not exceed 1–2 mU/min at 15–30-min intervals; use IV pump or microdrip device allowing precise control; piggyback into current IV fluid line or use separate infusion site
	Control of postpartum uterine bleeding	IV infusion: Add 10–40 U to 1 L of electrolyte or dextrose solution (10–40 mU/mL); give at rate sufficient to control uterine atony
		IM: 10 U after delivery of placenta
	Treatment of incomplete abortion	IV infusion: Add 10 U to 500 mL 0.9% sodium chloride or 5% dextrose; makes 20 mU/mL, infuse at 10–20 mU/min
	Stimulation of initial breast milk ejection	Nasal spray: Usually 1 spray in one or both nostrils 2–3 min before nursing or pumping breasts
RELATED DRUGS		
Ergonovine maleate		
(ERGOTRATE MALEATE)	Prevention, treatment of postpartum, postabortion bleeding	IM (preferred) or IV: 0.2 mg; if severe bleeding occurs and persists, may repeat dose q2–4h as needed; reserve IV administration for emergencies
	Control of late postpartum bleeding	Oral: Usually 0.2 or 0.4 mg q6–12h until danger of uterine atony, bleeding pass (about 48 hr)
Methylergonovine maleate		
(METHERGINE)	Control of routine management after delivery of placenta, management of postpartum uterine atony, hemorrhage, and in second stage of labor	Oral: 0.2 mg, tid or bid during puerperium for up to 1 week
		IM: 0.2 mg after delivery of placenta, delivery of anterior shoulder or during puerperium
		IV (emergencies only): 0.2 mg infused over at least 60 sec
		IM: As above; give only after delivery of anterior shoulder with full obstetric support present
	Abortifacients	
Carboprost tromethamine		
(PROSTIN/15M)	Termination of pregnancy, completion of incomplete abortions induced with other therapies	Deep IM: 250 µg initially; follow if needed with 250 µg at 1.5–3.5-hr intervals (may increase to 500 µg if several lower doses fail); administer only during 13th–20th week of gestation
	Control of refractory postpartum uterine bleeding	IM: Usually one 250-µg dose; may repeat at 15–90-min intervals as long as cumulative dose <2 mg
Dinoprostone		
(PROSTIN E2)	Evacuation of uterus to manage missed abortion, in utero fetal death up to 28 weeks of gestation; management of benign hydatiform mole	Vaginal suppositories: One suppository (20 mg) q3–5h as needed; administer only during 12th–20th week of gestation

(continued)

Table 49–C4 **Clinical Uses and Administration of Oxytocics, Abortifacients, and Uterine Relaxant (Ritodrine) (*Continued*)**

AGENT	CLINICAL USES	DOSAGE AND ROUTE OF ADMINISTRATION
	Uterine Relaxant	
PROTOTYPE		
Ritodrine hydrochloride (YUTOPAR)	Suppression of premature uterine contractions (premature labor) in pregnancies of 20 or more weeks gestation	IV: Dilute 150 mg in 500 mL 5% dextrose solution; infuse initially at 0.1 mg/min, increasing gradually at 10-min intervals to maintenance doses between 0.15–0.35 mg/min based on monitoring of uterine activity, maternal and fetal vital signs; continue for up to 12 hr, switch to oral route if longer treatment needed Oral: 10 mg q2h for first 24 hr; thereafter 10 or 20 mg q4–6h; begin first oral dose 30 min before stopping IV administration

Table 49–S3 **Major Side Effects of and Contraindications for Oxytocics and Prostaglandin Abortifacients***

BODY SYSTEM/ Side Effect	CONTRAINDICATION/ PRECAUTION	COMMENTS AND NURSING IMPLICATIONS
	Oxytocin	
CARDIOVASCULAR Edema, hypertension, and related consequences: stroke, heart failure, pulmonary edema, etc	Presence of these cardiovascular disorders, especially if severe, poorly controlled, or unstable	Usually caused by overdoses or prolonged infusions, with associated volume load; monitor accordingly, noting sudden or marked changes of maternal or fetal vital signs, symptomatic evidence of side effects; report changes at once, be prepared to stop oxytocin infusion or reduce dose temporarily; responses reflect both vasopressor activity, water-retaining (antidiuretic) activity of oxytocin
UTERUS Uterine pain, cramping; fetal distress; mechanical damage to fetus or mother's reproductive tract	Drug hypersensitivity; significant cephalopelvic disproportion; unfavorable fetal positions which must be converted before delivery, fetal distress where delivery is not imminent, hypertonic uterine patterns, in obstetric emergencies where benefit-risk ratio favors surgical intervention, contraindications to vaginal delivery	Withhold drug in presence of contraindications, if uterine tetany occurs before delivery, or other evidence of fetal distress occurs
	Ergonovine, Methylergonovine	
CENTRAL NERVOUS SYSTEM Headache, dizziness		Rule out hypertension, potential stroke, if severe headache occurs, especially if accompanied by other manifestations of stroke (paralysis or paresis; slurred speech, etc); see cardiovascular
RESPIRATORY Dyspnea		May reflect pulmonary edema; see cardiovascular
CARDIOVASCULAR Hypertension and related consequences (eg, stroke)	Hypertension; eclampsia/preeclampsia	Determine baseline blood pressure, monitor closely after drug is given; assess for signs of possible stroke: headache, paralysis or paresis; slurred speech, etc; notify physician at once; α-adrenergic blockers (eg, phentolamine; see Chapter 15) may be required if severe hypertension develops; if IV administration has been ordered, inject slowly, assess very closely
Paresthesias; reduced extremity blood flow; pallor; ischemia	Peripheral vascular disease (eg, Raynaud's)	Assess limb color, temperature periodically in all patients
Myocardial ischemia and its consequences (angina, infarction, arrythmias, heart failure, potential pulmonary edema)	Severe ischemic heart disease; Prinzmetal's (vasospastic) angina generally contraindicates ergonovine, may contraindicate methylergonovine; eclampsia, unless given postpartum in cases in which maternal blood pressure has lowered or normalized	Assess history carefully before giving these drugs; start ECG monitoring at once, be prepared to administer emergency drugs (eg, nitroglycerin for angina, antiarrhythmics, etc); report all untoward cardiovascular responses at once, withhold further ergot administration; oral methylergonovine preferred to other routes, and to ergonovine given by any route, for patients with positive cardiovascular history

(continued)

Table 49–S3 **Major Side Effects of and Contraindications for Oxytocics and Prostaglandin Abortifacients* (*Continued*)**

BODY SYSTEM/ Side Effect	CONTRAINDICATION/ PRECAUTION	COMMENTS AND NURSING IMPLICATIONS
Thromboembolism	History of thromboembolism	Caused mainly by peripheral blood stasis (from vasoconstriction) plus immobility during puerperium; minimized by encouraging ambulation as permitted by condition; assess for thrombosis and embolism, especially in immobile patients
GASTROINTESTINAL Nausea, vomiting		Advise patient to expect these side effects; offer comfort measures, administer antiemetics if ordered and not contraindicated by current condition or history
UTERUS See oxytocin	Pregnancy, induction of labor, threatened spontaneous abortion	Refuse to give ergonovine or methylergonovine during Stage 2 of labor unless child's anterior shoulder has been delivered *and* patient is in a room with full obstetric facilities and support personnel; other precautions as for oxytocin when used postpartum
OTHER Suppressed lactation	Drug hypersensitivity	Caused by suppression of prolactin levels, least likely to occur with oral methylergonovine; advise women who must receive one of these drugs of possible lactation difficulties, inquire about terminating drug therapy as soon as safe, based on assessment of bleeding
Prostaglandin Abortifacients		
CENTRAL NERVOUS SYSTEM Drowsiness, dizziness, anxiety, apprehension, etc		Offer reassurance, comfort measures; blood pressure measurements important to assess cause of syncope
Fever		Assess to help determine whether an expected drug-induced hypothalamic effect (occurs shortly after drug administration; no unusual pelvic pain or purulent vaginal discharge), or reflection of pelvic inflammation; if antipyretic treatment is indicated, acetaminophen may be preferred to minimize antiplatelet effect, which could increase uterine bleeding
EYE Ocular pain		Assess for, report eye pain at once for further evaluation; may reflect underlying glaucoma
RESPIRATORY Cough, dyspnea, wheezing, bronchoconstriction or bronchospasm	Asthma, COPD (especially if severe or poorly controlled)	Monitor accordingly, report severe symptoms or distress at once; bronchodilators, oxygen may be necessary, should be immediately available during initial treatment; anaphylaxis (respiratory difficulty, cardiovascular collapse, etc) may occur

(continued)

Table 49–S3 **Major Side Effects of and Contraindications for Oxytocics and Prostaglandin Abortifacients* (*Continued*)**

BODY SYSTEM/ Side Effect	CONTRAINDICATION/ PRECAUTION	COMMENTS AND NURSING IMPLICATIONS
CARDIOVASCULAR Arrhythmias; hypertension; hypotension sufficient to cause syncope; heart failure; angina	Active cardiovascular disease	Rule out contraindications, then monitor accordingly for changes; assess for blood loss as possible cause of hypotension; high-risk or symptomatic patients should have ECG monitoring, frequent checks of heart rate, blood pressure, etc
GASTROINTESTINAL Nausea, vomiting, diarrhea	Active hepatic disease	Incidence drug-dependent, most common with dinoprostone, occurs more often than any other prostaglandin-induced side effects (eg, vomiting in up to two-thirds of patients receiving dinoprostone); offer comfort measures, administer antiemetics as ordered; anticipate diarrhea lasting for several days; assess for fluid/electrolyte imbalances from severe or persistent vomiting, diarrhea
GENITOURINARY/ UTERUS Pain, tenderness, cramping; pelvic inflammation or infection; uterine rupture or perforation	Acute pelvic inflammatory disease	Assess for, report, have patient report, unusually intense or persistent side effects; assess for excessive uterine bleeding, purulent or foul-smelling discharge, fever, to help detect pelvic damage, infection, inflammation
OTHER Muscle, joint aches, pain; chills	Drug hypersensitivity	Assess for underlying infection; administer oral analgesic/antipyretic (preferably acetaminophen unless ordered otherwise) as directed

*Some side effects and related contraindications for ergonovine and methylergonovine are caused by their α-adrenergic blocking actions, and other effects. See Chapter 15 for more details.

See Chapter 14 for more information about ritodrine.

Table 49–12 Interactions Between Oxytocics, Abortifacients, and Other Agents

AGENT	RESULT OF INTERACTION	COMMENTS AND NURSING IMPLICATIONS
Potential Interactant with All Oxytocics, Abortifacients		
Aspirin, ibuprofen, indomethacin, other prescription or nonprescription nonsteroidal antiinflammatory drugs (see Chapter 52)	Increased risk of postpartum or postabortion bleeding	These drugs inhibit platelet aggregation, could increase risk or severity of uterine bleeding postpartum or postabortion; prostaglandin synthesis inhibitors may delay natural labor, cause premature closure of fetal ductus arteriosus (especially indomethacin); recommend acetaminophen for self-administration to relieve mild pain, fever; discourage use of OTC aspirin or ibuprofen for at least 2 weeks before anticipated delivery or scheduled abortion; assess for recent use of these interactants before scheduled procedures; regardless of potential interaction, use of these (or most) drugs during pregnancy should be discouraged because of potential adverse effects
Interactants with All Oxytocics		
All drugs that elevate blood pressure (eg, sympathomimetics, OTC or by prescription)	Increased risk of hypertension, stroke, heart failure in mother; fetal distress; cerebral hemorrhage	Discourage self-administration of sympathomimetics with vasoconstrictor activity (most cold, flu, allergy, weight-loss aids) before scheduled or anticipated delivery; assess for such use in pretreatment interview; monitor blood pressure closely if interactant was taken; if vasopressors must be administered during oxytocics therapy (to treat hypotension caused by uterine hemorrhage, or as ingredients in peripartum local anesthetics), anticipate need for reduced doses, extra cautious monitoring for excessive effect

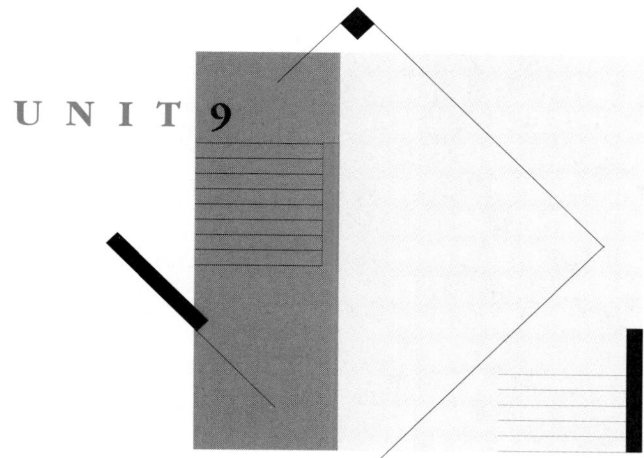

Drugs That Affect the Immune System

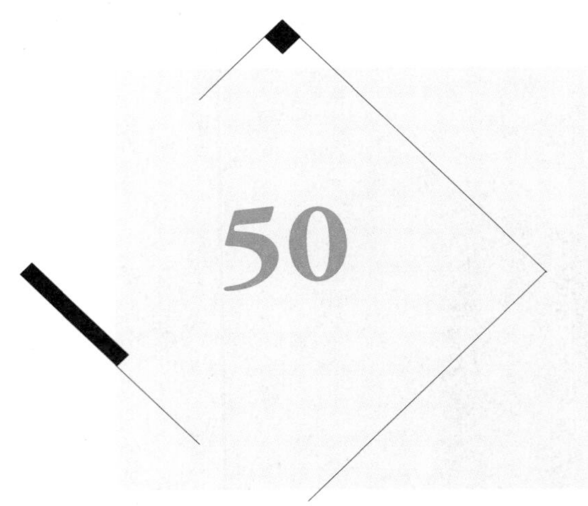

Structure and Function of the Immune System

Through inflammatory and immune reactions, the immune system protects the body against foreign invasion and assault. This system is activated following injury, or after entry of microorganisms or other foreign substances into the body. Inflammatory responses do not recognize specific invaders; instead, any alien substance is attacked and destroyed. In contrast, the immune response is selectively triggered by specific particulate matter (antigens). To function properly, the immune system must distinguish native (self) from foreign (nonself) proteins. This self-tolerance facilitates the direction of cytotoxic activities against nonself matter only.

Many types of pathologic disorders can occur when the immune system malfunctions. Inadequate responsiveness allows life-threatening malignancies and infections to thrive. An inability to differentiate self from nonself provides an autoimmune basis for disorders such as rheumatoid arthritis and systemic lupus erythematosus. Individual sensitivity to specific proteins results in hypersensitivity responses of varying severity. Normal immune system function can threaten the survival of transplanted tissues.

A variety of pharmacologic agents, to be discussed in this unit, are used to manage disorders of inflammatory and immune reactivity. Antihistamines (Chapter 51) may be effective in reducing some of the symptoms of allergic reactions. Corticosteroids (discussed in Chapter 45) and nonsteroidal antiinflammatory drugs (Chapter 52) have actions that ameliorate the pain and swelling of disorders such as rheumatoid arthritis and osteoarthritis. Immunostimulants provide protection against infectious diseases, and immunosuppressants can alleviate symptoms of autoimmune diseases and prevent rejection of grafted tissues (Chapter 54).

To comprehend immunopharmacology, it is necessary to understand the nature of inflammatory and immune responses. The complexity of the immune system has become apparent only in recent years, with the development of technologies such as recombinant DNA and cell cloning, which have made available sufficient amounts of components for study. This chapter outlines the individual components and the intricate interactions of the immune system, to provide a basis for subsequent study of the actions of immunomodulating drugs.

Immune System Components

The immune system consists of organs, circulating cells, and soluble substances called mediators. Bone marrow gives rise to the mobile cellular elements: lymphocytes, macrophages, and granulocytes (neutrophils, eosinophils, and basophils), all of which are generated from undifferentiated stem cells. The thymus gland is important for maturation of certain lymphocytes, a process that seems to involve the initial interactions with proteins, interactions that are essential to recognition of both antigen and self.

The mobile cells of the immune system travel throughout the body in the systemic circulation. Some take up residence in lymph nodes and the spleen. Specialized lymphoid cells are also found in skin, the tonsils, and along the intestinal tract. Lymph ducts (lymphatics) gather up wandering cells and accompanying interstitial fluid and return this accumulation, called lymph, to the venous blood. Nodes found along the system of lymphatic ducts filter foreign material from lymph, and provide one of the many opportunities for antigens to encounter responsive leukocytes. In a similar manner, foreign substances can be removed from blood by the spleen.

The highly specialized cells of the immune system participate in diverse ways in inflammatory and immune responses. Neutrophils (polymorphonuclear leukocytes) are capable of engulfing foreign matter (phagocytosis) and destroying it by means of intracellular lysosomal enzymes. Basophils, and the closely related mast cells found in skin and the respiratory and gastrointestinal (GI) tracts, are the source of histamine, heparin, and other biochemical participants in inflammatory and allergic reactions. Eosinophils are attracted especially to sites of allergic reactions, where they release enzymes that inactivate many of the mediators of hypersensitivity. Eosinophils are also phagocytotic.

Macrophages are long-lived cells that can proliferate and synthesize cytolytic enzymes in the course of an inflammatory response. Fixed macrophages are found in many tissues, including the liver (Kupffer cells), bone marrow, lymphatic ducts, the central nervous system (CNS), body cavities, lungs, and along the walls of blood vessels in the spleen.

In contrast to the granulocytes and macrophages, which can respond to nonspecific invaders, the lymphocytes are leukocytes that respond to specific antigens and give rise to immune responses. B lymphocytes develop in bone marrow; T lymphocyte precursors migrate from bone marrow to the thymus for differentiation into mature cells. Since the B and T cells are an integral part of the immune response, they are discussed together later in this chapter.

Specialized lymphocytes, known as killer cells and natural killer cells, have direct cytolytic activity. They appear to secrete proteins that erode pores into targeted cell membranes, destroying membrane integrity and allowing an influx of interstitial fluid and disruption of intracellular electrolyte balance. Natural killer cells are adept at destroying neoplastic cells, and appear to be defective in persons with acquired immunodeficiency syndrome (AIDS).

Mediators

The cells of the immune system synthesize and interact with a large number of biochemical mediators (called *lymphokines* or *cytokines*) that are essential to inflammatory and immune responses. Table 50–1 summarizes some of the more thoroughly investigated lymphokines. Interleukins, interferons, and hematopoietic colony-stimulating factors in particular have demonstrated potential usefulness as pharmacotherapeutic agents.

Interleukins

Interleukins are polypeptides secreted by leukocytes to influence actions of other leukocytes. Interleukin-1 (IL-1), originally called *lymphocyte-activating factor,* is secreted by cells such as macrophages that "present" antigen to T cells to initiate the immune response. Interleukin-1 is a major cofactor for T cell activation and B cell proliferation, and also enhances neutrophil activity.

Interleukin-2 (IL-2), previously called *T cell growth factor,* is released from activated T lymphocytes. This lymphokine stimulates further proliferation of T cells, and facilitates the activities of B cells, cytotoxic T cells, and natural killer cells. Since IL-2 enhances activity against malignant cells, it has been used to activate leukocytes for experimental treatment of cancer. The immunosuppressant drugs cyclosporine and FK506 appear to reduce the synthesis of IL-2. At least seven other interleukins have been identified and are being studied.

Interferons

Interferons, secreted by cells that have been invaded by viruses, diffuse to nearby cells and protect them against viral assault. Interferons also suppress the growth of malignant cells, and have been used clinically to prevent viral infections in organ transplant recipients and to suppress the proliferation of malignancies, including renal cell carcinoma, Kaposi's sarcoma, and hairy-cell leukemia (Chapter 59).

Colony-Stimulating Factors

Secreted by a variety of cells, colony-stimulating factors (also called *hematopoietic factors*) promote the production, differentiation, and activity of blood cells, including granulocytes and macrophages. These substances

Table 50–1 Selected Lymphokines

Lymphokine	Source	Major Actions
Interleukins		
Interleukin 1 (IL-1)	Macrophages, possibly other cells	Cofactor for T and B lymphocyte proliferation; endogenous pyrogen; stimulates secretion of IL-2 by T lymphocytes
Interleukin 2 (T cell growth factor)	T lymphocytes	T lymphocyte proliferation; activation of natural killer cells
Interleukin 3	T lymphocytes	Promotes development of granulocytes, macrophages, T and B lymphocytes, and many cell types
Interleukin 4	T lymphocytes	Costimulant for B lymphocyte proliferation; enhances development of T lymphocytes, granulocytes, macrophages, etc, and expression of MHC II antigens
Interleukin 5	T lymphocytes	B lymphocyte activation; expression of IL-2 receptors; eosinophil differentiation
Interleukin 6	Fibroblasts, monocytes, T and B lymphocytes, and other cells	Influences proliferation and differentiation of T and B lymphocytes; induces IL-2 receptors on T cells; synergistic with IL-1
Interleukin 7	Thymus, spleen	Growth of T and B lymphocytes
Other lymphokines		
B cell growth factor (BCGF)	T lymphocytes	Cofactor for B lymphocyte proliferation
Eosinophil chemotactic factors (ECF)	Basophils and mast cells	Chemotactic for eosinophils
Gamma interferon	T lymphocytes	Activation of suppressor T lymphocytes
Macrophage-activating factor (MAF)	T and B lymphocytes	Enhances macrophage activity
Macrophage-inhibitory factor (MIF)	T lymphocytes	Retains macrophages at inflammatory site
Neutrophil chemotactic factors	Basophils and mast cells	Chemotactic for neutrophils
Platelet-activating factor (PAF)	Basophils and mast cells	Platelet aggregation; activation of neutrophils

(Table 50–2) show possible efficacy in restoring immune function in persons who have received myelosuppressant therapy and in reducing the severe anemia that can accompany administration of zidovudine (RETROVIR, AZT; see Chapter 57) to AIDS patients.

Antibodies

Antibodies, or immunoglobulins (Ig), are secreted by "plasma" cells produced by B lymphocytes in response to an antigen–antibody interaction. The Y-shaped antibody molecule (Fig. 50–1) consists of four polypeptide chains bound together by disulfide bridges. The variable terminals of the molecule (the forked part of the Y) constitute the antigen-binding fragment (Fab) of the antibody. Great diversity, achieved through complex gene recombinations and mutations, provides the body with antibodies that are capable of highly specific interactions with thousands of different antigens. The specificity of antigen–antibody recognition is one of the

Table 50–2 **Colony-Stimulating (Hematopoietic) Factors**

Factor	Generic Name	Trade Name
Granulocyte colony-stimulating factor (G-CSF)	Filgastrim	Neupogen
Granulocyte-macrophage colony-stimulating factor (GM-CSF)	Sargramostin	Leukine Prokine
Erythrocyte-stimulating factor	Erythropoietin	Epogen
Macrophage colony-stimulating factor (M-CSF)		
Multicolony stimulating factor (interleukin 3 or multi-CSF)		

major characteristics that distinguishes the immune response from the inflammatory response.

The opposite terminal of the antibody molecule (the stem of the Y, or the Fc region) is critical for the initiation of immune responses subsequent to the antigen–antibody interaction. The structure of this region is constant within each of the major classes of antibody. Immunoglobulin G, the most plentiful antibody within the circulatory system, has a vital role in immune responsiveness, as will be discussed shortly. Immunoglobulin A, secreted by mucosal cells, protects against microbial entry through mucous membranes of the respiratory, GI, and genitourinary tracts. Immunoglobulin E molecules bind to receptors on mast cells and basophils and are essential for cell degranulation and release of the mediators of immediate hypersensitivity reactions. The exact roles of IgD and IgM have not been clearly defined.

Complement

The complement system is a series of nine glycoproteins, synthesized mainly in hepatocytes, that circulate in an inactive state in plasma and lymph. Activation of this system by either of two (classic and alternative) pathways results in the release of several fragments that modulate inflammatory events. Some complement components facilitate the phagocytic action of leukocytes by adhering to (opsonizing) antigen–antibody complexes. A chain of several complement components forms a "membrane-attack complex," which channels through the cell membrane of invading microorganisms, causing cytotoxic disruption of ion and fluid balance in a manner similar to that of "killer" lymphocytes. Fragments called *anaphylatoxins* provoke mast cell and basophil degranulation, resulting in a response resembling anaphylaxis. Inhibitors in plasma closely regulate and localize the actions of complement.

The classic pathway of complement activation occurs only after an antigen–antibody interaction. In contrast, the alternative pathway is set into motion by proteolytic enzymes, plasma factors such as properdin, and fragments of microbial cell walls and membranes. Thus, complement components can be functional in the early stages of microbial invasion when antibody production is just getting under way.

Deficiencies in the complement system allow the development of frequent severe infections similar to those observed in persons who lack endogenous IgG (agammaglobulinemia). The absence of complement-inhibitory factors fosters the occurrence of angioneurotic edema, an anaphylactoid swelling of many body tissues.

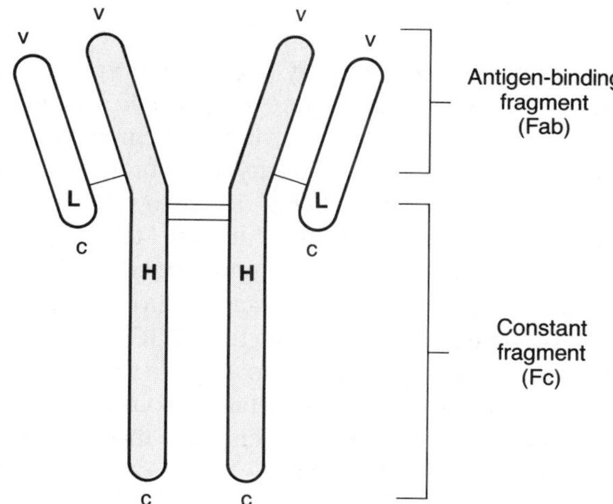

Figure 50–1

Antibody structure. Heavy (H) and light (L) chains have both variable (V) and nonvariable or constant (C) regions. The variable terminals of the chains constitute the antigen-binding fragment (Fab), capable of highly specific interaction with antigen. The constant fragments (Fc) are uniform throughout each of the five major classes of antibody.

(*Source:* Adapted from Porth CM: *Pathophysiology: Concepts of Altered Health States,* 2nd ed. Lippincott 1986, page 135.)

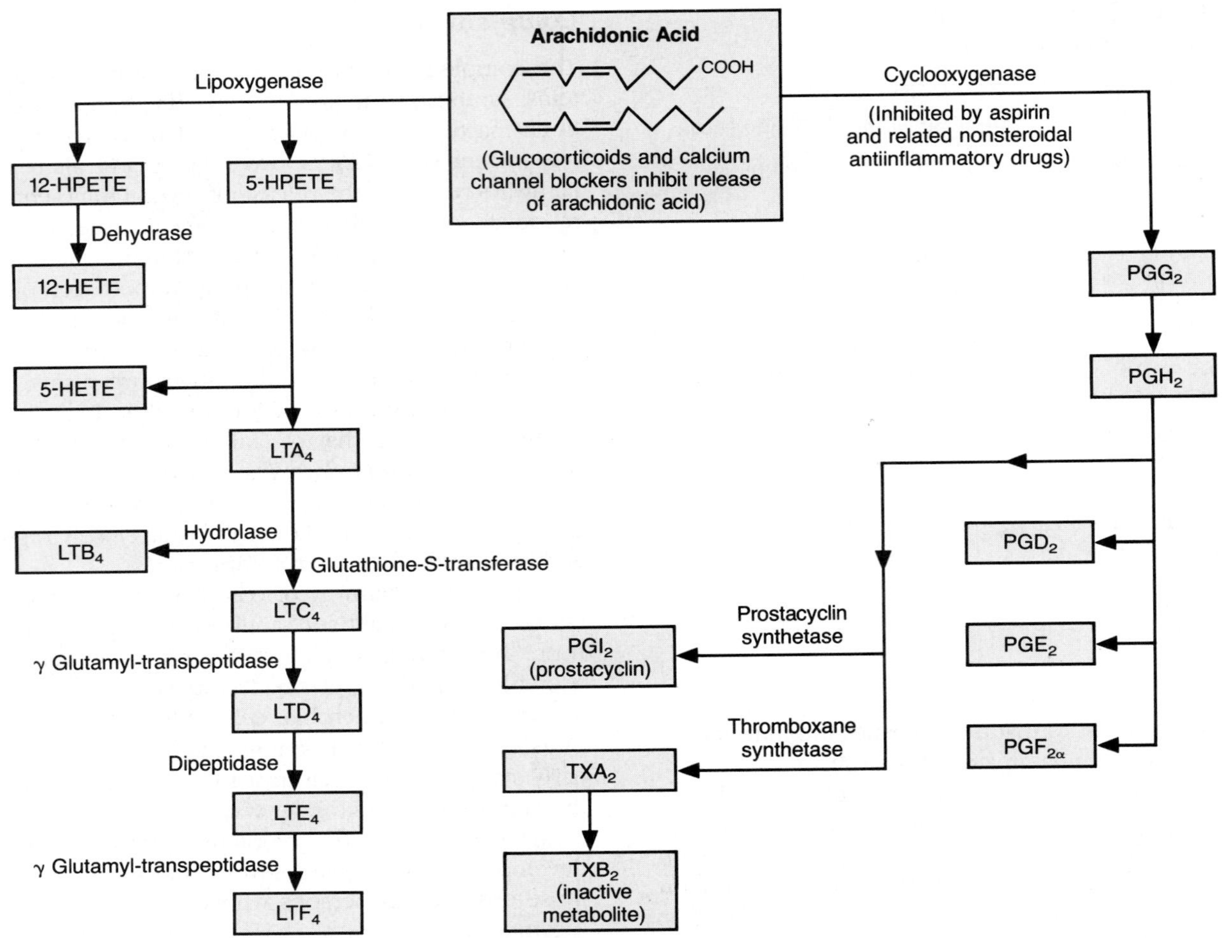

Figure 50–2

The arachidonic acid cascade. Arachidonic acid is liberated by phospholipases from cell membranes, and enters two enzymatic pathways to yield numerous mediators of inflammatory and immune responses. See Table 50–3 for major actions of selected arachidonic acid metabolites.

Prostaglandins

In the course of inflammatory and immune reactions, phospholipase enzymes liberate arachidonic acid from the membranes of many cells, including neutrophils, basophils, and mast cells. This fatty acid enters into two discrete enzymatic pathways (Fig. 50–2) to yield several mediators that have a variety of effects (Table 50–3). Among the prostaglandins (PG) synthesized by the enzyme cyclooxygenase (or prostaglandin synthetase) are intermediary metabolites such as PGG_2 and PGH_2 (called endoperoxides); PGI_2 (prostacyclin); and thromboxanes (TxA and TxB), which have proinflammatory actions on blood vessels, platelets, and movement of leukocytes. The antiinflammatory action of aspirin, indomethacin, and related drugs (Chapter 52) is due at least in part to their efficacy as cyclooxygenase inhibitors. However, PGs that evolve later in the cyclooxygenase cascade (PGE_2 and $PGF_{2\alpha}$, the "stable" prostaglandins) can have suppressant effects on inflammation. In fact, the actions of prostaglandins are frequently in opposition to each other. For example, PGI_2 is a vasodilator and inhibitor of platelet aggregation (it has "antiplatelet" activity), whereas TxA is a vasoconstrictor and promotes platelet aggregation.

The second pathway of arachidonic acid metabolism, via an enzyme called lipoxygenase, yields leukotrienes (LT) and hydroperoxy acids (HPETE and HETE). The leukotrienes are potent inducers of bronchoconstriction and vascular permeability. Leukotriene C_4 and LTD_4 were for many years called "slow-reacting substance of anaphylaxis" (SRS-A). HPETE and HETE ap-

Table 50–3 Actions of Major Arachidonic Acid Metabolites Related to Inflammatory, Immune Reactions

Substance	Actions
Arachidonic acid	Vasodilation, increased capillary permeability, pyrogenesis, hyperalgesia, platelet aggregation, chemotaxis
HETE	Chemotaxis, enhanced mast cell and basophil degranulation
HPETE	Vasoconstriction, enhanced mast cell and basophil degranulation
Leukotrienes	Increased capillary permeability, chemotaxis, bronchoconstriction
PGD_2	Bronchoconstriction, increased capillary permeability, antiplatelet
PGE_2	Pyrogenesis, hyperalgesia, vasodilation, bronchodilation
$PGF_{2\alpha}$	Bronchoconstriction
PGG_2	Vasoconstriction, platelet aggregation
PGH_2	Vasoconstriction
PGI_2	Vasodilation, hyperalgesia, antiplatelet, antichemotactic
TxA_2	Vasoconstriction, platelet aggregation

pear to have a role in promoting degranulation of mast cells and basophils. Arachidonic acid metabolism also yields several oxygen metabolites that can be cytotoxic.

Major Histocompatibility Complex

T lymphocytes respond only to antigen in close association with native proteins that are unique to each person's genetic makeup. These unique proteins are encoded by specific gene sequences called the major histocompatibility complex (MHC). There are two classes of MHC molecules, which are synthesized in almost the same extent of diversity as antibodies and T cell receptors. Major histocompatibility complex class I (MHC I) is found on the surface of almost all mammalian cells, while MHC class II proteins are present only on B lymphocytes, macrophages, and certain other specialized immune system cells. Only those cells that possess MHC II can be "antigen-presenting" cells for T helper cells. In contrast, cytotoxic T cells are activated by antigen plus MHC I; thus, almost any type of cell that has been virally invaded can become a target for destruction.

The Inflammatory Response

Inflammation is a physiologic sequence of events that acts to eliminate invading pathogens, to limit cellular destruction, and to aid in tissue repair. A variety of stimuli, including mechanical injury, severe heat or cold, invading microorganisms, and excessive exposure to X-rays and sunlight, can trigger an inflammatory response.

Injured cells initiate an inflammatory response by releasing or activating vasodilatory and chemotactic substances. The plasma enzyme kallikrein synthesizes bradykinin, which induces vasodilation with enhanced vascular permeability, liberates arachidonic acid from cell membranes, and causes pain by stimulating nerve fibers. Histamine, released from mast cells, also causes pain, vasodilation, and increased capillary permeability. Complement is activated early in the inflammatory response.

Large numbers of mobile cells are attracted to the site of injury. Neutrophils line up (marginate) along capillary walls and then emigrate into interstitial spaces. As these leukocytes phagocytize foreign matter and cellular debris, additional arachidonic acid is liberated. Neutrophils induce release of serotonin (5-hydroxytryptamine; 5-HT) from platelets; this vasoactive substance further enhances circulation at the site of inflammation.

If the inflammatory response is prolonged, lymphocytes and macrophages become more numerous and active at the site. Phagocytes and fibrin surround the inflamed area, forming an abscess that contains dead and damaged tissue, leukocytes, and invading foreign matter, often in a purulent liquid called pus.

The varied actions occurring at the site of inflammation give rise to four cardinal signs of this response. Increased flow of blood following capillary dilation induces warmth (calor) and redness (rubor). Leakage of plasma and cells from highly permeable capillaries causes edema and swelling (tumor). Pain (dolor) is the result of the actions of histamine and bradykinin, as well as increased pressure on nerve endings as swelling occurs. A fifth characteristic, loss of function, can ensue from cellular damage and destruction caused by biochemical mediators and lysosomal enzymes released during the inflammatory response.

The Immune Response

Many microorganisms, which are often able to survive neutrophil attack during the inflammatory reaction, become subject to a more specific immune response mediated by T and B lymphocytes. Cellular immune responses, effective predominantly against foreign and malignant cells and intracellular viruses, are dependent mainly on T cells. Humoral responses, most effective against extracellular microorganisms, are dependent on the secretion of antibody by B cells. It must be noted, however, that both types of cells, through complex interactions, participate in all immune responses.

An immune response begins when an antigen, or foreign particle, encounters on the surface of a B lymphocyte an antibody to which it can selectively bind. The antigen cross-links with, or bridges, two molecules of antibody on the B cell surface. The B cell then engulfs and fragments ("processes") the antigen. Portions of antigen return to the B cell surface and are displayed in association with MHC II proteins; the B cell thus acts as an "antigen-presenting" cell. T lymphocytes have membrane receptors that are very similar to antibodies in their ability to recognize specific antigen fragments, but only when that antigenic material is in close association with MHC II proteins. When T cell receptors interact with the antigen–MHC II complex on B cell surfaces, the T cells are activated to proliferate and secrete lymphokines, which enhance B cell activation (see Table 50–1).

B cell activation is facilitated by membrane receptors for lymphokines as well as for other mediators such as complement fragments and interferon. Stimulated B cells rapidly mature and divide into two types of cells, plasma cells and memory cells. The short-lived plasma cells produce copious amounts of antibody, which opsonizes the triggering antigen and promotes its removal by phagocytic cells. Memory cells are more persistent, providing "immunity" or resistance to subsequent encounters with the specific antigen by mounting a more rapid and vigorous response.

Activated T lymphocytes, vitally important to the progression of the immune response, proliferate to yield three subclasses of cells. T helper cells secrete lymphokines that influence the actions of many cellular participants in the immune response. T suppressor cells, as their name implies, release substances that inhibit immune reactivity and are thought to be essential for maintenance of self-tolerance. Cytotoxic T cells respond to antigen plus MHC I protein, as previously described.

Immunity

Immunity refers to the immune system's ability to attack and destroy specific alien invaders. The specificity of the antigen–antibody interaction, combined with the ability of the immune system to "remember" previously encountered invaders, provides the basis for immunity to infectious diseases. *Natural* or *innate immunity* is permanent immunity that is present at birth. Resistance to disease that develops as a result of exposure to the infectious agent is *acquired immunity,* which often persists for a lifetime. Either naturally occurring pathogens or modified microorganisms administered in the form of vaccines and toxoids will induce active acquired immunity by triggering an immune response with subsequent production of memory B cells. Thus, persons who have either had an infectious disease or been inoculated against one will not develop disease if they are reexposed to the causative microorganism.

To produce passive acquired immunity, antibodies extracted from the blood of actively immune persons are administered to nonimmune persons. Called antisera or gamma globulins (because they consist mainly of IgG), these agents provide immediate but temporary resistance to disease (Chapter 54). Passive immunity is present during the first few months of life, as a result of placental transfer of maternal IgG.

Disorders of the Immune System

Immunologic disorders can be grouped into

- hypersensitivity states,
- autoimmune diseases, and
- immunodeficiency states.

Hypersensitivity represents an "overreaction" of the immune system. Autoimmune diseases occur when the immune system fails to distinguish foreign from native molecules. In immunodeficiency, components of the immune system are absent or ineffective.

Hypersensitivity or Allergic States

Most large molecules—proteins in particular—have the potential to provoke an immune response (to act as antigens). Smaller molecules (haptens) can combine with proteins to form antigenic substances. Hypersensitivity involves abnormal immune responses triggered by individual reactivity to allergens (allergenic antigens).

For hypersensitivity to develop, an initial or sensitizing exposure to an allergen must occur. On subsequent exposures, hypersensitivity reactions may occur rapidly (immediate hypersensitivity, allergy) or may develop more gradually (delayed hypersensitivity). Four types of hypersensitivity reactions have been described; generally, types I, II, and III reactions are antibody-mediated, while type IV reactions are lymphocyte-dependent. However, like all immune system responses,

Table 50–4 Mediators of Immediate Hypersensitivity*

Mediator	Actions
	Preformed
Eosinophil and neutrophil chemotactic factors	Chemotactic for eosinophils and neutrophils
Heparin	Interaction with proteases
Histamine	Vasodilation, increased capillary permeability, bronchoconstriction
Proteases	Increased capillary permeability, chemotaxis (?)
	Newly Synthesized
Leukotrienes	Increased capillary permeability, bronchoconstriction, chemotaxis
PGD_2	Increased capillary permeability, bronchoconstriction
Platelet-activating factor	Platelet aggregation, increased capillary permeability, bronchoconstriction, chemotaxis

*A partial list. Most of these mediators are synthesized in, and released from, mast cells.

hypersensitivity reactions involve the complex interactions of many components.

Immediate hypersensitivity (type I) reactions develop rapidly in response to allergen interactions with IgE antibodies bound to the basophils and mast cell surfaces. Degranulation of these cells releases numerous mediators, both preformed and newly synthesized (Table 50–4), and reactions ranging from rashes and seasonal rhinitis to asthma and anaphylactic shock can occur. Many drugs can act as haptens and induce the development of allergies. The use of various drugs, such as epinephrine, corticosteroids, cromolyn sodium, and antihistamines, in the management of allergic reactions is discussed in other chapters of this book.

Cytotoxic (type II) hypersensitivity is mediated by complement-activating antibodies that facilitate cell destruction. In type III hypersensitivity, soluble antigen–antibody complexes ("immune complexes") escape from the circulatory system, activating complement and attracting neutrophils that subsequently induce cellular damage.

Serum sickness is an example of type III hypersensitivity that can be provoked by drugs such as penicillins, hydantoins, thiazides, and non-human–derived antisera. The extravasation of immune complexes induces glomerulonephritis, fever, rashes, myocarditis, and arthralgia, which are characteristic of this gradually evolving (seven to ten days) syndrome. The symptoms of acute serum sickness are usually completely reversible on drug termination, although continuous exposure to the allergenic substance can result in tissue destruction.

Type IV (delayed) hypersensitivity is a slowly developing (over 24 to 48 hours) immune response mediated by extravasation of activated T lymphocytes and macrophages. An example is contact hypersensitivity in response to plant resins (eg, "poison ivy"), topical drugs (eg, sulfonamides), or cosmetic constituents. Rejection of transplanted tissue is also a form of delayed hypersensitivity.

Autoimmune Disorders

Aberrant immune reactivity, in which the immune system's ability to distinguish between self and nonself is lost, leads to autoimmune disorders that are characterized by tissue destruction.

The exact mechanisms that allow native proteins to trigger the immune system are not known. Theories suggesting viral or drug-induced modifications of cellular proteins, exposure of previously sequestered antigens, or failure of T repressor cells to down-regulate immune reactivity have all been proposed. Currently, the favored theory is one of cross-reaction—that is, foreign substances structurally similar to native proteins may induce immune reactions that fail to distinguish between the two antigens. For example, rheumatic heart disease occurs when an immune response mounted against *Streptococcus A* proceeds to damage antigenically similar myocardial cells.

Rheumatoid arthritis, systemic lupus erythematosus, multiple sclerosis, insulin-dependent diabetes, Crohn's disease, nephrotic syndrome, psoriasis, Hashimoto's thyroiditis, myasthenia gravis, ulcerative colitis, and pernicious anemia are among the disorders that may arise from autoimmune reactions. Immunosuppressant drugs are occasionally of some use in treating these illnesses, although drug-induced inhibition of the immune system can foster the development of life-threatening infections and malignancies.

Immunodeficiency Diseases

The importance of the immune system to health and survival becomes apparent in persons who are immunodeficient. Lack of immunity can be congenital or acquired. Malnutrition, renal disease, exposure to radiation, and many drugs, most notably the myelosuppressant antineoplastics, interfere with immune responsiveness.

Because of the marked degree of interaction and interdependence among elements of the immune system, the absence of just one component can result in severely compromised defense against pathogens. Deficiencies in B and T lymphocytes, antibodies (IgG and IgA), phagocytosis, and complement have been identified. In *severe combined immunodeficiency syndrome,* a congenital absence of both B and T lymphocytes, survival beyond the first few months after birth is possible only in a sterile environment or with lymphocyte replacement achieved by bone marrow transplantation. AIDS occurs when a human T leukemia retrovirus (HIV, previously labeled HTLV-III) specifically depletes helper T cells. Subsequent failure of immunity allows the development of lethal "opportunistic" infections and neoplasms.

Annotated Bibliography

Claman NH: The biology of the immune response. *JAMA* 1992; 268:2790–2796. *Outlines the components of the immune response. (This entire issue of JAMA is devoted to the immune system, covering such topics as autoimmune diseases, allergy to drugs, and immunopharmacology.)*

Cohen IR: The self, the world and autoimmunity. *Sci Am* 1988; 258(4):34–42. *Gives a brief overview of the immune system, with emphasis on lymphocyte activity, then proposes a possible mechanism for self vs nonself discrimination.*

Gawlikowski J: White cells at war. *Am J Nurs* 1992;92(3):44–51. *Describes the functions of immune-system cells, and how to use counts and differentials as diagnostic indicators.*

Granulocyte colony-stimulating factors. *Med Lett Drugs Ther* 1991; 33:61–63. *Summarizes the clinical uses and adverse effects of these agents.*

Groopman JE, Molina JM, Scadden DT: Hematopoietic growth factors: Biological and clinical applications. *N Engl J Med* 1989;321: 1449–1459. *Describes biologic activity, clinical applications, and toxicity of the hematopoietic (or colony-stimulating) growth factors.*

Metcalf D: Control of granulocytes and macrophages: Molecular, cellular, and clinical aspects. *Science* 1991;254:529–533. *Presents characteristics, actions, and potential clinical usefulness of the colony-stimulating factors.*

Mizel SB: The interleukins. *FASEB J* 1989;3:2379–2388. *Describes the origins and actions of interleukins 1 through 7.*

Old LJ: Tumor necrosis factor. *Sci Am* 1988;258(5):59–75. *Describes the work leading to the isolation of tumor necrosis factor, then outlines the inflammatory reaction, with emphasis on the numerous actions of this factor.*

Smith KA: Interleukin-2. *Sci Am* 1990;262(3):50–57. *An overview of the immune response, with emphasis on the role of interleukin 2 and its receptor.*

von Boehmer H, Kisielow P: How the immune system learns about self. *Sci Am* 1991;265(4):74–81. *Summarizes the intricate interactions of the cells and factors of the immune system, then focuses on killer and helper T cells in proposing a mechanism of self vs nonself discrimination.*

Weller PF: The immunobiology of eosinophils. *N Engl J Med* 1991;324:1110–1118. *Describes the intracellular contents and cell surface receptors of eosinophils, as well as the activation of these cells by various cytokines and their participation in inflammatory and immune reactions.*

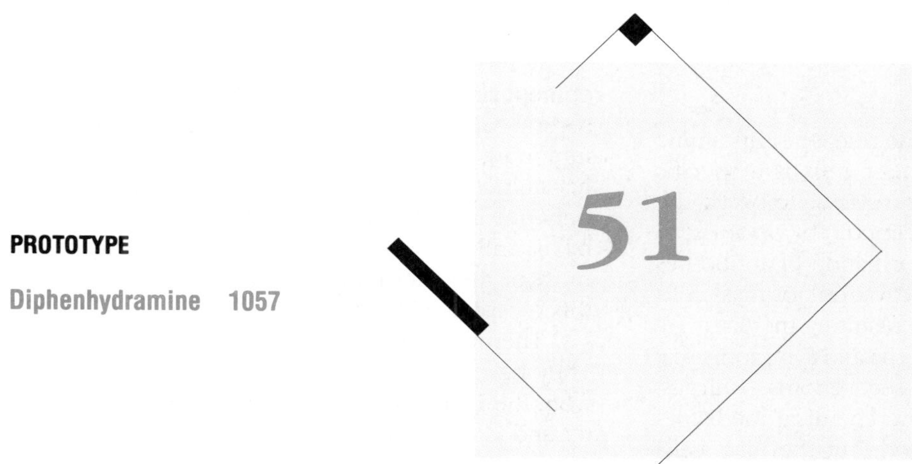

PROTOTYPE

51

Histamine and Histamine Receptor Antagonists

Various cells in the body synthesize, store, and release several very active chemicals called **autacoids**. Autacoids can be thought of as locally active hormones: when they are released from cells, they travel only a very short distance to exert effects on nearby cells. Their effects occur after they interact with specific receptors on target cell membranes. This local action distinguishes autacoids from other hormones, such as thyroid hormone or insulin, that are carried by the bloodstream to exert effects throughout the body, including sites quite far from where they were released.

This description of autacoids makes them sound very much like neurotransmitters. The two autacoids that are discussed in this chapter—histamine and serotonin—are found in some nerve cells, where they do act as neurotransmitters. However, as noted shortly, these substances are also released from other cell types. Whether they are released from nerves or other cells, their biologic actions are important to both the normal and abnormal function of key body processes.

Part I of this chapter focuses on perhaps the most important autacoid, histamine. Part II discusses the actions and uses of the many drugs that are used to inhibit one or more of histamine's actions. Some of these drugs—the antihistamines—are familiar to most healthcare workers in one way or another. The chapter ends with coverage of another autacoid, serotonin, and the drugs used to alter its actions.

I. Histamine

Location of Endogenous Histamine

Histamine is found in many tissues, but in small amounts. However, various cells in the lungs, the gastric mucosa, the skin and parts of the central nervous system (CNS) contain larger and more biologically important amounts of histamine.

Most histamine in the tissues is synthesized, stored in, and then released from, *mast cells.* As noted in Chapter 50, mast cells also contain other biologically active mediators that may be released along with histamine. Some histamine is also found in *basophils,* which are cells found in the bloodstream. From a biologic or therapeutic viewpoint, the histamine in mast cells is probably much more important.

Major reference tables appear beginning on page 1070.

Histamine Release

The most common stimulus for the release of histamine and other mediators found in mast cells is a specific antigen. For this type of *immune response* to occur, the mast cells must be prepared ("primed") by prior exposure to antigens that cause the formation of antibodies on the mast cell surface. The "activation" of mast cells in this type of response, and the resulting mediator release, accounts for many of the signs and symptoms that occur with allergies to pollens, insect venoms, or drugs. In antigen–antibody reactions, the chemical mediators in the mast cells may be released, but the mast cells themselves remain intact. This is sometimes called specific mast cell activation, because it depends on the presence of specific antigens and antibodies.

Antigen–antibody reactions are important and common, but they are not the only way by which histamine and other mediators can be released from mast cells. Some drugs, such as morphine (Chapter 21) and the neuromuscular blocker curare (Chapter 17) can trigger mediator release through a nonallergic process. This has been called nonspecific mast cell activation. Other stimuli that cause mediator release owing to mast cell damage or destruction include local trauma (eg, lacerations) and various forms of radiation, such as X-rays, ultraviolet rays, and infrared radiation (heat). Some animal venoms and substances released from plants can also activate mast cells in this way.

The reaction following mast cell activation and histamine release can vary, depending on where and how much histamine and other mediators are released. It can be localized and very mild (pruritus [itching] restricted to a small site on the skin), or generalized and potentially fatal (anaphylaxis). A minute amount of antigen is enough to trigger a massive response in some individuals. Most severe allergic reactions are not due to histamine alone, but involve all the mast cells' mediators.

Blockade of Histamine's Effects

There are two major ways to inhibit histamine's effects. One is to block histamine release. This can be done with the drug cromolyn sodium, which is discussed briefly at the end of the chapter and in detail in Chapter 38. The second and more common approach is to block the target cell receptors with which histamine interacts. The drugs that act in this manner are the *antihistamines.*

Histamine Receptors

Histamine acts as an *agonist* on specific histamine receptors, similar to the way acetylcholine (ACh) and epinephrine act on their specific receptors. There are several subclasses of histamine receptors; the two most important are called H_1 and H_2. Both types respond to histamine, but drugs classified as antihistamines block only one subtype, not both. Most of the effects caused by histamine are due to its actions on H_1 receptors, and most of the available antihistamines specifically block this receptor subtype.

There are four approved H_2-receptor blockers. They have properties and uses that are very different from the H_1 blockers, as described briefly in this chapter and in more detail in Chapter 40.

Absorption, Distribution, Metabolism, and Excretion

Histamine is not effective when given orally because it is inactivated in the gastrointestinal (GI) tract. In those few instances in which it is used as a drug, it must be injected. Histamine is distributed throughout the body, but does not cross the blood–brain barrier. The enzyme histaminase metabolizes histamine.

Pharmacologic Effects

Histamine's effects vary considerably in different animal species. Only the major effects in humans are discussed here. They are summarized in Table 51–1, which also shows the histamine receptor type—H_1 or H_2—that is involved. In general, whether histamine is given as a drug or released from mast cells, the effects are similar.

Pulmonary Effects

Histamine is a potent bronchoconstrictor. This effect is mediated by H_1 receptors. It accounts for the wheezing associated with common allergies and for the marked respiratory difficulty that occurs in severe asthma or anaphylaxis.

Vascular Effects

Histamine constricts venules and dilates arterioles. This increases fluid pressure in the affected capillary beds, producing local edema and what has been called "capillary dilation." The vascular responses are mainly mediated by H_1 receptors. (The H_1 blockers do not completely prevent the effects, so H_2 receptors may also be involved.)

Histamine's actions on the blood vessels cause a classic response called the *Triple Response of Lewis.* It can be produced by injecting a small amount of hista-

Table 51–1 | Major Pharmacologic Effects of Histamine and Histamine Antagonists

Organ or System Affected	Histamine	H_1 Antagonists
Respiratory tract	Bronchoconstriction, increased secretions (H_1)	Slight bronchodilation in the presence of histamine; decreased but thickened secretions (partly an antimuscarinic action)
Blood vessels	Arteriolar dilation, decreased blood pressure; venular constriction, increased intracapillary pressure, local edema (mainly H_1)	Slight antagonism of arteriolar dilation, venular constriction, in presence of histamine; possible capillary-stabilizing effect
Heart	Increased rate, force of contraction (H_2)	Rate may increase owing to antimuscarinic action
GI tract	Increased gastric acid secretion (H_2)	None (only H_2 receptors involved)
Adrenal medulla	Increased epinephrine release (H_1 and H_2?)	Negligible; may inhibit epinephrine release in presence of large amounts of histamine
Mucous glands	Increased secretions (H_1)	Decreased, thickened secretions (partly an antimuscarinic action)
Central nervous system	Exact action unknown; possible role in central regulation of cardiovascular system, body temperature (receptor type[s] unclear)	Usually drowsiness, sedation (partly an antimuscarinic action)
Peripheral nerves	Stimulation of sensory nerves (receptor type[s] unclear)	Local anesthetic effect (probably not due to antagonism of histamine's actions)

mine under the skin, but a simple mosquito bite causes a similar and more familiar effect.

1. First, a small red spot appears. It is caused by increased local blood flow as arteriolar dilation allows more blood to flow into the affected capillary bed and venular constriction reduces the blood's ability to leave. This lasts a minute or so.
2. Next, a bright red flare surrounds the area. This probably reflects reflex vasodilation that occurs when released histamine stimulates nearby nerve endings. Histamine also stimulates peripheral sensory nerves to cause itching or pain.
3. A white wheal develops in the center of the affected area. This is probably due to increased intracapillary pressure that forces plasma to leak out of the capillaries, causing local edema.

Generalized arteriolar dilation owing to histamine release can often be seen as the skin flushing that occurs when morphine is given to some patients. It is most pronounced in the upper chest, neck, and face—areas of the body in which histamine concentrations in the skin are highest. The profound hypotension that accompanies anaphylactic shock is the most graphic example of widespread, systemic release of histamine and resulting vascular effects.

Vascular effects of histamine in the lungs during anaphylaxis can cause pulmonary edema. The related fluid accumulation interferes with the blood's ability to take up oxygen and eliminate carbon dioxide, and intensifies the problems caused by bronchoconstriction.

Cardiac Effects

Histamine acts directly on the heart to stimulate rate and contractile force. These effects are mediated by H_2 receptors. When massive and widespread histamine release occurs, as in anaphylaxis, hypotension activates the baroreceptor reflex, which stimulates the sympathetic nervous system. That causes further cardiac stimulation, possibly to dangerous levels.

Gastric Effects

Histamine, through actions on the H_2 receptor, is probably the most important physiologic stimulus for gastric acid secretion. This is one of the few known *physiologic* roles for histamine outside the CNS, but it also contributes to the development of peptic ulcer disease.

Central Nervous System Effects

Histamine is found in various parts of the brain. Some is located in mast cells associated with cerebral blood vessels, outside the blood–brain barrier. This pool of histamine probably helps control local blood vessel tone.

Histamine is also located in certain nerve endings in the brain, where it may function as a neurotransmitter. This histamine may help regulate such processes as heart and circulatory function, body temperature control, water intake, and emesis. Injected histamine will not cause these latter CNS effects because the drug cannot cross the blood–brain barrier.

Other Effects

Histamine increases lacrimal fluid and mucus secretion. The related signs, watery eyes and runny nose (rhinorrhea), are common in allergic reactions.

Histamine stimulates the adrenal medulla, causing epinephrine release. This effect contributes to histamine's cardiac and vascular effects and accounts for one of the drug's clinical uses. The epinephrine-releasing effect also explains why histamine is contraindicated in persons with pheochromocytomas (tumors of the adrenal medulla).

Clinical Indications and Administration

Histamine's only uses are for diagnosing achlorhydria, pernicious anemia (one cause of achlorhydria), and pheochromocytoma (Table 51–C).

Diagnosis of Achlorhydria

Achlorhydria involves inadequate production of hydrochloric acid in the stomach. One test for achlorhydria is based on histamine's ability to stimulate acid secretion. In brief, a baseline sample of gastric juice is assayed for acidity, a low dose of histamine is injected subcutaneously (SC), and samples of gastric juice are again collected and assayed. Patients with achlorhydria show little or no increased acid secretion after histamine injection.

Unwanted stimulation of H_1 receptors can cause serious pulmonary and vascular effects, and the dose of histamine may not stimulate acid secretion sufficiently. Alternative tests were therefore developed. One is the *augmented histamine test.* It involves pretreating the patient with the antihistamine diphenhydramine (p 1057), then injecting a larger dose of histamine. This test is more conclusive, but still not risk-free.

Diagnosis of Pheochromocytoma

The pheochromocytoma test is based on histamine's ability to release epinephrine from the tumor cells. The drug is given intravenously (IV). In a normal individual, the dose that is given would cause little, if any, effect. In a person with pheochromocytoma, the release of large amounts of epinephrine from the tumor causes a large increase in blood pressure and heart rate.

This test is also very risky, because the positive response is an increase in blood pressure and heart rate in patients who, because of their tumor, already have increased blood pressure and heart rate. Safer and more conclusive tests are available, so histamine tests usually are a last choice.

NURSING IMPLICATIONS

Diagnostic tests involving histamine are performed by a physician. The nurse should review the patient's chart to rule out contraindications, obtain baseline vital signs, and be prepared to deal with adverse reactions (discussed later). Become familiar with scheduled times for sampling and preparing blood, urine, or other body fluids for laboratory assay.

Side Effects, Adverse Reactions, and Contraindications

Common but relatively mild side effects of histamine include flushing of the upper torso and face, pruritus, headache ("histamine headache") caused by cerebral vasodilation, wheezing, decreased blood pressure, and increased heart rate. Severe responses are extensions of the above effects; these are discussed in the next section as overdoses.

Histamine administration is contraindicated in persons with

- asthma or obstructive lung disease, because of the risk of fatal bronchospasm;
- pheochromocytoma, because of the risk of serious hypertension and cardiac stimulation from massive epinephrine release; and
- individuals with most other cardiovascular abnormalities, including ischemic heart disease, severe hypertension or hypotension, tachycardias or arrhythmias, and hyperthyroidism, all of which might be aggravated by histamine's effects.

NURSING IMPLICATIONS

Closely monitor blood pressure, pulse, and adequacy of ventilation during the diagnostic use of histamine, and for at least one hour after. Anticipate serious adverse responses, and have the appropriate emergency drugs and other means to monitor and support vital signs readily available.

Overdose and Toxicity

Overdoses of histamine alone are rare because histamine is seldom used as a drug. However, the signs and symptoms of true histamine toxicity are not very different from what occurs during anaphylaxis, which is relatively common. The major ones include severe bronchoconstriction, hypotension, tachycardia, and cardiac arrhythmias. If not treated soon and successfully, death may occur from asphyxia, cardiovascular collapse ("anaphylactic shock"), or both. Other signs and symptoms such as headache, urticaria, and pruritus occur, but they are not very important compared with the cardiopulmonary problems.

Persons experiencing anaphylaxis may also develop impaired blood clotting owing to release of heparin, the anticoagulant, which is one of the many substances found in mast cells and basophils.

A true histamine overdose is due to histamine alone, whereas anaphylaxis is due to the effects of histamine plus many other mast cell mediators. The most important first measures are to establish and maintain a patent airway (intubation, as needed), to maintain blood oxygenation (oxygen therapy, given routinely), and to normalize blood pressure and cardiovascular status in general.

The drug treatment of choice is epinephrine, injected SC (see Chapter 14 for doses). Epinephrine acts as a physiologic antagonist of histamine and most other mast cell mediators. It counteracts bronchoconstriction by directly dilating the bronchioles, raises blood pressure by constricting arterioles, and tends to lower heart rate once the baroreceptors sense an increase in blood pressure. However, epinephrine may aggravate tachycardias or arrhythmias through its direct cardiac-stimulating effects, and antiarrhythmic drug therapy may be needed.

Antihistamines, particularly diphenhydramine, can be used *adjunctively* to manage less serious responses such as pruritus and urticaria, but only *after* giving epinephrine to stabilize life-threatening changes of vital signs. Antihistamines cannot be used instead of epinephrine, especially for anaphylaxis, because they will not antagonize the dangerous effects of other mast cell mediators.

Corticosteroids may be used adjunctively to reduce inflammation and edema.

NURSING IMPLICATIONS

Whenever there is a risk of anaphylaxis, and whenever histamine is to be administered, epinephrine, diphenhydramine, and corticosteroids must be immediately available and ready to inject. Anticipate intubation and mechanical ventilation to ensure a patent airway and adequate gas exchange. Focus monitoring on cardiac and pulmonary status and on neurologic function, which could be altered by shock or cerebral anoxia. Auscultate breath sounds to assess the severity of bronchoconstriction and airway secretions. Monitor blood pressure and the electrocardiogram (ECG) continuously until vital signs stabilize.

II. Antihistamines (H_1 Blockers)

The drugs that are called antihistamines in casual conversation are competitive antagonists of histamine at the H_1 receptor. However, these drugs do far more than would be imagined from simply analyzing the term "antihistamine." They produce many other important effects, some of which are clinically useful, and some of which contraindicate their use for certain patients.

There are six major chemical classes of the older ("first-generation") H_1 blockers, and each contain several drugs. A miscellaneous group contains two H_1 blockers, terfenadine and astemizole.

All the drugs in all the groups cause generally similar effects, but the groups and their member drugs differ in terms of the intensities of these effects, as discussed on page 1064. These differences are clinically important.

PROTOTYPE

Diphenhydramine

Diphenhydramine (BENADRYL) belongs to the *ethanolamine* class of H_1 blockers. However, it is generally considered the prototype of *all* H_1 blockers.

Absorption, Distribution, Metabolism, and Excretion

Diphenhydramine and most other H_1 blockers are absorbed well from the GI tract, and they are usually given orally. They are distributed throughout the body, entering the CNS, the placental circulation, and maternal milk, and are metabolized in the liver. Diphenhydramine's duration of action is about four hours, although special timed-release formulations of some H_1 blockers are available to provide a longer-lasting effect.

Diphenhydramine and some related drugs can induce the hepatic drug-metabolizing enzyme systems, similar to the way barbiturates can. Thus, with repeated use, the duration of action may become shorter, and drug interactions may occur.

Pharmacologic Effects

In addition to the predicted effects of blocking H_1 receptors (see Table 51–1), the antihistamines have activity as antiemetics, local anesthetics, and sedatives.

Also, many antihistamines, including diphenhydramine, have antimuscarinic activity. That is, these drugs block muscarinic receptors for ACh, just like atropine. These many properties account for the effects of antihistamines on various organ systems.

Respiratory Effects

Diphenhydramine and other H_1 antagonists block the bronchoconstrictor actions of histamine, but *not* the effects of other mediators that may be released during anaphylaxis or an asthma attack. This is why H_1 blockers are not effective primary treatments for either of these conditions.

The antihistamines reduce (dry) respiratory tract mucus secretions. Part of this effect is due to their ability to block histamine receptors, and part is due to antimuscarinic effects.

Vascular Effects

Diphenhydramine and related H_1 antagonists block only part of the arteriolar dilator and venous constrictor actions of histamine (since these effects are mediated by both H_1 and H_2 receptors). These actions contribute to the relief of pruritus that H_1 blockers provide for insect bites, urticaria, and contact dermatitis such as poison ivy.

Central Nervous System Effects

Diphenhydramine and most related antihistamines usually cause sedation, but CNS stimulation may occur with some drugs or with very high doses of most antihistamines. Central nervous system effects are often unwanted and so are considered side effects.

Most H_1 blockers have antiemetic activity, but the clinical usefulness of some antihistamines (including diphenhydramine) for treatment of motion sickness or drug-induced nausea and vomiting is limited by the intense sedation they cause. Other antihistamines cause useful antiemetic effects and little or no sedation. They are identified below.

Local Anesthetic Effects

Diphenhydramine causes local anesthetic actions on peripheral nerves (see Chapter 18) if the local concentration near sensory nerves is sufficiently high. This effect also contributes to the drug's antipruritic action.

Other Effects

Diphenhydramine and most other antihistamines cause mydriasis and cycloplegia, tachycardia, and mild decreases of GI and urinary tract activity. These responses are caused by the drug's intense peripheral atropine-like activity, and in most cases they are unwanted side effects.

Clinical Indications and Administration

Most antihistamines are used to alleviate signs and symptoms of acute or chronic allergic states. In these instances, their ability to block histamine receptors is most important. Diphenhydramine and some of the others have special uses, often unrelated to allergy, that make use of their diverse properties. Dosages are noted in Table 51–C.

Management of Allergic Disorders

Oral antihistamine administration is preferred for most systemic allergic reactions such as hay fever or generalized drug-induced problems. Injection, IV (preferred) or intramuscular (IM), is indicated when oral administration is not feasible or when immediate actions are required, as in anaphylaxis.

Diphenhydramine reduces the cutaneous and sys-

TRENDS AND CONTROVERSIES IN PHARMACOLOGY

From R_x to OTC—Is It Wise?

Diphenhydramine was, until not so long ago, available only by prescription. It is now available over-the-counter (OTC) and there is still some controversy about the wisdom of deregulating it. The recommended adult dose—25 mg—is considered therapeutic in many instances.

Many people who self-medicate believe that a "mere" doubling of the dose of any drug will increase or speed the desired effects—relief of cold or allergy symptoms in this case. A 50 mg dose of diphenhydramine is sufficient to cause intense ataxia or sedation, or even sleep, in many people. Consuming a small amount of alcohol, even with the usual 25 mg dose, is liable to cause much more intense effects. The risk of excessive effects with an ethanolamine, the class to which diphenhydramine belongs, is probably greater than for any other class of antihistamines sold without prescription. Although nonprescription diphenhydramine is advertised for relief of cold and allergy symptoms, some knowledgeable members of the lay public realize its marked sedative activity. Thus, the drug can become popular but inappropriate self-medication for relief of simple anxiety, "nervous tension," or insomnia. Indeed, 25 mg doses of diphenhydramine are advertised as allergy relief medication, while the very same dose of the very same drug is marketed, under different names and with very different packaging, as a sleep aid.

Other antihistamines that may become available OTC, terfanidine (SELDANE) and astemizole (HISMANAL), have been found to induce potentially lethal arrhythmias, such as ventricular tachycardia, and convulsions in a few isolated cases. These adverse effects may not pose a significant risk to the general population, but risks are nonetheless increased in the context of inappropriate administration and overdosage.

Often, because drugs are available without prescription, they are considered safe by the public—and indeed they are when used properly. However, it is important for nurses to provide accurate information about the proper use of OTC drugs.

temic signs and symptoms of allergic states in which histamine is the major cause of symptoms. This includes urticaria (localized skin edema), angioneurotic edema, many forms of allergic or contact dermatitis, allergic conjunctivitis, certain allergic drug reactions, reactions to plasma or blood transfusions, pollinosis, and hay fever. The H_1 blockers also play an important role in managing urticaria pigmentosa (systemic mastocytosis), a condition in which there is an overabundance of mast cells and histamine release, usually in localized areas of the skin.

Diphenhydramine dries respiratory secretions, thereby reducing rhinorrhea, postnasal drip, and wheezing.

Antihistamines are indicated only for upper respiratory tract problems and should not be used for asthma or lower respiratory tract disorders.

Topical antihistamine preparations are available for managing mild allergic reactions in which signs and symptoms are limited to the skin. They should be used for only a few days. Prolonged use increases the risk of drug-induced rash. They should not be applied to large areas of the body or to broken (cut, blistered, or oozing) skin. Also, topical antihistamines should not be administered on mucous membranes.

Antihistamines in OTC Cough and Cold Remedies

Antihistamines are common ingredients in nonprescription cough, cold, allergy, and hay fever remedies. Some products contain only an antihistamine, while others may contain one or more of the following additional ingredients: a sympathomimetic decongestant; another antimuscarinic; aspirin or acetaminophen; and alcohol.

Although an antihistamine alone is a reasonable treatment for true allergies such as hay fever, antihistamines or combination products containing them are not rational treatments for cold or flu symptoms, in which histamine plays a very minor role. None of these products "cure" the cold or flu. When (or if) they work, the relief is due mainly to their atropine-like actions.

Sedative effects may also help the user sleep with less interference by annoying symptoms. However, they may also interfere with daytime activities.

Sedation

The marked CNS-depressant actions of diphenhydramine and a few related drugs have led to their use as sedatives, even for patients who have no "allergic" problems. Over-the-counter sleep aids contain an antihistamine—diphenhydramine, or the related drugs doxylamine or pyrilamine—as the "active" ingredient.

NURSING IMPLICATIONS

It is important for the nurse, and the prospective user, to be aware of the ingredients in OTC products. "Shotgun" therapies with multiingredient products increase the risk of side effects, adverse responses in contraindicating conditions, and drug–drug interactions. Recommend products containing only an antihistamine for minor allergy symptoms. As discussed in Chapter 14, sympathomimetic nasal drops or sprays are generally preferred for decongestant effects in persons with mild cold or flu symptoms.

Some OTC cold and allergy relief products contain 25 mg diphenhydramine per tablet or capsule, and nothing more. Other OTC products contain exactly the same amount of the same drug, and nothing else, yet they are advertised as sleep aids. Either product can be used for either purpose, regardless of how it is labeled. Even so, these products may not cost the same—sleep aids, for example, often cost more than an antihistamine.

There is a more important lesson, however: a person taking a product that contains diphenhydramine to alleviate annoying allergy symptoms during the day is also taking an effective dose of a drug meant to make the person sleepy. There are obvious risks, and the patient should be made aware of them before using the product. The information is on the package label, but you cannot trust everyone to read or understand it.

Treatment of Motion Sickness

Diphenhydramine can be used to prevent or treat motion sickness or nausea and vomiting owing to other causes. However, excessive sedation limits such use for many ambulatory individuals. A derivative of diphenhydramine, dimenhydrinate (DRAMAMINE), and several antihistamines in other chemical classes have excellent anti-motion sickness activity and cause much less sedation. The use of antihistamines and other antiemetic drugs is discussed in Chapter 42.

Management of Parkinsonism

The atropine-like actions of diphenhydramine in the extrapyramidal tract of the brain are used to alleviate various signs and symptoms of parkinsonism. Antihistamines such as diphenydramine may be particularly useful when sedation is desirable or the patient cannot tolerate side effects of other antiparkinson drugs (see Chapter 25).

Local Anesthesia

Because diphenhydramine has good local anesthetic activity but does not cross-react with traditional local anesthetics (see Chapter 19), it can be used as an alternative agent for anesthetizing the skin in patients with questionable histories of allergic reactions to the preferred agents. A 1% solution of diphenhydramine can be infiltrated into the desired region. Diphenhydramine should not be used when other local anesthetics can be used safely instead.

Side Effects, Adverse Reactions, and Contraindications

Diphenhydramine may be classified as a histamine receptor blocker, but its side effects are very similar to those noted in Chapter 13 for atropine and its CNS-depressant relative, scopolamine—both of which are classified as antimuscarinics (ACh receptor blockers). Table 51–S summarizes diphenhydramine's key side effects. Because of the similarities with atropine, the information noted below and in Table 51–S should be compared with that given for atropine (Table 13–S). Only highlights of diphenhydramine's side effects are presented here. Responses that are more common in or more important for children or the elderly are noted in separate sections below.

Central Nervous System Side Effects

Central nervous system depression, ranging from drowsiness or ataxia to sleep, is one of the most common side effects. These are desired effects when diphenhydramine is given to aid or cause sleep. They are unwanted, however, when the person receiving the drug wishes or needs to be fully awake and alert. Some individuals may experience paradoxical CNS "stimulation" with low doses. This is very similar to what occurs with low doses of alcohol or other sedatives (see p 349 and Fig. 22–2). (As noted in the section on overdoses and toxicity, CNS stimulation—seizures in particular—is a common response in serious antihistamine intoxication.)

Peripheral (Atropine-like) Side Effects

Diphenhydramine causes a host of side effects that readily show its ability to block ACh receptors well.

- Dry mouth, blurred vision (cycloplegia), and photophobia owing to mydriasis are the most common and sometimes most annoying side effects in the periphery. The most important related contraindication is glaucoma.
- Mucus secretions are reduced and thickened. Antihistamines are therefore generally contraindicated for persons with asthma.
- Sweating is decreased. This may make the patient susceptible to fever and heat stroke when the person engages in strenuous activity or is in a hot environment.
- Motility of the GI and urinary tracts is decreased. The related contraindications are constipation, paralytic ileus, or gut blockage; and prostatic hypertrophy, urinary tract obstruction, and other conditions that can be worsened by decreased urinary tract activity.
- Heart rate may increase. Use care, and monitor accordingly, if the patient already has an increased heart rate or a tachyarrhythmia or is hyperthyroid.

Cutaneous Side Effects

Paradoxically, topical antihistamine preparations that can be used to treat skin rashes (eg, those caused by poison ivy) can also act as skin "sensitizers." They can prolong or intensify existing skin eurptions or cause rashes themselves. The best way to minimize these side effects is to follow label directions about doses, the duration of therapy, and the need to apply the medications sparingly.

Regardless of the precautions that are taken, the application site(s) should be assessed often. Treatment should be stopped and drug therapy reevaluated by a physician when antihistamine-induced skin reactions occur.

In general, all the side effects noted for diphenhydramine also apply to the related H_1 blockers that are summarized later. The major difference with the other drugs is that one or more side effects may be more or less intense than those caused by equivalent therapeutic doses of diphenhydramine. When side effects become bothersome or dangerous, it may be possible either to reduce the dose of the current drug or to switch to another antihistamine.

NURSING IMPLICATIONS

If the side effects are bothersome and are caused by an OTC antihistamine, consult with a pharmacist or review product information in sources such as the *Handbook of Nonprescription Drugs* or *Drug Facts and Comparisons*. You may be able to recommend an alternative drug or product that causes the same symptomatic relief yet fewer side effects (provided that there is no true contraindication to the use of the alternative). When side effects are caused by the use of OTC combination drug products, which can contain many active drugs (eg, decongestants, analgesics, and alcohol), you should also consult the above sources. Often it is possible to "target" the patient's main complaints and recommend a single-ingredient product that might cause fewer problems. Sometimes, the cause may be an ingredient other than the antihistamine. In either case, review the product label with the patient, and be prepared to discuss the potential values and dangers of the medication.

Notify the physician if disturbing side effects were caused by a prescription antihistamine.

Regardless of whether side effects are caused by prescription or OTC medications, careful monitoring is essential. *Guidelines noted for atropine's side effects (p 185) apply to diphenhydramine and nearly all the other antihistamines.* If continued therapy is needed, dosages cannot be reduced, or alternative drugs cannot be used, nondrug measures (eg, sunglasses for photophobia, frequent sips of water for dry mouth) or dietary modifications (eg, adequate hydration) are usually the best initial approach.

If possible, avoid using still more drugs with systemic effects (eg, laxatives) to combat side effects (such as constipation) caused by one preparation. If other drugs do seem indicated, they should be prescribed by a physician. Nonprescription topical medications such as ocular or oral lubricants are acceptable but costly.

◆ Use During Pregnancy and Lactation

Diphenhydramine and other antihistamines are not recommended for use during pregnancy unless the benefits to the mother clearly outweigh potential risks to the fetus. Generally, such use should be limited to acute adjunctive management of serious allergic symptoms, particularly anaphylaxis.

The once common practice of prescribing antihistamines with antiemetic activity for morning sickness is no longer recommended owing to the risk of fetal malformations. Women who receive antihistamines should refrain from breast-feeding while they are taking the drug.

◆ Use in Children

Children tend to develop what appears to be CNS stimulation more often than older individuals, even with therapeutic doses of some antihistamines. However, the CNS stimulation may also reflect overdose. Unless you can determine the cause (eg, through *reliable* information from parents or guardians who may be administering the drug to a child), recommend immediate evaluation of the child in an emergency department.

◆ Use in the Elderly

Paradoxical CNS stimulation or ataxia caused by diphenhydramine and related drugs is common in the elderly. The presence of contraindicating conditions such as glaucoma or prostatic hypertrophy increases the risk of serious problems caused by side effects of antihistamines. Likewise, the use of other medications can increase the risk of drug interactions. Thus, pretreatment assessment of the medical and medication history must be particularly thorough for older patients. Extra vigilance is also essential once treatment has begun.

Even when there are no true contraindicating conditions in the elderly individual, the ability of antihistamines to cause many side effects at once can significantly interfere with normal daily living activities and wellness. Secondary problems can also occur. For example, dry mouth can make eating and swallowing difficult and unsafe and can potentially lead to anorexia, nutritional deficiencies, and diminished bowel or bladder function. Blurred vision combined with sedation or ataxia can make ordinary tasks such as walking or driving dangerous.

In general, advice concerning the administration of atropine to elderly individuals (p 176) applies fully to antihistamines. When side effects pose a problem and drug therapy must be continued, nondrug measures to alleviate the consequences of side effects are the best initial approach. Discourage patients from self-prescribing yet other systemic drugs (eg, laxatives) to combat problems caused by the antihistamine.

Interactions with Other Drugs

There are no specific interactions that involve diphenhydramine and the related first–generation antihistamines. However, one should expect increased side effects when an antihistamine is administered with any other medication that also causes atropine-like effects (see Chapter 13) or CNS depression, including alcohol. It is important to note that the antipsychotics and antidepressants are examples of rather commonly used drugs that cause both CNS depression and atropine-like effects. As a result, careless combined use with an antihistamine can lead to many extra problems at once.

Persons taking an antihistamine, even in OTC products, should be explicitly advised to avoid consuming alcohol. Owing to the potential risks of excessive CNS depression, some health-care providers question the wisdom of combining an antihistamine and alcohol in medications.

NURSING IMPLICATIONS

A thorough review of the patient's history and chart greatly reduces the risk of interactions between prescribed interactants. Give thorough instructions to outpatients, and include a list of medications to avoid, to reduce the risk of interactions with OTC drugs. Be sure to warn patients against consuming alcohol while taking an antihistamine.

Instruct the patient to inform health-care providers of all medications recently or currently being taken. Ask specifically about OTC product use.

Overdose and Toxicity

Overdoses of H_1-type antihistamines are fairly common, mainly because these drugs are available OTC and are widely used. Overdoses can also be fatal. The signs and symptoms, and the interventions used to treat them, are very similar to those associated with overdoses of atropine or scopolamine. That information is discussed fully in Chapter 13 (p 178 and Table 13–S); only highlights are presented here. Obviously, the consequences of poisoning, and treatment methods, vary if other drugs or alcohol were consumed also.

Signs and Symptoms

Major changes affect both the CNS and peripheral structures under control of the autonomic nervous system. They reflect a typical "antimuscarinic syndrome" (Appendix C).

In adults, the antihistamines cause progressive CNS depression: ataxia, sedation, delirium, and then coma as blood levels rise. Alcohol intensifies the CNS depression and speeds its progress. Seizures (status epilepticus) eventually occur, and they are the usual cause of death. The seizures are often triggered by a very high fever. Children respond somewhat differently. They tend to show signs of agitation, irritability, and excitement first. Seizures, coma, and fever may occur shortly thereafter.

Peripheral effects reflect atropine-like blockade of parasympathetic influences. They include

- tachycardia, possibly with arrhythmias, hypotension, and cardiovascular collapse;
- a marked decrease in gut and urinary tract motility (eg, constipation and urinary retention);
- an absence of lacrimal, mucus, sweat, and salivary secretions; and blurred vision and mydriasis.

Treatment

Initial measures are aimed at removing unabsorbed drug from the gut with induced emesis, gastric lavage, and so on. (See Appendix C; be aware that emetic drugs may not work if the overdose involved an antihistamine with significant antiemetic actions.) Thereafter, treatment is symptomatic and supportive. The goals are to normalize vital signs; reduce an elevated body temperature with physical means (eg, with sponge baths), *never* with an antipyretic drug; and treat seizures that may occur, usually with IV diazepam. The antidote for severe or life-threatening atropine poisoning, physostigmine (ANTILIRIUM; p 159), can be used for antihistamine poisonings as well.

Physostigmine counteracts many of the peripheral and central actions of diphenhydramine and other H_1 blockers, including seizures. Physostigmine should be used only for severe poisoning in adults, and only as a last resort in children.

NURSING IMPLICATIONS

Anticipate the need for anticonvulsant drugs, emergency intubation, and bladder catheterization in any severely ill adult and in all children. Sponge baths or a hypothermia blanket will reduce fever and thus may help prevent seizures, particularly in children. Monitor fluid intake and output, especially urine output.

If poisoning was due to a nonprescription product, try to identify the brand name and other relevant information (amount; time taken; other substances such as alcohol used, etc); this can help the treatment team provide better care.

Related Drugs

There are over a dozen other H_1-receptor blocking drugs. The older drugs constitute the majority of the related agents. They are much like diphenhydramine in their actions, uses, side effects, and drug interactions. There are two newer approved H_1 blockers that can be called "second-generation" antihistamines. They are very similar to diphenhydramine and the rest, except for a few important differences: they cause little or no CNS depression, they cause some unique and important side effects, and they cause important and potentially significant interactions with drugs that are not likely to interact with diphenhydramine and the rest. The older drugs are discussed first.

Older ("First-Generation") H_1 Blockers

Most of the currently available antihistamines have been around for many years. They can be grouped according to their chemical class. Table 51–2 compares and contrasts the various antihistamine classes with respect to their pharmacologic profiles. Table 51–C lists the approved uses for each drug, along with usual dosages. Some drugs are available in immediate-acting dosage forms, whereas others are marketed in extended-acting (sustained-release) formulations as well. Some drugs are available OTC, alone or in combination with other medications, whereas others are available by prescription only.

Like diphenhydramine, two of the related drugs are ethanolamines, but they are not used often. The rest are classified as alkylamines, ethylenediamines, piperazines, phenothiazines, or piperidines. Agents in each of the groups are given orally. All the related antihistamines share diphenhydramine's ability to block the effects of histamine on the H_1 receptors. However, they differ in how well or how effectively they do so; that is, they differ in potency, which affects the dose. They also differ in terms of pharmacokinetics (absorption, metabolism, etc.), which affects the dosing interval.

The drugs in the various antihistamine classes can also cause all the other desired effects or side effects noted for diphenhydramine: CNS depression, atropine-like actions, the ability to control nausea and vomiting, and so on. Once again, however, drugs in the different groups vary in the intensity of one or more of those effects with proper or excessive dosages.

Table 51–2 Overview of the Major Classes of H_1 Antagonists

Group	Examples	Major Properties of Comments
Alkylamines	Brompheniramine Chlorpheniramine Dexchlorpheniramine Triprolidine	a. Effective H_1 antagonists b. Mild sedative action; produce CNS stimulation more commonly than other antihistamine groups c. Moderate antimuscarinic actions d. Found in many prescription and OTC antihistamines marketed for cold and allergy symptoms e. Lack useful antiemetic effects
Ethanolamines	Carbinoxamine Clemastine Diphenhydramine	a. Moderate H_1-blocking activity b. Produce marked sedation c. Significant antimuscarinic activity d. GI side effects uncommon e. Excellent antiemetic activity, but use often limited by sedation
Ethylenediamines	Pyrilamine Tripelennamine	a. Effective H_1 antagonists b. Variable sedative, antimuscarinic actions (usually mild) c. Produce moderate GI upset d. Lack useful antiemetic activity
Piperazines	Cyclizine Hydroxyzine	a. Effective H_1 antagonists b. Sedation modest, variable c. Used mainly for antiemetic effects (see Chapter 42) d. Teratogenic—absolutely contraindicated during pregnancy
Phenothiazines	Methdilazine Promethazine Trimeprazine	a. Potent H_1 blockade b. Marked sedative activity; used mainly when sedation is desired c. Marked antimuscarinic actions d. Most effective as antiemetics e. See Chapter 23 for use of promethazine as antipsychotic, other actions
Piperidines	Azatadine Cyproheptadine Diphenylpyraline Phenindamine	a. Moderate H_1-blocking action b. Slight sedative activity c. Moderate antimuscarinic effects d. Lack useful antiemetic activity
Miscellaneous	Astemizole Terfenadine	a. Good antihistaminic activity b. Little or no sedation c. Little or no antimuscarinic effect d. No antiemetic activity e. Potentially arrhythmogenic f. Unique interaction with ketoconazole

Because of those differences, the desired effects/side effects profile of an individual agent (or antihistamine group) is important when choosing the one "best" agent, out of many, to match the needs of a particular patient. For example, when the clinical goal is to control emesis, the clinician chooses an antihistamine that has more antiemetic activity than the others. When the goal includes minimizing CNS depression, a drug that usually causes less CNS depression than the rest is better. The pharmacologic profiles also affect, to some extent, the severity of particular responses that might occur with an overdose. Nevertheless, the descriptions of diphenhydramine's actions generally apply to the related, older antihistamines.

"Second-Generation" H_1 Blockers

Astemizole (HISMANAL) and terfenadine (SELDANE) are the newer approved antihistamines. They are available OTC in Canada, but currently only by prescription in the United States. A similar drug that is likely to be approved soon is loratidine (CLARITIN).

Astemizole and terfenadine became quite well known and widely used because they do not cause CNS depression. Thus, they are not likely to cause bothersome or potentially dangerous sedative effects that can interfere with daytime activities or potentiate the sedative effects of other drugs. In addition, these drugs have much less atropine-like activity than older antihistamines such as diphenhydramine. That means fewer bothersome side effects and potential dangers for persons for whom antimuscarinic effects are contraindicated. Because these drugs can block histamine-induced bronchoconstriction without causing significant airway plugging, there is a growing interest in using these drugs to treat allergy-mediated asthma—a disorder for which older alternatives are contraindicated.

The second-generation antihistamines are receiving still more attention and interest. As their use increases, the awareness of some serious and potentially fatal unwanted effects and drug interactions is also growing. These drugs can cause cardiac arrhythmias, which seem to occur mainly when high doses—not necessarily toxic doses—are taken. The arrhythmia risk may be greater, and may occur at lower doses, when these drugs are given to persons who have a history of arrhythmias, tachycardia, or other conditions that favor disturbances in heart rate or rhythm. Exercise, because it increases heart rate, may be one of the factors that increases the risk.

Finally, terfenadine can cause serious interactions when administered with ketoconazole, an antifungal agent. The risk may also apply to astemizole and the newer, yet to be approved agents as well.

NURSING IMPLICATIONS

Instruct all patients not to exceed recommended terfenadine or astemizole dosages, and question medication orders calling for them. Avoid the interaction with ketoconazole.

Histamine H_2 Receptor Blockers

None of the antihistamines discussed so far can inhibit histamine's ability to stimulate gastric acid secretion—a function that is very important in a variety of GI disorders. The reason is that these drugs block H_1 receptors, whereas acid secretion is mediated by the H_2 subtype.

There are now four drugs that specifically block the H_2 receptor and have no effect on the H_1 type. The drugs are cimetidine (TAGAMET), the prototype H_2 blocker; and the related drugs famotidine (PEPCID), nizatidine (AXID), and ranitidine (ZANTAC). They are approved exclusively for managing peptic ulcer disease (gastric ulcers, duodenal ulcers, or both), and some are indicated for other gut disorders in which their ability to inhibit gastric acid secretion is clinically important.

The H_2 blockers are discussed in more detail in Chapter 40 (pp 801–804, and Tables 40–C, 40–S, and 40–I). To summarize some of the key ways in which they differ from diphenhydramine and the rest of the H_1 antagonists, the H_2 blockers

- have no clinically useful ability to block H_1 receptors and therefore cannot be substituted for an H_1 blocker for such uses as allergy control;
- cause little CNS depression, and none that is clinically useful;
- have no atropine-like actions and so do not share the related side effects or contraindications;
- do not have antiemetic or local anesthetic properties;
- cause very different side effects and toxicities; and
- interact with drugs that ordinarily do not interact with H_1 blockers.

Combined Use of H_1 and H_2 Blockers

The H_1-type antihistamines alone may be useful adjuncts for anaphylaxis, but they do not block all the unwanted effects caused by massive release of histamine (and other mediators). Cardiac stimulation, arrhythmias, and some vascular effects of histamine are examples of important consequences of anaphylaxis that are mediated by H_2 receptors.

Because both types of histamine receptors are involved, the use of both H_1 and H_2 blockers in this potentially life-threatening emergency is growing. Currently, these drugs do not replace epinephrine as the drug treatment of choice. Nevertheless, it is important to realize that such combinations are being evaluated and that for certain patients they may prove to be effective adjuncts to other therapies.

The combination of H_1 and H_2 blockers may also prove useful for managing other serious disorders that involve excessive histamine release, such as systemic mastocytosis (urticaria pigmentosa).

Mast Cell Stabilization and Prevention of Histamine Release

The antihistamines act by blocking the effects of histamine that has been released from mast cells and basophils. Another pharmacologic approach to reducing the effects of histamine is to prevent its release. This is accomplished by the drug cromolyn sodium (INTAL; NASALCROM). Its uses are limited to prophylaxis of bronchial asthma and seasonal allergies, as discussed in Chapter 38.

Cromolyn "stabilizes" the mast cell membrane. In doing so it blocks the release of histamine and other mast cell mediators that is triggered by an antigen. Cromolyn does not antagonize the effects of histamine or other mediators once they are released from mast cells or basophils, nor does it have any of the other actions noted for either H_1 or H_2 blockers.

III. Serotonin

Serotonin (5-hydroxytryptamine, or "5-HT") is an autacoid that is derived from the amino acid tyrosine. Most of the body's serotonin stores are located in enterochromaffin cells in the intestine. The rest is found in platelets and in the CNS. Serotonin acts through specific serotonin receptors (at least four subtypes have been identified) to produce its effects. Serotonin is not used clinically, but drugs that antagonize its effects are.

Serotonin stimulates intestinal muscle and is believed to help regulate GI motility. It is a powerful bronchoconstrictor in asthmatic persons. Serotonin released from platelets may have a role in hemostasis. Serotonin found in brain neurons probably acts as a neurotransmitter, but its precise physiologic roles are not known. It was thought to affect mood and behavior; serotonin deficiencies were thought to contribute to symptoms of schizophrenia. This concept was based partly on observations that the serotonin antagonist lysergic acid diethylamide (LSD) produced hallucinations and schizophrenic behavior.

Perhaps the most clinically important effects of serotonin are on blood vessels. Serotonin constricts some blood vessels and dilates others. The most obvious vascular effects of serotonin are seen in the *carcinoid syndrome,* which is a tumor of the serotonin-rich enterochromaffin cells in the gut. Persons with this disorder usually show marked skin flushing and vascular headache owing to cutaneous and cerebral vasodilation.

Serotonin Antagonists

Several drugs, including the illegal hallucinogen LSD, block some of serotonin's effects. However, only two antiserotonin agents are used clinically: methysergide and cyproheptadine. Cyproheptadine also has antihistaminic activity and is generally used like most other H_1 blockers to manage allergy symptoms. Therefore, it is not discussed here.

Methysergide

Methysergide (SANSERT) is an ergot alkaloid. It is chemically related to the oxytocic (uterine-stimulating) drugs methyl ergonovine and ergonovine maleate, and to ergotamine, a potent vasoconstrictor and α-adrenergic blocker (see Chapter 15).

Methysergide is absorbed after oral administration. It is indicated for prophylaxis of severe or frequent vascular headaches (migraine headaches) that do not respond to other therapies such as ergotamine or propranolol. Part of its benefits in this situation are due to its ability to block serotonin-induced cerebral vasodilation. It may also act through its ability to block α-adrenergic receptors, inhibit vasomotor control centers in the CNS, or directly constrict the cerebral blood vessels. Methysergide will not stop an ongoing headache.

Therapy is usually begun with a three-week trial period. If the drug was taken as directed but does not reduce the frequency or severity of headaches, methysergide administration should probably be stopped. If the drug is effective, therapy should be stopped for three to four weeks after six months of continual administration to reevaluate the patient and the need for continued drug treatment.

Methysergide is not used for routine treatment of vascular headaches because of its potentially serious adverse effects, especially when it is given chronically. The major problem is connective tissue fibrosis, often occurring in the lungs, aorta, mitral valve, or retroperitoneal areas. It is contraindicated in patients with fibrotic disease (for example, pulmonary fibrosis or mitral valve disease).

Even when used acutely, the drug's vasoconstrictor actions may cause hypertension, so it is contraindicated in patients with cardiac disease or hypertension. Reduced blood flow to the extremities may cause paresthesias, muscle cramps during exercise, or, at the extreme, ischemia and gangrene; peripheral vascular diseases such as thrombophlebitis, Raynaud's disease, and atherosclerosis are related contraindications.

Other side effects involve the GI tract (nausea, vomiting, diarrhea); the CNS (dizziness, drowsiness, or mild LSD-like hallucinations); and the cardiovascular system (edema and weight gain). Most of the acute effects are reversed when the drug is discontinued or the dose is reduced.

Methysergide and β-adrenergic blockers interact,

and combined therapy usually should be avoided. The β-blockers leave the vasoconstrictor effects of methysergide unopposed. The outcome could be a generalized increase of blood pressure (possibly severe, with stroke resulting) or more local effects that lead to decreased blood flow to the extremities. The latter is a particular problem in persons who have peripheral vascular disease. A significant reduction of blood flow could lead to tissue damage and tissue death (necrosis).

NURSING IMPLICATIONS

Stress to the patient the need for keeping follow-up appointments for evaluation. Encourage the patient to keep a diary documenting the frequency and severity of headaches during treatment; the occurrence of paresthesias, muscle weakness, pain on exercise, or other evidence of reduced peripheral blood flow; and daily body weight, which might indicate edema owing to heart, kidney, or liver dysfunction.

Teach migraine sufferers stress-avoidance and stress-management techniques. These important nondrug measures may reduce the number or severity of headaches.

Assessment involves checking blood pressure, peripheral pulses, and skin color and temperature, and examining for signs of vascular insufficiency. Lung, heart, and peripheral pulse sounds should be evaluated to help detect organ fibrosis (bruits, clicks, or murmurs).

SUMMARY OF NURSING IMPLICATIONS

◆ Assessment

Identify underlying conditions that increase the risk of adverse reactions; for histamine: asthma, cardiovascular disease, pheochromocytoma; for all first-generation antihistamines (older H_1 blockers, such as diphenhydramine): all conditions in which atropine is contraindicated; for second-generation antihistamines (astemizole, terfenadine): arrhythmias.

Establish baseline vital signs before diagnostic use of histamine.

Review recent and current medications for possible drug interactions with diphenhydramine or other antihistamines.

Assess for history of prior adverse or unusual reactions to antihistamines.

◆ Nursing Diagnoses

Ineffective breathing pattern related to bronchoconstriction, excessive mucus secretions from histamine (as from an allergic response).

Decreased cardiac output related to hypotension from histamine's effects.

Ineffective breathing pattern related to thick mucus and tight chest from adverse antihistamine effects.

Knowledge deficit related to prescribed drug therapy.

Sensory/perceptual alterations: dizziness, drowsiness, blurred vision, photophobia related to antihistamines.

Urinary retention related to antihistamines.

Noncompliance related to unpleasant drug effects: dry mouth, blurred vision, GI distress.

◆ Planning/Implementation

Administer drug dose accurately, noting exact time.

Monitor vital signs before diagnostic testing with histamine during administration, and for one hour thereafter.

Have emergency drugs (epinephrine, diphenhydramine, corticosteroids), oxygen, and cardiopulmonary support devices ready for use during diagnostic testing with histamine.

Administer antihistamines with meals or snack if GI distress occurs.

Assist with ambulation if dizziness or ataxia occurs.

Check peripheral pulses, skin color, temperature, and blood pressure regularly if patient is taking methysergide.

Obtain daily body weights for patients taking methysergide; periodically assess for edema caused by renal, cardiac, or hepatic dysfunction.

Assess patients taking methysergide for indications of lung fibrosis.

◆ Patient and Family Teaching

Teach the patient/family:

About diagnostic procedures, so they can anticipate how they will feel and understand expected desired responses and side effects (eg, flushing, tachycardia).

To avoid exposure to known allergens, excessive fatigue, or tension, all of which may increase need for antihistamines in allergy patients.

To avoid alcohol and other CNS depressants during antihistamine therapy (prescribed or self-prescribed).

To avoid driving or performing tasks requiring mental alertness and unimpaired vision while taking antihistamines.

How to relieve dry mouth: sips of water, use of sugarless gum or hard candies.

To wear sunglasses to alleviate problems owing to photophobia.

Not to increase drug dose if symptoms are not relieved.

To use topical antihistamines sparingly and for only a few days, unless directed otherwise by physician.

To recognize and report adverse antihistamine/antimuscarinic effects (eg, wheezing, constipation, urinary retention, ocular pain).

Not to use OTC preparations without the advice of a physician or pharmacist; recommend single-ingredient products for relieving minor allergy symptoms.

To keep flavorful medications out of reach of children to prevent accidental overdose.

◆ Evaluation

The patient/family will:

Have stable vital signs during testing with histamine.

Experience relief of symptoms; achieve therapeutic effects of drug.

Experience minimal or no adverse drug effects: no complaints referable to major organs/organ systems (eg, cardiovascular, pulmonary, GI, urinary tract, eyes).

Annotated Bibliography

Bryant BG, Lombardi TP: Cold and allergy products. In: Feldmann EG, ed. *Handbook of Nonprescription Drugs.* 9th edition. Washington, DC, American Pharmaceutical Association, 1990:133–206. *Arguably the best all-in-one source of information about medications for which billions of dollars are spent each year—some needlessly or with added health risk. Formulations for some products may have changed slightly, but the underlying information is timeless.*

Caro JP, Dombrowski SR: Sleep aid and stimulant products. In: Feldmann EG, ed. *Handbook of Nonprescription Drugs.* 9th edition. Washington, DC, American Pharmaceutical Association, 1990: 225–242. *Good teaching tips, and more, for the patient who wishes to use an OTC sleep aid.*

Gadomski A, Horton L: The need for rational therapeutics in the use of cough and cold medicine in infants. *Pediatrics* 1992;89(4 Pt 2):774–776. *Suggests that health-care workers need to do a better, more rational job when considering giving these medications to ill children.*

Gengo FM, Manning C: A review of the effects of antihistamines on mental processes related to automobile driving. *J Allergy Clin Immunol* 1990;86(6 Pt 2):1034–1039. *One key message from this study is that mental and motor impairments due to antihistamines can last much longer than their obvious sedative effects.*

Greco PJ, Ende J: Pruritus: A practical approach. *J Gen Intern Med* 1992;7(3):340–349. *Contains excellent tables and figures to help you understand better the proper assessment and treatment needed to manage this common complaint.*

Greco PJ, Ende J: An office-based approach to the patient with pruritus. *Hosp Pract [Off]* 1992;27(5A):121–128. *A practical discussion of how the "typical" outpatient with pruritus is optimally managed.*

Hutton N, Wilson MH, Mellits ED, et al: Effectiveness of an antihistamine–decongestant combination for young children with the common cold: A randomized, controlled clinical trial. *J Pediatr* 1991;118(1):125–130. *Study concluding that, based on clinical trial results, there is no clinically significant improvement in symptoms of upper respiratory tract infection, and no significant placebo effect, in young children for whom an antihistamine–decongestant is prescribed.*

Kaliner MA: Nonsedating antihistamines: Pharmacology, clinical efficacy and adverse effects. *Am Fam Physician* 1992;45(3):1337–1342. *A short but worth-reading comparison of newer antihistamines, such as terfenadine, with the older agents.*

Krause HF: Pharmacology of upper respiratory allergy. *Otolaryngol Clin North AM* 1992;25(1):135–150. *Will help you understand the indications, benefits, and potential adverse effects of several drug groups, including antihistamines, decongestants, steroids, and mast cell stabilizers, with the goal of providing the best total patient care.*

Lieberman P: The use of antihistamines in the prevention and treatment of anaphylaxis and anaphylactoid reactions. *J Allergy Clin Immunol* 1990;86(4 Pt 2):684–686. *Reviews the pathophysiology of anaphylaxis—including drug-induced anaphylaxis—to help explain a growing role for combinations of H_1 and H_2 blockers in its treatment.*

Lorenz, W, Ennis M, Doenicke A, Dick W: Perioperative uses of histamine antagonists. *J Clin Anesth* 1990;2(5):345–360. *Identifies high-risk operative patients who, in the authors' opinion, are candidates for prophylactic therapy with H_1 and H_2 blockers. Important reading: allergy-related reactions occur in nearly one-third of surgical patients.*

Meade V: Patients need advice as array of cold products grows. *Am Pharm* 1991;31(12):24–25. *Good insight into problems arising from the multitude of OTC cold remedies. Having more options isn't necessarily better.*

Middleton DB: An approach to pediatric upper respiratory infections. *Am Fam Physician* 1991;44(5 Suppl):33S–40S, 46S–47S. *Identifies the limitations of antihistamines when treating the most common of all pediatric illnesses.*

Rafferty P: Antihistamines in the treatment of clinical asthma. *J Allergy Clin Immunol* 1990;86(4 Pt 2):647–650. *Look for a growing role of second-generation antihistamines, which lack unwanted atropine-like actions that pose dangers in asthma, in this common pulmonary disorder.*

Ryhal BT, Fletcher MP: The second-generation antihistamines: What makes them different? *Postgrad Med* 1991;89(6):87–88, 91–94, 99. *A useful update on antihistamine therapy. Addresses a key question that relates to old versus new antihistamines: Should one prescribe a drug to gain a desired therapeutic effect or merely to avoid causing unacceptable side effects?*

Sause RB, Mangione RA: Cough and cold treatment with OTC medicines. *J Pract Nurs* 1991;41(3):15–25. *Read this short paper before you self-medicate with one of these common remedies or recommend one to someone else.*

Simons FE, Simons KJ: Second-generation H_1-receptor antagonists. *Ann Allergy* 1991;66(1):5–16, 19. *Helps you understand how the "new" and "older" antihistamines differ so that you'll have a better understanding of when, how, and why one is used instead of another.*

Tarnasky PR, Van Arsdel PP Jr: Antihistamine therapy in allergic rhinitis. *J Fam Pract* 1990;30(1):71–80. *Antihistamines are the mainstay of allergic rhinitis therapy, but is a particular drug best for all patients? Read this to learn how to determine whether a rational choice has been made.*

Veerman MW, Marcadis ML: Nonprescription drug use in children. In: Feldmann EG, ed. *Handbook of Nonprescription Drugs.* Washington, DC, American Pharmaceutical Association, 1990:1021–1032. *Good coverage of the formulations, use, and misuse of all the common OTC medication groups, including cough and cold remedies, for children.*

Vitale M, Fields-Blache C, Luterman A: Severe itching in the patient with burns. *J Burn Care Rehabil* 1991;12(4):330–333. *This "special topics" article addresses a common clinical problem in burn patients and how to manage it.*

Woolbert LF: Do antihistamines and decongestants prevent otitis media? *Pediatr Nurs* 1990;16(3):265–267. *Succinctly summarizes data suggesting that antihistamines and decongestants are not as effective in treating otitis media as believed.*

Wormser H: Poison ivy and poison oak products. In: Feldmann EG, ed. *Handbook of Nonprescription Drugs.* 9th edition. Washington, DC, American Pharmaceutical Association, 1990:931–944. *Good insight into the values—and limitations—of topical antihistamine-containing OTCs for these and other allergy-mediated skin reactions.*

Table 51–C Clinical Uses and Administration of Histamine, Antihistamines, and Antiserotonin Agents*

AGENT	CLINICAL USES†	DOSAGE AND ROUTE OF ADMINISTRATION‡
	Agonists	
PROTOTYPE		
Histamine phosphate		
	Diagnosis of pernicious anemia, achlorhydria	SC: 27.5 μg/kg
		Augmented histamine test: Pretreat patient with 50 mg diphenhydramine IM, then inject 40 μg/kg histamine
	Diagnosis of pheochromocytoma	IV: 10 μg initially; if no pressor response occurs, inject 50 μg
	First-Generation Antihistamines (H_1-Receptor Blockers)	
PROTOTYPE		
Diphenhydramine		
(BENADRYL, others)	Allergy symptoms	25–50 mg every 6–8 hr (before meals, at bedtime)
		Children > 10 kg: 12.5–25 mg tid or qid (or 5 mg/kg/24 hr), not to exceed 300 mg/day
		IV or deep IM: 10–50 mg (400 mg/day maximum)
		Children: 5 mg/kg/day (300 mg/day maximum) in 3–4 divided doses
	Cough due to colds, allergies	25 mg q4h (150 mg/24 hr maximum)
		Children 6–12 yr (syrup only): 12.5 mg q4h (75 mg/24 hr maximum)
		2–6 yr: 6.25 mg q4h (25 mg/24 hr maximum)
	Treatment, prophylaxis (oral only) of motion sickness	25–50 mg tid or qid
		Children >20 lbs: 12.5–25 mg 3–4 times daily
		Give first dose 30 min before travel; repeat before meals and at bedtime for duration of travel
	Prompt treatment of motion sickness, emesis	IV or deep IM: 10–50 mg
		(100 mg if needed; 400 mg maximum)
		Children: 5 mg/kg/24 hr in 4 divided doses
	Parkinson's disease, drug-induced parkinsonism (extrapyramidal reactions)	50 mg tid or qid
		Children >20 lbs: 12.5–25 mg tid or qid or 5 mg/kg/day (300 mg/day maximum)
		IV or deep IM: 10–50 mg; 100 mg if needed, 400 mg/day maximum
		Children: 5 mg/kg/day in 4 divided doses (300 mg/day maximum)
(NYTOL, other OTC products, or prescription)	Sleep aid/hypnotic	50 mg at bedtime

(continued)

*Antihistamines used mainly for managing motion sickness (eg, cyclizine, meclizine), and their dosages, are discussed in Chapter 42.
† "Allergy symptoms" denotes use for treatment of perennial and seasonal allergic rhinitis, or for urticaria.
‡ Dosages are for oral administration to adults unless noted otherwise. Antihistamines found only in multiingredient cold/allergy/cough products are *not* listed.

Table 51–C | Clinical Uses and Administration of Histamine, Antihistamines, and Antiserotonin Agents* (*Continued*)

AGENT	CLINICAL USES†	DOSAGE AND ROUTE OF ADMINISTRATION‡
RELATED DRUGS		
Azatidine maleate		
(OPTIMINE)	Allergy symptoms	Adults, children ≥ 12 yr: 1–2 mg bid
Brompheniramine maleate		
(DIMETANE, others)	Allergy symptoms	Adults, children ≥ 12 yr: 4 mg q4–6h or 8–12 mg sustained-release product q8–12h (24 mg/24 hr maximum)
		Children 6–12 yr: 2 mg q4–6h (12 mg/24 hr maximum, immediate-acting dosage form only)
	Acute control of allergy symptoms	IM, SC, or slow IV: Adults, children ≥ 12 yr: 10 mg, repeat in 12 hr if needed
		Children < 12 yr: 0.5 mg/kg/day in 3–4 divided doses
Chlorpheniramine maleate		
(CHLOR-TRIMETON, others)	Allergy symptoms	Adults, children > 12 yr: 4 mg q4–6h (24 mg/day maximum) or 8–12 mg sustained-release product q8–12h
		Children 6–12 yr: 2 mg q4–6h (12 mg/day maximum) or 8 mg sustained-release product at bedtime
	Acute allergic reactions, anaphylaxis	IM, SC, or slow IV: Adults: 10–20 mg single dose; give IV only for anaphylaxis
Clemastine fumarate		
(TAVIST)	Allergy symptoms	Adults, children > 12 yr: 1.34 mg bid to 2.68 mg tid; use 2.68-mg dosage only for allergic skin reactions
Cyproheptadine hydrochloride		
(PERIACTIN)	Allergy symptoms, urticaria caused by cold weather	Initially 4 mg tid; maintenance doses usually 4–20 mg/day
		Children: 0.25 mg/kg/day in 2–3 divided doses
Dexchlorpheniramine maleate		
(POLARAMINE, others)	Allergy symptoms	2 mg q4–6h or 4–6 mg timed-released product at bedtime or q8–10h during day
		Children 6–11 yr: 1 mg q4–6h or 4 mg timed-release product at bedtime; 2–5 yr: 0.5 mg (immediate-acting dosage form only) q4–6h
Doxylamine		
(in UNISOM, other OTCs)	Sleep aid	25 mg before bedtime

(*continued*)

Table 51–C | **Clinical Uses and Administration of Histamine, Antihistamines, and Antiserotonin Agents* (*Continued*)**

AGENT	CLINICAL USES†	DOSAGE AND ROUTE OF ADMINISTRATION‡
RELATED DRUGS		
Hydroxyzine		
(VISTARIL)	Relief of pruritus	25 mg tid or qid
		Children > 6 yr: 50–100 mg/day in divided doses; < 6 yr: 50 mg/day in divided doses
	Anxiety relief	May start with IM administration 50–100 mg qid, then switch to some dosages orally
		Children > 6 yr: 50–100 mg/day in divided doses; < 6 yr: 50 mg/day in divided doses; may start with IM administration
	Acute psychiatric emergencies, including acute alcoholism	IM: 50–100 mg immediately; repeat q4–6h as needed
	Acute control of nausea, vomiting; preoperative or postoperative sedation, emesis control	IM: 25–100 mg
		Children: 1.1 mg/kg
	Pre- or postpartum adjunct	IM: 25–100 mg
Methdilazine HCl		
(TACARYL)	Allergy symptoms	8 mg bid–tid
		Children > 3 yr: 4 mg bid–tid
Phenindamine tartrate		
(NOLAHIST)	Allergy symptoms	Adults, children > 12 yr: 25 mg q4–6h (150 mg/24 hr maximum)
		Children 6–12 yr: 12.5 mg q4–6h (75 mg/24 hr maximum)
Promethazine HCl		
(PHENERGAN, many others, including combination products)	Allergy symptoms	25 mg at bedtime or 12.5 mg before meals and at bedtime
		Children: 25 mg at bedtime or 6.25–12.5 mg tid (may use 25 mg rectal suppository when oral route not feasible)
	Severe or acute allergic reactions	IV or deep IM (preferred): 25 mg, repeat in 2 hr if needed
	Motion sickness	25 mg bid; initially 30–60 min before travel, repeated in 8–12 hr if needed; then, 25 mg on awakening and before evening meal
		Children: 12.5–25 mg bid (oral or rectal)
	Nausea, vomiting (eg, perioperatively)	Rectal: 25 mg; repeat 12.5–25 mg as necessary q4–6h
		IV or deep IM: 12.5–25 mg if needed, q4h or longer)
		Children: 0.5 mg/lb
	Sedation	Oral, IV, or deep IM: 25–50 mg
		Children: Oral, rectal, IV, or deep IM: 12.5–25 mg

(*continued*)

Table 51–C | **Clinical Uses and Administration of Histamine, Antihistamines, and Antiserotonin Agents* (*Continued*)**

AGENT	CLINICAL USES†	DOSAGE AND ROUTE OF ADMINISTRATION‡
RELATED DRUGS		
	Preoperative adjunct (with narcotic or antimuscarinic, if ordered)	50 mg evening before surgery Children: 12.5–25 mg
	Postoperative sedation and analgesic adjunct	Oral, IV, or deep IM: 25–50 mg Children: 12.5–25 mg
	Labor and delivery	IV or deep IM: 50 mg in early labor, 25–75 mg during full labor (with reduced dosages of narcotic or other drugs as needed)
Pyrilamine maleate (NISAVAL, others)	Allergy symptoms	25–50 mg tid or qid
Trimeprazine (TEMARIL)	Allergy symptoms	2.5 mg qid or 5 mg sustained-release product q12h Children > 3 yr: 2.5 mg at bedtime or tid if needed (children > 6 yr may take 5 mg sustained-release form once daily); 6 mos–3 yr: 1.25 mg at bedtime or tid
Tripelennamine HCl (PBZ)	Allergy symptoms	25–50 mg q4–6h or 100 mg sustained-release product AM and PM Children, infants: 5 mg/kg/day (300 mg/day maximum) in 4–6 divided doses
Triprolidine HCl (ACTIFED, others)	Allergy symptoms	Adults, children > 12 yr: 2.5 mg q4–6h Children 6–12 yr: 1.25 mg q4–6h For adults or children, do not exceed 4 doses/24 hr
Second-Generation Antihistamines (H_1-Receptor Blockers)		
Astemizole (HISMANAL)	Allergy symptoms	Adults, children ≥ 12 yr: 10 mg once daily at least 2 hr after a meal
Terfenadine (SELDANE)	Allergy symptoms	Adults, children ≥ 12 yr: 60 mg bid Children 6–12 yr: 30–60 mg bid; 3–6 yr: 15 mg bid

(*continued*)

Table 51–C **Clinical Uses and Administration of Histamine, Antihistamines, and Antiserotonin Agents* (*Continued*)**

AGENT	CLINICAL USES[†]	DOSAGE AND ROUTE OF ADMINISTRATION[‡]
	H_2 Blockers	
Cimetidine (TAGAMET), *Famotidine* (PEPCID), *Nizatidine* (AXID), *Ranitidine* (ZANTAC)	Peptic ulcer disease, gastroesophageal reflux	See Table 40–C, p 811
	Histamine Antirelease Agent	
Cromolyn (INTAL; NASALCROM)	Prophylaxis of asthma, allergy symptoms (see Chapter 38)	See Table 38–C, p 781
	Antiserotonin Agent	
Methysergide (SANSERT)	Prophylaxis of severe, frequent, and refractory vascular headache (migraine and related headaches)	4–8 mg/day, with meals

Table 51–S Major Side Effects of and Contraindications for Major Antihistamines (H_1 Antagonists)

BODY SYSTEM/ Side Effect	CONTRAINDICATION/ PRECAUTION	COMMENTS AND NURSING IMPLICATIONS
First-Generation Antihistamines (Diphenhydramine, others)		
CENTRAL NERVOUS SYSTEM Drowsiness, sedation, ataxia, paradoxical stimulation		Caution patients taking diphenhydramine and most other antihistamines to avoid operating car or hazardous machinery, and tasks in which mental acuity or good coordination are essential; avoid use of other CNS depressants, including alcohol, unless on physician's advice; geriatric or pediatric patients may experience paradoxical excitement or confusion with recommended doses
Extrapyramidal side effects (abnormal involuntary limb or muscle movements)		Most likely with high doses of promethazine, other phenothiazine antihistamines; assess for abnormal involuntary movements (extrapyramidal side effects)
EYE Cycloplegia (paralysis of accommodation); day blindness due to mydriasis; corneal irritation due to decreased lacrimation	Glaucoma	From antimuscarinic actions; rule out glaucoma; instruct patient to report eye pain at once; recommend sunglasses for pain caused by bright sunlight; may recommend artificial tears for corneal irritation
RESPIRATORY Dyspnea; tightness of chest; wheezing; mucus plugging of airways	Bronchial asthma, other lower respiratory tract disorders, including emphysema	Counsel asthma patients not to use antihistamines, even those available OTC
CARDIOVASCULAR Tachycardia, hypotension	Cardiovascular disease (use with caution; usually not an absolute contraindication)	Monitor heart rate, blood pressure, pulse of hospitalized patients, especially with history of cardiovascular disease
GASTROINTESTINAL OR GENITOURINARY Constipation; diarrhea; urinary hesitancy, retention, or frequency	Obstructive bowel or bladder disorders; prostatic hypertrophy	Monitor patient or have patient report difficulty in defecation, decreased bowel movements, diarrhea, difficult or frequent urination
SKIN Drug-induced rash (with topical administration)		Topical antihistamines meant for short-term use on relatively small body surface areas; do not apply to broken or oozing skin; report new rashes at once
Second-Generation Antihistamines (Astemizole, Terfenadine)		
CARDIOVASCULAR Cardiac arrhythmias, potentially serious (astemizole, terfenadine)	Arrhythmias	May be triggered by exercise; monitor; do not exceed recommended dosages

Table 51–I **Major Interactions Between Histamine Antagonists and Other Agents**

AGENT	RESULT OF INTERACTION	COMMENTS AND NURSING IMPLICATIONS
Interactions Involving Virtually All H_1 Blockers		
CNS depressants: alcohol, barbiturates, benzodiazepines, Chapter 22); antipsychotics (Chapter 23); antidepressants (Chapter 24); centrally acting antiparkinson drugs (Chapter 25); centrally acting antihypertensives (Chapter 33)	Excessive, potentially serious CNS depression	Monitor accordingly when interactants have been prescribed; otherwise, teach patient to identify and avoid potential interactants, especially OTC medications and alcohol
Antimuscarinic (atropine-like) drugs, including antipsychotics, antidepressants, centrally acting antiparkinson drugs (See Table 13-2 for complete listing)	Risk of excessive or toxic antimuscarinic effects	See general guidelines for CNS depressants, above
Additional Interaction Involving Terfenadine, Possibly Astemizole		
Ketoconazole (Chapter 57)	Risk of serious cardiac arrhythmias, cardiotoxicity	Avoid interaction
Interactions Involving H_2 Blockers (eg, Cimetidine)		
	See Table 40–I, p 814	
Interactions Involving Cromolyn Sodium		
	None; See Chapter 38	
Interactions Involving Methysergide		
β-adrenergic blockers (eg, propranolol; Chapter 15)	Hypertension, potential stroke; peripheral tissue ischemia, tissue damage	Beta blockade leaves vasoconstrictor effects of methysergide unopposed; avoid interaction; combined use requires careful assessment of BP, heart rate; assess distal pulses, skin color, and temperature as indicator of reduced extremity blood flow; may need to reduce dose of one of the interactants or discontinue altogether; discontinue β-blocker slowly, with great care (see p 237)

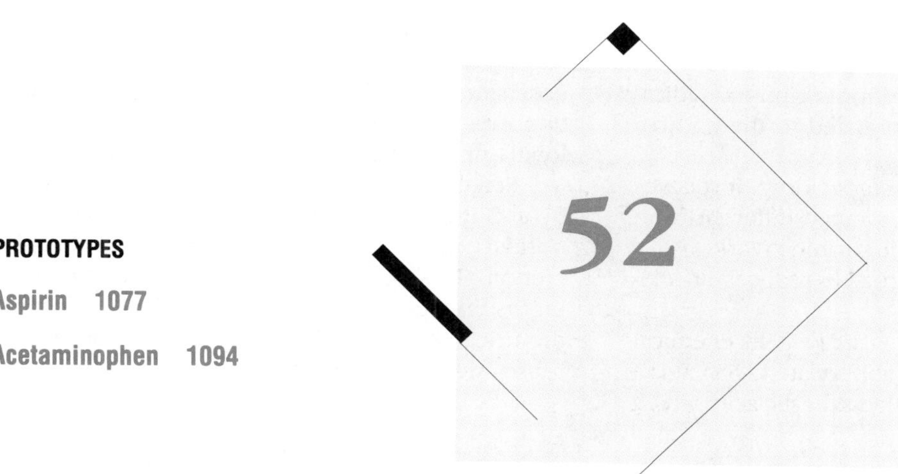

PROTOTYPES

Antiinflammatory and Analgesic/Antipyretic Drugs

Pain, inflammation, and fever are common symptoms of many ailments. Some or all of these symptoms can be relieved by inexpensive over-the-counter (OTC) drugs—aspirin, ibuprofen, and acetaminophen—or prescription drugs related to them. These drugs are the focus of this chapter.

The chapter considers not only the pharmacologic properties and clinical uses of these drugs and the groups to which they belong, but also issues related to the considerable confusion and misunderstanding the lay public has about them. The latter information is just as important as the former: it is often up to the nurse to help patients, friends, and family members make educated choices about buying these drugs and using them properly and safely. The chapter also gives insight into how to avoid, recognize, and help manage overdoses of these often misused OTC drugs.

Part I of the chapter focuses on aspirin—an inexpensive and old drug that is nevertheless still very effective, clinically useful, and potentially dangerous. Part II discusses other drugs, nearly all of which are prescription agents, that share many of aspirin's properties. In general, all the drugs discussed in Parts I and II modify disease symptoms, rather than the cause of the disease itself.

Part III focuses on other prescription drugs that are used mainly for arthritis. They differ from aspirin and its relatives in that they appear to modify the underlying pathology of arthritis, rather than merely masking signs and symptoms. Thus, they can be called disease-modifying antirheumatic drugs.

Part IV discusses acetaminophen. For years it was the only approved nonprescription aspirin substitute, and it is still a widely used and often misused OTC medication.

I. Nonsteroidal Antiinflammatory Drugs

PROTOTYPE

Aspirin

Aspirin can be classified in four main ways.

1. Aspirin is a *nonsteroidal antiinflammatory drug* (*NSAID*). It serves as the prototype of a very large

Major reference tables appear beginning on p. 1100.

group of prescription and nonprescription medications that are chemically unrelated to the corticosteroids.
2. Aspirin is a *nonnarcotic analgesic* drug. It relieves pain, but in a manner that is much different from that by which drugs such as morphine work.
3. Aspirin is an *antipyretic* drug. It reduces an elevated body temperature.
4. Aspirin is also classified as a *salicylate.* Its chemical name is acetylsalicylic acid (abbreviated ASA). It is a derivative of a substance called salicylic acid, which has few medical uses.

Absorption, Distribution, Metabolism, and Excretion

Characteristics of aspirin's absorption, distribution, and elimination are important for understanding how to administer the drug. They also help explain key concepts that relate to the drug's ability to interact with other medications, and to cause prolonged toxicity with overdoses.

Aspirin is almost always given orally. (It can be administered per rectum, but absorption through the rectal mucosa is unpredictable. An aspirin-like drug, sodium salicylate, can be given intravenously. That drug and administration route are also seldom used.) Aspirin is absorbed well from the gastrointestinal (GI) tract. In the normally acidic environment of the stomach, aspirin molecules are mainly in the nonionized (uncharged) form, so they are readily absorbed through the gastric mucosa and into the bloodstream. When gastric pH is raised (made less acidic), as by administering an antacid or "buffer," more of the aspirin molecules are converted to the ionized (charged) form. Ionized molecules are absorbed less well (see Chapter 4, p 52), so aspirin absorption is slowed. A large amount of aspirin is also absorbed across the large surface area of the intestines.

Aspirin is highly bound to plasma proteins (eg, albumin) as it is carried through the bloodstream. Aspirin binding to these proteins is strong, and the drug can easily displace other drugs that tend to bind to these proteins.

Aspirin's half-life is about 15 minutes when usual therapeutic doses are given. Aspirin is quickly converted to salicylate in the bloodstream; salicylate is then quickly excreted by the kidneys. When toxic doses of aspirin are taken, however, the body's ability to excrete salicylate is overwhelmed. Aspirin's half-life can be greatly prolonged, to as long as 20 hours, in such overdose situations. This variable, dose-dependent elimination rate is further addressed in the discussion of the longlasting toxicity associated with aspirin poisoning.

Renal salicylate excretion is increased dramatically by alkalinizing the urine. Increasing urine pH from a normal value of about 6 to about 8 quadruples excretion. This has considerable implications for treating aspirin poisoning, as discussed below. Acidifying the urine reduces salicylate excretion, but this seldom causes significant problems.

NURSING IMPLICATIONS

There are many different formulations and brands of oral aspirin. Most of them are more alike than different (see p 1086).

Pharmacologic Effects

Aspirin causes its major effects mainly by inhibiting an enzyme called *cyclooxygenase,* which plays a key role in the synthesis of *prostaglandins.* Prostaglandins are a family of very active chemicals derived from lipids in cell membranes, and they participate in a host of physiologic and pathophysiologic processes.

Two "regular strength" aspirin tablets (325 mg, or 5 grains, each), cause no *noticeable* effect in a normal individual. However, these doses of aspirin can cause clinically significant relief of pain, inflammation, and fever, plus other effects noted shortly. These effects involve suppression of symptoms and signs of some pathophysiologic process. In general, however, aspirin does not "cure" the underlying disease or pathology.

Analgesia

Aspirin relieves pain (an **analgesic** effect), but it is chemically and pharmacologically unrelated to morphine and other narcotics (Chapter 21), and is thus a nonnarcotic analgesic.

Aspirin works best to relieve mild-to-moderate musculoskeletal or neural pain. Aspirin acts on peripheral sensory nerves. It works by inhibiting the formation or reactivity of prostaglandins and kinins, which are the chemical stimuli of sensory nerves. Aspirin doses needed to relieve severe pain or visceral pain (eg, that following surgery of the internal organs) are usually toxic doses and usually not nearly as effective as a narcotic. Aspirin does not cause physical dependence, nor does it participate in cross-dependence with narcotics (Chapter 21, p 330).

Aspirin can relieve pain even when the pain is not caused by inflammation, as with a simple headache. However, when inflammation is also present, aspirin's ability to inhibit inflammation contributes to its overall pain-relieving effects.

Antiinflammatory Actions

Aspirin inhibits key parts of the inflammatory response that are mediated by prostaglandins. Overall, suppressed inflammation reduces swelling and redness and can restore relatively pain-free motion to an affected joint. The drug affects the mobility and activation of leukocytes, which are key players in the inflammatory response, in ways that are not fully understood. Other actions of aspirin on the inflammatory response also occur.

Antipyretic Actions

Aspirin lowers an elevated body temperature (an **antipyretic** effect). It crosses the blood–brain barrier and inhibits formation of fever-causing (pyrogenic) substances—prostaglandins, kinins, and others—that raise the hypothalamic "thermostat" during fever. Aspirin also promotes heat loss by dilating peripheral blood vessels, leading to diaphoresis. Aspirin does not affect typical causes of fever, such as bacteria and viruses. The drug will not lower normal body temperature. As noted later, toxic blood levels of aspirin can cause fever.

Antiplatelet Actions

Aspirin doses as low as 80 mg (one-fourth of a standard aspirin tablet) inhibit platelet aggregation—the ability of platelets to stick to one another. The antiplatelet effect is due to aspirin's ability to inhibit the synthesis of thromboxane A_2, a part of the prostaglandin synthesis pathway that causes platelets to aggregate. This effect is longlasting. Just one 325-mg aspirin tablet can double bleeding time for about a week, the typical lifetime of platelets. If aspirin therapy is stopped, normal platelet function will not return fully until the body can synthesize new, functional platelets.

The actions of aspirin on platelets can be clinically useful. It can also be unwanted, in other situations. See below, and Chapter 35 (p 717), for more information.

High doses of aspirin inhibit the synthesis of prostaglandin I_2 (PGI_2; also known as prostacyclin) in the endothelial cells. Prostaglandin I_2 normally keeps platelets from sticking to the normal, undamaged blood vessel lining. When its synthesis is inhibited, as by aspirin, platelets can stick abnormally on the endothelium, leading to obstructed blood flow.

Effects on Renal Uric Acid Excretion

Low doses of aspirin (1–2 g/day or less) decrease uric acid excretion by the kidneys. In contrast, doses of more than about 5 grams per day increase uric acid excretion; this is called a **uricosuric** effect. As discussed later, aspirin plays no role in the management of gout.

Clinical Indications and Administration

In most cases, plain, buffered, or enteric-coated aspirin can be used interchangeably for a variety of therapeutic purposes.

Symptomatic Relief of Mild Pain, Inflammation, or Fever

Aspirin is commonly used for its analgesic, antiinflammatory, and antipyretic effects. The usual recommended adult dose for managing mild pain, inflammation, or fever is 650 mg every four hours. The total daily dose should not exceed 4 grams unless treatment is supervised by a physician.

Aspirin products for pediatric use contain 80 mg of aspirin per unit dose and are taken every four hours. Pediatric doses are given in Table 52–1. Aspirin is a potentially dangerous drug for children. This is discussed further in the side effects section.

Arthritic Disorders

Aspirin is one of the oldest and most effective drugs for reducing pain and inflammation of arthritis due to causes other than gout. Antiarthritic doses can range anywhere from 4 to 10 grams per day. These dosages obviously are much higher than those indicated for relief of simple pain and fever, and they usually cause side effects. Such doses should be prescribed by a physician, who should also monitor the patient's therapy.

Prophylaxis of Recurrent Myocardial Infarction and Stroke

Aspirin's antiplatelet effects are useful for reducing the risk of death, nonfatal myocardial infarction, or both, in patients with a previous myocardial infarction or un-

TRENDS AND CONTROVERSIES IN PHARMACOLOGY

How Important Is the Fever Response?

The ability to raise body temperature is one characteristic of a well-functioning immune system. However, most people regard fever only as a dangerous symptom that necessitates a call or visit to their health care provider. Antipyretics are frequently prescribed, yet nurses should recognize such treatment may be directed toward reducing anxiety in patients, families, and caregivers; it "often lacks a compelling medical rationale" (Styrt and Sugarman, 1990).

Fever alone is not an indication for treatment. Most evidence indicates that temperatures in the usual range of fever may activate and strengthen host defenses. Many pathogens may be more susceptible at febrile body temperature, although prolonged, severe temperature elevations (above about 42°C) are clearly detrimental to effective host defenses.

Before the development of antibiotics, benefits of hyperthermia or "fever therapy" were reported in the treatment of infections, and syphilis was actually treated by the induction of malarial fevers. Current evaluation of the value of fever in the outcomes of infection has been difficult due to heterogeneity of disorders and the presence of concurrent antibiotic and antipyretic therapy. Interestingly, neonates and elderly individuals appear to exhibit smaller febrile responses and have less effective responses to infection than persons of intermediate ages—although this should not be interpreted as a cause-and-effect relationship. Existing information suggests that patients should, when possible, be permitted to use this important defense mechanism. Drugs that blunt the febrile responses should not be used routinely—but only after careful consideration (Cunha, 1985).

It is important to remember that the degree of fever does not reflect the severity of infection. Children are more likely than adults to run very high fevers, regardless of the underlying cause. And in cases of overwhelming sepsis, hypothermia—rather than hyperthermia—is often observed. A person's behavior may be a more accurate guide than body temperature to the severity of infection (Younger and Brown, 1985).

A real concern for many health care providers—and parents—is that a child with a high fever is likely to experience a seizure. It is generally agreed that the prevalence of seizures during febrile illness in children under the age of 5 years is only about 2–4%. Although high fevers in children do cause a low incidence of single, acute seizures—and some children do experience another—the episode almost never results in chronic seizures or any other permanent illness. High fevers are thought to be more likely to induce seizures. However, antipyretic therapy does not appear to prevent seizure recurrence, and studies have not addressed whether it will prevent the initial occurrence of seizures (Styrt and Sugarman, 1990). Fevers are not generally associated with neurological damage in adults.

While a fever itself does not necessarily require treatment, the associated discomfort may. Aspirin (although not when a viral illness is suspected in children), acetaminophen, ibuprofen, and other antipyretics may be useful as comfort measures. In some cases sponging with tepid water may be soothing, although it may not have a significant effect on body temperature. Alcohol sponging is not recommended because its rapid evaporation increases the risk of shivering, which in turn increases metabolism rate, temperature, and patient discomfort. For infants, nursing, rocking, holding, or singing can be comforting. Many adults find massage refreshing. Avoid problems that exacerbate fever, such as dehydration. Keep the feverish person well hydrated and dressed for comfort.

Cunha BA: Significance of fever in the compromised host. *Nurs Clin North Am* 1985; 20(1):163–169.

Styrt B, Sugarman B: Antipyresis and fever. *Arch Int Med* 1990; 150: 1589–1597.

Younger JB, Brown BS: Fever management: rational or ritual? *Pediatr Nurs* 1985;11(1): 26–29.

stable angina. Some physicians routinely administer an aspirin tablet early in the emergency management of patients with a suspected or known heart attack. The goal is to prevent further clotting that might further obstruct a coronary artery. Aspirin is also indicated for reducing the risk of stroke in high-risk males with a history of frequent transient ischemic attacks.

Prophylactic aspirin therapy for thrombotic disorders may be lifelong unless adverse responses occur (see p 717 for more information).

Table 52–1 Recommended Pediatric Analgesic-Antipyretic Dosages for Aspirin and Acetaminophen*

Age	Weight in lb (kg)	Aspirin† (mg)	Acetaminophen‡ (mg)
Up to 3 months	———	NR	40
4–11 months	———	NR	80
1–2 yr	———	NR	120
2–3 yr	24–35 (10.6–15.9)	162	160
4–5 yr	36–47 (16–21.4)	243	240
6–8 yr	48–59 (21.5–26.8)	324	320
9–10 yr	60–71 (26.9–32.3)	405	400
11 yr	72–95 (32.4–43.2)	486	480
12–14 yr	≥96 (≥43.3)	648	Adult dose
>14 yr	———	Adult dose	Adult dose

*Base dose on body weight when possible. If recommended doses fail to relieve pain after 5 days, or fever after 3 days, seek treatment from a physician.

†Give aspirin dose every four hours. Alternatively, use 10 to 15 mg/kg per dose every four hours, up to 60 to 80 mg/kg per 24 hours. Based on 81 mg per aspirin pediatric tablet. See Table 52–C1 for aspirin doses for juvenile rheumatoid arthritis.

‡May repeat acetaminophen dose four to five times daily (5 doses per 24 hours, maximum), or estimate as 10 mg/kg per dose.

NR Not recommended unless treatment is under advice and supervision of a physician.

NURSING IMPLICATIONS

Regardless of the reason for which aspirin is self-prescribed, it is important to stress the importance of following recommended doses and other instructions on the package label. Instruct patients to seek professional care if recommended doses, taken for three or four days in a row, fail to provide adequate relief or if symptoms worsen. See Aspirin Formulations (p 1086) for more tips and advice.

Side Effects, Adverse Reactions, and Contraindications

Aspirin causes many side effects, but the severity, frequency, and potential clinical importance vary from patient to patient. Table 52–2 compares aspirin's side effects with those caused by other selected NSAIDs.

Gastrointestinal Problems

Salicylates and virtually all other NSAIDs irritate the gastric mucosa. Many individuals who take aspirin experience no stomach upset, but others may experience intolerable nausea or GI pain and be unable to take the drug at all.

In all patients, usual doses of aspirin increase fecal occult blood loss by 2 to 6 mL per day. This added blood loss is inconsequential for most patients but may cause problems in patients with coagulation abnormalities, anemias, or periodic bleeding (eg, from menstruation or ulcers). The NSAIDs can inhibit healing of existing ulcers, and at high doses taken long-term they can cause ulcers. Thus, aspirin and the other NSAIDs are relatively contraindicated for persons with ulcers or a history of ulcer disease.

If aspirin (or other NSAID) therapy is necessary, prophylactic, adjunctive, antiulcer therapy is often recommended for high-risk patients. Giving antacids is one preventive approach, but the new gastric cytoprotective drug misoprostol (CYTOTEC) is gaining favor for this purpose (see Chapter 40, p 804).

Antiplatelet Effects

Aspirin's antiplatelet effects may be therapeutically useful for some patients. However, the very same effects may cause excessive or abnormal bleeding. Aspirin is absolutely or relatively contraindicated in patients with hemophilia, prothrombin or vitamin K deficiencies, severe liver disease (in whom clotting factor formation may be decreased), or anemias. Antiplatelet effects also increase the bleeding risk in persons with ulcers, regardless of the potential causes of the ulcers. To avoid unexpected or severe intraoperative or postoperative bleeding, advise patients not to take aspirin less than one week before elective surgery, if possible.

Hyperuricemia

Hyperuricemia—and, possibly, the development of acute gout—is another potential problem with aspirin use. This is particularly true with the relatively low doses listed on package labels—dosages that are likely to reduce uric acid excretion by the kidneys. Aspirin is generally contraindicated for persons with hyperuricemia or frank gout. Most other NSAIDs do *not* share aspirin's effect on uric acid levels and are therefore preferred alternatives for hyperuricemic patients.

Hypersensitivity Reactions

Aspirin may cause hypersensitivity reactions. The risk seems to be greatest in persons with a history of allergy-

Table 52–2 Approximate Frequency of Side Effects Produced by Selected Rapidly Acting NSAIDs (Antiarthritic Doses)

Drug	GI Distress (Dyspepsia)	GI Bleeding	Rash	Headache	Tinnitus	Other Effects
Placebo	++	–	–	+	–	Drowsiness, dizziness
Aspirin (plain)	++++	+*	++	+	++++	—
Fenoprofen	+++	+	++	++	–	—
Ibuprofen	+++	+*	+	+	–	Sodium, water retention
Indomethacin	++++*	+*	+	+++*	–	Blood dyscrasias, corneal changes
Naproxen	+	+*	+	++	–	—
Sulindac	++	+*	+	+	+	—
Tolmetin	+++	+*	+	–	–	—

Incidence code: –, rare
+, <5%
++, <10%
+++, <25%
++++, 25%–40%

*Can be a severe or potentially dangerous response

mediated asthma or recurrent urticaria. Some hypersensitive persons develop little more than wheezing; others experience severe respiratory symptoms, including intense bronchoconstriction and, possibly, anaphylaxis and death. (In asthmatics, bronchoconstriction occurs because aspirin inhibits the synthesis of a bronchodilator prostaglandin, PGE_2.) Other aspirin-hypersensitive patients mainly develop rashes or hives rather than bronchoconstriction, but they too may experience hypotension.

Just one aspirin tablet can trigger severe responses in some people. For them, all forms and doses of aspirin are contraindicated. Most other NSAIDs cause similar adverse responses in aspirin-hypersensitive patients (they cross-react), so those drugs are also contraindicated. The aspirin-like drugs choline salicylate, sodium salicylate, and salicylamide (see below) are less likely to cross-react, but they should be used cautiously; the potential risks are still present.

NURSING IMPLICATIONS

Patients who are at added risk of problems related to GI bleeding should have their stool checked periodically for occult and visible blood. Other tests, including blood tests, may be indicated. The appearance of black, tarry stools ("coffee-ground stools") is a good indicator of gastric bleeding, as it signals the presence of coagulated blood. Often the cause is the use of aspirin or a related NSAID.

If any check of the stool for occult blood shows increased levels, always inquire specifically about the use of aspirin or related NSAIDs. When taking a patient's medication history, ask explicit questions about the use of *any* OTC drugs.

◆ Use During Pregnancy and Lactation

Pregnant women should not take aspirin, or any other NSAID, unless specifically told to do so by, and can be followed by, a physician. Maternal aspirin use has been linked to low birth weight, intracranial hemorrhage in premature infants, stillbirths, and neonatal deaths.

The risks during the last three months of pregnancy may be especially significant. The NSAIDs can inhibit the contraction of uterine muscle, which is a process that is regulated in part by prostaglandins. The potential outcome is a delay or prolongation of labor. Aspirin's antiplatelet effects also increase the risks of maternal or neonatal bleeding at delivery, especially if a dose has been taken within a week of parturition.

In addition, prostaglandins help keep the fetal ductus arteriosus open before delivery. Inhibiting prostaglandin synthesis may cause premature closure of the ductus; the outcome can be lethal to the fetus. (The powerful NSAID indomethacin, discussed later, is used specifically for closing the ductus postpartum when it has failed to close spontaneously.)

Salicylates are excreted in breast milk, so breast-feeding is not recommended during long-term, high-dose (antiarthritic) aspirin therapy.

All the precautions noted above are correct and should be reinforced to pregnant women. However, new evidence from clinical studies indicates that giving 80 to 160 mg aspirin per day during the second and third trimesters significantly reduces maternal and neonatal morbidity and mortality associated with pregnancy-induced hypertension or preeclampsia. This is experimental therapy that should be supervised closely by a knowledgeable physician. (See Chapter 33, p 659, for information about the more traditional drugs that can be used for managing high blood pressure during pregnancy.)

◆ Use in Children

Aspirin should not be administered to children with febrile illness, chickenpox, influenza, or other known or possible viral infections, because of an increased incidence of Reye's syndrome. (Anyone less than or equal to the age of 16 years is considered at risk; some clinicians feel aspirin should be avoided up to age 21 years or so when these illnesses are present). Although rare, Reye's syndrome is a very serious condition characterized initially by vomiting and lethargy. It can progress to delirium and coma. About one-third of the affected patients die; some who survive are left with permanent neurologic impairments.

Aspirin use in children less than 2 years old should be supervised by a physician.

As noted later (p 1085), dehydrated children are more susceptible to aspirin toxicity.

◆ Use in the Elderly

Older adults are more likely to be taking medications that interact with aspirin; see below. Extra care is required.

Interactions with Other Drugs

The key interactants with aspirin include

- oral anticoagulants (eg, warfarin; may cause excessively prolonged prothrombin time, increased risk of bleeding);
- heparin, the prototype injectable anticoagulant (may cause excessive bleeding);
- streptokinase and other thrombolytic drugs (may cause excessive bleeding);
- oral hypoglycemic agents (may cause risk of hypoglycemia); and
- phenytoin (may cause increased CNS depression).

Most of these interactions arise because of aspirin's ability to displace the interactant from plasma protein binding sites, thereby increasing the drug's free (active) blood levels. When the interactant is another drug that affects some aspect of blood clotting processes—oral or injectable anticoagulants, or a thrombolytic drug—aspirin's antiplatelet effects add to the risk of excessive bleeding.

Changes of gut or urine pH may cause interactions. Ammonium chloride and other drugs (or foods) that acidify the urine interact to reduce renal aspirin excretion. This could increase the risk of aspirin toxicity. Sodium bicarbonate and other drugs that alkalinize the urine significantly increase salicylate excretion and could reduce aspirin's efficacy. (These interactants can be useful in managing aspirin overdoses, as noted below.)

Aspirin reduces the actions of the uricosuric drugs probenecid (BENEMID) and sulfinpyrazone (ANTURANE), which are used to treat hyperuricemia (Chapter 53, p 1116).

The gastric-irritating actions of all NSAIDs potentiate the similar effects caused by other ulcerogenic drugs, such as alcohol and corticosteroids.

Salicylates may antagonize the antiarthritic effects of other NSAIDs (see below). Thus, combined therapy usually should be avoided.

NURSING IMPLICATIONS

Just one aspirin tablet can cause serious interactions with some other drugs. It is important to instruct patients at risk to avoid aspirin altogether unless therapy is supervised by the physician, needed dosage adjustments can be made, and responses to the drugs can be monitored.

Aspirin and Alcohol

The combined use of aspirin and alcohol deserves special mention because aspirin is a common—and potentially dangerous—lay remedy for alcohol hangovers. Aspirin is one of the worst drugs for managing alcohol hangover, especially on a frequent basis. It may relieve a headache, but it adds to the gastric irritation that alcohol causes. Frequent alcohol and aspirin use or abuse may cause gastric bleeding, owing to the ulcerogenic effects of both agents. In addition, aspirin's antiplatelet effects inhibit the processes that otherwise would keep bleeding to a minimum. The aspirin-alcohol interaction is particularly dangerous for individuals who have a history of peptic ulcer disease and habitually abuse alcohol and aspirin.

Ibuprofen (further discussed below), the only other NSAID aspirin alternative available OTC, is no less risky than aspirin itself for persons who consume excessive amounts of alcohol. Acetaminophen (eg, TYLENOL), which is not an NSAID, is not much safer for alcohol abusers (see Part IV of this chapter).

Overdose and Toxicity

Aspirin overdoses can cause severe and sometimes fatal toxicity. The reasons for the frequency of aspirin toxicity are the same as those for many other OTC drugs: no prescription is needed to buy or use it; many people consider the drug to be safe and harmless; and many people persist in believing that if the correct dose works, increasing the dose considerably will make the drug work considerably better or faster.

Mild Toxicity

Mild aspirin intoxication is called *salicylism*. The syndrome often occurs with long-term use of antiarthritic doses of aspirin. Signs and symptoms of salicylism include several or all of the following:

- tinnitus (ringing or buzzing in the ears);
- headache;
- dizziness, drowsiness, or confusion;
- paresthesias;
- ventilatory stimulation; and
- GI distress.

There is no specific treatment for salicylism, other than reducing the aspirin dose or stopping treatment altogether. If blood salicylate levels are stable, the patient is experiencing the desired therapeutic effect (eg, inflammation relief), and there are no other problems, there may be no need to treat salicylism at all.

Salicylate Poisoning

The usual lethal dose of aspirin, taken at once, is from 5 to 8 grams for a small child, or from 10 to 30 grams for adults. Lower doses may cause toxicity if the patient is already ill.

Signs and Symptoms

Only laboratory tests can prove aspirin poisoning, but a skilled observer can recognize key signs and symptoms. *The most dangerous consequences are alterations of respiration; alterations in fluid, electrolyte, and acid–base balance; shock; and seizures from high fever.* The following discussion and Figure 52–1 highlight the sequence of signs and symptoms of salicylate poisoning in adults. Peculiarities of poisoning in children are noted later. Knowing what might happen and the sequence of changes to expect will help you greatly in assessing patients and anticipating and planning treatments.

Ventilatory Stimulation

Rising salicylate concentrations stimulate the brain's medullary respiratory center. Ventilatory rate increases much more than depth. These changes lower blood carbon dioxide concentration and increase pH. *Respiratory alkalosis* has developed.

Compensated Respiratory Alkalosis

The kidneys attempt to normalize blood pH by increasing bicarbonate excretion, which alkalinizes the urine and increases aspirin elimination. This results in a stage called *compensated respiratory alkalosis*. As bicarbonate is lost, sodium, potassium, and water are also lost. (Patients who take large doses of aspirin for arthritis and experience salicylism are in this stage. As long as aspirin intake does not increase markedly or suddenly, they may tolerate this stage quite well.)

Additional Peripheral and Central Effects

If blood salicylate levels continue to rise, blood gases and electrolytes become dangerously altered. Severe dehydration may occur because of water lost through expired air, the skin, and the urine. Vomiting and diarrhea worsen fluid and electrolyte loss, leading to hyponatremia, hypokalemia, and increased hematocrit. Oliguria and renal failure eventually develop. If the aspirin overdose is acute, the patient may appear excited, confused, or delirious at this time.

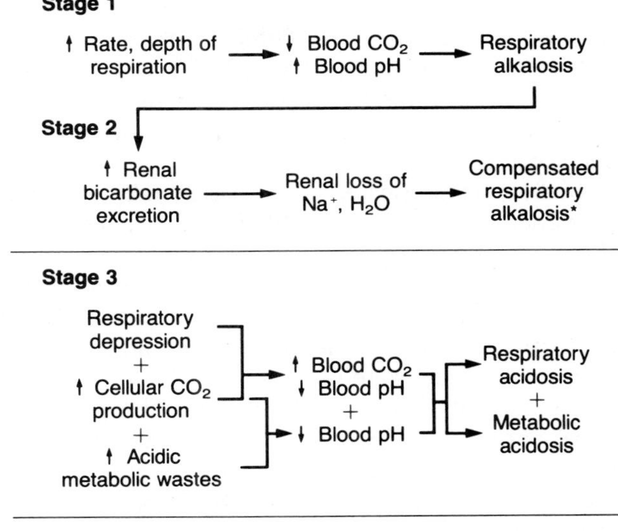

Figure 52–1

Patients pass through these "stages" of aspirin poisoning as blood salicylate levels rise. Severely ill children usually reach the emergency room in advanced stages. The changes of respiration, blood pH, and carbon dioxide (CO_2) levels provide the reason frequent laboratory tests and close patient monitoring are needed to treat the poisoned individual properly.

Respiratory Depression Plus Respiratory and Metabolic Acidosis

As more aspirin and its metabolites enter the brain, the respiratory center becomes depressed, and blood carbon dioxide levels rise. *Respiratory acidosis* has developed. High salicylate levels stimulate inefficient cell matabolism, increasing oxygen consumption and the production of carbon dioxide and lactic acid by the body cells. The outpouring of lactic acid and other acidic metabolites, combined with high levels of acidic aspirin metabolites, causes *metabolic acidosis.*

Stimulated cell metabolism also elevates body temperature, often to 104°F or more. The combination of respiratory and metabolic acidosis causes blood pH to fall dramatically, and the patient's condition quickly worsens.

Final Stages

The patient becomes comatose as acid–base and ventilatory status continue to worsen. The electroencephalogram becomes abnormal, and seizures follow. Death may occur from respiratory arrest during seizures or because of hypotension and cardiovascular collapse. A combination of aspirin-induced gastric erosion and inhibited platelet function may cause hemorrhage, another potential cause of death.

Treatment

No physician's office or clinic has the facilities for proper diagnosis of salicylate poisoning, let alone those needed for proper treatment. Do not waste time with a "wait-and-see" approach. Get the patient to a hospital emergency department as quickly as possible, even if an overdose is only suspected.

There are three key parts to the management of aspirin poisoning:

1. Prevent further systemic absorption of any drug left in the stomach.
2. Hasten the elimination of absorbed salicylate.
3. Provide symptomatic, supportive treatment.

There is no antidote for aspirin poisoning. Inducing emesis, lavaging the gastric contents, and administering activated charcoal are the main initial measures to reduce further absorption of the drug from the gut. Syrup of ipecac, an emetic (Chapter 42), can and should be used at home as an initial first-aid measure—provided that the patient is conscious and has intact gag reflexes. (See Appendix C for more information on the management of poisoning emergencies.)

Correcting blood gases, fluid, and electrolytes and lowering body temperature may be necessary. Doing these procedures depends, of course, on the availability of facilities and personnel for measuring blood gases and electrolytes, detecting fluid loss or dehydration, and following up on laboratory test results and vital signs. To prevent febrile seizures, reduce an elevated temperature by sponging the patient with lukewarm water or using a hypothermia blanket. *Never give an antipyretic drug to lower a fever in an aspirin-poisoned patient.*

Initially, establish venous access for all patients, if only as a precautionary measure. Often this serves as the route for administering fluids and electrolytes to correct abnormalities. The composition of the intravenous (IV) fluid is chosen to correct serum electrolytes (sodium and potassium in particular) and pH. Treatment should be guided by blood tests, which will continue to be useful in modifying therapy as the patient's condition changes.

Sodium bicarbonate, given parenterally, can be very beneficial. By increasing blood pH, it helps redistribute salicylate from the brain into the bloodstream; simultaneously, it helps correct the metabolic and respiratory acidosis that occurs with severe aspirin poisoning. In addition, it alkalinizes the urine and thereby increases salicylate excretion.

Mannitol, the osmotic diuretic, may be given to "force" diuresis. The diuretic acetazolamide (DIAMOX) may help increase salicylate excretion because it alkalinizes the urine, especially when bicarbonate is also given. (These diuretics are discussed in Chapter 32, pp 619–622.)

Intravenous fluids—possibly in large amounts—may be needed to correct dehydration, normalize hematocrit, maintain blood pressure, and prevent renal failure. The composition of the fluid should be adjusted to help correct electrolyte and acid–base problems as well as those that involve dehydration.

If hemorrhage occurs, vitamin K, platelets, or whole blood should be given. In severe poisoning, peritoneal dialysis, hemodialysis, or exchange transfusion may be needed.

Oxygen should be administered routinely, and mechanical ventilation should be used as needed. *Barbiturates, diazepam, or opiates should not be used to manage stimulated ventilation or central nervous system (CNS) function.* If the aspirin dose was actually low, ventilatory stimulation may be self-limiting, and drug therapy unnecessary. However, if a high dose was taken, depressant drugs such as these will suppress respiration and cortical function even further. In addition, their CNS depressant effects can obscure important diagnostic signs. However, diazepam *should* be administered if seizures occur.

Stimulants (eg, methylphenidate, amphetamines, aminophylline) should *not* be used to manage respiratory or CNS depression. These drugs increase the risk or severity of seizures.

Aspirin Poisoning in Children

Adults who have taken a toxic dose of aspirin may arrive at the emergency room with any of the above stages predominating. However, children are very sensitive to salicylates. They tend to pass quickly through the early stages and reach the hospital with advanced poisoning that is much more difficult to treat. The following scenario shows what can happen.

Assume a child has a serious *bacterial* illness for which aspirin might initially be indicated. The infection causes fever, aches and pains, GI upset, and the anorexia that often accompanies such an illness. Aspirin is given. It may alleviate some of the symptoms, but because the drug has no antibacterial action, the infection grows worse. The child may lose fluids owing to aspirin's diaphoretic effect, and the illness may trigger vomiting or diarrhea, which adds to fluid and electrolyte loss and imbalance. Because of the illness, the child ingests less fluids and nutrients, adding to the current problems. More aspirin is given, the child becomes worse, more aspirin is given, and so on.

By the time the child gets proper medical attention, the child may be suffering from a severe illness and fever and fluid and electrolyte imbalances owing to the combined effects of the illness and aspirin toxicity. Successful treatment may be very difficult.

NURSING IMPLICATIONS

Good preventive teaching includes stressing to parents or other responsible adults the need to control aspirin use and its accessibility to children. The risk of a serious overdose can be minimized by keeping only small amounts of aspirin, properly locked away, in the home. Urge parents or guardians to seek professional health care if a child does not improve after a few days of treatment with recommended doses of aspirin.

Oral Aspirin Formulations

There are many brand-name aspirin products and many different aspirin formulations. Some are advertised as having some definite significant advantage over a competing brand or formulation. All the alternatives cost more than the "plain generic" aspirin tablet. Before you read the following sections, it is important to understand that when plain aspirin is contraindicated for the patient—whether because of diseases such as peptic ulcer disease or asthma, or because of the use of an interacting drug—the other products usually are contraindicated too.

Generic or Store-Brand Aspirin versus Brand-Name Products

The major difference between brand-name and generic aspirin products is cost.

Half-Strength and Extra Strength Aspirins

Some products, such as HALFPRIN, contain only 165 mg aspirin. These have been used for pediatric administration and in adults for indications such as antiplatelet effects, for which a full 325-mg dose is not needed.

Other aspirin products contain anywhere from 500 to 975 mg per tablet. These may offer some convenience to the patient, especially those for whom high doses of aspirin are prescribed. For example, they can take one 975-mg tablet instead of three 325-mg dosages. However, there is the potential risk of an accidental overdose unless the patient reads the label carefully or is otherwise aware of the difference in the amount of drug per tablet. Many of these products are called "extra strength," "maximum strength," or such; some are labeled "arthritis strength." Still other products are labeled simply "aspirin" yet contain significantly more drug than other aspirin products. Nevertheless, the user may not know that the amount of drug is the only difference between these products and standard aspirin.

Buffered and Effervescent Aspirin

The buffers in buffered aspirin products are one or more antacids. These products are formulated as tablets (eg, BUFFERIN), which must be swallowed whole, or in effervescent tablets (eg, ALKA-SELTZER WITH ASPIRIN), which must be dissolved in water first.

The antacid may reduce the incidence or severity of GI distress for patients who experience these problems in response to plain aspirin—especially if the upset is mild. For persons who experience no GI upset with plain aspirin, adding buffers does little more than increase cost. The presence of a buffer does not make these products safe for persons with peptic ulcer disease or any other disease or drug therapy that would contraindicate plain aspirin itself. The buffer may increase the dissolution of the aspirin tablet (certainly true with effervescent tablets) and may increase the drug's absorption rate. However, the effect is rarely clinically important.

Effervescent aspirins contain sodium bicarbonate. Depending on the number of tablets taken and the duration of administration, enough bicarbonate can be absorbed to cause metabolic alkalosis. The sodium load can cause significant problems for persons who must restrict their sodium intake, such as those with heart failure, edema, or hypertension.

The use of buffered or enteric-coated aspirin should not be condemned if the patient or physician feels that it causes less GI distress. These formulations may even be preferred for high-dose or chronic therapy.

Enteric-Coated Aspirin

Some aspirin products (eg, ECOTRIN, plus other brand-name and generic products) are enteric-coated tablets. The coating does not dissolve in the acidic environment of the stomach, thereby protecting the gastric mucosa from the aspirin underneath. The coating dissolves in the duodenum, and the aspirin is absorbed from the intestines. Like buffered aspirins, enteric-coated aspirins seem to reduce gastric distress. Some physicians specifically recommend them for patients who will be taking large doses of aspirin on a long-term basis, as for arthritis. This may be a wise choice. However, the coating is probably unimportant for persons who experience no GI distress and who consume small amounts of aspirin infrequently.

Timed-Release Aspirin

Timed-release aspirin products reduce the frequency with which each dose must be administered. Typically, these products are administered every eight hours. Some are available OTC; some require a prescription. Overall, however, these formulations are no better, clinically, than other aspirin formulations.

Chewable Aspirin

The chewable formulations are aspirin gum (eg, ASPERGUM) and chewable tablets (eg, BAYER CHILDREN'S ASPIRIN). At comparable dosages, these formulations are no more effective or safe than nonchewable aspirin products. Some persons feel that these products are best for managing a sore throat, because the salivary juices that contain the drug bathe the throat. There is no good evidence to support this belief; to alleviate the pain, the drug must be swallowed, absorbed, and distributed to sites of action. There is also some evidence that contact between the drug and the mucosal surfaces in the throat can add to the irritation.

NURSING IMPLICATIONS

For the majority of situations in which aspirin is to be taken at regular intervals and plain aspirin is not contraindicated, the advertised differences are not clinically significant; virtually any aspirin product works just as well as any other. Cheaper is generally better, because the only major difference is cost.

Combinations of Aspirin with Other Drugs

Several OTC and prescription products contain aspirin plus other analgesics or antipyretics, but an important question is whether they are more effective than single ingredient products. There is good evidence that aspirin potentiates the analgesic actions of codeine and other codeine-like narcotics, and some conflicting evidence that caffeine (as in ANACIN) increases aspirin's analgesic actions. Otherwise, there is no definite advantage to combining aspirin with other drugs such as acetaminophen or with other salicylates (see below). All the combination products are more expensive than plain aspirin.

Related Salicylates

Other Salicylates for Internal Use

Several other salicylates are available, some in OTC medications marketed for relief of mild pain or fever. They can be compared with aspirin in the following general ways:

- None is more effective than plain aspirin for relief of pain, inflammation, or fever.
- Most produce fewer mild adverse GI side effects than aspirin, but they are nevertheless generally contraindicated in ulcer patients.
- Some are somewhat less likely to cause bronchoconstriction in asthmatic patients, but they should be administered with great care, if at all, to such persons.
- Some salicylates inhibit platelet aggregation less than aspirin, but they cannot be substituted for aspirin for desired antiplatelet effects.
- All the alternatives can cause aspirin-like toxicity and drug–drug interactions, including interactions with oral anticoagulants.
- Most are *not* indicated for pediatric use.
- They are more expensive than plain aspirin.

Choline, Magnesium, and Potassium Salicylate

Choline salicylate (ARTHROPAN) or potassium salicylate (an ingredient in PABALATE-SF) can be used instead of aspirin for pain and inflammation. They cause less of a sodium load than sodium salicylate.

Magnesium salicylate (eg, MAGAN) is indicated for the management of arthritis, bursitis, and other musculoskeletal disorders. It should not be taken by patients with renal disease because of the increased risk of magnesium intoxication.

Salicylamide

This drug, used for relief of minor pain, is available OTC. It is said to have some sedative properties; for this reason, it is found in some sleep aids. However, the salicylamide doses in these products are probably subtherapeutic in terms of hypnotic effects.

Salsalate

Salsalate (DISALCID; salicylsalicylic acid) is indicated for symptomatic relief of rheumatoid arthritis, osteoarthritis, and related disorders. It is a prescription drug. It seems to cause less bronchoconstriction in patients who are hypersensitive to aspirin.

Sodium Salicylate

Sodium salicylate (eg, PABALATE) is also OTC analgesic. It is less effective than an equal dose of aspirin for relieving pain or fever. High doses may cause hypernatremia or other problems for patients with hypertension or heart failure. One advantage of sodium salicylate for some patients is that it does not inhibit platelet aggregation.

Salicylates for Topical Use

Two other salicylates, salicylic acid and methyl salicylate, differ markedly from aspirin in terms of uses and toxicities. They are administered topically, on relatively small areas of intact skin. They should never be taken internally or applied to sites other than intact skin.

Salicylic Acid

Salicylic acid is a **keratolytic** (skin-eroding) agent used to dissolve corns, calluses, and warts. It should not be applied to large areas of the skin, because some drug can be absorbed. Ingestion of salicylic acid can cause serious erosive mucosal damage in mouth, esophagus, and gut. Adverse systemic effects from internal use are much less a concern than the mucosal damaging effects.

Methyl Salicylate

Methyl salicylate (oil of wintergreen) is an ingredient in several topical OTC medications advertised to relieve minor muscle and joint aches and pains. When applied to the skin, these medications cause a feeling of warmth or slight burning that obscures the pain and discomfort caused by the underlying condition. This is called a **counterirritant** effect. These drugs also cause local vasodilation, which may provide some relief. True irritation or tissue damage can occur when excessive amounts of methyl salicylate are applied to the skin (especially broken or abraded skin) or to mucosal surfaces.

Systemic effects can result from percutaneous absorption if excessive amounts of medicines containing methyl salicylate are applied to the skin. However, the most serious danger is due to ingestion of one of these products or to ingestion of methyl salicylate itself. (Methyl salicylate can be bought, in its pure form, in some pharmacies. It is used as a flavoring for candies and as an air freshener.) Less than a teaspoon of pure methyl salicylate (which can be purchased without a prescription) can kill a child. Methyl salicylate poisoning is relatively easy to diagnose, owing to the characteristic wintergreen breath odor.

NURSING IMPLICATIONS

Never apply dressings, especially occlusive dressings, over sites where medications containing methyl salicylate have been applied. Serious skin burns, which have in some cases necessitated skin grafting or even limb amputation, have occurred when this warning was not given or followed. Similarly, instruct patients who use these products to avoid contact between the application site and warm or (especially) hot water (as from a bath or shower) for a day or so. Such contact can also cause burns.

Methyl salicylate, especially in its pure form, smells like candy. Children, mistaking it for candy, may ingest this poison. Advise people who purchase methyl salicylate and have children in the house to keep it out of the child's reach. Better yet, advise them to discard any unused product.

Bismuth Subsalicylate

Bismuth subsalicylate is the active ingredient in PEPTO-BISMOL, a well-known remedy for nausea, diarrhea, and other common GI maladies. It works locally, in the gut, but some of the drug can be absorbed. Bismuth subsalicylate is not indicated for any of the systemic or topical uses noted for aspirin or the other salicylates. It is mentioned here only to note that patients who are at risk from adverse effects of aspirin can experience the same adverse effects to this medication. With the exception of peptic ulcer disease (see Chapter 40, p 806, for more information), bismuth subsalicylate is contraindicated in all the situations for which aspirin is contraindicated. Bismuth subsalicylate can also cause all the drug interactions mentioned for aspirin.

II. Other Rapidly Acting Nonsteroidal Antiinflammatory Drugs

Therapy for arthritic disorders may start with aspirin or another salicylate, but other NSAIDs may be used instead. Quite often, one of these alternatives will be used instead of aspirin. These agents are called rapidly acting NSAIDs because their effects appear promptly—usually as fast as the effects of aspirin, and much faster than the other drugs, such as gold salts, discussed on p 1092. These other NSAIDs are *not* salicylates. However, they share many of the side effects, contraindications, and drug–drug interactions noted for aspirin and other salicylates. They belong to different chemical classes, but all act by inhibiting prostaglandin synthesis.

What follows is a general overview of the NSAIDs that are not salicylates. Additional features of selected agents are highlighted thereafter.

Indications

Nearly all the NSAIDs are indicated for managing rheumatoid arthritis and osteoarthritis. Only a few are appropriate for treating juvenile arthritic conditions, however. Some are also indicated for treating bursitis, ankylosing spondylitis, or mild-to-moderate pain or inflammation from other causes. A few of these drugs are indicated for treating gout, which should not be treated with aspirin. (Another drug that can be classified as an NSAID is colchicine. However, colchicine is used only for gout. Because of that limited use, colchicine is discussed separately in Chapter 53, which deals exclusively with gout and its treatment.)

These alternative NSAIDs differ in terms of equally effective doses (ie, potencies) and recommended administration schedules. The approved uses and dosages for these drugs are summarized in Table 52–C1. All these drugs are given orally for their antiinflammatory actions. Two drugs, indomethacin and ketorolac, are available in injectable dosage forms. These formulations have special uses, which are discussed separately in short sections devoted to each drug.

All the alternatives that share aspirin's indications for inflammatory disorders are more expensive than plain aspirin—some much more expensive when equivalent doses are compared. However, many of them need to be given only once or twice daily; this simple administration schedule can improve compliance, which could be especially important—some arthritis patients may need to take 30 or so aspirin tablets throughout the day, each day.

None of these drugs should be prescribed for simple headache, mild musculoskeletal pain, or other situations (eg, tennis elbow) in which aspirin, nonprescription strength ibuprofen, or acetaminophen would suffice.

Side Effects, Contraindications, and Drug Interactions

All the NSAIDs typically cause less mild GI distress than aspirin. For most of these drugs, GI side effects (nausea, vomiting, pain, etc) are the most common. The incidence and severity of the GI responses to the other NSAIDs may be somewhat lower than those to aspirin. Nevertheless, *all* these drugs are ulcerogenic and therefore share the related contraindication—peptic ulcer disease—noted for aspirin.

Other side effects also differ in intensity from those caused by aspirin (see Table 52–2), but they are generally of the same type. Some of the NSAIDs, such as indomethacin (INDOCIN), share aspirin's antiplatelet effects but do not share aspirin's use as an antiplatelet drug. Most of these drugs do not significantly increase serum uric acid levels; therefore, for persons with gout or hyperuricemia, they are suitable alternatives to aspirin. Otherwise, they share identical relative and absolute contraindications, including the dangers for persons with asthma. Most of the other NSAIDs participate in virtually the same drug–drug interactions noted for aspirin—including potentially serious interactions with anticoagulants. Some of the alternative NSAIDs cause interactions that are not caused by aspirin (see Table 52–11).

Selected Nonsteroidal Antiinflammatory Drugs

Ibuprofen

Ibuprofen is the only prescription NSAID currently available in an OTC formulation also. Prescription strength ibuprofen (MOTRIN, RUFEN) comes in unit doses of 300 to 800 mg. Nonprescription ibuprofen (sold as ADVIL, HALTRAN, MIDOL 200, NUPRIN, many others, and generics) comes in 200-mg unit doses. Pediatric oral suspensions (eg, CHILDREN'S ADVIL; PEDIAPROFEN), currently available only by prescription, contain 100 mg per 5 mL. Ibuprofen does not increase the risk of Reye's syndrome. In routine use for fever, inflammation, or pain, ibuprofen may be no more efficacious than aspirin; however, ibuprofen does appear to be superior for relieving discomfort of primary dysmenorrhea.

Side effects (other than hyperuricemia), contraindications, and drug interactions should be considered equivalent to those for aspirin, and at-risk patients should be made aware of this. High-dose ibuprofen therapy may cause sodium and water retention, so the drug should be used cautiously in patients with hypertension or cardiac disease. With chronic, high-dose use, there is a risk of serious nephropathy. The magnitude of this renal damage and the attention given to it by health professionals are growing as the use (and misuse) of ibuprofen by the lay public increases.

NURSING IMPLICATIONS

The confusion among the lay public about generic and brand-name aspirin products also applies to ibuprofen. (Indeed, even some health care professionals are ill-informed about ibuprofen products.) All the current OTC ibuprofen products contain exactly the same amount of the same active drug. Nothing is different, other than the packaging, the color of the coating on the tablet or capsule, and cost. Ibuprofen products advertised for managing menstrual discomfort, for example, are no more or less effective (or safer) for that or other conditions than other generic or brand-name OTC ibuprofen products. In addition, the same number of milligrams of OTC ibuprofen is no different from the same dose of a prescription product. Once again, if the drug is not contraindicated, buying the least expensive ibuprofen product is the wisest choice.

Indomethacin

Indomethacin (INDOCIN) is one of the most powerful inhibitors of prostaglandin synthesis, and one of the most powerful and effective NSAIDs. For all practical purposes, all the side effects and drug interactions noted for aspirin apply to indomethacin. Compared to aspirin, however, indomethacin tends to cause more frequent and severe headache. Moreover, long-term use may cause cloudiness of the cornea of the eye, leading to visual impairments.

A parenteral dosage form of indomethacin, given IV, is indicated only for closing a patent (open) ductus arteriosus in newborns. Oral indomethacin is sometimes the chosen starting NSAID for arthritic conditions in which full doses of aspirin are ineffective or are not tolerated well by the patient. It is often preferred to colchicine (see Chapter 53, pp 1113–1115) for treating acute gout and for gout prophylaxis. There are two main oral dosage formulations of indomethacin: an immediate-acting dosage form (the "standard" formulation, much like that used for the other NSAIDs) and a sustained-release form. Antiinflammatory therapy should start only with the immediate-acting dosage form, because the slow-release products are absorbed more slowly; that is, they take longer to reach effective blood levels. However, once symptoms are controlled well with the faster-acting formulation, some patients can switch to proper dosages of a low-release product for maintenance therapy.

NURSING IMPLICATIONS

Patients on maintenance therapy with a sustained-release antiinflammatory drug such as indomethacin should have a supply of the immediate-acting dosage form on hand to use for symptom flare-ups. Consult with the physician about this, and provide instructions for appropriate use to patients for whom both formulations are prescribed.

Ketorolac Tromethamine

Ketorolac tromethamine, marketed as TORADOL, is unique in several ways. It is an NSAID, but it is indicated only for managing pain. Ketorolac is the first and so far the only NSAID approved in the United States for short-term parenteral (intramuscular [IM]) use. An oral dosage form is also available.

Ketorolac's analgesic efficacy, based on several studies on patients with moderate-to-severe pain, is at least equivalent to that afforded by usual IM doses of morphine or meperidine. No other NSAID appears to be as potent for pain in that regard. Analgesia caused by ketorolac appears to last longer than that caused by narcotics such as morphine, but ketorolac's onset of action is somewhat slower. In addition, ketorolac controls pain without the CNS or respiratory depression caused by narcotics. Side effects and drug interactions appear to be similar to those expected with short-term use of other NSAIDs.

Since ketorolac is not approved for uses other than pain control, it is not a substitute for other NSAIDs when the primary goal is to suppress inflammation, for example.

NURSING IMPLICATIONS

Do not administer parenteral ketorolac for more than five days straight. The oral dosage form is indicated for "limited use," but the actual duration of therapy is not specified.

Phenylbutazones

Phenylbutazone and a very similar drug, oxyphenbutazone, are NSAIDs that are being withdrawn from use in the United States because of their ability to interact with many drugs and to cause serious and sometimes fatal effects on blood cell formation, the liver, and the kidneys. These drugs are still available in some countries, where they are used mainly for severe, refractory arthritic conditions and acute gout. If your patient is receiving phenylbutazone or oxyphenbutazone, review the package insert, and consult with a knowledgeable pharmacist.

III. Slow-Acting/Disease-Modifying Antirheumatic Drugs

For many years, the most common general therapy plan for arthritis was one called the "pyramid approach." The base of the pyramid involved rest, exercise, physical therapy, and the use of aspirin or other NSAIDs. These foundations were not necessarily effective all the time, and they relieved only symptoms, not the underlying disease. However, these measures often worked well and tended to cause relatively little harm, in comparison with other drugs, to the patient.

The tip of the pyramid—the drug therapies usually implemented late or last—consisted of the *slow-acting antirheumatic drugs* (*SAARD*s). These drugs are so named because their onsets of action develop slowly, often after several months of continued treatment. Specific examples of SAARDs are the gold salts, hydroxychloroquine, and penicillamine. There is no overall prototype.

There were two main reasons, or beliefs, for using the slow-acting drugs only when NSAIDs did not work or could not be tolerated by the patients:

- *A slow onset of action.* This was a disadvantage for patients seeking a prompt return of function, symptom relief, and an overall improvement in their quality; and it made for a long wait by caregivers wanting to assess the progress of treatment.

- *Toxicities that were considered to be relatively serious and were sometimes fatal.* Detecting these toxicities required frequent evaluation, including laboratory tests (and tissue biopsies) that were expensive, time-consuming, and sometimes stressful to the patient. Also, many of the toxic reactions to these slow-acting drugs tended to develop slowly and be cumulative (with repeated dosing), longlasting, and quite serious. Without proper testing, the reactions could not be detected early enough. In short, there was concern that, for some patients, these drugs could do more harm than good.

Prescribing practices for rheumatoid arthritis, as well as the overall view of the pyramid approach or philosophy, are changing somewhat for four main reasons:

- Based on hard data, the toxicities of some of these drugs may be no more frequent or severe than those caused by high doses of some NSAIDs—the traditional first-line antiarthritic agents.
- Knowledge about how to monitor therapy has increased, especially with regard to assessing for adverse effects so that they can be halted or reversed.
- There is a growing appreciation that arthritis is more than a collection of pathophysiologic changes, annoying symptoms, and reduced life quality. In its advanced stages, the disorder can cause significant morbidity and mortality. More aggressive treatment may be needed for many patients.
- More importantly, the slow-acting rheumatic agents appear to stop (or even reverse) the underlying pathophysiology of arthritis, not just alleviate signs and symptoms. Thus, a newer and perhaps more descriptive name for these agents is *disease-modifying antirheumatic drugs—DMARDs.*

As a result, for many patients the SAARDs or DMARDs are now used much earlier, and more aggressively, in the therapy of rheumatoid arthritis. Nevertheless, these agents should be prescribed and supervised only by a physician who is very familiar with their actions and toxicities and who can provide the necessary monitoring.

In general, treatment should start with low drug dosages, built up gradually to recommended maintenance doses based on the patient's desired responses and the potential for unwanted responses. None of these drugs should be given to pregnant women or those who wish to breast-feed their infants.

What follows is a brief description of the traditional DMARDs: the gold salts, hydroxychloroquine, and penicillamine. Toxicities unique to each group are identified.

Gold Salts

Gold salts stop or partially reverse joint destruction in about 60% of patients taking recommended doses. The exact ways by which gold salts work are not known for sure. The injectable drugs are gold sodium thiomalate (MYOCHRYSINE) and aurothioglucose (SOLGANAL).

Another gold salt, auranofin (RIDAURA), is given orally. Auranofin is often tried first because of its convenient and acceptable administration route; because the risks of acute toxic reactions (see below) are much lower than those with injectable gold; and because maintenance dosages can sometimes be used to start treatment. Therapy usually is started and then maintained with a maximum daily dose of 6 mg. If improvement does not occur after six months of treatment, a three-month trial of 9 mg per day can be given. The drug should be discontinued if there is still no improvement.

Patients may be started on parenteral gold and then switched to auranofin. There are no pediatric doses for auranofin.

Diarrhea (potentially severe) occurs in about 40% of patients taking oral gold. It is the most common side effect of auranofin and may be alleviated by reducing the dose. Diarrhea is less common and severe with parenteral gold. *All* gold salts can cause longlasting, painful, pruritic skin rashes and oral lesions (stomatitis), but they are more common with parenteral therapy.

The injectable gold salts may cause an acute reaction, a *nitritoid crisis,* so called because it resembles the effects of a large dose of nitroglycerin. Nitritoid crisis is characterized by flushing, a feeling of warmth and lightheadedness, and possibly profound hypotension. Thus, parenteral gold therapy must begin with a small test dose to assess for this response. If the initial low doses are tolerated (and blood tests are normal), treatment continues with a series of weekly to monthly injections until a cumulative (total) dose of 1 gram has been given. Signs of improvement should appear after a cumulative dose of about 0.5 gram (six to 10 weeks). About two-thirds of patients show improvement after receiving a total of 1 gram. Therapy must be stopped at once if there is any indication of blood dyscrasias or renal dysfunction.

The most serious adverse effect of *any* gold salt is fatal bone marrow suppression. Pretreatment blood tests are essential before therapy starts, and they should be performed before giving each subsequent dose. Evidence of bone marrow suppression contraindicates therapy (initial or continued) with these drugs. Renal damage may also occur.

All gold salts are contraindicated in patients with renal or hepatic disease; a history of infectious hepatitis or hematologic disorders; or uncontrolled and severe diabetes, heart failure, or hypertension. Gold salts should not be used with radiation therapy or with any drug that is liable to cause blood dyscrasias—including all other DMARDs.

Overdoses of any gold salt can exaggerate the hematologic effects noted above and cause renal damage. The heavy metal chelator dimercaprol (British Anti-Lewisite, or BAL for short) can be used adjunctively to treat acute overdoses. Otherwise, management is symptomatic and supportive.

NURSING IMPLICATIONS

Assess all patients receiving any slow-acting antirheumatic drug for evidence of bone marrow depression before therapy is started and periodically thereafter. Be aware that none of these drugs are indicated for pregnant women, and the drugs should be administered to women of childbearing age only with emphatic instructions to report pregnancy at once. Advise all patients not to expect symptomatic relief (such as decreased morning stiffness) for a month or so after treatment starts.

Inject gold salts into the gluteus, with the patient lying down and remaining in the recumbent position for at least 10 minutes after injection. Use proper technique to avoid accidental IV injection. Assess for evidence of the nitritoid crisis, and measure blood pressure frequently during this time.

Advise patients taking auranofin to *expect* diarrhea during early therapy, even if they are switched from parenteral therapy to this drug.

Assess periodically for evidence of renal and hepatic dysfunction. All patients should be monitored for excessive diarrhea and resulting fluid and electrolyte imbalances and for rashes or stomatitis, regardless of which gold salt is used.

Hydroxychloroquine Sulfate

Hydroxychloroquine (PLAQUENIL) has been used for years as an antimalarial drug. It is also indicated for severe acute or chronic rheumatoid arthritis and for some forms of systemic lupus erythematosus. Most arthritis patients start to get some symptom relief after one to three months of therapy.

Hydroxychloroquine's major toxicity is dose-dependent ocular damage, including retinal pigmentation or retinopathy, corneal deposits, alterations of the ciliary body, and an overall loss of visual acuity. Some of these toxicities may be irreversible, so hydroxychloroquine therapy should be stopped at the first sign of them. However, ocular damage may progress even after hydroxychloroquine therapy is stopped.

Other adverse responses include dermatologic reactions, blood dyscrasias, and GI distress. Hydroxychloroquine increases digoxin serum levels and may increase the risk of digoxin toxicity.

NURSING IMPLICATIONS

Administer hydroxychloroquine with meals or a glass of milk to reduce GI upset. Stress the need for periodic and comprehensive ophthalmic evaluation before hydroxychloroquine therapy is started and every three months during treatment. Other NSAIDs or corticosteroids may be used concurrently.

D-Penicillamine

D-Penicillamine (CUPRIMINE; DEPEN) is a heavy metal chelator that is used to treat Wilson's disease (copper poisoning) and poisoning with mercury, lead, or iron. It is also indicated for treating advanced rheumatoid arthritis, especially cases that cannot be managed with other NSAIDs or DMARDs (eg, gold). Penicillamine is given orally for arthritis.

Penicillamine therapy usually is started with low doses, increased at one- to three-month intervals until the maintenance dose (500–750 mg) is reached. Most patients show obvious improvement after two to three months of treatment. In general, if daily doses of 750 mg to 1 gram fail to give adequate relief after several months of treatment, penicillamine therapy should be stopped. Penicillamine can be administered with salicylates or other rapidly acting NSAIDs. There are no recommended pediatric doses. The drug should be taken on an empty stomach, between meals, because food interferes with absorption.

The most serious adverse responses to penicillamine are blood dyscrasias (including fatal aplastic anemia and agranulocytosis) and renal damage (probably an autoimmune reaction), which can lead to the nephrotic syndrome.

NURSING IMPLICATIONS

Administer penicillamine on an empty stomach at least one hour before meals or two hours after, and at least one hour apart from any drug, food, or milk. Stress the need for frequent blood tests and urinalyses during penicillamine therapy.

Corticosteroids

Corticosteroids are important adjuncts to the therapy of severe arthritic conditions. These drugs have other uses, and they are discussed more fully in Chapter 45.

Corticosteroids are perhaps the most efficacious antiinflammatory drugs available, but they seldom provide longlasting relief in arthritis. In addition, prolonged systemic administration causes significant side effects. Therefore, corticosteroids are best used on a short-term basis for acute flare-ups of arthritic disease.

The preferred route of administration is by local (intraarticular) injection into one or two affected joints. Parenteral therapy typically involves aspirating the joint and instilling 25 or 50 mg of hydrocortisone, or equivalent doses of a related steroid. This administration route reduces the chance of systemic side effects that occur when these drugs are given orally. However, frequent intraarticular injection increases the risk of infection if careful aseptic technic is not used, and local steroid effects may cause joint degeneration and weakening of tendons and ligaments.

Systemic corticosteroid therapy (eg, with a drug such as methylprednisolone) may be appropriate in a few instances. One involves young adults with severe erosive rheumatoid disease complicated by life-threatening cardiac or pulmonary problems. Other candidates include middle-aged persons for whom traditional therapies have failed and aggressive and immediate use of steroids may be the only way to prevent total disability. Geriatric patients who develop rheumatoid arthritis late in life are also candidates for oral steroids. Often they do not tolerate traditional NSAIDs well, but if their acute inflammatory disease progresses rapidly they may develop more severe systemic problems, become bedridden, debilitated, and die. Even for these patients, gradual reduction and eventual withdrawal of steroids should be a therapeutic goal.

The major problem with starting oral corticosteroid therapy is how eventually to stop it safely. As discussed in Chapter 45, systemic steroids cause many side effects during administration, and others occur during withdrawal. Adrenal cortex suppression, one important unwanted effect, can be reduced but not prevented by alternate-day therapy.

Corticosteroids are ulcerogenic and are contraindicated in patients with peptic ulcer disease. They cause sodium and water retention, and so are also contraindicated in patients with congestive heart failure or hypertension.

Other Treatments Directed at the Immune System

Other medications are approved, or are being studied, as DMARDs. They inhibit one or more parts of the immune system. They include azathioprine (IMURAN; Chapter 54), methotrexate (FOLEX, MEXATE; Chapter 59), cyclophosphamide (CYTOXAN, NEOSAR; Chapter 59), and sulfasalazine (Chapter 56). A variety of *biologic response modifiers* (eg, gamma interferon and monoclonal antibodies against certain activated lymphocytes) are also being tested (see Chapter 59). Refer to the cited chapters for more information about these drugs.

IV. Acetaminophen

Acetaminophen is the only approved member of a group of drugs called para-aminophenol derivatives. (It is sometimes called APAP, an abbreviation of its chemical name, N-acetyl para-aminophenol.) Acetaminophen is chemically unrelated to salicylates. Along with ibuprofen, it is the only OTC aspirin substitute. Some familiar trade names are TYLENOL, DATRIL, and PANADOL.

PROTOTYPE

Acetaminophen

Absorption, Distribution, Metabolism, and Excretion

Acetaminophen is completely absorbed from the GI tract. It is metabolized in the liver, and the metabolites are excreted in the urine. Acetaminophen crosses the blood–brain and placental barriers. Acetaminophen absorption is variable when the drug is given as a rectal suppository. Unlike aspirin, it is not extensively bound to plasma proteins.

Pharmacologic Effects

Acetaminophen, like aspirin, causes most of its therapeutic effects by inhibiting enzymes involved in prostaglandin synthesis. However, acetaminophen presumably differs from NSAIDs in how well it inhibits those enzymes and the specific types of cells it acts on. As a result, acetaminophen causes some aspirin-like effects, but not others.

Analgesia and Antipyresis

Acetaminophen has analgesic and antipyretic actions similar to those of aspirin. Acetaminophen is essentially equipotent to aspirin for relief of fever or pain *that is not due to inflammation.* Thus, two regular aspirin tablets, 325 mg each, are essentially equivalent in potency to two acetaminophen tablets (usually 300 mg each).

Major Differences Between Acetaminophen and Aspirin and Other Nonsteroidal Antiinflammatory Drugs

As virtually every television watcher knows, acetaminophen (at usual doses) lacks an important therapeutic effect of aspirin (or ibuprofen), but it is "gentler on the stomach." What follows here is a list that addresses these and other differences between aspirin and acetaminophen.

Acetaminophen, at usual recommended doses,

- lacks appreciable antiinflammatory actions. It may alleviate pain associated with inflammation, but not to the same degree as aspirin or another NSAID;
- does not inhibit platelet aggregation or interact appreciably with other antiplatelet or anticoagulant drugs; it does not share aspirin's platelet-related clinical uses;
- does not alter uric acid excretion or serum urate levels, nor does it antagonize the effects of uricosuric drugs;
- rarely causes gastric upset or irritation and does not seem to intensify gastric irritation caused by alcohol. However, acetaminophen is not a wise choice as a hangover remedy for alcohol abusers, as noted in the drug interactions section (p 1096).
- is not likely to trigger bronchoconstriction or other adverse effects in persons who are hypersensitive to aspirin or other NSAIDs;
- does not interact with drugs that interact with aspirin, because, in part, acetaminophen does not displace other drugs from plasma protein binding sites;
- does not increase the risk of Reye's syndrome in children with viral infections, as does aspirin (but not ibuprofen);
- does not cause salicylism or a poison syndrome like that of aspirin. As noted shortly, however, acetaminophen can, by a different mechanism, cause fatal toxicity when overdoses are taken.

Clinical Indications and Administration

Acetaminophen is used to alleviate fever or mild pain. It is preferred for patients who cannot tolerate or should not take aspirin (or ibuprofen). The usual adult and pediatric analgesic or antipyretic doses of acetaminophen are similar to those for aspirin (Table 52–C1). Many pediatric dosage forms are available (see Nursing Implications, immediately below.)

Acetaminophen can be used for arthritis, but it is not as effective as an NSAID. High acetaminophen doses should not be used routinely, as is aspirin when it is used for arthritis.

NURSING IMPLICATIONS

Advise patients with gout, asthma, or peptic ulcer disease, and those taking drugs that interact with aspirin, that acetaminophen is preferable for relieving simple pain and fever. When answering patients' questions about the choice between aspirin and acetaminophen, inform them that acetaminophen does lack aspirin's antiinflammatory effect.

To reduce the risks of accidental toxicity, make patients aware of the differences between standard strength (usually 325 mg) and extra strength acetaminophen preparations (which usually contain 500 mg).

Teach parents or guardians that some pediatric acetaminophen preparations contain different concentrations or amounts of the drug. Most chewable tablets contain 80 mg; other products contain up to 160 mg. These strength differences are especially important for liquid products, many of which look alike and have similar brand names. Accidental substitution of one for another could cause underdoses or serious overdoses if the volumes are not adjusted properly. Some acetaminophen liquid preparations contain alcohol; recommend alcohol-free products as necessary.

Side Effects, Adverse Reactions, and Contraindications

Therapeutic doses of acetaminophen cause no major side effects when taken for short periods of time. A small number of patients develop a rash, and even fewer develop serious mucosal lesions and drug fever.

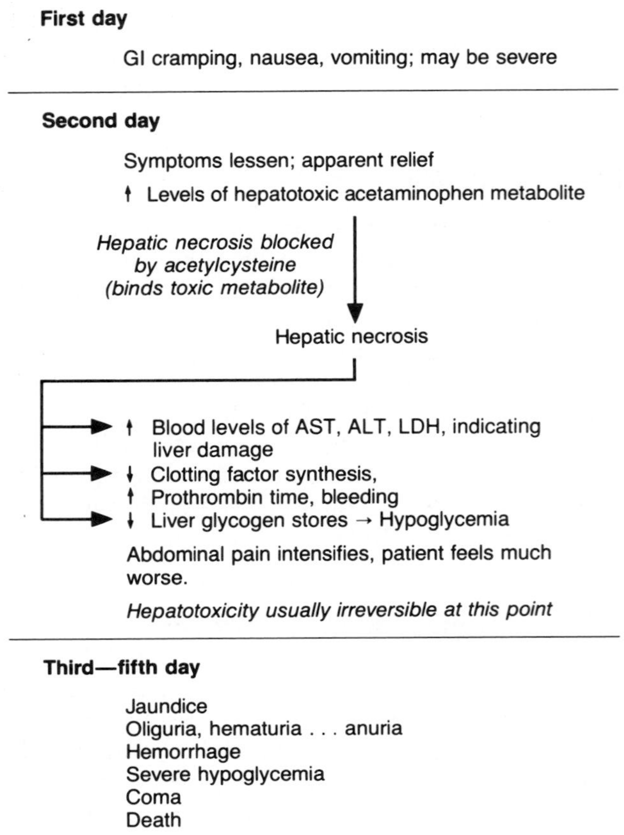

First day

GI cramping, nausea, vomiting; may be severe

Second day

Symptoms lessen; apparent relief

↑ Levels of hepatotoxic acetaminophen metabolite

Hepatic necrosis blocked by acetylcysteine (binds toxic metabolite)

Hepatic necrosis

→ ↑ Blood levels of AST, ALT, LDH, indicating liver damage

→ ↓ Clotting factor synthesis, ↑ Prothrombin time, bleeding

→ ↓ Liver glycogen stores → Hypoglycemia

Abdominal pain intensifies, patient feels much worse.

Hepatotoxicity usually irreversible at this point

Third—fifth day

Jaundice
Oliguria, hematuria . . . anuria
Hemorrhage
Severe hypoglycemia
Coma
Death

Figure 52–2

Typical sequence of acetaminophen intoxication.

Patients with known allergy or hypersensitivity to aspirin or other NSAIDs usually tolerate acetaminophen well. The greatest concerns come with excessive and long-term acetaminophen use. These are discussed in the section on overdoses and toxicity and in the section dealing with analgesic use and renal disease, below.

NURSING IMPLICATIONS

If acetaminophen does not provide the expected relief after about three days of therapy, consult a physician. Acetaminophen should be used cautiously for arthritis in children under 12 years of age, because high and potentially toxic doses are needed for symptom relief. These conditions are best treated with NSAIDs.

Interactions with Other Drugs

Table 52–11 summarizes the relatively few important drug interactions that involve acetaminophen. The drug's relative lack of drug interactions, in comparison with those involving NSAIDs, is a clear benefit for many patients who take other medications. However, at very high doses (eg, 900 mg or more every four hours, which are seldom recommended), acetaminophen can potentiate the actions of oral anticoagulants.

Acetaminophen and Alcohol

As noted above, acetaminophen does not potentiate alcohol's gastric toxicity. However, important problems can result from combined and excessive or prolonged use of the two drugs. Alcohol (like barbiturates; see Chapter 22, p 348) stimulates the liver's major drug metabolizing enzyme system. In doing so, alcohol increases the formation of an acetaminophen metabolite that is responsible for potentially fatal acetaminophen liver toxicity. Thus, acetaminophen should not be used as a "cure" for alcohol-induced hangover, nor should persons take both drugs on a long-term basis.

Overdose and Toxicity

Acetaminophen is a widely used drug, and overdoses are relatively common. However, the signs, symptoms, and treatment of acetaminophen toxicity differ dramatically from those of aspirin poisoning. *The major danger of acute acetaminophen poisoning is fatal liver damage* (hepatic necrosis). Single doses of 25 grams or more, taken at one time, are generally fatal to adults; less than half that dose can kill a child. Figure 52–2 outlines the sequence of signs and symptoms that occur with a fatal acetaminophen overdose.

Signs and Symptoms

Severe GI cramping, nausea, and vomiting occur in the early stages of acetaminophen poisoning. They usually last from 12 to 24 hours. Many patients then experience apparent "relief" during the second day, even though they may have ingested a lethal dose. This feeling of wellness may be interpreted as recovery or as an indication that nothing worse will happen. That is not the case, and such a false assumption may prevent the victim from seeking needed medical care.

During the second day after the overdose, urine output begins to fall, hematuria occurs, and pain develops in the right upper quadrant of the abdomen and worsens as liver damage progresses.

Blood levels of key enzymes indicative of hepatic damage (eg, AST, ALT) rise. Three to five days after ingestion, hepatic necrosis is essentially irreversible. Abdominal pain increases, jaundice and anuria occur, and impaired blood coagulation develops because hepatic clotting factor synthesis is reduced (as evidenced by increased prothrombin times). Hypoglycemia, coma, and death follow.

Hepatotoxicity is caused by an acetaminophen metabolite. When safe doses of the drug are taken, liver cell components that are rich in sulfhydryl (—SH) groups can react with and detoxify the metabolite. However, if these cellular constituents are overwhelmed by high levels of the acetaminophen metabolite, the liver cells themselves are attacked and damaged.

Treatment

Acetaminophen poisoning is harder to treat successfully than aspirin poisoning. As with any oral poisoning, the first goals are to remove unabsorbed drug from the GI tract and to prevent further absorption (by emesis, lavage, etc). With high-dose, acute intoxication, this alone may not save the patient's life, especially if no other medical care is given.

Blood tests to measure acetaminophen levels and half-lives are performed. The results help predict how serious the outcome may be and whether hepatotoxicity is apt to be lethal. In general, if plasma acetaminophen levels are too high or the half-life is too prolonged, the prognosis is not good.

Whereas there is no antidote for aspirin poisoning, there *is* an antidote for acetaminophen poisoning: N-acetylcysteine (MUCOMYST). This medication is also used as a mucus-thinning (mucolytic) drug for several pulmonary disorders. N-Acetylcysteine reacts with the hepatotoxic acetaminophen metabolite, reducing the interaction between the metabolite and liver cells. It works best when given within 10 to 12 hours after acetaminophen ingestion, and it should always be given as soon as possible. (The MUCOMYST package insert contains the information used to predict the clinical outcome, based on acetaminophen half-lives and blood levels.)

NURSING IMPLICATIONS

Expect that blood will be drawn to measure acetaminophen levels and that MUCOMYST treatment will be ordered. However, do question medication orders calling for withholding MUCOMYST treatment until blood test results are known. The waiting time for laboratory results, which can be long, can mean the difference between life and death. The physician should order the start of MUCOMYST treatment ***without waiting for blood test results.*** MUCOMYST is relatively safe, and its administration can be stopped if tests indicate a safe acetaminophen level.

MUCOMYST is supplied as a 20% solution that should be diluted to 5% (one part drug, three parts diluent) before use. Prepare each diluted dose immediately before use. Dilute it in cola, a citrus-flavored soft drink, or citrus juice to help mask the drug's terrible taste. (Water can be used as the diluent if the patient cannot swallow the drug and a nasogastric tube must be used.) Discard diluted and unused MUCOMYST if prepared more than one hour earlier. Undiluted drug in containers that have been opened to remove a dose can be recapped and stored in a refrigerator for up to four days.

The patient first receives an oral loading dose of 140 mg MUCOMYST per kilogram of body weight. Thereafter, they receive 17 maintenance doses of 70 mg/kg each, separated by four hours. This protocol can be stopped earlier if blood tests indicate a nontoxic acetaminophen level. If the patient vomits any of the doses within one hour of administration, repeat the dose, and don't count it as part of the sequence. Never give N-acetylcysteine by any route other than orally when treating acetaminophen overdoses.

Once MUCOMYST is administered, withhold further treatment with activated charcoal or emetics; they reduce acetylcysteine absorption. Avoid giving diuretics, antihistamines, CNS depressants, or antidiarrheal agents. Supportive care includes management of hypoglycemia, maintenance of fluid and electrolyte balance, and administration of vitamin K or plasma as required.

Monitor vital signs, blood chemistry, liver marker enzymes, coagulation profiles, and acetaminophen levels frequently until the patient is fully recovered.

Concerns About Analgesic Use and Chronic Renal Disease

For years before acetaminophen gained such widespread use, the most popular OTC aspirin alternative or additive was a drug called phenacetin. It was often found in a combination product known as APCs: aspirin, phenacetin, and caffeine. Phenacetin overuse was eventually linked to a high incidence of renal damage and renal failure, some cases of which were fatal.

Now there is evidence that acetaminophen may also pose a risk of renal damage when used chronically in high doses. Interestingly, one of phenacetin's major metabolites is acetaminophen, so the question now is whether acetaminophen was responsible for the kidney damage attributed to phenacetin. (There is also growing concern about ibuprofen-induced nephrotoxicity.) Based on current information, there is a definite risk of analgesic-induced nephrotoxicity in persons

- taking analgesic combination products;
- with preexisting renal dysfunction;
- with chronic renal vascular insufficiency (as may accompany congestive heart failure [CHF], or as might be induced by the causative drugs themselves);
- with reductions of blood volume, as may occur with dehydration or diuretic use, which might concentrate the drugs or their metabolites in the urine.

Over-the-counter analgesic products now have label warnings for a variety of potential problems, but none that address the risks of renal damage. Because of the potential dangers, advise patients not to use high doses of OTC analgesics for prolonged periods of time, unless they can be provided with proper, frequent monitoring.

SUMMARY OF NURSING IMPLICATIONS

◆ Assessment

Identify nature of patient's pain; describe involved joints or areas; not limitation of motion.

Determine ability to complete activities of daily living.

Establish baseline vital signs and laboratory values.

Review history for contraindications: bleeding tendencies, chronic renal failure, impaired liver function, child with influenza or chickenpox, allergies.

Review patient's medication list for potential drug–drug interactions with aspirin, ibuprofen, and most prescription antiinflammatory drugs: oral anticoagulants, furosemide, antacids, steroids, probenecid, alcohol.

Assess for signs of blood dyscrasias (abnormal bruising or bleeding or sudden flu-like symptoms) with antiinflammatory drugs.

◆ Nursing Diagnoses

Pain related to gastric irritation from ASA, NSAIDs, or DMARDs.

Knowledge deficit related to prescribed drug therapy, disease condition.

Ineffective breathing pattern related to salicylate poisoning and respiratory depression.

High risk for impaired skin integrity (pruritis, erythema) related to DMARDs.

Altered oral mucous membranes related to DMARD therapy.

Diarrhea related to adverse effects of gold therapy.

Sensory/perceptual alterations: visual (blurring and diplopia) and auditory (tinnitus) related to adverse drug effects (salicylates, hydroxychloroquine).

Activity intolerance related to joint stiffness, pain or fatigue.

◆ Planning/Implementation

Monitor for adverse effects; report hives, dizziness, GI bleeding, respiratory difficulty, and/or abnormal bruising with aspirin; visual changes with indomethacin or hydroxychloroquine; weight gain, edema, fatigue, or dyspnea with phenylbutazone, ibuprofen, or systemic steroids; oral lesions with gold salts; proteinuria or hematuria with penicillamine.

Observe for salicylism in patients who self-prescribe or receive high doses of aspirin: tinnitus, headache, dizziness, confusion, paresthesias.

Give medications with meals or a full glass of milk to reduce GI upset.

Encourage range-of-motion exercises and physical therapy in patients with arthritic conditions.

Use acetaminophen to relieve mild pain or fever in patients at risk with aspirin use; provide patient with list of acceptable drugs.

Prepare for suspected overdose of acetaminophen: gastric lavage; blood samples for analysis; oral administration of N-acetylcysteine (MUCOMYST).

Monitor vital signs, blood chemistry and coagulation profiles, fluid and electrolyte status, and urine output if overdose occurs.

Discard MUCOMYST within one hour after diluted, after four days if open but undiluted.

◆ Patient and Family Teaching

Teach the patient/family:

To seek medical help if symptoms are not relieved after several days or severe symptoms occur.

Not to use aspirin unless directed by a physician if pregnant; if gout or hyperuricemia are present; or if the patient is hypersensitive.

To avoid use of aspirin or aspirin-containing products for teenagers or younger children with chickenpox or flu-like signs, symptoms, or illness.

To seek immediate evaluation and treatment of possible overdoses, especially with children.

To keep methyl salicylate– or salicylic acid–containing drugs safely locked and out of reach of children.

The superiority and low cost of plain aspirin; the use of enteric or buffered aspirin for GI upset when appropriate; the benefits and safety of acetaminophen for patients who cannot take aspirin; the inability of acetaminophen to relieve inflammation; and the risk of sharing antiarthritic drugs with other individuals.

◆ Evaluation

The patient/family will:

Experience reasonable relief of presenting symptoms: pain reduced; temperature lowered or within normal limits; mobility increased.

Deny adverse or toxic drug effects (eg, ringing in the ears, visual changes, occult bleeding in stool or urine, increased respiratory rate).

Comply with teaching program: take drug as prescribed; incorporate nondrug therapies; avoid known drug interactants; return for follow-up evaluation.

Annotated Bibliography

Brooks PM, Needs CJ: Antirheumatic drugs in pregnancy and lactation. *Baillieres Clin Rheumatol* 1990;4(1):157–171. *Useful information about how to maximize desired effects while minimizing risks to the fetus or nursing infant when arthritis therapy is needed.*

Fink CW: Medical treatment of juvenile arthritis. *Clin Orthop* 1990;(259):60–69. *Describes the use of NSAIDs and other therapies for children with arthritis; includes coverage of the clinical course during treatment, assessment, potential unwanted effects, and therapeutic limitations.*

Fischetti LF: Interaction between nonsteroidal antiinflammatory drugs and high-dose methotrexate: A literature review. *J Pediatr Oncol Nurs* 1990;7(1):14–6. *Succinct coverage of an important and potentially toxic drug interaction; explains why educating nursing staff, patients, and families is so important.*

Fries JF: Reevaluating the therapeutic approach to rheumatoid arthritis: The "sawtooth" strategy. *J Rheumatol Suppl* 1990;22:12–15. *One of the early papers stressing the potential need to modify traditional arthritis therapy, which nearly always started with an NSAID and saved disease-modifying agents until late in the treatment plan; identifies six principles that form the basis for a new treatment philosophy and approach.*

Furst DE: Rheumatoid arthritis. Practical use of medications. *Postgrad Med* 1990;87(3):79–92. *Worthwhile reading for its content on all the key drugs, plus a valuable holistic approach that considers rest, exercise, and therapy; family involvement; and participation of the patient in care.*

Furst DE: Toxicity of antirheumatic medications in children with juvenile arthritis. *J Rheumatol Suppl* 1992;33:11–15. *Uses clinical examples to discuss the toxicity of nonsteroidal antiinflammatories and disease-modifying antirheumatic drugs—alone and in combination—in children.*

Gray MA: Nonsteroidal antiinflammatory agents. *Orthop Nurs* 1991; 10(4):63–70, 78. *Reviews the key drugs, with an eye on their use in orthopedics.*

Holt L, Holt S, Saleeby G, Todd M: Gastroduodenal injury from nonsteroidal anti-inflammatory drugs: Risk management issues. *Gastroenterol Nurs* 1991;14(3):124–126. *Practical advice about a common adverse effect of long-term NSAID therapy.*

Houston MC: Nonsteroidal anti-inflammatory drugs and antihypertensives. *Am J Med* 1991;90(5A):42S–47S. *Excellent coverage of the effects of NSAIDs on blood pressure, interactions with antihypertensive drugs, and high-risk groups (eg, the elderly, blacks). The consequences can be serious and affect many more people than you might imagine.*

Katz WA: Challenging the pyramid: A new look at therapeutic approaches for rheumatoid arthritis. Patient selection. *J Rheumatol Suppl* 1990;25:39–41. *Identifies goals of arthritis therapy, criteria to be used in drug selection, and the common drug choices and clinical outcomes—in a way that differs from what has been done for many years.*

Kean WF, Buchanan WW: Pregnancy and rheumatoid disease. *Baillieres Clin Rheumatol* 1990;4(1):125–140. *Discusses not only drug therapy and its impact on the mother and fetus, but also how the physiologic and pathophysiologic changes of pregnancy and rheumatoid diseases affect one another.*

Levinson JE, Wallace CA: Dismantling the pyramid. *J Rheumatol Suppl* 1992;33:6–10. *A hard look at arthritis therapy in the recent past—the pyramid approach—and proposals about how and why treatment plans should change.*

Reeves-Swift R: Rational management of a child's acute fever. *MCN* 1990;15(2):82–85. *Good information for you to learn and then pass on to parents and guardians.*

Schenkier S, Golbus J: Treatment of rheumatoid arthritis: New thoughts on the classic pyramid approach. *Postgrad Med* 1992;91(1):285–286, 289–292. *Current perspective on the changing trends in arthritis therapy.*

Soscia PN, Zurier RB: Drug therapy of rheumatic diseases during pregnancy. *Bull Rheum Dis* 1992;41(2):1–3. *Short, but with invaluable information for treating the patient who has arthritis and is also pregnant.*

Spilman P, Whelton A: Nonsteroidal antiinflammatory drugs: Effects on kidney function and implications for nursing care. *ANNA J* 1992;19(1):19–26. *Covers pathophysiology, comprehensive nursing assessment, and patient education about risks of renal dysfunction caused by OTC and prescription NSAIDs.*

Sterling LP: Rheumatoid arthritis: Current concepts and management. Part 2. *Am Pharm* 1990;NS30(9):49–54. *A good review with emphasis on the uses and potential dangers of the disease-modifying antirheumatic drugs (DMARDs).*

Vissering TR: Pharmacologic agents for pain management. *Crit Care Nurs Clin North Am* 1991;3(1):17–23. *Discusses narcotic and nonnarcotic analgesic drug selection and use criteria, monitoring, and outcomes from a nursing perspective.*

Table 52–C1 Clinical Uses and Administration of Salicylates, Other Rapidly Acting NSAIDs, and Acetaminophen*

AGENT	CLINICAL USES	DOSAGE AND ROUTE OF ADMINISTRATION
PROTOTYPE		
Aspirin	Minor aches, pain, fever	325–650 mg q4h as needed; some extra-strength products recommend 500 mg q3h, or 1000 mg q6h
		Children: see Table 52–1, p 1081
	Arthritis, other rheumatic conditions	3.2–6 g/day in divided doses
		Children: 60–110 mg/kg/day in divided doses (every 6–8 hr)
	Acute rheumatic fever	5–8 g/day in divided doses, then titrate
		Children: 100 mg/kg/day (divided doses) for 2 weeks, then 75 mg/kg/day for 4–6 weeks
	Transient ischemic attacks in men	650 mg bid or 325 mg qid
	Myocardial infarction	300–325 mg/day
RELATED DRUGS		
Choline salicylate		
(ARTHROPAN)	Minor pain and inflammation, as in arthritis	Adults, children >12 yrs: 870 mg q3–4h; for arthritis, may start with 870–1740 mg up to 4 times daily
Magnesium salicylate		
(MAGAN, ORIGINAL DOAN'S)	Rheumatoid arthritis, osteoarthritis, bursitis	650 mg q4h or tid
Potassium salicylate		
(in PABALATE SF enteric-coated)	As for magnesium salicylate	600 mg (2 tablets) q2–6h
Salicylamide	Minor pain	200–400 mg q4h while symptoms persist
Salsalate		
(DISALCID)	As for magnesium salicylate	3000 mg/day in divided doses
Sodium salicylate		
(PABALATE)	Minor pain, aches, fever	325–650 mg q4h
Sodium thiosalicylate		
(TUSAL, others)	Acute gout	IM (preferred) or IV: 100 mg q3–4h for 2 days, then 100 mg/day until symptom-free
	Muscular pain	IM or IV: 50–100 mg/day or every other day
	Rheumatic fever	IM or IV: 100–150 mg q4–8h for 3 days, then 100 mg bid until symptom-free

(continued)

*Note: Unless stated otherwise, all administration routes are oral, and dosages are for adults.

Table 52–C1 **Clinical Uses and Administration of Salicylates, Other Rapidly Acting NSAIDs, and Acetaminophen* (*Continued*)**

AGENT	CLINICAL USES	DOSAGE AND ROUTE OF ADMINISTRATION
Other Rapidly Acting Nonsteroidal Antiinflammatory Drugs		
Diclofenac sodium		
(VOLTAREN)	Rheumatoid arthritis	150–200 mg/day in divided doses
	Osteoarthritis	100–150 mg/day in divided doses
	Ankylosing spondylitis	25 mg qid with extra dose at bedtime if needed
	Reduction of eye inflammation after cataract extraction	Topical: Instill 1 drop in eye qid starting 24 hr after surgery; continue for 2 weeks
Diflusinal		
(DOLOBID)	Mild-to-moderate pain	Initially 1000 mg followed by 500 mg q8–12h
	Rheumatoid or osteoarthritis	500–1000 mg/day in 2 doses
Etodolac		
(LODINE)	Osteoarthritis	Initially 800–1200 mg/day in 2–4 doses; adjust to usual maintenance of 600–1200 mg/day (1200 mg/day maximum or 20 mg/kg maximum for patients ≤60 kg)
	Acute pain	200–400 mg q6–8h as needed; maximum doses as noted above
Fenoprofen calcium		
(NALFON)	Rheumatoid or osteoarthritis	300–600 mg tid or qid
	Mild-to-moderate pain	200 mg q4–6h
Flurbiprofen		
(ANSAID)	Rheumatoid arthritis or osteoarthritis	200–300 mg/day in 2–4 divided doses; give no more than 100 mg/dose
Flurbiprofen sodium		
(OCUFEN)	Inhibition of intraoperative miosis in eye surgery	Topical: Instill 1 drop in conjunctival sac every half-hour, starting 2 hr preoperatively (ie, 4 doses total)
Ibuprofen		
(MOTRIN, other prescription names, products)	Rheumatoid arthritis or osteoarthritis	1.2–3.2 g/day in 3–4 divided doses
		Children: 30–40 mg/kg/day in 3–4 divided doses
	Mild-to-moderate pain	400 mg q4–6h as needed
	Primary dysmenorrhea	400 mg q4h as needed
	Fever reduction in children	Oral suspension: 5 mg/kg if baseline temperature ≤39.2°C (102.5°F), 10 mg/kg for higher starting temperatures, q4–6h
(ADVIL, NUPRIN, other OTC products)	Self-medication for minor aches, pain, fever, dysmenorrhea	200 mg q4–6h while symptoms last; may use 400 mg if fever or pain persists; limit 1.2g/24 hr; limit use to 10 days for pain, 3 days for fever, then notify physician
Indomethacin		
(INDOCIN)	Moderate-to-severe rheumatoid arthritis, ankylosing spondylitis	Oral, rectal: 25 mg bid or tid, increase if tolerated and needed to 25–50 mg/day (at weekly intervals), 150–200 mg/day maximum; may need to increase daily dosage by 25–50 mg for acute rheumatoid arthritis flare-ups

(continued)

Table 52–C1 **Clinical Uses and Administration of Salicylates, Other Rapidly Acting NSAIDs, and Acetaminophen* (*Continued*)**

AGENT	CLINICAL USES	DOSAGE AND ROUTE OF ADMINISTRATION
Other Rapidly Acting Nonsteroidal Antiinflammatory Drugs		
	Acute painful shoulder	Oral, rectal: 75–150 mg/day in 3–4 divided doses
	Acute gouty arthritis	Immediate-acting oral dosage forms only: 50 mg tid until pain tolerable, then discontinue rapidly, may use sustained-release form for maintenance therapy
	Closure of patent ductus arteriosus in selected premature infants	IV: 3 doses of 0.1–0.25 mg/kg (age-dependent) 12–24 hr apart
(INDOCIN-SR)	Maintenance therapy for above indications (except acute gout, patent ductus arteriosus)	May substitute 75-mg capsule once daily for 25 mg tid immediate-acting form, or twice daily instead of 50 mg tid; start treatment with immediate-acting dosage form
Ketoprofen		
(ORUDIS)	Rheumatoid arthritis or osteoarthritis	Initially 75 mg tid or 50 mg qid; average maintenance dose 150–300 mg in 3 or 4 doses; reduce initial dose by ⅓–½ in elderly patients or those with impaired renal function; maintenance 150–300 mg/day in 3–4 doses: take with antacids, food, or milk
Ketorolac tromethamine		
(TORADOL)	Acute pain	10 mg as needed q4–6h; do not exceed chronic doses of 10 mg qid; limit to 40 mg/day when and after switching to oral from IM
		IM: 30–60 mg initially, then half the loading dose q6h as needed up to 150 mg/day maximum on first day, then 120 mg/day; limit to 5 days treatment
Meclofenamate sodium		
(MECLOMEN)	Mild-to-moderate pain	50 mg q4–6h
	Excessive menstrual blood loss, primary dysmenorrhea	100 mg tid for up to 6 days, starting at onset of menstruation
	Rheumatoid arthritis, osteoarthritis	Adults, children ≥14 yr: Initially 100–200 mg/day in 3–4 divided doses, usual maintenance 200–400 mg/day in 3–4 divided doses
Mefenamic acid		
(PONSTEL)	Acute pain, primary dysmenorrhea	Adults, children ≥14 yr: 500 mg, then 250 mg q6h as needed, with food, usually for ≤1 week (acute pain), 2–3 days for dysmenorrhea (start at bleeding/symptom onset)
Nabumetone		
(RELAFEN)	Rheumatoid arthritis or osteoarthritis	1000-mg single dose with or without food; maintenance 1500–2000 mg/day in 1 dose or 2 divided doses

(continued)

Table 52–C1 **Clinical Uses and Administration of Salicylates, Other Rapidly Acting NSAIDs, and Acetaminophen*** **(*Continued*)**

AGENT	CLINICAL USES	DOSAGE AND ROUTE OF ADMINISTRATION
Naproxen		
(ANAPROX)	Rheumatoid arthritis, osteoarthritis, ankylosing spondylitis	250–500 mg bid; may increase to 1500 mg/day for limited periods
	Juvenile arthritis	About 10 mg/kg/day in 2 divided doses
	Acute gout	750 mg, then 250 mg q8h until attack subsides
	Mild-to-moderate pain, primary dysmenorrhea, acute tendinitis and bursitis	500 mg, then 250 mg q6–8h, up to 1250 mg/day maximum
Naproxen sodium		
(NAPROSYN)	Rheumatoid arthritis, osteoarthritis, ankylosing spondylitis	275–550 mg bid; may increase to 1650 mg/day for limited periods
	Acute gout	825 mg, then 275 mg q8h until attack subsides
	Mild-to-moderate pain, primary dysmenorrhea, acute tendinitis and bursitis	550 mg, then 275 mg q6–8h, up to 1375 mg/day maximum
Piroxicam		
(FELDENE)	Rheumatoid arthritis or osteoarthritis	20 mg once daily, or 10 mg bid
Sulindac		
(CLINORIL)	Rheumatoid arthritis, osteoarthritis, ankylosing spondylitis	150 mg bid, then individualize to no more than 400 mg/day
	Acute painful shoulder, acute gouty arthritis	200 mg bid, usually for 1–2 weeks (painful shoulder), 1 week (gout)
Suprofen		
(PROFENAL)	Inhibition of intraoperative miosis in eye surgery	Topical: Instill 2 drops in conjunctival sac on day of surgery at 3, 2, 1 hr before surgery, may use 2 drops q4h during waking hours on day before surgery
Tolmetin sodium		
(TOLECTIN)	Rheumatoid arthritis or osteoarthritis	400 mg tid, preferably with one dose in AM and PM; maintenance usually 600–1800 mg/day in 3 divided doses
		Children ≥2 yr: 20 mg/kg/day in 3–4 divided doses to start; maintain at 15–30 mg/kg/day in divided doses
	Acetaminophen	
(DATRIL; PANADOL; TYLENOL; others)	Symptomatic relief of minor fever, pain	325–650 mg q4–6h, not to exceed 4 g in 24 hr; see Table 52–1, p. 1081, for pediatric doses
		Rectal suppositories: 650 mg q4–6h (6 suppositories/24 hr maximum)
		Children 6–12 yr: 325 mg q4–6h (2.6 g/24 hr maximum)
		3–6 yr: 120 mg q4–6h (720 mg/24 hr maximum) <3 yr: Consult physician

Note: Unless stated otherwise, all administration routes are oral, and dosages are for adults.

Table 52–S1 Major Side Effects of and Contraindications for Salicylates and Other Rapidly Acting NSAIDs

BODY SYSTEM/ Side Effect	CONTRAINDICATION/ PRECAUTION	COMMENTS AND NURSING IMPLICATIONS
CENTRAL NERVOUS SYSTEM		
Dizziness; confusion; paresthesias; tinnitus		Usually a sign of salicylism; dizziness, confusion, and neuromuscular changes may also occur in patients with poor renal function who take magnesium salicylate
Drowsiness		Mainly with ingestion of high doses of salicylamide
Headache		May be common and intense with indomethacin, less problematic with others; may require discontinuation of use, may cause noncompliance; alternative drugs preferred
BLOOD		
Excessive or abnormal bruising, bleeding; petechial hemorrhage; epistaxis	Impaired blood coagulation; hemophilia; anemias; use of anticoagulant, antiplatelet, or fibrinolytic drugs	Monitor prothrombin time and fecal occult blood levels in high-risk patients; avoid aspirin, other rapidly acting NSAIDs in persons with hemophilia, thrombocytopenia, anemias, other bleeding disorders
RESPIRATORY		
Wheezing, tightness of chest, bronchoconstriction	Bronchial asthma; history of hypersensitivity to aspirin, other NSAIDs	Absolute contraindication with prior untoward response; assess all patients, particularly with asthma history, for wheezing or more severe respiratory difficulty; all rapidly acting NSAIDs may cross-react
CARDIOVASCULAR		
Edema; hypertension; worsening of heart failure	History of heart failure or hypertension (rare)	Mainly with sodium salicylate, high doses of buffered aspirin, ibuprofen
Premature closure of fetal ductus arteriosus	Pregnancy, especially last trimester	Avoid all NSAIDs, particularly in last trimester
GASTROINTESTINAL		
Nausea, vomiting, abdominal pain; increased fecal blood loss; possible GI hemorrhage	Presence or history of peptic ulcer disease; chronic, high-dose alcohol consumption	Incidence, severity highly variable; buffered or enteric-coated aspirin may reduce mild GI distress, are nevertheless contraindicated in peptic ulcer disease; avoid all aspirin products, other NSAIDs, for alcohol hangover
SKIN		
Urticaria	History of aspirin-induced urticaria; aspirin hypersensitivity	Usually indicates hypersensitivity to aspirin, other NSAIDs; avoid use; most rapidly acting NSAIDs cross-react
REPRODUCTIVE		
Prolonged or inhibited labor and delivery; postpartum bleeding	Pregnancy	Avoid drug use

Table 52–11 Major Interactions Involving Salicylates, Other Rapidly Acting NSAIDs, and Acetaminophen

AGENT	RESULT OF INTERACTION	COMMENTS AND NURSING IMPLICATIONS
Interactions Involving Aspirin, Most Other Salicylates		
Acetazolamide (Chapter 32)	Increased blood levels, effects, potential toxicity of both interactants	Avoid interaction if possible; otherwise, monitor accordingly; may need to monitor plasma salicylate levels during combined use
Alcohol (Chapter 22)	Additive risk/severity of gastric irritation, ulceration, bleeding	Discourage frequent combined use; separate use of interactants by at least 12 hr; buffered or enteric-coated aspirins or nonacetylated salicylates (eg, choline salicylate) may have somewhat lower interaction risk
Anticoagulants, oral (eg, warfarin; Chapter 35)	Increased anticoagulant effects, risk of bleeding, possibly serious	Salicylates displace anticoagulant from plasma proteins, simultaneously inhibit platelet aggregation; avoid interaction; otherwise, monitor coagulation, and teach patient how to assess for signs of interaction; discourage unsupervised self-medication with aspirin; acetaminophen preferred for OTC pain, fever relief
Corticosteroids (Chapter 45)	Decreased salicylate levels, effects	Monitor clinical response(s) during combined therapy; may need to increase salicylate dose when starting systemic steroids and to reduce it again when steroids discontinued
Heparin (Chapter 35)	Increased bleeding risk	Greater than additive effects on clotting pathways; avoid interaction if possible; otherwise, monitor blood studies, responses accordingly
Insulin (Chapter 46)	Increased or excessive hypoglycemia	Salicylates increase pancreatic insulin release; of most concern in patients with non–insulin-dependent diabetes who are taking insulin; if interaction unavoidable, monitor blood glucose levels, assess (and teach patient) for hypoglycemia; combined use may necessitate/allow reduced insulin dosages
Methotrexate (Chapter 59)	Increased methotrexate effects, potential toxicity	Avoid interaction; otherwise, anticipate need to reduce methotrexate dose and to treat methotrexate toxicity aggressively
Probenecid, sulfinpyrazone (Chapter 53)	Decreased uricosuric effects, persistent hyperuricemia, increased frequency of gout attacks	Avoid combined use; advise patients to avoid all aspirin dosages, forms, except on physician's advice; recheck for aspirin use when uricosurics seem ineffective; recommend acetaminophen, ibuprofen for OTC fever, pain relief
Valproic acid (Chapter 26)	Increased valproate blood levels, effects; possibly excessive/toxic	Avoid interaction; if unavoidable, assess for excessive effects; monitor anticonvulsant blood levels more frequently than otherwise
Interactions Involving Most Prescription NSAIDs (and OTC Ibuprofen)		
β-Adrenergic blockers (eg, propranolol; Chapter 15)	Decreased antihypertensive effects of β blocker	Important interaction with ibuprofen (including OTC), indomethacin, piroxicam; avoid combined use if possible; otherwise, monitor BP closely; naproxen allegedly does not interact, may be preferred
Diuretics, loop (eg, furosemide, Chapter 32)	Decreased diuretic effects	Monitor accordingly; may need to increase diuretic dosage during combined therapy
Lithium (Chapter 24)	Increased lithium levels, potential toxicity	Monitor for excessive lithium effects; anticipate need to check lithium blood levels every 4–5 days until stable when adding or discontinuing NSAID; may need to lower lithium dosage

(continued)

Table 52–I1 Major Interactions Involving Salicylates, Other Rapidly Acting NSAIDs, and Acetaminophen (*Continued*)

AGENT	RESULT OF INTERACTION	COMMENTS AND NURSING IMPLICATIONS
Additional Interactions Involving Indomethacin		
Angiotensin converting enzyme (ACE) inhibitors (eg, captopril; Chapter 33)	Reduced antihypertensive effects of ACE inhibitors	Indomethacin inhibits prostaglandin synthesis in kidney, which is important to BP lowering by ACE inhibitor; avoid interaction; otherwise, monitor BP closely; other antihypertensives may be preferred, but see β blockers above in general interactions section
Interactions Involving Acetaminophen		
Alcohol (Chapter 22)	Increased risk of acetaminophen hepatotoxicity	Risk greatest with chronic alcohol consumption, excessive acetaminophen use (especially overdoses); ethanol stimulates metabolic formation of hepatotoxic acetaminophen metabolite; teach patients to limit use of both drugs
Hydantoins (eg, phenytoin; Chapter 26)	Increased hepatotoxicity risk; hydantoin effects possibly reduced	Mechanism as for alcohol–acetaminophen interaction; risk greatest with acetaminophen overdose; little concern when both drugs used in proper therapeutic doses, but monitor for decreased anticonvulsant control
Sulfinpyrazone (Chapter 53)	Hepatotoxicity risk as with hydantoins	See hydantoins

Table 52–C2 | Clinical Uses and Administration of Slow-Acting Antirheumatic Drugs

AGENT	CLINICAL USES	DOSAGE AND ROUTE OF ADMINISTRATION
	Gold Salts	
Auranofin		
(RIDAURA)	Active rheumatoid arthritis	Oral: Initially 6 mg once daily or 3 mg bid; after 6 months may increase dose to 3 mg tid if needed
Aurothioglucose		
(SOLGANAL)	Active rheumatoid arthritis	IM (gluteus): Adults: weekly injections: 10 mg (1st), 25 mg (2nd and 3rd), 50 mg (4th and later) up to cumulative dose of 0.8–1 g; may continue for stable patients at 50 mg, eventually at 3- to 4-week intervals
		Children 6–12 yr: One-fourth adult dose, adjusted to body weight; not to exceed 25 mg/dose
Gold sodium thiomalate		
(MYOCHRYSINE)	Active rheumatoid arthritis	IM (gluteus): Adults: weekly injections of 10 mg (1st), 25 mg (2nd), 25–50 mg (3rd and later) up to cumulative dose of 1 g; if patient responds, may continue 25–50 mg every other week to every 3–4 wks
		Children: Proportional to adult dose; 10 mg initially, then 1 mg/kg (50 mg maximum for any one dose) per adult schedule
	Others	
Azathioprine		
(IMURAN)	Severe, active rheumatoid arthritis	Oral (adults only): Initially 1 mg/kg once daily or 0.5 mg/kg bid; if needed, increase dose 6–8 weeks after starting treatment, then every 4 weeks; limit increases to 0.5 mg/kg, total daily dose to <2.5 mg/kg
	Other indications	See Chapter 54
Hydroxychloroquine sulfate		
(PLAQUENIL SULFATE)	As for azathioprine	Oral (adults only): Initially 400–600 mg with meals or milk; if possible, reduce to 200–400 mg/day after 4–12 weeks
Methotrexate		
(RHEUMATREX)	As for azathioprine	Oral (adults only): 7.5 mg once weekly or 2.5 mg for 3 doses 12 hr apart per week; may increase weekly dosage, but not to exceed 20 mg/wk
	Other indications	See Chapter 54
D-Penicillamine		
(CUPRIMENE, DEPEN)	As for azathioprine	Oral (adults only): Initially 125–250 mg/day, increase by 125 mg/day at 1- to 3-month intervals; usual maintenance dose 500–750 mg/day

Table 52–S2 Major Side Effects of and Contraindications for Slow-Acting Antirheumatic Drugs

BODY SYSTEM/ Side Effect	CONTRAINDICATION/ PRECAUTION	COMMENTS AND NURSING IMPLICATIONS
Azathioprine		
BLOOD Leukopenia and/or thrombocytopenia, increased risk of infection or bleeding tendencies	Leukemias, bleeding tendencies; use of anticoagulants, other drugs that suppress bone marrow	Monitor closely for signs of platelet depression (excessive bleeding) or immunosuppression (flu-like symptoms, etc); stress need for periodic blood tests
Gold Salts		
BLOOD Blood dyscrasias, bleeding tendencies, immune suppression	Radiation therapy; other drugs that affect blood-forming tissues (other SAARDs, chemotherapeutic agents, immunosuppressants)	Complete blood tests required before and periodically during therapy; assess for abnormal bruising, bleeding, flu-like symptoms, anemia; avoid concomitant use of other drugs that suppress blood-forming tissues
CARDIOVASCULAR Nitritoid crisis (with parenteral gold): facial flushing, warmth; severe hypotension, tachycardia; dizziness or lightheadedness due to hypotension	History of ischemic heart, brain, or extremity disorders	Most likely on first dose; is main reason for administering small initial test dose; have patient in supine position during and for at least 10 min after drug injection; close monitoring of vital signs mandatory; have devices and drugs for cardiopulmonary resuscitation, support available; not likely to occur with orally administered gold (auranofin)
GASTROINTESTINAL Painful buccal lesions		May be severe, persist after gold therapy discontinued
Diarrhea	Ulcerative colitis, other severe GI disorders	May be severe, more likely to occur with auranofin (oral gold); monitor all patients for GI bleeding, regardless of gold salt selected
RENAL, HEPATIC Organ damage	Renal or hepatic disease; hepatitis	Assess for jaundice, abdominal pain, proteinuria or hematuria, etc
SKIN Skin rashes, possibly pruritic or severe		May be severe, longlasting; often warrants discontinuation of therapy; more likely with injectable gold
Hydroxychloroquine		
EYE Chloroquine retinopathy: decreased acuity; retinal and/or corneal deposits	Visual impairment	Dose-dependent; frequent ophthalmic examinations required
BLOOD Blood dyscrasias	See gold salts	See gold salts

(continued)

Table 52–S2 | Major Side Effects of and Contraindications for Slow-Acting Antirheumatic Drugs (*Continued*)

BODY SYSTEM/ Side Effect	CONTRAINDICATION/ PRECAUTION	COMMENTS AND NURSING IMPLICATIONS
Methotrexate		
See Table 59–5		
D-Penicillamine		
BLOOD Blood dyscrasias	See gold salts	See gold salts
RENAL Glomerular damage, possibly leading to nephrotic syndrome	Renal disease	Frequent urinalysis and measurement of body weight (to detect edema) necessary

Table 52–I2 | Major Interactions Between Slow-Acting Antirheumatic Drugs and Other Agents

AGENT	RESULT OF INTERACTION	COMMENTS AND NURSING IMPLICATIONS
Interactions Involving Gold Salts		
None		
Interactions Involving Hydroxychloroquine		
Digoxin (Chapter 31)	Increased digoxin blood levels, effects; possible toxicity	Monitor digoxin levels during combined therapy; may need to reduce digoxin dosages
Interactions Involving Methotrexate		
See Table 59–I		
Interactions Involving D-Penicillamine		
Antacids, esp. aluminum-containing (Chapter 30)	Reduced or absent penicillamine effect	Avoid interaction or space administration of interactants as much as possible; teach patients accordingly; administer penicillamine on empty stomach (food also decreases absorption)
Digitalis (digoxin, digitoxin; Chapter 31)	Reduced digitalis effect	Separate administration by as much as possible, and teach patients; assess for decreased digitalis effects; may need to remeasure digitalis blood levels and adjust dosages when starting or stopping penicillamine
Iron salts, oral (Chapter 61)	Reduced penicillamine absorption, effects	Avoid combined use; separate administration by as much as possible; teach patients who may self-prescribe iron-containing vitamin/mineral supplements

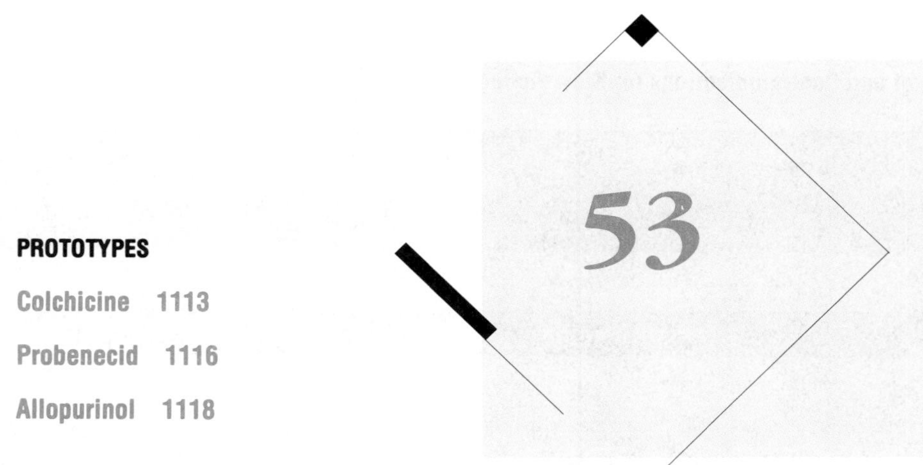

PROTOTYPES

Drugs for Gout and Other Hyperuricemic States

This chapter discusses the three major groups of drugs that are used to treat gout, a common metabolic disorder, and its underlying cause, *hyperuricemia*. First, however, some features of the disorder itself are reviewed.

Biochemistry and Pathophysiology of Hyperuricemia and Gout

The breakdown of DNA, RNA, and adenosine triphosphate (ATP) is part of the normal turnover of cells within the body. It provides a constant source of metabolites called purines, which include adenosine, inosine, and hypoxanthine. Toward the end of the purine breakdown pathway, hypoxanthine is converted to xanthine by an enzyme called *xanthine oxidase*. Xanthine oxidase then converts xanthine to uric acid (Fig. 53–1).

Uric acid circulates in the bloodstream in the form of the somewhat soluble sodium salt, sodium urate (or urate, for short). Uric acid is eventually excreted by the kidneys. A healthy person on a normal diet excretes

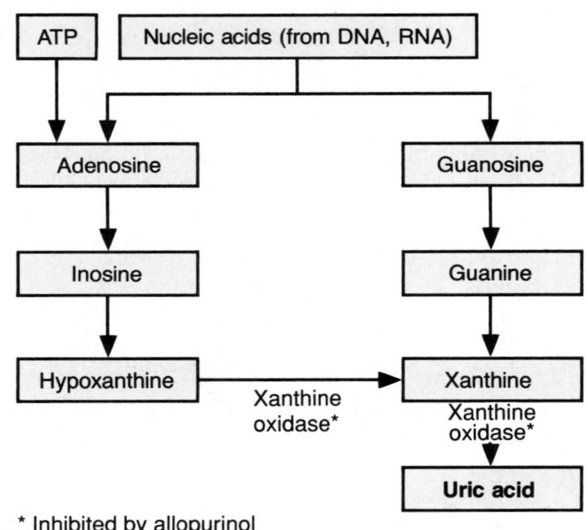

Figure 53–1

Overview of uric acid synthesis. Xanthine oxidase is the critical enzymatic step in the formation of uric acid from the more soluble purine precursors adenosine, inosine, hypoxanthine, and xanthine. Xanthine oxidase activity is inhibited by allopurinol.

Major reference tables appear beginning on p. 1122.

Table 53–1 Serum Uric Acid Levels and the Incidence of Gout in Males

Serum Uric Acid Level* (mg/100 mL)	Approximate Incidence of Gout (%)
<6	1
6.0–6.9	5
7.0–7.9	20
8.0–8.9	30
>9	90

*Normal range of serum uric acid levels: males—2.1–7.5 mg/100 mL; females—2.0–6.6 mg/100 mL. Data apply to persistent (untreated) elevations of serum urate.

about 0.4 to 0.8 grams of uric acid in the urine every 24 hours. Normal serum uric acid levels are between 2.1 and 7.5 mg/dL (100 mL) in men, and 2.0 to 6.6 mg/dL in women. Hyperuricemia is an increase of serum urate levels above normal. In simplest terms, it occurs because of increased uric acid production, reduced renal uric acid excretion, or both.

Uric acid is not directly toxic to cells. It causes problems because it is poorly soluble in body fluids, especially fluids that have a low (ie, acidic) pH value. If the uric acid concentration rises too high, it comes out of solution and precipitates (crystallizes), causing the signs and symptoms of gout. The higher the serum urate concentration and the longer it is elevated, the more likely that gouty symptoms will appear (Table 53–1).

Classification of Hyperuricemia and Gout

Hyperuricemia and gout are classified as primary or secondary. Primary hyperuricemia usually involves a genetically based metabolic disorder that causes excessive uric acid production. Lesch-Nyhan syndrome, which causes profound and eventually lethal effects in young children born with the disorder, is an example. Secondary hyperuricemia is more common. It involves hyperuricemia due to other causes, such as renal disease (decreased urate excretion), leukemias, and other disorders that cause uric acid overproduction at rates that cannot be handled by the kidneys. As noted later, drugs also can cause hyperuricemia or further increases of already elevated uric acid levels.

The typical person with gout is male and about 50 years old. He may have had hyperuricemia for several years but be symptom-free. He is apt to be overweight and have other cardiovascular risk factors, such as hypertension, atherosclerosis, or hyperlipidemias. Premenopausal women and prepubertal males or females are affected by gout much less often.

Progression and Consequences of Hyperuricemia

Asymptomatic Hyperuricemia

A person may be hyperuricemic but have no signs or symptoms of the disorder for many years. During that time the increase in serum uric acid levels may go completely undetected unless the blood is tested for it. This condition is called *asymptomatic hyperuricemia* (Fig. 53–2).

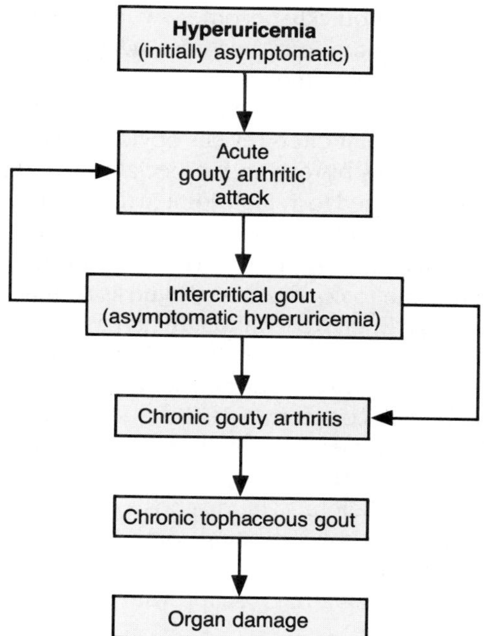

Figure 53–2

Progression of hyperuricemia and gout. Patients with hyperuricemia may be asymptomatic until uric acid crystals precipitate in the joints, leading to an acute gout attack. With or without treatment, symptoms may subside, leading to another asymptomatic period (intercritical gout) with persistent hyperuricemia. With time, gouty arthritis, chronic tophaceous gout, and potentially fatal organ damage may occur.

However, if uric acid levels rise sufficiently high, eventually an *acute gout (gouty arthritic) attack* will occur. These attacks usually come on suddenly and often are triggered by illness, trauma, strenuous exercise, high alcohol intake, or a combination of these factors. A common feature of many of these triggers is dehydration, which concentrates uric acid in the body fluids. Hyperuricemia becomes clinically important when symptoms appear.

Acute Gout

Most patients with an acute gout attack develop *podagra* as the first sign. Podagra is acute inflammation of a joint in one of the great toes. It eventually appears in nearly 90% of patients with gout. Unlike most other arthritic attacks, which usually affect several joints at once, the first gouty arthritic attack almost always involves only one joint initially—usually one of the great toes. Thus, gout is considered a *monoarticular* arthritis. The appearance of a single inflamed joint, especially in the great toe, is an important characteristic in the diagnosis of gout.

The microscopic uric acid crystals that form in the synovial fluid work like sandpaper to destroy the smooth lubricated joint surfaces that normally allow pain-free motion. Leukocytes are attracted to the inflamed area. They engulf the crystals and release a variety of inflammatory substances, some of which are acidic. Local pH falls, favoring more uric acid crystallization. The joint quickly becomes swollen, red, and immobile. Moving the joint becomes nearly unbearable; even gently touching the area causes excruciating pain. A comparison of the affected joint with the corresponding unaffected joint often reveals obvious deformity.

The patient's history and, especially, the signs and symptoms localized to a single joint in the great toe make the diagnosis of gout relatively simple and straightforward in well over 90% of cases. However, further testing is usually done to confirm the diagnosis so that proper treatment can be started. Although increased serum uric acid levels are the cause of gout, a blood test does not confirm the diagnosis. During the attack, much of the excess urate is concentrated in the joint. As a result, serum uric acid levels during the attack are normal, subnormal, or (at most) only slightly elevated. Thus, blood tests are rarely helpful. The diagnosis of gout is almost always confirmed by aspirating some fluid from the affected joint and examining it for the presence of uric acid crystals using a microscope with a special (polarized) light source.

NURSING IMPLICATIONS

Question orders to draw nothing more than a blood sample for the purpose of confirming the diagnosis of acute gout. Do anticipate that the physician will aspirate the joint. This is a fear- and anxiety-provoking procedure for the patient, who is already in extreme pain and distress. Explain why the procedure will be done, allay anxiety as best as possible, and be sure to check whether appropriate premedications (usually an injectable narcotic, such as meperidine, and an antiemetic, such as hydroxyzine) have been ordered and administered first. Do not be surprised if the physician does not inject a local anesthetic (eg, lidocaine) into the area around the joint before it is aspirated; in the presence of severe inflammation and a very low local pH, safe doses of local anesthetics are not likely to work well (see Chapter 19, p 291).

Intercritical Gout

If left untreated, the acute gout attack may subside spontaneously. (However, few patients can tolerate the intense pain without seeking medical attention.) Whether the attack stops on its own or with appropriate drug therapy, the patient subsequently enters another asymptomatic period. Blood tests will almost certainly reveal hyperuricemia again. The period following one gout attack and possibly preceding another is called *intercritical gout* (literally meaning between crises, or acute attacks). If the patient is not treated and urate levels remain high, the acute attacks will return more frequently. The patient can develop more gout attacks, eventually, developing *chronic gouty arthritis,* with permanent deformity and immobility of the joint.

Tophaceous Gout

When hyperuricemia is sufficiently severe and longlasting, uric acid crystals can form in soft tissues, including the skin and organs. This is called *tophaceous gout,* and it is a serious condition. In some skin sites where these deposits, called *tophi,* commonly form, such as the earlobes, you may be able to feel the gritty or sandy nodules as you palpate the tissues; you may be able to see larger deposits.

Gouty arthritis may be painful and disabling; end-organ damage can be fatal. Uric acid crystal deposits can form in the kidney tubules or the renal vascular supply. The urine in the distal tubules is normally an acidic environment, which favors uric acid crystallization. As a result, the distal tubules are often an initial site of kidney damage. Urate crystal formation in the coronary arteries can cause heart failure, infarction, or arrhythmias. Drugs can interrupt these processes, both acutely and chronically. When symptoms of hyperuricemia occur, drug therapy is always indicated.

Drug Therapy

There are three main drugs or drug groups used to treat gout.

- Antiinflammatory drugs. The prototype antiinflammatory drug for gout is *colchicine.*
- Uricosuric drugs, which by definition increase uric acid excretion. The prototype is *probenecid.*
- Uric acid synthesis inhibitors. There is only one approved drug classified this way: *allopurinol.*

Drugs are given during an acute attack specifically to alleviate pain and inflammation as quickly as possible. The long-term goal is to prevent chronic gouty arthritis and organ damage. This is done by continuing antiinflammatory drugs for a while and then giving other medications that lower serum urate levels, either by increasing uric acid excretion or decreasing its synthesis. As noted below, uricosuric drugs or uric acid synthesis inhibitors are often given too soon.

There is no question about the importance of treating acute gout or any hyperuricemic state in which symptoms have occurred. However, many clinicians feel that asymptomatic hyperuricemia—urate elevations in patients who have had no related symptoms—should not be treated with drugs. Although the drugs discussed below are relatively safe and free from side effects, for persons with no symptoms of hyperuricemia the risks of using drugs may be greater than the risks of no therapy at all.

I. Antiinflammatory Drugs

Historically, colchicine has been considered the prototype antiinflammatory drug for gout because it is efficacious and because, for all practical purposes, it is not effective or suitable for managing other inflammatory states. Its use for acute gout is declining considerably, but colchicine is still important for gout prophylaxis.

PROTOTYPE

Colchicine

Absorption, Distribution, Metabolism, and Excretion

Colchicine is absorbed well from the gastrointestinal (GI) tract. Some of the drug is metabolized in the liver. The metabolites are excreted in the bile and then eliminated from the body in the feces. Renal excretion of unmetabolized colchicine is particularly important, and renal dysfunction requires dosage reductions.

Pharmacologic Effects

Therapeutic doses of colchicine suppress inflammation, indirectly relieving pain. Colchicine probably works by inhibiting the ability of leukocytes to migrate to, and release their noxious mediators at, sites of inflammation. Colchicine is not nearly as effective as a traditional antiinflammatory drug for arthritis pain not caused by gout. In fact, the effect of colchicine is so specific that if joint pain and inflammation decrease after a full dose of the drug is administered the odds are great that the symptoms were due to gout.

Colchicine does not lower serum urate levels; it has no effect on urate formation or urate excretion.

Clinical Indications and Administration

Colchicine is available for oral or intravenous (IV) administration. The drug is available alone and as a fixed-dose oral combination with another antigout drug, probenecid (marketed as COLBENEMID; see p 1116). Only plain colchicine should be used to treat acute gout. Dosages are provided in Table 53–C. The dose may have to be titrated until symptoms are relieved or GI side effects occur.

Colchicine works best for acute gout when the first dose is given as soon as possible after the onset of symptoms. With oral therapy, dramatic relief usually occurs after the first or second dose, and most patients are symptom-free within 48 hours. Relief comes hours faster with IV administration.

Unfortunately, the high and frequently repeated doses of colchicine needed to stop an acute gout attack usually cause intolerable GI side effects (see below and Table 53–S). Some other nonsteroidal antiinflammatory drugs (NSAIDs, eg indomethacin; see Chapter 52, and p 1115) work just as well and nearly as quickly as colchicine; moreover, they cause fewer severe side effects. Therefore, few physicians now use colchicine for acute gout.

Oral colchicine is still considered acceptable for the prophylaxis of attacks during the intercritical period, mainly because maintenance doses (see Table 53–C) are somewhat lower than those used for acute treatment and because the drug does not need to be administered so frequently. As a result, side effects usually are somewhat less severe. Hyperuricemic patients undergoing elective surgery who have had gout but are currently symptom-free may receive colchicine prophylactically for a few days before and after the operation.

The other antigout drugs—probenecid or allopurinol—may also be indicated during the intercritical period. These are discussed shortly.

NURSING IMPLICATIONS

Given the availability of other, more tolerable antiinflammatory drugs, you should double-check orders calling for oral or parenteral colchicine for an acute attack. Always question orders calling for administration of the colchicine-probenecid combination product when the patient has acute gout; the preparation is not indicated for acute symptoms. Check the preoperative patient's history, and inquire whether colchicine prophylaxis is indicated.

Some physicians give colchicine IV for acute gout because the incidence of GI upset is less than that associated with oral therapy. This is still risky. There have been cases of serious cardiovascular reactions with single doses and of fatal bone marrow suppression following repeated IV administration. Follow these guidelines to reduce dangers, and refuse to give the drug if they cannot be met:

- Never give more than 2 mg of colchicine IV to start.
- Always inject the dose over at least 2 to 5 minutes.
- Never give more than 4 mg during any 24-hour period.
- Never give more than 4 mg to treat any one gout attack.
- Do not repeat IV colchicine therapy for several weeks.
- Do not give any colchicine, by any route, for 7 days after the patient has received a full course (4 mg) of IV colchicine.

To avoid severe local tissue damage and pain, be sure the needle or catheter is in a vein lumen. Follow the injection with a sterile saline flush.

Side Effects, Adverse Reactions, and Contraindications

Without question, GI side effects are the most common side effects with oral colchicine. Intense abdominal pain or cramping, nausea, vomiting, or diarrhea often occurs when full therapeutic doses are used to treat an acute attack. When diarrhea is severe yet continued colchicine therapy is advisable, antidiarrheal drugs (eg, opiates) may be needed.

Colchicine is contraindicated in patients with a history of peptic ulcer disease or GI bleeding. (These disorders relatively contraindicate the use of all NSAIDs, but the risks with colchicine appear to be greater.)

Renal dysfunction reduces colchicine elimination, increases blood levels, and increases the risk of side effects or toxicity. Thus, dosage reductions may be needed. Urinary levels of colchicine that are too high may cause renal tubular damage. This can arise from overdoses or from renal dysfunction, but it can also occur with usual doses given to patients whose renal function is good but who are dehydrated. Overall, avoid giving the drug in these situations.

High oral doses or IV doses that are too great or too fast can cause serious cardiovascular reactions. These usually are reflections of overdose (see below).

NURSING IMPLICATIONS

Ensure adequate hydration and monitor urine output if possible. Explain to patients the need to ingest adequate amounts of fluids. Advise them to report intolerable GI pain, diarrhea, vomiting, or signs of GI or renal damage (bloody vomitus or stool; black, tarry stools; discolored or bloody urine).

◆ Use During Pregnancy and Lactation

Colchicine crosses the placental barrier and may cause fetal malformations or death. Pregnant women should therefore not take colchicine. Termination of pregnancy should be considered if conception occurs during colchicine therapy and therapy cannot be stopped.

◆ Use in Children

There is no information on the safety or effectiveness of colchicine in children.

◆ Use in the Elderly

Decreased renal function may lead to the accumulation of colchicine in the bloodstream; anticipate the need for reduced dosages. Be aware that excessive fluid and electrolyte loss owing to severe diarrhea or vomiting—which are risks for any patient—may pose greater dangers in the elderly.

Interactions with Other Drugs

Colchicine does not participate in clinically significant interactions with other drugs. However, owing to the risk of vascular damage and bleeding, administer colchicine with care and proper monitoring to patients receiving oral or injectable anticoagulants.

Overdoses and Toxicity

Eight milligrams of colchicine (only twice the maximum daily dose), taken at once, can cause serious toxicity. If the overdose was taken orally, GI problems occur first. Severe nausea, vomiting, and diarrhea, which are common with full therapeutic doses of colchicine, are likely to be accompanied by loose, bloody stools caused by GI bleeding or true hemorrhage. Intense abdominal cramping is likely.

Regardless of the administration route, colchicine overdoses may cause serious damage to the vascular endothelium, leading to hemorrhage, shock (cardiovascular collapse), or eventually both. Since colchicine is excreted in the urine, hematuria and serious damage to the renal vasculature can occur. Renal damage eventually leads to oliguria and renal failure.

The combined GI and vascular effects lead to dehydration and hypotension. Fluid and electrolyte changes may cause muscle paralysis. The patient generally remains conscious throughout this ordeal and then becomes delirious and has seizures. Fatal respiratory depression or arrest can occur during the seizures.

Treatment of colchicine overdoses is supportive and addresses symptoms. There is no antidote. Oral overdoses are managed first by inducing emesis or performing gastric lavage to reduce further drug absorption (Appendix C).

Regardless of the overdose route, treatment may require hemodialysis or peritoneal dialysis to reduce colchicine blood levels; IV fluid administration to correct dehydration; vasopressors and fluids to counteract shock; and ventilatory support. Morphine or atropine can be used to alleviate severe cramping, but they are not antidotes; they will not improve cardiovascular or renal status, and morphine can intensify depressed ventilation.

Other Antiinflammatory Drugs as Colchicine Alternatives

Indomethacin, an NSAID, is the most commonly used alternative to colchicine for the treatment of acute gout and for maintenance therapy. However, some other NSAIDS are also indicated for gout. (See Chapter 52 and Table 52–C, for more information and dosages.) Some physicians also use corticosteroids, which also exert antiinflammatory activity, for gout. The choice usually depends on unique characteristics of the patient and on physician preferences and experience.

Aspirin should not be used for treating gout or for prophylactic therapy. As noted in Chapter 52, this prototype NSAID can reduce renal uric acid secretion and interact with the uricosuric drugs that are important in long-term management of hyperuricemia. In essence, aspirin is contraindicated for persons with hyperuricemia.

NURSING IMPLICATIONS

Some NSAIDS that are approved for gout—eg, indomethacin—are available in both immediate-acting and sustained-release oral formulations. Question medication orders calling for sustained-release forms for treating an ongoing gout attack. They act much too slowly to be of help in the acute setting. If a sustained-acting preparation is prescribed for maintenance therapy (an acceptable option), be sure the patient has a supply of the immediate-acting preparation on hand in case of an acute flare-up; be sure the patient understands when and how to use it.

Advise patients with a history of gout or hyperuricemia not to use aspirin—even for relief of mild headache, fever, or pain—without a physician's approval.

II. Increasing Uric Acid Excretion: Uricosuric Drugs

Uricosuric drugs are defined as drugs that increase renal excretion of uric acid. They play important adjunctive roles in management of chronic hyperuricemia. Probenecid (BENEMID) is the prototype; the related drug is sulfinpyrazone (ANTURANE). These agents provide one important way to accomplish the second major objective of gout therapy, the reduction of serum urate levels.

PROTOTYPE

Probenecid

Absorption, Distribution, Metabolism, and Excretion

Probenecid (BENEMID), which is given orally, is rapidly absorbed from the GI tract. It is extensively metabolized in the liver and excreted by the kidneys. Alkalinizing the urine increases the excretion of probenecid and reduces its effectiveness. Urinary acidification does not alter probenecid elimination markedly.

Pharmacologic Effects

Low (subtherapeutic) blood levels of probenecid inhibit renal excretion of uric acid by reducing tubular secretion of urate. Therapeutic doses increase urate excretion by inhibiting uric acid's tubular reabsorption. With continued administration of full therapeutic doses, serum urate levels gradually fall toward normal.

Probenecid and the related drug sulfinpyrazone have no antiinflammatory activity and do not inhibit uric acid synthesis.

Clinical Indications and Administration

Hyperuricemia

Probenecid is indicated for the management of hyperuricemia, such as that associated with gout or gouty arthritis. It is particularly useful when laboratory tests indicate that the patient is excreting lower than normal amounts of uric acid in the urine—ie, when decreased uric acid excretion appears to be the major problem. Desired outcomes are an increased 24-hour urine output, a significant reduction or normalization of serum urine levels, a reduced frequency and severity of arthritic attacks, and a decreased risk of tophaceous gout or organ damage. Probenecid dosages are listed in Table 53–C.

Several months of probenecid therapy may be needed before urate levels fall satisfactorily. Antiinflammatory drug therapy should be continued during this time. Probenecid therapy may need to be continued for years or, in some cases, for the rest of the patient's life.

Probenecid is available by itself and as a fixed-dose combination with colchicine (500 mg probenecid and 0.5 mg colchicine per tablet, marketed as COLBENEMID). It is essential to repeat that the probenecid–colchicine combination should *not* be used as initial therapy of acute gout. Plain colchicine or another antiinflammatory drug should be used first. The antiinflammatory drug should always be available to the patient for treating acute gout flare-ups.

Uricosuric drug therapy should not be started until gout attacks can be stopped completely, for at least two months, by the use of a suitable antiinflammatory drug alone. Only then is it acceptable to start a uricosuric drug. If uricosuric therapy is started too soon, gout attacks may recur or become more severe. If a gout attack develops during uricosuric therapy, the uricosuric drug should be temporarily stopped (or the dose reduced) and antiinflammatory drug therapy restarted (or the dose increased). The same rules apply to the use of allopurinol, which is discussed below.

NURSING IMPLICATIONS

Be aware that guidelines about when to start uricosuric therapy are often overlooked, mainly because physicians know that gout is caused by hyperuricemia and that elevated serum uric acid levels can be reduced with a uricosuric drug. Question medication orders calling for administration of a uricosuric drug or a probenecid–colchicine combination to a patient with current or recent gout that has not been controlled with antiinflammatory drugs first. Question orders calling for a uricosuric or uricosuric–antiinflammatory combination to treat an ongoing gout attack.

Whenever uricosuric drug therapy is started, assess more closely for a return of gout attacks. Have the patient notify the physician immediately if they occur so that proper antiinflammatory drug therapy can be restarted or modified.

Adjunct to Penicillin Therapy

Probenecid can be used adjunctively with penicillins—usually ampicillin—to manage uncomplicated gonorrhea or gonococcal infections. Such disorders require very high antibiotic levels for effective treatment. Probenecid is used because it inhibits renal penicillin (ampicillin) excretion, thereby increasing blood levels and prolonging the antibiotic's half-life. Fixed-dose combination products of probenecid and ampicillin (eg, POLYCILLIN-PRB, PROBAMPACIN) are available. Probenecid can also be used as an adjunct to cephalosporin therapy.

Side Effects, Adverse Reactions, and Contraindications

Probenecid is relatively safe. It may cause GI distress in a few patients and should be used cautiously in patients with a history of peptic ulcer disease. Drug rash occurs in a small number of patients and may indicate hypersensitivity to probenecid and the possibility of future anaphylactoid reactions. Probenecid is therefore contraindicated for these patients.

Paradoxically, worsening of gout is an important potential side effect of uricosuric drugs used to treat hyperuricemia. When therapy is started, the low blood levels of drug can decrease renal excretion of urate. Simultaneously, the drug can displace uric acid from tissue sites into the bloodstream. Both effects temporarily increase serum urate levels and thus can increase the risk or severity of a gout attack. This is one reason why antiinflammatory drug should be given for several months first. Worsening of gout or increases of blood uric acid levels can also occur during chronic uricosuric drug therapy if the dose is subtherapeutic, either because of improper prescribing or (more often) poor compliance.

Uricosuric drugs can also increase the risk of the formation of urate stones in the renal tubules. This is most likely to occur in patients with severe hyperuricemia, patients with poor renal function, or both. Either condition relatively contraindicates uricosuric drug use. The reason for this adverse effect is simple: Even when serum uric acid levels are high, the uric acid concentration in the blood is relatively dilute owing to a large blood volume. However, uricosuric drugs effectively move large amounts of uric acid from the blood into a much smaller volume of acidic urine; that is, uric acid is concentrated in the urine, increasing the likelihood of crystallization.

To reduce the chance of kidney damage, all patients who receive uricosuric drugs should be well hydrated. They should be encouraged to drink sufficient water to maintain a urine output above 2 liters per day. Some patients may also need to take a urinary alkalinizer, such as sodium bicarbonate (3–8 g per day) or potassium citrate (7.5 g per day), if the risk of urinary stone formation seems great. Urinary alkalinization increases uric acid solubility and so reduces the risk of stone formation. It also increases the delivery of probenecid to its renal sites of action.

Patients with poor renal function or a history of kidney stones should not receive uricosuric drugs. Allopurinol, a drug discussed shortly, should be used instead.

NURSING IMPLICATIONS

Encourage patients to measure their daily urine output and drink enough water to maintain the desired output of 2 to 3 liters per day. Explaining, in simple terms, the reason for doing this promotes compliance. Advise patients to report sudden decreases of urine output, discoloration of the urine (which may indicate hematuria), or flank pain (which may indicate development of renal stones).

Be aware that giving sodium bicarbonate to maintain urate solubility may cause significant problems for patients with hypertension or heart failure; monitor accordingly. Potassium citrate may cause hyperkalemia and arrhythmias, particularly in digitalized patients and those taking potassium-sparing diuretics.

◆ Use During Pregnancy and Lactation

Use probenecid in pregnant women only when the expected benefits outweigh the potential risks. Breast-feeding probably should be discouraged.

◆ Use in Children

Probenecid is used in children mainly as an adjunct to penicillin or cephalosporin therapy. Dosages are based on body weight. Probenecid should not be administered to children less than two years old.

◆ Use in the Elderly

Evaluate for renal impairment, which may require reducing the initial and maintenance doses of probenecid. Maintain adequate hydration as for all patients, but be aware that alkalinizing the urine, which may reduce the risk of urate stone formation, may pose greater systemic risks to the elderly patient.

Interactions with Other Drugs

The therapeutically desirable interaction between probenecid and penicillin or cephalosporin antibiotics was noted above. However, there are several other interactions in which the outcome is unwanted or potentially toxic (Table 53–1).

The most common interaction involves probenecid with aspirin or other salicylates. These antiinflammatory drugs can significantly antagonize the ability of probenecid to lower serum uric acid levels. The interaction occurs with all aspirin formulations (eg, plain, buffered, and enteric-coated) and apparently with any dose of aspirin. More information on this is given in Chapter 52.

Probenecid also interacts with dyphylline (a theophylline-like drug), methotrexate (used for some cancers, arthritis, and psoriasis), and zidovudine (used for AIDS and AIDS-related complex) by decreasing their renal excretion. In doing so, probenecid increases their blood levels. The interaction can increase the therapeutic effects, or allow a dosage reduction, of the interactant. However, a more likely outcome is an increased risk of toxicity caused by the interactant.

NURSING IMPLICATIONS

Be sure patients with hyperuricemia are instructed to avoid using aspirin or aspirin-containing medications, even for relief of simple headache or fever. Aspirin use should be prescribed and monitored by a physician. When an over-the-counter (OTC) remedy is indicated, ibuprofen or acetaminophen are preferred because they do not interact with probenecid.

Overdoses and Toxicity

There are few reports of overdose-related probenecid toxicity. The major problems to be expected are GI, and they can usually be managed by discontinuing drug administration. Treatment is symptomatic and supportive.

Related Drug

Sulfinpyrazone

Sulfinpyrazone (ANTURANE) is the other approved uricosuric drug (see Table 53–C for dosages). Like probenecid, sulfinpyrazone is used for managing hyperuricemia. However, sulfinpyrazone differs from the prototype in some clinically important ways, and those differences usually make the prototype the first choice.

Unlike probenecid, sulfinpyrazone inhibits platelet aggregation. Therefore, it should be used cautiously in patients who have bleeding disorders or are taking any drugs that interfere with blood coagulation.

Sulfinpyrazone is more likely than probenecid to cause gastric distress. Taking the drug with meals or a glass of milk reduces this problem. Nevertheless, the risk of gut irritation relatively contraindicates sulfinpyrazone use for patients with active peptic ulcers. The drug should be used cautiously in patients with healed ulcers.

The interaction between probenicid and salicylates (aspirin) noted above applies to sulfinpyrazone, but other probenecid interactions do not. However, sulfinpyrazone interacts with still other drugs that do not interact with the prototype. They are

- acetaminophen, especially at excessive or toxic doses. Sulfinpyrazone stimulates the formation of a hepatotoxic acetaminophen metabolite.
- oral hypoglycemic drugs. Sulfinpyrazone can inhibit the metabolic inactivation of such drugs as tolbutamide, increasing the risk of excessive lowering of blood glucose levels.
- warfarin. There is a significantly increased risk of excessive bleeding, owing to sulfinpyrazone's ability to inhibit warfarin metabolism and platelet aggregation.

Nursing implications related to sulfinpyrazone administration are listed in Tables 53–S and 53–I. See Table 53–C for dosages.

III. Inhibition of Uric Acid Synthesis: Allopurinol

Reducing serum urate levels is a desirable long-term objective for the patient with gout, but drugs such as probenecid may cause dangerous renal effects if the patient has severe hyperuricemia or poor kidney function. Allopurinol (LOPURIN; ZYLOPRIM) can be used for these, and other, patients. Like a uricosuric, allopurinol lowers blood urate levels. However, it does so in a very different manner. There are no related drugs approved for use in the United States.

PROTOTYPE

Allopurinol

Absorption, Distribution, Metabolism, and Excretion

Allopurinol is readily absorbed after oral administration. The drug is metabolized, but renal excretion is the main way by which the drug is eliminated from the body.

Pharmacologic Effects

Allopurinol inhibits uric acid synthesis by inhibiting xanthine oxidase, the enzyme that eventually forms uric acid from its metabolic precursors. Allopurinol itself is a weak inhibitor of xanthine oxidase. However, one of allopurinol's metabolites, called oxypurinol (or alloxanthine) is a more powerful and longlasting xanthine oxidase inhibitor.

It takes about a week of continuous allopurinol therapy before blood uric acid levels start to show measurable falls, and usually several months of treatment are needed to reach and maintain normal serum urate levels. Over the long run, renal excretion of uric acid falls because there is less uric acid that needs to be eliminated from the bloodstream.

Allopurinol has no antiinflammatory or uricosuric activity.

Clinical Indications and Administration

Allopurinol has several clinical uses. Dosages are listed in Table 53–C; they should be reduced if the patient has reduced renal function.

When the gout patient has severe hyperuricemia or impaired renal function, allopurinol is preferred to a uricosuric drug. Allopurinol reduces the amount of uric acid delivered to the kidneys and so reduces the risk of renal complications. (In contrast, a uricosuric drug increases the amount of urate that is excreted and so could increase the risk of renal damage owing to excessive urine levels of uric acid.)

When allopurinol is to be used for a patient who has had a gout attack, treatment should start in the same way in which uricosuric drug therapy is started: symptoms should be controlled first with an antiinflammatory drug, and once the patient has remained symptom-free allopurinol therapy can begin.

When allopurinol therapy is started, tissue deposits of uric acid may dissolve, redistribute into the bloodstream, and then reform in the joints. This can trigger a gout attack, necessitating the administration of an antiinflammatory drug (or a higher dose if one is already being used). Starting with a low dose of allopurinol (eg, 100 mg per day) and increasing it slowly seems to reduce the risk of such problems. A few gout patients may require colchicine, a uricosuric drug, and allopurinol. Long-term allopurinol therapy is usually needed, and serum uric acid levels are likely to rise once again when allopurinol therapy is stopped.

A related indication for allopurinol is the prophylaxis of renal calcium oxalate stones in patients who excrete unusually large amounts of uric acid. Such individuals may or may not have had a prior gout attack.

Allopurinol also plays an important adjunctive role in preventing hyperuricemia and its consequences—and renal damage in particular—for high-risk patients who receive drugs that increase urate levels. Such drugs include thiazide and high-ceiling diuretics and drugs used to treat malignancies such as leukemias (see below). Dosages are given in Table 53–C.

Lastly, allopurinol is an important adjunctive drug in oncology and cancer therapy. In patients with leukemias, for example, the overproduction and turnover of white blood cells release large amounts of uric acid into the bloodstream. Administration of chemotherapeutic drugs that kill massive numbers of blood cells can raise urate levels even more. The potential outcomes include not only gout, but also renal damage. Thus, allopurinol is often given prophylactically before a course of cancer therapy.

NURSING IMPLICATIONS

The need to maintain adequate hydration and monitor urine output applies to allopurinol as well as to uricosuric drugs. Urinary alkalinization may also be needed until serum uric acid levels fall sufficiently. A urinary alkalinizer is usually indicated if the patient is also taking a uricosuric drug and if there are no other contraindications. It is wise for gout patients to have a supply of an antiinflammatory drug available to take, as directed by the physician, if a gout attack occurs. Advise the patient to notify the physician promptly if an attack does develop.

Assess for indicators of renal dysfunction (eg, increase serum creatinine levels); anticipate the need to reduce allopurinol dosages if renal dysfunction is present.

Be aware that thiazide diuretics are being evaluated for prophylaxis of calcium oxalate stones. On the positive side, they reduce renal calcium and urate excretion and modestly alkalinize the urine. All these actions help reduce stone formation. However, these drugs can cause unwanted increases of serum urate (and calcium) levels, thereby triggering a gout attack.

Side Effects, Adverse Reactions, and Contraindications

Allopurinol is safe for and well tolerated by most patients. The drug occasionally causes drowsiness. Patients who experience this should be cautioned against operating hazardous machinery or motor vehicles. Minor GI distress may occur; it can be alleviated by taking allopurinol after meals. Severe diarrhea should be evaluated by a physician.

There are rare reports of hypersensitivity and hepatotoxic reactions to allopurinol. Some reactions have been fatal. Skin rashes are usually the first indication of such an adverse response. Allopurinol therapy should be stopped, and not restarted, if they appear. Other manifestations include elevations of blood urea nitrogen (BUN) levels and liver enzymes (alkaline phosphatase, AST, ALT). During therapy, follow the results of the test for renal function. Rises of serum creatinine or BUN levels may indicate allopurinol-induced renal problems.

Interactions with Other Drugs

Allopurinol can inhibit the metabolic detoxification of thiopurine anticancer drugs (eg, azathioprine, 6-mercaptopurine), a process that depends on xanthine oxidase activity. Unless the dose of the thiopurine is reduced (substantial dosage reductions are usually indicated; see Table 53–1), serious toxicity can occur.

Allopurinol also seems to increase the allergenicity of ampicillin and perhaps that of other penicillins. The usual outcome is an increased risk of penicillin-induced rash. Usual management involves discontinuing allopurinol, reducing the allopurinol dose, or using noninteracting drugs instead.

Overdoses and Toxicity

There are few reports of serious allopurinol overdose. Treatment is symptomatic and supportive.

IV. Other Considerations and Nursing Implications for Hyperuricemic Patients

Several things can be done to help drug therapy of hyperuricemia and gout work better. Some of these are nondrug measures. Some may dramatically reduce the consequences of hyperuricemia, reduce the frequency of gout attacks, and even reduce the dosages of drugs that might be used.

Diet

Stringent restriction of dietary protein intake to reduce uric acid production was common until the development of effective drugs for reducing serum urate levels. However, it is often unreasonable to expect patients to eat a mainly vegetarian diet; proper drug therapy is more acceptable and effective. Nevertheless, most patients should be instructed to eat meat in moderation and to avoid purine-rich foods (liver, sweetbreads, brains, sardines, and anchovies) completely.

Encourage overweight patients to lose weight in accordance with their physician's recommendations. That may help lower urate levels and usually benefits cardiovascular disorders that the patient may have concurrently.

Alcohol

Alcohol consumption should also be stopped. Alcohol can increase serum uric acid levels by acting as a cell poison and by causing dehydration, which can concentrate uric acid in the blood. A drinking binge is apt to precipitate a gout attack in a previously asymptomatic hyperuricemic patient.

Hydration

Dehydration, regardless of the cause, can dramatically worsen the condition of the hyperuricemic patient. A liberal daily intake of water is almost always indicated, particularly if the patient is physically active and in a hot environment.

Noncompliance and Iatrogenic Factors

Other common causes for therapeutic failure include inadequate patient follow-up and failure of the physician to continue therapy with uricosuric drugs or allopurinol for an adequate time. Because many hyperuricemic adults have other disorders, such as heart disease, multiple drug therapy may also contribute to a poor response. This situation increases the need for close patient monitoring of urate levels and the responses to other drugs.

SUMMARY OF NURSING IMPLICATIONS 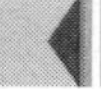

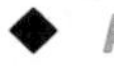

Assessment

Assess activity level (or limitations) and ability to complete activities of daily living.

Note appearance of involved joint(s).

Establish baseline laboratory values (eg, CBC, sedimentation rate, urinalysis, etc) as reference for drug-induced changes.

Obtain a complete nursing history to include use of OTC or prescription medications that may precipitate hyperuricemia or may contraindicate or interact with antigout drugs.

Review dietary pattern for food sources high in purines.

◆ Nursing Diagnoses

Pain related to joint inflammation (acute gout attack).

Impaired physical mobility related to swollen, tender, inflamed joints (acute gout and gouty arthritis).

Activity intolerance related to pain.

Knowledge deficit related to prescribed antigout drugs or interacting drugs to be avoided.

Ineffective individual coping related to chronic illness.

Noncompliance related to drug side effects, dietary restrictions.

Diarrhea related to antigout medications.

◆ Planning/Implementation

Dilute IV colchicine as directed; use proper injection technique to prevent extravasation; question IV use of colchicine for more than 24 hours.

Apply cold compresses and administer analgesics (other than aspirin) if extravasation occurs.

Monitor patients for edema, weight gain, hypertension, or other indications of heart failure or high blood pressure when taking sodium bicarbonate as a urinary alkalinizer; hyperkalemia if potassium salts are used; hypoglycemia in diabetic patients taking uricosuric drugs; abnormal bleeding in patients taking sulfinpyrazone; gastric/epigastric pain with any antigout drug.

Administer antigout drugs with meals or a full glass of milk to reduce GI distress.

Institute passive and active range of movement exercises, and ambulate patient as soon as possible as acute gout attack resolves and activity is tolerated.

◆ Patient and Family Education

Teach the patient/family:

To keep a diary listing frequency and severity of gout attacks and response to drugs and diet, for review at subsequent medical visits.

To avoid alcohol and purine-rich foods and strenuous exercise in hot environments.

To drink at least ten 8-oz. glasses of water per day, unless directed otherwise by physician.

To avoid aspirin and use acetaminophen or ibuprofen instead for minor pain or fever.

To expect nausea, vomiting, or diarrhea with colchicine and to report severe GI effects (eg, intractable vomiting, diarrhea, bloody or black tarry stools) at once.

To report flank or back pain, hematuria, or decreased urine output, which may indicate renal urate stones.

To report skin rashes while taking allopurinol at once.

That drug and dietary therapy of hyperuricemia or gout may be lifelong to reduce the chance of adverse effects, including potentially serious organ damage.

◆ Evaluation

The patient/family will:

Resume self-care; be able to complete activities of daily living; ambulate unassisted.

Express relief from joint pain and immobility.

Report no redness or swelling of joints.

Maintain optimal fluid intake.

Manage medication program correctly: take drug(s) at prescribed times with food and/or fluid as indicated; avoid interacting drugs; recognize side effects, and report as necessary.

Experience minimal or no drug-induced side effects.

Annotated Bibliography

Abramson SB: Treatment of gout and crystal arthropathies and uses and mechanisms of action of nonsteroidal anti-inflammatory drugs. *Curr Opin Rheumatol* 1992;4(3):295–300. *Reviews current controversies in the treatment of gout with NSAIDs and discusses the recent literature on how these drugs may cause their beneficial actions.*

Agudelo CA, Wise CM: Gout and hyperuricemia. *Curr Opin Rheumatol* 1991;3(4):684–691. *Explores reasons why usually "straightforward" therapy may need to be changed when gout is not your patient's only medical condition.*

Groff GD, Franck WA, Raddatz DA: Systemic steroid therapy for acute gout: A clinical trial and review of the literature. *Semin Arthritis Rheum* 1990;19(6):329–336. *Discusses the potential benefits of short corticosteroid "bursts" for acute gout, especially for cases in which NSAIDS are contraindicated or not fully effective.*

Roubenoff R: Gout and hyperuricemia. *Rheum Dis Clin North Am* 1990;16(3):539–550. *Emphasizes epidemiology but is important for considering gout risk factors and how gout itself may be a risk factor for coronary heart disease, Western society's number-one cause of death.*

Wolfe F: Gout and hyperuricemia. *Am Fam Physician* 1991;43(6): 2141–2150. *Good coverage of key points on gout diagnosis and treatment, including the declining use of colchicine for acute gout, avoidance of treating asymptomatic hyperuricemia, and the limitations of dietary therapy.*

Yeomans AC: Assessment and management of gouty arthritis. *Nurse Pract* 1991;16(4):18, 21, 25–26. *Reviews causes, consequences, diagnosis, and treatment of this metabolic disorder; good nursing perspective.*

Table 53–C | **Clinical Uses and Administration of Major Drugs Used to Treat Hyperuricemia and Gout**

AGENT	CLINICAL USES	DOSAGE AND ROUTE OF ADMINISTRATION
	Antiinflammatory Drug	
PROTOTYPE		
Colchicine	Acute gout	Oral: 1–1.2 mg initially, then 0.5–1.2 mg every 1–2 hr until pain is relieved
		IV: 1–2 mg initially, then 0.5 mg q6h if needed, up to maximum of 4 mg in any 24-hr period
	Gout prophylaxis	Oral: 0.5–0.6 mg/day, 3–4 times a week or daily (depending on attack frequency, severity)
	Prophylaxis before elective surgery	Oral: 0.5–0.6 mg tid for 3 days before and 3 days after surgery
Other antiinflammatory drugs		See Chapter 52
	Uricosuric Drugs	
Probenecid (BENEMID)	Hyperuricemia	Oral: Initially 0.25 mg bid for 1 week, then 0.5 mg bid thereafter
	Adjunct to penicillin or cephalosporin therapy	Oral: 2 g/day in divided doses. Children 2–14 yr: Initially 25 mg/kg (or 0.7 g/m^2); maintenance: 40 mg/kg/day (1.2 g/m^2/day) in 4 doses; use adult dose for children >50 kg; not recommended for children <2 yr old
	Uncomplicated gonorrhea (adjunct)	Oral: One 1-g dose, followed 30 min later by 4.8 million units procaine penicillin G (IM)
	Uncomplicated gonococcal infections (eg, urethral, cervical)	Oral: 1 g plus suitable penicillin
	Neurosyphilis	Oral: 500 mg qid, with aqueous penicillin G (2–4 million units/day) for 10–14 days
RELATED DRUG		
Sulfinpyrazone (ANTURANE)	Hyperuricemia	Oral: Initially 100–200 mg bid with meals or milk; maintenance doses 200–800 mg/day in 2 doses
	Xanthine Oxidase Inhibitor	
PROTOTYPE		
Allopurinol (LOPURIN; ZYLOPRIM)	Hyperuricemia	Oral: 200–600 mg/day, depending on severity; divide doses >300 mg. Children <6 yr: 150 mg/day; children 6–10 yr: 300 mg/day
	Gout prophylaxis	Oral: 100 mg/day; increase weekly by 100 mg/day as needed to reach desired serum urate level
	Prophylaxis of renal damage during aggressive cancer chemotherapy trials	Oral: 600–800 mg once daily for 2–3 days
	Prophylaxis of recurrent renal calcium oxalate stones	Oral: 200–300 mg/day in 1 or 2 doses

Table 53–S **Major Side Effects of and Contraindications for Drugs Used for Hyperuricemia and Gout**

BODY SYSTEM/ Side Effect	CONTRAINDICATION/ PRECAUTION	COMMENTS AND NURSING IMPLICATIONS
	Colchicine	
GASTROINTESTINAL Nausea, vomiting, diarrhea	Peptic ulcer disease	May be severe; forewarn patients that doses used to treat ongoing arthritic attacks usually produce these side effects; diarrhea may be managed with paregoric; instruct patient to report bloody or profuse diarrhea at once
RENAL Abdominal, back, or flank pain	Poor renal function	Colchicine is concentrated in urine, may cause renal damage; encourage liberal daily water intake; have patient report pain, bloody urine at once
VASCULATURE Vascular irritation, necrosis		Due to improper IV administration; avoid extravasation; apply cold packs, give analgesics should this occur
BLOOD Blood dyscrasis	Blood dyscrasias	Occurs mainly with excessive or unduly prolonged IV administration of colchicine; question medication orders for more than 2 days of colchicine administration
	Probenecid, Sulfinpyrazone	
GASTROINTESTINAL Nausea, vomiting, diarrhea	Peptic ulcer disease	Encourage patients to report these to physician at once; GI distress most likely to occur with sulfinpyrazone; may be managed by taking drug with meals, milk
RENAL Increased risk of renal uric acid stones	Severe hyperuricemia; poor renal function, low creatinine clearance	Encourage liberal daily water intake to maintain urine output >2 L/day; encourage patient to measure urine output, report signs or symptoms of renal stones (pain, decreased urine output, urine discoloration); observe for side effects of urinary alkalinizing drugs if prescribed
SKIN Rash	History of hypersensitivity reaction to current or related drug (eg, hypersensitivity to phenylbutazone warrants cautious use of sulfinpyrazone)	Rash may indicate hypersensitivity reaction; have patient see physician at once; therapy is likely to be changed, discontinued
BONE AND JOINT Increased risk of gout attacks		Colchicine or other antiinflammatory drug therapy must be maintained when starting uricosuric drug therapy to prevent, treat acute attacks
	Allopurinol	
CENTRAL NERVOUS SYSTEM Drowsiness		A variable side effect; give appropriate precautions to patients who experience noticeable or bothersome sedation
SKIN Rash		See probenecid; potentially serious sign; notify physician at once
BONE AND JOINT Increased risk of acute gout attacks		See probenecid above; use antiinflammatory drug during initial therapy with allopurinol

Table 53–I **Major Interactions Between Antigout Drugs and Other Agents**

AGENT	RESULT OF INTERACTION	COMMENTS AND NURSING IMPLICATIONS
Interactions Involving Colchicine		
	None	
Interactions Involving Probenecid		
Aspirin, other salicylates (Chapter 52)	Decreased uricosuric effects	Avoid interaction; advise patients wishing to use OTC drugs to relieve mild pain or fever to use ibuprofen or acetaminophen instead
Dyphylline (Chapter 38)	Reduced dyphylline excretion, increased risk of toxicity	Avoid interaction; unlike dyphylline, other theophyllines are eliminated by hepatic metabolism and do not interact
Methotrexate (Chapter 59)	Reduced methotrexate excretion, increased blood levels and risk of toxicity	Avoid interaction; otherwise, anticipate need to reduce methotrexate dose, and monitor blood levels; prolonged leucovorin rescue (p 1309) may be needed to reduce toxicity risk
Zidovudine (Chapter 57)	Increased risk of zidovudine side effects	Monitor accordingly if interaction unavoidable
Interactions Involving Sulfinpyrazone		
Acetaminophen (Chapter 52)	Increased risk of acetaminophen hepatotoxicity	Risk greatest when high or toxic acetaminophen doses (overdoses) are taken; low doses, occasional use of acetaminophen not contraindicated if patient has good liver function
Aspirin	See probenecid, above	
Hypoglycemic drugs, oral (eg, tolbutamide, Chapter 46)	Reduced hypoglycemic drug metabolism; increased risk of excessive hypoglycemia	Monitor accordingly if combined therapy needed; may need to reduce hypoglycemic drug dose; interaction may not apply to newer oral hypoglycemics (glipizide, glyburide)
Warfarin (Chapter 35)	Reduced warfarin metabolism, significantly increased risk of excessive effects (eg, bleeding or hemorrhage)	Probable need to reduce warfarin dose; essential to monitor coagulation profiles during combined use
Interactions Involving Allopurinol		
Ampicillin (Chapter 56)	Increased risk of ampicillin-induced skin rash	Monitor accordingly; rash usually requires reducing allopurinol dose or switching to alternative drug(s)
Thiopurines (eg, azathioprine, 6-mercaptopurine; Chapter 54)	Increased desired or toxic effects of thiopurine	Monitor for toxicity; anticipate need to limit starting thiopurine dose to as little as 25% of usual during combined therapy

PROTOTYPES

DPT Triple Antigen 1126

Immune Serum Globulin 1132

Azathioprine 1135

Cyclosporine 1137

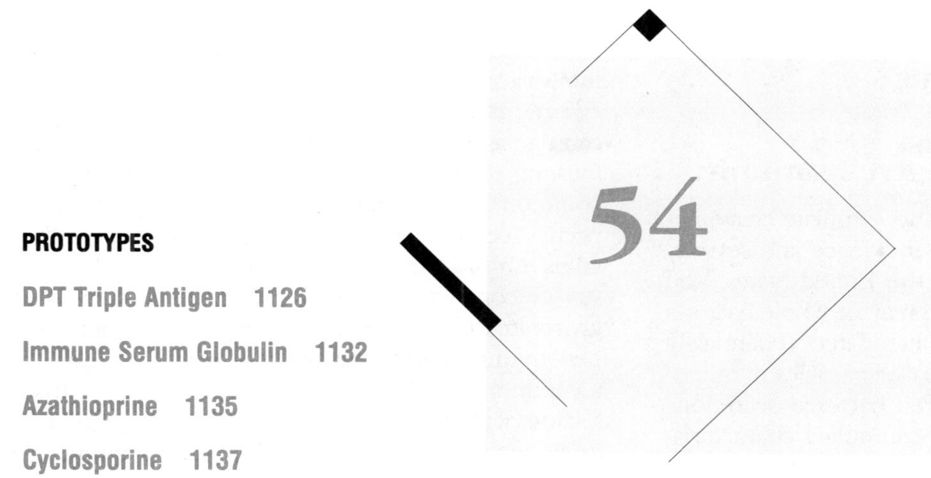

Immunostimulant and Immunosuppressant Drugs

Drugs or other biologic products that affect the immune system can be generally categorized as either immunostimulants or immunosuppressants. *Immunostimulant* drugs can be further categorized as those that produce active immunity and those that produce passive immunity. As discussed in Chapter 50, active immunity can be acquired either from natural exposure to pathogens—that is, having and recovering from an illness caused by a pathogen—or from administration of a pathogen in the form of a vaccine or toxoid. The prototype drug that produces active immunity is the DPT triple antigen vaccine. Passive immunity is immediate but temporary protection against diseases, provided by antibodies from the blood of other persons or animals. Called antisera or immune globulins, these preparations are administered to nonimmune individuals who have been exposed to infectious antigens. The prototype drug producing passive immunity is immune serum globulin.

Although an active immune system is usually desirable for protection against infectious diseases and neoplasms, it is sometimes advantageous to reduce the effectiveness of the immune response. Drugs that interfere with the formation and activity of immune system cells are called *immunosuppressants.* They are used to ameliorate rejection of organ transplants or destruction of normal body tissues by aberrant immune reactivity (autoimmune disease). Some immunosuppressant drugs are cytotoxic; the prototype for this class is azathioprine. Other immunosuppressants are more specific and affect only T lymphocytes. The prototype for the T cell suppressors is cyclosporine. Corticosteroids may also be used as immunosuppressants. These drugs are discussed in detail in Chapter 45, so only a brief discussion of their administration for suppression of organ transplant rejection or for autoimmune disease is presented here.

At the end of the chapter, a brief presentation of acquired immunodeficiency syndrome (AIDS) and the drugs currently used in its treatment is provided. Because of the rapidly changing status of drugs available for the treatment of AIDS, it is especially important to be aware of the current literature to amplify this discussion.

Major reference tables appear beginning on p. 1144.

I. Immunostimulants

Drugs That Produce Active Immunity

The use of vaccines and toxoids to stimulate active immunity has greatly reduced the incidence and severity of many infectious diseases in the United States. The antigenic component of *vaccines* may be whole bacteria or viruses that are killed or attenuated (chemically treated to reduce their virulence), or particles of microorganisms. *Toxoids* are denatured bacterial secretions (toxins) that retain their immunostimulant characteristics. Administration of vaccines and toxoids provokes an immune response identical to that which occurs during natural bacterial or viral infections, usually without the hazards that accompany the actual disease.

Although the development of active immunity requires the presence of an immune system that is capable of an adequate response, many vaccines and toxoids are given to persons who are immunodeficient, either as a result of diseases such as leukemia or AIDS or of administration of immunosuppressant agents. Vaccines and toxoids are contraindicated in persons who have severe infectious illnesses. Administration of passive immunity agents such as immune serum globulins, including those in blood products, can suppress the expected response to some vaccines and toxoids.

Because they are biologic preparations, vaccines and toxoids can provoke allergic responses. Agents derived from human sources generally are safer than those obtained from other animal species. Adequate means for resuscitation, including epinephrine injection, must always be immediately available when these agents are administered. Biologic preparations are susceptible to spontaneous decomposition; manufacturers' instructions for storage, reconstitution, and use must always be followed carefully.

A summary of the agents used to produce active immunity, and their dosages and administration, adverse effects, and contraindications, is provided in Table 54–C1/S1.

PROTOTYPE

DPT Triple Antigen

Many vaccines are available to provide protection against a variety of infectious diseases. Some are given routinely to young children, to establish immunity early in life. One such preparation is DPT, a "triple antigen" that contains diphtheria toxoid, tetanus toxoid, and pertussis vaccine. Diphtheria is caused by the bacillus *Corynebacterium diphtheriae,* which secretes a toxin that can damage heart and nerve tissue and produce a suffocating pharyngeal membrane. Diphtheria is now uncommon in the United States, although outbreaks do occur. Tetanus, caused by the toxic secretion of the bacillus *Clostridium tetani,* is characterized by muscle spasm, convulsions, and dyspnea. The tetanus bacillus grows in soil and frequently contaminates puncture or penetrating injuries. Pertussis (whooping cough), once a common childhood disease, is a respiratory tract infection of *Bordetella pertussis* bacteria. Sequelae of pertussis include pneumonia and central nervous system (CNS) damage. This disease is usually most severe in infants and young children.

Pharmacologic Effects

The DPT vaccine activates the immune system to synthesize and release antibodies to diphtheria and tetanus toxins and to pertussis bacteria, and to develop "memory cells" that will initiate a similar response if these antigens are again encountered. Immunity to diphtheria and tetanus lasts approximately 10 years, at which time a "booster" or recall inoculation is necessary. Readministration of diphtheria and tetanus toxoid is advisable during outbreaks of diphtheria or following a deep injury that may be contaminated with *C. tetani.* Reimmunization (or initial immunization) with pertussis vaccine of persons older than 6 years is not recommended since this disease is less common and less severe in older children and adults. In addition, administration of pertussis vaccine to persons older than 6 years is more frequently accompanied by adverse reactions. A vaccine without pertussis (Pediatric Diphtheria and Tetanus Toxoids; DT) is available for use in children with contraindications to the pertussis component. Tetanus and Diphtheria Toxoids for Adult Use (TD) contains the same amount of tetanus toxoid as the pediatric vaccine but a much smaller amount of diphtheria toxoid. Adults are often more sensitive to diphtheria toxoid; the use of a smaller dose reduces the incidence and severity of adverse effects.

Clinical Indications and Administration

DPT is used in infants and children up to 6 years to induce active immunity against diphtheria, pertussis, and tetanus. The recommended schedule of administration is three 0.5-mL doses at 4- to 8-week intervals—at ages two, four, and six months—followed by a fourth dose one year after the third (at 15 to 18 months of age). A triple antigen preparation (DTaP) containing acellular pertussis vaccine is recommended for the fourth (and fifth) doses. This vaccine appears to cause less severe adverse effects.

The sequence of inoculations can be instituted later than 2 months of age, with the precaution that the triple antigen DPT is contraindicated after the seventh birthday. Interruption of the schedule of injections does not require restarting the series; immunity will be provided if the remaining doses are administered. If the fourth dose of the series was given before the fourth birthday, a booster dose is usually given between 4 and 6 years of age, when the child enters school.

NURSING IMPLICATIONS

Shake vials of DPT vigorously before withdrawing each dose of antigen. Inject DPT by the intramuscular (IM) route, preferably in the deltoid or lateral thigh muscles. Use different sites for each injection. Inadvertent intravenous (IV) injection must be avoided; aspirate gently into the syringe to assure that the injection will not be into a blood vessel. As for all IM injections, avoid injection sites that are close to major nerve trunks. Provide parents or guardians with a complete record of all immunizations, and advise them to keep this available for reference.

Side Effects, Adverse Reactions, and Contraindications

Children may experience a fever and be irritable following immunization. Acetaminophen doses appropriate to the child's age are usually given for this. Occasional serious neurologic responses have occurred after DPT administration. These have usually been attributed to the pertussis component and always contraindicate further administration of pertussis vaccine. Pediatric diphtheria and tetanus toxoids can usually be administered to complete the series of inoculations. These severe reactions most frequently occur within 24 to 48 hours following antigen administration and include convulsions, fever above 40.5°C (105°F), crying, or screaming of greater than three hours' duration, marked alterations of consciousness, and shock-like collapse. Permanent CNS damage and deaths have occasionally occurred. Some instances of sudden infant death syndrome (SIDS) have been attributed to pertussis vaccine.

It is not possible to determine before administration which children will react adversely. The benefit to most children appears to outweigh the risk of similar serious consequences that can result from spontaneous pertussis infection. However, the severity of the sequelae and the financial liability of the vaccine's manufacturers have jeopardized the future availability of this product.

Allergic reactions, including anaphylactic shock, can occur after administration of DPT or any other biologic preparation. However, the most common adverse effects are usually mild. Localized erythema with or without tenderness, fever of 100° to 102°F, anorexia, vomiting, fretfulness, and drowsiness can occur. Occasionally, a nodule may persist for several days or weeks at the injection site, and abscess formation and lymph node enlargement have been reported. Neurologic complications have also been attributed to the tetanus toxoid content of the preparation.

The DPT vaccine should not be administered to children older than 6 years of age, to children with history of or familial tendency toward CNS disorders, or to children who have exhibited any neurologic adverse effects following a dose of DPT. (TD is available for use in children beyond the seventh birthday or those sensitive to pertussis vaccine.)

Symptoms of hypersensitivity to any component of the DPT antigen contraindicate further use. Most active immunologic agents, including DPT, are contraindicated in the presence of illnesses (eg, fever, acute infections, or leukemia) or drugs (eg, corticosteroids or antineoplastics) that can alter the immune system's responsiveness. The DPT vaccine is usually not administered during outbreaks of poliomyelitis. The presence of coagulation disorders that contraindicate IM injection of any drug precludes the use of DPT.

NURSING IMPLICATIONS

Obtain a thorough history, including allergies and drug use, before administering any drug. Carefully observe patients receiving vaccines or other biologic preparations for adverse responses, especially anaphylaxis. Inform parents or guardians of the possible adverse effects, and question them on return visits about their occurrence. Withhold any vaccine if reported effects suggest sensitivity to any of its components.

Before administration of DPT or any biologic preparation, have a syringe containing epinephrine 1:1000 readily available for use in case anaphylaxis occurs.

Publicity surrounding potential adverse effects of the pertussis component of DPT has resulted in the refusal by some parents to immunize their children against pertussis; as a result, the incidence of the disease is increasing. Advise parents that their children are more likely to contract spontaneous pertussis, with its serious consequences, than to suffer a serious complication from the immunization.

Interactions with Other Drugs

The DPT vaccine is usually not administered simultaneously with any other immunostimulant except oral poliomyelitis vaccine (see the section on related drugs and Table 55–I1). Drugs that suppress immune responsiveness will interfere with the ability of DPT and other vaccines to induce protection against disease, and may increase the risk of antigen-induced adverse reactions. Antibodies present in blood or plasma transfusions, or immune serum globulin administered within the previous three months, can inactivate the antigenic component of many vaccines.

Related Drugs

Poliovirus Vaccine

Poliomyelitis is a viral infection of the CNS that can result in paralysis of skeletal muscles, including those involved in respiration. Vaccines developed during the 1950s have markedly decreased the incidence of this disease. Trivalent oral poliovirus vaccine (TOPV; Sabin; ORIMUNE) is recommended for use in all children from 2 months to 18 years of age. The vaccine is routinely given at ages 2, 4, and 15 to 18 months (at the same time as DPT antigen), with an optional sixth-month dose. A booster dose is recommended on entry to school. Children may be started on a course of immunization at any age, however. Six to eight weeks should separate the first two doses, with the third dose six to 12 months later. Trivalent oral poliovirus vaccine may be recommended for adults at increased risk of contracting poliomyelitis, such as during epidemics or travel to areas where the virus is endemic.

The TOPV contains live attenuated virus of all three types known to produce poliomyelitis. It must be administered orally. (An inactivated poliovirus vaccine, Salk vaccine, is available for parenteral administration in special circumstances.) The oral vaccine induces intestinal immunity, which reduces survival of the virus. Following vaccination, poliovirus is excreted in the feces and by the pharyngeal route for six to eight weeks. Rarely, the vaccine has caused paralytic poliomyelitis in inoculated persons or close contacts. Other adverse effects have not been reported.

Trivalent oral poliovirus vaccine is contraindicated in persons with suppressed immune responses or those who reside with others who are immunodeficient. Inactivated virus vaccine is preferred under these circumstances. Trivalent oral poliovirus vaccine must be withheld during acute or debilitating illness, in the presence of vomiting or diarrhea, or in the presence of active respiratory infection. Although administration of vaccines is usually not recommended during pregnancy, TOPV can be given if the risk of poliomyelitis threatens the mother and the fetus.

The vaccine, supplied in single-dose pipettes, can be administered directly or can be taken mixed with milk or chlorine-free water or on bread or a sugar cube. The preparation, cultured in monkey kidney cells, contains sorbitol and up to 25 μg of the antibiotics neomycin and streptomycin; allergic reactions can occur.

NURSING IMPLICATIONS

The TOPV is red to yellow in color. Follow manufacturers' directions for storage and use carefully. Warn patients, parents, or guardians of the possibility of vaccine-related paralytic poliomyelitis. Never administer the vaccine by any route other than oral.

Measles, Mumps, and Rubella Vaccines

Vaccines for measles, mumps, and rubella ("German measles") are routinely administered to children in the United States. These are available as single agents and in combinations (M-M-R II) that facilitate administration by reducing the required number of injections. Each of the three vaccines contains live attenuated virus. Administration is recommended for children at 15 months of age. Before that age, residual maternal circulating antibodies interfere with the ability of the child's immune system to respond adequately to the vaccine. When circumstances lead to inoculation of infants younger than 1 year old, revaccination after 15 months of age is usually recommended. However, infants vaccinated at an earlier age may fail to develop an adequate response when subsequently reimmunized. The presence of upper respiratory infections at the time of inoculation may also result in an inadequate immune response.

Rubella is especially hazardous in pregnant women. The virus induces fetal damage and congenital abnormalities. Rubella virus vaccine, or any preparation that includes this antigen, is contraindicated during pregnancy. Nonimmune children of pregnant women should be vaccinated to prevent them from acquiring the disease and subsequently exposing other family members. Adolescent girls and women of childbearing age should be tested for susceptibility to rubella, and those who are not immune can be inoculated with rubella virus vaccine if they are not pregnant. Women must be warned of the possible risk to the fetus if pregnancy occurs sooner than three months after immunization. Women can be inoculated against rubella immediately following childbirth. However, rubella virus is excreted in breast milk and may induce mild symptoms of disease in the infant.

Measles and mumps vaccines are derived from chick embryo cell cultures and should not be given to persons who have exhibited severe reactions following ingestion of eggs. Inoculation appears to be safe in persons who have had milder reactions to eggs. Hypersensitivity to the antibiotic neomycin, which is present in these vaccines, also contraindicates vaccine administration.

Adverse reactions to these vaccines given either singly or in combination include fever, rash, general malaise, localized reactions such as burning or stinging at the injection site, and regional lymph node enlargement. Children may experience febrile seizures. Occasionally, measles virus vaccine may cause nervous system disorders such as encephalitis, ocular palsies, and Guillain-Barré syndrome. Rubella inoculation can cause arthritis and polyneuritis, especially in women and adolescent girls. These painful reactions can persist for months or years. It should be noted that many of the adverse responses to measles, mumps, rubella, and other vaccines can also develop as sequelae to natural occurrences of these infections.

Measles, mumps, and rubella vaccines can be combined with each other but should not be given within one month before or after any other immunostimulants. Exceptions are the occasional simultaneous administration of these three antigens plus DPT and TOPV when there is concern that the individual may not return for further health care, and at age 15 months to 18 months to reduce the number of health-care visits necessary for children during the second year of life. The measles, mumps, and rubella vaccines are believed to provide lasting immunity, and no booster dose is recommended.

NURSING IMPLICATIONS

Combined measles, mumps, and rubella vaccine is reconstituted with the diluent supplied by the manufacturer. Preservatives and other additives that may be present in other generally available diluents can inactivate the viruses present in the vaccine. Shake the vial after addition of the diluent, and administer the entire volume of a single-dose vial (approximately 0.5 mL) into the upper arm.

Hepatitis B Vaccine

Hepatitis B vaccine (HEPTAVAX-B, ENGERIX-B, RECOMBIVAX-HB) contains a subviral antigen. Immunization against hepatitis B is recommended for persons who are at significant risk of contracting this infection, which predisposes patients to development of chronic liver dysfunction, cirrhosis, and hepatocellular cancer. Hepatitis B inoculation is now recommended for all neonates and adolescents, as well as health-care personnel at risk of exposure to infected blood, patients requiring hemodialysis or frequent infusions of blood or blood products, persons confined to prison or to institutions for the mentally disabled.

Two doses of 20 μg (1 mL) each are given one month apart, with a booster injection five months later. Persons who are immunodeficient or require dialysis, and children younger than 10 years, require lower doses (see Table 54–C1/S1). RECOMBIVAX also is given in lower doses. Immunity usually persists for at least three years; booster doses can be given. Persons who have serious active infections should not receive hepatitis B vaccine unless the immediate risk of hepatitis is significant. The vaccine has been used safely and effectively in children.

The most frequent adverse reactions to the vaccine are transient localized responses. Fever, malaise, nausea, and fatigue have been reported. Persons who have been exposed to hepatitis B may receive hepatitis B immune globulin (discussed later) concurrently with vaccine. The recombinant DNA hepatitis B vaccines (RECOMBIVAX and ENGERIX) may produce more rapid immunity than the plasma-derived HEPTAVAX.

NURSING IMPLICATIONS

Administration is usually by the IM route. The deltoid is the recommended site for greatest absorption. Subcutaneous injection can be used in persons with coagulation disorders, but intravenous injection must be avoided.

Influenza Vaccines

Influenza is a viral infection of the respiratory tract that can lead to secondary diseases such as pneumonia and bronchitis. Influenza virus type A is responsible for most occurrences of the disease. The virus frequently mutates, and the antigen content of influenza vaccines varies each year in accordance with Public Health Service observation of infectious agents responsible for outbreaks of disease. Vaccines contain either whole or split virus.

Immunization against influenza is especially recommended for persons with chronic metabolic, cardiovascular, or pulmonary disease; persons who have extensive contact with high-risk patients; immunodeficient persons; and persons who are older than 64 years. Because of the apparent association between influenza, salicylates, and Reye's syndrome, children receiving chronic aspirin therapy also should be immunized.

Because of the viral and vaccine variations, susceptible persons should be reimmunized each year, preferably in November so that protection will last through the winter and early spring "flu season." A single dose of either whole or split virus vaccine is administered to persons older than 12 years. Split virus vaccine is given to children between the ages of 6 months and 12 years (see Table 54–C1/S1). Pregnant women may receive vaccine after the first trimester. The vaccine contains small amounts of the antibiotic gentamicin and of egg protein, and is contraindicated in persons with allergy to aminoglycosides or anaphylactic hypersensitivity to eggs.

Adverse responses, which occur more frequently in children, include localized reactions, fever, and malaise. Neurologic disorders such as Guillain-Barré syndrome have occurred. Influenza vaccine may delay the metabolism of warfarin and theophylline, which necessitates observation for signs of drug toxicity.

Amantadine (SYMMETREL), also effective as an antiparkinson drug (see Chapter 25), can be given orally to prevent influenza A. Persons at immediate risk of developing influenza can receive this drug concurrently with the influenza vaccine. Administered for two weeks, amantadine will provide protection during the time required for active immunity to develop. For persons with contraindications to receiving the vaccine, amantadine may be administered prophylactically throughout the "flu season."

Haemophilus influenzae type b is a severe form of infection that occurs most frequently in young children. It can lead to meningitis and permanent CNS damage, arthritis, pneumonia, epiglottitis, and osteomyelitis. A majority of victims are under 18 months of age. Two vaccines are recommended for use in infants. HibTITER is given at 2, 4, 6, and 15 months, or PedvaxHIB can be given at 2, 4, and 12 months. Injections can be given at the same time that DPT is administered. Modified injection schedules are available for children who receive the first dose after 7 months of age.

Rabies Vaccine (Human Diploid-Cell Strain, Subvirion Antigen)

Rabies is a slowly developing (one to three months' incubation) viral infection of the CNS that is usually fatal. Most human cases are transmitted from animals through exposure to saliva. The incidence of rabies among many wild species has increased in recent years, particularly in the eastern United States. Persons at high risk of exposure to the rabies virus (veterinarians and assistants, certain laboratory workers, and persons traveling in countries where rabies is widespread) should receive preexposure immunization.

All persons exposed to rabies through bites or contact of mucous membranes or broken skin with saliva or other potentially infectious material must receive immediate treatment to prevent the development of rabies. Once the symptoms of the infection appear, the disease is usually no longer amenable to treatment and is rapidly fatal. If the animal is subsequently proven to be rabies-free, the course of inoculation can be discontinued.

Human diploid-cell rabies vaccine contains inactivated particles of virus grown in human diploid-cell strain cultures, as well as small amounts of human serum albumin and the antibiotics neomycin, gentamicin, and amphotericin B. Preexposure immunization is induced by administering 1 mL IM on days 0, 7, and 28. Persons at continued high risk of exposure should have serum antibody levels measured every six months and should receive booster inoculations as required. Other persons at risk may need booster doses every two years if rabies antibody levels become inadequate.

Postexposure treatment with rabies vaccine is begun as soon as possible, regardless of the patient's preexposure immunity. Nonimmune persons receive a series of five 1-mL doses, administered over one month (see Table 54–C1/S1), with the first dose administered as soon as possible after exposure. Nonimmune persons also receive one dose of human rabies immune globulin or of equine antirabies serum. Previously immunized persons receive one dose of vaccine immediately and a second dose three days later. Rabies vaccine of human diploid-cell origin is given only by the IM route.

Adverse effects of human diploid-cell rabies virus include localized pain and itching, headache, nausea, and dizziness. More serious reactions include allergy (both immediate and delayed responses) and occasional neurologic disturbances. Because of the extreme risk of developing rabies, vaccine administration may be continued despite serious adverse reactions. Assistance in managing patients can be obtained from state health departments or the Centers for Disease Control.

Pregnancy is not a contraindication to postexposure treatment of women possibly exposed to rabies virus. Human diploid-cell rabies vaccine has been used safely and effectively in children.

Some adverse reactions can be alleviated with antipyretic and antiinflammatory drugs. However, corticosteroids should not be administered, and other immunosuppressant agents should be avoided during therapy, because they can reduce the effectiveness of the antirabies treatment.

NURSING IMPLICATIONS

Because of the seriousness of rabies infection, its prevention in persons known or suspected to be exposed to the virus will usually take precedence over all other medical treatment except that which is also essential to survival. In some persons, such as those requiring corticosteroids and those exhibiting allergic reactions, astute observation and care will be necessary. All persons directly exposed to rabies must be treated as soon as possible and must receive the full course of therapy indicated. Persons who have been bitten may require tetanus toxoid and antibiotics to control the threat of other infections.

Rabies vaccine, reconstituted in sterile water and injected immediately, is colorless to faintly pink. The deltoid or buttocks are frequently used for IM injections. (Daily injections under the skin of the abdomen are not required for postexposure immunotherapy with the human form of the rabies vaccine.) Check injection sites for local erythema, swelling, and itching, and report adverse or untoward responses, or rabies symptoms to the physician. Antihistamines and aspirin or acetaminophen may be ordered. Injection sites must avoid blood vessels and major nerve trunks. Allergic reactions to vaccine components, including the antibiotics, are possible. A means for resuscitation must be immediately available.

BCG Vaccine

An increased incidence of tuberculosis among immunocompromised and other persons, as well as the emergence of drug-resistant *Mycobacterium* strains, has heightened the importance of protection against this potentially debilitating disease. BCG vaccine is used to induce active immunity to tuberculosis in persons who are at risk of contracting this disease and who are tuberculin-negative when skin-tested. One form of the vaccine, for intradermal injection, contains a dried living culture of the tubercle bacillus Calmette-Guerin. Another form, for percutaneous administration with a multiple puncture tine, contains a live culture of the tubercle bacillus. Dosages are noted in Table 54–C1/S1. Because BCG vaccine is not always effective, the tuberculin skin test should be repeated two to three months after vaccination. Persons who again test negative and are at continued risk of tuberculosis should be reinoculated.

The usual response to either route of administration is a local skin reaction that appears within seven to ten days when the intradermal preparation is used, and within ten days to two weeks after percutaneous administration. A small scar usually persists after intradermal administration but is less likely with the percutaneous administration route. With either route, there is a low incidence of adverse effects such as malaise, fever, and lymph node inflammation. Administration of BCG vaccine occasionally induces tuberculosis. The BCG vaccine is contraindicated in immunodeficient persons, persons who have been vaccinated against smallpox, persons taking antitubercular drugs, and in burn patients. The vaccines should not be administered during pregnancy unless there is almost certain risk that the patient will be exposed to infective tuberculosis.

The BCG vaccine occasionally is administered to stimulate immune cytotoxic responses in cancer patients. For this use it can be given intradermally or injected directly into solid tumors. Intravesicular administration is beneficial in persons with urinary bladder cancer. Intralesional injections are associated with more serious adverse reactions.

NURSING IMPLICATIONS

Reconstitute the BCG vaccine preparation intended for intradermal injection by adding 1 mL sterile water to each ampule. Avoid shaking the container once the vaccine has been reconstituted, and administer immediately. The vaccine for percutaneous administration should be reconstituted with 1 mL sterile, preservative-free water per ampule, and mixed vigorously. This vaccine should be used within eight hours of reconstitution. Both preparations should be stored in a refrigerator, protected from light, before reconstitution.

Pneumococcal Vaccine

Pneumococcal infection is a major cause of pneumonia, meningitis, and otitis media. The fatality rate among immunodeficient persons and the elderly is high.

Pneumococcal vaccine (PNEUMOVAX; PNU-IMUNE 23) contains antigenic capsular polysaccharides from 23 bacteria types that account for 90% of pneumococcal infections. Many of these strains have developed drug resistance, so vaccination to prevent infection is recommended for high-risk populations, including the elderly; persons with diabetes or chronic cardiovascular, pulmonary, hepatic, or renal disease; persons with sickle cell anemia and other immunologic deficits; and institutionalized persons. Vaccination before age 65 (eg, as early as age 55) may result in a more vigorous protective response by the immune system.

A single 0.5 mL dose of pneumococcal vaccine is given IM or subcutaneously (SC). Persons at high risk for pneumoccocal pneumonia and also for rapid decline in antibody production may benefit from repeat doses of vaccine. Administration to children younger than 2 years old is contraindicated because this age group does not produce an adequate immune response to the vaccine. Persons who are severely immunodeficient also may not produce effective antibody levels. Pneumococcal vaccine is contraindicated in persons receiving immunosuppressive therapy.

NURSING IMPLICATIONS

Avoid intradermal or IV injection of pneumococcal vaccine. Anticipate a low-grade fever on the first day after immunization. Most patients complain of soreness, redness, and induration at the injection site for a couple of days. Institute comfort measures appropriate for these side effects.

Additional Agents

Cholera, plague, hepatitis A, and typhoid vaccines are available for administration to persons at risk of exposure to these diseases. Vaccines that reduce metastasis of cancer cells may be developed. A varicella (chickenpox) vaccine is under study, and an experimental AIDS vaccine appears to have slowed disease progression in some persons with early HIV infection.

Drugs Providing Passive Immunity

Passive immunity against infectious disease is conferred by transferring antibodies to persons who lack endogenous active immunity. Antibody preparations are derived from biologic sources, so many of the same precautions noted for active immunity agents apply. Following administration, close observation for symptoms of anaphylaxis is required, and adequate means for resuscitation must be immediately available.

A summary of the agents used to provide passive immunity, their dosages and administration, adverse effects, and contraindications is provided in Table 54–C1/S1.

PROTOTYPE

Immune Serum Globulin

Clinical Indications and Administration

Immune serum globulin (gamma globulin, IgG) is the concentrated IgG antibody fraction of serum obtained from large pools of human blood. It is used to prevent or reduce the severity of various infectious diseases, including measles, varicella (chickenpox), hepatitis A and B, and poliomyelitis, in recently exposed persons and in those who are deficient in endogenous IgG. Some persons with idiopathic thrombocytopenic purpura (ITP) will respond to IV immune serum globulin with a rapid temporary increase in platelets, which can be beneficial by controlling excessive bleeding.

Immune serum globulin is available in both IM and IV preparations. Administration should be instituted as soon as possible following exposure to infectious agents. The usual dosages vary, depending on the infectious agent, and whether the patient is immunoglobulin-deficient. Dosages are summarized in Table 54–C1/S1.

NURSING IMPLICATIONS

Intramuscular preparations must not be injected into a blood vessel. Vials must be used soon after opening, and should be discarded if the contents are turbid. Immune serum globulin for IV administration should be diluted in D_5W and infused through a separate line.

Side Effects, Adverse Reactions, and Contraindications

Although immune serum globulin is derived from human blood, some persons exhibit allergic reactions to it. Persons who lack endogenous IgA may produce anti-IgA antibody. Avoid IV administration to these persons. Severe allergic responses usually contraindicate subsequent administration of immune serum globulin. However, some persons who experience severe reactions following IM injection may be able to tolerate cautious IV administration.

Headache is the most frequently observed adverse effect. Nausea, chills, fever, and a flu-like syndrome of joint pain and fatigue may occur. Commonly, severe pain at the IM injection site will persist for several hours. Although usually reserved for use in immunodeficient patients, the IV route may also be preferred in persons with small muscle mass or coagulation disorders that make IM injection hazardous. Intravenous administration can cause marked hypotension, which responds to a reduction in the infusion rate. The effects of immune serum globulin on the fetus have not been determined.

NURSING IMPLICATIONS

Adverse reactions necessitate slowing or stopping drug administration. Warm soaks and aspirin or acetaminophen may help to relieve the systemic discomforts. Acetaminophen should be used for children because of the link between aspirin, viral illness, and Reye's syndrome.

Interactions with Other Drugs

Immune serum globulin can interfere with the expected immune response to active immunity agents such as vaccines; administration of the two types of immunostimulants should be separated by at least three months (see Table 54–I1).

Related Drugs

Hepatitis B Immune Globulin

Some preparations of immune globulins contain concentrated antibodies to specific infections. Hepatitis B immune globulin (H-BIG; HEP-B-GAMMAGEE) is prepared from the plasma of persons having elevated levels of antibody to the hepatitis B surface antigen (HBsAg, Australia antigen). The antigen itself is not present in the globulin preparation, and transmission of hepatitis B has not been reported with its use. The immune globulin should be administered IM as soon as possible (preferably within 24 hours, but no later than seven days) after exposure to the infection by accidental needle-stick or oral contact with blood from persons known to have or suspected of having hepatitis B. Infants born to women who test positive for hepatitis B surface antigen also should receive hepatitis B immune globulin. Dosages are noted in Table 54–C1/S1.

The most frequent adverse effects are localized pain and tenderness at the injection site. To reduce the risk of anaphylaxis, hepatitis B immune globulin is never administered IV. Persons with IgA deficiency may develop antibodies and subsequent allergic reactions to this component of hepatitis B immune globulin. Coagulation disorders that make IM injection hazardous preclude the administration of this globulin unless the risk from hepatitis B infection is serious.

NURSING IMPLICATIONS

In addition to precautions required for administration of any biologic preparation, take great care to avoid inadvertent IV injection. Intramuscular injection in infants should be into the lateral thigh muscle, avoiding small muscle masses in areas traversed by major nerve trunks.

Rabies Immune Globulin

As described earlier, treatment of rabies exposure in nonimmune persons includes administration of a passive immunity agent as well as a vaccine. Two rabies antisera are available. Rabies immune globulin (HYPERAB; IMOGAM) and equine antirabies serum are derived, respectively, from the plasma of humans and of horses inoculated with rabies vaccine. The human immune globulin is preferred to the equine because of its lower potential for evoking severe allergic reactions. The immune globulin is administered once, at the same time as the first dose of rabies vaccine, to provide immediate protection during the time required for the development of active immunity. To inactivate viruses that remain localized at the site of injury, one half the dose of 20 IU/kg is infiltrated around the bite wound or area of exposure and the remainder is injected IM. Immune globulin is not given to persons who have high circulating levels of rabies antibody. Localized soreness and slight fever are the most frequently observed side effects.

NURSING IMPLICATIONS

Thoroughly clean the bite wound or area of exposure with soap and water before infiltrating the globulin. Since the rabies immune globulin can inactivate the rabies vaccine, a separate syringe and injection site should be used for each.

Rh_o(D) Immune Globulin

Rh_o(D) immune globulin (RhoGAM) contains anti-Rh_o(D) antibody derived from human plasma, and is used to prevent Rh sensitization in Rh-negative persons exposed to Rh-positive blood cells. Rh-negative women may be exposed at the time of delivery or abortion of an Rh-positive fetus. They may also be exposed if abdominal trauma or amniocentesis occurs during pregnancy. Rh_o(D) immune globulin should be administered whenever it is known or suspected that Rh-positive fetal blood cells have entered the circulation of an Rh-negative woman. Usually, a single IM dose of 300 μg of antibody is adequate unless the woman is exposed to a volume greater than 15 mL of fetal blood. However, if antibody administration occurs earlier than 18 weeks of gestation, a second dose should be given at 26 to 28 weeks. Antibody given at the end of pregnancy must be administered within 72 hours of delivery of an Rh-positive infant. When mismatched blood has been transfused, multiple doses of antibody may be required. Each 300-μg dose will suppress the immune response to approximately 15 mL of blood.

Rh_o(D) immune globulin is contraindicated in persons who have experienced a severe reaction to human globulin. The most common adverse effects are slight fever, myalgia, and discomfort at the injection site. Administration during pregnancy does not appear to affect the fetus adversely.

NURSING IMPLICATIONS

Multiple vials of Rh_o(D) may be administered at different sites at one time, or they may be divided and injected at intervals within 72 hours of the transfusion or fetomaternal exchange.

Antitoxins

Antitoxins are antibodies that have been extracted from the serum of horses inoculated with bacterial toxins. These antibodies, when injected into infected humans, combine with circulating toxins and prevent them from interacting with body tissues. Antitoxins are frequently used in the treatment of botulism, diphtheria, and tetanus.

Botulism Antitoxin

Botulism occurs after ingestion of improperly preserved foods contaminated with *Clostridium botulinum* bacteria. The bacterial toxins bind irreversibly to presynaptic cholinergic nerve membranes and cause paralysis by preventing acetylcholine release from the nerve terminals. Fatal respiratory and cardiac arrest can occur. Supportive care and administration of botulism antitoxin (available from the Centers for Disease Control) reduce the incidence of fatalities. The antitoxin does not displace toxin already bound to nerve terminals but will neutralize toxin in the circulatory system.

Antitoxin should be administered as soon as possible (within 24 hours) after ingestion of contaminated food, even before a definitive diagnosis is available and before symptoms appear in persons who may have ingested the bacteria. Table 54–C1/S1 summarizes usual dosages and preferred administration routes and schedules.

The most frequent adverse effects of botulism antitoxin are anaphylaxis and serum sickness, a slowly developing allergic response characterized by fever, urticaria, joint pain, and enlarged lymph glands. Persons should be tested for sensitivity to the antitoxin, especially if hypersensitivity to proteins of equine origin is known or suspected. If symptoms are not immediately life-threatening, persons allergic to the preparation may be desensitized in accordance with a schedule of increasing doses provided by the manufacturer.

Skin testing with the antitoxin has caused fatal reactions, and persons who test negatively may respond adversely when the full dose of antitoxin is given. To decrease the risk of anaphylaxis, it is recommended that epinephrine be given together with the antitoxin. Another adverse reaction is hyperthermia with chills and mild respiratory difficulty developing within 20 to 60 minutes after administration.

Diphtheria Antitoxin

Diphtheria antitoxin is used to prevent and treat diphtheria. Dosages and administration routes (see Table 54–C1/S1) depend on whether the antitoxin is used for prophylaxis or for treatment of symptomatic disease.

Tetanus Antitoxin

Tetanus antitoxin is used in the treatment of tetanus, and can provide passive immunization if human tetanus immune globulin is not available. In cases of known or suspected exposure to the causative agent, persons at significant risk of developing tetanus may receive both tetanus antitoxin and tetanus toxoid, the latter to induce active immunity. Administration of both immunizing agents (if both are indicated) should begin as soon as possible after exposure to the infection.

NURSING IMPLICATIONS

Question patients regarding allergies or previous injections of "serum," and test them for sensitivity to the individual antitoxin preparation. Patients who react positively may be desensitized by administering gradually increasing doses of antitoxin. Since anaphylaxis can occur, epinephrine and means for resuscitation must be immediately available during sensitivity testing, desensitization, and administration of full doses. Follow manufacturers' directions for administration of antitoxins. Record the type and location of the injury if the patient is to receive tetanus antitoxin, a description of symptoms or exposure to diphtheria, or any indications of muscle or respiratory involvement from botulism contamination. Serum sickness can develop, particularly after administration of large doses of antitoxin. Localized pain, redness, and itching may occur seven to ten days after injection. Instruct the patient to report immediately any signs or symptoms indicating development of the bacterial infection after receiving antitoxin.

Additional Agents

Interferons are gradually acquiring clinical usefulness. Alpha interferon, derived by recombinant DNA technology, has some efficacy in hairy-cell leukemia, AIDS-related Kaposi's sarcoma, condyloma (genital warts), chronic hepatitis C, and, possibly, chronic hepatitis B. Gamma interferon reduces the incidence of infections in persons with chronic granulomatous disease. Interferons commonly cause a flu-like syndrome. With prolonged treatment, psychiatric symptoms, hair loss, and thyroid changes may develop.

In persons having nonmyeloid cancers, colony-stimulating (hematopoietic) factors (see Table 50–2) are used to promote production and activity of neutrophils, monocytes, and macrophages when chemotherapeutic agents have caused myelosuppression. (There is the possibility that myeloid malignancies may be stimulated by these agents). Granulocyte-macrophage colony-stimulating factor (GM-CSF) also enhances recovery of cell-producing myeloid activity following bone marrow transplant. These factors are naturally occurring substances that are now produced with recombinant DNA techniques.

Side effects of granulocyte colony-stimulating factor (G-CSF) include bone pain, enlarged spleen, and alterations in serum uric acid, lactate dehydrogenase, and alkaline phosphatase. GM-CSF can produce transient fever and a "capillary leak syndrome" that may lead to pleural or pericardial fluid accumulation.

II. Immunosuppressants

The immune reactions that usually protect against invasion by undesirable foreign matter may also lead to failure of organ transplants and destruction of normal cells. An overzealous immune response can threaten the survival of the individual who requires replacement of a nonfunctional heart, kidney, or liver. In addition, if the immune system loses the ability to distinguish "self" from "nonself," autoimmune diseases such as those listed in Chapter 50 may result.

To reduce unwanted immune reactivity, immunosuppressant drugs are administered. Immunosuppressant drugs include cytotoxic agents such as azathioprine, which depresses bone marrow activity, T cell suppressors such as cyclosporine, and adrenal corticosteroids. Along with suppression of the normal immune response, however, each of these groups of drugs carries the risk of unopposed infections and malignancies.

Because of the special hazards of immunosuppressant therapy and the disorders it alleviates, these drugs should be administered only by physicians who are skilled in their use, and only in facilities equipped for full cardiopulmonary resuscitation. Nurses must continuously and thoroughly assess patients for indications of adverse reactions, especially for any signs of seriously compromised immunity or developing infections. Patients must always be fully informed of possible adverse effects.

A summary of the immunosuppressant drugs, their dosages and administration, adverse side effects, and contraindications is presented in Table 54–C2/S2.

Cytotoxic Immunosuppressants

PROTOTYPE

Azathioprine

Absorption, Distribution, Metabolism, and Excretion

Azathioprine (IMURAN) is well absorbed from the gastrointestinal (GI) tract, yielding peak serum concentrations in one to two hours. Azathioprine is biotransformed to 6-mercaptopurine, which is inactivated, largely by the enzyme xanthine oxidase, in the liver. The plasma half-life is less than five hours. Although renal clearance does not appear to participate in the drug's inactivation, doses are usually reduced in patients with impaired kidney function.

Pharmacologic Effects

Azathioprine and 6-mercaptopurine are purine analogs that enter into cellular pathways that use the natural purines adenosine and guanine, disrupting the synthesis of DNA and RNA and other processes vital to cellular growth and survival. Bone marrow function in particular is suppressed; the resultant leukopenia may be the primary mechanism of azathioprine's immunosuppressant action.

Clinical Indications and Administration

Azathioprine is primarily used to prevent rejection of renal transplants. It is also approved for use in severe degenerative rheumatoid arthritis that is refractory to other forms of therapy.

Azathioprine is usually administered orally, although IV administration is often used to initiate therapy. A single daily dose of 3 to 5 mg/kg (IV or oral) is started one to three days before transplant surgery. Azathioprine is diluted with sterile saline or dextrose and infused over 30 to 60 minutes (although injection time can vary from five minutes to eight hours). Oral doses may be divided into smaller amounts and administered after meals to reduce nausea and vomiting. Drug doses should be reduced to maintenance levels of between 1 and 3 mg/kg per day as soon as possible. The risk of serious adverse drug effects precludes the use of toxic amounts to prevent graft rejection.

Side Effects, Adverse Reactions, and Contraindications

The major adverse effects of azathioprine and the other cytotoxic immunosuppressant agents are leukopenia and subsequent infections, thrombocytopenia, nausea and vomiting, hepatotoxicity, hair loss (alopecia), and induction of neoplasms, including myelogenous leukemia and solid tumors. Potential allergic reactions include pancreatitis that induces abdominal pain and vomiting. The incidence of toxicity is high in renal transplant recipients. Because of the potential for serious adverse effects, the potential benefits of azathioprine (or other cytotoxic drugs) must be carefully considered in relation to the risks. Hypersensitivity to azathioprine contraindicates its use.

NURSING IMPLICATIONS

Inform patients of all the possible adverse effects of azathioprine. Blood counts and hepatic function tests are performed before the start of therapy and periodically thereafter. Close observation for signs of infection (eg, fever or sore throat) and for bruising and abnormal bleeding from thrombocytopenia are required. Patients must be protected from sources of infection, and serious infections must be treated with appropriate antiinfective therapy. In addition, patients receiving immunosuppressant therapy after renal transplantation must be observed for signs of rejection, such as decreased urine output or weight gain.

Azathioprine's potential for severe toxicity necessitates that patients receiving it report any adverse effects. Dosage reduction or termination may be required, even if the consequences include transplant rejection or recurrence of arthritis symptoms.

Instruct patients to take the drug in divided doses or after meals to reduce GI distress. Emotional support and assistance in dealing with hair loss may also be important.

◆ Use During Pregnancy and Lactation

Azathioprine is generally contraindicated during pregnancy. However, transplant recipients who are pregnant may take azathioprine after the first trimester if benefits clearly outweigh risks. Although normal infants have been born to women who received azathioprine during pregnancy, congenital immunologic aberrations have occurred. The drug is mutagenic and teratogenic in laboratory animals. Discuss methods of contraception with the patient if necessary.

Interactions with Other Drugs

Allopurinol (ZYLOPRIM), used to reduce serum and urine levels of uric acid, inhibits the xanthine oxidase pathway of azathioprine inactivation. When these drugs are given concurrently, azathioprine must be reduced to one quarter to one third the usual dose (Table 54–12). Azathioprine is usually combined with corticosteroids and occasionally with antithymocyte globulin in transplant recipients, which increases the risk of serious infection. Interactions most likely to apply to the use of azathioprine for refractory arthritis are discussed in Chapter 52.

NURSING IMPLICATIONS

Instruct patients to make all health-care providers aware of current therapy with azathioprine and to avoid nonprescription drugs unless recommended by a physician.

Overdose and Toxicity

The primary manifestations of azathioprine toxicity are nausea, alopecia, pancreatitis, and immunosuppression. Azathioprine is rapidly metabolized; thus, most toxic effects are reversible when doses are reduced or administration is stopped. Because the drug is not extensively bound to plasma proteins (approximately 30%), dialysis can be of some benefit in removing azathioprine from the circulatory system.

Related Drugs

Methotrexate and Cyclophosphamide

Both methotrexate and cyclophosphamide are cytotoxic drugs that are used primarily to treat neoplasms (see Chapter 59), but they have also been used investigationally to treat a variety of autoimmune disorders that do not respond to more conventional therapies. Of the two drugs, only methotrexate (FOLEX; MEXATE; RHEUMATREX) has an FDA-approved indication for its immunosuppressant actions—management of advanced, refractory rheumatoid arthritis (see Table 54–C2/S2). Additional information for cyclophosphamide and methotrexate is presented in Chapter 59.

T Cell Suppressors

PROTOTYPE

Cyclosporine

Cyclosporine (cyclosporin A; SANDIMMUNE), a naturally occurring substance derived from a soil fungus, has immunosuppressant action that is more selective than that of the cytotoxic agents.

Absorption, Distribution, Metabolism, and Excretion

Cyclosporine is insoluble in water; thus, for oral administration it is prepared in alcohol and olive oil, and for IV administration in alcohol and polyoxyethylated castor oil. GI absorption is slow and incomplete and is further reduced in patients with malabsorption disorders. Peak plasma concentrations occur in three to four hours. Approximately 50% of the drug is distributed in erythrocytes; as a result, drug levels in whole blood will be significantly higher than those in plasma. Cyclosporine binds extensively (90%) to plasma proteins. Cyclosporine's average half-life is 19 hours (with a range of 10 to 27 hours). It is metabolized by several enzymatic pathways—hydroxylation in particular—and is excreted in the bile. Less than 10% is excreted unchanged in the urine.

Pharmacologic Effects

Cyclosporine interferes with T lymphocyte activity, reducing the proliferation of T helper and cytotoxic T cells and suppressing the synthesis of the lymphokines IL-2, interferon, and macrophage inhibitory and chemotactic factors. T suppressor cells appear to be less affected by cyclosporine. B lymphocytes retain considerable activity, thus humoral immunity is less affected than are T cell–mediated responses. Cyclosporine enhances transplant survival with less risk of occurrence of infectious disease.

Clinical Indications and Administration

Cyclosporine is administered to recipients of heart, kidney, or liver transplants, and has also been effective in graft-versus-host disease following bone marrow transplants, in which T lymphocytes from the transplanted marrow mobilize an immune response against the recipient's tissues. Cyclosporine may delay cell damage in some autoimmune disorders. Oral administration is preferred. Treatment is begun 4 to 12 hours before transplant surgery. Daily maintenance doses usually are 5 to 10 mg/kg. When the oral route is unsuitable, reduced doses of cyclosporine (see Table 54–C2/S2) can be given IV, with a switch to oral administration as soon as possible.

NURSING IMPLICATIONS

Mix cyclosporine for oral administration in a glass tumbler with water, milk, or orange juice, at room temperature. Assess the patient's personal preference and the possibility of allergy to milk or citrus to determine the most suitable diluent. Diluted drug should be consumed at once. The amount of fluid must be sufficient to make the drug palatable, especially for children, yet small enough to be consumed quickly. Advise patients to use the pipette supplied by the manufacturer to measure the drug solution. To ensure that the complete dose is consumed, rinse the glass container used for drug administration with a small amount of the beverage used to dilute the drug, and have the patient drink the rinse immediately. Oral doses administered shortly before surgery should be mixed with water.

Side Effects, Adverse Reactions, and Contraindications

The major adverse reaction to cyclosporine is nephrotoxicity, which produces elevations of serum creatinine that are difficult to distinguish from those caused by graft rejection. Rejection usually occurs within the first month following surgery. Subsequent symptoms of deteriorating kidney function necessitate a reduction in the cyclosporine dose while the patient is observed for return of optimal renal activity. Graft rejection and drug-induced dysfunction may be present simultaneously.

Drug-induced hypertension may necessitate antihypertensive drug administration, especially to cardiac transplant patients. Hepatotoxicity manifested as elevated plasma levels of enzymes and bilirubin has occurred. Hyperkalemia, hirsutism, venous thrombosis, gingival hyperplasia, fluid retention, and neurotoxicity ranging from tremor to convulsions have been reported.

The incidence of opportunistic infections during cyclosporine therapy is lower than that observed with other immunosuppressive agents. However, the risk of viral invasion, including reactivation of Epstein-Barr (EB) virus and infectious mononucleosis, is significant. Lymphomas (malignancies of lymphoid tissue) induced by EB virus have occurred in persons receiving cyclosporine as well as other immunosuppressive therapy, although a direct causal relationship has not been established. Cyclosporine is not usually myelosuppressive, yet anemia, leukopenia, and thrombocytopenia can develop.

Anaphylactic reactions have occurred with IV administration of cyclosporine. Any sign of allergic response requires that cyclosporine infusion be stopped immediately and any necessary treatments instituted. The allergen appears to be the polyoxyethylated castor oil, since persons who have shown hypersensitivity during IV administration have subsequently tolerated oral doses with no allergic manifestations. Allergy to cyclosporine or to drug vehicle (eg, alcohol or oil) precludes its administration.

NURSING IMPLICATIONS

Determine baseline laboratory values for formed elements of blood (ie, complete blood counts), blood urea nitrogen (BUN), serum creatinine, bilirubin, and liver enzymes before drug therapy is begun. Continue monitoring these values throughout therapy, with adjustment of drug dosage in accordance with any changes in bone marrow, renal, or hepatic function. Adverse effects are generally dose-related and will remit with a dose reduction.

Circulating levels of drug should be monitored by radioimmunoassay (RIA); recommended values measured 24 hours following the last dose are 250 to 800 ng/mL for whole blood and 50 to 300 ng/mL for plasma.

When the IV route is used, have a 1:1000 epinephrine solution and other means for resuscitation immediately available. Patients must be under continuous observation for at least the first half hour of administration and at frequent intervals thereafter. Report decreased urinary output, fatigue, bruising or bleeding, and signs of infection to the physician.

Carefully instruct patients in the administration of cyclosporine and the importance of strict compliance, follow-up appointments and laboratory tests, and observation for signs of adverse drug effects or transplant rejection.

◆ Use During Pregnancy and Lactation

High doses of cyclosporine are embryotoxic in laboratory animals; thus, this drug should be administered during pregnancy only if the benefit to the mother clearly outweighs the potential risks to the fetus. Drug doses should be just sufficient to suppress transplant rejection. Cyclosporine is excreted in breast milk and is contraindicated in nursing mothers.

◆ Use in Children

Although extensive studies in children have not been performed, cyclosporine has been safely and effectively administered to children as young as 6 months of age.

Interactions with Other Drugs

Adrenocorticosteroid therapy should always accompany cyclosporine administration, to enhance immunosuppression. Although other immunosuppressant agents should be avoided, some transplant centers add azathioprine to this drug regimen. The major drug interactions are listed in Table 54–12. Ketoconazole (NIZORAL) increases plasma levels of cyclosporine and may therefore be used beneficially to reduce required doses of cyclosporine significantly.

Overdose and Toxicity

There has been very little experience with cyclosporine overdoses. The "size" of an overdose could vary greatly, because absorption of and sensitivity to the drug vary greatly among people. Blood levels are usually monitored. Symptoms would be primarily those of hepatic or renal failure. Long-term consequences have not been reported. Because oral cyclosporine is absorbed slowly, evacuation of gastric contents up to two hours following ingestion should be attempted. Supportive measures and alleviation of symptoms of transient nephrotoxicity and hepatotoxicity may be required.

Related Drugs

Muromonab-CD3

Muromonab-CD3 (ORTHOCLONE OKT3) is a monoclonal antibody obtained from murine (mouse) cell lines. It binds to the CD3 surface antigen on T lymphocytes and suppresses cellular activity. It does not suppress bone marrow function. Muromonab-CD3 is used to reverse acute renal transplant rejection, including some episodes that are refractory to other therapy. The drug is administered as a 5 mg bolus IV injection once daily for 10 to 14 days.

The untoward responses to muromonab-CD3 include expected responses to any immunosuppressant, as well as some that are unique to this drug. The former include the risk of severe infections because of drug-induced suppression of T lymphocyte function. Infections with herpes simplex, cytomegalovirus, *Staphylococcus epidermidis,* and *Pneumocystis carinii* are among those frequently observed in persons receiving muromonab-CD3. As with other immunosuppressants, there is an increased risk of development of malignancies, including lymphoma.

Three unique adverse syndromes are liable to occur within the first 30 minutes to six hours after administering the first dose of muromonab-CD3. For each there are predrug assessments or treatments that can help avoid or minimize the untoward response, and precautions that should be taken to help correct a potentially severe reaction. Some of these syndromes may involve allergic responses to the protein in the drug preparation. Such responses are not only potentially dangerous, but also may reduce the drug's efficacy and safety during subsequent therapy.

One syndrome is characterized by high fever, chills, and malaise. It is prevented by attempting to normalize body temperature (if elevated before muromonab-CD3 administration) with acetaminophen. Corticosteroid pretreatment may also be indicated. Muromonab-CD3 should not be administered to patients with body temperatures above 37.8°C (100°F). If fever occurs after muromonab-CD3 administration, acetaminophen and physical means to reduce body temperature are indicated.

Another syndrome is characterized by pulmonary edema that may be severe and life-threatening, and may require intubation, mechanical ventilation, and oxygen therapy. Adjunctive use of parenteral corticosteroids, antihistamines, or both may be required. Abnormal chest X-rays, dyspnea, evidence of heart failure, or sudden weight gain over the pretreatment period (eg, more than a 3% increase during the week prior to muromonab-CD3 administration) contraindicate the use of this drug.

If pretreatment chest X-rays and body weight are normal, patients may nevertheless experience respiratory difficulty that is not associated with pulmonary edema. Administration of parenteral corticosteroids, antihistamines, or both may be indicated if this occurs. If symptoms become severe, additional symptomatic and supportive therapy may be required.

Muromonab-CD3 is contraindicated in persons with prior allergic or hypersensitivity reactions to this drug or to other products derived from murine cell lines.

NURSING IMPLICATIONS

Muromonab-CD3 is supplied in ampules that must be kept refrigerated before use. Withdraw the proper dose into a syringe using aseptic technique and an in-line filter (0.2 to 0.22 μm pore size). Discard the filter and holder, and inject the drug IV, administering the total dose in less than one minute. Do not infuse the drug or add it to other drug solutions or infusions.

Do not administer muromonab-CD3 if there is a relevant history of allergy or the presence of factors (in particular, abnormal chest X-rays, fever, weight gain) that might indicate significant risks of early and possibly severe untoward responses. Do not administer the drug unless necessary drugs and facilities for cardiopulmonary resuscitation and treatment of anaphylaxis are immediately available. Lymphocyte levels should be determined before muromonab-CD3 administration and periodically thereafter. Assess all patients receiving this drug for signs of desired effects as well as for indications of immediate untoward responses and for late developing evidence of immunosuppression (eg, infection).

Muromonab-CD3 has been used successfully and safely in children as young as 2 years of age. Its effects on the fetus are unknown, and so its use during pregnancy is recommended only when the anticipated benefits exceed the potential risks. Muromonab-CD3 is a protein that is degraded in the GI tract. Therefore, its administration to lactating mothers should not adversely affect nursing infants.

Antithymocyte Globulin

Antithymocyte globulin (lymphocyte immune globulin; ATGAM) is purified gamma globulin extracted from the blood of horses immunized with human T lymphocytes. Administered to human beings, it reduces the number of functional T lymphocytes in the circulatory system. Antithymocyte globulin is used as adjunctive therapy with other immunosuppressants (azathioprine or corticosteroids, for example) to reverse or delay the onset of renal transplant rejection. It is also used to alleviate aplastic anemia when bone marrow transplantation is not appropriate. Aplastic anemia, characterized by bone marrow failure and a reduction in all formed blood elements (pancytopenia), may be an autoimmune disease.

Antithymocyte globulin is administered only by the IV route. Dosages are summarized in Table 54–C2/S2. Administration may begin within 24 hours before or after transplant surgery to delay rejection onset, or it may be withheld until rejection is diagnosed.

Although highly purified, antithymocyte globulin can contain small amounts of antibodies to other blood elements and can induce hemolysis and thrombocytopenia. Transfusions of erythrocytes or platelets may be necessary. Severe leukopenia or thrombocytopenia in transplant recipients requires termination of drug therapy.

Patients should be skin-tested for hypersensitivity before administration of antithymocyte globulin. Systemic allergic responses contraindicate its use. Localized reactions dictate extreme caution. Some patients who do not react to skin-testing may still develop severe allergic responses to therapeutic doses. Drug infusion must be terminated immediately if any symptoms suggestive of anaphylaxis appear.

The most frequently reported adverse effects include chills and fever, dermatologic reactions, arthralgia, myalgia, diarrhea, and nausea. Some of the milder adverse affects can be alleviated with antipyretics, mild analgesics, or antihistamines. Thrombophlebitis may occur. The safety of antithymocyte globulin during pregnancy and lactation has not been determined. A small number of children, both transplant recipients and patients with aplastic anemia, have been safely treated with antithymocyte globulin.

NURSING IMPLICATIONS

Use saline to dilute antithymocyte globulin; dextrose-containing and acidic solutions will inactivate the drug. Invert the IV solution container when adding drug to prevent contact with air. Use an in-line micropore filter, and infuse into a central vein, to reduce the risk of thrombophlebitis. Have injectable epinephrine available in case of anaphylaxis. Monitor vital signs every four hours, and notify the physician if body temperature rises during therapy. Administer antipyretics, analgesics, or antihistamines as ordered.

Additional Agents

An investigational agent, FK-506, has action similar to that of cyclosporine. FK-506 has been effective in suppressing liver, kidney, heart and other transplant rejection reactions, including some in persons unresponsive to or intolerant of other immunosuppressant agents. The major adverse effects are those of cyclosporine: hypertension, nephrotoxicity, infections, and occasional diabetes. FK-506 can be given IV or orally; hepatic and renal function, serum concentration of drug, and rejection status must be monitored.

Thalidomide has been granted orphan drug status for studies as an immunosuppressant that affects T lymphocyte activity. It is reported to ameliorate lepromatous leprosy, discoid lupus erythematosus, and rheumatoid arthritis as well as graft-versus-host disease. Although this drug appears to have few side effects, it must overcome a tremendous legacy as a teratogen in order to be widely accepted.

Corticosteroids

The adrenal glucocorticoids are useful as immunosuppressant agents. These drugs are discussed in detail in Chapter 45, and only their immunosuppressant effects will be discussed here. In particular, prednisone, prednisolone, and methylprednisolone are used. Their immunosuppressive effects are of longer duration, and they have less mineralocorticoid (sodium-retaining) activity than cortisone and hydrocortisone.

The exact immunosuppressive mechanism of corticosteroids is not known, but they alter cellular action in several ways. They reduce circulating levels of lymphocytes (T cells in particular), eosinophils, and monocytes; and they suppress the accumulation of lymphocytes and macrophages at the site of inflammatory reactions. Corticosteroids also reduce production of cytotoxic mediators.

The immunosuppressant action of corticosteroids makes them useful in reversing organ transplant rejection and in alleviating symptoms of lupus erythematosus, polymyositis, rheumatoid arthritis, and other disorders that appear to have an autoimmune component. Corticosteroids can also be applied topically on the eye to suppress corneal transplant rejection.

Severe disease states usually require daily divided-dose administration of corticosteroids. Two thirds of the dose of a drug such as prednisone is given just after awakening, and the remainder is given later in the day, to mimic the normal circadian fluctuations of corticosteroid release.

Once the pathologic response is controlled, doses should be reduced to a level just sufficient to maintain remission. The total daily maintenance dose should be administered in the early morning on alternate days. This regimen usually will provide a good therapeutic response with few adverse effects. The transition from one dosage schedule to the other must be gradual. Sudden decreases in the amounts of exogenous glucocorticoids can leave the patient with dangerously low levels of hormone. See Chapter 45 for more information about corticosteroid withdrawal and problems of iatrogenic suppression of the hypothalamic-pituitary-adrenal axis.

As discussed in Chapter 45, corticosteroid administration produces many side effects and adverse reactions. Patients receiving these drugs for an immunosuppressive effect must be monitored carefully. Infection presents a particularly difficult problem, because large doses of corticosteroids may conceal its signs and symptoms. The contraindications and drug interactions discussed in Chapter 45 apply also to the use of corticosteroids to suppress a transplant rejection reaction or to control an autoimmune disorder.

Acquired Immunodeficiency Syndrome

Immune system deficiencies take several forms (decreased levels of circulating antibodies, absence of gamma globulins, inadequate numbers of lymphocytes) and can arise from various causes (genetic aberrations, malnutrition, neoplasms, extensive burns, use of certain drugs). Acquired immunodeficiency syndrome (AIDS), first recognized in the United States in 1981, is a failure of the immune system that predisposes the patient to the development of fatal opportunistic infections and cancers. AIDS is caused by a retrovirus called HTLV-III (human T lymphotropic virus type III) or HIV (human immunodeficiency virus). Such viruses use the enzyme reverse transcriptase to encode their genetic makeup into the DNA of the cells they invade. When the infected cells subsequently proliferate, they reproduce the virus.

The AIDS retrovirus attacks in particular the T4 or helper cells of the immune system. Characteristic of this immune deficiency is a marked decrease in the number of T4 cells, while T8 (or suppressor lymphocyte) cell numbers remain unchanged. The deficiency in T helper cells greatly hinders the mobilization of immune responses, which may be further impeded by the overabundant activity of the suppressor cells.

Many drugs are used in the treatment of AIDS patients, most of them in attempts to control infections and to alleviate the symptoms of the syndrome. Drugs such as zidovudine (RETROVIR or AZT), dideoxyinosine (DDI, VIDEX), and dideoxycytidine (DDC), which inhibit reverse transcriptase, currently offer the most promise for successful treatment or palliation. Their success will probably depend on identifying AIDS patients before damage to the immune system has become extensive and irreversible. Unfortunately, zidovudine may cause severe bone marrow depression, resulting in anemia, thrombocytopenia, and granulocytopenia. See Chapter 57 for more information on antiviral drugs.

The discovery of the causative virus has spurred attempts to develop an AIDS vaccine. Emphasis has centered on the use of subviral antigens, since a whole-virus vaccine might have an unacceptably high risk of inducing AIDS itself. However, several strains of the virus have been identified, and an effective vaccine would have to provoke sufficient antibody formation to protect against all infectious agents.

SUMMARY OF NURSING IMPLICATIONS

◆ Assessment

Obtain a complete nursing history, noting allergies, state of health, and current or previous drug use.

Establish baseline laboratory determinations that may be altered by drug administration (blood count, hepatic and renal function).

Note skin-test reaction prior to drug administration; accurately measure reaction.

Identify potential risks for infection before and during immunosuppression.

Check skin and mucous membranes for intact condition needed to resist infection.

Recognize indications of hypersensitivity or other severe reactions requiring termination of drug therapy.

Assess patient's and family's ability to cope and comply with long-term therapy.

Determine adequacy of rest and nutrition status to prevent a lack of immunocompetency.

◆ Nursing Diagnoses

Knowledge deficit related to immunotherapy, long-term care needs, or importance of immunizations.

Fear related to possible transplant rejection, disease progression, or death.

Altered family processes related to chronic illness.

Self-care deficit related to physical condition (eg, immunosuppressed, arthritic).

Body image disturbance related to drug effects (eg, alopecia with azathioprine).

High risk for impaired skin integrity related to drug hypersensitivity (eg, rash).

High risk for injury related to bleeding tendencies and decreased resistance to infection with immunosuppressants.

Impaired gas exchange related to an allergic reaction from drug therapy.

◆ Planning/Implementation

Follow manufacturers' instructions for storage, reconstitution, and use of biologic preparations to prevent spontaneous decomposition.

Administer drugs precisely; IV use is generally contraindicated; avoid IM injections near major nerve trunks or blood vessels, particularly in children or others with small muscle mass and in persons with coagulation defects.

Prepare for possible cardiopulmonary resuscitation; have epinephrine available.

Monitor laboratory tests throughout drug treatment.

Observe closely for signs of developing infections and neoplasms during immunosuppressant therapy.

Provide the patient with a complete record of all immunizations.

◆ Patient and Family Education

Teach the patient/family:

Possible adverse effects and drug interactions.

To return for full course of therapy, follow-up physician visits, and/or laboratory appointments.

To avoid sources of infection (eg, persons with upper respiratory infection).

◆ Evaluation

The patient/family will:

Experience minimal to no serious side effects; chills, low-grade fever, malaise, if present, will resolve in 24 to 48 hours.

Show no signs of respiratory distress from an allergic reaction.

Maintain positive self-concept: participate in family/social activities as physical condition permits.

Remain free of infection during immunotherapy; avoid sources of infection.

Verbalize anger, anxiety, depression, or understanding of changes in situation.

Identify need for support and counseling.

Perform self-care to optimal level or accept need for assistance.

Demonstrate ability to follow prescribed regimen; administer medication accurately; return for physician and laboratory appointments.

Annotated Bibliography

Anastasi JK, Rivera JL: AIDS drug update: DDI and DDC. *RN* 1991; 54(11):41–43. *Focuses on new reverse transcriptase inhibitors.*

Boitard C, Bach JF: Long-term complications of conventional immunosuppressive treatment. *Adv Nephrol* 1989;18:335–354. *Focuses on neoplastic and infectious complications of therapy with cyclophosphamide, azathioprine, and cyclosporine.*

Buckley RH, Schiff RI: The use of intravenous immune globulin in immunodeficiency diseases. *N Engl J Med* 1991;325:110–117. *In-depth discussion of the preparation, clinical uses, adverse reactions, and other risks pertaining to the IV use of this biologic agent.*

Centers for Disease Control: General recommendations on immunization. *JAMA* 1989;262:22–26; 187–191; 339–340. *Covers in detail the administration schedules, precautions, and contraindications for immunization.*

Creekmore SP, Longo DL: Biologic response modifiers: Interferons, interleukins, and other cytokines. *Resident Staff Physician* 1988; 34(8):23–31. *Reviews the use of several cytokines, including tumor necrosis factor and lymphokine-activated killer cells, in the treatment of neoplasms.*

Drugs for AIDS and associated infections. *Med Lett Drugs Ther* 1991; 33:95–102. *Update on anti-HIV drugs and antiinfective agents used against opportunistic infections and neoplasms.*

Dudjak LA, Fleck AE: BRMs (biological response modifiers): New drug therapy comes of age. *RN* 1991;54(10):42–48. *Summarizes approved and investigational uses, mechanisms of action, and nursing management of adverse effects of interferons, hematopoietic factors, interleukin 2, and tumor necrosis factor. Includes a brief summary of the immune response.*

Finter NB, et al: The use of interferon-α in virus infections. *Drugs* 1991;42:749–765. *Discusses the clinical use of interferon in a variety of viral infections.*

Hollingshead LM, Goa KL: Recombinant granulocyte colony-stimulating factor (rG-CSF): A review of its pharmacological properties and prospective role in neutropenic conditions. *Drugs* 1991; 42:300–330. *Presents the pharmacologic actions, adverse effects, and potental therapeutic uses of this stimulant of granulocyte proliferation and action.*

Jost EE, Peter G: New developments in childhood immunizations. *Drug Ther* 1990;20(1):51–67. *Discusses new vaccines and reviews current recommendations for administration.*

Jurgrau A: Why aren't we protecting our children? *RN* 1990;53(11): 30–35. *Reviews the basics of childhood immunizations. Includes timetable for all vaccinations, and review questions.*

Kelly P: Counseling patients with HIV. *RN* 1992;55(2):54–58. *Discusses all aspects of treatment, including pharmacotherapy, of HIV-positive persons.*

Lieschke GJ, Burgess AW: Granulocyte colony-stimulating factor and granulocyte-macrophage colony-stimulating factor (Two parts). *N Engl J Med* 1992;327:28–35 and 99–106. *Details the clinical pharmacology of these agents.*

Mayer DK: Biotherapy: Recent advances and nursing implications. *Adv Oncol Nurs* 1990;25:291–308. *Presents an overview of clinical experience with several biologic response modifiers, including colony-stimulating factors, lymphokines, and effector cells. Emphasizes nursing management of patients receiving these agents.*

Pezze JL, Whiteman K: Transplantation's newest weapon: FK 506. *Am J Nurs* 1991;91(10):40–42. *Discusses actions, administration, and adverse effects of this investigational drug.*

Table 54–C1/S1 **Immunostimulant Dosages, Adverse Effects, and Contraindications**

Drug	Dosage	Adverse Effects	Contraindications*
		Drug Conferring Active Immunity	
BCG vaccine	Percutaneous: Apply 0.2 to 0.3 mL to cleaned skin, apply multiple-puncture disc Intradermal: 0.1 mL (or 0.05 mL for children <3 months old)	Skin lesion at injection site, malaise, fever, inflammation of lymph nodes; rarely, disseminated BCG infection and death	Tuberculin-positive skin test; immunodeficiency; presence of burns; administration of antituberculosis drugs
DPT triple antigen	IM: Three 0.5-mL doses at 4–8-week intervals or at ages 2, 4, and 6 months, followed by a fourth dose 1 year after the third or at 15–18 months of age, and a dose on entry to school (Tetanus and diphtheria toxoids should be given every 10 years for life)	Neurologic sequelae attributed to pertussis, occasional permanent CNS damage and death; hypersensitivity reactions; localized erythema with or without fever; anorexia; drowsiness	Severe reactions 24–48 hr following DPT preclude further administration of pertussis: fever above 40.5°C (105°F), crying of greater than 3 hours' duration, marked alterations of consciousness, shock-like collapse. Pertussis component contraindicated in persons older than 6 years and in children with history or familial tendency to CNS disorders; allergy to any component(s) of the preparation; immunodeficiency; outbreaks of poliomyelitis; coagulation disorders that contraindicate IM injection
Haemophilus influenzae type B vaccine	IM, single-dose vial; at ages 2, 4, 6, and 15 months.	Mild localized reaction, mild fever, irritability, vomiting, diarrhea	Unknown
Hepatitis B vaccine (HEPTAVAX, ENGERIX, RECOMBIVAX)	IM: Two 1.0-mL doses 1 month apart, third dose 6 months after the first. Children under 10 years: 0.5 mL per dose. Persons who are immunodeficient or who require dialysis: 2 mL per dose (smaller volumes for RECOMBIVAX)	Localized reactions, fever, malaise, nausea, fatigue	History of allergic response to the vaccine
Influenza type A vaccine	IM: All persons over 12 years: Split or whole vaccine, 0.5 mL; 3–12 years: Split vaccine, two 0.5-mL doses; 6–35 months: Split vaccine, two 0.25-mL doses, reimmunize annually (eg, each November); administer to high-risk pregnant women after first trimester	Localized reactions, fever, malaise, neurologic disorders including Guillain-Barré syndrome	Allergy to any component (eg, egg protein, aminoglycoside antibiotics); acute febrile illness
Measles, mumps, and rubella vaccines (M-M-R II)	SC: One 0.5-mL dose at 15–18 months of age	Fever, rash, malaise, localized burning or stinging upon injection, regional lymph node enlargement, febrile convulsions in children, encephalitis, Guillain-Barré syndrome, arthritis and polyneuritis in girls and women	Ages under 15 months; rubella vaccine during pregnancy; fever, infectious disease; hypersensitivity to any component(s) of the vaccine (severe hypersensitivity reactions to eggs preclude administration of measles and mumps vaccines)

(continued)

*Most vaccines and toxoids are contraindicated during pregnancy, although significant risk of serious diseases (eg, rabies or poliomyelitis) permits their administration.

Table 54–C1/S1 **Immunostimulant Dosages, Adverse Effects, and Contraindications (*Continued*)**

Drug	Dosage	Adverse Effects	Contraindications*
Pneumococcal vaccine (PNEUMOVAX)	IM or SC: 0.5 mL	Localized reaction, fever	Age under 2 years
Poliovirus vaccine (TOPV, Sabin)	Oral: Two 0.5-mL doses 6–8 weeks apart, followed by a third dose 6–12 months later; a booster dose given on entry into school is recommended	Rare cases of paralytic poliomyelitis to vaccinees or close contacts	Immunodeficiency in patient or close contacts; acute or debilitating illness; vomiting, diarrhea; hypersensitivity
Rabies vaccine (IMOVAX)	IM: Preexposure: 1 mL on days 0, 7, and 28; postexposure: 1 mL on days 0, 3, 7, 14, and 28; a sixth dose may be given 3 months after the first	Localized reactions, headache, nausea, dizziness, hypersensitivity, neurologic disorders	
Drug Conferring Passive Immunity			
Botulism antitoxin	IV/IM: Usually 1 vial (21,500 IU) diluted 1:10 with saline, given by slow IV injection; give second vial (undiluted) IM, with additional IM doses 2–4 hr later if symptoms worsen; reduced doses may be sufficient for asymptomatic patients	Anaphylaxis, serum sickness	Allergic persons can be desensitized to permit administration
Diphtheria antitoxin	IM (or IM/IV): For prophylaxis in nonimmune, exposed persons: Usually 10,000 U; for symptomatic diphtheria: 20,000–120,000 U, depending on disease stage, symptom severity, usually with half of dose given IV, balance IM; use only IM route in patients with allergy to diphtheria antitoxin	See botulism antitoxin	See botulism antitoxin
Hepatitis B immune globulin (H-BIG, HEP-B-GAMMAGEE)	IM: Adults with known or suspected exposure: Usually 0.06 mL/kg (or 3–5 mL total); give second dose 1 month after exposure. Infants born to hepatitis B–positive women: 0.5 mL as soon as possible after delivery, repeated at 3 and 6 months of age	Localized reactions, hypersensitivity	Allergy, coagulation disorders that preclude IM injection
Immune serum globulin	IM: for hepatitis A, usually 0.02 mL/kg; hepatitis B, 0.06 mL/kg; measles, 0.25 mL/kg; for Ig-deficient patients, 1.2 mL/kg initially, then 0.66 mL/kg every 3–4 weeks, or more often if needed IV: For Ig-deficient patients: 2–4 mL/kg once monthly; infuse at rate of 0.01–0.02 mL/kg/min (or 0.02–0.04 mL/kg/min if tolerated based on lack of side effects)	Headache, nausea, chills, fever, flu-like syndrome, severe pain at IM injection site, marked hypotension with IV administration	Allergy

(continued)

Table 54–C1/S1 **Immunostimulant Dosages, Adverse Effects, and Contraindications (*Continued*)**

Drug	Dosage	Adverse Effects	Contraindications*
Rabies immune globulin (IMOGAM)	IM: 10 IU/kg: infiltrate wound with another 10 IU/kg	Localized reactions, fever	
Rh_o (D) immune globulin (RhoGAM)	IM: 300 μg per 15 mL blood exposure	Localized reactions, fever, myalgia	Allergy
Tetanus antitoxin	Routes vary: For suspected exposure, 1500–5000 U, depending on body weight, IM or SC. For symptomatic patients, usually 50,000–100,000 U with a portion given IV, balance given IM	See botulism antitoxin	See botulism antitoxin

Table 54–I1 **Major Interactions Between Immunostimulants and Other Agents**

AGENT	INTERACTANT	RESULT OF INTERACTION
All agents used to induce active immunity	Immunosuppressant drugs: corticosteroids, agents for passive immunity, others (see text)	Suppression of immune system response to antigens, failure to develop adequate active immunity; immunostimulant administration usually ineffective, not recommended, in presence of immunosuppressant drugs unless anticipated benefits outweigh potential dangers of not immunizing patient
BCG vaccine	Antitubercular drugs	Interactants inactivate antigen and prevent immune response; interaction may be used when BCG vaccine overdoses occur
Hepatitis B vaccine	Hepatitis B immune globulin	A desired interaction; use drugs concurrently to prevent or ameliorate disease symptoms in persons exposed to hepatitis B virus
Immune serum globulins	Agents for inducing active immunity (all)	Immune serum globulins suppress response to antigens, resulting in failure to develop adequate active immunity
Influenza type A vaccine	Anticoagulants, oral	Inhibited anticoagulant metabolism, excessive prolongation of prothrombin time, risk of bleeding; if vaccine must be given during oral anticoagulant therapy, monitor accordingly; frequent coagulation studies may be required for a short time after administration of vaccine
Rabies vaccine	Rabies immune globulin	A desired interaction used to suppress rabies infection to nonimmune persons upon exposure to rabies

Table 54–C2/S2 Immunosuppressant Indications, Dosages, Adverse Effects, and Contraindications

Drug	Indication	Dosage	Adverse Effects	Contraindications*
Antithymocyte globulin (lymphocyte immune globulin; ATGAM)	To delay or reverse renal transplant rejection (adjunct to other immunosuppressants)	IV: Adults: 10–30 mg/kg per day for 14 consecutive days, then on alternate days for a total of 21 doses in 4 weeks; infuse dose over at least 4 hr through in-line filter, preferably into central vein. Children: 5–25 mg/kg using adult schedule	Chills, fever, arthralgia, myalgia, nausea, diarrhea, other "flu-like" signs symptoms; skin rashes; other manifestations of mild to severe allergic reactions; thrombophlebitis; thrombocytopenia, hemolysis	Allergic response to antithymocyte globulin; skin-testing prior to administering full therapeutic dose is recommended; monitor response to all doses closely; systemic allergic responses contraindicate further use; localized reactions require extreme care with further administration
	Alleviation of aplastic anemia when bone marrow transplantation is not feasible	IV: 10–20 mg/kg per day for 8–14 days, then on alternating days for a total of up to 21 doses; infuse slowly as noted above		
Azathioprine (IMURAN)	Prevention of renal transplant rejection	Oral: Initially 3–5 mg/kg/day, reduced as soon as possible to maintenance dose of 1–3 mg/kg/day; may be administered in divided doses after meals	Leukopenia, increased risk of infection; thrombocytopenia; nausea, vomiting; alopecia; induction of neoplasms (solid tumors, myelogenous leukemias)	Pregnancy; allergy to azathioprine
		IV: Dosages as noted for oral administration, diluted in sterile saline or dextrose, infused slowly (usually over 30–60 min)		
Cyclosporine (SANDIMMUNE)	Prevention of heart, liver, or kidney transplant rejection	Oral (preferred): Initially, 15 mg/kg given 4–12 hr before operation; thereafter give 15 mg/kg once daily for 1–2 weeks postoperatively, reduce by 5% per week to usual daily maintenance dose of 5 to 10 mg/kg	Nephrotoxicity or other manifestations of impaired renal function; hepatotoxicity; hypertension, esp. in heart transplant patients; immunosuppression	Allergy to cyclosporine or polyoxyethylated castor oil (in IV formulation); care in pregnancy, breast-feeding
		IV (when oral administration is not feasible): 5–6 mg/kg (or about 1/3 typical oral dose) infused over 2–6 hr; switch to oral administration as soon as possible		
FK-506	Rescue or primary therapy in rejection of various transplants	Oral: 0.15 mg/kg bid, adjusted to apparent rejection or toxicity	Similar to those of cyclosporine; possibly less severe	Unknown
		IV: 0.1 mg/kg infused over 24 hr		

(continued)

Table 54–C2/S2 **Immunosuppressant Indications, Dosages, Adverse Effects, and Contraindications (*Continued*)**

Drug	Indication	Dosage	Adverse Effects	Contraindications*
Methotrexate (FOLEX; MEXATE; RHEUMATREX)	Advanced refractory psoriasis; refractory rheumatoid arthritis (see test dose, below)	Oral, IM, or IV: Usually 10–25 mg given once weekly (not to exceed 50 mg/week). Divided oral maintenance dose schedule: give 2.5 mg at 12-hr intervals for 3 doses per week, or at 8-hr intervals for 4 doses per week. (*Note:* May administer 2.5 mg daily for 5 consecutive days, followed by at least 2 consecutive drug-free days, but risk of serious liver damage increases)	Hepatotoxicity; diarrhea; ulcerative stomatitis; intestinal perforation, hemorrhagic enteritis See Chapter 59 for more details	Hepatic dysfunction; renal dysfunction; pregnancy or childbearing age; serious untoward reaction to test dose (see below)
	Test dose (required before use for psoriasis)	IM or IV: 5–10 mg, injected 1 week before giving full therapeutic doses		
Muromonab-CD3 (ORTHOCLONE OKT3)	Treatment of acute renal transplant rejection	IV: give 5 mg bolus once daily for 10–14 days	Acute (first dose) reactions: Severe pulmonary edema; fever, chills; dyspnea, other manifestations of severe untoward respiratory effects. Other (later) effects: Immunosuppression, including risk of infections; predisposition to lymphomas, other malignancies	Allergy to muromonab-CD3 or other products of murine origin; evidence of fluid overload (eg, heart failure, abnormal chest X-ray, weight gain >3% during week before starting therapy, or during therapy); cautious use during pregnancy

Table 54–12 **Major Interactions Between Immunosuppressants and Other Agents***

AGENT	INTERACTANT	RESULT OF INTERACTION
Azathioprine	Allopurinol	Allopurinol inhibits azathioprine metabolism, increases risk of immunosuppressant toxicity; reduce azathioprine dose to ¼ to ⅓ of usual if combined therapy is necessary
	Corticosteroids or antithymocyte globulin	Combined therapy, as often required for transplant patients, increases risks of infection from immunosuppression; monitor frequently and closely for pertinent signs and symptoms
Cyclosporine	Aminoglycoside antibiotics, other nephrotoxic drugs	Increased risk of nephrotoxicity; avoid concomitant administration, guideline applies to all other nephrotoxic drugs
	Amphotericin B	Decreases hepatic metabolism of cyclosporine, increases blood levels, may increase the risk of side effects or toxicity; monitor accordingly
	Cimetidine	Reduces cyclosporine metabolism; related H_2 blockers famotidine and ranitidine less likely to interact, may be preferred
	Digoxin	Cyclosporine elevates plasma levels of digoxin
	Disulfiram	Acute and potentially serious reaction caused by alcohol (in both oral and IV preparations); disulfiram therapy should be discontinued several weeks before starting cyclosporine therapy, and before surgery for which cyclosporine would be used
	Erythromycin	Enhances gastrointestinal absorption of cyclosporine
	Ketoconazole	See amphotericin B; may be used to reduce required cyclosporine doses.
	Metoclopramide	See erythromycin
	Phenobarbital	Stimulates hepatic metabolism of cyclosporine, reduces blood levels, may compromise effectiveness; monitor cyclosporine blood levels and therapeutic response if interaction is unavoidable
	Phenytoin	See phenobarbital
	Rifampin	See phenobarbital
	Sulfamethoxazole plus trimethoprim (co-trimoxazole)	When given IV, stimulates cyclosporine metabolism; see precautions noted for phenobarbital
FK506	Cyclosporine	Additive toxicity
	Corticosteroids	Additive immunosuppression allows lower doses of corticosteroids to be effective
Muromonab-CD3	Immunosuppressants, other: azathioprine, corticosteroids, cyclosporine	Increased risk of infection; monitor accordingly; reduce doses of corticosteroids or azathioprine during combined therapy; reduce or discontinue cyclosporine; maintenance doses of other immunosuppressants should be resumed about 3 days before last anticipated muromonab-CD3 dose

*See Chapter 59 for interactions involving methotrexate and cyclophosphamide

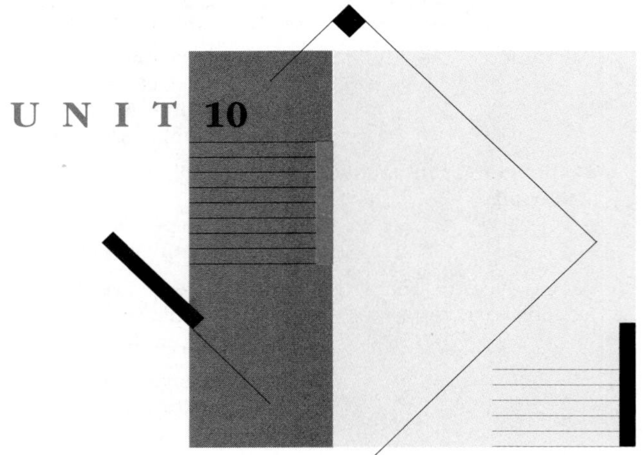

Antimicrobial Agents

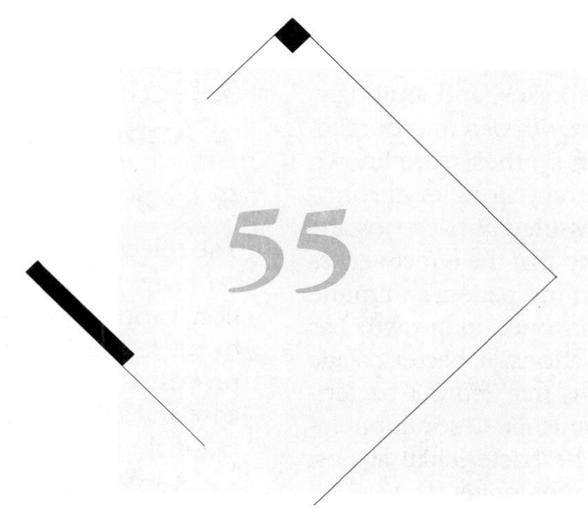

Principles of Antimicrobial Therapy

Antimicrobial therapy is a complex and challenging field of medicine. The emergence of new or resistant pathogens, combined with research and marketing efforts by the pharmaceutic industry, has led to the development of a vast array of antimicrobial agents—drugs used to treat bacterial, fungal, or viral infections. In addition, advances in treatment areas such as organ transplantation and cancer chemotherapy have increased the number of patients who are susceptible to infections and are placed on increasingly complex combinations of antibiotics.

Nurses are presented with many challenges when caring for a patient with an infectious process. They must become familiar with the use, misuse, dosing regimens, and side effects of the many antimicrobial agents available.

The goal of this chapter is to provide the nurse with the general principles of antimicrobial therapy, including the diagnostic approach to infectious diseases, the selection of the proper drug and its administration, monitoring for side effects, and patient education. Although much of the discussion focuses on antibacterial drug therapy, the same general principles apply also to antifungal and antiviral therapy, which are discussed in Chapter 57.

There are too many antimicrobial drugs to learn each one in great detail. This chapter provides a general overview of antimicrobial agents, their mechanisms of action, and their adverse reactions. Chapters 56 and 57 address the specific classes of antimicrobials and their role in the treatment of infections caused by bacteria, fungi, parasites, viruses, and other microorganisms.

The many and diverse antimicrobials now available make it possible to cure many types of infections. However, it is important to realize that these agents are used as adjunctive therapy. In many instances, antibiotics alone cannot provide the cure. Maintenance of an intact immune system, appropriate debridement of wounds, irrigation, and proper surgical technique are as important as the selection and use of the proper antimicrobial agent.

Pharmacologic Effects and Mechanisms of Antimicrobial Action

The effective use of an antimicrobial agent will destroy the infecting organism or inhibit its growth. Antibiotics that are capable of killing the organism are known as **bactericidal** agents. Common examples include the penicillins, cephalosporins, and aminoglycosides. Agents that inhibit the growth of a microorganism, usually by inhibiting protein synthesis, are known as **bacteriostatic** agents. The tetracyclines, erythromycin, and chloramphenicol are classified as bacteriostatic agents. It is essential to understand that the effectiveness of a bacteriostatic agent relies on the patient's immune system to eradicate the organism once its growth has been inhibited. In selected situations, a bacteriostatic agent used at high concentrations may exhibit bactericidal action against specific organisms. Chloramphenicol, for example, is thought to be bactericidal against organisms that commonly cause meningitis.

Antimicrobial agents exert their activity on bacteria, fungi, and viruses by one of five basic mechanisms.

1. *Inhibition of cell wall synthesis.* The disruption of bacterial cell wall synthesis will cause the organism to become osmotically unstable. This causes the cell to lyse, which destroys the organism. The penicillins and cephalosporins act in this way.
2. *Inhibition of protein synthesis.* Some antimicrobial agents cause the formation of abnormal proteins or inhibit protein synthesis, by irreversibly binding to ribosomal subunits. Antimicrobials that are capable of inhibiting protein synthesis can be either bacteriostatic or bactericidal, for reasons that are not well understood. The aminoglycosides, for example, inhibit protein synthesis and are considered bactericidal. Chloramphenicol, tetracyclines, and erythromycin also inhibit bacterial protein synthesis, but at usual doses they are considered to be bacteriostatic agents.
3. *Disruption or alteration of membrane permeability.* Some antimicrobials, primarily the antifungal agents, will bind to specific cell wall components. This alters the permeability of the cell wall, which results in leakage and loss of intracellular molecules that are essential for microbial cell function.
4. *Inhibition of nucleic acid synthesis.* Rifampin is an example of a drug that inhibits RNA synthesis in some bacteria. Antiviral agents such as idoxuridine exert their activity by inhibiting viral DNA or RNA synthesis.
5. *Inhibition of other specific biochemical pathways.* The sulfonamides are examples of an antibiotic agent's ability to competitively inhibit metabolic pathways that are critical to the survival of some microbes of susceptible bacteria. Some antituberculosis agents also have this ability. Antibiotics that work in this manner are usually bacteriostatic.

Selection and Administration of Antimicrobial Agents

Selection

The selection of a specific antimicrobial agent depends on many factors, including the suspected site of infection, various host factors, and the organism most likely to cause the infection. An organized, orderly thought process is necessary when diagnosing an infectious disease and selecting antibiotic therapy that is effective and rational.

A working knowledge of the organisms most commonly associated with various sites of infection will greatly aid the selection of an antibiotic. For example, a high percentage of urinary tract infections are caused by gram-negative organisms, and the majority of these are caused by *Escherichia coli.* Most cases of childhood meningitis are caused by one of three different organisms, allowing immediate selection of antibiotics that target these organisms and will effectively treat this life-threatening infection. Hospitals gather statistics on infections acquired by patients during hospitalization. This identifies trends regarding which organisms are most likely to cause infections in a particular hospital setting, as well as their antibiotic susceptibilities.

The ability of an antibiotic to reach or penetrate the site of infection is extremely important in the antibiotic selection process. The most potent antibiotic can be useless if concentrations at the infection site are inadequate. For example, many cephalosporins are very active against organisms that frequently cause meningitis. However, some cephalosporins penetrate poorly into the cerebrospinal fluid and so are ineffective if used to treat meningitis. Successful treatment of urinary tract infections is accomplished by using antibiotics that are present in high amounts in the urine. Most cases of osteomyelitis require four to six weeks of therapy because of the very low bone concentration achieved by most antibiotics.

Initial Approach to the Patient

Early assessment of a patient with a possible infection includes gathering relevant data about the history of the illness, signs and symptoms, prior therapy, and a drug allergy history.

A thorough *history* of the present illness is very important. Facts such as onset of illness (sudden or insidious), or possible exposures to an infectious agent, can be extremely helpful in identifying the offending organism. Concurrent diseases, especially those that are chronic, may predispose a patient to particular types of infections and also to particular organisms. For example, the organisms most likely to cause pneumonia in a patient with a history of chronic pulmonary disease are different from those likely to cause pneumonia in a young, otherwise healthy adult. Therefore, the proper antibiotic for these patients may be quite different.

The *signs and symptoms* of an infection are fairly typical. A high fever, sometimes accompanied by chills, will be associated with most infections. The elderly and infants, however, may not respond with a fever; instead, an elevated heart rate and general malaise may be the only symptoms. Signs of inflammation, such as redness, heat, and especially pain, are usually present at the infection site and are evident in infections of the skin and skin structures. Localized pain, accompanied by fever, may give a good indication of the type of infection and the organisms likely to be present.

The patient's own ability to combat an infection can also affect the antibiotic choice. An elevated white blood cell count is a typical finding in most infections. This is usually accompanied by a "left shift," which is an elevation in the more immature forms of the white blood cells, often called "bands."

A more urgent finding would be a very small number of white blood cells, or neutropenia, which would indicate that the patient is unable to fight an infection adequately. The neutropenic patient will require antibiotics that have bactericidal actions to successfully treat the infection. Other life-threatening infections, such as endocarditis or meningitis, require bactericidal therapy to eradicate the infection. Bacteriostatic agents can be used to treat infections of lesser severity or when the patient has an intact immune system.

Isolation and Identification of the Organism

The cornerstone of any attempt to make an accurate diagnosis is to isolate and identify the offending organism, and determine its susceptibility to various antimicrobial drugs. The nurse should be aware of the various methods of collecting data needed to confirm a diagnosis.

Appropriate cultures should be obtained before starting antibiotic therapy. If the organism cannot be identified immediately, antibiotic therapy must initially be directed at common pathogens causing the suspected infection. Once the specific organism is identified, therapy should be changed, if needed, to the most specific, least toxic antimicrobial to which the organism is sensitive. In some cases, the offending organism is so predictable (for example, strep throat or a urinary tract infection in an otherwise healthy individual), that treatment will begin immediately and is changed only if the cultured organism is different from what was expected.

The simplest and most frequently used method of identifying an infecting organism is Gram's stain. It is inexpensive and can rapidly confirm an infection and narrow the list of possible organisms. Organisms that hold the initial purple stain are called gram-positive organisms; those that do not hold the original stain, but stain red during the counterstain, are known as gram-negative organisms. A specific shape of bacteria will also be noted on the Gram's stain. Bacteria that take on a round appearance are called *cocci;* others have a rod-like appearance and are appropriately called *rods.* Four different combinations can occur: gram-positive cocci and rods, and gram-negative cocci and rods. Other microorganisms, such as fungi or viruses, require special staining procedures for identification; this will not be addressed in this chapter.

The organism thought to cause the infection can be identified further by culturing and growing the bacteria on various growth media. Specimens for culture can be collected from most sites and body fluids. Sputum, urine, wound, and blood cultures are a few examples. Good collection technique is important to avoid contamination with the body's normal bacterial flora, which could lead to an incorrect diagnosis. Other, more invasive, collection techniques are available if contamination is a potential problem.

Antibiotic Combinations

Antibiotic combinations are used when a synergistic action is desirable, development of resistance is a problem, mixed infections are present, or the nature of the infection is unknown.

Antibiotic synergism occurs when the antibacterial activity of two antibiotics together is at least four times greater than that of either antibiotic used alone. The synergistic use of antibiotics is important in the treatment of infections caused by *Pseudomonas* and *Enterococcus* because these organisms typically do not respond to treatment with a single antibiotic.

Combination therapy is routinely used to treat tuberculosis, because of the tendency for rapid resistance to develop when only one drug is used.

A physician may elect to use more than one antibiotic when the site of infection is unknown and a broad range of infecting organisms is possible. Antibiotics with primarily gram-positive activity are combined with antibiotics aimed at gram-negative organisms. Antibiotics directed at anaerobic bacteria, fungi, or viruses may also be included. The development of newer antibiotics with a wide range of antibacterial activity will reduce the need for multiple antibiotic treatment. Some infections, especially those involving the pelvic or peritoneal area, may be caused by more than one organism and may require the use of more than one antibiotic.

Administration

Antimicrobials can be administered by different routes, the most common being intravenous (IV), intramuscular (IM), and oral. The choice of administration route depends on several factors, including the severity of the infection, patient convenience, cost, and the particular antibiotic selected.

Intravenous Administration

Intravenous administration requires the most nursing care. This route is selected when high concentrations of the antibiotic must reach the site of infection. This is especially important in treating meningitis or osteomyelitis, or other situations in which only a small percentage of the antibiotic will reach the infection site. Other instances where parenteral therapy is necessary are when patients are unable to take oral medications, when antibiotic of choice is only available as an injectable product, or when oral absorption is poor.

NURSING IMPLICATIONS

Patients who receive antibiotics IV require a significant amount of nursing care. Accurate and timely antibiotic administration will help ensure a successful recovery. In addition, antibiotics whose doses are individualized using pharmacokinetic calculations—chiefly the aminoglycosides—depend highly on accurate IV administration. Erratic administration or missed doses can lead to an inadequate response or the development of resistant organisms.

Some hospitalized patients require two or three different antibiotics, each of which can be scheduled for administration at various times. It is vital to carefully double-check all medications to make sure that the right antibiotic is given at the right time.

Drug incompatibilities are always a potential problem when giving IV antibiotics, especially for patients receiving multiple antibiotics. This problem is minimized by thoroughly flushing the IV tubing with normal saline or another compatible IV fluid to remove the remaining antibiotic before the next one is given. Consult a pharmacist for more information about incompatibility.

Many injectable antibiotics can cause phlebitis at the injection site. It is important, therefore, to monitor for the typical signs of phlebitis: pain, redness, heat, and edema located at or near the injection site. Many patients, especially the elderly, would not be able to tolerate an antibiotic if given in concentrated form. Most antibiotics are diluted in 50 to 100 mL of normal saline or 5% dextrose before administration. Some antibiotics may require even further dilution. For children or other patients who may be fluid restricted, dilute the drug in the minimum recommended volume (consult product information) and infuse it over the recommended time. Change intravenous sites every 48 to 72 hours to minimize the incidence of phlebitis.

Intramuscular Administration

The IM route is an acceptable alternative for most antibiotics if IV access is difficult. It is also the required route of administration for certain penicillin products available as sustained release suspensions.

NURSING IMPLICATIONS

Intramuscular administration is less convenient and often more unpleasant for the patient than oral administration, mainly because of pain. Many antibiotics irritate muscle tissue, just as they cause phlebitis with the IV route. Some pain can be reduced by mixing the antibiotic with a local anesthetic such as lidocaine. Be sure to avoid using a local anesthetic that contains a vasoconstrictor (eg epinephrine).

Some antibiotics, such as vancomycin, should never be given IM because they can cause severe muscle necrosis. It is important to ascertain before administration that the drug is indicated for IM use.

To ensure proper blood concentrations, give antibiotics deep into a large muscle mass such as the gluteal or deltoid muscles. Rotate the injection site frequently to avoid severe muscle damage. Avoid the use of IM injections in situations where blood flow is poor, such as in shock or other hypoperfusion states.

Oral Administration

Many common infections, such as urinary tract and respiratory tract infections, can be treated by oral antibiotic administration. Patients prefer this route because it is less expensive, more convenient, and free from the pain or worry caused by injections.

NURSING IMPLICATIONS

The general disadvantages of oral antibiotics include unpleasant taste, gastrointestinal (GI) upset, occasional diarrhea, and resulting poor compliance. Patients are more likely to miss one or several doses when relied on to take oral antibiotics. Some patients will mistakenly stop taking their antibiotic when they begin to feel better. This may result in a failure to adequately eradicate the infection, and a relapse may occur.

Many antibiotics are available as oral suspensions; some are unpleasant tasting, which can be a problem for children. Further comments about potential problems associated with self-administration of oral antibiotics are presented later in the section on general nursing implications.

General Side and Adverse Effects of Antimicrobials

Antibiotics, for the most part, are relatively safe. However, they are not without toxic effects, some of which can prolong illness or even threaten life. Some adverse reactions that are unique to a specific class or classes will be discussed in later chapters. General side effects common to all classes are discussed here.

Allergic Reactions

The most common adverse effect of antibiotics is an allergic reaction. An allergy to an antibiotic can be manifested in many ways, ranging from a generalized rash to severe, life-threatening anaphylactic shock. In general, the penicillins are the most common cause of allergic reactions, but the cephalosporins and sulfonamides are also common offenders.

The management of allergic reactions will vary depending on the severity of the reaction and the infection being treated. Many rashes are mild and can be treated by discontinuing the offending drug and using antihistamines to treat discomfort. In some cases, a mild rash will be tolerated if a patient's infection necessitates treatment with a particular antibiotic.

Anaphylactic reactions are life-threatening and require immediate care. Symptoms include hypotension, bronchoconstriction, laryngeal edema, and possible cardiovascular collapse.

Superinfection

Superinfections are infections that occur while the patient is receiving, or has recently received, antimicrobial therapy. They occur when the body's normal bacterial flora have been altered by the use of an antibiotic, allowing proliferation of selected bacteria that are typically resistant to the current antibiotic. Superinfections may be localized or systemic, and some may be extremely difficult to treat.

Patients are most susceptible to developing superinfections when they are placed on antibiotics that have a broad spectrum of antimicrobial activity, which theoretically will cause a greater disruption of the normal flora, or when they receive a combination of antibiotics. Other risk factors include antibiotics that concentrate in the bile, which in turn will concentrate in the large intestine.

A specific example of a superinfection is the condition known as pseudomembranous colitis. When exposed to any of a number of broad-spectrum antibiotics, bowel flora are markedly suppressed. This causes overgrowth of an organism called *Clostridium difficile,* a toxin-producing bacteria resistant to many antibiotics. Severe, sometimes life-threatening, diarrhea may occur. Another common example is the development of vaginal candidiasis in women who have received broad-spectrum antibiotics. This is common in young women who have received chronic tetracycline therapy to treat acne.

Other Common Adverse Reactions

Diarrhea, vomiting, and other manifestations of GI upset may reflect not only superinfection, worsening of an underlying disorder, or local intolerance to the administered drug. The consequences can be mild and annoying, or serious because of fluid and electrolyte imbalances that could aggravate imbalances caused by the disorder for which antibiotics were prescribed.

Many antibiotics are available as sodium salts. In addition, the broad spectrum penicillins, such as ticarcillin, contain large amounts of sodium. Patients who require sodium restriction may experience sodium and fluid overload if given one of these agents. Weight gain; increased blood pressure; evidence of edema, pulmonary, or cardiac disorders; and other manifestations of sodium and fluid overload may occur. Likewise, other antibiotic salts or preparations, such as those containing potassium, may cause special problems for selected patients.

NURSING IMPLICATIONS

Allergic reactions to antibiotics (and many other drugs) are commonly—usually incorrectly—called "hypersensitivity" reactions. Hypersensitivity reactions involve a heightened response to a usually safe and effective dose of a drug. The incidence and severity of true hypersensitivity reactions may be reduced by lowering the dose. With antibiotics and other allergy-provoking substances, a true antigen–antibody reaction triggers the synthesis and release of noxious pathologic mediators. Even minuscule amounts of the offending drug can trigger a fatal reaction.

A thorough and accurate drug history should uncover prior "allergic" responses. However, information received from the patient or family may not be reliable. For example, a history of a generalized rash could be a manifestation of an underlying disease rather than a drug-induced response. Prior GI upset, vomiting, or diarrhea often represent local drug intolerance or superinfection, and rarely represent true allergy. Helping identify the true nature of an untoward response is an important nursing role. It could allow the safe administration of a needed antibiotic drug, or prevent the inadvertent use of a drug that might cause serious harm.

Be aware that in cases of documented antibiotic allergy, *the offending drug, drugs in the same chemical class, or even some agents from other classes that cross-react* should not be administered, regardless of the dose or administration route, unless the anticipated benefits clearly outweigh the potential risks. In such instances, always have ready for use parenteral epinephrine, antihistamines, and corticosteroids; oxygen; and facilities for full cardiopulmonary resuscitation. Even if the history is only questionable, emergency drugs and facilities should be readily available.

Chart all documented patient allergies; affix warning labels to the front of the patient's chart, and annotate other patient summaries. Advise patients with such allergies to notify all future health-care providers of their allergy, and to carry or wear appropriate identification to alert others in case of emergency. Assess patients for, and have them assess for and report, indicators of allergic reactions (hives or rashes; flushing or diaphoresis; dizziness or palpitations as might be caused by hypotension; dyspnea or other forms of respiratory distress; fever; arthralgias or myalgias).

Be aware that anyone may develop antibiotic allergies—even persons with no known prior therapeutic antibiotic administration history—through exposure to trace amounts of these drugs in the environment, vaccines, and foods. Nurses, pharmacists, and physicians may develop antibodies to antibiotics through occupational exposure. They are at higher risk of developing allergic reactions when receiving these drugs for therapeutic purposes. Meticulous dispensing and administration techniques are important to avoid repeated, direct contact (even with the skin) with antibiotics, especially high-risk agents such as the penicillins. Avoid handling these drugs if there is a question of allergies to them.

Be aware of the signs, symptoms, and risks of superinfections. Their potentially serious complications emphasize the need to ensure that the patient is taking the most specific antibiotic possible, and the need to avoid using a "shotgun" approach.

Assess patients for worsening of other underlying conditions during antibiotic administration. Such changes include fluid and electrolyte loss caused by diarrhea or vomiting, other imbalances caused by the antibiotic salt or formulation, and inadequate nutrient intake caused by drug-induced GI upset and nausea.

◆ Use During Pregnancy and Lactation

Women who are pregnant or nursing pose a special problem when selecting the proper antimicrobial agent. All antimicrobials cross the placenta to some degree, thus exposing the fetus to potential adverse effects. Since data on the teratogenic potential of antibiotics is limited, the benefits of antibiotic therapy must be weighed against the risk of harm to the fetus. Tetracyclines, for example, should not be used in pregnant or nursing mothers because of their ability to disrupt bone and tooth formation in the fetus. Additional data regarding the teratogenic potential of specific antibiotics will be detailed in Chapters 56 and 57.

◆ Use in Children and the Elderly

Age-dependent differences in common infecting organisms, as well as differences in drug absorption, distribution, metabolism and excretion, and toxicities, make age another important factor to consider in antibiotic therapy. The metabolism and excretion of antibiotics often are reduced in neonates and often diminish in the elderly. Therefore, antibiotics that rely on healthy kidneys for elimination may be toxic in a neonate or elderly patient. Conversely, the immature liver of a neonate may be unable to inactivate an antibiotic such as chloramphenicol, leading to life-threatening side effects. Specific examples of the importance of age considerations are presented in the next two chapters.

General Assessment of Desired Antimicrobial Drug Responses

Specific patient monitoring parameters are discussed in greater depth when each class of antibiotics is addressed. However, some general monitoring parameters are pertinent to all patients receiving any antibiotic.

The patient's response to antibiotic treatment is the major way to assess for drug efficacy or therapeutic failure. Assess for a reduction in fever, a decrease in inflammation of local infections, a reduction in the white blood cell count, and a generalized improvement in the patient's well-being. An inadequate response may occur for a number of reasons. The suspected organism may be resistant to the antibiotics prescribed, the dosage may be inadequate, or only minimal concentrations of antibiotic may be reaching the infection site. A reevaluation of the patient's therapy may be necessary if an adequate response is not seen within 48 hours.

Patient Education

A patient must receive thorough counseling regarding the proper administration of an antibiotic to ensure proper treatment. This is especially true with oral antibiotics, since they are usually self-administered without direct supervision.

The single most important concept to stress to patients is the importance of finishing all the prescribed amount of antibiotic. Antibiotics are typically prescribed to be taken for a period of five to 14 days. Most infections, however, will begin to resolve within 24 to 48 hours, and symptoms will decrease. Once patients begin to feel better they may stop taking the antibiotic before the infection is completely eliminated. This may lead to a recurrence of the infection and risks the development of resistant organisms.

Ideally, antibiotics should be taken around-the-clock at evenly spaced intervals. While this can be controlled when the patient is hospitalized, it may be impractical when the patient is home. An antibiotic given every six hours would require that doses are taken late at night and then early in the morning. This is obviously disruptive, and few patients will adhere to such a schedule. It is much easier to ensure that a patient takes the antibiotic four times a day at times that are easily identifiable and acceptable, such as with meals (if appropriate) and at bedtime.

The absorption of many antibiotics can be altered by food. For example, some penicillins and cephalosporins are more completely absorbed on an empty stomach and should be given at least one hour before meals. However, this is not always practical. Although erythromycin absorption is optimal when the drug is taken on an empty stomach, it can cause extreme irritation to the stomach unless taken with food. In such cases it would be better to sacrifice some drug absorption than to neglect taking the drug because of discomforting side effects.

Because of convenience and cost, some patients receive IV antibiotics at home to treat certain chronic infections. The primary care nurse should be extensively involved in teaching the patient and family the proper technique for preparing and administering these drugs.

PROTOTYPES

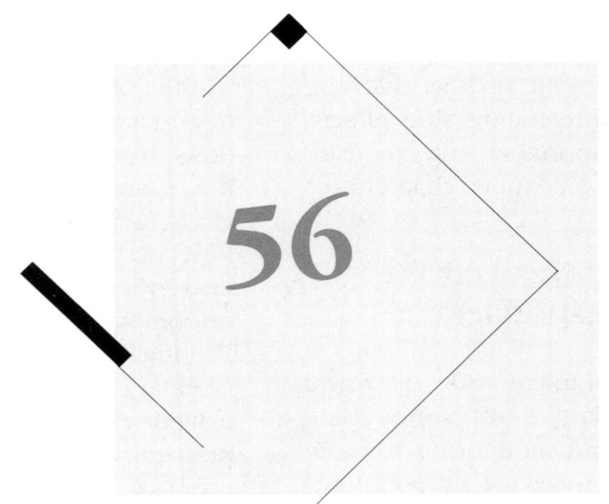

Antibiotics

This chapter focuses on eight major classes of antibiotics that are widely used to treat most of the common bacterial infections. They are the

- penicillins,
- cephalosporins,
- aminoglycosides,
- tetracyclines,
- erythromycins,
- sulfonamides
- quinolones, and
- chloramphenicol.

In each case, the information centers on a prototype agent. However, some of the groups have subclasses, each of which contains important related drugs with special properties and uses.

The chapter concludes with discussions of several other antibiotics that either stand alone in terms of their chemical class, or have other properties that distinguish them from agents in the eight major groups. Nevertheless, they too are important drugs. Table 56–1 identifies the common bacteria for which the drugs discussed in this chapter are used.

Drugs that exert their primary activities against microorganisms other than common bacteria will be discussed in Chapter 57. They include drugs used to manage tuberculosis (caused by mycobacteria), because the traditional antitubercular drugs differ from those used to treat the more common bacterial infections.

The reader is strongly encouraged to read or review the introductory material presented in Chapter 55; it presents many of the general guidelines for antimicrobial therapy, including ways to assess for desired and adverse antimicrobial drug effects. That information is not repeated in this chapter.

I. Penicillins

A. Natural Penicillins

PROTOTYPE

Penicillin G

Penicillin G (PENTIDS; PFIZERPEN; others) is the prototype of the natural penicillins, which are derived by fermentation from strains of *Penicillium* mold. Penicillin

Major reference tables appear beginning on p. 1205.

Table 56–1 Classification of Common Bacteria

Gram-Positive Cocci	Gram-Positive Rods	Gram-Negative Cocci	Gram-Negative Rods
Staphylococcus aureus	*Clostridium difficile*	*Branhamella catarrhalis*	*Acinetobacter*
Staphylococcus epidermidis	*Clostridium tetani*	*Neisseria gonorrheae*	*Bacteroides fragilis*
Streptococcus pneumoniae	*Corynebacterium diphtheriae*	*Neisseria meningitidis*	*Enterobacter cloacae*
Streptococcus pyogenes	*Listeria monocytogenes*		*Escherichia coli*
Streptococcus faecalis (Enterococcus)			*Haemophilus influenzae*
Streptococcus viridans			*Klebsiella pneumoniae*
			Proteus mirabilis
			Providencia stuartii
			Pseudomonas aeruginosa
			Serratia marcescens

G was identified and named by Alexander Fleming in 1928. Commercial isolation and clinical use began in 1939. It was one of the few antibiotics available during World War II. Because of its low cost and toxicity, and its great clinical efficacy against many gram-positive organisms, penicillin G remains one of the most important antibiotics currently marketed. Other natural derivatives of penicillin G have been developed to enhance or prolong absorption or reduce toxicity, but they have the same spectrum of clinical activity. Although newer penicillins often will effectively treat penicillin-susceptible organisms, penicillin G and its natural derivatives remain the drugs of choice for susceptible organisms.

Absorption, Distribution, Metabolism, and Excretion

Penicillin G is not absorbed well following oral administration because most of it is hydrolyzed by gastric acid. Only 15% to 30% of the administered dose is absorbed when given to a fasting patient. Administration with meals further reduces oral absorption of penicillin G. Decreased gastric acidity, such as occurs in the neonate or elderly, increases oral absorption. Peak serum concentrations are reached 30 to 60 minutes following oral administration, and serum levels are detectable for up to 6 hours.

Penicillin G is readily absorbed following intramuscular (IM) administration, achieving peak serum concentrations in 15 to 30 minutes. However, since the drug must be given every 6 hours, and the injections are painful, IM penicillin G is generally reserved for patients, such as neonates, in whom reduced renal excretion permits less frequent dosage.

The potassium or sodium salts of penicillin G can be given intravenously (IV). They achieve high serum concentrations rapidly, but effective blood levels last only 3 to 6 hours, so frequent administration is required.

Penicillin G achieves effective antibiotic levels throughout the body when proper doses are given. It does not cross the blood–brain barrier well unless the meninges are inflamed. Moderate drug levels in the cerebrospinal fluid are reached in this condition.

Penicillin G is eliminated by both hepatic degradation to inactive metabolites and renal excretion of unchanged drug and its metabolites. Renal excretion is mainly by active tubular secretion. Probenecid blocks this tubular secretion, and that drug can be used to prolong blood penicillin G levels in a few clinical circumstances in which high blood levels must be maintained. Renal clearance is reduced in neonates and other patients with diminished renal function. This can prolong to several hours the normal serum half-life of 0.4 to 0.9 hour. Since penicillin G has a very low toxicity, its dose seldom needs to be adjusted unless the patient has severe renal dysfunction. The usual adjustment is less frequent administration.

Pharmacologic Effects

Penicillins exert a bactericidal effect on susceptible organisms by interfering with the formation of critical proteins in the bacterial cell wall. Altered cell wall formation makes the bacterium susceptible to destruction by osmotic processes and through actions of self-destructive enzymes (called *bacterial autolysins*) located within certain bacteria.

Bacterial enzymes at penicillin's target sites, known as *penicillin-binding proteins,* vary greatly among bacterial species. They account, in part, for the variable effectiveness of penicillins and their synthetic derivatives against differing bacterial species, and in some cases even bacterial subgroups.

Penicillins are most effective against gram-positive bacteria. Gram-negative bacteria, which are less responsive, possess a lipopolysaccharide coat that blocks penetration of penicillins into the organism. This limited ability to penetrate gram-negative bacteria is shared by other natural penicillins and by the penicillinase-resistant penicillins. The aminopenicillins and extended-spectrum penicillins, discussed later, appear to have activity against gram-negative bacteria because they can penetrate these outer membranes.

Some bacteria are resistant to certain penicillins because they synthesize an enzyme that destroys the beta-lactam ring of the penicillin molecule, a part of the molecule that is critical for antibiotic activity. The enzyme, also called *beta-lactamase* or *penicillinase,* can also inactivate some of the cephalosporin antibiotics that are discussed later.

Some important penicillins are resistant to inactivation by penicillinase. Other penicillins are able to penetrate gram-negative bacteria, and are therefore useful in infections caused by these organisms. These drugs are identified and discussed later.

Clinical Indications and Administration

Penicillin G is used to treat infections caused by susceptible aerobic gram-positive cocci, including most streptococcal organisms (except some enterococci) and nonpenicillinase-producing *Staphylococcus,* gram-positive bacilli (*Bacillus anthracis, Corynebacterium diphtheriae*), gram-negative cocci (*Neisseria meningitidis*), anaerobes (anaerobic cocci, *Clostridia*), spirochetes (*Treponema pallidum, Leptospira*), and *Actinomyces israelii.* Penicillin G is generally considered the drug of choice for these organisms because it exerts highly specific antibiotic action against them and is relatively nontoxic to the host. The drug can also be used for prophylaxis of rheumatic fever, bacterial endocarditis, and pneumococcal infections in susceptible patients.

The potassium and sodium salts of penicillin G are used for parenteral therapy; these products are sometimes called "crystalline penicillin." Penicillin G potassium is used most often and is usually the form implied when the physician does not explicitly state the salt to be used. Typical dosages are listed in Table 56–C1.

Penicillin G is usually given IV in high doses to treat infections such as meningitis, pneumonia, septicemia, and endocarditis. Because of local pain and the need for frequent dosing, IM injection should be reserved for patients with reduced renal function, such as neonates. However, the procaine and benzathine preparations, which are specifically intended for IM use, are generally preferred for these patients, since they provide longer durations of action and injections are less painful.

Penicillin G is seldom given orally because it is absorbed poorly and must be given on an empty stomach, which may cause gastrointestinal (GI) upset. For most indications in which oral penicillin therapy is desired, penicillin V (discussed later) is preferred. Penicillins are potent skin-sensitizing agents and should not be administered topically.

NURSING IMPLICATIONS

When administering penicillin G IV, be certain that the correct salt (usually potassium) is used. If frequent IM administration is required, alternative penicillins may be preferred. If oral penicillin G is indicated, give it on an empty stomach. Penicillin V is preferred to circumvent the problems of poor absorption and GI upset. Avoid topical application of penicillin G.

Side Effects, Adverse Reactions, and Contraindications

Penicillin G and the other natural penicillins are relatively nontoxic antibiotics. Their margin of safety is much greater than that of most other antibiotics. Major adverse effects are rare and usually involve hypersensitivity reactions. Overdosage or administration of high doses of penicillin G may be associated with adverse neurologic, hematologic, and renal effects, especially in patients with compromised renal function. Table 56–S1 summarizes the adverse reactions and contraindications of the natural penicillins.

Allergic Reactions

Allergic reactions are the most common and potentially serious adverse effects caused by penicillin G and all other penicillins. They usually result from prior exposure to a penicillin used therapeutically, but may also occur in the settings described in Chapter 55 (p. 1156). The penicillins cross-react: a patient who experiences an allergic reaction to one penicillin will react to *any* other penicillin. There is also some cross-reactivity between penicillins and cephalosporin antibiotics.

Allergic reactions to penicillins usually involve urticarial, erythematous, or maculopapular (morbilliform) rashes, often accompanied by pruritus. The overall incidence of dermatologic reactions is 2% to 4% of all patients receiving these drugs. Urticaria usually occurs within the first 3 days of penicillin therapy; other skin reactions usually do not develop until 48 hours or more after therapy has started. Some of the skin reactions may be serious.

In some patients, the only manifestation of an allergic reaction to penicillin is fever, chills, or eosinophilia. A Coombs'-positive hemolytic anemia may also occur, but is seen mainly when high doses are given IV. Serum sickness–like reactions (fever, arthralgia, myalgia, rash, lymphatic or splenic enlargement) occur in at least 1% of patients receiving penicillins. These symptoms usually resolve when penicillin treatment is stopped, but they may last for several weeks.

The most sudden and serious allergic reaction caused by penicillins is anaphylaxis and all of its life-threatening consequences: bronchospasm, laryngeal edema, stridor, cyanosis, and circulatory collapse. The reaction may be preceded by nausea and vomiting, diaphoresis, and dizziness. Anaphylaxis usually occurs within 30 minutes of administration of these antibiotics. The overall incidence is 0.05% of patients receiving the drug. Parenteral administration of penicillins is most likely to cause anaphylaxis.

Any allergic reaction to a penicillin requires immediate discontinuation of the drug and related antibiotics. Mild reactions may require administration of antihistamines or corticosteroids. Anaphylactoid reactions may be fatal and so require immediate subcutaneous (SC) or IV administration of epinephrine; oxygen therapy; maintenance of a patent airway; and treatment with corticosteroids. Similar treatments are used to treat allergic reactions caused by virtually all antibiotics.

Because penicillins are the drugs of choice for many infections, physicians often feel compelled to use them, even in patients with suspected "hypersensitivity" to them. Since the reported incidence of penicillin allergy is high, physicians have tried to reduce the incidence or severity of such reactions by pretreating susceptible patients with antihistamines or corticosteroids. This practice seldom prevents a serious reaction and should be discouraged.

If the patient with a history of penicillin allergy has a life-threatening infection, and the clinician feels that penicillin must be used, penicillin desensitization may be attempted. Increasing doses of the penicillin derivative are given frequently, initially intracutaneously or intradermally in very small doses, progressing to SC or IM administration, and finally to IV therapy until the desired dosage is reached. This procedure is thought to gradually bind circulating antibody, which would normally result in the allergic manifestations when exposed to a full dose, and cause a gradual rather than a precipitous release of histamine. It is important to note that therapy cannot be interrupted once therapeutic doses are initiated. Otherwise, sufficient antibody may accumulate to cause a severe reaction on reinitiation of the medication. This is a high-risk procedure that requires close supervision and immediate availability of adequate support systems to treat anaphylactoid reactions that may occur.

If penicillin allergy is suspected, penicillin skin testing can be accomplished using intradermal skin test antigens (eg, penicilloyl-polylysine [PRE-PEN]) and the penicillin, or minor determinant derivatives of it. It is important to note that failure to react to a skin test does *not* rule out the possibility of an allergic reaction, since this test results in many false-negatives.

Hematologic Side Effects

In addition to eosinophilia or Coombs'-positive hemolytic anemia, discussed earlier, leukopenia and thrombocytopenia have occasionally been reported with penicillin therapy. These are usually dose-dependent, and usually resolve after therapy is stopped. Large IV doses of penicillin G may occasionally cause bleeding by interfering with coagulation and platelet function, especially in patients with impaired renal function.

Renal Side Effects

Acute interstitial nephritis, with fever, proteinuria, hematuria, and occasionally eosinophilia and eosinophiluria, has been reported with high IV doses used for long periods. They are reversible on discontinuation of therapy. High doses of penicillin G potassium may cause severe hyperkalemia, manifested as hyperreflexia, seizures, coma, and possibly arrhythmias. Hyperkalemia may be fatal, especially when the drug is given rapidly to patients with renal impairment. Similarly, penicillin G sodium may cause hypernatremia that can aggravate congestive heart failure or hypertension and cause hypokalemic, hypochloremic metabolic alkalosis.

Nervous System and Local Side Effects

Penicillin G and its derivatives are tissue irritants. High concentrations of penicillins can cause central nervous system (CNS) reactions such as confusion, delirium, or seizures. Discontinuation of the drug reverses most CNS side effects, usually within 12 to 72 hours. However, seizures may persist and be unresponsive to anticonvulsant drugs. If refractory status epilepticus occurs, the outcome will probably be death.

Intrathecal or brain intraventricular injection of pencillins causes severe neurologic irritation. These administration routes are inappropriate.

Intramuscular therapy with penicillin G is very irritating to the muscles and can cause sterile abscesses; IV therapy can cause phlebitis and thrombophlebitis.

Jarisch–Herxheimer Reaction

Patients receiving penicillin G for syphilis or other spirochetal infections, including Lyme disease, may experience a syndrome called the Jarisch–Herxheimer reaction. It is characterized by headache, fever, hypertension, diaphoresis, chills, myalgia and arthralgia, tachycardia, and lethargy. This response is thought to be due to the release of pyrogens or endotoxins from the microorganisms in response to penicillin's action on them. It usually occurs within 12 hours after penicillin treatment is begun and subsides within 24 hours. It does not necessitate discontinuation of penicillin therapy, and requires no treatment.

Gastrointestinal Side Effects

Oral administration of penicillins can cause nausea or epigastric distress, vomiting, and diarrhea. Sore mouth or tongue (**stomatitis**, **glossitis**), or black hairy tongue may also occur.

NURSING IMPLICATIONS

Patients with a history of allergic reactions to any penicillin derivative should be considered potentially allergic to all penicillins. Clearly document in the medical record a patient's history of penicillin allergy, and encourage the patient to carry penicillin allergy identification and notify all caregivers of this allergy.

Observe all patients who receive injectable penicillins for at least 30 minutes. Have epinephrine, antihistamines, and corticosteroids, as well as ventilatory assistance readily available when injectable penicillins are administered. Observe patients for the development of rash, fever, arthralgias or myalgias, nausea and vomiting, diaphoresis, dizziness, and respiratory distress; if these occur, discontinue the drug and notify the physician. Instruct all patients to call the physician if rash or other evidence of an allergic reaction develops.

Report bleeding and laboratory or clinical evidence of anemia or impaired leukocyte function (infection, pallor) to the physician. Assess patients receiving high-dose IV penicillin G for fever, proteinuria, or hematuria; for laboratory evidence of eosinophilia, eosinophiluria, and sodium or potassium imbalance based on blood tests; and for symptoms of hypokalemia (weakness, arrhythmias), hyperkalemia (arrhythmias, seizures, coma), and hypernatremia (worsening of congestive heart failure, edema, increasing body weight, dyspnea, hypertension). Report such changes to the physician at once.

Administer IV penicillin G potassium over at least 30 minutes, especially in patients with impaired renal function; verify that the dosage schedule ordered is appropriate for the patient's renal status.

Observe patients receiving high-dose IV penicillin therapy for evidence of neurologic reactions (delirium, seizures). Observe IV sites for evidence of phlebitis or thrombophlebitis.

Reassure patients with spirochetal illnesses such as syphilis that the Jarisch–Herxheimer reaction is common and that therapy need not be stopped. Report severe reactions to the physician.

◆ Use During Pregnancy and Lactation

The natural penicillins cross the placenta and are excreted in breast milk. Although the concentrations of the drugs may be low in the fetal circulation or in breast milk, the amounts may be sufficient to sensitize the infant or cause the infant GI distress. These potential risks to the infant must be weighed against potential benefits to the mother of penicillin therapy. Penicillin may reduce estriol levels in serum; the estriol test, which is used to measure pregnancy well-being, cannot be used during penicillin therapy or for 10 to 14 days after therapy is stopped.

◆ Use in Children

Penicillin dosages are adjusted according to age, weight, and the severity of infection.

◆ Use in the Elderly

Prolonged penicillin therapy in debilitated elderly patients may result in superinfections of *Proteus, Pseudomonas,* or *Candida.* The plasma half-life is elevated in the elderly owing to decreased renal elimination. While toxicity is generally low with penicillin G, degenerative disease and concurrent drug therapies increase the risk of adverse effects.

Interactions with Other Drugs

Clinically significant drug interactions with penicillin G and other natural penicillins are summarized in Table 56–I1. Few major interactions occur with the natural penicillins.

Penicillins, and especially the extended-spectrum penicillins (discussed later), inactivate aminoglycoside antibiotics, thereby inhibiting their antibacterial activity. This drug interaction and its therapeutic consequences will almost certainly occur if parenteral formulations of penicillins and aminoglycosides are physically mixed together (eg, in the same syringe or IV bag) before or during administration. It may also occur in the patient's bloodstream following proper and separate administration of these drugs. The risk appears to be greatest for patients with renal impairment who are receiving high doses of extended-spectrum penicillins. Moreover, penicillins and aminoglycosides may interact in a blood sample, particularly if it is not assayed promptly. This interaction would lead to an underestimate of aminoglycoside blood levels, and could result in an inappropriate dosage increase of the aminoglycosides, which are potentially dangerous drugs.

Overdose and Toxicity

Penicillin G has a large margin of safety. The principal effects of penicillin overdoses are neurologic reactions similar to, but usually more severe than, those discussed as side and adverse effects.

Hemodialysis, but not peritoneal dialysis, can effectively lower blood levels of penicillin G, although this or other emergency interventions are seldom necessary. The ability of an antibiotic (whether penicillin or other agents specified in this chapter) to be removed by dialysis is important for two major reasons. First, dialysis can be used to lower blood levels rapidly in cases of severe antibiotic toxicity. Second, if a patient is being dialyzed to help manage other medical conditions, and requires administration of a dialyzable antibiotic, changes in the antibiotic dosage regimen (increased or more frequent doses, for example) may be required.

Nursing implications to minimize adverse effects, discussed earlier, apply also to penicillin overdoses.

Related Penicillins

The benzathine and procaine salts of penicillin G were developed to provide longer durations of action than are achieved with the other penicillin G salts. These drugs have identical mechanisms of antibiotic action, and, unless stated otherwise, are equivalent to penicillin G. General side effects, adverse reactions, contraindications, and nursing implications are similar to those noted for penicillin G. Unique aspects of each drug are summarized here.

Benzathine Penicillin G

Benzathine penicillin G (BICILLIN L-A; PERMAPEN) is marketed as a suspension for IM use only. The advantage of benzathine penicillin G injection is that a single dose provides low but effective blood levels for 1 to 4 weeks, and usually needs to be given only once monthly (see Table 56–C1 for dosages). It is usually used for prophylaxis of rheumatic fever or for treatment of minor infections such as streptococcal pharyngitis in patients who are not likely to comply with daily long-term penicillin G or V therapy. It is also used to treat syphilis.

Intramuscular administration of benzathine penicillin G may cause prolonged injection-site pain. Inadvertent intravascular administration may cause severe neurovascular reactions, blood vessel occlusion, or neurologic changes such as delirium, bizarre behavior, or sensory disturbances.

Procaine Penicillin G

The procaine salt of penicillin G (CRYSTICILLIN; WYCILLIN; others) is also used for IM administration when prolonged antibiotic effects are required. Its duration of action is longer than that of oral penicillin G, and it causes less injection-site pain when given IM. It is a useful alternative to oral or IV penicillins for infections that respond to only moderately high serum levels (pneumococcus, streptococcus). This product is contraindicated in patients with a history of hypersensitivity reactions to procaine and related local anesthetics (Chapter 19).

Benzathine and Procaine Penicillin G Combinations

Products that combine the benzathine and procaine salts of penicillin G are available (BICILLIN C-R; BICILLIN C-R 900/300). They are given IM. Some physicians prefer these products to benzathine penicillin G alone because they provide moderately high serum levels for about 24 hours, followed by prolonged low blood levels. These properties may be useful in the initial phase of therapy of susceptible infections (see benzathine penicillin G).

NURSING IMPLICATIONS

The benzathine and procaine salts of penicillin G (and their combinations) should be administered only IM into large muscle masses. Be sure to aspirate prior to injection to avoid intravascular injection. Observe for hypersensitivity, neurovascular, and local occlusive reactions following injection; report such reactions to the physician. Check the history for prior allergic or hypersensitivity reactions to procaine before giving procaine penicillin G.

Penicillin V

Penicillin V potassium (BEEPEN-VK; BETAPEN-VK; LEDERCILLIN VK; others) is the preferred penicillin for oral therapy because it is more resistant to destruction by stomach acid than penicillin G and other natural penicillins, and so is more reliably absorbed. The oral absorption of penicillin V products is slowed by food, so administration on an empty stomach (between meals) is preferred. However, if this causes GI distress, the drug can be taken with food with little risk of reducing antibiotic effectiveness. Dosages are listed in Table 56–C1.

B. Penicillinase-Resistant Penicillins

Some strains of bacteria, such as *Staphylococcus aureus* and *Staph. epidermidis,* are resistant to the penicillins discussed thus far because they synthesize an enzyme, penicillinase, that damages a critical part of the penicillin molecule necessary for antibiotic activity. To overcome this resistance, several penicillinase-resistant penicillins have been developed. They are used almost exclusively to treat infections caused by penicillinase-producing organisms.

These antibiotics are similar to penicillin G in their mechanisms of action, toxicities and side effects, usage in pregnancy and during lactation, and drug interactions. The following discussion is limited to their differences from penicillin G.

PROTOTYPE

Methicillin

Absorption, Distribution, Metabolism, and Excretion

Methicillin sodium (STAPHCILLIN) is very sensitive to inactivation by gastric acid, and so cannot be given orally. When given IM, peak serum concentrations occur within 30 to 60 minutes; therapeutic levels last 4 to 6 hours. When methicillin is administered IV, therapeutic levels may last only 2 to 3 hours. Regardless of the parenteral route used, the drug must be given at least every 6 hours, and often every 4 hours, for most indications.

Methicillin and related penicillinase-resistant penicillins achieve adequate levels in most biologic fluids when recommended doses are given. However, they cross the blood–brain barrier poorly in the absence of meningeal inflammation, and only moderately when the meninges are inflamed.

About 30% to 50% of methicillin molecules in the bloodstream are bound to plasma protein; related penicillins are more extensively bound, ranging from 70% to 90% for nafcillin to as high as 99% for oxacillin, cloxacillin, and dicloxacillin.

Methicillin is eliminated completely by renal excretion without prior hepatic metabolism. Patients with impaired renal function and children with immature kidney function require reduced doses or less frequent administration. Other penicillinase-resistant penicillins depend more on hepatic metabolism and require adjustments for patients with reduced liver function. Penicillinase-resistant penicillins are only minimally removed by peritoneal dialysis and hemodialysis.

Clinical Indications and Administration

Methicillin and related antibiotics are the drugs of choice for treating suspected or proven staphylococcal infections of soft tissue and bone, and for septicemia, in which penicillin resistance owing to penicillinase production is common. They are also indicated for prophylaxis of staphylococcal infections that are likely to occur in surgical or traumatic wounds.

The penicillinase-resistant antibiotics are clearly effective for treating infections caused by penicillin-sensitive organisms that do not produce penicillinase, but they are seldom prescribed for them because alternative drugs are cheaper, less toxic, and equally effective. Methicillin is given only IM or IV; the dosages are listed in Table 56–C1.

Two primary reasons account for failure of methicillin or related agents to control an infection. One is the presence of staphylococcal abscesses, which these drugs do not penetrate well. Such abscesses usually must be drained to prevent persistent infection. The other main reason for therapeutic failure is that some strains of *Staphylococcus* are said to be "methicillin-resistant." (Methicillin-resistance is a misnomer, because such bacteria are resistant to *all* penicillinase-resistant penicillins.)

If methicillin or related drugs fail to control a proven staphylococcal infection, alternative antibiotics such as vancomycin should be considered promptly.

NURSING IMPLICATIONS

When administering methicillin sodium IM, inject it deep into a large muscle mass and rotate sites; pain following injection is common. Intravenous administration should be slow; at least over 30 minutes, and preferably 1 hour.

Side Effects, Adverse Reactions, and Contraindications

Most side effects of methicillin sodium are similar to those already discussed for penicillin G. Methicillin is less likely than penicillin to cause new hypersensitivity reactions, but it is nevertheless contraindicated for patients with a history of penicillin reactions or allergy.

Chronic high-dose therapy with penicillins may cause acute interstitial nephritis, which appears to be a hypersensitivity reaction. The risk appears to be greatest for methicillin sodium. (Nephritis also may occur with oxacillin or ampicillin therapy, but is rarely associated with nafcillin.) Interstitial nephritis presents as fever, rash, eosinophilia and eosinophiluria (which may be early indicators of toxicity), proteinuria, hematuria, pyuria, and progressive deterioration of renal function. Discontinuation of therapy will usually reverse this reaction.

Methicillin and other penicillinase-resistant penicillins can cause neutropenia and may cause agranulocytosis. Methicillin sodium and other penicillinase-resistant penicillins have been associated with transient, asymptomatic elevations of serum alkaline phosphatase, alanine aminotransferase (ALT), and aspartate aminotransferase (AST) levels.

NURSING IMPLICATIONS

Monitor patients receiving high parenteral doses of methicillin for 5 days or more for the development of fever, rash, eosinophilia or eosinophiluria, proteinuria or hematuria, and for deteriorating renal function. If these occur, therapy should be discontinued if possible; the use of other drugs known to cause this reaction, such as ampicillin, oxacillin, or nafcillin, should be avoided. Patients who have experienced this reaction are at risk to develop it again on subsequent use of methicillin.

Be aware that transient elevations in hepatic enzymes are possible during therapy with methicillin and other penicillinase-resistant penicillins.

Related Penicillinase-Resistant Penicillins

The following drugs are similar to methicillin in clinical effectiveness, uses, and toxicities. They differ in their extent of protein binding, which may influence their tissue distribution. Compared with methicillin, all related drugs except nafcillin are eliminated mainly by renal excretion. Nafcillin elimination depends on both renal and hepatic function.

Oral dosage forms of these agents are poorly absorbed and must be administered on an empty stomach, even though this is likely to cause GI distress. Oral liquids are poorly tolerated by children because of poor taste and GI upset.

Cloxacillin Sodium

Cloxacillin sodium (CLOXAPEN; TEGOPEN) is an oxacillin derivative that is available in capsules or as a liquid for oral administration.

Dicloxacillin Sodium

Dicloxacillin sodium (DYCILL; DYNAPEN; others) is an oral oxacillin derivative. It achieves higher serum concentrations than either oxacillin or cloxacillin.

Nafcillin Sodium

Nafcillin sodium (NAFCIL; NALLPEN; UNIPEN) is available in both oral and parenteral dosage forms. Most clinicians discourage oral administration because nafcillin is absorbed poorly and is inactivated in the liver so quickly that blood levels are erratic and usually low.

Intramuscular injections are very painful and should be given deep into large muscle masses. Rotate IM injection sites when repeated injections are needed.

Intravenous administration of nafcillin is more likely than other penicillin derivatives to cause phlebitis. To reduce this problem, nafcillin solutions should be well diluted and administered into a large vein; infuse the total dose over about 1 hour.

Oxacillin Sodium

Oxacillin sodium (BACTOCILL; PROSTAPHILIN) is available in both oral and parenteral dosage forms. It is less well absorbed than cloxacillin and dicloxacillin but is less highly protein-bound. The parenteral dosage forms can be given IM or IV, but they irritate the surrounding tissues and can cause local reactions that are similar to, but less severe than, those described for nafcillin. Intravenous administration of oxacillin can also cause hepatic dysfunction that resembles hepatitis. Discontinuation of the drug is recommended; this usually reverses the reaction. Nafcillin sodium can be safely substituted if hepatic dysfunction occurs. Like methicillin, IV administration of oxacillin can cause interstitial nephritis.

C. Aminopenicillins

The penicillins discussed thus far are more effective against gram-positive organisms than against gram-negative bacteria. Adding an amino group to the penicillin molecule increases bactericidal effectiveness against gram-negative organisms. However, these drugs—called aminopenicillins—are not penicillinase-resistant. Aminopenicillins are similar to penicillin G in their mechanisms of action, toxicities and side effects, usage during pregnancy and lactation, and drug interactions. The prototype aminopenicillin is ampicillin.

PROTOTYPE

Ampicillin

Absorption, Distribution, Metabolism, and Excretion

Peak serum concentrations of ampicillin (OMNIPEN; POLYCILLIN; PRINCIPEN; others) are attained 1 to 2 hours following oral administration. Potentially therapeutic levels will usually persist for 6 to 8 hours.

Only about 30% to 55% of an administered oral dose is absorbed when given on an empty stomach, and less is absorbed when it is taken with food. Following IM injection, peak levels are attained at about 1 hour, and potentially therapeutic levels persist for 6 to 8 hours, while IV administration usually results in potentially therapeutic levels for approximately 6 hours.

With appropriate dosages, ampicillin and other aminopenicillins achieve adequate levels in most biologic fluids. Distribution into the cerebrospinal fluid is low with intact meninges, but moderate when the meninges are inflamed.

Ampicillin is primarily excreted unchanged by renal tubular secretion. A small fraction is metabolized by the liver. Renal clearance is reduced in neonates, geriatric patients, and patients receiving probenecid; such patients will usually require reduced doses. Ampicillin (and the related drug amoxicillin) are removed by hemodialysis but minimally by peritoneal dialysis.

Clinical Indications and Administration

Ampicillin is administered orally (as the anhydrous or trihydrate derivatives), IM, or IV (as the sodium salt) to treat infections caused by susceptible strains of *Listeria monocytogenes, Salmonella, Shigella, Escherichia coli, Haemophilus influenzae, Neisseria gonorrhoeae, Proteus mirabilis,* and enterococci. Ampicillin also is effective in the treatment of meningitis caused by pneumococci or meningococci, although penicillin is the preferred therapy if these organisms are positively identified. It is also used in prophylaxis for bacterial endocarditis during GI or genitourinary (GU) tract surgery or other invasive procedures in patients at risk.

Because penicillin is less toxic, less expensive, and more specific, it is usually preferred over the aminopenicillins for treatment of susceptible gram-positive infections, even though they are usually susceptible to aminopenicillins. Dosages of ampicillin and other aminopenicillins are listed in Table 56–C1.

NURSING IMPLICATIONS

If ampicillin is being used to treat urinary tract infections, keep the patient well hydrated and give the drug with a full glass of water; concentration of the urine may reduce the bactericidal effect of ampicillin. Administer IM doses of ampicillin sodium deep into large muscle masses and rotate injection sites; pain following injection is common. Intravenous administration should occur over at least 30 minutes, and preferably over 1 hour.

Side Effects, Adverse Reactions, and Contraindications

Most side effects and adverse reactions of ampicillin, and the relevant nursing implications, are similar to those discussed for the natural penicillins (Table 56–S1). However, ampicillin and other aminopenicillins may also cause an apparently nonimmunologic reaction in up to 10% of patients. It is characterized by the development of a generalized erythematous or maculopapular rash (often described as "measles-like" or a "fine red rash") beginning on the trunk and spreading peripherally, usually occurring after 3 to 14 days of therapy. The reaction will often subside, even when therapy is continued, and is generally not considered indicative of penicillin allergy. This reaction will occur *predictably* in patients with infectious mononucleosis (it usually occurs when a physician attempts to treat the sore throat—common in mononucleosis—with one of these antibiotics). Since the presence of a widespread rash is generally distressing to the patient, use of aminopenicillins in patients with suspected mononucleosis is relatively contraindicated.

Ampicillin-induced rash also occurs frequently in patients with cytomegalovirus and respiratory tract viral infections. Patients with lymphatic leukemia, reticulosarcoma, and other lymphomas are at increased risk of this reaction as well.

Ampicillin and other aminopenicillins can cause neutropenia or agranulocytosis. These effects are usually reversible following discontinuation of therapy. Ampicillin and amoxicillin can cause bleeding by interfering with platelet aggregation and clotting. In rare instances, ampicillin and amoxicillin have been reported to cause acute interstitial nephritis similar to methicillin.

Pain at IM ampicillin injection sites is common; phlebitis with the use of IV ampicillin is rare. Moderate increases in AST have occasionally been reported with aminopenicillin therapy, especially in infants.

Nausea, vomiting, and epigastric pain are reported by approximately 2% of patients receiving oral aminopenicillins. Sore mouth and black hairy tongue also are occasionally associated with therapy. Orally administered ampicillin, presumably because of its poor absorption, may cause diarrhea. The overall incidence is about 20%, with a greater frequency in children and the elderly. Oral administration of other aminopenicillins causes diarrhea less often, but the incidence is still clinically significant. Severe diarrhea may require discontinuation of the offending drug and substitution of an alternative but appropriate antibiotic. Pseudomembranous colitis has been reported with ampicillin and amoxicillin. Nausea and diarrhea occasionally occur in patients receiving IV ampicillin.

NURSING IMPLICATIONS

Observe for and report rash, mouth soreness, tongue discoloration, nausea, vomiting or epigastric distress, and diarrhea. In severe cases of GI distress, discontinuation of the drug may be necessary. Inform patients that a "measles-like" or erythematous rash occurring during ampicillin therapy is not a drug allergy and does not necessitate discontinuing the drug.

◆ Use During Pregnancy and Lactation

While aminopenicillins readily cross the placenta, effects on the fetus are usually minimal. Ampicillin and amoxicillin are commonly used during pregnancy, especially to treat urinary tract infections. Ampicillin may reduce estriol levels in blood and urine; these measurements normally are indicative of pregnancy well-being, but they cannot be used during therapy with ampicillin or for 10 to 14 days following its discontinuance.

Use caution when administering aminopenicillins to nursing mothers, since the drugs appear in breast milk and may cause diarrhea or other adverse effects, such as rash, in the nursing infant.

Interactions with Other Drugs

There is an increased risk of nonallergic, macropapular rash in hyperuricemic patients receiving both aminopenicillins and the uric acid–lowering drug allopurinol.

Overdose and Toxicity

The principal effects of aminopenicillin overdose are neurologic reactions (see penicillin G, p 1162 and Table 56–S1).

Related Aminopenicillins

Unless stated otherwise, information discussed for ampicillin applies to these agents. For dosage and administration, side effects and contraindications, and drug interactions, see Tables 56–C1, 56–S1, and 56–I1, respectively.

Amoxicillin Trihydrate

Amoxicillin trihydrate (AMOXIL; POLYMOX; others) is an ampicillin derivative that is better absorbed orally, achieving serum concentrations at least twice as high as equal doses of oral ampicillin. Amoxicillin is normally given every 8 hours, instead of every 6 hours as ampicillin must be. This may improve patient compliance.

Amoxicillin shares the same clinical indications as oral ampicillin, except for *Shigella,* for which ampicillin is preferred. Amoxicillin is generally preferred to oral ampicillin for most indications in which oral therapy is acceptable because the incidence of diarrhea is less and it can be given with food if necessary. Amoxicillin is often used for acute otitis media in children.

Amoxicillin Trihydrate and Clavulanate Potassium

Amoxicillin, like other aminopenicillins, is inactivated by organisms that synthesize penicillinase. Clavulanic acid is a chemical with a β-lactam structure. It has little antibiotic activity, but will irreversibly bind and inhibit the action of many bacterial β-lactamase enzymes.

The proprietary drug AUGMENTIN is a combination of amoxicillin trihydrate and clavulanate potassium. It is given orally. Potassium clavulanate extends the spectrum of this combination to affect bacteria that produce β-lactamase and that otherwise would be resistant. Some AUGMENTIN products contain amoxicillin and potassium clavulanate in a 4:1 ratio (eg, the "500" tablet contains 500 mg of amoxicillin and 125 mg of potassium clavulanate). The "250" tablet, however, contains 250 mg and 125 mg, respectively, of amoxicillin and potassium clavulanate. Thus, two "250" tablets should not be substituted for a "500" tablet because the total amount of potassium clavulanate will be doubled.

AUGMENTIN is useful in the treatment of infections caused by susceptible β-lactamase–producing strains of *Staph. aureus, Branhamella catarrhalis, E. coli,* and *H. influenzae.* AUGMENTIN should not be used to treat infections caused by other amoxicillin-sensitive organisms that do not produce penicillinase, since this brand-name combination product is more expensive and potentially more toxic than amoxicillin alone.

The amoxicillin-clavulanate combination has a broader antibiotic spectrum than amoxicillin alone, but it is also more likely to cause GI distress and diarrhea. Use in pregnancy should be restricted, when possible, since fetal effects of clavulanic acid have not been clearly established.

Ampicillin Sodium/Sulbactam Sodium

The inactivation of ampicillin by specific bacterial enzymes can be prevented by the inclusion of a chemical called sulbactam into the ampicillin molecule. This extends the antibacterial spectrum of ampicillin to include a number of otherwise resistant gram-negative and anaerobic organisms. The therapeutic agent that results is marketed as UNASYN.

The major use for UNASYN is in treating gynecologic or intraabdominal infections. The drug is given parenterally. Diarrhea occurs more often than with ampicillin alone.

Bacampicillin Hydrochloride

Bacampicillin hydrochloride (SPECTROBID) is an oral derivative of ampicillin that is rapidly absorbed following oral administration and is hydrolyzed to ampicillin. Its clinical uses are identical to those of oral ampicillin. Since bacampicillin is well absorbed, achieving much higher antibiotic levels than are obtained with oral ampicillin, it can be administered every 12 hours. This less-frequent dosing schedule may improve compliance.

Bacampicillin tablets can be administered with food, but the manufacturer states that the suspension should not be. Diarrhea is less frequent than that reported with ampicillin because of extensive absorption.

D. Extended-Spectrum Penicillins

PROTOTYPE

Ticarcillin

Ticarcillin disodium (TICAR) is the prototype of a group of antibiotics that are structurally related to ampicillin but have a greater spectrum of activity against gram-negative organisms, particularly *Pseudomonas.* Structural differences in the side chains of these antibiotics may explain why they more readily penetrate the outer membranes of gram-negative bacteria, allowing access to target enzymes (penicillin-binding proteins). Extended-spectrum penicillins may also be more resistant to inactivation by β-lactamase produced by gram-negative bacteria. These antibiotics are, however, susceptible to inactivation by penicillinase produced by gram-positive organisms such as *Staphylococcus.* The indanyl disodium salt of carbenicillin, a related drug, is the only extended-spectrum penicillin that is orally effective.

The extended-spectrum penicillins are similar to penicillin G in their mechanisms of action, toxicities and side effects, usage during pregnancy and lactation, and drug interactions.

Absorption, Distribution, Metabolism, and Excretion

Peak serum concentrations of ticarcillin disodium given IM occur within 30 to 75 minutes after administration, with potentially therapeutic levels persisting for up to 8 hours when given IM or IV.

Ticarcillin and other extended-spectrum penicillins reach adequate levels in most body fluids when proper doses are given. Ticarcillin levels in the cerebrospinal fluid are low in the absence of meningeal inflammation, and only moderate when they are inflamed.

Ticarcillin is mainly excreted unchanged by the kidneys, and the drug concentrates in the urine. Because elimination depends on renal function, neonates, the elderly, and patients with renal disease may need a reduced dosage. Probenecid reduces renal clearance of the drug. Ticarcillin blood levels can be lowered significantly by hemodialysis and slightly by peritoneal dialysis.

Pharmacologic Effects

Ticarcillin and other extended-spectrum penicillins exert bactericidal effects in a manner identical to that of other penicillins. Their unique structure allows them to penetrate gram-negative bacteria well and to resist inactivation by some gram-negative bacterial β-lactamases.

Clinical Indications and Administration

Ticarcillin and other extended-spectrum penicillins are primarily used to treat infections caused by *Pseudomonas aeruginosa, Proteus* species (especially indole-positive strains), and certain strains of *E. coli* and *Enterobacter*. They are commonly used in combination with aminoglycoside antibiotics to treat *Pseudomonas* infections, since these two groups of antibiotics appear to have synergistic antibiotic activity against the organism. Other clinical uses include mixed bacterial infections, alone or combined with other antibiotic therapy; and empiric therapy of febrile granulocytopenic patients. Ticarcillin dosages are listed in Table 56–C1.

Side Effects, Adverse Reactions, and Contraindications

Most side effects of ticarcillin, and the relevant nursing implications, are similar to those discussed for the natural penicillins (Table 56–C1).

Severe hypersensitivity reactions are less frequent with extended-spectrum penicillins than with the natural penicillins. Ticarcillin and other extended-spectrum penicillins can cause neutropenia, anemia, and granulocytopenia. These effects are usually reversible following discontinuation of therapy. All the extended-spectrum penicillins have been associated with abnormal platelet function and inhibition of clotting; bleeding has occurred in patients with renal dysfunction, especially when the drug is given chronically in high doses. Intravenous ticarcillin has been associated with bleeding, in some cases, in the absence of renal impairment. Hypernatremia can occur with use of these antibiotics, since they contain significant amounts of sodium and are administered in relatively high doses.

Intramuscular therapy causes pain on injection, and IV injections can cause phlebitis and thrombophlebitis. Oral carbenicillin indanyl disodium causes dose-related nausea and vomiting, diarrhea, and abdominal cramping, and has an unpleasant bitter taste. On occasion, these reactions may occur even with parenteral administration of extended-spectrum penicillins. Several cases of pseudomembranous colitis also have been associated with oral carbenicillin therapy.

NURSING IMPLICATIONS

To reduce the incidence of pain with IM injection, slow the rate of injection or add a local anesthetic such as lidocaine. Inject the drug deeply into a large muscle mass, and rotate injection sites. To avoid phlebitis and thrombophlebitis with IV injection, administer the drug slowly, preferably over 30 minutes to 2 hours. Administer oral carbenicillin with a full glass of water on an empty stomach.

Tablets of carbenicillin indanyl disodium are film-coated and therefore should not be crushed, which makes them totally unpalatable. If the patient cannot swallow the relatively large tablet, the physician should consider a different route of administration or a different antibiotic.

Neutropenia or granulocytopenia may present as increased susceptibility to infection, sore throat, or lassitude; report these symptoms to the physician. Bleeding is a significant risk in patients receiving high parenteral doses of extended-spectrum penicillins; it is usually evident within three to 12 days after initiation of therapy. Monitor and report GI upset, vomiting, diarrhea, or cramping, as well as patient complaints of bitter taste that preclude compliance.

Overdose and Toxicity

The principal effects of ticarcillin overdose are neurologic reactions, diarrhea, and increased risk of bleeding (see section on side effects).

Related Extended-Spectrum Penicillins

The antibiotics related to ticarcillin are azlocillin, carbenicillin, mezlocillin, and piperacillin. They are largely similar to ticarcillin, but differ in their elimination routes, the extent of their gram-negative spectrum and resistance to *Pseudomonas,* and relative cost. All but one of these related drugs are only given parenterally. Each delivers less sodium per average dose than ticarcillin. However, as noted in the discussion of ticarcillin, any of these alternatives can cause hypernatremia.

Carbenicillin, like ticarcillin, is primarily excreted unchanged in the urine. Azlocillin, mezlocillin, and piperacillin also depend on some hepatic metabolism; patients receiving one of these three agents require only minor dosage adjustments in the presence of renal impairment.

Whereas approximately 15% to 35% of *Pseudomonas* isolates are resistant to ticarcillin or carbenicillin, only 5% to 15% are reported resistant to mezlocillin, and less than 10% are resistant to azlocillin or piperacillin. This is important, for prolonged or frequent use of an antibiotic, either in a particular patient or in a particular institution, may result in resistance to that antibiotic. For example, a patient with cystic fibrosis often will be chronically colonized with *Pseudomonas.* Initially, ticarcillin might effectively suppress clinical exacerbations of *Pseudomonas* pneumonia. However, with long-term and recurrent use of this antibiotic, patients often become colonized with resistant *Pseudomonas,* at which time azlocillin, mezlocillin, or piperacillin must be used instead. Except for activity against *Pseudomonas,* mezlocillin has a broader coverage of gram-negative organisms than other drugs in this group.

Because of relative cost and the risk of developing resistance, many clinicians reserve azlocillin, mezlocillin, and piperacillin for treatment of infections by organisms resistant to less expensive extended-spectrum penicillins.

Information about dosages and administration, side effects and contraindications, and drug interactions is presented in Tables 56–C1, 56–S1, and 56–I1, respectively.

Azlocillin Sodium

Azlocillin sodium (AZLIN) is less active than piperacillin or mezlocillin against Enterobacteriaceae. It is more effective than mezlocillin, or ticarcillin against *P. aeruginosa,* and is approximately equipotent with piperacillin against this organism.

Carbenicillin Indanyl Sodium

Carbenicillin indanyl sodium (GEOCILLIN) is formulated as an oral tablet that achieves therapeutic concentrations of carbenicillin only in the urinary tract. This drug is sometimes used for urinary tract infections caused by organisms susceptible to the extended-spectrum penicillins, and is used for prostatitis. Gastrointestinal upset is the primary adverse effect.

Mezlocillin Sodium

Mezlocillin sodium (MEZLIN) has greater activity against Enterobacteriaceae than any other extended-spectrum penicillin. It is generally more active against *P. aeruginosa* than ticarcillin, but less so than azlocillin or piperacillin. Many clinicians reserve mezlocillin for treatment of organisms resistant to ticarcillin, especially where Enterobacteriaceae are common infecting organisms (for example, abdominal and pelvic infections). Mezlocillin may cause interstitial nephritis.

Piperacillin Sodium

Piperacillin sodium (PIPRACIL) is more effective than azlocillin against Enterobacteriaceae. It is more active than mezlocillin and ticarcillin against *P. aeruginosa,* and is approximately equipotent with azlocillin against this organism.

Ticarcillin Disodium and Clavulanate Potassium

TIMENTIN is a parenteral combination of ticarcillin disodium with the potassium salt of clavulanic acid, the β-lactamase inhibitor discussed earlier (see AUGMENTIN). Clinical uses include susceptible β-lactamase–producing strains of *Staph. aureus, Citrobacter, Enterobacter, E. coli, H. influenzae, Klebsiella, Pseudomonas,* and *Serratia.* Use of this combination in other infections otherwise susceptible to extended-spectrum penicillins, especially those susceptible to ticarcillin alone, is discouraged because of cost and the risk of toxicity from an additional drug. There may be a slightly increased incidence of GI complaints with the ticarcillin–clavulanate combination.

II. Cephalosporins and Related Beta-Lactam Antibiotics

Cephalosporins are the second major class of antibiotics. They are derived from cephalosporin C, which is produced from the fungus *Cephalosporium acremonium*. Cephalosporins share a close structural similarity with the penicillins, including the presence of a β-lactam ring, but have added chemical side groups that give them unique properties.

Nevertheless, both penicillins and cephalosporins share many properties, including mechanisms of action, adverse effects, and a limited risk of cross-sensitivity (allergic) reactions.

The cephalosporins and related β-lactam antibiotics (other than penicillins) are divided into three groups, or "generations," based on their spectrums of activity.

The first commercially available cephalosporins—the *first-generation cephalosporins*—have activity against a number of gram-positive organisms, including *Staph. aureus* and *epidermidis,* as well as some gram-negative bacteria. *Second-generation cephalosporins* have extended gram-negative activity (*not* including *Pseudomonas*) but reduced gram-positive effectiveness. All *third-generation cephalosporins,* which are the most recent group of cephalosporins to be marketed, have extended activity against gram-negatives, including *Pseudomonas* for most, with reduced gram-positive effectiveness.

The general properties of cephalosporins and related β-lactams are discussed for cefazolin, the prototype of the first-generation cephalosporins.

A. First-Generation Cephalosporins

PROTOTYPE

Cefazolin

Cefazolin sodium (ANCEF; KEFZOL; ZOLICEF) is representative of the first-generation cephalosporins. The primary uses of this group are in the therapy of gram-positive coccal infections and some gram-negative bacterial infections. Their lower cost and greater specificity for susceptible organisms make these drugs the preferred cephalosporins for most infections caused by gram-positive organisms.

Absorption, Distribution, Metabolism, and Excretion

Cefazolin is poorly absorbed from the GI tract and therefore is only given IM or IV. Peak serum concentrations occur 1 to 2 hours after IM injection. Effective blood levels last about 8 hours with IM or IV use, making a dosage interval of every eight hours possible in many patients. All first-generation cephalosporins distribute well to most tissues except the cerebrospinal fluid; therefore, none are used for CNS infections such as meningitis. Cefazolin and most other first-generation cephalosporins are excreted unchanged in the urine. For most of these agents, renal impairment, including that evident in neonates and the elderly, usually necessitates giving reduced doses, prolonging the dosage interval, or both. Oral probenecid may be used to prolong the activity of most cephalosporins. Cephalosporin blood levels can be reduced by peritoneal dialysis or hemodialysis.

Pharmacologic Effects

Cefazolin, and most other cephalosporins and cephalosporin-like β-lactam antibiotics, exert mainly bactericidal effects on susceptible organisms. Their mechanism of action is similar, if not identical, to that described for penicillin (inhibition of bacterial cell wall synthesis). Indeed, they appear to bind to "penicillin-binding proteins." Like the situation with penicillin resistance, resistance to cephalosporins may be due to the lack of such binding proteins in some bacterial strains, or due to the production of bacterial enzymes (β-lactamase; penicillinase) that destroy the drugs' critical β-lactam structures. Organisms initially sensitive to cephalosporins may develop resistance shortly after therapy is started. This newly acquired resistance may be due to the ability of the cephalosporin to induce the bacteria to synthesize chemicals that block permeability of the antibiotic, or to induce β-lactamase production.

The usual spectrum of activity of cefazolin sodium includes gram-positive cocci, including penicillinase-producing and nonpenicillinase-producing *Staph. aureus* and *epidermidis,* group A β-hemolytic streptococci, group B streptococci and *Streptococcus pneumoniae,* and a few gram-negative bacteria such as some strains of *E. coli, Klebsiella pneumoniae, Proteus mirabilis,* and *Shigella.* Cefazolin sodium has very limited activity or clinical utility outside of use in treating infections caused by susceptible gram-positive cocci, and in prophylaxis against infection by these organisms during surgical procedures.

Clinical Indications and Administration

Cefazolin sodium is administered IM or IV to treat infections caused by susceptible gram-positive and gram-negative bacteria. Dosages of this and other cephalosporins are listed in Table 56–C2. Cefazolin sodium causes less pain on IM injection and requires less frequent administration than other first-generation parenteral cephalosporins, and is less expensive and usually more specific against susceptible gram-positive organisms than second- or third-generation agents. It is therefore often considered the first-generation cephalosporin of choice for parenteral therapy of infections caused by susceptible gram-positive bacteria such as *Staph. aureus, Strep. pneumoniae,* or group A or B streptococci involving the respiratory, biliary, or urinary tracts; skin, bone, and joints; or in septicemia or serious intraabdominal infection caused by these organisms.

Cefazolin can occasionally be used to treat susceptible gram-negative infections (usually strains of *E. coli, Klebsiella pneumoniae,* or *Proteus mirabilis*) involving these organ systems. It is also used in the short-term prophylaxis of surgical wound infection in patients undergoing certain obstetric, gynecologic, cardiovascular, orthopedic, or biliary tract surgeries. Since surgical wound infections are most frequently caused by organisms that are sensitive to first-generation cephalosporins, such as *Staph. aureus* or *epidermidis,* cefazolin is usually the preferred cephalosporin.

First-generation cephalosporins are inappropriate treatments for CNS infections.

Side Effects, Adverse Reactions, and Contraindications

Cefazolin sodium and other first-generation cephalosporins are relatively nontoxic. Their major adverse effects are usually allergic reactions. They also may cause adverse neurologic, hematologic, renal, hepatic, and GI effects. Table 56–S2 summarizes the adverse reactions and contraindications of the cephalosporins.

Allergic Reactions and Cross-Reactivity

Allergic reactions may occur in up to 5% of patients receiving a cephalosporin. Patients who are allergic to one cephalosporin should be considered allergic to all others. There is some risk of cross-allergy between cephalosporins and penicillins; individuals who exhibit anaphylactoid reactions to one group should probably avoid the other group as well. Minor allergic reactions (for example, skin rash) caused by penicillins do not contraindicate cephalosporin use, but do require caution and close monitoring of the patient.

Signs and symptoms of allergic reactions to cephalosporins include urticaria, rash (maculopapular, erythematous, or morbilliform), fever and chills, eosinophilia, serum sickness–like reactions (see penicillin G), edema, genital and anal pruritus, exfoliative dermatitis, angioedema, and occasionally anaphylaxis (see penicillin G). Anaphylactoid reactions usually occur within 30 minutes of administration; other reactions may be delayed.

If allergic reactions occur during therapy, cephalosporin administration should be discontinued. Supportive therapy and drugs appropriate to the severity of the reaction may be needed, as discussed for penicillin G.

Other Adverse Effects

Neutropenia, leukopenia, and thrombocythemia or thrombocytopenia are occasionally reported with cefazolin and other cephalosporin therapy, resulting in reduced response to therapy or bleeding or bruising. False-positive direct and indirect Coombs' tests can occur, especially with high cephalosporin doses and in patients with renal impairment. Nephrotoxicity is generally a rare complication of cefazolin, cephalexin, and cephalothin therapy. It is most likely to occur in patients over 50 years of age and in patients with renal impairment, especially when other nephrotoxic drugs are being used. Use reduced doses in patients with renal impairment.

Transient increases in serum bilirubin, lactate dehydrogenase (LDH), ALT, AST, and alkaline phosphatase levels have been reported with cephalosporins. Nervous system reactions (headache and dizziness, malaise, and fatigue) are infrequent with cephalosporins. They should be reported to the physician at once.

Do not administer cefazolin or other cephalosporins by intrathecal or cerebral intraventricular injection. Intrathecal administration causes neurologic reactions similar to those caused by penicillin G, including seizures. Intramuscular injection can cause local pain, which can be reduced by injecting the drug into a large muscle mass and rotating injection sites. Intravenous administration can cause phlebitis or thrombophlebitis, which is usually mild and can be reduced by reducing the infusion rate of the drug, diluting the drug well, and rotating injection sites.

While more common with other cephalosporins that are administered orally, adverse GI effects such as diarrhea, including pseudomembranous colitis, oral candidiasis (thrush), nausea, vomiting, and GI upset can occur with parenteral administration of cefazolin and other cephalosporins.

Overgrowth of nonsusceptible organisms may occur with prolonged therapy, especially monilial vaginitis (*Candida*).

NURSING IMPLICATIONS

All the precautions that apply to penicillin allergy apply to cephalosporins. Monitor patients for abnormal bruising or bleeding caused by reduced platelet counts. Consider the possibility that false-positive Coombs' tests may be caused by cephalosporin therapy. Observe patients for evidence of nephrotoxicity (creatinine, BUN, proteinuria, oliguria) while receiving cefazolin, cephalexin, or cephalothin, especially in the elderly, in patients with renal impairment, and in patients receiving other nephrotoxic drugs. Be certain that the dose ordered is appropriate for the patient's renal status. Hepatic effects are usually mild and reversible on discontinuation of therapy. Report evidence of hepatic toxicity to the physician.

Monitor for and report significant diarrhea, thrush, nausea, vomiting, or GI upset to the physician. Severe diarrhea may be life-threatening.

Observe for and report any evidence of superinfection or failure of therapy.

◆ Use During Pregnancy and Lactation

Cefazolin and other cephalosporins are detectable in the fetus and in breast milk. While no evidence of fetal harm has been documented, these antibiotics should be used in pregnancy only if clearly indicated. Cephalosporins should be used in nursing mothers only if the benefit clearly outweighs the risk of adverse effects, such as diarrhea or rash, in the infant.

Interactions with Other Drugs

There are very few clinically significant drug interactions involving cefazolin and other cephalosporins (Table 56–I2). Renal toxicity of some cephalosporins may be increased by concomitant use of other nephrotoxic agents such as aminoglycosides or vancomycin. Probenecid inhibits renal excretion of cephalosporins, including cefazolin, which may be therapeutically useful in some circumstances. In addition, most cephalosporins may cause false-positive results with urinary glucose tests using cupric sulfate (eg, Benedict's solution or CLINITEST); glucose oxidase methods, used on most urine glucose test strips (eg, CLINISTIX, TES-TAPE), are not affected.

Overdose and Toxicity

Cephalosporin overdoses are seldom serious, and usually involve an increased risk of the adverse effects that may occur when therapeutic doses are given. Peritoneal dialysis or hemodialysis may be effective adjuncts for managing severe symptomatic cephalosporin toxicity.

Related First-Generation Cephalosporins

The drugs discussed in the following sections are largely similar to cefazolin but differ in their routes of administration or dosage frequency. Adverse GI effects are much more common with oral cephalosporins than with parenteral dosage forms. Major uses of oral first-generation cephalosporins include urinary tract, skin, and soft tissue infections caused by susceptible organisms (see cefazolin). Because of greater palatability and reduced GI adverse effects, these cephalosporins are often used instead of penicillinase-resistant penicillins for oral therapy of staphylococcal infections.

Renal excretion is the primary route of elimination of these antibiotics; patients with renal impairment usually require dosage adjustments. Information on dosage and administration, side effects and contraindications, and drug interactions is presented in Tables 56–C2, 56–S2, and 56–I2, respectively.

Cefadroxil

Cefadroxil (DURICEF; ULTRACEF) is an orally effective cephalosporin that is well absorbed following administration, even with food, which may reduce GI distress. It has a longer half-life than other oral first-generation cephalosporins and can be administered once or twice daily, which may improve patient compliance.

Cephalexin

Cephalexin (KEFLEX; KEFLET) is an oral cephalosporin with a shorter half-life than cefadroxil. It usually must be given four times a day, but may be given less frequently for very susceptible skin infections. Cephalexin suspension is usually well tolerated by children and has proven more palatable in taste tests than cefadroxil. Food slows its absorption but does not affect the total amount absorbed, so it can be administered with meals, if necessary, to decrease adverse GI effects.

Cephalothin Sodium

Cephalothin sodium (KEFLIN) is a parenteral first-generation cephalosporin with a spectrum of activity and clinical uses similar to cefazolin. Cephalothin has a shorter half-life than cefazolin, and thus must be administered more frequently, usually every 4 to 6 hours. It causes more venous irritation than cefazolin with IV administration, and more pain with IM injection.

Cephapirin Sodium

Cephapirin sodium (CEFADYL) is a parenteral first-generation cephalosporin with uses, dosage schedules, and adverse effects that are very similar to cephalothin sodium. Cephapirin is usually better tolerated for IM injection than cephalothin, and is reported to cause less severe phlebitis with IV use. Cephapirin can be injected IM every 8 hours, rather than every 4 to 6 hours, if IM injections cause excessive pain.

Cephradine

Cephradine (ANSPOR; VELOSEF) is the only first-generation cephalosporin currently marketed that is available for both oral and parenteral administration. Indications for oral use are similar to cefadroxil; parenteral uses are similar to cefazolin. Cephradine is well absorbed orally; food delays absorption, but does not change the total amount absorbed. Pain occurs with IM injection, and mild phlebitis may occur with IV use. It is usually given every 6 hours to treat severe infections, but a 12-hour interval between doses may be acceptable for minor infections.

B. Second-Generation Cephalosporins

The second-generation cephalosporin antibiotics are useful in treating infections caused by specific gram-negative or anaerobic bacteria, especially when activity against gram-positive organisms is also needed. These antibiotics should be reserved for specific clinical situations in which the goal is to cover specific organisms not covered by first-generation cephalosporins, such as *Bacteroides* or *H. influenzae.* Cefoxitin sodium is considered most representative of these drugs, even though its chemical structure is not identical to most other cephalosporins, and it is more properly called a cephamycin or β-lactam antibiotic.

PROTOTYPE

Cefoxitin

Absorption, Distribution, Metabolism, Excretion

Cefoxitin sodium (MEFOXIN) is inadequately absorbed when given orally. It is available only for IM or IV injection. Peak serum concentrations occur 20 to 30 minutes after IM injection, and persist at potentially therapeutic levels for only about 4 hours.

The drug distributes well to most tissues, but not to cerebrospinal fluid. This failure to enter the CNS well, and the resulting lack of effectiveness for treating CNS infections, applies to all second-generation cephalosporins except cefuroxime. Unlike most other second-generation cephalosporins, cefoxitin may achieve appreciable biliary concentrations, which may be useful for treating biliary tract infections. Cefoxitin is eliminated primarily by renal excretion of unchanged drug. Renal impairment usually necessitates dosage reduction. Oral probenecid may prolong the activity of cefoxitin and related antibiotics.

Cefoxitin is removed by hemodialysis but not significantly by peritoneal dialysis. Removal of cefoxitin by hemodialysis may affect dosing schedules in patients undergoing this procedure.

Clinical Indications and Administration

Dosages and routes of administration of this and other cephalosporins are listed in Table 56–C2.

The major clinical use for cefoxitin is in therapy of mixed aerobic-anaerobic bacterial respiratory, abdominal, gynecologic, and skin infections, and in prophylaxis in surgery involving the abdominal or pelvic regions. Second-generation cephalosporins have activity in vitro against *H. influenzae* and (except cefaclor) against some strains of other gram-negative bacteria such as *Enterobacter, E. coli, Klebsiella, Neisseria, Proteus,* and *Serratia* that are resistant to first-generation cephalosporins. Cefoxitin and the related drugs cefotetan and cefmetazole are often effective against *Bacteroides* and other anaerobes such as *Clostridium, Peptococcus,* and *Peptostreptococcus.* Cefoxitin is usually considered the parenteral cephalosporin of choice for use in infections caused by susceptible anaerobes. Second-generation cephalosporins do *not* have activity against enterococci, *Pseudomonas, Listeria monocytogenes,* or methicillin-resistant staphylococci.

The usual spectrum of activity of cefoxitin sodium includes gram-positive cocci and gram-negative organisms as outlined for cefazolin. However, activity against these gram-positive organisms is usually less than equal doses of first-generation cephalosporins. Because of their lower cost and greater specificity, first-generation cephalosporins or penicillins should be used for infections caused by susceptible organisms (for example, streptococci and staphylococci) and for specific prophylaxis against them.

Side Effects, Adverse Reactions, and Contraindications

Cefoxitin sodium and other second-generation cephalosporins have side effects and toxicities (see Table 56–S2) that are very similar to cefazolin. Pain occurring with IM injection can be reduced by administering cefoxitin with 0.5% or 1% lidocaine.

Interactions with Other Drugs

Clinically significant drug interactions with cefoxitin are similar to those occurring with cefazolin (see Table 56–I2).

Related Second-Generation Cephalosporins

Cefaclor

Cefaclor (CECLOR) is orally effective. It has an antibiotic spectrum of activity similar to first-generation agents, and its efficacy against gram-negative organisms other than *H. influenzae* is relatively poor.

Cefaclor can be used to treat any infection in which cefadroxil is indicated, but this is seldom done because cefaclor is usually more expensive and liable to cause more side effects.

Cefaclor's major use is to treat soft tissue infections in which *H. influenzae* are common, such as acute otitis media, cellulitis, or pneumonia, when alternative antibiotics such as amoxicillin cannot be used owing to contraindications, treatment failure, or resistance (documented or suspected).

Renal impairment usually does not necessitate dosage adjustment for cefaclor. Food does not interfere with its absorption, which enables administration with meals to reduce GI upset.

Serum sickness–like reactions (see penicillin G) occur more frequently with cefaclor than with other cephalosporins. These usually occur during or after a second course of cefaclor therapy. Since cefaclor is frequently used for otitis media in children, serum sickness occurs most often in this population.

Cefamandole Nafate

Cefamandole nafate (MANDOL) is a parenteral second-generation cephalosporin with a spectrum of activity and clinical uses similar to cefoxitin. Notable differences from cefoxitin are

- its efficacy against anaerobes is less;
- it is not clinically useful in gonorrhea;
- staphylococcal coverage may be slightly improved, and;
- *Enterobacter* coverage is increased.

Cefamandole is usually administered every 4 to 8 hours.

Cefamandole kills gut bacteria that normally synthesize vitamin K, a vitamin essential for formation of clotting factors in the liver. It may also interfere with vitamin K activity. Thus, cefamandole may cause hypoprothrombinemia and increased bleeding tendencies. Clinically significant hypoprothrombinemia is most likely to occur in patients with preexisting vitamin K deficiency or severe renal or hepatic impairment; elderly, debilitated, or malnourished patients; or patients who have had extensive gastrointestinal surgery. Such predisposed patients may require prophylactic vitamin K therapy.

Concomitant use of alcohol, even the amounts typically found in many medications, may cause a disulfuram-like reaction (flushing, tachycardia, nausea, headache) in some patients (see Table 56–I2 and Chapter 22).

Cefmetazole Sodium

Cefmetazole sodium (ZEFAZONE) is a parenterally administered second-generation cephalosporin with activity similar to cefoxitin. It is slightly more active against staphylococci than cefoxitin, but less so than first-generation cephalosporins. It contains the same side-chain that has been associated with bleeding tendencies during therapy with cephalosporins such as cefamandole.

Cefonicid Sodium

Cefonicid sodium (MONOCID) is given IM or IV. It has a long half-life that permits once-daily dosing. Its activity is very similar to cefoxitin, but it is not used for gonorrhea and lacks anaerobe coverage.

Ceforanide

Ceforanide (PRECEF) is an IM or IV second-generation cephalosporin that can be given every 12 hours because of its long half-life. Its activity is similar to cefoxitin, but it lacks anaerobe coverage, is considered less active against *H. influenzae,* and lacks approval for therapy of gonorrhea. Ceforanide may cause falsely elevated serum or urine creatinine levels when the Jaffe method is used. This altered test result could lead to an erroneous diagnosis of renal dysfunction.

Cefotetan Disodium

Cefotetan disodium (CEFOTAN) is a parenterally administered β-lactam (cephamycin) antibiotic. Nevertheless, it is generally considered as a second-generation cephalosporin because its spectrum of activity is similar to that of cefoxitin. Compared with cefoxitin, cefotetan is less potent against gram-positive bacteria, more active against Enterobacteriaceae, and equally or slightly less effective against *Bacteroides fragilis.* Cefotetan also has a longer half-life and is effective when given only once or twice daily, and so it is an alternative to cefoxitin.

Like ceforanide, cefotetan may falsely elevate serum or urine creatinine levels. The drug is removed by both peritoneal dialysis and hemodialysis; patients undergoing dialysis may require administration of additional doses. Intramuscular doses may be mixed with lidocaine to reduce pain.

Cefuroxime Sodium

Cefuroxime sodium (CEFTIN, ZINACEF) is the only second-generation cephalosporin that achieves significant levels in cerebrospinal fluid although it is no longer recommended for treatment of meningitis. It is given parenterally. It has a spectrum of activity similar to cefamandole but is less susceptible to inactivation by β-lactamases. Cefuroxime is active against *N. gonorrhoeae* and *N. meningitidis* and some strains of *E. coli, Enterobacter,* and *Klebsiella* that are resistant to cefamandole. In addition to having clinical uses similar to cefamandole, cefuroxime can be used parenterally to treat gonorrhea.

Oral cefuroxime has uses similar to cefaclor, and can be used to treat urinary tract infections caused by *E. coli* and *K. pneumoniae.* Oral absorption is enhanced by administration with food.

Cefuroxime has been reported to cause decreased hemoglobin and hematocrit levels in up to 10% of patients, and causes hepatic effects similar to cefoxitin as well as transient bilirubin elevation. Monitor patients for signs of anemia or jaundice.

C. Third-Generation Cephalosporins

PROTOTYPE

Cefotaxime

The first- and second-generation cephalosporins, while moderately expensive, are effective in treating a variety of infecting organisms. However, they have important limitations that are not shared by cephalosporins classified as third-generation agents, of which cefotaxime sodium is the most representative.

Most of the third-generation cephalosporins cross the blood–brain barrier, reaching potentially therapeutic levels when the meninges are inflamed. This is a distinct advantage over all other cephalosporins when CNS infections must be treated.

In addition, the third-generation agents are generally more effective than other cephalosporins against gram-negative bacteria, are effective against many strains of *E. coli* and *Enterobacter* that are reportedly resistant to second-generation cephalosporins, and most have some activity against *Pseudomonas* and *Bacteroides fragilis.*

Limitations of third-generation cephalosporins include greater cost; lower efficacy against gram-positive bacteria; and lack of effectiveness against enterococci, and *Listeria monocytogenes.*

Absorption, Distribution, Metabolism, and Excretion

Cefotaxime sodium (CLAFORAN), like all third-generation cephalosporins except cefixime (see p 1177), is inadequately absorbed after oral administration. They are only available in IM or IV dosage forms. Following injection, peak serum concentrations of cefotaxime are obtained rapidly but become very low by 8 hours after dosing. Cefotaxime appears in the bile in concentrations that are 15% to 75% of serum levels. The drug concentrates in the gallbladder to up to three times serum levels, which makes this a useful antibiotic in treatment of biliary tract infections.

Cefotaxime is eliminated primarily through renal excretion of unchanged drug and a less active metabolite. Patients with renal impairment who receive any third-generation cephalosporin except cefoperazone (discussed later) usually require lower doses or less frequent administration. Occasionally this interaction may have therapeutic benefit. Cefotaxime is removed by hemodialysis but not significantly by peritoneal dialysis.

Clinical Indications and Administration

Cefotaxime sodium is administered IM or IV to treat serious infections of the GU and lower respiratory tracts, intraabdominal and pelvic cavities, bones and joints, and skin and soft tissues caused by susceptible gram-positive and gram-negative bacteria, including some anaerobes. It is effective against gram-positive cocci and gram-negative organisms as outlined for cefazolin, but is less potent against gram-positive organisms than equal doses of first-generation cephalosporins. Cefotaxime is often active against strains of *E. coli, Klebsiella, Enterobacter, Neisseria, Serratia,* and *Proteus* that are resistant to first- and second-generation agents. Cefotaxime has moderate activity against *Pseudomonas* and may be active against some anaerobes such as *Bacteroides fragilis.*

Clinical activity against *H. influenzae, N. meningitidis,* pneumococcus, and *Enterobacter* makes cefotaxime useful for therapy of meningitis, especially in neonates, in whom *Enterobacter* infections are common and difficult to treat with other antibiotics. It is also used to treat septicemia caused by susceptible organisms. While cefotaxime may be effective in gram-positive soft tissue infections, first-generation cephalosporins or penicillins are usually preferred because they are more effective, cheaper, and less likely to induce resistance.

Cefotaxime has been used to treat uncomplicated gonorrhea, including gonorrhea caused by penicillinase-producing strains. It is not considered first-choice therapy in *Pseudomonas* infections, since activity against this organism is only moderate. Cefotaxime is approved for use in infection prophylaxis for GI and pelvic surgery, but use of a first- or second-generation cephalosporin is usually preferred, depending on the surgical site.

Dosages of cefotaxime and other cephalosporins are listed in Table 56–C2.

Side Effects, Adverse Reactions, and Contraindications

Cefotaxime sodium and other third-generation cephalosporins have toxicities that are very similar to cefazolin (see Table 56–S2).

Third-generation cephalosporins may induce resistance in some gram-negative organisms; a patient who initially responds to therapy may later relapse. Use of other beta-lactam antibiotics along with third-generation cephalosporins may increase the risk of resistance development. If signs and symptoms of infection persist or become worse, the physician should reassess therapy.

Interactions with Other Drugs

Clinically significant drug interactions are similar to those occurring with cefazolin (see Table 56–I2). Unlike most cephalosporins, cefotaxime does not interfere with urinary glucose tests that use cupric sulfate (eg, Benedict's solution or CLINITEST).

Related Third-Generation Cephalosporins

All the drugs discussed in the following sections are classified as third-generation cephalosporins, either because of cephalosporin structure and antibiotic spectrum of activity, or because of β-lactam structure and antibiotic spectrum similar to true cephalosporins. All third-generation cephalosporins except cefixime are available for IM or IV administration only. With the exceptions noted later, all have the same spectrum of activity, clinical uses and limitations, and toxicities as cefotaxime. Dosages, toxicities, and drug interactions are listed in Tables 56–C2, 56–S2, and 56–I2, respectively.

Cefixime

Cefixime (SUPRAX) is the only orally effective third-generation cephalosporin. It is given once daily. Cefixime is considered third-generation because of broad gram-negative coverage. It is not clinically useful for anaerobic, staphylococcal, or *Pseudomonas* infections. Uses are similar to cefaclor and oral cefuroxime.

Cefoperazone Sodium

Cefoperazone sodium (CEFOBID) has a long half-life, which permits a 12-hour dosing schedule. It has less activity against most enteric gram-negative bacilli than other third-generation cephalosporins, but has increased activity against *Pseudomonas*. It may be clinically useful in *Pseudomonas* infections; however, other antipseudomonal antibiotics, such as extended-spectrum penicillins, aminoglycoside antibiotics, or both, are usually more effective and therefore preferred.

Cefoperazone is excreted principally in the bile, and so it may be useful in the treatment of susceptible organisms infecting the biliary tract. Renal impairment does not markedly affect cefoperazone elimination. However, very high dosages should be avoided in patients with significant renal impairment. Hepatic impairment reduces biliary excretion of cefoperazone, but usually not enough to necessitate a dosage alteration unless the total daily dose exceeds 4 g in adults. Hemodialysis removes very little cefoperazone. Like cefamandole, cefoperazone can cause bleeding and disulfuram-like reactions with alcohol.

Ceftazidime

Ceftazidime (CEPTAZ; FORTAZ; TAZICEF; TAZIDIME) has greater activity against *Pseudomonas* and some other Enterobacteriaceae than other currently marketed cephalosporins. Activity against gram-positive bacteria and *Bacteroides* is lower than with cefotaxime.

The primary clinical use of ceftazidime is to treat *Pseudomonas* and other infections caused by Enterobacteriaceae, often in combination with other antibiotics such as aminoglycosides. Because of reduced activity against gram-positive organisms and anaerobes, ceftazidime should not be used alone when these are potential infecting organisms.

Lidocaine can be added to IM injections to reduce pain if necessary. Peritoneal dialysis and hemodialysis remove ceftazidime. Renal impairment necessitates administering reduced doses.

Ceftizoxime Sodium

Ceftizoxime sodium (CEFIZOX) is similar to cefotaxime in activity and clinical uses. However, it is more active against *Serratia* and slightly more active against *Bacteroides*. It also has a slightly longer half-life than cefotaxime and so is given every eight hours. It is partially removed by peritoneal dialysis and hemodialysis. Renal impairment necessitates a dosage reduction.

Ceftriaxone Sodium

Ceftriaxone sodium (ROCEPHIN) is a preferred drug for gonorrhea, but is otherwise similar to cefotaxime in terms of antibiotic activity and clinical uses. The major differences, compared with cefotaxime, are a longer half-life, allowing administration every 12 to 24 hours, and the ability to mix it with lidocaine to reduce IM injection pain. Ceftriaxone is not removed by peritoneal dialysis or hemodialysis. Renal impairment necessitates a dosage reduction.

III. Aminoglycosides

The aminoglycosides are an important group of antibiotics with good efficacy against a number of gram-negative bacteria. They derived their name because a critical part of their structure is an aminosugar. All aminoglycosides share common mechanisms of action, metabolism, and toxicities. Although several effective aminoglycosides were introduced into clinical use many years ago, many of them are used much less frequently than other antibiotics (aminoglycosides and other classes), or have only a few specific uses, because of unique properties or limitations. Gentamicin sulfate is the prototype because of its broad gram-negative activity (including many *Pseudomonas* species), widespread use, and comparatively low cost.

PROTOTYPE

Gentamicin

Absorption, Distribution, Metabolism, and Excretion

Gentamicin (GARAMYCIN; JENAMICIN) and other aminoglycosides are poorly absorbed following oral administration. Although only approximately 5% of an administered dose may be absorbed, this may be sufficient to cause adverse systemic effects in patients with renal dysfunction. Gentamicin, when injected IM, achieves peak plasma concentrations in 30 minutes to 2 hours, and measurable levels usually last 8 to 12 hours. Serious illness may reduce absorption from IM administration sites because of reduced muscle blood flow. For these patients IV administration is therefore preferred. This achieves higher blood levels more rapidly, and measurable blood levels last about 8 hours. (As discussed later, the preferred IV administration technique is controversial.) Gentamicin may also reach substantial plasma levels following local instillation of large doses into the lung, peritoneal cavity, joints, or wounds, or when applied liberally to denuded skin.

Gentamicin and other aminoglycosides are widely

distributed throughout most extracellular fluids, except for the cerebrospinal and ocular fluids. Tissue accumulation of the drug is slow, but progressive, and may account for the toxic effects on the ear and on renal function that usually develop during prolonged therapy (see pp 1180–1182).

Gentamicin and other aminoglycosides are excreted unchanged by glomerular filtration. This process is the major determinant of the drug's half-life, which affects not only the therapeutic response but also the risk of adverse effects caused by these potentially toxic drugs. The usual half-life of gentamicin in an adult with normal renal function is 2 to 4 hours. This value is prolonged, often to 4 to 12 hours, in patients with underdeveloped renal function, such as neonates who are gestationally immature or have low body weight, or decreased kidney function owing to disease or advanced age. Such patients usually require reduced doses or increased dosage intervals. Children older than 6 months of age often have aminoglycoside half-lives that are shorter than those in adults. Fever or pathologic fluid accumulations, such as ascites, will lower plasma aminoglycoside concentrations and shorten their half-lives. As body temperature or fluid accumulation change during therapy, dosage adjustments may be needed as discussed later.

Hemodialysis readily lowers plasma aminoglycoside levels; peritoneal dialysis has variable effects. Plasma level monitoring is recommended for patients undergoing dialysis to determine dosing requirements. Hemodialysis may be useful in reducing toxic gentamicin levels.

Pharmacologic Effects

Gentamicin and other aminoglycosides exert bactericidal effects on susceptible gram-positive and gram-negative organisms and mycobacteria. The effect presumably occurs because the aminoglycosides attach to a portion of the bacteria's ribosomes, leading to the synthesis of proteins that cannot maintain bacterial viability.

This antibacterial mechanism is relevant to combined therapy with aminoglycosides and other antibiotics. For example, aminoglycosides and penicillins exert synergistic bactericidal effects through actions on different bacterial functions that are essential to organism viability. Combined use of antipseudomonal aminoglycosides and penicillins is common, rational, and clinically useful in patients with *Pseudomonas* infections.

In contrast, since aminoglycosides (and all bactericidal antibiotics) act only on actively growing bacteria, their effects will be reduced significantly if bacterial growth is inhibited, as occurs when bacteriostatic antibiotics such as erythromycin or tetracycline are given. This combination would be theoretically irrational.

As is true of all bactericidal antibiotics, the effects of aminoglycosides are not diminished significantly in patients with compromised immune systems.

Resistance to gentamicin and other aminoglycosides may be caused by reduced bacterial cell wall permeability to these antibiotics; changes in drug binding to the ribosomes; or the presence of transferable resistance factors (also called *R-factors*), which may enzymatically inactivate the aminoglycoside. Differences in susceptibility to these R-factor–associated enzymes account for most of the difference in resistance to the commonly used systemic aminoglycosides. The related drug amikacin is rarely inactivated by R-factors.

Clinical Indications and Administration

Gentamicin and other aminoglycosides are effective against most aerobic gram-negative bacteria. Indeed, gentamicin and the related drugs amikacin, netilmicin, and tobramycin are among the most effective antibiotics for treating infections caused by gram-negative bacilli. Infections caused by *Acinetobacter, Citrobacter, Enterobacter, E. coli, Klebsiella, Proteus, Providencia, Pseudomonas, Salmonella, Serratia,* and *Shigella,* as well as gram-positive infections caused by *Staph. aureus* and *Staph. epidermidis,* may all respond to therapy with one of these agents. Aminoglycosides are relatively ineffective against most anaerobic bacteria. They are effective against some gram-positive bacteria.

Unlike penicillins and cephalosporins, some of the aminoglycosides are administered locally. Local administration includes irrigation of surgical sites; ophthalmic and otic instillation; and even oral administration, because very low systemic absorption largely confines the drug's actions to the gut. In any case, the drug is used to treat or prevent infections in the area exposed to the drug. Most aminoglycosides can be administered IM or IV to treat systemic or urinary tract infections.

Systemic Uses

Gentamicin and similar antipseudomonal aminoglycosides are administered IM or IV to treat serious infections such as septicemias and bone, skin, soft tissue, respiratory tract, abdominal, pelvic, and urinary tract infections caused by susceptible strains of gram-negative bacilli. Although aminoglycosides may be effective in some gram-negative infections, less toxic alternatives are usually preferred.

Typical dosages for gentamicin and other aminoglycosides are listed in Table 56–C3. Peak plasma concentrations of 6 to 8 μg/mL are considered optimal for most susceptible bacteria. An exception is *Pseudomonas,* for which many clinicians recommend plasma levels of 8 to 10 μg/mL. At higher doses, it is especially important to monitor peak plasma gentamicin concentrations, because levels that exceed 12 μg/mL are considered potentially toxic, regardless of the drug's intended use.

Aminoglycosides are commonly used in combination with other antibiotics that either expand the therapeutic coverage or have additive or synergistic effects against specific bacteria.

Combinations with penicillins or cephalosporins may be used to treat septicemia, and are occasionally used to treat meningitis (realizing that aminoglycoside penetration into the cerebrospinal fluid is low and intraventricular or intrathecal administration may be needed to obtain adequate levels). Penicillin or ampicillin plus gentamicin or streptomycin has been used to treat enterococcal endocarditis and may sometimes be used for endocarditis caused by *Strep. viridans,* the most common cause of subacute bacterial endocarditis. The penicillin or ampicillin plus gentamicin or streptomycin combinations may also be used as prophylactic therapy when enterococcus is a potential pathogen during invasive procedures in a patient at risk for bacterial endocarditis. In this case, a peak plasma level of gentamicin of 4 to 6 μg/mL is considered adequate. Combining gentamicin with clindamycin may be useful in mixed anaerobic-aerobic bacterial infections, as may occur in the abdominal or pelvic areas.

Local Uses

Topical gentamicin sulfate cream or ointment may be used for skin infections with susceptible organisms; however, widespread or extensive use should be discouraged since these infections are usually minor and liberal use of these antibiotics increases the risk of resistance development. Gentamicin sulfate ophthalmic ointment or solution may be useful in the therapy of superficial eye infections caused by susceptible organisms. Parenteral solutions of gentamicin sulfate and similar aminoglycosides can be given orally to treat intestinal infections, and by inhalation to suppress *Pseudomonas* pneumonia in patients with cystic fibrosis.

NURSING IMPLICATIONS

Expect improvement in the extent of skin, ophthalmic, or otic infections within 2 to 3 days after starting topical aminoglycoside therapy; notify the physician if the infection does not improve or if it actually worsens.

Plasma level monitoring is becoming much more common to assure adequacy of therapy and to avoid potentially toxic levels. The times of drug administration and serum sampling should be accurately documented to permit accurate calculation of dosage alterations. When possible, infusions should be administered in a manner that will assure delivery of the entire dose to the patient over about 30 minutes; draw post-dose ("peak") blood samples 30 minutes after completion of the infusion. Intermittent infusion times may be as long as 2 hours per dose.

Do not mix other drugs in the same syringe with an aminoglycoside.

Side Effects, Adverse Reactions, and Contraindications

Of the antibiotics in common use, the aminoglycosides are most likely to cause serious toxic effects in the kidney and ear, and may cause muscle weakness or paralysis. Since many of these adverse effects are believed to be dose-related, plasma aminoglycoside levels should be monitored to minimize the risks.

Major systemic adverse effects may also occasionally occur with local uses of these agents if significant renal impairment exists. This is especially true when treating large denuded areas, such as abraded skin, GI tract ulcers, or extensive surgical irrigation. There is also a risk of systemic allergic reactions with *any* administration route. Adverse reactions and contraindications are summarized in Table 56–S3. Many of the important adverse reactions caused by aminoglycosides may be triggered or worsened by interacting drugs that may be required for managing the patient's overall condition.

Nephrotoxicity

When plasma aminoglycoside levels are high and sustained (for example, if gentamicin concentrations never fall below 2 μg/mL), the drug accumulates in cells of the renal tubules. Eventually, these cells die, leading to decreased glomerular filtration and an overall fall of renal excretory function. Renal damage is most likely to occur in the elderly, any patient with dehydration (including that which may accompany diuretic therapy) or impaired renal function, or in patients who are receiving other nephrotoxic drugs (see the section on drug interactions).

Nephrotoxicity can be detected with laboratory tests: serum creatinine and BUN levels rise, urine specific gravity and creatinine clearance fall, proteinuria occurs, and cells or casts may be present in the urine. Early damage may progress to clinically obvious late kidney damage (weight gain, edema, or oliguria), and may, on rare occasions, progress to frank renal failure. Early evidence of renal damage may not occur until the patient has received at least 5 days of aminoglycoside therapy. Nephrotoxicity is usually slowly reversible when aminoglycoside therapy is stopped.

The best way to avoid nephrotoxicity is to avoid excessive aminoglycoside blood levels by adjusting doses properly, and by keeping the patient well hydrated.

Ototoxicity

When given in high doses (peak plasma levels exceeding 12 μg/mL), aminoglycosides can accumulate to toxic levels in the sensory cells of the inner ear, destroying cells responsible for hearing, balance, or both. Factors that predispose the patient to ototoxicity include previous hearing or balance disorders, advanced age, or concomitant use of other ototoxic drugs such as high-ceiling diuretics (eg, furosemide). The type of ototoxicity that is most likely to occur seems to depend on the aminoglycoside. Gentamicin, tobramycin, and streptomycin are more likely to initially cause vestibular toxicity, with dizziness, nystagmus, or ataxia, although hearing loss may occur as well. Amikacin and neomycin are more likely to cause auditory impairment.

A common early manifestation of auditory toxicity is high-frequency hearing loss that is detectable only with audiometric tests. This may progress to frank hearing deficits or even deafness.

Recommendations for hearing tests are summarized in the next Nursing Implications section.

Neuromuscular Effects

Gentamicin and other aminoglycosides produce varying degrees of skeletal neuromuscular blockade. The intensity of this response is dose-related and usually self-limiting. Mild signs include general muscular weakness, but if doses are sufficiently high it may progress to hypoventilation and respiratory paralysis.

Patients with myasthenia gravis are extremely sensitive to the neuromuscular blocking effects of the aminoglycosides and should receive these drugs only when absolutely necessary, with close monitoring of adverse neuromuscular responses. Hypocalcemia is also a risk factor, so plasma calcium levels should be measured and normalized before giving aminoglycosides.

Neuromuscular blocking drugs, general anesthetics, and aminoglycosides act synergistically at the neuromuscular junction. Aminoglycoside administration to a patient who has recently received one of these drugs may cause significant or prolonged muscle weakness or paralysis, and possibly apnea. Administration of calcium salts is the most effective way to overcome neuromuscular blockade caused by an aminoglycoside. Acetylcholinesterase inhibitors (eg, neostigmine), which are traditionally used to reverse muscle paralysis caused by other neuromuscular blockers, have extremely variable effectiveness in this situation.

Allergic Reactions

Gentamicin and other aminoglycosides can cause allergic reactions. Rash, urticaria, generalized burning, fever, and eosinophilia are most common; agranulocytosis and anaphylaxis have been reported, but are rare. A prior allergic reaction to an aminoglycoside contraindicates subsequent use of these agents. Cross-sensitivity among the aminoglycosides has been reported; no cross-allergy occurs with other antibiotic classes.

Other Adverse Effects

Gentamicin and other aminoglycosides can (rarely) cause other neurotoxic reactions, including headache, paresthesias, lethargy, visual disturbances, and acute organic brain syndrome. Intrathecal administration of gentamicin (which is rarely required) can cause local inflammatory reactions. Local reactions to parenteral injection of these antibiotics include pain and induration, thrombophlebitis, sterile abscesses, and subcutaneous atrophy or fat necrosis.

NURSING IMPLICATIONS

Periodically assess plasma levels to ensure that they drop below 2 μg/mL before the next dose, and that post-dose levels do not exceed 12 μg/mL. This helps reduce the risk of nephrotoxicity and ototoxicity. Serum creatinine should be assessed prior to therapy and periodically during therapy (at least weekly in the absence of evidence of renal impairment; more frequently if it exists). Assess urine for protein and casts. When indicated, creatinine clearances can be determined.

Monitor the patient's weight for fluid retention and urinary output, which could signal oliguria. Be aware that fluid retention and oliguria occur relatively late in the course of nephrotoxicity, and should rarely occur if other precautions are taken earlier. Patients should maintain adequate hydration to decrease the risk of nephrotoxicity.

Assess for complaints of tinnitus, vertigo, or "fullness in the ears." Report balance disorders or hearing difficulty to the physician at once. Audiometric testing is recommended at the following times: before starting aminoglycoside therapy; at weekly intervals during therapy; and at 3 weeks after treatment if treatment for more than 14 consecutive days is anticipated or needed, or if the patient has one or more of the following risk factors for ototoxicity:

- age over 60 years;
- prior aminoglycoside therapy;
- concomitant therapy with other ototoxic drugs;
- elevated peak plasma aminoglycoside levels;
- markedly elevated serum creatinine levels; or
- preexisting auditory deficits.

Explain to patients why this testing is important.

Use extreme caution in administering aminoglycosides to patients who have myasthenia gravis, hypocalcemia, or have recently received neuromuscular blocking or anesthetic agents. Assess for respiratory depression.

If any allergic response occurs during aminoglycoside therapy, the drug should be discontinued and the allergy noted in the patient's record. Patients with a history of allergy or hypersensitivity to any aminoglycoside should probably not receive the same agent again, and other aminoglycosides should be used only with extreme caution. Use caution in handling these antibiotics yourself, since sensitization can occur if skin is exposed repeatedly to these agents.

◆ Use During Pregnancy and Lactation

All aminoglycosides cross the placental barrier and enter the fetal circulation, and there are potential fetal risks. However, most of these drugs are appropriate for administration during pregnancy if the mother has a serious or life-threatening illness for which possible benefits outweigh possible fetal risks. Use of a related aminoglycoside, streptomycin, during pregnancy has been associated with several cases of congenital deafness; it appears to be the least suitable aminoglycoside for use during pregnancy. Since small amounts of aminoglycosides are found in breast milk, the physician and nursing mother should consider therapeutic or feeding alternatives to reduce possible risks to the infant. Assess infants being breast-fed by mothers receiving aminoglycosides for evidence of GI superinfection or malabsorption.

◆ Use in Children

The volume of diluent should be less in infants and children.

◆ Use in the Elderly

Elderly patients (particularly those over 70 years) with decreased renal function are at greater risk for adverse effects from gentamicin.

Interactions with Other Drugs

Clinically significant drug interactions involving gentamicin or other aminoglycosides are summarized in Table 56–13. Interactions with general anesthetics, neuromuscular blocking agents, and ototoxic or nephrotoxic drugs were discussed earlier.

There are several other important interactions involving aminoglycosides. Concomitant oral administration of aminoglycosides (eg, neomycin) and orally administered digitalis glycosides may interfere with the absorption and clinical effect of digitalis.

Any drug with antiemetic or anti–motion sickness activity may mask aminoglycoside-induced vestibular ototoxic symptoms. Such interactants include not only prescribed and nonprescribed drugs (for example, dimenhydrinate [DRAMAMINE]) given specifically to suppress nausea, vomiting, or motion sickness, but also drugs such as the antipsychotics, which also suppress these symptoms.

Orally administered aminoglycosides may reduce the number of vitamin K–producing gut flora. If administered in conjunction with oral anticoagulants, which inhibit hepatic synthesis of vitamin K–dependent blood clotting factors, prolonged or abnormal bleeding, and possibly hemorrhage, may occur.

The ability of extended-spectrum penicillins to inactivate aminoglycosides in vivo and in vitro was noted earlier (p 1163).

NURSING IMPLICATIONS

Monitor closely patients receiving gentamicin in conjunction with other nephrotoxic drugs (for example, amphotericin B or cephalothin) for evidence of nephrotoxicity. Ensure adequate hydration for all patients; monitor fluid intake and output if the patient is hospitalized, and report indicators of renal dysfunction so therapy can be changed or other tests can be ordered as needed.

When aminoglycosides are administered with ototoxic diuretics, assess closely for vestibular or auditory deficits, and recommend audiometric testing when appropriate. Be aware that diuretic therapy may increase the risk of dehydration and increased aminoglycoside blood levels, thereby increasing the risk of ototoxicity and other dose-related adverse responses. To reduce the risk of ototoxicity, regardless of whether the patient is taking another ototoxic interactant, question medication orders calling for the administration of drugs with antiemetic activity. If such drugs must be administered, frequent monitoring of aminoglycoside blood levels becomes very important, and audiometric tests may be the only way to detect early hearing loss. Advise outpatients to avoid use of nonprescription antiemetic or anti–motion sickness drugs without a physician's approval during aminoglycoside therapy.

If you are responsible for the immediate postoperative care of a patient who has recently received an aminoglycoside, or for whom one is ordered, check the operative summary to determine whether neuromuscular blockers or inhaled general anesthetics were used. If the patient is on a ventilator, anticipate the need for prolonged ventilatory support. If the patient is breathing spontaneously, monitor the adequacy of ventilatory rate and depth closely and frequently, and have parenteral calcium and some form of ventilatory support available for prompt use if needed.

Monitor patients taking oral aminoglycosides and digitalis preparations for signs of worsening heart failure (weight gain, venous distention, dyspnea) that may indicate reduced digitalis absorption; monitoring of digitalis blood levels may be needed.

Monitor patients receiving oral aminoglycosides and oral anticoagulants for signs of additive effects on coagulation (eg, excessive or abnormal bruising or bleeding). Reduced anticoagulant doses may be required during aminoglycoside therapy, but the dose may need to be increased again once antibiotic treatment has stopped.

Overdose and Toxicity

The major problem with acute aminoglycoside overdose is neuromuscular blockade, which may require assisted ventilation. Ototoxicity and nephrotoxicity are the major problems associated with chronic overdoses. They, and the related nursing implications, were discussed earlier.

Related Aminoglycosides

Related aminoglycosides include

- amikacin, netilmicin, and tobramycin, which have uses similar to gentamicin but are less likely to induce resistance;
- streptomycin, which is used primarily to treat tuberculosis; and
- neomycin, which is too toxic for systemic use but is used as a topical antibiotic, and orally for reduction in intestinal bacteria to reduce ammonia formation in hepatic coma or before intestinal surgery.

For all these drugs, routes of elimination and toxicities associated with systemic use are generally similar to gentamicin. Information about dosage and administration, side effects and contraindications, and drug interactions is presented in Tables 56–C3, 56–S3, and 56–I3, respectively.

Amikacin Sulfate

Amikacin sulfate (AMIKIN) is currently the aminoglycoside with the broadest coverage of *P. aeruginosa.* It is also effective against some gram-negative bacilli that are resistant to other aminoglycosides. Many hospitals and physicians restrict use of amikacin to infections resistant to other aminoglycosides, to reduce the risk of emergence of strains resistant to this antibiotic. Amikacin is administered IM or IV; dosages are given in Table 56–C3. Intravenous doses should generally be infused over not more than 30 minutes. Continued therapy should be based on plasma levels, as discussed for gentamicin. However, with amikacin desired peak levels should be 15–30 μg/mL and predose (trough) levels should not exceed 8 μg/mL. Doses for children, based on plasma levels, will often be higher than those for adults. Toxicities related to elevated peak and predose plasma levels are similar to gentamicin.

Neomycin Sulfate

Neomycin sulfate (MYCIFRADIN; NEOBIOTIC) causes such severe systemic toxicity that it is not recommended for systemic therapy, despite being marketed for this use.

Neomycin tablets or oral solutions are administered to reduce bowel flora prior to gut surgery, or to reduce bacterial ammonia formation in patients with hyperammonemia. A laxative effect is expected. Oral use in the presence of bowel obstruction is contraindicated.

Neomycin is also contained in solutions used for surgical irrigation, usually combined with other antibiotics such as polymyxin B. It is also a common ingredient in many antibiotic creams and ointments (often combined with polymyxin B and bacitracin) that are administered on the skin. However, neomycin is a potent topical contact sensitizing agent that should not be used indiscriminately. Ophthalmic and otic combination products, which often also contain polymyxin B and gramicidin, can cause similar reactions. Wear gloves when administering these products.

Oral absorption of neomycin, or absorption from irrigation or topical applications, is minimal, but may result in systemic toxicity if large amounts are administered for prolonged periods. In addition, the likelihood of toxicity is increased in patients with severe renal impairment. Renal and otic function must be monitored closely during therapy.

Netilmicin Sulfate

Netilmicin sulfate (NETROMYCIN) has uses and toxicities very similar to gentamicin. The drug is given by the IM or IV route. It is effective against some gentamicin-resistant gram-negative bacilli and *Staph. aureus.* Nursing implications are similar to those noted for gentamicin.

Streptomycin Sulfate

Streptomycin sulfate is used mainly to treat tuberculosis. It is given IM in combination with other antitubercular drugs. It is also effective as a single agent in the treatment of plague and tularemia; and in combination with other antiinfectives to treat brucellosis, glanders, granuloma inguinale, and chancroid. Streptomycin is used concomitantly with penicillin G or ampicillin to treat enterococcal and streptococcal (viridans group) endocarditis. Streptomycin is effective against a number of gram-negative bacillary infections, but less toxic, more effective alternatives exist. Therefore, its use for these situations is limited.

Nephrotoxicity is less common with streptomycin than with other systemic aminoglycosides, but ototoxicity, especially vestibular toxicity, is greater. Neonatal deafness has occurred because of placental transfer of streptomycin.

Tobramycin Sulfate

Tobramycin sulfate (NEBCIN) is similar to gentamicin in dosage, desired serum concentrations, uses, and toxicities. It is more effective than gentamicin against *P. aeruginosa,* but is slightly more expensive. To reduce induction of tobramycin-resistant strains, this drug should probably be reserved for gentamicin-resistant infections. Tobramycin is claimed to be less nephrotoxic than gentamicin, but this is controversial.

IV. Tetracyclines

The tetracyclines were the first broad-spectrum antibiotics. These agents, which were originally obtained from cultures of *Streptomyces,* are active against many gram-positive and gram-negative bacteria, and also against *Rickettsia, Chlamydia, Mycoplasma,* spirochetes, *Mycobacterium,* and *Balantidium.* The prototype is tetracycline.

PROTOTYPE

Tetracycline Hydrochloride

Absorption, Distribution, Metabolism, and Excretion

Approximately 75% of an oral dose of tetracycline (ACHROMYCIN-V; SUMYCIN; others) is absorbed if given on an empty stomach. Absorption can be reduced by more than half if the drug is given with food or any dairy product. Peak levels are usually attained between 1 and 4 hours after ingestion. No parenteral preparations are available.

Tetracycline is readily distributed to all tissues other than the cerebrospinal fluid. The drug binds to newly formed bone and teeth. Tetracycline is concentrated in bile and is eliminated in urine and, to a lesser extent, in feces.

The usual serum half-life of tetracycline in patients with normal renal function is 6 to 12 hours; the value may be extended to as long as 5 days in patients with impaired renal function.

Pharmacologic Effects

The tetracyclines usually exhibit a bacteriostatic action, but can become bactericidal to certain organisms when present at high concentrations. The effects are usually due to inhibited bacterial protein synthesis. Tetracyclines may also alter the bacterial cell membrane, causing leakage of critical metabolites.

However, the mechanism of action appears to differ for tetracycline effects on *Propionibacterium acnes,* the causative organism responsible for the primary clinical use of these drugs, acne vulgaris. In this instance tetracyclines appear to reduce the organism's ability to form essential free fatty acids from triglycerides, which reduces the organism's ability to cause acne lesions.

Many common bacteria have developed resistance to tetracycline.

Clinical Indications and Administration

Tetracyclines are the drugs of choice for rickettsial infections (including Rocky Mountain spotted fever, typhus, Q-fever, rickettsialpox), Lyme disease, and for most chlamydial infections. Tetracyclines reduce both the duration and severity of mycoplasmal pneumonia. These agents are the most commonly used oral medications in the treatment of acne. Dosages are summarized in Table 56–C4.

Uncommon uses of tetracycline include infections caused by the gram-negative organisms *Brucella, Bartonella bacilliformis,* and *Calymmatobacterium granulomatis.* Tetracyclines have also been used in treatment of cholera, Vincent's infection, pneumonic plague, chancroid, rat-bite fever, and pertussis.

Syphilis can sometimes be treated with tetracycline in patients allergic to penicillins. Tetracyclines are used in other spirochetal infections as well. They may also be used in bronchitis and for resistant malaria. Since tetracyclines are bacteriostatic, use in immunosuppressed patients is relatively contraindicated.

Tetracycline can be applied topically for skin infections and as an ophthalmic preparation to treat eye infections caused by organisms listed previously.

NURSING IMPLICATIONS

Give oral tetracyclines on an empty stomach 1 hour before or 2 hours after meals with a full glass of water. The related drugs doxycycline and minocycline may be given with food or milk.

Side Effects, Adverse Reactions, and Contraindications

Gastrointestinal Side Effects

The most common side effects caused by tetracycline involve the gastrointestinal tract (Table 56–S4). They may be diverse, usually representing local irritation or superinfection. Oral involvement may involve stomatitis, black hairy tongue, or overgrowth of the oral tissues with *Candida.* Sore throat and hoarseness may occur. Gastric burning and other forms of lower GI tract upset, as well as nausea and vomiting, are fairly common. Rare side effects include flatulence, anogenital inflammation (often fungal in origin), systemic candidal infections, and pseudomembranous colitis.

Allergic Reactions

Allergic reactions rarely occur with tetracycline, and a history of such reactions is the only true contraindication to use of these drugs. These reactions usually appear as an erythematous or maculopapular rash, but may be more severe. Serum sickness–like reactions, with fever, headache, and arthralgia, can occur. If patients are hypersensitive to one tetracycline, they are probably allergic to all tetracyclines. The procaine contained in IM preparations may also be responsible for allergic reactions.

Dermatologic Side Effects

Photosensitivity reactions manifested as sunburn on sun-exposed areas occur most frequently with the related drug demeclocycline, but can occasionally occur with doxycycline, oxytetracycline, or tetracycline itself. Nail growth or color may be altered.

Renal Side Effects

Tetracyclines may be nephrotoxic on rare occasion; therapy can cause increased BUN concentrations and increased urinary nitrogen excretion with or without elevations in serum creatinine. Although renal changes are usually clinically insignificant in patients with normal renal function, progressive azotemia may develop in patients with renal impairment who receive tetracycline, demeclocycline, or oxytetracycline. (This is not a problem with doxycycline or minocycline.) Although rare with preparations currently marketed, outdated or otherwise deteriorated tetracycline may cause a reversible Fanconi-like syndrome, characterized by nausea and vomiting; lethargy; acidosis; excessive urinary loss of fluid, glucose, amino acids, protein, and phosphate; and hypokalemia.

Other Adverse Effects

Fatty liver is occasionally reported with high doses of tetracycline, and it is sometimes fatal. It occurs most often during pregnancy. Patients who are receiving other hepatotoxic drugs or who have preexisting hepatic or renal impairment are especially at risk for hepatotoxicity. Tetracycline use to treat brucellosis or spirochetal infections may cause a Jarisch–Herxheimer reaction (see penicillin). Neurologic side effects include lightheadedness, dizziness, vertigo, and fatigue. Intravenous administration may cause phlebitis.

NURSING IMPLICATIONS

Ideally, administer oral tetracyclines at least 1 hour before or 2 hours after meals. Tetracycline-induced GI upset may tempt many patients to take the antibiotic with meals. However, food interferes with drug absorption. In particular, milk, other dairy products or calcium-rich foods, and antacids will significantly reduce tetracycline absorption. Therefore, encourage patients to avoid taking tetracyclines with these "interactants"; in general, encourage them to limit the amount of *any* food consumed with these drugs. Advise patients that eating a few crackers with between-meal doses may alleviate stomach upset.

Report superinfection, usually presenting as tongue discoloration, thrush, diarrhea, or anorectal irritation or infection, at once. Encourage meticulous hygiene of the skin, mouth, and perianal area, to reduce the risk of superinfections.

Be aware that tetracyclines occasionally cause a variety of skin reactions, including rashes, that may be reported by the patient as an allergy. These usually are hypersensitivity reactions, not allergies; unless they can be diagnosed more completely, they should not be documented as true allergic reactions, and they do not contraindicate future use of the drug.

Encourage patients to avoid needless exposure to the sun, through the use of appropriate clothing and sunscreens, to reduce the risk of photosensitivity reactions.

Stress to all patients the need to not only complete the prescribed course of therapy, but also to discard any unused tetracycline. Outdated tetracyclines have been linked to the occurrence of additional adverse effects.

◆ Use During Pregnancy and Lactation

Ordinarily, tetracyclines should not be administered during pregnancy or to women who are breast-feeding their infants. Tetracyclines can affect the developing fetus, causing abnormal skeletal development and other untoward responses. Sufficient amounts of the drug can be ingested via breast milk to cause tooth enamel hypoplasia and permanent tooth discoloration. The only major exception for these guidelines is when a serious infection must be treated (for example, rickettsial infections, including Rocky Mountain spotted fever), and there are no less toxic alternatives. As noted earlier, pregnancy also increases the risk of serious liver dysfunction in women receiving high tetracycline doses.

◆ Use in Children

Impaired skeletal development and tooth calcification and permanent tooth staining, relatively contraindicate administration of tetracyclines to children less than 8 years old. The incidence and severity of these untoward responses increase as the duration of therapy increases. Of all the tetracyclines, doxycycline is the least likely to cause adverse dental effects. Exceptions noted in the section on pregnancy and lactation apply also to pediatric use.

◆ Use in the Elderly

Tetracyclines are generally considered safe for elderly patients. Reinforce the importance of taking the drug at the prescribed time, of timing the dose properly with respect to meals or interacting drugs (discussed later), and of not stopping treatment until the course of therapy is completed.

Interactions with Other Drugs

Minerals such as calcium, iron, aluminum, and zinc can substantially reduce absorption of tetracyclines by chelation. Thus, concomitant oral administration of vitamins with minerals, medicinal iron supplements, antacids, or kaolin-pectin containing antidiarrheals (as well as foods high in these minerals, such as milk) should be avoided. Drug administration should occur at least 1 hour before or 2 hours after administration of such interacting substances. The bactericidal effects of aminoglycosides and penicillins may be impaired by concomitant administration of tetracyclines, which are bacteriostatic antibiotics. The effects of anticoagulants are potentiated by tetracyclines, either by impairing the utilization of prothrombin or by tetracycline-induced reduction of vitamin K–producing intestinal flora. Prothrombin times should be monitored more closely if anticoagulants are used with tetracyclines. Antiepileptic agents can increase the metabolism of tetracyclines and thus lessen their effectiveness. See Table 56–14 for a summary of drug interactions.

Overdose and Toxicity

The primary manifestations of tetracycline overdosage are GI effects and possibly fatal hepatotoxicity.

Related Tetracyclines

There is little difference in clinical indications among the tetracyclines. The choice usually depends on cost, patient tolerance of particular agents, ease and frequency of administration, adverse effects, and the status of the patient's renal function. Use in pregnant women and children under 8 years is discouraged for all of the related agents. Tables 56–C4, 56–S4, and 56–I4 summarize dosages, adverse effects and contraindications, and drug interactions for these antibiotics.

Chlortetracycline Hydrochloride

Chlortetracycline hydrochloride (AUREOMYCIN) is marketed only as ophthalmic and topical ointments that are used for skin and eye infections caused by tetracycline-susceptible organisms.

Doxycycline

Doxycycline (DORYX; DOXY; VIBRAMYCIN; others) is available in calcium, hyclate, and monohydrate salts. Oral absorption is more complete than with tetracycline and is less affected by food. Indeed, oral doxycycline should be given with food and fluid to avoid GI and esophageal side effects. Doxycycline is usually given orally, but a parenteral formulation of doxycycline hyclate can be administered IV if oral administration is not feasible.

Of all the tetracyclines, doxycycline is excreted the least by the kidneys and is therefore considered the tetracycline of choice for patients with renal impairment.

Doxycycline is prescribed by many physicians to prevent "travelers' diarrhea" in individuals traveling for short periods of time to areas where this affliction commonly occurs. This is not an approved use, and the drug itself can cause diarrhea and may result in the development of resistant organisms.

Doxycycline is often used for chlamydial disease and pelvic inflammatory disease; it is an alternative treatment for syphilis.

Minocycline Hydrochloride

Minocycline hydrochloride (MINOCIN), like doxycycline, has good oral absorption and even better tissue distribution. Minocycline commonly causes CNS side effects, including dizziness, drowsiness, and fatigue; and especially vertigo (evident most often when high doses are used in women).

Minocycline is excreted less by the kidneys than most other tetracyclines and may therefore be a better choice than other tetracyclines (except doxycycline) in patients with renal dysfunction.

Oxytetracycline

Oxytetracycline (TERRAMYCIN; URI-TET; others) is similar to tetracycline in absorption, clinical indications, and dosage. It is given orally or IM, but not IV.

V. Erythromycins

Erythromycins are isolated from *Strep. erythreus.* They are clinically important and widely used because of their broad antibiotic spectrum, their usefulness in treating infections that do not respond well to other common antibiotics, and their relatively low incidence of serious adverse effects or toxicity. Erythromycin base ("erythromycin") is the prototype. Five erythromycin salts are available, all of which have similar pharmacologic properties and clinical uses.

PROTOTYPE

Erythromycin

Absorption, Distribution, Metabolism, and Excretion

Erythromycin base (E-BASE; E-MYCIN; ERYC; ERY-TAB; others) is available for oral administration. Orally administered erythromycin is inactivated by gastric acid, so it is formulated as tablets or capsules in which the drug is protected by a film- or enteric-coating. These should be administered on an empty stomach unless they are sustained release formulations or if the package insert indicates they can be administered with food. Peak serum concentrations occur 1 to 4 hours after oral administration. The serum half-life is about 2 hours, which usually necessitates administration four times a day.

Erythromycin is partially metabolized by the liver, but the drug is mainly excreted unchanged in the bile; small amounts appear in the urine. Renal impairment may prolong the half-life but does not necessitate a dosage change. Hemodialysis removes small amounts of erythromycin.

Erythromycin distributes well to most body tissues and fluids other than the cerebrospinal fluid, where concentrations are, at most, only 10% of serum levels.

Topical erythromycin ointment and solution, and ophthalmic ointment, are marketed for treatment of local infections.

Pharmacologic Effects

Erythromycin is a bacteriostatic antibiotic. It inhibits bacterial protein synthesis, much like the tetracyclines do. Erythromycin is more effective against gram-positive bacteria than against gram-negative bacteria, because it is better able to penetrate the cell wall of gram-positive organisms and thus achieve higher concentrations in them.

Clinical Indications and Administration

Erythromycin has a very broad spectrum of activity, broader even than that of penicillin G. It is used against gram-positive cocci, gram-positive bacilli, some gram-negative cocci, and a few bacilli. Additionally, erythromycin inhibits the growth of *Chlamydia, Actinomyces, Mycoplasma,* rickettsiae, *Treponema,* and *Entamoeba.* Clinical uses and dosages are listed in Table 56–C5.

Erythromycin is the drug of choice for oral therapy of respiratory tract infections caused by *Mycoplasma pneumoniae, Corynebacterium diphtheriae,* and *Bordetella pertussis.* Additionally, it is the drug of choice in Legionnaires' disease and chancroid. A common but unapproved use is in oral treatment of acne. When combined with sulfisoxazole, erythromycin is used against *H. influenzae.* Erythromycin is used as an alternate drug in numerous streptococcal infections, as well as *Chlamydia,* Lyme disease, and *Treponema.*

When an erythromycin-sensitive infection requires immediately high serum levels and parenteral therapy is indicated, or when oral erythromycin administration is not possible, the gluceptate or lactobionate salts of the drug are used. These parenteral erythromycins are given IV; IM administration causes too much local pain and tissue irritation. See the Related Drugs section for more information about these erythromycin salts.

Erythromycin gel, ointment or solution is used topically for acne, and an ophthalmic ointment is used for susceptible eye infections.

NURSING IMPLICATIONS

Before giving the drug, check the physician's order carefully, as similarities exist between generic and trade name preparations of erythromycin, which may result in the wrong form being given. Oral forms should generally be taken on an empty stomach or immediately before meals unless the package insert indicates they may be given with food. Absorption of erythromycin estolate and erythromycin ethylsuccinate is not significantly altered by food. Enteric-coated preparations may be given with food. Give the drug with a full glass of water; do not offer acidic fruit juice. Administer parenteral forms by slow IV infusion to prevent pain along the vein.

Side Effects, Adverse Reactions, and Contraindications

The erythromycins are one of the least toxic antibiotics; they rarely cause any serious adverse reactions. The most frequent side effect with orally administered erythromycins is GI upset (Table 56–S5): cramping and diarrhea; heartburn, stomatitis, and anorexia; and, rarely, pseudomembranous colitis. High-dose therapy has caused reversible hearing loss.

Erythromycins may cause hepatotoxicity, usually manifested as cholestatic jaundice. However, the incidence is low when erythromycin base is used. As noted later, the incidence is higher when some of the salts are used.

Allergic reactions are usually mild and characterized by rashes and urticaria; however, some severe anaphylactic reactions have occurred. Anaphylactic reactions represent the only true contraindication for erythromycin base therapy.

NURSING IMPLICATIONS

Gastric upset during erythromycin therapy is common. If the patient does not tolerate a particular erythromycin product, an alternative product, usually a different salt, may be tolerated better. Additionally, enteric-coated forms given with food reduce GI distress. Such reactions are commonly identified by patients as "allergy" to erythromycin; true allergy to erythromycins is rare and does not present as gastric burning or intolerance.

◆ Use During Pregnancy and Lactation

Safe use of erythromycin during pregnancy has not been established. However, the drug has been used to treat urogenital chlamydial infections and syphilis during pregnancy. Erythromycin crosses the placenta and achieves levels in breast milk approximately 50% of maternal serum levels. Because of relatively low toxicity, this is often clinically acceptable; however, GI upset may occur in breast-fed infants and should be assessed for.

◆ Use in the Elderly

The incidence of serious adverse effects from antibiotics in elderly patients is probably lowest with erythromycin. Transient auditory impairment associated with high-dose therapy has been seen in the elderly and in patients with renal insufficiency. Use erythromycin cautiously when daily doses exceed 4 g and the patient is over 50 years old.

Interactions with Other Drugs

Erythromycin inhibits the hepatic metabolism of several drugs, including theophylline, carbamazepine, and methylprednisolone (Table 56–I5). Through poorly understood mechanisms, cyclosporine may accumulate in the body when coadministered with erythromycin. Increased pharmacologic effects of warfarin, bromocriptine, and digoxin associated with reduced clearance may necessitate lower doses of these agents.

Overdose and Toxicity

Erythromycin overdoses will usually only increase the side effects noted above. They are treated symptomatically, with appropriate supportive care.

Related Erythromycins

Erythromycin derivatives have similar clinical indications but differ in routes of administration, tolerance of oral administration, and toxicities. Information on dosages, side effects and contraindications, and interactions with other drugs is given in Tables 56–C5, 56–S5, and 56–I5, respectively.

Erythromycin Estolate

Erythromycin estolate (ILOSONE) shares the indications of erythromycin base. The estolate salt is absorbed better than the base, and it is one of the two salts that can appropriately be administered with meals to reduce GI upset (the other is the ethylsuccinate salt). The suspension is the most palatable erythromycin liquid. The risk of hepatotoxicity, which appears to be a form of allergic reaction, is greater with the estolate than with any other erythromycin preparation. Cholestatic jaundice may occur, generally after 1 to 2 weeks of therapy, and especially with advancing age. Many consider erythromycin estolate inappropriate for therapy in adults. It has also produced hepatitis. Hepatic dysfunction is reversible after discontinuation of therapy, although it may take several weeks to resolve. It is probably best not to use this drug if therapy is to last more than 10 days or if repeated courses of treatment are planned or likely to be needed.

Erythromycin Ethylsuccinate

Erythromycin ethylsuccinate (E.E.S.; ERY PED) is less bioavailable than other oral erythromycin preparations; for example, a dose of 400 mg of this salt is equivalent to a dose of 250 mg of other oral erythromycins. It may cause hepatotoxic reactions. Erythromycin ethylsuccinate should probably be given with meals to reduce GI upset, which is fairly common.

Erythromycin Gluceptate and Erythromycin Lactobionate

Erythromycin gluceptate (ILOTYCIN GLUCEPTATE) and erythromycin lactobionate (ERYTHROCIN LACTOBIONATE-IV) are the only forms of erythromycin available for IV use. They are used when the oral route is not possible or when severe infections require immediate high serum levels. These erythromycins are best given by continuous infusion; however, intermittent infusion is acceptable if the interval between infusions is no less than 6 hours (to avoid prolonged periods of subtherapeutic serum levels). These drugs cause considerable venous irritation.

Erythromycin Stearate

Erythromycin stearate (ERAMYCIN; ERYTHROCIN STEARATE; others) is an oral preparation that is poorly absorbed when administered with meals. It should therefore be administered on an empty stomach. Erythromycin stearate has the same clinical uses, doses, and dosing schedule as erythromycin base.

VI. Sulfonamides

The sulfonamides were the first safe systemic antibacterial agents available. Since then, sulfonamide use has declined somewhat, although they are still widely used because of their low cost and high efficacy. Sulfisoxazole is considered the prototype, even though the related drug sulfamethoxazole is used more often for many indications.

PROTOTYPE

Sulfisoxazole

Sulfisoxazole (GANTRISIN) is a short-acting antibiotic. It is used most often to treat urinary tract infections, but it has many other uses as well.

Absorption, Distribution, Metabolism, and Excretion

Sulfisoxazole is rapidly and completely absorbed after oral administration. Peak plasma concentrations occur in 2 to 4 hours. The drug distributes to all body tissues, but it is largely confined to the extracellular fluids. It is extensively bound to plasma proteins. Sulfisoxazole readily enters the cerebrospinal fluid, reaching concentrations there that are about 10% to 20% of plasma levels.

About one third of the absorbed dose is metabolized in the liver. The metabolites have no antibiotic activity, but they may still contribute to some of the drug's toxic effects.

Overall, about 95% of the absorbed dose is excreted in the urine within 24 hours of administration, and urinary concentrations of active drug may be twice as high as corresponding blood levels. Compared with many other sulfonamides, sulfisoxazole is relatively soluble in the urine. The presence and activity of sulfisoxazole in the urine is important not only for the drug's use in treating urinary tract infections, but also for some of the drug's potentially adverse renal effects.

Pharmacologic Effects

Sulfisoxazole usually exerts bacteriostatic activity, but high urinary concentrations may be bactericidal. Sulfisoxazole and the other sulfonamides inhibit bacterial growth by interfering with the enzymatic conversion to folic acid of para-aminobenzoic acid (PABA), an essential nutrient for some microorganisms. Microorganisms that do not synthesize folic acid are resistant to sulfonamides.

Clinical Indications and Administration

Sulfisoxazole (and, in particular, the related drug sulfamethoxazole) is commonly used to treat urinary tract infections caused by *E. coli, Klebsiella, Enterobacter, Proteus,* and *Staph. aureus* (Table 56–C6). The sulfonamides can be administered alone, but they are also available in proprietary products that contain a tetracycline, a phenazopyridine (a urinary analgesic), or both. Products containing phenazopyridine are particularly useful for the first 2 days of treatment of urinary tract infections because the phenazopyridine helps reduce urinary pain, burning, and frequency. Sulfisoxazole or another sulfonamide should be used alone for the remainder of therapy. Too many combination products are available to discuss each one separately.

Sulfisoxazole is also used in acute otitis media, usually in combination with erythromycin. This combination is usually active against *H. influenzae,* including ampicillin-resistant strains. Sulfisoxazole is also available in combination with other agents in vaginal creams for the treatment of *H. vaginalis* vaginitis, but such combinations are generally considered ineffective.

NURSING IMPLICATIONS

Oral sulfisoxazole preparations should be taken on an empty stomach, 1 hour before or 2 hours after meals, with a full glass of water (unless ordered otherwise). Check the physician's order for oral sulfisoxazole carefully. The manufacturers recommend a loading dose to start therapy, but because the drug is absorbed rapidly (and reaches high urinary concentrations rapidly), the loading dose may be unnecessary.

Encourage patients not to miss a dose; for most sulfonamides, a missed dose should be taken as soon as the oversight is realized. Advise patients to take these drugs at easily remembered times (eg, with respect to meals or bedtime, as suitable for each drug). Stress the need for the patient to complete the entire prescribed course of therapy.

Side Effects, Adverse Reactions, and Contraindications

Sulfisoxazole (and the related sulfonamides) cause many side effects that affect nearly every organ system (Table 56–S6). However, these drugs are usually well tolerated, and only about 3% of patients require discontinuation of the drug because of adverse reactions.

Minor and relatively common side effects affecting the GI tract include nausea, vomiting, and diarrhea. Altered liver enzymes have occurred occasionally during the first few days of therapy. Central nervous system side effects include dizziness, drowsiness, or ataxia; neuropsychiatric changes, such as depression or psychosis, have occurred occasionally.

Sulfonamide therapy is associated with three more important untoward responses: allergy, crystalluria, and bone marrow toxicity. The syndrome of kernicterus—important for the fetus and neonate—is discussed separately later.

Allergic Reactions

Allergic reactions are common. The manifestations of the reaction are diverse, as with other antibiotic classes, and range from rashes, pruritus, and urticaria, to more severe responses including exfoliative dermatitis and Stevens–Johnson syndrome. Many of the allergy-related skin rashes are photosensitive.

The sulfonamides participate in cross-sensitivity with other drugs having a sulfa structure, of which the thiazide diuretics and the oral hypoglycemic drugs (sulfonylureas) are perhaps the most important and common. Any of these agents is contraindicated for persons with a history of an allergic reaction to another. Allergic reactions appear to occur more frequently in persons with acquired immunodeficiency syndrome (AIDS).

Crystalluria

Sulfonamides are poorly soluble in the urine, and may crystallize in the renal tubules if their concentration becomes too high. This condition is called *crystalluria,* and it may cause serious renal damage. It is a concentration-dependent (dose-dependent) effect. For any given dose, the risk of crystalluria increases as the urine volume, or urine pH, falls. The risk can be reduced by reducing the dose, maintaining adequate urine output (at least 1.5 L per day for an adult), and alkalinizing the urine if needed (as by administering sodium bicarbonate).

Administering small doses of two or three sulfonamides, rather than a large dose of one agent, also reduces the risk of crystalluria. This is the basis for prescribing one of the sulfonamide combination products. Renal impairment and urinary tract obstruction are among the common conditions that contraindicate sulfonamide use.

Bone Marrow Toxicity

Sulfonamides exert a direct toxic effect on bone marrow. This can cause several serious hematologic reactions, including aplastic anemia, thrombocytopenia, agranulocytosis, and their consequences. Hemolytic anemia is common in patients with a glucose-6-phosphate dehydrogenase deficiency.

NURSING IMPLICATIONS

Obtain a thorough medication history before administering sulfonamides, to help identify prior allergies to these antibiotics and to structurally related drugs. Instruct patients to discontinue the drug at once, and to notify their physician, at any sign of allergy, including mild skin rashes. Instruct adult patients who receive sulfonamides to drink at least eight full glasses of water each day to reduce the risk of crystalluria. Monitor fluid intake and output of hospitalized patients receiving these drugs. Periodic checks of urine pH are advised for hospitalized patients. Administer sodium bicarbonate or other urinary alkalinizers as ordered. Assess periodically for evidence of bone marrow depression and its consequences (bruising, bleeding; fever and other evidence of systemic infection, and so on). Complete blood counts before treatment and periodically during therapy are advised if sulfonamide therapy lasting more than 2 weeks is anticipated. Because of the risk of photosensitivity, advise patients to wear suitable clothing and sunscreens if they cannot avoid exposure to sunlight or other ultraviolet light sources.

◆ Use During Pregnancy and Lactation

Sulfonamides can displace bilirubin from plasma protein–binding sites in the fetal circulation or neonatal circulation. The resulting hyperbilirubinemia can cause severe and permanent neurologic changes (*kernicterus*) in the child. Therefore, sulfonamides should not be used during pregnancy (especially near or at term), nor during breastfeeding.

◆ Use in Children

The risk of kernicterus contraindicates the use of sulfonamides in children less than 2 months of age, whether administered directly or ingested via breast milk.

◆ Use in the Elderly

Impaired renal function and the resulting risks of crystalluria are the major general concerns associated with sulfonamide use in the elderly. Monitory therapy closely for evidence of side effects or toxicity.

Interactions with Other Drugs

The sulfonamides, to varying degrees, bind to plasma proteins. As a result, they may displace, or be displaced by, other protein-bound drugs. The expected result is an intensification of the actions of the displaced drug; the actual response may be difficult to predict.

The most common, clinically significant interactions appear to involve oral anticoagulants (particularly warfarin: increased risk of bruising, bleeding, and other consequences of excessive anticoagulation); phenytoin (increased risk of phenytoin side effects or toxicity); and oral hypoglycemic drugs (increased risk of hypoglycemia). In general, these interactants should be avoided. If the interaction is unavoidable, close monitoring and possible dosage reductions of the drug(s) are essential. Sulfonamides may also increase blood levels of methotrexate, and increase the risk of toxicity unless methotrexate dosages are reduced. The cause of the sulfonamide–methotrexate interaction is unknown. Drug interactions involving sulfonamides are summarized in Table 56–I6.

Overdose and Toxicity

Overdoses of any sulfonamide can cause serious problems, or even death. In general, the untoward effects on the GI, renal, central nervous, and hematopoietic systems, noted earlier, occur and intensify. Severe neuritis, hepatic damage, and blood dyscrasias may occur. Serious responses may be preceded by a high fever.

Management involves immediate discontinuation of sulfonamide administration (and induced emesis as used for other overdoses; see Appendix C), and symptomatic and supportive care. Give liberal amounts of oral or parenteral fluids to promote diuresis and reduce the risk of crystalluria if the patient has reasonably normal renal function. Urinary alkalinization may be indicated. Anticipate renal failure and the need to treat it. Antibiotics other than sulfonamides may be needed to prevent or combat infections when agranulocytosis occurs and the body's defenses are compromised. Blood transfusions or blood component therapy may be required to control excessive bleeding or hemorrhage caused by thrombocytopenia.

Related Sulfonamides

Several other sulfonamides are available as single-entity products or as fixed-dose combinations of a sulfa with one or more drugs. Dosages are summarized in Table 56–C6. In general, these drugs share most or all of the properties noted for sulfisoxazole, but indications vary. Importantly, they share the risks of allergy, crystalluria, bone marrow toxicity, and the production of kernicterus.

Single-Entity Sulfonamides

Sulfamethoxazole

Sulfamethoxazole (GANTANOL; URI-BAK) shares all sulfisoxazole's indications. The main advantage of this oral sulfonamide is its long half-life, which usually allows twice-daily dosing. This improves patient compliance, and so sulfamethoxazole has largely replaced sulfisoxazole for most clinical indications. Sulfamethoxazole is also a component in several fixed-dose combination products that are discussed later.

Sulfasalazine

Sulfasalazine (AZULFIDINE) has only one indication: treatment of ulcerative colitis. It is the only sulfonamide antibiotic approved for this use. The drug is given orally. Enteric-coated sulfasalazine tablets cause less GI distress than regular tablets or the oral suspension. There are rare reports of reversible oligospermia, and resulting infertility, in males treated with sulfasalazine.

Sulfonamide Combination Products

Co-trimoxazole and the proprietary drug PEDIAZOLE contain a sulfonamide plus one or two other drugs. All precautions noted for sulfisoxazole apply to these medications.

Co-trimoxazole

Co-trimoxazole ("TMP-SMZ"; BACTRIM; SEPTRA; others) is a combination of sulfamethoxazole and trimethoprim in a 5:1 ratio. Both agents are bacteriostatic antiinfectives that work by antagonizing folic acid production. However, these agents exert their activity on different steps of the folic acid production pathway, and when given together they act synergistically to cause a bactericidal effect. Trimethoprim, used alone to treat urinary tract infections, is discussed in Chapter 57.

The combination of sulfamethoxazole and trimethoprim expands the antimicrobial spectrum of the sulfonamides. Most strains of gram-positive and gram-negative organisms are susceptible, including *Staph. aureus, Strep. pneumoniae, Strep. pyogenes, E. coli, Enterobacter, Klebsiella, Proteus, Serratia, Shigella,* and *Acinetobacter.*

Co-trimoxazole is available as tablets or a suspension for oral use, and as a sterile solution for IV administration. The dosage (see Table 56–C6) is based on the amount of trimethoprim in the combination. Regular-strength BACTRIM and SEPTRA tablets, and related brand-name products, contain 80 mg trimethoprim and 400 mg sulfamethoxazole. Double-strength tablets (BACTRIM DS and SEPTRA DS, for example) contain twice the amount of each ingredient. Co-trimoxazole oral suspensions contain, in each 5 mL, 40 mg of trimethoprim and 200 mg of sulfamethoxazole.

Co-trimoxazole is well absorbed from the GI tract, with serum levels approximating those obtained with IV administration. Co-trimoxazole is widely distributed to most body tissues and fluids, including the cerebrospinal fluid. Both components in co-trimoxazole are metabolized in the liver and excreted in the urine as active drug and inactive metabolites. Renal impairment necessitates the use of reduced doses.

Co-trimoxazole is a very useful drug for a wide variety of infections. It is used in acute, uncomplicated urinary tract infections, although other less expensive agents such as ampicillin or sulfamethoxazole should be used first. Co-trimoxazole is usually reserved for the treatment of chronic or recurrent urinary tract infections because resistance does not readily develop. Co-trimoxazole is frequently used in acute otitis media in children and is especially useful in treating infections caused by ampicillin-resistant strains of *H. influenzae* or *Branhamella catarrhalis.* It is effective in the treatment or prophylaxis of acute exacerbations of chronic bronchitis, commonly seen in patients with chronic obstructive pulmonary disease. Co-trimoxazole is considered to be the drug of choice for the treatment of infections caused by *Pneumocystis carinii,* a protozoan that is the frequent cause of pneumonia in patients who are severely immunosuppressed, such as cancer patients receiving intensive chemotherapy or patients suffering from AIDS. It is also used prophylactically for patients with chronic immunosuppression to prevent the development of *Pneumocystis* infections. Other uses of co-trimoxazole include infections caused by *Nocardia,* and enteritis caused by *Shigella.*

Side effects caused by co-trimoxazole use are similar to those associated with other sulfonamides (Table 56–S6). Hypersensitivity reactions are the most common, and appear to occur more frequently in patients with AIDS. Pain and phlebitis may occur when the product is given IV.

The precautions and contraindications for co-trimoxazole are the same as for other sulfonamides.

NURSING IMPLICATIONS

Intravenous co-trimoxazole can cause phlebitis at the injection site and may cause tissue damage if the solution extravasates. The solution is usually diluted in 75 to 125 mL of fluid and should be infused over at least 60 minutes.

Sulfisoxazole plus Erythromycin

The proprietary product PEDIAZOLE, dispensed as a suspension for oral administration, contains sulfisoxazole and erythromycin ethylsuccinate. It is used exclusively for treating acute otitis media in children. Nursing implications for both the sulfonamides and the erythromycins apply to this product.

VII. Quinolones

The quinolones (less often referred to by their more formal name, fluoroquinolones) are derivatives of nalidixic acid, an antimicrobial drug used only to treat urinary tract infections (see Chapter 57, p 1239). The chemical process that creates the quinolones gives them increased antibiotic potency against gram-negative organisms, and a broader spectrum of activity that covers more gram-positive organisms and *Pseudomonas.* Quinolones are the newest group of antibiotics, and they are receiving more attention than the older antibiotics, mainly because they possess many desirable properties. (However, see the Nursing Implications section under related drugs.) These relate to

- pharmacokinetic properties, including good oral absorption and easy access to diverse body tissues;
- a broad spectrum of bactericidal activity, with clinical usefulness in a variety of infections; and
- relatively few significant or common side effects, adverse responses, true toxicities, or drug–drug interactions.

The first quinolone to be used in the United States was norfloxacin, but another agent that is perhaps more well known is ciprofloxacin. It will be considered as the prototype.

PROTOTYPE

Ciprofloxacin

Absorption, Distribution, Metabolism, and Excretion

Ciprofloxacin (CIPRO) can be given orally or by IV infusion. The drug is absorbed well from the gut, regardless of whether it is taken in the fasting state or with meals. Blood levels after oral dosing come close to those achieved when the drug is given IV. Ciprofloxacin is widely distributed throughout the body, and it appears to enter most body tissues well. Entry into the cerebrospinal fluid is not very great, however.

Ciprofloxacin is metabolized, but renal elimination of the drug seems to be very important: decreased renal function (rather than liver function) is the major determinant of whether and by how much dosages might need to be reduced. The plasma half-life of orally administered ciprofloxacin is normally about 4 hours, but therapeutic blood levels last long enough to permit twice-daily dosing.

Pharmacologic Effects

Ciprofloxacin and the other quinolones inhibit a microbial enzyme, called *DNA gyrase,* that is necessary for the infecting organisms to replicate their DNA.

Clinical Indications and Administration

Ciprofloxacin is given orally or IV to treat systemic or urinary tract infections caused by some gram-positive and most gram-negative aerobic isolates, including *Pseudomonas,* that are resistant to other (and usually less expensive) drugs. Ciprofloxacin and oflaxacin currently are the only oral antibiotics available to treat *Pseudomonas* infections outside the urinary tract. The drug is effective against most bacterial cases of diarrhea, and is often used for empiric therapy of diarrhea. Dosages are listed in Table 56–C7.

Bacterial resistance has developed during ciprofloxacin therapy; in some cases it can be reversed by discontinuing the drug.

Side Effects, Adverse Reactions, and Contraindications

In general, most patients who receive a quinolone experience few side effects. Nausea is the most common side effect (Table 56–S7). Other GI side effects include nonspecific GI upset, abdominal pain, and vomiting. These are more likely to occur in elderly patients or when high doses of ciprofloxacin are given.

Central nervous system side effects include headache, irritability, dizziness, and confusion. Seizures or psychosis have been reported; the risk seems greatest in patients with preexisting seizure disorders or other brain dysfunctions, such as cerebral atherosclerosis. For patients who are taking theophylline, or who consume large amounts of caffeine, the ability of ciprofloxacin to inhibit the metabolism of these substances may contribute to some of the CNS side effects (see Drug Interactions section).

Crystalluria (crystalline deposits of ciprofloxacin in the urine) is possible, but is unlikely to occur if maximum recommended dosages are not exceeded and the patient is kept well hydrated.

Hypersensitivity reactions (eg, rash, edema, flushing, fever) can occur. Some of the skin reactions are photosensitive. Nephrotoxicity (possibly related to crystalluria) or hepatotoxicity occasionally occurs. Bone marrow suppression and eosinophilia are rare hematologic complications.

◆ Use During Pregnancy and Lactation

In animal studies, quinolones have been shown to cause defects in cartilage development; similar effects may occur in humans. Thus, do not give these drugs to pregnant or nursing women unless expected benefits clearly outweigh potential risks, and no safer alternatives are effective or can be used.

◆ Use in Children

Quinolones should not be administered to children less than 18 years old.

◆ Use in the Elderly

Reduced renal function usually requires reduced dosages. Maintain adequate hydration as permitted by other disorders the elderly patient may have.

NURSING IMPLICATIONS

General guidelines with respect to side effects include ensuring that recommended maximum dosages are not exceeded; the patient is kept well hydrated; excessive exposure to sunlight is avoided to reduce the risk of photosensitive skin reactions; and routine blood tests to assess liver, kidney, and bone marrow function (eg, complete blood counts) are done periodically. The serum creatinine level is the most commonly used indicator of renal function for making quinolone dosage adjustments. Manufacturers' data (eg, in package inserts) give explicit directions about how to adjust the dose based on creatinine levels.

Interactions with Other Drugs

Interactions involving ciprofloxacin are summarized in Table 56–I7. Antacids, sucralfate, and oral iron salts (and possibly zinc salts) can inhibit quinolone absorption and effectiveness. Ciprofloxacin inhibits the metabolism of methylxanthines (eg, theophylline), and may do the same to oral anticoagulants and cyclosporine. Blood levels and effects of these interactants can rise to potentially toxic levels if their dosages are not reduced.

NURSING IMPLICATIONS

Monitor accordingly for the potential outcomes of the interactions between quinolones and other drugs. Be aware that several key interactants are available without prescription. The interaction with methylxanthines also may involve caffeine, which is often consumed in large amounts in coffee, many cola beverages, and chocolates. Inquire about how much caffeine-containing beverages and foods your patient is taking, especially if signs of CNS stimulation (owing to excessive blood caffeine levels) occur during ciprofloxacin therapy. In addition, assess for the patient's use of antacids and multivitamin–mineral supplements (many products contain iron, zinc, or both). Advise patients who use or who may wish to use these OTC interactants to get their physician's approval and directions first. See Table 56–I7 for additional nursing implications.

Overdose and Toxicity

Very little information is available about overdoses with quinolones. Treatment of acute overdoses involves standard first-aid measures (induced emesis, etc; see Appendix C) followed by symptomatic, supportive care. Hemodialysis or peritoneal dialysis can be used for severe ciprofloxacin overdose.

Related Quinolones

All the related quinolones are given orally. They share the same mechanism of action noted for ciprofloxacin, and also share generally similar side effects and adverse responses. Thus, precautions noted for ciprofloxacin apply. Major differences for some of these include clinical indications; interactions with food (which affects timing of administration with respect to meals); and the degree of renal dysfunction needed to require a dosage reduction.

Lomefloxacin, Norfloxacin, and Ofloxacin

Ofloxacin (FLOXIN) shares the many clinical uses noted for ciprofloxacin. There are fewer indications for the other related agents. Lomefloxacin (MAXAQUIN) is used only to treat susceptible organisms that cause urinary tract or lower respiratory tract infections. It can also be given preoperatively, as prophylaxis against urinary tract infections caused by urethral surgery. Norfloxacin (NOROXIN) is used only for treating urinary tract infections and uncomplicated urethral or cervical gonorrhea.

These drugs are given orally, and are not indicated for children. Dosages are summarized in Table 56–C7. Renal dysfunction requires reducing the dose of these drugs, as noted for ciprofloxacin. Of all the related drugs, ofloxacin appears to depend most on renal status. Modest reductions of creatinine clearance that might not require changing the dose of another quinolone usually will require giving less ofloxacin. (See package inserts for details.)

Overall, side effects and adverse responses noted for ciprofloxacin apply to these alternatives. Interactants that interfere with ciprofloxacin absorption (eg, antacids) also interfere with the related agents. The related quinolones seem to interact less than the prototype with methylxanthines and oral anticoagulants. Assume that all the general precautions concerning use and assessment, noted for ciprofloxacin, apply to these related drugs.

NURSING IMPLICATIONS

Monitor patients closely for side effects and adverse responses, especially with the newer quinolones (eg, lomefloxacin) and others that will certainly be marketed in the future. Some of these newly approved drugs are in wide use, but perhaps not enough time has passed to give a full appreciation of potential adverse effects that can arise in general practice. A good example is another quinolone, temafloxacin, which was marketed as OMNIFLOX. Within months after it was approved and began being prescribed, a disturbing number of serious adverse effects were reported. The drug was quickly withdrawn from the market.

VIII. Chloramphenicol

PROTOTYPE

Chloramphenicol

Chloramphenicol is a synthetic antibiotic, originally isolated from *Streptomyces venezuelae,* that is structurally different from all other antibiotics. Different forms of the drug are available for oral, topical, or parenteral administration. All dosage forms are highly active against many strains of *H. influenzae, Salmonella typhi, Rickettsia,* and *Chlamydia,* which represent the major clinical uses of this antibiotic.

Serious toxicity limits the use of chloramphenicol to treat severe infections that cannot be treated with other antibiotics, whether owing to resistance or contraindication.

Absorption, Distribution, Metabolism, and Excretion

Only free chloramphenicol, found in chloramphenicol capsules, is absorbed well from the GI tract. Similarly, only the free drug is pharmacologically active. The oral suspension contains the palmitrate ester of the drug. It is rapidly hydrolyzed (metabolized) in the gut to free chloramphenicol, which is then absorbed. Peak plasma concentrations usually occur within 1 to 3 hours after oral administration. This process occurs slowly in neonates, in whom absorption of free drug from the liquid preparation may be slow and erratic.

The sodium succinate salt of chloramphenicol is used for IV therapy. This salt is also inactive and must be hydrolyzed to yield active drug. This is accomplished by esterases in the kidneys, liver, and lungs. Some of the inactive ester in the bloodstream is excreted by the kidneys prior to activation. As a result, serum concentrations of active drug may actually be lower following IV administration than after oral administration, provided the patient has normal renal and hepatic function. Thus, and unlike the situation with most drugs, oral doses of chloramphenicol can be lower than IV doses to maintain similar plasma levels. Intramuscular administration of chloramphenicol sodium succinate is not recommended because of poor absorption.

A topical cream, an ophthalmic solution and ointment, and an otic solution are available for local infection. Absorption of chloramphenicol from these sites is minimal, but on rare occasions it may be sufficient to cause allergic reactions or bone marrow suppression.

Chloramphenicol is widely distributed to most body tissues. Concentrations in the cerebrospinal fluid may reach as high as 90% of plasma levels. This property makes the drug particularly useful for treating CNS infections such as meningitis.

Chloramphenicol is inactivated primarily in the liver by conjugation with glucuronic acid. The kidneys excrete the inactive glucuronide and a small amount of free chloramphenicol. Plasma half-lives in adults with normal hepatic function range from about 1 to 4 hours. Patients with underdeveloped or impaired hepatic function, including newborn infants, may accumulate toxic blood levels of chloramphenicol unless the dose is reduced. Renal impairment does not significantly prolong the half-life. Hemodialysis has only a slight ability to reduce chloramphenicol plasma concentrations; peritoneal dialysis has no effect.

NURSING IMPLICATIONS

Do not administer chloramphenicol IM. For patients other than neonates, question medication orders calling for increased chloramphenicol doses when switching from IV to oral administration.

Pharmacologic Effects

Chloramphenicol usually causes bacteriostatic effects, except when very high doses are given or when the infecting bacteria are very susceptible to the drug. The main antimicrobial effect involves inhibition of protein synthesis. However, this effect is also responsible for the drug's dose-related toxicity: chloramphenicol may also inhibit protein synthesis significantly in rapidly proliferating mammalian cells, such as bone marrow.

Clinical Indications and Administration

Chloramphenicol is active against many gram-positive aerobic bacteria, including streptococci, and many gram-negative aerobic bacteria, including *H. influ-*

enzae, N. meningitidis, Salmonella, and *Shigella* (Table 56–C8). It is also active against *Rickettsia, Chlamydia,* and *Mycoplasma,* as well as many anaerobic bacteria such as *Bacteroides.*

Systemic chloramphenicol should be used only for serious or life-threatening infections in which less toxic antiinfectives are ineffective or contraindicated. The drug can be used to treat severe cases of typhoid fever and rickettsial infections such as Rocky Mountain spotted fever; *H. influenzae* meningitis, and in life-threatening pneumococcal and meningococcal infections. Chloramphenicol is considered an alternative treatment for meningitis in children who cannot receive, or do not respond to, a third-generation cephalosporin such as cefotaxime or ceftriaxone. In this instance, chloramphenicol is usually used in conjunction with ampicillin. In addition, chloramphenicol is occasionally an alternative drug for treating anaerobic bacterial infections.

When used for life-threatening infections, IV administration is usually necessary; oral therapy should be started as soon as possible.

Chloramphenicol topical cream, ophthalmic ointment and solution, and otic solution are used to treat susceptible infections of the skin, eyes, or ears, when less toxic alternatives cannot be used.

The duration of chloramphenicol therapy should not exceed 14 days in most cases, to reduce the risk of adverse effects.

NURSING IMPLICATIONS

Neonates and patients with renal or hepatic disease usually require lower dosages; monitor plasma concentrations closely to avoid overdosage and dose-related toxicity. Dilute IV doses to a concentration of 100 mg/mL of sterile water for injection, and inject them over at least 1 minute. Have patients take oral medication on an empty stomach unless GI upset occurs.

Side Effects, Adverse Reactions, and Contraindications

Chloramphenicol causes fewer minor side effects than most other antibiotics, and allergic reactions such as rashes are uncommon (Table 56–S8). However, chloramphenicol is more likely than any other antibiotic to cause *serious and potentially fatal* adverse responses. Some are dose-related and usually occur when therapy is prolonged or when serum chloramphenicol levels exceed 25 μg/mL. Others may occur regardless of the dose. All these problems provide good reasons why chloramphenicol should never be used unless the patient has a severe infection that cannot be treated with a safer antibiotic.

Hematologic Side Effects

Chloramphenicol causes two types of bone marrow suppression. The most serious blood dyscrasia is *irreversible* and *not dose-related.* In this instance, bone marrow depression leads to pancytopenia (aplastic anemia). Although it occurs rarely (the estimated occurrence is about 1 in 40,000 uses of the drug), the mortality rate is high. This is a prime example of why the drug should not be used for trivial purposes.

Some clinicians avoid oral therapy since aplastic anemia is believed to be caused only by oral administration. However, the manufacturer warns that IV therapy probably also carries this risk. The place of oral chloramphenicol in therapy remains controversial.

Reversible, dose-dependent bone marrow suppression is more common and is especially likely to occur with prolonged chloramphenicol therapy or when blood levels exceed 25 μg/mL. The usual initial manifestation is reticulocytopenia with decreased serum iron-binding capacity, which increases serum iron levels. Reticulocytopenia commonly progresses to anemia, leukopenia, thrombocytopenia, or combinations of these problems.

Regardless of the type of blood dyscrasia, immunosuppression makes the patient susceptible to severe and possibly life-threatening infections. Similarly, all patients who experience decreased platelet numbers are susceptible to potentially serious or fatal bleeding tendencies.

Gray Baby Syndrome

Chloramphenicol can cause a type of circulatory collapse in premature and newborn infants. It is called the *gray baby syndrome* because of the patient's appearance. The greatest risk arises when chloramphenicol therapy is started during the first 48 hours of life. Although less common, it has occurred in children up to 2 years of age, and has also occurred in infants whose mothers received chloramphenicol during late pregnancy or labor.

The syndrome usually develops 2 to 9 days after starting chloramphenicol therapy, presenting with feeding difficulties, abdominal distention, vomiting, pallid cyanosis, circulatory collapse, and respiratory irregularity. It is frequently fatal. The reaction is attributed to the accumulation of toxic drug levels because of an inability of the infant to conjugate chloramphenicol in the liver or excrete the unconjugated drug. Early discontinuation of the drug may completely reverse this reaction.

Other Adverse Reactions

Allergic reactions, presenting as fever, rashes, and skin or mucosal hemorrhage, are very uncommon with chloramphenicol. Nevertheless, chloramphenicol is contraindicated in individuals with known allergy to it. It should be used in patients who have previously experienced severe toxic reactions only when it is essential.

Chloramphenicol can also occasionally cause GI upset and superinfection. Peripheral and optic neuritis have occurred with high-dose, long-term therapy.

NURSING IMPLICATIONS

Monitor plasma concentrations to maintain levels below 25 μg/mL. Question orders calling for therapy that exceeds 14 days. In general, prescriptions for chloramphenicol should not be refillable. Appropriate laboratory monitoring (WBC, reticulocyte counts, RBC and indices, serum iron or iron binding capacity, platelets) should be done before, during, and after therapy. Report significant changes to the physician. Monitor for bleeding, sore throat, oral mucosal lesions, pallor, and lassitude as evidence of bone marrow suppression, and report these to the physician.

While chloramphenicol use in the United States is appropriately restricted to serious infections, it is often available without prescription to international travelers in products such as cold preparations. Question patients being worked up for bone marrow suppression about recent international travel; try to identify any drug products purchased during such travel, since some may contain chloramphenicol.

Assess for allergic reactions and GI complaints and for visual and sensory deficits, especially in patients on high doses for long periods. Report any of these responses to the physician at once.

◆ Use During Pregnancy and Lactation

Chloramphenicol crosses the placenta and is excreted in breast milk. It should be used with extreme caution in pregnancy, near term, and in nursing mothers, to avoid toxic accumulation in the fetus or child.

◆ Use in Children

Recommend plasma monitoring to maintain levels less than 25 μg/mL in neonates and young infants. Base initial dosage on recommendations found in Table 56–C8.

Interactions with Other Drugs

Chloramphenicol inhibits the hepatic metabolism of phenytoin, oral hypoglycemic drugs, and oral anticoagulants. In each case, the potential outcome is an elevated blood level of the interactant, and possibly toxicity, unless the interactant's dose is reduced.

Barbiturates stimulate hepatic metabolism of chloramphenicol, and combined therapy may cause subeffective antibiotic blood levels. If the barbiturate interaction cannot be avoided, the chloramphenicol dose may need to be increased. Clinically significant interactions of chloramphenicol with other drugs are summarized in Table 56–I8.

IX. Miscellaneous Antibiotics

A few clinically useful antibiotics do not belong to a particular class. Dosages and indications, plus a synopsis of other pertinent information, are summarized in Table 56–C9.

Azithromycin

Azithromycin (ZITHROMAX) is an oral azalide antibiotic. It is given once daily for streptococcal pharyngitis and chlamydial cervicitis and urethritis. Gastrointestinal upset is the most frequent adverse effect, occurring much less often than with the structurally similar erythromycins.

Aztreonam

Aztreonam (AZACTAM) is a beta-lactam derivative that differs in structure from other beta-lactams. It is the first drug in the class of antibiotics known as the *monobactams.* It is useful for parenteral treatment of gram-negative–aerobic infections, including penicillinase-producing *H. influenzae;* as well as some *P. aeruginosa* isolates. Adverse effects are similar to those caused by penicillins. A possible advantage of aztreonam could be its use in patients who are allergic to penicillins and cephalosporins, since cross allergenicity is rare. Superinfection caused by gram-positive cocci may occur.

Bacitracin

Bacitracin is an antibiotic with a limited antibacterial spectrum. It is primarily effective against gram-positive organisms. Its use has essentially been replaced by the penicillins and cephalosporins. Bacitracin is used as a topical powder or ointment for superficial skin infections, and as an ophthalmic ointment for eye infections caused by *Staphylococcus*. The primary adverse effect from topical use is local allergic reactions.

Clarithromycin

Clarithromycin (BIAXIN) is an oral macrolide antibiotic similar to erythromycin. It is used for respiratory tract, skin, and soft tissue infections, and may be useful against pathogens such as *Helicobacter pylori,* which may be a cause of peptic ulcer disease and gastritis (Chapter 40), and atypical *Mycobacteria*. Adverse effects, primarily involving gastrointestinal upset, are less frequent than with erythromycin.

Clindamycin

Clindamycin (CLEOCIN) is a lincosamide antibiotic with activity primarily against gram-positive and anaerobic bacteria.

Clindamycin is active when given orally or IV. The absorption of clindamycin from the GI tract is virtually complete. It is distributed to many body tissues, and appears to have a high affinity for bone tissue. Clindamycin does not obtain appreciable levels in the cerebrospinal fluid. The serum half-life is 2 to 3 hours. The drug is metabolized to a great extent by the liver, so doses may need to be reduced in the presence of hepatic impairment.

Clindamycin is very effective in treating infections caused by *Bacteroides* species. Respiratory tract infections (lung abscesses, empyema), pelvic infections, and intraabdominal infections in which anaerobic bacteria are involved respond well to clindamycin. Clindamycin has been used in combination with the aminoglycosides for mixed aerobic–anaerobic infections. Clindamycin may also be used as an alternate to the penicillins for the treatment of various gram-positive infections. It is not often used for this purpose, however, because of the availability of less toxic, less expensive agents, such as erythromycin. Clindamycin is often used in osteomyelitis caused by gram-positive organisms because of its excellent penetration into bone tissue.

Clindamycin phosphate topical gel, lotion, and solution (CLEOCIN T) are used topically for the treatment of acne vulgaris.

The major side effect associated with oral or IV clindamycin use is diarrhea. Pseudomembranous colitis can occur with both the oral and parenteral products, and should be closely watched for. The disorder can occur within a few days after clindamycin therapy is started, or several weeks after completion of therapy. Carefully assess patients for diarrhea, and question them about stool frequency, consistency, and the presence of blood. The drug should be discontinued, if possible, if diarrhea develops; notify the physician.

Clindamycin may cause a generalized rash. Other adverse reactions include transient increases in liver enzymes, thrombophlebitis, and rare bone marrow toxicities.

There are no definite contraindications to using clindamycin. Use extra caution in patients with a history of GI tract disease, especially colitis. Patients with severe renal or hepatic impairment will require reduced dosages.

Imipenem-Cilastatin

Imipenem-cilastatin sodium (PRIMAXIN) is a recently released drug belonging to a new class of antibiotics known as the *carbapenems*. Imipenem possesses the broadest and most potent antibacterial activity of all antibiotics currently available. Its spectrum of activity includes most gram-positive, gram-negative, and anaerobic bacteria.

Imipenem is rapidly excreted in the urine, and can be inactivated by a renal enzyme. For this reason, the drug is combined with the enzyme inhibitor cilastatin, which allows imipenem to attain therapeutic concentrations in the urine. Therapeutic concentrations of imipenem can be found in a variety of tissues, including the cerebrospinal fluid.

Imipenem is useful in the treatment of polymicrobial systemic and urinary tract infections, especially those caused by organisms resistant to the third-generation cephalosporins, the aminoglycosides, and the extended-spectrum penicillins.

Common side effects associated with imipenem use include nausea and vomiting associated with rapid infusion rates or the administration of greater than a 1-g dose. The incidence of diarrhea, allergic reactions, and phlebitis is similar to that with other agents. Recently, considerable concern has been expressed over the apparent increased incidence of myoclonic seizures in patients receiving imipenem. Further study indicates that seizures are more likely to occur in patients with renal impairment in whom the dose of imipenem has not been adjusted, and in patients with a prior history of seizure activity. Renal, hepatic, and hematologic toxicities occur occasionally. A dosage reduction is required only with severe renal impairment.

Mupirocin

Mupirocin (BACTROBAN) is an important antibiotic with only one major use. It is the only antibiotic considered appropriate for topical therapy of impetigo caused by *Staphylococcus aureus,* β-hemolytic *Streptococcus,* and *Strep. pyogenes.* Mupirocin ointment is the only formulation available. Local reactions occasionally occur. Mupirocin's effects during pregnancy or lactation are unknown; it should be used with caution during pregnancy, and breast-feeding should be interrupted temporarily if therapy is required.

Spectinomycin

Spectinomycin hydrochloride (TROBICIN) is active against a wide variety of organisms, but its use is limited to treating infections caused by *N. gonorrhea.* Spectinomycin should be reserved for use in patients who are allergic to penicillins, cephalosporins, and tetracyclines, or for those gonococcal strains that are multiply resistant. Spectinomycin is administered by deep IM injection.

The primary adverse effect of spectinomycin is pain on injection. Rash, pruritus, fever, and vomiting have been occasionally reported.

Vancomycin

Vancomycin hydrochloride (VANCOCIN; VANCOLED) is a bactericidal antibiotic used primarily to treat serious *Staphylococcus* infections. Its use has been steadily increasing with the development of *Staphylococcus* that is resistant to conventional therapy.

Vancomycin is poorly absorbed from the GI tract. Following IV administration—the most common administration route—it is distributed to a wide variety of body tissues. There is some penetration into the cerebrospinal fluid. The serum half-life is approximately 6 hours. The drug is eliminated almost entirely by the kidneys; therefore, doses may need to be decreased in patients with renal impairment.

Vancomycin is used to treat a wide variety of infections caused by susceptible organisms, including those responsible for osteomyelitis, endocarditis, pneumonia, and septicemia. It is considered to be the drug of choice for infections caused by *Staphylococcus* species in patients who have a penicillin and cephalosporin allergy or in whom resistance to the antistaphylococcal penicillins has developed. Vancomycin is also the primary choice for methicillin-resistant *Staph. epidermidis* infections, which frequently cause prosthetic heart valve infections and septicemia in immunocompromised patients. Intravenous vancomycin is used for prophylaxis of bacterial endocarditis in penicillin-allergic patients who undergo dental or selected surgical procedures.

Administer IV vancomycin over at least 1 hour. Dilute the drug in a minimum of 100 mL of fluid, because it can be irritating to the veins. Some other undesirable side effects may occur if the drug is administered faster than over 1 hour (see below). Never give vancomycin by the IM route because of its locally irritating effects.

Because oral vancomycin is not absorbed by the GI tract, it can be administered orally to treat pseudomembranous colitis, caused by *Clostridium difficile* overgrowth, usually resulting from the use of broad-spectrum antibiotics. Vancomycin is available as an oral solution and capsules; the capsules are preferred whenever possible because the solution has an unpleasant taste.

The most serious adverse effects associated with vancomycin use are ototoxicity and nephrotoxicity. These occur most commonly in patients with renal failure, those who receive prolonged therapy, or those receiving other ototoxic or nephrotoxic drugs, such as the aminoglycosides.

Ototoxicity is associated with peak serum levels of greater than 80 μg/mL. Damage to the auditory branch of the eighth cranial nerve may result in partial or complete hearing loss. Patients may experience tinnitus before hearing loss. Nephrotoxicities were commonly associated with impurities found in earlier formulations of the drug. The incidence of nephrotoxic effects has decreased with the development of a more pure product. However, some studies have suggested that nephrotoxicity may occur even with the newer formulation.

Because of vancomycin's ability to cause ototoxicity and nephrotoxicity, use extra caution in patients with renal impairment or previous hearing loss. Frequent blood concentrations and baseline audiometric studies should be performed for high-risk patients.

Rapid IV administration of vancomycin may result in a hypotensive reaction known as the "red neck syndrome." The reaction involves a sudden drop in blood pressure, accompanied by a rash on the face, neck, chest, and upper extremities. Hypotension may be severe. The reaction occurs most often when vancomycin dose is infused in 10 minutes or less. The reaction is seldom seen with infusions of at least 1 hour, but may still occur. If the reaction occurs, the infusion should be stopped immediately. Subsequent doses should be given over 1 or more hours. Antihistamine therapy may need to be administered to alleviate or prevent symptoms.

Other side effects are a throbbing pain in the back and neck muscles, chills, fever, and neutropenia. Allergic reactions occur in 5% to 10% of the patients; the drug is contraindicated in patients with a history of allergy to vancomycin.

SUMMARY OF NURSING IMPLICATIONS

◆ Assessment

Determine and document in detail previous history of allergic reactions or side effects.

Review current drug regimen for possible interactants with antibiotics.

Establish baseline physical assessment data (vital signs, clinical signs and symptoms, laboratory data) to determine consequences and effectiveness of drug therapy.

Identify contraindications to drug therapy from patient's past history and present clinical condition.

◆ Nursing Diagnoses

Knowledge deficit related to administration and management of prescribed drug therapy.

Diarrhea related to adverse drug effects.

Altered nutrition: less than body requirements related to gastrointestinal distress from medication.

Ineffective breathing pattern: wheezing related to allergic drug reaction.

High risk for impaired skin integrity related to rash, itching from antibiotic therapy.

Altered tissue perfusion related to clotting and blood dyscrasia from adverse drug effects.

High risk for injury related to superinfection secondary to adverse drug effects.

Sensory/perceptual alterations: auditory (ototoxicity) related to adverse drug effect.

Fluid volume excess related to nephrotoxic drug effects (decreased renal function).

Noncompliance related to unpleasant drug side effects.

◆ Planning/Implementation for Penicillins

Observe patient for at least 30 minutes after administration of the first dose of parenteral penicillin; have emergency resuscitation equipment available.

Report any reaction occurring with oral medication immediately.

Use careful technique in the preparation and administration since penicillins may cause sensitivity reactions through personal contact; avoid handling if hypersensitivity is known.

Monitor for and report GI upset and diarrhea.

Consult individual product information on administering with food (eg, penicillinase-resistant penicillin should not be given with food).

Give IM injections into large muscle masses and rotate injection sites to reduce pain; mix with local anesthetic such as lidocaine to reduce irritation if possible.

Give IV penicillin over at least 30 minutes; a slow rate and reduced dosage are indicated if renal impairment is present, in neonates, and in the elderly.

Observe for and report neurologic changes in patients with renal impairment.

Observe for and report adverse effects: bleeding, infections, sore throat, fever, hematuria, oliguria, increased BUN and creatinine levels, hyperkalemia, and hypernatremia.

If patient is receiving treatment for syphilis, provide symptomatic care and reassurance during first 24 hours after initiating therapy; drug response (fever, hypertension, diaphoresis, chills, myalgia, arthralgia, tachycardia, and lethargy) does not constitute allergic reaction.

Maintain adequate hydration and urinary output when administering penicillin for urinary tract infections.

Observe for treatment failure due to drug–drug interaction: tetracycline interferes with the activity of penicillin; admixing penicillin with aminoglycoside injection will inactivate aminoglycoside.

Probenecid decreases renal clearance of most penicillins; may be used concurrently to enhance effectiveness of penicillin.

Concurrent administration of antifungal agents may be necessary to combat overgrowth of *Candida* in the mouth, vagina, or on the skin, especially in immunocompromised patients.

◆ Patient and Family Teaching with Penicillins

Teach the patient/family:

To report rash, fever, arthralgias, signs of anemia or hepatitis, respiratory difficulty, nausea, vomiting, diaphoresis indicating hypersensitivity; discontinue therapy if allergy occurs.

About the possible development of a nonallergic rash that occurs within 3 days when taking aminopenicillins; does not indicate allergy to any medication.

About foods high in potassium to assist with diet needs if hyperkalemia present; provide list.

◆ Planning/Implementation with Cephalosporins

Observe patient for at least 30 minutes after administration of the first dose of parenteral cephalosporin; have emergency resuscitation equipment available.

Use care in preparing medication; sensitivity reactions can occur through personal contact; avoid handling if hypersensitivity is known.

Monitor for GI upset, diarrhea, and, less frequently, pseudomembranous colitis, particularly with oral cephalosporins.

Administer with food to reduce GI upset if necessary.

Give IM injections into large muscle masses and rotate sites to minimize pain; with excessive pain lidocaine may be indicated.

Give IV infusions over 30 minutes to reduce incidence of phlebitis or thrombophlebitis; report if symptoms of irritation occur.

Be certain dose ordered is appropriate for patient's renal status; elderly, neonates, and those with known renal impairment require dosage adjustment.

Monitor AST, ALT, alkaline phosphatase, and bilirubin for transient increases; report to physician; elevations are usually mild and reversible.

Recognize signs of vitamin K deficiency, particularly in elderly, debilitated, or malnourished patients or patients with severe renal impairment.

Maintain adequate hydration when receiving drug for a urinary tract infection; monitor renal function closely if patient is receiving cephalosporin and another known nephrotoxic agent (eg, aminoglycosides).

Be aware that false-positive test results may occur with indirect and direct Coombs' and urine glucose tests; test blood glucose if possible; report to physician suspected false-positive results.

◆ Patient and Family Teaching with Cephalosporins

Teach the patient/family:

To avoid alcohol ingestion; disulfiram-like reactions (flushing, tachycardia, nausea, headache) may occur with cefamandole and cefoperazone.

To report immediately any reaction occurring with oral medication (rash, fever, arthralgias, respiratory difficulty, nausea, vomiting, diaphoresis).

◆ Planning/Implementation with Aminoglycosides

Maintain hydration to reduce risk of ototoxicity and nephrotoxicity.

Observe for rash or anaphylactic reactions; report immediately and withhold additional doses.

Unless otherwise instructed, draw peak level blood samples 30 minutes after completion of infusion; record time of infusion and blood draw.

Monitor for fluid retention or oliguria, increasing serum creatinine and BUN, proteinuria, urinary casts, decreased creatinine clearance; report to physician; nephrotoxicity is usually reversible upon discontinuation of drug.

Report complaints of hearing, auditory (tinnitus, roaring sounds), or vestibular (dizziness, ataxia, nystagmus) deficits to the physician; early changes may be reversible; may develop following discontinuation of therapy.

Expect a laxative effect, usually with oral therapy, but severe diarrhea is undesirable and may indicate superinfection, and should be reported.

Avoid excessive dosage of oral and topical aminoglycosides to reduce risk of systemic absorption and toxicity.

Withhold medication and notify physician if local irritation or rash occurs.

Wear gloves if possible when applying topical preparations.

Observe for hypoventilation or apnea if high doses are being given; support ventilation as required.

Do not mix parenteral aminoglycosides with other drugs.

◆ Patient and Family Teaching with Aminoglycosides

Teach the patient/family:

To avoid excessive exposure to sunlight, since topical application may cause photosensitivity reactions.

◆ Planning/Implementation with Tetracyclines

Notify physician if rash develops; withhold further medication pending assessment.

Avoid administration with milk or other foods high in calcium or iron, and with antacids, which impair absorption; give tetracycline 1 hour before or 2 hours after interacting medications or meals whenever possible; may give with small amounts of food (low in calcium) if nausea and abdominal distress occur.

Observe for and report evidence of superinfection (eg, tongue discoloration, candidal infections, or diarrhea).

Monitor for and report signs of renal toxicity (elevated BUN or creatinine or changes in urine output).

Observe for and report signs of hepatic toxicity; lightheadedness, dizziness, vertigo, and fatigue.

Give IM injections into large muscle masses; rotate injection sites.

Monitor closely for potentiation of anticoagulant effects when given with tetracycline; report bleeding.

Be aware that anticonvulsants may decrease levels of doxycycline; another tetracycline may be indicated.

◆ Patient and Family Teaching with Tetracyclines

Teach the patient/family:

To practice meticulous hygiene of skin, mouth, and perianal area.

To be aware of the possibility of changes in nail growth or coloration during therapy.

To avoid sun exposure, especially with demeclocycline, since phototoxic reactions can occur.

◆ Planning/Implementation with Erythromycins

Monitor for and report: significant evidence of hepatic dysfunction; changes in mental function; hearing loss.

Dilute IV preparations according to manufacturer's recommendations; give slowly into a large vein; observe closely for phlebitis; sites may need to be changed frequently; switch to oral preparations as soon as possible.

Do not give erythromycin IM because of severe tissue irritation.

Monitor for increased effects from digoxin, theophylline, carbamazepine, warfarin, triazolam, or cyclosporine if given with erythromycin.

◆ Patient and Family Teaching with Erythromycins

Teach the patient/family:

To give enteric-coated oral tablets and capsules with meals to reduce GI upset.

Report any reaction occurring with oral medication.

◆ Planning/Implementation with Sulfonamides

Observe IV sites for phlebitis, especially when giving co-trimoxazole; dilute drug in 75–125 mL of fluid and infuse over at least 60 minutes.

If giving oral anticoagulants and a sulfonamide concurrently, observe for the sudden appearance of bruising or blood in the urine or stool; the anticoagulant dose should be reduced; monitor coagulation test results.

Assess patients taking oral hypoglycemics concurrently for hypoglycemia; anticipate dosage reduction; monitor blood glucose levels closely.

◆ Patient/Family Teaching with Sulfonamides

Teach the patient/family:

Not to miss a dose or several doses; to take missed doses as soon as they remember; to schedule drug administration at a time that is easy to remember, such as bedtime or mealtime.

To take drug with at least a full glass of water to prevent the development of crystalluria; maintain at least 1.5 L daily water intake.

◆ Planning/Implementation with Quinolones

Give drug orally or IV; do not exceed maximum dosages.

Maintain hydration to prevent crystalluria.

Monitor for side effects (nausea, headache, rash); particularly observe elderly.

◆ Patient/Family Teaching with Quinolones

Teach the patient/family:

To drink sufficient fluids (6–8 glasses) daily.

To avoid excessive caffeine ingestion as it may result in CNS stimulation.

To minimize exposure to sunlight, which causes skin reactions.

To return for follow-up blood tests to assess liver, kidney, and bone marrow status.

◆ Planning/Implementation with Chloramphenicol

Maintain peak plasma levels of 25 μg/mL or less to reduce risk of toxicity.

Reduce dosage in neonates and young infants because hepatic drug clearance is reduced; observe for signs of gray baby syndrome (poor feeding, abdominal distention, pallid cyanosis, irregular respirations, hypotension); report immediately.

Question orders calling for prolonged therapy of more than 14 days at high dosages, because of increased risk of bone marrow suppression (presents as reticulocytopenia and anemia).

Monitor for bleeding, sore throat, mucosal lesions, pallor, or lassitude; report immediately.

Recognize visual deficits, peripheral numbness, nausea, vomiting, or enterocolitis as potential adverse reactions.

When giving concurrently with barbiturates, oral sulfonylurea hypoglycemics, phenytoin, or dicoumarol, monitor for decreased or increased drug effects.

Avoid prolonged topical, otic, and ophthalmic therapy to reduce risk of absorption and systemic toxicities, including bone marrow suppression.

◆ Patient/Family Teaching with Chloramphenicol

Teach the patient/family:

To monitor for and report bleeding, sore throat, lassitude.

To take only amount prescribed and for time prescribed.

◆ Planning/Implementation with Vancomycin

Administer IV in minimum of 100 mL solution over at least 1 hour; never give IM.

Observe for hypotensive reaction (red neck syndrome) with rapid infusion; administer over longer period (2–3 hours) if this occurs.

Use capsules when possible when drug is given orally to eliminate unpleasant taste.

Monitor for signs of ototoxicity (tinnitus, hearing loss) and nephrotoxicity (oliguria); establish baseline blood values and audiometric studies.

Observe for allergic reactions (rash, chills, itching); have antihistamine available.

◆ Patient/Family Teaching with Vancomycin

Teach the patient/family:

To report any change in hearing or kidney function, hematuria.

To take adequate fluids (2000 mL) daily to prevent kidney damage.

◆ Evaluation

The patient/family will:

Experience a reduction in or complete loss of symptoms of infection; maintain vital signs, laboratory data within normal limits.

Tolerate drug therapy with minimal side effects (eg, gastric distress controlled and subsides).

Show no signs of toxic effects; hearing and renal function within normal parameters; no respiratory difficulty.

Take medication until gone or otherwise advised by physician to prevent reinfection.

Comply with drug regimen (eg, proper dose, frequency, method of administration, and storage of medication).

Return for follow-up examinations and laboratory testing (urine, blood chemistry) as indicated.

Wear medication allergy identification tag if advised.

Annotated Bibliography

Anti-infective agents. In: AHFS Drug Information 92. *American Hospital Formulary Service.* Bethesda, MD, American Society of Hospital Pharmacists, 1992. *This is an unreferenced but concise, objective review of the antiinfective agents reviewed in this chapter; a very valuable resource. Updated annually.*

Bennett WM: Guide to drug dosage in renal failure. *Clin Pharamcokinet* 1988;15:326–354. *A well-referenced tabulation of the effects of renal disease on drug dosing; discusses many drugs other than antibiotics as well.*

Dajani AS, Bisno AL, Chung KJ, et al: Prevention of bacterial endocarditis. Recommendations by the American Heart Association. *JAMA* 1990;264:2919–2922. *Recommended regimens of prevention of bacterial endocarditis.*

Sexually transmitted diseases treatment guidelines 1989. *MMWR* 1989; 38(5–8):1–42. *Guidelines for treatment of sexually transmitted diseases.*

Walsh ML, Johnson CC: Update on antimicrobial agents. *Nurs Clin North Am* 1991;26:341–360. *Reviews trends in antimicrobial therapy and their impact on nursing practice.*

Zaske D: Aminoglycosides. In: Evans WE, Schentag, JJ, Jusko WJ, eds. *Applied Pharmacokinetics.* Second ed. Spokane, WA: Applied Therapeutics, 1986:331–381. *A referenced, comprehensive discussion of factors related to aminoglycoside toxicity and to therapeutic drug monitoring for these antibiotics.*

Table 56–C1 | **Clinical Uses and Administration of Penicillins**

AGENT	CLINICAL USES	DOSAGE AND ROUTE OF ADMINISTRATION
	Natural Penicillins	
PROTOTYPE		
Penicillin G		
(PFIZERPEN)	Systemic infections caused by susceptible gram-positive, nonpenicillinase-producing cocci; *Meningococcus;* some anaerobes; and in treating syphilis	IM and IV: Adults, children >12 years: 5–40 million U/d in 4–6 equal divided doses. Children 1 month –12 years: 25,000–400,000 U/kg/d in 4–6 equal divided doses. Infants < 1 month: 50,000–250,000 U/kg/d in 2–6 equal divided doses depending on weight, age, and severity of disease. *Note:* Usual IM dosage schedule in neonates is q8–12h Always infuse IV doses over 1–2 h; give IM injections into large muscle masses, rotate sites
RELATED DRUGS		
Penicillin G benzathine		
(BICILLIN L-A; PERMAPEN)	Susceptible gram-positive infections such as *Streptococcus*	IM: Adults: 1.2 million U. Infants, children <27 kg (60 lbs): 300,000–600,000 U, given once. Older children: 900,000 U
	Rheumatic fever prophylaxis	IM: 1.2 million U once monthly or 600,000 U every 2 weeks Inject deep into large muscle mass; avoid intravascular injection; do not massage injection site
Penicillin G procaine		
(CRYSTACILLIN; PFIZERPEN-AS; WYCILLIN)	Systemic infections caused by susceptible gram-positive bacteria	IM: Adults: 0.6–1.2 million U/d in 1 or 2 doses. Children: 25,000–50,000 U/kg/d as a single dose (not to exceed recommended adult maximum)
	Syphilis	IM: 600,000 U qd for 8 d (15 d if late or latent). Neurosyphilis may require 2.4 million U/d for 10–14 d with probenecid 500 mg q6h. Congenital: 50,000 U/kg/qd for at least 10 d (maximum dose 600,000 U/d) Do not give IV; inject deep into large muscle mass; avoid intravascular administration; do not massage injection site
Penicillin V, Penicillin VK		
("Phenoxymethyl penicillin," BEEPEN VK; BETAPEN VK; LEDERCILLIN VK; PEN V; PEN-VEE K; ROBICILLIN VK; SK-PENICILLIN VK; V-CILLIN K; VEETIDS; generic products)	Infections caused by susceptible gram-positive bacteria	Oral: Adults and children >12 years: 125–250 mg (200,000–400,000 U) q6h–q8h or 500 mg (800,000 U) bid–tid. Children <12 years: 15–56 mg (25,000–90,000 U)/kg/d in 3–6 divided doses
	Rheumatic fever prophylaxis	Oral: 250 mg bid
	Prophylaxis of pneumococcal infections	Oral: Adults and children >5 years: 250 mg bid. Children <5 years: 125 mg bid

(continued)

Table 56–C1 **Clinical Uses and Administration of Penicillins (*Continued*)**

AGENT	CLINICAL USES	DOSAGE AND ROUTE OF ADMINISTRATION
Penicillinase-Resistant Penicillins		
PROTOTYPE		
Methicillin sodium (STAPHCILLIN)	Suspected or proven infections caused by penicillinase-producing *Staph. aureus* or *epidermidis* and for surgical prophylaxis for these organisms	IM and IV: Adults: 4–12 g/d in 4–6 equal divided doses. Children >1 month: 100–300 mg/kg/d in 4–6 equal divided doses. Children <1 month: 25–50 mg/kg/q8h–q12h during first 2 weeks, q6h–q8h during weeks 2–4. Administer IV doses over 30 min and IM doses into large muscle masses, rotating sites
RELATED DRUGS		
Cloxacillin sodium (CLOXAPEN; TEGOPEN)	Suspected or proven infections caused by penicillinase-producing *Staph. aureus* or *epidermidis*	Oral: Adults and children >20 kg: 1–4 g/d in 4 equal divided doses. Children <20 kg: 50–100 mg/kg/d (sometimes more) in 4 equal divided doses (maximum 4 g/d) on empty stomach
Dicloxacillin sodium (DYCILL; DYNAPEN; PATHOCIL)	Same as cloxacillin	Oral: Adults and children >40 kg: 1–2 g/d in 4 equal divided doses. Children <40 kg: 12.5–100 mg/kg/d in 4 equal divided doses. Administer on empty stomach
Nafcillin sodium (NAFCIL; NALLPEN; UNIPEN)	Same as methicillin	IM and IV: Adults: 2–12 g/d in 4–6 equal divided doses. Children >1 month: 50–200 mg/kg/d in 4–6 equal divided doses. Children <1 month: neonatal doses of 50 mg/kg/d in 2 equal divided doses are suggested; >7 days of age, up to 200 mg/kg/d in 3 equal divided doses is suggested. Administer IV doses over 1 hr, IM doses into large muscle masses, rotating sites
Oxacillin sodium (BACTOCILL; PROSTAPHLIN)	Same as methicillin	Oral: Adults, children >40 kg: 2–6 g/d in 4–6 equal divided doses. Children <40 kg: 50–100 mg/kg/d in 4–6 equal divided doses IM and IV: Adults, children >40 kg: 1–12 g/d in 4–6 equal divided doses. Children <40 kg: 50–200 mg/kg/d in 4–6 equal divided doses. Children <1 month: 25–50 mg/kg q8h–q12h if <7 days old, q6h–q8h 7–28 days old. Administer IV over ≥30 min, IM into large muscle masses, rotating sites; administer oral doses on empty stomach

(continued)

Table 56–C1 Clinical Uses and Administration of Penicillins (*Continued*)

AGENT	CLINICAL USES	DOSAGE AND ROUTE OF ADMINISTRATION
Aminopenicillins		
PROTOTYPE		
Ampicillin, ampicillin trihydrate (D-AMP; OMNIPEN; POLYCILLIN; PRINCIPEN; TOTACILLIN)	Systemic and urinary tract infections caused by susceptible *Listeria, Salmonella, Shigella, E. coli, H. influenzae, N. gonorrhoeae, Proteus mirabilis,* and enterococci; penicillin is preferred for sensitive gram-positive organisms	Oral: Adults and children >20 kg: 1–4 g/d in 4 equal divided doses. Children <20 kg: 25–100 mg/kg/d in 4 equal divided doses IM and IV: Adults and children >40 kg: 1–12 g/d in 4–8 equal divided doses. Children <40 kg: 25–400 mg/kg/d in 4–8 equal divided doses (maximum daily dose is 12 g). Children <1 month: 50–300 mg/kg/d in 2–4 equal divided doses, based on age
	Subacute bacterial endocarditis prophylaxis	Oral, IM, and IV: Consult current American Heart Association guidelines (subject to frequent change) Administer IV over at least 30 min, IM into large muscle masses, rotating sites; give orally on empty stomach. IV doses must be further diluted or administered within 1 h of reconstitution
RELATED DRUGS		
Amoxicillin trihydrate (AMOXIL; BIOMOX; POLYMOX; TRIMOX; WYMOX)	Systemic and urinary tract infections caused by ampicillin-susceptible organisms, except *Shigella*	Oral: Adults, children >20 kg: 250–500 mg q8h. Children <20 kg: 20–40 mg/kg/d in 3 equal divided doses
	Prophylaxis of subacute bacterial endocarditis	Oral: Consult current American Heart Association guidelines (subject to frequent change) Administer with food to reduce GI upset
Amoxicillin trihydrate and clavulanate potassium (AUGMENTIN)	Systemic and urinary tract infections caused by susceptible beta-lactamase–producing organisms such as *Branhamella catarrhalis, E. coli, H. influenzae, Klebsiella,* and *Staph. aureus*	Oral: Adults, children >40 kg: 250–500 mg amoxicillin content q8h. Children <40 kg: 20–40 mg amoxicillin content/kg/d in 3 equal divided doses. Administer with meals to decrease GI upset. All products except 250-mg (nonchewable) tablets have 4 : 1 amoxicillin:clavulanate ratio; 250 mg tablets are 2 : 1. 250-mg nonchewable tablets cannot be used interchangeably with other products
Ampicillin sodium and sulbactam sodium (UNASYN)	Systemic infections caused by susceptible β-lactamase–producing organisms such as *E. coli, Klebsiella, Enterobacter, Bacteroides,* and *Staph. aureus*	IM and IV: Adults, children >12 years: 1.5 (1 g ampicillin and 0.5 g sulbactam)–3 g q6h. No approved pediatric dose
Bacampicillin hydrochloride (SPECTROBID)	Systemic and urinary tract infections where oral ampicillin therapy is appropriate	Oral: Adults, children >25 kg: 400 mg–1.6 g q12h. Children <25 kg: 12.5–25 mg/kg q12h

(continued)

Table 56–C1 **Clinical Uses and Administration of Penicillins (*Continued*)**

AGENT	CLINICAL USES	DOSAGE AND ROUTE OF ADMINISTRATION
	Extended-Spectrum Penicillins	
PROTOTYPE		
Ticarcillin disodium (TICAR)	Systemic infections caused by susceptible gram-negative aerobic bacilli (*P. aeruginosa, Proteus mirabilis, E. coli*)	IM and IV: Adults, children >1 month: 50–300 mg/kg/d in 3–6 equal divided doses. Neonates under 2 kg: 75 mg/kg q12h, increasing to q8h when 7 days old. Neonates over 2 kg: 75 mg/kg q8h, increasing to 100 mg/kg q8h when 7 days old Give IV over at least 30 min. Give IM into large muscle masses, rotate sites; add lidocaine if needed
RELATED DRUGS		
Azlocillin sodium (AZLIN)	Same as ticarcillin	IV: Adults: 100–350 mg/kg/d in 4–6 equal divided doses (maximum 24 g/d). Children: 300–450 mg/kg/d in 4–6 equal divided doses (maximum 24 g/d). Administer by injection over 5 min or infuse over 30 min
Carbenicillin indanyl sodium (GEOCILLIN)	Urinary tract infections caused by susceptible gram-negative aerobic bacilli	Oral: Adults: 382–764 mg 4 times daily
Mezlocillin sodium (MEZLIN)	Same as ticarcillin	IM and IV: Adults, children >12 years: 100–350 mg/kg/d in 4–6 equal divided doses (maximum 24 g/d). Children >1 month: 50 mg/kg q4h. Children <1 month: 75 mg/kg q12h if <7 days, 75 mg/kg q8h (under 2 kg) or q6h (over 2 kg) if >7 days. Give IV doses over 3–5 min by injectionor 30 min by infusion; give IM doses into large muscle masses, rotate sites; add lidocaine if needed
Piperacillin sodium (PIPRACIL)	Same as ticarcillin	IM and IV: Adults: 100–400 mg/kg/d in 4–6 equal divided doses (maximum 24 g/d). Children <12 years: Dosage not established; 75–300 mg/kg/d in children over 1 month is suggested. Doses for cystic fibrosis may be higher. Give IV over 3–5 min by injection or 30 min by infusion; give IM doses into large muscle masses, rotate sites; add lidocaine if needed
Ticarcillin disodium/clavulanate potassium (TIMENTIN)	Systemic and urinary tract infections caused by susceptible beta-lactamase–producing organisms such as *Staph, aureus, Citrobacter, Enterobacter, E. coli, H. influenzae, Klebsiella, Pseudomonas,* and *Serratia*	IV: Adults >60 kg: 3.1 g q4h–q8h. Adults and children >12 years weighing <60 kg: 200–300 mg ticarcillin equivalent/kg/d q4h–q6h. Infuse over 30 min

Table 56–S1 **Major Side Effects of and Contraindications for Penicillins**

BODY SYSTEM/ Side Effect	CONTRAINDICATION/ PRECAUTION	COMMENTS AND NURSING IMPLICATIONS
CENTRAL NERVOUS SYSTEM Irritability; delirium, confusion, seizures		Most common at high doses, especially in presence of renal impairment; monitor closely, and adjust dose for renal impairment; seizures often unresponsive to anticonvulsants; avoid intrathecal, intraventricular injections
BLOOD Leukopenia, thrombocytopenia, impaired coagulation; neutropenia or agranulocytosis with penicillinase-resistant penicillins (see also immune system)		Monitor for, report anemia, infection, leukopenia, bleeding; bleeding most often associated with extended-spectrum penicillins, occasionally with high-dose penicillin G
Transient, asymptomatic elevation of alkaline phosphatase, ALT, AST with penicillinase-resistant penicillins		Hepatitis-like reaction possible with parenteral oxacillin; monitor for and report hepatic enzyme elevation in patients receiving penicillinase-resistant penicillins, especially oxacillin
GASTROINTESTINAL Nausea, vomiting, epigastric distress, diarrhea, pseudomembranous colitis, glossitis, stomatitis		Monitor for, report gastric distress, diarrhea, sore mouth; especially seen with oral administration; pesudomembranous colitis may occur with broad-spectrum agents (eg, ampicillin)
RENAL Acute interstitial nephritis; hyperkalemia with potassium salts; hypernatremia, sometimes with hypokalemia and alkalosis, with sodium salts		Interstitial nephritis most often associated with methicillin, oxacillin, sometimes other penicillins given at high doses over long time; assess for, report fever, proteinuria, hematuria, or lab evidence of eosinophilia or eosinophiluria; discontinue the antibiotic; be aware that structurally similar antibiotics may cause the same reaction if substituted (eg, in methicillin-induced nephritis, switching to oxacillin may continue reaction). Assess for, report hyperkalemia when administering potassium salts (eg, penicillin G potassium), especially in renal disease, or hypernatremia with sodium salts (eg, ticarcillin disodium, oxacillin sodium). Hypernatremia may worsen congestive heart failure

(continued)

Table 56–S1 | Major Side Effects of and Contraindications for Penicillins (*Continued*)

BODY SYSTEM/ Side Effect	CONTRAINDICATION/ PRECAUTION	COMMENTS AND NURSING IMPLICATIONS
IMMUNE Hypersensitivity reactions; rashes (urticarial, erythematous, morbilliform), fever, chills, eosinophilia, Coombs'-positive hemolytic anemia; serum sickness–like reactions; anaphylaxis; hepatitis (hypersensitivity reaction to carbenicillin, oxacillin)	Known hypersensitivity to any penicillin	Monitor for and immediately report rash, fever, muscle or joint complaints, respiratory difficulty; observe patients for 30 minutes following parenteral doses; have emergency supplies immediately available; skin testing for suspected allergy can be done but yields frequent false-negatives; desensitization may be required in allergic individuals who must receive penicillin; do not miss doses in desensitized patients; desensitization offers protection only during the immediate course of therapy. Use caution in handling penicillins, avoid handling if severely hypersensitive or truly allergic. Ampicillin and derivatives sometimes cause morbilliform or maculopapular rash, usually 3–14 days after start of therapy, especially in patients with infectious mononucleosus or cytomegalovirus infections; this does not indicate allergy, will often subside with continued therapy; observe for and report evidence of hepatitis in patients receiving oxacillin
LOCAL Pain on IM injection, sterile abscesses; phlebitis, thrombophlebitis with IV administration; superinfection (especially with extended-spectrum penicillins)		See text and Table 56–S1 for proper injection, infusion guidelines; assess for pain, etc; assess for, report evidence of superinfection, especially when using extended-spectrum penicillins
OTHER Jarisch–Herxheimer reaction in patients treated with penicillin for spirochetal infections, usually syphilis		Reaction common, usually within 12 hr after first dose, subsiding within 24 hr: headache, fever, hypertension, lethargy, muscle and joint pain, tachycardia; report severe reactions to the physician

Table 56–I1 | Major Interactions Between Penicillins and Other Agents

AGENT	RESULT OF INTERACTION	COMMENTS AND NURSING IMPLICATIONS
Aminoglycosides	Decreased aminoglycoside levels	Extended-spectrum penicillins slowly inactivate aminoglycosides; avoid physically admixing in IV solutions; monitor aminoglycoside plasma levels, adjust aminoglycoside dose or dosage interval as required; follow laboratory-recommended procedures for handling samples for aminoglycoside level determinations with combined therapy
Tetracyclines	Penicillins can be antagonized by concomitant administration of bacteriostatic antibiotics such as tetracyclines, leading to potential treatment failure	Adequate doses of each agent should be used, start penicillins prior to tetracyclines; and observe the patient for failure of therapy. When possible, based on bacterial sensitivity results, only one drug (preferably the penicillin) should be continued long-term.

Table 56–C2 Clinical Uses and Administration of Cephalosporins

AGENT	CLINICAL USES	DOSAGE AND ROUTE OF ADMINISTRATION*
	First-Generation Cephalosporins	
PROTOTYPE		
Cefazolin sodium (ANCEF; KEFZOL; ZOLICEF)	Infections caused by susceptible gram-positive cocci, including *Staph. aureus* and *epidermidis,* group A and B streptococci, and pneumococcus and for some *E. coli, Klebsiella pneumoniae,* and *Proteus mirabilis* infections involving the respiratory, biliary, or urinary tract, skin, bone, and joints, and in septicemia or serious intraabdominal infection; also used in surgical prophylaxis	IM and IV: Adults: 250 mg–1.5 g q6h–q12h (usually given q8h). Children >1 month: 25–100 mg/kg/d in 3 or 4 equal divided doses (up to maximum adult dose)
RELATED DRUGS		
Cefadroxil (DURICEF; ULTRACEF)	Urinary tract, skin, and soft tissue infections caused by susceptible organisms (see cefazolin)	Oral: Adults: 1–2 g/d in 1 or 2 doses. Children: 30 mg/kg/d in 1 or 2 doses (up to adult maximum dose)
Cephalexin (KEFLEX; KEFLET)	Same as cefadroxil	Oral: Adults: 1–4 g/d in 2–4 equal divided doses. Children: 25–100 mg/kg/d in 2–4 equal divided doses (up to maximum adult dose)
Cephalothin sodium (KEFLIN)	Same as cefazolin, but not recommended for biliary tract infections	IM and IV: Adults: 2–12 g/d in 4–6 equal divided doses. Children: 80–160 mg/kg/d in 4–6 equal divided doses
Cephapirin sodium (CEFADYL)	Same as cephalothin	IM and IV: Adults: 2–12 g/d in 4–6 equal divided doses. Children >3 months: 40–80 mg/kg/d in 4 equal divided doses
Cephradine (ANSPOR; VELOSEF)	Same oral uses as cefadroxil, parenteral uses as for cephalothin	Oral: Adults: 1–4 g/d in 2–4 equal divided doses. Children >9 months: 25–100 mg/kg/d in 2–4 equal divided doses (up to adult maximum dose) IM and IV: Adults: 2–8 g/d in 4 equal divided doses. Children >1 year: 50–100 mg/kg/d in 4 equal divided doses (up to adult maximum dose)

(continued)

*Renal impairment may require reduced cephalosporin doses or prolonged dosage intervals. Except where noted, administer IV doses as 3- to 5-minute injections or infuse over about 30 minutes. Administer IM injections deep into a large muscle mass, rotating sites to reduce pain. Administer oral doses with meals if necessary to reduce GI distress.

Table 56–C2 Clinical Uses and Administration of Cephalosporins (*Continued*)

AGENT	CLINICAL USES	DOSAGE AND ROUTE OF ADMINISTRATION*
Second-Generation Cephalosporins		
PROTOTYPE		
Cefoxitin (MEFOXIN)	Infections caused by susceptible gram-positive and gram-negative bacteria and anaerobes. Major clinical uses are in *Bacteroides fragilis, N. gonorrhoeae, H. influenzae, E. coli, Klebsiella,* and *Proteus* infections of respiratory, biliary, and urinary tracts and in septicemia and intraabdominal, pelvic, skin, and soft tissue infections caused by these organisms. Also used for anaerobe prophylaxis in abdominal or pelvic surgery	IM and IV: Adults: 3–12 g/d in 3 or 4 equal divided doses. Children > 3 months: 80–160 mg/kg/d in 4–6 equal divided doses (up to 12 g/d). Add lidocaine to IM injections, if necessary, to reduce pain
	Gonorrhea	IM: 2 g once, with 1 g oral probenecid
RELATED DRUGS		
Cefaclor (CECLOR)	Infections caused by susceptible gram-positive and gram-negative bacteria; major clinical use is in soft tissue infections where *H. influenzae* and gram-positive cocci are common pathogens	Oral: Adults: 750 mg–1.5 g/d in 2 or 3 equal divided doses. Children >1 month: 20–40 mg/kg/d in 2 or 3 equal divided doses (maximum 1 g/d)
Cefamandole naftate (MANDOL)	Infections caused by susceptible gram-positive and gram-negative bacteria, especially *Enterobacter* and *H. influenzae*	IM and IV: Adults: 1.5–12 g/d in 3–6 equal divided doses. Children >1 month: 50–150 mg/kg/d in 3–6 equal divided doses
Cefmetazole sodium (ZEFAZONE)	Same as cefoxitin	IM and IV: Adults: 4–8 g/d in 2–4 equal divided doses
Cefonicid sodium (MONOCID)	Same as cefoxitin (except *not* approved for gonorrhea or anaerobe coverage)	IM and IV: Adults: 500 mg–2 g qd. No approved pediatric dose
Ceforanide (PRECEF)	Same as cefoxitin (except *not* approved for gonorrhea or anaerobe coverage, may be less active against *H. influenzae*)	IM and IV: Adults: 0.5–1 g q12h. Children >1 year: 20–40 mg/kg/d in 2 equal divided doses

(continued)

Table 56–C2 | **Clinical Uses and Administration of Cephalosporins (*Continued*)**

AGENT	CLINICAL USES	DOSAGE AND ROUTE OF ADMINISTRATION*
Cefotetan disodium (CEFOTAN)	Same as cefoxitin (except less gram-positive bacterial coverage, more active against Enterobacteriaceae)	IM and IV: Adults: 1–6 g/d in 1 dose or 2 equal divided doses. Children: Dosage not established (40–60 mg/kg/d in 2 equal divided doses is suggested). Add lidocaine to IM injections, if necessary, to reduce pain
Cefuroxime sodium (CEFTIN, ZINACEF)	Same as cefamandole but more active against *N. gonorrhoeae, N. meningitidis,* and some *Enterobacter, E. coli,* and *Klebsiella*	IM and IV: Adults: 750 mg–1.5 g q6h–q8h. Children >3 months: 50–240 mg/kg/d in 3 or 4 equal divided doses
	Uncomplicated gonorrhea	IM: 1.5 g once, with 1 g oral probenecid
	Urinary tract infections caused by *E. coli* or *K. pneumoniae* and other uses same as for cefaclor	Oral: Adults, children >12 years: 125–500 mg q12h. Children <12 years: 125–250 mg q12h
Third-Generation Cephalosporins		
PROTOTYPE		
Cefotaxime sodium (CLAFORAN)	Serious systemic, urinary tract, and skin infections caused by susceptible gram-positive and gram-negative bacteria, including some anaerobes; especially useful in *Enterobacter* infections; meningitis in newborns and children.	IM and IV: Adults, children >50 kg: 3–12 g/d in 2–6 equal divided doses (usually 4). Children >1 month, <50 kg: 50–180 mg/kg/d in 4–6 equal divided doses (maximum 12 g/d). Neonates: 50 mg/kg q12h (0–7 days old) or q8h (1–4 weeks old)
	Uncomplicated gonorrhea	IM: 1 g once
RELATED DRUGS		
Cefixime (SUPRAX)	Same as cefaclor, except no *Staphylococcal* coverage	Oral: Adults, children >50 kg or 12 years: 400 mg/d in 1–2 doses. Children 6 months–12 years: 8 mg/kg/d in 1 or 2 doses
Cefoperazone sodium (CEFOBID)	Serious systemic, urinary tract, and skin infections with spectrum similar to cefotaxime but greater *Pseudomonas* coverage, less coverage of other enteric gram-negative bacilli; not approved for meningitis	IM and IV: Adults, children >12 years: 2–12 g/d in 2–4 equal divided doses (usually 2). Children: dosage not established. Administer IV as infusion over about 30 min; add lidocaine to IM injection, if necessary, to reduce pain

(continued)

Table 56–C2 Clinical Uses and Administration of Cephalosporins (*Continued*)

AGENT	CLINICAL USES	DOSAGE AND ROUTE OF ADMINISTRATION*
Ceftazidime		
(CEPTAZ; FORTAZ; TAZICEF; TAZIDIME)	Serious systemic, urinary tract, and skin infections; spectrum similar to cefotaxime, but less gram-positive bacterial and *Bacteroides* coverage, greater activity against *Pseudomonas* and some other Enterobacteriaceae	IM and IV: Adults, children >12 years: 500 mg–6 g/d in 2 or 3 equal divided doses. Children 1 month–12 years: 30–50 mg/kg q8h (maximum 6 g/d). Neonates (≤4 weeks): 30 mg/kg q12h. Add lidocaine to IM injection if necessary
Ceftizoxime sodium		
(CEFIZOX)	Serious systemic, urinary tract, and skin infections; spectrum and uses similar to cefotaxime, but more active against *Serratia,* slightly more active against *Bacteroides*	IM and IV: Adults: 1–12 g/d in 2 or 3 equal divided doses. Children >6 months: 50–200 mg/kg/d in 3 or 4 equal divided doses (maximum 12 g/d)
	Uncomplicated gonorrhea	IM: 1 g once
Ceftriaxone sodium		
(ROCEPHIN)	Serious systemic, urinary tract, and skin infections; spectrum similar to cefotaxime	IM and IV: Adults, children >12 years: 1–4 g/d in 1 dose or 2 equal divided doses. Neonates, children <12 years: 50–100 mg/kg/d in 2 equal divided doses (maximum 4 g/d). Add lidocaine to IM injection if necessary
	Uncomplicated gonorrhea (for other uses in gonorrhea, consult current literature)	IM: 250 mg once

Table 56–S2 **Major Side Effects of and Contraindications for Cephalosporins**

BODY SYSTEM/ Side Effect	CONTRAINDICATION/ PRECAUTION	COMMENTS AND NURSING IMPLICATIONS
CENTRAL NERVOUS SYSTEM Headache, dizziness, fatigue; CNS irritation		Assess for, report reactions; avoid intrathecal or intraventricular administration
BLOOD Neutropenia, leukopenia, thrombocytosis, thrombocytopenia; false-positive Coombs' tests; anemia and agranulocytosis (rare); hypoprothrombinemia with possible bleeding with cefamandole, moxalactam, cefoperazone		Assess for, report evidence of bone marrow suppression; be aware that false-positive Coombs' tests may occur, especially at high doses; monitor PT in patients receiving cefamandole, moxalactam, or cefoperazone, report bleeding; prophylactic vitamin K administration may prevent this (at risk: geriatric, debilitated, renally impaired, or GI surgery patients)
GASTROINTESTINAL Nausea, vomiting, GI upset, oral candidiasis, diarrhea, possibly pseudomembranous colitis		Most common with oral cephalosporins, can occur with parenteral dosages; monitor for and report gastric distress, diarrhea; report severe diarrhea immediately
HEPATIC Transient increases in ALT, AST, and alkaline phosphatase; hyperbilirubinemia; increased LDH hepatomegaly (cephradine)		Usually mild and reversible; assess for, report any side effects
RENAL Nephrotoxicity: rare except in the elderly, in renal impairment, or when used with other nephrotoxic drugs (aminoglycosides, vancomycin)		Assess for, report evidence of nephrotoxicity (creatinine, BUN, proteinuria, oliguria), especially in high-risk patients; reduce dosage in renal impairment

(continued)

Table 56–S2 | **Major Side Effects of and Contraindications for Cephalosporins (*Continued*)**

BODY SYSTEM/ Side Effect	CONTRAINDICATON/ PRECAUTION	COMMENTS AND NURSING IMPLICATIONS
IMMUNE Hypersensitivity reactions; urticaria, rash, fever, eosinophilia, serum sickness–like reactions, genital or anal pruritus, exfoliative dermatitis, angioedema, anaphylaxis	Known hypersensitivity to any cephalosporin; relatively contraindicated if severely penicillin-allergic	Assess for, report immediately any rash, fever, urticaria, joint or muscle pain, genital or anal pruritus, or respiratory difficulty; observe patients for 30 min following parenteral doses; have emergency supplies immediately available; serum sickness–like reactions most common with cefaclor; discontinuation of cefaclor and use of antihistamine or corticosteroid may be required; cross-allergy with penicillins may occur; avoid cephalosporin use if severely penicillin-allergic, and use cautiously with history of less severe penicillin-allergic reactions
LOCAL OR GENERALIZED EFFECTS IM injection pain; phlebitis, thrombophlebitis with IV administration; superinfection		See text, Table 56–S2, for parenteral administration guidelines; assess for, report evidence of superinfection

Table 56–I2 | **Major Interactions Between Cephalosporins and Other Agents**

AGENT	RESULT OF INTERACTION	COMMENTS AND NURSING IMPLICATIONS
Alcohol	Disulfiram-like reaction: nausea, hypotension, tachycardia, flushing	Avoid alcohol, including that found in medications, toiletries, elixirs, other alcohol-containing products, if patients receiving cefamandole, cefotetan, or cefoperazone; report reactions to physician
Aminoglycosides (and potentially vancomycin)	Increased risk of nephrotoxicity	Avoid concomitant use when possible, assess for nephrotoxicity when used together; adjust dosages in renal impairment

Table 56–C3 **Clinical Uses and Administration of Aminoglycosides**

AGENT	CLINICAL USES	DOSAGE AND ROUTE OF ADMINISTRATION
PROTOTYPE		
Gentamicin sulfate		
(GARAMYCIN; JENAMICIN)	Serious gram-negative bacillary infections (including *Pseudomonas*) such as sepsis and pulmonary, abdominal, pelvic, bone, joint, skin, soft tissue, and urinary tract infections and some infections caused by *Staph. aureus*	IM and IV: Adults: 3–5 mg/kg/d in 3 or 4 divided doses. Children: 6–7.5 mg/kg/d divided q8h. Infants and neonates (>1 week old): 7.5 mg/kg/d divided q8h. Neonates (≤1 week): 5 mg/kg/d divided q12h (extreme immaturity may require as little as 2.5 mg/kg q24h). Impaired renal function usually requires reduced doses or increased dosage interval to maintain appropriate peak and predose levels. Patients with extensive burns and cystic fibrosis may require higher doses
	CNS infections caused by susceptible organisms	Intrathecal: Adults: 4–8 mg qd. Infants >3 months: 1–2 mg qd
RELATED DRUGS		
Amikacin sulfate		
(AMIKIN)	Serious gram-negative bacillary infections and some infections caused by *Staph. aureus* (see gentamicin) resistant to other aminoglycosides	IM and IV: Usually 15 mg/kg/d in 2 or 3 divided doses; adjust to maintain recommended levels. Neonates <2 weeks of age, patients with renal impairment, may require lower doses or longer intervals; burns and cystic fibrosis may necessitate higher doses
Neomycin sulfate		
(MYCIFRADIN; NEOBIOTIC)	Adjunctive treatment of hepatic encephalopathy	Oral: Adults: 4–12 g/d for 5 or 6 days in 4 equal divided doses. Children: 50–100 mg/kg/d. Chronic disease may require up to 4 g/d indefinitely
	Preoperative reduction of gut flora	Oral: Adults: 1 g hourly for 4 doses, then q4h for 5 doses; *or* following cathartic therapy for 2 days, give 1 g at 1 PM, 2 PM, and 11 PM on day prior to surgery with equal oral doses of erythomycin base
	Diarrhea caused by enteropathogenic *E. coli*	Oral: 50 mg/kg/d in 4 equal divided doses for 2 or 3 days (maximum adult dosage is 3 g)
(NEOSPORIN G.U. IRRIGANT)	Bladder irrigation	1 mL per 1 L 0.9% sodium chloride; instill 1–2 L/d for up to 10 days (contains polymyxin B)
Netilmicin sulfate		
(NETROMYCIN)	Serious infections caused by susceptible gram-negative bacilli and by *Staph. aureus*	IM and IV: Adults: 4–6.5 mg/kg/d in 2 or 3 equal divided doses. Children and infants: 5.5–8 mg/kg/d in 2 or 3 equal divided doses. Neonates <6 weeks: 4–6.5 mg/kg/d in 2 equal divided doses. Infuse IV dose over 30 min. Base subsequent dosage adjustments on serum level

(continued)

Table 56–C3 **Clinical Uses and Administration of Aminoglycosides (*Continued*)**

AGENT	CLINICAL USES	DOSAGE AND ROUTE OF ADMINISTRATION
Streptomycin sulfate	Tuberculosis	IM: Adults: 15 mg/kg/d (up to 1 g maximum/d) as single daily dose; dosage is discontinued or reduced after about 3 months to 25 mg/kg 2 or 3 times per week. Children: 20–40 mg/kg qd. Give only with other antitubercular drugs
	Enterococcal endocarditis	IM: Adults: 1 g q12h for 2 weeks, then 500 mg q12h for 4 weeks. Usually given with concurrent penicillin therapy
	Streptococcal endocarditis (viridans group)	IM: Adults: 1 g q12h for 1 week, then 500 mg q12h for 1 week; reduce dose for elderly; usually given with concurrent penicillin. Monitor closely for vestibular toxicity
Tobramycin sulfate		
(NEBCIN)	Serious systemic infections and urinary tract infections caused by susceptible gram-negative bacilli and serious systemic infection caused by *Staph. aureus*	IM and IV: Adults: 3–5 mg/kg/d in 3 or 4 equal divided doses. Infants and children: 6–7.5 mg/kg/d in 3 or 4 equal divided doses. Neonates <1 week old: Up to 4 mg/kg/d divided in 2 equal doses

Table 56–S3 | Major Side Effects of and Contraindications for Aminoglycosides

BODY SYSTEM/ Side Effect	CONTRAINDICATION PRECAUTION	COMMENTS AND NURSING IMPLICATIONS
CENTRAL NERVOUS SYSTEM Optic neuritis; organic brain syndrome; peripheral neuritis; pain		Rare; assess for, report to physician
HEARING, BALANCE Auditory toxicity; high-frequency hearing loss progressing to deafness if aminoglycoside is not discontinued; vestibular toxicity; dizziness, ataxia; usually irreversible	Higher risk, more caution required in presence of one or more of the following: advanced age; dehydration; renal dysfunction; excessive doses, continuous therapy >10 days–2 weeks	Maintain adequate hydration, monitor blood levels, anticipate need for dosage adjustments; report signs, symptoms of hearing changes, vestibular dysfunction; stress need for baseline and follow-up tests for high-risk patients (see left), plus those taking other ototoxic drugs (eg, furosemide) or with preexisting hearing or balance dysfunction
BLOOD Granulocytopenia, agranulocytosis, thrombocytopenia, anemia		Rare; observe for referable symptoms such as lassitude, petechiae, and pallor, and report to physician
GASTROINTESTINAL AND HEPATIC Increased AST, ALT, LDH, serum bilirubin; hepatomegaly, anorexia, nausea, vomiting, superinfection with oral use (neomycin especially)	Oral neomycin and kanamycin contraindicated in intestinal obstruction owing to absorption to toxic levels	Rare; assess for, report to physician
RENAL Acute tubular necrosis with resulting azotemia and sometimes oliguria; usually reversible on discontinuation of therapy	See *hearing, balance* above for general risks, precautions; added risks: concurrent renal dysfunction, use of nephrotoxic drugs (eg, amphotericin B)	Baseline tests of renal status (eg, urinalysis, creatinine, BUN), follow-up testing, advised for high-risk patients; explain need to patients; monitor accordingly, report changes to physician at once; be aware that oliguria is a late-developing sign of renal dysfunction
NEUROMUSCULAR Potential neuromuscular blockade, hypoventilation, apnea	Relatively contraindicated in patients receiving neuromuscular blocking agents unless giving respiratory support	Monitor respiratory rates closely, especially in the elderly; after receiving general anesthetics or neuromuscular blocking agents; or in hypocalcemic patients; be prepared to assist ventilation; IV administration of calcium salts may reverse this
IMMUNE Hypersensitivity reactions; rash, anaphylaxis, skin rash from contact sensitivity from neomycin and streptomycin	Known hypersensitivity to the antibiotic; caution required when using other aminoglycosides (cross-allergy may occur)	Avoid use in patients with known allergy; monitor for rash, anaphylaxis, and notify physician if these occur; avoid personal contact with neomycin or streptomycin to avoid contact allergy

Table 56–13 Major Interactions Between Aminoglycosides and Other Agents

AGENT	RESULT OF INTERACTION	COMMENTS AND NURSING IMPLICATIONS
Amphotericin B (Chapter 57), cephalothin	Increased risk of nephrotoxicity	Additive nephrotoxicity; maintain hydration and monitor closely for nephrotoxicity
Anticoagulants (oral) (Chapter 35)	Increased prothrombin time (PT), leading to bleeding	Caused by decreased vitamin K–producing gut bacteria and decreased vitamin K absorption; monitor PT, assess for bleeding; anticoagulant dosage reduction may be required
High-ceiling diuretics (eg, furosemide; Chapter 32)	Increased risk of ototoxicity	When combined therapy is required, monitor dosages closely to use lowest possible dosage for the shortest period; monitor closely for vestibular symptoms, hearing deficits
Digitalis glycosides (oral; Chapter 31)	Decreased digitalis absorption, reduced blood levels and effects	Monitor digitalis levels and anticipate need to adjust dosage; assess for symptoms of loss of digitalis control (congestive heart failure, etc)
Dimenhydrinate, other antiemetic drugs (Chapter 42)	Masking of vestibular ototoxicity	Interactants may mask vestibular symptoms of ototoxicity; if combined use cannot be avoided, monitor for vestibular and auditory dysfunction more closely
Extended-spectrum penicillins	Decreased aminoglycoside levels	See Table 56–12
Methoxyflurane (Chapter 20), neuromuscular blocking agents (succinylcholine, tubocurarine, etc; Chapter 17)	Hypoventilation or respiratory paralysis	Enhanced neuromuscular blockade; administer aminoglycosides with extreme caution during surgery and the immediate postoperative period; monitor respiratory function; treatment with parenteral calcium salts may reverse this; be prepared to support ventilation

Table 56–C4 **Clinical Uses and Administration of Tetracyclines**

AGENT	CLINICAL USES	DOSAGE AND ROUTE OF ADMINISTRATION
PROTOTYPE		
Tetracycline (ACHROMYCIN V; PANMYCIN; ROBITET; SUMYCIN)	*Rickettsia,* uncommon gram-positive bacteria, *Chlamydia, Mycoplasma,* gonorrhea, spirochetes, bronchitis, acne	Oral: 1–2 g/d in 2–4 doses Ophthalmic: 1–2 cm of ointment or 1 or 2 drops of suspension instilled onto affected eye(s) 2–4 times daily Topical: Apply ointment sparingly to infected skin 2 or 3 times daily. Apply solution morning and evening for acne
RELATED DRUGS		
Doxycycline (DOXY; DOXYCHEL; DORYX; VIBRAMYCIN; VIBRA-TABS)	Same uses as tetracycline; consult package literature for specific dosage recommendations	Oral: Adults: 50–100 mg q12h. Children >8 years: 2.2 mg/kg once or twice daily IV: Adults: 100–200 mg/d. Children >8 years: 2.2 mg/kg once or twice daily. Infuse over at least 1 h
Minocycline (MINOCIN)	Same as tetracycline	Oral and IV: 100 mg q12h or 50 mg q6h
Oxytetracycline (TERRAMYCIN; URI-TET)	Same as tetracycline	Oral: 250–500 mg q6h IM: 250 mg/qd or 300 mg q8h–q12h

Table 56–S4 | **Major Side Effects of and Contraindications for Tetracyclines**

BODY SYSTEM/ Side Effect	CONTRAINDICATION/ PRECAUTION	COMMENTS AND NURSING IMPLICATIONS
CENTRAL NERVOUS SYSTEM Vertigo, dizziness		Most common with minocycline
BLOOD Leukopenia, others		Monitor CBC if treatment is prolonged
GASTROINTESTINAL Nausea, vomiting, burning, diarrhea, pseudomembranous colitis		Do not give tetracyclines with meals, except minocycline and doxycycline; report evidence of severe GI distress
HEPATIC Hepatotoxicity	Known liver dysfunction	Monitor for signs of liver toxicity
SKIN Hypersensitivity; photosensitivity	Known allergies	Check for allergies; assess for rash; cross-allergy exists among tetracyclines; caution patients about sun exposure, especially with demeclocycline; rare with minocycline
TEETH Binds to, stains, developing teeth	Pregnancy, age under 8 years	

Table 56–I4 | **Major Interactions Between Tetracyclines and Other Agents**

AGENT	RESULT OF INTERACTION	COMMENTS AND NURSING IMPLICATIONS
Aminoglycosides	Decreased effect of aminoglycoside	Do not give concomitantly
Antacids (Chapter 40)	Decreased tetracycline absorption, effects	Give 1 hour before or 2 hours after tetracycline
Anticoagulants, oral (Chapter 35)	Potentiated anticoagulant effects, risk of excessive bleeding	Monitor prothrombin times and for bleeding; administer vitamin K, if needed, during prolonged tetracycline therapy
Kaolin-pectin (Chapter 40)	Decreased tetracycline absorption, effects	Avoid concurrent use
Minerals	Decreased tetracycline absorption, effects	Give 1 hour before or 2 hours after tetracycline
Penicillins	See Table 56-I1	
Additional Interactions Involving Doxycycline		
Carbamazepine (Chapter 26)	Increased doxycycline metabolic inactivation, decreased effects	Increase doxycycline dose or use other tetracycline
Phenobarbital (Chapter 22)	See carbamazepine	
Phenytoin (Chapter 26)	See carbamazepine	

Table 56–C5 Clinical Uses and Administration of Erythromycins

AGENT	CLINICAL USES	DOSAGE AND ROUTE OF ADMINISTRATION
PROTOTYPE		
Erythromycin base (E-BASE; E-MYCIN; ERYC; ERY-TAB; ERYTHROMYCIN FILMTABS; ILOTYCIN; PCE DISPERTAB; ROBIMYCIN; RP-MYCIN)	Infections caused by susceptible *Mycoplasma pneumoniae, Corynebacterim diphtheriae, Legionella pneumophila, Bordetella pertussis, H. influenzae, H. ducreyi, Strep. pyogenes, Strep. viridans, Strep. pneumoniae, Listeria monocytogenes, Ureaplasma urealyticum, Campylobacter fetus* (subsp. *jejuni*), *Borrelia burgdorferi, Chlamydia trachomatis,* and *Treponema pallidum*	Oral: Adults: 250 mg q6h or 333 mg q8h. More than 4 g/d may be needed in some infections. Children: 30–50 mg/kg/d in 4 equal divided doses or 0.9–3 g/m^2/d in 4 equal divided doses. For preoperative intestinal antisepsis, see Table 56–C3, NEOMYCIN SULFATE)
RELATED DRUGS		
Erythromycin estolate (ILOSONE)	Same as erythromycin base	Oral: Adults: 250 mg q6h. May need more than 4g/d in some infections. Children: see erythromycin base
Erythromycin ethylsuccinate (E.E.S., ERY PED)	Same as erythromycin base	Oral: Adults: 400 mg q6h. More than 4g/d may be needed in some infections. Children: see erythromycin base
Erythromycin gluceptate (ILOTYCIN GLUCEPTATE)	Same as erythromycin base	IV: 1–4 g/d, 15–20 mg/kg/d, or 300–600 mg/m^2/d in 4 equal divided doses or as a continuous infusion
Erythromycin lactobionate (ERYTHROCIN LACTOBIONATE-IV)	Same as erythromycin base	IV: See erythromycin gluceptate
Erythromycin stearate (ERAMYCIN; ERYTHROCIN STEARATE; WYAMYCIN S)	Same as erythromycin base	Oral: See erythromycin estolate

Table 56–S5 **Major Side Effects of and Contraindications for Erythromycins**

BODY SYSTEM/ Side Effect	CONTRAINDICATIONS/ PRECAUTION	COMMENTS AND NURSING IMPLICATIONS
EAR Hearing Loss		Use caution in elderly, with prolonged usage, or high dose
GASTROINTESTINAL Nausea, diarrhea, cramps, colitis		May give estolate or ethylsuccinate salts with food if nausea is intolerable
HEPATIC Hepatotoxicity; cholestatic jaundice	Hepatic dysfunction	Monitor accordingly; patients, especially with erythromycin estolate; avoid use in adults if possible
SKIN Allergic reactions	Do not give if hypersensitive	Monitor for rash or urticaria

Table 56–I5 **Major Interactions Between Erythromycins and Other Agents**

AGENT	RESULT OF INTERACTION	COMMENTS AND NURSING IMPLICATIONS
Bromocriptine (Chapter 25)	Elevated bromocriptine levels	Monitor for bromocriptine toxicity; possibly reduce bromocriptine dose
Carbamazepine (Chapter 26)	Elevated carbamazepine levels	Monitor carbamazepine levels, assess for toxicity
Cyclosporine (Chapter 54)	Increased cyclosporine effects	Possibly lower dose
Digoxin (Chapter 31)	Elevated digoxin levels	Monitor digoxin levels, assess for toxicity
Theophylline (Chapter 38)	Elevated theophylline levels	Monitor theophylline levels, assess for toxicity
Warfarin (Chapter 35)	Increased warfarin effect	Monitor clotting times

Table 56–C6 Clinical Uses and Administration of Sulfonamides

AGENT	CLINICAL USES	DOSAGE AND ROUTE OF ADMINISTRATION
PROTOTYPE		
Sulfisoxazole (GANTRISIN)	Various (see text)	Oral: Adults: Initially, 2–4 g; maintain with 4–8 g/d given in 4–6 divided doses. Children >2 months: Initially, 75 mg/kg/d; maintain with 150 mg/kg/d (4 g/m²/d) in 4–6 divided doses, up to 6 g/d maximum
Single-Entry Sulfonamides		
Sulfamethoxazole (GANTANOL; URI-BAK)	As for sulfisoxazole	Oral: Adults: Initially, 2 g, then 1 g bid (mild-to-moderate infections) or tid (severe infections). Children <2 months: Initially, 50–60 mg/kg, then 25–30 mg/kg bid (not to exceed 75 mg/kg/d)
Sulfasalazine (AZULFIDINE)	Ulcerative colitis	Oral: Adults: Usually start with 3–4 g/d in several evenly divided doses after meals; usual maintenance dose is 500 mg qid. Children >2 months: Initially, 40–60 mg/kg/d in 3–6 divided doses; maintenance dose usually 30 mg/kg/d in 4 divided doses
Sulfonamide Combination Products		
*Co-trimoxazole** ("TMP-SMZ"; trimethoprim + sulfamethoxazole; BACTRIM; COTRIM; SEPTRA; SULFATRIM; UROPLUS)	Acute otitis media; urinary tract infections; shigellosis; bronchitis	Oral: Adults: 160 mg TMP bid for 10–14 (7 d for shigellosis). Children: 8 mg/kg/d TMP 12h for 10 d (5 d for shigellosis)
	Severe urinary tract infections; shigellosis	IV: Adults, children: 8–10 mg/kg/d in 2–4 evenly divided doses for 5 d (shigellosis) or 14 d (UTI)
	P. carinii pneumonitis	Oral: Adults, children: 20 mg/kg/d TMP in 4 divided doses
		IV: 15–20 mg/kg/d TMP in 3 or 4 divided doses
Sulfisoxazole plus erythromycin ethylsuccinate† (ERYZOLE; PEDIAZOLE)	Acute otitis media in children	Oral: 1.25 mL/kg/d in equal divided doses qid for 10 d; do not exceed 10 mL/dose for any child

*Dosages are expressed in terms of trimethoprim (TMP) content; because of the fixed ratio in the combination, the sulfamethoxazole dose (mg) will be five times the TMP dose; the minimum age for pediatric therapy is 2 months for all indications.

†Contains (per 5 mL reconstituted suspension) the equivalent of 600 mg sulfisoxazole, 200 mg erythromycin; not indicated for children <2 months old.

Table 56–S6 **Major Side Effects of and Contraindications for Sulfonamides**

BODY SYSTEM/ Side Effect	CONTRAINDICATION/ PRECAUTION	COMMENTS AND NURSING IMPLICATIONS
CENTRAL NERVOUS SYSTEM Occasional drowsiness, dizziness; psychosis or depression (uncommon)		Monitor accordingly
BLOOD Agranulocytosis, thrombocytopenia, aplastic anemia, hemolytic anemia	Blood dyscrasias, care with concurrent therapy with other marrow-suppressant drugs or therapies; glucose-6-phosphate dehydrogenase (G6PD) deficiencies	Obtain baseline hematologic data if possible, especially if treatment is likely to last >2 weeks; monitor CBC periodically during prolonged therapy; risk of hemolytic anemia great in patients with G6PD deficiencies; avoid use
GASTROINTESTINAL Nausea, vomiting, diarrhea		Seldom requires discontinuation; give with full glass of water
HEPATIC Potential hepatic dysfunction or elevation of blood levels of marker enzymes		Usually slight, occurs within first few days of treatment; monitor accordingly
RENAL Crystalluria, resulting renal tubular damage	Severe renal dysfunction	Patient should be well hydrated before and during therapy, goal is urine output of 1.5 L/d; urinary alkalinization (as with sodium bicarbonate) reduces risk of crystalluria, may be required adjunctive therapy; assess urine output, urine pH, adjust pH (or reduce sulfonamide dose) as needed
Yellow-orange urine discoloration		Occurs in alkaline urine with sulfasalazine *only;* advise patient that this is expected, to avoid alarm; skin discoloration may occur also
SKIN Photosensitivity		May or may not be allergy-related; assess accordingly; advise patient to wear suitable protective clothing, sunscreens, if exposure to sunlight or strong ultraviolet sources cannot be avoided
REPRODUCTIVE Oligospermia, infertility		Uncommon, but reversible; occurs only with sulfadiazine
IMMUNE Allergic reactions: rashes, urticaria, serum sickness, Stevens–Johnson syndrome; anaphylaxis	Allergy to sulfonamides, drugs with sulfa structures (thiazide diuretics, sulfonylurea oral-hypoglycemic drugs, etc)	Check history thoroughly before treatment starts; reactions may be severe; agent should be discontinued at once, physician notified, at first sign of any allergic reaction (see also skin)

Table 56–16 Major Interactions Between Sulfonamides and Other Agents

AGENT	RESULT OF INTERACTION	COMMENTS AND NURSING IMPLICATIONS
Anticoagulants, oral (Chapter 35)	Increased anticoagulant effects	Sulfonamides displace these drugs from plasma proteins; risk appears to be highest with warfarin; if interaction is unavoidable, assess for bruising, bleeding petechiae, etc; assess urine color for evidence of renal bleeding, which could be caused by a combination of crystalluria (renal tubular damage) and increased anticoagulant effect; anticipate need to reduce anticoagulant dose during combined therapy, increase upon sulfonamide discontinuation; coagulation studies usually required
Oral hypoglycemic drugs (sulfonylureas; Chapter 46)	Hypoglycemia	Caused by displacement of interactant from plasma proteins, reduced renal clearance of hypoglycemic; monitor blood glucose levels more often, assess for evidence of hypoglycemia, if interaction is unavoidable; probably less likely to occur or be severe with newer oral hypoglycemics, glipizide and glyburide
Methotrexate (Chapter 59)	Increased risk of methotrexate side effects	Monitor methotrexate levels if possible; reduce dose of methotrexate if levels are high or toxicity occurs
Phenytoin (Chapter 26)	Increased risk of phenytoin side effects	Sulfonamides displace phenytoin from plasma proteins; if interaction cannot be avoided, assess for excessive drowsiness, ataxia, etc; reduced phenytoin doses may be indicated, but phenytoin blood levels should be measured to ensure adequate anticonvulsant coverage

Table 56–C7 | **Clinical Uses and Administration of Quinolones***

AGENT	CLINICAL USES	DOSAGE AND ROUTE OF ADMINISTRATION
PROTOTYPE		
Ciprofloxacin (CIPRO)	Systemic or urinary tract infections (UTIs) caused by gram-negative aerobes and *Staphylococcus* resistant to less expensive but otherwise suitable antibiotics	IV: Uncomplicated UTIs: 200 mg q12h; other infections: 400–750 mg q12h, depending on type, severity of infection Oral: Uncomplicated UTIs: 250 mg q12h; severe UTIs or systemic infections: 500–750 mg q12h; give with full glass of water
RELATED DRUGS		
Lomefloxacin (MAXAQUIN)	Treatment of acute bacterial flare-ups of chronic bronchitis	Oral: 400 mg qd for 10 d
	Treatment of uncomplicated UTIs (cystitis)	Oral: 400 mg qd for 10 d
	UTIs with complications	Oral: 400 mg qd for 14 d
	Preoperative prophylaxis of early postoperative UTIs	Oral: 400 mg 2–6 hr before surgery (single dose)
Norfloxacin (NOROXIN)	UTIs	Oral: 400 mg bid for 3–21 d, depending on severity, cause of infection
	Uncomplicated gonorrhea	Oral: 800 mg, single dose
Ofloxacin (FLOXIN)	As for ciprofloxacin	Oral: 200–400 mg q12h for 3 days to 6 weeks, depending on nature and site of infection
	Acute, uncomplicated gonorrhea	Oral: 400 mg, single dose

*Quinolones are indicated only for adults and children >18 years old; dosages apply only to patients with normal renal function.

Table 56–S7 | **Major Side Effects of and Contraindications for Quinolones**

BODY SYSTEM/ Side Effect	CONTRAINDICATION/ PRECAUTION	COMMENTS AND NURSING IMPLICATIONS
CENTRAL NERVOUS SYSTEM Headache, dizziness	Caution in patients with history of seizures, CNS dysfunction	Seizures, psychosis have occurred; monitor accordingly
GASTROINTESTINAL Nausea, diarrhea, abdominal pain or discomfort		Nausea is not common side effect of quinolones
SKIN Photosensitivity		Reactions can be severe; advise patient to avoid excessive sunlight exposure, notify physician if skin rashes, other changes, occur
OTHER Hypersensitivity reactions, anaphylaxis	Prior reaction to any quinolone	May be serious or fatal; assess accordingly, advise patient to discontinue drug at once, notify physician, with appearance of any risk sign, symptom

Table 56–I7 | **Major Interactions Between Quinolones and Other Agents**

AGENT	RESULT OF INTERACTION	COMMENTS AND NURSING IMPLICATIONS
Antacids (Chapter 40)	Decreased oral quinolone absorption, effects	Avoid combined use if possible; otherwise give antacids at least 6 h before or 2 hr after the antibiotic; discourage self-prescribing of antacids (eg, to reduce quinolone GI upset) without physician's approval, instructions for proper use
Anticoagulants, oral (Chapter 35)	Potentially excessive anticoagulation	Monitor coagulation profiles during combined therapy, assess for possible excessive anticoagulant effects
Cyclosporine (Chapter 54)	Potentially increased blood levels, toxic effects of interactant	Monitor for evidence of interaction, anticipate need to check cyclosporine levels, if combined therapy cannot be avoided
Iron salts (Chapter 61)	Decreased oral absorption, effects, of quinolones	Avoid combined use if possible; check for use of OTC nutrient products (eg, multivitamin–mineral supplements) when taking medication history, notify physician of use; advise patients who may wish to use iron supplements to notify physician first
Sucralfate (Chapter 40)	As for antacids	Avoid concurrent use
Theophylline (Chapter 38)	Reduced theophylline metabolism, increased blood levels, risk of toxicity	If combined therapy is needed, monitor theophylline blood levels, assess for excessive effects; anticipate need to reduce theophylline dose; interaction affects caffeine: assess for excessive caffeine intake if patient shows signs of excessive CNS stimulation; encourage moderation of coffee, cola intake (unless decaffeinated) during quinolone therapy
Zinc salts (Chapter 61)	As for iron salts	As for iron salts

Table 56–C8 Clinical Uses and Administration of Chloramphenicol

AGENT	CLINICAL USES	DOSAGE AND ROUTE OF ADMINISTRATION
Chloramphenicol, chloramphenicol palmitate, chloramphenicol sodium succinate		
(CHLOROMYCETIN)	Severe, life-threatening infections caused by susceptible organisms where other therapy cannot be used due to resistance or contraindication	IV and Oral: Adults, children: 50–100 mg/kg/d in 4 equal divided doses. Neonates: 25 mg/kg/d in up to 4 equal divided doses if <2 weeks of age; 50 mg/kg/d in 4 equal divided doses if >2 weeks of age. Adjust dosage as needed to maintain plasma concentrations of 5–20 μg/mL; avoid levels over 25 μg/mL. Reduce dosage in presence of renal or hepatic disease

Table 56–S8 Major Side Effects of and Contraindications for Chloramphenicol

BODY SYSTEM/ Side Effect	CONTRAINDICATION/ PRECAUTION	COMMENTS AND NURSING IMPLICATIONS
CENTRAL NERVOUS SYSTEM Optic neuritis, peripheral neuritis		Related to long-term, high-dose therapy; assess for visual deficits, complaints of peripheral numbness
BLOOD Non–dose-related, irreversible bone marrow suppression; dose-related, reversible bone marrow suppression		Monitor CBC closely; dose-related suppression often presents with reticulocytopenia and anemia; report any major changes in laboratory studies, bleeding, sore throat, mucosal ulcerations, pallor, or lassitude to physician; maintain plasma levels less than 25 μg/mL
GASTROINTESTINAL Nausea, vomiting, superinfection (enterocolitis)		Rare; assess for and report to physician
IMMUNE Hypersensitivity reactions; fever, rash, skin or mucosal hemorrhage	Known hypersensitivity to chloramphenicol or previous history of severe toxic reactions	Avoid use; monitor for fever, rash, skin or mucosal hemorrhage, and report to physician immediately
OTHER Gray baby syndrome: cardiovascular collapse and possibly death due to accumulation of excessively high blood levels	Caution: pregnancy, breastfeeding	Use initial doses no higher than those recommended in Table 56–C8, adjust dosage as needed to maintain plasma levels no higher than 25 μg/mL in neonates and young infants. Observe for and report poor feeding, abdominal distention, pallid cyanosis, hypotension, or respiratory irregularities immediately

Table 56–I8 **Major Interactions Between Chloramphenicol and Other Agents**

AGENT	RESULT OF INTERACTION	COMMENTS AND NURSING IMPLICATIONS
Barbiturates	Increased chloramphenicol metabolism	Monitor plasma concentrations of chloramphenicol and adjust dosage as necessary; observe for decreased chloramphenicol effectiveness
Phenytoin, oral sulfonylurea hypoglycemic agents (tolbutamide, chlorpropamide)	Decreased hepatic clearance of these interactants may lead to excessive plasma levels and toxicity	Observe serum levels of phenytoin and for nystagmus, ataxia, or sedation; blood glucose response or for hypoglycemia with sulfonylureas; reduce dose as indicated

Table 56–C9 **Clinical Uses and Administration of Miscellaneous Antibiotics**

AGENT	CLINICAL USES	DOSAGE AND ROUTE OF ADMINISTRATION	COMMENTS AND NURSING IMPLICATIONS
Azithromycin			
(ZITHROMAX)	Streptococcal pharyngitis, chlamydia	Oral: 250–500 mg qd	
Aztreonam			
(AZACTAM)	Systemic or urinary tract infections caused by gram-negative aerobes	IM or IV: For UTIs: 0.5–1 g q8h–q12h. For systemic infections: 1–2 g q6h to q12h. No established pediatric dose	Adverse effects like those for penicillin. Some cross allergy with penicillin or cephalosporin. Reduce dosage in renal impairment
Clarithromycin			
(BIAXIN)	Upper and lower respiratory tract infections, skin and soft tissue infections, *H. pylori,* atypical *Mycobacteria*	Oral: 250–500 mg bid	
Clindamycin			
(CLEOCIN)	Anaerobic pulmonary infections, mixed infections in the abdomen and pelvis	IV: 600 mg–4.8 g/d given in 2–4 divided doses. Children: 15–40 mg/kg/d in 3 or 4 divided doses Oral: 150–450 mg q6h Children: 8–25 mg/kg/d in 3 or 4 divided doses	Observe for diarrhea; question patients about stool frequency, consistency, and appearance
Imipenem and cilastatin sodium			
(PRIMAXIN)	Alternate choice for treating infections caused by multiply resistant organisms	IV: Adults: 1–4 g/d in 3 or 4 divided doses. Children: up to 25 mg/kg q6h. Reduce dosage in presence of renal failure	Seizures can occur, especially in elderly patients with severe renal impairment
Spectinomycin hydrochloride			
(TROBICIN)	Gonococcal infections resistant to penicillins, cephalosporins, and tetracyclines	IM: Adults: 2 g administered as a single dose. Children: 40 mg/kg as a single dose	Injection is painful; allergic reactions are possible

(continued)

Table 56–C9 Clinical Uses and Administration of Miscellaneous Antibiotics (*Continued*)

AGENT	CLINICAL USES	DOSAGE AND ROUTE OF ADMINISTRATION	COMMENTS AND NURSING IMPLICATIONS
Vancomycin hydrochloride (VANCOCIN; VANCOLED)	*Staphylococcus* infections, especially with penicillin allergy or antistaphylococcal penicillin resistance; methicillin-resistant *Staph. epidermidis;* prophylaxis of bacterial endocarditis	IV: Adults: Dilute in minimum of 100 mL of parenteral fluid and infuse 500 mg q6h–q8h or 1 g q12h; avoid infusing total dose in less than 1 hr Children: 40 mg/kg/d in 4 divided doses	Potential ototoxicity and nephrotoxicity, especially with high-dose, long-term therapy or in presence of renal failure; severe hypotension, upper extremity flushing (red neck syndrome) may occur with rapid IV injection; infuse over at least 1 h, monitor closely
	Pseudomembranous colitis caused by *C. difficile*	Oral: Adults: Usually 125–500 mg tid or qid. Children: 40 mg/kg/d in 3 or 4 divided doses. Do not exceed 2 g/d total	

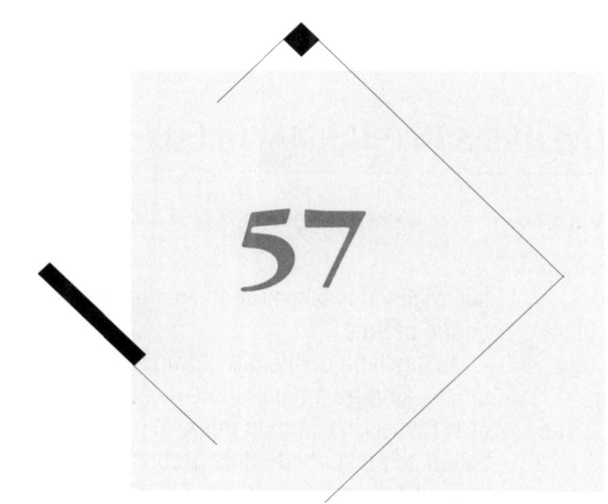

PROTOTYPES

Miscellaneous Antiinfective Agents

This chapter discusses antiinfective agents that do not fit easily into the drug categories presented in the previous chapter. Two of the sections focus on bacterial disorders that are unique, either because of the causative organism or because of the limited usefulness of drugs used to treat them: tuberculosis and urinary tract infections. Since some of the traditional antibiotics discussed in Chapter 56 play a role in the therapy of these disorders, material about them will not be repeated here. The rest of the chapter discusses the treatment of infections caused by fungi, viruses, *helminths* (worms), and protozoa. There are many causes of infectious diseases, and many drugs available to treat them. As a result, what follows is selective and limited to the major representative drugs.

I. Antitubercular Drugs

Tuberculosis (TB) is a bacterial infection caused by the organism *Mycobacterium tuberculosis.* The infection occurs primarily in the lungs, but can also affect the meninges, bones, peritoneum, and the genitourinary tract. Until recently, the incidence of tuberculosis in the United States (approximately 12 cases per 100,000) had been declining. The recent slight increase in the incidence of TB is thought to be due primarily to the high incidence of TB found in Southeast Asian refugees admitted to this country. The increased incidence of intravenous drug abuse and acquired immunodeficiency syndrome (AIDS) are also contributing to the rise of TB cases. In addition, a group of *Mycobacterium* known as "atypical mycobacterium" is increasing in incidence in the AIDS population. Some of the more common organisms include *Mycobacterium avium* complex and *M. kansasii.*

Tuberculosis presents in one of two major ways. The usual preferred starting treatment depends on the findings. One manifestation is simply an infection in which *M. tuberculosis* is present in the body, but no clinical symptoms or other significant physical findings can be identified. The asymptomatic infection is treated with only a single agent, isoniazid. Isoniazid is the cornerstone of all antitubercular drug therapies. The drug will be considered as a prototype.

Symptomatic TB usually presents as hemoptysis, fatigue, weight loss, productive chronic cough, and night sweats. Pulmonary involvement often predominates.

Regardless of the absence or presence of symptoms, or the drug(s) selected, treatment is prolonged—usually from 9 months to 3 years. This lengthy course is

Major reference tables appear beginning on p. 1257.

TRENDS AND CONTROVERSIES IN PHARMACOLOGY

Tuberculosis—No Longer a Conquered Disease?

The development of antibiotics revolutionized the treatment of tuberculosis and led to the closure of the sanitoriums that were once so important to prevent the spread of *Mycobacterium tuberculosis* infection. Tuberculosis has represented one of the best examples of a "conquered" disease—one that no longer poses a threat to the public health. Until 1985, reports of new cases of tuberculosis decreased by about 5% annually in the United States. But in 1986, for the first time since disease reporting was initiated in 1953, this pattern changed. There was an increase in the number of new cases reported, and this trend continues (Lordi and Reichman, 1991).

Persons can be exposed to tuberculosis without becoming infected and can be infected, as evidenced by a positive skin test, without developing active disease. Clinically active disease develops in about 10% of persons with tuberculosis infection. This rate is significantly higher when the immune system is compromised, as in patients receiving immunosuppressant therapy or with immune system disorders. However, both prevention and treatment of clinically active disease can be accomplished successfully if an effective regimen is taken for an adequate period of time.

In any type of infection, drug resistance—and treatment failure—can occur when patients do not take medication as prescribed—this problem is termed acquired resistance. Infection with drug resistant organisms in previously untreated patients is referred to as primary resistance. Surveys by the Centers for Disease Control (CDC) from 1975–1986 noted relatively stable rates of primary resistance, although there were large differences according to race and ethnicity, and the occurrence of acquired resistance increased significantly over the period from 1982–1986 (Snider et al, 1991). Both types of resistance were approximately twice as frequent in foreign-born patients as compared to those born in the United States.

For a variety of reasons, including cost constraints, drug resistance surveillance was discontinued in 1986. Recent reports of outbreaks of multiple drug-resistant tuberculosis among patients with HIV infection have led the CDC to reconsider this step and to encourage health care providers and local health departments to begin surveillance of the problem (Snider et al 1991). Although immunosuppressed patients, such as persons with AIDS, may be at greatest risk, evidence suggests that drug resistance is related to epidemiological factors rather than to the presence of HIV-related conditions (Monno et al, 1991).

An increasing incidence of drug-resistant tuberculosis poses a threat to the health of immunocompromised patients and may ultimately pose a threat to the health of the general population. In view of this problem, nursing actions to reduce the spread of infection and to ensure that patients take medications as prescribed become increasingly important. Effective patient education, early detection of compliance problems, and appropriate public health referrals are among the interventions needed to deal with this problem.

Lordi GM, Reichman LB: Treatment of tuberculosis. *Am Fam Phys* 1991; 44:219–224.

Monno L, Carbonara S, Costa D: Emergence of drug-resistant *Mycobacterium tuberculosis* in HIV-infected patients. *Lancet* 1991; 337:852.

Snider DE, Cauthen GM, Farer LS et al; Drug-resistant tuberculosis. *Ann Rev Resp Dis* 1991; 144:732.

needed because the sites of infection are usually poorly vascularized and so antitubercular drugs do not reach them well. In addition, the causative organism can rapidly become resistant to one agent. Thus, other reasons why it is common to find a patient with TB taking two or three drugs are to prevent the development of resistance and to eradicate the organism as quickly as possible. Although multiple-drug therapy may be needed, it is associated with an increased risk of serious side effects.

PROTOTYPE

Isoniazid

Isoniazid ("INH"; NYDRAZID; others), because of its efficacy and comparatively low toxicity, is the drug of choice in treating TB. When an infection of *M. tuberculosis* without clinical evidence of disease is detected, INH alone, given for 12 months, will prevent development of symptomatic disease in a high percentage of patients.

Absorption, Distribution, Metabolism, and Excretion

Isoniazid is absorbed well from the gastrointestinal (GI) tract, although absorption may be somewhat impaired when it is given with food. Levels in the cerebrospinal fluid and breast milk are similar to plasma levels.

Isoniazid undergoes hepatic metabolism via a process known as acetylation. The rate of acetylation is greatly influenced by genetic factors and has much individual variation. For example, most Japanese, Chinese, Eskimos, and American Indians are "rapid acetylators," and they usually metabolize the drug very rapidly. Approximately 50% of Caucasians and blacks are "slow acetylators." The rate of INH metabolism may influence the incidence of toxicity or poor therapeutic responses in some rapid acetylators who receive twice-weekly treatment, but this has not been well substantiated by controlled studies.

One half to three quarters of absorbed INH is excreted by the kidneys as active drug and inactive metabolites.

Pharmacologic Effects

Isoniazid is bacteriostatic against actively growing bacteria but, in high concentrations, becomes bactericidal. Isoniazid's mechanism of action against *M. tuberculosis* is uncertain.

Clinical Indications and Administration

Isoniazid is used both for prophylaxis of TB in individuals who are at risk, and for treatment in patients with clinical disease (Table 57–C1).

Prophylaxis

Exposure to *M. tuberculosis,* and the presence of the organism in the body, is determined by a skin test that involves administration of a purified protein derivative (PPD) obtained from a human-type strain of the organism. The actual test procedures and their interpretation vary, but the general approach involves intradermal injection of the PPD or multiple skin puncture (with a multiple tine disk). Positive, negative, or questionable outcomes are based on the dermal response, assessed 48 to 72 hours later. Depending on the test used, a positive finding might be indicated by a particular size or amount of vesiculation or induration (skin hardness) surrounding the administration site(s). Questionable results generally require repeated testing. Positive results require a more comprehensive diagnostic workup. As with any test, false-positive or false-negative results may occur.

Isoniazid prophylaxis is used only in high-risk groups because it may cause serious hepatic damage. High-risk groups include

1. household members or other close contacts of a patient with active TB;
2. positive skin test reactors who are less than 35 years of age; and
3. positive skin test reactors who are receiving immunosuppressive therapy or who have leukemia or Hodgkin's disease.

Treatment

When INH is used to treat clinical TB, it is usually used in combination with other antitubercular agents. Treatment varies according to the severity of illness, the susceptibility of the organism to a specific agent, and the individual practitioner's preference. The most widely used regimen is a combination of the first-line agents, INH and rifampin, both given daily. Another combination frequently used is INH plus ethambutol. Either regimen is usually continued for 18 to 24 months.

Triple-drug therapy is used when the disease is extensive, extrapulmonary, or life-threatening. The triple-drug combinations used most often are isoniazid-ethambutol-rifampin or isoniazid-rifampin-pyrizinamide. Isoniazid and rifampin are considered to be first-line antitubercular agents. When a third drug is added, it is usually given only for the first 2 to 3 months of therapy.

Recent investigations suggest that a 9-month course of treatment with INH plus rifampin has been successful in adults with previously untreated, uncomplicated tuberculosis. After 2 months of daily therapy, patients who are unreliable in self-administering medications can be successfully treated with INH and rifampin on a twice-weekly basis under supervised conditions.

A fixed-dose combination product that contains 150 mg of INH plus 300 mg of rifampin (marketed as RIFAMATE) is available for patients who respond to separate administration of these two antitubercular drugs at dosages available in the proprietary product. It is not indicated for prophylactic use or to start treatment of symptomatic tuberculosis.

NURSING IMPLICATIONS

Oral INH preparations are best administered on an empty stomach at least 1 hour before or 2 hours after meals, and as a single daily dose. Advise the patient that intramuscular (IM) administration may cause pain or discomfort at the injection site. Reinforce the importance of continuous therapy for the prescribed period of time.

Side Effects. Adverse Reactions, and Contraindications

The most frequent side effects caused by INH (Table 57–S1) involve the nervous system. Dose-related peripheral neuropathy is the most common toxic effect; it results from the inhibition of pyridoxine's metabolism in nervous tissues. Neuropathy is manifested by numbness and tingling in the extremities, and occurs most frequently in malnourished, diabetic, and alcoholic patients. Neuropathy is easily treated with oral pyridoxine (vitamin B_6). Some practitioners advocate prophylaxis for patients at risk of developing neuropathy by initiating pyridoxine (25 mg/d) at the same time INH is started.

Hepatic side effects are common, especially with combination-drug antitubercular therapy. Approximately 10% to 15% of patients will exhibit signs of impaired liver function while receiving INH alone. The incidence of liver damage in patients on a combination of INH and rifampin increases approximately twofold. Patients receiving INH should undergo routine monitoring of liver function, including checking for discoloration of the skin and the sclera of the eye. Severe and sometimes fatal hepatitis may occur even after many months of therapy. Patients over 35 years of age and alcoholic patients are at the greatest risk of developing hepatitis. Any patient with a history of INH-induced hepatic injury should not be given INH again.

Hematologic abnormalities such as agranulocytosis, thrombocytopenia, and aplastic anemia have occurred. As with all antiinfective agents, allergic responses can occur, usually manifested as skin eruptions and fever. Isoniazid is contraindicated in patients with a history of hypersensitivity or allergy to this drug.

Nausea and vomiting occur from gastric irritation. The incidence can be reduced by giving INH with meals or by dividing the total daily dose into three equal doses.

Endocrine disturbances such as hyperglycemia and gynecomastia have occurred.

NURSING IMPLICATIONS

Be aware that effective treatment of tuberculosis is prolonged and often requires combination therapy. Both these factors increase the risk of side effects and create compliance problems.

Patients who have demonstrated compliance problems with their drug regimen may benefit from higher doses administered two or three times per week under supervision. The higher doses given may also predispose patients to particular types of side effects. When appropriate, use of the fixed-dose INH-rifampin product may improve compliance.

Monitor patients' liver function tests periodically during INH therapy. The onset of scleral discoloration may be the first sign of liver damage. Assess for and instruct the patient to report loss of appetite, fatigue, malaise, weakness, darkening of urine, or nausea and vomiting. Have patients weigh themselves weekly and report any significant weight loss.

◆ Use During Pregnancy and Lactation

Prophylactic therapy in the mother should be weighed against possible risks to the fetus. Chemoprophylaxis may be indicated during pregnancy if the woman is a recent tuberculin converter or tuberculin reactor with inactive disease. All other pregnant women who are candidates for therapy should be treated during the postpartum period. Breast-fed infants should be observed for adverse effects.

◆ Use in the Elderly

The risk of severe and sometimes fatal hepatitis is highest in patients 50 to 64 years old.

Interactions with Other Drugs

The primary interactions involving isoniazid are summarized in Table 57–I1. Isoniazid may increase the effects of the anticonvulsants phenytoin and carbamazepine by decreasing their metabolism. Corticosteroids may increase INH clearance. Combinations of INH and rifampin can increase the risk of hepatotoxicity. Isoniazid may act as an MAO inhibitor, causing a hypertensive crisis in the presence of foods or drugs that have sympathomimetic activity. (See Chapter 00 for more information about MAO inhibitors.)

NURSING IMPLICATIONS

Instruct patients to avoid tyramine-rich foods (for example, cheddar cheese, fermented sausages, yeast extracts, and red wines).

Overdose and Toxicity

Isoniazid overdose results in nausea, vomiting, slurred speech, and visual disturbances. Large overdoses can result in respiratory and CNS depression. Seizures have occurred with INH doses over 80 mg/kg.

Other Antitubercular Drugs

Several other drugs are used, usually along with INH, for prophylaxis or treatment of TB. The dosages of these agents are summarized in Table 57–C1, and side effects and contraindications in Table 57–S1; important interactions with other drugs are noted in Table 57–I1. Rifampin is considered by most authorities to be a first-line adjunct to INH. Second-line drugs are ethambutol, pyrazinamide, and streptomycin. The remainder are generally used for patients who have failed to respond to preferred drugs.

First-Line Antitubercular Drug

Rifampin

Rifampin (RIFADIN; RIMACTANE) is also a first-line drug for initial therapy of symptomatic TB. It is always given with other antitubercular agents (usually isoniazid, ethambutol, or both). The drug can be given orally (on an empty stomach) or by IM or IV injection.

Rifampin also has excellent activity against *Staphylococcus aureus* and *Neisseria meningitidis*. It has been used prophylactically to prevent the spread of meningococcal meningitis, but is not indicated for the treatment of active infection because resistance occurs quickly. Rifampin has also been used in combination with vancomycin to treat infections caused by methicillin-resistant *Staph. aureus*.

The most frequent side effects associated with rifampin are GI disturbances. Headache, drowsiness, dizziness, visual disturbances, and fever have also occurred, especially during the first weeks of therapy. Rifampin and its metabolites will impart a red-orange color to urine, feces, sputum, tears, and sweat; it is important to warn the patient that this may occur and that it is not serious. However, soft contact lenses may be permanently discolored. Rifampin has caused elevations in the serum levels of liver enzymes and bilirubin. Hypersensitivity or true allergic reactions are characterized by a flu-like syndrome, with occasional thrombocytopenia and hemolytic anemia. They are usually associated with high-dose intermittent therapy.

Rifampin interacts with many drugs (see Table 57–I1), because it stimulates the liver's microsomal drug-metabolizing enzymes. The usual result is diminished blood levels and activities of other drugs that are inactivated in the liver. Interactions with oral anticoagulants, systemic corticosteroids, digitoxin, oral contraceptives, and certain β-adrenergic blockers are particularly important.

Second-Line Antitubercular Drugs

Ethambutol

Ethambutol (MYAMBUTOL) is an orally effective drug used in the initial therapy of TB, in combination with the first-line agents INH and rifampin. Ethambutol is typically added as a third agent in situations where resistant organisms are suspected, such as when the patient has immigrated from or resides in an area of high-level drug resistance, or has a history of previous TB treatment.

Ethambutol may cause ophthalmic disorders, especially optic neuritis that manifests as changes in visual acuity or color perception. The severity of the neuritis is related to the dosage and the duration of therapy. Patients who receive ethambutol should undergo monthly tests for visual acuity. Instruct patients to inform their physician if any change in visual or color perception (eg, red-green color blindness) is noticed. Other side effects include dermatitis, headache, and GI disturbances.

Ethambutol should be used with caution in patients with impaired renal function and in patients with a history of ocular defects (for example, cataracts or diabetic retinopathy). The safe use of ethambutol in pregnancy has not been established. The drug is not recommended for use in children under 13 years of age.

Pyrazinamide

Pyrazinamide can be combined with first-line agents when a highly resistant organism is suspected. It is always used with at least one other antitubercular agent. It is given orally.

One of pyrazinamide's principal adverse effects is hepatotoxicity. It appears to be dose-related, and may vary from mild, abnormal hepatic cell function evidenced only by elevated hepatic enzymes, to a progressive fulminating jaundice and death. Pyrazinamide should never be used in the presence of existing hepatic damage.

Another major adverse effect of this agent is an elevation of uric acid levels, leading to acute gouty attacks. Use it with caution in patients with history of gout.

Streptomycin

Streptomycin, an aminoglycoside antibiotic, is used in the initial treatment of tuberculosis when resistance is suspected or when the disease is considered severe. The drug is given by IM injection two to three times per week, adjusted for age and renal function. See Chapter 55 (p 1184) for more information.

Third-Line Antitubercular Drugs

Aminosalicylate Sodium

Aminosalicylate ("PAS"; P.A.S.; TEEBACIN) is used in cases of documented resistance or when specific contraindications to other agents exist. It is always given in combination with other agents. It should be taken with meals to avoid the common complaint of GI upset.

Powder and tablet forms are unstable under certain temperatures, moisture, and light conditions. The drug should not be given if purplish or brownish. If aminosalicylic acid is used with rifampin, doses of each agent should be separated by at least 8 hours, as PAS will inhibit rifampin absorption. Aminosalicylate sodium may inhibit the absorption of iron, folic acid, and vitamin B_{12}, requiring supplemental administration of one or more of these compounds. Hypersensitivity or allergic reactions, including fever, urticaria, and pruritus, have been reported.

Capreomycin

Capreomycin (CAPASTAT) is used to treat pulmonary TB when other agents fail. It is administered by deep IM injection daily during the acute stages of the infection. Thereafter, it can be given two to three times per week. Nephrotoxicity and ototoxicity are the major side effects. Acute renal tubular necrosis occurs frequently.

Cycloserine

Cycloserine (SEROMYCIN) is used in combination with other antitubercular agents in documented cases of treatment failure or in infections caused by unusual strains of *Mycobacterium*. This agent is given once a day; doses should be reduced by 50% to 75% in patients with renal impairment.

Central nervous system toxicity, manifested by psychoses, delirium, confusion, headache, and seizures, is a concern with cycloserine use; the risk of toxicity is increased when cycloserine is administered together with INH. The addition of pyridoxine may minimize these effects.

Ethionamide

Ethionamide (TRECATOR-S.C.) is used to treat TB that has failed to respond to treatment with standard agents. It should be taken with food if GI upset is a problem. Many patients are bothered by the drug's metallic taste. Hepatitis occurs in 5% of patients taking ethionamide; therefore, it should be used with caution in patients with liver dysfunction. Peripheral neuropathies similar to those caused by INH have occurred. The neurotoxic effect is enhanced by INH or cycloserine; therefore, such combinations should be used cautiously. The prophylactic use of pyridoxine is recommended.

II. Miscellaneous Urinary Tract Antiinfective Agents

The agents discussed in this section include miscellaneous antimicrobials that are used mainly for urinary tract infections (UTIs). Their use is usually limited to prophylactic therapy in patients with chronic UTI to reduce recurrent infections. Because these agents are not structurally similar, no prototype agent is identified. The sulfonamide antibiotics, also widely used for treating UTIs, were discussed in Chapter 56.

Effective use of any of the urinary antiinfectives for a chronic UTI may require therapy lasting 6 months to a year. Encourage patients to remain compliant with the prescribed regimen and to take doses at times that are easily identifiable, such as with meals and at bedtime.

Methenamine

Methenamine (MANDELAMINE; HIPREX) exerts its antibacterial effect by being hydrolyzed to formaldehyde in the presence of acidic urine. Optimal hydrolysis and antibacterial activity occur when the urine pH is 5.5 or less. The drug is not effective in alkaline urine.

Methenamine (and formaldehyde) are bactericidal. The drug is effective against most gram-positive and gram-negative organisms, including *Escherichia coli, Proteus, Klebsiella,* and *Pseudomonas.* Methenamine is readily absorbed from the GI tract, but is ineffective in the treatment of systemic infections because insignificant amounts of formaldehyde reach the circulatory system.

Methenamine is available as the hippurate salt or as the shorter-acting mandelate salt. Also available are fixed-dose combination products containing a methenamine salt and antispasmodics (belladonna alkaloids), analgesics (salicylates or phenazopyridine), or urinary acidifiers (sodium or potassium phosphates). The inclusion of a urinary acidifier in some of these products attests to the fact that urine pH must be low for methenamine to work.

Methenamine, and products containing it, are used for prophylaxis or chronic suppression of recurrent UTIs. They are less toxic than alternatives such as co-trimoxazole or single-entity sulfonamides (see Chapter 56), and so are particularly useful for patients requiring long-term therapy. The drug is administered orally. Typical dosages are summarized in Table 57–C2. Refer to manufacturers' data or other references for dosages of the many methenamine-containing proprietary products.

The most common adverse effects (Table 57–S2) of methenamine are GI disturbances; nausea, vomiting, and diarrhea, probably owing to formation of small amounts of formaldehyde. Administration of the drug with meals, or use of methenamine mandelate enteric-coated tablets, will minimize this unwanted reaction.

Hypersensitivity reactions are rare. Methenamine hippurate tablets contain tartrazine dye, which can cause allergic reactions, especially in patients with asthma.

Methenamine is relatively contraindicated in patients with renal or hepatic impairment, gout, and severe dehydration. Its safe use during pregnancy has not been established. Foods or drugs that alkalinize the urine (milk and citrus products; sodium bicarbonate; acetazolamide) will antagonize the effects of methenamine and should be avoided. Ordinarily, sulfonamides should not be used concomitantly.

Acidifying the urine to maximize the effects of methenamine will increase the risk of sulfonamide-induced crystalluria; conversely, alkalinizing the urine to prevent crystalluria will antagonize the effects of methenamine.

NURSING IMPLICATIONS

Measure urine pH before administering methenamine. If it is 5 or less, it is not necessary to add a urine-acidifying agent. If urine acidification is necessary and a product that lacks an acidifying substance has been prescribed, cranberry juice taken once or twice a day is an excellent way to reduce urine pH. Instruct patients to avoid excessive intake of fruits, juices (other than cranberry), and milk products that may alkalinize the urine (Table 57–I2). Methenamine should be taken with food to minimize GI upset.

Assess patients for a history of tartrazine dye allergy or asthma before administering methenamine hippurate.

Methenamine mandelate oral suspensions are formulated in a vegetable oil base. Because of the risk of aspiration and resulting lipid pneumonitis, such products should be used with great care, if at all, in children, debilitated patients, or the elderly.

Nalidixic Acid

Nalidixic acid (NEGGRAM) is used to treat or prevent UTIs caused by gram-negative organisms. Its spectrum of activity includes *E. coli, Klebsiella, Proteus,* and *Enterobacter* (see Table 57–C2).

Nalidixic acid is used only to treat chronic UTIs caused by susceptible organisms. Its clinical utility is severely limited by many side effects and the rapid development of resistant organisms.

Nitrofurantoin

Nitrofurantoin is effective in UTIs caused by susceptible gram-negative and gram-positive organisms, including *E. coli, Klebsiella, Enterobacter,* and *Enterococcus.*

Nitrofurantoin is available in microcrystal and macrocrystal formulations (FURADANTIN; MACRODANTIN, respectively) for oral administration. The macrocrystal is simply a larger size particle that allows for a slower dissolution and absorption, which will minimize GI upset. The macrocrystal formulation is therefore preferred. The microcrystal formulation is rarely used unless an oral suspension is needed.

Nitrofurantoin has been used to treat both acute and chronic UTIs. In the initial treatment of UTI it is usually reserved for patients with an allergic history to the penicillins, cephalosporins, and sulfonamides. Nitrofurantoin is not effective in the treatment of systemic infections, because it concentrates in the urine and does not reach adequate serum concentrations. Dosages are summarized in Table 57–C2.

The side effects of nitrofurantoin are summarized in Table 57–S2. Gastrointestinal upset is the most frequent adverse effect. It can be minimized by use of the macrocrystal product and by taking the drug with food. Reducing the dose may also help.

Peripheral neuropathies have occurred and can be severe. Symptoms include paresthesia of the lower extremities, which may lead to muscle weakness and eventually muscle wasting. Elderly patients, patients with renal impairment, and diabetics may be predisposed to this reaction. Significant renal dysfunction contraindicates nitrofurantoin use.

Nitrofurantoin can cause acute or chronic pulmonary reactions. Acute reactions involve sudden dyspnea, chills, chest pain, fever, and cough and are sometimes mistaken for the flu. Skin reactions such as urticaria and pruritus may accompany the pulmonary effects. The reaction may occur immediately in patients sensitized by prior nitrofurantoin administration, or may occur after approximately 3 weeks in a patient receiving the drug for the first time. Chronic pulmonary reactions occur in patients receiving chronic nitrofurantoin therapy for 6 months or more.

NURSING IMPLICATIONS

Use nitrofurantoin cautiously in patients with renal impairment, diabetes, or other debilitating diseases that increase the risk of peripheral neuropathies. Monitor patients receiving chronic nitrofurantoin therapy for pulmonary reactions.

Question patients who have previously received nitrofurantoin about prior pulmonary reactions or the onset of flu-like symptoms. Instruct patients to recognize the onset of these symptoms and to immediately discontinue the use of this drug and notify their physician.

Withhold nitrofurantoin and notify the physician if the patient reports numbness, tingling, or weakness in the extremities.

Check with the physician regarding fluid intake. Drug effectiveness depends on drug concentration in the urine, which may be diminished by forcing fluids. Advise patients that brown or rust-yellow coloring of the urine is not harmful, and is expected.

Trimethoprim

Trimethoprim (PROLOPRIM; TRIMPEX) is an antiinfective that is active against most common gram-negative organisms, including *Acinetobacter, Enterobacter, E. coli, Klebsiella,* and *Proteus.* It acts by interfering with folic acid synthesis in susceptible bacteria. The drug was mentioned in Chapter 56 as an ingredient in co-trimoxazole, which also contains the sulfonamide sulfamethoxazole.

Trimethoprim is almost completely absorbed from the GI tract. The drug is metabolized in the liver and is excreted in the urine as metabolites and active drug. It is widely distributed throughout the body. High concentrations are found in the prostate gland.

Trimethoprim is indicated for the treatment and prevention of acute and chronic UTIs in both men and women (see Table 57–C2). It has been particularly effective in the treatment and prevention of recurrent UTIs in men, which are usually caused by chronic prostate infections.

Allergic reactions, usually a rash or pruritus, are the most frequently reported side effects (see Table 57–S2). Occasional GI disturbances have also been reported. Trimethoprim, used alone or in combination products such as co-trimoxazole (see Chapter 56, p 1193, and Table 56–C6), may elevate blood levels of phenytoin and related hydantoin anticonvulsants. If combined therapy is essential, monitor for evidence of the interaction (eg, excessive sedation or ataxia; increased serum anticonvulsant levels).

III. Antifungal Agents

Systemic fungal infections are relatively rare compared with bacterial infections. However, fungal infections can be difficult to treat; they typically appear in patients who are immunosuppressed, especially patients with AIDS or organ transplant recipients. Fortunately, a number of antimicrobial agents are effective against a wide variety of infections caused by pathogenic fungi. Mucocutaneous fungal infections are much more common. Vaginal fungal infections occur more frequently than other types of vaginal infection, especially in sexually active women during childbearing years and in diabetic or prediabetic women. Table 57–C3 summarizes the antifungal drugs and their key properties and dosages.

PROTOTYPE

Amphotericin B

The prototype agent for this group of antimicrobials is amphotericin B (FUNGIZONE), not only because it is considered the drug of choice for many severe systemic fungal infections, but also because proper use requires a considerable number of nursing interventions owing to its toxic effects.

Absorption, Distribution, Metabolism, and Excretion

Amphotericin B is poorly absorbed when taken orally and is therefore given only IV or topically. Very little is known about its biologic fate. Small amounts of the drug are excreted in the urine, even several weeks after the drug is discontinued.

Pharmacologic Effects

Amphotericin B can be either fungistatic or fungicidal, depending on the susceptible organism and the drug concentration. Amphotericin B works by binding to sterols in the fungal cell membrane, which alters cell wall permeability.

Clinical Indications and Administration

Amphotericin B, given IV, is considered the drug of choice for treating most systemic fungal infections, including aspergillosis, blastomycosis, *Candida,* coccidiomycoses, cryptococcosis, and histoplasmosis. However, the drug is very toxic when given by injection, and so should be used primarily for treating progressive and potentially fatal infections. Topical amphotericin B is used to treat mucocutaneous *Candida* infections, but other topical antifungals are prescribed more frequently.

The IV dosages (Table 57–C3) and administration methods for amphotericin B are designed to minimize the drug's toxicities. The overall approach is to first administer a small test dose to assess the patient's ability to tolerate it. Therapy then continues daily with incremental dosage increases until a maximum daily dose of 1 mg/kg is reached. This dose is continued for the duration of treatment. Each dose must be infused slowly, ideally over 4 to 6 hours, to reduce untoward responses further. If the patient tolerates the drug well, the infusion time can be shortened to a minimum of 30 minutes. Patients who develop severe renal impairment (discussed later) may require alternate-day dosing with 1.5 mg/kg.

Most fungal infections respond slowly to amphotericin B, and require a total (cumulative) dose of 2 to 4 g. Since the daily dosage must be increased gradually to minimize toxicity, the entire treatment course can be lengthy—4 to 8 weeks.

NURSING IMPLICATIONS

Use strict aseptic technique to prepare and handle parenteral amphotericin B. The drug contains no preservative or bacteriostatic agent. Do not use an in-line filter when reconstituting the drug, because the filter will remove drug particles. Reconstitute the drug only with preservative-free sterile water to prevent precipitation. Dilute the reconstituted drug in 5% dextrose only. An in-line filter can be used for the IV infusion (mean pore diameter must be at least 1.0 μm), and an infusion pump is recommended. Amphotericin B is light-sensitive: protect the solution from light during administration.

Side Effects, Adverse Reactions, and Contraindications

Parenteral amphotericin B has a significant side effect profile (Table 57–S3). Many of the untoward responses occur acutely during drug infusion; others are more common with long-term therapy. All require frequent monitoring and appropriate interventions. They underscore the need to avoid using parenteral amphotericin B unless a fungal infection is strongly suspected or documented, the patient can receive close medical supervision, and the patient's prognosis is poor unless the drug is given.

Almost all patients will experience a combination of the following side effects on initial administration of amphotericin B: headache, chills, fever, malaise, muscle and joint pain, anorexia, weight loss, nausea, and vomiting. The cause of these reactions is unknown. The febrile reaction and shaking chills can be quite dramatic and cause a great deal of stress for the patient and the nurse. Severe reactions may require stopping the infusion until it subsides. Premedicating the patient approximately 30 minutes before the infusion begins may minimize these reactions in some patients. A wide variety of premedications has been used, including aspirin, acetaminophen, diphenhydramine, meperidine, and corticosteroids. Not exceeding the recommended infusion rate also reduces the incidence of fever and chills. The reaction will often diminish as therapy is continued.

Intravenous amphotericin B can cause severe thrombophlebitis at the injection site. When possible, administration through a central line is preferred. If a peripheral line is used, the use of a scalp vein needle, frequent change of injection sites, or the addition of small amounts of heparin to the solution may be helpful.

SPOTLIGHT ON NURSING RESEARCH

Most adults receiving amphotericin B for systemic fungal infections experience uncontrollable shivering that produces discomfort, exhaustion, and dread of future therapy. Intravenous meperidine is used to suppress shivering but may lead to additional problems including dizziness, respiratory depression, nausea, and hypotension. This study examined the effectiveness of extremity wraps as a nursing intervention to reduce the incidence, intensity, and duration of amphotericin B-induced shivering in 40 adult cancer patients who had previously experienced this side effect. As a pyrogen, amphotericin B elevates the thermostatic set point. This elevation increases the gradient between skin and set point temperatures, providing a stimulus for febrile shivering. In this study, it was postulated that protection of skin sensors from heat loss with extremity wraps would reduce the stimulus for shivering.

Subjects that gave informed consent to participate were randomly assigned to treatment or control groups. Prior to amphotericin B infusion, the extremities of treatment group subjects were wrapped with terry cloth towels from groin to toes and from the axilla to fingertips. All subjects were monitored using the same protocol by trained data collectors, and routine care, which included the use of intravenous meperidine, was given by the nursing staff.

Visual and tactile observations of shivering were scored on a rank ordered scale. The scale of shivering stages ranged from stage zero, which represented no shivering, to stage 4, which denoted strong generalized contractions including extremities. Subjects were observed continuously throughout the 3 to 5 hour infusion period, and the time of each shivering episode was carefully recorded.

The occurrence of shivering activity during amphotericin B infusion varied, but 78% of all subjects experienced symptoms ranging from mild masseter tremors to generalized rigors. Shivering was less intense among the treatment group. Only 9 of 20 treatment group subjects as compared to 17 of 20 control group subjects experienced severe shivering (stages 3 and 4). The total duration of shivering was also significantly less, with a mean duration of 10.95 minutes in the treatment group versus 21.95 minutes in the control group. Although treatment group subjects tended to receive less meperidine, the total amount of meperidine received did not differ significantly between treatment (mean = 50 mg) and control (mean = 68.75 mg) groups.

The results of this study suggest that extremity wraps may reduce incidence, intensity, and duration of shivering induced by amphotericin B therapy. Although the use of extremity wraps did not reduce the administration of intravenous meperidine, anecdotal data indicated that nurses often gave intravenous meperidine as a premedication for anxiety or general discomfort rather than as a specific treatment for drug-induced shivering.

As the author notes, the ability to make generalizations from the present work are limited by small sample size, and by lack of standardization in amphotericin B dosage and meperidine administration. However, pilot work done on a small scale can provide important information to justify and to refine subsequent investigation. Currently, a major study is in progress that will provide further evaluation of the effectiveness of extremity wraps as a low cost nursing intervention to reduce amphotericin B-induced shivering.

Holtzclaw BJ: Effects of extremity wraps to control drug-induced shivering: A pilot study. *Nurs Res* 1990; 39:280–283.

Nephrotoxicity will occur in most patients, to some degree, as therapy continues. This will elevate BUN and serum creatinine levels, and may cause severe hypomagnesemia and renal tubular acidosis. Significant hypokalemia almost always occurs. Renal damage is related to the total dose received during a course of therapy. Renal function usually improves within a few months after therapy is completed, although some permanent damage will remain. The nephrotoxic risk may be reduced by slowly titrating the daily dose to the 1 mg/kg maximum. Alternate-day dosing can be used for patients who have evidence of renal damage but require continued treatment. Recently, the use of pentoxyfylline (Chapter 35) has shown some promise in reversing renal damage.

Monitor serum potassium and magnesium levels closely. A significant decrease in both electrolytes is common. Large amounts of potassium supplements, as much as 100 to 200 mEq/d, may be necessary to keep potassium levels near normal.

A normocytic, normochromic anemia occurs in most patients who receive long-term amphotericin B. This anemia is reversible when therapy is completed, although transfusions of packed red cells are occasionally necessary.

Cardiovascular toxicities, such as hypotension, ventricular fibrillation, and even cardiac arrest, are rare and are usually associated with rapid drug administration. However, hypokalemia increases the risk of cardiac complications.

NURSING IMPLICATIONS

Become familiar with the proper administration procedures, and the potential untoward effects, to help make parenteral amphotericin B therapy more tolerable and safer for the patient. Be sure that any pretreatment medication orders have been written and carried out before giving amphotericin B. Consult with the physician first to determine the preferred intervention(s) to be used in the event of a serious adverse reaction.

Administer IV amphotericin B over a minimum of 4 hours to reduce the incidence of fever, chills, and cardiovascular problems. If the drug cannot be given via a central line, check frequently for the development of phlebitis at and near the injection site.

Monitor temperature and all vital signs regularly, at at least 1- to 2-hour intervals, and especially during the test and first therapeutic doses. Monitor red cell counts, renal function, and serum electrolyte levels routinely during parenteral amphotericin therapy. In particular, anticipate and assess for hypomagnesemia and hypokalemia, based on both blood tests and signs and symptoms of these electrolyte deficiencies (for example, muscle weakness, lethargy, confusion, electrocardiographic or other cardiac irregularities). Anticipate the need for daily potassium supplementation to prevent symptomatic hypokalemia.

Interactions with Other Drugs

Table 57–I3 summarizes the major interactions between amphotericin B and other drugs. The most important concerns arise from combined use with other nephrotoxic drugs (for example, flucytosine or aminoglycoside antibiotics), other potassium-depleting drugs (systemic corticosteroids, potassium-wasting diuretics), and drugs for which toxicity is increased by hypokalemia (digitalis, neuromuscular blockers, and skeletal muscle relaxants). Amphotericin B is physically incompatible with most other drugs, and so should not be admixed with them (except with small amounts of heparin, as discussed earlier).

Other Antifungal Drugs

Other antifungal drugs are generally less toxic than amphotericin B. They are used mainly when the risks of using the prototype clearly outweigh the likely benefits. Some are used instead of amphotericin B, and others are used adjunctively. Dosages are summarized in Table 57–C3; side effects and contraindications are listed in Table 57–S3; and important drug interactions are noted in Table 57–I3.

Clotrimazole

Clotrimazole is a broad-spectrum antifungal drug. It is poorly absorbed from the GI tract, and is used only for local effects.

Clotrimazole oral lozenges (MYCELEX) are used to treat oropharyngeal candidiasis. Clotrimazole solution, lotion, or cream (LOTRIMIN; others) are indicated for treating various cutaneous worm infestations such as tinea versicolor. Vaginal creams and tablets are available for treating vaginal candidiasis. Several clotrimazole products for cutaneous uses are available over-the-counter.

NURSING IMPLICATIONS

Forewarn patients that clotrimazole lozenges have an unpleasant taste, yet they must be allowed to dissolve slowly in the mouth, over about 15 to 30 minutes, to obtain the maximum effect. Discourage patients from chewing or swallowing the product.

Fluconazole

Fluconazole (DIFLUCAN) is a broad-spectrum antifungal agent that is effective when given by oral or IV routes. The drug is widely distributed to most body tissues, including the cerebrospinal fluid. Oral fluconazole is almost completely absorbed from the GI tract. Oral administration is always preferred over the IV route if the patient can tolerate oral medications.

Fluconazole has been used primarily in the treatment of oropharyngeal candidiasis in immunocompromised adults with AIDS or malignancy; and has been used in combination with amphotericin B to treat *Cryptococcal neoformans* meningitis, which has been found in patients with AIDS. It has also been used as long-term maintenance therapy, since the incidence of relapse of cryptococcal meningitis is high. Because fluconazole causes fewer side effects than IV amphotericin B, it should be considered the drug of choice for susceptible fungal infections that can be treated orally.

Fluconazole is very well tolerated. Common side effects include nausea, vomiting, rash, and mild elevations in liver enzymes. It is currently not recommended for use in children because of limited safety data. Fluconazole can potentially interact with other drugs that undergo extensive liver metabolism, such as oral anticoagulants and hypoglycemics.

Flucytosine

Flucytosine (ANCOBON) is an orally effective antifungal agent. The drug is well absorbed from the GI tract and is widely distributed in various body tissues.

Flucytosine's main use is in combination with amphotericin B to treat meningitis caused by *Cryptococcus neoformans*. It is also an alternate choice for the treatment of serious *Candida* infections that may be unresponsive to amphotericin B.

Although less toxic than amphotericin B, flucytosine does cause some serious side effects. Adverse GI effects include nausea, vomiting, diarrhea, and abdominal bloating. Bone marrow depression, resulting in leukopenia, anemia, or thrombocytopenia, severely limits this drug's effectiveness. Complete blood counts should be frequently monitored.

The patient may need to take as many as eight or ten flucytosine capsules at one time, despite the obvious inconvenience and uncertainty of taking so many at once. Advise the patient that such doses are correct. If the patient has difficulty swallowing the tablets, prepare a suspension from the capsules.

Flucytosine is teratogenic. It should not be administered to pregnant women or to women in their childbearing years.

Griseofulvin

Griseofulvin (GRISACTIN; others) is used to treat some common fungal disorders of the skin. It is primarily reserved for treating ringworm infestations caused by susceptible organisms that may not be responsive to topical antifungal agents. It is especially effective for fungal infections involving the keratinized structures (primarily the nails, soles, and palms). Treatment of fungal nail infection may require therapy for as long as 1 year.

Griseofulvin is administered orally. The drug has been formulated as microsize and ultramicrosize preparations, which enhance absorption.

Griseofulvin seldom causes serious side effects. Headache occurs frequently, especially during early therapy. Gastrointestinal side effects, such as nausea and vomiting, may also occur. Encourage patients to take the drug on a full stomach to increase absorption.

Itraconazole

Itraconazole (SPORANOX) is a broad-spectrum antifungal agent that is only administered by the oral route. It should be administered with food. While effective against many superficial and systemic fungal infections, it appears particularly useful in neutropenic and immunosuppressed patients with systemic fungal infections, especially aspergillus.

Common side effects include gastrointestinal distress, headache, and rash. It is currently not recommended for use in children because of limited data.

Itraconazole drug interactions are not yet well defined, but appear to be similar to fluconazole. It should not be used with terfenidine because of potential cardiovascular toxicity.

Ketoconazole

Ketoconazole (NIZORAL) is active against most pathogenic fungi and has been used for a wide variety of infections in which oral administration is preferred. The drug is also available as a topical cream.

The most frequent side effects associated with ketoconazole are nausea and vomiting. The drug can inhibit testosterone synthesis at high doses: decreased libido, impotence, gynecomastia, and decreased sperm counts have been reported in males who have received chronic, high-dose therapy. Hepatotoxicity is rare and usually reversible. Several cases of ketoconazole-induced hepatitis have been reported in children. It is important to note that ketoconazole requires gastric acidity in order to be dissolved and absorbed. Therefore, any drug that raises gastric pH, such as antacids or H_2 antagonists such as cimetidine, will significantly decrease absorption. Ketoconazole should not be used in elderly patients since a significant number of patients may experience achlorhydria (low gastric acid output).

Patients with a history of liver disease or who are receiving other hepatotoxic agents should not receive ketoconazole therapy unless absolutely necessary. The drug is teratogenic in rats, therefore, its use in pregnant females should be considered only if the benefits outweigh the potential risks.

Miconazole

Miconazole (MONISTAT) is structurally related to ketoconazole. Like ketoconazole, it is active against a wide variety of fungi. Its primary use is to treat vaginal candidiasis, for which it is administered as a vaginal cream or suppository. Miconazole is also available in an IV formulation for systemic fungal infections that are unresponsive to amphotericin B, or as an alternate choice for patients who cannot tolerate amphotericin B. Topical creams, powders, and lotions (eg, MICATIN) are available over-the-counter to treat athlete's foot, jock itch, and ringworm infestations.

Topical miconazole is relatively free of side effects, although some local irritation may occur. Intravenous administration can cause thrombophlebitis. Anaphylaxis and cardiac or respiratory arrest can occur if the drug is administered rapidly. This reaction is most likely caused by the preservative in the IV preparation rather than by the drug itself. A test dose should be administered to determine the patient's tolerance of the drug.

Nystatin

Nystatin (MYCOSTATIN; others) is used primarily as a topical agent to treat *Candida* infections. It is available as an oral suspension, pastille (lozenge), tablet, vaginal suppository, and a topical cream.

Because the drug is poorly absorbed, it should not be used to treat systemic fungal infections. However, the lack of absorption makes oral nystatin useful for treating intestinal candidiasis. The oral suspension is frequently used as treatment or prophylaxis of oral candidiasis, which often develops in patients who are receiving immunosuppressive therapy. The infection usually involves the oral mucosa and esophagus, resulting in lesions that can be extremely painful. Instruct patients to use the suspension as a mouthwash, swishing thoroughly in order to coat the mouth, then swallowing to protect the esophagus. The suspension may be placed directly on the lesions with a cotton swab if the patient is unable to cooperate with instructions. The taste of oral preparations often makes compliance a problem.

Topical nystatin cream is used to treat superficial fungal infections of the skin.

Adverse reactions are rare with topical nystatin, although occasional GI upset may occur with high doses.

Tolnaftate

Tolnaftate (TINACTIN) is available as an over-the-counter product and is used in the treatment of athlete's foot, jock itch, and ringworm. It is available as a topical cream, spray, lotion, or powder. It has minimal side effects, although local irritation may occur.

IV. Antiviral Agents

The viruses are a diverse group of organisms that can cause illnesses as minor as the common cold or as serious as acquired immunodeficiency syndrome (AIDS).

Chemotherapy against viral diseases has been much less successful than against bacterial diseases. The difficulty in treating viral disease is due to the facts that the virus inhabits the host cell and that viral replication is usually complete before clinical symptoms appear. In addition, many viral infections are self-limiting and do not require chemotherapy. The exception is in the immunocompromised host, in whom untreated viral infections can be fatal.

Most drugs capable of viracidal action would also kill host cells. For this reason specific antiviral agents that inhibit the viral replication process were developed.

Many different antiviral agents are available, and it is difficult to identify a prototype. Acyclovir is considered to be one of the most useful drugs in treating selected viral diseases and so will be discussed in depth.

PROTOTYPE

Acyclovir

Acyclovir (ZOVIRAX) inhibits many viruses, but its principal clinical use is against herpes simplex virus types 1 and 2 (HSV1 and HSV2) and herpes zoster (shingles). Acyclovir is considered to be the most effective antiviral agent for the treatment of serious herpes infections, and it has gained widespread use.

Absorption, Distribution, Metabolism, and Excretion

Acyclovir is available in topical, parenteral, and oral preparations. The oral form is slowly and incompletely absorbed from the GI tract, reaching peak serum levels in about two hours. Less than one third of an oral dose is absorbed. The absorption is not altered by food. Acyclovir that reaches the bloodstream is eliminated unchanged, mainly by renal excretion. Topical dosage forms are not absorbed appreciably.

Pharmacologic Effects

Although metabolism is not important for eliminating acyclovir from the body, it has an important role in the drug's viracidal actions. Acyclovir is preferentially taken up by cells infected with the herpes simplex virus. The drug then passes into the viruses themselves, where it is converted to an active cytotoxic metabolite, acyclovir triphosphate, a nucleotide analogue. The metabolite acts mainly by inhibiting viral DNA polymerase and DNA replication. Acyclovir's preferential uptake and metabolism in infected cells accounts for its selective antiviral action, and therefore its relatively lesser toxicity for noninfected human cells.

Clinical Indications and Administration

Acyclovir is the drug of choice for the treatment of infections caused by herpes simplex (Table 57–C4). Acyclovir decreases the severity and duration of herpes infections. It is not a cure for herpes infections, and does not appear to reduce the incidence of recurrent herpes infections in most patients.

The parenteral (IV) formulation of acyclovir is used to treat initial and recurrent mucosal, cutaneous, and systemic HSV1 and HSV2 infections in immunocompromised patients, and in the initial treatment of severe episodes of genital herpes. Acyclovir should not be given as IM or SC injections because it can cause muscle necrosis.

Acyclovir is given orally in some patients for initial treatment and prevention of recurrent genital herpes infections. Patients are selected for oral therapy based on the severity of the disease and their ability to comply with the regimen. Chronic therapy for the prevention of recurrent disease lasts up to 6 months.

Topical therapy with acyclovir ointment is indicated for initial treatment of genital herpes infections.

Acyclovir has not been shown to be effective in the treatment or prevention of herpes labialis infections, also known as "cold sores." Widespread use of the drug for this indication should be discouraged because of the expense and the possibility of developing resistance.

NURSING IMPLICATIONS

Advise patients that although acyclovir decreases the severity and duration of genital herpes infections, it is not curative, and episodes may recur.

Administer IV acyclovir over at least 1 hour to prevent renal dysfunction and to minimize the occurrence of phlebitis. Concentrations of 7 mg/mL or lower are recommended. Check the infusion rate every 5 to 10 minutes if a rate-controlled infusion pump is not used.

Oral and topical acyclovir must be administered frequently while the patient is awake. Encourage patients to adhere strictly to the prescribed regimen to maximize the chance of a successful treatment outcome.

Apply topical acyclovir sparingly, directly on the lesions. Use a finger cot or rubber gloves to apply the ointment to prevent further spread of the infection.

Owing to the emotional involvement surrounding herpes infections, encourage patients to receive counseling regarding the disease itself.

Side Effects, Adverse Reactions, and Contraindications

Few side effects have been identified with acyclovir therapy (Table 57–S4). Renal dysfunction has been observed. It can be minimized by avoiding IV bolus administration and by ensuring adequate hydration of the patient, particularly within the first 2 hours following infusion, when urine concentration of the drug is the greatest. Patients who receive chronic acyclovir therapy frequently report headache. Nausea, vomiting, and diarrhea are common with oral therapy. Rare psychiatric and neurologic changes have occurred. Use acyclovir with caution in patients with either existing renal or CNS abnormalities. Acyclovir is contraindicated in patients with a history of hypersensitivity or allergy to it.

NURSING IMPLICATIONS

Measure fluid intake and output every 8 hours to coincide with each drug administration. Follow the prescriber's guidelines for ensuring adequate hydration to minimize nephrotoxicity (IV fluid volumes and delivery rates, for example). Be sure renal function tests are performed periodically. Assess frequently for acyclovir's common CNS and GI tract side effects.

◆ Use During Pregnancy and Lactation

Acyclovir should not be given by systemic routes to pregnant women unless the anticipated benefits outweigh potential risks to the fetus. It is not known whether acyclovir is excreted in breast milk; administer cautiously to women who wish to breast-feed their infants.

◆ Use in Children

The safety and efficacy of acyclovir for children have not been established.

Interactions with Other Drugs

Probenecid may decrease renal excretion of acyclovir, leading to a prolonged half-life and increased risk of side effects of the antiviral agent (Table 57–I4).

Overdose and Toxicity

The major risk of acyclovir overdose is renal damage caused by precipitation of the sparingly soluble drug in the urine. Renal damage is not likely to occur unless inappropriately high doses are given IV, especially to patients with renal dysfunction or dehydration, or if the drug is given too rapidly as an IV bolus (avoid). If there is evidence of renal damage (increased BUN or creatinine levels, diminished urine output), giving sufficient volumes of parenteral fluids to maintain brisk urine output should help. Otherwise, hemodialysis may be required to lower blood levels of the drug.

Other Antiviral Drugs

Amantadine

Amantadine (SYMMETREL) is active against influenza A virus. It is used in both the prevention and treatment of respiratory infections caused by this virus (see Table 57–C4). Amantadine is used most commonly in individuals who have not been immunized and are at high risk of serious morbidity from influenza, such as patients with pulmonary, metabolic, or cardiovascular disorders. It may also be given to immunized individuals who have impaired immune systems, to individuals who are otherwise healthy but are in frequent close contact with affected patients (eg, health-care personnel), or to patients in institutional settings, such as nursing homes, in which an outbreak of influenza A has occurred. Amantadine is also used to treat Parkinson's disease, as discussed in Chapter 25.

Amantadine is about 80% effective in preventing influenza A infections. If it is given 24 to 48 hours after the onset of symptoms, a reduction in symptoms will usually occur. Amantadine should be given as soon as possible after exposure and continued for 10 days. Treatment for up to 90 days has been used in patients when vaccination is not possible.

Most side effects associated with amantadine use are manifested as CNS or psychic disturbances; they are usually dose-related and are reversible (see Table 57–S4). Nervousness, irritability, fatigue, psychoses, confusion, slurred speech, and headache have all been reported. Patients who receive the drug for a prolonged period may experience a condition called *livedo reticularis,* a bluish mottling of the skin on the legs and arms. The side effects and nursing implications of amantadine are discussed further in Chapter 25.

Because of its multiple CNS toxicities, amantadine should not be used in patients with a history of psychiatric disturbances or epilepsy. Warn patients who receive amantadine of the various CNS side effects that may occur, and to avoid driving or operating heavy machinery.

Didanosine

Didanosine (VIDEX), commonly referred to as DDI, is used as an orally administered alternative to zidovudine in the treatment of the human immunodeficiency virus. It is used primarily in patients who are unable to tolerate, or have become refractory to, zidovudine. It has also been used in combination with zidovudine to allow the use of lower, better tolerated doses of the latter. Side effects include rash, oral mucositis, fever, and, rarely, pancreatitis.

Foscarnet

Foscarnet (FOSCAVIR) is active against many viruses, but is primarily used to treat AIDS-related retinitis caused by cytomegalovirus (CMV). It has also been used to treat other CMV infections, such as pneumonitis and gastroenteritis. Foscarnet is generally reserved to treat ganciclovir-resistant cases.

Foscarnet is given IV only, and it is relatively toxic. Some renal impairment will occur in most patients. Decreases in serum electrolytes (chiefly calcium, phosphate, magnesium, and potassium) have been observed and should be carefully monitored. The decrease in ionized calcium may be related to the drug's infusion rate. Monitor patients for signs and symptoms of tingling, numbness in the extremities, and possible tetany. Other side effects include possible seizures, anemia, and granulocytopenia.

Ganciclovir

Ganciclovir (CYTOVENE) is structurally related to acyclovir. It is active against many viruses. Its principle use is to treat CMV retinitis in patients with AIDS. It has also been successfully used to treat CMV pneumonitis and gastroenteritis. Ganciclovir may also be effective in treating herpes infections that are resistant to acyclovir.

Ganciclovir is poorly absorbed, and so it is administered by the IV route. Side effects are common and should be closely monitored. The most common side effects are neutropenia and thrombocytopenia. Central nervous system side effects range from headaches to seizures.

Ganciclovir is considered potentially carcinogenic and teratogenic. It should not be used in pregnancy, and appropriate antineoplastic precautions should be used to prepare and administer the drug.

Idoxuridine

Idoxuridine (STOXIL; HERPLEX) is a topical antiviral agent used to treat herpes simplex keratitis.

Ribavirin

Ribavirin (VIRAZOLE) is a relatively new antiviral agent used specifically for respiratory tract infections caused by respiratory syncytial virus (RSV) in infants and small children (see Table 57–C4). The drug is given as an inhaled aerosol using special nebulization equipment. Ribavirin can worsen the respiratory status of some patients. Ventilatory difficulties are especially problematic for patients requiring mechanical ventilation because the drug can precipitate in, and then occlude, the ventilator tubes. Ribavirin is very expensive and is reserved for treating documented RSV infections at medical centers with the proper nebulizing equipment.

Vidarabine

Vidarabine (VIRA-A) is an antiviral used primarily in the treatment of herpes simplex encephalitis. It is given IV for this indication (see Table 57–C4 for dosages). Clinical trials indicate that the response rate improves when the drug is administered as soon as the disease is suspected. For most cases, acyclovir is preferred to vidarabine. Vidarabine has been shown to be clinically useful in the treatment of herpes zoster infections in the immunocompromised host. Vidarabine is also available as an ophthalmic ointment for the treatment of herpes simplex keratitis and keratoconjunctivitis.

The most common side effects associated with parenteral vidarabine are nausea, vomiting, and diarrhea. These side effects usually diminish after 1 to 4 days. Thrombophlebitis at the injection site is common and may be reduced by decreasing the infusion rate, further diluting the drug, and changing IV sites. Central nervous system side effects, such as headache, dizziness, hallucinations, and tremors, can occur and are usually dose-related. The ophthalmic ointment may cause sensitivity to bright light.

Zidovudine

Zidovudine (also known as azidothymidine, AZT, Compound-S; marketed as RETROVIR) is the newest antiviral agent. It was developed specifically to control AIDS. This orally and IV administered drug is used for selected patients with HIV infection, symptomatic AIDS, or the AIDS-related complex (ARC) with *Pneumocystis carinii* infections or lymphocytopenia. The drug is not a cure for AIDS, nor will it control opportunistic infections liable to develop in these patients, and so adjunctive therapy may be required. Compliance can be a problem because the drug must be taken every 4 hours around the clock; it is essential to stress to the patient the need for compliance.

The most common general side effects caused by zidovudine include nausea, vomiting, diarrhea; headache and fever; listlessness; and skin rashes. Zidovudine is potentially nephrotoxic, and should not be administered with other nephrotoxic drugs. The risk of granulocytopenia is increased by coadministration of drugs that inhibit zidovudine's metabolism, of which the list may be long. Aspirin and, in particular, acetaminophen, are thought to interact in this way. Since these are over-the-counter drugs that might be self-administered, be sure to caution the patient against using them without prior approval.

The major dose-limiting toxicities of zidovudine are serious anemia or granulocytopenia. Either may require not only reduced dosages or discontinuation of therapy, but also, if the reaction is severe, blood transfusions. Thus, frequent assessment and blood tests are necessary during zidovudine therapy.

V. Anthelminthic Drugs

Parasitic infections by worms and flukes (helminths) are treated by a group of antiinfective agents known as the anthelminthics. Three major groups of helminths are responsible for these infestations: cestodes (tapeworm), nematodes (roundworm, hookworm, larva migrans, whipworm, pinworm, and threadworm), and flukes (schistosomes). One third of the world's population has a helminth infestation, although many of the affected individuals have no clinical evidence of the disorder. Helminthiasis is traditionally associated with inhabitants of underdeveloped countries, but the disorders have become more widespread because of immigration and increased travel to these regions. Helminth infections can cause malnutrition, tissue damage, and production of toxic by-products.

The anthelminthic drugs are oral products that are minimally absorbed through the GI tract. This allows for a high local concentration of drug, which is desirable since infestations are localized in the GI tract. The lack of absorption also tends to localize side effects to the gut, although not entirely. The selection of an anthelminthic is based on the most effective agent for a particular parasite, as well as patient preference. Dosages for these drugs are summarized in Table 57–C5, and side effects are listed in Table 57–S5. Scant information is available about specific drug–drug interactions involving anthelminthic drugs, and so there is no table for this.

Mebendazole

Mebendazole (VERMOX) is one of the drugs of choice for pinworm, roundworm, threadworm, and hookworm infestations. Because of its very broad spectrum of activity it is often considered the agent of choice in mixed helminthic infections. Few adverse reactions occur with this agent, although cramping and fever have been reported.

Niclosamide

Niclosamide (NICLOCIDE) is one of the drugs of choice for treating tapeworm infections because it is highly effective and generally well tolerated. A one-time dosage is usually sufficient in all but dwarf tapeworm infestations, which require 7 days of therapy. Nausea and abdominal pain are occasionally reported.

Piperazine

Piperazine (VERMIZINE) is an alternative to pyrantel and mebendazole for treating roundworm and pinworm infestations. It is particularly effective against roundworm, and is less toxic than pyrantel and mebendazole. However, compared with pyrantel, piperazine is more inconvenient to administer because multiple doses are needed.

Nausea, vomiting, and mild diarrhea are the most common piperazine-induced side effects. Several CNS reactions, including ataxia, headache, and vertigo, have been reported. Usually, such symptoms reflect neurotoxicity as the result of overdosage or impaired excretion. Nystagmus or blurred vision may occur. Cataracts have been reported, but are not likely to occur with short-term treatment. A history of seizure disorders contraindicates piperazine use. In addition, the drug should not be administered to patients taking antipsychotic drugs, which could increase the risk of seizures or extrapyramidal side effects. Piperazine and pyrantel are mutually antagonistic and so should not be used together.

Pyrantel

Pyrantel (ANTIMINTH) is commonly used in a number of worm infestations. It is considered to be one of the drugs of choice for both pinworms and roundworms, owing to its high degree of effectiveness and its low toxicity. It has a cure rate of 90% to 100% after only one dose. In addition, pyrantel is clinically useful against hookworm infestations.

Pyrantel appears to paralyze the parasite by stimulating the release of acetylcholine, after which the normal peristaltic activity of the host's gut expels the organism.

Adverse reactions to pyrantel are infrequent and usually consist of mild GI disturbances such as nausea, vomiting, anorexia, diarrhea, and cramping. It may cause drowsiness, dizziness, and headache. A transient increase in serum concentrations of AST, which indicates hepatic side effects, has been observed. Patients with hepatic dysfunction should be treated with caution. Allergy to pyrantel is the only absolute contraindication to use of this drug.

Encourage patients to take the entire dosage as a single dose. The use of pyrantel in pinworm infestations must be accompanied by meticulous hygiene, cleaning, and disinfecting to avoid further infections. Administer pyrantel with milk, juice, or food.

Quinacrine

Quinacrine (ATABRINE) has a wide spectrum of activity and is used to treat tapeworm infections, giardiasis, and malaria. Quinacrine may impart a yellow stain to the skin or urine. Dizziness, headache, and vomiting are also frequently reported side effects. Sodium bicarbonate may be taken with each dose to minimize GI upset. Quinacrine should not be administered to pregnant women.

Thiabendazole

Thiabendazole (MINTEZOL) is prescribed for a number of helminth infestations, including pinworm, threadworm, roundworm, hookworm, and whipworm. Gastrointestinal upset commonly occurs 3 to 4 hours after ingestion. Thiabendazole may cause dizziness and drowsiness sufficient to require assistance with ambulation and caution when performing tasks requiring full mental alertness and coordination.

General Nursing Implications for Anthelminthic Drugs

Pinworms can be spread from person to person. Consequently, an entire family may need treatment. Meticulous handwashing before and after patient contact is essential, particularly after disposing of feces or urine or changing linens. Advise patients to wash their hands before eating and after bowel movements, to clean fingernails daily, to keep nails short to discourage biting, and to keep fingers out of the mouth. Instruct patients to change and wash underwear, bed linens, night clothes, and towels daily, and to clean and disinfect toilet facilities each day. To check for the presence of eggs in the stool to determine treatment effectiveness, wrap cellophane tape around a tongue blade or finger, sticky side out. Press against the anal area, and then on to a glass slide for microscopic examination. Have the patient collect the specimen in the early morning before getting out of bed.

VI. Antimalarial Drugs

Malaria is an infectious disease caused by four species of the genus *Plasmodium*. It is responsible for approximately one million deaths each year. It is commonly found in Asia, Africa, and Latin America. The incidence of malaria in the United States is comparatively low, but has increased recently as travel to endemic areas has increased.

Malaria is transmitted by the bites of infected female mosquitoes or by exposure to infected blood. Affected patients typically experience high fever, chills, and rigor. A prodromal period of one to several days during which the patient may complain of malaise, headache, and myalgias, may precede the acute onset of symptoms.

Malaria therapy is divided into prevention and treatment. Prevention can be subdivided into chemoprophylaxis (while in endemic areas) and attack prevention (after departure from endemic areas). Treatment can be subdivided into therapy of uncomplicated attacks, treatment of severe illness, and prevention of relapses.

PROTOTYPE

Chloroquine

Absorption, Distribution, Metabolism, and Excretion

Chloroquine (ARALEN) is absorbed rapidly and nearly completely from the GI tract. Its bioavailability is greater when it is administered with food. This agent is widely distributed throughout the body and accumulates in major organs. Drug concentrations in the CNS may be ten to thirty times higher than plasma concentrations, and levels in other organs, such as the liver, may be hundreds of times higher than blood levels. Unfortunately, the drug also concentrates in the eye and skin by binding to melanin, which leads to disturbing side effects. Chloroquine has a half-life of 3 to 5 days. As much as 70% of chloroquine is excreted in the urine unchanged. Chloroquine that concentrates in tissues is slowly released back into the bloodstream, and then excreted in the urine. The drug can be detected in the patient's urine for months or years after treatment has ended.

Pharmacologic Effects

Chloroquine appears to kill the *Plasmodium* organism by interfering with its ability to replicate DNA and to transcribe its genetic code as needed for protein synthesis.

Clinical Indications and Administration

Chloroquine is used in the prevention and treatment of malaria from *Plasmodium vivax, P. malariae, P. ovale,* and susceptible strains of *P. falciparum*. It is considered the drug of choice in most types and phases of prevention and treatment of malaria except for prophylaxis in areas where resistant strains of *P. falciparum* have been reported.

Chloroquine phosphate is used for oral administration; the hydrochloride salt is formulated for IM injection. The usual dose of chloroquine for suppression or prophylaxis of malaria is 300 mg of chloroquine base (the dosage standard), which is equivalent to 500 mg of chloroquine phosphate, once weekly. Ideally, therapy should be started 1 to 2 weeks before entering an endemic area, and continued for 6 to 8 weeks after leaving. Pediatric doses, dosages for treating malaria, and other related information are presented in Table 57–C6. Chloroquine phosphate is also marketed as a fixed-dose combination product that contains the related antimalarial drug primaquine phosphate. This product, marketed as ARALEN PHOSPHATE WITH PRIMAQUINE PHOSPHATE, is used for prophylaxis of malaria in all endemic areas, regardless of the *Plasmodium* species that are present.

Side Effects, Adverse Reactions, and Contraindications

Chloroquine-related side effects are summarized in Table 57–S6. The drug causes mild GI upset that usually can be minimized by administering the drug with food. It also causes many ocular side effects. Some, such as impaired accommodation and resulting blurred vision, are usually mild and readily reversible when treatment stops. As many as 70% of patients have developed corneal inclusions, keratopathy, or ocular edema during prolonged chloroquine therapy. These effects, although more severe, are reversible as well. The most severe ocular problem is retinopathy. If not detected early it can progress further, potentially leading to blindness, even if chloroquine therapy is stopped. Chloroquine is contraindicated for patients who have incurred serious ophthalmic responses from prior use of the drug.

Chloroquine may bleach scalp and body hair pigments after several months of use. It may cause pruritus that is usually unresponsive to antihistamines. It may also exacerbate psoriasis or cause an attack. A history of psoriasis contraindicates chloroquine use. Rare side effects include blood dyscrasias, hypotension, and electroencephalographic changes. A history of hypersensitivity or allergy to chloroquine contraindicates further use.

Chloroquine is potentially hepatotoxic; dosages should be reduced in patients with hepatic impairment.

NURSING IMPLICATIONS

Rule out major contraindications before administering chloroquine (especially prior allergies or severe ocular changes), and check the patient's history for hepatic dysfunction that might require dosage reductions.

Instruct patients to take their weekly chloroquine doses on the same day each week, with meals, to obtain the best effect and fewest GI side effects. Advise them to complete the entire prescribed course of treatment. Encourage all patients to receive ophthalmologic examinations every 3 months during chloroquine therapy, and to notify a physician at once if any visual changes occur.

◆ Use During Pregnancy and Lactation

Chloroquine is contraindicated during pregnancy. Encourage women receiving the drug to use effective contraceptive methods, and to report possible pregnancy at once. Women receiving this drug should not breast-feed their infants.

◆ Use in Children

Children are particularly sensitive to overdoses of chloroquine. Even relatively small doses have caused fatalities. Children should not be given parenteral doses except in severe cases of malaria that do not respond to other drugs.

Encourage patients to keep the medication out of reach of small children and to supervise the administration of doses to children. Instruct the patient to notify a physician or poison control center immediately if accidental ingestion has occurred and to induce emesis immediately.

Interactions with Other Drugs

Antacids and antidiarrheal drugs that act as adsorbents (for example, kaolin and pectin, bismuth salts) interfere with absorption of oral chloroquine, and should not be administered concomitantly. Chloroquine has quinidine-like properties (see Chapter 30) and can displace digoxin from tissue binding sites, causing digoxin toxicity. These interactions, and related nursing implications, are summarized in Table 57–I6.

Overdose and Toxicity

Chloroquine overdoses cause symptoms quickly, and death has occurred in as little as 2 hours. Initial symptoms include headache, drowsiness, and visual disturbances. Seizures, cardiovascular collapse, and respiratory arrest may occur. Standard interventions, such as induced emesis and gastric lavage, should be started promptly (see Appendix C). Activated charcoal should be administered in an amount equal to five times the amount of chloroquine that was ingested (if known). Acidifying the urine with ammonium chloride helps promote chloroquine excretion. Otherwise, treatment is symptomatic and supportive.

Related Drugs

Hydroxychloroquine Sulfate

Hydroxychloroquine sulfate (PLAQUENIL) is a chloroquine derivative with similar actions and effects. It is slightly more potent than chloroquine (see Table 57–C6), and is as effective as chloroquine for suppressing or preventing malaria and for treating uncomplicated attacks. All nursing implications noted for chloroquine apply also to hydroxychloroquine. Hydroxychloroquine is also used to treat refractory rheumatoid arthritis, as discussed in Chapter 52.

Primaquine Phosphate

Primaquine phosphate is structurally similar to chloroquine and hydroxychloroquine, but is sufficiently different to act in a different way. Primaquine destroys the parasite's mitochondria, thereby disrupting major metabolic pathways essential for the parasite's life. It is an orally effective drug that is indicated only for curing infections from *P. vivax,* and for preventing relapses of malaria caused by that strain. It is contraindicated in patients who are receiving quinacrine or who have received quinacrine recently.

Pyrimethamine

Pyrimethamine (DARAPRIM) is an orally effective folic acid antagonist used for prophylaxis of malaria caused by susceptible plasmodia. It can also be used to treat acute malaria attacks, but is best reserved as an adjunct to chloroquine, quinine, or quinacrine. A proprietary pyrimethamine-sulfadoxine preparation (FANSIDAR) is available for treatment or prophylaxis of malaria. Pyrimethamine is also indicated for treatment of toxoplasmosis, for which it is used adjunctively with a sulfonamide.

Quinine Sulfate

Quinine sulfate (QUINAMM; others) is a cinchona alkaloid that is closely related to the antiarrhythmic drug quinidine. It is used to treat falciparum malaria that is resistant to chloroquine and quinacrine, usually adjunctively with pyrimethamine and a sulfonamide or tetracycline antibiotic. Its side effects and drug interactions are similar to those for quinidine (see Chapter 30). The drug is absolutely contraindicated during pregnancy. Quinine sulfate also has skeletal muscle–relaxant properties, and is used to treat nocturnal leg cramping, an indication that is completely unrelated to its antimalarial activity (see Chapter 17).

VII. Miscellaneous Antiprotozoal Drugs

Two miscellaneous drugs—metronidazole and pentamidine—are antiprotozoal agents that differ chemically and pharmacologically from all other agents discussed thus far.

Metronidazole

Metronidazole (FLAGYL) is classified as an amebicidal drug, but it has many other clinically useful indications.

At least 80% of an orally administered dose of metronidazole is absorbed. Peak plasma concentrations occur 1 to 3 hours after administration. The absorption rate and peak plasma concentrations are decreased when the drug is given with meals, although total absorption is not affected. The drug is widely distributed to most body tissues including the cerebrospinal fluid.

The plasma half-life of metronidazole is around 6 to 8 hours, values that are prolonged by hepatic dysfunction but not by renal dysfunction. Metronidazole's metabolites may darken the urine to a reddish-brown color.

The metabolites of metronidazole are bactericidal, trichomonacidal, and amebicidal, presumably because they disrupt DNA synthesis in the invading organisms.

Metronidazole's broad spectrum of activity is reflected in its many uses, most of which are approved. Dosages for each use are summarized in Table 57–C6; oral administration is used for most indications. Metronidazole's most common use is to treat trichomoniasis, a sexually transmitted disease caused by *Trichomonas vaginalis.* All individuals who have had recent sexual contact with an infected patient should be treated with the drug. A single 2-g dose is the treatment of choice because it is convenient and usually effective. Daily treatment with lower dosages for 7 consecutive days may be slightly more effective, but only if total compliance can be ensured.

Metronidazole is the drug of choice for treating acute amebic dysentery (intestinal amebiasis) and liver abscesses caused by *Entamoeba histolytica.* The best response is obtained when it is used adjunctively with another amebicidal agent such as iodoquinol. It is also the drug of choice for vaginitis caused by *Gardnerella vaginalis.*

Metronidazole is used to treat giardiasis, an intestinal disorder caused by a protozoal parasite called *Giardia lamblia,* for which it is slightly less effective but better tolerated than the alternative drug, quinacrine. It has been used as an equally effective but less expensive alternative to oral vancomycin for treating pseudomembranous colitis.

Because of its great efficacy against most gram-negative anaerobic bacteria, metronidazole is frequently used in combination with an aminoglycoside to treat mixed aerobic/anaerobic infections in the peritoneum and pelvic region. It is also effective for treating lower respiratory and CNS infections caused by anaerobic bacteria. The parenteral (IV) dosage form can be used for these indications, but oral therapy may be suitable and should be started as soon as possible if parenteral administration is used first.

The most common side effect caused by metronidazole is GI distress (nausea, vomiting, and anorexia) (see Table 57–S6). The drug sometimes causes a metallic taste. Central nervous system effects include dizziness, vertigo, syncope, and ataxia; such mental changes as depression, confusion, and irritability have been reported. The most common peripheral neurologic side effects—numbness and paresthesias—seem to reflect a reversible peripheral neuropathy. Preexisting neurologic problems necessitate cautious use of metronidazole.

Other untoward responses affect the genitourinary tract, and include urethral burning, dysuria, incontinence, and dryness of the vagina. Metronidazole may cause allergic reactions, including urticaria, erythematous rash, and pruritus. Some patients also develop joint pain, fever, and congestion. Prior allergic responses to the drug contraindicate further use. There have been rare reports of metronidazole-induced pseudomembranous colitis.

Animal studies have revealed a carcinogenic potential for metronidazole. Although there are no comparable human data, the drug should be used only when absolutely necessary.

Metronidazole inhibits alcohol metabolism in a manner similar to disulfiram (Chapter 22), and may cause a disulfiram-like adverse reaction (see Table 57–I6). Symptoms include mild flushing, headache, vomiting, sweating, and abdominal cramps. The reaction is unpredictable and does not occur in all individuals. Metronidazole can potentiate the activity of oral anticoagulants, so concomitant use of these agents should be avoided. Cimetidine inhibits the metronidazole metabolism, resulting in higher plasma concentrations and an increased risk of side effects or toxicity.

There have been few reports of serious overdoses caused by metronidazole. The expected manifestations are nausea, vomiting, and ataxia, which are treated symptomatically and supportively.

NURSING IMPLICATIONS

Encourage patients being treated for trichomoniasis to identify recent sex partners so they can be contacted for treatment. Advise patients to avoid sexual intercourse during trichomoniasis treatment, but to have the male partner wear a condom if intercourse is continued.

One metronidazole formulation for IV use is supplied ready-to-use. Another is a freeze-dried powder that must be reconstituted, diluted in an IV solution, and then neutralized before administration because of its very low pH. If the powder is used, be sure to consult the manufacturer's procedure and follow all steps in proper sequence.

Reduce dosages in patients with hepatic dysfunction or neurologic disorders.

Assist patients with ambulation if they experience dizziness, vertigo, or other untoward CNS responses. Suggest that the patient suck hard candy if the drug-induced metallic taste is bothersome. Metronidazole may darken the urine; reassure the patient that this is not of concern.

Instruct patients not to use alcohol while they are taking metronidazole and for 1 week after discontinuing the drug. This includes any medications that contain any amount of alcohol, including over-the-counter medications. Instruct patients who take oral anticoagulants concomitantly with metronidazole to check for abnormal bruising or the presence of blood in the urine or stool.

◆ Use During Pregnancy and Lactation

Metronidazole should not be administered during the first trimester, and should be used in later stages only for trichomoniasis that cannot be symptomatically relieved with other measures. Metronidazole levels in breast milk are comparable to plasma levels, and so breast-feeding should be discouraged if the drug must be administered. The mother should express and discard the milk during therapy, and resume breast-feeding 1 to 2 days after treatment has stopped.

◆ Use in Children

Treatment of amebiasis is the only indication for which the safety and effectiveness of metronidazole for children has been established. Anticipate a much longer half-life in children less than 1 year of age.

Other Amebicides

There are several alternatives or adjuncts to metronidazole for treating amebiasis, but they are rarely used. One—chloroquine—has already been discussed. Carbarsone, iodoquinol (diiodohydroxyquin; various trade names) and paromomycin (HUMATIN) are orally effective drugs used to treat intestinal amebiasis. Emetine is a parenteral agent used adjunctively with other amebicides for intestinal or extraintestinal amebiasis. Table 57–C6 summarizes typical dosages of these agents; important side effects and related contraindications are summarized in Table 57–S6. Little is known about interactions between these drugs and other agents.

Pentamidine

Pentamidine (PENTAM 300) is an antiprotozoal agent that is active against *P. carinii,* the organism responsible for some cases of pneumonia in immunosuppressed patients especially patients with AIDS. The drug is given by IM or IV injection, or by inhalation (via a nebulizer).

Very little is known about pentamidine's pharmacokinetics, other than that it is rapidly excreted unchanged in the urine.

Pentamidine is used almost exclusively as an alternative to co-trimoxazole for the treatment of *P. carinii* pneumonia (see Table 57–C6). Co-trimoxazole is the current drug of choice because it is less toxic.

Pentamidine can substantially alter blood pressure and has caused severe hypotension when administered either IM or IV. If the IV route is used, the drug should be given over 60 minutes. Nephrotoxicity is common, with some reports indicating a 25% incidence. Elevations of both serum creatinine and BUN levels occur usually after the second week of therapy. Renal insufficiency is usually reversible, but if acute renal failure occurs the drug should be discontinued at once. Both hyperglycemia and hypoglycemia have occurred. Hypoglycemic reactions can be severe. Blood glucose levels should be measured daily. Although side effects caused by pentamidine are potentially serious, there are no contraindications to its use in patients with documented *P. carinii* pneumonia. Health-care workers have expressed concern about the possible exposure to nebulized pentamidine, especially because there are no good data about the drug's potential teratogenecity. Since this risk is not clearly elucidated, it is currently recommended that exposure to aerosolized pentamidine by pregnant health-care workers be avoided.

NURSING IMPLICATIONS

Pentamidine injections are painful and may cause sterile abscesses. Change the injection site each day, and observe for signs of inflammation at previous injection sites.

SUMMARY OF NURSING IMPLICATIONS

◆ Assessment

Obtain a complete nursing history to include information regarding past and present illnesses that may be contraindications to antiinfective therapy.

Review current medication usage for potential drug–drug interactions with prescriptive or over-the-counter preparations, or episodes of hypersensitivity reactions.

Obtain physical and psychologic data necessary to determine drug effectiveness and consequences of therapy (eg, site of infection, appearance of infected area, renal function, baseline vital signs, laboratory results, understanding of present condition, emotional response to condition).

◆ Nursing Diagnoses

Pain related to gastrointestinal upset or superinfections.

High risk for impaired skin integrity related to rash, redness.

Sensory/perceptual alteration: visual related to blurring, optic neuritis, or color perception change from adverse drug effects.

Sensory/perceptual alteration: auditory related to ringing in ears or ototoxicity from drug side effects.

Knowledge deficit related to current drug regimen.

Diarrhea related to drug therapy.

Altered nutrition: less than body requirements related to gastric upset.

Altered urinary elimination: pain or burning related to adverse drug effects.

High risk for fluid volume deficit related to insufficient intake with urinary antiinfectives.

Noncompliance related to untoward side effects and strict administration schedule.

Ineffective individual coping related to chronic or recurrent infections.

Altered tissue perfusion related to liver or renal failure, or blood dyscrasias associated with toxic drug effects.

◆ Planning/Implementation with Antituberculosis Drugs

Monitor liver function tests periodically while giving isoniazid and rifampin; observe for jaundice in the sclera of the eye.

Give pyridoxine to treat and prevent peripheral neuropathies associated with isoniazid therapy.

Avoid administering streptomycin by IV route if possible; auditory and vestibular toxicities are more likely to occur.

◆ Patient and Family Teaching with Antituberculosis Drugs

Teach the patient/family:

To expect a reddish-orange color to most body secretions with rifampin; it is not harmful and the drug should be continued.

To have periodic ophthalmologic examinations while receiving ethambutol.

To report immediately changes in vision or color perception.

◆ Planning/Implementation with Urinary Antiinfective Drugs

Check urine pH before giving mandelamine: if 5 or less, urine acidifying agent is not necessary (eg, ascorbic acid); if needed, cranberry juice once or twice a day may be used.

Give mandelamine, nalidixic acid, and nitrofurantoin with food to avoid GI upset.

◆ Patient and Family Teaching with Urinary Antiinfective Drugs

Teach the patient/family:

To comply with prescribed regimen, which may last 6 months to a year.

To avoid excessive intake of fruits, juices (other than cranberry), and milk products, which may cause alkalinization of urine while taking mandelamine.

To notify physician at once if neurologic side effects develop with nalidixic acid and nitrofurantoin.

To avoid prolonged exposure to sun; to use a sunscreen of 15 or greater to avoid photosensitivity reactions with nalidixic acid.

To recognize "flu-like" symptoms that may be a reaction to nitrofurantoin; to discontinue drug immediately and notify physician.

◆ Planning/Implementation with Antifungal Drugs

Anticipate adverse responses in virtually every patient receiving amphotericin B.

Always mix amphotericin B with 5% dextrose or sterile water; mixing with saline will result in precipitation; do not mix with other drugs.

Premedicate as ordered at least 30 minutes prior to giving amphotericin B, to minimize febrile reactions.

Give slowly over 4 to 6 hours to minimize the initial adverse effects; use a rate-controlled infusion pump to prevent inadvertent rapid administration.

Monitor laboratory tests to determine nephrotoxic effects of drug.

Give potassium supplements based on test results when giving amphotericin B chronically; observe for signs and symptoms of hypokalemia (muscle weakness, lethargy, and confusion).

Further dilution of amphotericin B, frequent changing of IV sites, and addition of small amounts of heparin may reduce severe phlebitis.

Give griseofulvin with food to minimize adverse GI effects and to increase absorption.

Give IV miconazole over 1 hour to avoid severe cardiovascular effects.

Monitor for bone marrow suppression with flucytosine.

◆ Patient and Family Teaching with Antifungal Drugs

Teach the patient/family:

The importance of maintaining drug regimen even if response is slow.

To report a worsening of infection to physician; may indicate treatment failure.

On the proper administration of vaginal creams and tablets, and proper use of lozenges.

◆ Planning/Implementation with Antiviral Drugs

Give IV acyclovir over 1 hour to prevent renal dysfunction and minimize occurrence of phlebitis.

Apply topical acyclovir sparingly directly on lesions; use finger cot or rubber gloves to prevent further spread of infection.

Monitor renal function tests periodically.

Observe for headache, dizziness, lethargy, nausea, vomiting, and diarrhea.

Never give vidarabine IM or SC; thrombophlebitis is common with IV administration; dilute in as much fluid as possible and use an in-line filter.

Restrict use of ribavirin to severe respiratory syncytial virus infections; give via special nebulization equipment.

◆ Patient and Family Teaching with Antiviral Drugs

Teach the patient/family:

That the possibility of recurrent infections still exists after treatment with an antiviral agent.

To adhere to the prescribed regimen.

To seek counseling regarding herpes infection because of the emotional consequences.

◆ Planning/Implementation with Anthelminthic Agents

Recognize symptoms of parasitic infection in high-risk groups (eg, recent foreign travel, immigration from a Third World country).

◆ Patient and Family Teaching with Anthelminthic Agents

Teach the patient/family:

The importance of compliance and dependability when self-administering drugs; determine patient preferences (eg, suspension or tablets).

To recognize major side effect of GI distress.

Essential hygiene measures to prevent spread and reinfection.

◆ Planning/Implementation with Antimalarial Drugs

Drug should be taken weekly with meals on the same day each week for the best effect.

◆ Patient and Family Teaching with Antimalarial Drugs

Teach the patient/family:

To keep medication out of reach of small children, as toxic reactions are more severe in children; to supervise administration of medication to children; to notify physician or poison control center immediately if accidental ingestion occurs; to induce emesis immediately.

To have frequent (every 3 months) ophthalmologic examinations while receiving antimalarial agents (chloroquine and hydroxychloroquine); be aware of changes in vision and to notify physician if this occurs.

◆ Planning/Implementation with Miscellaneous Antiinfective Drugs

Change injection site each day when giving pentamidine; observe for signs of inflammation at previous injection sites.

◆ Patient and Family Teaching with Miscellaneous Antiinfective Drugs

Teach the patient/family:

To avoid alcohol while taking metronidazole and for 1 week after discontinuing therapy (includes elixirs and over-the-counter medications).

To identify any recent sexual contacts who should be treated for an infection with metronidazole.

To observe for bruising or blood in the urine or stool if an anticoagulant and metronidazole are taken concurrently.

◆ Evaluation

The patient/family will:

Show evidence of resolving infection: vital signs and temperature within normal limits; relief from clinical signs and symptoms.

Eat and drink sufficient quantities to enhance drug effectiveness and promote healing.

Experience minimal to no adverse drug effects: skin free of redness, rash, yellow color; stool of normal frequency and consistency; voiding sufficient amounts.

Report reasonable comfort during recovery and drug therapy.

Participate in prescribed drug regimen; discuss consequences of noncompliance with drug therapy.

Respond appropriately to visual and auditory stimulation; experience no visual or hearing deficit.

Verbalize frustration with situation; participate in decisions to manage infection; take precautions to prevent spread or recurrence of infection.

Annotated Bibliography

Anti-infective agents. In: McEvoy GK, McQuarrie GM, eds. *American Hospital Formulary Service.* Bethesda, MD, American Society of Hospital Pharmacists, 1991. *This is an unreferenced but concise, objective review of the antiinfective agents reviewed in this chapter; a very valuable resource. Updated annually.*

Drugs for AIDS and associated infections. *Med Lett* 1991;33(855): 95–102. *A concise review of the unique infections and the drugs used in treating patients with AIDS.*

Table 57–C1 | Clinical Uses and Administration of Antitubercular Drugs*

AGENT	CLINICAL USES	DOSAGE AND ROUTE OF ADMINISTRATION
	First-Line Drugs	
Isoniazid		
(INH; NYDRAZID; others)	Chemoprophylaxis of TB (see text for description of candidates)	Oral: Adults: 300 mg/d for 1 year. Children: 10 mg/kg/d for 1 year
	Initial or adjunctive treatment of TB	Oral (preferred) or IM: Adults: 5 mg/kg/d for 9–24 months. Children: 10–20 mg/kg/d for 9–24 months
Rifampin		
(RIMACTANE)	Initial treatment of TB, in conjunction with isoniazid	Oral: Adults: 600 mg. Children: 10–20 mg/kg/d
	Second-Line Drugs	
Ethambutol		
(MYAMBUTOL)	Alternative to rifampin for initial treatment of TB; alternatively, third drug in combination with isoniazid plus rifampin in cases of suspected resistance	Oral: Adults and children: 15 mg/kg/d as a single dose; for retreatment, start with 25 mg/kg/d for 60 days, reduce to 15 mg/kg/d thereafter; give at same time each day with food
Pyrazinamide	Tuberculosis treatment after prior failures, adjunctively with other antitubercular drugs	Oral: Adults and children: 20–35 mg/kg/d in 3 or 4 divided doses
Streptomycin	Used in combination with isoniazid and rifampin or ethambutol for prior treatment failures or suspected resistance	IM: Adults: 0.5–1 g 3 times weekly. Children: 20–40 mg/kg/d 3 times weekly. Reduce dosage in presence of renal dysfunction
	Third-Line Drugs	
Aminosalicylate sodium		
(P.A.S.; TEEBACIN)	Adjunctive therapy of TB	Oral: Adults 12–16 g/d in 2 or 3 divided doses. Children: 200–400 mg/kg/d in 3 or 4 divided doses
Capreomycin		
(CAPASTAT)	Refractory TB	IM: Adults: 1 g/d, then reduce to 1 g 3 times weekly after acute symptoms are controlled; inject deeply into large muscle; not recommended for children
Cycloserine		
(SEROMYCIN)	Adjunctive therapy of TB (refractory or caused by unusual *Mycobacterium* strains)	Oral: Adults: 0.5–1 g/d. Children: 5–15 mg/kg/d
Ethionamide		
(TRECATOR-S.C.)	As for aminosalicylate	Oral: Adults: 0.5–1 g/d in up to 3 divided doses. Children: 10–20 mg/kg/d, up to 705 mg/d, in divided doses

*Listed by group in usual order of preference, alphabetically within groups.

Table 57–S1 Major Side Effects of and Contraindications for Antitubercular Drugs*

BODY SYSTEM/ Side Effect	CONTRAINDICATION/ PRECAUTION	COMMENTS AND NURSING IMPLICATIONS
Aminosalicylate Sodium		
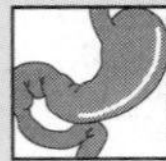 **GASTROINTESTINAL** Nausea, vomiting		Administer drug with meals
Capreomycin		
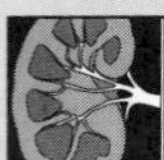 **RENAL** Evidence of renal dysfunction, including acute tubular necrosis		Monitor renal function periodically; obtain baseline renal function data
Cycloserine		
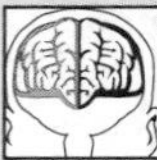 **CENTRAL NERVOUS SYSTEM** Psychoses, delirium, confusion, seizures		Assess carefully and frequently; instruct family to report any mental changes; adjunctive use of pyridoxine may be beneficial, suggesting cause is vitamin B_6 deficiency
Ethionamide		
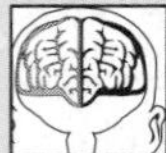 **CENTRAL NERVOUS SYSTEM** Paresthesias, peripheral neuritis		Risk increases with concomitant isoniazid therapy (avoid); concomitant use of pyridoxine is recommended
Isoniazid		
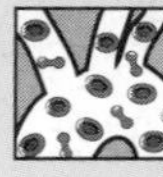 **BLOOD** Agranulocytosis, thrombocytopenia, aplastic anemia, other blood dyscrasias		Assess for indicators (bruising, bleeding, fever, sore throat, etc); recommend complete blood counts, coagulation studies, if dyscrasias are suspected
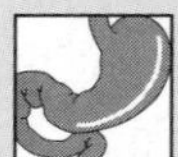 **GASTROINTESTINAL** Nausea, vomiting		Administer drug with meals, dividing daily dose into three equal parts reduces incidence, severity
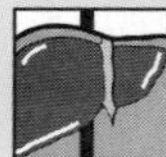 **HEPATIC** Elevated serum levels of marker enzymes of liver dysfunction (eg, increased AST, ALT, etc); jaundice	Prior hepatic damage caused by isoniazid	Check markers of liver status before treatment and periodically thereafter; assess for evidence of hepatic dysfunction (eg, jaundice, scleral yellowing)
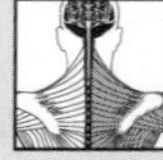 **NEUROMUSCULAR** Paresthesias, other evidence of peripheral neuropathy		Most common in patients with vitamin B_6 deficiencies (alcoholism, malnutrition, diabetes mellitus); easily treated or prevented with pyridoxine (vitamin B_6); assess accordingly

(*continued*)

Table 57–S1 | Major Side Effects of and Contraindications for Antitubercular Drugs* (*Continued*)

BODY SYSTEM/ Side Effect	CONTRAINDICATION/ PRECAUTION	COMMENTS AND NURSING IMPLICATIONS
	Pyrazinamide	
METABOLIC Elevated serum uric acid levels	Care in patients with hyperuricemia, gout	Acute gout attacks may occur during therapy; advise patient to report any joint pain, swelling, or redness
HEPATIC Elevated serum levels of marker enzymes of liver dysfunction; jaundice		Monitor accordingly, including by regular liver function tests; see isoniazid
	Rifampin	
CENTRAL NERVOUS SYSTEM Headache, visual disturbances, drowsiness		Usually subsides after first few weeks of therapy; instruct patients to notify physician if continual or severe
GASTROINTESTINAL Nausea, vomiting		Administer drug wtih meals
HEPATIC See isoniazid		
OTHER "Flu-like" symptoms		Incidence appears to be greatest in patients receiving high-dose rifampin on intermittent basis (20%–50% incidence); significance, cause unknown, nevertheless requires prompt notification of physician
Reddish-orange discoloration of sweat, tears, urine, feces		Forewarn patient that this is common but is not cause for alarm

*See Table 56–S3 for side effects related to streptomycin use.

Table 57–I Major Interactions Between Selected Antitubercular Drugs and Other Agents

AGENT	RESULT OF INTERACTION	COMMENTS AND NURSING IMPLICATIONS
Interactions Involving Aminosalicylate Sodium		
Vitamins (Chapter 61)	Nutritional deficiencies	Aminosalicylate interferes with absorption of iron, folic acid, B_{12}; multivitamin plus iron supplements generally recommended during therapy
Interactions Involving Isoniazid		
Carbamazepine (Chapter 26)	Increased carbamazepine blood levels, possible toxicity	Isoniazid inhibits carbamazepine metabolism; if interaction cannot be avoided, anticipate need to lower carbamazepine dose, preferably based on blood level measurements; assess accordingly
Phenytoin (Chapter 26)	Increased phenytoin blood levels, possible toxicity	As for carbamazepine
Rifampin	Increased risk of hepatotoxicity	Is often necessary to administer both drugs, but each is hepatotoxic; risk increased through synergistic actions; monitor liver function tests periodically; ensure that patients understand signs, symptoms of hepatitis (jaundice, etc) so they can report adverse effects at once
Interactions Involving Rifampin		
Anticoagulants, oral (Chapter 26)	Decreased anticoagulant blood levels, effect	Rifampin stimulates hepatic metabolism of oral anticoagulants (and other drugs listed as interactants); anticipate need to increase oral anticoagulant dose during combined therapy, and reduce its dose (to reduce risk of bleeding tendencies) when rifampin therapy is stopped; use coagulation studies to assist dosage adjustments
Corticosteroids (oral or parenteral; Chapter 35)	Decreased corticosteroid blood levels, effect	Anticipate need to increase corticosteroid dose (perhaps by as much as 100%) during combined treatment, and to reduce steroid dose at end of rifampin therapy
Digitoxin (Chapter 45)	Decreased digitoxin blood levels, effect	Assess for worsening of heart failure; anticipate need to increase digitoxin dose during combined therapy; digitoxin blood levels should be measured as a dosage guide; probably less likely to affect digoxin, which depends less on hepatic metabolism for elimination
Isoniazid	See isoniazid-rifampin above	
Oral contraceptives (Chapter 31)	Decreased contraceptive blood levels, effect	Contraceptive failure has occurred; have patient assess for evidence of inadequate effects (eg, breakthrough bleeding, spotting); if these occur have patient begin alternative or additional contraceptive methods at once and notify physician promptly for further evaluation, dosage adjustments, other advice
Propranolol, metoprolol (Chapter 15)	Decreased β blocker blood levels, effect	Assess for inadequate β blockade based on use for which β blocker was given (angina, hypertension, tachycardia, etc); β blocker dose may need to be increased during combined therapy, and reduced again at its end; interaction probably less important for other β blockers, which do not depend so much on hepatic metabolism for elimination

*Drugs are listed alphabetically by generic name. Other antitubercular drugs, for which there are no common, major interactions, are not listed.

Table 57–C2 | Clinical Uses and Administration of Miscellaneous Urinary Tract Antiinfectives

AGENT	CLINICAL USES	DOSAGE AND ROUTE OF ADMINISTRATION*
Methenamine hippurate (HIPREX; UREX)	Treatment of chronic urinary tract infections	Adults: 1 g bid. Children 6–12 years: 500 mg–1 g bid
Methenamine mandelate (MANDELAMINE; others)	As for methenamine hippurate	Adults: 1 g after meals and at bedtime. Children 6–12 years: 500 mg at times noted for adults. Children <6 years old: 250 mg per 30 lbs of body weight at times noted for adults
Nalidixic acid (NEGGRAM)	As for methenamine salts	Adults: Usually 1 g qid for 1 or 2 weeks; may reduce to half this dose for long-term treatment; give with food to reduce GI upset. Children 3 months–12 years: Initially, 55 mg/kg/d in 4 equal divided doses; reduce to 33 mg/kg/d for long-term therapy; contraindicated in children <3 months old
Nitrofurantoin (FURADANTIN; MACRODANTIN)	Treatment of acute or chronic urinary tract infections	Adults: 50–100 mg qid (with meals and at bedtime) for initial treatment; may reduce to 50–100 mg hs for long-term therapy. Children: Initially 5–7 mg/kg/d in 4 equal divided doses; may reduce to 1 mg/kg/d for long-term therapy; contraindicated in children <1 month old See Chapter 56
Trimethoprim (PROLOPRIM; TRIMPEX)	Initial treatment of urinary tract infections	Adults, children: 100 mg q12h or 200 mg qd, usually for 10 days; reduce dose in patients with renal impairment

*All drugs are administered orally.

Table 57–S2 Major Side Effects of and Contraindications for Selected Urinary Tract Antiinfective Drugs

BODY SYSTEM/ Side Effect	CONTRAINDICATION/ PRECAUTION	COMMENTS AND NURSING IMPLICATIONS
Methenamine		
GASTROINTESTINAL Nausea, vomiting, diarrhea		Administer with meals
IMMUNE Allergic reactions from tartrazine dye in HIPREX	Asthma, tartrazine dye sensitivity	Use alternative products
Nalidixic Acid		
CENTRAL NERVOUS SYSTEM Headache, malaise, vertigo, syncope; peripheral neuritis; rare psychosis or seizures	Care in patients with history of seizures, psychosis	Minor CNS side effects are common, should subside in 48 hr; patients should report severe or persistent side effects at once
EYE Visual disturbances, including altered color perception, impaired ability to focus eyes		Advise patient to wear sunglasses if bright lights are disturbing; most visual side effects occur with each increased dose, disappear with dosage reduction or discontinuation
SKIN Photosensitive rashes		Probably an allergic response from even brief sun exposure, may last weeks to months; advise patients to avoid sun exposure, wear appropriate clothing, sunscreens
Nitrofurantoin		
RESPIRATORY Acute or gradual dyspnea, other manifestations of respiratory impairment	Similar prior response to nitrofurantoin	Onset and severity vary; assess for adequate pulmonary function, especially during prolonged therapy; chart untoward pulmonary responses so drug will not be administered again
GASTROINTESTINAL Nausea, vomiting		Administer with milk or meals; macrocrystal product (eg, MACRODANTIN) causes less GI intolerance
NEUROMUSCULAR Lower extremity paresthesias		Risk higher in elderly patients, diabetics, persons with renal impairment; assess accordingly and anticipate need to reduce dose

Table 57–S2 **Major Side Effects of and Contraindications for Selected Urinary Tract Antiinfective Drugs (*Continued*)**

BODY SYSTEM/ Side Effect	CONTRAINDICATION/ PRECAUTION	COMMENTS AND NURSING IMPLICATIONS
Trimethoprim		
GASTROINTESTINAL Nausea, vomiting, other manifestations of GI intolerance; glossitis		Occurs in about 1 of 20 patients
SKIN Rashes		Usually occurs between weeks 1 and 2 of treatment, could reflect allergy; advise patient to report at once for further evaluation

Table 57–I2 **Major Interactions Between Selected Urinary Tract Antiinfective Drugs and Other Agents**

AGENT	RESULT OF INTERACTION	COMMENTS AND NURSING IMPLICATIONS
Methenamine		
Sulfonamides (Chapter 56)	Crystalluria from acidic urine pH needed for methenamine activity	Avoid interaction; sulfonamides more likely to crystallize in acidic urine, which is necessary for methenamine action; conversely, alkalinizing urine to reduce risk of sulfonamide-induced crystalluria counteracts methenamine's effects
Urinary alkalinizers (milk products, citrus juices, sodium bicarbonate, acetazolamide)	Reduced or abolished effect of methenamine	Avoid interaction; instruct patient about common foods, beverages, drugs to avoid
Nalidixic Acid		
Anticoagulants, oral (Chapter 35)	Increased risk of excessive anticoagulant effect	If interaction is unavoidable, monitor accordingly for signs, symptoms of excessive anticoagulation (bruising, bleeding, hematuria, etc); caused by displacement of anticoagulant from plasma protein–binding sites
Trimethoprim		
Phenytoin (Chapter 26)	Increased risk of phenytoin side effects (drowsiness, ataxia, etc)	Trimethoprim may reduce metabolism of phenytoin, other hydantoin anticonvulsants; monitor accordingly during combined therapy

Table 57–C3 **Clinical Uses and Administration of Major Antifungal Drugs***

AGENT	CLINICAL USES	DOSAGE AND ROUTE OF ADMINISTRATION
Amphotericin B		
(FUNGIZONE)	Pulmonary, urinary, meningeal, and disseminated candidiasis, histoplasmosis, aspergillosis, cryptococcosis, coccidiosis, blastomycosis (severe infections)	IV: Administer 1 mg test dose over 1–2 hr; if tolerated give 5 mg in 250 mL of 5% dextrose (only) over 4–6 hr; increase daily dose by 5 mg increments until maximum of 1 mg/kg is reached; see precautions in Table 57–S3
	Cutaneous or mucocutaneous candidal infections	Topical: Apply cream, lotion, or ointment liberally to lesions bid–qid; treatment usually lasts 1–3 weeks
Clotrimazole		
(MYCELEX)	Oral candidiasis	Oral (lozenge): One lozenge 5 times daily for 14 days; allow lozenge to dissolve slowly in mouth
(GYNE-LOTRIMIN; MYCELEX-G; others)	Vaginal candidiasis	Intravaginal: One tablet daily for 7 days, or one 500-mg tablet as single dose
(LOTRIMIN; MYCELEX; others)	Topical (cutaneous) treatment of candidiasis, tinea pedis (athlete's foot), versicolor, other susceptible infections—available as an OTC product	Topical (cream, lotion, solution): Massage into affected area and surrounding skin twice daily (morning and evening)
Fluconazole		
(DIFLUCAN)	Oral, esophageal, urinary candidiasis, adjunct to amphotericin for meningitis caused by *Cryptococcus neoformans;* also adjunct to amphotericin for severe aspergillosis infections	IV or Oral: 200 mg as single dose on first day, then 100 mg qd; for more serious infections, 400 mg initially, then 200 mg qd; no dosage recommendations for children
Flucytosine		
(ANCOBON)	Adjunct to amphotericin B for meningitis caused by *Cryptococcus neoformans*	Oral: Adults, children: 50–150 mg/kg/d in 4 divided doses; reduce dose in presence of renal failure; as many as 10 capsules may be required for each dose; prepare suspension for patients with difficulty swallowing
Griseofulvin		
(FULVICIN; GRISACTIN; others)	Ringworm infections of skin, nails, hair	Oral: Adults: 330–375 mg qd of ultramicrosize tablet (or 500 mg–1 g/d for microsize tablet). Children: 7.3 mg/kg/d of ultramicrosize tablet (or 10–11 mg/kg/d of microsize)
Itraconazole		
(SPORANOX)	Severe systemic fungal infections	Oral: Adults: 200 mg qd or bid; loading doses of 200 mg tid are sometimes used for the first 3 days; no dosage recommendations for children

(continued)

Table 57–C3 Clinical Uses and Administration of Major Antifungal Drugs* (*Continued*)

AGENT	CLINICAL USES	DOSAGE AND ROUTE OF ADMINISTRATION
Ketoconazole		
(NIZORAL)	Pulmonary histoplasmosis, other systemic fungal infections; ringworm infections for which griseofulvin is ineffective or unsuitable	Oral: Adults: 200–400 mg (depending on severity of infection, response), qd. Children: 3.3–6.6 mg/kg qd
	Tinea corporis, cruris, versicolor caused by responsive organisms	Topical: Apply to lesion and surrounding skin qd or bid
Miconazole		
(MONISTAT 3; MONISTAT 7)	Vaginal candidiasis	Intravaginal: One intravaginal tablet qd for 3 days, or 1 full applicator of cream qd for 7 days
	Severe systemic fungal infections (alternative to amphotericin B)	IV: Adults: 1.8–3.6 g/d in 3 divided doses, each infused over 30–60 min; doses may need to be titrated in 200-mg increments. Children: 20–40 mg/kg/d in divided doses not to exceed 15 mg/kg per infusion
	Fungal meningitis	Intrathecal: Usually 20 mg, qd (as supplement to IV therapy)
	Severe fungal infections of urinary bladder	Intravesicular: Instill 200 mg into bladder (as supplement to IV therapy)
(MICATIN; MONISTAT-DERM)	Tinea pedis, cruris, versicolor; cutaneous candidiasis, other common cutaneous fungal infections—available as OTC product	Topical: Apply powder, cream, lotion or spray to affected area(s) bid; treatment usually lasts 2–4 weeks, depending on nature, response of organism
Nystatin		
(MYCOSTATIN; NILSTAT; others)	Cutaneous or mucocutaneous candidal infections	Topical: Apply cream, ointment or powder bid or tid until healing is complete
	Vaginal candidiasis	Intravaginal: Usually 1 tablet daily for 2 weeks
	Oropharyngeal candidiasis	Oral (suspension or troche): Adults, children: Usually 400,000–600,000 U qid (eg, 5–10 mL of most oral suspension as dispensed); swish half of each dose on one side of mouth for at least 1 min, repeat on other, before swallowing; may apply directly to lesion(s). Infants: Usually 200,000 U qid, divided as noted above
	Intestinal candidiasis	Oral: Usually 1 or 2 tablets (500,000 U each) tid, swallowed

*Arranged alphabetically by generic name.

Table 57–S3 | **Major Side Effects of and Contraindications for Selected Antifungal Drugs***

BODY SYSTEM/ Side Effect	CONTRAINDICATION/ PRECAUTION	COMMENTS AND NURSING IMPLICATIONS
Amphotericin B		
GENERAL Febrile reactions, chills, muscle and joint pain, nausea, vomiting		Anticipate potentially severe response with several of the listed symptoms in most patients; premedicate (analgesics, antihistamines, corticosteroids, etc) as ordered; advise patient that untoward responses are common; ensure patient has received and tolerated test dose before giving full therapeutic doses
CARDIOVASCULAR Hypotension, tachycardia; arrhythmias (including possible ventricular fibrillation); cardiac enlargement		Uncommon unless drug is infused too rapidly; monitor all patients closely, preferably including ECG; report significant changes of vital signs, ECG at once; do not give full dose faster than over 4–6 hr
Phlebitis at peripheral infusion sites		Infusion into central venous catheter preferred to avoid peripheral venous irritation; if peripheral sites are used, change/rotate every 48–72 hr
RENAL Renal damage manifest as reduced creatinine excretion, increases of serum creatinine, BUN, etc; possible renal tubular acidosis; hypokalemia, hypomagnesemia		Some renal dysfunction occurs in most patients; monitor frequently; assess for signs, symptoms of hypokalemia, hypomagnesemia (eg, confusion, lethargy, muscle weakness); severe responses may require every-other-day administration
Flucytosine		
BLOOD Blood dyscrasias (eg, leukopenia, anemia, thrombocytopenia)		Perform baseline blood tests (CBC, coagulation studies, etc) for comparison with frequent repeat tests during treatment; report significant deviations from baseline, or other evidence of dyscrasias (bleeding, fever, flu-like symptoms, etc); instruct patient about symptoms that require prompt notification of physician
GASTROINTESTINAL Nausea, vomiting, diarrhea, bloating		Recommend taking capsules (many required per dose) a few at a time to reduce incidence of GI upset

Table 57–S3 Major Side Effects of and Contraindications for Selected Antifungal Drugs* (*Continued*)

BODY SYSTEM/ Side Effect	CONTRAINDICATON/ PRECAUTION	COMMENTS AND NURSING IMPLICATIONS
Griseofulvin		
CENTRAL NERVOUS SYSTEM Headache, fatigue, dizziness, insomnia		Frequent, especially during early therapy; usually subside with continued use; advise patient to notify physician if persistent, intolerable; advise avoidance of tasks made dangerous by drowsiness, dizziness, etc (eg, motor vehicle operation)
BLOOD Blood dyscrasias		See flucytosine for patient information
GASTROINTESTINAL Nausea, vomiting		Administer drug on full stomach
IMMUNE Skin rashes, urticaria, other mild or serious manifestations of allergy/hypersensitivity		Relatively common, usually mild; monitor for incidence, severity of response; some rashes are photosensitive, best prevented by avoidance of sunlight, wearing protective clothing, sunscreens, etc.
Ketoconazole		
CENTRAL NERVOUS SYSTEM See griseofulvin		Usually mild, uncommon
ENDOCRINE Decreased libido, impotence, gynecomastia, especially in males		Caused by drug-induced reduction of serum testosterone levels, is reversible upon discontinuation; advise patient to report severe symptoms
GASTROINTESTINAL Nausea, vomiting, etc		Administer with food, but avoid concomitant use of antacids or H_2 blockers (within 2 hr of ketoconazole administration; drug action requires low gastric pH); notify physician if GI upset is prolonged or intolerable
HEPATIC Hepatotoxicity		Has been fatal in rare cases; monitor accordingly, advise patients of potential risk, need to monitor
Miconazole		
CARDIOVASCULAR Thrombophlebitis, transient hypotension, arrhythmias		Infuse drug no faster than recommended

*Includes only drugs for which oral or parenteral dosage forms are available, and for which important side effects occur; listed alphabetically.

Table 57–13 Major Interactions Between Antifungal Drugs and Other Agents*

AGENT	RESULT OF INTERACTION	COMMENTS AND NURSING IMPLICATIONS
Interactions Involving Amphotericin B		
Corticosteroids, systemic (Chapter 45)	Increased risk of symptomatic hypokalemia	If interaction is unavoidable, monitor serum potassium levels, assess for evidence of hypokalemia (including ECG) closely, be prepared to administer potassium supplements
Digitalis (Chapter 31)	Increased risk of arrhythmias, other manifestations of digitalis toxicity (mainly cardiac)	Hypokalemia is major cause of digitalis toxicity; therefore, risk is increased by amphotericin B; monitor ECG, digitalis blood levels during combined therapy; applies to all digitalis glycosides
Diuretics, potassium-wasting (thiazides, high-ceiling; Chapter 32)	Hypokalemia	See corticosteroids; anticipate need for potassium supplementation or potassium-sparing diuretics
Flucytosine	Increased therapeutic effect, increased risk of nephrotoxicity	Monitor renal function with extra care
Miconazole	Reduced therapeutic effect of each	Are mutually antagonistic; avoid combined use
Nephrotoxic drugs (eg, aminoglycoside antibiotics, cyclosporine, other nephrotoxic drugs)	Increased risk of nephrotoxicity	Avoid combined use if possible
Skeletal muscle relaxants (eg, tubocurarine; Chapter 17)	Prolonged muscle paralysis (esp. apnea)	Caused by amphotericin B–induced hypokalemia, hypomagnesemia; anticipate prolonged recovery from neuromuscular blockade, need for mechanical ventilatory support; monitor spontaneous ventilatory status closely; monitor accordingly in patients receiving oral skeletal muscle relaxants
Interactions Involving Fluconazole		
Anticoagulants, oral (Chapter 35)	Increased anticoagulant effect	Anticoagulant doses may need to be reduced; prothrombin times monitored
Cyclosporine (Chapter 54)	Increased cyclosporine levels	Monitor cyclosporine concentrations and adjust accordingly
Phenytoin (Chapter 26)	Increased phenytoin levels	May result in significant phenytoin toxicity; monitor levels carefully and adjust doses accordingly
Interactions Involving Griseofulvin		
Anticoagulants, oral (Chapter 35)	Decreased anticoagulant effect	Increased anticoagulant doses may be required (based on coagulation studies) during combined therapy, subsequent dosage reduction when combined therapy stops
Interactions Involving Itraconazole		
Terfenadine (Chapter 51)	Increased terfenadine cardiac effects	May cause significant cardiovascular toxicity; deaths reported; avoid combined use
Other drugs	See fluconazole above	New drug; interaction profile not clearly established

Table 57–13 | Major Interactions Between Antifungal Drugs and Other Agents* (*Continued*)

AGENT	RESULT OF INTERACTION	COMMENTS AND NURSING IMPLICATIONS
Interactions Involving Ketoconazole		
Alcohol (Chapter 22)	Disulfiram-like reaction (flushing, hypotension, palpitations, headache, etc)	Encourage patient to avoid intake of all forms of alcohol (beverages, foods, medications, etc) during ketoconazole therapy and for 1–2 weeks thereafter
Antacids (Chapter 40)	Decreased ketoconazole effect	Ketoconazole requires low gastric pH for effectiveness; avoid administering antacids less than 2 hr after administering ketoconazole; advise patient of interaction, as antacids might be self-prescribed to combat GI upset
Anticoagulants, oral (Chapter 35)	Increased anticoagulant effects	Anticoagulant doses may need to be reduced during combined therapy, increased again at its end; monitor accordingly
Antihistamines (H_2 blockers, eg, cimetidine; Chapter 40)	See antacids	
Cyclosporine (Chapter 54)	Increased risk of nephrotoxicity	Both drugs are nephrotoxic; ketoconazole may increase cyclosporine blood levels, further increasing risk; avoid interaction
Hypoglycemics, oral (Chapter 46)	Increased risk of hypoglycemia, possibly severe	Both drugs may lower blood glucose levels independently or through interaction; avoid combined use if possible; if not, monitor blood glucose levels carefully, advise patient to anticipate and assess for evidence of hypoglycemia; interaction may apply to insulin as well
Phenytoin (Chapter 26)	Increased or decreased effect of one or both interactants	Monitor for effects of both interactants; outcome unpredictable
Rifampin	Reduced ketoconazole blood levels, effect	Avoid interaction
Terfenadine (Chapter 51)	See itraconazole	
Interactions Involving Miconazole		
Amphotericin B	See amphotericin B	
Anticoagulants, oral (Chapter 35)	See ketoconazole	
Cyclosporine (Chapter 54)	See ketoconazole	
Phenytoin (Chapter 26)	See ketoconazole	
Rifampin	See ketoconazole	

*Includes only drugs for which oral or parenteral dosage forms are available, and for which important interactions occur, listed alphabetically.

Table 57–C4 Clinical Uses and Administration of Antiviral Drugs*

AGENT	CLINICAL USES	DOSAGE AND ROUTE OF ADMINISTRATION
Acyclovir		
(ZOVIRAX)	Treatment of severe systemic infections caused by herpes simplex types 1 and 2	IV: Adults: 5 mg/kg q8h for 5–7 days, infused over 1 hr or more. Children: 250 mg/m^2 as noted for adults
	Initial treatment, prevention of recurrences of genital herpes (selected adults)	Oral: Initially, 200 mg q4h during waking hours for 10 days, then 200 mg 3–5 times daily for up to 6 months. For herpes zoster, 800 mg q4h, 5 times daily for 7–10 days
	Initial treatment of genital herpes infections	Topical: Apply ointment 6 times daily for 1 week
	Treatment of herpes zoster (shingles)	
Amantadine		
(SYMMETREL)	Prophylaxis, treatment of influenza A infections	Oral: Adults: Usually 100 mg bid for 10 days, started within 24–48 hr after symptom onset or immediately after exposure (reduce in presence of renal failure)
	Parkinsonism	See Chapter 25
Didanosine		
(VIDEX, "DDI")	Treatment of advanced HIV infection in patients intolerant of zidovudine, or when zidovudine is no longer effective	Oral: Adults: 125–300 mg bid; dose based on weight. Children: 25–100 mg bid based on body surface area
Foscarnet		
(FOSCAVIR)	Treatment of CMV retinitis in patients with AIDS	IV: Induction therapy: 60 mg/kg q8h for 2–3 weeks; maintenance: 120 mg/kg bid
Ganciclovir		
(CYTOVENE)	Treatment of CMV retinitis in immunocompromised patients; has also been used for other CMV infections, such as pneumonitis and gastroenteritis	IV: Adults, children: Induction therapy: 5 mg/kg q12h for 2–3 weeks; maintenance: 5 mg/kg/d for duration of immunosuppression
Idoxuridine		
(HERPLEX; STOXIL)	Treatment of herpes simplex keratitis	Topical: Ointment: Apply 5 times daily (eg, q4h). Drops: Apply every hour while awake, every 2 hr during night; both therapies usually given for 3–5 days after healing to prevent recurrences
Ribavirin		
(VIRAZOLE)	Treatment of respiratory tract infections caused by respiratory syncytial virus	Inhaled (via nebulizer): Given for 12–18 hr per 24 hr for 3–7 days
Vidarabine		
(VIRA-A)	Treatment of herpes simplex encephalitis	IV: Adults, children: 15 mg/kg/d, infused over 12–24 hr through in-line membrane filter; reduce dosage in presence of renal impairment
	Ocular manifestations of herpes (conjunctivitis, keratitis, etc)	Topical (ophthalmic ointment): Apply 0.5 in. every 3 hr (5 times daily) for at least 7 days after complete healing of lesion(s)

Table 57–C4 | **Clinical Uses and Administration of Antiviral Drugs*** (*Continued*)

AGENT	CLINICAL USES	DOSAGE AND ROUTE OF ADMINISTRATION
Zidovudine (azidothymidine; "AZT"; RETROVIR)	Symptomatic management of selected patients with symptomatic AIDS or AIDS-related complex	Oral: Initially 200 mg (or about 3 mg/kg) q4h around the clock; continue as needed or until evidence of anemia or leukocytopenia develops, when dose may need to be reduced or therapy stopped until bone marrow recovery

*Arranged alphabetically by generic name.

Table 57–S4 | **Major Side Effects of and Contraindications for Systemically Administered Antiviral Drugs**

BODY SYSTEM/ Side Effect	CONTRAINDICATION/ PRECAUTION	COMMENTS AND NURSING IMPLICATIONS
	Acyclovir	
CENTRAL NERVOUS SYSTEM Headache		Tends to occur with long-term oral therapy, but often diminishes with time
GASTROINTESTINAL Nausea, vomiting, diarrhea		More common with oral acyclovir; administer drug with meals to reduce severity
RENAL Elevations of serum creatinine, BUN; other evidence of transient renal dysfunction		Mainly a problem with IV acyclovir, can be minimized by avoiding bolus administration, keeping patient well hydrated
	Amantadine	
CENTRAL NERVOUS SYSTEM Nervousness, fatigue, confusion, slurred speech, headache	History of psychiatric disturbances	Are reversible when drug is discontinued; occurs frequently in the elderly
SKIN Livedo reticularis		Occurs with prolonged therapy; primarily as used for parkinsonism; see Chapter 25 for more details
	Ribavirin	
RESPIRATORY Worsened respiratory status; pulmonary bacterial infections; ventilator dependence		Assess frequently for diminishing ventilatory capacity, possible need for ventilatory assistance; because ribavirin can occlude mechanical ventilator tubes, including the endotracheal tube, frequent assessment of tube patency, adequacy of ventilation is essential if the ventilator-supported patient must receive this drug
CARDIOVASCULAR Hypotension, cardiac arrest		Monitor blood pressure closely, report any sudden decreases at once

Table 57–S4 | **Major Side Effects of and Contraindications for Systemically Administered Antiviral Drugs (*Continued*)**

BODY SYSTEM/ Side Effect	CONTRAINDICATION/ PRECAUTION	COMMENTS AND NURSING IMPLICATIONS
	Vidarabine	
CENTRAL NERVOUS SYSTEM Headache, dizziness, tremors		If severe, reducing the dose may be helpful
GASTROINTESTINAL Nausea, vomiting, diarrhea		Usually diminishes within 1–4 days; make sure patient remains well hydrated, especially if newborn
OTHER Thrombophlebitis at injection site		Dilute drug in 100–200 mL of fluid, administer via central line if possible; if given in peripheral vein, rotate administration sites frequently
	Zidovudine	
CENTRAL NERVOUS SYSTEM Headache, fever, listlessness		
BLOOD Anemia, granulocytopenia		May be sufficiently severe to require discontinuation of drug or transfusions; frequent assessment, blood tests recommended during therapy; risk increased by other drugs that inhibit zidovudine metabolism (Table 57–I4): avoid if possible
GASTROINTESTINAL Nausea, vomiting, diarrhea		
RENAL Nephrotoxicity	Concurrent use of nephrotoxic drugs; impaired renal function (care)	Assess for diminished urine output; periodic tests indicating renal status (creatinine, BUN) may be warranted

Table 57–14 Major Interactions Between Systemically Administered Antiviral Drugs and Other Agents

AGENT	RESULT OF INTERACTION	COMMENTS AND NURSING IMPLICATIONS
Acyclovir		
Probenecid (Chapter 53)	Reduced renal clearance of acyclovir	Interaction may be beneficial if there is need to increase serum acyclovir levels
Amantadine		
All drugs with antimuscarinic (atropine-like) activity (Chapter 13)	Increased risk of atropine-like side effects	Avoid possible interaction if possible; see Chapter 25 for more details
Vidarabine		
Allopurinol (Chapter 53)	May reduce vidarabine metabolism	Monitor for excessive vidarabine effects if interaction is unavoidable
Zidovudine		
Other nephrotoxic or cytotoxic agents (eg, aminoglycosides, amphotericin B, vinca alkaloids)	Increased risk of zidovudine side effects or toxicity, especially on kidneys, blood	Monitor renal status, hematologic profiles closely if an interactant must be administered
Aspirin, indomethacin, possibly most other nonsteroidal anti-inflammatory drugs; acetaminophen (Chapter 52); probenecid (Chapter 53)	Increased risk of zidovudine toxicity	Monitor accordingly, advise patient to avoid using nonprescription drugs (especially acetaminophen) during zidovudine therapy

Table 57–C5 Clinical Uses and Administration of Major Anthelminthic Drugs

AGENT	CLINICAL USES	DOSAGE AND ROUTE OF ADMINISTRATION*
Mebendazole		
(VERMOX)	Pinworm	Adults, children: 1 100-mg dose; tablets may be swallowed, crushed, chewed, or mixed with food
	Roundworm, threadworm, hookworm	Adults, children: 100 mg bid for 3 days
Niclosamide		
(NICLOCIDE)	Tapeworm	Adults: 1 2-g dose. Children: 1–1.5 g; for adults or children with dwarf tapeworm infestations, continue treatment for 1 week
Piperazine		
(VERMIZINE)	Roundworm	Adults: 3.5 g/d for 2 days. Children: 75 mg/kg/d for 2 days
	Pinworm	Adults: 2.5 g/d for 7 days. Children: 65 mg/kg/d for 7 days; always administer on empty stomach
Pyrantel		
(ANTIMINTH)	Roundworm, pinworm	Adults, children: 1 dose of 11 mg/kg (equivalent to 1 mL per 10 lb of body weight of supplied product), taken with milk, juice, or food; ensure entire dose is taken all at once
Quinacrine		
(ATABRINE)	Dwarf tapeworms	Adults, children: Initially, 3 300-mg doses spaced by 20 min on empty stomach; purge 1.5 hr later; then give 100 mg tid for next 3 days
	Other tapeworm infestations	Adults, children: Initially, 200-mg doses spaced by 10 min; administer sodium bicarbonate and purges/enemas
	Giardiasis	Adults: 100 mg tid after meals for 5–7 days. Children: 7 mg/kg at times noted for adults
Thiabendazole		
(MINTEZOL)		For all indications: Adults: 1.5 g bid. Children: 22 mg/kg bid; administer with food, chew tablets thoroughly before swallowing
	Pinworm	Administer for 1 day, repeat in 1 week
	Hookworm, threadworm	Treat for 2 consecutive days
	Whipworm	Treat for 4 consecutive days

*All doses are administered orally.

Table 57–S5 Major Side Effects of and Contraindications for Anthelminthic Drugs

BODY SYSTEM/ Side Effect	CONTRAINDICATION/ PRECAUTION	COMMENTS AND NURSING IMPLICATIONS
All		
GASTROINTESTINAL Nausea, vomiting, diarrhea	Severe dehydration or malnutrition	Attempt to correct severe fluid-electrolyte imbalances, nutritional status before routine treatment with anthelminthics; avoid administering antidiarrheal drugs, which would help retain parasite in gut; incidence, severity depend on drug, patient, severity of infection
Mebendazole		
GASTROINTESTINAL Abdominal cramping, occasional fever		
Piperazine		
CENTRAL NERVOUS SYSTEM Ataxia, headache, vertigo; extrapyramidal signs and symptoms; seizures	History of seizure disorders	
EYE Blurred vision, nystagmus, occasional cataracts		Cataracts not likely to occur unless treatment is prolonged
Pyrantel		
CENTRAL NERVOUS SYSTEM Headache, drowsiness, dizziness		
HEPATIC Transient elevations of marker enzymes of hepatic status (eg, AST, ALT)		Use with care in patients with liver dysfunction, regardless of the cause
SKIN Rash		Usually harmless

Table 57–S5 Major Side Effects of and Contraindications for Anthelminthic Drugs (*Continued*)

BODY SYSTEM/ Side Effect	CONTRAINDICATION/ PRECAUTION	COMMENTS AND NURSING IMPLICATIONS
Quinacrine		
CENTRAL NERVOUS SYSTEM Dizziness, headache, transient psychosis		Use with care in elderly patients, patients with history of psychosis
EYE Visual disturbances		Recommend periodic eye examinations for patients on long-term therapy
GASTROINTESTINAL Yellow staining of expelled worms in stool		Examine stool, looking for yellow-colored worms as evidence of expected drug action
HEPATIC Transient elevations of marker enzymes of hepatic status (eg, AST, ALT)		Use with care in patients with liver dysfunction, regardless of the cause
RENAL Yellow discoloration of urine		Expected, harmless
SKIN Yellow discoloration		Expected, harmless
Thiabendazole		
CENTRAL NERVOUS SYSTEM Anorexia, dizziness		Common and most likely to occur 3 to 4 hr after administration; assist ambulation, advise avoidance of hazardous tasks
GASTROINTESTINAL Nausea, vomiting		Incidence, onset, similar to those noted for anorexia and dizziness

Table 57–C6 Clinical Uses and Administration of Selected Antiprotozoal-Antimicrobial Drugs*

AGENT	CLINICAL USES	DOSAGE AND ROUTE OF ADMINISTRATION
Carbarsone (generic)	Intestinal amebiasis	Oral: Adults: 500–750 mg/d in divided doses for 10 days or for lesser time if there is evidence of arsenic toxicity. Children: Total (not daily) dose of 75 mg/kg, given over 10 days in 3 divided doses each day
Chloroquine HCl or phosphate (ARALEN)	Malaria caused by susceptible strains of *Plasmodium*	
	Malaria suppression (prophylaxis)	Oral: Adults: 500 mg of phosphate salt once weekly on same day each week. Children: 8.3 mg/kg phosphate salt once weekly, but not to exceed adult dose. Adults, children: Start treatment 2 weeks before entering endemic areas, continue for 6–8 weeks after leaving; oral therapy preferred; if prophylactic therapy is not started before exposure, double initial dose, give in 2 divided doses of 6 hr apart
	Treatment of uncomplicated malaria attacks	Oral: Adults: 1 g of phosphate salt initially, then 500 mg at 6, 24, 48 hr after initial dose. Children: 6.25 mg/kg phosphate salt at times noted for adults
	Treatment of severe malaria attacks or when initial oral therapy is not feasible or suitable	IM: Adults: 200–250 mg of HCl salt (4–5 mL of supplied product); repeat in 6 hr, continue for 3 days until approximately 1.875 g has been administered; do not exceed 1 g HCl in first 24 hr; begin oral therapy as soon as possible. Children: Initially, 6.25 mg/kg HCl, repeated in 6 hr; avoid exceeding 12.5 mg/kg HCl in first 24 hr
	Treatment of extraintestinal amebiasis (usually adjunctive with intraintestinal amebicide)	Oral (Adults only): 1 g phosphate salt daily for 2 days, then 500 mg daily for at least 2–3 weeks IM (Adults only): 200–250 mg of HCl salt for 10–12 days
Emetine (generic)	Intestinal, extraintestinal amebiasis	Deep SC (preferred) or IM: Adults: Usually 65 mg/d in single or 2 divided daily doses for 10 days, not to exceed cumulative dose of 650 mg; with acute fulminating dysentery, give only long enough to control diarrhea. Children <8 years: <10 mg/d; 8 years <20 mg/d; use only for severe amebiasis refractory to other amebicides
Hydroxychloroquine sulfate (PLAQUENIL)	Malaria, as for chloroquine	
	Malaria suppression	Oral: Adults: 400 mg weekly at times noted for chloroquine. Children: Approx. 6.25 mg/kg weekly, as noted for chloroquine
	Malaria treatment	Oral: Adults: 800 mg initially, then 400 mg at times noted for chloroquine. Children: 13 mg/kg initially, then 6.25 mg/kg at times noted for chloroquine
	Rheumatoid arthritis, lupus erythematosus	See Chapter 52

(continued)

Table 57–C6 Clinical Uses and Administration of Selected Antiprotozoal-Antimicrobial Drugs* (*Continued*)

AGENT	CLINICAL USES	DOSAGE AND ROUTE OF ADMINISTRATION
Iodoquinol		
(diiodohydroxyquin; various trade names)	Acute, chronic intestinal amebiasis	Oral: Adults: 650 mg bid or tid for 20 days; give after meals. Children: 40 mg/kg/d in 3 divided doses for 20 days
Metronidazole		
(FLAGYL; others)	Acute amebic dysentery (intestinal amebiasis)	Oral: Adults: 750 mg tid for 5–10 days; often administered with oral iodoquinol, 650 mg tid for 20 days. Children: Usually 35–50 mg/kg in divided doses
	Amebic liver abscess	Oral: Adults: 500 or 750 mg for 5–10 days. Children: 35–50 mg/kg/d, in 3 divided doses each day, for 10 days
	Giardiasis (alternative to quinacrine)	Oral: Adults: 250 mg tid for 7 days
	Vaginitis caused by *Gardnerella vaginalis*	Oral: Adults: 500 mg bid for 7 days. Children: 15 mg/kg/d for 5 days
	Trichomoniasis	Oral (preferred): Single dose of 2 g, or 2 1-g doses taken on same day. Alternative: 250 mg tid for 7 days; allow 4–6 weeks to elapse between re-treatments
	Treatment of various infections caused by gram-negative anaerobes	IV: Initially 15 mg/kg, infused over 1 hr; maintenance dose 7.5 mg/kg q6h; do not exceed 4 g/24 hr; treatment usually lasts 7–10 days; start oral therapy as soon as possible Oral: 7.5 mg/kg q6h
Paromomycin		
(HUMATIN)	Acute, chronic intestinal amebiasis	Oral: Adults, children: 25–35 mg/d in 3 divided doses with meals for 5–10 days
	Management of hepatic coma	Oral: Adults: 4 g/d in divided doses at regular intervals for 5 or 6 days
Pentamidine isethionate		
(PENTAM 300)	Treatment of *P. carinii* pneumonia	IM or IV: Adults, children: 4 mg/kg qd; solution should be 100 mg/mL in sterile water for IM injection; for IV use, dilute drug in sterile water so total dose is in 50–150 mL 5% dextrose solution, infuse over 60 min; treatment usually lasts 14 days
Primaquine phosphate	Treatment or prevention of *P. vivax* malaria	Oral: Adults: 1 tablet (26.3 mg) daily for 14 days or 3 tablets once weekly for 8 weeks. Children: Roughly 0.5 mg/kg/d for 14 days or 1 mg/kg/d weekly for 8 weeks. Begin primaquine administration during last 2 weeks of treatment with chloroquine or related drug, or after a course of suppression (prophylaxis) with chloroquine, etc

Table 57–C6 Clinical Uses and Administration of Selected Antiprotozoal-Antimicrobial Drugs* (*Continued*)

AGENT	CLINICAL USES	DOSAGE AND ROUTE OF ADMINISTRATION
Quinacrine HCl		
(ATABRINE)	Suppression of malaria	Oral: Adults: 100 mg/d for 1–3 months. Children: 50 mg/d
	Treatment of malaria	Oral: Adults, children >8 years: 200 mg q6h for 5 doses, then 100 mg tid for 6 days; give with 1 g sodium bicarbonate each time. Children 4–8 years: 200 mg tid on day 1, then 100 mg q12h for 6 days. Children 1–4 years: 100 mg tid on day 1, then 100 mg qd for 6 days
	Other indications	See Table 57–C5
Quinine sulfate		
(QUINAMM; others)	Treatment of chloroquine-resistant *P. falciparum* malaria	Oral: Adults: 650 mg q8h for 10–14 days. Children: 25 mg/kg/d, in divided doses q8h for 10–14 days. For adults, children: use adjunctively with pyrimethamine and sulfadiazine or a tetracycline

*Listed alphabetically by generic name.

Table 57–S6 Major Side Effects of and Contraindications for Selected Antiprotozoal-Antimicrobial Drugs*

BODY SYSTEM/ Side Effect	CONTRAINDICATION/ PRECAUTION	COMMENTS AND NURSING IMPLICATIONS
Carbasone		
CENTRAL NERVOUS SYSTEM Neuritis, seizures		May reflect overdosage (arsenic toxicity); hemorrhagic encephalitis, seizures may occur; discontinue immediately, treat symptomatically, supportively, administer arsenic chelator dimercaprol (BAL; see Appendix C)
EYE Visual disturbances	Altered vision	See CNS
CARDIOVASCULAR Hypotension, shock		Possible arsenic toxicity; see CNS
GASTROINTESTINAL Nausea, vomiting, diarrhea exceeding that before treatment; resulting fluid, electrolyte imbalances		Potential indicator of arsenic poisoning; see CNS
HEPATIC Hepatitis, hepatic necrosis	Liver disease	Assess, may progress to coma and death; may reflect arsenic poisoning
RENAL Renal damage, failure	Renal disease	
SKIN Pruritus, other minor rashes; severe responses such as exfoliative dermatitis (fatal)	Prior allergic response to carbasone, other arsenic compounds	Assess closely; discontinue drug at once, avoid repeat exposure to it; response could be fatal
Chloroquine, Hydroxychloroquine		
EYE Blurred vision, corneal inclusions, keratopathy, ocular edema, retinopathy	Visual impairments (unless no other antimalarial treatment is available)	Frequent ophthalmic examinations are essential; advise patient to report any visual disturbances or alterations at once
BLOOD Hemolysis, hemolytic anemia; falls of hemoglobin, hematocrit, red cell count	Care in patients with glucose-6-phosphate dehydrogenase deficiency	Periodic complete blood counts are recommended during prolonged therapy

(*continued*)

Table 57–S6 Major Side Effects of and Contraindications for Selected Antiprotozoal-Antimicrobial Drugs* (*Continued*)

BODY SYSTEM/ Side Effect	CONTRAINDICATION/ PRECAUTION	COMMENTS AND NURSING IMPLICATIONS
GASTROINTESTINAL Anorexia, nausea, vomiting, diarrhea, cramping		Administer with meals
SKIN Pigmentary changes of skin and hair (usually seen as bleaching); aggravation of psoriasis		Bleaching usually occurs after several months of use
Emetine		
CENTRAL NERVOUS SYSTEM Headache, dizziness		Common; may be accompanied by other complaints (see GI)
CARDIOVASCULAR Hypotension, various rate and rhythm disturbances	Cardiac disease other than amebic abscesses	Are the most severe toxic effects of this drug; monitor accordingly, with special emphasis on ECG changes indicative of myocardial ischemia
GASTROINTESTINAL Nausea, vomiting		Occur in one third to one half of patients, often accompanied by dizziness, headache; monitor for onset, severity, notify physician accordingly; important to determine whether caused by drug or underlying disease
NEUROMUSCULAR Muscle weakness, pain, weakness, stiffness		Assess closely, as these may be early warnings of serious toxicity
Iodoquinol		
EYE Optic neuritis, atrophy		Assess visual status; usually associated with prolonged therapy, which should be avoided
ENDOCRINE Thyroid enlargement		Iodoquinol is an iodine compound, may interfere with thyroid function, thyroid function tests; see iodine/iodides, Chapter 48
GASTROINTESTINAL Nausea, vomiting, diarrhea		Assess carefully to determine whether drug- or disease-related; anticipate some degree of GI distress

Table 57–S6 | **Major Side Effects of and Contraindications for Selected Antiprotozoal-Antimicrobial Drugs*** (*Continued*)

BODY SYSTEM/ Side Effect	CONTRAINDICATION/ PRECAUTION	COMMENTS AND NURSING IMPLICATIONS
	Metronidazole	
CENTRAL NERVOUS SYSTEM Vertigo, syncope, confusion		Infrequent with oral administration; dizziness may involve orthostatic hypotension, advise patient to avoid standing suddenly
GASTROINTESTINAL Nausea, vomiting, anorexia; metallic taste		Administer drug with food
GENITOURINARY Urethral burning, vaginal dryness		Advise patient to notify physician if symptoms become severe or intolerable
	Paromomycin	
	See aminoglycosides, Chapter 56	
	Pentamidine	
	No contraindications in patients with documented P. carinii *pneumonia*	
ENDOCRINE Hypoglycemia or, less often, hyperglycemia	Care in patients with diabetes mellitus	Monitor blood glucose levels daily; hypoglycemia can be severe, fatal
BLOOD Blood dyscrasias (various, but especially leukopenia, thrombocytopenia)	Care in patients with abnormal hematologic or coagulation profiles	Perform baseline CBC, coagulation studies, repeat periodically during therapy; may be life-threatening
CARDIOVASCULAR Severe hypotension	Care in hypotensive or hypertensive patients or disorders that can be worsened by marked blood pressure changes	Can occur with IM or IV injections; if IV route is used, be sure to infuse entire dose no faster than over 60 min; symptomatic hypotension may require treatment with parenteral fluid boluses; may be life-threatening
Arrhythmias (potentially fatal)	Care in patients with history of arrhythmias	Record ECG before and then periodically during and after therapy
RENAL Elevated serum creatinine, BUN, other evidence of potential or actual renal failure	Care in patients with renal dysfunction	Tends to occur by second week of therapy; monitor renal function, urine output daily; stop drug at once if acute renal failure occurs or seems imminent; incidence of some degree of renal dysfunction is as high as 1 in 4 patients

(*continued*)

Table 57–S6 | Major Side Effects of and Contraindications for Selected Antiprotozoal-Antimicrobial Drugs* (*Continued*)

BODY SYSTEM/ Side Effect	CONTRAINDICATION/ PRECAUTION	COMMENTS AND NURSING IMPLICATIONS
SKIN Sterile abscesses, inflammation, pain at injection site (IM)		Rotate injection sites frequently; assess previous sites for inflammation, abscesses
	Primaquine	
	See chloroquine	
	Pyrimethamine	
CENTRAL NERVOUS SYSTEM CNS stimulation, seizures		Usually results from overdosage (therapeutic dosages for toxoplasmosis are borderline toxic); assess accordingly; never exceed recommended dosages for malaria; anticonvulsant therapy, folinic acid (leucovorin) usually required if seizures occur
GASTROINTESTINAL Anorexia, vomiting, glossitis		Administer with meals
BLOOD Anemias, other blood dyscrasias (especially in patients with glucose-6-phosphate dehydrogenase deficiencies, who are at higher risk of hemolytic anemia)		Most likely to occur with high doses needed for treating toxoplasmosis, best monitored with twice-weekly CBC; discontinuation of drug and/or administration of folinic acid (leucovorin) may be indicated
	Quinacrine	
	See Table 57–S5	
	Quinine Sulfate	
	See quinidine, Chapter 30, Table 30–S	

*Arranged alphabetically by generic name.

Table 57–16 Major Interactions Between Antimalarials and Other Antiprotozoal Drugs and Other Agents

AGENT	RESULT OF INTERACTION	COMMENTS AND NURSING IMPLICATIONS
Interactions Involving Chloroquine, Hydroxychloroquine, Related Aminoquinolines		
Antacids; antidiarrheals (eg, kaolin-pectin; Chapters 34, 41)	Decreased absorption of antimalarial drug	Avoid combined use
Digoxin (Chapter 31)	Increased risk of digoxin toxicity	Chloroquine and hydroxychloroquine are related to quinidine, may displace digoxin from tissue binding sites, reduce digoxin renal clearance; assess for evidence of digitalis toxicity if combined therapy cannot be avoided
Interactions Involving Metronidazole		
Alcohol (Chapter 22)	Alcohol intolerance (disulfiram-like reaction): headache, hypotension, chest pain, etc	Incidence, severity unpredictable; mechanism identical to that involving alcohol and disulfiram; advise patients to avoid consuming any beverage, food, or medication containing alcohol for up to 1 week after discontinuing metronidazole
Anticoagulants, oral (Chapter 35)	Increased risk of excessive anticoagulant effect	If interaction cannot be avoided, monitor prothrombin times closely, assess for evidence of impaired clotting (bruising, bleeding, etc), which may have sudden onset; anticipate need to reduce anticoagulant dose during combined therapy
Cimetidine (Chapter 40)	Increased risk of metronidazole side effects	Cimetidine inhibits metronidazole metabolism, causing blood levels to rise; interaction less likely to occur with related antihistamines famotidine, nizatidine, rantidine, which may be preferred if combined therapy is essential
Disulfiram (Chapter 22)	Severe, acute psychotic reaction, confusion, etc	Avoid combined use
Phenobarbital, phenytoin, related drugs (Chapters 22, 26)	Diminished action of metronidazole	Avoid combined use if possible; interactant increases metronidazole metabolism; increased metronidazole doses may be required; monitor accordingly
Interactions Involving Pyrimethamine		
	None reported	
Interactions Involving Quinine Sulfate		
	See Quinidine, Chapter 30, Table 30–S	

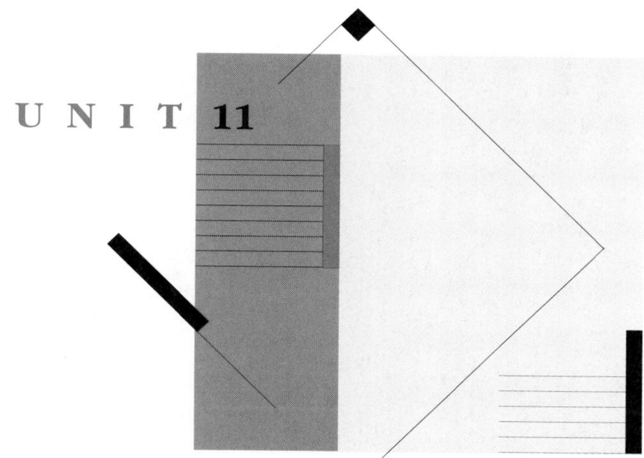

Chemotherapy of Neoplastic Diseases

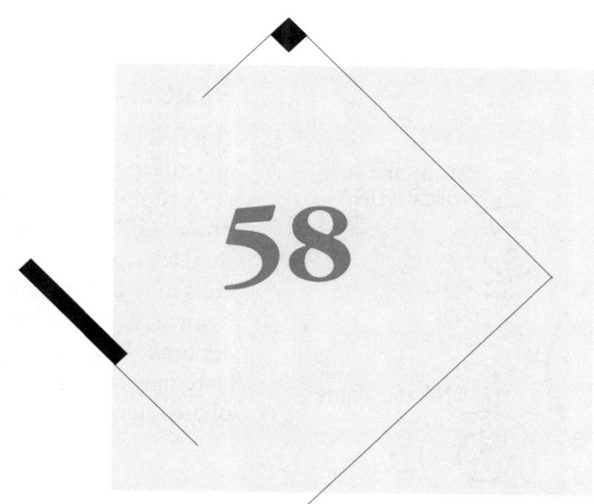

Cell Growth, Neoplasia, and Principles of Cancer Chemotherapy

Cancer is a complex group of diseases that requires specialized skills for detection, diagnosis, and treatment. Fifty years ago the five-year survival rate was one in five. Today, 50% of patients will be alive five years after diagnosis. Much of the improvement in survival rates is attributable to the use of chemotherapy. Drug treatment is used alone and in combination with surgery, radiation, and biotherapy to achieve cure, control (prevent continued growth), or palliation (control of symptoms) of cancer. Even when cure is not possible, control will prolong survival, and palliation can relieve symptoms and restore physical function.

Most of the drugs used in cancer treatment are highly toxic chemicals that can be harmful to both tumors and normal tissues. In addition, the therapeutic value of these agents depends on their ability to *selectively* kill tumor cells. This selectivity is often due to differences between the growth characteristics of tumors and those of normal host tissues. Therefore, understanding the reasons for therapeutic successes and failures depends on knowing how tumors and host tissues grow and how these growth patterns change over time.

Normal Cell Growth

All tissues and tumors are mixtures of cells in different growth states. In mature, normal tissues, most cells are highly specialized. Having achieved a state of permanent **quiescence** (dormancy), they will never divide. Other cells ("stem" cells) are less differentiated, and still retain the potential to divide when it is necessary to replace cells lost as a result of injury or aging. Because the need for replacement is usually low, most stem cells are also quiescent at any given time. When the need does arise, some of these stem cells leave quiescence and begin the division process known as the **cell cycle**.

The cell cycle consists of four sequential phases called G_1, S, G_2, and M. When cells make the transition from quiescence into the cycle, they initially enter the G_1 phase (Fig. 58–1). The length of G_1 varies greatly among tumor types, and ranges from several hours to a few days. It appears that there are one or more "restriction points" during G_1, at which cell division is delayed until conditions are right to proceed further. One of the main activities that occurs in G_1 is the production of enzymes needed for DNA replication. When this process is complete, cells progress into S phase and begin DNA **synthesis** (hence the designation "S"). S phase

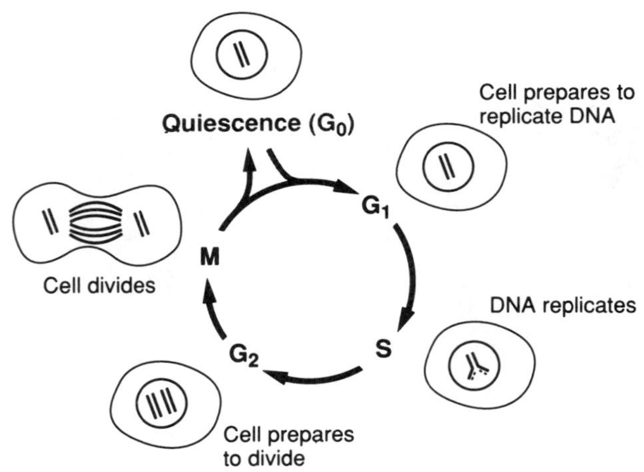

Figure 58–1

The cell cycle. Once a cell is committed to divide, it begins an ordered sequence of events. Cells in G_1 phase prepare for DNA replication. The synthesis of new DNA occurs in S phase. Cells in G_2 phase produce components necessary for mitosis, which constitutes M phase. After mitosis is complete, cells may initiate another division cycle or may go into a dormant state called "quiescence." Entering quiescence is conceptually equivalent to leaving the cell cycle, although this state may represent merely an indefinite elongation of G_1 phase. Hence, quiescence sometimes is referred to as "G_0."

also varies in length (10–20 hours), although not as much as G_1. Once DNA replication is finished, cells enter G_2 phase (2–10 hours), during which they begin to make components necessary for the segregation of chromosomes and cell division. These events take place during mitosis (M phase, 0.5–1 hour). At the end of mitosis the cycle is complete and two identical daughter cells are formed, each of which finds itself back in G_1 phase. These cells may stay in the cycle and go on to divide again, or they may leave the cycle and reenter quiescence.

A parameter used to describe the relative degree of proliferation in various tissues is the **growth fraction**. It is defined as the fraction of the total cell population that is in any phase of the cell cycle at the time of measurement. Although the growth fraction of most normal tissues is ordinarily quite low (eg, $\leq$ 0.01, or 1%), tissues that regularly experience substantial turnover, such as blood and epithelium, can have much higher growth fractions (0.01–0.10, or 1% to 10%).

It is uncertain how the body controls its growth processes and what causes cells to stop growing once normal tissue size has been reached. Some type of mechanism controls cell growth, limits cell size and shape, and regulates the effects of body hormones and growth stimulating factors. The discovery of these mechanisms may lead to an understanding of how cancer is caused, as well as how cancer may be prevented or cured.

Tumor Cell Growth

In normal tissues the transition of cells into and out of the cell cycle is tightly controlled, resulting in an equilibrium between cell death and the production of new cells. One fundamental difference between normal and cancerous cells is the loss of this control. As a result, the growth fraction of tumors is higher than would be necessary to just replace dying cells. The net effect is that the total number of cells in the tumor (and, therefore, the size of the tumor) increases steadily over time. This difference in growth fraction also is thought to be the basis for selective cell kill by anticancer drugs. The primary biochemical effect of most of these drugs is interference with one or more steps involved in progression through the cell cycle. Inhibition of DNA synthesis during S phase is the most common way in which anticancer drugs affect the cell cycle.

One property of tumors that makes them difficult to treat is that their growth patterns change significantly over time (Fig. 58–2). Tumors have their highest growth fraction during the early stages of development. At this point the tumors are still relatively small and all of their cells have good access to blood-borne nutrients and oxygen. Because of these favorable growth conditions, the number of cells in such a tumor increases exponentially. As the tumor expands, it begins to outgrow its blood supply and eventually reaches a point where many of its cells go into quiescence or die due to lack of nutrients and oxygen. The growth fraction at this stage is much lower than it was during early growth; it may be not much different than that of normal tissues. This decreases the ability of chemotherapeutic agents to target selectively the tumor population. It is a serious problem in practice because most tumors are not detected until they have reached this late stage of growth. Indeed, with current technologies that usually are used, tumors weighing less than about one gram cannot be detected. However, these small, undetectable, and still rapidly growing tumors contain an estimated one billion (10^9) cells (see Fig. 58–2).

Cancer cells differ from normal cells in other ways, including *loss of contact inhibition, lack of adhesion,* and *inability to differentiate fully.* Contact inhibition is

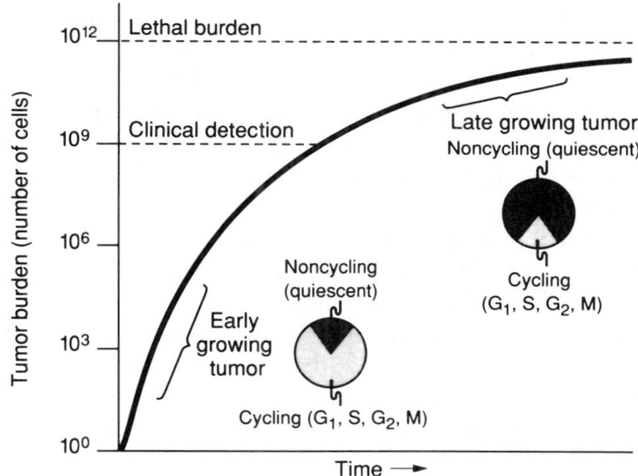

Figure 58–2

Changes in tumor cell growth over time. Early in the development of a solid tumor, its cell number and mass increase exponentially. The fraction of cycling cells (growth fraction) is relatively high during this time. Later, as the tumor outgrows its blood supply, the rate of growth, the growth fraction, and tumor response to drug therapy, decrease. Most tumors already have reached this late phase of growth by the time they are detected clinically—when the cell number exceeds one billion (10^9), yet cell mass is barely more than one gram.

one of the processes that regulates normal cell growth. During growth, when normal cells come in direct contact with other cells, they stop moving and growing. Cancer cells have lost this contact inhibition and grow without control. Normal cells tend to adhere to one another to form clumps of tissue of one cell type. This lack of adhesion in cancer cells contributes to their ability to break off and **metastasize**, or move about the body. Because of these altered growth properties, tumors often are called **neoplasms**, which literally means "new growths."

Differentiation is a process in which cells mature and become specialized to form specific structures or perform specific functions. A well-differentiated cell has unique properties and a prescribed function. An undifferentiated cell is immature and cannot carry out specialized functions. Cancer cells tend to be less differentiated and are often referred to as **anaplastic**. Anaplastic cells lack both the structural organization and the useful functions of a normal cell. The replacement of normal tissue cells with anaplastic cells of cancer is responsible for the physiologic dysfunctions that accompany cancer. For example, the bone marrow contains stem cells that may differentiate into one of three different types of blood cells. Leukemia, a cancer of the blood-forming tissue, results in white blood cells that are undifferentiated, immature, and cannot perform the needed functions to prevent infection.

Tumor Cell Kill

In general, the more intense the drug treatment, the greater the tumor cell kill. Such intense therapy is achieved either by administering anticancer drugs repetitively or at high doses. The usual relationship between drug treatment and cell kill is logarithmic, rather than linear (Fig. 58–3). For example, if a certain dose

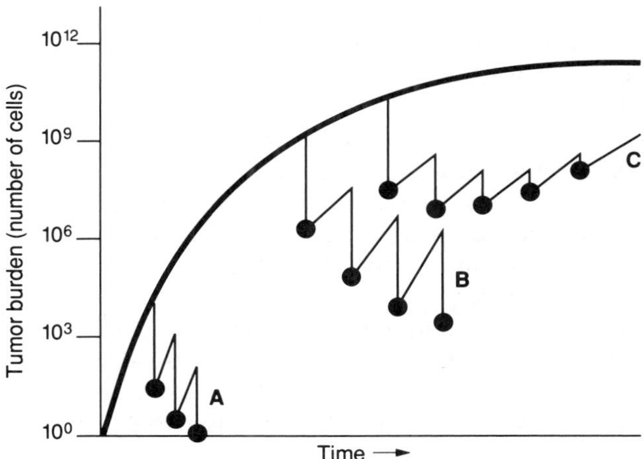

Figure 58–3

Log cell kill. The thick curve shows expected progression of a solid tumor without treatment. Vertical lines indicate tumor shrinkage due to treatment. Thin curves represent tumor regrowth between treatments.

A). If treatment is started early (e.g., at a tumor burden of ≈ 10^4 cells), then treatments with a therapy that produced 99.9% tumor cell kill (i.e., 3 log unit reduction in cell number) would eradicate the tumor after a few treatment cycles.

B). When treatment is started at a later stage, the absolute number of cells killed in each treatment cycle is much greater than in A, but the fraction killed remains the same. Therefore, many cycles of treatment would be needed to eliminate the tumor completely. Also, patient tolerance may limit the frequency with which therapy is administered, allowing significant regrowth between treatment cycles.

C). Resistant tumor cells often arise during the course of treatment. As a result, the effectiveness of a particular treatment regimen may decrease with each successive treatment cycle. Ultimately, the course of tumor progression may be almost the same with treatment as without.

of an anticancer drug kills 90% of the cells in a tumor, it will reduce the fraction of live tumor cell from 1.0 to 0.1, or one log unit (10^{-1}). After the second treatment, the total tumor burden will be reduced from 0.1 to 0.01—another one log-unit fall. This reduction in the number of live tumor cells continues with continued dosing.

To put this in a different perspective, consider that when treatment starts with a drug that kills 90% of tumor cells, the tumor contains 10^9 cells. (As noted in Fig. 58–2, this is roughly the minimum number of cells that can be detected in a typical tumor.) After the first dose, 10^8 live cells are left. After the second dose, 10^7 live cells remain. Thus, nine consecutive treatment courses would be required to reduce the tumor down to one (10^0) cell.

In practice, it is necessary to allow time between courses of drug therapy for patients to recover from the drug's toxic side effects. The tumor is likely to begin regrowing during these intervals. The ultimate success of chemotherapy therefore depends, in part, on how great the cell kill is with each treatment round, and on how often treatment can be given.

Resistance

Another major difficulty in chemotherapy is that some tumor cells are either naturally resistant to the drugs used to treat them, or they acquire such resistance over time. Natural resistance is an initial unresponsiveness of cancer cells to chemotherapeutic agents. The failure to respond to a drug may be owing to a low growth fraction or the location of the tumor in a site that has poor blood perfusion or minimal drug penetration. Acquired resistance occurs after the start of therapy and may be the result of the presence and growth of resistant cell lines. As the individual is exposed to progressive doses of chemotherapy, the likelihood increases that tumor cells will undergo a spontaneous mutation that creates resistance. Chemotherapy preferentially kills sensitive cells, leaving behind the resistant cells to continue growing.

Insufficient uptake of the drug into the tumor cell, insufficient activation of the drug, or inactivation of the drug by the tumor, are all responsible for chemotherapy failures. Cancer cells also may decrease their need for certain metabolic products or may use alternate metabolic pathways to meet their nutrient needs. Thus, they can continue growing even though the drug is still exerting its usual metabolic effects. Some cancer cells are able to repair drug-induced DNA defects before the damage is lethal. Cancer cells may also develop spontaneous mutants that have simultaneous resistance to multiple classes of chemotherapy agents (pleiotropic resistance).

Strategies for Drug Treatment

The information we have learned about tumor biology is, in large part, the basis for designing strategies for administering chemotherapy. One major use for this data is to help decide which drugs should be used in combination with each other.

Although some patients with cancer obtain excellent results from a single antineoplastic agent, most cancers are treated with a combination of drugs. Combination chemotherapy produces better responses and can increase the disease-free intervals and survival rates. Combination chemotherapy is also used to prevent or delay failures owing to resistance. Exposing the tumor to several drugs with different modes of action helps diminish the problem of drug resistance. The goals of combination chemotherapy are to provide the maximum cell kill without producing excessive toxicity, to inhibit the effects of natural resistance, and to prevent or slow the emergence of new, resistant, cell lines.

Several principles guide the selection of specific agents used in combination anticancer therapy. Each drug used as part of the combination must have established activity against the particular cancer being treated. Agents are selected because they have different types of toxicities, or because their toxicities occur at different times or to different degrees. Some drugs work synergistically to enhance the effects of another drug, providing a greater therapeutic benefit than if each drug were given alone.

In addition to the choice of chemotherapeutic agents, the timing of their delivery also is determined by certain properties of tumors, host tissues, and the drugs themselves. Some antineoplastic drugs (Chapter 59) are only active against cells that are in a particular phase of the cell cycle. Methotrexate and 5-fluorouracil, which preferentially kill S-phase cells, are examples of such "phase-specific" drugs. Phase-specific drugs often are given by continuous infusion regimens over a long period of time (from several hours to days or even weeks) so that as many tumor cells as possible will pass through the critical cell cycle phase while the drug is present. Other drugs (such as the alkylating agent, cyclophosphamide) kill cells with about equal efficiency no matter where they are in the cell cycle. They are called "cycle-specific" agents. Cycle-specific drugs commonly are given as bolus doses or short infusions.

As mentioned earlier, large tumors with low growth fractions are especially difficult to treat with chemotherapy. One way to increase the effectiveness of both phase-specific and cycle-specific drugs against these tumors is to remove as much of the tumor mass as possible, by surgery or radiation therapy, before drug treatment. This stimulates quiescent cells to be *recruited* back into the cell cycle, and increases the likelihood of benefit from chemotherapy.

When two or more drugs are used in combination they may be administered in varying sequences and intervals. The drug combination, given over a specified period of time, is referred to as a treatment cycle. A common treatment cycle lasts three to six weeks. When the patient recovers from the expected toxicities of a treatment, the cycle is repeated. Repeated cycles may be used for periods of four to 12 months. As long as the patient tolerates the drug side effects, therapy may continue indefinitely using drug combinations to obtain the desired responses.

Dose Determination

The ideal dose of a chemotherapeutic agent is one that kills a maximum number of cancer cells. In practice, the dose that kills the most cancer cells could be lethal to the patient. In practice, therefore, drug doses must be selected to allow the highest possible doses to be given, while producing tolerable toxicity. The preferred method to determine the correct dose is based on the patient's body surface area, although doses may also be based on body weight. The use of body surface area minimizes individual variations in size at different weights, and provides a useful index to standardize doses for adults and children.

Drug doses may be modified if the drugs in a combination have overlapping toxicities, if the patient has previously received treatment with chemotherapy or radiation therapy (which can reduce the bone marrow's ability to recover from insult), or if the patient has any organ dysfunction. Doses should be reduced, or the drug withheld, when toxicities affect an impaired organ's ability to metabolize or excrete the drug. The patient's general health and nutritional status also influence the drugs and doses selected. Weakened or debilitated patients poorly tolerate the toxicities of chemotherapy, and suffer increased morbidity and mortality because of it.

Proper dosage calculation and administration are important because few antineoplastic drugs have antidotes that could be used to treat toxicity from overdose.

General Nursing Responsibilities Related to Handling and Administering Chemotherapeutic Agents

Special precautions must be used in the handling and administration of chemotherapeutic agents. Antineoplastic agents are mutagenic, and in some cases carcinogenic, so the nurse must take protective measures to reduce personal exposure. Safety measures should focus on protecting the skin, eyes, and respiratory tract of personnel handling the drugs. Wear latex gloves and a long-sleeved protective garment with a closed front and cuffs during antineoplastic drug mixing and administration. Mix the drugs in a biologic safety cabinet that is vented, to prevent aerosol contact with the skin and respiratory tract. Take care to eliminate internal pressure or vacuum in vials, to reduce aerosol formation. To prevent accidental ingestion of contaminated substances, do not eat or drink in areas where drugs are mixed and administered.

During administration, special care is needed to prevent drug spills during priming of intravenous (IV) tubings. Handle spills with extra caution to prevent exposure. Wear protective eyewear and use disposable cleaning materials when wiping spills. Dispose as hazardous waste any leftover drug or administration materials (vials, IV needles, tubing).

Establish venous access immediately before drug administration. The preferred method of administration for drugs given by the bolus technique is through the sidearm of a running IV infusion. Take extra care to determine the patency of the vein when giving drugs known to be vesicants. Vesicants can cause soft tissue damage if they extravasate. Check the IV line for blood return every one to two minutes during bolus administration of vesicants.

As a general rule, never mix antineoplastic agents together or with other drugs unless compatibility has been proved. When several antineoplastic agents are to be administered at the same time, they should be given in sequence.

General Nursing Responsibilities Related to Common Side Effects of Chemotherapeutic Agents

One of the major roles of the nurse caring for the cancer patient is to monitor and assess the toxic effects of the chemotherapeutic agents. The nurse can also teach patients self-care strategies that will help control and

SPOTLIGHT ON NURSING RESEARCH

With the shift in the administration of chemotherapy to outpatient settings, patients and their families have assumed increasing responsibilities for identifying and managing associated side effects. To help them deal with these responsibilities, nurses and other health care providers need to give information about effective strategies for managing the side effects of cytotoxic drugs. Many types of self-care activities are commonly suggested, but their usefulness to patients has not been established.

These investigators wanted to find out more about patients' experiences in dealing with chemotherapy. They developed a self-care diary so patients could record specific side effects along with the types and effectiveness of activities used to manage them. Each of 18 different side effects was listed in conjunction with a number of possible self-care activities. Space was also provided for patients to add comments to the diary.

Fifty-five adult oncology clinic patients at the beginning of a treatment cycle participated in the study. Subjects agreed to complete and return the self-care diary at two and five days after receiving chemotherapy. When completing the diary, subjects described the severity of the side effects they experienced using a 5 point scale. The efficacy of identified self-care activities was also rated on a 5 point scale.

The number of side effects reported by subjects averaged 5.6 and side effects were described as moderately severe. Most subjects (81%) identified fatigue as a problem. Sleeping difficulty, nausea, and decreased appetite were each experience by about one-half of the subjects. Changes in taste and smell and hair loss were somewhat less common—reported by approximately one-third.

Subjects reported using multiple strategies to deal with the symptoms they experienced. For example, obtaining extra sleep and distraction were the most common approaches used to manage fatigue, and they were moderately effective. Subjects reporting difficulty sleeping indicated that the strategies used—ignoring the problem and watching TV or reading—were only somewhat effective. Although many activities were initiated to treat nausea, taking antiemetic medication was used most often and was the most helpful—providing "quite a bit of relief."

A recognized limitation of this work was the heterogeneity of the sample. Subjects with various types of cancer receiving different chemotherapy drugs were included. Therefore, it is difficult to draw conclusions about specific patterns of side effects and the efficacy of specific self-care activities used to treat them. Also, because most subjects had received prior treatment, self-care activities previously found to be ineffective were probably not reported. As the authors conclude, however, this study demonstrates that the self-care diary can be used effectively to obtain patients' reports about the occurrence and management of side effects associated with chemotherapy. Only about 10 to 20% of subjects did not return their diaries, supporting the diary's ease of use for chemotherapy patients.

Nail LM, Jones LS, Greene D, Schipper DL, Jensen R: Use and perceived efficacy of self-care activities in patients receiving chemotherapy. *Oncol Nurs Forum* 1991;18:883–887.

minimize the side effects of chemotherapy. The first step in administering antineoplastic agents is to educate the patient and the family about their use. Many individuals have misconceptions about these drugs and their potential side effects.

Using knowledge of the drugs and their expected effects, the nurse is in the best position to detect changes that may indicate the appearance of drug side effects. The nurse may independently institute many measures to increase patient safety and comfort. Along with these nursing measures, drug therapy is frequently used to alleviate or reduce the side effects of antineoplastic agents.

Because of their nonselective nature, many chemotherapeutic agents share several side effects. These agents not only kill cancer cells, but they also exert their cytotoxic effect on normal dividing cells. Any tissue that has a high growth fraction is susceptible to destruction by chemotherapy. The normal cells and tissues that are the most vulnerable are the bone marrow, the epithelial cells of the gastrointestinal (GI) tract, hair follicles, gonadal tissue, and the developing fetus. Cells in a wound may also be affected, leading to delayed wound healing.

Myelosuppression

The suppression of bone marrow function by chemotherapy is known as **myelosuppression**. It is the major dose-limiting toxicity for most of the chemotherapeutic agents. Depending on the drug and its dose, leukopenia, thrombocytopenia, and anemia may occur. As with cancer cells, a certain proportion of the dividing blood cells will be damaged and a reduced number of new cells will be available for release into the circulation. The point at which the blood counts drop to their lowest level is known as the nadir. One important component of the white blood cell (WBC) count is the number of circulating granulocytes. When the absolute granulocyte count drops below 1000/mm^3 (normal, 2500 to 6000/mm^3), the patient is at increased risk for infection. A platelet count below 20,000/mm^3 (normal, 150,000 to 350,000/mm^3) places the patient at risk for uncontrolled bleeding. Platelet transfusions to prevent spontaneous bleeding may be necessary when the platelet count falls below 10,000/mm^3.

Conservative measures to help the patient with thrombocytopenia include preventing injury and avoiding invasive procedures and intramuscular (IM) injections. Instruct patients to use an electric razor for shaving, to avoid heavy lifting or straining, and to refrain from sports. Acetaminophen should be used instead of aspirin, which inhibits platelet aggregation. Any evidence of petechiae or frank bleeding should be reported, as it requires immediate attention.

A reduced number of red blood cells can result in impaired cardiovascular and pulmonary function, and can interfere with physical activity and produce fatigue. Most chemotherapeutic agents cause the blood count to reach its nadir seven to 14 days after treatment. Recovery can be expected 14 to 28 days after treatment.

Implement measures to prevent infection while the patient is myelosuppressed. Careful personal hygiene and frequent handwashing should be routine. Instruct patients to avoid crowded areas that might bring them in contact with infections, and to avoid contact with children who might be infected with viral illnesses such as influenza or varicella. Infections require prompt medical attention. Any temperature above 38°C (100°F) should be reported and investigated for a cause. Patients should also report any symptoms of a cold, chills or sweating, frequent or painful urination, vaginal discharge or itching, or other signs of infection. Early antibiotic treatment of infections can lower the otherwise high morbidity and mortality associated with infections in myelosuppressed cancer patients.

The treatment of anemia usually involves increased rest, avoiding strenuous activity, and eating a well-balanced diet. Red cell transfusions are indicated if conservative measures do not improve symptoms, if the patient experiences bleeding, or if cardiovascular symptoms occur.

Gastrointestinal Disturbances

Destruction of the epithelial lining of the GI tract can cause several problems. Cell loss in the mouth can cause stomatitis and ulceration. Mouth care can help minimize the development of oral lesions. Instruct the patient to brush the teeth after each meal using a soft nylon-bristle toothbrush. Flossing the teeth is advised, as long as the platelet count is above 50,000/mm^3 and flossing does not cause pain. Rinsing the mouth with one quarter-strength hydrogen peroxide, or a baking soda and water solution (one tsp in 500 mL), soothes and cleanses the mouth. Have the patient rinse the mouth after each meal and every four hours while awake. If mouth lesions develop, oral rinsing should be increased to every two hours. A sponge-tipped applicator can be used in place of a toothbrush to reduce discomfort. Topical or systemic analgesics, oral protective agents, antifungal agents, or antibiotics may be needed if inflammation is severe.

Chemotherapy-induced diarrhea can be minimized or prevented by eating a diet high in calories and protein and low in fat and fiber. Foods or beverages that might irritate or stimulate the GI tract should be avoided: strong spices and herbs; fatty foods; raw vegetables; fresh or dried fruits; gas-producing foods; whole grain products; alcohol; and tobacco. Diarrhea may be managed with over-the-counter (OTC) or prescription antidiarrheal drugs. Encourage the patient to drink eight to ten glasses of fluid daily to prevent dehydration, and to consume foods and fluids that restore sodium and potassium to the body. Meals are best taken as small frequent feedings, avoiding extremely hot or cold fluids that can irritate the GI tract.

Most nausea and vomiting caused by chemotherapy is self-limiting and resolves within 24 to 48 hours after drug administration. Some individuals may develop anticipatory nausea and vomiting (occurring prior to therapy) as a result of conditioning to the stimulus of drug administration. Antiemetics can often relieve or reduce nausea and vomiting. Antiemetics are usually given four to 12 hours before chemotherapy and continued every four to six hours for 12 to 48 hours. Refer to Chapter 42 for additional information about antiemetics.

Several other strategies may also reduce nausea and vomiting. Eating bland crackers or drinking flat cola is effective for some patients. Foods that are cold or served at room temperature are usually better tolerated, since the odor of hot foods is thus reduced. Patients with nausea and vomiting should avoid highly seasoned foods and choose instead bland foods and clear liquids. Any sights, sounds, or odors that stimulate nausea should be avoided. Many patients benefit from having someone else prepare their food. Distraction, relaxation, self-hypnosis, and guided imagery help some individuals overcome nausea and vomiting. Advise patients to plan their activities so that they are asleep when episodes of nausea are anticipated.

Alopecia

Some drugs damage the hair follicles by preventing production of DNA needed for hair growth. Partial or complete alopecia may result over a period of several days or weeks. Changes and loss of the hair are usually first noted two to three weeks after the first drug treatment. Alopecia has no physiologic consequences, but is psychologically distressing to many patients. Forewarn patients to expect hair loss, and encourage them to purchase a wig, hairpiece, or head covering in preparation.

Reproductive Disturbances

Cancer chemotherapy can decrease gonadal function. This can lead to oligospermia (decreased sperm number) or azoospermia (absence of sperm) in men, and to amenorrhea in women. These effects are most often seen with the alkylating agents or when combination chemotherapy includes alkylating agents. The use of alkylating agent chemotherapy accelerates the onset of menopause, especially in older women. Younger women may tolerate longer periods of exposure and higher doses of drugs before amenorrhea becomes irreversible. In males, sex drive and capability are not affected, but recovery from azoospermia may take years and complete recovery is not guaranteed. Men may be counseled to deposit sperm in a sperm bank if permanent sterility is anticipated. Other reproductive options may be available to patients who experience permanent sterility. Discuss the possibility of sterility with patients of child-bearing age and their families, and obtain informed consent before initiating treatment.

All the antineoplastic agents have negative effects on the developing fetus. Chemotherapy has the potential to cause teratogenic and mutagenic changes in exposed ova and sperm. Stillbirths and birth defects owing to chromosomal damage are possible. Since gonadal function during chemotherapy is uncertain, birth control measures should be taken. Birth control should be used during chemotherapy and for two years following completion of treatment, to allow the ova and sperm to recover from the drug effects. In most cases, reproductive potential after chemotherapy is not predictable. Help the patient and sexual partner by openly discussing their concerns and anxieties, and by making available accurate information about reproductive potential.

Hyperuricemia

Hyperuricemia is a common response to cancer and cancer chemotherapy. It is most often seen with leukemia, lymphoma, or widespread metastatic cancer when the number of cancer cells is high. Aggressive chemotherapy can lead to rapid cell destruction. The release of dead cells into the bloodstream produces large amounts of metabolites that eventually form uric acid. If blood uric acid levels rise too high, symptoms of gout may occur. There is also an increased risk of uric acid precipitation in the urine, where the substance is excreted. If uric acid precipitates form in the kidney tubules, serious and potentially permanent renal damage may result. To prevent hyperuricemia in patients with leukemia, the drug allopurinol (Chapter 53) may be given before a course of chemotherapy to inhibit uric acid synthesis. In other cancer patients receiving chemotherapy, rising uric acid levels are an indication to use allopurinol. Using allopurinol along with measures to keep the patient well hydrated and producing adequate amounts of dilute urine reduces the risk of urate stone formation and renal damage.

Fatigue

Fatigue, caused by many factors, is commonly experienced by cancer patients. Chemotherapy increases fatigue through accumulation of waste products from cell destruction. Other causes of fatigue in the cancer patient are anemia, malnutrition, disruptions in sleep and rest, pain, emotional stress, anxiety, and depression. Teach patients to take frequent rest periods and to pace their activity level to available energy. Advise mild to moderate exercise, if tolerated. Drinking extra fluids, up to eight to 10 glasses per day, will help eliminate cellular waste products from the blood and reduce the risk of renal impairment. A well-balanced diet will provide the necessary nutrients to maintain optimal activity levels. Routine activities such as household tasks should be minimized or eliminated to conserve energy for other activities.

The nurse also has an important role in minimizing the emotional distress of cancer and its treatment. Keeping the patient informed and prepared for the common side effects of chemotherapy is important for effective coping.

Response to Chemotherapy

The therapeutic responses to antineoplastic agents are usually not immediate. Drug-induced side effects and toxicities will usually appear before any judgment can be made about the success of the agent in treating the cancer. Both subjective and objective data must be used to assess the response to cancer therapy. A subjective response is based on the patient's personal opinion of whether the chemotherapy has helped. Patients may be questioned about how they feel, if pain or other symptoms have changed, if activity levels and strength are altered, and about their general sense of well-being.

Objective responses are more reliable measures of responses to antineoplastic agents. The findings of diagnostic tests and physical examination are compiled to determine if an objective response has occurred. Examples of objective responses include reductions in tumor size or changes in laboratory values toward normal. A complete response is said to occur if there is complete disappearance of any tumor that was measurable by physical, radiologic, or biochemical examination. The duration of this response must be one month or longer. A partial response is defined as a reduction in the size of any measurable tumor by at least 50% and the absence of any new tumor growth. When no change occurs in the size of existing tumor, or the measurable disease shrinks by less than 50%, no response has occurred.

Remission, stable disease, and progressive disease are other terms used to describe patients' responses to chemotherapy. A remission usually describes an improvement in the patient's condition, and the term is sometimes used interchangeably with complete response. Stable disease means that the clinical findings have not changed. This may apply to patients who have had partial or no responses if there is no change over a period of time. Progressive disease is diagnosed when there is a 50% increase in the amount of tumor present or tumor appears in any new areas of the body.

It is usually necessary to repeat a course of drug therapy two or three times to evaluate the patient's response. Since there are intervals between drug administrations, several weeks to months may elapse before a response can be evaluated. This can be a very stressful time for patients and their family members who are anxious to hear the results of treatment. The nurse can teach the patient how a response is evaluated and provide emotional support during this time.

SUMMARY OF NURSING IMPLICATIONS

◆ Assessment

Obtain baseline data on health status before administering antineoplastic agents: height, weight, activity level, nutritional status, blood profile, and organ function, to determine patient's tolerance to drug dose.

Determine the emotional and psychological impact of illness on the patient and family.

◆ Nursing Diagnoses

Anxiety related to anticipated drug effects.

Diarrhea related to gastrointestinal side effects of drug.

High risk for injury related to susceptibility to infection.

Altered nutrition: less than body requirements related to stomatitis, mouth ulceration, nausea, vomiting.

Body image disturbance related to alopecia.

Fear related to disease process.

Pain related to drug side effects or disease progression.

High risk for impaired skin integrity related to drug extravasation.

Knowledge deficit related to prescribed chemotherapeutic agent and regimen.

Altered oral mucous membrane.

◆ Planning/Implementation

When giving antineoplastic agents IV, ensure patency of line and good blood return; observe for tissue effects if extravasation occurs, be prepared to intervene.

Follow institutional policies for mixing, administering, and disposing of chemotherapeutic agents and contaminated equipment.

Give medications for pain and infection as indicated.

Give antiemetics prior to chemotherapy and for 12 to 48 hours after to minimize nausea and vomiting.

Prior to chemotherapy, discuss changes in reproductive functioning that can occur; establish method of birth control to be used since gonadal function after therapy is uncertain.

◆ Patient and Family Teaching

Teach the patient/family:

About antineoplastic agents to be used; side effects of drugs to expect; self-care measures to manage myelosuppression; to avoid and prevent infection; to report temperature above 100°F; to avoid injuries that might lead to bleeding.

To practice frequent mouth care to minimize discomfort and potential for infection from drug-induced stomatitis; use oral rinses of quarter-strength hydrogen peroxide or baking soda in water, and brush after meals with soft bristle brush.

About foods that are low in residue, high in calories and protein, and low in fat and fiber to minimize and prevent diarrhea; to avoid spiced foods and beverages; to drink eight to ten glasses of fluid, take antidiarrheal agents, and eat small frequent feedings if diarrhea present.

To eat bland foods and drink clear liquids if nausea is present; distraction, relaxation, self-hypnosis, and guided imagery may be useful with nausea.

That frequent rest periods, mild to moderate exercise, and eating a balanced diet may help combat fatigue.

To expect hair loss; purchase wig before loss occurs.

◆ Evaluation

The patient/family will:

Show a positive response to chemotherapy (eg, reduction in tumor size, laboratory values return toward normal).

Tolerate drug side effects; comfort measures will be effective.

Maintain sufficient fluid and food intake; maintain body weight.

Verbalize correct administration of medication and recognition of side effects to report.

Identify effective and ineffective coping patterns used to deal with anxiety and fear; be receptive to support and encouragement from family/significant others.

State the early signs of infection or allergic reactions.

Annotated Bibliography

Baird SB, McCorkle R, Grant M (eds): *Cancer Nursing: A Comprehensive Textbook.* Philadelphia, Saunders, 1991. *As implied by the title, this is a complete, detailed source for information on all aspects of oncology nursing.*

Cassidy J, Macfarlane DK: The role of the nurse in clinical cancer research. *Cancer Nurs* 1991;14:124–131. *A concise introduction to the conduct of clinical trials of anticancer drugs.*

Carnevali DL, Reiner, AC: *The Cancer Experience: Nursing Diagnosis and Management.* Philadelphia, Lippincott, 1990. *Focuses on the effect of cancer and cancer treatment on patients' daily lives.*

Chabner BA, Collins JM (eds): *Cancer Chemotherapy: Principles and Practice.* Philadelphia, Lippincott, 1990. *Detailed information about the biochemical actions of agents used in cancer chemotherapy.*

DeVita VT, Hellman S, Rosenberg SA (eds): *Cancer: Principles and Practice of Oncology.* Philadelphia, Lippincott, 1989. *A comprehensive resource on the diagnosis, treatment, and management of all cancers.*

Pratt WB, Ruddon RW, Ensminger WD, Maybaum J: *The Anticancer Drugs.* New York, Oxford University Press, 1993. *This recently revised edition provides a concise summary of the basic and clinical aspects of cancer chemotherapy, as well as introductory material on cancer biology.*

Hydzik CA: Late effects of chemotherapy. Implications for patient management and rehabilitation. *Nurs Clin North Am* 1990;25(2): 423–446. *Focuses on cardiac, reproductive, neurologic, pulmonary, and renal complications that may occur well after chemotherapy courses have been completed, and how they may affect the cancer survivor's quality of life.*

Jenkins J, Hubbard S: History of clinical trials. *Semin Oncol Nurs* 1991;7(4):228–234. *Reviews the steps involved in bringing anticancer drugs from the laboratory to the bedside, and how clinical trials can affect the nurse.*

Lilley LL: Side effects associated with pediatric chemotherapy: Management and patient education issues. *Pediatr Nurs* 1990;16(3): 252–255, 272. *A brief but valuable review of key issues for nurses whose cancer patients are children.*

Lynch M, Yanes L: Flowsheet documentation of chemotherapy administration and patient teaching. *Oncol Nurs Forum* 1991;18(4): 777–783. *Developing a standard of care for chemotherapy-related knowledge deficits and patient teaching allowed the authors to modify therapy flowsheets to include information that goes beyond traditional drug-dose–time data. The outcome is an asset to both health care providers and patients.*

Miaskowski C: Chemotherapy update. *Nurs Clin North Am* 1991; 26(2):331–339. *Discusses basics of tumor cell kinetics, and the basis for individual and multidrug resistance, and shows how this information led to new developments in chemotherapy. "Nurses must remain knowledgeable about these concepts to understand the mechanisms underlying the administration of various combinations of cancer chemotherapy."*

Skeel RT: *Handbook of Cancer Chemotherapy.* Boston, Little, Brown and Company, 1991. *A complete pocket summary of clinical data on anticancer drugs.*

Tucker R, Rahr V: Nursing care of the patient with non-Hodgkin's lymphoma. A case study. *Cancer Nurs* 1990;13(4):229–234. *Despite a focus on lymphoma, this paper provides information that applies generally to cancer treatment protocols, and provides a background for nursing assessment and interventions.*

Wiseman KC, Wachs JE: Policies and practices used for the safe handling of antineoplastic drugs. *AAOHN J* 1990;38(11):517–523. *Discusses risks to health care providers caused by anticancer drugs, and shows that adequate protective measures often are not implemented.*

Yarbro JW (ed): Cancer in the elderly. *Sem Oncol* 1989;16:1–84. *A series of articles concerning chemotherapy for elderly patients.*

PROTOTYPES

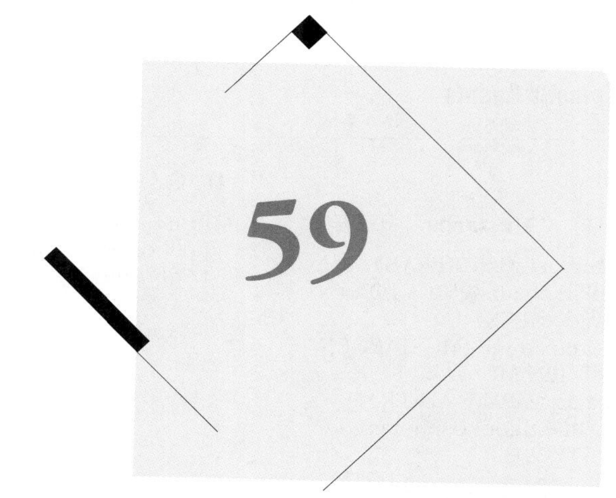

Antineoplastic Drugs

Most types of drugs are designed to treat disease states either by correcting the functions of abnormally behaving cells or by adjusting the functions of normal cells to counteract the underlying pathology. In contrast, the mechanisms responsible for the abnormal growth of cancer cells are so poorly understood that it is usually more effective to try to kill tumor cells than to rehabilitate them. For this reason, the majority of antineoplastic agents are highly toxic chemicals that destroy cancer cells as well as some normal cells.

The specific drugs prescribed are selected based on their mechanisms of action, effects on the cell cycle, toxicities, and effectiveness against a specific tumor type. Although the drugs may be administered as single agents, in most cases a combination of drugs is used for maximum effectiveness. The doses of these drugs are highly individualized, and the nurse must be familiar with the drug and its many uses; care must be taken to administer the drugs in the correct doses, as they have toxic side effects. Only specially trained nurses who are familiar with the uses, actions, and side effects of the antineoplastic agents should be involved in their administration.

The biochemical properties of anticancer drugs are diverse, so it is usually helpful to subdivide these drugs into classes based on either their mechanisms of action or, in the case of natural products, on the source from which they were obtained (Table 59–1). Because DNA replication is central to the process of cellular proliferation, many of these drugs are intended to disrupt the synthesis, structure, or function of DNA. One class, the alkylating agents, consists of chemicals that attach themselves to DNA through a covalent bond. This creates a structural defect that is difficult to repair. Another group, the **antimetabolites**, interferes with the synthesis of new DNA either by preventing production of necessary DNA precursors or by substituting for these precursors during DNA synthesis. Still others inhibit replication by antagonizing the function of proteins responsible for maintaining chromatin structure and organization. Finally, several agents, such as hormones and substances affecting the immune system, have actions unrelated to DNA.

Within each class most drugs have similar biochemical actions, pharmacokinetics, side effects, and contraindications. However, the clinical indications, dos-

Major reference tables appear beginning on p. 1321.

Table 59–1 Classes of Antineoplastic Agents

Drug Class	Agent
Alkylating agents	**Mustards**
	Chlorambucil (LEUKERAN)
	Cyclophosphamide* (CYTOXAN)
	Ifosfamide (IFEX)
	Mechlorethamine (MUSTARGEN; NITROGEN MUSTARD)
	Melphalan (L-PAM; ALKERAN)
	Triethylene thiophosphoramide (THIOTEPA)
	Nitrosoureas
	Carmustine (BCNU, BiCNU)
	Lomustine (CCNU, CeeNU)
	Streptozocin (STREPTOZOTOCIN; ZANOSAR)
	Other Covalent DNA-Binding Drugs
	Busulfan (MYLERAN)
	Carboplatin (PARAPLATIN, "CBDCA")
	Cisplatin (PLATINOL)
Antitumor antibiotics	Bleomycin (BLENOXANE)
	Dactinomycin (ACTINOMYCIN-D)
	Daunorubicin (CERUBIDINE)
	Idarubicin (IDAMYCIN)
	Doxorubicin* (ADRIAMYCIN)
	Mitomycin (MITOMYCIN-C; MUTAMYCIN)
	Mitoxantrone (NOVANTRONE)
	Plicamycin (MITHRACIN)
Antimetabolites	Cytarabine (ARA-C; CYTOSAR-U)
	Floxuridine (5-FUDR)
	5-Fluorouracil (5-FU; ADRUCIL)
	Fludarabine (FLUDARA)
	6-Mercaptopurine (6-MP)
	Methotrexate* (MTX, FOLEX)
	6-Thioguanine (THIOGUANINE)
Plant alkaloids	Etoposide (VP-16, VEPESID)
	Taxol
	Vinblastine (VELBAN)
	Vincristine* (ONCOVIN)
Hormonal/ antihormonal agents	**Estrogens**
	Diethylstilbestrol (DES)
	Ethinyl estradiol (ESTINYL)
	Androgens
	Fluoxymesterone (HALOTESTIN)
	Methyltestosterone
	Testolactone (TESLAC)
	Testosterone propionate (ANDROLAN)
Hormonal/ antihormonal agents (*Continued*)	**Progestins**
	Hydroxyprogesterone caproate (PRODROX)
	Medroxyprogesterone acetate (PROVERA; DEPO-PROVERA)
	Megestrol acetate (MEGACE)
	Adrenocorticosteroids
	Cortisone acetate
	Dexamethasone (DECADRON)
	Hydrocortisone sodium succinate (SOLU-CORTEF)
	Methylprednisolone sodium succinate (SOLU-MEDROL)
	Prednisone
	Antiandrogens
	Flutamide (EULEXIN)
	Antiestrogens
	Tamoxifen (NOLVADEX)
	Antiadrenals
	Aminoglutethimide (CYTADREN)
	Gonadotropin-Releasing Hormones
	Goserelin (ZOLADEX)
	Leuprolide (LUPRON)
Miscellaneous agents	Asparaginase (L-ASPARAGINASE; ELSPAR)
	Dacarbazine (DTIC)
	Hydroxyurea (HYDREA)
	Mitotane (LYSODREN)
	Procarbazine (MATULANE)
	Biologic Response Modifiers
	Interferon (INTRON, ROFERON)
	Levamisole (ERGAMISOL)

*Prototype.

ages, and factors related to the administration of each drug must be considered separately because the individual drugs vary significantly from one another with respect to these properties.

I. Alkylating Agents

An alkylator can be defined as a chemical that attaches itself to another molecule by making a single covalent carbon-carbon ("alkyl") bond. The alkylating agents (Table 59–C1) comprise the oldest and largest group of antineoplastic drugs. The first ones to be used clinically were derived from highly corrosive chemicals called "mustards," which were employed as chemical warfare agents in World War I. When researchers noted that exposure to one such compound (nitrogen mustard) caused atrophy of lymphoid and myeloid tissue, they decided to test its effects on tumors of lymphoid and myeloid origin. Therapy with nitrogen mustard, now called mechlorethamine, was so successful that development of a whole series of other alkylators followed. Based on chemical structure, the two major subgroups of alkylators in use today are the **mustards** and the **nitrosoureas**. Of these, the most commonly administered alkylator is the mustard derivative, cyclophosphamide.

PROTOTYPE

Cyclophosphamide

Absorption, Distribution, Metabolism, and Excretion

Cyclophosphamide ("CTX"; CYTOXAN) is given as an oral or intravenous (IV) agent. It is rapidly absorbed from the gastrointestinal (GI) tract. Cyclophosphamide must undergo metabolic activation in the liver before it can be cytotoxic. The drug and its metabolites are excreted in the urine. It is well distributed throughout the body, with small amounts found in breast milk, sweat, and saliva. Doses should be decreased if the patient has decreased liver or kidney function.

NURSING IMPLICATIONS

Take protective measures to reduce exposure to urine containing the metabolites of cyclophosphamide and all other alkylating agents. Follow federal and state guidelines, and institutional policies to reduce exposure to cytotoxic agents. Wear gloves while handling excreta, and take care to prevent splashes or spills. The waste may be disposed of in the usual fashion in the public sewer system.

Pharmacologic Effects

Clinically active alkylating agents typically contain two or more active sites with which they can form bonds to DNA and other macromolecules. In many instances only one of these sites is able to react with DNA, resulting in damage to one of the two strands in the DNA duplex. Such single-strand lesions are potentially harmful, but most cells contain enzyme systems that can repair this kind of damage relatively efficiently. Less frequently, a single alkylator molecule will react simultaneously with both DNA strands, forming an unnatural bridge (or "cross-link") between them. Cross-links are much more difficult to repair. The presence of only a few (perhaps even one) of these lesions is sufficient to disrupt the balance of cellular processes during division, and to cause cell death. These cross-linking reactions can occur during any phase of the cell cycle, and alkylators therefore are not considered to be phase-specific drugs. However, because the consequences of cross-link formation are not seen unless the cell begins to replicate, cross-links do affect cycling cells more than noncycling cells. Alkylating agents are therefore said to be "cycle-specific" in their action.

Clinical Indications and Administration

Cyclophosphamide is indicated for the treatment of cancers of the breast, lung, testes and endometrium, Hodgkin's disease, non-Hodgkin's and Burkitt's lymphomas, multiple myeloma, neuroblastoma, retinoblastoma, rhabdomyosarcoma, Ewing's sarcoma, mycosis fungoides, and leukemias (see Table 59–C1). It also has a potent immunosuppressant effect that is sometimes used to treat autoimmune diseases, and to obliterate bone marrow intentionally, in preparation for a bone marrow transplant.

Cyclophosphamide is used in combination chemotherapy according to various administration schedules. When IV doses over 500 mg are used in a single treatment course, IV hydration (300 to 400 mL of normal saline) is recommended before drug administration. Additional fluid (100 to 200 mL over 20 to 30 minutes) is given after infusing the drug. When cyclophosphamide is given orally, morning or early afternoon administration is recommended so the drug and its metabolites will not remain in the bladder overnight.

NURSING IMPLICATIONS

If cyclophosphamide is being used as part of a combination chemotherapy protocol, give it before or after the other agents as ordered. Do not mix it with any other drugs.

Side Effects, Adverse Reactions, and Contraindications

Nausea and vomiting are common side effects of cyclophosphamide, especially when the drug is used in high doses or as an oral agent (Table 59–S). Nausea usually begins about six hours after drug administration and lasts about four hours. Cyclophosphamide may be contraindicated in patients with a poor nutritional status that could be exacerbated by nausea and vomiting.

Thrombocytopenia is mild in comparison to leukopenia. The nadir for the white blood cells (WBCs) occurs at 8 to 14 days, and recovery is evident by 18 to 25 days.

Alopecia occurs in up to 50% of patients; the usual onset is three weeks after the start of therapy. A high fluid output is needed to prevent sterile hemorrhagic cystitis, an infrequent but potentially lethal effect of cyclophosphamide. Increased urine output reduces the amount of time that the drug metabolites are in contact with the bladder mucosa.

Cyclophosphamide is carcinogenic and may cause secondary malignancies. Kidney and bladder tumors have occurred in patients receiving long-term cyclophosphamide therapy. The drug also has been associated with sterility in both men and women.

Cyclophosphamide and other alkylating agents have myelosuppressive effects, and so should be given in reduced doses or withheld when the blood counts are below normal.

NURSING IMPLICATIONS

Nursing interventions for the common side effects were discussed in Chapter 58. Monitor blood counts before drug administration to determine that the patient has enough reserve to withstand the effects of treatment. Repeat blood counts at the expected nadir to determine the patient's potential for infection and bleeding.

◆ Use During Pregnancy and Lactation

Discuss adequate methods of contraception with the patient because of the mutagenic potential of cyclophosphamide. Congenital malformations may occur if the drug is taken during the first trimester. Because the drug is excreted in breast milk, breastfeeding should be stopped during cyclophosphamide therapy.

Interactions with Other Drugs

Cyclophosphamide, like many other anticancer drugs (Table 59–I), alters the gastric mucosa and reduces the ability of some drugs to be absorbed through it. The interaction is particularly important for orally administered digoxin. With long-term combined therapy, reduced digoxin absorption can lead to a worsening of heart failure signs and symptoms. These should be assessed, and digoxin blood levels should be monitored closely as needed.

Cyclophosphamide also prolongs the skeletal muscle-relaxing effects of succinylcholine. The effects of a single succinylcholine dose, which can include respiratory paralysis, normally last less than one minute. More prolonged effects owing to the interaction with cyclophosphamide can place the patient at greater risk of prolonged hypoxia and potential brain damage. Therefore, anticipate the consequences of the interaction and be prepared to maintain a patent airway and ventilate the patient until adequate spontaneous ventilation returns.

NURSING IMPLICATIONS

The potential clinical significance of the interaction between oral digoxin and cyclophosphamide (or many other anticancer drugs) appears to depend on the digoxin formulation. Digoxin formulated as a capsule that contains liquid drug (eg, LANOXICAPS) normally is absorbed nearly 100%. Its absorption is affected little, if at all, by anticancer drug therapy. In contrast, digoxin administered as a tablet normally is absorbed much less completely (see Table 31–2). Anticancer drugs have greater impact on the absorption of that formulation. Check the dosage form that the patient is taking to get some idea about the potential risk for the interaction. Since different digoxin dosage forms differ in terms of absorption, one formulation cannot be interchanged for another without changing the dose. Do not make such changes unless the physician writes an order for the change.

Overdose and Toxicity

Like other antineoplastic drugs, cyclophosphamide has a very narrow margin of safety. No precise toxic dose can be specified. Effective therapy may require doses

SPOTLIGHT ON NURSING RESEARCH

The nausea and vomiting induced by chemotherapy have many sequelae that affect patients' physiological and psychological well being. Not surprisingly, attention has been given to the development of both pharmacologic and nonpharmacologic strategies for managing these side effects.

In this study, clinicians examined the effectiveness of patient-controlled antiemetic therapy in chemotherapy patients. Experience with patient-controlled analgesia suggests that it can provide effective pain relief with less medication and fewer side effects than nurse-administered therapy. Based on parallels that can be drawn between symptoms of nausea and pain, the investigators hypothesized that volunteer subjects receiving patient-controlled antiemetic therapy (PCAE) would experience the same amount of nausea and vomiting but would require less medication and would experience less sedation than subjects receiving nurse-controlled antiemetic therapy (NCAE).

Twenty adults receiving chemotherapy for the first time were randomly assigned to either experimental (PCAE) or control (NCAE) groups by pharmacy staff. A variety of moderately emesis-causing chemotherapeutic agents were used, although cyclophosphamide was administered most often. Antiemetic therapy consisted of a combination of IV metoclopramide (REGLAN) and diphenhydramine (BENADRYL).

The study was carried out in a double-blind fashion: neither subjects nor data collectors could identify the method by which antiemetic therapy was administered. Informed consent was obtained from all subjects. Subjects in the NCAE group received the antiemetic drugs by nurse-administered, intermittent minibag infusions and received a normal saline placebo when they depressed the control button of a patient-controlled pump. In the PCAE group, antiemetic drug treatment was given in IV boluses by patient-controlled pump, and subjects also received intermittent minibag infusions of normal saline from the nurse. It is important to note that the double-blind approach used in this study minimizes bias in data collection and helps to avoid confounding effects related to subjects' (and nurses') beliefs about the effectiveness of experimental treatments.

Nausea, vomiting, and sedation level were evaluated at 1, 12, and 24 hours after chemotherapy. Self-reports of nausea were measured on an analog scale ranging from "not at all nauseated" to "extremely nauseated." Vomiting and sedation level were evaluated using instruments developed for the study. All subjects were premedicated by the nurse with IV lorazepam (ATIVAN) and dexamethasone (DECADRON) before chemotherapy, and dexamethasone was repeated every 3 hours for 3 doses after chemotherapy. Metaclopramide and diphenhydramine premedications were administered IV by either minibag or PCA pump.

The findings indicated that both methods of administering antiemetic therapy provided effective symptom control. NCAE and PCAE subjects reported only mild nausea. The highest average nausea rating was 11.2, and only one study subject vomited. Symptomatic control of nausea and vomiting did not differ between groups. As hypothesized, the average amount of antiemetic medication received was significantly less in PCAE as compared to NCAE subjects. Contrary to expectations, sedation level was not significantly less in PCAE versus NCAE subject groups, although accurate measurement of sedation was difficult.

Research can be a cumulative process with studies building on each other. This study indicates that patient-controlled administration of intravenous antiemetic therapy is safe and effective for treatment of acute nausea and vomiting associated with chemotherapy. As the investigators point out, after therapeutic effectiveness has been demonstrated, subsequent work can add patients' perceptions of control as an influencing variable on the outcomes of patient-controlled antiemetic treatment.

Edwards JN, Herman J, Wallace BK, Pavy MD, Harrison-Pavy J: Comparison of patient-controlled and nurse-controlled antiemetic therapy in patients receiving chemotherapy. *Res Nurs Health* 1991; 14: 249–257.

that are clearly capable of causing toxicity. Toxicities may lead to treatment delays or dosage reductions, and may necessitate discontinuing the drug. Drug toxicity can cause significant morbidity, and may even be fatal.

Few antineoplastic agents have antidotes. Therefore, an overdose can create a life-threatening situation that may not be reversible. The treatment of overdoses and severe toxicities is primarily supportive. For example, if bone marrow depression occurs, the patient may be transfused with blood products to counteract anemia and thrombocytopenia. Antibiotics, antiemetics, and total parenteral nutrition are other therapies that can be used to support patients with severe or life-threatening responses to anticancer drugs.

To prevent cystitis in patients receiving high doses of cyclophosphamide, coadminister 2-mercaptoethane sulfonate (MESNA). MESNA is converted in the urine to a substance that can interact with and inactivate the reactive, toxic metabolites of cyclophosphamide that accumulate in the bladder.

Other Mustards

Although cyclophosphamide is used to treat a variety of neoplastic diseases, the other mustards are used selectively, against only one or a few tumor types. Other alkylating agents are busulfan, carmustine, chlorambucil, ifosfamide, lomustine, mechlorethamine, melphalan, streptozocin, and triethylene thiophosphoramide (see Table 59–C1 for dosages). Carmustine, lomustine, and streptozocin are often subgrouped as *nitrosoureas.* They are discussed on the next page.

Chlorambucil

Chlorambucil (LEUKERAN) is useful for indolent malignancies that require long-term management, such as chronic lymphocytic leukemia (CLL). The drug also has activity against lymphomas, choriocarcinoma, and ovarian and breast cancer.

Most patients tolerate chlorambucil very well. Myelosuppression, as evidenced by neutropenia, thrombocytopenia, and lymphopenia, is seen with prolonged use. As with cyclophosphamide, other toxicities and secondary malignancies may be seen following prolonged use or when high doses are used.

Ifosfamide

Ifosfamide (IFEX), like its analog, cyclophosphamide, requires metabolic activation to become reactive enough to form DNA lesions and kill cells. It is administered by short IV infusion and is used to treat testicular and lung carcinomas and some soft-tissue sarcomas. Myelosuppression is usually the dose-limiting toxicity for ifosfamide, although hemorrhagic cystitis is more common and more severe with this drug than with cyclophosphamide. Because of this problem, the protective agent MESNA must be coadministered with ifosfamide (see Table 59–C1). Vigorous hydration also should be maintained in patients receiving this drug.

Mechlorethamine

Mechlorethamine (nitrogen mustard; MUSTARGEN) is the parent agent of the classic alkylating agents. It is highly reactive in aqueous solution and rapidly inactivated by body fluids. The drug is given IV and within minutes penetrates cells through an active transport mechanism. Mechlorethamine is most commonly used for the treatment of Hodgkin's disease and the non-Hodgkin's lymphomas. It is also used to treat lung cancer and as a topical agent for cutaneous T cell lymphoma (mycosis fungoides).

Mechlorethamine is a powerful vesicant that can cause induration and eventual necrosis if infiltrated into soft tissues. Since it is not stable in solution, it should be administered within 30 minutes of dilution. Leukopenia and thrombocytopenia occur 10 to 14 days after administration. Nausea and vomiting occur in more than 70% of patients treated with mechlorethamine. Alopecia and temporary or permanent sterility are other common side effects.

Melphalan

Melphalan ("L-PAM"; ALKERAN) enters cells by active transport and preferentially localizes in tumors that actively use phenylalanine or tyrosine. This makes melphalan active against lymphomas; breast, testicular, and ovarian cancers; and multiple myeloma. When the drug is given orally, it is mainly excreted in the stool over five to six days. Most of the drug is highly metabolized before excretion. Rates of absorption after oral administration vary. Absorption may be enhanced by ingesting the drug on an empty stomach. The IV route is used in investigative cancer treatment.

Myelosuppression is the most common side effect of melphalan. Leukopenia and thrombocytopenia occur 14 to 21 days after drug administration when intermittent administration is used. Some drug schedules are designed to achieve significant degrees of bone marrow suppression as evidence of this drug's effectiveness. A nadir of 3000 to 3500 lymphocytes/mm^3 usually is considered to be optimal. Although melphalan has been used in low continuous doses, there is a trend away from this schedule since it is thought to induce leukemia.

Triethylene Thiophosphoramide

Triethylene thiophosphoramide (THIOTEPA) is an alkylating agent used in the treatment of superficial papillary tumors of the bladder. It is used as a topical agent, instilled into the bladder via an indwelling catheter and held there for two hours. The patient needs to be frequently repositioned during this time to distribute the drug to all the bladder mucosa. The drug treatment is repeated weekly.

Triethylene thiophosphoramide may cause myelosuppression, with the nadir appearing in seven to 28 days. Blood counts should be obtained and reviewed before each treatment.

Nitrosoureas

The nitrosoureas, carmustine, lomustine, and streptozocin, have a very different core chemical structure than mustards. However, they share with mustards the capacity to form cross-links between DNA strands. Because the nitrosoureas are relatively lipophilic, they penetrate the blood-brain barrier well and are therefore often the agents of choice in the treatment of brain tumors. They are also effective for lymphomas, malignant melanomas, and cancers of the GI tract.

Carmustine

Carmustine ("BCNU"; BiCNU) is rapidly distributed throughout the body after IV administration. It is given as a single dose or for two consecutive days, and repeated every six to eight weeks. Since carmustine can cause myelosuppression, which reaches its nadir at four to six weeks, more frequent drug administration is contraindicated. Leukopenia and thrombocytopenia may be severe and protracted, especially for patients who have received prior chemotherapy. Bone marrow toxicity may also be cumulative, with longer periods of time required for bone marrow recovery between doses.

Carmustine is diluted with alcohol and sterile water, and may cause burning, pain, or both at the injection site or along the vein. This can be reduced by further diluting the drug with 0.9% sodium chloride or 5% dextrose and giving the drug as an infusion over 30 minutes. Carmustine is sensitive to light and has limited stability once diluted. Wrap the infusion container with a protective covering (aluminum foil is effective), and discard any solution that is not used within two hours of mixing.

Nausea and vomiting are common side effects. They occur two to four hours after injection and last four to six hours. Antiemetics are frequently helpful to prevent or reduce these effects. Pulmonary fibrosis, evidenced by dyspnea, tachypnea, decreased breath sounds, rales, and nonproductive cough, has been observed after six months of use or when carmustine is given with bleomycin or chest irradiation. Pulmonary fibrosis is an indication to stop drug administration. To prevent pulmonary fibrosis, cumulative doses should not exceed 1000 to 1200 mg/m^2.

Lomustine

Lomustine ("CCNU"; CeeNU) is used for the palliative management of primary or metastatic brain tumors and advanced Hodgkin's disease. Its mechanism of action is similar to carmustine's, but it is effective when given orally. It is usually administered as a single oral dose at six-week intervals. Nausea and vomiting often occur two to six hours after the drug is taken. Since absorption is rapid, occurring within 30 to 60 minutes, drug efficacy should not be reduced by later vomiting.

As with carmustine and other alkylating agents, the most frequent toxicity associated with lomustine is bone marrow suppression. A delayed and potentially cumulative myelosuppression can occur. Thrombocytopenia occurs at 26 to 34 days and has a duration of six to 10 days. Leukopenia reaches its nadir at 41 to 46 days, and lasts nine to 14 days. A reexamination of the blood counts before subsequent drug administration is essential for safe therapy.

Streptozocin

Streptozocin (STREPTOZOTOCIN; ZANOSAR) is a weak alkylating agent that causes cross-linking of DNA and interferes with enzymatic pathways for glyconeogenesis. It is used in the treatment of malignant pancreatic islet-cell tumors. The drug is excreted in the urine. Streptozocin is given IV. Usually it is given twice a week for four or more weeks, repeated every six weeks. Local pain and burning may be reduced by infusing the drug slowly over one hour or more. The nurse may also place an icepack above the injection site to decrease nerve sensation and enhance comfort during drug infusion. Almost all patients experience some degree of nausea and vomiting one to four hours after drug infusion. These side effects do not seem to be alleviated by antiemetics.

Streptozocin differs from the other alkylating agents because myelosuppression is rare. Ten percent of patients experience diarrhea and abdominal cramping, which usually can be controlled effectively with antidiarrheals. Check the stools for occult blood that may reflect GI tract ulceration. Many patients (45% to 65%) experience renal dysfunction from streptozocin, characterized by proteinuria, decreased glomerular filtration, increased BUN, hypophosphatemia, glycosuria, and renal tubular acidosis. Kidney function tests and urinary protein concentrations must be monitored closely.

Other Covalent DNA-Binding Drugs

The last group of drugs discussed in this section are those that form covalent bonds to DNA, but are not mustards or nitrosoureas. The first one, busulfan, can accurately be termed an alkylator, although it belongs to a different chemical class than the other drugs mentioned so far. The other two, cisplatin and carboplatin, are not really alkylators, because they form carbon-platinum bonds instead of carbon-carbon bonds. However, because these carbon-platinum bonds result in DNA cross-links, they have some similarities to the alkylators and therefore are included here.

Busulfan

Busulfan (MYLERAN) is used to treat chronic myelogenous leukemia (CML) since it has selective affinity for the granulocytic cell lines. At low doses, busulfan affects the granulocytes, while sparing platelets and lymphocytes. At higher doses, total bone marrow depression results.

The drug is administered orally over several weeks. A decreased maintenance dose then is used to depress the WBC count. If the leukocyte count falls below 15,000/mm^3, therapy should be discontinued and not restarted until blood counts indicate that the bone marrow has recovered and is producing mature white cells. Since blood counts are used to monitor therapy, monitoring is very important so that busulfan can be discontinued before a potentially fatal leukopenia occurs.

Cisplatin

Cisplatin (PLATINOL) is a platinum metal complex that inhibits DNA synthesis by forming intrastrand and interstrand cross-links. It is cell cycle phase–nonspecific. It is primarily excreted in the urine as different platinum compounds.

Cisplatin is indicated in the treatment of cancers of the testes, ovary, cervix, head and neck, lung, esophagus, prostate, and bladder. It is also used to treat lymphomas, sarcomas, myeloma, and osteosarcoma. Cisplatin doses vary widely. It is given IV either as a single dose or every day for five days. Administration is repeated every three to four weeks. Inadequate bone marrow or kidney function are indications to reduce the dosage.

Renal toxicity is the major dose-limiting side effect of cisplatin. It can be prevented by ensuring adequate renal function and hydration prior to giving the drug. Fluids should be given in amounts that maintain a urine output of 100 to 150 mL/hour before drug administration. These fluids may be taken by mouth, but it is usually necessary to give supplementary IV fluids. A bolus injection of mannitol (12.5 to 50 g) is frequently given along with the fluids to ensure diuresis. Once the fluids have been given, the drug is administered IV over 20 minutes to 24 hours, depending on the cisplatin dose and desired schedule.

In addition to nephrotoxicity, cisplatin can cause severe nausea and vomiting, mild to moderate myelosuppression, decreased serum magnesium, tinnitus, hearing loss, and anaphylactic reactions. Nausea and vomiting are pronounced, usually starting within the first hour of treatment and lasting eight to 12 hours after the drug is infused. This effect may be less severe if longer infusion times are used. High doses of metoclopramide, dexamethasone, or both appear to be the most useful treatments for reducing nausea and vomiting. The nadir of white cells and platelets occurs two to four weeks after the drug is given. Bone marrow recovery is usually complete by the third week. Hypomagnesemia can be treated by giving supplemental magnesium. Other serum electrolytes, such as potassium, phosphorus, and calcium, occasionally need replacement.

Cisplatin can cause ototoxicity. It is characterized by high-frequency hearing loss and tinnitus; the effect is dose-related and can be prevented by using adequate hydration and diuresis. However, diuretic therapy should be planned carefully and monitored closely. Loop diuretics (eg, furosemide; LASIX) are also potentially ototoxic. Combined use with cisplatin can, therefore, increase the risk or severity of hearing damage. See Chapter 32 for more information about the ototoxicity of these diuretics, and the drugs and administration conditions that increase the potential for this adverse effect.

Cisplatin is also one of several anticancer drugs (see Table 59–1) that can interact with phenytoin, a widely used anticonvulsant. The outcome of the interaction is a gradual but potentially significant lowering of phenytoin blood levels, leading to reduced control of seizure disorders for which the anticonvulsant is given. Monitoring the anticonvulsant's blood levels more frequently, and using this information to help adjust the phenytoin doses, can help reduce the risk of further seizures.

Anaphylactoid reactions to cisplatin are unusual but potentially serious responses. They occur within minutes after the drug is started in a patient who has received at least one previous dose. Wheezing, flushing, hypotension, and tachycardia occur. Immediate administration of epinephrine may be needed to prevent vascular collapse and bronchospasm. Antihistamines and corticosteroids are useful adjuncts. In patients who have experienced this reaction, cisplatin may be used again with caution if pretreatment with antihistamines and corticosteroids is given.

Carboplatin

Carboplatin (PARAPLATIN, "CBDCA") is structurally and mechanistically similar to cisplatin. It is a small molecule consisting of a central platinum atom surrounded by four substituents, and it forms DNA cross-links as a crucial part of its cytotoxic action. Unlike cisplatin, two of the substituents in carboplatin contain carbon. In general, the spectrums of clinical response of, and resistance to carboplatin are very much like those of cisplatin. Current indications for carboplatin include treatment of ovarian and endometrial carcinomas.

The main differences between carboplatin and cisplatin are the side effects of these drugs. Myelosuppression is the dose-limiting toxicity for carboplatin, with very little (if any) of the renal, neurologic, or ototoxicities seen with cisplatin. Carboplatin is eliminated almost completely by renal excretion. Forced diuresis is not as critical with carboplatin as it is with cisplatin, although renal function must be monitored carefully with both drugs and dose adjustments must be made if creatinine clearance drops significantly.

II. Antitumor Antibiotics

The antitumor antibiotics are byproducts of the fermentation process of microorganisms. The toxic action of these drugs on human cells makes them inappropriate for treating infections. Antitumor antibiotics act on cancer cells by interfering with the synthesis of DNA, RNA, or both. The exact mechanism of action differs for each drug in the category. With the exception of bleomycin, each of the antitumor antibiotics is cell cycle phase–nonspecific. Doxorubicin is considered the prototype.

PROTOTYPE

Doxorubicin

Absorption, Distribution, Metabolism, and Excretion

Following IV administration, doxorubicin (ADRIAMYCIN) is rapidly dispersed in plasma and tissues. The drug is metabolized primarily in the liver. Most of the metabolized drug is excreted in the bile, but a small amount (5% to 6%) is excreted in the urine. This small amount is enough to color the urine pink to red for several days after injection.

Pharmacologic Effects

Doxorubicin has many biochemical actions, and its major mechanism of cytotoxicity may not be the same in all cells. Because it is a flat, lipophilic molecule, it can slide in between the base pairs of DNA molecules and generally disrupt their functions. Doxorubicin also can inhibit the activity of enzymes responsible for winding and unwinding complex DNA structures (topoisomerases), resulting in DNA single- and double-strand breaks. Because it has the capacity to form free radicals, doxorubicin also can cause DNA strand breaks by directly interacting with the DNA sugar-phosphate backbone.

Resistance to doxorubicin largely occurs via the multiple-drug resistance mechanism mentioned in Chapter 58. This phenomenon is due to the action of a protein embedded in the outer membranes of tumor and normal cells, which acts as a one-way pump, removing certain kinds of molecules from the intracellular fluid. Although this protein is normally present in many kinds of cells at a low level of activity, treatment of tumor cells with anticancer drugs often causes the gene coding for the pump protein to be amplified considerably. The tumor cells in which this amplification takes place are then able to eliminate not only the drug that induced the amplification, but some other drugs, as well. Unfortunately, this amplification does not occur in most normal cells. Consequently, once this amplification happens in tumor cells, it is no longer possible to administer a high enough concentration of drug to kill them without causing tremendous damage to host tissues.

Clinical Indications and Administration

Doxorubicin is effective against a wide variety of cancers, and is frequently used in combination chemotherapy. It is used in the treatment of cancers of the breast, lung, thyroid, and ovaries, and in soft tissue sarcomas, acute leukemias, and lymphomas (Table 59–C2).

The drug is administered IV as a bolus. It has also been given by intracavitary instillation into the bladder and peritoneum, by intraarterial injection, and by continuous IV infusion. Precautions must be taken to prevent extravasation of doxorubicin.

NURSING IMPLICATIONS

Wear gloves when handling and preparing doxorubicin powder or solution to prevent skin reactions. If contact occurs, wash immediately with soap and water. Determine patency of the IV catheter before administering the drug. If the IV bolus (push) method is being used, give 5 to 10 mL of normal saline first to verify needle position. If there is any question regarding needle placement, do not give the drug because severe tissue necrosis may occur.

Side Effects, Adverse Reactions, and Contraindications

Side effects of doxorubicin are summarized in Table 59–S. The dose-limiting toxicities of doxorubicin are bone marrow suppression and cardiotoxicity. All myeloid tissue is affected, but platelets and leukocytes are affected most. Evidence of bone marrow depression may be evident seven to 10 days after drug administration, with the nadir occurring at three weeks.

Cardiotoxicity is a serious toxic response to doxorubicin. The mechanism of cardiotoxicity is unknown, but it is clear that it is very likely to occur with total *lifetime* doxorubicin doses greater than 550 mg/m^2. This cumulative dose should never be exceeded. Patients with known cardiac disease should be treated cautiously, if at all, with this drug.

Early manifestations of an adverse cardiac response include altered heart rate and rhythm caused by conduction defects, and signs and symptoms of heart failure. With time, irreversible cardiomyopathy may occur. Diuretics and digitalis—traditional drugs for heart failure—may provide symptomatic relief, although they do not reverse cardiac damage.

Nausea, vomiting, alopecia, and stomatitis are common side effects of doxorubicin therapy. Alopecia is almost universally seen in patients treated with this drug. Complete loss of scalp, axillary, and pubic hair occurs two to five weeks after treatment is started. Men also lose their facial and chest hair.

An unusual side effect of doxorubicin is its ability to cause radiation "recall," a reactivation of tissue reactions in areas of previously irradiated skin. Radiation recall presents as erythema followed by dry desquamation. More severe skin reactions may progress to blistering and wet desquamation.

With the exception of bleomycin, all the antitumor antibiotics have vesicant properties. If inadvertently extravasated into soft tissue, induration, painful erythema, and necrosis may occur.

NURSING IMPLICATIONS

It is imperative to keep an accurate record of all doxorubicin doses administered, and the total cumulative amount, so the recommended lifetime total of 550 mg/m^2 is not exceeded. Teach the patient to keep skin affected by radiation recall clean and dry, and to avoid all mechanical and chemical irritants. These include tight-fitting clothing, lotions, powders, and other topical preparations. If extravasation occurs, apply cold packs to the site for up to 50 minutes each hour for 24 hours after extravasation.

◆ Use During Pregnancy and Lactation

Safe use of doxorubicin during pregnancy has not been established. The potential benefits should clearly outweigh the risks before using the drug.

◆ Use in Children

Increased pigmentation of the soles, palms, and nailbeds may be more common in children. These effects are reversible.

◆ Use in the Elderly

The prevalence of cardiac disease in the elderly requires careful evaluation before doxorubicin administration, and frequent assessment of cardiac status if the drug is used.

Interactions with Other Drugs

Doxorubicin is incompatible with 5-fluorouracil, dexamethasone, hydrocortisone sodium phosphate, aminophylline, cephalothin sodium (KEFLIN), and sodium heparin; never mix it with these agents.

NURSING IMPLICATIONS

Always flush the IV line before and after drug administration. Never mix doxorubicin with other drugs, not only to prevent drug incompatibilities but also to minimize the possibility of extravasation.

Overdose and Toxicity

Doxorubicin overdoses lead to exaggerated toxic effects. One potential acute toxic reaction is a life-threatening arrhythmia that occurs during or within a few hours of drug administration. Progressive and fatal cardiac failure is the major long-term toxicity.

Related Drugs

The other antitumor antibiotics are bleomycin, dactinomycin, daunorubicin, idarubicin, mitomycin, mitoxantrone, and plicamycin (see Table 59–C2 for dosages).

Bleomycin

Bleomycin (BLENOXANE) is active against many cancers. It has been successfully used to treat squamous carcinoma of the head and neck, cervix, vulva, skin, penis, and rectum, the lymphomas, testicular cancer, mycosis fungoides, lung cancer, and melanoma. Bleomycin does not cause significant myelosuppression, so it is frequently combined with other drugs used to treat these cancers.

Up to 70% of bleomycin is excreted by the kidneys. The drug may be given via the IV, intramuscular (IM), or subcutaneous (SC) routes, or as a regional arterial perfusion. It also has been given as an intracavitary instillation in the treatment of malignant effusions. Intramuscular or SC administration may cause burning, pain, or both at the injection site.

Bleomycin causes a febrile reaction in 60% of patients. About four to 10 hours after the drug is given, temperature rises to 103°F to 105°F, and may remain elevated for up to 48 hours. Fever may be accompanied by chills, sweating, dehydration, and hypotension. Acetaminophen and antihistamines such as diphenhydramine usually are effective in controlling this reaction. The prophylactic use of antipyretics is advised.

About 50% of patients experience cutaneous reactions to bleomycin. These reactions usually are manifested as hyperpigmentation and hyperkeratosis, mainly on the palms and fingers. Cutaneous reactions are related to the total dose given, but not to the route or schedule of administration. The reactions may be severe enough to require that the drug be discontinued. Alopecia may occur within several weeks of therapy, but the hair will regrow within months after therapy is stopped. Myelosuppression with bleomycin is rare; nausea, vomiting, and anorexia are usually mild and self-limiting.

A serious late effect of bleomycin is pulmonary toxicity. The drug causes pneumonitis with dry cough, dyspnea, rales, and lung infiltrates that can progress to pulmonary fibrosis. Pulmonary function is impaired and permanent lung tissue damage can occur. Long-term inhalation of oxygen, or inhalation of gas mixtures containing high oxygen concentrations, can worsen damage to the alveoli.

Patients should have pulmonary function tests and chest radiograms before starting bleomycin; these tests should be repeated routinely after treatment. Since pulmonary toxicity is seen more frequently in persons older than 70 years, those who have had previous radiation therapy to the chest, and when the total lifetime dose exceeds 400 units, the drug should be used with caution in these circumstances. Some clinicians recommend stopping treatment with bleomycin when the total cumulative dose reaches 300 units.

Dactinomycin

Dactinomycin (ACTINOMYCIN D; COSMEGEN) is used to treat testicular tumors, melanoma, choriocarcinoma, Wilm's tumor, neuroblastoma, retinoblastoma, rhabdomyosarcoma, Ewing's sarcoma, and Kaposi's sarcoma. The drug is given IV; the dosage varies depending on the tumor being treated, the treatment protocol, and the patient's age.

Dactinomycin can cause reversible alopecia and a variety of cutaneous manifestations. About 50% of patients experience skin hyperpigmentation and hyperkeratosis, especially on the palms and fingers. The drug interacts with radiation and produces "recall" skin reactions. This can occur even if the radiation occurred several months before dactinomycin administration. As a safety precaution, reduce dactinomycin doses when radiation has been used previously or is being used simultaneously.

The dose-limiting toxicities of dactinomycin are myelosuppression, nausea, and vomiting. All the myeloid tissue is affected, but the effect is most pronounced on platelets and leukocytes. Evidence of bone marrow depression may be evident seven to 10 days after drug administration, with the nadir at three weeks. Vomiting is often severe, beginning within a few hours of drug administration and lasting four to 20 hours. Antiemetics are effective for preventing or treating this response.

Daunorubicin

Daunorubicin (DAUNOMYCIN) is used mainly to treat acute myelocytic and lymphocytic leukemias. The drug is given IV as a bolus injection.

Daunorubicin is metabolized in the liver, necessitating reduced doses in the presence of abnormal liver function. Patients with known cardiac disease should be treated with caution since daunorubicin displays cardiac toxicities like those of doxorubicin. A total lifetime dose of 550 mg/m^2 is recommended. Other side effects are similar to those of doxorubicin.

Idarubicin

Idarubicin (IDAMYCIN) is an analog of daunorubicin and shares many properties with that drug, including its primary indication for treatment of acute leukemias. Idarubicin is somewhat less soluble than daunorubicin, and therefore is administered in larger volumes of fluid. Although cardiotoxicity of idarubicin might be less than that of daunorubicin (in relation to its other toxicities), this has not been demonstrated conclusively.

Mitomycin

Mitomycin (MITOMYCIN-C; MUTAMYCIN) is active against adenocarcinomas of the stomach, pancreas, colon, and breast. It is largely metabolized by the liver, with only 10% to 30% excreted unchanged in the urine. It is administered IV, preferably using a bolus; care must be taken to avoid extravasation. When given in combination with other antineoplastic agents, the doses of each drug must be reduced. Mitomycin also has been used at various doses for hepatic intraarterial infusion to treat liver cancer and cancers metastatic to the liver. Intracavitary instillation also is used.

Mitomycin is relatively well tolerated, although some patients do report nausea and vomiting. The major side effect is myelosuppression, which can be cumulative with successive doses. The leukocyte and platelet counts reach their nadir four to six weeks after the first dose. With a second dose myelosuppression may last as long as eight weeks. It is often necessary to reduce the total dose by 50% or more by the third treatment cycle. Mitomycin also can cause pulmonary fibrosis and renal toxicity, evidenced by increases in the BUN and creatinine levels. A rare drug-induced hemolytic uremic syndrome also has been reported. The clinical picture includes renal toxicity progressing to renal failure and cardiopulmonary insufficiency.

Mitoxantrone

Mitoxantrone (NOVANTRONE) is a synthetic antineoplastic agent categorized as an anthracenedione. It is structurally similar to doxorubicin and daunorubicin, but causes fewer severe GI side effects. The drug is used in combination with other agents for the initial treatment of acute nonlymphocytic leukemia. Effectiveness is being tested for the treatment of breast cancer and non-Hodgkin's lymphoma. Following IV administration, the drug is rapidly distributed in the blood and tissues. Mitoxantrone excretion is primarily hepatobiliary and renal. The safety of giving mitoxantrone to patients with hepatobiliary insufficiency has not been established, so caution is advised for this population.

Mitoxantrone's side effects include myelosuppression and cardiotoxicity. Leukopenia occurs within 10 days of administration, with recovery of the blood counts by 21 days. Thrombocytopenia and anemia also may occur. Supportive therapy with blood and blood products may be necessary. Functional cardiac changes such as congestive heart failure and arrhythmias are possible. Cardiac function should be monitored periodically since cardiotoxicity is an indication to stop treatment. The effects of mitoxantrone on cardiac function are not fully understood because patients with leukemia often exhibit depressed cardiac function owing to anemia, fever, infection, and hemorrhage. The drug should be used cautiously in patients with reduced cardiac function and patients who have received cardiotoxic drugs or mediastinal radiation therapy.

Nausea and vomiting are usually mild and transient. Stomatitis and alopecia may occur occasionally. Mitoxantrone is not a vesicant, and will rarely cause tissue necrosis if extravasated. For the first 24 hours after administration, the urine will be colored blue-green by the drug's metabolites.

Plicamycin

Plicamycin (MITHRACIN) is most commonly used for its hypocalcemic effect, which makes it useful in the treatment of malignant hypercalcemia (elevated serum calcium owing to a cancerous process). Serum calcium is lowered through decreased bone reabsorption of calcium and interference with parathyroid hormone production. This effect may last seven to 21 days. Plicamycin has been used to treat testicular cancer, but it is rarely used for this indication today because other drugs are more effective.

Plicamycin causes myelosuppression, nausea, anorexia, vomiting, and diarrhea. Myelosuppression is usually a mild depression of platelet and WBC counts, and of hemoglobin content. Most patients experience nausea and vomiting within six hours of receiving plicamycin. This reaction can persist for 12 to 24 hours, and is usually controlled well with antiemetics. Rapid infusion of plicamycin increases the incidence and severity of adverse GI effects; decreasing the rate of infusion does the opposite.

Plicamycin's major toxic side effect is hemorrhage secondary to depression of clotting factors and thrombocytopenia. One third of patients treated for testicular cancer have developed coagulation abnormalities. Monitor platelet counts and coagulation studies (prothrombin time and partial thromboplastin time), and observe patients for epistaxis, ecchymoses, petechiae, and facial flushing. Persistent epistaxis and facial flushing are signs to discontinue the drug, even in the absence of coagulopathy.

Plicamycin can impair liver and kidney function. The liver enzymes AST (SGOT) and LDH rise sharply after drug administration. Continued elevation of LDH is an indication to stop the drug. Over one half of patients experience proteinuria and increased serum creatinine and urea nitrogen levels. Electrolyte disturbances may also occur. Thus, appropriate tests to detect these untoward responses are important to ensure that the patient is tolerating successive doses.

III. Antimetabolites

The antimetabolites are a group of drugs that exert their major effect during the synthetic (S) phase of the cell cycle. These cell cycle phase–specific drugs are structural analogs of naturally occurring metabolites needed for DNA and RNA synthesis. They work by substituting for purines or pyrimidines in normal metabolic pathways for nucleic acid synthesis. When the antimetabolites are incorporated into DNA or RNA molecules, they form defective molecules that are unable to synthesize proteins needed to maintain cellular function. These agents are most effective in rapidly growing tumors.

Antimetabolites can be divided into three groups: the folate antagonists, the purine antagonists, and the pyrimidine antagonists. The most common folate antagonist, as well as the most frequently used antimetabolite, is methotrexate. Purine antagonists include fludarabine, 6-mercaptopurine, and 6-thioguanine. Cytarabine, 5-fluorouracil, and floxuridine are examples of pyrimidine antagonists.

PROTOTYPE

Methotrexate

Absorption, Distribution, Metabolism, and Excretion

Methotrexate ("MTX"; FOLEX; MEXATE) is absorbed rapidly, regardless of the administration route. The drug is actively transported into body cells, and reaches equilibrium concentrations in most cells within 30 minutes. About 50% to 60% of the drug in the blood is bound to plasma proteins. The majority of methotrexate molecules in the blood are excreted unchanged in the urine by both glomerular filtration and renal tubular secretion. A very small amount is metabolized to inactive products.

When given in conventional doses, methotrexate does not cross the blood–brain barrier in concentrations high enough to have an antineoplastic effect. To achieve effective concentrations in the cerebrospinal fluid (CSF), the drug can be given by the intrathecal route or at high doses by another parenteral route. The usual half-life in the CSF is 12 to 18 hours, but may be up to 48 hours. Over time, the drug slowly diffuses into the general circulation after intrathecal injection.

Pharmacologic Effects

Methotrexate exerts cytotoxicity by inhibiting the enzyme dihydrofolate reductase. This enzyme is necessary to keep folates in a chemical state suitable for their use in cell metabolism. Once inside the cell, methotrexate binds tightly to dihydrofolate reductase and blocks the reduction of dihydrofolate into a usable form. Without available folates, synthesis of thymidine and purines needed for DNA synthesis cannot occur. In order for methotrexate to be fully effective, a sufficient quantity must get into and remain in the target cells. Once the drug enters the cells, the body responds by increasing dihydrofolate synthesis in an attempt to compete with the methotrexate for binding sites.

The effects of methotrexate can be reversed by administering a reduced folate to take up binding sites. *Leucovorin calcium,* a reduced form of folic acid, is commonly used to prevent methotrexate toxicity to the bone marrow and GI tract epithelium occurring when methotrexate is given in high doses. This treatment is called *leucovorin "rescue."* If leucovorin is not given or is taken incorrectly, severe methotrexate-induced toxicities, and even death, can result.

Clinical Indications and Administration

Methotrexate is most commonly used in combination with other antineoplastic agents against a wide variety of cancers (Table 59–C3). It is very active in treating acute lymphoblastic leukemia (ALL), trophoblastic tumors such as choriocarcinoma and hydatidiform mole, Burkitt's lymphoma, lymphosarcoma, and mycosis fungoides. When given in high doses, it is also active against osteogenic sarcoma, carcinoma of the head and neck, multiple myeloma, lymphomas, and cancers of the lung, breast, testes, cervix, and ovary.

The range of doses for methotrexate varies widely. The usual dose for patients with normal renal function is 25 to 40 mg/m^2 given IV once a week. High-dose therapy (100 to 7500 mg/m^2) may be given if followed by leucovorin. The drug also may be given orally, IM, SC, intraarterially, or intrathecally. The method for giving IV methotrexate depends on the dose. Doses less than 150 mg can be given safely as a bolus. Doses between 150 and 500 mg should be infused over 20 minutes. When doses over 500 mg are used, infusions up to 24 hours should be used. For intrathecal doses, and IV doses over 500 mg, a preservative-free solution should be used. Preservative used in the liquid-reconstituted vials can irritate and damage the meninges.

Before giving high doses, determine that the patient has adequate renal function. Blood urea nitrogen and creatinine levels should be obtained routinely for all patients receiving methotrexate, regardless of the dose. A 24-hour creatinine clearance measurement is also desirable before therapy is initiated to determine that the kidney can excrete methotrexate. If the renal function is normal, methotrexate may be given in high doses after hydrating the patient and alkalinizing the urine. These steps are necessary to prevent precipitation of methotrexate in the renal tubules. Hydration is accomplished with IV fluids, sometimes in combination with oral fluids. Sodium bicarbonate is given to obtain a urine pH above 7.0. Sodium bicarbonate usually is administered in doses of 3 g every three hours for the 12 hours preceding therapy. It may be continued for 48 hours after the drug is given and increased in dose if urine pH does not stay above 7.0. Six to 24 hours after the methotrexate is given, a leucovorin rescue is initiated: leucovorin is given IV or orally in doses of 6 to 100 mg/m^2 over 36 to 48 hours. Blood levels of methotrexate sometimes are measured to determine the precise timing and dose of leucovorin.

NURSING IMPLICATIONS

The nurse is responsible for monitoring fluid intake and output and urine pH, and for timing methotrexate, sodium bicarbonate, and leucovorin administration. When high-dose methotrexate therapy is administered to outpatients, it is very important to evaluate their ability to understand the treatment and to comply with directions.

Rheumatoid Arthritis and Psoriasis

Oral methotrexate (eg, RHEUMATREX) also is indicated for managing severe rheumatoid arthritis, particularly that which has not responded to more traditional and relatively safer nonsteroidal antiinflammatory drugs (see Chapter 52 for more on this topic). The usual starting dosage is a once-weekly course of three 2.5 mg doses, spaced 12 hours apart, for a total of 7.5 mg per week. Alternatively, a single 7.5 mg dose can be given once a week. Treatment may continue for one to two years, depending on the patient's response to the drug. Similar dosages can be used for treating severe, refractory psoriasis. When used for these indications, methotrexate provides only symptom relief for the duration of therapy. The underlying pathology continues during therapy, and symptoms should be expected to occur once methotrexate therapy stops.

NURSING IMPLICATIONS

The methotrexate dosages for arthritis and psoriasis are lower than those typically used to treat cancers, and the treatment plan essentially involves once-weekly administration. Nevertheless, all the key side effects, precautions, drug interactions, and other considerations noted below for this anticancer drug apply to these other indications.

Side Effects, Adverse Reactions, and Contraindications

Myelosuppression, nausea, anorexia, and stomatitis are common side effects of methotrexate (see Table 59–S). The nadir for myelosuppression is usually six to nine days after therapy starts. Nausea occurs frequently, but is usually mild to moderate, and can be alleviated by antiemetics. Vomiting is not common, even when large doses of methotrexate are used. Stomatitis may appear as an early sign of drug toxicity. This can progress to bleeding ulcerations of the mouth and GI tract lining. If stomatitis is seen during prolonged methotrexate infusion, the drug should be discontinued; this helps prevent severe diarrhea, hemorrhagic enteritis, and intestinal perforation.

High doses or prolonged use of methotrexate cause alopecia, and may cause tubular necrosis and hepatic fibrosis. Be alert for a nonproductive cough, fever, and cyanosis, which may indicate the rare appearance of pneumonitis. These symptoms are reversible and will usually disappear within a week without treatment.

Intrathecal use of methotrexate may cause headache, vomiting, and fever. These effects are treated symptomatically with analgesics, antiemetics, and antipyretics. Neurotoxicity after three or four intrathecal doses is common in adults and in patients with active meningeal leukemia. The patient may exhibit motor dysfunction, cranial nerve palsies, coma, or seizures. These are indications to discontinue methotrexate.

Methotrexate-induced dermatologic manifestations include erythematous rashes, pruritus, urticaria, photosensitivity, and hyperpigmentation. Acute sunburn may result from photosensitivity, so advise patients to avoid exposure to the sun or to use an effective sunscreen agent if exposure is unavoidable.

Methotrexate is generally contraindicated in patients with impaired renal function. It may be used at reduced doses with caution, but should never be administered in high doses to these patients. Malignant effusions in the pleural space or abdomen are contraindications to methotrexate use. Methotrexate can be slowly distributed into these third-space fluids, and will also exit slowly from them. This will prolong exposure of the drug as it reenters the systemic circulation. When the patient has an effusion, the fluid should be evacuated before methotrexate administration, or frequent drug levels should be obtained for monitoring.

NURSING IMPLICATIONS

Ensure that the patient has been fully informed of all drug risks and is instructed to report immediately any adverse reactions.

◆ Use During Pregnancy and Lactation

Methotrexate can cause fetal death and congenital abnormalities, and so is contraindicated during pregnancy.

◆ Use in Children

Long-term use of methotrexate has caused lower extremity bone pain in children.

◆ Use in the Elderly

Age-related effects on renal function affect use of methotrexate. Whenever possible, creatinine clearance, rather than serum creatinine levels, should be used to monitor drug dosage in elderly patients.

Interactions with Other Drugs

Probenecid, sulfonamide antibiotics, or salicylates (eg, aspirin and many drugs related to it), can increase the therapeutic efficacy of methotrexate. However, they also can rapidly lead to serious and potentially fatal bone marrow depression if combined treatment is not planned and monitored properly. Nonsteroidal anti-inflammatory (NSAI) drugs that are not salicylates (eg, indomethacin, ibuprofen; see Chapter 52) are also potential interactants. All of these interactants appear to reduce renal excretion of methotrexate. In addition, sulfonamides may increase free methotrexate blood levels by displacing methotrexate from plasma protein binding sites. If one of these interactions occurs, prolonged treatment with leucovorin may be necessary to prevent death.

Like many anticancer drugs, methotrexate can lower blood levels and the effectiveness of phenytoin significantly.

NURSING IMPLICATIONS

The interaction between methotrexate and salicylates—and possibly other interacting NSAI drugs—can pose a potential therapeutic dilemma. When methotrexate is used for arthritis, salicylates or other NSAI drugs are almost always tried first. These interactants may be continued during methotrexate therapy for increased symptom relief. Nevertheless, the potential for increased methotrexate toxicity is real. Therefore, frequent monitoring is essential.

Aspirin and ibuprofen (eg, ADVIL, NUPRIN, MIDOL-200, MOTRIN) are available over-the-counter. In addition, many other nonprescription medications are, or contain, salicylates (eg, PEPTO-BISMOL contains bismuth subsalicylate). Thus, teach patients who are taking methotrexate, regardless of the indication, to avoid self-prescribing these medications. Review the information in Chapter 52, or data in references such as *Drug Facts & Comparisons* or the *Handbook of Nonprescription Drugs,* to help with your patient teaching.

Recommend acetaminophen (eg, DATRIL, TYLENOL) for temporary relief of minor fever or pain; it does not interact with methotrexate. However, advise patients who do not experience expected relief after taking acetaminophen to notify their physician at once.

Overdose and Toxicity

Fatal toxicities can occur when the usual side effects of methotrexate are exaggerated by poor excretion, prolonged drug exposure, or failure to follow prescribed leucovorin rescue therapy. The appearance of toxicities before a course of methotrexate has been completed indicates the need to stop therapy. Leucovorin may be administered as an antidote, but it will not alleviate the signs of toxicity already present. Methotrexate therapy should not be restarted until toxicities are resolved, and then only reduced doses are advised.

Related Drugs

Other commonly used antimetabolites are cytarabine, floxuridine, fludarabine, 5-fluorouracil, 6-mercaptopurine, and 6-thioguanine.

Cytarabine

Cytarabine (ARA-C; CYTOSAR-U) is a pyrimidine analog that inhibits DNA polymerase and DNA synthesis. It is most effective against cancers with a high growth fraction and is used in the treatment of acute myelogenous leukemia and in the acute phase of chronic myelogenous leukemia.

Cytarabine penetrates cells very quickly, but the drug is rapidly inactivated by liver enzymes. This accounts for the short plasma half-life, about 10 minutes, and the low efficacy of oral therapy. A continuous IV infusion helps to maintain therapeutic blood levels by overcoming problems caused by rapid hepatic metabolism. The intrathecal route is also useful in the management of meningeal leukemia or carcinomatosis. Preservative-free diluent should be used for intrathecal injections. The SC route may be used for maintenance therapy when remission is achieved.

Common side effects of cytarabine are nausea, vomiting, and myelosuppression. Nausea and vomiting appear in up to 50% of patients, and are more frequent with higher doses. Vomiting can be protracted, and is controlled poorly by antiemetics. Stomatitis may occur. Myelosuppression usually occurs seven to 14 days after the drug is given and appears to be related to the dose, duration, and frequency of cytarabine administration. Anemia is common, and may require blood transfusion to replace red cells.

Floxuridine

Floxuridine (5-FUDR) is indicated for continuous intraarterial chemotherapy of advanced adenocarcinomas of the GI tract, including the pancreas, liver, and biliary tract. Its metabolite can bind selectively with the enzyme necessary for the formation of thymidine, an essential building block for DNA synthesis. RNA synthesis is also inhibited when floxuridine metabolites are incorporated into RNA.

Floxuridine is given at a low dose as a continuous infusion over days or weeks. (High doses should be reserved for direct infusion into the liver, where immediate detoxification can occur.) This prevents high circulating blood levels and the development of systemic toxicities. When given by this method, myelosuppression is rare, but anorexia, abdominal cramps, pain, and diarrhea may still appear. Gastritis is common and may be prevented with prophylactic use of antacids. Chemical hepatitis is a rare but severe complication of floxuridine administration. Elevated alkaline phosphatase and bilirubin levels, with jaundice, can occur. Chemical hepatitis is an indication to discontinue the drug. The therapy should be reinstituted cautiously using reduced doses.

Fludarabine

Fludarabine (FLUDARA) is an unusual antimetabolite in that it contains modifications in both the sugar and purine-base portions of its structure. The biologic activity of fludarabine is thought to be primarily a consequence of its incorporation into DNA. It has demonstrated impressive activity against chronic lymphocytic leukemia, yielding a response rate in excess of 80% in patients who had not been treated previously with chemotherapy. These responses also appear to be longer lasting than the ones resulting from other drug protocols. Because fludarabine is not very soluble in aqueous solutions, it usually is administered as a more soluble prodrug, fludarabine phosphate ("FAMP"), which is converted rapidly to the active form of the drug. FAMP currently is given by IV injection or infusion, although an oral dosage form may be available soon. Moderate to severe myelosuppression is often the dose-limiting toxicity. In addition, severe neurotoxicities can occur, usually with a delayed onset of three to six weeks. These side effects can include blindness, coma, and paralysis.

5-Fluorouracil

5-Fluorouracil ("5-FU"; ADRUCIL) is the most commonly used pyrimidine antimetabolite. Its mechanism of action is the same as floxuridine's. 5-Fluorouracil is indicated for treating carcinoma of the stomach, colon, pancreas, liver, bladder, prostate, breast, and ovary. The topical preparation (EFUDEX) is effective against basal cell carcinoma of the skin.

5-Fluorouracil can be administered IV, intraarterially, or topically. The doses and schedules for administration vary according to the cancer being treated and the route for administration. When giving this drug topically, wear gloves and use a spatula to apply the medication to prevent unnecessary skin exposure.

Myelosuppression, nausea, vomiting, stomatitis, esophagitis, diarrhea, alopecia, maculopapular rashes, and photosensitivity are all side effects of 5-fluorouracil. Neutropenia and thrombocytopenia are common, with the nadir occurring in nine to 14 days. Premedication with antiemetics can usually prevent nausea and vomiting. Stomatitis may often be severe and the drug should be discontinued if it appears during therapy. Stomatitis may be preceded by a beefy, tender, or painful tongue or a generalized sore mouth. Its first appearance is usually as small, shallow ulcerations on the inner surface of the lower lip. These can quickly advance to ulcerations throughout the mouth and GI tract. Dermatologic reactions include alopecia (most common with five-day courses); a maculopapular rash, which sometimes occurs on the extremities or the trunk; and erythema or increased skin pigmentation when the skin is exposed to sunlight. Advise patients to avoid prolonged exposure to the sun and to use topical sunscreen preparations. The rash is rarely serious and can be treated with steroids, antihistamines, or both.

6-Mercaptopurine

6-Mercaptopurine ("6-MP"; MERCAPTOPURINE) is a purine analog that inhibits the formation of adenine and guanine nucleotides needed for the final synthesis of DNA and RNA. It is indicated for the treatment of ALL and is occasionally used for chronic myelogenous leukemia. It is also used as an immunosuppressive agent to prepare patients for bone marrow transplantation and in the treatment of autoimmune diseases such as Crohn's disease, ulcerative colitis, and rheumatoid arthritis.

6-Mercaptopurine is given orally, but gastrointestinal absorption is erratic. Less than 20% of the dose reaches the systemic circulation because most of the drug is metabolized in the gut and liver by the enzyme xanthine oxidase.

Nausea and vomiting are uncommon; stomatitis is seen only when doses exceed the normal range. Liver toxicity may occur, presenting as reversible cholestatic jaundice. Routine liver function tests are recommended to allow for early detection of hepatotoxicity. Routine blood and platelet counts are also indicated for monitoring myelosuppression. The blood counts can continue to fall after therapy is discontinued, so continue to monitor them.

The most important drug interaction in which 6-mercaptopurine participates involves allopurinol. It is a drug that often is used to treat or prevent elevated serum uric acid levels associated with gout, malignancies, and cancer chemotherapy. Allopurinol inhibits xanthine oxidase, an enzyme that is responsible for not only the metabolic inactivation of 6-mercaptopurine, but also for uric acid synthesis. If both drugs are to be administered, the mercaptopurine dose should be reduced by about 75%. If that is not done, unmetabolized mercaptopurine can accumulate in the bloodstream, posing a great risk of serious or potentially fatal bone marrow suppression.

6-Thioguanine

6-Thioguanine (THIOGUANINE) is indicated for the treatment of acute and chronic myelogenous leukemia and ALL. The mechanisms of action and excretion are the same as that of 6-mercaptopurine. 6-Thioguanine is catabolized differently, however, and is unaffected by allopurinol use. Since oral absorption is erratic, investigators are examining its effectiveness when given IV. Myelosuppression is the major dose-limiting side effect of 6-thioguanine. Other side effects are infrequent and similar to those of 6-mercaptopurine.

IV. Plant Alkaloids

Vincristine, vinblastine, taxol, and etoposide are drugs that affect the overall structure of chromosomes and the nucleus, but not as a result of direct interactions with DNA. They are plant derivatives that each have different therapeutic uses and toxicities. Vincristine is considered the prototype.

PROTOTYPE

Vincristine

Absorption, Distribution, Metabolism, and Excretion

Vincristine (ONCOVIN) is derived from the periwinkle plant (*Vinca rosea*). It is rapidly distributed to body tissues after IV injection. The half-life is short; over 50% of the drug is cleared within 20 minutes of administration. The drug is metabolized in the liver and excreted in the bile and feces. Insignificant amounts of the drug enter the CSF.

Pharmacologic Effects

Vincristine is described as a mitotic poison. It arrests cells that are undergoing mitosis at the stage of metaphase, thereby inhibiting cell division. This action is thought to be due to vincristine's ability to interfere with the assembly of the spindle fibers of the mitotic apparatus.

Clinical Indications and Administration

Vincristine is indicated in the treatment of acute leukemia, lymphoma, Wilm's tumor, neuroblastoma, rhabdomyosarcoma, and cancers of the brain, testes, breast, and cervix (Table 59–C4). It is given as an IV injection on a weekly basis. The upper limit of the adult dose is 2.0 mg, but larger doses are used investigationally. Children may tolerate doses up to 2.0 mg/m² without the neurotoxicity seen in adults. Since excretion is dependent on the liver, the dose should be decreased in the presence of liver disease.

Side Effects, Adverse Reactions, and Contraindications

The side effects of vincristine are summarized in Table 59–S. Neurotoxicity is the most common dose-limiting side effect; it presents most frequently as a peripheral neuropathy after three or four doses. The patient may complain of numbness, weakness, myalgia, and cramping, which may progress to severe motor difficulties that interfere with even simple daily living activities.

Damage to nerves in the GI tract may cause constipation or paralytic ileus. These effects will reverse when vincristine is discontinued, but they can take months to years to resolve completely.

Myelosuppression may occur, but it is usually mild in comparison to other antineoplastic agents. Alopecia is common, but reversible when the drug is discontinued. Rare side effects are jaw pain; a metallic taste; mental depression; and stimulation of antidiuretic hormone release, which can lead to hyponatremia, fluid retention, and decreased urine output.

Vincristine is a potent vesicant and should be administered with care to prevent extravasation. The manufacturer recommends that extravasation be treated by injecting hyaluronidase (a proteolytic enzyme) and applying heat to the area. There is little clinical evidence that this is more beneficial than simply applying ice to the area.

Neurotoxicity may be more frequent and severe in patients who have underlying neurologic problems, or those who are weak or bedridden before treatment. Since the motor deficits associated with severe vincristine toxicity are rarely completely reversible, the drug should not be used in individuals who already have neurologic deficits. If vincristine is used in the presence of liver disease, dose reduction is advised.

NURSING IMPLICATIONS

Completely and frequently assess the patient's motor abilities. Ask the patient to describe any numbness or tingling of the finger. or toes, clumsiness in hand movement, or difficulty in climbing stairs, as an aid to identify sensory and motor changes. Bowel symptoms may require the use of stool softeners, mild laxatives, or enemas for relief. Most patients benefit from a structured bowel regimen to prevent constipation, including increased dietary fiber and fluid as well as stool softeners and laxatives when appropriate.

◆ Use During Pregnancy and Lactation

Vincristine can cause fetal harm when given to a pregnant woman.

◆ Use in the Elderly

Elderly patients are particularly sensitive to vincristine's neurotoxic effects.

Interactions with Other Drugs

Vincristine is one of the anticancer drugs that reduces the absorption and therapeutic effects of some oral digoxin formulations.

Overdose and Toxicity

A vincristine overdose can cause severe and potentially irreversible neurotoxicity. High doses also increase the risk of myelosuppression.

Related Drugs

Etoposide

Etoposide ("VP-16"; VEPESID) comes from the American mandrake (May-apple) plant. Its major biochemical effect is to inhibit the enzyme (topoisomerase II) that is primarily responsible for untangling DNA in preparation for cell replication. This inhibition results in DNA strand breaks and, eventually, cell death. The drug has been used by oral and IV routes in the treatment of lymphomas; acute nonlymphocytic leukemia; cancers of the testes, bladder, prostate, liver, and uterus; small cell carcinoma of the lung; and rhabdomyosarcoma. Excretion is mainly via bile, and to a lesser extent in the urine. Etoposide usually is given three to five times over a five-day period. Dose reductions are advised in the presence of liver dysfunction, but are not necessary for renal failure.

Etoposide's major side effects are myelosuppression (leukopenia, thrombocytopenia), nausea, vomiting, and temporary alopecia. Leukopenia is usually more pronounced than thrombocytopenia. It has a nadir at 14 to 16 days and recovery occurs by days 20 to 22. Minor nausea and vomiting are common, and can be effectively managed with antiemetics. Hypotension may occur, but can be minimized by infusing the dose over 30 to 60 minutes.

Taxol

Taxol is derived from the bark and leaves of the Pacific yew. In phase II clinical trials, it has shown promise in the treatment of ovarian carcinomas (especially in patients in whom chemotherapy has failed) and also may have some use against melanomas. Development of this drug has been slowed by the limited availability of the plant source and the lack of a chemical synthesis route.

Curiously, the major biochemical effect of taxol is just the opposite of the vinca alkaloids; that is, taxol makes microtubules unnaturally stable and hard to dissociate, whereas the vincas destabilize microtubules. Both types of disruption apparently lead to the same endpoint, however: selective inhibition of cellular functions related to proliferation. Taxol is extremely lipophilic and requires a polyoxyethylated castor oil vehicle (Cremophor EL). The drug is provided in a mixture of this vehicle with anhydrous ethanol (1:1) and must be diluted with large volumes of NaCl or dextrose solution for administration. Taxol is relatively unstable in this solution and must be administered soon after preparation. Because of problems with leaching of plasticizers, the drug solution should not contact plastic tubing or bags except for polyolefin vessels or polyethylene-lined tubing.

The major dose-limiting toxicity of taxol is neutropenia. Hypersensitivity reactions, characterized by hypotension, dyspnea, bronchospasm, and urticaria also were observed with great frequency in early trials. It is not clear whether these reactions are due to the drug itself or to the vehicle. Prophylactic treatment with dexamethasone and antihistamines is recommended to minimize this problem. Gastrointestinal mucositis and some neurologic toxicities also have been found on treatment with taxol.

Vinblastine

Vinblastine (VELBAN) works in the same way as vincristine, but has different side effects. It is useful in the treatment of the lymphomas; cancers of the testes, head and neck, breast, and kidneys; and Kaposi's sarcoma. The drug is given by IV on a weekly basis. Some treatment guidelines call for starting the drug at a low dose, and increasing the dose weekly as long as leukopenia is not a problem.

Myelosuppression is vinblastine's major side effect. The nadir of leukopenia usually occurs in four to 10 days, with bone marrow recovery occurring within one to two weeks. The duration of leukopenia appears to be dose-related and is highly predictable. Thrombocytopenia can occur, but is usually mild when moderate doses are used. Although vinblastine can cause neurotoxicity, this side effect is seen most often in patients treated with high doses or for long periods of time. Alopecia, skin rashes, photosensitivity, and severe stomatitis are potential side effects. As with vincristine, vinblastine can cause severe necrosis of soft tissue if it extravasates.

V. Hormonal and Antihormonal Agents

Many cancers arise from tissues that respond to hormones normally produced in the body. Altering the hormonal environment can interfere with the growth of such tumors. Cancer therapy with hormones may involve giving estrogens, androgens, progestins, adrenocorticosteroids, or antihormonal agents (Table 59–C5). Treatment is designed to antagonize, in one of several ways, the hormones that stimulate the growth of the tissue where the cancer originated. For example, in prostate cancer, where tumor growth could be stimulated by androgens, the treatment is estrogen therapy. The information given here pertains to the use of these agents for cancer treatment. See Chapters 45, 48, and 49 for a broader discussion of the hormones and their side effects.

The anticancer actions of the hormonal agents are not completely understood. They may act by interfering with the uptake and use of steroids needed for cell growth. Before natural hormones can produce a physiologic or cancer-promoting response, they must bind to steroid receptors found in the cell cytoplasm. The goal of anticancer hormonal therapy is either to block the receptor proteins and prevent a needed hormone from stimulating the cell, or to create biologic antagonistic activity. This treatment keeps more cancerous cells in the resting phase and decreases the growth fraction of the tumor. Since they have no direct cytotoxic effect, hormonal agents cannot cure cancer.

Estrogens

Estrogens are used to treat advanced prostate cancer and advanced breast cancer that has not responded to other treatments. The treatment of breast cancer with estrogen is restricted to postmenopausal women, since estrogen can exacerbate disease symptoms in premenopausal women. The most common estrogens for cancer are diethylstilbestrol (STILPHOSTROL) and ethinyl estradiol (ESTINYL). Both these drugs are given orally. They cause nausea and occasional vomiting, although nausea usually subsides within one to two weeks of starting therapy. Sodium retention can lead to hypertension and congestive heart failure. Therefore, monitor blood pressure and cardiac status periodically, especially when renal or cardiac disease is present. Other potential side effects are feminization and gynecomastia in males, and vaginal bleeding and breast tenderness in females. Low-dose irradiation to the breasts has been used successfully in males to prevent breast tissue growth.

Androgens

Androgens play an important role in the palliative treatment of breast cancer in women. Common drugs used for this purpose are fluoxymesterone (HALOTESTIN), methyltestosterone (ANDROID; TESTRED), testolactone (TESLAC), and testosterone propionate (ANDROLAN). The benefits of androgens are most often seen in women with breast cancer who have shown a response to other endocrine manipulations or who test positive for the presence of steroid receptors. These drugs are generally well tolerated. Common side effects are fluid retention, nausea and vomiting, and virilization. Fluoxymesterone can cause obstructive jaundice. A small number of women with bone metastases experience an acute tumor "flare" when androgen therapy is begun. This is characterized by a sudden increase in bone pain, which subsides as treatment continues. Androgens are contraindicated in men who have breast cancer.

Progestins

Progestins are used in the treatment of advanced endometrial cancer that is not responsive to surgery or radiation therapy. They are sometimes used to treat renal, prostate, and breast cancers. The most commonly used progestins are hydroxyprogesterone caproate (PRODROX), medroxyprogesterone acetate (PROVERA; DEPO-PROVERA), and megestrol acetate (MEGACE). Since these drugs are metabolized in the liver, they must be used cautiously in patients with liver dysfunction. Progestins may cause vaginal bleeding, mild fluid retention, and hypercalcemia in patients with bone metastases.

Adrenocorticosteroids

Adrenocorticosteroids are synthetic compounds derived from cortisol, a natural adrenal cortical hormone. They are used to treat acute and chronic lymphocytic leukemias, Hodgkin's and non-Hodgkin's lymphomas, myeloma, and selected breast cancers. These drugs somehow stop DNA synthesis and inhibit mitosis and cellular protein synthesis. Adrenocorticosteroids are also used for their weak antihypercalcemic effect and suppression of inflammatory edema found with bone and brain metastases. Patients may also benefit from the euphoria and appetite stimulation that are side effects of these drugs. This group of agents includes cortisone acetate, dexamethasone (DECADRON), hydrocortisone sodium succinate (SOLU-CORTEF), methylprednisolone sodium succinate (SOLU-MEDROL), and prednisone. Fluid retention, GI upset, hypertension, hyperglycemia, glycosuria, and increased susceptibility to infection are the side effects of their use. See Chapter 45 for further information.

Antihormone Agents

The antihormone drugs fall into one of four general classes: antiestrogen, antiandrogen, antiadrenal, and gonadotropin-releasing agents. Tamoxifen (NOLVADEX) is an antiestrogen used to treat advanced breast cancer in postmenopausal women who test positive for estrogen receptors, and as adjuvant therapy for pre- and postmenopausal women with breast cancer. Patients commonly experience side effects similar to menopausal symptoms. The flushing, hot flashes, nausea, and vomiting are usually not severe enough to discontinue therapy, and subside within a few weeks of starting tamoxifen. Some patients may experience an acute "flare" of bone and tumor pain that requires analgesics.

This is temporary and usually is an indication of response to therapy.

Flutamide (EULEXIN) is a nonsteroidal compound that competitively antagonizes androgen binding to the androgen receptors. The metabolite, α-hydroxyflutamide, binds to the receptor significantly better than the parent drug, and is probably the more active form of the two. Flutamide is administered orally for the treatment of prostatic carcinomas. Side effects are relatively mild and include mastodynia, gynecomastia, hot flashes, hepatotoxicity, and some impotence and loss of libido.

Aminoglutethimide (CYTADREN) is an antiadrenal agent used to treat metastatic breast cancer and adrenocortical cancer. It blocks the synthesis of glucocorticoids, mineralocorticoids, and estrogens, and inhibits their availability for stimulation of tumor growth. The drug is given orally with supplemental hydrocortisone. Adrenal insufficiency, skin rash, mild nausea and vomiting, and lethargy are the most common side effects.

Leuprolide (LUPRON) and goserelin (ZOLADEX) are gonadotropin-releasing hormone analogs used to treat prostate cancer. Although they frequently cause hot flashes, their use is associated with less gynecomastia, breast tenderness, nausea, vomiting, and peripheral edema than diethylstilbestrol. These drugs suppress luteinizing hormone and androgen levels and are used for this effect in the treatment of prostate cancer. They are given daily as an SC injection as long as there is a response. Patients may experience transient bone pain.

VI. Miscellaneous Agents

Several other drugs that do not fit into the classification schemes described thus far are commonly used in cancer care. Each of the drugs has unique properties and must be considered individually. The miscellaneous agents are L-asparaginase, dacarbazine, hydroxyurea, mitotane, and procarbazine. Dosages are summarized in Table 59–C6.

L-Asparaginase

L-Asparaginase (ELSPAR) is an enzyme that inhibits tumor cells, such as those in acute lymphoblastic leukemia, from using the amino acid asparagine to produce DNA and RNA. L-Asparaginase is used to treat lymphoma and some refractory myeloblastic leukemias. The drug is given IM three times a week for three weeks.

Nausea, vomiting, urticaria, and fever are common side effects. Antiemetics, antihistamines, steroids, and antipyretics are indicated for their management. An anaphylactic reaction of rapid onset may occur. As a precaution, a test dose of the drug (2.0 IU) should be given as an intradermal injection before administration of full doses. The test dose should be repeated if more than seven days elapse between full doses. Antihistamines and corticosteroids are used in the treatment of mild to moderate allergic reactions. Epinephrine must be used for true allergic reactions such as anaphylaxis. Malaise and altered liver function tests are common reactions that reverse when therapy is stopped.

Dacarbazine

Dacarbazine (DTIC) functions as an alkylating agent, but acts mainly on nucleic acids (especially DNA) of cancer cells. It is used to treat malignant melanoma, Hodgkin's disease, and soft tissue sarcomas. Dacarbazine is given as an IV injection or infusion for five days every four weeks or as a one-time dose every three or four weeks. Since the drug is metabolized in the liver and excreted by the kidneys, adequate hepatic and renal function are prerequisites to dacarbazine therapy. Dacarbazine can cause burning or pain at the injection site, which may be decreased by applying ice above the site. The drug can cause tissue necrosis if it extravasates, and precautions must be taken to avoid this.

The usual side effects of dacarbazine are myelosuppression and flu-like symptoms. The nadir of the white cell and platelet counts is 21 to 25 days after drug administration. Anemia is possible. Over 90% of patients experience severe nausea and vomiting, which may last from one to 12 hours; the severity decreases with subsequent dacarbazine doses. Pretreatment with antiemetics is of limited value but should be used. Patients benefit most by limiting food and fluids for several hours before treatment.

Hydroxyurea

Hydroxyurea (HYDREA) is a urea derivative that selectively destroys granulocytes. It is indicated for the treatment of chronic myelogenous leukemia, cancers of the colon, ovary, head and neck, and melanoma. It is cell cycle phase–specific in the S phase, in which it inhibits DNA synthesis.

Hydroxyurea, given orally, is rapidly absorbed from the GI tract. The usual dose is based on lean body weight. The presence of obesity or fluid retention should be taken into account when determining the correct dose. The drug is metabolized in the liver and 50% is excreted in the urine. Renal dysfunction requires a dosage reduction.

The major side effect of hydroxyurea is bone marrow depression; its onset and severity are dose-dependent. High doses can cause a rapid drop of the WBC count within 24 hours; leukopenia is seen most often within 10 days. Nausea and vomiting are mild or moderate and well controlled with antiemetics.

Mitotane

Mitotane (LYSODREN) has a direct cytotoxic effect on adrenal cortical cells. In doing so it decreases steroid secretion and alters the peripheral metabolism of steroids. The only cancer treated with mitotane is adrenocortical carcinoma.

Nausea and vomiting occur in up to 75% of patients, but can be avoided by starting mitotane at low doses and gradually increasing to a maintenance dose. Diarrhea, lethargy, somnolence, and vertigo are less common side effects, which respond to discontinuing the drug and restarting at lower doses. Stress, shock, and infection can precipitate acute adrenal insufficiency while using this drug. Patients should be aware that mitotane can cause adrenal insufficiency (eg, intolerance of stress; infections; altered psyche or libido) and be prepared to obtain early medical care if it occurs.

Procarbazine

Procarbazine (MATULANE) is a hydrazine derivative used in combination with other drugs to treat Hodgkin's disease, lung cancer, and brain tumors. It probably inhibits the synthesis of proteins, RNA, and DNA by working like an alkylating agent. The drug is given orally each day for 10 to 20 days (usually two weeks). It may be taken as a single daily dose or in divided doses throughout the day.

The side effects of procarbazine include myelosuppression, nausea and vomiting, and altered reproductive potential. Myelosuppression occurs two to three weeks after the drug is stopped. In some cases this reaction may prevent further treatment with the drug. Nausea and vomiting are common; they respond to the use of antiemetics such as metoclopramide and diphenhydramine. Azoospermia and amenorrhea are almost universal outcomes when the drug is used in high doses. There are reports of individuals parenting children after using procarbazine, but the majority of patients do not regain normal reproductive function. Since this drug is commonly used in the treatment of Hodgkin's disease in young individuals, this side effect has important consequences. Procarbazine is a potent carcinogen and may cause acute leukemia.

Procarbazine inhibits monoamine oxidase (MAO). If the patient ingests a catecholamine-releasing drug such as ephedrine or pseudoephedrine, commonly found in cough, cold, and allergy remedies, or foods such as some beers, wines, and cheeses containing tyramine (also a catecholamine-releaser), a serious or fatal hypertensive crisis may occur (see Chapters 14 and 24). Alcohol may interact to cause profound central nervous system (CNS) depression. Instruct patients taking this anticancer drug to avoid interacting drugs and foods.

VII. Biologic Response Modifiers

The biologic response modifiers (BRMs) are biologic and chemical agents that enhance the function of the immune system. Since the origins and actions of these agents differ from the typical antineoplastic agents, they are considered to be distinct from chemotherapy. There are many BRM agents including interferons, interleukin-2 (IL-2), lymphokine-activated killer (LAK) cells, transforming growth factor, tumor necrosis factor, colony stimulating factor, and monoclonal antibodies. These agents can activate and augment the body's immune mechanisms, interfere with cancer cells' ability to survive or metastasize, stop the transformation of normal cells into cancer cells, or have a direct cytotoxic effect on cancer cells.

With the exception of alpha interferon and levamisole, all these agents are investigational. Nevertheless, they hold great promise for future use in the diagnosis and treatment of cancer. In addition to administering these agents, nurses are responsible for explaining to patients and families how they work and offering realistic hope about their usefulness.

Interferons

The **interferons** include alpha, beta, and gamma interferons. Alpha interferons have been studied more than the others, and are commercially available for the treatment of hairy cell leukemia. They can enhance the actions of fluorouracil in experimental systems, and also may do so in patients with colorectal cancer. Alpha interferon (INTRON, ROFERON) is given SC or IM in doses of 3 to 6 million units three times per week; this dosage is continued for long-term maintenance. Initial side effects include flu-like symptoms, fever, chills, muscle aches, loss of appetite, and nausea. These adverse effects may be reduced or prevented by giving acetaminophen before and after drug administration. Tolerance to the side effects develops after the first few interferon doses. A history of cardiovascular disease contraindicates alpha interferon use, which has been associated with acute cardiac failure, arrhythmias, and ischemia in such patients. Beta interferon is similar in activity and toxicity to alpha interferon. Gamma interferon has not been found to elicit antitumor responses. However it does activate macrophages that can engulf tumor cells, and so clinical investigations are continuing to examine the usefulness of this agent.

Interleukin-2

Interleukin-2 (IL-2) is a lymphokine that is produced by the body's helper T cells, an important component of the immune response. Genetic engineering has allowed the production of IL-2 in sufficient amounts for investigational use. Interleukin-2 is being studied for its efficacy and toxicity as a single agent, as well as in combination with LAK cells, which attack cancer cells but not normal cells. Most clinical trials with IL-2 focus on the treatment of renal cell cancer and melanoma. Interleukin-2 has significant side effects, some of which can be ameliorated by prophylaxis with acetaminophen, indomethacin, and meperidine. When administering IL-2, carefully observe for adverse neurologic, renal, hematologic, hepatic, and cutaneous effects. The addition of LAK cells increases the antitumor effects of IL-2, but experimental regimens that combine these two agents have caused life-threatening toxicities.

Levamisole

Levamisole (ERGAMISOL) is an immunostimulant that has, paradoxically, been used to treat rheumatoid arthritis. It is used in combination with fluorouracil for treating carcinoma of the colon, although the mechanism by which levamisole enhances fluorouracil action is unclear. Levamisole is given orally over several weeks, during or before the course of fluorouracil therapy. Toxicities attributed to levamisole include nausea, vomiting, diarrhea, stomatitis, a flu-like syndrome, and some CNS effects.

Monoclonal Antibodies

Monoclonal antibodies (MoAbs) are proteins that can be directed toward specific target cells in the body. Monoclonal antibodies targeted for cancer cells can be grown using modern tissue culture techniques. This makes MoAbs useful in diagnostic testing to find small numbers of cancer cells or to carry antitumor agents or radioactive particles directly to them. Side effects of MoAbs include fever, chills, headache, flushing, and anaphylaxis. Newer methods of producing MoAbs are being developed to eliminate this problem.

SUMMARY OF NURSING IMPLICATIONS

◆ Assessment

Establish baseline assessment data to include information on previous treatment; current blood profiles; liver and kidney function; activity level; and nutritional status. Abnormal findings may indicate withholding drug or lowering dose.

Complete an initial physical assessment of cardiac and respiratory function, motor and sensory status, and body weight.

Review patient history for conditions known to increase risk to patient (eg, liver or kidney dysfunction, cardiac or pulmonary disease).

◆ Nursing Diagnoses

Knowledge deficit related to drug therapy.

Anxiety related to drug side effects.

Constipation or diarrhea related to adverse drug effects.

Altered nutrition: less than body requirements related to nausea and vomiting.

Ineffective individual coping related to disease process and adverse drug effects.

High risk for impaired skin integrity related to drug extravasation, radiation recall (doxorubicin), or other adverse effects of specific drugs.

Altered oral mucous membrane.

◆ Planning/Implementation

Closely monitor blood counts for evidence of myelosuppression; if present, notify physician and take steps to prevent infection, injury, and bleeding; provide well-balanced diet and frequent rest periods.

Assist patient in managing nausea and vomiting from cisplatin, cyclophosphamide, doxorubicin, and others; give antiemetics, offer distraction; teach relaxation techniques and guided imagery.

Give frequent mouth care if stomatitis is present; use quarter-strength hydrogen peroxide or baking soda in water, analgesics, and antifungal agents.

Monitor for evidence of dyspnea, tachypnea, decreased breath sounds, rales, nonproductive cough, or fever indicating pulmonary (or cardiac) toxicity.

Monitor for cardiotoxicity (arrhythmias, evidence of heart failure) with doxorubicin and daunorubicin.

Monitor for pulmonary toxicity with bleomycin.

Observe for skin reactions from drug therapy (eg, hyperpigmentation, hyperkeratosis, dermatitis, nail damage).

Monitor intake and output, encourage intake of fluids, and monitor changes in BUN or creatinine levels; renal toxicity more likely with cisplatin, cyclophosphamide, and methotrexate.

Give large amounts of fluids and oral or IV sodium bicarbonate to alkalinize urine and prevent urinary precipitation with high doses of methotrexate.

Note complaints of numbness and tingling in hands and feet or general weakness with vincristine; withhold drug if motor weakness is present.

Have epinephrine injection available in case of drug hypersensitivity and anaphylaxis; have antihistamines and corticosteroids available for possible adjunctive use.

Apply ice and give antihistamines for severe urticaria with flare reaction of doxorubicin.

◆ Patient and Family Teaching

Teach the patient/family:

To purchase wigs or head covering to decrease psychologic distress with alopecia.

To avoid sun exposure and wear protective sunscreens when sun is unavoidable, to prevent aggravation of hyperpigmentation (eg, with methotrexate); to avoid tight-fitting clothing and any mechanical or chemical irritants.

About possible effects on reproductive function leading to sterility; men may want to consider sperm banking prior to chemotherapy.

About drug side effects; encourage early reporting if cardinal signs of toxicity occur (eg, cardiac, pulmonary, renal, or neurotoxicity).

About possible feminization with estrogens and masculinization with androgens, which can be psychologically distressing; hot flashes and fluid retention may also occur.

About importance of carefully following guidelines for drug doses and methods of administration.

◆ Evaluation

The patient/family will:

Respond positively to antineoplastic drug therapy; tumor size reduces; laboratory values within normal limits.

Manage drug side effects: comfortable; able to eat a balanced diet; maintain body weight.

Comply with prescribed drug and medical regimen; return for follow-up laboratory tests and physician visits.

Cope effectively with anxiety and fears; seek counseling if needed.

Annotated Bibliography

Cawley MM: Recent advances in chemotherapy. Administration and nursing implications. *Nurs Clin North Am* 1990;25(2):377–391. *Insight into what has happened, and is likely to occur, with anticancer drugs and combinations, treatment regimens, and dosing schedules; emphasizes how these developments affect nursing roles and responsibilities.*

Chabner BA, Collins JM (eds): *Cancer Chemotherapy: Principles and Practice.* Philadelphia, Lippincott, 1990. *This book contains detailed information about the biochemical actions of agents used in cancer chemotherapy.*

DeVita VT, Hellman S, Rosenberg SA (eds): *Cancer: Principles and Practice of Oncology.* Philadelphia, Lippincott, 1989. *A detailed resource on the diagnosis, treatment, and management of all cancers.*

Fischetti LF: Interaction between nonsteroidal anti-inflammatory drugs and high-dose methotrexate: A literature review. *J Pediatr Oncol Nurs* 1990;7(1):14–16. *Worthwhile for its coverage of how OTC drugs can increase the risk of serious toxicity caused by a common anticancer and antirheumatic drug, and how this can be prevented with proper nursing and patient education.*

Gullatte MM, Graves T: Advances in Antineoplastic Therapy. *Oncol Nurs Forum* 1990;17:867–876. *A short article summarizing for nurses clinical information about new and investigational anticancer drugs and their implications.*

Holmes S: The oral complications of specific anticancer therapy. *Int J Nurs Stud* 1991;28(4):343–360. *Adverse effects of anticancer drugs in and on the oral cavity are diverse and important. The author reviews these problems, the drugs that cause them, and key nursing measures that can prevent or minimize unwanted outcomes, and highlights areas for future research.*

Lobert S, Correia JJ: Antimitotics in cancer chemotherapy. *Cancer Nurs* 1992;15(1):22–33. *Explains the mechanism of action of these cell cycle–specific drugs in a way that will help the nurse understand and anticipate their common adverse effects, and plan nursing interventions for them.*

Pratt WB, Ruddon RW, Ensminger WD, Maybaum J: *The Anticancer Drugs.* New York, Oxford University Press, 1993. *This recently revised edition provides a concise summary of the basic and clinical aspects of cancer chemotherapy, as well as introductory material on cancer biology.*

Skeel RT: *Handbook of Cancer Chemotherapy.* Boston, Little, Brown and Company, 1991. *A complete pocket summary of clinical data on anticancer drugs.*

Yarbro JW (ed): Cytokines as Modulators of Cytotoxic Drugs in Experimental and Clinical Hematology and Oncology. *Semin Oncol* 1992;19 (suppl. 4):1–103. *This collection of articles provides an overview of current approaches to the clinical uses of biologic response modifiers in cancer chemotherapy.*

Table 59–C1 Clinical Uses and Administration of Alkylating Agents

AGENT	CLINICAL USES	DOSAGE AND ROUTE OF ADMINISTRATION	COMMENTS AND NURSING IMPLICATIONS
PROTOTYPE			
Cyclophosphamide (CYTOXAN)	Acute and chronic lymphocytic leukemia; cancers of breast, lung, ovary, cervix; Ewing's sarcoma; Hodgkin's disease; multiple myeloma; neuroblastomata; non-Hodgkin's lymphoma; rhabdomyosarcoma; sarcomas	IV: 500–1500 mg/m² every 3 weeks in single or divided doses; reconstitute IV drug with sterile water Oral: 60–120 mg/m² daily for 14 days every 28 days	Hemorrhagic cystitis prevented by fluid intakes of 2 L for 3 or 4 days; some patients report "metallic taste" in mouth during injection; hard candy may reduce sensation
RELATED DRUGS (MUSTARDS)			
Chlorambucil (LEUKERAN)	Chronic lymphocytic leukemia; lymphomas; choriocarcinoma; cancers of breast, ovary, testes	Oral: 4–10 mg/daily for 3–6 weeks	
Ifosfamide (IFEX)	Testicular and lung cancers, bony and soft-tissue sarcomas	IV: 1.2 g/m²/daily for 5 days, every 3 weeks	Must be used with MESNA and adequate hydration to prevent hemorrhagic cystitis
Mechlorethamine (MUSTARGEN)	Lung cancer, Hodgkin's disease, non-Hodgkin's lymphoma, mycosis fungoides	IV: 1.6–6 mg/m² every 3–4 weeks; reconstitute with 10 mL of sterile water and use immediately	Protect skin and eyes when mixing and administering; prevent extravasation
Melphalan (ALKERAN)	Cancers of breast, ovary, testes; malignant melanoma; multiple myeloma	Oral: 6–10 mg daily, 2–4 mg daily for maintenance	Drug schedule may be designed to achieve myelosuppression; give drug on empty stomach
Triethylene thiophosphoramide (THIOTEPA)	Cancers of breast, bladder, ovary	IV, IC: 16–32 mg/m² or 8 mg/m² daily for 4–5 days Intravesical: 60–90 mg dissolved in 60–100 mL sterile water for bladder instillation once a week for 4 weeks	
Nitrosoureas			
Carmustine (BiCNU)	Brain tumors, lymphomas, multiple myeloma, lung cancer	IV: 75–100 mg/m² daily for 2 days, 200 mg/m² once every 6 weeks	Administer over 30 minutes to decrease local irritation; protect solution from light

(continued)

Table 59–C1 Clinical Uses and Administration of Alkylating Agents (*Continued*)

AGENT	CLINICAL USES	DOSAGE AND ROUTE OF ADMINISTRATION	COMMENTS AND NURSING IMPLICATIONS
Lomustine			
(CeeNU)	Brain tumors, lymphomas, melanoma, renal and lung cancer	Oral: 70 mg/m^2 every 3 weeks or 130 mg/m^2 every 6 weeks	Administer on an empty stomach
Streptozocin			
(STREPTOZOTOCIN; ZANOSAR)	Carcinoid; Zollinger-Ellison syndrome; Hodgkin's disease; colon, liver, pancreatic cancer	IV: 500–1500 mg/m^2/week for 4 or more weeks: 500 mg/m^2 on day 1 and 5, repeated every 6 weeks	Give slowly over 1 hour; place ice pack above injection site to reduce local irritation
Other Covalent DNA-Binding Drugs			
Busulfan			
(MYLERAN)	Chronic myelogenous leukemia, polycythemia vera	Oral: 4–8 mg/daily, 1–3 mg daily for maintenance	Causes cumulative myelotoxicity; discontinue when WBC reaches 15,000/mm^3
Carboplatin			
(PARAPLATIN, "CBDCA")	Ovarian, cervical, lung, esophageal, head and neck, bladder, and testicular cancers	IV: 300–400 mg/m^2 every 4 weeks	
Cisplatin			
(PLATINOL)	Cancers of ovary, testes, bladder, lung, esophagus, cervix, prostate; lymphomas, myeloma; melanoma; osteosarcoma	IV: 50–120 mg/m^2 every 3–4 weeks: 15–40 mg/m^2 daily for 5 days, repeat every 3–4 weeks	Hydration and diuretics before therapy

Key: IA=intraarterial; IC=intracavitary.

Table 59–C2 | Clinical Uses and Administration of Antitumor Antibiotics

AGENT	CLINICAL USES	DOSAGE AND ROUTE OF ADMINISTRATION	COMMENTS AND NURSING IMPLICATIONS
PROTOTYPE			
Doxorubicin (ADRIAMYCIN)	Cancer of the breast, bladder, thyroid, lung, ovary; acute leukemia; sarcoma; neuroblastoma; lymphomas; Ewing's sarcoma	IV, IC: 60–90 mg/m every 3 weeks; also given in low daily doses and by continuous infusion	Prevent extravasation. Incompatible with sodium heparin. Maximum lifetime dose 550 mg/m^2
RELATED DRUGS			
Bleomycin (BLENOXANE)	Cancers of the head and neck, penis, testes, vulva, cervix, esophagus, lung, skin, anus; lymphomas; sarcomas; melanoma	IV, IM, SC, IC: 10–20 units/m^2 once or twice weekly	IM or SC doses may cause pain or burning at site. Give test dose (3–5 units) before first administration and observe for anaphylaxis. Maximum lifetime dose 300–400 units.
Dactinomycin (ACTINOMYCIN-D, COSMEGEN)	Testicular cancer, melanoma, choriocarcinoma, Wilm's tumor, neuroblastoma, retinoblastoma, rhabdomyosarcoma, Ewing's sarcoma, Kaposi's sarcoma	IV: 15–30 μg/kg/week or 10–15 μg/kg/day for 5 days every 3 weeks	Reduce dose if radiation is used; prevent extravasation
Daunorubicin DAUNOMYCIN, CERUBIDINE)	Acute myelocytic and lymphocytic leukemia	IV: 30–60 mg/m^2/day for 2 to 3 days every 3 to 4 weeks	Prevent extravasation; place ice pack above injection site to reduce local irritation. Incompatible with sodium heparin. Maximum lifetime dose 550 mg/m^2
Idarubicin (IDAMYCIN)	Acute lymphocytic leukemia	IV: 12 mg/m^2/day for 3 days by slow injection	
Mitomycin (MITOMYCIN C, MUTAMYCIN)	Cancer of the gastrointestinal tract, breast, lung, cervix, bladder	IV, IA, IC: 10–20 mg/m^2 every 6-8 weeks: 2 mg/m^2 for 5 days, skip 2 days, and readminister for 5 days	Prevent extravasation
Mitoxantrone (NOVANTRONE)	Acute nonlymphocytic leukemia	IV: 12 mg/m^2 for 3 days, may be repeated for 2 days after 3 weeks	Use with caution in patients with abnormal liver or cardiac function
Plicamycin (MITHRACIN)	Testicular cancer Malignant hypercalcemia	IV: 25–50 μg/kg on alternate days for 8 doses IV: 15–25 μg/kg for 3 days	Prevent extravasation

Key: IA=intraarterial; IC=intracavitary; IT=intrathecal.

Table 59–C3 Clinical Uses and Administration of Antimetabolites

AGENT	CLINICAL USES	DOSAGE AND ROUTE OF ADMINISTRATION	COMMENTS AND NURSING IMPLICATIONS
PROTOTYPE			
Methotrexate			
(FOLEX)	Cancer of breast, lung, head and neck, testes, ovary, cervix; choriocarcinoma; medulloblastoma; acute lymphocytic and myeloblastic leukemia; mycosis fungoides; osteogenic sarcoma; rhabdomyosarcoma	Oral: 2.5–30 mg daily IV, IM: 25–40 mg/m^2 once or twice weekly every 2–4 weeks; 100–7500 mg/m^2 high dose with leucovorin rescue IT: 6–15 mg every 2–5 days	Length of time for IV injection should be increased as dose increases. High-dose therapy potentially lethal without rescue
RELATED DRUGS			
Cytarabine			
(ARA-C; CYTOSAR-U)	Acute myelogenous leukemia, acute phase of chronic myelogenous leukemia, cancer of head and neck	IV, SC: 100–150 mg/m^2 for 5–10 days IT: 20–30 mg/m^2 in 10 mL sterile saline	Use preservative-free saline to prepare IT dose
Floxuridine			
(5-FUDR)	Cancer of the stomach, liver, colon, pancreas, biliary tract	IA: 0.1–0.6 mg/kg daily as continuous infusion every 2 to 6 weeks	Drug is concentrated, give only IA
Fludarabine			
(FLUDARA)	Chronic lymphocytic leukemia	IV: 25 mg/m^2/day for 5 days, repeated every 4 weeks (given as prodrug FAMP)	Consider discontinuing if neurotoxicity occurs
5-Fluorouracil			
(5-FU; ADRUCIL; EFUDEX)	Cancers of breast, colon, bladder, liver, pancreas, stomach, ovary, cervix, prostate; basal and squamous cell skin cancers	IV, IA: 12 mg/kg for 3–5 days every 4 weeks, or 15 mg/kg (maximum 1 g) weekly for 6 weeks, or 15 mg/kg for 6 days Topical: Apply cream to tumor twice a day for 3–6 weeks	Wear gloves when applying cream. May be given as continuous infusion
6-Mercaptopurine			
(MERCAPTOPURINE; 6-MP)	Acute lymphocytic and acute and chronic myelogenous leukemia	Oral: 2.5 mg/kg daily for weeks to months	Reduce dose if allopurinol is given concurrently
6-Thioguanine			
(THIOGUANINE)	Acute lymphocytic and acute and chronic myelogenous leukemia	Oral: 80–100 mg/m^2 daily for 5–10 days every 1 to 4 weeks	Administer between meals

Key: IA = intraarterial; IT = intrathecal

Table 59–C4 Clinical Uses and Administration of Plant Alkaloids

AGENT	CLINICAL USES	DOSAGE AND ROUTE OF ADMINISTRATION	COMMENTS AND NURSING IMPLICATIONS
PROTOTYPE			
Vincristine (ONCOVIN)	Acute leukemia; lymphomas; cancers of brain, testes, breast, cervix; Wilm's tumor	IV: 0.4–1.4 mg/m^2 weekly; upper limit of single dose in adults is 2.0 mg	Prevent extravasation
RELATED DRUGS			
Etoposide ("VP-16"; VEPESID)	Lymphomas; acute nonlymphocytic leukemia; cancers of lung, testes, bladder, prostate, liver, uterus; rhabdomyosarcoma	IV: 50–100 mg/m^2 3–5 times over 5 days every 3 to 4 weeks	Rapid administration may cause hypotension
Taxol	Ovarian carcinoma, melanoma	IV: 200 mg/m^2 every 3 weeks, administered as 3 consecutive freshly prepared 8-hr infusions	Prevent anaphylactic reaction by prophylaxis with dexamethasone and antihistamines
Vinblastine (VELBAN)	Lymphomas; cancers of testes, breast, kidney, head and neck; Kaposi's sarcoma	IV: 2.5–6.0 mg/m^2 weekly for weeks to months	Prevent extravasation

Table 59–C5 Clinical Uses and Administration of Hormonal and Antihormonal Agents

AGENT	CLINICAL USES	DOSAGE AND ROUTE OF ADMINISTRATION
	Estrogens	
Diethystilbestrol (STILPHOSTROL)	Breast cancer	Oral: 5 mg 3 times daily
	Prostate cancer	Oral: 1–3 mg once daily
Ethinyl estradiol (ESTINYL)	Breast cancer	Oral: 1 mg 3 times daily
	Prostate cancer	Oral: 0.1 mg 3 times daily
	Androgens	
Fluoxymesterone (HALOTESTIN)	Breast cancer	Oral: 10–40 mg daily
Testolactone (TESLAC)	See fluoxymesterone	Oral: 250 mg 4 times daily
Testosterone propionate (ANDROLAN)	See fluoxymesterone	IM: 50–100 mg 3 times weekly
Methyltestosterone (ANDROID; TESTRED)	See fluoxymesterone	Oral: 50–200 mg daily

(continued)

Table 59–C5 Clinical Uses and Administration of Hormonal and Antihormonal Agents (*Continued*)

AGENT	CLINICAL USES	DOSAGE AND ROUTE OF ADMINISTRATION
Progestins		
Hydroxyprogesterone caproate (PRODROX)	Breast, endometrial, renal cancers	IM: 1000–1500 mg weekly
Medroxyprogesterone acetate (PROVERA; DEPO-PROVERA)	See hydroxyprogesterone	Oral: 400–800 mg twice weekly IM: 1000–1500 mg weekly
Megestrol acetate (MEGACE)	See hydroxyprogesterone	Oral: 40–80 mg 4 times daily
Adrenocorticosteroids		
Cortisone acetate	Acute and chronic lymphocytic leukemias; lymphomas; multiple myeloma; breast cancer	Oral: 20–100 mg daily
Dexamethasone (DECADRON)	See cortisone	Oral: 0.5–4 mg daily
Hydrocortisone sodium succinate (SOLU-CORTEF)	See cortisone	IV: 100–500 mg daily
Prednisone	See cortisone	Oral: 15–100 mg daily
Methylprednisolone sodium succinate (SOLU-MEDROL)	See cortisone	IM, IV: 10–125 mg daily
Antiandrogen		
Flutamide (EULEXIN)	Prostate cancer	Oral: 250 mg 3 times daily
Antiestrogen		
Tamoxifen (NOLVADEX)	Breast cancer	Oral: 10–20 mg twice daily
Antiadrenal		
Aminoglutethamide (CYTADREN)	Breast cancer	Oral: 250–500 mg 4 times daily
Gonadotropin-Releasing Hormone		
Leuprolide (LUPRON)	Prostate cancer	SC: 1 mg daily
Goserelin (ZOLADEX)	Prostate cancer	SC: 3.6 mg monthly

Table 59–C6 Clinical Uses and Administration of Miscellaneous Chemotherapeutic Agents

AGENT	CLINICAL USES	DOSAGE AND ROUTE OF ADMINISTRATION	COMMENTS AND NURSING IMPLICATIONS
Asparaginase			
(L-ASPARAGINASE; ELSPAR)	Acute lymphoblastic leukemia, lymphoma	IM: 6000 IU/m^2 for 3 days for 3 weeks	Give test dose to check for sensitivity
Dacarbazine			
(DTIC)	Melanoma, Hodgkin's disease, sarcomas	IV: 150–250 mg/m^2/day for 5 days every 4 weeks, or 800–900 mg/m^2 every 3–4 weeks	Apply ice at injection site or slow rate of infusion to decrease irritation; prevent extravasation
Hydroxyurea			
(HYDREA)	Acute leukemias; chronic myelogenous leukemia; cancers of ovary, colon, head and neck; melanoma	Oral: 500–3000 mg daily for weeks to months	Reduce dose for renal dysfunction
Mitotane			
(LYSODREN)	Adrenocortical cancer	Oral: 2–16 g/day in 3 or 4 doses for weeks to months	Begin at lower dose and increase gradually to prevent nausea and vomiting
Procarbazine			
(MATULANE)	Lymphomas, cancers of lung and brain	Oral: 50–200 mg daily for 10–20 days every 4 weeks	Do not give with drugs and foods containing monoamine oxidase (MAO)

Table 59–S Common Side Effects of the Antineoplastic Agents*

	Myelo-Suppression	Mucositis	Nausea and Vomiting	Alopecia and Skin Reactions	Other
L-Asparaginase	0	–	0	+	Anaphylaxis; CNS toxicity; hyperpyrexia
Bleomycin	0	0	0	+	Anaphylaxis; hyperpyrexia; pulmonary toxicity
Busulfan	+	–	0	–	Pulmonary toxicity
Carmustine	+	+	+	–	Cardiac, hepatic, and pulmonary toxicity; skin necrosis
Chlorambucil	+	–	0	–	
Cisplatin	+	–	+	–	Anaphylaxis; ototoxicity; renal toxicity; peripheral neuropathy
Cyclophosphamide	+	–	+	+	Hemorrhagic cystitis
Cytarabine	+	+	+	+	CNS and pulmonary toxicity with high doses

(continued)

Table 59–S **Common Side Effects of the Antineoplastic Agents* (*Continued*)**

	Myelo-Suppression	Mucositis	Nausea and Vomiting	Alopecia and Skin Reactions	Other
Dacarbazine	+	–	+	–	Anaphylaxis; hypotension; skin necrosis
Dactinomycin	+	+	+	+	Skin necrosis
Daunorubicin	+	+	+	+	Cardiotoxicity; hepatic toxicity; skin necrosis
Doxorubicin	+	+	+	+	Cardiotoxicity; hepatic toxicity; skin necrosis
Etoposide	+	0	+	+	Anaphylaxis; hypotension
Floxuridine	+	+	+	+	Diarrhea, gastritis; hepatic toxicity
Fludarabine	+	0	0	–	CNS toxicity at high doses
5-Fluorouracil	+	+	+	+	Diarrhea; cerebellar ataxia
Hydroxyurea	+	0	+	0	
Idarubicin	+	–	+	+	Hepatic toxicity; diarrhea
Ifosfamide	+	–	+	–	Hemorrhagic cystitis; CNS toxicity
Lomustine	+	+	+	0	Hepatic and renal toxicity
Mechlorethamine	+	–	+	+	Skin necrosis
Melphalan	+	0	0	–	
6-Mercaptopurine	+	+	0	0	Hepatic toxicity
Methotrexate	+	+	+	+	CNS toxicity (intrathecal); hepatic toxicity; pneumonitis; renal toxicity
Mitomycin	+	+	+	+	Pulmonary and renal toxicity; skin necrosis
Mitotane	–	+	+	0	Adrenal insufficiency; CNS toxicity
Mitoxantrone	+	0	0	0	Cardiotoxicity
Plicamycin	+	+	+	–	Hepatic and renal toxicity; skin necrosis
Procarbazine	+	0	+	–	MAO inhibition
Streptozocin	0	0	+	+	Diarrhea; abdominal cramps; renal toxicity
Taxol	+	0	+	+	Anaphylaxis
6-Thioguanine	+	+	0	0	Hepatic toxicity
Triethylene thiophosphoramide	+	–	+	–	
Vinblastine	+	+	0	+	Skin necrosis
Vincristine	–	–	–	+	Skin necrosis; hepatic toxicity; neurotoxicity

*Key: + = Common; 0 = occasional; – = uncommon

Note: Long-term use of any antineoplastic agent may lead to sterility and the development of secondary malignancies.

Table 59–I **Major Drug Interactions Involving the Anticancer Drugs**

INTERACTANT	RESULT OF INTERACTION	COMMENTS AND NURSING IMPLICATIONS
Bleomycin		
Digoxin, oral (Chapter 31)	Reduced digoxin absorption and effects	Monitor congestive heart failure patients for evidence of worsening heart failure; digoxin dosage increase may be needed, especially when not using liquid-containing digoxin capsules; occurs because of gut mucosal damage by bleomycin drug
Oxygen	Increased risk of bleomycin pulmonary toxicity	Monitor accordingly if long-term oxygen therapy is needed
Phenytoin, other hydantoins (Chapter 26)	Reduced phenytoin blood levels, effects	Monitor clinical response to phenytoin, use frequent measurements of blood levels to guide dosage increases that may be needed; interaction occurs because anticancer drug increases phenytoin metabolism or reduces absorption from gut
Carboplatin		
Phenytoin	See bleomycin: phenytoin	
Carmustine		
Cimetidine (Chapter 40)	Increased risk of bone marrow suppression or true carmustine toxicity	Avoid interaction unless no alternatives can be used; interaction probably less likely or serious with cimetidine alternatives (eg, famotidine, nizatidine, ranitidine), which may be preferred
Digoxin, oral	See bleomycin: digoxin	
Phenytoin	See bleomycin: phenytoin	
Cisplatin		
Bleomycin	Increased risk of ototoxicity	Avoid combination if possible; otherwise perform hearing tests often to detect problem early
Furosemide, other loop diuretics (Chapter 32)		
Phenytoin	See bleomycin: phenytoin	
Cyclophosphamide		
Digoxin	See bleomycin: digoxin	
Succinylcholine (Chapter 17)	Prolonged neuromuscular blockade, impaired ventilation	Anticipate interaction and need for prolonged monitoring and ventilatory assistance
Cytarabine		
Digoxin	See bleomycin: digoxin	
Doxorubicin		
Digoxin	See bleomycin: digoxin	

(continued)

Table 59–I Major Drug Interactions Involving the Anticancer Drugs (*Continued*)

INTERACTANT	RESULT OF INTERACTION	COMMENTS AND NURSING IMPLICATIONS
Floxuridine		
Cimetidine	May increase risk of excessive cytotoxicity	Monitor accordingly, cimetidine may need to be discontinued; see interactions above involving cimetidine and carmustine
5-Fluorouracil		
Calcium leucovorin	Increased cytotoxic, toxic effects	Some protocols use this combination; monitor for excessive effects
Hydrochlorothiazide, similar diuretics (Chapter 32)	Potential increased risk of fluorouracil toxicity	Use alternative diuretics or antihypertensive drugs; monitor accordingly if combined use is unavoidable
6-Mercaptopurine		
Allopurinol (Chapter 53)	Significant risk of severe bone marrow depression	Avoid interaction if possible; if unavoidable, starting doses of mercaptopurine should be only 25% to 33% of usual
Anticoagulants, oral (Chapter 35)	Potential antagonism of anticoagulant effects	Monitor accordingly if interaction unavoidable; closer monitoring of coagulation parameters needed, increased anticoagulant dose possibly necessary
Methotrexate		
Phenytoin	See bleomycin: phenytoin	
Probenecid (Chapter 53)	Reduced methotrexate excretion, potentially rapid onset of major toxicity	Combined therapy usually requires reduced methotrexate dose, prolonged leucovorin rescue; monitor methotrexate blood levels closely during combined therapy
Salicylates (aspirin, all related drugs, Chapter 52)	See probenecid	
Sulfonamide antibiotics and medications containing sulfas (eg, trimethoprim-sulfamethoxazole Chapter 56)	Increased risk of potentially fatal bone marrow suppression	More frequent blood tests indicated
Procarbazine		
Digoxin	See bleomycin: digoxin	
Ethanol (Chapter 22)	Rapid but transient facial flushing	Discourage alcohol use
Vinblastine		
Phenytoin	See bleomycin: phenytoin	
Vincristine		
Digoxin	See bleomycin: digoxin	

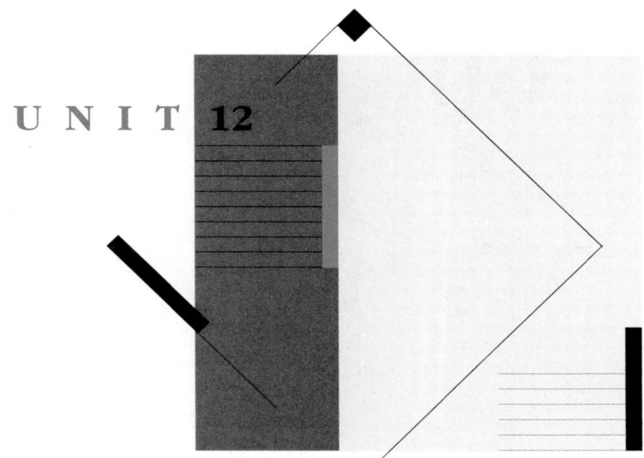

Fluids and Nutrients

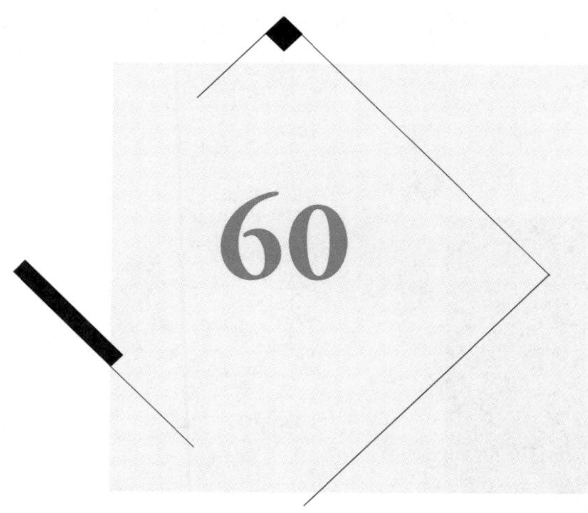

Fluid Balance

This chapter describes the administration of blood, blood products, fluids, and electrolyte solutions. These products and solutions must be viewed as drugs, and all the considerations of drug administration apply. The nurse who administers them must always analyze the dosage, method of administration, side effects, contraindications, drug interactions, and possible toxicity. This is true both for intravenous products, such as plasma or electrolyte solutions, and for oral fluid and electrolyte solutions. Improper administration can lead to serious outcomes.

Blood and Blood Products

The administration of whole blood, blood cell concentrates, plasma and plasma components, and blood substitutes is often necessary. Blood is a heterogeneous mixture of cells in a fluid (plasma) that contains different chemicals, proteins, and other essential factors. Identifying blood components has led to the isolation and purification of many of these, some of which have been commercially prepared for administration to patients. As an example, clotting factors are found in the blood in minute amounts. Some of them have been commercially produced and are available to patients with hemophilia.

Whenever whole blood is administered, all blood components will also be administered. Some blood components could cause reactions owing to various antigens attached to the cell membrane of the blood cells, immunoglobulins in the plasma, or microbial contaminants, such as the hepatitis virus, or human immunodeficiency virus (HIV), which causes acquired immunodeficiency syndrome (AIDS).

Whole Blood

Whole blood is not used frequently since purified blood component preparations that are less likely to cause side effects are now available. Also, the components can be more effective and are more easily administered.

The most common indication for whole blood administration is for blood volume replacement in acute blood loss. However, patients often receive concentrates such as packed red cells, to replace erythrocytes, or blood volume expanders or plasma, to replace vascular fluid volume. Whole blood may be used to prepare patients for surgery and in the treatment of hepatic coma. Whole blood is also used for exchange transfusion in the treatment of erythroblastosis fetalis. In this procedure, the infant's entire blood volume is slowly replaced with donor whole blood to remove the immature erythrocytes and circulating immune factors that cause the disease. This condition has been seen infrequently since the introduction of routine administration of Rh_o immune globulin (RhoGAM) to Rh-negative mothers. Occasionally donor blood is transfused before organ transplantation, as this procedure may improve graft survival.

Administration Techniques

Whole blood is a viscous suspension that must be administered intravenously (IV). Whole blood is generally anticoagulated with citrate and stored in plastic bags. The entire blood administration set is treated to prevent coagulation, and the blood is usually administered through a large bore (18 gauge or larger) needle in a hand or antecubital fossa vein. Blood is filtered through a 170 to 220 μm pore-sized filter. Warmers are often used to keep blood at body temperature before administration. Whole blood is prepared in 500 mL units; in general, one unit of normal-hematocrit whole blood will contribute at least 1 gram of hemoglobin per 100 mL of the recipient's blood.

NURSING IMPLICATIONS

Many of the precautions used with the administration of whole blood apply also to the administration of other blood components. Identify the donor blood type in the same manner as for careful medication administration, using three checks. Usually, two nurses or licensed personnel check the blood before administration. Blood should be administered with normal saline unless sodium is contraindicated for the patient. Dextrose and blood can cause red cell clumping.

Assessment of the patient during blood administration is imperative. Remain with the patient for the first 10 to 15 minutes of blood administration. Observe closely, and take vital signs every five minutes for the first 10 minutes and then every 15 minutes as indicated. Monitor intake and output; a urinalysis should be performed routinely. Do not allow a unit of whole blood to hang longer than four hours, as clotting can occur.

Side Effects or Complications

Volume Overload

Several serious complications can occur during the administration of whole blood. One concern is the potential for fluid volume excess, which can be caused by too-rapid circulatory filling, or by giving an excessive amount of whole blood. Blood delivery should be monitored according to the patient's cardiovascular response. Obviously, patients who have experienced a life-threatening hemorrhage will be able to handle several units of blood, even when administered rapidly. At greatest risk from volume overload are patients who, because of age or disease, already have a compromised cardiovascular system.

NURSING IMPLICATIONS

The nursing assessment for signs of circulatory overload should focus on the cardiovascular system. Monitor for such signs as a rapid, bounding pulse, flushing of the skin, increasing blood pressure, and heart failure with dyspnea and pulmonary edema. Careful monitoring of the IV flow rate is an important nursing responsibility.

Transfusion Reaction

A serious side effect of blood administration is an incompatibility reaction that can be fatal if not immediately recognized and treated. Blood is normally "typed and cross-matched" before it is transfused, because the donor blood type must be compatible with the patient's blood type. Whenever possible, as in the case of elective surgery, autologous blood should be used to avoid transfusion reactions or infections. Patients can donate blood up to 42 days before use.

Blood type is determined by cell membrane antigens on erythrocytes. For example, an individual with type A blood possesses type A antigens; such blood contains antibodies that will react with the B antigen. If type B blood is administered, the recipient's B-reactive antibodies will lyse the donor B-antigen–bearing erythrocytes. A potentially massive blood agglutination reaction will ensue. Type O erythrocytes contain neither A nor B antigens, and therefore the blood has antibodies against both A and B blood types. However, the titer of antibodies is low, and becomes so diluted by the recipient's blood that type O blood is considered acceptable donor blood for patients with any blood type; it is considered "the universal donor." In type AB blood, the erythrocytes contain both A and B antigens, and therefore no antibodies against either of these types are present. For that reason, type AB blood is called the "universal recipient."

One of the first signs of incompatibility may be a rapid fever spike or chest and abdominal pain. As cells lyse and cell stroma and hemoglobin complexes agglutinate inside the circulatory system, blood vessels become obstructed, leading to ischemia of tissues such as the kidneys, heart, and brain. Pain, dyspnea, and shock can develop rapidly. Hemolysis can also occur, liberating free hemoglobin into the plasma. Hemoglobin liberated by the reaction can form complexes that may obstruct the glomerulus, leading to renal failure.

NURSING IMPLICATIONS

Incompatibility can almost always be avoided by careful blood typing. If a transfusion reaction is going to occur, it usually does so during the administration of the first 50 mL of blood. Teach the patient and any family at the bedside the signs and symptoms of transfusion reaction, and instruct them to report such signs immediately. If a transfusion reaction occurs, stop the transfusion immediately, notify the physician, maintain the IV site with the priming solution (normal saline), monitor vital signs, and reassure the patient. If an adverse response is suspected, save the blood administration set and return it to the laboratory for analysis.

Infection

Another complication that can follow blood transfusion is infection. Many infectious agents can be transmitted from donor blood to the recipient (eg, mononucleosis, malaria, and syphilis). Those of most common and greatest concern are the hepatitis virus and the human immunodeficiency virus (HIV).

Hepatitis is a serious viral liver infection that can occur in three forms: A, B, and C. Hepatitis B and C viruses are blood-borne, and can be transmitted through needles, blood, or any other material contaminated with infected blood. Blood donors are carefully screened to prevent this possibility, and blood is tested for the presence of a particular hepatitis B antigen so that contaminated blood will not be used. A new test for hepatitis C on donor blood is now available, so that the risk of posttransfusion hepatitis should be less than 1% in the future.

The risk of contracting AIDS through infected donor blood dropped greatly after 1985, when investigators began doing routine serologic testing for antibodies to HIV with a very accurate testing method known as enzyme-linked immunosorbent assay (ELISA). Based on ELISA, about three in 10,000 donors test HIV-positive. Most of these are false-positives. Nevertheless, such blood is always discarded. False-negative ELISA readings are not common. Sources place the incidence between one in 40,000 to one in 250,000 donors.

Blood from paid donors generally poses a higher risk of transmitting hepatitis and other transmissible infections. Intensive interviews and careful histories of blood donors and elimination of those with risk factors is routine in all blood banks.

NURSING IMPLICATIONS

The best way to avoid infection is to know the origin of the donor blood. Many people donate their own blood in advance of elective surgery. Family members also may donate blood ahead of time. No apparent immediate responses will be detectable if infected blood is transfused because the incubation time before manifestation of the disease is so long. Blood is always collected and stored under completely sterile conditions, and the general risk of infectious contamination is thus very small. However, if the nurse suspects that the blood to be administered is not sterile, or if it appears contaminated, the blood should be saved for examination and not administered.

Nurses administering blood products need be mindful not only of their patients' safety, but also of their own. Exercise great caution when handling blood and blood administration material. The Centers for Disease Control (CDC) recommends wearing gloves while handling blood or blood products.

Packed Red Cells

Usually, when a patient requires blood, packed red cells rather than whole blood are administered. A smaller volume of packed red cells is needed to normalize the hemoglobin and hematocrit values, thus reducing the risk of fluid volume overload. Frozen and thawed red cells may be used instead of fresh red blood cells. Packed red cells are used mainly for anemias, in which blood volume is normal. In this situation, a concentrate of erythrocytes is more appropriate than whole blood. The packed red cell suspension has a high hematocrit (70%–80%), and therefore is more viscous and prone to sludging. It may be mixed with normal saline for easier administration. Otherwise, all precautions noted for whole blood apply to packed red cells.

Leukocyte Preparations

Occasionally, a patient will require the administration of white blood cells. The patient's own white cells may be removed from whole blood, and the remaining constituents reinfused or discarded. The white cell suspension may be irradiated or treated with a chemical and then reinfused into the patient. Recently, leukocytes have been removed and treated with interleukin 1, which transforms certain white cells into very intense phagocytic "killer cells" that are more capable of attacking malignant cells. While experimental, these types of natural immunologic adjuvant approaches can be expected to become more common. Another approach is to separate granulocytes from donor blood through a continuous filtering system to prepare a concentrated granulocyte suspension. This suspension can then be administered to patients who are profoundly neutropenic, such as occurs with some leukemias and with septicemia. A great danger in granulocyte transfusion is an incompatibility reaction, which can occur in an even more deadly form than occurs with whole blood. The same nursing precautions as used with whole blood apply to patients receiving leukocyte preparations.

Platelet Preparations

Blood clotting is incomplete in the absence of platelets. Platelets are prepared in units, and one unit generally increases the platelet count 5000 to 10,000 μL in an average adult. Indications for platelet transfusion include platelet deficiency syndromes (such as idiopathic thrombocytopenic purpura), bone marrow failure resulting in thrombocytopenia, and cancer (particularly leukemia). Platelets are much more immunologically tolerated than other blood cells, but they nevertheless should be of a compatible blood type. Some patients may require matching tissue types, as occasionally a patient has antibodies against nonmatching donor platelets. The platelet life span is only about seven days, and so repeated platelet administration may be needed to control bleeding or to increase the platelet count significantly. As with granulocytes, platelets may be separated from whole blood (plateletpheresis), and a platelet concentrate prepared and transfused into the recipient. Nursing precautions during platelet administration include the usual assessments for possible incompatibility reactions, as well as monitoring for cessation of bleeding, when appropriate.

Coagulation Factors

Concentrates of coagulation factors are available for administration to factor-deficient individuals. This is usually done during a bleeding episode. The usual factor preparation is a cryoprecipitate (obtained after freezing and thawing blood), which contains factor VIII, von Willebrand's factor, fibrinogen, and factor XIII. Lyophilized factor VIII is used for classic hemophilia. Concentrates of fibrinogen, prothrombin, and factors VII, IX, and X are also available. Many hemophiliacs are now self-administering factor VIII concentrate at home, which reduces the cost and inconvenience of hospital therapy. However, self-administration increases the risk of infection, improper dosage, and venous damage. An important nursing function is educating the family and patient so that safe and proper at-home administration can continue. Most hemophiliacs have, on the average, 10 or more bleeding episodes a year. There has been a trend toward prophylactic factor VIII administration to some patients, and home health care and education become even more important in these situations.

Plasma and Plasma Expanders

Many clinical conditions call for plasma, plasma substitutes, and blood expanders rather than whole blood or cellular components. Plasma has certain advantages that make it easier to administer than whole blood. It is pooled from the blood donations of several individuals, it can be used in patients of any blood type, and it can be frozen, freeze-dried, or used fresh. It is readily available when large amounts are needed suddenly, and contains all the natural clotting factors that may be depleted during hemorrhage. Plasma is administered in 500-mL units for shock, bleeding, and burns. A disadvantage of using plasma is the higher risk of transmitting blood-borne infections than with whole blood administration. The use of plasma for blood volume replacement has decreased because of the availability of plasma substitutes and expanders such as albumin or dextrans.

Plasma Substitutes

Several products can be used instead of plasma. Human albumin solutions, prepared as either 5% or 25% solutions, can be used to treat shock or hypoalbuminemic patients. Albumin is pasteurized, so there is no risk of viral contamination. One hundred milliliters of a 25% albumin solution is roughly equivalent to a unit of plasma. Another choice for plasma expansion is plasma protein fraction, which is prepared from human plasma and contains mostly albumin. Other preparations frequently used in shock and circulatory volume deficit include dextran solutions, hetastarch, hydroxyethyl starch, and modified fluid gelatin polypeptides. All accomplish the same purpose. Because their molecular weights are similar to albumin, the solutions mimic the osmotic effect of albumin in the vascular compartment, and

Table 60–1 | Electrolyte Composition of Fluids

Solution	Calories (Kcal/30 mL)	HCO_3^- (mEq/L)	Na^+ (mEq/L)	Ca^{2+} (mEq/L)	K^+ (mEq/L)	Mg^{2+} (mEq/L)	Cl^- (mEq/L)	Predominant Carbohydrate
Water								
PEDIALYTE (oral electrolyte solution)	6.0		30.0	4.0	20.0	4	30.0	Dextrose
LYTREN (oral electrolyte solution)	9.0 (isotonic)		30.0	4.0	25.0	4	25.0	Glucose
5% glucose in water	6.0							Glucose
10% glucose in water	12.0							Glucose
PEPSI-COLA	13.2	7.3	6.5		0.8			Sucrose
COCA-COLA	14.4	13.4	0.4		12.0			Sucrose
Ginger ale	10.0	3.6	3.5					Sucrose
GATORADE	5.5		23.0		3.0		17.0	Glucose Sucrose
Lemon-lime soda	9.6		7.5	0.3	0.2			
Broth, beef (canned)	6.0		55.0					
Tea, unsweetened	0.25					Trace		

increase intravascular colloid osmotic pressure. This causes interstitial fluid to be mobilized into the blood. Dextran is a polysaccharide and is available in a dextran-70 form and a dextran-40 form (the numbers refer to 1/1000 of the average molecular weight). Dextran-70 is used most commonly in shock, as it is long-acting. It also may be used prophylactically during surgery. Contraindications to the use of dextran include renal failure, severe dehydration, pregnancy, and cardiac failure. Nurses should evaluate patients receiving any plasma expander for cardiac and pulmonary congestion, and should monitor renal function. Dextran stimulates histamine release, which may cause an anaphylactoid reaction. Therefore, conditions such as asthma contraindicate dextran use. Slight bleeding tendencies may also occur. Patients should be typed and cross-matched before dextran is administered, as its presence may interfere with test accuracy.

Hetastarch is made from cornstarch, and in a 6% solution will approximate the colloid osmotic properties of albumin. It is usually given in amounts of 0.5 to 1.5 L. Its major advantage is that it is less likely than dextran to cause an allergic reaction. It does produce some side effects, however, including a mild bleeding tendency, nausea and vomiting, myalgia, and parotid gland swelling.

Fluid and Electrolyte Replacement

Oral Fluids

Many clinical conditions require fluid and electrolyte replacement. Whenever possible, the oral route is the most desirable. Oral fluid replacement is possible in states of dehydration in which the patient is conscious and capable of drinking. Thirst is usually a dominant drive in states of fluid volume deficit, owing to hypothalamic thirst center activation and the oral sensation of dryness.

Most patients with a fluid volume deficit require hypotonic fluid replacement. When excess water and electrolyte loss is from an insensible route (eg, respiration or excessive sweating), or from vomiting or diarrhea, the patient will require replacement of hypotonic fluid through the administration of hypotonic fluids. In many fluid volume deficit states there is also a net loss of body electrolytes that must be replaced. Most fluids that are regularly consumed by healthy humans are hypotonic. Appropriate oral fluids for common dehydration states include PEDIALYTE for infants and small children and GATORADE (usually diluted) for adults. Other common oral fluids are the "clear" fluids: tea, apple juice, jello, broth, and Popsicles. Table 60–1 lists the electrolyte

Table 60–2 Fluid and Weight Loss in Dehydration

	DEHYDRATION		
	Mild	Moderate	Severe
Infants	5% (50 mL/kg)	10% (100 mL/kg)	15% (150 mL/kg)
Adults	3% (30 mL/kg)	6% (60 mL/kg)	9% (90 mL/kg)

composition of some of these fluids. Clear fluids are usually prescribed if the patient has gastrointestinal distress or dysfunction. Otherwise, any fluids that the patient requests may appropriately satisfy tonicity requirements. In many situations, extracellular fluid that remains after fluid loss stays isotonic, and the patient may consume plain water in response to the thirst drive. This will fulfill volume needs, but electrolyte replacement will need to be achieved through intake of other fluids or food.

NURSING IMPLICATIONS

An important area of nursing intervention is to offer fluids to patients. A patient with any type of infection is usually helped by extra fluid. This is particularly true for urinary tract infections in which large volumes of urine will dilute and wash out the microorganisms. Patients with viral illnesses also benefit from copious fluid intake. Febrile patients lose extra insensible water, as do those inspiring dry air. Patients who are being prepared for surgery (before becoming fluid-restricted) and patients experiencing severe metabolic stress usually need extra fluid. The choice of fluid depends on many factors, but the patient's preferences must always be considered. Help the patient select the type of fluid to be administered, and assist the patient if necessary. Furthermore, accurate record-keeping of intake and output and assessment of hydration status are required.

Many serious dehydration states could be avoided by proper fluid administration. Teach patients and families about the signs of fluid imbalance and types and amounts of fluid to offer.

Intravenous Fluids

Intravenous fluids are often required for hospitalized patients. This may be necessary only to keep a vein available, so small amounts of a solution such as 5% dextrose in water can be administered. A patient may have suffered a fluid deficit that is too great to replace orally, or may be unable to drink needed fluids. The first category of IV fluids to be discussed is that given to patients suffering from fluid volume deficit and dehydration. Possible causes of dehydration include:

1. Gastrointestinal loss (diarrhea, vomiting, suction, fistula);
2. Tissue fluid loss (burns, inflammation);
3. Renal disease (nephrosis, diuretic phase of renal failure);
4. Hormonal imbalance (diabetes insipidus, diabetes mellitus);
5. Excessive insensible loss (hyperpnea, fever, hypermetabolism); and
6. Diaphoresis (as from exercise).

Table 60–2 depicts the classification of dehydration severity. This is a critical assessment for the nurse to make before any fluids are administered. The nature and amount of the fluid to be administered depend on thorough patient assessment. Nursing assessment, medical examination, and laboratory tests determine the type and extent of dehydration. Most dehydration is of the isonatremic (or isotonic) type. Less than 20% of cases are hypernatremic dehydration; hyponatremic dehydration is rare. Sodium is the major extracellular fluid (ECF) cation, and contributes most to the osmotic pressure of the ECF. When sodium is in the range of 136–144 mEq/L, the ECF stays isotonic, and there is osmotic balance between the cells and the ECF.

A person who becomes dehydrated, losing large amounts of fluid and electrolytes, usually suffers an isotonic loss, and the serum sodium stays in the normal range. A net fluid and electrolyte loss from the ECF and the intracellular fluid occurs, but the osmotic balance is maintained. This person presents the classic clinical picture of dehydration—dry skin and mucous membranes, decreased skin turgor, decreased urine output, weight loss, and activation of the sympathetic nervous system when the degree of dehydration approaches 5%. Five percent body water loss is approximately 50 mL water lost per kilogram of body weight.

Table 60–3 | **Composition of Common IV Solutions (mEq/L)**

Solution	Na^+	Cl^-	K^+	Ca^{2+}	Mg^{2+}	PO_4^{3-}	HCO_3^-
0.9% saline	154	154					
Ringer's lactate	130	109	4	3			28
IONOSOL D	140	103	10	5	3		55
IONOSOL G	63	150	17				
IONOSOL T	40	40	35			15	20
IONOSOL MB	25	22	20		3	3	
IONOSOL DM	80	64	36	5	3		60
IONOSOL B	59	52	25		6	13	25

In this situation, the goal is to repair fluid and electrolyte balance. The "repair fluid" should therefore be isotonic, since this is what the patient appears to have lost, and the maintenance fluid should be hypotonic to replace the normal everyday fluid losses. Therefore, the patient will require the administration of a hypotonic and electrolyte-containing fluid of sufficient volume to fulfill both repair and maintenance needs. Examples of fluids that might be appropriate to use for dehydration are listed in Table 60–3. The volume administered must be regulated. Central venous pressure greater than 12 cm H_2O could indicate the development of hypervolemia.

The occasional case of hypernatremic dehydration will be accompanied by fewer signs of tissue fluid deficit and less activation of the sympathetic nervous system. In fact, the degree of dehydration may approach 10% (100 mL/kg water loss), which is severe, before sympathetic nervous system activation is apparent. However, because the ECF is hypertonic, there will be a fluid shift from the cells into the ECF, causing cellular dehydration and shrinking. The patient usually suffers extreme thirst and nervous system irritability. The therapy is administration of fluid that will dilute the ECF. A solution containing 0.18% sodium chloride in 5% dextrose can be given at the rate of 150 mL/kg per day. The patient also usually requires other electrolytes such as potassium.

Hyponatremic dehydration may occur when there has been excessive diaphoresis, and in states of severe malnutrition. Occasionally it is seen as the result of excessive sodium and water loss during diuretic therapy, and after diarrhea. In this type of dehydration cells are swollen, owing to the osmotic loss of water from the ECF into cells. There is proportionately greater fluid loss from the vascular compartment, so sympathetic activation occurs earlier than in isotonic dehydration. Repair and maintenance fluids are given in the form of a hypertonic solution of 3% or 5% sodium chloride along with isotonic fluid such as Ringer's lactate. The hypertonic saline solution must be administered slowly and cautiously to prevent fluid shifts that could result in adverse cardiovascular or renal effects.

NURSING IMPLICATIONS

Administration of any solution directly into the vascular system requires careful nursing assessment. Observe for fluid overload (edema, distended neck veins, respiratory congestion or difficulty). Observe for signs of systemic infection, air or catheter embolism (sudden drop in blood pressure; cyanosis; weak, rapid pulse; loss of consciousness), or hypersensitivity reactions. Nursing assessment of the dehydrated patient is crucial since seizures or other neuromuscular abnormalities may occur. Weigh the patient daily and measure intake and output.

Inspect the solution for particulate matter, and the bag or bottle for cracks or punctures. Do not use if contamination is suspected. The infusion rate must be calculated carefully; it is not appropriate to "catch up" if the rate falls behind. Check the infusion site for infiltration, infection, hematoma, and thrombophlebitis. Ensure that all IV solutions are labeled, particularly if additives are present. Record accurately administration of IV fluids, as you would do with any medication.

Use extra caution when infusing fluids in the elderly patient. Infuse fluids slowly, as the older patient may have inadequate cardiovascular and renal reserves. Assess vital signs frequently and watch for signs of pulmonary edema or cardiovascular distress. Elderly patients have poorer, less elastic veins than younger patients. Select needle size carefully. A scalp vein is often best. Evaluate veins for sclerosis or fragility. Use a contour splint rather than an armboard to support an infusion in an arm.

Electrolyte Solutions

Potassium

Electrolyte and acid–base abnormalities accompany many dehydration states. The choice of IV fluid and the need for supplements to be added to the fluid are dictated by patient assessment and by clinical laboratory data, when available. Potassium deficit is often observed, so the addition of potassium chloride, acetate, or phosphate to IV fluids is common. Potassium chloride is generally used for uncomplicated hypokalemia. Potassium phosphate is also appropriate and is used when alkalosis is not present. Potassium acetate is the choice for hypokalemia accompanied by renal tubular acidosis, since patients with this condition usually are acidotic and have hyperchloremia.

NURSING IMPLICATIONS

A major precaution in the administration of potassium is assessment of renal function. The kidneys normally excrete potassium, which is toxic to many systems above the normal serum value of 3.5 to 5.5 mEq/L. Small amounts of potassium, either ingested orally or given IV, can cause large changes in ECF potassium if renal function is not adequate. For example, the usual daily dietary potassium intake is 100 mEq. Without renal excretion, this 100 mEq would be diluted in the ECF to a concentration of approximately 6.8 mEq/L, indicating hyperkalemia. Before administering potassium, evaluate whether normal renal function is present through history, assessment, and careful recording of urine output. Hyperkalemia may be lethal, causing neuromuscular and cardiac dysfunction. Monitor the electrocardiogram during potassium administration. Dilute commercially available potassium solutions to concentrations under 80 mEq/L and administer them at a rate not to exceed 10 mEq/hour. If higher hourly infusion rates are needed for some reason, infuse the solution into a central vein to minimize vascular irritation.

The major causes of hypokalemia are potassium-wasting diuretics, laxatives, stress, diarrhea or vomiting, and dietary or intravenous deficiency. Patients taking diuretics are at great risk for potassium deficit, and are at even greater risk if they are taking digitalis. These patients usually develop both an ECF and an ICF potassium deficit and may slowly develop a low serum potassium level, which can cause physiologic disruptions. Without potassium replacement, fatal cardiac arrhythmias or respiratory muscle weakness may occur.

Calcium

Hypocalcemia is defined as a serum calcium level below 8.5 mg/dL. It can occur as a result of hyperphosphatemia, hypoalbuminemia, parathyroid disease, vitamin D deficiency, gastrointestinal malabsorption syndromes, neoplasia, pancreatitis, and alkalosis. A common pharmacologic cause of hypocalcemia is administration of high doses of furosemide or other loop diuretics. The rapid infusion of citrated blood can also cause hypocalcemia because citrate will bind free calcium.

The signs and symptoms of hypocalcemia reflect the normal role of calcium in neuromuscular function. A severe hypocalcemic state is tetany, which is characterized by extreme electrochemical irritability of neuromuscular activity. Pharmacologic intervention in states of hypocalcemia is therefore aimed at decreasing neuromuscular irritability and increasing the serum and ECF calcium levels. This is usually achieved by administering calcium IV in the form of calcium gluconate, chloride, or gluceptate. Calcium chloride is used in cardiac resuscitation. Calcium gluceptate is the usual salt used for hypocalcemia caused by parathyroid disease, hyperphosphatemia, or vitamin B deficiency. Calcium chloride and gluconate are available in 10% solutions. The usual dosage of the chloride solution for treating hypocalcemia is 0.5 to 1 g per day. Calcium gluconate, available in 5 to 20 mL volumes, must be given no faster than 0.5 mL/minute. With all calcium salt solutions, take care when mixing them in other salt solutions. For example, calcium will precipitate if mixed with sulfates, tartrate, phosphates, or carbonates.

NURSING IMPLICATIONS

Assess the integrity of the IV site, since calcium can cause serious local tissue irritation or necrosis. Start oral calcium supplements as soon as possible, and monitor serum calcium levels so that the dosage can be adjusted. Possibly fatal arrhythmias can occur with concurrent calcium and epinephrine administration. Calcium must be administered very cautiously in digitalized patients. Nursing assessment should focus on cardiac function (heart rate and rhythm; blood pressure) and on the neuromuscular system (deep tendon reflexes, level of consciousness, muscle strength and tone, Chvostek's and Trousseau's sign, contraction of muscle groups, irritability or tetany).

Phosphate

Phosphate solutions are used adjunctively to manage hypercalcemia. There is an inverse relationship between calcium and phosphate within the body, such that hypercalcemia is accompanied by hypophosphatemia. Hypercalcemia occurs when the ECF calcium concentration is greater than 12 mg/dL. Causes include malignancy, hyperparathyroidism, hypervitaminosis D, renal disease, prolonged immobilization, chronic administration of high doses of aluminum-containing antacids, and many bone diseases. Serum calcium levels may need to be reduced quickly if they are 16 to 17 mg/dL. Phosphates may be administered in this situation to bind excess calcium in the ECF, thereby lowering serum calcium levels. The usual IV form is potassium phosphate, available in a concentration of 3 mmols phosphate/L, which must be diluted before use. The amount to be given is determined by the degree of hypercalcemia. Potassium phosphate should be used with extra care in patients with renal or cardiac disease, or in digitalized patients, because of its potassium content.

When milder hypercalcemia is present, serum calcium may be lowered by administering a large volume of normal saline, plus the diuretic furosemide, which increases renal calcium excretion. Thiazide diuretics should not be used because they reduce renal calcium excretion and worsen hypercalcemia.

Phosphate solutions are also used as urinary acidifiers to help prevent calcium stones in the urinary tract, and to treat hypophosphatemia. Oral phosphate preparations (potassium phosphate, monobasic and dibasic potassium phosphate) are available. Drug interactions with oral phosphates include binding by concurrently administered aluminum- or magnesium-containing antacids. If other potassium-containing medications are being administered, or if potassium-sparing diuretics are being used, there is a danger of hyperkalemia. Another interaction might occur in patients taking salicylates, which are not excreted well in acidified urine. Therefore, salicylate toxicity is a potential outcome. Phosphates should be administered cautiously to digitalized patients, patients with chronic renal disease, or patients with any condition in which serum potassium or phosphate levels are high.

NURSING IMPLICATIONS

Nursing concerns in cases of hypercalcemia include assessment of the neuromuscular system, responses to pharmacologic therapy, side effects of potassium phosphate (muscle cramps, arrhythmia, thirst, oliguria, headache, or gastrointestinal disturbances), and patient education. If oral phosphate preparations are used, encourage patients to take the medication after meals, and monitor the possible need for potassium or calcium restriction.

Magnesium

Magnesium, a divalent cation, is normally present in the serum at the concentration of 1.5 to 2.5 mEq/L. Magnesium activates many enzymatic reactions, and in some ways is similar to calcium in its effects on neuromuscular activity. Magnesium acts at synapses to inhibit acetylcholine release. It is a central nervous system depressant when large doses are given parenterally. (This action accounts for its common use as an anticonvulsant in eclampsia.) Another use for parenteral magnesium is in hypomagnesemic states that can occur during hyperalimentation therapy, in alcoholics, and in starvation and malabsorption states. Occasionally a patient may suffer a magnesium deficit as a result of diuresis. Treatment for these conditions consists of intramuscular (IM) or IV administration of magnesium sulfate. The usual IM dose is 1 to 5 g, given as a 25% to 50% solution every 4 to 6 hours. For IV infusion, magnesium sulfate is used at a dose of 4 g per 250 mL of 5% dextrose, given no faster than 4 mL/min.

NURSING IMPLICATIONS

Iatrogenic magnesium excess can occur. Assess for signs of this through careful neurologic evaluation, particularly of deep tendon reflexes. If they become depressed, withhold further magnesium. Evaluate renal function through measurement of fluid intake and urine output, since normal renal function is required for excess magnesium excretion.

◆ Use in the Elderly

Elderly patients, who are likely to have age-related decreases of renal function and are thus at increased risk of magnesium toxicity, require special care during magnesium administration.

Solutions Used to Treat Acid–Base Imbalances

Sodium Bicarbonate

The use of fluid and electrolyte therapy in disturbances of acid–base balance is common. Body pH must be kept within a very narrow range to preserve normal physiologic functions. Various homeostatic buffering mechanisms preserve the pH of the extracellular fluid. When these systems fail or become inadequate, and alkalosis or acidosis occur, intervention is necessary. Acidosis, a state defined by a decrease of serum pH to a value below 7.35, can be of either metabolic origin, such as occurs in diabetic ketoacidosis, or respiratory origin, as might occur in respiratory disease. In any cause of acidosis, hydrogen ion accumulates, and as the pH falls many normal regulatory processes begin to fail.

Intravenous therapy for metabolic acidosis consists of hydration fluids if necessary, and the administration of sodium bicarbonate or sodium lactate, either of which buffers the excess acid. Lactate is used as a buffer because it is converted in the liver to bicarbonate. Sodium bicarbonate itself is available in solutions ranging from 4% to 8.4%. The usual dosage for the treatment of metabolic acidosis is 1 mg/kg of body weight. The patient's response is used to assess and guide therapy. Metabolic alkalosis may occur because of overzealous treatment with bicarbonate. Sodium bicarbonate usually is given in cases of cardiac arrest, as well as in other types of metabolic acidosis. Sodium bicarbonate is also occasionally used to alkalinize the urine in salicylate and barbiturate intoxication, for which it is administered IV at a dosage of 2 to 5 mEq/kg of body weight.

NURSING IMPLICATIONS

The nursing assessment of hydration status, cardiovascular function, nervous system activity, evidence of compensatory responses, and laboratory findings will aid in determining how well the patient is responding. Metabolic acidosis may occur in many situations. Therefore, assessment and treatment of the underlying condition are imperative. Sodium bicarbonate should not be mixed with epinephrine, which is inactivated at alkaline pH.

Ammonium

The prototype ammonium salt is ammonium chloride, used in the treatment of metabolic alkalosis. Causes of metabolic alkalosis include vomiting, excessive nasogastric suction loss, steroid administration, and Cushing's syndrome. Obviously, the cause of the alkalotic condition must be identified and treated. However, metabolic alkalosis is usually accompanied by hypochloremia, and the bicarbonate concentration will tend to rise, resulting in a buffer base excess. There will be increased renal reabsorption of bicarbonate, accompanied by a net loss of hydrogen ion and sodium ion. Therefore, the provision of chloride will correct the imbalance and restore both the pH and the bicarbonate concentration toward normal. Chloride is administered as either ammonium chloride, potassium chloride, or sodium chloride. Ammonium chloride can be used as a urinary acidifier to hasten renal elimination of amphetamines in amphetamine overdoses, and it can be used to treat metabolic alkalosis caused by excessive doses of furosemide or related high-ceiling diuretics. The usual replacement dosage is estimated by measuring serum chloride levels. Ammonium salts are not metabolized well in the presence of liver damage, and should be given carefully to patients with renal disease.

NURSING IMPLICATIONS

Assess for ammonium toxicity, which may be manifested by arrhythmias and bradycardia, diaphoresis, muscle twitching, and vomiting.

SUMMARY OF NURSING IMPLICATIONS 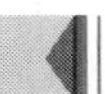

◆ Assessment

Establish baseline vital signs, laboratory values (K^+, Ca^{2+}), and physical assessment data (cardiac and neuromuscular status) to evaluate effectiveness of therapy.

Ensure patient has been typed and cross-matched to avoid incompatibility reactions; check Rh and ABO match of blood with patient data.

Assess the integrity of the IV site and surrounding tissue for infiltration, thrombosis, infection, or thrombophlebitis.

Determine patient's knowledge level and readiness for health education concerning parenteral fluids.

◆ Nursing Diagnoses

Fluid volume deficit related to dehydration.

High risk for injury related to incompatibility reaction or infection.

Altered nutrition: less than body requirements related to hypocalcemia.

Impaired physical mobility related to neuromuscular weakness from electrolyte imbalance (Ca^{2+} or K^+).

Decreased cardiac output related to arrhythmias from electrolyte imbalance (Ca^{2+} or K^+).

Dysreflexia related to electrolyte imbalance.

◆ Planning/Implementation

Verify with another licensed person Rh and ABO compatibility before giving blood.

Stay with the patient for 10 to 15 minutes after beginning transfusion; monitor for signs and symptoms of transfusion reaction (ie, abdominal pain, rash, spiking fever, anxiety, oliguria, shortness of breath, and, ultimately, shock).

Immediately stop the transfusion and notify physician at once if an incompatibility reaction is suspected.

Record intake and output; save urine specimen for analysis.

Calculate fluid administration rate accurately; do not "catch up" if infusion falls behind.

Observe for possible fluid overload with IV therapy.

Label all solutions carefully and completely in accord with agency guidelines.

Do not give fluids containing potassium until adequate renal function has been determined if dehydration or shock is present.

Monitor for electrolyte imbalances when giving electrolyte-containing solutions; if they occur as a result of fluid administration, stop administration and notify physician.

Observe for cardiac arrhythmias when electrolytes (with or without other drugs) are given.

Encourage patient to take oral fluids if dehydration being treated; allow patient choice of fluids.

◆ Patient and Family Teaching

Teach the patient/family:

The purpose of therapy, reactions to report, and desired outcomes of blood administration.

◆ Evaluation

The patient/family will:

Experience no adverse transfusion effects (eg, no chills, rash, anxiety, increased temperature).

Maintain normal body weight, indicating adequate hydration.

Show a return of laboratory values to normal level (eg, hemoglobin, hematocrit, Ca^{2+}, K^+).

Maintain normal sinus rhythm; no arrhythmias.

Annotated Bibliography

Churchill WH, Kurtz SR: *Transfusion Medicine.* Cambridge, MA, Blackwell Scientific Publications, 1988. *A current textbook addressing blood and blood products administration and complications, and management of patients requiring blood and blood products.*

Gahart B: *Intravenous Medication.* Seventh ed. St. Louis, Mosby, 1991. *A compendium of IV drugs that describes dosages, dilutions, rates of administration, actions, indications and uses, precautions, side effects, contraindications, incompatibilities, and antidotes. Designed for quick reference in both acute care and community health settings.*

N.I.T.A., the Journal of the National Intravenous Therapy Association. *Contains useful articles on all aspects of intravenous therapy, particularly aimed at nurses.*

Plumer A, Cosentino F: *Principles and Practices of Intravenous Therapy.* Fourth ed. Boston, Little, Brown, 1987. *A textbook that provides much practical information for nurses administering intravenous fluids, medications, and blood and blood products. Reviews general aspects of physiologic rationale for fluid and electrolyte therapy, and discusses in depth nursing care, legal implications, risk management, and quality assurance issues.*

Roberts M: Fluid resuscitation in the adult trauma patient. *Orthopaed Nurs* 1989:8(6):41–47. *A review article addressing the special fluid needs of the critically ill trauma patient.*

Rutherford C: Fluid and electrolyte therapy: Considerations for patient care. *J Intraven Nurs* 1989:12(3):173–183. *A general review of nursing concerns related to fluid and electrolyte administration.*

Transfusion nursing: Trends and practices for the '90s. Choosing blood components and equipment. *Am J Nurs* 1991; 91(6): 42–46, 53–56. *A current, state-of-the-art, practical guide for the practicing nurse.*

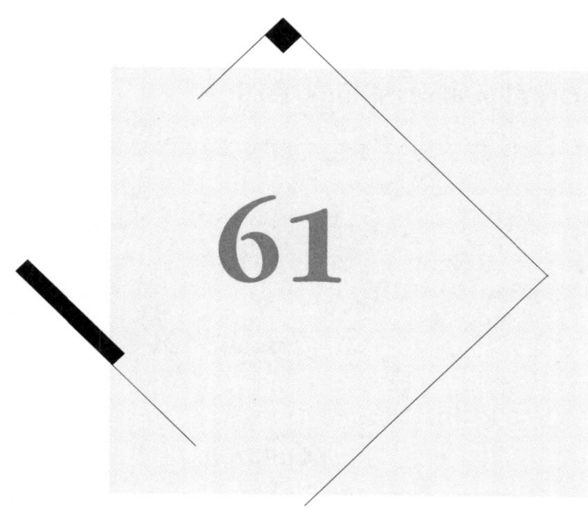

Nutrition

Good nutrition is essential for normal body function, resistance to infection, and tissue repair. Nutritional deficiencies occur when there is inadequate nutrient intake or absorption, abnormal nutrient use, or increased need. The first part of this chapter provides an overview of the biologic roles of common vitamins and minerals; situations that might require the administration of supplements; and nursing implications related to deficiency states and replacement therapy for each nutrient. The National Research Council, National Academy of Sciences (NRC/NAS) has established guidelines on the amounts of vitamins and minerals that should be ingested—recommended daily allowances (RDAs). These guidelines were last published in 1989 (Table 61–1). Students should refer to a nutrition text for more information about this topic, and for details about RDAs.

The nutrient requirements (and therefore the RDAs) for healthy individuals vary according to age, sex, and such factors as pregnancy and lactation. Separate sections of the chapter are devoted to these general issues. Other important factors that affect the RDAs are illness, lifestyle habits (smoking and alcohol consumption, for example), and drugs. These factors are noted in discussions of individual nutrients.

Major reference tables appear beginning on p. 1366.

The second part of the chapter discusses two special methods of nutrient therapy—enteral and parenteral nutrition—that may be needed in selected clinical situations.

Vitamins

Vitamins are organic compounds necessary for normal growth, development, and body maintenance. The body uses vitamins to synthesize coenzymes, which participate in essential physiologic processes. Vitamins are divided into two broad categories: fat-soluble and water-soluble. Vitamins A, D, E, and K are the fat-soluble vitamins; vitamin C and the B complex vitamins (thiamin, riboflavin, niacin, pyridoxine, folic acid, and cyanocobalamin) are the water-soluble vitamins.

Table 61–2 summarizes the major physiologic roles of the vitamins discussed in this chapter, and lists major signs of their respective deficiency states. Typical dosages for various indications, mainly those used for replacement therapy, are summarized in Table 61–C1. Although vitamins are essential for good health, administration of supplements may cause side effects, particularly if overdoses are given. This information is summarized in Table 61–S1. Other drugs that the patient may be taking, whether prescribed or self-prescribed,

Table 61–1 Recommended Dietary Allowances[a] (RDA), 1989

Age (years)	Weight (kg)	Weight (lb)	Height (cm)	Height (in)	Protein (g)	Vitamin A (μg RE)[b]	Vitamin D (μg)[c]	Vitamin E (mg α-TE)[d]	Vitamin K (μg)
						FAT-SOLUBLE VITAMINS			
					Infants				
0.0–0.5	6	13	60	24	13	375	7.5	3	5
0.5–1.0	9	20	71	28	14	375	10	4	10
					Children				
1–3	13	29	90	35	16	400	10	6	15
4–6	20	44	112	44	24	500	10	7	20
7–10	28	62	132	52	28	700	10	7	30
					Males				
11–14	45	99	157	62	45	1000	10	10	45
15–18	66	145	176	69	59	1000	10	10	65
19–24	72	160	177	70	58	1000	10	10	70
25–50	79	174	176	70	63	1000	5	10	80
51 +	77	170	173	68	63	1000	5	10	80
					Females				
11–14	46	101	157	62	46	800	10	8	45
15–18	55	120	163	64	44	800	10	8	55
19–24	58	128	164	65	46	800	10	8	60
25–50	63	138	163	64	50	800	5	8	65
51 +	65	143	160	63	50	800	5	8	65
					Pregnant				
					60	800	10	10	65
					Lactating				
			1st 6 months		65	1300	10	12	65
			2nd 6 months		82	1200	10	11	65

[a]The allowances are intended to provide for individual variations among most normal persons as they live in the United States under usual environmental stresses. Diets should be based on a variety of common foods in order to provide other nutrients for which human requirements have been well defined.
[b]Retinal equivalents: 1 retinol equivalent = 1μg retinal or 6 μg β-carotene.
[c]As cholecalciferol; 10 μg cholecalciferol = 400 IU vitamin D.
[d]α-TE = α-Tocopherol equivalent; 1 mg d-α tocopherol = 1α-TE.

may cause vitamin deficiencies. Still others may interact with a vitamin supplement. Selected drug interactions are listed in Table 61–I1.

Fat-Soluble Vitamins

Vitamin A

Vitamin A is essential for normal function of the retina. In the form of **retinal,** it combines with opsin (the red pigment in the retina) to form rhodopsin (visual purple), which is necessary for visual adaptation to darkness. Other forms (retinol, retinoic acid) are necessary for bone and epithelial tissue growth, reproduction, steroid metabolism, cholesterol synthesis, and embryonic development.

Vitamin A combines with lipid compounds and bile to form micelles that are actively absorbed through the duodenum and jejunum. Micelles are then carried by the bloodstream to the liver for metabolism. Vitamin A compounds—retinol, retinyl esters, and retinoic acid—bind with plasma proteins, are transported to target tissues, and are stored in the liver. Normal adult liver

WATER-SOLUBLE VITAMINS							MINERALS						
Vitamin C (mg)	Thiamin (mg)	Riboflavin (mg)	Niacin (mg NE)[e]	Vitamin B_6 (mg)	Folate (μg)	Vitamin B_{12} (μg)	Calcium (mg)	Phosphorus (mg)	Magnesium (mg)	Iron (mg)	Zinc (mg)	Iodine (μg)	Selenium (μg)
						Infants							
30	0.3	0.4	5	0.3	25	0.3	400	300	40	6	5	40	10
35	0.4	0.5	6	0.6	35	0.5	600	500	60	10	5	50	15
						Children							
40	0.7	0.8	9	1.0	50	0.7	800	800	80	10	10	70	20
45	0.9	1.1	12	1.1	75	1.0	800	800	120	10	10	90	20
45	1.0	1.2	13	1.4	100	1.4	800	800	170	10	10	120	30
						Males							
50	1.3	1.5	17	1.7	150	2.0	1200	1200	270	12	15	150	40
60	1.5	1.8	20	2.0	200	2.0	1200	1200	400	12	15	150	50
60	1.5	1.7	19	2.0	200	2.0	1200	1200	350	10	15	150	70
60	1.5	1.7	19	2.0	200	2.0	800	800	350	10	15	150	70
60	1.2	1.4	15	2.0	200	2.0	800	800	350	10	15	150	70
						Females							
50	1.1	1.3	15	1.4	150	2.0	1200	1200	280	15	12	150	45
60	1.1	1.3	15	1.5	180	2.0	1200	1200	300	15	12	150	50
60	1.1	1.3	15	1.6	180	2.0	1200	1200	280	15	12	150	55
60	1.1	1.3	15	1.6	180	2.0	800	800	280	15	12	150	55
60	1.0	1.2	13	1.6	180	2.0	800	800	280	10	12	150	55
						Pregnant							
70	1.5	1.6	17	2.2	400	2.2	1200	1200	320	30	15	175	65
						Lactating							
95	1.6	1.8	20	2.1	280	2.6	1200	1200	355	15	19	200	75
90	1.6	1.7	20	2.1	260	2.6	1200	1200	340	15	16	200	75

[e]NE = niacin equivalents; 1 NE = 1 mg of niacin or 60 mg of dietary tryptophan.

Adapted from the National Research Council, National Academy of Sciences; Recommended Dietary Allowances. 10th ed. Washington, DC: National Academy of Sciences, 1989.

stores are sufficient to provide two years' requirements of vitamin A. Small amounts of vitamin A are also found in fat deposits and in the lungs and kidneys. Vitamin A metabolites are excreted in feces and urine.

Therapeutically, vitamin A is used to treat deficiency symptoms, such as night blindness (nyctalopia), hyperkeratosis, xerophthalmia, keratomalacia, muscular weakness, retarded growth, and epithelial tissue atrophy that can increase susceptibility of these tissues to infections and cancers. Because vitamin A and the other fat-soluble vitamins require dietary fat, pancreatic lipase, and bile salts for absorption, conditions interfering with fat absorption also interfere with uptake of these vitamins, and may lead to deficiency states. Such conditions include biliary or pancreatic disease, celiac sprue, colitis, cirrhosis, and regional enteritis. Water-miscible preparations of vitamin A are absorbed more readily than oil-based solutions. Prolonged ingestion of mineral oil, or prolonged steatorrhea, may interfere with intestinal absorption of vitamin A and other fat-soluble vitamins. Oral contraceptives significantly increase plasma vitamin A levels.

Tretinoin (vitamin A acid; RETIN-A), isotretinoin (ACCUTANE), and etretinate (TEGISON) are vitamin

Table 61–2 Physiologic Roles and Deficiency Syndromes for Common Vitamins

Nutrients	Functions	Signs of Deficiency
	Fat-Soluble Vitamins	
Vitamin A (retinol)	Essential for formation and maintenance of epithelial cells; essential for normal function of retina and synthesis of rhodopsin (visual purple)	Night blindness; xerosis and softening of the cornea; dry, bumpy skin
Vitamin D (calciferol)	Necessary for calcium and phosphorus absorption and metabolism; important for formation of normal teeth and bones	Rickets in children; osteomalacia in adults
Vitamin E (α-tocopherol)	Antioxidant that protects red blood cells from hemolysis; used in epithelial tissue maintenance and prostaglandin synthesis	Increased hemolysis of red blood cells, macrocytic anemia, increased capillary fragility
Vitamin K (eg, phytonadione)	Essential for formation of prothrombin and other clotting factors by liver	Hypoprothrombinemia; hemorrhagic disease in newborns
	Water-Soluble Vitamins	
Vitamin C (ascorbic acid)	Essential for collagen formation; promotes healing of wounds and fractures; reduces susceptibility to infections; promotes iron absorption; necessary for conversion of folic acid to folinic acid, tryptophan to serotonin, and cholesterol to bile salts. May play a role in resistance to certain types of cancer	Scurvy—petechiae and ecchymoses, joint pain, delayed wound healing, gingivitis, bleeding gums, loss of teeth
Vitamin B_1 (thiamine)	Coenzyme in carbohydrate metabolism; essential for normal nerve function	Beri beri—peripheral neuropathy, muscle cramping, paresthesias, muscle degeneration, and heart failure
Vitamin B_2 (riboflavin)	Coenzyme in cellular metabolism and respiration; essential for healthy eyes	Red conjunctivae; fissures at corners of mouth, around nose and ears, and on tongue; magenta tongue
Vitamin B_3 (niacin)	Coenzyme in carbohydrate and amino acid metabolism; essential for synthesis of fatty acids and cholesterol and conversion of phenylalanine to tyrosine	Pellagra—cracks in skin and lips; red lesions of hands, feet, face, and neck; dementia
Vitamin B_6 (pyridoxine)	Coenzyme in protein metabolism and several other enzymatic reactions; necessary for the formation of norepinephrine, epinephrine, tyramine, dopamine, and serotonin	Seborrheic dermatitis, cheilosis, peripheral neuritis, and convulsions
Vitamin B_9 (folic acid)	Essential for DNA synthesis and normal maturation of red blood cells	Megaloblastic and macrocytic anemia; reduced platelet levels
Vitamin B_{12} (cyanocobalamin)	Coenzyme in protein metabolism; essential for red blood cell formation and maintenance of myelin sheaths of nerves	Pernicious anemia, progressive neuropathy owing to demyelination

A–like compounds. They are not used as vitamin supplements, and so only a few comments about each will be made. Tretinoin is widely used as a prescription acne medication. Clinical studies have led to growing interest in the drug as a way to reverse skin wrinkling associated with aging or sun exposure, and as a means of preventing the progression of precancerous skin lesions. Erythema is a common side effect of this drug. Use of isotretinoin is limited to severe, refractory acne because of its relatively high risk of causing corneal opacities, inflammatory bowel disorders, benign intracranial hypertension, and elevated serum triglyceride levels. Isotretinoin is a strong teratogen and so is absolutely contraindicated during pregnancy. Etretinate, also absolutely contraindicated during pregnancy, is used to treat various forms of severe, refractory psoriasis. It, too, frequently causes adverse effects on virtually all major body systems, including the skin and special senses.

NURSING IMPLICATIONS

Good food sources of vitamin A include yellow and green leafy vegetables and yellow fruits, liver, fish (cod and halibut), and vitamin A–fortified margarine and milk.

Caution patients taking a vitamin A supplement about the importance of not exceeding the RDA. Overdose or excessive ingestion can result in hypervitaminosis A. Instruct patients to report symptoms of overdose—irritability, headache, fatigue, anorexia, and flaking skin with yellow discoloration. Overdoses are treated by discontinuing vitamin A supplementation immediately and instituting symptomatic and supportive treatment.

Vitamin A preparations should be stored in tightly closed, light-resistant containers.

Vitamin D

Vitamin D compounds regulate the absorption of calcium and phosphate from the small intestine, mineral resorption in bone, and reabsorption of phosphate from the renal tubules. Vitamin D actually functions as a hormone, working in concert with parathyroid hormone and calcitonin to regulate calcium homeostasis. (Review Chapter 47 for information about this link with parathyroid function.)

The term vitamin D encompasses two related substances, ergocalciferol (D_2) and cholecalciferol (D_3). Ergocalciferol is a plant-derived vitamin that is used to fortify common foods such as milk, cereals, and breads, and in human beings, can serve all the roles of vitamin D_3. Ergocalciferol and cholecalciferol are absorbed from the jejunum and ileum. Absorption of these fat-soluble substances requires bile. Cholecalciferol is formed in the skin following ultraviolet light activation of provitamin D_3. Vitamin D_3 is then metabolized in the liver to calcifediol, which is the major transport form of the vitamin. Enzymes in the kidney convert calcifediol to calcitriol (1,25 dihydroxyvitamin D_3), which is responsible for the biologic effects attributed to the vitamin/hormone. Similar metabolic steps transform provitamin D_2 and vitamin D_2 to the active form. Vitamin D is stored in the liver, adipose tissue, and skin, and is excreted in the bile and, eventually, in the feces.

The major manifestation of vitamin D deficiency in children is rickets; in adults, the most common deficiency disorder is osteomalacia. The major consequence of hypervitaminosis D is hypercalcemia and its associated complications.

Both vitamins D_2 and D_3 are available for therapeutic use, as are three other substances with vitamin D–like activity. All these substances require adequate dietary calcium intake (or calcium supplements, if needed) for proper actions. Ergocalciferol (D_2), noted earlier as a food additive, is also indicated as a supplement for managing hypophosphatemia, hypoparathyroidism, and refractory rickets (so-called vitamin D–resistant rickets). Oral and parenteral (IM) dosage forms are available. Cholecalciferol (D_3), administered orally, is used to treat or prevent vitamin D deficiencies. Although it is available in over-the-counter (OTC) preparations, its use should be guided by a health-care professional. A vitamin D supplement may be indicated if fortified food sources are not available or cannot be consumed in amounts sufficient to prevent deficiency. In particular, infants, rapidly growing children, and pregnant, lactating, or postmenopausal women require adequate daily vitamin D intake.

Calcifediol (CALDEROL) and calcitriol (ROCALTROL) are administered orally to treat hypocalcemia in patients on long-term renal dialysis, and to manage various manifestations of hyperparathyroidism. Dihydrotachysterol ("DHT"; HYTAKEROL), a drug with about three times the potency of vitamin D_2, is used to treat acute or chronic tetany.

NURSING IMPLICATIONS

Good food sources of vitamin D include fish liver oils; fortified milk, butter, and margarine; salmon, sardines, and herring; and egg yolk. Vitamin D toxicity develops only when dosages far exceed the RDA, acutely or with chronic ingestion. Signs and symptoms of toxicity include nausea, anorexia, weakness, and thirst. Hypercalcemia, hyperphosphatemia, osteomas, and calcification of soft tissues (heart, lungs, and kidneys) may occur. The most serious consequence is renal damage.

Monitor serum levels of calcium, phosphorus, magnesium, and alkaline phosphatase, as well as urea and urinary calcium for abnormalities. Use of magnesium-containing antacids, cholestyramine, mineral oil, or laxatives interferes with intestinal absorption of vitamin D. Phenytoin and barbiturates increase the metabolic inactivation of vitamin D, possibly resulting in hypocalcemia and clinical osteomalacia or rickets. Patients in chronic renal failure who receive vitamin D preparations should avoid taking magnesium-containing antacids and laxatives because renal dysfunction increases the risk of magnesium intoxication.

Vitamin D decomposes on exposure to light and air; therefore, store these vitamin preparations in tightly closed, light-resistant containers.

Vitamin E

Vitamin E, also known as α-tocopherol, is an antioxidant. In this role it protects against oxidative breakdown of all cell membranes (as occurs as part of aging), and protects red blood cells from hemolysis. Vitamin E is also important to epithelial tissue maintenance and prostaglandin synthesis. In normal individuals, vitamin E is readily absorbed from the intestinal tract and enters the circulatory system via the lymphatics. Vitamin E is stored mainly in fatty tissues, with smaller amounts found in liver, muscle, and pituitary and adrenal glands. Vitamin E is metabolized in the liver and excreted in the bile and feces.

The only approved use for vitamin E supplements is for correcting deficiencies of the vitamin caused by inadequate dietary intake. It has been used to correct hemolytic anemia and to relieve edema and dermatitis occurring in low-birth-weight premature infants fed artificial formulas containing iron and high concentrations of polyunsaturated fatty acids.

Prolonged, excessive use of vitamin E can cause muscle weakness, fatigue, diarrhea, creatinuria, and thrombophlebitis. High-dose intake may also cause hemorrhage in vitamin K–deficient persons.

NURSING IMPLICATIONS

Advise patients that the best natural food source of vitamin E is wheat germ. Other good sources include vegetable oils, green leafy vegetables, nuts, dairy products, eggs, cereals, meats, and liver. Vitamin E supplements are available as drops, capsules, and tablets. If tablets or capsules are prescribed (or self-prescribed), advise the patient to swallow them whole. The products should be stored in a tightly closed container and protected from light.

Requirements for vitamin E may be increased by concomitant therapy with large doses of antibiotics, iron, mineral oil, or isoniazid. These medications interfere with vitamin E absorption. As applies to all fat-soluble vitamins, advise patients not to use mineral oil except under the advice and supervision of a health-care professional.

Vitamin E has been touted to enhance sexuality and to slow the aging process. These claims have not been verified scientifically, but this lack of support has not stifled the public's interest in products that might improve sexual performance or delay getting older. Because of the potential dangers of hypervitaminosis E, discourage excessive use of vitamin E.

Recent experimental studies have shown that vitamin E may reduce or prevent tissue or organ damage caused by toxic oxygen metabolites. These oxidants are thought to play important roles in cellular damage caused by ischemia (as might occur during shock, heart attacks, or when organs are briefly stored before transplantation), certain drugs (for example, the anticancer drug doxorubicin, and the defoliant paraquat, which is sprayed on marijuana plants to kill them, yet is an important cause of poisoning when contaminated marijuana is smoked), and damaging radiation (from X-rays, sunlight, and atomic weapons). Although vitamin E currently has no approved role in such situations, be aware that these uses may become important in the near future.

Vitamin K

Naturally occurring vitamin K is synthesized by intestinal flora. Vitamin K is absorbed rapidly from the upper part of the small intestine. Absorption is facilitated by bile salts. Chylomicrons transport vitamin K to the liver, where it is metabolized. Vitamin K is stored in limited amounts in the liver, skin, muscles, and kidneys, and is excreted in the feces and urine.

Vitamin K has an important role in hepatic synthesis of active blood clotting factors: prothrombin (factor II); proconvertin (factor VII); plasma thromboplastin component (factor IX); and Stuart factor (factor X). Refer to Chapter 35 for more information on clotting factors.

Vitamin K is used clinically to treat hypoprothrombinemia caused by conditions that limit vitamin K absorption or synthesis, including prolonged and excessive steatorrhea, obstructive jaundice, biliary fistulae, celiac sprue, colitis, hepatic damage, and antibacterial therapy. Vitamin K is also indicated for oral anticoagulant–induced prothrombin deficiency, and for the prevention and treatment of hemorrhagic disease of the newborn (as caused by administration of barbiturates or phenytoin as anticonvulsants to pregnant women with epilepsy; see Chapters 22 and 26).

Several forms of vitamin K are available, each differing in solubility and rapidity and duration of effect. Phytonadione (K_1; marketed as AQUAMEPHYTON; KONAKION; MEPHYTON) and menadione (K_3) are fat-soluble synthetic analogs of vitamin K. Menadiol sodium diphosphate (K_4; marketed as SYNKAYVITE) is a water-soluble precursor that is converted to menadione in the body. For treatment of hemorrhage caused by oral anticoagulant-induced hypoprothrombinemia, phytonadione (K_1) is preferred to K_3 or K_4 because of its more rapid onset and prolonged effect. Vitamin K *does not* counteract the action of heparin. Phytonadione has a greater margin of safety than the other synthetic analogs in the prevention and treatment of hemorrhagic disease in the newborn.

NURSING IMPLICATIONS

Vitamin K–rich foods include green leafy vegetables, cauliflower, soybeans, beef liver, and tomatoes.

When vitamin K is administered to correct coagulation disorders, monitor the complete blood count (CBC), serum prothrombin time (PT), and partial thromboplastin time (PTT). Assess for bleeding (ecchymosis, petechiae, hematuria). Be prepared to administer fresh whole blood, plasma (or its derivatives), platelet concentrates, or other blood components, if there is no response to vitamin K. Assess for anaphylaxis, which has been reported after parenteral administration of vitamin K.

Anticipate the need for prepartum coagulation tests in women receiving barbiturates or phenytoin during pregnancy (as for epilepsy), and the need to perform similar tests on their newborns. Also anticipate the need for prepartum administration of vitamin K to the mother, and postpartum to the child.

Unless there is a serious bleeding disorder that can be remedied by vitamin K, question orders calling for the administration of vitamin K to patients with elevated serum prothrombin levels or severe liver disease, or patients receiving oral anticoagulants.

Water-Soluble Vitamins

Vitamin C

Vitamin C (ascorbic acid) is essential for the formation of hydroxyproline and hydroxylysine, which are necessary for collagen synthesis and for the promotion of wound and fracture healing. It also reduces the susceptibility to infection, promotes iron absorption, and is necessary for the conversion of folic acid to folinic acid, of tryptophan to serotonin, and of cholesterol to bile salts. Like vitamin E, ascorbic acid serves as an antioxidant.

Vitamin C is absorbed throughout the jejunum, and transported in the bloodstream (especially by white blood cells) to important storage and use sites, including the liver, brain, and adrenal glands. Vitamin C is not metabolized. It is excreted in urine and breast milk.

The major consequence of vitamin C deficiency is scurvy. Its common signs and symptoms include petechiae and ecchymoses; joint pain; gingival bleeding or inflammation; loss of teeth; and delayed wound healing. Vitamin C is indicated for the prevention and treatment of scurvy (relatively uncommon in Western cultures), and for lesser degrees of diagnosed vitamin C deficiency (called a scorbutic state) that may be more common. These are the only approved uses. Oral therapy is preferred unless signs and symptoms of scurvy are severe or the patient cannot take oral medications. Vitamin C has been used as a urinary acidifier, particularly in the management of overdoses of basic drugs such as amphetamines and tricyclic antidepressants. It has also been used as an adjunct to the management of febrile states, chronic illnesses, infections, burns, and delayed bone fracture or wound healing. Very high doses (megadoses) of vitamin C have been promoted as able to prevent or speed the relief of symptoms of the common cold. No conclusive and universally accepted evidence supports this notion, and blood levels of the vitamin that exceed the kidney's ability to reclaim them are lost in the urine. Nevertheless, vitamin C supplements are used extensively by the lay public.

NURSING IMPLICATIONS

Fresh fruits (especially citrus) and vegetables (particularly potatoes) are abundant dietary sources of vitamin C.

Assess dietary, drug, and lifestyle histories of patients with symptoms of vitamin C deficiency. Causes of increased vitamin C requirements to which assessment should be directed include hyperthyroidism, smoking, and any intense or prolonged stress, including fever, severe or diffuse infections, burns, or recent surgery.

Unless there is a true vitamin C deficiency state, avoid the use of high doses of vitamin C supplements in persons taking oral contraceptives (increased contraceptive blood levels), high doses of aspirin (decreased renal aspirin excretion, increased risk of toxicity), oral anticoagulants (usually a decreased anticoagulant effect), barbiturates (decreased renal excretion, increased risk of excessive effects of the barbiturate), and sulfonamide antibiotics (increased renal excretion, risk of crystalluria).

Counsel patients against taking high doses of vitamin C and iron supplements. Vitamin C increases iron absorption and may increase the risk of iron toxicity. If patients ask about the value of vitamin C for preventing the common cold, advise them that there simply is no good answer about the benefits or potential risks.

Advise pregnant women to avoid exceeding the vitamin C RDA during pregnancy. Although controversial, evidence suggests that children born to women taking high doses of vitamin C may adapt to high levels of the vitamin, and may show deficiency symptoms after delivery.

Vitamins B

There are six B vitamins, and they generally work in concert. Deficiencies of a single B vitamin are relatively uncommon, so assessment should focus on multiple deficiencies, as should therapy. Alcoholism is probably the most common cause of B-vitamin deficiencies.

Thiamine (B_1)

Thiamine functions as a coenzyme in carbohydrate metabolism, and is essential for normal nerve function. Thiamine is absorbed throughout the jejunum and ileum, and is transported via the blood cells as cocarboxylase and via the serum as free B_1. It is distributed in small amounts to the heart, liver, kidneys, and brain, and is excreted in the urine as pyrimidine, a metabolite.

Beri beri is the classic example of thiamine deficiency. It is characterized by a variety of neurologic deficits affecting both the peripheral and central nervous systems, including muscular weakness, anorexia, neuritis, and dyspnea. A variant is "wet" beri beri, in which the typical signs and symptoms of beri beri are accompanied by tachycardia, palpitations, and other signs and symptoms of high-output cardiac failure that resemble (but are not caused by) longstanding hyperthyroidism. Wernicke's encephalopathy (nystagmus, ataxia, confusion, and other neurologic deficits) is another consequence of thiamine deficiency. Common causes of this disorder include long-term, excessive alcohol consumption, and starvation (including that from anorexia nervosa).

Beri beri, neuritis, Wernicke's encephalopathy, and evidence of milder degrees of thiamine deficiency are the major indications for the use of thiamine supplements. The vitamin usually is given orally, but parenteral formulations for IM use are available when more immediate effects are necessary.

NURSING IMPLICATIONS

Good dietary sources of thiamine include yeast, whole or enriched grain products, legumes (peas and dried beans), and meats (especially pork, but also beef).

Consider thiamine deficiency when assessing patients with peripheral neuropathy, muscle cramping, paresthesias, muscle degeneration, nystagmus, and heart failure (particularly with an absence of congestive or low-output failure signs and symptoms; heart failure may progress to low-output failure, or circulatory collapse, if the deficiency is severe and acute). Consider thiamine deficiency in anorexic patients or those who habitually ingest excessive amounts of alcohol, and in pregnant women (who may experience cardiovascular complications of deficiency). Attempt to ensure that dietary thiamine intake during pregnancy is adequate, based on assessment of the patient's diet.

If thiamine must be administered parenterally, use only the IM route except in emergencies. For example, beri beri complicated by cardiac failure may require initial IV administration. Never mix parenteral formulations of thiamine with alkaline solutions (barbiturates, carbonates, citrates) or solutions containing sulfites. Assess all patients receiving thiamine parenterally for anaphylactoid reactions, including facial flushing, pruritus or other skin reactions, dyspnea, and hypotension.

Riboflavin (B_2)

Riboflavin is a coenzyme for both flavin mononucleotide (FMN) and flavin adenine dinucleotide (FAD). These are crucial metabolic components in biochemical pathways that release energy from carbohydrates, fats, and proteins. Riboflavin is also essential for maintaining normal vision.

Riboflavin is absorbed readily from the jejunum and ileum. It is actively transported into the bloodstream and distributed to all tissues. Highest concentrations are found in the heart, lungs, and kidneys.

Riboflavin is indicated for the prevention and treatment of riboflavin deficiencies, which include symptoms such as fissures at the angles of the mouth (cheilosis), nose, and ears; visual disturbances; glossitis; and dark, red tongue. It is also indicated, in conjunction with nicotinic acid, to treat pellagra. The vitamin is given orally.

NURSING IMPLICATIONS

Good food sources of riboflavin include organ meats, fortified milk or milk products, and green leafy vegetables.

Assess for multi-B-vitamin deficiencies when riboflavin deficiencies are suspected.

Anticipate, and advise patients to expect, that riboflavin supplement therapy may cause the urine to turn a bright yellow color. Assess for this. Riboflavin supplements are administered orally, and should be ingested with food to enhance absorption.

Store riboflavin preparations in suitable containers that protect the drug from light and air.

Nicotinic Acid (B_3)

Nicotinic acid (niacin) functions with riboflavin as a coenzyme in the metabolism of carbohydrates, proteins, and lipids. Nicotinic acid is actively absorbed from the gastrointestinal (GI) tract, transported mainly as a coenzyme in red cells, and stored in the heart, liver, and muscles.

Pellagra is the major manifestation of nicotinic acid deficiency, and the major vitamin-related indication for nicotinic acid replacement therapy. In this situation, nicotinic acid is used along with other B-complex vitamins. The vitamin usually is given orally, but parenteral dosage forms (for subcutaneous [SC], IM, or slow IV injection) are available. An alternative drug form is nicotinamide (also called niacinamide), which is converted in the body to nicotinic acid. This product is less likely than nicotinic acid to alter serum lipid profiles or to cause hypotension.

Nicotinic acid dramatically affects serum lipid levels, and the drug is used to treat hypertriglyceridemia and hypercholesterolemia. This use is discussed in Chapter 36.

NURSING IMPLICATIONS

Good dietary sources of nicotinic acid include meats (especially organ meats such as liver, heart, and kidney), wheat germ, and legumes. Milk and eggs contain only small amounts of nicotinic acid, but they are excellent sources of tryptophan, a precursor that is converted readily to nicotinic acid.

Monitor patients for the suspected signs and symptoms of nicotinic acid deficiency, including dementia and lesions of the face and extremities (redness, dryness, cracking).

Anticipate that persons with diabetes or prediabetic conditions may have increased requirements of insulin or oral hypoglycemic drugs to compensate for nicotinic acid-induced hyperglycemia, glycosuria, and ketonuria.

Assess patients taking isoniazid for evidence of nicotinic acid deficiency.

Pyridoxine (B_6)

Pyridoxine is a cofactor for several amino acid-metabolizing systems, including transaminases, decarboxylases, and dehydratases. It also serves as a coenzyme in carbohydrate metabolism, and is necessary for the formation of biogenic amines (norepinephrine, epinephrine, dopamine, and serotonin). Pyridoxine is absorbed from the jejunum and ileum, degraded in the liver, and circulated in the bloodstream. It is stored in small amounts in skeletal muscle as phosphorylase, and is excreted in the urine.

Pyridoxine is used to treat deficiency states resulting from inadequate dietary intake, certain drug-induced causes, inborn errors of metabolism (particularly those causing seizures or anemias that are responsive to B_6), and impaired GI absorption. It is also indicated for the prevention or treatment of peripheral neuritis induced by drugs such as hydralazine, isoniazid, or oral contraceptives. Pyridoxine is given orally or parenterally (IV, IM) for treatment of severe isoniazid poisoning.

The most common and important interaction involving pyridoxine is with levodopa, which is used to treat parkinsonism. As discussed in Chapter 25, pyridoxine stimulates the gastrointestinal conversion of the drug, levodopa, to dopamine. When this conversion occurs, dopamine cannot enter the central nervous system and exert its desired antiparkinson effects, and so its therapeutic effect is reduced or abolished. A similar antagonism may apply to the proprietary drug combination SINEMET, which contains both levodopa and carbidopa.

NURSING IMPLICATIONS

Good dietary sources of pyridoxine include yeast, wheat germ, whole-grain cereals, liver, legumes, green vegetables, and bananas.

Assess all patients taking hydralazine, isoniazid, oral contraceptives, or penicillamine for evidence of pyridoxine deficiency. In particular, assess for seborrheic dermatitis, cheilosis, peripheral neuritis, and seizures.

Advise patients receiving levodopa for parkinsonism to avoid ingesting more than 5 mg of pyridoxine per day. Thus, not only pyridoxine itself but also most multivitamins, which contain this substance, must be avoided. If parkinsonism patients require vitamin supplements, consult the physician about a prescription for products such as LAROBEC, which are vitamin B_6–free and specifically indicated for persons taking levodopa. B vitamins other than B_6 are not contraindicated.

Folic Acid (B_9)

Folic acid (folacin, folate, or pteroylglutamic acid) is essential for DNA synthesis and normal maturation of red blood cells. Folic acid is absorbed through the proximal jejunum, is transported as prefolic acid A in the bloodstream, and is stored in small amounts in the liver as polyglutamates. Folate is excreted in the urine.

Folic acid is indicated for treatment of megaloblastic anemias caused by celiac sprue, nutritional deficits, and pregnancy, infancy, or childhood. The agent is not indicated for treating aplastic, normocytic, or pernicious anemias. The usual route of administration is oral (tablets), but products for parenteral (IV, IM, SC) administration are available for use when gastrointestinal absorption of oral dosage forms is impaired severely.

Folinic acid (leucovorin) is a folic acid analog that can be used for treating the anemias noted in the previous paragraph. It is also indicated to prevent or treat cytotoxicity caused by the anticancer drug methotrexate, which acts as a folate antagonist. See Chapter 59 for more information about this drug and its use.

NURSING IMPLICATIONS

Foods rich in folic acid include yeast, whole-grain cereals and breads, bran, green leafy vegetables, asparagus, legumes, nuts, and fruits.

Assess patients with megaloblastic or macrocytic anemia, or thrombocytopenia, for folic acid deficiency as a possible cause.

The anticonvulsants phenytoin and barbiturates (and chemically related anticonvulsants; see Chapter 26) may interact with folic acid supplements. The result may be poor seizure control caused by a decreased anticonvulsant blood level, or signs and symptoms of folate deficiency caused by the anticonvulsant. Impaired folate use or folate deficiencies may also be caused by chronic alcohol ingestion, methotrexate, oral contraceptives, triamterene, or trimethoprim. Monitor accordingly if any of these interactants are being used.

Cyanocobalamin (B_{12})

Cyanocobalamin serves as a coenzyme in protein metabolism. It is essential for erythrocyte formation and for maintenance of the myelin sheaths of nerves. Absorption of dietary cyanocobalamin requires the presence of gastric acid and intrinsic factor, a gastric glycoprotein. Gastric acid cleaves the vitamin from meat proteins, to which it is bound, and intrinsic factor carries the vitamin to the terminal ileum, the major site of B_{12} absorption. The liver is the principal storage site of B_{12}; small amounts are stored in the lungs, kidneys, and adrenal glands. The vitamin is excreted in bile and breast milk.

Malabsorption syndromes, diminished gastric acid secretion (including achlorhydria), and lack of intrinsic factor are the most common causes of cyanocobalamin deficiencies in persons eating normal diets. Inadequate dietary intake seldom is the cause of deficiency in adults unless they consume a strictly vegetarian diet, or have greatly increased vitamin B_{12} demands imposed by such conditions as malignancies, pregnancy, thyrotoxicosis, hemolytic anemia, hemorrhage, or severe liver or kidney failure. Severe vitamin B_{12} deficiency can cause permanent nervous system damage. Pernicious anemia is another serious consequence.

Oral cyanocobalamin is indicated only for managing simple nutritional vitamin B_{12} deficiencies in otherwise healthy persons. Two major preparations are available for parenteral use: crystalline cyanocobalamin (B_{12}, for IM or SC administration) and crystalline hydroxocobalamin (also called vitamin B_{12a}; for IM injection only). Parenteral forms must be used in cases of malabsorption syndromes or deficits of gastric acid or intrinsic factor, which would render oral dosage forms ineffective. Such instances include gastric or intestinal surgery (especially gastrectomy), gluten enteropathy, and celiac sprue. Tapeworm infestations, intestinal bacterial overgrowth, tumors of the GI tract or accessory organs (the pancreas, for example), and certain drugs (discussed later) also may reduce oral cyanocobalamin absorption, necessitating parenteral use.

Another use for cyanocobalamin, injected IM, is as part of Schilling's test, which helps diagnose pernicious anemia. A small dose of radioactive B_{12} is given orally, along with a parenteral dose of regular cyanocobalamin. The amount of radioactivity in the urine is measured as an index of B_{12} absorption. If the value is low, but is increased when the test is repeated with simultaneous administration of intrinsic factor, pernicious anemia can be suspected.

NURSING IMPLICATIONS

Good food sources of vitamin B_{12} include organ and muscle meats, shellfish, salmon, sardines, and milk and other dairy products.

Administer oral vitamin B_{12} with meals, since food increases intrinsic factor release and thereby facilitates vitamin absorption. Do not administer oral B_{12} supplements when malabsorption is suspected or known. Never inject a parenteral dosage form IV. Assess patients for the major signs of vitamin B_{12} deficiency (neuropathies, pernicious anemia).

Table 61–3 | **Physiologic Roles and Deficiency Syndromes for Common Minerals**

Nutrient	Functions	Signs of Deficiency
Calcium	Required for bone and tooth formation; essential for blood coagulation, transmission of nerve impulses, muscle contraction; activator of several enzymes, including ATPase, lipase	Rickets, osteomalacia, osteoporosis, tetany
Iodine	Integral part of thyroid hormones (thyroxine, triiodothyronine), which regulate rate of cellular oxidation	Thyroid diseases, including goiter; See Chapter 47
Iron	Constituent of hemoglobin and myoglobin; involved in O_2–CO_2 transport; constituent of enzyme systems involved in energy production	Iron deficiency anemia—hypochromic microcytic anemia
Magnesium	Mineralization of bones and teeth; component of many enzymes; with calcium, moderates nerve impulse transmission and muscular contraction	Anorexia, growth failure, ECG and neuromuscular changes
Phosphorus	Mineralization of bones and teeth; essential to absorption of glucose and derivation of energy from foodstuffs; constituent of DNA, RNA; component of phosphates and phospholipase enzymes	Neuromuscular, skeletal, hematologic, and renal dysfunction from decreased synthesis of ATP and other organic compounds
Zinc	Essential component of many enzymes (eg, carbonic anhydrase, lactate dehydrogenase, alkaline phosphatase); helps in wound healing	Delayed wound healing, taste alterations, growth failure, dermatitis, hair loss

Therapy with histamine H_2 receptor blockers (cimetidine, others) for peptic ulcer disease may interfere with oral vitamin B_{12} absorption by inhibiting gastric acid secretion. Colchicine, neomycin, alcohol, and slow-release oral potassium supplements may also interfere with B_{12} absorption. Assess patients taking these interactants for evidence of a deficiency state.

Minerals

Minerals are inorganic elements involved in a wide variety of physiologic functions (Table 61–3). They serve as structural materials in bones, teeth, cell membranes, and connective tissue. They also function in the regulation of enzyme metabolism, and maintenance of acid–base balance, blood osmotic pressure, and nerve and muscle activity.

Among the major nutritionally essential minerals are sodium, potassium, calcium, phosphorus, and magnesium. Sodium, the primary cation in extracellular fluid, and potassium, the primary intracellular cation, are discussed in Chapter 60. The trace minerals include iron, zinc, and iodine.

Most of the information about minerals discussed in the following sections is summarized in Table 61–6 (roles and deficiency syndromes), Table 61–C2 (uses and doses), Table 61–S2 (side effects and contraindications), and Table 61–I2 (interactions with foods and other drugs).

Calcium

Calcium is required for bone and tooth mineralization and formation, blood clotting mechanisms, nerve impulse transmission, neurotransmitter storage and release, and muscle contraction. It also regulates vitamin B_{12} absorption and amino acid uptake.

Calcium is absorbed through the small intestine and transported through the blood, largely bound to plasma proteins. Its absorption and metabolic fate are critically linked to the availability and actions of vitamin D, calcitonin, and parathyroid hormone, as noted earlier and in Chapter 47. By far, bone and teeth are the major stores of body calcium. The ion is excreted mainly in the feces, with small amounts eliminated in the urine, saliva, and breast milk.

Therapeutically, calcium is used most frequently as a nutritional supplement when dietary calcium intake is inadequate, particularly during childhood, adolescence, pregnancy, lactation, menopause, and old age. Other uses include treatment of hypocalcemia associated with hypoparathyroidism, chronic renal insufficiency, malabsorption syndromes, vitamin D deficiency, rickets, and osteomalacia. Oral administration usually is preferred, but parenteral calcium salts (particularly chloride) may be indicated for severe or acute deficiencies, when oral administration is not feasible or effective, or for such other indications as cardiac arrest or hyperkalemia. The use of calcium carbonate as an antacid is discussed in Chapter 40.

Hypocalcemia may be caused by systemic corticosteroids, barbiturates, laxatives/cathartics, and neomycin, all of which interfere with calcium absorption; or by furosemide and other high-ceiling diuretics, and prolonged, excessive alcohol consumption, which increase renal calcium elimination. Hypercalcemia may be caused by combination oral contraceptives (increase intestinal calcium absorption) or by thiazide diuretics (decrease renal calcium excretion). Hypercalcemia may increase the risk of digitalis toxicity. The greatest risks of hypercalcemia are in persons taking calcium supplements without supervision.

Disodium EDTA (not calcium EDTA) may be used to treat acute, life-threatening hypercalcemia. Use of this calcium chelator requires constant intensive-care monitoring.

NURSING IMPLICATIONS

Milk and other dairy products are the most abundant sources of calcium. Other dietary sources include leafy green vegetables, salmon (especially with bones left in), clams, and oysters. However, discourage the administration of whole cow's milk to newborn infants, because its calcium–phosphorus ratio favors calcium excretion.

Assess patients with possible hypocalcemia for expected signs and symptoms: neuromuscular hyperexcitability, paresthesias, muscle spasms (including laryngospasm), and arrhythmias. Be aware that certain foods interfere with calcium absorption and may increase the risk of hypocalcemia in susceptible persons. They include spinach, rhubarb, chocolate (containing oxalic acid, a calcium chelator); bran and whole-grain cereals (containing phytic acid); and zinc-rich foods (nuts, seeds, sprouts, legumes, and tofu). It may be necessary to avoid or reduce the intake of these foods during hypocalcemic states.

If oral dietary calcium supplements are indicated, the product should be taken with meals. Patients taking such products should be instructed to drink ample amounts of fluid and to eat foods high in fiber to prevent constipation, which is the major adverse GI effect of calcium salts. Since vitamin D is required for calcium absorption, also ensure that the patient's dietary intake of that vitamin is adequate but not excessive.

Advise patients to whom calcium supplements are given to avoid excessive intake of dairy products, which may cause hypercalcemia, an increased risk of constipation, and possible systemic alkalosis (the milk-alkali syndrome; see Chapter 40). Give similar advice to persons wishing to self-medicate with calcium supplements, which are being advertised intensively, especially for older women. Depending on the patient, such use can be either harmless and no better than a balanced diet and exercise, or it can be dangerous if excessive or done in the presence of interacting drugs. Recommend evaluation by a physician if a person suspects a need to take self-prescribed calcium supplements.

Assess patients who take calcium supplements for signs and symptoms of hypercalcemia: constipation; thirst and polyuria; lethargy and muscle weakness; urinary difficulty or flank or back pain that might indicate renal calcium calculi; and altered pulse. Electrocardiographic monitoring, as well as laboratory measurements of serum calcium levels, may be necessary.

If parenteral calcium salts are indicated, inject the drug only IV, because they are tissue irritants. Cardiac monitoring is strongly advised whenever calcium salts are injected.

Phosphorus

A component of all tissues, phosphorus is essential for bone and tooth mineralization; regulation of calcium metabolism; and synthesis of proteins, fats, and carbohydrates. It is also a constituent of DNA and RNA, and is a component of phosphatase and phospholipase enzymes.

Like calcium, phosphorus is absorbed through the small intestine, transported bound to plasma proteins, and excreted in feces. About 80% of the body's phosphorus is deposited in bones and teeth. The other 20% is active metabolically and is found within cells and in extracellular fluid.

Phosphorus-containing supplements for dietary replacement generally contain both the sodium and phosphorus salts. Some are sodium-free. Uses include management of hypophosphatemia, calcium–phosphorus ratio imbalance, and hyperparathyroidism. Phosphorus administration lowers urinary calcium levels and reduces the risk of urinary calcium stone formation.

NURSING IMPLICATIONS

The best food sources of phosphorus are milk and milk products.

Common signs and symptoms of hypophosphatemia include generalized weakness, hyperventilation, and decreased serum phosphate levels. Assess accordingly.

Hyperphosphatemia, most likely to occur with excessive use of phosphorus-containing supplements, is assessed by measurements of blood phosphate and calcium levels.

Phosphorus supplements, depending on their formulation, contain sufficient amounts of potassium, sodium, or both, to cause problems in selected patients. Potassium phosphate may cause hyperkalemia, particularly in patients taking potassium-sparing diuretics. Sodium phosphate may cause or aggravate heart failure, edema, or hypertension, especially in patients taking systemic corticosteroids or most antihypertensive drugs (unless accompanied by a diuretic). Plain potassium phosphate generally is preferred for patients at risk of added sodium loads.

Closely monitor antacid use during phosphorus supplement therapy. High-dose, prolonged therapy with antacids containing only aluminum salts (seldom used) can cause hypophosphatemia. Most of the popular antacid products, especially those prescribed for ulcer disease or self-administered for GI upset, contain both aluminum and magnesium salts. They may significantly interfere with the absorption of phosphorus supplements. To reduce the chance of this interaction, advise patients to separate ingestion of antacids and the supplement by at least one hour.

Assess patients taking oral phosphorus supplements for diarrhea. If it occurs and becomes severe, the phosphorus dosage may need to be reduced or discontinued altogether.

Magnesium

Magnesium is involved in bone and tooth mineralization and is a component of many enzymes. In conjunction with calcium, magnesium moderates nerve impulse transmission and muscle contraction.

Magnesium is absorbed readily from the GI tract, and all but the small amounts required by the body are excreted in the urine if renal function is normal. Most of the body's magnesium stores are in bones. Muscle, soft tissue, and body fluids contain relatively small amounts.

Simple magnesium deficiency, and the need for magnesium supplementation, is relatively uncommon. The incidence of hypomagnesemia, and the need for magnesium supplements, increases during pregnancy, chronic alcoholism, malnutrition, or diarrhea; after intestinal bypass surgery; and with repeated nasogastric suctioning. Diuretics (particularly thiazides or ethacrynic acid) or ammonium chloride may cause hypomagnesemia by enhancing renal magnesium excretion. Hypomagnesemia is one of the most common causes of seizures in chronic alcoholics, and the most common cause of seizures in eclampsia.

Magnesium gluconate or a complex with amino acids is administered orally as a supplement for mild deficiencies. Magnesium oxides and hydroxides (milk of magnesia), administered orally, exert antacid and laxative effects. Although they are used appropriately for such effects, they are more often misused through self-medication. Side effects and contraindications of oral magnesium supplements are the same as those that apply to the use of magnesium as an antacid or laxative. Refer to Chapters 40 and 41 for more information. Magnesium sulfate is given parenterally for seizures caused by acute hypomagnesemia, as in eclampsia or alcoholism. This use, and the related precautions, are discussed in Chapter 26.

NURSING IMPLICATIONS

Good sources of magnesium include whole-grain cereals, legumes, leafy green vegetables, and bananas.

Assess patients at high risk of magnesium deficiency for the common acute signs and symptoms: seizures, tetany, muscle twitching or cramps; hypertension and tachycardia; and anorexia. Delayed growth may occur with chronic magnesium deficiency in children.

Assess patients (especially the elderly) for impaired renal function, which generally contraindicates safe use of magnesium for any purpose other than emergencies.

Periodically assess patients receiving any drug form of magnesium for signs of hypermagnesemia: muscle weakness, flaccid paralysis, depressed or absent reflexes; extreme thirst; lethargy and confusion; hypocalcemia; depressed cardiac and respiratory function.

Anticipate and assess for diarrhea, the most common side effect of oral magnesium preparations, regardless of the reason for which they were given.

Have calcium gluconate ready for injection when giving parenteral magnesium salts. It may help counteract adverse effects caused by an accidental magnesium overdose.

Iron

Iron is used mainly for the synthesis of heme, the essential protein of hemoglobin, which is responsible for transporting and releasing oxygen and carbon dioxide. It is also a critical component of several enzyme systems involved in energy production in all body cells.

Iron is absorbed through the duodenum and jejunum. Once in the bloodstream, iron is transported mainly by transferrin, an iron-binding protein, and is distributed to all tissues and to storage sites in the bone marrow, liver, and spleen. Iron is eliminated in the feces.

Iron deficiency is the most common mineral deficiency. Iron supplements are indicated for treating hypochromic microcytic (iron deficiency) anemia that occurs after hemorrhage or in persons with inadequate dietary iron intake. It is used prophylactically during periods of increased need, such as during pregnancy, infancy, and childhood, mainly for its effects on the blood (a hematinic effect). Pregnancy is perhaps the most common situation in which dietary iron intake is inadequate, and for which supplementation is indicated.

Ferrous sulfate is the most commonly administered iron preparation when oral therapy is indicated. Other formulations for oral use include the fumarate and gluconate salts, complexes with polysaccharides, and those containing vitamin C (which enhances iron absorption) or other vitamins. The dosage form (tablets, capsules, suspensions, elixirs, drops), the chemical form, and the dosage all affect the amount of iron that is absorbed. The fumarate salt contains the most available iron (on a per-milligram basis), with the gluconate salt containing the least. Gastrointestinal intolerance may limit many patients' willingness to take some iron supplements. Sustained-release or enteric-coated iron supplements are available to reduce this problem, but they delay the release and absorption of iron, thereby lowering the desired effects unless dosage adjustments are made.

When oral administration is not feasible but iron supplementation is necessary, an iron-dextran complex (IMFERON; others) is available. It is given by IM or IV injection or infusion. Iron loss caused by hemorrhage is the most common use for this formulation.

NURSING IMPLICATIONS

Foods rich in iron include organ meats (liver, heart, kidney), brewer's yeast, wheat germ, egg yolk, beans, fruit, and oysters.

Assess patients for common signs and symptoms of iron deficiency: headaches, dizziness, dyspnea after mild exertion, pallor, and listlessness. Many of these reflect anemia, which should be evaluated further with common blood tests.

Prenatal care for all pregnant women should include a diet history and routine blood tests to assess for iron deficiency and the need for supplemental iron administration.

Food (especially eggs, milk products, chocolate, and beverages containing caffeine) interferes with absorption of oral iron supplements. Ideally, the supplements should be taken on an empty stomach or with citrus juices, which contain vitamin C (enhances iron absorption). However, gastrointestinal upset may necessitate the administration of iron supplements with food. This is permissible as long as the dietary interactants that interfere with iron absorption are avoided.

Liquid iron preparations may stain the teeth. Such products should be well diluted before ingestion, and administered through a straw or with a dropper placed on the back of the tongue. This is especially important for children.

Advise patients taking solid dosage forms of iron to swallow it whole.

Administer parenteral iron formulations using a Z-track technique to avoid leakage into subcutaneous tissues.

Assess for, and advise patients to expect, darkening of the stools, diarrhea or constipation; GI upset; and possible nausea and vomiting. Notify the physician if these side effects become severe or intolerable.

Most antacids bind iron in the GI tract and inhibit iron absorption. If concurrent therapy is indicated, space administration of the interactants by at least one to two hours. The same precaution applies to patients taking tetracycline antibiotics, because iron binds the tetracycline and inhibits its absorption. Monitor for signs and symptoms of iron deficiency in patients receiving chloramphenicol. This antibiotic may interfere with the use of blood-borne iron by erythrocytes.

Assess all patients taking iron for evidence of overdose: nausea, vomiting, and other signs of GI distress; and altered bowel motility (usually constipation).

Iron poisoning, often caused by ingestion of iron supplements used by adults, is a relatively common cause of fatalities in children. Iron supplements should be kept in a place that cannot be reached by children. Advise persons responsible for administering iron supplements to children of the expected signs of overdose, and caution them not to exceed recommended doses.

If overdoses of oral iron preparations occur, induce vomiting immediately. The iron chelator, deferoxamine (desferrioxamine; DESFERAL), is indicated for treating severe iron poisoning. See Appendix C for more information.

Zinc

Zinc is a trace mineral that is essential for normal cell growth and wound healing. Zinc is poorly absorbed from the GI tract, but with adequate dietary intake sufficient amounts reach the bloodstream. Zinc concentrates in bones, muscles, eyes, hair, teeth, and the pancreas and liver. Some is also bound to albumin and other serum proteins. Zinc, including that which is administered orally as a supplement and not used by the body, is secreted in the small bowel and eliminated in the feces. Parenteral zinc is eliminated in the feces and in the urine.

The major manifestations of zinc deficiency are delayed wound healing, alterations of the special senses (taste, smell, vision), growth failure (children), and such skin disorders as alopecia and acrodermatitis enterohepatica (a syndrome characterized by diarrhea, steatorrhea, and pustules around the body orifices and on the hands, feet, and head). Zinc supplements can be administered orally (sulfate or gluconate salts) to prevent or treat zinc deficiency, or parenterally (chloride or sulfate; IV) for acute and severe deficiencies.

Other zinc salts are found in a variety of prescription or OTC products. They are used topically to treat such diverse problems as acne, athlete's foot, diaper rash, jock itch, and ocular irritation.

NURSING IMPLICATIONS

Zinc-rich food sources include seafoods, meats, nuts, seeds, bean sprouts, and legumes (including soy products).

Patients with suspected or known systemic zinc deficiency, and those requiring systemic zinc supplement therapy, should avoid (if possible) drugs or foods that may cause further zinc deficiencies: bran and dairy products (decreased absorption). On the other hand, alcohol, corticosteroids, most diuretics, most oral contraceptives, and D-penicillamine increase zinc absorption and can lead to zinc toxicity.

Apply topical zinc products sparingly to avoid skin damage, which may be caused by the product's ability to interfere with evaporation of sweat gland secretions.

Iodine

Iodine's major biologic role is in the synthesis of thyroid hormones. See Chapter 47 for more information.

Age-Related Alterations in Vitamin and Mineral Requirements

The recommendations of the NRC/NAS (see Table 61–1) indicate age-related differences in vitamin and mineral RDAs for infants, children (ages one to 10 years), and male and female adults. Ideally, persons in many of these groups can meet the RDAs through adequate diet, with no need for supplementation. However, common factors such as disease, drug therapy, smoking, alcohol consumption, and also financial capabilities (ie, the ability to purchase proper foods), affect whether diet alone will be sufficient to prevent deficiencies. The need for vitamin or mineral supplements must be assessed on an individual basis, and only after a thorough evaluation has been made. The availability and intensive advertising of many OTC vitamin and mineral supplements may make it more difficult to ensure proper use.

Pregnancy and Lactation

Adequate dietary intake of vitamins and minerals is important to the pregnant woman and the developing fetus. For virtually all vitamins and minerals, the RDAs for pregnant and lactating women are higher than the RDAs for otherwise healthy, age-matched nonpregnant women. As long as the criteria of adequate diet, freedom from disease, and the lack of other factors that increase nutrient demand apply, proper diet alone may be sufficient. If the adequacy of maternal intake cannot be ensured, cautious use of supplements prescribed by a physician may be appropriate. Obtaining pertinent information about nutritional status should be a part of prenatal care and evaluation, and of postnatal care of both the mother and infant. Routine administration of vitamin or mineral supplements, with the aim of exceeding pregnancy-related RDAs, should be avoided during a normal pregnancy unless the anticipated benefits exceed the potential risks. Vitamins A, C, D, K, and niacin, in particular, must be administered cautiously during pregnancy. Iron is one exception to the rule of general avoidance. The consensus opinion is that the increased iron requirements during pregnancy cannot be met by even the best of "average" American diets, nor by the mother's iron stores. Thus, it is relatively common to prescribe a daily iron supplement of 30 to 60 mg during pregnancy. Maternal iron requirements during lactation are no different from those existing before pregnancy. However, it may be necessary to continue iron supplement administration for two to three months after delivery to replenish stores that were depleted prepartum.

Children

Physical growth and maturation, combined with increased physical activity, obviously increase nutrient requirements. Here, too, adequate diet and good health usually eliminate the need for supplementation. Nevertheless, a careful and complete assessment, including the child's health and dietary history, is necessary for determining whether a particular individual needs supplementation. Until parenting experience is gained or professional advice and evaluation can be provided, many parents become concerned over their child's selective food preferences and eating patterns. Nurses should help the parents assess whether a dietary problem actually exists.

The availability and mass marketing of nutrient supplements for children often conveys the impression that there is a real need to administer such products to all children. Many nurses, nurse practitioners, physicians, and registered dietitians—including those specializing in pediatrics—feel that for otherwise healthy children with balanced diets, such products are unnecessary but probably harmless if the manufacturer's recommended daily dose is not exceeded. However, nurses must stress to parents the potential dangers of both acute and long-term overdoses. Parents often overlook the fact that children may equate these drugs with candy. This is not surprising, since many of the popular vitamin-mineral supplements are in the form of flavorful, colorful tablets shaped like familiar and friendly cartoon characters or animals. Nurses should make parents aware of this possibility, not only to avoid vitamin and mineral overdoses, but also to avoid a child's impression that all drugs are candy.

Adults and the Elderly

For most healthy males and healthy nonpregnant females, the RDAs for many vitamins and minerals remain relatively constant after the age of 15 years. This does not mean that daily requirements for individuals are unchanging. Age-related increases in nutrient requirements most often are associated with the elderly population. However, health-care providers should understand that increased nutrient requirements of the "older population" may actually begin in younger adults, a fact often overlooked during assessment and treatment.

It is during the younger adult years that lifestyle patterns such as poor dietary intake, smoking, consumption of alcohol and other drugs, and the exposure to increased physical and emotional stress develop. Such factors, which may persist into the later years of life, can have dramatic impact on nutritional needs and overall health.

A host of factors affect nutritional status in the elderly, including limited financial resources; depression; anorexia; altered taste or smell, which reduces the pleasure of eating; poorly fitting dentures or other physical problems that make eating difficult; and an inability to prepare meals. Many of these problems are common accompaniments of aging, age-related disorders, or the drugs used to treat such disorders. Physiologic alterations of nutrient absorption, distribution, metabolism, and elimination add other problems. All these factors may require a higher dietary nutrient intake to achieve the RDAs and maintain optimal well-being. Most healthy elderly persons do not need to take vitamin and mineral supplements. However, institutionalized or chronically ill elderly patients are at substantial risk for deficiencies and do require supplements. Commonly deficient nutrients in these individuals include vitamins A, D, B_1, B_2, folic acid, calcium, and iron. All elderly persons should be advised to avoid taking excessive doses of vitamin A or D, either of which can be toxic. The use of nonprescription drugs (laxatives, antacids, and so on) also should be evaluated closely, and restricted as necessary, as part of the overall treatment plan.

Patients, regardless of age, may have misconceptions about the use of vitamins and mineral supplements. Several problems related to supplement use can occur:

1. Taking large amounts of vitamins and minerals is likely to result in adverse or toxic effects.
2. Risking interactions among the supplements themselves or with prescription or OTC drugs can result in untoward responses.
3. Buying expensive supplements may reduce the amount of money available for purchasing food.
4. Using dietary supplements may give a false sense of security, potentially impairing adequate food intake or masking an underlying nutritional deficit.

Enteral Nutrition

When oral intake does not meet nutritional needs, enteral or parenteral nutrition may become necessary. Enteral nutrition is the administration of liquid nutritional products orally or through nasogastric, nasoduodenal, nasojejunal, gastrostomy, esophagostomy, or jejunostomy tubes. Parenteral nutrition is the administration of nutrients by the IV route. If the GI tract is functional and accessible, enteral nutrition is preferred to parenteral nutrition for several reasons. First, nutrient use is improved because the gut and portal system process nutrients in the normal fashion. Second, enteral nutrition is less costly than parenteral nutrition and is associated with fewer complications. Third, enteral feedings preserve gut structure and function, so that normal absorptive, secretory, and barrier functions are maintained. The development of narrow-bore feeding tubes that produce less discomfort; the use of new gut access techniques that permit noninvasive tube placement; and the recent availability of gravity infusion pumps that prevent accidental bolus infusions, are among the other reasons that make enteral nutrition the preferred method.

The composition and nutritional values of enteral formulas vary greatly (Table 61–4). Nutrient sources and osmolarity are major considerations in formula selection. In addition, caloric and lactose contents may vary. A clinical dietitian can assist in choosing the formula that best meets a patient's requirements.

The digestive and absorptive capacities of the GI tract must be considered when selecting nutrient sources. Nutrients may be present in their simplest forms—glucose, crystalline amino acids, medium-chain triglycerides—which require little or no digestion; or they may occur in more complex forms—polysaccharides, milk solids, corn oil—which must be digested. Patients with impaired digestive capabilities (for example, pancreatitis or bile duct obstruction) or impaired absorptive capacity (for example, Crohn's disease) may require feedings containing simple nutrient sources. However, if the GI tract is fully functional, these formulas are not necessary. Rather, a more complete formula, with intact proteins, complex carbohydrates, and a higher percentage of fat, is appropriate. In general, nutrients in simpler form are less palatable and should be administered through a straw or feeding tube. Vitamin, mineral, and electrolyte contents also vary. Most commercial formulas are designed to meet the RDA for vitamins in approximately 2 liters of formula.

The **osmolality** of normal body fluids is about 300 milliosmoles (mOsm)/kg. Enteral products that have an **osmolarity** greater than body fluids are hyperosmolar; they cause water to be drawn into the GI tract if given too rapidly, and may result in "dumping syndrome"—characterized by abdominal discomfort and diarrhea. Most tube feedings are hyperosmolar, although several products are isoosmolar. In general, the closer an enteral feeding is to isoosmolar, the lower the potential for hyperosmolar complications.

Enteral products usually provide 1 kilocalorie (kcal)/mL when given undiluted. In other words, a volume of 1000 mL is required to provide 1000 kcal. Several newer formulas contain 1.5 or 2.0 kcal/mL and can be used when energy needs are high. As a rule, the higher the caloric content of a formula, the higher the osmolarity. Therefore, the advantages of higher caloric content versus increased risk for hyperosmolar complications must be carefully weighed.

Lactose, the predominant disaccharide of milk, must be broken down into monosaccharides by the enzyme lactase in order to be absorbed. Certain intestinal diseases such as celiac sprue and regional enteritis can result in insufficient lactase levels. Also, over half of all adults in the United States have a primary lactase deficiency, which results in lactose intolerance. Symptoms of lactose intolerance are bloating, gas, abdominal cramping, and diarrhea. Although some enteral formulas are lactose-free, several contain skim or whole milk that may produce these symptoms.

Clinical Uses and Administration

Enteral nutrition is used for patients with functioning GI tracts who cannot take food by mouth, cannot meet nutritional requirements with ordinary diets, or both. Common indications for enteral nutrition include central nervous system disorders, dysphagia/anorexia, cancer cachexia, burns, sepsis, mechanical obstructions of the head and neck region, and early postoperative feeding.

Three general categories of enteral products are commercially available: nutritionally complete, specialized, and supplements (see Table 61–4). Nutritionally complete formulas supply protein, carbohydrate, fat, vitamins, and minerals in sufficient quantities to maintain the nutritional status of an individual receiving no other source of nourishment. The formulas in this category vary greatly in composition. Some formulas, such as the defined or elemental formulas, require minimal digestion and are clear liquids with minimal residue. Others, such as polymeric formulas and blenderized feedings, require full digestive and absorptive abilities and contain varying amounts of residue and lactose.

Specialized formulas have been developed for use in patients with specific metabolic abnormalities. Formulas that are low in protein and electrolytes are used in nondialyzed patients with renal disease. Formulas with high branched-chain amino acid content have been prepared for patients with hepatic insufficiency, since these patients cannot use large quantities of non-branched–chain amino acids.

Supplements or modular components provide one single nutrient or a combination of nutrients in quantities *insufficient* to maintain nutritional status. Such for-

Table 61–4 Examples of Enteral Nutrition Products*

Product	Form	Kcal/mL	Osmolality (mOsm)	Lactose	Comments
		Nutritionally Complete			
ENRICH	L, F	1.1	480	–	Fiber-supplemented, for constipation or diarrhea
ENSURE PLUS	L, F	1.5	600	–	Concentrated; good for fluid-restricted patients
ISOCAL HCN	L, U	2.0	690	–	High calorie; good for fluid-restricted patients
OSMOLITE	L, U	1.0	300	–	Isotonic; low levels of sodium and potassium
SUSTACAL	L, F	1.0	620	–	High protein
SUSTACAL PUDDING	Pd, F	1.6	NA	+	High calorie
TWOCAL HCN	L, F	2.0	690	–	Concentrated formula; good or patients with high energy needs
VITAL HN	P, F	1.0	500	+	Partially hydrolyzed formula
VIVONEX TEN	P, U	1.0	630	–	Elemental diet, flavor packets available; good for malabsorption and radiation enteritis
			Specialized		
AMIN-AID	P	2.0	700	–	Low protein; for renal dysfunction
HEPATIC-AID III	P	1.1	560	–	For liver dysfunction; high in branched-chain amino acids
PORTAGEN	P	1.0	320	–	For fat malabsorption; high in medium-chain triglycerides
			Supplements		
MCT OIL	L	7.7		–	Used for fat malabsorption; contains no essential fatty acids
MICROLIPID	P	4.5		–	Contains long-chain and medium-chain fatty acids
POLYCOSE LIQUID	L	2.0		–	Glucose polymers; supplements calories
PROPAC	P	2.0		–	Whey protein; supplements protein

*Key: L = liquid; F = flavored; U = unflavored; Pd = pudding; P = powder; NA = not available; + = present; – = absent.

mulas should be used only to supplement nutritional intake.

Tube feeding can be administered by several methods. The least preferred technique is bolus delivery, which involves the rapid administration of enteral formula by syringe. With this method, the patient is fed a volume of 300 to 400 mL of liquid four to six times daily. Feedings using this technique permit the rapid infusion of a large, hyperosmolar bolus of liquid, which may be poorly tolerated and may result in abdominal cramping, diarrhea, or dumping.

Enteral feedings into the stomach are most often administered by intermittent infusion. With this method, the prescribed volume of formula is administered over a 30- to 60-minute interval. Some of the problems associated with bolus delivery are eliminated, but tolerance may still be poor in some patients.

Continuous infusion is the preferred method of enteral delivery for critically ill patients or patients with intestinal tubes. Formula is delivered by continuous drip over 8 to 24 hours, using a pump or other controller to avoid accidental bolus delivery. Generally, enteral feedings should be initiated at isoosmolar concentrations at a rate of 50 mL per hour. If the patient tolerates the feeding, the rate, and then the concentration, can gradually be increased over 24 to 48 hours. If the feeding is not tolerated, the rate or concentration should be reduced to levels tolerated by the patient, then gradually increased again.

Complications and Contraindications

Most mechanical and metabolic complications associated with enteral nutrition are preventable with proper tube placement, correct formula selection and administration, and careful monitoring. Some problems with tube insertion, such as misplacement in the trachea or perforation of the duodenum, can be lethal. Proper tube placement should always be confirmed by X-ray examination. The development of soft, pliable, small-bore tubes has decreased the incidence of GI irritation and perforation.

Aspiration is another very dangerous complication of enteral feeding. Weak, debilitated, and comatose patients are especially at risk. Routinely checking for gastric distention and gastric residuals, and elevating the head of the bed at all times to an angle greater than 30 degrees, reduces the risk of aspiration.

Electrolyte imbalances, glycosuria, and dehydration may be minimized by administering water and by closely monitoring serum electrolytes, osmolality, blood urea nitrogen (BUN), and intake and output.

Diarrhea is the most common complication of tube feedings. It can result when one or a combination of factors is present, including administration of hyperosmolar solutions, fecal impaction, hot or cold formula, bacterial contamination of formula or delivery sets, lactose intolerance, low serum albumin, low fiber content of formula, or concurrent drug therapy. Most diarrhea attributable to tube feedings can be prevented or controlled. Ongoing assessment to rule out these factors prevents or alleviates diarrhea in tube-fed patients. The related problems of abdominal cramps, distention, nausea, and vomiting are usually avoided when feedings are administered by continuous drip, rather than as a bolus.

Tube feedings are contraindicated in patients with intestinal obstruction, severe malabsorption, fistulae, or other clinical conditions for which total bowel rest is indicated.

NURSING IMPLICATIONS

The patient who is unable to take food by mouth, or cannot meet nutritional requirements, should be assessed for the advisability of enteral feedings. Consult the dietitian, physician, and pharmacist to determine proper formula selection and administration method. Once tube feedings are initiated, assess nutritional status parameters for adequacy of nutritional supplementation. Monitor and document all intake and output, daily weights, calorie counts, and laboratory values for serum glucose, electrolytes, and BUN concentrations. Explain to the patient and family the purpose and plans for tube feeding, and instruct them to report signs and symptoms of intolerance.

Follow recommended policies and procedures for tube feeding administration. Avoid bacterial contamination by washing your hands before preparing the formula and by replacing the entire administration system every 24 to 48 hours (or according to institutional protocol). Provide oral and nasal hygiene. Confirm tube placement and patency prior to feeding. Check for gastric distention and residuals, and delay feeding when indicated. Elevate the head of the bed to an angle of 30 degrees or greater at all times to prevent regurgitation and aspiration. Document consistency and frequency of bowel movements.

Any medications to be added to enteral products should be evaluated for compatibility. Syrups that are strongly acidic (pH 4 or below; eg, iron preparations) can cause gelling or rapid coagulation of the nutritional product. Elixirs, suspensions, granule formulations, effervescent tablets, and other solid dosage forms are possible alternatives.

Observe for mechanical, metabolic, and gastrointestinal complications. Advise the patient to exercise and move about as much as possible to ensure maximum use of enteral nutrients. If home tube feedings are required, be certain the patient and family thoroughly understand all aspects of therapy. Advise them of the availability and potential need for home health care nurses.

◆ Use in Children

To prevent nausea and regurgitation, feedings should not be administered faster than 5 mL every five to 10 minutes in premature and small infants or 10 mL per minute in older infants and children.

◆ Use in the Elderly

Because aspiration is potentially lethal, patients who are unconscious, obtunded, or have neuromuscular impairments should receive postpyloric

Table 61–5 Examples of Parenteral Nutrition Solutions

Central Venous Nutrition Solution		Peripheral Venous Nutrition Solution	
Each 1000 mL container provides:		**Each 1000 mL container provides:**	
	1010 kcal total calories		285 kcal total calories
Crystalline amino acids	4.25%	Crystalline amino acids	2.75%
Dextrose	25%	Dextrose	5%
Sodium	35 mEq	Sodium	35 mEq
Potassium	30 mEq	Potassium	30 mEq
Calcium	4.7 mEq	Calcium	4.7 mEq
Magnesium	5 mEq	Magnesium	5 mEq
Phosphorus	30 mEq	Phosphorus	30 mEq
Chloride	35 mEq	Chloride	35 mEq
Acetate	67.5 mEq	Acetate	50 mEq
1850 mOsm/L	Total volume = 1040 mL	710 mOsm/L	Total volume = 1020 mL

Note: Vitamins are automatically added and consist of 2 units of MVI-12 daily. Trace elements are an automatic daily additive for patients on CVN, and provide the AMA recommendations for metabolically stable adult patients. Trace elements may be ordered for addition to PVN also, and as single entities when needed.

Adapted from *Parenteral Nutrition Product Listings.* Chicago, IL, Rush-Presbyterian–St. Luke's Medical Center Department of Pharmacy (revised 7/86).

(jejunal or intestinal) feedings rather than gastric feedings. Severe dehydration may occur if insufficient water is given with concentrated feedings.

Parenteral Nutrition

Parenteral nutrition is used to provide nutrients through a peripheral or large central vein. Parenteral solutions contain water, amino acids, a source of non-protein calories (glucose or a combination of glucose and fat), electrolytes, vitamins, and trace elements (Table 61–5). Parenteral nutrition is indicated for patients who cannot receive adequate nutrients through the GI system to meet physiologic needs.

Several types of parenteral nutrition are commonly employed. *Central venous nutrition* (CVN) consists of parenteral nutrition solutions, administered through a large central vein, that contain 10% or greater glucose concentrations, 4.25% or greater amino acid concentrations, and electrolytes, vitamins, and trace elements. *Peripheral venous nutrition* (PVN) is peripheral vein administration of solutions consisting of glucose (5% to 10%), amino acids, electrolytes, vitamins, and trace minerals. *Total parenteral nutrition* (TPN) combines CVN or PVN with IV fat emulsion. *Home parenteral nutrition* (HPN) refers to parenteral nutrition provided in the home setting.

Minimum daily energy needs for a normal adult in the resting state are between 1400 and 1800 kcal. Patients who have undergone major surgery often require a minimum of 3000 kcal daily. Severely septic, traumatized, or burned patients may require 5000 to 10,000 kcal per day to satisfy energy requirements. Standard IV solutions of 5% glucose in water or saline contain only 170 kcal/L. Patients would require the infusion of many liters per day to meet minimal energy needs, which is not feasible. Thus, standard IV therapy cannot provide the patient with sufficient calories or protein to meet the body's daily requirements.

When energy demands are high, CVN, with or without IV lipid supplementation, is usually the most effective form of support; such solutions can be formulated with many calories in a relatively small volume (high caloric density). Central venous solutions are hypertonic (1700 mOsm/L) and contain approximately 1000 kcal/L. In patients with lower caloric needs, nutritional support through a peripheral vein, with or without IV fat emulsion, is generally considered. The osmolarity of PVN is about 700 mOsm/L, with a total caloric content of less than 300 kcal/L.

Fat emulsions are infused daily or twice weekly to prevent essential fatty acid deficiency and to boost caloric intake. These preparations are isoosmolar and may be infused either peripherally or centrally. Lipid solutions have been used in the United States since 1977 and are now available in 10% or 20% concentrations. The 10% solutions provide 1.1 kcal/mL, and the 20% solutions provide 2.2 kcal/mL.

An advantage of PVN is that a central venous catheter is not needed; therefore, there is a lower rate of sepsis. However, patients who need large amounts of protein and calories usually require CVN. The recent use of multilumen central catheters and venous access devices may minimize many of the complications associated with standard central venous catheters.

Clinical Uses and Administration

Indications for parenteral nutrition include gastrointestinal fistulae, short bowel syndrome, renal failure, inflammatory bowel disease, acute pancreatitis, complications of anorexia nervosa, burns, trauma, and other hypercatabolic states.

Parenteral nutrition solutions that have glucose as the major caloric source are generally hyperosmolar, and tend to cause phlebitis or thrombosis if infused through peripheral veins. For this reason, IV access to a large central vein is imperative. The high flow rate of the superior vena cava allows hypertonic parenteral nutrient solutions to be rapidly diluted in the bloodstream, thereby reducing the probability of phlebitis or thrombosis.

Hyperosmolar glucose solutions must be given slowly at first. Usually, 1 liter is given in 24 hours, using a constant drip infusion maintained by an infusion pump. Depending on patient tolerance and blood glucose, urine glucose, and electrolyte levels, the rate is gradually increased—typically over three to five days—until the patient is receiving the prescribed amount.

Hyperosmolar parenteral solutions should be administered at a steady rate. If the administration rate falls behind, the rate should be corrected rather than attempting to "catch up," since an excessive glucose load could result. At one time, hyperosmolar parenteral nutrition was discontinued slowly over two to three days to prevent rebound hypoglycemia. It is now considered safe to taper hyperosmolar parenteral nutrition for just one to two hours before discontinuing therapy.

The first dose of fat emulsion should be infused slowly to allow time to assess for potentially adverse reactions. Side effects from fat emulsion therapy include dyspnea, fever, chills, and pain in the chest and back owing to embolism. Hepatomegaly and other adverse reactions have been reported infrequently. The suggested starting rate is 1 mL per minute for 15 to 30 minutes. If no adverse effects are noted, the rate may be increased to a maximum of 125 mL per hour of the 10% fat emulsion or 60 mL per hour of the 20% fat emulsion. To prevent bacterial contamination, a single unit of lipid should not hang longer than 8 to 12 hours. Because they are too viscous, fat emulsions should not be administered through a filter.

Patient monitoring includes periodic evaluations of BUN, creatinine, electrolytes, calcium, phosphorus, magnesium, total protein, albumin, and prothrombin time, as well as liver function studies. Vital signs, infusion rate, intake and output, catheter care, daily weights, and blood glucose levels should also be monitored and documented on an ongoing basis.

Complications and Contraindications

With proper patient monitoring and careful technique, most complications of parenteral nutrition can be prevented. When complications do occur, they may be classified into three categories: technical, metabolic, and septic. *Technical complications* are the most common and are related to central catheter placement. Potential problems arising during central vein cannulation include pneumothorax, air embolus, catheter malposition, hemothorax, and hemopericardium.

Metabolic problems caused by parenteral nutrition include both hyperglycemia and hypoglycemia, glucosuria, various mineral and electrolyte abnormalities, and hepatic enzyme derangements. With improved administration techniques, infusion of appropriate amounts of nutrients, and better patient monitoring, these complications are less frequent.

Septic complications occur as the result of contaminated catheters, contaminated parenteral nutrition solutions, or both. Catheter sepsis is minimized by strict adherence to aseptic catheter care. Parenteral solution preparation under laminar air flow hoods, solution administration through micropore filters, daily administration set and tubing changes, and allowing parenteral solutions to hang no longer than 8 to 24 hours are among the procedures used to prevent contamination of parenteral nutrition solutions.

NURSING IMPLICATIONS

Assess patients for protein-calorie malnutrition or other conditions that may indicate a need for parenteral nutrition. Explain to the patient and the family the purpose, plan, and procedures for parenteral nutrition.

Once parenteral nutrition has been initiated, the therapeutic response to treatment must be assessed. Monitor and document vital signs, intake and output, daily weight, and blood glucose levels. BUN, creatinine, electrolytes, calcium, phosphorus, magnesium, prothrombin time, total protein, albumin levels, and liver function studies should be monitored periodically.

Follow recommended policies and procedures for administration of parenteral nutrition. Maintain the infusion flow at a specific rate. Provide routine mouth care. Begin infusion of fat emulsions slowly, and monitor for adverse effects during the first 30 minutes of infusion. Change dressings, tubing, filters, and solutions according to hospital policy.

Observe for technical, metabolic, and septic complications. If parenteral therapy is to be continued at home, give detailed instructions to both the patient and the family on infusion techniques and on signs and symptoms of complications. Discuss the psychosocial aspects of long-term dependency on parenteral nutrition solutions.

Use in Children

Liver disease is a complication seen in preterm infants begun on TPN at an early age. Parenteral fat emulsions should be given with extreme caution to low-birth-weight and premature infants. Death has occurred from poor clearance of lipids and increased serum levels of free fatty acids.

Use in the Elderly

Diminished cardiovascular function in the elderly may increase the risk of volume overload from hyperosmolar solutions or rapid infusion rates.

SUMMARY OF NURSING IMPLICATIONS

Assessment

Review patient history for existing medical conditions or concurrent drug therapy contraindicating use of supplements.

Establish baseline laboratory and physical assessment data indicating nutritional deficiency.

Obtain a complete nutritional history to determine dietary patterns, preferences, and deficiencies.

Nursing Diagnoses

Altered nutrition: less than body requirements related to inadequate intake, a specific disease condition, or a drug-nutrient interaction.

Knowledge deficit related to adequate dietary intake of essential nutrients or proper administration of vitamin/mineral supplements.

High risk for impaired skin integrity related to vitamin/mineral deficiency.

Ineffective individual coping: depression related to inability to take oral food and fluid.

Diarrhea related to enteral nutrition.

Altered growth and development related to vitamin/mineral deficiency.

Planning/Implementation

Monitor vital signs and laboratory values for indications of therapeutic or toxic effects.

Observe for signs and symptoms of deficiency, excess, or toxicity.

Administer supplement as indicated to enhance absorption and minimize adverse effects.

Follow recommended policies and procedures for enteral and parenteral feedings.

Observe for mechanical, metabolic, gastrointestinal, and/or septic complications associated with enteral and parenteral feedings.

Patient and Family Teaching

Teach the patient/family:

About dietary sources for a specific supplement; provide list.

The importance of not exceeding RDA of vitamin/mineral supplement unless prescribed.

About symptoms of overdose and the importance of reporting them.

About proper administration and storage of vitamin/mineral preparations.

To expect changes in urine and/or stool with certain supplements (eg, iron, riboflavin).

The purpose and plans for tube feedings.

About home tube feeding or home parenteral nutrition: preparation, handling, administration, and storage.

Evaluation

The patient will:

Maintain or regain normal body weight.

Ingest a diet containing adequate nutrients.

Tolerate enteral or parenteral feeding; no aspiration, minimal bowel changes, no volume overload or infection.

Show an increase in serum levels of essential nutrients.

Achieve a growth and development level consistent with age.

Annotated Bibliography

Committee on Dietary Allowances, Food and Nutrition Board: Recommended Dietary Allowances. Tenth Ed. Washington, DC, National Academy of Sciences, 1989. *This is the most current authoritative source for recommendations on the requirements for all major nutrients: vitamins, minerals, and trace elements; carbohydrates, fats, proteins/amino acids; and water and electrolytes. In addition to sections on these nutrients, and comments on the meaning and limitations of RDAs (established by this group), the document provides important and readable insights into altered nutrient requirements owing to age, pregnancy and lactation, drug therapy, and other factors likely to be encountered in patients.*

Edes TE, Walk BE, Austin JL: Diarrhea in tube-fed patients: Feeding formula not necessarily the cause. *Am J Med* 1990; 88:91–93. *When diarrhea occurs in enterally fed patients, the tube feeding usually is assumed to be responsible. This study reports a new and significant cause of diarrhea in tube-fed patients. Patients receiving tube feedings often are given liquid forms of medications. Many of these medicinal elixirs contain sorbitol, which may or may not be listed on the package inserts, in amounts sufficient to cause significant osmotic diarrhea.*

Eisenberg P: Enteral nutrition: Indications, formulas, and delivery techniques. *Nurs Clin North Am* 1989; 24(2):315–338. *Clearly written for nurses, this article addresses such important considerations as feeding formulas, feeding tube types, and administration methods. Most valuable are its comprehensive tables of enteral formulas, enteral tubes, and its discussion of the latest in feeding tubes and feeding routes.*

Horwath CC: Nutrition goals for older adults: A review. *Gerontologist* 1991; 31(6):811–821. *This well-written paper discusses specific nutrition education goals for older adults and high-risk groups within the elderly population. In formulating the goals, the authors review three important areas: current knowledge of dietary intake of older adults, the multiple influences (physical, behavioral, and socioeconomic) that affect eating habits in this age group, and the potential benefits of dietary and lifestyle changes in old age. Since elderly people are often at nutritional risk, nutrition education is a priority for this group.*

Kohn CL, Keithley JK: Enteral nutrition: Potential complications and patient monitoring. *Nurs Clin North Am* 1989; 24(2):339–353. *Although most complications associated with enteral nutrition are preventable, some are potentially lethal. This article discusses the etiologies of common enteral complications and research-based nursing interventions for avoiding, recognizing, and treating complications.*

Moore EE: Early postinjury enteral feeding: Attenuated stress response and reduced sepsis. *Contemp Surg* 1988; 32(2-A):1–40. *This is one of the first articles to demonstrate the use and benefits of enteral nutrition in the early postoperative period. Total parenteral nutrition previously was considered to be the choice of nutritional support in surgical patients. In the stressed postinjury state, however, aggressive enteral nutrition protects the gut barrier, reduces metabolic stress, maintains normal hepatic function, and decreases the risk of sepsis and multiple organ failure.*

Neuvonen PJ, Kivisto KT: The clinical significance of food-drug interactions: A review. *Med J Austral* 1989; 150:36–40. *This article focuses on the major mechanisms of food-drug interactions, as well as specific categories of drugs, such as nonsteroidal antiinflammatory, antineoplastic, cardiovascular, and antimicrobial agents, that have potential for clinically significant interactions.*

Nielsen FH: Trace and ultratrace elements in health and disease. *Comprehensive Therapy* 1991; 17(3):20–26. *In this article, the biologic roles, homeostatic regulation, and nutritional importance of trace and ultratrace elements are reviewed. Much of what is known about the trace and ultratrace elements is very new knowledge, with exciting implications for health maintenance and disease prevention.*

Urrows ST, Freston MS, Pryor DL: Profiles in osteoporosis. *AJN* 1991; 91(12), 33–37. *Osteoporosis, which is caused by an interplay of a variety of genetic, hormonal, nutritional, and genetic factors, is one of the most debilitating conditions faced by elderly people. This article discusses risk factors and ways to prevent or minimize the potentially devastating effects of osteoporosis. Most valuable are the tables characterizing calcium forms and supplement types.*

Veterans Affairs Total Parenteral Nutrition Cooperative Study Group: Perioperative total parenteral nutrition in surgical patients. *New Eng J Med* 1991; 325(8):525–532. *This important article reports the results of a multicenter randomized trial of perioperative parenteral nutrition support in malnourished patients undergoing major abdominal or thoracic surgery. This study refutes the efficacy of this therapeutic modality in reducing morbidity and mortality in patients with mild or moderate malnutrition. Severely malnourished patients may, however, benefit from perioperative parenteral nutrition.*

Table 61–C1 **Clinical Uses and Administration of Major Vitamins**

AGENT	CLINICAL USES	DOSAGE AND ROUTE OF ADMINISTRATION
	Fat-Soluble Vitamins	
Vitamin A		
(retinol; ACON; ALPHALIN; AQUASOL A; others)	Prophylaxis and treatment of vitamin A deficiency; treatment of skin diseases and visual deficiencies	Oral, IM: Adults: 15,000–100,000 IU/day; Children: 5000–35,000 IU/day
Vitamin D		
(calciferol; DELTALIN GELSEALS; DRISDOL; GELTABS)	Rickets, including refractory rickets; osteomalacia; familial phosphatemia; hypoparathyroidism	Oral, IM: Adults: 12,000 IU/day; Children 1000–500,000 IU/day
Calcifediol		
(CALDEROL)	Management of hypocalcemia or bone disease in patients on chronic renal dialysis	Oral: Initially 300–350 μg/week, given in daily or alternate-day divided doses; average maintenance dose is 50–100 μg daily, or twice that amount every other day
Calcitriol		
(ROCALTROL)	Hypocalcemia, as for calcifediol	Oral: usually 0.25 μg taken once daily
Dihydrotachysterol		
("DHT"; HYTAKEROL)	Adjunctive management of tetany	Oral: Usually 0.8–2.4 mg once daily for several days (until serum calcium levels approach desired levels; symptoms subside); average maintenance dose 0.6 mg/day; simultaneous calcium supplement therapy acceptable
Vitamin E		
(α-tocopherol; AQUASOL E; E-FEROL SUCCINATE; TOCOPHER; others)	Prevention of vitamin E deficiency that accompanies prolonged protein-calorie malnutrition or malabsorption syndromes	Oral, IM: Adults: 30–200 IU/day
Vitamin K_1		
(phytonadione; AQUAMEPHYTON; KONAKION; MEPHYTON)	Hypoprothrombinemia due to anticoagulant therapy, antibacterial therapy, or prolonged therapy with salicylates; conditions that cause inadequate intake, absorption, or synthesis of vitamin K (eg, extensive bowel resection, chronic diarrhea, excessive use of laxatives)	Oral, IM, SC: Adults: 1–50 mg/day
	Prevention of hemorrhagic disease in neonates	IM, SC: 0.5–2.0 mg immediately after birth
Vitamin K_3		
(menadione; HYKINONE); (menadione sodium bisulfate; and Vitamin K_4 SYNKAYVITE); (menadiol sodium diphosphate)	Hypoprothrombinemia from vitamin K deficiency induced by antibiotics, salicylates, obstructive jaundice, or biliary fistulae	Oral, IM: Adults: 5–15 mg/day; Children: 5–10 mg/day

(continued)

Table 61–C1 Clinical Uses and Administration of Major Vitamins (*Continued*)

AGENT	CLINICAL USES	DOSAGE AND ROUTE OF ADMINISTRATION
	Water-Soluble Vitamins	
Vitamin C		
(ascorbic acid; ASCORBICAP; CECON; CETANE; others)	Prophylaxis and treatment of vitamin C deficiency—scurvy; stress conditions such as wound healing, surgery, burns, and infection	Oral, IM, IV: Adults: 250–1000 mg/day; Children: 100–250 mg/day
Vitamin B_1		
(thiamine; BETALIN S; BETAXIN; BIAMINE)	Prophylaxis and treatment of thiamine deficiency—beri beri	Oral, IM, IV: Adults: 5–100 mg/day
Vitamin B_2		
(riboflavin; RIOBIN-50; LACTOFLAVIN)	Prevention and treatment of riboflavin deficiency; adjunct in the treatment of other vitamin B deficiencies, including beri beri and pellagra	Oral, SC, IM, IV: Adults: 2–20 mg/day
Vitamin B_3		
(niacin; NICOBID; NOVO-NIACIN)	Pellagra; hyperlipidemia	Oral, SC, IM, IV: Adults: 50–3000 mg/day
Vitamin B_6		
(pyridoxine; BESSIX; HEXA-BETALIN)	Prophylaxis and treatment of pyridoxine deficiency	Oral, SC, IM, IV: Adults: 10–20 mg/day
Vitamin B_9		
(folic acid; FOLACINE; FOLITE)	Folic acid deficiency; megaloblastic anemia	Oral, SC, IM, IV: Adults: 0.4–1.0 mg/day; Children: 0.1–0.4 mg/day
Vitamin B_{12}		
(cyanocobalamin; BERUBIGEN; BETALIN 12; KAYBOVITE; others)	Pernicious anemia	IM, SC: Adults: 30 μg/day for 5–10 days followed by maintenance dose of 100–250 μg/month

Table 61–S1 **Major Side Effects of and Contraindications for Common Vitamins**

VITAMIN SIDE EFFECT	CONTRAINDICATION	COMMENTS AND NURSING IMPLICATIONS
	Fat-Soluble Vitamins	
VITAMIN A (retinol) Overdose or excessive ingestion can cause hypervitaminosis A	Hypervitaminosis A or hypersensitivity to vitamin A	Observe for hypervitaminosis A—irritability, headache, fatigue, drowsiness, anorexia, flaking skin with a yellow discoloration
VITAMIN D (calciferol) Overdose results in toxicity; chronic ingestion causes osteomas and calcification of soft tissues, including heart, lungs, kidneys	Hypercalcemia, severe renal impairment, hyperphosphatemia, and hypervitaminosis A or D	Observe for hypervitaminosis D—nausea, anorexia, weakness, thirst, impaired renal function; monitor serum calcium, phosphorus, urea levels and urinary calcium
Hypercalcemia and hyperphosphatemia may occur		Monitor renal function
VITAMIN E (α-tocopherol) High doses may cause hemorrhage in vitamin K-deficient patients; prolonged excessive doses may cause muscle weakness, fatigue, diarrhea, creatinuria, or thrombophlebitis	Vitamin K deficiency	Monitor for side effects when large doses are administered
VITAMIN K_1 (phytonadione) Anaphylaxis reported after IV administration; less severe reactions include dizziness, flushing, hypotension	Elevated serum prothrombin levels; severe liver disease (eg, hepatitis, cirrhosis)	Observe for hypersensitivity reactions; monitor newborns for signs of hyperbilirubinemia; monitor CBC, serum prothrombin time (PT) and partial prothrombin time (PTT); fresh blood transfusions, frozen plasma, or other therapy may be required for lack of response to vitamin K
VITAMIN K_3 (menadione) Anemia due to hemolysis, polycythemia, and splenomegaly; renal and hepatic damage	Elevated serum prothrombin levels; severe liver disease	Synthetic vitamin K substitute; monitor CBC, PT, and PTT
Can cause hyperbilirubinemia, brain damage, death in neonates—especially premature neonates	Neonates	
	Water-Soluble Vitamins	
VITAMIN C (ascorbic acid) Large doses taken orally may cause gastric irritation and diarrhea; may cause kidney stones in high-risk individuals or hemolytic anemia in person with G-6-PD deficiency; rapid IV administration may cause syncope	Renal failure, G-6-PD deficiency, risk for kidney stone development	Monitor for signs of deficiency—petechiae, ecchymoses, joint pain, delayed wound healing, bleeding gums, gingivitis; monitor for pain and swelling at injection site; ascorbic acid requirements are increased in smokers and alcoholics, and in presence of fever, infections, other conditions that elevate metabolic rate

(continued)

Table 61–S1 Major Side Effects of and Contraindications for Common Vitamins (*Continued*)

VITAMIN SIDE EFFECT	CONTRAINDICATION	COMMENTS AND NURSING IMPLICATIONS
Water-Soluble Vitamins		
VITAMIN B_1 (thiamine) Toxic reactions after IV administration include muscular weakness and labored breathing, followed by death due to respiratory failure, anaphylactic reactions reported after IV administration, but are rare	Persons hypersensitive to thiamine	Observe for signs of hypersensitivity; use parenteral administration only in severe deficiency or when oral administration not feasible; alcohol and digitalis impair thiamine absorption
VITAMIN B_2 (riboflavin) Large doses may cause urine to turn bright yellow	None known	Riboflavin deficiency usually is related to B vitamin deficiency; vitamin B complex therapy usually required; monitor for discolored urine
VITAMIN B_3 (niacin) Large doses may irritate GI tract, alter liver function tests, induce hyperglycemia, aggravate hyperuricemia and gout; circulatory collapse has occurred after rapid IV administration; transient side effects include flushing, headache, hypotension within one hour of administration	Hypersensitivity, active ulcer disease, gastritis, severe liver disorders, diabetes mellitus	Assess for side effects after IV administration; observe for signs and symptoms of GI irritation; monitor hepatic function; monitor blood glucose levels in diabetic patients, who may require additional insulin
VITAMIN B_6 (pyridoxine) Paresthesia and somnolence; burning or pain at injection site	Hypersensitivity to pyridoxine; levodopa or levodopa/carbidopa therapy of parkinsonism	Observe for side effects pyridoxine significantly decreases effectiveness of levodopa: recommend vitamin B_6-free products.
VITAMIN B_9 (folic acid) May rarely cause hypersensitivity reactions, including rash, malaise, and bronchospasm; warmth and flushing reported after IV administration	Aplastic, normocytic, or other anemia, in which the causative factor is unknown (supplemental folic acid may mask symptoms of underlying disease process)	Drug (including alcohol) history may reveal whether folic acid deficiency is due to drug interaction; antineoplastic activity of folic acid antagonists will be blocked if folic acid is administered concurrently; not effective in treatment of pernicious, aplastic, or normocytic anemia
VITAMIN B_{12} (cyanocobalamin) Anaphylaxis, mild transient diarrhea, irritation and injection site pain	History of sensitivity to vitamin B_{12} or cobalt (vitamin B_{12} is the only vitamin that contains cobalt)	Give intradermal test with 0.1 μg before full-dose parenteral therapy is initiated; vitamin C destroys vitamin B_{12}; do not administer concurrently. an intestinal pH above 5.5 and intrinsic factor, a mucoprotein secreted by the stomach, must be present for absorption. Prednisone increases vitamin B_{12} absorption.

Table 61–I1 | **Major Interactions Between Vitamins and Other Agents**

VITAMIN	INTERACTANT	COMMENTS AND NURSING IMPLICATIONS
All	Antacids, cathartics, laxatives; cholesterol-binding resins (eg, cholestyramine)	Interfere with absorption of all orally administered vitamins; advise patients to avoid self-administration of interactants unless under physician's supervision; if any of these interactants must be administered, separate administration of nutrient by at least two hours if possible.
	Alcohol (chronic, high intake)	Alcohol abuse may increase requirements of many or most vitamins due to inadequate dietary intake, assess nutritional status closely, discourage excessive alcohol intake, recommend balanced diet and nutritional supplements as needed
All fat-soluble vitamins	Mineral oil	Do not take mineral oil chronically or with meals
Fat-Soluble Vitamins		
Vitamin D (calciferol)	Phenobarbital, related barbiturates (mainly those used for long-term seizure control); phenytoin	Stimulate metabolic inactivation of vitamin D; increase intake of foods rich in vitamin D
Vitamin E (α-tocopherol)	Iron supplements, some antibiotics, isoniazid	Interfere with vitamin E absorption; vitamin E supplements may be necessary
Vitamin K (phytonadione)	Oral anticoagulants	Vitamin K antagonizes inhibitory effect of oral anticoagulants on hepatic clotting factor synthesis; interaction often unwanted, leading to poor anticoagulant effect; interaction is clinically useful to help overcome hemorrhage caused by oral anticoagulant overdoses, and to manage hemorrhagic disorders in newborns of women receiving phenobarbital, phenytoin for seizures during pregnancy
Vitamin C (ascorbic acid)	Oral iron supplements	Vitamin C increases iron absorption, may favor toxicity; combined use should be supervised monitored accordingly
	Sulfonamide antibiotics	Increased antibiotic renal excretion, risk of crystalluria, renal damage
Water -Soluble Vitamins		
Vitamin B_6 (pyridoxine)	Hydralazine (long-term oral use, as for hypertension)	Likely to induce symptomatic B_6 deficiency, may require B_6 therapy for prophylaxis or treatment
	Isoniazid	See hydralazine
	Levodopa	B_6 stimulates conversion of levodopa to dopamine in gut, thereby preventing drug from entering brain and causing desired antiparkinson effect; discourage use of any supplement containing B_6 in such patients; if nutritional supplements are needed, prescribed products (eg, LAROBEC; B_6-free) are available; interaction may apply to levodopa-carbidopa combination product (SINEMET), does not apply to other B vitamins
Vitamin B_9 (folic acid)	Methotrexate	Antagonizes anticancer effect of methotrexate, other agents that act as folate antagonists; avoid inadvertent interactions; interaction therapeutically useful to antagonize side effects, toxicity, of methotrexate and related drugs (see Chapter 59)

(continued)

Table 61–11 **Major Interactions Vitamins Between and Other Agents (*Continued*)**

VITAMIN	INTERACTANT	COMMENTS AND NURSING IMPLICATIONS
Vitamin B_9 (folic acid)	Phenobarbital, phenytoin	Reduce blood levels, anticonvulsant effect possible; monitor accordingly (eg, anticonvulsant blood levels, desired effects); interaction may be unavoidable, as these anticonvulsants may induce folate (B_9) deficiency
Vitamin B_{12} (cyanocobalamin)	Sulfasalazine	Possible folate deficiency; monitor, assess for need for folate supplements
	Cimetidine, probably famotidine, ranitidine, nizatidine	Absorption of food-derived B_{12} requires gastric acid, the secretion of which is inhibited by these interactants; interaction less likely to apply to B_{12} supplements, which do not require release of vitamin from food proteins by acid

Table 61–C2 **Clinical Uses and Administration of Major Minerals**

AGENT	CLINICAL USES	DOSAGE AND ROUTE OF ADMINISTRATION
	Calcium	
Calcium carbonate		
(BIOCAL; CAL-SUP; CALTRATE; others)	Gastric irritation, mild calcium deficiency	Oral: Adults: 10–25 mEq 1–4 times daily
Calcium chloride	Tetany due to hypocalcemia; treatment of hypocalcemia caused by multiple blood transfusions containing citrate; as an adjunct in the treatment of cardiac arrest and profound cardiovascular collapse	See calcium carbonate
Calcium glubionate		
(NEO-CALGLUCON)	Hypoparathyroidism, osteoporosis, rickets	See calcium carbonate
Calcium gluconate	Same uses as calcium chloride	See calcium carbonate
Calcium lactate	Mild calcium deficiency	See calcium carbonate
	Iron	
Ferrous fumarate		
(FECO-T; FEMIRON; FEOSTAT; HEMOCYTE)	Prevention and treatment of iron-deficiency anemia	Oral: Adults: 50–100 mg 3 times daily; Children: 15–45 mg 3 times daily
Ferrous gluconate		
(FERGON; FERRALET; FERTINIC)	See ferrous fumarate	
Ferrous sulfate		
(FEOSOL; FER-IRON; FERO-GRAD; FEROSPACE)	See ferrous fumarate	
	Magnesium	
Magnesium carbonate	Antacid	See Chapter 40
Magnesium gluconate	Dysmenorrhea; hypomagnesemia	Oral: Adults: 500–1000 mg 2 or 3 times daily
Magnesium hydroxide		
(MILK OF MAGNESIA)	Antacid	See Chapter 40
	Laxative/cathartic	See Chapter 41
Magnesium sulfate	Injection: anticonvulsant; treatment of eclampsia; cardiac depressant (calcium antagonist)	Oral, IM, IV: Adults: 0.5–10.0 g/day
	Oral: laxative/cathartic	See Chapter 41

Table 61–S2 **Major Side Effects of and Contraindications for Major Minerals**

MINERAL/ SIDE EFFECT	CONTRAINDICATION	COMMENTS AND NURSING IMPLICATIONS
CALCIUM Acute hypercalcemia, muscle and joint pains, increased excitability of muscles and nerves that progresses to tetany, ECG changes, calcium precipitation in the urine, lethargy, confusion, vomiting, paralytic ileus, irritation at injection site	Hypercalcemia, hypercalciuria, renal calculi, severe renal impairment	Monitor serum calcium, electrolyte, and phosphate levels; check urine for signs of stones (precipitation); observe for signs of hypercalcemia. Administer calcium chloride by IV only; monitor IV site for irritation. Monitor heart during parenteral administration. The various forms and brands of calcium salts contain differing amounts of calcium. Use with caution in patients receiving high doses of vitamin D
MAGNESIUM Hypermagnesemia, especially in patients with impaired renal function; symptoms include depression, absence of deep tendon reflexes, heart block, respiratory paralysis, hypotension, flaccid paralysis, and cardiac arrest	Renal insufficiency, congestive heart failure, heart block	Monitor serum magnesium, electrolyte, and calcium levels. Keep calcium gluconate at the bedside when giving parenteral injections; it acts as an antidote in the event of magnesium sulfate overdose; monitor for signs and symptoms of hypermagnesemia. Record frequency and consistency of stool. An ingredient in many antacids (eg, GELUSIL, MAALOX, MYLANTA); patients with contraindicating conditions should take these only under physician's supervision
IODINE See Chapter 47		
IRON IV administration may cause headache, hypotension, nausea, allergy-like reactions; oral administration commonly causes nausea, constipation, or diarrhea. Iron usually darkens the stool	Hypersensitivity to iron; hemochromatosis, hemosiderosis	Monitor hematology profile. Administration with food may decrease GI distress; give oral liquid forms in water or fruit juice using straw or dropper to protect teeth from discoloration; do not administer iron with milk, eggs, caffeine-containing beverages, or chocolate. Monitor stool color, frequency, and consistency

Table 61–12 Major Interactions Between Minerals and Other Agents

MINERAL	INTERACTANT	COMMENTS AND NURSING IMPLICATIONS
All	Antacids, cathartics, laxatives	Interfere with absorption of all orally administered minerals, or may add excessive amounts of mineral supplements, based on ingredient(s): see individual interactants below; discourage use of antacids, laxatives, cathartics, unless therapy can be supervised, assessment for untoward effects is feasible
All cationic minerals (calcium, iron, magnesium, zinc)	Tetracyclines	These minerals bind tetracyclines in gut, dramatically reduce antibiotic absorption and effect; avoid interaction if possible, otherwise space administration of interactants (oral routes) by at least 2 hours; advise patient to avoid mineral supplements or mineral-rich foods (milk, etc) or medications (eg, antacids, laxatives) during combined therapy unless under physician's supervision
Calcium	Barbiturates (long-term, high-dose use)	May cause hypocalcemia
	Contraceptives, oral	Increase calcium absorption from gut, favoring hypercalcemia
	Corticosteroids (systemic, with long-term, high-dose use)	May cause hypocalcemia
	Digitalis	Increases risk of digitalis toxicity; may occur even with digitalis blood levels in therapeutic range; discourage self-prescribing of calcium supplements during combined therapy (especially important for elderly women, for whom OTC calcium supplements are advertised intensively); assess for evidence of digitalis toxicity (cardiac, extracardiac signs, symptoms) if calcium supplement therapy is prescribed
	Diuretics: high-ceiling (eg, furosemide)	Increase renal calcium excretion, may be a cause of hypocalcemia in some patients
	Diuretics: thiazides	Decrease renal calcium excretion, may cause hypercalcemia; interaction is best avoided, or combined use supervised and monitored closely
	Foods containing oxalate (chocolate, rhubarb, spinach); foods containing phytic acid (bran, whole-grain cereals); zinc-rich foods (legumes, nuts, seeds, sprouts, tofu)	If ingested in large amounts, may interfere with calcium absorption, decreasing effective treatment of calcium deficiency or causing deficiency; assess diet thoroughly, consult with nutritionist if food interaction is suspected
	Milk, other dairy products (large amounts)	Contain calcium, which, when ingested in high amounts with calcium supplements, increase risk of hypercalcemia; systemic alkalosis (milk-alkali syndrome) also may occur; see Chapter 40
Iodine	See Chapter 47	
Iron	Deferoxamine	Deferoxamine chelates ferric ion in blood, is indicated for iron poisoning or other forms of severe iron overload
	Eggs, milk; caffeine-containing beverages; chocolate	If oral iron supplements must be administered with meals to alleviate GI upset, avoid these substances; interaction is probably best established for eggs, milk, questionable with others
	Penicillamine	Iron binds penicillamine, antagonizes its effects, whether used for arthritis, cystinuria, or copper poisoning (eg, Wilson's disease); avoid use of oral iron supplements if therapy with this interacant is necessary
	Vitamin C	See Table 61–5

(continued)

Table 61–12 Major Interactions Between Minerals and Other Agents (*Continued*)

MINERAL	INTERACTANT	COMMENTS AND NURSING IMPLICATIONS
Magnesium	Alcohol (chronic, high intake)	A common cause of hypomagnesemia, which may trigger seizures
	Antacids (containing magnesium)	Concomitant high-dose use of magnesium-containing laxatives or antacids (milk of magnesia; most popular antacid combination products) increases risk of hypermagnesemia, excessive fluid and electrolyte loss via diarrhea; risk of magnesium intoxication particularly high in elderly patients, others with impaired renal function; discourage unsupervised use
	Diuretics: thiazides, high-ceiling agents	Increase renal magnesium excretion, may cause symptomatic deficiency
Phosphorus	Antihypertensive drugs (most except diuretics) Digitalis	Many oral phosphate supplements contain large amounts of sodium, which may counteract desired effects of antihypertensive drugs, digitalis; if combined therapy is required, recommend sodium-free supplements
	Corticosteroids, systemic	Systemic steroids cause renal sodium retention, risk of hypernatremia, heart failure, edema, hypertension if sodium-containing phosphorus supplements are used; sodium-free supplements usually preferred if interaction occurs or becomes significant
	Potassium supplements, potassium-sparing diuretics	Many oral phosphate supplements contain appreciable amounts of potassium, may increase risk of hyperkalemia, interactions with still other drugs (eg, digitalis) if administered with other sources of potassium or with potassium-sparing diuretics; if combined therapy is essential, monitor closely

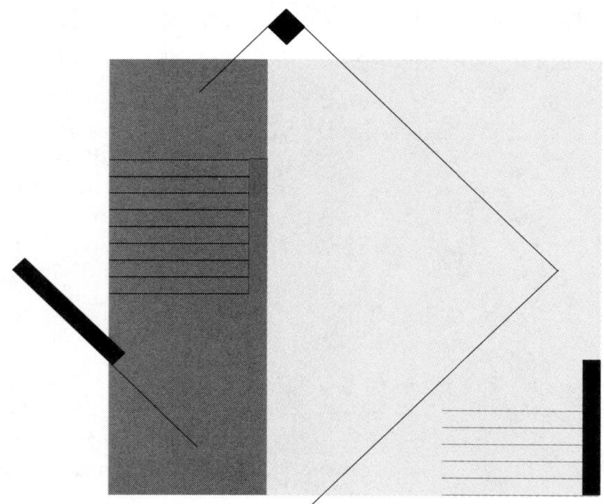

Appendixes

APPENDIX

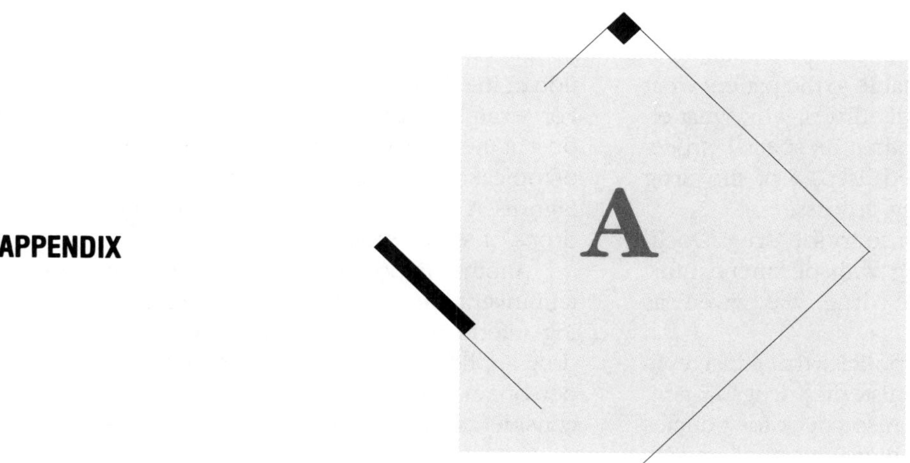

*Techniques of Drug Administration: An Overview**

Chapter 1—Nursing Roles and Responsibilities in Drug Therapy—identified several important topics related to the general issue of drug administration: fundamental nursing responsibilities; supply systems; common physical drug formulations; components of the medication order; routes of administration; and equipment necessary for proper drug administration. Other chapters identified special aspects of administration techniques to be used for the drugs discussed there, and identified consequences of the pharmacologic effects of specific drugs. This appendix focuses on some of the common problems associated with the act of administering a drug. It is not meant to be a comprehensive "how-to" guide for administration techniques, nor is it meant to replace the detailed administration information that is likely to be taught in other nursing courses or found in the texts used for such courses.

**Portions of this appendix have been adapted with permission from Kozier B, Erb G:* Techniques in Clinical Nursing. *Fourth ed. Addison–Wesley, Menlo Park, Calif., 1993.*

General Principles

Several nursing responsibilities always apply to drug administration, regardless of the drug and the route by which it will be administered.

- Ensure that the "five rights" of drug administration are followed:
  1. The right drug
  2. The right dose
  3. The right administration route
  4. The right patient
  5. The right time
- Know the expected actions of the drug. This includes knowing not only the desired effects (and why the drug is being given), but also likely manifestations of side effects, other adverse reactions, and toxicities. In addition, knowing when effects are likely to occur is as important as knowing which ones to expect.
- Ensure that necessary adjunctive nursing measures are provided before, during, and after the medication is administered.
- Before giving the drug, assess baseline data, such as vital signs, as appropriate. Having this information facilitates comparison with changes that occur once the drug's effects have begun.

- Explain in terms understandable to the patient what is to be administered (identify drug), why, what effects to expect, and what other or special procedures must be implemented as part of the drug administration or monitoring process.
- Evaluate the patient's response to the drug. Document this information along with pertinent information indicating that the drug was given as ordered.
- Check all applicable agency policies that affect techniques to be used for administering drugs in general, and for specific drugs. Also check for policies that contraindicate the administration of certain drugs (or their administration by certain routes) by nursing staff.

Topical Administration

There are many variations of the general term "topical administration." For example, drugs may be applied topically to the skin, or to mucous membranes either on a body surface (eg, the eye) or within an accessible body cavity (eg, the nares, the rectum, or the vagina). Even inhalation may be considered a route of topical administration for drugs given for their local effects in the respiratory passages. Although each variation of topical administration requires some specific techniques, several features common to all can be identified.

Compared to most other drug formulations, it is more difficult to measure the proper dose of topically applied agents such as ointments, creams, lotions, and so on. Thus, the situation differs from that which applies to oral or injectable liquids (for which calibrated cups or syringes are available), and for tablets, capsules, and other solid dosage forms (which contain fixed amounts of active ingredient). Drugs applied topically are not necessarily innocuous or without dose-related adverse effects. Careful measurement of dosages is necessary.

Some topically applied drugs are given intentionally for systemic effects—nitroglycerin is a good example. However, the vast majority are not, yet it often is assumed that such agents cause only local effects. As a result, potentially important or adverse systemic effects or contraindicating conditions, some of which are related to unwanted drug absorption, are often ignored or overlooked. The ability of beta blockers applied topically to the eye to cause fatal bronchoconstriction in some asthmatic patients attests to the importance of this. Thus, special techniques or positioning may be needed to maximize local drug effects while simultaneously reducing the risk of unwanted systemic actions if a portion of the dose is swallowed or absorbed in other ways. For example, gentle pressure over the nasolacrimal duct at the eye's inner canthus can minimize absorption of topical ocular preparations; positioning the head (see Figures A–1 and A–2) can do the same when nasal drops or sprays are administered.

Another important consideration is that topical drug administration can pose a relatively great risk of spreading infection or other contamination from the site of drug application to other areas of the patient, to nursing personnel, and to other individuals. These and other considerations are summarized in Table A–1.

Oral Administration

Although oral administration is the preferred route for many drugs, and medications given in this way are easy to administer and usually to take, some problems may arise. The vast majority of drugs administered orally (or sublingually or buccally) are given to produce systemic effects, which requires their absorption from the gastrointestinal (GI) tract or oral mucosa. Once a drug has been swallowed, it becomes difficult—although clearly not impossible—to retrieve it in case the wrong drug or the wrong dose was given, or if other problems arise.

The ability to swallow comfortably and safely is a crucial prerequisite for oral drug administration, and one that precludes use of this route for neonates, small children, and many elderly, ill, or debilitated patients (unless a nasogastric tube, for example, is used). Even for relatively normal and healthy persons, large tablets and capsules may present difficulties, whether because of insufficient amounts of salivary secretions or problems with coordinating swallowing reflexes. Liquids or powders meant to be dissolved or suspended in liquids may offer additional problems of poor taste, unpleasant consistency, the ability to stain teeth or damage the oral tissues, and more. Still other problems common to oral administration relate to interactions with foods or drugs that may be ingested concomitantly. There are several general ways to minimize these problems, one or more of which may be suitable for a particular medication, dosage form, or patient; they are summarized in Table A–2.

The availability of many drugs in several alternative physical forms for oral administration—tablets, capsules, and liquids, for example—often provides the ability to make appropriate substitutions for patients having problems taking certain formulations. The actual physical form that is used will affect some aspects of administering medications orally. In addition, the shape,

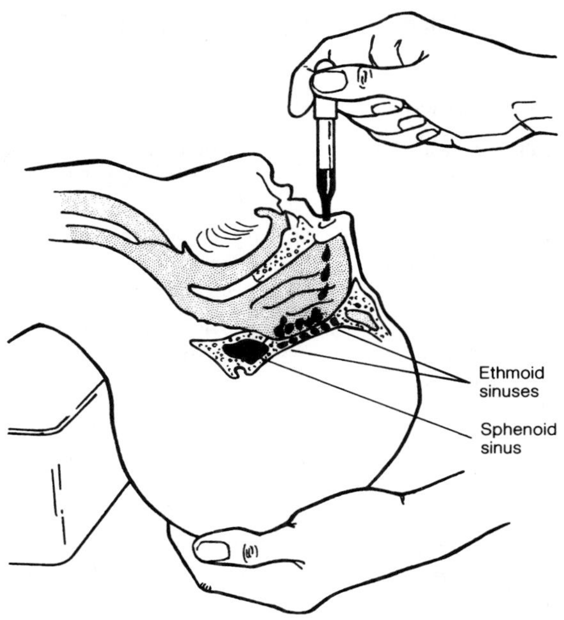

Figure A–1

Placing patient in a back-lying position, with the head over a pillow or edge of the bed on a lower plane (Protez position), helps direct medication towards ethmoid and sphenoid sinuses, maximizes drug action and minimizes contact with and absorption from other sites. Support back of head to avoid straining neck musculature. A simple back-lying position, with the back of the head *on* the plane of the bed, can be used to direct drug to the eustachian tube openings. Do not allow dropper to contact the patient.

(*Source:* Kozier B, Erb G, *Techniques in Clinical Nursing,* 4th ed., p. 846. Addison-Wesley, 1993).

color, size, and other properties of orally administered drugs provide the patient with a relatively easy way to recognize whether the medication has been administered before, if it is being given for the first time, and if the drug being given is the proper one. However it is essential to use the recognizable characteristics of orally administered drugs only as one additional way to determine that the proper agent and dose are being given. Never rely on appearance to the exclusion of other safeguards; never give the drug without other prior checks of the medication order and of the drug itself.

Parenteral Administration

Injectable drugs offer many advantages for situations in which other administration routes are unsuitable. Depending on the drug's formulation, and the method by which it is given, effects may be immediate or of gradual onset, short-lived or longlasting, desirable or unwanted. Although administering an injection eventually becomes a relatively simple task, and is a common nursing responsibility, it should not become so routine that the potential consequences are overlooked or proper technique is compromised. Injections are invasive procedures.

Several general assumptions can be made about parenteral administration compared with other administration routes. More nursing-centered skills and judgments may be needed to ensure that the drug is administered properly, so that the desired effects will occur and unwanted effects will not. Many drugs formulated for administration by other major routes have some inherent safeguards that somewhat reduce the chance that an improper route will be used. For example, it is impossible to inject a tablet or capsule (unless extraordinary and intentional measures are taken to dissolve it first), and highly unlikely that an ointment, cream, or lotion would be swallowed or injected (although clearly such topical products could be applied

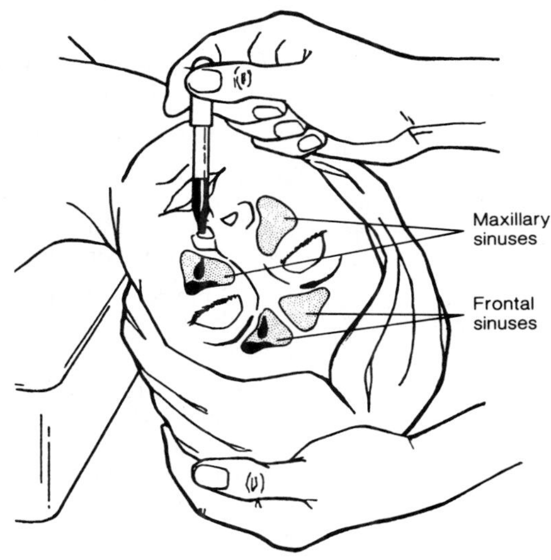

Figure A–2

Maximizing effects on maxillary or frontal sinuses. A position similar to that shown in Figure A–1, but with head turned toward the desired site of drug action (Parkinson position) directs drug to the maxillary and frontal sinuses. After allowing proper time for drug action, rotate head and repeat on the other side if indicated.

(*Source:* Kozier B, Erb G, *Techniques in Clinical Nursing,* 4th ed., p. 846. Addison-Wesley, 1993.

Table A–1 | Potential Problems Associated with Topical Drug Administration

Potential Problem	Solutions
Difficult to measure dose accurately and consistently	As appropriate for drug being used, use ruler or standardized dropper; try to dispense consistent thickness of drug ribbon when dispensing ointment from tube (as with nitroglycerin ointment)
Risk of unwanted systemic effects	Measure carefully to avoid exceeding recommended dose (amount, frequency of administration); follow directions carefully concerning liberal or sparing application of drug to skin or mucous membranes
	If drug is indicated for application to skin, avoid mucous membranes; avoid broken or inflamed skin or membranes unless drug is given specifically for effects on such structures
	With topical ophthalmic drops, use gentle pressure on inner canthus to localize drug effects and minimize systemic absorption
	With nasal instillations (drops or sprays), position patient's head properly to help localize drug to desired area(s) and minimize swallowing drug, which reduces contact with unwanted areas and maximizes desired drug actions (see Figs. A–1 and A–2)
Risk of patient or nursing contamination from drug administration or irrigation	Use nothing less than aseptic technique for applying drug to or irrigating intact, uninfected skin; use sterile technique otherwise; wear gloves as needed
	Use tongue blades for applying ointments or creams, gauze for lotions (plus gloves if there is risk of infection); sterile, disposable administration devices are often preferred
	Do not take multiple-dose containers (eg, stock jars of ointment or cream) used to dispense medication for several patients to patient's bedside; do not use same applicator device (tongue blade, gauze) for both removing drug and applying to patient, especially if the multiple-dose container will be used to dispense medication to more than one patient
	Avoid direct contact between patient and drug-dispensing container
	Advise outpatients not to share drug administration devices (droppers, nasal sprays, oral inhalers, etc)
	Clean droppers from multiple-use containers carefully before reinserting into container (for use by single patient only)
	Discard unused portion of drops in dropper; do not return to container
	For ocular administration or irrigation; clean eyelid and lashes gently with sterile cotton, moistened with sterile saline or irrigation solution, before applying medication or irrigating eye
	With ocular irrigations, position patient's head so that fluid drains away from inner canthus and nasolacrimal duct to reduce absorption, retention of contaminated fluid; irrigate from inner canthus towards outer canthus for same reason; wipe excess fluid in same direction
	When eye cups are being used for ocular irrigation (as for outpatient use), be sure container is clean and edges are smooth
	For otic administration or irrigation: clean pinna and external meatus first
	With otic irrigations, position patient's head to allow for proper fluid drainage, collection into basin; check for intact tympanic membrane, lack of foreign bodies in external ear canal; check for full fluid outflow during irrigation to prevent pressure build-up that might force fluid against or past tympanic membrane; allow fluid to flow and drain by gravity
	For oral inhalers, advise patients using multiple-dose inhalers to clean mouthpiece, spacers, etc., according to manufacturer's directions after each use, and to check for cleanliness before next use
	For vaginal drug administration or irrigation, use sterile supplies and technique for in-hospital procedures, and whenever there is local infection or an open wound. Clean the perineal area to avoid flushing microorganisms into the vagina before administration, and again after the procedure; collect and properly dispose of irrigating solution and other discharge; position properly to avoid drainage from anal, urethral openings toward vagina

Table A–2 | Potential Problems Associated with Oral Drug Administration

Potential Problem	Solutions
Swallowing	Patient should be in sitting position (assist as needed); if not possible, use lateral position; applies to all drugs, patients; minimizes swallowing difficulty, risk of aspiration
	Administer sufficient amount of water, juice, or other suitable beverage as appropriate for drug, patient. Even some liquid dosage forms may be easier to swallow if diluted to about 15 mL before administration
	Have patient suck a few ice chips or sip a small amount of water to moisten oral cavity and throat before administration
	Have patient place medication (solid dosage form) on back of tongue before taking water or other liquid
	Crush tablets and mix with small amount of soft food (eg, applesauce), if permitted. Check package insert before opening capsules for addition to food; ordinarily, capsules, enteric-coated tablets should not be opened or otherwise altered
	Ensure that drug powders (eg, cholestyramine resin, some oral potassium supplements, some laxatives) are fully dissolved or well-suspended in an adequate volume of suitable liquid. This facilitates swallowing and reduces risk of aspiration
	Ensure that tablets meant to be dissolved in liquid (eg, some oral potassium supplements) are dissolved completely before administration
	Identify whether other oral dosage forms that are easier to swallow may be substituted (eg, liquids for tablets or capsules)
	Inquire about use of alternative administration routes (eg, parenteral) if patient cannot safely or easily take oral medication, and other approaches fail
Medication has objectionable taste	Check to determine whether solid dosage form can be substituted
	Give medication with juice or bread, or mix with small amount of soft food, as appropriate, to mask poor taste
	Administer ice chips before giving drug, or ensure that liquid used to help swallow drug is well chilled
Liquid medication is damaging or irritating to teeth, oral tissues (eg, liquid iron- or iodine-containing medications)	Administer medication through a straw
	Have patient drink a glass of water or other suitable beverage after ingesting drug
Drug is causing erratic response or response of lesser- or greater-than-expected intensity	Assess for accidental or purposeful noncompliance; some patients may "cheek" drug or use other measures for intentional noncompliance (particularly problematic with antipsychotic drugs): witness ingestion of each dose to be sure it was swallowed; assess for anticipated short- and long-term drug effects as a way to help ensure drug has been taken; recommend use of acceptable liquid dosage form if intentional noncompliance is suspected or documented with tablets or capsules; a switch to parenteral administration may be necessary for some patients; recruit assistance of family members, other potential caregivers, for noncompliant outpatients
	Assess for use of interacting drugs (eg, antacids) or food; space administration of interacting substances appropriately, advise outpatients to do the same (provide written instructions)
Person self-administering drug has memory or physical problems	Recruit help of a responsible caregiver; modify a calendar with written indications of when drugs are to be taken; have patient mark administrations; recommend dated or compartmentalized containers to facilitate proper administration (made by the nurse, another caregiver, or purchased from commercial sources); have prescriptions dispensed in suitable containers if patient has difficulty opening childproof containers and risk of accidental poisoning by child is low

(continued)

Table A–2 Potential Problems Associated with Oral Drug Administration (*Continued*)

Potential Problem	Solutions
Patient forgets last dose was taken, takes another dose (common with sedatives or hypnotics, especially in elderly or confused patients)	Advise patient to keep medication well away from bedside, and to record in writing that drug was taken at proper time
Medication that must be self-administered during sleeping hours is missed (eg, some antibiotics)	Recommend use of alarm clock if no other caregivers are available
Medication for buccal or sublingual use is taken improperly	Teach proper administration methods, including need to allow tablet to dissolve completely without chewing; to avoid eating, drinking, or smoking while intact tablet is in place
Patient is a child or other person dependent on others for outpatient drug administration	Identify, coordinate roles of caregivers to avoid missed doses, accidental overdoses caused by duplication, and to assess effects of administered drug(s)

to the wrong site). The packaging used for noninjectable drugs also helps guide the administrator towards the proper route. Drugs formulated for injection usually are packaged in ways that help make it obvious that they are to be injected, and information on the label has been prepared carefully to minimize errors. Nevertheless, the containers for parenteral drugs often look alike; so do the substances contained in them, even though pharmacologically, chemically, and in other ways they may be very different. Each much be used in a special, careful way.

A very important problem is that the sites into which a needle is inserted and a drug eventually injected usually cannot be viewed directly. The skin hides the common desired sites for injection—subcutaneous tissues, muscle, and blood vessels—and for any given injection only one of these structures is the appropriate one. In addition, there are nearby nerves, bones, and other structures that must be avoided unless a special procedure is being done. Once a drug has been drawn into a syringe many other techniques must still be used properly, and so there is a great opportunity for more errors. In the best case of inappropriate injection, perhaps, the consequence may be no drug effect at all. In the worst case, the outcome may be fatal. Once a drug has been injected, it is largely irretrievable; the only ways to counteract a medication error may be to inject still other drugs or to impose measures that may be both discomforting to the patient and ineffective.

Nursing responsibilities for parenteral drug administration include not only selecting the right pharmacologic substance (the drug), but also selecting the correct drug formulation (physical form, composition, and concentration) from many potential alternatives. It is often necessary to prepare the drug (as by reconstitution, dilution, admixing, and so on) before use. The nurse has the obligation to identify the precise administration site, which may be affected by many patient-related factors, and to properly select and use administration supplies (needles, syringes, IV tubing, pumps, and so on). Done carefully and correctly, these precautionary measures will help minimize patient discomfort; avoid accidental introduction of drug into improper tissues or body compartments; and avoid tissue damage and infection (hematomas, nerve damage, necrosis and abscesses, extravasation, and so on).

There is also a greater need for the nurse to allay the patient's anxiety about pain, to assess desired and adverse responses closely and often, and to provide other comfort measures. All these considerations emphasize the importance of nursing measures and skillful technique. Many of the pitfalls are summarized in Table A–3. If patients will be self-administering injectable drugs (insulin for diabetes, for example), all the techniques and precautions generally considered to be part of the nurse's domain will have to be taught to them. Table A–4 summarizes typical syringe and needle recommendations for subcutaneous, intramuscular, and intravenous injections. Figures A–3 through A–8 identify some of the common injection sites.

Table A–3 | Potential Problems Associated with Parenteral Drug Administration

Potential Problem	Solutions
Local trauma at or surrounding injection site; other discomfort	Select needle of proper length and bore (gauge) based on administration route, drug, patient-related characteristics (age, muscle mass, amount of local body fat, etc)
	Ensure proper positioning of patient before injecting drug
	Identify alternative injection sites that might be associated with less postinjection pain or tissue damage
	Limit injection volume to amount appropriate for administration route: normally less than 2 mL for SC, less than 5 mL for IM; divide dose over two or more sites if necessary
	Systematically rotate injection sites when repeated injections are anticipated; use anatomic diagram inserted in patient's chart (or provided to outpatients) to facilitate proper sequential injections; when patient has been self-administering drug (eg, insulin), use sites normally inaccessible to patient; teach proper injection technique to outpatients who will be self-administering injections
	Avoid direct injection of cold drugs: allow to warm to room temperature first
	Use Z-track technique or "chase" drug with small air bubble (check agency policies) for IM injection of drugs that might irritate subcutaneous tissues
	Gently massage injection site after administration of most SC injections (except heparin), most IM injections (other than those employing Z-track); do not massage after intradermal injections
	Apply pressure over sites of IV push (bolus) administration to reduce hematoma formation
	Check for blood return into syringe before proceeding with injection; blood return is wanted with IV injections, but not with most other injection routes (eg, SC, IM)
	Depending on drug, suitably dilute when giving IV to avoid phlebitis, thrombosis, etc; inject at proper rate; flush indwelling catheters with sterile saline or other appropriate solution
	Monitor IV infusions for free flow; assess skin color, temperature, tone, distal pulses, for indications of extravasation, diminished blood/drug flow; inquire about adverse subjective responses, such as paresthesias, pain
	Assess injection site for redness, swelling, etc.; provide appropriate comfort measures
Infection, systemic or at injection site	Ensure sterility of drug to be dispensed or injected, and of syringe, needle, other supplies
	Use sterile technique to withdraw, reconstitute, or admix drug, and to administer it
	Select injection site that is free of obvious inflammation, irritation, burning, etc
	Disinfect drug container and injection site with alcohol wipe, other antiseptic (follow agency policy)
Effects appear erratic, excessive, less than expected, etc	Check for consistency of administration methods and dose
	Check expiration date to ensure that product is not outdated
	Ensure adequacy of storage conditions
	Check for proper color, clarity, freedom from precipitate (be aware that many products for parenteral administration are supplied in lightproof or other containers that make direct inspection difficult)
	Check for use of proper drug concentration: be aware that several drugs intended for parenteral use are available in different strengths, each intended for a specific route or use, and labeling may appear similar; double check label, and have label verified by another nurse (check institutional policies)
	Check for use of drug formulation suitable for intended route (eg, solution or suspension, aqueous or in oil, etc)
	Check for presence of additional drugs or additives (eg, epinephrine in local anesthetics, preservatives that might cause allergies in some products) that may be either wanted or contraindicated
	Use diluent supplied or recommended by manufacturer; prepare within allotted time before administration; reconstitute as described by manufacturer: depending on drug techniques for adding diluent and mixing (eg, rolling between the palms or vigorous shaking) will differ

(continued)

Table A–3 Potential Problems Associated with Parenteral Drug Administration (*Continued*)

Potential Problem	Solutions
	Check for physical, chemical compatibility before mixing drugs, adding drugs to IV fluid infusions; observe for changes in color, clarity, even when allegedly compatible substances are mixed; be aware that some drugs may be compatible but only for a limited time; be sure drug is administered within allotted time after preparation, mixing, etc.
	Check for compatibility, interactions between drug and administration device(s): for example, no plastic should contact paraldehyde solutions; avoid polyvinylchloride tubing sets with IV nitroglycerin: use IV sets provided by manufacturer, or be prepared to adjust dosage for drug binding to standard PVC sets
	Ensure that drug is not being injected into scarred, underperfused, or otherwise abnormal area
	Consider need for alternative injection site for same injection technique, or need to switch to other parenteral route
	Aspirate before injecting drugs not meant to be given IV; conversely, with intended IV injections, ensure return of venous blood before giving drug
	Select a syringe having a size appropriate for the anticipated total dose of drug; needlessly large syringes increase the measuring error
	Use calibrated pump with audible flow alarm for IV infusion of most drugs, especially when drug is potent, unusually toxic, has very short half-life, or patient is critically ill; do not rely on pump or its alarm as a way to lessen need for direct monitoring
	Check for use of interacting drugs, including pharmacologic or physiologic antagonists, incompatible substances
	Recommend specific syringes or injection aids to outpatients who must self-administer injections (eg, of insulin), especially if they have physical or visual impairments that might hinder administration of proper doses; teach essential aspects of administration techniques

Table A–4 Injection Site, Syringe, and Needle Recommendations for Common Parenteral Administration Methods

	Subcutaneous	Intramuscular	Intravenous
Common injection sites	Outer aspect of upper arm; anterior aspect of thighs; rotate systematically for repeated injections; see Figure A–3	Ventrogluteal (von Hochstetter's site): suitable because of relative lack of large nerves, blood vessels, fat; suitable for most age groups; see Figure A–4 Vastus lateralis; suitably thick and well developed in most adults, children; lacking major vessels and nerves; middle third of muscle preferred; see Figure A–5	Suitable, accessible peripheral vein for most injections, infusions (eg, cephalic or cubital vein of arm; dorsal vein of hand); when possible for ambulatory or conscious patient, and when not contraindicated, ask for patient's preference (eg, dominant or nondominant limb), avoid needless restrictions of ambulation, range of motion; for some critically ill patients requiring invasive monitoring, some highly irritating drugs, a central vein (eg, subclavian) may be required; always check agency policies concerning who may administer IV drugs and/or establish IV access; see Figure A–9
Alternative sites	Abdomen; ventrodorsal gluteal areas; scapular areas of upper back	Rectus femoris: convenient for self-administration, but injections tend to be painful; often reserved for infants, children, adults when other sites are contraindicated Dorsogluteal site: often convenient but also more difficult to locate, therefore less preferred; see Figure A–6	

(continued)

Table A–4 | Injection Site, Syringe, and Needle Recommendations for Common Parenteral Administration Methods (*Continued*)

	Subcutaneous	Intramuscular	Intravenous
Syringe		Deltoid: seldom preferred, is close to radial nerve, artery; see Figure A–7	
	Typically 2 mL or less	2 mL to 5 mL	If used, depends on volume of drug or fluid to be administered (nominally 5 or 10 mL for most intermittent injections; may be as large as 50 or 60 mL for such drugs as diazoxide given for acute blood pressure control)
Needle size and lengths	Typically 25 gauge Adults: Usually ⅝" for injections at 45-degree angle, ½" for 90-degree injections (or one half the width of a skin fold, if that method is used) Obese adults: May need up to 1" Children: Usually ⅜"	Adults: Large muscles (eg, gluteus medius): 20–23 gauge, ¼"–3"; small muscles (eg, deltoid): 23–25 gauge, ½"–1" Children: 22–25 gauge, ⅝"–1" may be suitable Oily suspensions generally require thicker needle	Typically 20 or 21 gauge × 1" or 1½" (or indwelling IV catheter for infusions, repeated IV injections); larger bore needles may be indicated for viscous drugs, large volumes that must be injected quickly, whole blood or blood cell fractions
Precautions	Aspirate before injecting to avoid accidental IV injection; massage gently after injecting to disperse, facilitate absorption of drug (except heparin or intradermal injections)	Aspirate before injecting; massage gently after injecting	Assess for free blood backflow (or draw back on syringe) before injecting or infusing Monitor for solution flow rate, distal pulses, skin color and temperature, etc, during infusions Use volume control device (eg, VOLUTROL), flow regulator, or infusion pump as needed or required by agency policy
Special techniques or considerations	*Heparin:* Avoid highly vascular or muscular areas to reduce hematoma risk, alterations in drug absorption rates; use ½", 25 or 26 gauge needle, 90-degree angle *Insulin:* See Chapter 46 (Fig. 46–2) for suggested injection sites, rotation patterns Intradermal (intracutaneous) injections generally use tuberculin syringe, 25 gauge × ½" needle; inject only small volumes (eg, 0.1 mL); common sites include inner lower arm, upper chest, subscapular region (see Fig. A–8); do not massage site upon needle removal	Methods to reduce damage to subcutaneous tissues upon IM injection include Z-track technique, inclusion of 0.2 mL of air in syringe to clear drug from needle, reduce risk of drug backleakage (often preferred for diphtheria, tetanus, pertussis vaccinations, singly or in combination); avoid massaging after injection of irritating drugs by these methods	Consult agency policies, other texts, for information about adding drugs to IV fluid in bottle or bag, use of piggyback technique or secondary IV set, need for inline filters, etc

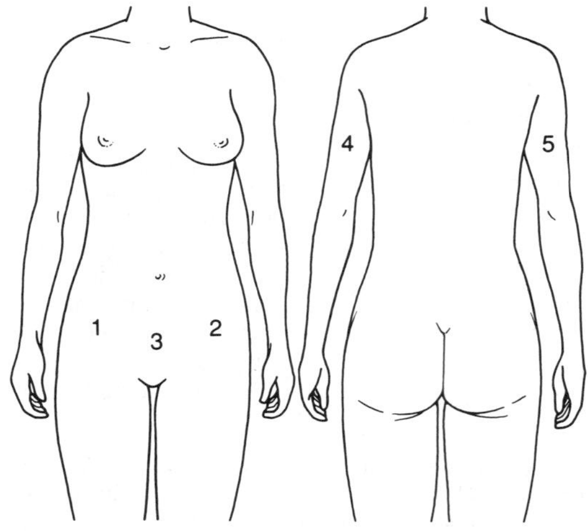

Figure A–3

Common subcutaneous injection sites. Limit injection volume to no more than 2 mL; a 25 gauge × ½ in. or ⅝ in. needle is generally used, depending on injection site and patient-related factors (eg, age, local body fat, etc.). See Fig. 46–2 for an injection site rotation sequence for insulin.

(*Source:* Alfaro-LeFevre R, Blicharz ME, Flynn NM, Boyer MJ, *Drug Handbook, A Nursing Process Approach,* p 12. Addison-Wesley, 1992).

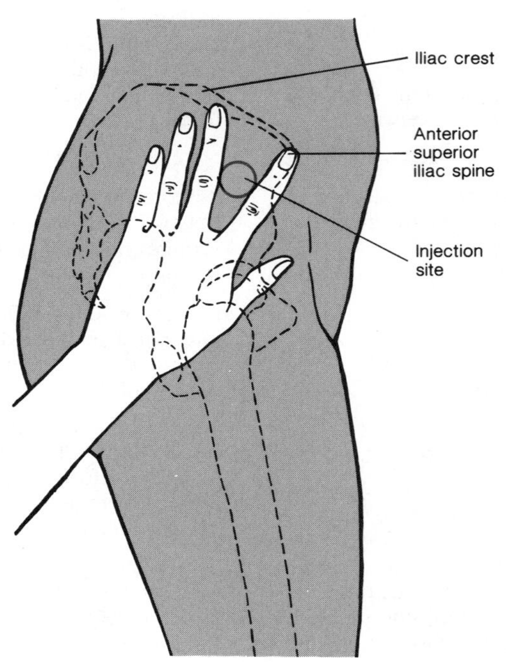

Figure A–4

Ventrogluteal (von Hochstetter's) site for IM injections is suitable for persons in most age groups, has relative lack of large nerves, blood vessels, and fat nearby. The patient's position can be a back- or side-lying position with the knee and hip flexed to relax the gluteal muscles.

(*Source:* Kozier B, Erb G, *Techniques in Clinical Nursing,* 3rd ed., p. 519. Addison-Wesley, 1989.)

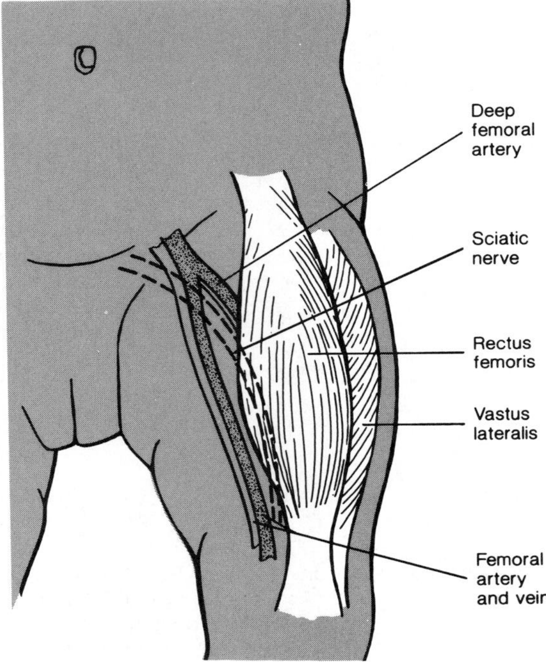

Figure A–5

The vastus lateralis and rectus femoris sites for IM injection. The vastus lateralis is preferred for infants because of its relative lack of nearby large blood vessels and nerves. The preferred site is the middle third of the muscle. The patient can be in a sitting or back-lying position. The rectus femoris is easy to reach for persons who self-administer IM injections, but the injections may be painful.

(*Source:* Kozier B, Erb G, *Techniques in Clinical Nursing,* 4th ed., p. 870, Addison-Wesley, 1993.)

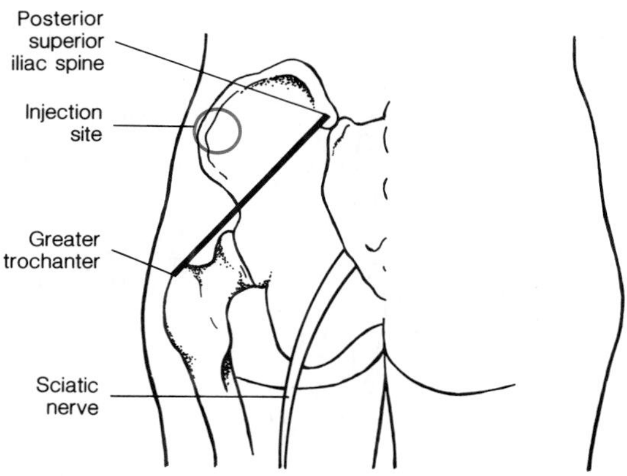

Figure A–6

The dorsogluteal site for IM injections is losing favor because of the difficulty involved in locating it accurately. Palpate the posterior superior iliac spine, then draw an imaginary line to the greater trochanter of the femur. The injection site will be lateral and superior to this line, well away from the sciatic nerve. The patient should be prone, with the toes pointing medially, or side-lying with the upper leg flexed at the thigh and knee and placed in front of the lower leg.

(*Source:* Kozier B, Erb G, *Techniques in Clinical Nursing,* 4th ed., p. 870. Addison-Wesley, 1993.)

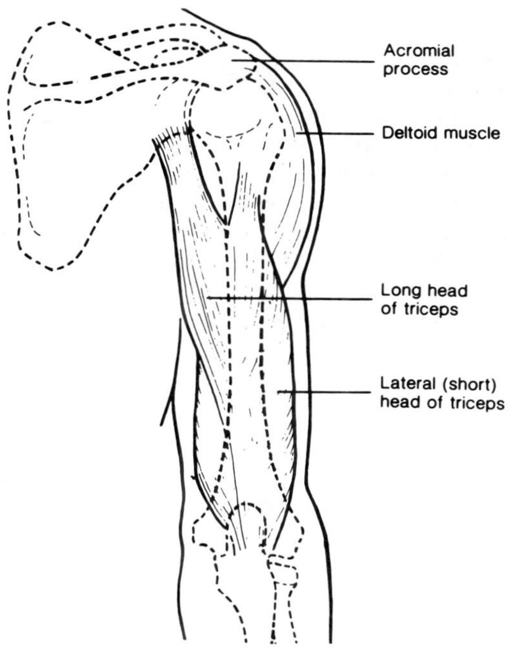

Figure A–7

The deltoid site for IM injections (posterior view of upper right arm). The deltoid is found on the lateral aspect of the arm. It is not used often because the muscle is relatively small and it is near the radial artery and nerve.

(*Source:* Modified from Kozier B, Erb G, *Techniques in Clinical Nursing,* 3rd ed., p. 521. Addison-Wesley, 1989.)

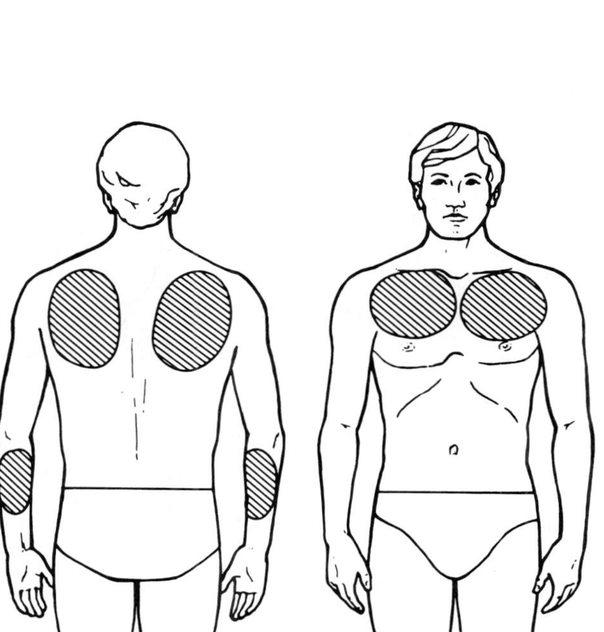

Figure A–8

Common intradermal (intracutaneous) injection sites. Intradermal injections are often used for administering vaccines or for allergy or tuberculin testing. Use a tuberculin syringe to measure and inject the small volumes that are administered—typically, 0.1 mL. To minimize pain and to avoid injecting into subcutaneous structures, a 25 gauge × ½ in. needle is generally used. Do not massage the site after withdrawing the needle.

(*Source:* Kozier B, Erb G, *Techniques in Clinical Nursing,* 4th ed., p. 864. Addison-Wesley, 1993.)

Figure A–9

Common venipuncture sites on the ventral surface of the arm, and dorsal surfaces of the hand and foot. These sites are best used for adolescents and adults. Infants do not have large veins in the antecubital fossa. Veins in the temporal scalp region, or the dorsal surfaces of the hand or foot, usually are used for prolonged IV infusions.

(*Source:* Modified from Kozier B, Erb G, *Fundamentals of Nursing,* 4th ed., p. 1064. Addison-Wesley, 1991.)

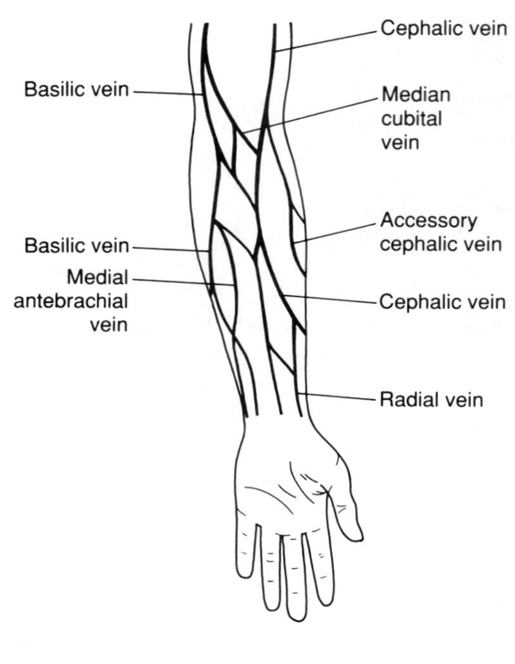

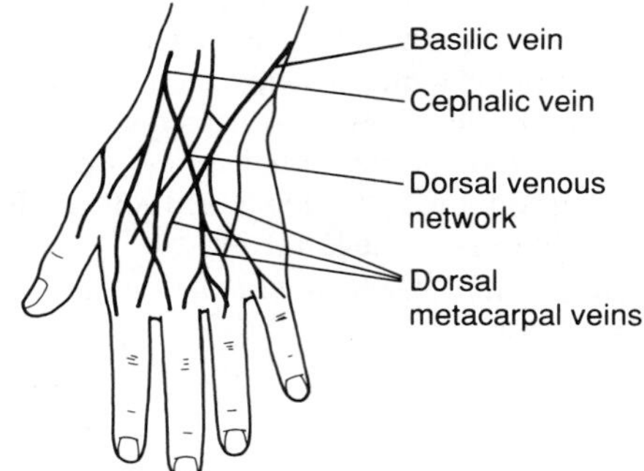

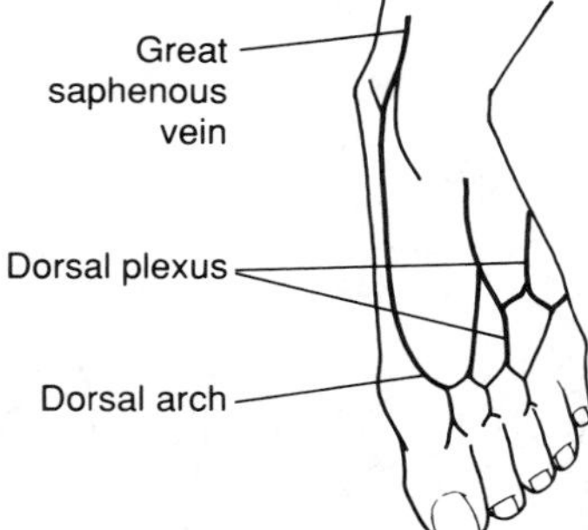

APPENDIX

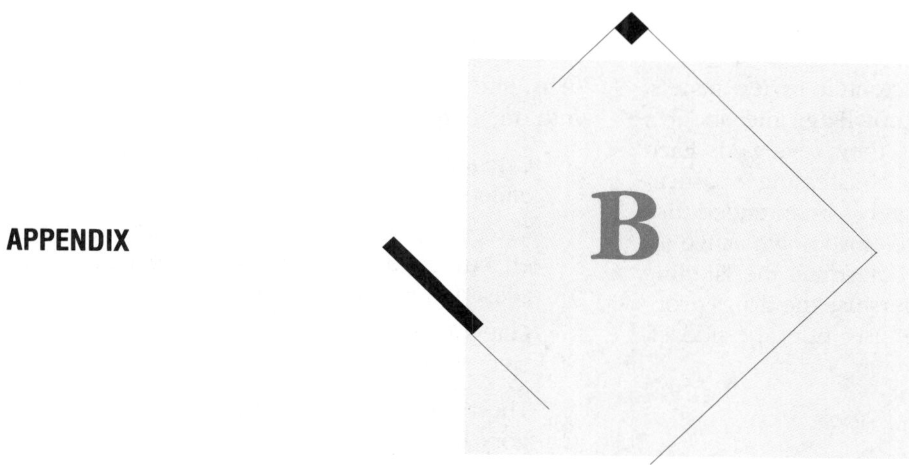

Over-the-Counter Drugs

Drugs available without prescription allow us to obtain, at relatively low cost, pharmacologically active substances to treat a variety of illness symptoms. They offer many advantages to consumers. However, if they are used improperly, they may cause several significant problems.

This appendix reviews the major classes of over-the-counter (OTC) drugs that have been discussed in the text. The discussion is limited to drugs or products that are taken orally or administered in another way, such as topically or by inhalation, that are likely to cause appreciable systemic absorption and, therefore, possible adverse responses. It identifies some of their potential advantages and risks, highlights the major active substances found in representative products (without specifying brand names), and summarizes the major disease or drug-related contraindications that are likely to apply.

The information should be useful for the nurse in the role of patient teaching, and should also help the nurse be a more knowledgeable consumer of nonprescription drugs.

Regulation and Evaluation of Nonprescription Drugs

Over-the-counter drugs, and the advertising claims made for them, are regulated by federal agencies. The two major criteria that any drug or product must meet—efficacy and safety—apply to prescription and OTC drugs alike. There are sufficient safeguards concerning effectiveness and safety that individuals in otherwise normal health may benefit from taking some of these drugs.

According to amendments to the 1938 Food, Drug, and Cosmetic Act, OTC drugs must be safe. In 1962 the Kefauver–Harris amendment mandated that prescription drugs must be both safe and effective. In 1972 the Food and Drug Administration (FDA), concerned with OTC drug safety and efficacy, contracted with the National Academy of Science/National Research Council (NAS/NRC) to review available drugs. NAS/NRC initially reviewed over 500 OTC drugs, and concluded that only about 15% could be judged effective. Later reviews of all available OTC drug preparations, of which there were an estimated half a million, indicated that they contained, over all, about 800 "active" ingredients.

Since a more complete review appeared to be essential, the FDA established 26 scientific review panels, each staffed by professionals knowledgeable about a particular group of drugs that they reviewed. Each panel was charged with the task of assessing a particular group of drugs, based largely on intended use (Table B–1), to identify standards for known active ingredients. Another goal was to determine the labeling that was needed to help consumers use the drugs properly (indications, directions for use, relevant side effects, and contraindications). The panels placed drugs into one of three categories:

Category I: drugs judged to be both safe and effective;

Category II: drugs judged to be *either* unsafe *or* ineffective, and which should not be included in nonprescription products; and

Category III: drugs for which there were insufficient data to judge safety or efficacy.

The panels indicated that products with drugs in Category II should be either removed from the market or reformulated so that only ingredients falling in Category I were available to the public. Interestingly, to comply with guidelines manufacturers can change the formulation of an OTC product, such as by deleting certain ingredients and replacing them with others, without changing the brand name. This often leads to confusion for both the health-care provider and the user. It also makes it essential for health-care providers to stay up to date by consulting frequently updated information sources, such as *Drug Facts & Comparisons.*

Some of the review panels also recommended that certain prescription drugs be reclassified so that they could be sold without prescription. Often, such recommendations have generated considerable controversy from the health-care community, consumer protection groups, the FDA, and even from members of the review panels. It will be important for the nurse to keep abreast of similar recommendations in the future, as more drugs become available to the public without prescription.

It is important to understand that the opinions of regulatory panels are not universally accepted. Some authorities claim that fewer than one third of available drugs (an even smaller fraction of drug *products*) meet both effectiveness and safety claims.

Table B–1 | FDA Over-the-Counter Dug Categories

Allergy treatment products (internal)*
Analgesics-antipyretics (internal)*
Antacids* and antiflatulents
Antidiarrheal products*
Antimicrobials
Antiperspirants
Antiarthritic products (see also analgesics, internal)*
Antitussives*
Bronchodilator/antiasthma products*
Cold remedies, decongestants*
Contraceptive products
Dandruff products
Dentifrices and other dental products (eg, analgesics, antiseptics)
Dermatologic products, miscellaneous
Emetics* and antiemetics
Hematinics
Hemorrhoidal products
Laxatives and cathartics*
Ophthalmic products
Oral hygiene drug products
Sleep aids and sedatives*
Stimulants*
Sunburn prevention/treatment products
Vitamin-mineral supplements*
Weight-loss aids*
Miscellaneous products (all OTC products not covered above)

*Drug categories denoted with an asterisk are discussed in Table B-3.

Implications for Nurses and Patients of Nonprescription Drug Availability and Use

Over-the-counter drugs offer an effective and convenient way to manage the symptoms of various illnesses. If comparable prescription drugs are available, an OTC preparation may also be much less costly. Judicious self-prescribing of an OTC drug for a simple malady may prevent the costs associated with a physician visit. Nevertheless, billions of dollars are spent on OTC drugs each year, much of that needlessly. Perhaps millions more are spent on medical therapy to undo the adverse effects of OTC drugs that are inappropriately administered.

Despite the existence of guidelines concerning OTC drugs, some products may do little more than no drug treatment at all. Indeed, for some medical problems, no-drug treatment is often the cheapest and safest approach to alleviating discomfort.

Some OTC products contain active ingredients with proven effectiveness, but the doses are generally considered to be subtherapeutic if the manufacturer's recommendations are followed. (Often, they are not.)

More important, however, is that virtually any OTC product has the potential to cause great harm to certain individuals. At one extreme, the negative aspects of purchasing and using an OTC drug may be no more than wasting money. At the other extreme, use of such a drug may place the individual at needless risk.

Several problems can be identified (Table B–2). In each case at least one nursing intervention can be used to prevent or remedy the problem. All these interventions rely on a solid knowledge of pharmacology and fundamental therapeutic principles: administration of the right drug, to the right patient, at the right time, in the right dose, and with the right administration route.

Encourage the consumer to contact the physician or pharmacist if there is any doubt about the applicability of a general recommendation. By demonstrating knowledge about OTC drug action and use, the nurse also serves as a good role model for others.

Table B–3 summarizes information about some of the major OTC drug groups.

Table B–2 | Problems Associated with OTC Drug Use

Problem	Nursing Intervention
Ingredients in OTC products may interact with other medications, whether prescribed by a physician or self-prescribed.	Discourage use of more than one OTC product unless under a physician's supervision. Recommend use of single-ingredient OTC products. Provide patients taking prescription drugs with explicit written lists of OTC drugs to avoid.
OTC drugs are contraindicated for patients with certain diseases, one or more of which may be unknown to the patient.	Provide written lists of OTC drugs to avoid.
The self-prescribing individual may, because of improper "diagnosis," use a drug that is inappropriate for the symptoms to be alleviated.	Inquire about the nature of symptoms so proper OTC drug, if indicated, may be selected. Help the individual understand the meaning of terms written on package labels.
The presence of "inactive" substances in an OTC product, such as alcohol, dyes, or preservatives, may cause adverse effects or interactions.	Become familiar with ingredients in OTC drugs. Since it is impossible to be aware of the active ingredients, diluents, or preservatives in all OTC drugs, have access to a current drug guide, and rely on the help of a pharmacist.
Self-prescribing OTC drugs may prevent an individual from seeking, or seeking soon enough, professional diagnosis of and treatment for a disorder that may be potentially serious.	Ask the individual to describe symptoms for which a drug is being taken. If the condition sounds serious, or if you have pertinent knowledge of the patient's history, recommend immediate medical evaluation. In general, if a product does not provide noticeable relief within 2 days of administration (as directed on the package label), advise consulting a physician.
OTC drugs may mask or alter symptoms of serious underlying problems, making professional diagnosis more difficult. They may increase the risk of surgical or drug therapy that would be relatively safe without the OTC product, or therapy that could be altered or delayed if drug intake were known.	Ask specifically about OTC drug use when taking a patient's history.
Symptoms may disappear spontaneously. Relief *in spite of* the drug can be misinterpreted as relief *because of* the drug; or, the placebo effect may occur. Such responses could foster further and needless use of a useless (or potentially dangerous) substance.	Provide knowledgeable but understandable information about the ability of a particular drug to alter symptoms. Teach patients that some disorders, such as the common cold or infrequent and acute diarrhea or constipation, resolve without drug therapy. Teach nondrug approaches that alleviate common, infrequent disorders.

(continued)

Table B–2 Problems Associated with OTC Drug Use (*Continued*)

Problem	Nursing Intervention
True relief may be obtained with use of a particular multiingredient OTC product. In reality, however, relief may be due to a single ingredient; the others are useless.	Knowledge of the single effective ingredient enables the consumer to buy the proper single-ingredient product, usually saving money and reducing the risk of interactions or adverse effects of other agents. Recommend a single-entity product that contains that ingredient.
An individual may self-administer more than one OTC product, perhaps products indicated for different purposes. Each product may share a common ingredient. Therefore, even if recommended doses of each product are taken, combined use may lead to inadvertent overdose of the common ingredient.	Discourage multiple-drug use. Help the individual select single-ingredient products to reduce the risk of ingesting the same active ingredient in several forms.
Extra money is spent buying a brand-name product, usually one that is vigorously advertised, rather than an equally effective store brand.	Advise individuals that there is little hard evidence to indicate that brand-name products are better than store brands.
The availability of a drug or product in the home exposes others, particularly small children, to risks of adverse effects or toxicity.	Advise persons with small children to buy no more drug than is likely to be needed for a couple of days. Recommend that all drugs be kept out of sight and reach of children. Encourage adults to inform children that medicines are not candy. When possible, purchase drugs packaged in child-proof containers.
Individuals often feel that if the recommended dose is effective, increasing the dose or the frequency of drug use will provide greater or faster relief.	Explain the importance of taking drugs as recommended on the label.
Individuals often select the proper pharmacologic agent, but not a formulation that is administered by the safest route.	If symptoms (eg, relief of nasal congestion) can be alleviated through local effects of a drug, teach patients that this route carries the lowest risk of adverse effects (eg, nasal spray or drops are preferred to orally administered drug), and so is preferred.
Individuals may consider that preparations of a particular drug that look alike are identical.	Some drugs, such as acetaminophen pediatric drops and elixirs, look similar but differ dramatically in terms of drug strength per volume. Provide explicit instructions to the person using or administering the drug about which product to use or give, and about which not to use. Acknowledging that two medicines that look alike are indeed different may help avoid confusion and a serious error.

Table B–3 | OTC Drug Ingredients, Side Effects, and General Contraindications

Typical Ingredient(s)	Chapter Reference	Common Side Effects	Major Contraindications	Major Drug Interactants	Comments
			Allergy Treatment Products (Internal)		
Antihistamines (eg, chlorpheniramine, diphenhydramine)	51	Dry mouth; blurred vision; photophobia; mild constipation; tachycardia; urinary retention	Glaucoma; prostatic hypertrophy; constipation or paralytic ileus; tachycardia; asthma	Other antimuscarinics; CNS depressants; MAO inhibitors; sympathomimetics	Periodic use may be acceptable for relief of seasonal allergy symptoms
Sympathomimetic decongestants (eg, phenylpropanolamine)	14	CNS stimulation; tachycardia or arrhythmias; hypertension; photophobia; hyperglycemia	Hypertension or tachycardia of any cause; glaucoma; pheochromocytoma	Antihypertensive drugs; MAO inhibitors; thyroid hormone supplements; insulin	Products containing only antihistamine preferred if symptoms known to be caused by allergic reaction; also see decongestants, below
			Analgesics–Antipyretics (Internal)		
Acetaminophen	52	Hepatotoxicity if excessive doses taken acutely or chronically	Hepatic dysfunction; OTC drug and alcohol abuse		Improper use, toxicity common; teach patient to follow label dosage instructions; recommend as preferred alternative to aspirin or ibuprofen for relief of pain or fever in persons for whom aspirin is contraindicated; acknowledge lack of anti-inflammatory activity; advise that inexpensive products are equieffective to expensive brand-name products; evaluate all suspected or known overdoses in hospital
Aspirin	52	Increased bleeding time (all doses); salicylism if high doses used; elevated serum uric acid levels	History of aspirin allergy; asthma; bleeding tendencies; gout or asymptomatic hyperuricemia; pregnancy, especially near term	Potentiates action of most highly protein-bound drugs, especially oral anticoagulants, hypoglycemics; antagonizes action of uricosuric drugs	Improper use, toxicity is common; teach pertinent side effects of interacting drugs, need to follow label doses; indicate that all products containing any form of aspirin are contraindicated as noted at left; cost-effectiveness relation noted for acetaminophen applies to aspirin; evaluate all suspected or known overdoses in hospital
Ibuprofen	52	See aspirin	See aspirin	See aspirin	See aspirin; cost-effectiveness relationship for various ibuprofen products same as for aspirin products; may be more effective for relief of dysmenorrhea; user should not exceed label dose without physician's approval; evaluate known or suspected overdoses in hospital

(continued)

Table B–3 | OTC Drug Ingredients, Side Effects, and General Contraindications (*Continued*)

Typical Ingredient(s)	Chapter Reference	Common Side Effects	Major Contraindications	Major Drug Interactants	Comments
			Antacids		
Usually contain aluminum and magnesium salts (single-ingredient antacids seldom appropriate when antacids are indicated)	40	Depends on composition of product: chronic use may cause hypophosphatemia, hypercalcemia, or osteomalacia owing to aluminum; risk of hypermagnesemia in persons with poor renal function; variable risk of constipation or diarrhea; sodium overload, heart failure, edema, hypertension unless product is sodium-poor or -free	Heart failure; edema; hypertension (for sodium-rich products taken frequently in high doses)	Reduced absorption of most orally administered drugs	Infrequent use generally safe in absence of contraindications, interacting drugs; use for ulcers should be supervised by physician
Calcium carbonate	40	Constipation; hypercalcemia; urinary calcium stones	Obstructive bowel disease; renal dysfunction, stones; hypercalcemia; most cardiovascular diseases	Reduces absorption of many other orally administered drugs, especially tetracycline antibiotics	Avoid frequent use of products containing only calcium as antacids; use as calcium supplements (eg, postmenopausal) is controversial
Magnesium salts (eg, milk of magnesia)	40, 41	Diarrhea, fluid and electrolyte loss; loss of spontaneous bowel function with habitual use; hypermagnesemia in patients with poor renal function	Preexisting diarrhea, fluid or electrolyte imbalances; renal failure; gut obstruction or perforation	Reduces absorption of many other orally administered drugs	Discourage routine or high-dose use; use of antacids containing magnesium alone is generally irrational; use for infrequent constipation seldom necessary
Sodium bicarbonate	40	Hypernatremia, increased blood pressure, edema, aggravation of heart failure; acid rebound	See side effects	Increased sodium load counteracts effects of antihypertensives, digitalis, diuretics	Discourage use; use for peptic ulcer disease generally irrational
			Antidiarrheal Products		
Kaolin + pectin; bismuth salts	41	Loss of spontaneous bowel function, constipation if used excessively		Increased or decreased absorption of many drugs given orally	Mild, infrequent diarrhea best left untreated or managed first by dietary changes

(continued)

Table B–3 OTC Drug Ingredients, Side Effects, and General Contraindications (*Continued*)

Typical Ingredient(s)	Chapter Reference	Common Side Effects	Major Contraindications	Major Drug Interactants	Comments
			Antiarthritic Products		
Oral: Aspirin, ibuprofen	52	See analgesics–antipyretics			
Topical: Methyl salicylate	52	Local irritation, burning, erythema at site of application; salicylate toxicity if ingested	Broken or abraded skin		May provide temporary symptomatic relief of minor musculoskeletal discomfort (eg, sprains); efficacy in true rheumatic condition doubtful; limit to infrequent, sparing use; discourage purchase of pure methyl salicylate (oil of wintergreen), which is highly toxic (4 mL lethal dose for children); evaluate all cases of oral ingestion in hospital
			Antitussives		
Antihistamines	51	See allergy treatment products			
Dextromethorphan	21				May be useful if cough is nonproductive or interferes with rest, sleep; prolonged cough or cough accompanied by dark or bloody sputum requires evaluation by physician
Sympathomimetics	14	See allergy treatment products			Allegedly work by reducing nasal secretions that trigger cough; questionable value
			Bronchodilator/Antiasthma Products		
Antihistamines	38, 51	See allergy treatment products; may worsen breathing problems owing to mucus plugging (anticholinergic action)			OTC products lack efficacy, safety; discourage use, recommend treatment by physician
Sympathomimetic bronchodilators	14, 38	See allergy treatment products			Questionable efficacy and safety of some oral OTC products; OTC epinephrine inhalers safe, effective if used as directed by physician

(continued)

Table B–3 | **OTC Drug Ingredients, Side Effects, and General Contraindications (*Continued*)**

Typical Ingredient(s)	Chapter Reference	Common Side Effects	Major Contraindications	Major Drug Interactants	Comments
			Cold Remedies, Decongestants		
Antihistamines	51	See allergy treatment products			May provide subjective relief; histamine thought to play no role in cold symptoms
Antimuscarinics	13	See bronchodilator/antiasthma products—antihistamines	Rhinitis		Best symptomatic relief, lowest risk of side effects, interactions, when long-acting sympathomimetic nasal sprays used; single-ingredient products preferred; discourage use of oral sympathomimetics
Sympathomimetic decongestants	14, 38	See allergy treatment products; rebound nasal congestion, rhinitis medicamentosa with nasal drops or sprays	Rhinitis		
			Emetics		
Syrup of ipecac	42	Aspiration of vomitus; hypotension, thready pulse, other expected consequences of vomiting; cardiac damage with frequent or high-dose use	Unconscious or semiconscious individual; ingestion of corrosive or volatile poisons		Syrup of ipecac should be in first-aid kit in all homes; instruct proper use; advise that any situation requiring emetic administration be followed by thorough professional evaluation of patient; discourage frequent use; excessive use may indicate anorexia nervosa, bulimia
			Laxatives and Cathartics		
All	41	Loss of spontaneous bowel function with chronic use; risk of laxative-antidiarrheal cycle	Gut obstruction, perforation, weakness of gut wall	Reduced absorption, effect of most other drugs given orally	Advise dietary modification for most cases of constipation (eg, adequate daily fluid intake, adding bulk-forming or fibrous food to diet); have patient report prolonged constipation (>2 days), abdominal pain, bloody or tarry stool, at once
Milk of magnesia, citrate of magnesia	41	See antacids—magnesium salts	See antacids	See antacids	Discourage frequent or prolonged use; have patient report GI pain at once; recommend taking product with ample water; discourage bedtime use to avoid sleep interference

(continued)

Table B–3 | OTC Drug Ingredients, Side Effects, and General Contraindications (*Continued*)

Typical Ingredient(s)	Chapter Reference	Common Side Effects	Major Contraindications	Major Drug Interactants	Comments
Bisacodyl, senna, phenolphthalein, other stimulants or irritants	41	See milk of magnesia	See milk of magnesia	GI irritation when antacids taken with enteric-coated bisacodyl tablets; reduced absorption of other drugs taken orally	See milk of magnesia
Docusate sodium, most other stool softeners	41	GI pain; fecal impactions	Dysphagia; others as for milk of magnesia	Reduced absorption of most other orally effective drugs; increased risk of toxicity of other laxatives taken simultaneously	Advise patient to mix product well with full glass of water; avoid frequent use or use with other laxatives
Mineral oil	41	Liquid pneumonitis from inhalation of liquid; anal irritation		Reduced absorption of most other orally effective drugs; reduced absorption of fat-soluble vitamins (A, D, E, K)	Discourage use without physician's approval; risk of aspiration probably greatest in very young children, the elderly, debilitated persons, persons with dysphagia
			Sleep Aids and Sedatives		
Antihistamines	22, 51	See allergy treatment products			Questionable efficacy if recommended doses used; teach nondrug aids to sleep (eg, avoiding late meals or use of alcohol, stimulants; value of reading or other quieting activity)
			Stimulants		
Caffeine	27	Nervousness, anxiety, insomnia, irritability; dyspepsia; tachycardia; fluid loss from diuresis	Peptic ulcer disease; tachycardia or cardiac arrhythmias of any cause; diabetes mellitus	May increase risk of toxicity in persons taking methylxanthines (eg, theophylline) for asthma	Use of stimulant drug products, even short-term, seldom justified; discourage exceeding recommended dose
			Vitamin Supplements		
Vitamin B_6 (pyridoxine)	61		Therapy of parkinsonism with levodopa or SINEMET	Stimulates peripheral metabolism, reduces efficacy of levodopa; counteracts effects of carbidopa in SINEMET; physician can prescribe LAROBEC (B_6-free multivitamin) if necessary	Advise persons with parkinsonism who are taking interacting drugs to avoid B_6 in all forms and products
			Weight-Loss Aids		
Phenylpropanolamine	14, 27	See allergy treatment products—sympathomimetics	See allergy treatment products	See allergy treatment products	Discourage long-term use, explain simplest and safest weight-loss principle: reduce calorie intake, increase physical activity, maintain good nutritional state; advise patient to seek professional advice if goal is to lose >20 pounds or >15% of current weight

APPENDIX

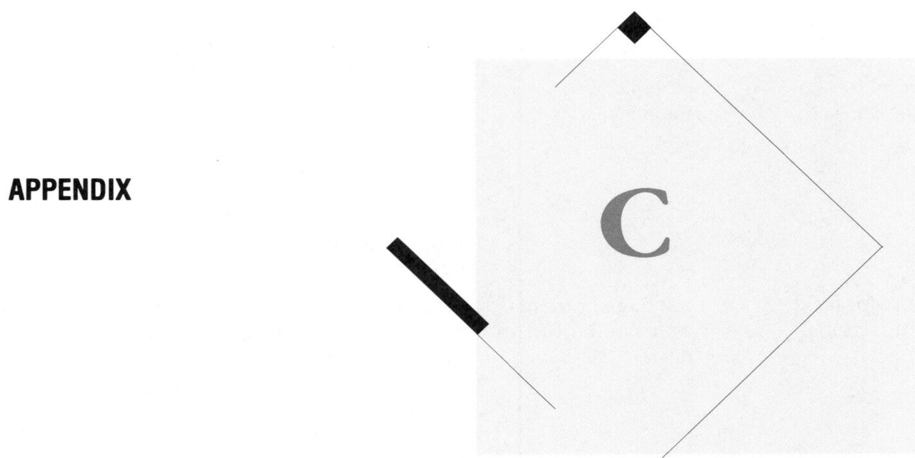

Management of Poisoning Emergencies

The saying "An ounce of prevention is worth a pound of cure" has never held more meaning than in reference to poisoning. In 1990, poison centers throughout the United States handled nearly 1.75 million poisoning exposures (Litovitz et al.: *Am J Emerg Med* 1991; 9: 461–507), of which only about 10% were intentional poisonings. Those numbers do not reflect the true magnitude of the problem, because most poisonings are not reported to poison centers that participate in periodic data collection and analysis. Statistics also show that with prompt recognition and skilled intervention, the risk of death from accidental poisonings can be relatively low.

Poisoning data provide insight into where the major problems lie, and where educational emphasis should be directed. Nearly 80% of poisonings, and a large percentage of fatalities, involve ingestion of a substance. Surprisingly, perhaps, most poison exposures involve ingestion of only a single substance, most frequently cleaning agents, analgesics, plants, and cosmetics. Most of these substances are found in or near the home, which is the most common site of poisoning. Fatalities are most often related to ingestion of antidepressant drugs, analgesics, sedative-hypnotics, street drugs, and to inhalation of carbon monoxide. Although the victims of poisoning are most likely to be children, the incidence of poisoning in the elderly is growing.

Nursing Interventions

Some nurses have the opportunity to care for poisoned individuals. All nurses should share with other health-care professionals and agencies the need to educate the public to prevent poisonings, especially those that are accidental. It appears that it is difficult for the public to comprehend the dangers, so educational efforts take on increased importance. Encourage parents or guardians of small children to survey their homes for hazardous substances stored in unsafe locations (eg, cleaning supplies, medications, automotive products, insecticides and pesticides, vitamins, and cosmetics); all medications should be stored in childproof containers, preferably in places that are locked or inaccessible to inquisitive children. Even alcoholic beverages, which have caused fatal poisonings in young children who have ingested only small amounts, should be stored properly. Tobacco products are also highly toxic for small children, and should be kept out of their reach.

Another important nursing intervention is thorough education of patients about the medications they are taking, whether prescribed by a physician or self-prescribed. This should include both written and verbal instructions about the proper use of prescription and nonprescription drugs, the anticipated beneficial effects, and information about adverse effects that require prompt notification of a health-care provider, emergency department, 911, or a poison center. Such teaching can reduce the incidence or dangers of poisoning owing to drug misuse, which can be defined as improper use of a substance when therapeutic or beneficial effects were intended.

Common examples of misuse include administration of a drug for the wrong purpose (eg, the patient or person administering the drug did not understand the indications or warnings on a medication package); administration of drugs to a child by both parents, each unaware of the other's actions; or the common misconception that a bigger dose of a drug provides better or faster relief of the symptom or disorder.

Teaching of the geriatric patient should consider age-related factors that contribute to drug misuse. Important considerations should focus

- on failing eyesight, which affects elderly patients' ability to read labels and to dispense the proper dose;
- failing memory, which hinders recall of verbal medication instructions and of recent ingestion of a drug;
- failing sense of taste, which otherwise might help a person realize he or she has swallowed a potentially hazardous substance;
- and psychologic and social changes that might predispose the elderly person to accidental or intentional overdose.

The prevalence of multiple diseases also places the elderly person at added risk. Age and disease generally make the elderly person less tolerant of drug-induced side effects and interactions. The problem is magnified by the fact that the elderly person takes, on the average, a greater than average number of medications.

Last, and for younger individuals in particular, counseling about the dangers of substance abuse and the need to resist peer pressure that casts drug abuse in a favorable light is essential.

Poison Centers

Poison centers recognized by the American Association of Poison Control Centers were established for the primary purpose of providing comprehensive, up-to-date poisoning management guidelines for both the general population and health-care facilities. Health-care professionals should familiarize themselves with the poison center in their area, and post its phone number where it can be found quickly. Regional poison centers also provide educational materials.

Most of these centers subscribe to the POISINDEX Information System, a detailed toxicology database designed to identify and provide ingredient information on commercial, industrial, pharmaceutical, and botanical substances. POISINDEX also provides detailed treatment and management protocols in the event of a toxicology problem owing to ingestion, absorption, or inhalation of known or unknown toxins. The system was developed in conjunction with the Rocky Mountain Poison and Drug Centers, Emergency Information Center, in Denver, Colorado, and has been published by Micromedex since 1974. The POISINDEX System is currently being used in well over a thousand hospital emergency/trauma departments and poison/drug centers throughout the world. It is updated every 90 days, so it provides health-care professionals with the most current resources for management of acute poisonings available.

Nurses are frequently approached with questions related to medication reactions or possible toxicity of a particular substance, even though that is not always their area of expertise. It is always prudent for any health-care provider to refer decision-making to others who are most knowledgeable in a particular area. In the case of poisoning, this means contacting the regional poison center for advice in *all* cases in which it is not absolutely certain that the ingestion was nontoxic. This advice protects the patient from the possibility of receiving misinformation in what could be a life-threatening situation, and protects the nurse from the possibility of litigation. All regional centers receive calls 24 hours a day, 7 days a week, and many have "800" numbers.

Management of Acute Poisoning

When faced with an emergency situation involving poisoning, health-care providers should always give priority to supporting vital functions. The responsibility to collect pertinent data about the patient and the possible cause of the poisoning should be delegated to others who are not needed to provide care.

It is repeated throughout the literature to "treat the patient, not the poison." This guideline is important. Treatment for most acute poisonings is symptomatic and supportive. The most important thing to remember is that there is always time to stabilize the patient before attempting to treat the toxic ingestion.

Cardiopulmonary resuscitation of a poisoned patient is the same as for any other critically ill patient. Use standard Basic or Advanced Life Support protocols as the patient's condition dictates. The "universal antidote"—a mixture of burnt toast, magnesium oxide (milk of magnesia), and tannic acid (tea)—is ineffective and possibly harmful, and should *never* be used. It could be considered negligent for a nurse or physician to use, or recommend the use of, this remedy.

Nursing care of the poisoned patient focuses on maintenance of ventilation; circulation; fluid, electrolyte, and acid–base balance; and removal or absorption of the poison. Monitor vital signs frequently. The patient with a decreased level of consciousness will require frequent neurologic assessment. At some point it should be ascertained whether the poisoning was suicidal, so that appropriate psychologic intervention may be obtained after recovery. The physician should perform a brief physical examination to rule out any associated illness or injury.

Ventilation

Many toxic ingestions lead to respiratory depression. Give special attention to maintaining a patent airway. Patients who are comatose, seizing, or have ingested or otherwise received a product with the potential to cause central nervous system (CNS) depression will most likely require endotracheal intubation. Intubation may also be necessary for persons with depressed or absent gag reflexes. Have supplemental oxygen and suction equipment readily available. Obtain a chest X-ray to rule out aspiration or pulmonary edema, which are common occurrences in many toxic ingestions. Position the lethargic patient on the left side with the head down (Trendelenburg position) to prevent aspiration in the event that emesis occurs spontaneously.

Circulation

Cardiac monitoring may be necessary. Many toxic ingestions precipitate cardiac arrhythmias. Obtain a 12-lead ECG for baseline information regarding cardiac status.

Fluid and Electrolyte Balance

Establish an IV with a large-bore catheter for all patients who have, or are at high risk for developing, unstable vital signs or decreased level of consciousness. This will provide venous access in the event the patient becomes hypotensive, and will also provide a means to administer adjunctive drugs or antidotes as needed. Ringer's lactate or 0.9% sodium chloride are the most frequently recommended IV fluids.

Blood should be drawn to determine acid–base status and fluid and electrolyte balance, to help identify the cause of poisoning, and to detect markers of organ damage. Laboratory studies may include a complete blood count, electrolyte levels, a complete assay to screen for common drugs or poisons, and measurements of levels of specific drugs (eg, acetaminophen, salicylates, narcotics, alcohol) or metabolites that might cause or indicate organ damage. Serial blood tests help establish trends indicating the progression of poisoning or the effectiveness of treatment. Save all initial samples of urine and emesis for toxicologic analysis.

Acid–Base Balance

An arterial blood gas sample and analysis may be ordered for the patient who presents in respiratory distress or has ingested a substance that may upset acid–base balance. This information not only helps guide respiratory therapy, but also provides added insight into underlying metabolic alterations and the status of vital organs such as the lungs and kidneys.

Neurologic Status

During initial assessment and intervention, pay special attention to the patient's response to verbal and painful stimuli. Standardized procedures and paradigms such as the Glasgow Coma Scale shown in Table C–1, will be used to assess neurologic status. Modified assessment tools are available for use with preverbal children.

Nearly every patient who presents with a decreased level of consciousness, or who is unconscious for unknown reasons, will be given an intravenous injection of the narcotic antagonist naloxone (NARCAN). The usual dose for adults or children is 2 mg, which can be sufficient to induce acute withdrawal in persons who are physically dependent on a narcotic. As a result, lower naloxone doses—for example, 0.2–0.4 mg—might be safer if the patient is known or suspected to be narcotic-dependent and his or her condition is not life threatening. Many patients will also receive the new benzodiazepine antagonist, flumazenil (MAZICON; 0.2 mg, IV, initially).

Naloxone and flumazenil are important. They serve not only as potential treatments for narcotic or benzodiazepine overdoses, respectively, but they also serve as useful diagnostic aids: a positive response to usual doses of naloxone indicates involvement of a narcotic in the poisoning, and a similar response to flumazenil implicates a benzodiazepine. It is important to monitor posi-

Table C–1 | Glasgow Coma Scale

Finding	Score
Eyes open	
Spontaneously	4
To speech	3
To pain	2
Not at all	1
Verbal response	
Oriented	5
Confused	4
Inappropriate	3
Incomprehensible	2
None	1
Motor response	
Obeys commands	5
Localizes pain	4
Flexion to pain	3
Extension to pain	2
None	1
Modified Glasgow Scale for Children	
Eyes open	
Spontaneously	4
To speech	3
To pain	2
Not at all	1
Best verbal response	
Coos, babbles	5
Irritable, cries	4
Cries in response to pain	3
Moans in response to pain	2
None	1
Best motor response	
Normal spontaneous movements	6
Withdraws to touch	5
Withdraws to pain	4
Abnormal flexion	3
Abnormal extension	2
None	1

With each neurocheck, total the response scores. A total of 7 or less indicates a comatose state. A change in total score represents a change in the patient's neurologic status. The patient's vital signs, pupillary reaction, grip strength, pressure resistance, and ability to move should also be evaluated with each neurocheck.

Source: Trauma Nursing Core Course (Provider) Manual. First ed. Chicago, IL, Emergency Nurses Association, Award Printing Corporation, 1986: III-10–III-11.

tive responses to naloxone or flumazenil closely and patiently, anticipating that the level of consciousness may fall once again after these antagonists are given. That is because these antidotes have durations of action that are shorter than those of many drugs whose effects they can counteract. Thus, repeated administration of the blockers, or substituting the long-acting narcotic antagonist naltrexone for naloxone, may be necessary until the patient recovers sufficiently. Currently, there is no approved benzodiazepine antagonist with a duration of action longer than flumazenil's.

Intravenous dextrose administration (25 g, it 50 mL of a 50% solution) is also common for persons with impaired consciousness, with or without seizures, and regardless of whether naloxone or flumazenil are given or whether they work. Persons with a history of alcoholism may also receive thiamine (vitamin B_1; 100 mg IM or IV), preferably before the glucose. Thiamine helps prevent or treat encephalopathy.

Seizures that may develop must be stopped pharmacologically. The usual drug of choice for seizures is diazepam, given intravenously. Recommended doses (Chapter 26) usually work well, and quickly, but drugs such as theophylline may cause seizures that are resistant to diazepam or most other anticonvulsants, such as phenobarbital. Poisoning with antimuscarinic (atropine-like) drugs may require administration of the specific antidote, physostigmine (see below), to stop seizures.

The nurse who is caring for a patient with refractory seizures should anticipate that the next step is likely to involve paralyzing the patient with a neuromuscular blocker (eg, tubocurarine; Chapter 17), or placing the patient under general anesthesia. Either approach will require intubating the patient. Whether typical anticonvulsants, neuromuscular blockers, or general anesthetics are used, oxygen administration is crucial. Planning for the potential need to paralyze or anesthetize the patient should involve prompt notification of appropriately trained personnel, such as an anesthesiologist or nurse-anesthetist. If seizures are caused or accompanied by fever, physically cooling the patient with ice or hypothermia blankets becomes an important nondrug adjunct.

Data Collection

While the emergency team stabilizes the patient, another member of the health-care team should attempt to identify the poison and obtain information about the patient and, if necessary, the family. Remember that in many cases involving drug ingestion, histories are notoriously inaccurate. Question significant others, if available, about the patient's:

- Age
- Weight
- Pertinent medical history: medications (currently or possibly taking), allergies, history of prior overdose

- Route of exposure: ingestion, parenteral, inhalation, or dermal
- Substance(s) involved: the specific product name, if available, and the manufacturer's phone number, if listed on the label. Determine whether the patient has ingested alcohol as well. Be aware that persons who have ingested a street drug may not really know what they have taken or may be hesitant to admit to ingestion for fear of prosecution. If a phone call precedes the emergency visit, always tell the caller to bring the medication or substance in, along with its container
- Amount: It is helpful to remember that a small child swallows approximately 5 mL; a 10-year-old, 10 mL; and an adolescent or adult, 15 mL. Always assume the largest amount that could have been ingested.
- Time of ingestion
- Symptoms
- First aid given

If the substance involved is unknown, a responsible individual should search the area where the patient was found for an empty container, drug paraphernalia, or any other possible clues. Determine what the patient was doing before the poisoning occurred. Check the patient's pockets; note any characteristic breath odor; check for needle marks; look for a medical alert tag. Identifying the poison and its basic pharmacologic and pharmacokinetic properties, and its target organs, is an important determinant for subsequent treatment. A drug taken in overdose amounts may act very differently than the same drug taken in therapeutic amounts. It may also act differently in the very young or very old, or in the chronically ill patient.

Toxic Syndromes

A syndrome is a collection of signs and symptoms that are characteristic of a particular disorder. The signs and symptoms of overdoses with many drugs or chemicals that are involved in poisonings may also fit a characteristic pattern that can be called a toxic syndrome. By carefully assessing vital signs and subjective indicators of a patient's condition (eg, behavior, the level of consciousness, reflexes), you may recognize the pattern. That information, in turn, can help guide proper and sometimes specific treatments aimed at normalizing vital signs and counteracting effects of the poison cause. Trying to fit a given patient's clinical findings into one of the toxic syndromes is not a fool-proof approach; it does not apply to every potential cause of poisoning; there is some overlap in terms of diagnosis, especially when several drugs have been taken: and it will not allow the caregiver to identify the exact drug or drugs that have caused the patient's problems. Nevertheless, it is a great help for providing proper care as soon as possible.

There are four main toxic syndromes. Their characteristics are summarized in Table C–2 and highlighted briefly below; the more common drugs and drug groups likely to cause the syndromes are listed in Table C–3. Specific antidotes, when available, are listed in Table C–4 along with other antidotes used for poisonings that do not fit into one of the syndromes.

The *anticholinergic/antimuscarinic syndrome* involves signs and symptoms you would expect to occur with overdoses of atropine (Chapter 11) or other drugs with atropine-like actions. Bizarre behavior, tachycardia, a significant absence of secretions (eg, lacrimal, salivary), inability to defecate or urinate, and fever, are among the hallmarks. Poisonings with drugs that cause this syndrome are relatively common, owing to the many prescription and nonprescription drugs that exert atropine-like activity. One of the specific interventions includes administration of physostigmine (ANTILIRIUM), the acetylcholinesterase inhibitor that causes a build-up of acetylcholine (ACh) and overcomes blockade of receptor sites by an atropine-like agent that has caused the poisoning.

The *cholinergic syndrome* is caused by parasympathomimetic (Chapter 12) or acetylcholinesterase-inhibitor (Chapter 13) drugs. It is characterized by many changes opposite to those seen in the anticholinergic syndrome. Here the problems are caused by an excess of ACh actions throughout the body. For example, tachycardia, a dramatic increase in secretions, and overstimulation of the gastrointestinal and urinary tracts, usually are very apparent. Stimulation or eventual paralysis of skeletal muscle is also prevalent. Other than the acetylcholinesterase inhibitors that are often used to treat myasthenia gravis, there are few drugs found in outpatient settings that cause the cholinergic syndrome. However, insecticide chemicals are a common nontherapeutic cause. Since the syndrome reflects an excess of ACh, blocking the ACh receptors with atropine will be an important part of treatment.

The *sedative/hypnotic/narcotic syndrome* reflects a generalized decrease in central nervous system activity—sedation to coma and death depending on the dose of the causative agent. With severe overdoses depression of cardiovascular and ventilatory function also appears. Ventilatory depression is a very common finding, even in early stages of poisoning, with narcotic overdoses.

The sedative/hypnotic/narcotic syndrome is very common, owing to the widespread use and abuse of

Table C–2 | **Toxic Syndromes**

Syndrome	CNS	Pupils	Cardiovascular	Respiratory	GI	Integumentary	Secretory	Other
Anticholinergic/antimuscarinic syndrome	Excitability, confusion, delirium, hallucinations, seizures, coma, hyperthermia	Mydriasis	Tachycardia, arrhythmias, ventricular tachycardia and fibrillation	Tachypnea, loss of secretions in pharynx, bronchi, and nasal passages	Decreased bowel sounds, constipation	Flushed, dry skin	Decreased salivary and sweat gland activity	Urinary retention
Cholinergic syndrome	Headache, restlessness, anxiety, coma, muscle weakness and fasciculations	Miosis, lacrimation	Bradycardia	Bradypnea, bronchospasm, increased secretions in pharynx, bronchi, and nasal passages	Abdominal cramping, diarrhea, vomiting	Flushed, moist skin	Increased salivary and sweat gland activity	Urinary incontinence; skeletal muscle fasciculations, tremor, hyperactivity, or paralysis
Narcotic, sedative-hypnotic syndrome*	Decreased level of consciousness, coma; hypothermia	Miosis	Tachycardia	Bradypnea, noncardiogenic pulmonary edema	Decreased bowel sounds			
Sympathomimetic	Delusions, paranoia; hyperreflexia; potential seizures	Mydriasis (with α agonists)	Tachycardia (with β agonists or combined α/β agonists) or bradycardia (with pure α agonists); arrhythmias (depending on drug); hypotension (with β agonists) or hypertension (with pure α agonists)			Piloerection (gooseflesh); diaphoresis	Decreased salivary, lacrimal secretions (with α agonists)	Fever

*Patients who have ingested an overdose of a sedative-hypnotic drug will generally present with most of the same symptoms listed under the narcotic syndrome; however, these patients will not respond to treatment with IV naloxone unless the ingestion also contained narcotics. Flumazenil injection can help identify poisoning with benzodiazepines.

barbiturates, benzodiazepines, narcotics (Chapter 21), and alcohol, the latter of which exerts barbiturate-like depressant effects throughout the body (Chapter 22). Naloxone (NARCAN) and flumazenil (MAZICON) are useful for narrowing the diagnosis and as antidotes during further treatment. Naloxone specifically blocks the effects of narcotics, and flumazenil specifically antagonizes the effects of benzodiazepines. These antidotes are especially useful if only one class of drugs is responsible for the poisoning. However, suicidal overdoses often include many CNS depressant drugs, which can limit the value of just one antidote as a diagnostic or treatment aid.

The *sympathomimetic syndrome* is the fourth ma-

Table C–3 Common Substances or Drug Classes Associated with "Toxic Syndromes"

Syndrome	Chapter Cross Reference
Anticholinergic/Antimuscarinic Syndrome	
Antidepressants (all "cyclics")	24
Antihistamines (H_1 blockers; includes many OTC allergy and cold remedies and sleep aids, which contain chlorpheniramine, diphenhydramine, doxylamine, pyrilamine, others)	51
Antiparkinson agents (antimuscarinics: benztropine, trihexyphenidyl)	25
Antipsychotics	23
Antispasmodics (antimuscarinics, opiates)	13, 21
Belladonna alkaloids	13
Mydriatics, topical (antimuscarinics: scopolamine, atropine, related ophthalmic solutions; does *not* include sympathomimetic mydriatics)	13
Plants including jimson weed (*Datura stramonium*), wild sage (*Lantana camara*), nutmeg (*Myristica fragrans*), and some mushrooms (*Amanita muscaria* and *Amanita pantherina*)	13
Cholinergic Syndrome	
Acetylcholinesterase inhibitors (includes edrophonium, neostigmine, physostigmine, and pyridostigmine, many of which are used for treating myasthenia gravis)	12
Insecticides: carbamates and organophosphates	12
Mushrooms (sp. *Clitocybe* and *Inocybe*)	12
Parasympathomimetics (eg, bethanechol, pilocarpine)	11
Narcotic, Sedative-Hypnotic Syndrome*	
Alcohol	22
Anticonvulsants	26
Benzodiazepines	22
Barbiturates	22
Chloral hydrate	22
Ethchlorvynol	22
Meprobamate	22
Methaqualone (illegal)	27
Methyprylon	22
Narcotics (includes morphine and all other prescription narcotics used for analgesia, antidiarrheal effects, etc, and illicit drugs such as heroin)	21
Sympathomimetic Syndrome*	
Amphetamines and related drugs	14, 27, 28
Cocaine	14, 27, 28
OTC decongestants, weight-loss aids	14
Caffeine, theophylline	38

*Differential diagnosis of narcotic overdose is based on a positive response (eg, improved ventilation, level of consciousness) to naloxone or to flumazenil (benzodiazepine overdose). A negative response indicates only that the causative agent may not have been a narcotic or benzodiazepine, and does not indicate the underlying drug class (eg, barbiturate, alcohol, other).

Table C–4 | Antidotes

Poison (Chapter Cross Reference)	Antidote
Acetaminophen (52)	N-Acetylcysteine (MUCOMYST)
Anticholinergics/antimuscarinics (13)	Physostigmine (ANTILIRIUM)
Anticoagulants, oral (35)	Vitamin K
Benzodiazepines (22)	Flumazenil (MAZICON)
Beta-adrenergic blockers (15)	Isoproterenol, glucagon
Calcium channel blockers (33, 34)	Calcium chloride
Cholinergics and acetylcholinesterase inhibitors (11, 12)	Atropine
Cyanide, nitroprusside sodium (33)	Amyl nitrate, then Sodium nitrite, then Sodium thiosulfate
Digoxin, digitoxin (31)	Digoxin immune (DIGIBIND, DIGIDOTE)
Heavy metals	
Arsenic, gold, lead, mercury	Dimercaprol ("BAL")
Iron	Deferoxamine (DESFERAL)
Lead	Calcium EDTA
Heparin (35)	Protamine sulfate
Methanol/ethylene glycol	Ethanol
Opiates, products containing opiates (eg, LOMOTIL) (21)	Naloxone (NARCAN)
Organophosphates or carbamate insecticides (12)	Atropine, pralidoxime

jor toxic syndrome. It is caused mainly by amphetamines, amphetamine-like drugs, and cocaine (Chapters 14, 27, 28), but may also occur with sympathomimetics found in decongestants and weight-loss aids (Chapter 14). High blood levels of theophylline and caffeine may also cause a sympathomimetic syndrome owing to their ability to release catecholamines. The overdose picture in this syndrome usually reflects significant CNS stimulation and behavior changes. Cardiovascular responses can range from bradycardia to tachycardia, and hypotension to hypertension, depending on the type of sympathomimetic drug (ie, its α- or β-agonist activity) that caused the poisoning. The cause of the poisoning, and the actual responses that occur, will influence how to treat the situation.

General Treatment Approaches for Poisoning by Ingestion

The general approach to managing a patient who has ingested a toxic substance or drug overdose includes prevention of absorption, enhancement of elimination, and the use of physiologic or pharmacologic antagonists, when available (Table C–3).

Prevention of Absorption

The poison victim's prognosis often depends on the promptness with which the poisons are eliminated from the gastrointestinal (GI) tract, or their ability to be absorbed from the gut is reduced. Methods for emptying the stomach include induced emesis and gastric lavage. Since many ingested drugs delay gastric emptying, emesis or lavage should probably be initiated after all toxic ingestions, unless otherwise contraindicated, regardless of the time interval between ingestion and treatment.

Induced Emesis

Syrup of ipecac is an effective means of producing emesis, and often its administration is safe. The dose for a child aged 6 months to 1 year is 10 mL; for children aged 1 to 10 years, 15 mL. Patients 10 years of age and older should receive 30 mL. In all instances, syrup of ipecac should be followed by liberal amounts of clear liquids. If vomiting does not occur within 20 minutes, and the patient is 1 year old or more, the same dose may be repeated once.

Many ingestions by individuals older than 6 months can be treated at home under the supervision of the poison center. Induced emesis should be initiated only under medical supervision in children under the age of 12 months, and ipecac generally should not be administered more than once to infants.

Home administration of ipecac to elderly or chronically ill persons is not recommended owing to the risk involved from prolonged vomiting and possible dehydration in a person who already may have fluid or electrolyte imbalances.

Inducing emesis in patients who have spontaneously vomited is controversial. Some studies have shown spontaneous emesis to be ineffective in removing the ingested substance, supporting the need for inducing emesis pharmacologically. Most of the literature recommends inducing emesis regardless of whether spontaneous emesis has occurred.

For any patient, if emesis does not occur, gastric lavage should be considered on an individual basis. It is important to realize that emetic drugs may not always work, and even if they do, they may not do so immediately. The precious minutes that may be wasted in waiting for vomiting to occur will delay the use of other interventions, such as administration of activated charcoal, that may be more effective or life-saving. Thus, judgment must be exercised on a case-by-case basis.

However, induced emesis is generally contraindicated in some situations, including:

- Ingestion of alkalis or acids, in which emesis increases the likelihood of gastric or esophageal perforation
- Ingestion of a rapidly acting CNS depressant (eg, cyanide) or convulsant (eg, strychnine); this is one instance in which waiting for induced emesis to occur is not only time-wasting but also potentially dangerous
- Ingestion of a petroleum distillate, unless advised by the poison control center. The major risk of this type of ingestion is aspiration. (The one area of agreement among authorities with regard to the use of ipecac in petroleum distillate ingestion seems to be that when the petroleum distillate is a carrier for a more toxic substance, emesis should be induced.)
- Presence of coma or seizures (including patients who are postictal), owing to a high risk for recurrent seizure activity
- Nontoxic ingestion
- Depressed or absent gag reflex (another relative contraindication, based on assessing the patient, that must be considered on an individual basis)

Gastric Lavage

Gastric lavage is generally used when induced emesis may be too slow to be effective, when two doses of ipecac fail to induce emesis, or when the patient is at increased risk of aspiration. A physician should evaluate the patient to determine whether endotracheal intubation is required prior to lavage. If indicated, a cuffed endotracheal tube should be used to provide the greatest protection against aspiration. The gastric tube should be at least 28 French to allow for removal of pill fragments; a 36-French tube is recommended. Orogastric insertion is preferred, but the largest possible nasogastric or orogastric tube should be used. Lavage should take place with the patient positioned on the left side with the head down (Trendelenburg) if they have not been intubated prior to lavage. The stomach contents should be aspirated prior to the lavage and saved for analysis by the toxicology lab. Warm tap water (10 to 20 L, administered in 200- to 300-mL aliquots) should be used for adults. Normal saline (5 to 10 L in 50-mL aliquots) should be used for children to reduce the risk of water intoxication. Instilling greater amounts of fluid at one time may distend the stomach and force the poison into the duodenum, where it may be more readily absorbed.

Lavage should continue until the returning fluids are clear, and all lavage fluids should be saved for possible analysis. After lavage has been completed, activated charcoal should be administered down the tube; the tube can then be removed. Because of the risk of perforating the GI tract while inserting the tube, gastric lavage is contraindicated in patients who have ingested alkalis or acids.

Activated Charcoal

Activated charcoal is the residue from the distillation of wood pulp. It forms a stable complex with (adsorbs) the poison, thus preventing systemic absorption of the toxicant. It should be given to all patients who have overdosed on medications that are adsorbed by it, after emesis or lavage is concluded. If the patient has been lavaged, activated charcoal should be instilled via the lavage tube before removing the tube. The usual dose of charcoal is approximately 1 to 2 g/kg. Most toxins can be adsorbed effectively by activated charcoal. Notable exceptions include alcohols, boric acid, corrosives, cyanide, DDT, N-methyl carbamate, ferrous sulfate, and malathion.

Repeated oral charcoal administration, in doses ranging from 20 to 50 g every 2 to 6 hours in adults, has been used successfully to enhance the elimination of theophylline, phenobarbital, and digoxin. (Pediatric doses have not been established, but one half the initial dose is recommended.) Saline cathartics or sorbitol may be given with the first dose (see below) and repeated until charcoal appears in the stool. The technique has led to improved recovery. Since research indicates that multiple-dose activated charcoal may have more widespread applicability, consult a poison center for the latest information concerning efficacy of this treatment for specific cases. Neither activated charcoal nor cathartics should be administered more than once if bowel sounds are absent.

Enhancement of Poison Elimination

Catharsis

The most commonly used method for enhancement of elimination is the administration of a cathartic after emesis is concluded, usually along with activated charcoal. Cathartics are given to hasten the passage of poisons through the GI tract, thus decreasing the absorption of poisons not removed by emesis or lavage. Cathartics are contraindicated in patients who have or may have GI bleeding, and in patients who have ingested a caustic substance. A standard commercial solution of magnesium citrate (0.5 mL/kg for children; 120 to 240 mL for adults) or a 10% solution of magnesium sulfate (Epsom salts; 2.5 mL/kg for children, 150 to 200 mL for adults) are the two most commonly used cathartics.

As noted earlier, repeated administration of cathartics may be indicated as adjuncts to multiple-dose administration of activated charcoal. The patient's age and medical history should be considered first, especially if cathartics containing magnesium are used, to reduce the risk of electrolyte imbalances (eg, hypermagnesemia) owing to impaired renal function. Diarrhea caused by multiple doses of any cathartic can lead to other fluid and electrolyte imbalances, especially in pediatric and geriatric patients.

Diuresis

Another method used to enhance the excretion of poisons is forced diuresis, with or without drug treatments to alter urine pH. The safety of forced diuresis has been established only for poisonings with salicylates or phenobarbital, the renal excretion of which is increased in alkaline urine. Alkaline diuresis may be produced by administering large amounts of IV fluids (eg, 5% dextrose-water) to keep urine flow at 3 to 6 mL/kg per hour, with the addition of two or three ampules of sodium bicarbonate to each liter of parenteral solution to keep urine pH at 7.5 or greater. Serum electrolytes must be monitored, and administration of supplemental potassium is usually indicated.

Mannitol or furosemide may be given to maintain urine flow. If mannitol is used, it should be administered in a volume of fluid that is appropriate for the patient's condition (eg, large volumes may be more acceptable in a hypotensive patient than in a normotensive patient), and, if possible, the composition of the fluid should be such that it will help normalize electrolyte imbalances that are either present or likely to arise as the result of subsequent treatment. Hypertension and precipitation of heart failure or pulmonary edema are potential problems when large amounts of mannitol are administered quickly.

If furosemide is used, take precautions to guard against hypotension or shock; the drug should be used with great care if the patient is already hypotensive. Parenteral administration of the urinary acidifiers ascorbic acid or ammonium chloride, previously recommended to enhance elimination of amphetamines, isoniazid, phencyclidine, strychnine, or any other agents, is no longer recommended.

Other Methods

Other special methods used to hasten drug elimination include hemodialysis, peritoneal dialysis, and hemoperfusion. The poison center can be a valuable resource when determining whether one of these more invasive procedures might be indicated in a particular patient. Patients requiring these treatments almost always require monitoring in an intensive-care unit.

Specific Antidotes

Pharmacologic, physiologic, or chemical antagonists (antidotes; see Table C–4) are available and effective for treating overdoses or poisonings caused by specific chemicals or drugs, or for substances that closely fit a particular toxic syndrome.

Also available are antidotes for heavy metals that may cause toxicity through oral ingestion or inhalation. The most important of these antidotes are dimercaprol, deferoxamine, and calcium disodium edetate. Dimercaprol (British Anti-Lewisite; BAL), given as a repository intramuscular injection, chelates arsenic, gold, lead, and mercury. Deferoxamine (also called desferrioxamine; DESFERAL), given intramuscularly or intravenously, chelates iron and is indicated for treating acute or chronic iron toxicity. Calcium disodium edetate (calcium EDTA; calcium disodium versenate) is indicated for acute or chronic lead poisoning.

Unfortunately, many poisons have no specific antidotes. Contact the regional poison center as soon as the poison is identified to determine whether an antidote exists and if it is indicated for use in a particular poison exposure. The availability of a specific antidote does not replace the need to monitor vital signs and to use measures to normalize them. As noted earlier, never use the "universal antidote."

Treatment Plans for Poisoning Through Other Routes

While ingestion is the most common route of poisoning, the nurse may be called on to treat patients who have been poisoned through other routes, such as dermal, ocular, or inhalation. The general management for the patient who has been exposed to a toxic substance through these routes is similar to that for cases involving ingestion, but each of these other routes also has additional and unique management aspects.

Dermal Exposure

It is possible to develop systemic toxicity from dermal exposure to some substances, most notably insecticides and toxins released from fires. Persons exposed to these substances should remove their clothes immediately and wash exposed skin areas, since residual insecticide spray on clothing may be continually absorbed. Two washings of exposed skin areas with soap and water should generally be sufficient to remove the poison.

Personnel involved in transporting and decontaminating these patients should wear protective clothing and gloves to prevent contaminating themselves. Discarded clothing from the patient and health-care personnel, and all gowns or dressings, should be treated as possible sources of contamination. They should be packaged in air-tight containers, clearly labeled, and disposed of according to local or poison center policy.

Ocular Exposure

Standard care for ocular exposure consists of copious irrigation with water or, if in a health-care facility, normal saline or other isotonic solution (eg, Ringer's lactate) for at least 15 minutes. Irrigation should be instituted immediately after exposure, before transport to the hospital (if possible), and without question upon arrival at the hospital while someone else contacts the poison center. Ocular exposure to strong alkalis requires irrigation for as long as 30 minutes. Neutral isotonic solutions are used regardless of the pH of the substance involved. A physician's evaluation is required if irritation or visual disturbance persists after irrigation is completed.

Inhalation Exposure

Persons who suffer inhalation exposure to toxic substances should be moved immediately to fresh air and given oxygen to inhale. On arrival at the emergency department they may require many of the same interventions instituted for a patient with exposure by ingestion, since many inhaled substances are quickly or extensively absorbed into the blood.

It is possible to experience local or systemic symptoms as late as 72 hours after some inhalation exposures. In addition, substances that irritate, inflame, or otherwise affect the respiratory tract may cause acute or slowly developing impairments of ventilation or gas exchange, leading to adverse responses far more serious than the systemic effects caused by early absorption of the poison. Therefore, close monitoring of the patient's status and careful assessment of ventilatory function and its consequences are essential during this time.

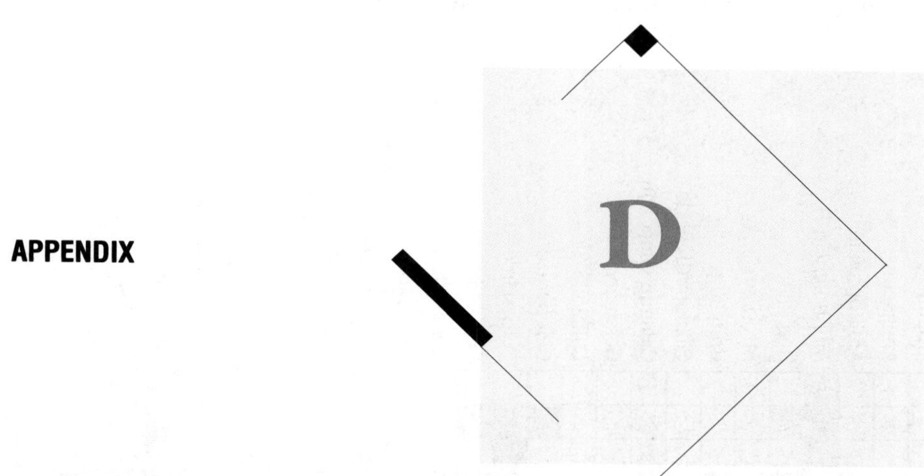

APPENDIX D

Physical and Chemical Compatibilities of Common Drugs and Fluids

TABLE D–1 **Compatibility of Drugs for Intravenous Administration**

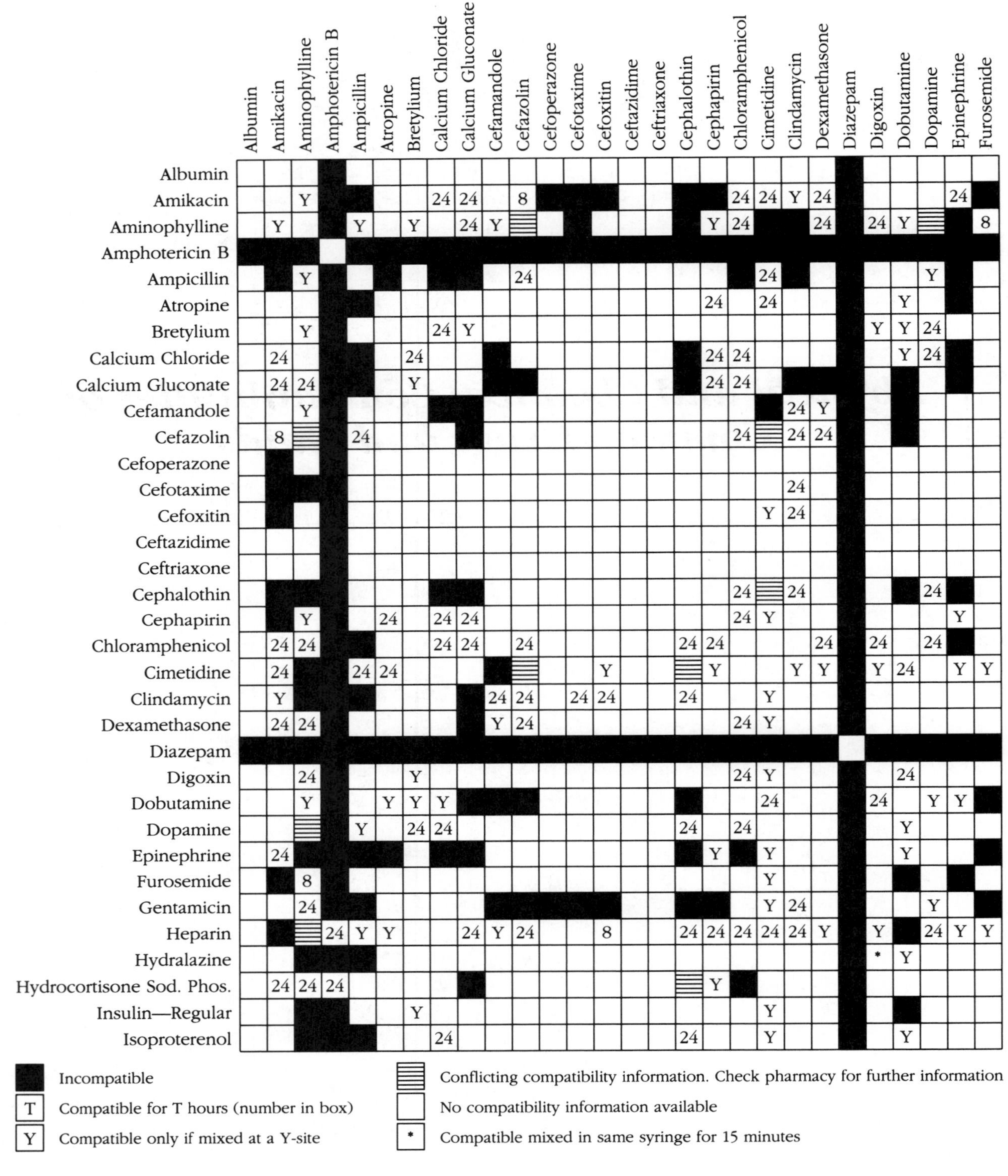

	Albumin	Amikacin	Aminophylline	Amphotericin B	Ampicillin	Atropine	Bretylium	Calcium Chloride	Calcium Gluconate	Cefamandole	Cefazolin	Cefoperazone	Cefotaxime	Cefoxitin	Ceftazidime	Ceftriaxone	Cephalothin	Cephapirin	Chloramphenicol	Cimetidine	Clindamycin	Dexamethasone	Diazepam	Digoxin	Dobutamine	Dopamine	Epinephrine	Furosemide
Albumin				■																			■					
Amikacin			Y	■	■			24	24		8	■	■	■			■	■	24	24	Y	24	■				24	■
Aminophylline		Y		■	Y		Y		24	Y	▤		■				■	Y	24	■	■	24	■	24	Y	▤	■	8
Amphotericin B	■	■	■		■	■	■	■	■	■	■	■	■	■	■	■	■	■	■	■	■	■	■	■	■	■	■	■
Ampicillin		■	Y	■		■		■	■		24								■	24	■		■			Y	■	
Atropine				■	■													24		24			■		Y		■	
Bretylium			Y	■				24	Y														■	Y	Y	24		
Calcium Chloride		24		■	■		24			■							■	24	24				■		Y	24	■	
Calcium Gluconate		24	24	■	■		Y			■	■						■	24	24		■	■	■		■		■	
Cefamandole			Y	■				■	■											■	24	Y	■		■			
Cefazolin		8	▤	■	24				■										24	▤	24	24	■		■			
Cefoperazone		■		■																			■					
Cefotaxime		■	■	■																	24		■					
Cefoxitin		■		■																Y	24		■					
Ceftazidime				■																			■					
Ceftriaxone				■																			■					
Cephalothin		■	■	■				■	■										24	▤	24		■		■	24	■	
Cephapirin		■	Y	■		24		24	24										24	Y			■				Y	
Chloramphenicol		24	24	■	■			24	24		24						24	24				24	■	24		24	■	
Cimetidine		24	■	■	24	24				■	▤			Y			▤	Y			Y	Y	■	Y	24		Y	Y
Clindamycin		Y	■	■	■				■	24	24		24	24			24			Y			■					
Dexamethasone		24	24	■					■	Y	24								24	Y			■					
Diazepam	■	■	■	■	■	■	■	■	■	■	■	■	■	■	■	■	■	■	■	■	■	■		■	■	■	■	■
Digoxin			24	■			Y												24	Y			■		24			
Dobutamine			Y	■		Y	Y	Y	■	■	■						■			24			■	24		Y	Y	■
Dopamine			▤	■	Y		24	24									24		24				■		Y			
Epinephrine		24	■	■	■	■		■	■								■	Y	■	Y			■		Y			■
Furosemide		■	8	■																Y			■		■		■	
Gentamicin			24	■	■					■	■	■	■	■			■	■		Y	24		■			Y		■
Heparin		■	▤	24	Y	Y			24	Y	24			8			24	24	24	24	24	Y	■	Y	■	24	Y	Y
Hydralazine			■	■	■																		■	*	Y			
Hydrocortisone Sod. Phos.		24	24	24					■								▤	Y	■				■					
Insulin—Regular			■	■			Y													Y			■		■			
Isoproterenol			■	■	■			24									24			Y			■		Y			

■ Incompatible

T Compatible for T hours (number in box)

Y Compatible only if mixed at a Y-site

▤ Conflicting compatibility information. Check pharmacy for further information

☐ No compatibility information available

* Compatible mixed in same syringe for 15 minutes

Gentamicin	Heparin	Hydralazine	Hydrocortisone Sod. Phos.	Insulin—Regular	Isoproterenol	Lidocaine	Magnesium Sulfate	Mannitol	Meperidine	Methyldopate	Methylprednisolone Sod. Succ.	Metoclopramide	Metronidazole	Mezlocillin	Morphine Sulfate	Multivitamins—12	Nafcillin	Nitroglycerin	Nitroprusside	Norepinephrine	Oxytocin	Penicillin G K^+	Pentobarbital	Phenobarbital	Phentolamine	Phenytoin	Piperacillin	Potassium Chloride	Procainamide	Propranolol	Ranitidine	Sodium Bicarbonate	Ticarcillin	Tobramycin	Trimethoprim-Sulfamethoxazole	Vancomycin	Verapamil
																												24									8
			24			24	Y	24	Y				24		Y					24	Y	8	24	24				24			Y	24				Y	Y
24			24			24				24		24	24					Y			24	Y	24	24			6	24	24			24					
	24		24																																		
	Y						Y		Y						Y	Y					Y							24			Y						Y
	Y								*			*			*		Y						*					Y									Y
				Y		24		24										Y										24	Y			24					Y
					24	24										24				24		24		24				24									Y
	24					24						Y				24				24		24		24				24	24					Y		24	Y
	Y							24	Y		Y				Y	Y					Y							24			Y						Y
	24						Y		Y						Y	Y					24	24		24				24			Y						Y
							Y								Y	Y					Y																
							Y		Y						Y						Y																Y
	8					24	Y	24	Y						Y	Y					Y										Y	24					Y
	24				24		Y		Y						Y	Y					Y							24			Y						
	24	Y					Y	8	Y						Y						Y	24	24	24				24				24					Y
	24					24	Y	24	Y	24			24		Y		24				24							24	24			24		24			Y
Y	24			Y	Y	Y			*		Y		24		*	Y	24			Y		Y						24				24				Y	Y
24	24						Y		Y		Y	24	24		Y						Y	24						24			Y	24		24			Y
	Y					24						24					24					24						Y			Y						Y
	Y	*				24																						Y			Y						Y
		Y			Y	Y	Y		Y						Y			Y		Y					Y			24	Y	Y				Y			Y
Y	24					24		24			Y							24		Y		6						24									Y
	Y					Y																						24			Y						Y
	Y							20										Y										Y			Y						Y
							Y		Y				24		Y	Y					Y										Y						Y
		Y			24	24	Y			24	24	24	24				24			24	Y			24			24	24	Y	Y		Y					Y
	Y																	Y										Y									
												24										24															Y
												24																24			Y						Y
	24						24																					24			Y						Y

Notes: **(1)** the compatibility guidelines indicated in this chart refer to the combination of these drugs in 5% dextrose, 0.9% sodium chloride, and mixtures of dextrose and sodium chloride only. **(2)** Always check to ensure that each of the drugs that you are combining is compatible with the IV solution that will be used as a diluent before mixing them. **(3)** The intravenous compatibility of drugs may depend on the order of mixing, the relative concentrations, the speed of mixing, or the agitation of the solution while mixing. **(4)** Preparing separate piggybacks for each individual drug is preferable to combining these drugs in the same solution. Separate piggybacks provide ease of dosage adjustment and avoid many concentration-dependent incompatibilities that can occur without any visible signs of precipitation or color change. **(5)** If any physical change is noted, ie, precipitate, color change, foaming, or haze, do not administer the solution. **(6)** No reliable data are available regarding the mixing of three or more drugs. **(7)** Drugs reported in the literature to be visually compatible are noted on this chart with a Y. **(8)** This list does not indicate all potential admixture incompatibilities. Always check first with the hospital pharmacy or drug information service.

Source: Modified with permission from data provided by The University of Michigan Hospitals Drug Information Service.

	Albumin	Amikacin	Aminophylline	Amphotericin B	Ampicillin	Atropine	Bretylium	Calcium Chloride	Calcium Gluconate	Cefamandole	Cefazolin	Cefoperazone	Cefotaxime	Cefoxitin	Ceftazidime	Ceftriaxone	Cephalothin	Cephapirin	Chloramphenicol	Cimetidine	Clindamycin	Dexamethasone	Diazepam	Digoxin	Dobutamine	Dopamine	Epinephrine	Furosemide
Lidocaine		24		■			24	24	24	≡	■			24			≡		24	Y		24	■	24	Y	24	Y	■
Magnesium Sulfate		Y		■	Y			≡	≡	≡	Y	Y	Y	Y			Y	Y	Y		Y		■		Y			
Mannitol		24		■			24			24				24				8	24				■			24		20
Meperidine		Y	■	■	Y	*				Y	Y	■	Y	Y			Y	Y	Y	*	Y		■		Y			■
Methyldopate			24	■															24				■					
Methylprednisolone Sod. Succ.			≡	≡					■	Y							≡		≡	Y	Y		■			Y		
Metoclopramide			24	■	■	*			Y								■		■	≡	24	24	■					
Metronidazole		24	24	■	≡					■	■			■			■		24	24	24		■			■		
Mezlocillin		■		■																			■					
Morphine Sulfate		Y	■	■	Y	*				Y	Y	Y	Y	Y			Y	Y	Y	*	Y		■		Y			
Multivitamins—12			■	■	Y			24	24	Y	Y	Y		Y			Y			Y			■					■
Nafcillin			■	■		Y													24			24	■		■			
Nitroglycerin			Y	■			Y																■		Y	24		Y
Nitroprusside	■	■	■	■	■	■	■	■	■	■	■	■	■	■	■	■	■	■	■	≡	■	■	■	■	■	■	■	■
Norepinephrine		24	■	■	■	■		24	24								≡	■		Y			■		Y	Y		■
Oxytocin		Y	24	■	Y					Y	24	Y	Y	Y			Y	Y	24		Y		■					
Penicillin G K+		8	Y	■				24	24		24						≡	24	■	Y	24	24	■		■	6	■	
Pentobarbital		24	24	■	■	*		≡	■		■						■	24	≡	■	■		■					
Phenobarbital		24	24	■	■			24	24		24						■	24		■	■	■	■					
Phentolamine				■																			■		Y			
Phenytoin	■	■	■	■	■	■	■	■	■	■	■	■	■	■	■	■	■	■	■	■	■	■	■	■	■	■	■	■
Piperacillin		■	6	■																			■					
Potassium Chloride	24	24	24	■	24	Y	24	24	24	24	24						24	24	24	24	24	Y	■	Y	24	24	24	Y
Procainamide			24	■			Y		24										24				■		Y			
Propranolol				■																			■		Y			
Ranitidine		Y		■	Y					Y	Y			Y			Y				Y	Y	■	Y			Y	Y
Sodium Bicarbonate		24	24	■	■	■	24	■	■				■	24			■	24	24	24	24		■		■	■		
Ticarcillin		■		■																			■					
Tobramycin				■					Y	■		■	■	■			■		24		24		■		24			■
Trimethoprim-Sulfamethoxazole				■																			■					
Vancomycin		Y	■	■					24										■	Y		■	■				■	
Verapamil	8	Y	≡	■	Y	Y	Y	Y	Y	Y	Y		Y	Y				Y	Y	Y	Y	Y	■	Y	Y	Y	Y	Y

■ Incompatible

T Compatible for T hours (number in box)

Y Compatible only if mixed at a Y-site

≡ Conflicting compatibility information. Check pharmacy for further information

No compatibility information available

* Compatible mixed in same syringe for 15 minutes

Gentamicin	Heparin	Hydralazine	Hydrocortisone Sod. Phos.	Insulin—Regular	Isoproterenol	Lidocaine	Magnesium Sulfate	Mannitol	Meperidine	Methyldopate	Methylprednisolone Sod. Succ.	Metoclopramide	Metronidazole	Mezlocillin	Morphine Sulfate	Multivitamins—12	Nafcillin	Nitroglycerin	Nitroprusside	Norepinephrine	Oxytocin	Penicillin G K+	Pentobarbital	Phenobarbital	Phentolamine	Phenytoin	Piperacillin	Potassium Chloride	Procainamide	Propranolol	Ranitidine	Sodium Bicarbonate	Ticarcillin	Tobramycin	Trimethoprim-Sulfamethoxazole	Vancomycin	Verapamil
	24											24						Y				24	24	24			24	24	24		Y			24			Y
Y	Y				24					24		24	Y			24	Y			24	24	Y					Y	24					Y	Y	Y	Y	Y
												24										10					24							24			Y
Y												*	Y														Y						Y	Y	Y	Y	Y
	24						24																					24				24					Y
	24											24								24		24						Y			Y						Y
	24		24	24		24	24	24	*		24				24	24												24									Y
24	24						Y		Y						Y						Y	24															
															Y																						
Y												24	Y	Y			Y					Y						24					Y	Y	Y	Y	Y
Y							24					24										Y					Y	24					Y				
	24						Y								Y					Y	Y							24									
		Y				Y																															Y
	24						24				24						Y								24			24			Y						Y
Y	Y						24						Y				Y										Y	24					Y	Y	Y	Y	Y
			24			24	Y	10			24		24		Y	Y												24	24		Y	6					Y
						24																						24									Y
	24					24																							24								Y
																				24																	Y
	24					24	Y	24	Y							Y					Y							24				24					
	24	Y		24	24	24	24			24	Y	24			24	24	24			24	24	24	24				24		24	Y	Y	24		24		24	
	Y					24																24		24				24								24	Y
	Y																											Y				24					Y
Y				Y	Y	Y					Y									Y		Y						Y				24				Y	
	Y									24												6					24	24		24							
							Y		Y						Y	Y					Y																Y
						24	Y	24	Y						Y						Y							24									Y
							Y		Y						Y						Y																
							Y		Y						Y						Y							24	24		Y						Y
Y	Y		Y	Y	Y	Y	Y	Y	Y	Y	Y	Y			Y			Y		Y	Y	Y	Y	Y	Y				Y	Y			Y	Y		Y	

Notes: **(1)** the compatibility guidelines indicated in this chart refer to the combination of these drugs in 5% dextrose, 0.9% sodium chloride, and mixtures of dextrose and sodium chloride only. **(2)** Always check to ensure that each of the drugs that you are combining is compatible with the IV solution that will be used as a diluent before mixing them. **(3)** The intravenous compatibility of drugs may depend on the order of mixing, the relative concentrations, the speed of mixing, or the agitation of the solution while mixing. **(4)** Preparing separate piggybacks for each individual drug is preferable to combining these drugs in the same solution. Separate piggybacks provide ease of dosage adjustment and avoid many concentration-dependent incompatibilities that can occur without any visible signs of precipitation or color change. **(5)** If any physical change is noted, ie, precipitate, color change, foaming, or haze, do not administer the solution. **(6)** No reliable data are available regarding the mixing of three or more drugs. **(7)** Drugs reported in the literature to be visually compatible are noted on this chart with a Y. **(8)** This list does not indicate all potential admixture incompatibilities. Always check first with the hospital pharmacy or drug information service.

Source: Modified with permission from data provided by The University of Michigan Hospitals Drug Information Service.

TABLE D–2 Compatibility of Drugs for Intramuscular Injection

	Atropine	Chlorpromazine	Cimetidine	Codeine	Dexamethasone	Diphenhydramine	Droperidol	Fentanyl	Glycopyrrolate	Hydrocortisone	Hydromorphone	Hydroxyzine	Meperidine	Methylprednisolone	Metoclopramide	Morphine	Pentazocine	Pentobarbital	Prednisolone	Prochlorperazine	Promethazine	Scopolamine
Atropine		C*	C	O	O	C*	C*	C*	C	O	C*	C*	C*	O	C*	C*	C*	C*	O	C*	C*	C*
Chlorpromazine	C*		O	C	O	C*	C*	C*	C	O	C*	C*	C*	I	C*	C*	C*	I	O	C*	C*	C*
Cimetidine	C	O		O	O	O	O	O	O	O	O	O	O	O	O	O	O	I	O	O	O	O
Codeine	O	C	O		O	O	O	O	C	O	O	C	C*	O	O	O	O	I	O	C	I	O
Dexamethasone	O	O	O	O		I	O	O	C	I	C	O	O	O	O	O	O	O	C	I	I	O
Diphenhydramine	C*	C*	O	O	I		C*	C*	C	I	C*	C*	C*	I	C*	C*	C*	I	C	C*	C*	C*
Droperidol	C*	C*	O	O	O	C*		C*	C	O	O	C*	C*	O	C*	C*	C*	I	O	C*	C*	C*
Fentanyl	C*	C*	O	O	O	C*	C*		C	I	C*	C*	C*	I	C*	C*	C*	I	O	C*	C*	C*
Glycopyrrolate	C	C	O	C	C	C	C	C		O	C	C	C	I	O	C	I	I	O	C	C	C
Hydrocortisone	O	O	O	O	I	I	O	I	O		O	O	O	O	O	O	O	I	C	I	I	O
Hydromorphone	C*	C*	O	O	O	C*	O	C*	C	O		C*	I	O	O	O	C*	C*	O	I	C*	C*
Hydroxyzine	C*	C*	O	C	O	C*	C*	C*	C	O	C*		C*	O	C*	C*	C*	I	C	C*	C*	C*
Meperidine	C*	C*	O	C*	O	C*	C*	C*	C	O	I	C*		O	C*	I	C*	I	O	C*	C*	C*
Methylprednisolone	O	I	O	O	O	I	O	I	I	O	O	O	O		C	O	I	O	O	O	O	O
Metoclopramide	C*	C*	O	O	C	C*	C*	C*	O	C	O	C*	C*	C		C*	C*	O	O	C*	C*	C*
Morphine	C*	C*	O	O	O	C*	C*	C*	C	O	O	C*	I	O	C*		C*	I	O	C*	C*	C*
Pentazocine	C*	C*	O	O	O	C*	C*	C*	I	O	C*	C*	C*	O	C*	C*		I	O	C*	C	C*
Pentobarbital	C*	I	I	I	O	I	I	I	I	I	C*	I	I	O	O	I	I		C	I	I	C*
Prednisolone	O	O	O	O	C	C	O	O	O	C	O	C	O	O	O	O	O	C		I	I	O
Prochlorperazine	C*	C*	O	C	I	C*	C*	C*	C	I	I	C*	C*	O	C*	C*	C*	I	I		C*	C*
Promethazine	C*	C*	O	I	I	C*	C*	C*	C	I	C*	C*	C*	I	C*	C*	C*	I	I	C*		C*
Scopolamine	C*	C*	O	O	O	C*	C*	C*	C	O	C*	C*	C*	O	C*	C*	C*	C*	O	C*	C*	

Key: **C** = physically compatible; **C*** = compatible or stable, but only for 15 minutes; **I** = incompatible; **O** = no data regarding compatibility.

Note: It is recommended that the following medications not be combined (mixed) with other drugs in the same syringe: Amobarbital; Benztropine; Chlordiazepoxide; Diazepam; Haloperidol; Pentobarbital; Phenobarbital; Phenytoin; Ritodrine; Secobarbital.

Modified, with permission, from The Formulary of The University of Michigan Hospitals, 1992.

APPENDIX

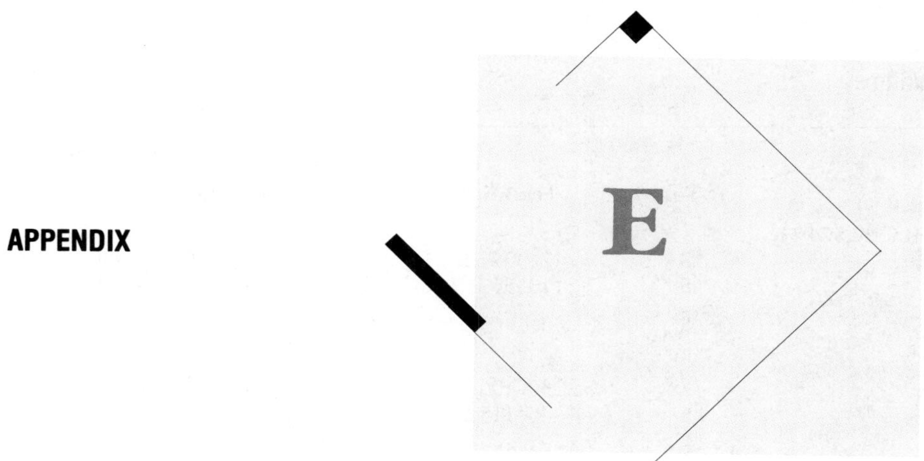

*Selected Laboratory Values**

**Adapted from* Lagerquist SL (ed): *Addison-Wesley's Nursing Examination Review,* 4th ed., 1991, and Jordan CD, Flood JG, Laposta M, Lewandrowski KB: Normal Reference Laboratory Values, *N Engl J Med* 327(10): 718–724, 1992.

Table E–2 | General Chemistry Values

		Normal Values	
Substance	**Sample***	**Traditional Units†**	**SI Units†**
Alanine aminotransferase (ALT; formerly SGPT)			
Females	S	7–30 U/L	0.12–0.50 kat/L
Males	S	10–55 U/L	0.17–0.91 kat/L
Albumin	S	3.1–4.3 g/dL	31–43 g/L
Alkaline phosphatase			
Females	S	30–100 U/L	0.50–1.67 μkat/L
Males	S	45–115 U/L	0.75–1.92 μkat/L
Amylase	S	53–123 U/L	0.88–2.05 nkat/L
Aspartate aminotransferase (AST; formerly SGOT)			
Females	S	9–25 U/L	0.15–0.42 μkat/L
Males	S	10–40 U/L	0.17–0.67 μkat/L
Bicarbonate	WB, S	22–26 mEq/L	22–26 mmol/L
Bilirubin, direct	S	0.0–0.4 mg/dL	0–7 μmol/L
Bilirubin, total	S	0.0–1.0 mg/dL	0–17 μmol/L
Calcium	S	8.5–10.5 mg/dL	2.1–2.6 mmol/L
	U	0–300 mg/day	0–7.5 mmol/day
Calcium, ionized	P	1.14–1.30 mmol/L	Same
Carbon dioxide content, total	S	24.0–30.9 mmol/L	Same
Carbon dioxide partial pressure (arterial $PaCO_2$)	WB	35–45 mm Hg	4.7–6.0 kPa
Chloride	P, S	100–108 mmol/L	Same
	U	10–200 mmol/L	Same
Cholesterol, total	S	<200 mg/dL	<5.18 mmol/L
Cholesterol, HDL	S	<35 mg/dL	<0.91 mmol/L
Cholesterol, LDL	S	<130 mg/dL	<3.36 mmol/L
Creatine kinase (CK)	S		
Females		40–150 U/L	0.67–2.50 μkat/L
Males		60–400 U/L	1.00–6.67 μkat/L
Creatinine	S	0.6–1.5 mg/dL	53–133 μmol/L
	U	15–25 mg/kg/day	0.13–0.22 mmol/kg/day
Glucose, fasting	P	70–110 mg/dL	3.9–6.1 mmol/L
Iron	S	50–150 μg/dL	9.0–26.9 μmol/L
Lactic dehydrogenase (LDH)	S	110–210 U/L	1.83–3.50 μkat/L
Lactic acid	P	0.5–2.2 mmol/L	Same
Magnesium	S	1.5–2.0 mEq/L	0.8–1.0 mmol/L
Osmolality	S	280–296 mOsm/kg water	280–296 mmol/kg
pH, arterial	WB	7.35–7.45 pH units	Same
Phosphorus, inorganic	S	2.6–4.5 mg/dL	0.84–1.45 mmol/L
	U	1g/day (avg.)	32 mmol/day (avg)
Potassium	S	3.5–5.0 mmol/L	Same
Protein, total	S	6.0–8.0 g/dL	60–80 g/L
	U	<165 mg/day	<0.165 g/day

(continued)

Table E–2 | General Chemistry Values (*Continued*)

Substance	Sample*	Normal Values Traditional Units†	SI Units†
Sodium	S	135–145 mmol/L	Same
Triglycerides, fasting	S	40–150 mg/dL	0.45–1.69 mmol/L
Urea nitrogen (BUN)	S	8–25 mg/dL	2.9–8.9 mmol/L
Uric acid	S		
Females		2.3–6.6 mg/dL	137–393 μmol/L
Males		3.6–8.5 mg/dL	214–506 μmol/L
Hematology and Coagulation			
Bleeding Time		2–9.5 min	Same
Differential blood count	WB		
Neutrophils		45–74%	0.45–0.74
Lymphocytes		16–45%	0.16–0.45
Monocytes		4–10%	0.04–0.10
Eosinophils		0–7%	0.00–0.07
Basophils		0–2%	0.00–0.02
Erythrocyte count	WB	$4.15–4.9 \times 10^6/mm^3$	$4.15–4.9 \times 10^{12}/L$
Erythrocyte sedimentation rate	WB		
Females		1–30 mm/hr	Same
Males		1–13 mm/hr	Same
Hematocrit	WB		
Females		37–48%	0.37–0.48
Males		42–52%	0.42–0.52
Hemoglobin	WB		
Females		12–16 g/dL	7.4–9.9 mmol/L
Males		13–18 g/dL	8.1–11.2 mmol/L
Partial thromboplastin time, activated (APTT)	P	24–37 sec	Same
Platelet count	WB	$150–350 \times 10^3/mm^3$	$150–350 \times 10^9/L$
Prothrombin time (PT)	P	8.8–11.6 sec	Same

*Samples: P, plasma; S, serum; U, urine; WB, whole blood.

†Traditional units are reported in most texts and laboratory reports. SI Units are units of the new Système international d'Unités. SI units are based mainly on the metric system, in which (for example) amounts of a substance in a sample are stated in moles per liter, rather than in weight per (other) volume of sample. One goal of implementing the use of SI units is to standardize the reporting of laboratory values worldwide, but this has not gained universal acceptance yet, mainly because some units are very unfamiliar to persons who need to use them. Values listed above, regardless of the units in which they are reported, may depend on the testing method used to analyze a sample. Consult your clinical laboratory for the units and testing methods used by your facility.

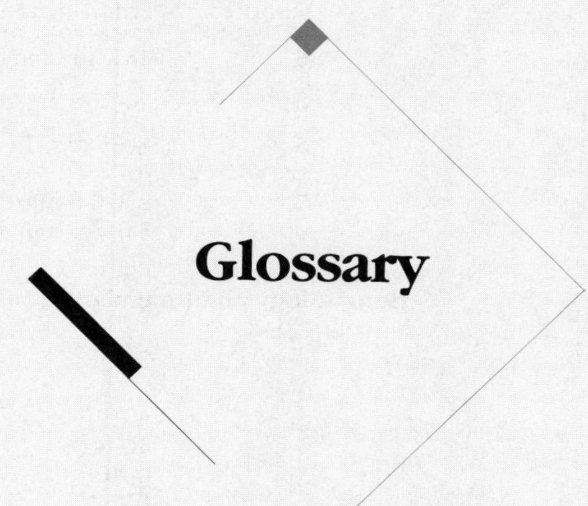

Glossary

absorption: the process by which a drug passes from its site of administration into the bloodstream; absorption, and the factors that modify it, do not apply to drugs administered directly into the bloodstream (for example, by intravenous routes)

abstinence syndrome: See *withdrawal syndrome*

accommodation: the process of focusing the eye

acidosis: a condition characterized by a below normal blood pH, as caused by loss of base (such as bicarbonate) or accumulation of acid; its origin may be respiratory (as from hypoventilation) or metabolic (as from excessive diarrhea or the administration of certain drugs)

acute: of sudden onset or short duration (usually several hours or less)

addiction: a condition characterized by uncontrolled drug seeking or use, and often accompanied by physical and/or psychologic dependence

additive effect: a term used to describe the combined (interacting) effects of two drugs that act simultaneously to produce the same type of response by the same mechanism of action; the total effect equals that which would be expected by simply adding the intensity of each drug's effects $(1 + 1 = 2)$

adjunctive: used as an additional and often necessary part of therapy or treatment with some other drug or nondrug intervention

adrenergic: acting like, or resembling the effects of, epinephrine, norepinephrine, or activation of the sympathetic nervous system; often used synonymously with the term sympathomimetic; the term *noradrenergic,* which was used to describe a drug acting like norepinephrine, is used less frequently

adsorption: the attachment or binding of one substance (eg, a drug molecule) to another structure or substance

adverse effect: an unwanted, undesirable, and possibly harmful side effect of a drug that occurs regardless of whether the drug dose is excessive. See *side effect*

afferent: directed or leading to a center (eg, to the central nervous system)

affinity: an indicator of a drug molecule's tendency to bind to its receptor; on a logarithmic dose–response curve for an agonist (cf.), the ED_{50} reflects the drug's affinity; a drug with a lower ED_{50} than another agonist for the same receptor has the greater affinity

afterload: the pressure that the heart's ventricles must overcome to expel blood into the circulatory system during systole (ie, systolic blood pressure)

agonist: a drug that interacts with a receptor and alters the cell's function(s) to cause an effect, usually an increase or decrease in the cell's predrug level of activity; agonists have both affinity and efficacy (cf.)

akathisia: a subjective condition characterized by restlessness, jitteriness, uneasiness, an inability to sit or lie quietly, and resulting disturbed daily activity or sleep; often induced by antipsychotic drugs as an adverse response

akinesia: abnormal absence or infrequency of motor activity

alkaloid: a particular type of organic chemical (including drugs), usually derived from a plant, that has biologic (pharmacologic) activity

alkalosis: a condition characterized by an excessively high blood pH, as caused by loss of acid or accumulation of base (such as bicarbonate); its origin may be respiratory (as from hyperventilation) or metabolic (as from excessive vomiting or the administration of certain drugs)

allergic response: an adverse response to a foreign chemical (including a drug), resulting from previous exposure to that or a related chemical, that is mediated by an antigen–antibody reaction

alopecia: partial or complete loss of body (usually scalp) hair

analeptic: characterized by general central nervous system stimulation; a drug generally administered to stimulate respiration or overall wakefulness

analgesic: characterized by relief of pain, but not necessarily accompanied by generalized central nervous system depression or loss of consciousness; a drug that relieves pain

anaphylaxis: a severe, often life-threatening, form of antigen–antibody reaction (cf. *allergic response*) to a drug or other foreign substance to which a patient has previously been exposed; frequent signs and symptoms include marked hypotension (shock), severe bronchoconstriction and respiratory difficulty, and mild-to-severe dermatologic reactions (skin rashes)

anesthetic: characterized by a reversible loss of sensation, including pain; general anesthetic drugs produce loss of sensations and loss of consciousness; local anesthetic drugs produce sensory loss (usually analgesia) at or surrounding the region where the drug is applied or injected

anorexia: loss of or lack of appetite for food

anoxia: complete lack of oxygen; the extreme of hypoxia (cf.)

antagonism: See *drug antagonism*

antagonist: a drug molecule that interacts with a cell receptor but either produces no effect or inhibits or blocks the response of an agonist; antagonists have affinity for a receptor but cause no response (ie, have no efficacy) in the absence of an agonist; sometimes called a receptor blocker

antibiotic: a chemical substance that either kills or inhibits the growth of microorganisms; traditionally defined as a substance produced by one microorganism that can alter the growth, reproduction, or viability of another microorganism. See *bactericidal; bacteriostatic*

antibody: a substance in the body tissues or fluids that interacts with specific foreign substances (cf. antigen) that enter the body; an essential component of the immune response that plays a role in host defenses, allergy, and anaphylaxis

anticholinergic: producing blockade of receptors for acetylcholine; see *antimuscarinic*

antidote: a drug or drug mixture that is used to counteract the effects of a poison or another drug, particularly when toxicity occurs

antigen: a substance that, when introduced into the body, can trigger the formation of specific antibodies; antigens are generally proteins

antimuscarinic: producing atropine-like actions—that is, blockade of the muscarinic subtype of acetylcholine receptors; also see anticholinergic

antipsychotic: producing effects that suppress the psychiatric manifestations of a severe mental disorder such as schizophrenia or other psychoses

antipyretic: fever-reducing

anuria: lack of urine production and excretion

anxiolytic: able to relieve minor anxiety or simple emotional tension; a drug that relieves anxiety; sometimes used synonymously with the term minor tranquilizer

aqueous: water-soluble, or dissolved in water or a water-based solution

arrhythmia: any irregular elecrical activity of the heart, often accompanied by changes of heart rate or rhythm; absence of rhythm; often used synonymously with dysrhythmia; bradyarrhythmias are characterized by abnormally low rates and rhythm, and tachyarrhythmias by unusually high rates and rhythm

arrhythmogenic: capable of causing an arrhythmia

asthenia: diminished or absent strength or energy; weakness

asymptomatic: lacking, or causing no, symptoms

ataxia: abnormal coordination of muscle movements, particularly voluntary muscle movements; may be due to diseased muscles or nerves, but is frequently produced as a side effect of drugs, particularly those that depress the central nervous system

atopic: allergy-related

autacoid: a substance, synthesized and released by cells, that exerts biologic effects at or very near the site of release; a local hormone (eg, histamine)

autonomic: self-controlling or involuntary; usually applied to the sympathetic and parasympathetic nervous systems or sympathetic or parasympathetic drugs

azotemia: the abnormal presence or excessively high concentration of urea, proteins, and related nitrogen-containing substances in the blood, frequently caused by kidney disease, excessive fluid loss, or muscle wasting

bactericidal: capable of killing bacteria

bacteriostatic: capable of inhibiting the growth or multiplication of bacteria

bioassay: assessment (description, measurement) of a drug's effects in a living system, such as a whole animal or isolated tissue, and comparison of the drug's activity to that of a standardized preparation

bioavailability: the amount of an administered dose of drug that can be absorbed (usually after oral administration) to produce a pharmacologic effect; a term that implies that although identical doses of chemically identical drugs may be administered, factors related to the manufacture of one product may enable it to be more completely absorbed and better able to produce the intended effects

biochemical antagonism: the process by which one drug decreases the amount of another drug available to produce its actions; often caused by the ability of one drug to change the metabolism of a second drug

bioequivalence: the ability of two or more drugs to produce responses that are identical in kind and intensity

biotransformation: metabolism

blood dyscrasia: any disorder characterized by abnormal numbers or types of cellular blood components (eg, red cells, white cells, platelets, and their precursors)

bolus: a large amount; when applied to parenteral drug administration, a single and usually large volume of liquid drug that is injected more or less at once, often rapidly

brady- (prefix): slow

bradycardia: a heart rate that is below normal limits

buccal: pertaining to the fleshy, interior portion of the cheeks; a route of drug administration in which a tablet is placed between the cheek and gums to allow for dissolution and systemic absorption. See *sublingual*

capsule: an oral dosage form in which a drug, in solid or liquid form, is enclosed in a gelatinous container

carcinogenic: capable of producing changes of cell growth control and causing the affected cells to become cancerous

cardioselective: literally, affecting only the heart; when applied to certain beta-adrenergic drugs, indicates preferential effects on $beta_1$ receptors

catecholamine: a class of organic chemicals with a particular structure, exemplified by epinephrine, norepinephrine, and dopamine; a specific class of drugs that produces sympathomimetic actions; often but not necessarily synonymous with adrenergic or sympathomimetic drug

chemical antagonism: the inhibition or inactivation of a drug's activity by its chemical interaction with another drug

chemotherapy: the use of drugs, including antibiotics and anticancer agents, for the purpose of killing or inhibiting the growth of specific living cells or organisms in the body

cholinergic: acting like acetylcholine; usually used to describe the type of effects or responses produced by a particular drug or group of drugs, including acetylcholine-like agonists and inhibitors of acetylcholinesterase, that act on two types of acetylcholine receptors—muscarinic and nicotinic (cf.); often used synonymously with the term parasympathomimetic or cholinomimetic

cholinomimetic: cholinergic; mimicking the effects of acetylcholine

chromatopsia: visual disturbances characterized by alterations in the apparent color of objects

chronic: of long duration, and often of slow onset

chronotropic: characterized by a change of rate; usually applied to heart rate: a positive chronotropic effect is an increase of heart rate, a negative chronotropic effect is a decrease

cinchonism: a syndrome caused by overdoses of the antiarrhythmic drug quinidine, a cinchona alkaloid

coma: a state of profound central nervous system depression from which the patient cannot be aroused by external stimuli

competitive antagonism: a type of pharmacologic antagonism in which the antagonist binds reversibly with the same receptor as an agonist, thereby inhibiting the agonist's actions in a way that can be overcome by increasing the agonist's dose; often used synonymously with surmountable antagonism. See also *noncompetitive antagonism*

compliance: willingness or ability of the patient to carefully follow specific guidelines or instructions for therapy, whether with drugs or otherwise, as set forth by a health-care provider

concomitant: accompanying or given with something else; occurring at the same time

congener: a drug that belongs to a particular group of compounds having very similar chemical structures; a chemical analogue

contraindication: a situation in which a drug should not be given, whether for prophylaxis, diagnosis, or treatment: *absolute contraindication:* a situation in which a drug must not be given under any circumstances because of the risk of severe or possibly fatal consequences; *relative contraindication:* a situation in which a drug ordinarily should not be given, but it may be given if the potential benefits of the drug outweigh its potential risks

controlled substance: a drug whose use, prescribing, and dispensing are regulated or restricted by one or more federal, state, or local laws

counterirritant: a topically applied drug that produces mild pain, warmth, or cold, and in doing so obscures underlying pain of pathologic origin or distracts the patient from the underlying pain

cross-dependence: the ability of one drug to substitute for another drug that has produced physical dependence, maintaining the signs and symptoms of dependence produced by the first, and not producing a withdrawal (abstinence) syndrome

cross-sensitivity: the phenomenon in which exposure to a drug may produce an allergic reaction in an individual previously exposed to a different but chemically related drug

cyanosis: a bluish discoloration of the skin and mucous membranes caused by inadequately oxygenated blood

cycloplegia: paralysis of accommodation (cf.) caused by inability of the ciliary muscle of the eye to alter the shape of the lens to focus on objects; often induced by anticholinergic/antimuscarinic (atropine-like) drugs that permit the eye to focus on distant objects, but cause blurred vision when looking at near objects

delirium: a mental disturbance characterized by excitement, restlessness, incoherence, illusions, and hallucinations

depot: a storage site; a site in the body that tends to accumulate an administered drug

depot preparation: a pharmaceutical preparation made to be injected or implanted in the body to release drug slowly into the circulation

depressor: characterized by a decrease of pressure; usually applied to blood pressure (vasodepressor)

diaphoresis: sweating or excessive perspiration

diffusion: the process by which drugs passively cross biologic membranes down their concentration gradient (from the region of highest concentration to the region of lowest concentration), without the need for metabolic energy (eg,

ATP) to drive drug movement; the primary process by which most drugs cross membranes

digitalis: a general term referring to one or more cardiac-stimulating glycosides, such as digoxin or digitoxin

digitalize: to administer an effective dose of digitalis (cf.), usually for starting therapy (ie, to give a loading dose of digitalis)

diplopia: double vision

direct-acting: the ability of an agonist to directly stimulate target cells (effectors), producing an effect that is independent of reflexes or release of other mediators; often applied to sympathomimetic drugs such as epinephrine. Cf. *indirect-acting; mixed-acting*

distribution: the process by which a drug is circulated throughout the body by the bloodstream to produce its systemic effects

diuretic: characterized by increased production and excretion of urine; a drug that increases urine output, usually through increased sodium excretion

dopaminergic: involving or resembling the effects of dopamine; a nerve that synthesizes, stores, and releases dopamine

dose: the amount of drug administered

dose–response curve: the graphic representation showing the response to a drug (on the ordinate, or Y-axis) as it relates to the drug's dose (on the abscissa, or X-axis); *graded dose–response curve:* a dose–response curve in which the intensity of the response is plotted against the dose; *log dose–response curve:* a dose–response curve in which the drug dose is plotted on a logarithmic scale; *quantal dose–response curve:* a dose–response curve in which the effect is expressed as an all-or-none response (eg, the percentage of individuals showing a certain predetermined, measurable response)

drug: any chemical capable of interacting with a living system and altering its activity

drug antagonism: any interaction between two drugs in which the combined effects of the two are less than expected by simply adding the individual effects produced by each alone (2 + 2 = 3). See *biochemical antagonism; chemical antagonism; pharmacologic antagonism; physiologic antagonism*

drug dependence: a condition in which the drug-taker has either a psychologic or physiologic need or desire to continue taking the drug in order to maintain a sense of apparent well-being. See *physical dependence; psychologic dependence*

drug resistance: a condition of decreased responsiveness to a usually effective dose of a drug, due to known or unknown causes (cf. *drug tolerance*)

drug tolerance: decreased responsiveness to a drug that develops after previous or repeated administration of a drug or its congeners; tolerance is characterized by the need to increase subsequent drug doses in order to produce the same intensity or duration of effects that were produced before tolerance developed. See *tachyphylaxis*

dyscrasia: any abnormal, morbid condition in which there is an imbalance between normal components. See *blood dyscrasia*

dyskinesia: impaired function of voluntary muscle groups, outwardly appearing as irregular, incomplete, or abnormal movements

dyspepsia: gastric or esophageal pain or other unpleasant responses caused, for example, by excessive gastric acid; "acid indigestion"

dysphagia: difficulty or discomfort in swallowing

dysphoria: a feeling of unrest or uneasiness, often intense; sometimes produced by drugs that have prominent central nervous system effects. Cf. *euphoria*

dyspnea: difficult or labored breathing

dysrhythmia: See *arrhythmia*

ectopic: located or originating away from its normal position

ED_{50}: See *median effective dose*

edema: accumulation of abnormally large amounts of fluid in the extracellular (intercellular) spaces of the body,

effector: the cell, tissue, or organ upon which a drug exerts its effects; more specifically, the cell with specific receptors for an agonist, whose function is changed by that agonist; the target of drug action

efferent: directed or leading away from a center (eg, from the central nervous system)

efficacy: the ability of a drug to produce a biologic response; the property that distinguishes agonists (which have affinity and efficacy) from their antagonists (which have affinity but no efficacy); an indicator of the maximum intensity of a drug's effects

elixir: a clear, sweetened, aromatic drug preparation in which the active ingredient is usually dissolved in a water-alcohol solution. See *tincture*

embolus: a thrombus (cf.) that has become dislodged and is free-floating; it may become lodged in a smaller blood vessel, thereby obstructing blood flow; any small free-floating mass (air, fat, cell debris) that lodges in a vessel and obstructs blood flow

emesis: vomiting

emetic: tending to cause vomiting

empiric: based on tradition, experience, or assumption rather than on direct proof of a cause and effect relationship

endocytosis: the process by which drugs or other substances are actively taken up by a cell, usually inside membrane-bound vesicles

endogenous: normally present within the body; the opposite of exogenous (cf.)

enteral: given in or by way of the alimentary tract (eg, by mouth or into the stomach, intestines, or rectum). Cf. *parenteral*

enteric coating: a special coating around a drug tablet or other oral dosage form to prevent its dissolution in the stomach, thereby preventing gastric inactivation of the active drug or irritation of the gastric mucosa

enterohepatic recirculation: the process by which an absorbed drug is excreted via the bile into the gastrointestinal tract and then reabsorbed into the circulation at a more distal site in the gut

essential hypertension: hypertension of unknown etiology

etiology: the cause of a disease or abnormal function

euphoria: a sense of well-being, comfort, or pleasure; an exaggerated and sometimes abnormal sense of well-being that is often produced by drugs that have prominent central nervous system effects. Cf. *dysphoria*

excipient: inert ingredients added to a drug formulation to give it a consistency or form suitable for administration

excretion: the process by which drugs or their metabolites are removed from the body, usually in the urine, feces, or other substances that are eventually eliminated from the body

exocytosis: the process by which substances such as neurotransmitters are actively expelled, usually in membrane-bound vesicles, from intracellular storage sites to the extracellular space

exogenous: from a source outside of the body; not normally found in the body; the opposite of endogenous (cf.)

extract: a concentrated, orally administered form of a drug that is derived from animal or plant source. See *fluid extract*

extraneuronal: outside a nerve

extrapyramidal: brain tracts that control involuntary motion of skeletal muscle

extravasation: discharge, escape, or seepage into the surrounding tissues of a drug that is being injected or infused into a vessel

febrile: characterized by an above-normal body temperature; feverish

first-pass effect: rapid and almost complete hepatic metabolism of a drug, leading to very low blood levels in the systemic circulation, as the drug is delivered to the liver via the hepatic portal vein after oral administration and absorption from the gut

fixed-dose combination: a commercial or proprietary combination of two or more drugs in a single dosage form, usually used to manage a condition for which the individual drugs would normally be administered

fluid extract: an alcoholic solution of a drug that is derived from animal or plant sources; more concentrated than an extract

ganglion: a group of nerve cell bodies and the nerve endings that form synapses with them, located outside the central nervous system

generic: a term used to designate the common or officially assigned name for a drug, as opposed to the proprietary (cf.) or "brand" name given by the drug manufacturer

glycoside: a compound (drug), usually isolated from a plant, that contains a sugar as part of the molecule; glucoside

graded dose–response curve: See *dose–response curve*

gynecomastia: enlargement of the breasts, in either males or females

hallucination: a sensory change in which an individual hears, sees, tastes, smells, or feels things that do not exist; adj: hallucinogenic. Cf. *illusion*

hapten: a small chemical molecule that can bind to a larger molecule, thereby forming a substance with antigenic properties

hormone: a chemical substance secreted by cells in one part of the body that can influence the growth, development, or other functions of cells distant from the hormone source

hydrophilic: tending to dissolve or accumulate in an aqueous, rather than a lipid, environment; water-soluble

hydrophobic: tending to exclude water; tending to dissolve or accumulate in a lipid, rather than an aqueous, environment. Cf. *lipophilic*

hygroscopic: tending to accumulate water

hypercalcemia: elevated serum calcium levels

hypercalciuria: excessive calcium excretion in the urine, often leading to the formation of stones (calculi) that can obstruct and damage the renal tubules

hyperkalemia: elevated serum potassium levels

hyperplasia: an increase in the number of normal cells in a tissue. See *hypertrophy; neoplasia*

hypersensitivity: an unusually intense response to a dose of a drug that normally causes only a mild or modest effect in other individuals; inappropriately used to indicate a severe allergic reaction to a drug. See *idiosyncrasy*

hypertension: arterial blood pressure that is unsatisfactorily high; unrelated to emotional "tension"

hypertrophy: excessive growth or enlargement of a tissue or organ, caused by disease or, sometimes, by prolonged, excessive stimulation of its function, and characterized by an increase in the size, but not number, of its constituent cells. See *hyperplasia; neoplasia*

hyperuricemia: elevated levels of uric acid in the blood, often leading to the development of gout and related arthritic diseases

hypnotic: causing sleep from which the patient can be awakened; a drug that induces sleep; a drug used to treat insomnia; See *sedative*

hypokalemia: abnormally low blood potassium levels

hyponatremia: abnormally low blood sodium levels

hypotension: arterial blood pressure that is unsatisfactorily low or below the blood pressure that is normal for a particular patient. See *orthostatic hypotension*

hypovolemia: a state of fluid depletion or diminished blood volume, as may occur with excessive vomiting, diarrhea, diuresis, hemorrhage, or inadequate fluid intake

hypoxia: inadequate supply of oxygen to a tissue or organ, despite maintenance of blood flow to that structure. See *anoxia; ischemia*

iatrogenic: caused by treatment given by a health-care provider for a particular medical condition; usually applied to adverse consequences or conditions arising as the result of treatment of another disorder

idiopathic: having an unknown cause

idiosyncrasy: an unusual, atypical, or unexpected response to a drug, whether in intensity or in characteristics, that is usually caused by underlying genetic factors; adj: idiosyncratic

illusion: a distorted sensory image of something that really exists; cf. *hallucination*

indication: a condition for which a drug is appropriately given, whether for prophylaxis, diagnosis, or treatment. Cf. *contraindication*

indirect-acting: a response that is not caused by a direct effect of a drug on an effector; usually applied to sympathomimetic drugs that cause effects by stimulating release of norepinephrine from nerves, which then causes the eventual effect on target cells

infarction: an area of local tissue damage and eventual tissue death usually caused by reduced blood flow to that area, as by local hemorrhage, coagulation, or other physical blockage of the blood vessel

infusion: the slow administration of a fluid or drug, usually into a vein, propelled either by gravity or by a pump; cf. *injection*

injection: the administration of a fluid or drug, as into a vein or artery, forced by pressure as from a syringe; injections usually imply delivery rates faster than those achieved with infusions (cf.)

inotropic: characterized by a change of the force of muscle contraction; usually applied to the contractile force of the heart; a *positive inotropic effect* is an increase of force; a *negative inotropic effect* is a decrease of force

insomnia: the inability to fall asleep and/or stay asleep; abnormal sleep patterns

instillation: the act of dropping a liquid into or onto a body cavity or opening (eg, the urinary bladder, conjunctival sac, or ear canal)

insufflation: the act of blowing a powder, vapor, or gas into a body cavity such as the lungs

intraneuronal: inside a nerve

intrinsic activity: efficacy; the ability of a drug to produce a biologic response

intrinsic sympathomimetic activity (ISA): a term applied to certain beta-adrenergic blocking drugs to indicate that, at low doses or in the presence of low sympathetic tone, they cause weak sympathetic stimulating effects

ionized: electrically charged; not neutral

ischemia: reduction of tissue or organ blood flow (and hence oxygen and nutrient delivery) to levels that are not adequate to maintain function or viability, potentially producing infarction or necrosis; complete lack of blood flow to a tissue or organ. See *necrosis*

junctional: at the meeting place of two structures; when applied to nerves, at the junction between a nerve and a structure that it innervates. See *postjunctional; prejunctional*

kaliuretic: characterized by increased potassium loss in the urine; potassium-wasting

keratolytic: capable of dissolving the outer layers of the skin

lag period: the time between the onset of drug administration and the appearance of a specified, usually the desired, effect

LD_{50}: See *median lethal dose*

liniment: an oily liquid, containing one or more active ingredients, that is applied to the skin

lipophilic: liking or preferring a lipid (fat) environment; tending to dissolve or accumulate in a lipid, rather than an aqueous, environment; fat-soluble

loading dose: the initial dose of a drug given to produce a certain level or concentration of drug in the blood, usually quickly; the loading dose is usually higher than subsequent doses (see *maintenance dose*), and it may be given by a route of administration different from that used for subsequent doses; sometimes used synonymously with priming dose; the digitalizing dose, when applied to digoxin or digitoxin

log dose–response curve: See *dose–response curve*

lozenge: a flat, round, or oval drug preparation that is meant to be held in the mouth, where it dissolves and releases the drug; a troche

maintenance dose: the dose of drug given repeatedly in order to maintain effective and relatively constant blood concentrations and, therefore, relatively constant biologic effects

malignant: tending to become progressively and often quickly worse, and to result in death

margin of safety: the relationship between the dose of a drug needed to cause desired therapeutic responses and that which causes a serious adverse effect such as death; in practical terms, an indicator of the likelihood that an excessive dose will cause toxicity or death, compared to a comparable overdose with a similar drug having a higher or lower margin of safety. Cf. *therapeutic index*

median effective dose ED_{50}: the dose of drug required to produce half the maximal response or effect; for a population or group of subjects, the smallest dose needed to produce a stated effect in half the population. Cf. *median lethal dose*

median lethal dose (LD_{50}): the smallest dose needed to kill half of a population or group of subjects receiving the drug

metabolism: the processes by which a drug is chemically modified within the body to convert it to more or less active compounds that are generally more easily excreted; synonymous with biotransformation

metered dose: a precise dose of drug that is automatically dispensed from a multidose container (eg, a pressurized container); commonly used for inhaled bronchodilators

micturition: urination

milliequivalent (mEq): the amount of a drug, salt, or ion equal to one one-thousandth of its molecular or atomic weight (for ions, divided by the valence or number of charges) when expressed in grams (for example, the atomic weight of sodium ion, which has a valence of +1, is 23, so 1 mEq is 0.023 g, or 23 mg; calcium has an ionic weight of 40 and a valence of +2, so 1 mEq is 20 mg)

miosis: constriction of the pupil of the eye; drugs that constrict the pupil are called *miotic* drugs

mixed-acting: the ability of an agonist (usually a sympathomimetic) to produce its effects by a combination of two primary mechanisms, one involving direct interaction with its receptor, the other involving indirect actions owing to release of other agonists by the drug

morbid: diseased, ill, or sick; sometimes used synonymously with moribund

muscarinic: related to or resembling the actions of the alkaloid muscarine; a specific subclass of cholinergic receptor that, by definition, is stimulated by acetylcholine or related agonists but is specifically blocked by atropine. See *nicotinic*

mutagenic: capable of causing alterations of gene structure, often resulting in abnormal cell growth and multiplication, and sometimes resulting in carcinogenic or teratogenic effects

mydriasis: dilation of the pupil of the eye; drugs used to dilate the pupil are called mydriatic drugs

narcotic: clouding the mind; in practice, having both analgesic and sedative action; a controlled substance with analgesic and sedative activity; an opiate or morphine-like drug

nebulizer: a drug-dispensing device that atomizes (finely disperses) a liquid drug for inhalation

necrosis: tissue death, often due to inadequate blood flow (cf. *ischemia*)

neoplasia: new and abnormal cell growth, as in a tumor. See *hyperplasia; hypertrophy*

neuroeffector junction: the anatomic or functional region of communication between a nerve ending and the effector cell that is affected by the nerve's transmitter; the synaptic connection between a preganglionic nerve and one or more postganglionic nerves; the site of neurotransmitter release

neurogenic: forming neural tissue; caused by nerves or abnormal nerve activity

neuroleptic: producing effects that resemble disorders of the nervous system, especially the central nervous system

neurolytic: able to destroy nervous tissue; often applied to such drugs as phenol and alcohol, which are used for permanent regional analgesia (local anesthesia) in persons with severe, intractable pain

neuronal: pertaining to nerves. See *extraneuronal; intraneuronal*

neurotransmitter: a chemical substance (eg, acetylcholine, norepinephrine) that is synthesized and released by a nerve ending and that then acts as an agonist on the effector cell (nerve, muscle, or gland) located adjacent to it

nicotinic: related to or resembling the actions of the alkaloid nicotine; a specific subclass of cholinergic receptor that, by definition, is stimulated by acetylcholine or other cholinergic drugs but is specifically blocked by curare and curare-like drugs. See *muscarinic*

noncompetitive antagonism: a type of pharmacologic antagonism in which an antagonist interacts more or less irreversibly with receptors for an agonist, inhibiting the agonist's actions in a way that cannot be overcome with even marked increases of the agonist's dose; sometimes used synonymously with unsurmountable antagonism. See *competitive antagonism; pharmacologic antagonism*

nonionized: neutral; not electrically charged

ointment: a semisolid preparation of one or more drugs, usually applied topically to the skin. See *paste*

oliguria: the production and excretion of diminished volumes of urine

ophthalmic: pertaining to the eye

opiate: having both analgesic and sedative actions; morphine-like; a synthetic or naturally occurring drug with morphine-like actions; synonymous with opioid. See *narcotic*

orphan drug: a drug, often a new drug, for which clinical indications are rare

orthostatic hypotension: a fall of blood pressure that occurs upon prolonged standing in one place without movement, frequently causing symptoms of dizziness or fainting (syncope); also applied to hypotension that occurs on changing suddenly from a supine to a standing position

otic: pertaining to the ear

parasympatholytic: acting like atropine (ie, as a muscarinic receptor blocker) to inhibit the effects normally caused by parasympathetic nervous system stimulation or administration of parasympathomimetic drugs

parasympathomimetic: mimicking the responses that would occur when the parasympathetic nervous system is stimulated. See *cholinergic*

parent drug: the original chemical form of a drug that was administered, from which the body may produce various metabolites

parenteral: given by a route other than through the alimentary tract (ie, by intravenous, subcutaneous, or intramuscular routes). See *enteral*

paresthesia: an abnormal sensation such as burning, tingling, or numbness, usually sensed in the extremities

partition coefficient: in pharmaceutics, a number that indicates the relative ability of a drug to separate into two different environments, such as oil and water; for example, drugs with a high lipid:water partition coefficient are better able to diffuse through lipid membranes or be stored in fatty tissue than drugs with a lower partition coefficient

paste: a preparation similar to an ointment, but thicker and stiffer, and usually less able to penetrate the skin

pathognomonic: a sign or symptom that is so uniquely characteristic of a disease, pathologic condition, or drug effect that it can be used as the basis for a differential diagnosis

percutaneous: through the skin; a route of absorption in which a drug, usually formulated as an ointment, paste, or liniment, is applied to the skin for subsequent diffusion into deeper structures and, possibly, absorption into the systemic circulation

pharmacodynamics: the study of how drugs interact with cells or other body structures to produce their characteristic responses

pharmacogenetics: the study of hereditary (genetic) factors that account for subject-to-subject differences in the response to drugs

pharmacokinetics: the study of distribution, metabolism, and excretion, as they influence the amount of drug available to produce a biologic effect, with emphasis on drug actions as a function of time (onset, duration of action, and so on)

pharmacologic antagonism: the process by which one drug—the antagonist—interferes with the action of another—the agonist—by preventing the latter drug from combining with its receptor. See *competitive antagonism; noncompetitive antagonism*

pharmacologic dose: the amount (dose) of a drug needed to cause a specified, usually desired, response; a dose producing blood levels of a substance higher than those found normally within the body. Cf. *physiologic dose*

pharmacology: a broad discipline studying the physical, chemical, physiologic, and biochemical actions of drugs, whether experimentally or in clinical settings

pharmacopoeia: a book, usually quite large, that lists and describes various chemicals used in therapeutics, usually including their formulas, tests for their purity, and chemical properties

pharmacy: the science or discipline dealing with the preparing, compounding, and dispensing of drugs

pheochromocytoma: a tumor, usually of the adrenal medulla, that produces and releases into the bloodstream large amounts of epinephrine and norepinephrine; a tumor of any tissue that is capable of synthesizing and releasing catecholamines

photophobia: ocular pain, discomfort due to light; generally caused by drugs that dilate the pupil or prevent miosis

photosensitive: affected or worsened by exposure to light

physical dependence: a type of drug dependence characterized by altered physiologic states, and caused by repeated administration of a drug; physical dependence can only be demonstrated by abruptly discontinuing administration of the drug or reducing its dose, or by giving a specific antagonist that blocks effects of the drug, either of which induces a characteristic withdrawal (abstinence) syndrome

physiologic antagonism: a type of antagonism in which two agonists, acting at different sites and by different mechanisms, produce opposite effects that tend to counteract or balance the effects of each other; used synonymously with functional antagonism

physiologic dose: the dose of a drug or hormone that produces blood levels equivalent to those normally found within the body

placebo: a substance presumed to be without biologic activity that, nevertheless, produces a response; a substance given to psychologically appease or gratify a patient, perhaps leading the patient to believe that the medication will cure or relieve illness or symptoms; an inactive substance given as a "control" during the clinical evaluation of new drugs claimed to produce therapeutic effects, for the purpose of determining whether the new drug produces effects that are statistically different from those observed when no active drug (the placebo) is given

plasma: the protein-rich blood fraction obtained after sedimenting the blood cells before coagulation has taken place. See *serum*

plateau principle: the principle stating that giving fixed doses of a drug at regular times will eventually produce a more or less steady blood level and effect once rates of drug absorption equal rates of drug elimination

polyuria: excessive production and excretion of urine. See *anuria; oliguria*

postjunctional: at the distal site of the meeting place between two structures; when applied to nerves, usually equivalent to postsynaptic

postsynaptic: located at, on, or in the distal nerve at a synapse; located at or on the structure (eg, muscle, gland) that is innervated by a nerve

postural hypotension: See *orthostatic hypotension*

potency: the relative dose of a drug needed to produce an effect of a given intensity, compared to the dose of another drug that produces the same effect, of the same intensity, and by a similar mechanism of action

potency factor: the ratio of the ED_{50} values of two drugs that have the same efficacy; the drug with the lower ED_{50} is the more potent drug; the factor is the reciprocal of the ED_{50} values, with the more potent drug's ED_{50} being in the denominator

potentiation: a type of drug interaction occurring when one drug, which is without measurable effect, intensifies the actions of a second drug which when given alone can produce an effect $(0 + 2 = 3)$

powder: a finely ground solid preparation of one or more drugs

prejunctional: at the proximal site of the meeting place between two structures; when applied to nerves, usually equivalent to presynaptic

pressor: characterized by an increase of pressure; usually applied to blood pressure

presynaptic: located at, on, or in the proximal nerve at a synapse

priming dose: See *loading dose*

prodrug: a drug that is inactive in the form in which it is administered, and gains biologic activity upon metabolism

prophylaxis: prevention

proprietary: when applied to drugs, the brand name or trade name assigned by a drug company to the particular product that it sells; each proprietary drug also has a generic name (cf.) for each active ingredient

prototype: for a group of drugs, the agent that pharmacologically is most representative of all other drugs in the group; the best example of a group of drugs

pruritus: itching

psychologic dependence: a type of drug dependence characterized by an emotional need or desire to continue taking the drug in order to maintain a feeling of well-being

psychosis: a severe disturbance of normal thought, reasoning, behavior, or interpersonal relationships, such as in schizophrenia

psychotomimetic: causing psychosis-like symptoms; hallucinogenic

pyrogen: a fever-causing substance, often one released by bacteria

quantal dose–response curve: See *dose–response curve*

rebound: a response, occurring after abrupt discontinuation of a drug, that is characterized by an "overshoot" of a parameter (eg, blood pressure) beyond pretreatment levels

receptor: a specific structure on the cell membrane or in the cell with which specific agonist or antagonist drug molecules interact

refractory: not readily altered by therapy; characterized by a loss or lack of responsiveness to a drug, as might be due to progressing disease, development of tolerance, or physiologic changes produced by the drug itself

rhinitis: irritation and inflammation of the nasal passages; *rhinitis medicamentosa:* rhinitis caused by administration of drugs, usually locally on the nasal passages (eg, with sympathomimetic decongestant nasal drops or sprays), and particularly when used improperly

rhinorrhea: a watery, mucous discharge from the nose; runny nose

salicylism: a syndrome (cf.) of aspirin (salicylate) intoxication

sedative: causing drowsiness; a drug that causes drowsiness, usually by central nervous system depression, at doses that are generally insufficient to produce sleep (hypnosis); a drug that produces sedation

selectivity: the ability of a drug to produce one particular effect, or to affect a particular structure, rather than causing many or widespread effects. See *specificity*

serum: that part of the blood that is left after separating blood cells and other elements once the blood has clotted. See *plasma*

sialorrhea: excessive salivation

side effect: an effect of a drug, either beneficial, deleterious, inconsequential, pleasant, or unpleasant, that is secondary to the desired effect for which the drug was given; frequently used to denote adverse or unpleasant drug effects

sign: any objective (eg, observable, measurable) evidence of disease or response to a drug

solution: a preparation of one or more chemicals completely dissolved in a liquid carrier (eg, aqueous solutions are those in which the carrier is water)

somatic: pertaining to the body or periphery, as opposed to the mind or brain

specificity: the ability of a drug to produce its actions by a single mechanism of action or at a single site; selectivity

spirit: a concentrated alcoholic solution of a volatile substance

sublingual: under the tongue; a route of drug administration in which the dosage form, usually a tablet, lozenge, or troche, is placed under the tongue for subsequent dissolution and systemic absorption. See *buccal*

summation: a type of drug interaction in which two drugs, given together and producing the same type of effect, produce a response with an intensity that is the sum of their individual effects. See *additive effect*

superinfection: an overgrowth of bacteria different from those causing an original infection for which antibiotic drugs were prescribed, resulting in a secondary infection for which other antibiotic drugs must be given

suppository: a preparation of one or more drugs mixed in a base (eg, glycerin) that dissolves gradually at body temperature, releasing the drug for local effects or systemic absorption, as through mucous membranes

surmountable antagonism: See *competitive antagonism*

suspension: a preparation containing finely divided particles of solid drug floating in a liquid carrier; aqueous suspensions are those in which the carrier is water

sustained-release: a drug product, usually given orally in tablet or capsule form, that is formulated to dissolve and be absorbed slowly, thereby providing a relatively constant and long-lasting effect; timed-release

sympatholytic: acting to inhibit activation or effects of the sympathetic nervous system; acting like an adrenergic (alpha or beta) receptor blocker or antagonist

sympathomimetic: mimicking the responses that occur when the sympathetic nervous system is stimulated; eg, a sympathomimetic drug. See *adrenergic*

symptom: any functional evidence, often subjective or perceived by the patient, of a disease or drug response

synapse: the junction between one nerve and another, across which a neurotransmitter (cf.) diffuses; the junction between a nerve and another structure (eg, muscle, gland) that is regulated by that nerve

syncope: fainting, usually owing to a sudden hypotensive event

syndrome: a set of signs or symptoms, often characteristic of a particular disease or drug action, that occur together

synergism: a type of drug interaction in which the combined effects of two drugs given simultaneously is greater than the algebraic sum of the individual effects of these two drugs ($2 + 2 = 5$); synergism often occurs when the two drugs produce the same effect, but do so by different mechanisms of action, or when one drug alters the absorption, distribution, metabolism, or excretion of the other

syrup: an aqueous solution of drug containing sugar or flavorings to disguise unpleasant-tasting drugs

systemic: generalized; pertaining to or affecting all or most of the body

tablet: a powdered drug formulation compressed into a hard small form; may be made with special coatings (eg, enteric coatings) to ease swallowing or prevent early dissolution and absorption

tachycardia: a heart rate faster than normal

tachyphylaxis: a type of tolerance to a drug that occurs very quickly, often after the first one or few doses

tardive: occurring late or after prolonged therapy; often applied to dyskinesias that occur with long-term antipsychotic drug therapy

teratogenic: capable of producing birth defects in the developing fetus

therapeutic: having curative, healing, or otherwise beneficial actions

therapeutic dose: the amount (dose) of a drug that is necessary to produce the desired pharmacologic action; a pharmacologic or physiologic dose

therapeutic index: a relatively crude index of the relative safety of a drug, defined as the ratio of the LD_{50} to the ED_{50}, usually measured experimentally; when comparing two drugs, the one with the higher therapeutic index is relatively safer. See *margin of safety*

thrombocytopenia: abnormally low numbers of platelets (thrombocytes) in the blood, usually leading to impaired blood clotting

thrombolytic: capable of dissolving a blood clot. See *thrombus*

thrombus: a plug or clot of blood that forms on and remains at its site of origin on a blood vessel wall; when dislodged, a thrombus becomes an embolus

timed-release: See *sustained-release*

tincture: a drug preparation, usually derived from plants, in which the active ingredient is dissolved in alcohol or a water–alcohol (hydroalcoholic) solution. See *elixir*

tinnitus: ringing of the ears

tolerance: a diminished response to a particular drug that occurs, over time, with repeated administration of that drug, and requires administration of increased doses of the drug to achieve the same intensity of effect as could be produced before the development of tolerance. See *tachyphylaxis*

tone: the degree of tension or activity normally present under resting conditions; often applied to muscle or nerve activity

topical: on the skin or other body surface with which a drug has direct contact

toxic: harmful to the well-being or life of the organism or its constituent parts

transdermal: through the skin; percutaneous; a specific drug delivery system, such as a patch that contains active drug, that enables gradual but controlled absorption of the active substance through the skin

troche: See *lozenge*

unit: a measurement of drug dosage expressed in terms of the ability to produce a certain biologic response of specified intensity, rather than on the amount (volume or weight) of the drug

unit dose: usually a single dose of a drug, prepared and packaged by a hospital pharmacy or manufacturer for delivery to the patient-care setting and administration to a specific patient

untoward effect: an adverse, unwanted, unpleasant, or dangerous side effect

uricosuric: characterized by increased excretion of uric acid by the kidneys; a drug that increases renal uric acid excretion

urticaria: a vascular reaction of the skin, usually caused by an allergic process, that is characterized by the appearance of wheals or hives that may itch and produce a fluidy discharge

varicosity: a swelling; when applied to adrenergic nerves, the site at which neurotransmitter is synthesized, stored, and released

vasoactive: having effects on the blood vessels, usually to cause vasodilation or vasoconstriction

vasodepressor: a drug that decreases blood pressure; vasodilator; depressor

vasopressor: a drug that increases blood pressure; vasoconstrictor; pressor

visceral: pertaining to any organ in one of the major body cavities, especially the abdomen

withdrawal syndrome: specific behavioral and physiologic changes, often intense, produced by suddenly discontinuing administration or markedly reducing the dose of a drug that causes physical dependence (eg, morphine, heroin, and other opiates); signs and symptoms usually are characteristic for the drug or drug group that has caused dependence; also called abstinence syndrome

xerostomia: excessive dryness of the mouth caused by inadequate saliva secretion; may be a side effect of drugs with anticholinergic actions

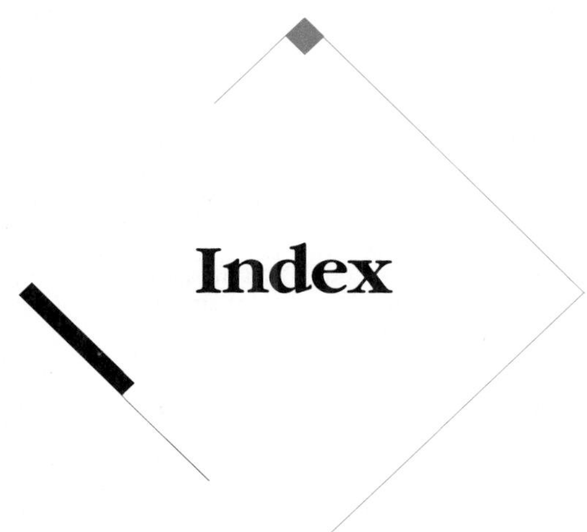

Index

NOTE: Drugs are listed under their generic names. Trade names are provided with a cross reference to the generic drug. Prototype drugs are in bold face type, and related drugs are cross referenced to the appropriate prototype. A *t* following a page number indicates tabular material and an *f* following a page number indicates an illustration.

D